clindamycin	I	N	N	C	C	C	N	C	C
doxycycline	CFC	N	I	I	C	C	N	C	C*
erythromycin	C	N	N	I	C	C	N	N	C
fluconazole	C	N	N	C	C	C	N	C	N
foscarnet	C	I	C	C	N	C	N	N	N
ganciclovir	N	N	N	N	N	N	N	I	N
gentamicin	C	N	CFC	I	C	C	N	C	C
imipenem/cilastatin	N	N	N	C	I	N	N	C	C**
metronidazole	C	N	N	C	C	C	N	N	C
mezlocillin	N	N	N	C	C	C	N	I	N
moxalactam	N	N	N	C	C	C	N	N	N
nafcillin	C	I	N	C	C	C	N	N	
netilmicin	C	N	N	I	N	N	N	N	
ofloxacin	N	N	N	N	N	N	N	N	
penicillin G	I	N	I	C	C	C	N	N	
pentamidine	N	N	N	N	N	N	N	N	
piperacillin	C	N	N	C	C	C	N	I	
tobramycin	C	N	I	I	C	C	N	N	
trimethoprim/sulfa-methoxazole	N	N	N	C	C	C	N	N	
vancomycin	C	N	N	I	C	C	N	C	

C = Compatible at Y-site; C* = Compatible at Potassium conc. < 80 mEq/L; C** = Compatible at Potassium conc. ≤ 20 mEq/L; CFC = Compatibil
fluid and/or concentration; I = Incompatible at Y-site; N = No information available; NN = No information available, probably should NOT mix.

APPLETON & LANGE

nurses drug guide 2000

Billie Ann Wilson, APRN, PhD
Professor and Director, Nursing Department
Loyola University
New Orleans, Louisiana

Margaret T. Shannon, APRN, PhD
Professor and Dean, Division of Nursing
Our Lady of Holy Cross College
New Orleans, Louisiana

Carolyn L. Stang, PharmD
Drug Information Specialist
Chicago, Illinois

Appleton & Lange
Stamford, Connecticut

www.appletonlange.com

00 01 02 03 04 / 10 9 8 7 6 5 4 3 2 1

Prentice Hall International (UK) Limited, *London*
Prentice Hall of Australia Pty. Limited, *Sydney*
Prentice Hall Canada, Inc., *Toronto*
Prentice Hall Hispanoamericana, S.A., *Mexico*
Prentice Hall of India Private Limited, *New Delhi*
Prentice Hall of Japan, Inc., *Tokyo*
Simon & Schuster Asia Pte. Ltd., *Singapore*
Editora Prentice Hall do Brasil Ltda., *Rio de Janeiro*
Prentice Hall, *Upper Saddle River, New Jersey*

ISBN: 0-8385-7115-8

ISSN 1062-9092
ISBN: 0-8385-7115-8

9 780838 571156 90000

Acquisitions Editor: Patricia E. Casey
Editorial Assistant: Elisabeth Church Garofalo
Production Editor: Elizabeth Ryan
Cover Designer: Janice Barsevich Bielawa

PRINTED IN THE UNITED STATES OF AMERICA

CONTENTS

To

Alvin, Theresa, Ellen, and

Michael, Bob, Mary Elizabeth, and Richard

without whom this work would not have been possible

♦

ABOUT THE AUTHORS

Billie Ann Wilson is currently Professor and Director of the Department of Nursing at Loyola University in New Orleans, Louisiana. Prior to entering nursing, she taught natural and physical sciences at the secondary and collegiate levels. She holds a Bachelor of Science in Biology from Boston College, a Master of Science in Biology from Purdue University, a Bachelor of Science in Nursing from Northwestern State University of Louisiana, a Master of Nursing from Louisiana State University Medical Center, and a PhD in Curriculum and Instruction from the University of New Orleans.

Margaret T. Shannon is currently Professor and Dean of the Division of Nursing at Our Lady of Holy Cross College, New Orleans, Louisiana. Her educational preparation includes a Bachelor of Science in Chemistry and a Master of Science in Chemistry, both from Saint Louis University; a Master of Arts in Teaching Biology from Saint Mary's College, a Bachelor of Science in Nursing from Northwestern State University of Louisiana, a Master of Nursing from Louisiana State University Medical Center, and a PhD in Curriculum and Instruction from the University of New Orleans. Prior to entering nursing, she taught physical science, natural science, and mathematics at the secondary and collegiate levels.

Carolyn L. Stang is currently a drug information specialist in Chicago, Illinois. She has worked in hospital and community pharmacies, home health care, and the pharmaceutical industry. Dr. Stang has been a freelance medical writer and an assistant professor at Rutgers University College of Pharmacy. She holds a Bachelor of Science in Pharmacy from The Ohio State University and a Doctor of Pharmacy from the University of Tennessee, Memphis, and completed a fellowship in Family Medicine at the Medical University of South Carolina, Charleston.

PREFACE

Nurses Drug Guide 2000 is a current and reliable reference designed to provide the information needed to make appropriate decisions regarding drug administration. New to this edition are user-friendly charts of ocular medications, low-molecular weight heparins, and oral and nasal corticosteroids (Appendix A). All drugs listed on these charts may be located in the body of the text under their alphabetized generic names and in the index. Also new to this edition, pediatric and geriatric dosages as well as adult dosages are listed in the Route and Dosage section for each drug.

This text contains a valuable administration tool, a list of oral drug dosage forms that should not be crushed. This "do-not-crush" list is found in Appendix E. The 2000 edition of the *Nurses Drug Guide* also includes 43 new FDA-approved drugs, and a disk (inside the back cover) that may be used to print monographs of commonly dispensed drugs.

In the Administration section of each drug monograph, complete and comprehensive information for IV drugs includes directions for reconstitution, dilution, methods of administration, and rate of injection or infusion. Thus, this *Guide* eliminates the need for additional resources for IV drug administration. Also important for IV drug administration, and listed in individual drug monographs, is Y-site compatibility. Charts are conveniently located inside the front cover (antibiotic drugs) and after the index (non-antibiotic drugs) in this book.

The Nursing Implications section of each drug monograph is formatted in an easy-to-use manner so that all pertinent information needed by nurses is listed under three headings: Administration, Assessment & Drug Effects, and Patient &

Family Education. Under these headings, the reader can quickly and easily identify needed information and incorporate it into the appropriate steps of the nursing process. *Therapeutic effectiveness* of the drug can be determined by monitoring improvement in the condition for which the drug is prescribed, and by using the Assessment and Drug Effects section of the Nursing Implications.

The authors recognize that the decision-making process related to drug administration is a cyclical one. For example, assessments are made both prior to and after drug administration. Thus, nursing diagnoses and interventions may change as a result of an *achieved therapeutic effect, therapeutic failure, manifestation of an adverse effect,* or *demonstration of a learning need.* The authors believe that users of this reference will find that the clear and logical design of the drug monographs facilitates decision-making and supports the nursing process.

The disk at the back of this *Nurses Drug Guide 2000* runs on Windows-based computers. It is designed to assist nurses in providing drug information and nursing implications for patients in hospitals, clinics, and all community settings. Monographs of the most commonly prescribed and dispensed drugs and prototype drugs are available on the disk and may be printed for convenient use by students and nurses. Appropriate information can be retrieved for patients.

The authors wish to acknowledge Phyllis Peterson, RN, MN, and Joanne Bullard, RN, MN, at Our Lady of Holy Cross College, and Debora Panepinto for their assistance in the preparation of this book. Most of all, we wish to express our appreciation to our past and present students who have provided the inspiration for this work. It is for these individuals and all who strive for excellence in patient care that this work was undertaken.

Billie Ann Wilson, APRN, PhD
Margaret T. Shannon, APRN, PhD
Carolyn L. Stang, PharmD

HOW TO USE THIS BOOK

In this *Guide,* all drugs are listed alphabetically according to generic names. Each drug is, however, indexed by both its generic and trade names. Trade names followed by a maple leaf (✦) indicate that the drug is available only in Canada. If a drug is not listed in the alphabetical section, it may be a combination drug, which by definition is made up of more than one generic component. These *combination drugs* are found by their trade names in the index and in a separate Appendix F of the *Guide,* which lists the generic components and the amount of each generic drug.

THERAPEUTIC EFFECTIVENESS

Therapeutic effectiveness of the drug can be determined by monitoring improvement in the condition for which the drug is prescribed, and by using the Assessment and Drug Effects section of the Nursing Implications.

The information needed for safe and effective drug administration is given for each drug in the alphabetical listing. The reader should review all the information provided. Occasionally, the reader will be referred to the Glossary, Appendix G. This glossary of key terms, clinical conditions, and associated signs and symptoms provides valuable information regarding common assessment findings related to therapeutic effectiveness or ineffectiveness of specific drugs.

Drugs have multiple uses or indications; therefore, it is important to know why a drug is being prescribed for a client. Therapeutic effectiveness of the drug may be determined by monitoring for improvement in the condition for which the drug is prescribed.

While some advanced practice nurses and other health professionals now have prescriptive privileges, physician is used throughout this book to designate the prescriber of medications.

For each drug, the following information is provided where pertinent:

CLASSIFICATION The classifications used in this book are based on the classification scheme used by the American Hospital Formulary Service (AHFS), which classifies drugs by pharmacologic and therapeutic category. This enables the nurse to identify different classes of drugs that have similar therapeutic implications or that primarily affect the same physiologic system. In general, all drugs in a class will have similar actions, uses, side effects, and nursing implications. Therefore, we have selected certain drugs representative of a class—**prototype drugs**—and have discussed them in more detail than the other drugs in that class. In addition, throughout the generic listing the names of prototype drugs are highlighted in color-tinted boxes. In-depth information on those drugs not extensively discussed may be obtained by referring to the prototype drug. When a drug belongs to a class that has a designated prototype, that prototype is identified directly below the drug classification. The table on pages xiii to xviii outlines the classification scheme and lists the drug considered representative for each class.

PREGNANCY CATEGORY Drugs may be described as category A, B, C, D, or X according to risk–benefit ratio for the mother and fetus, with A being the lowest and X the highest risk. If the FDA pregnancy category is known, it will be indicated. Refer to Appendix D for a more complete description of pregnancy categories.

SCHEDULE In the United States, controlled substances, such as narcotics, are classified as belonging to one of five schedules (I to V) according to abuse potential, with I having the highest and V the lowest potential for abuse. Refer to Appendix B for a more complete description of each schedule. The Canadian controlled substances classification scheme is given in Appendix C.

ACTIONS/PHARMACODYNAMICS This entry describes the mechanism by which the specific drug produces physiologic and biochemical changes at the cell, tissue, or organ level.

USES The therapeutic applications of each drug are described in terms of normal (labeled) use and unlabeled use. An unlabeled use is literally one that does not appear on the drug label or in the manufacturer's literature on the use of the drug. The unlabeled use is, nevertheless, an accepted use for the drug supported by the medical literature.

ROUTE & DOSAGE Route is specified as SC, IM, IV, PO, PR, nasal, ophthalmic, vaginal, topical, aural, intradermal, or intrathecal; doses are listed separately for adult, geriatric, child, and infant for those with reduced renal function (creatinine clearance), and according to use. This information is highlighted with shading for quick reference.

PHARMACOKINETICS This section lists information about onset, peak, and duration of drug action. It also lists the mechanisms of metabolism and elimination when known.

CONTRAINDICATIONS & PRECAUTIONS Many drugs are contraindicated and therefore should not be used in specific pathophysiologic conditions, during pregnancy, or with particular drugs or food. In other cases, the drug should be used with great caution because of a greater than average risk of untoward effects.

ADVERSE/SIDE EFFECTS Virtually all drugs have adverse or side effects that may be bothersome to some individuals but not to others. In this entry, adverse/side effects are listed according to systems or organs with the most common printed in italics and those that are life-threatening underlined.

DIAGNOSTIC TEST INTERFERENCES This entry describes the effect of the drug on various diagnostic tests and alerts the nurse to possible misinterpretations of test results.

DRUG INTERACTIONS Individual drugs, drug classes, and foods that interact with the drug under discussion are listed. Drugs may interact to inhibit or enhance one another; thus, drug interactions may improve the therapeutic response, lead to therapeutic failure, or produce specific untoward reactions. Only drugs that have been shown to cause clinically significant interactions with the drug under discussion are listed.

INCOMPATIBILITIES Solutions and drug additives physically incompatible with the drug under discussion are listed. Therefore, these solutions and drug additives should not be mixed in solution with the drug. The table on the inside front cover contains information related to the compatibility of antibiotic drugs administered by intravenous Y-site. At the back of the book after the index is a table containing information about the compatibility of nonantibiotic drugs administered via an intravenous Y-site. Additional drugs that should not be administered together are listed in the monographs.

NURSING IMPLICATIONS Nursing implications are listed under three headings: **Administration, Assessment & Drug Effects,** and **Patient & Family Education**. Before administering a drug, the nurse should read all three sections to determine (1) the appropriate administration techniques, (2) the assessments that should be made before and after administration of the drug and indicators of drug effectiveness, and (3) essential patient or family education related to the drug.

Classification	Prototype
ANTIGOUT AGENT	Colchicine (p. 362)
ANTIHISTAMINES	
ANTIHISTAMINES (H_1-RECEPTOR ANTAGONIST)	Diphenhydramine Hydrochloride (p. 464)
ANTIPRURITIC	Hydroxyzine Hydrochloride (p. 696)
ANTIVERTIGO AGENT	Meclizine Hydrochloride (p. 843)
ANTIINFECTIVES	
AMEBICIDE	Emetine Hydrochloride (p. 510)
ANTHELMINTIC	Mebendazole (p. 838)
ANTIBIOTICS	
AMINOGLYCOSIDE	Gentamicin Sulfate (p. 633)
ANTIFUNGAL	Fluconazole (p. 592)
BETA-LACTAM	Imipenem-Cilastatin Sodium (p. 706)
CEPHALOSPORIN	
FIRST GENERATION	Cephalothin Sodium (p. 272)
SECOND GENERATION	Cefonicid Sodium (p. 244)
THIRD GENERATION	Cefotaxime Sodium (p. 250)
CLINDAMYCIN	Clindamycin Hydrochloride (p. 337)
MACROLIDE	Erythromycin (p. 532)
PENICILLIN	
AMINOPENICILLIN	Ampicillin (p. 77)
ANTIPSEUDOMONAL PENICILLIN	Mezlocillin Sodium (p. 918)
NATURAL PENICILLIN	Penicillin G Potassium (p. 1075)
TETRACYCLINE	Tetracycline Hydrochloride (p. 1341)
ANTILEPROSY (SULFONE) AGENT	Dapsone (p. 403)
ANTIMALARIAL	Chloroquine Hydrochloride (p. 293)
ANTIPROTOZOAL	Metronidazole (p. 912)
ANTITUBERCULOSIS AGENT	Isoniazid (p. 747)
ANTIVIRAL	Acyclovir (p. 14)

*Based on the American Hospital Formulary Service Pharmacologic–Therapeutic Classification
†Prototype drugs are highlighted in tinted boxes in this book.

Classification	Prototype
ANTIRETROVIRAL AGENTS	
NUCLEOSIDE REVERSE TRANSCRIPTASE INHIBITOR	Zidovudine (p. 1477)
NONNUCLEOSIDE REVERSE TRANSCRIPTASE INHIBITOR	Nevirapine (p. 984)
PROTEASE INHIBITORS	Saquinavir Mesylate (p. 1257)
QUINOLONE	Ciprofloxacin Hydrochloride (p. 324)
SULFONAMIDE	Sulfisoxazole (p. 1314)
URINARY TRACT ANTIINFECTIVE	Trimethoprim (p. 1422)
VACCINE	Hepatitis B (p. 676)
ANTINEOPLASTICS	
ALKYLATING AGENT	Cyclophosphamide (p. 382)
ANTIBIOTIC	Doxorubicin Hydrochloride (p. 493)
ANTIMETABOLITE	Fluorouracil (p. 600)
CAMPTOTHECIN	Topotecan Hydrochloride (p. 1394)
AROMATASE INHIBITOR	Anastrozole (p. 85)
HORMONE, ANTIESTROGEN	Tamoxifen Citrate (p. 1325)
MITOTIC INHIBITOR	Vincristine Sulfate (p. 1462)
NITROGEN MUSTARD	Mechlorethamine Hydrochloride (p. 840)
ANTITUSSIVES, EXPECTORANTS, & MUCOLYTICS	
ANTITUSSIVE	Benzonatate (p. 142)
EXPECTORANT	Guaifenesin (p. 656)
MUCOLYTIC	Acetylcysteine (p. 11)
AUTONOMIC NERVOUS SYSTEM AGENTS	
ADRENERGIC AGONISTS (SYMPATHOMIMETICS)	
ALPHA-ADRENERGIC AGONIST	Methoxamine Hydrochloride (p. 889)
ALPHA- AND BETA-ADRENERGIC AGONIST	Epinephrine (p. 519)
BETA-ADRENERGIC AGONIST	Isoproterenol Hydrochloride (p. 749)
ADRENERGIC ANTAGONISTS (SYMPATHOLYTICS)	
ALPHA ANTAGONISTS (BLOCKING AGENT)	Prazosin Hydrochloride (p. 1159)
BETA ANTAGONISTS (BLOCKING AGENT)	Propranolol Hydrochloride (p. 1193)
ERGOT ALKALOID	Ergotamine Tartrate (p. 530)
$5\text{-}HT_1$ SEROTONIN AGONIST	Sumatriptan (p. 1318)

Classification	Prototype
ANTICHOLINERGICS (PARASYMPATHOLYTICS)	
ANTIPARKINSONISM AGENT	Levodopa (p. 785)
ANTIMUSCARINIC, ANTISPASMODIC	Atropine Sulfate (p. 110)
CHOLINERGICS (PARASYMPATHOMIMETICS)	
CHOLINESTERASE INHIBITOR	Neostigmine Bromide (p. 979)
DIRECT-ACTING CHOLINERGIC	Bethanechol Chloride (p. 153)
SKELETAL MUSCLE RELAXANTS	
CENTRAL ACTING	Cyclobenzaprine Hydrochloride (p. 380)
DEPOLARIZING	Succinylcholine Chloride (p. 1304)
NONDEPOLARIZING	Tubocurarine Chloride (p. 1438)
BENZODIAZEPINE ANTAGONIST	Flumazenil (p. 597)
BLOOD DERIVATIVE, PLASMA VOLUME EXPANDER	Normal Serum Albumin, Human (p. 1013)
BLOOD FORMERS & COAGULATORS	
ANTICOAGULANT	Heparin Sodium (p. 671)
ANTIPLATELET AGENT	Ticlopidine (p. 1371)
GLYCOPROTEIN IIb/IIIa INHIBITOR	Abciximab (p. 1)
HEMATOPOIETIC GROWTH FACTOR	Epoetin Alpha (Human Recombinant Erythropoietin) (p. 523)
HEMOSTATIC	Aminocaproic Acid (p. 46)
IRON PREPARATION	Ferrous Sulfate (p. 583)
THROMBOLYTIC ENZYME	Streptokinase (p. 1297)
BRONCHODILATORS (RESPIRATORY SMOOTH MUSCLE RELAXANT)	
XANTHINE	Theophylline (p. 1348)
5-LIPOXYGENASE INHIBITOR	Zafirlukast (p. 1458)
CARDIOVASCULAR AGENTS	
ANGIOTENSIN II RECEPTOR ANTAGONIST	Losartan Potassium (p. 817)
ANGIOTENSIN-CONVERTING ENZYME INHIBITOR	Captopril (p. 212)
ANTIARRHYTHMIC	Procainamide Hydrochloride (p. 1171)
ANTILIPEMICS	
BILE ACID SEQUESTRANT	Cholestyramine Resin (p. 312)
HMG-CoA REDUCTASE INHIBITOR (STATIN)	Lovastatin (p. 818)

Classification	Prototype
CALCIUM CHANNEL BLOCKER	Nifedipine (p. 991)
CARDIAC GLYCOSIDE	Digoxin (p. 451)
CENTRAL-ACTING ANTIHYPERTENSIVE	Methyldopa (p. 896)
NITRATE VASODILATOR	Nitroglycerin (p. 999)
NONNITRATE VASODILATOR	Hydralazine Hydrochloride (p. 679)
RAUWOLFIA ALKALOID	Reserpine (p. 1128)

CENTRAL NERVOUS SYSTEM (CNS) AGENTS

Classification	Prototype
ANALGESICS, ANTIPYRETIC	
NARCOTIC (OPIATE) AGONIST	Morphine Sulfate (p. 944)
NARCOTIC (OPIATE) AGONIST-ANTAGONIST	Pentazocine Hydrochloride (p. 1085)
NARCOTIC (OPIATE) ANTAGONIST	Naloxone Hydrochloride (p. 965)
NONNARCOTIC	Acetaminophen (p. 5)
NONSTEROIDAL ANTIINFLAMMATORY DRUG (NSAID)	Ibuprofen (p. 699)
SALICYLATE	Aspirin (p. 99)
ANESTHETIC	
GENERAL	Thiopental Sodium (p. 1356)
LOCAL (ESTER TYPE)	Procaine Hydrochloride (p. 1171)
ANTICONVULSANT	
BARBITURATE	Phenobarbital (p. 1100)
BENZODIAZEPINE	Diazepam (p. 431)
GABA INHIBITOR	Valproic Acid Sodium (p. 1445)
HYDANTOIN	Phenytoin (p. 1115)
SUCCINIMIDE	Ethosuximide (p. 559)
ANXIOLYTIC, SEDATIVE-HYPNOTIC	
BARBITURATE	Secobarbital (p. 1262)
BENZODIAZEPINE	Lorazepam (p. 815)
CARBAMATE	Meprobamate (p. 862)
PSYCHOTHERAPEUTIC	
ANTIDEPRESSANT	
SELECTIVE SEROTONIN-REUPTAKE INHIBITOR	Fluoxetine Hydrochloride (p. 602)
MONOAMINE OXIDASE INHIBITOR	Phenelzine Sulfate (p. 1096)
TRICYCLIC	Imipramine Hydrochloride (p. 708)
ANTIMANIC	Lithium Carbonate (p. 805)
ANTIPSYCHOTIC	
BUTYROPHENONE	Haloperidol (p. 667)
PHENOTHIAZINE	Chlorpromazine (p. 301)
UNCLASSIFIED	Clozapine (p. 357)

Classification	Prototype
RESPIRATORY & CEREBRAL STIMULANT	
AMPHETAMINE	Amphetamine Sulfate (p. 71)
XANTHINE	Caffeine (p. 190)

ELECTROLYTIC & WATER BALANCE AGENTS

Classification	Prototype
DIURETIC	
LOOP	Furosemide (p. 623)
OSMOTIC	Mannitol (p. 833)
POTASSIUM-SPARING	Spironolactone (p. 1293)
THIAZIDE	Hydrochlorothiazide (p. 681)
REPLACEMENT SOLUTION	Calcium Gluconate (p. 202)

EYE, EAR, NOSE, & THROAT (EENT) PREPARATIONS

Classification	Prototype
CARBONIC ANHYDRASE INHIBITOR	Acetazolamide (p. 7)
CYCLOPLEGIC	Cylopentolate Hydrochloride (p. 382)
MIOTIC (ANTIGLAUCOMA AGENT)	Pilocarpine Hydrochloride (p. 1122)
MYDRIATIC	Homatropine Hydrobromide (p. 678)
VASOCONSTRICTOR, DECONGESTANT	Naphazoline Hydrochloride (p. 968)

GASTROINTESTINAL AGENTS

Classification	Prototype
ANORECTANT	Diethylpropion Hydrochloride (p. 446)
ANTACID, ADSORBENT	Aluminum Hydroxide (p. 35)
ANTIDIARRHEAL	Diphenoxylate Hydrochloride with Atropine Sulfate (p. 467)
ANTIEMETIC	Prochlorperazine (p. 1177)
ANTIEMETIC (5-HT_3 ANTAGONIST)	Ondansetron Hydrochloride (p. 1026)
ANTISECRETORY (H_2-RECEPTOR ANTAGONIST)	Cimetidine (p. 320)
BULK LAXATIVE	Psyllium Hydrophilic Mucilloid (p. 1203)
PROKINETIC AGENT (GI STIMULANT)	Metoclopramide Hydrochloride (p. 906)
PROTON PUMP INHIBITOR	Omeprazole (p. 1025)
SALINE CATHARTIC	Magnesium Hydroxide (p. 828)
STIMULANT LAXATIVE	Bisacodyl (p. 158)
STOOL SOFTENER	Docusate Calcium (p. 479)

Classification	Prototype
GOLD COMPOUND	Aurothioglucose (p. 116)
HORMONES & SYNTHETIC SUBSTITUTES	
ADRENAL CORTICOSTEROID	
GLUCOCORTICOID	Prednisone (p. 1163)
MINERALOCORTICOID	Fludrocortisone Acetate (p. 595)
ANDROGEN/ANABOLIC STEROID	Testosterone (p. 1336)
ANTIDIABETIC	
INSULIN	Insulin Injection (p. 720)
SULFONYLUREA	Tolbutamide (p. 1385)
ESTROGEN	Estradiol (p. 539)
GONADOTROPIN-RELEASING HORMONE ANALOG	Leuprolide Acetate (p. 783)
OXYTOCIC	Oxytocin Injection (p. 1050)
PITUITARY (ANTIDIURETIC)	Vasopressin Injection (p. 1451)
PROGESTIN	Progesterone (p. 1181)
THYROID AGENTS	
ANTITHYROID AGENT	Propylthiouracil (p. 1197)
THYROID	Levothyroxine Sodium (p. 793)
VITAMIN D ANALOG	Calcitriol (p. 197)
IMMUNOMODULATOR	Interferon Alfa-2a (p. 730)
IMMUNOSUPPRESSANT	Cyclosporine (p. 386)
MONOCLONAL ANTIBODY: INTERLEUKIN-2 RECEPTOR ANTIBODY	Basiliximab (p. 132)
LUNG SURFACTANT	Beractant (p. 151)
MAST CELL STABILIZER	Cromolyn Sodium (p. 374)
PROSTAGLANDIN	Dinoprostone (p. 463)
REGULATOR, BONE METABOLISM (BIPHOSPHONATE)	Etidronate Disodium (p. 561)
SKIN & MUCOUS MEMBRANE AGENTS	
ANTIACNE (RETINOID)	Isotretinoin (p. 756)
ANTIINFLAMMATORY STEROID	Hydrocortisone (p. 684)
PEDICULICIDE	Permethrin (p. 1091)
PSORALEN	Methoxsalen (p. 890)
SCABICIDE	Lindane (p. 799)

ABCIXIMAB (c7E3 Fab)

(ab-cix'-i-mab)
Trade name: ReoPro
Prototype for classifications: ANTITHROMBOTIC; ANTIPLATELET; GLYCOPROTEIN IIB/IIIA INHIBITOR
Pregnancy category: C

ACTIONS/PHARMACODYNAMICS A human–murine monoclonal antibody Fab (fragment antigen binding) fragment, abciximab binds to the glycoprotein IIb/IIIa (GPIIb/IIIa) receptor sites of platelets. The drug inhibits platelet aggregation by preventing fibrinogen, von Willebrand's factor, and other molecules from adhering to GPIIb/IIIa receptor sites of the platelets.

USE Adjunct to aspirin and heparin for the prevention of acute cardiac ischemic complications in patients undergoing percutaneous transluminal coronary angioplasty (PTCA).

ROUTE & DOSAGE

PTCA
Adult: **IV** Starting 10–60 min prior to start of angioplasty, 0.25 mg/kg bolus over 5 min followed by continuous infusion of 10 μg/min for next 12 h.

PHARMACOKINETICS **Onset:** >90% inhibition of platelet aggregation within 2 h. **Duration:** approximately 48 h. **Elimination:** half-life: 30 min.

CONTRAINDICATIONS & PRECAUTIONS **Contraindicated in:** Active internal bleeding; GI or GU bleeding within 6 wk; history of CVA within 2 y or a CVA with severe neurologic deficit; administration of oral anticoagulants unless PT < 1.2 times control; thrombocytopenia (< 100,000 cells/ml); recent major surgery or trauma; intracranial neoplasm, aneurysm, severe hypertension; history of vasculitis; use of dextran before or during PTCA; hypersensitivity to abciximab or to murine proteins. **Cautious use in:** pregnancy (category C); patients weighing < 75 kg; elderly; history of previous GI disease; recent thrombolytic therapy; PTCA within 12 h of MI; unsuccessful PTCA; PTCA procedure lasting > 70 min.

ADVERSE/SIDE EFFECTS **Hematologic:** *bleeding*, including intracranial, retroperitoneal, and hematemesis; thrombocytopenia.

DRUG INTERACTIONS ORAL ANTICOAGULANTS, NSAIDS, **dipyridamole, ticlopidine, dextran** may increase risk of bleeding.

INCOMPATIBILITY It is recommended that abciximab be infused through a separate IV line.

NURSING IMPLICATIONS

Administration
- Do not shake vial. Discard if visible opaque particles are noted.
- Use a nonpyrogenic low-protein-binding 0.2- or 0.22-μm filter when withdrawing drug into a syringe from the 2 mg/ml vial and when infusing as continuous IV.
- Administer bolus dose over 5 min.
- For continuous IV infusion, inject 4.5 ml of drug into 250 ml of sterile 0.9% NaCl or D5W. Infuse at 17 ml/h (10 μg/min) via an infusion pump; add no other drugs to the solution or IV line.
- Discard any unused drug at the end of the 12-h infusion as well as any unused portion left in vial.
- Store vials at 2–8C (36–46F).

Assessment & Drug Effects
- Before, during, and after treatment, closely monitor Hgb, Hct, platelet count, PT, APTT, and acti-

vated clotting time. Monitor every 2–4 h during first 24 h.
- Monitor for bleeding, especially the elderly and patients weighing less than 75 kg (165 lb) or having a history of GI disease, recent thrombolytic therapy, or failed or prolonged (> 70 min) PTCA.
- Carefully monitor all potential bleeding sites (e.g., catheter insertion, needle puncture, or cutdown sites; GI, GU, or retroperitoneal sites).
- Monitor for hypersensitivity, which may occur anytime during administration.
- Use of unnecessary invasive procedures and devices should be avoided or minimized to reduce risk of bleeding.
- When femoral artery access is used, elevate the head of the bed ≤ 30° and keep limb straight. Following sheath removal, apply pressure for 30 min.
- Stop infusion immediately if bleeding or hypersensitivity occurs.

ACARBOSE

(a-car′-bose)

Trade name: Precose

Classifications: ANTIDIABETIC AGENT; α-GLUCOSIDASE INHIBITOR

Pregnancy category: B

ACTIONS/PHARMACODYNAMICS Acarbose is one of a new class of oral α-glucosidase inhibitors. It inhibits or delays the absorption of sugars from the intestinal tract. The inhibitory effect of acarbose varies according to which enzymes are involved; from most to least inhibited are glucoamylase, sucrase, maltase, and isomaltase. Lactase is not affected by acarbose. Acarbose reduces blood sugar by interfering with carbohydrate absorption from the GI tract.

USE As monotherapy or in combination with a sulfonylurea in patients with Type 2 NIDDM. **Unlabeled use:** in combination with insulin and metformin in patients with Type 1 NIDDM.

ROUTE & DOSAGE

Diabetes Mellitus

Adult: **PO** Initiate with 25 mg q.d. to t.i.d. with meals; may increase q4–8wk up to 50–100 mg t.i.d. with meals; max: 150 mg/d for ≤ 60 kg, 300 mg/d for > 60 kg.

PHARMACOKINETICS Absorption: only 0.5–2% is absorbed intact from GI tract. After degradation by intestinal bacteria, up to 35% of dose may be absorbed. **Peak:** peak blood glucose reduction approx 70 min after dose. **Metabolism:** metabolized in GI tract by intestinal bacteria and digestive enzymes. **Elimination:** half-life: 2 h; 35% excreted in urine, 51% excreted in feces, and 5% excreted in air as CO_2.

CONTRAINDICATIONS & PRECAUTIONS Contraindicated in: inflammatory bowel disease, colon ulcers, partial bowel obstructions, or predisposition for obstruction; patients < 18 y; nursing mothers. **Cautious use in:** GI distress or liver disorders, pregnancy (category B).

ADVERSE/SIDE EFFECTS CNS: sleepiness, weakness, dizziness, headache, vertigo (CNS effects may be due to poor diabetic control). **Endocrine:** hypoglycemia (especially in combination with sulfonylureas and insulin). **GI:** *diarrhea, flatulence, abdominal distention,* borborygmi, increased liver function tests. **Hematologic:** anemia (especially iron deficiency). **Skin:** erythema, exanthema, urticaria.

DRUG INTERACTIONS SULFONYLUREAS may increase hypoglycemic effects. Drugs that induce hyperglycemia (e.g., THIAZIDES, CORTICOSTEROIDS, PHENOTHIAZINES, ESTROGENS, **phenytoin, isoniazide**) may decrease effectiveness of acarbose.

NURSING IMPLICATIONS

Administration

- Drug should be removed from foil wrapper immediately before administration.
- Drug should be taken with the first bite of each of the three main meals.
- Store according to manufacturer's directions.

Assessment & Drug Effects

- Monitor fasting and postprandial blood sugar and glycosylated hemoglobin to determine therapeutic effectiveness.
- Periodically monitor liver enzymes and Hct and Hgb.

Patient & Family Education

- Instruct to take drug with the first bite of each of three main meals daily.
- Advise to report abdominal distress; dietary adjustment or dosage reduction may be warranted.
- Instruct to monitor weight and report significant changes.

ACEBUTOLOL HYDROCHLORIDE

(a-se-byoo'toe-lole)

Trade names: Monitan♣, Sectral

Classifications: AUTONOMIC NERVOUS SYSTEM AGENT; BETA-ADRENERGIC ANTAGONIST (BLOCKING AGENT, SYMPATHOLYTIC); CARDIOVASCULAR AGENT; ANTIHYPERTENSIVE; ANTIARRHYTHMIC

Prototype: Propranolol

Pregnancy category: B

ACTIONS/PHARMACODYNAMICS $Beta_1$-selective adrenergic blocking agent with mild intrinsic sympathomimetic activity (partial beta-agonist activity). Exhibits antiarrhythmic activity (class II antiarrhythmic agent). Produces negative chronotropic and inotropic activity; i.e., decreases exercise-induced heart rate, inhibits reflex orthostatic tachycardia, and decreases cardiac output at rest and during exercise. Decreases both systolic and diastolic BP at rest and during exercise.

USES Mild to moderate hypertension. Stepped-care approach to antihypertensive therapy as step 1 or step 2 drug. Management of recurrent stable ventricular arrhythmias. **Unlabeled uses:** supraventricular arrhythmias, chronic stable angina pectoris.

ROUTE & DOSAGE

Hypertension

Adult: **PO** 400–800 mg/d in 1–2 divided doses (max 1200 mg/d).
Geriatric: **PO** 200–400 mg/d (max 800 mg/d).

Ventricular Arrhythmias

Adult: **PO** 200 mg b.i.d. increased to 600–1200 mg/d.

Angina Pectoris

Adult: **PO** 300–400 mg t.i.d.

Adjust for Renal Impairment

Cl_{cr} <50 ml/min: reduce dose by 50%; <25 ml/min: reduce dose by 75%.

PHARMACOKINETICS Absorption: well absorbed after PO administration; undergoes extensive first-pass metabolism in liver with an average bioavailability of 40%. (In geriatric patients, bioavailability increases twofold.) **Peak:** 3 h. **Distribution:** minimally into CSF; crosses placenta; is excreted in breast milk. **Metabolism:** metabolized in liver to diacetolol with activity equipotent to parent compound. **Elimination:** half-life: acebutolol 3–4 h, metabolite 8–13 h; 50–60% excreted via bile into feces, and 30–40% excreted in urine.

CONTRAINDICATIONS & PRECAUTIONS Contraindicated in: overt CHF, second- or third-degree AV block, severe bradycardia, cardiogenic shock. Safety during pregnancy (category B), lactation, or in children <12 y not established. **Cautious use in:** impaired cardiac function, well-compensated CHF, mesenteric or peripheral vascular disease; patients undergoing major surgery involving general anesthesia; renal or hepatic impairment; labile diabetes mellitus; hyperthyroidism; bronchospastic disease (asthma, emphysema); avoid abrupt withdrawal.

ADVERSE/SIDE EFFECTS CNS: *fatigue,* dizziness, insomnia, drowsiness, confusion, fainting, decreased libido. **CV:** *bradycardia,* hypotension, CHF. **GI:** nausea, *diarrhea, constipation,* flatulence. **Respiratory:** bronchospasm, pulmonary edema, dyspnea. **Sensitivity reactions:** antinuclear antibodies (ANA) (10–30% of patients). **Other:** <u>agranulocytosis</u>, impotence, hypoglycemia (may mask symptoms of a hypoglycemic reaction).

DRUG INTERACTIONS OTHER HYPOTENSIVE AGENTS, DIURETICS increase hypotensive effect; with **albuterol, metaproterenol, terbutaline,** or **pirbuterol** there is mutual antagonism with acebutolol; NSAIDS blunt hypotensive effect; decreases hypoglycemic effect of **glyburide;** increases bradycardia and sinus arrest with **amiodarone.**

DIAGNOSTIC TEST INTERFERENCE See **propranolol.**

NURSING IMPLICATIONS

Administration

- Check apical pulse before administration. If slower than 60 bpm, consult physician.
- Store at 15–30C (59–86F).

Assessment & Drug Effects

- Monitor BP and cardiac status throughout therapy. Report bradycardia and hypertension to physician.
- Monitor I&O ratio and pattern. Report changes to physician, e.g., dysuria, nocturia, oliguria, weight change.
- Monitor for signs and symptoms of CHF, especially peripheral edema, dyspnea, activity intolerance (see Signs & Symptoms, Appendix G).
- In long-term therapy, incidence of drug-induced positive ANA titer is high, especially in women and in the elderly. Complaints about persistent lupuslike symptoms (myalgia, arthritis, arthralgia) suggest ANA sensitivity and should be reported to the physician. Discontinuation of drug therapy usually reverses symptoms.
- If patient is also receiving a catecholamine-depleting drug (e.g., reserpine), observe for marked bradycardia or hypotension. Acebutolol prevents compensatory tachycardia; therefore patient may experience vertigo, syncope, or orthostatic changes in BP.

Patient & Family Education

- Teach patients how to check their

pulse before they take medication. Advise patient to notify physician if pulse is below 60.

- Warn patient that CNS adverse effects are the most common, e.g., insomnia, drowsiness, confusion.
- Warn patient not to drive or operate equipment requiring alertness and manual skills until response to drug is known.
- Caution patient not to increase, decrease, omit, or discontinue drug regimen without advice from the physician.
- Abrupt withdrawal may exacerbate angina or precipitate MI in patient with heart disease or thyroid storm in patient with thyrotoxicosis.
- Contact physician promptly at the first signs or symptoms of CHF (see Appendix G).
- Advise diabetics that drug may mask symptoms of hypoglycemia (see Appendix G) and may potentiate insulin-induced hypoglycemia.
- Avoid use with OTC oral cold preparations and topical nasal decongestants containing alpha-adrenergic agonists (e.g., phenylephrine). An exaggerated hypertensive reaction is a potential hazard.
- Following gradual withdrawal over 2 wk, patient should temporarily limit physical activity.

ACETAMINOPHEN, PARACETAMOL

(a-seat-a-mee′noe-fen)

Trade names: Abenal ♣, A'Cenol, Acephen, Anacin-3, Anuphen, APAP, Atasol ♣, Campain ♣, Datril Extra Strength, Dolanex, Exdol ♣, Halenol, Liquiprim, Panadol, Pedric, Robigesic ♣, Rounox ♣, Tapar, Tempra, Tylenol, Valadol

Prototype for classifications: CNS AGENT; NONNARCOTIC ANALGESIC, ANTIPYRETIC

Pregnancy category: B

ACTIONS/PHARMACODYNAMICS Unlike aspirin, acetaminophen has little effect on platelet junction, does not affect bleeding time, and generally produces no gastric bleeding. Produces analgesia by unknown mechanism, perhaps by action on peripheral nervous system. Reduces fever by direct action on hypothalamus heat-regulating center with consequent peripheral vasodilation, sweating, and dissipation of heat.

USES Fever reduction. Temporary relief of mild to moderate pain. Generally as substitute for aspirin when the latter is not tolerated or is contraindicated.

ROUTE & DOSAGE

Adult: **PO** 325–650 mg q4–6h (max 4 g/d). **PR** 650 mg q4–6h (max 4 g/d).
Child: **PO** *Neonate,* 10–15 mg/kg q6–8h; *0–3 mo,* 40 mg q4–6h; *4–11 mo,* 80 mg q4–6h; *1–2 y,* 120 mg q4–6h; *2–3 y,* 160 mg q4–6h; *4–5 y,* 240 mg q4–6h; *6–8 y,* 320 mg q4–6h; *9–10 y,* 400 mg q4–6h; *11–12 y,* 480 mg q4–6h. **PR** *2–5 y,* 120 mg q4–6h (max 720 mg/d); *6–12 y,* 325 mg q4–6h (max 2.6 g/d).

PHARMACOKINETICS **Absorption:** rapid and almost complete absorption from GI tract; less complete absorption from rectal suppository. **Peak effect:** 0.5–2 h. **Duration:** 3–4 h. **Distribution:** well distributed in all body fluids; crosses placenta. **Metabolism:** extensively metabolized in liver. **Elimination:** half-life: 1–3 h;

90–100% of drug excreted as metabolites in urine; excreted in breast milk.

CONTRAINDICATIONS & PRECAUTIONS Hypersensitivity to acetaminophen or phenacetin. **Contraindicated in:** children <3 y, unless directed by a physician; repeated administration to patients with anemia or hepatic disease. Safe use during pregnancy (category B) or in nursing women not established. **Cautious use in:** arthritic or rheumatoid conditions affecting children <12 y; alcoholism; malnutrition; thrombocytopenia.

ADVERSE/SIDE EFFECTS Negligible with recommended dosage; rash. **Acute poisoning:** anorexia, nausea, vomiting, dizziness, lethargy, diaphoresis, chills, epigastric or abdominal pain, diarrhea; onset of hepatotoxicity—elevation of serum transaminases (ALT, AST) and bilirubin; hypoglycemia, hepatic coma, acute renal failure (rare). **Chronic ingestion:** neutropenia, pancytopenia, leukopenia, thrombocytopenic purpura. ***Hepatotoxicity in alcoholics:*** renal damage.

DIAGNOSTIC TEST INTERFERENCE Acetaminophen may cause (1) false increases in ***urinary 5-HIAA*** (5-hydroxyindoleacetic acid) by-product of serotonin; (2) false decreases in ***blood glucose*** (by glucose oxidase–peroxidase procedure); (3) false increases in ***urinary glucose*** (with certain instruments in glucose analyses); and (4) false increases in ***serum uric acid*** (with phosphotungstate method).

DRUG INTERACTIONS **Cholestyramine** may decrease acetaminophen absorption. With chronic coadministration, BARBITURATES, **carbamazepine, phenytoin,** and **rifampin** may increase potential for chronic hepatotoxicity. Chronic, excessive ingestion of **alcohol** will increase risk of hepatotoxicity.

NURSING IMPLICATIONS

Administration

- May be crushed and taken with fluid of patient's choice. Chewable tablets should be thoroughly chewed and wetted before they are swallowed.
- Coadministration with a high-carbohydrate meal may significantly retard absorption rate.
- Store in light-resistant containers at room temperature, preferably between 15–30C (59–86F), unless otherwise directed.

Assessment & Drug Effects

- With high doses or long-term therapy, periodic tests of hepatic, renal, and hematopoietic function are advised.
- Individuals with poor nutrition or who have ingested alcohol over prolonged periods are prone to hepatotoxicity even from moderate acetaminophen doses.
- Abuse potential is high; psychological dependence can occur. Withdrawal following long-term use has been associated with restlessness and excitement in some patients.
- Most poisonings result from suicide attempts or accidental ingestion.

Patient & Family Education

- Caution patient about taking other medications containing acetaminophen without medical advice.
- Overdosing and chronic use can cause liver damage and other toxic effects.
- Acetaminophen should not be used for self-medication of pain for more than 10 d in adults or 5 d in children, without consulting a physician. It should not be used for fever persisting longer than 3 d and never for fever over 39.5C

(103F) or for recurrent fever without medical direction. No more than 5 doses in 24 h should be given to children unless prescribed by physician.

ACETAZOLAMIDE

(a-set-a-zole'a-mide)

Trade names: Acetazolam ♣, Ak-Zol, Apo-Acetazolamide ♣, Dazamide, Diamox, Diamox Sequels

ACETAZOLAMIDE SODIUM

Trade name: Diamox Parenteral

Prototype for classifications: EYE PREPARATION: CARBONIC ANHYDRASE INHIBITOR; DIURETIC; CNS AGENT; ANTICONVULSANT

Pregnancy category: C

ACTIONS/PHARMACODYNAMICS Diuretic effect is due to inhibition of carbonic anhydrase activity in proximal renal tubule, preventing formation of carbonic acid. Inhibition of carbonic anhydrase in eye reduces rate of aqueous humor formation with consequent lowering of intraocular pressure. This effect is independent of systemic acid–base balance and diuretic action. Mechanism of anticonvulsant action unknown but is thought to involve inhibition of CNS carbonic anhydrase, which retards abnormal paroxysmal discharge from CNS neurons.

USES Seizures: absence or petit mal, generalized tonic-clonic (grand mal), and focal; reduction of intraocular pressure in open-angle glaucoma and secondary glaucoma; preoperative treatment of acute closed-angle glaucoma; drug-induced edema and as adjunct in treatment of edema due to congestive heart failure; acute high-altitude sickness. **Unlabeled uses:** to prevent uric acid or cystine renal calculi; to treat acute pancreatitis, premenstrual syndrome (PMS), metabolic alkalosis, and hypokalemic and hyperkalemic forms of familial periodic paralysis; to increase secretion of phenobarbital or lithium; hydrocephalus.

ROUTE & DOSAGE

Glaucoma

Adult: **PO** 250 mg 1–4 times/d; 500 mg sustained release b.i.d. **IM/IV** 500 mg; may repeat in 2–4 h.
Child: **PO** 8–30 mg/kg/d in 3 doses. **IM/IV** 5–10 mg/kg q6h.

Epilepsy

Adult: **PO** 8–30 mg/kg/d in 1–4 doses.
Child: **PO** Same as for adult.

Edema

Adult: **PO** 250–375 mg every AM (5 mg/kg).
Child: **PO/IM/IV** 5 mg/kg or 150 mg/m^2 every AM.

High Altitude Sickness

Adult: **PO** 250 mg q8–12h *or* 500 mg sustained release q12–24h, starting 24–48 h before climb and continuing for 48 h at high altitude.

Hydrocephalus

Neonates/Infants: **PO/IV** 5 mg/kg q6h; may increase by 25 mg/kg/d to max of 100 mg/kg/d.

Renal Impairment

Cl_{cr} 10–50 ml/min: dose q12h.
Cl_{cr} < 10 ml/min: use not recommended.

PHARMACOKINETICS Absorption: well absorbed from GI tract. **Onset:**

1 h regular release; 2 h sustained release; 2 min IV. **Peak effect:** 2–4 h reg; 8–18 h sustained; 0.25 min IV. **Duration:** 8–12 h reg; 18–24 h sustained; 4–5 h IV. **Distribution:** distributed throughout body, concentrating in RBCs, plasma, and kidneys; crosses placenta. **Elimination:** half-life: 2.4–5.8 h; excreted primarily in urine.

CONTRAINDICATIONS & PRECAUTIONS **Contraindicated in:** hypersensitivity to sulfonamides and derivatives (e.g., thiazides), marked renal and hepatic dysfunction; Addison's disease or other types of adrenocortical insufficiency; hyponatremia, hypokalemia, hyperchloremic acidosis; prolonged administration to patients with hyphema or chronic noncongestive angle-closure glaucoma. Safe use during pregnancy (category C) or in nursing mothers not established. **Cautious use in:** history of hypercalciuria; diabetes mellitus, gout, patients receiving digitalis, obstructive pulmonary disease, respiratory acidosis.

ADVERSE/SIDE EFFECTS **CNS:** paresthesias, sedation, malaise, disorientation, depression, fatigue, muscle weakness, flaccid paralysis. **GI:** anorexia, nausea, vomiting, weight loss, dry mouth, thirst, diarrhea. **Hematologic/electrolyte imbalance (as for other sulfonamides):** bone marrow depression with agranulocytosis, hemolytic anemia, aplastic anemia, leukopenia, pancytopenia. Increased excretion of calcium, potassium, magnesium, and sodium; metabolic acidosis; hyperglycemia; hyperuricemia. **Renal:** glycosuria, urinary frequency, polyuria, dysuria, hematuria, crystalluria. **Other:** exacerbation of gout, hepatic dysfunction.

DIAGNOSTIC TEST INTERFERENCE False-positive ***urinary protein*** determinations; falsely high values for ***urine urobilinogen;*** depressed ***iodine uptake*** values (exception: hypothyroidism).

DRUG INTERACTIONS Renal excretion of AMPHETAMINES, **ephedrine, flecainide, quinidine, procainamide,** TRICYCLIC ANTIDEPRESSANTS may be decreased, thereby enhancing or prolonging their effects. Renal excretion of **lithium** is increased. Excretion of **phenobarbital** may be increased. **Amphotericin B** and CORTICOSTEROIDS may accelerate potassium loss. DIGITALIS GLYCOSIDES may predispose persons with hypokalemia to digitalis toxicity; puts patients on high doses of SALICYLATES at high risk for salicylate toxicity.

NURSING IMPLICATIONS

Administration

- Diuretic dose administered in morning to avoid interrupted sleep.
- May be taken with food or meals to minimize GI upset.
- Tablet (not sustained release form) may be softened in 2 tsp of hot water and added to 2 tsp of honey or syrup to disguise bitter taste. Avoid syrups containing alcohol or glycerin. Alternatively, tablet(s) may be crushed and suspended in syrup (250–500 mg/5 ml syrup). The drug does not dissolve in fruit juices. Prepare just before administration.
- IV preparation: Reconstitute each 500-mg vial with at least 5 ml of sterile water for injection.
- IV administration: May be given by direct IV at a rate of 500 mg or fraction thereof over 1 min. Acetazolamide may be added to compatible IV fluids and administered as a continuous infusion over 4–8 h.
- IV administration to neonates, infants, and children: Verify correct

IV concentration and rate of infusion/injection with physician.
- Parenteral solution use within 24 h of reconstitution is strongly recommended by manufacturer. (Each 500-mg vial should be reconstituted with at least 5 ml sterile water for injection before use.)
- Store oral preparations at 15–30C (59–86F) unless otherwise directed.

Assessment & Drug Effects
- Observe for mild to severe metabolic acidosis.
- Monitor I&O and body weight.
- Weigh under standard conditions before drug therapy is initiated and daily thereafter.
- Potassium loss tends to be greatest during early therapy.
- Observe for and advise patient to report signs of hypokalemia or metabolic acidosis (see Appendix G).
- Blood pH, blood gases, urinalysis, CBC, and serum electrolyte determinations are recommended initially and at periodic intervals during prolonged drug therapy or during concomitant therapy with other diuretics or digitalis.

Patient & Family Education
- Do not accept brand interchange unless approved by physician.
- Adequate fluid intake (1.5–2.5 L/24 h) should be maintained to reduce risk of kidney stones.
- Report numbness, tingling, burning, and other paresthesias, drowsiness, and visual problems.
- Report sore throat or mouth, unusual bleeding, fever, skin or renal problems.
- When acetazolamide is given in high doses or for prolonged periods, patient may need potassium-rich diet and potassium supplement.

ACETOHEXAMIDE

(a-seat-oh-hex'a-mide)

Trade names: Dimelor♣, Dymelor

Classifications: HORMONE; SULFONYLUREA ANTIDIABETIC

Prototype: Tolbutamide

Pregnancy category: C

ACTIONS/PHARMACODYNAMICS
Promotes increased effectiveness of endogenous insulin. More potent and has longer action than tolbutamide, but actions, uses, precautions, and adverse reactions are similar. Lowers blood glucose by stimulating pancreatic beta cells to secrete insulin.

USES Mild to moderately severe stable type II diabetes, NIDDM (noninsulin-dependent diabetes mellitus). Also reduces insulin requirements in select patients with type I diabetes, IDDM (insulin-dependent diabetes mellitus). Preferred by some clinicians for patients who also have gout.

ROUTE & DOSAGE

Glycemic Control
Adult: **PO** 250 mg/d before breakfast; may be increased by 250–500 mg q5–7d (max 1.5 g/d); doses >1 g should be given before breakfast and dinner.

PHARMACOKINETICS Absorption: rapidly absorbed from GI tract. **Onset:** 1 h. **Peak:** 2–4 h. **Duration:** 12–24 h. **Distribution:** breast milk. **Metabolism:** metabolized in liver to active metabolite. **Elimination:** half-life: 5–6 h; 80–95% eliminated in urine; 15% in bile.

CONTRAINDICATIONS & PRECAUTIONS Contraindicated in: hypersensitivity to sulfonylureas; severe impairment of hepatic, renal, thyroid, or other endocrine function; as sole therapy for IDDM and in diabetes complicated by ketosis, acidosis, coma, infection, trauma, hyperglycemia, and glycosuria associated with primary renal disease. Safe use during pregnancy (category C), in nursing mothers, and in children not established. **Cautious use in:** renal insufficiency, history of hepatic porphyria.

ADVERSE/SIDE EFFECTS Generally dose-related. **GI:** nausea, vomiting, epigastric fullness, anorexia, stomach pain or discomfort, heartburn, diarrhea. **Hematologic:** agranulocytosis, aplastic anemia, severe hypoglycemia, thrombocytopenia. **Hypersensitivity:** erythema, urticaria, pruritus, rash, photosensitivity. **Other:** headache, dizziness.

DIAGNOSTIC TEST INTERFERENCE ***Serum uric acid*** levels may be appreciably reduced.

DRUG INTERACTIONS **Alcohol** may elicit disulfiram reaction; **warfarin, aspirin** and other SALICYLATES, **chloramphenicol, clofibrate, fenfluramine, guanethidine,** MAO INHIBITORS, **oxytetracycline, phenylbutazone, probenecid, sulfinpyrazone**, and SULFONAMIDES may enhance hypoglycemic effects; with **diazoxide** there is mutual antagonism and effects of both drugs are reduced; thiazide diuretics may exacerbate hyperglycemia, resulting in need for increased acetohexamide doses; **phenytoin** may decrease effects of acetohexamide; beta-adrenergic blockers may mask symptoms of hypoglycemia.

NURSING IMPLICATIONS

Administration

- Administer daily dose before breakfast.
- Doses in excess of 1 g are normally divided and given before breakfast and dinner.
- Store at 15–30C (59–86F) unless otherwise directed.

Assessment & Drug Effects

- Blood and urine glucose concentrations should be closely monitored during first 24 h after therapy is initiated.
- The elderly, malnourished, and debilitated patients and those with impaired hepatic or renal function or adrenal or pituitary insufficiency require close monitoring because they have a tendency to develop an exaggerated hypoglycemic response to acetohexamide, which may be difficult to recognize.
- Patients are usually given at least a 7-d trial period to determine therapeutic response. Favorable response is indicated by reduction in diabetes hyperglycemia symptoms (see Appendix G).
- Monitor for signs and symptoms of hypoglycemia (see Appendix G), which indicate a need for dosage adjustment.
- Periodic tests of liver function are recommended, i.e., bilirubin, cholesterol, AST, ALT.
- Dermatologic reactions tend to be transient and frequently subside even with continuation of therapy. However, if they persist or are severe, discontinuation of drug may be necessary.

Patient & Family Education

- Patient should ingest some form of sugar such as orange juice, sugar cube, table sugar (dissolved in water), corn syrup, or honey if symptoms of hypoglycemia develop, and seek medical assistance.
- During conversion from one antidiabetic agent to another, pa-

tient should check urine for glucose and ketones (acetone) at least 3 times a day and report to physician as directed. Blood glucose monitoring may also be prescribed.

- Caution patient not to take any other medication unless approved or prescribed by physician.
- Alcoholic beverages may produce a disulfiram-type reaction (see Signs & Symptoms, Appendix G).
- Advise patient to avoid prolonged direct exposure to sun to prevent photosensitivity reaction.

ACETYLCYSTEINE

(a-se-til-sis'tay-een)

Trade names: Airbron✤, Mucomyst, Mucosol, *N*-Acetylcysteine

Prototype for classifications: MUCOLYTIC; ANTIDOTE

Pregnancy category: B

ACTIONS/PHARMACODYNAMICS Probably acts by disrupting disulfide linkages of mucoproteins in purulent and nonpurulent secretions, thereby lowering viscosity and facilitating their removal.

USES Adjuvant therapy in patients with abnormal, viscid, or inspissated mucous secretions in acute and chronic bronchopulmonary diseases, and in pulmonary complications of cystic fibrosis and surgery, tracheostomy, and atelectasis. Also used in diagnostic bronchial studies and as an antidote for acute acetaminophen poisoning. **Unlabeled uses:** as an ophthalmic solution for treatment of dry eye (keratoconjunctivitis sicca); as an enema to treat bowel obstruction due to meconium ileus.

ROUTE & DOSAGE

Mucolytic

Adult: **Inhalation** 1–10 ml of 20% solution q4–6h *or* 2–20 ml of 10% solution q4–6h.
Direct instillation 1–2 ml of 10–20% solution q1–4h.
Infant: **Inhalation** 1–2 ml 20% solution or 2–4 ml of 10% solution 3–4 times/d.
Child: **Inhalation** 3–5 ml of 20% solution or 6–10 ml of 10% solution 3–4 times/d.

Acetaminophen Toxicity

Adult: **PO** 140 mg/kg followed by 70 mg/kg q4h for 17 doses (use a 5% solution).
Child: **PO** Same as for adult.

PHARMACOKINETICS **Onset:** 1 min after inhalation or instillation. **Peak:** 5–10 min. **Metabolism:** deacetylated in liver to cysteine and subsequently metabolized.

CONTRAINDICATIONS & PRECAUTIONS **Contraindicated in:** hypersensitivity to acetylcysteine; patients at risk of gastric hemorrhage. Safe use during pregnancy (category B) and in nursing mothers not established. **Cautious use in:** patients with asthma, the elderly, debilitated patients with severe respiratory insufficiency.

ADVERSE/SIDE EFFECTS **CNS:** dizziness, drowsiness. **GI:** nausea, *vomiting,* stomatitis. **Respiratory:** bronchospasm, rhinorrhea, burning sensation in upper respiratory passages, epistaxis. **Hepatoxicity:** urticaria.

NURSING IMPLICATIONS

Administration

- The 20% solution may be diluted with NS or water for injection. The

10% solution may be used undiluted.

- Acetylcysteine may be given by direct instillation into tracheostomy (1–2 ml of 10–20% solution).
- Treatments commonly administered when patient arises, before meals, and prior to retiring at night.
- For maximum effect, instruct patient to clear airway, if possible, coughing productively prior to aerosol administration.
- Once opened, vial can be stored in refrigerator to retard oxidation; use within 96 h. However, dilutions should be freshly prepared and used within 1 h; does not contain an antimicrobial agent. A light purple color apparently does not significantly impair its mucolytic effectiveness.
- Unopened vial should be stored at 15–30C (59–86F), unless otherwise directed.

Assessment & Drug Effects

- Have suction apparatus immediately available. Increased volume of respiratory tract fluid may be liberated; suction or endotracheal aspiration may be necessary to establish and maintain an open airway. Elderly and debilitated patients require close monitoring to prevent aspiration of excessive secretions.
- Bronchospasm is most likely to occur in patients with asthma, and it may happen unpredictably. If it occurs, drug should be discontinued immediately.
- Unpleasant odor of drug (rotten egg odor of hydrogen sulfide) and excess volume of liquefied bronchial secretions may cause nausea and possibly vomiting, particularly when face mask is used. Odor becomes less noticeable with continued inhalation.

Patient & Family Education

- Instruct patient to immediately report difficulty with clearing the airway or any other respiratory distress.
- Advise patient to report nausea, as an antiemetic may be indicated.

ACITRETIN

(a-ci-tree′tin)

Trade name: Soriatane

Classifications: SKIN AND MUCOUS MEMBRANE AGENT; ANTIACNE; RETINOID

Prototype: Isotretinoin

Pregnancy category: X

ACTIONS/PHARMACODYNAMICS Highly toxic metabolite of retinol (vitamin A). Mechanism of action of acitretin is unknown.

USE Treatment of severe psoriasis.

ROUTE & DOSAGE

Psoriasis
Adult: **PO** 10–50 mg q.d. with main meal.

PHARMACOKINETICS **Absorption:** rapidly absorbed from GI tract, optimal absorption when taken with food. **Peak:** 2–5 h. **Distribution:** crosses placenta, distributed into breast milk. **Metabolism:** metabolized active metabolite, *cis*-acitretin. **Elimination:** half-life: 49 h acitretin, 63 h *cis*-acitretin; excreted in both urine and feces.

CONTRAINDICATIONS & PRECAUTIONS **Contraindicated in:** pregnancy (category X), sensitivity to parabens, lacatation. **Cautious use in:** patients with impaired hepatic function, hepatitis, diabetes mellitus, obesity, alcoholism, history of pancreatitis, hypertriglyceridemia, hypercholesterolemia, coronary artery disease, retinal disease, degenerative joint disease.

ADVERSE/SIDE EFFECTS Body as whole: *hyperesthesia, paresthesias, arthralgia, progression of existing spinal hyperostosis, rigors,* back pain, hypertonia, myalgia, fatigue, hot flashes, increased appetite. **CNS:** headache, depression, insomina, somnolence. **CV:** flushing, edema. **GI:** *dry mouth, increased LFTs, increased triglycerides and cholesterol,* hepatitis, gingival bleeding, gingivitis, increased saliva, stomatitis, thirst, ulcerative stomatitis, abdominal pain, diarrhea, nausea, tongue disorder. **Ocular:** blurred vision, blepharitis, conjunctivitis, decreased night vision/night blindness, eye pain, photophobia. **Respiratory:** sinusitis. **Skin:** *alopecia, skin peeling, dry skin, nail disorders, pruritus, rash, cheilitis, skin atrophy, paronychia,* abnormal skin odor and hair texture, cold/clammy skin, increased sweating, purpura, seborrhea, skin ulceration, sunburn. **Other:** *rhinitis, epistaxis, xerophthalmia,* earache, taste perversion, tinnitus.

DRUG INTERACTIONS Combination with ethanol can create etretinate (see p. 566), which has a significantly longer half-life than acitretin; interferes with the contraceptive efficacy of progestin-only oral contraceptives.

NURSING IMPLICATIONS

Administration

- Administer as single dose with main meal because food enhances absorption.
- Store at 15–25C (59–77F) and protect from light. After opening bottle, avoid exposure to high temperatures and humidity.

Assessment & Drug Effects

- Therapeutic effectiveness is indicated by improvement in psoriasis lesions. Transient worsening of psoriasis may occur in early therapy.
- Lab tests: before initiating therapy and at 1- to 2-wk intervals until response to drug is known, lipid profile and liver function tests should be done. Blood glucose should be monitored periodically.
- Monitor diabetics for loss of glycemic control.
- Monitor for/immediately report S&S of pancreatitis.

Patient & Family Education

- Therapeutic effect may not be evident for 2–3 mo.
- Patients must be fully informed regarding common adverse effects.
- If visual problems develop, discontinue drug and report immediately to physician.
- Dry eyes may decrease tolerance for contact lenses.
- Avoid concurrent alcohol intake as it increases risk of hepatotoxicity and hypertriglyceridemia.
- Do not donate blood for 3 y following therapy.
- Avoid excessive exposure to sunlight or UV light.
- Women must be fully informed regarding risk of serious fetal deformities; two forms of effective contraception must be used for 1 mo before and at least 3 y following therapy.
- Females should avoid alcohol during and for 2 mo following therapy.

ACRIVASTINE/PSEUDOEPHEDRINE

(a-cri-vas′teen)

Trade name: Semprex-D (combination with pseudoephedrine)

Classifications: ANTIHISTAMINE; H_1-RECEPTOR ANTAGONIST; DECONGESTANT
Prototype: Diphenhydramine
Pregnancy category: B

ACTIONS/PHARMACODYNAMICS Acrivastine is an H_1-receptor histamine antagonist. It is effective in allergic rhinitis and dermatologic disorders by controlling histamine-mediated symptoms. Pseudoephedrine is a sympathomimetic amine that, like ephedrine, produces decongestion of the respiratory tract mucosa through its action on sympathetic nerve endings.

USE Seasonal and perennial allergic rhinitis with nasal congestion.

ROUTE & DOSAGE

Allergic Rhinitis
Adult: **PO** 1 tab (8 mg acrivastine/ 60 mg pseudoephedrine) t.i.d.

PHARMACOKINETICS **Absorption:** rapidly absorbed from GI tract. **Onset:** 1 h. **Duration:** approx 12 h. **Metabolism:** metabolized in liver. **Elimination:** half-life: 1.5 h; approx 65% excreted unchanged in urine.

CONTRAINDICATIONS & PRECAUTIONS **Contraindicated in:** Hypersensitivity to acrivastine, triprolidine, pseudoephedrine, or ephedrine; severe hypertension or severe coronary artery disease; patients on MAO inhibitor drugs; nursing mothers. **Cautious use in:** renal insufficiency, hypertension, DM, ischemic heart disease, increased intraocular pressure, hyperthyroidism, BPH, GI disorders, elderly, pregnancy (category B). Safety and effectiveness in children < 12 y have not been established.

ADVERSE/SIDE EFFECTS **CNS:** headache, vertigo, dizziness, insomnia, jitteriness, *drowsiness*. **GI:** nausea, diarrhea, dry mouth, dyspepsia.

DRUG INTERACTION **Alcohol** may increase psychomotor impairment.

NURSING IMPLICATIONS

Administration
- The drug should not be given to patients with a creatinine clearance of 48 ml/min or less.
- Store at 15–25C (59–77F); protect from light and moisture.

Assessment & Drug Effects
- Monitor for dizziness, sedation, urinary obstruction, and hypotension, especially the elderly.
- Assess for significant drowsiness, which may necessitate drug discontinuation.

Patient & Family Education
- Advise not to use this drug in combination with other OTC antihistamines or decongestants.
- Advise caution with hazardous activities until reaction to the drug is known.
- Warn against concurrent use of alcohol or other CNS depressants.

ACYCLOVIR
(ay-sye′-kloe-ver)
Trade names: Acycloguanosine, Zovirax

ACYCLOVIR SODIUM
Prototype for classifications: ANTIINFECTIVE; ANTIVIRAL
Pregnancy category: C

ACTIONS/PHARMACODYNAMICS Synthetic acyclic purine nucleoside analog, derived from guanine. Reduces viral shedding and formation of new lesions and speeds healing time. Acyclovir triphosphate preferentially interferes with DNA synthesis of herpes simplex virus types 1 and 2 (HSV-1 and HSV-2) and varicella-zoster virus, thereby inhibiting viral replication. Demonstrates antiviral activity against herpes virus simiae (B virus), Epstein-Barr (infectious mononucleosis), varicella-zoster and cytomegalovirus. Does not eradicate the latent herpes virus.

USES Parenterally for treatment of initial and recurrent mucosal and cutaneous herpes simplex virus (HSV-1 and HSV-2) infections in immunocompromised adults and children and for severe initial episodes of herpes genitalis in immunocompetent (normal immune system) patients. Used orally for treatment of initial episodes of genital herpes, for management of selected patients with severe recurrent episodes, and for prophylaxis to reduce frequency and severity of recurrent infections. Also used orally in varicella-zoster (chickenpox) in immunocompetent children and adolescents. Used topically for initial episodes of herpes genitalis and in non-life-threatening mucocutaneous herpes simplex virus infections in immunocompromised patients. **Unlabeled use:** for treatment of eczema herpeticum caused by HSV localized and disseminated herpes zoster.

ROUTE & DOSAGE

Genital Herpes Simplex

Adult: **PO** 200 mg q4h 5 times/d, or 400 mg t.i.d. × 7–10 d. **IV** 5 mg/kg q8h.
Child: **IV** <12 y: 250 mg/m^2 q8h, or 80 mg/kg/d in 2–5 doses.

Herpes Simplex Immunocompromised Patient

Adult: **IV** 15 mg/kg/d divided q8h × 5–7 d.
Child <1 y: **IV** 15–30 mg/kg/d divided q8h × 7–14 d.
Child ≥ 1 y: **IV** 750–1500 mg/m^2/d or 15–30 mg/kg/d divided q8h × 7–14 d.

Prophylaxis for Genital Herpes Simplex

Adult: **PO** 200 mg 2–5 times/d *or* 400 mg t.i.d. or 800 mg b.i.d.
Child: **PO** 80 mg/kg/d in 2–5 divided doses.

Herpes Zoster

Adult: **PO** 800 mg q4h 5 times/d.
Child: **PO** 80 mg/kg/d in 5 divided doses.

Herpes Simplex Encephalitis

Adult: **IV** 15 mg/kg q8h × 14–21 d.
Child: **IV** Same as for adult.
Premature neonate: **IV** 20 mg/kg/d divided q12h × 14–21 d.
Neonate: **IV** 30 mg/kg/d divided q8h × 14–21 d.

Varicella Zoster

Child/Adolescent: **PO** 20 mg/kg (max 800 mg) q.i.d. × 5 d initiated within 24 h of onset of rash.

Adjustment for Renal Impairment (all indications)

Cl_{cr} 25–50 ml/min: same dose q12h; 10–25 ml/min: same dose q24h.

PHARMACOKINETICS Absorption: oral dose is 15–30% absorbed. **Peak effect:** 1.5–2 h after oral dose. **Distribution:** distributes into most tissues with lower levels in the CNS; crosses placenta. **Metabolism:** drug is primarily excreted unchanged. **Elimination:** half-life: 2.5–5 h; renally eliminated; also excreted in breast milk.

CONTRAINDICATIONS & PRECAUTIONS **Contraindicated in:** rapid or bolus injection of acyclovir—infuse over 1 h. Safe use during pregnancy (category C) and in children not established. **Cautious use in:** nursing mother, renal insufficiency, dehydration.

ADVERSE/SIDE EFFECTS (generally minimal and infrequent). **CNS:** *headache,* light-headedness, lethargy, fatigue, tremors, confusion, seizures, dizziness. **GI:** *nausea, vomiting, diarrhea.* **Renal:** glomerulonephritis, renal tubular damage, acute renal failure. **Skin:** rash, urticaria, pruritus, burning, stinging sensation, irritation, sensitization. **Other:** inflammation or phlebitis at IV injection site, sloughing (with extravasation), <u>thrombocytopenic purpura/hemolytic uremic syndrome.</u>

DRUG INTERACTIONS **Probenecid** decreases acyclovir elimination; **zidovudine** may cause increased drowsiness and lethargy.

INCOMPATIBILITIES **Solution/additive:** bacteriostatic water for injection, albumin, hetastarch, **dopamine, dobutamine.** **Y-site:** Foscarnet, TPN.

NURSING IMPLICATIONS

Administration

Oral

- Absorption of oral acyclovir is not affected by food.
- Store capsules in tight, light-resistant containers at 15–30C (59–86F) unless otherwise directed.

Parenteral (IV)

- Reconstitute by adding 10 ml sterile water for injection to 500-mg vial (provides concentration of 50 mg/ml). Note: Solutions containing benzyl alcohol are toxic to neonates. Shake well to ensure complete dissolution of drug. This solution should be used within 12 h.
- To reduce risk of renal injury and phlebitis, final concentration should be 7 mg/ml or less. Infuse over at least 1 h. Once prepared, diluted solution should be used within 24 h.
- Manufacturer approves use of standard commercially available electrolyte and glucose solutions for infusion solution; incompatible with blood products and protein-containing solutions.
- IV administration: Parenteral solution is intended for IV infusion only and must be administered over a period of at least 1 h to prevent renal tubular damage. Rapid or bolus IV and IM or SC administration must be avoided.
- Monitor IV flow rate carefully; infusion pump or microdrip infusion set preferred. Usual rate of administration is a single dose over 60 min. Observe infusion site during and for a few days following infusion.
- IV administration to neonates, infants, children: Verify correct IV concentration and rate of infusion with physician.
- Keep patient adequately hydrated during first 2 h after infusion to maintain sufficient urinary flow and thus prevent precipitation of drug in renal tubules.
- Consult physician about amount and length of time oral fluids need to be pushed after IV drug treatment.
- Refrigeration of reconstituted solution may cause precipitation; however, crystals will redissolve at room temperature.
- Store acyclovir powder and reconstituted solutions at controlled room temperature preferably at 15–30C (59–86F) unless otherwise directed by manufacturer.

Topical

- Thorough hand washing is needed before and after treatment of lesions and after handling and disposition of secretions. Virus is killed by soap and water.
- Use liquid soap for hand washing to prevent cross-contamination.
- Apply topical preparation with finger cot or surgical glove to prevent further self-infection as well as spread of virus to others. Use sufficient ointment to completely cover lesions.
- Store at 15–25C (59–78F) unless otherwise directed.

Assessment & Drug Effects

- Monitor I&O ratio and pattern, especially after IV administration. Note: Unusual tiredness and weakness suggest poor hydration as well as early renal failure.
- Baseline and periodic renal function studies should be done. This is particularly important with IV administration. Elevations of BUN and serum creatinine and decreases in creatinine clearance indicate need for dosage adjustment, discontinuation of drug, or correction of fluid and electrolyte balance.
- Prophylactic use of the oral drug will require careful monitoring for possible long-term side effects and for viral resistance to acyclovir and is generally given for no longer than 6 mo pending complete evaluation of the benefits and dangers of prolonged use of acyclovir.
- Notify physician if local reactions to topical drug are pronounced or annoying and if no improvement is noted within 1 wk.
- Pregnant patients should be followed closely to detect reinfection.
- Patients with history of neurologic problems, drug related or otherwise, are reportedly more prone to manifest acyclovir-induced neurologic symptoms.
- Immunocompromised patients receiving prolonged or repeated therapy have developed drug resistance.
- Concomitant use with other nephrotoxic drugs and preexisting renal disease may cause acute renal failure.

Patient & Family Education

- Therapy is most effective when started as soon as possible after onset of signs and symptoms.
- Even after the HSV infection is controlled, latent virus can be activated by such stimuli as stress, trauma, fever, exposure to sunlight, sexual intercourse, menstruation, treatment with immunosuppressive drugs.
- Warn patient to refrain from sexual intercourse if either partner has signs or symptoms of herpes infection.
- Acyclovir is not a cure for herpetic infections. HSV-1 virus (cold sore or fever blister) remains latent for patient's lifetime and may emerge intermittently to cause symptoms.
- Caution patient not to exceed recommended dosage, frequency of drug administration, or specified duration of therapy. Urge patient to contact physician if relief is not obtained or side effects appear.
- Women with genital herpes reportedly are at a high risk level for developing cervical cancer. Urge patient to have periodic Papanicolaou (Pap) smears to detect early cervical changes.

Topical Application

- Cleanse affected areas with soap and water 3 or 4 times daily; dry well. Hair dryer may be helpful. Wear loose-fitting clothing and absorbent (e.g., cotton) undercloth-ing.

- Avoid drug contact in or around eyes. Any unexplained eye symptoms (e.g., redness, pain) should be reported immediately. Untreated infection can lead to corneal keratitis and blindness.
- Avoid use of OTC emollient creams or ointments unless specifically prescribed by physician. These agents tend to delay healing and may even spread lesions.
- Topical applications do not prevent transmission to other individuals and do not prevent recurrence.

ADAPALENE

(a-da'pa-leen)

Trade name: Differin

Classifications: SKIN AND MUCOUS MEMBRANE AGENT; ANTIACNE; RETINOID

Prototype: Isotretinoin

Pregnancy category: C

ACTIONS/PHARMACODYNAMICS Adapalene is a topical retinoid-like compound that modulates cellular differentiation, keratinization, and inflammatory processes related to the pathology of acne vulgaris. Topical adapalene may normalize the differentiation of epithelial follicular cells, resulting in decreased acne formation.

USE Topical treatment of acne vulgaris.

ROUTE & DOSAGE

Acne

Adult: **Topical** Apply once daily to affected areas in evening.

PHARMACOKINETICS **Absorption:** minimal absorption through intact skin. **Elimination:** excreted primarily in bile.

CONTRAINDICATIONS & PRECAUTIONS **Contraindicated in:** hypersensitivity to adapalene or any of the components of the gel, irritating topical products, and sunburn. **Cautious use in:** pregnancy (category C), nursing mothers. Safety and effectiveness in children < 12 y not established.

ADVERSE/SIDE EFFECTS Skin: *erythema, scaling, dryness, pruritus, burning*, skin irritation, stinging, sunburn, acne flares.

NURSING IMPLICATIONS

Administration

- Apply a thin film to clean skin, avoiding eyes, lips, mucous membranes, cuts, abrasions, eczematous or sunburned skin.
- Do not apply to skin recently treated with preparations containing sulfur, resorcinol, or salicylic acid.
- Store at 20–25C (68–77F).

Assessment & Drug Effects

- During early weeks of therapy, an apparent worsening of acne may occur but therapy should not be stopped. Therapeutic results occur after 8–12 wk of treatment.
- Cutaneous reactions (e.g., erythema, scaling, pruritus) are common and normally diminish after first month of therapy.

Patient & Family Education

- Apply only as directed; excessive application will not result in faster healing but will cause marked redness, peeling, and discomfort.
- Minimize exposure to sunlight and sunlamps, and use sunscreen and protective clothing as needed.

ADENOSINE

(a-den'o-sin)

Trade names: Adenocard, Adenoscan

Classifications: CARDIOVASCULAR AGENT; ANTIARRHYTHMIC

Prototype: Procainamide

Pregnancy category: C

ACTIONS/PHARMACODYNAMICS

Slows conduction through the atrioventricular (AV) and sinoatrial (SA) nodes. Can interrupt the reentry pathways through the AV node. Depresses left ventricular function, but effect is transient due to short half-life.

USES Conversion to sinus rhythm of paroxysmal supraventricular tachycardia (PSVT) including PSVT associated with accessory bypass tracts (Wolff-Parkinson-White syndrome). "Chemical" thallium stress test. **Unlabeled uses:** afterload-reducing agent in low-output states; to prevent graft occlusion following aortocoronary bypass surgery; to produce controlled hypotension during cerebral aneurysm surgery.

ROUTE & DOSAGE

Supraventricular Tachycardia

Adult: **IV** 6 mg rapid IV bolus (over 1–2 s); may repeat in 1–2 min with 12 mg IV push × 2 (total of 3 doses); max recommended dose is 12 mg; injection should be given directly into the vein or as proximal as possible in the IV line and followed by a rapid saline flush.

Neonate/Infant/Child: **IV** 0.05 mg/kg; may increase dose by 0.05 mg/kg q2min to max of 0.25 mg/kg or 12 mg/dose.

PHARMACOKINETICS Absorption: rapid uptake by erythrocytes and vascular endothelial cells after IV administration. **Onset:** 20–30 s. **Metabolism:** rapid uptake into cells; degraded by deamination to inosine, hypoxanthine, and adenosine monophosphate. **Elimination:** half-life: 10 s; route of elimination unknown.

CONTRAINDICATIONS & PRECAUTIONS Contraindicated in: AV block, preexisting second- and third-degree block or sick sinus rhythm without pacemaker, since a heart block may result. Also contraindicated in atrial flutter, atrial fibrillation, and ventricular tachycardia because the drug is ineffective. **Cautious use in:** asthmatics, pregnancy (category C), hepatic and renal failure.

ADVERSE/SIDE EFFECTS *Transient facial flushing,* transient dyspnea, atrial fibrillation or flutter, irritability in children.

DRUG INTERACTIONS Dipyridamole can potentiate the effects of adenosine; **theophylline** will block the electrophysiologic effects of adenosine; **carbamazepine** may increase risk of heart block.

NURSING IMPLICATIONS

Administration

- For rapid bolus IV, administer directly into vein. If given by IV line, administer as proximally as possible, and follow with a rapid saline flush.
- Adenosine must be given as a rapid bolus IV over 1–2 s.
- The solution must be clear at time of use. Since it contains no preservatives, discard used portion.
- If high-level block develops after one dose, do not repeat dose.
- Store at room temperature 15–30C (59–86F). Do not refrigerate, as crystallization may occur. If crys-

tals do form, dissolve by warming to room temperature.

Assessment & Drug Effects

- Because of the short half-life (10 s), adverse side effects are generally self-limiting.
- Use a hemodynamic monitoring system during administration.
- Monitor BP and heart rate q15–30s for several minutes after administration.
- An ECG is recommended to confirm efficiency of adenosine.
- Potential for bronchospasms in asthma patients is thought to exist. Monitor carefully.
- At the time of conversion to normal sinus rhythm, PVCs, PACs, sinus bradycardia, and sinus tachycardia, as well as various degrees of AV block, are seen on the ECG. These usually last only a few seconds and resolve without intervention.

Patient & Family Education

- Inform patient that facial flushing may occur.

ALBENDAZOLE

(al-ben′da-zole)

Trade name: Albenza

Classifications: ANTIINFECTIVE; ANTHELMINTIC AGENT

Prototype: Mebendazole

Pregnancy category: C

ACTIONS/PHARMACODYNAMICS Albendazole is a broad-spectrum oral anthelmintic agent. It is the only anthelmintic drug active against all stages of the helminth life cycle (ova, larvae, and adult worms). Its mechanism of action is unclear, but it appears to cause selective degeneration of cytoplasmic microtubules in the intestinal cells of the helminths and larvae. It ultimately causes decreased ATP production in the helminths, resulting in energy depletion, which kills the worms.

USES Treatment of neurocysticercosis caused by the larval form of pork tapeworm (*Taenia solium*), hydatid disease caused by the larval form of dog tapeworm (*Echinococcus granulosus*).

ROUTE & DOSAGE

Neurocysticercosis

Adult & Child >6 y: **PO** Weight <60 kg: 15 mg/kg/d divided b.i.d. with meals × 8–30 d (max 800 mg/d); weight ≥60 kg: 400 mg b.i.d. with meal × 8–30 d.

Hydatid Disease

Adult & Child > 6 y: **PO** Weight < 60 kg: 15 mg/kg/d divided b.i.d. with meals (max 800 mg/d); weight ≥ 60 kg: 400 mg b.i.d. with meal for 28-d cycle, then 14 d without drug. Repeat regimen for 3 cycles.

PHARMACOKINETICS Absorption: poorly absorbed from GI tract, absorption enhanced with a fatty meal. **Peak:** 2–5 h. **Distribution:** 70% bound to plasma proteins; widely distributed throughout body including cyst fluid and CSF; secreted into animal breast milk. **Metabolism:** metabolized in liver to active metabolite, albendazole sulfoxide. **Elimination:** half-life: 8–12 h; excreted in bile.

CONTRAINDICATIONS & PRECAUTIONS Contraindicated in: hypersensitivity to the benzimidazole class of compounds or any components of albendazole; pregnancy (category C). **Cautious use in:** retinal lesions, nursing mothers.

ADVERSE/SIDE EFFECTS CNS: *headache*, dizziness, vertigo, increased intracranial pressure, meningeal signs, alopecia (reversible), fever. **GI:** *abnormal liver function tests*, abdominal pain, nausea, vomiting. **Hematologic (rare):** <u>leukopenia</u>, <u>granulocytopenia</u>, <u>pancytopenia</u>, <u>agranulocytosis</u>. **Skin:** rash, urticaria. **Other:** hypersensitivity reactions.

DRUG INTERACTIONS Cimetidine, dexamethasone, praziquantel increase albendazole levels.

NURSING IMPLICATIONS

Administration

- Give with meals.
- Patients treated for neurocysticercosis should receive appropriate steroid and anticonvulsant therapy as required.
- Maximum total daily dose should not exceed 800 mg.
- Store at 20–25C (68–77F).

Assessment & Drug Effects

- At start of each 28-day cycle and q2wk during cycle, monitor total WBC count, absolute neutrophil count, and liver function tests.
- Withhold drug and notify physician if WBC count falls below normal or liver enzymes are elevated.

Patient & Family Education

- Take with meals.
- Women of childbearing age should avoid becoming pregnant during and for at least 1 mo after therapy.

ALBUTEROL

(al-byoo'ter-ole)

Trade names: Novosalmol ♣, Proventil, Proventil HFA, Proventil Repetabs, Salbutamol, Ventolin, Ventolin Rotocaps, Volmax

Classifications: AUTONOMIC NERVOUS SYSTEM AGENT; BETA-ADRENERGIC AGONIST (SYMPATHOMIMETIC); BRONCHODILATOR (RESPIRATORY SMOOTH MUSCLE RELAXANT)

Prototype: Albuterol

Pregnancy category: C

ACTIONS/PHARMACODYNAMICS

Synthetic sympathomimetic amine and moderately selective $beta_2$-adrenergic agonist with comparatively long action. Has more prominent effect on $beta_2$ receptors (particularly smooth muscles of bronchi, uterus, and vascular supply to skeletal muscles) than on $beta_1$ (heart) receptors. Minimal or no effect on alpha-adrenergic receptors. Inhibits histamine release by mast cells. Produces bronchodilation, regardless of administration route, by relaxing smooth muscles of bronchial tree. This decreases airway resistance, facilitates mucus drainage, and increases vital capacity.

USES To relieve bronchospasm associated with acute or chronic asthma, bronchitis, or other reversible obstructive airway diseases. Also used to prevent exercise-induced bronchospasm. **Unlabeled uses:** as adjunct in treatment of refractory heart failure and to stimulate intracellular transport of potassium in hyperkalemic familial periodic paralysis.

ROUTE & DOSAGE

Bronchospasm

Adult: **PO** 2–4 mg 3–4 times/d; 4–8 mg sustained release 2 times/d. **Inhaled** 1–2 inhalations q4–6h.
Child: **PO** 2–6 y, 0.1–0.2 mg/kg t.i.d. (max 4 mg/dose); 6–12 y, 2 mg 3–4 times/d; 2–6 y, 0.1 mg/kg 3 times/d. **Inhaled** 6–12 y, 1–2 inhalations q4–6h.

PHARMACOKINETICS Onset: inhaled: 5–15 min; PO 30 min. **Peak effect:** inhaled: 0.5–2 h; PO 2.5 h. **Duration:** inhaled: 3–6 h; PO 4–6 h (8–12 h with sustained release). **Metabolism:** metabolized in liver; may cross the placenta. **Elimination:** half-life: 2.75 h; 76% of dose eliminated in urine in 3 d.

CONTRAINDICATIONS & PRECAUTIONS Contraindicated in: safe use not established during pregnancy (category C) and in nursing mothers; use of oral syrup in children <2 y. **Cautious use in:** cardiovascular disease, hypertension, hyperthyroidism, diabetes mellitus, hypersensitivity to sympathomimetic amines or to fluorocarbon propellant used in inhalation aerosols.

ADVERSE/SIDE EFFECTS CNS: *tremor*, anxiety, nervousness, restlessness, convulsions, weakness, headache, hallucinations. **CV:** palpitation, hypertension, hypotension, bradycardia, reflex tachycardia. **Eye:** blurred vision, dilated pupils. **GI:** nausea, vomiting. **Other:** muscle cramps, hoarseness, hypersensitivity reaction.

DIAGNOSTIC TEST INTERFERENCE Transient small increases in ***plasma glucose*** may occur.

DRUG INTERACTIONS With **epinephrine,** other SYMPATHOMIMETIC BRONCHODILATORS, possible additive effects; MAO INHIBITORS, TRICYCLIC ANTIDEPRESSANTS potentiate action on vascular system; BETA-ADRENERGIC BLOCKERS antagonize the effects of both drugs.

NURSING IMPLICATIONS

Administration

- Tablets and syrup should be stored between 2 and 30C (36 and 86F) in tight, light-resistant container.
- Store canisters between 15 and 30C (59 and 86F) away from heat and direct sunlight.

Assessment & Drug Effects

- Most common adverse effect associated with oral drug is fine tremor in fingers, which may interfere with precision handwork. Keep physician informed of any unusual symptoms.
- Children 2–6 y old appear to be more prone to experience CNS stimulation (hyperactivity, excitement, nervousness, insomnia), tachycardia, GI symptoms. Report promptly to physician.
- If drug-induced insomnia is a problem, consult physician about giving last albuterol dose several hours before bedtime.

Patient & Family Education

- Patient should receive explicit directions for correct use of medication and inhaler. Periodically check adequacy of patient's technique. Avoid contact of drug with eyes.
- If patient is also receiving beclomethasone (Vanceril) inhalation treatments, albuterol should be administered 20–30 min before, to allow deeper penetration of beclomethasone into lungs, unless otherwise directed by physician.
- Caution patient not to increase number or frequency of inhalations without advice of physician.
- Significiant subjective improvement in pulmonary function should occur within 60–90 min after drug administration. Advise patient to notify physician if albuterol fails to provide relief, as this can signify worsening of pulmonary function. Reevaluation of patient's condition and therapy may be indicated.
- Since albuterol can cause dizziness

or vertigo, caution patient to take necessary precautions.

- Emphasize dangers of self-prescribed OTC drugs without physician approval. Many medications (e.g., cold remedies) contain sympathomimetics that may intensify albuterol action.

ALCLOMETASONE DIPROPIONATE

(al-clo-met′a-sone)

Trade name: Alclovate

Classifications: SKIN AGENT; ANTI-INFLAMMATORY; STEROID

Prototype: Hydrocortisone

Pregnancy category: C

See Appendix A.

ALENDRONATE SODIUM

(a-len′dro-nate)

Trade name: Fosamax

Classifications: REGULATOR, BONE METABOLISM; BONE RESORPTION INHIBITOR, BIPHOSPHONATE

Prototype: Etidronate

Pregnancy category: C

ACTIONS/PHARMACODYNAMICS Alendronate is an aminobiphosphonate that inhibits osteoclast-mediated bone resorption. Antiresorption mechanism is not fully understood. Alendronate does, however, localize preferentially to resorption sites of active bone turnover and has minimal to no interference with bone mineralization. It is used in treatment of disorders characterized by increased bone resorption.

USES Prevention and treatment of osteoporosis in postmenopausal women, Paget's disease.

ROUTE & DOSAGE

Osteoporosis—Treatment
Adult: **PO** 10 mg once/d (max 40 mg/d).

Osteoporosis—Prevention
Adult: **PO** 5 mg q.d.

Paget's Disease
Adult: **PO** 40 mg once/d for 6 mo.

PHARMACOKINETICS Absorption: 0.5–1% absorbed from GI tract (absorption significantly decreased by calcium and food). **Onset:** 3–6 wk. **Duration:** 12 wk after discontinuation. **Distribution:** rapid skeletal uptake. **Metabolism:** not metabolized. **Elimination:** half-life: up to 10 h; up to 50% excreted unchanged in urine.

CONTRAINDICATIONS & PRECAUTIONS Contraindicated in: hypersensitivity to alendronate or other biphosphonates, severe renal impairment Cl_{Cr} 35 ml/min hypocalcemia, abnormalities of esophagus (strictures or achalasia), inability to stand or sit upright for 30 min. **Cautious use in:** renal impairment, CHF, hyperphosphatemia, liver disease, fever or infection, active upper GI problems, pregnancy (category C).

ADVERSE/SIDE EFFECTS Endocrine: hypocalcemia. **GI:** esophageal irritation and *ulceration, nausea, vomiting, abdominal pain, dyspepsia,* diarrhea, constipation, flatulence. **Other:** arthralgias, myalgias, headache, rash.

DRUG INTERACTIONS Calcium and food (especially dairy products) reduce alendronate absorption.

NURSING IMPLICATIONS

Administration

- Hypocalcemia must be corrected before alendronate may be administered.

- Ideally, drug should be given 30 min before the first medication, food, or beverage of the day. Give with 8 oz of plain water.
- Do not administer within 2 h of calcium-containing foods, beverages, or medications.
- Patient should avoid lying down for 30 min after taking drug.
- Store according to manufacturer's directions.

Assessment & Drug Effects
- Monitor albumin-adjusted serum calcium, serum phosphate, serum alkaline phosphatase, fasting and 24-h urinary calcium, and serum electrolytes.
- Periodically monitor renal and liver functions. Drug should be discontinued if the creatinine clearance is less than 35 ml/min.

Patient & Family Education
- Advise to carefully follow directions for taking drug correctly with respect to foods, beverages, and other drugs.
- Advise to report fever especially when accompanied by arthralgia and myalgia.

ALFENTANIL HYDROCHLORIDE

(al-fen'ta-nill)

Trade name: Alfenta

Classifications: CNS AGENT; NARCOTIC (OPIATE) AGONIST ANALGESIC; GENERAL ANESTHETIC

Prototype: Morphine

Pregnancy category: C

Controlled substance: Schedule II

ACTIONS/PHARMACODYNAMICS Narcotic agonist analgesic with rapid onset and short duration of action. Brief duration is advantageous for short surgical procedures but necessitates incremental injections or continuous infusion for long operations. CNS effects of alfentanil appear to be related to interaction of drug with opiate receptors. Tolerance to analgesic effects of alfentanil infusion has not been observed.

USES Major component of balanced anesthesia; analgesic, analgesic supplement, and primary anesthetic for induction of anesthesia when endotracheal and mechanical ventilation are required.

ROUTE & DOSAGE

Anesthesia Induction

Adult: **IV** 8–20 μg/kg for surgery lasting < 30 min; maintenance anesthesia can be maintained with incremental doses of 3–5 μg/kg *or* a continuous infusion of 0.5–1 μg/kg/min (total dose of 8–40 μg/kg).

PHARMACOKINETICS **Onset:** 2 min. **Duration:** injection 30 min; continuous infusion 45 min. **Distribution:** crosses placenta. **Metabolism:** completely metabolized in liver. **Elimination:** half-life: 46–213 min; excreted in breast milk.

CONTRAINDICATIONS & PRECAUTIONS **Contraindicated in:** safe use during pregnancy (category C), in children <12 y, or during lactation not established. **Cautious use in:** elderly, history of pulmonary disease.

ADVERSE/SIDE EFFECTS **CV:** hypotension, hypertension, tachycardia, bradycardia. **GI:** *nausea,* vomiting, anorexia, constipation, cramps. **Respiratory:** <u>apnea, respiratory depression</u>, dyspnea. **Other:** dizziness; thoracic muscle rigidity; euphoria, drowsiness, flushing, diaphoresis; extremities feel heavy and warm.

DRUG INTERACTIONS BETA-ADRENERGIC BLOCKERS increase incidence of bradycardia; CNS DEPRESSANTS such as BARBITURATES, TRANQUILIZERS, NEUROMUSCULAR BLOCKING AGENTS, OPIATES, and INHALATION GENERAL ANESTHETICS may enhance the cardiovascular and CNS effects of alfentanil in both magnitude and duration when administered with alfentanil; enhancement or prolongation of postoperative respiratory depression also may result from concomitant administration of any of these agents with alfentanil.

NURSING IMPLICATIONS

Administration

- Alfentanil is available in concentrations of 500 μg (as HCl) per milliliter. When 20 ml of alfentanil is added to 230 ml of compatible IV solution, the resulting concentration is 40 μg/ml.
- IV preparation: Compatibility has been demonstrated in solution (concentration range: 25–80 μg/ml) with normal saline, 5% dextrose in normal saline, D5W, and lactated Ringer's.
- Store at 15–30C (59–86F). Avoid freezing.

Assessment & Drug Effects

- If a narcotic antagonist has been administrated to overcome residual effects of alfentanil, observe patient frequently for symptoms of increased sympathetic stimulation (arrhythmias) and for evidence of depressed postoperative analgesia (tachycardia, pain, pupillary dilation, spontaneous muscle movement).
- Monitor vital signs at regular intervals during recovery period: check for bradycardia, especially if patient is also taking a beta blocker.
- When alfentanil is used as a postoperative analgesic, many patients experience dizziness, sedation, nausea, and vomiting.
- Adequacy of spontaneous ventilation must be evaluated carefully during postoperative period. Monitor chest wall movement and quality of respirations.
- Drug's narcotic effects wear off quickly with neglible residual effects.

Patient & Family Education

- If drug is used for patient-controlled analgesia, instruct patient to report unpleasant side effects.

ALLOPURINOL

(al-oh-pure′i-nole)

Trade names: Alloprin ♣, Apo-allopurinol ♣, Lopurin, Novopurinol ♣, Purinol ♣, Zyloprim

Classification: ANTIGOUT AGENT

Prototype: Colchicine

Pregnancy category: C

ACTIONS/PHARMACODYNAMICS Allopurinol reduces endogenous uric acid by selectively inhibiting action of xanthine oxidase, enzyme responsible for converting hypoxanthine to xanthine and xanthine to uric acid (end product of purine catabolism). Thus, urate pool is decreased by the lowering of both serum and urinary uric acid levels, and hyperuricosuria is prevented. Has no analgesic, antiinflammatory, or uricosuric actions.

USES To control primary hyperuricemia that accompanies severe gout and to prevent possibility of flare-up of acute gouty attack; to prevent recurrent calcium oxalate stones; prophylactically to reduce severity of hyperuricemia associated with antineoplastic and radiation therapies, both of which greatly increase plasma uric acid levels by promoting nucleic acid degradation. **Unlabeled use:** to reduce hyperuricemia secondary to Lesch–Nyhan syndrome, polycythemia vera, G6PD deficiency, sarcoidosis, and therapy with thiazides or ethambutol.

ROUTE & DOSAGE

Hyperuricemia

Adult: **PO** 100 mg/d; may increase by 100 mg/wk (max 800 mg/d); doses >300 mg/d should be divided.
Child: **PO** *≤10 y,* 10 mg/kg/d in 2–3 divided doses (max 800 mg/d); *>10 y,* same as adult.

Secondary Hyperuricemia

Adult: **PO** 200–800 mg/d for 2–3 d or longer; doses >300 mg/d should be divided.
Child: **PO** *6–10 y,* 100 mg t.i.d.; *<6 y,* 50 mg t.i.d.

Adjustment for Renal Impairment

Cl_{cr} 80 ml/min: 250 mg/d; 60 ml/min: 200 mg/d; 40 ml/min: 150 mg/d; 20 ml/min: 100 mg/d; 10 ml/min: 100 mg q2d; 0 ml/min: 100 mg q3d.

PHARMACOKINETICS Absorption: 80–90% absorbed from GI tract. **Onset:** 24–48 h. **Peak:** 2–6 h. **Metabolism:** 75–80% metabolizes to the active metabolite oxypurinol. **Elimination:** half-life: 1–3 h (half-life of oxypurinol: 18–30 h); slowly excreted in urine; excreted in breast milk.

CONTRAINDICATIONS & PRECAUTIONS Contraindicated in: hypersensitivity to allopurinol; as initial treatment for acute gouty attacks; idiopathic hemochromatosis (or those with family history); children (except those with hyperuricemia secondary to neoplastic disease and chemotherapy). Safe use during pregnancy (category C) and in nursing mothers not established. **Cautious use in:** impaired hepatic or renal function, history of peptic ulcer, lower GI tract disease, bone marrow depression.

ADVERSE/SIDE EFFECTS CNS: drowsiness, headache, vertigo. **GI:** nausea, vomiting, diarrhea, abdominal discomfort, indigestion, malaise. **Hematologic** (rare): <u>agranulocytosis</u>, <u>aplastic anemia</u>, <u>bone marrow depression</u>, thrombocytopenia. **Skin:** urticaria or pruritus, pruritic maculopapular rash, toxic epidermal necrolysis. **Other:** hepatotoxicity.

DIAGNOSTIC TEST INTERFERENCE Possibility of elevated blood levels of ***alkaline phosphatase*** and ***serum transaminases*** (AST, ALT), and decreased blood ***Hct, Hgb, leukocytes.***

DRUG INTERACTIONS Alcohol may inhibit renal excretion of uric acid; **ampicillin, amoxicillin** increase risk of skin rash; enhances anticoagulant effect of **warfarin;** toxicity from **azathioprine, mercaptopurine, cyclophosphamide** increased; increases hypoglycemic effects of **chlorpropamide;** THIAZIDES increase risk of allopurinol toxicity and hypersensitivity (especially with impaired renal function).

NURSING IMPLICATIONS

Administration

- Best tolerated when taken following meals; tablet may be crushed and taken with fluid or mixed with food.
- When used with antineoplastic therapy, allopurinol should be prescribed 1 or 2 d before chemotherapy begins.

- Store at 15–30C (59–86F) in a tightly closed container.

Assessment & Drug Effects

- Baseline CBC and liver and kidney function tests should be performed before therapy is initiated and then monthly, particularly during first few months of therapy.
- Aim of therapy is to lower serum urate level gradually to about 6 mg/dl. Serum uric acid levels should be evaluated at least every 1–2 wk to check adequacy of dosage. A sudden decrease in serum uric acid can precipitate an acute gouty attack.
- Acute gouty attacks are most likely during first 6 wk of therapy, possibly because of mobilization of urates from tissue deposits. Concurrent prophylactic therapy with colchicine may be prescribed, for the first 3–6 mo of therapy.
- Monitor I&O ratio and pattern. Decreased renal function causes drug accumulation.
- Urinary pH should be checked at regular intervals. Excessive alkalinity can make uric acid stones more difficult to dissolve.
- The elderly and patients with renal disorders tend to have a higher than usual incidence of renal stones and drug toxicity including dermatologic (hypersensitivity) problems.
- A life-threatening toxicity syndrome has occurred 2–4 wk after initiation of therapy, commonly in patients with impaired renal function, and is generally accompanied by malaise, fever, and aching, a diffuse erythematous, desquamating rash, hepatic dysfunction, eosinophilia, and worsening of renal function. Report immediately to physician the onset of rash or fever. Drug should be withdrawn.
- Therapeutic response is indicated by normal serum and urinary uric acid levels (usually by 1–3 wk), gradual decrease in size of tophi, absence of new tophaceous deposits (after approximately 6 mo), with consequent relief of joint pain and increased joint mobility.

Patient & Family Education

- It is advisable to maintain fluid intake sufficient to produce urinary output of at least 2000 ml/d (fluid intake of at least 3000 ml/d). Instruct patient to report diminishing urinary output, cloudy urine, unusual color or odor to urine, pain or discomfort on urination.
- Instruct patient to report promptly the onset of itching or rash, especially if ampicillin is prescribed concurrently.
- A skin rash, which may appear after 1–5 wk (and reportedly even after 2 y) of therapy, is the most common adverse reaction and is an indication to stop drug therapy.
- Physician may advise patient to limit high purine foods, e.g., organ meats (e.g., kidney, liver), anchovies, sardines, salmon, meat soups, gravies, dried peas and beans, asparagus, cauliflower, mushrooms, spinach, peppers.
- For treatment of oxalate stones, advise patient to abstain from high oxalate foods: tea, chocolate, rhubarb, spinach, nuts, beets, figs, peppers.
- Advise patient to minimize exposure and to shield eyes from ultraviolet or sunlight. Ultraviolet light may stimulate the development of cataracts. Patients should be examined periodically for lens changes.
- Caution patient to avoid driving or performing other complex tasks

until reaction to drug has been evaluated.

- Allopurinol is generally continued indefinitely; patient should remain under medical supervision. The drug can cause severe adverse reactions.

ALPHA$_1$-PROTEINASE INHIBITOR (HUMAN)

(pro′ten-ase)
Trade name: Prolastin
Classification: ENZYME INHIBITOR
Pregnancy category: C

ACTIONS/PHARMACODYNAMICS Alpha$_1$-proteinase inhibitor (α_1-PI; α_1-antitrypsin) is extracted from plasma and used in patients with panacinar emphysema who have α_1-antitrypsin deficiency. α_1-Antitrypsin deficiency is a chronic, hereditary, and usually fatal autosomal recessive disorder that results in a slowly progressive, panacinar emphysema.

USES Indicated for chronic replacement therapy in patients with α_1-antitrypsin deficiency and demonstrable panacinar emphysema.

ROUTE & DOSAGE

Adult: **IV** 60 mg/kg once weekly administered at a rate of ≥0.08 ml/kg/min.

PHARMACOKINETICS Distribution: crosses placenta; distributed into breast milk. **Metabolism:** undergoes catabolism in the intravascular space; approximately 33% is catabolized per day, with estimated production levels of 34 mg/kg/d. **Elimination:** half-life: 4.5–5.2 d.

CONTRAINDICATIONS & PRECAUTIONS Contraindicated in: individuals with selective IgA deficiencies. **Cautious use in:** patients with significant heart disease or other conditions that may be aggravated with slight increases in plasma volume. During pregnancy, use only when clearly needed and when the potential benefits outweigh the potential hazards to the fetus. Safety and efficacy in children has not been established.

ADVERSE/SIDE EFFECTS Hematologic: leukocytosis. **CNS:** dizziness, fever (may be delayed). **Other:** hepatitis B if not immunized.

NURSING IMPLICATIONS

Administration

- Reconstitute with sterile water for injection supplied by manufacturer to yield a concentration of 20 mg/ml.
- Administer within 3 h after reconstitution. Give alone, without mixing with other agents. If necessary, it may be diluted with normal saline.
- Administer properly diluted drug by direct IV injection at rate of at least 0.08 ml/kg/min.
- Administration by intermittent or continuous infusion not recommended.
- Hepatitis B vaccine should be administered prior to utilizing this drug.
- Refrigerate unreconstituted drug at 2–8C (35–46F). Do not refrigerate after reconstitution. Discard unused solution.

Assessment & Drug Effects

- Monitor serum α_1-PI level. Minimum serum concentration level should be 80 mg/ml.
- Assess respiratory status (rate, dyspnea, lung sounds) prior to any therapy.
- Caution should be used in patients at risk for circulatory overload.

Patient & Family Education

- Advise patient to avoid smoking and notify physician of any changes in respiratory pattern.

ALPRAZOLAM

(al-pray′zoe-lam)

Trade name: Xanax

Classifications: CNS AGENT; BENZODIAZEPINE ANXIOLYTIC; SEDATIVE-HYPNOTIC

Prototype: Lorazepam

Pregnancy category: D

Controlled substance: Schedule IV

ACTIONS/PHARMACODYNAMICS CNS depressant. Mode of action not known but appears to act at the limbic, thalamic, and hypothalamic levels of the CNS. It is associated with significantly less drowsiness. Has antidepressant as well as anxiolytic actions.

USES Management of anxiety disorders or for short-term relief of anxiety symptoms. Also used as adjunct in management of anxiety associated with depression and agitation and for panic disorders, such as agoraphobia.

ROUTE & DOSAGE

Anxiety Disorders

Adult: **PO** 0.25–0.5 mg t.i.d. (max 4 mg/d).
Geriatric: **PO** 0.125–0.25 mg b.i.d.

Panic Attacks

Adult: **PO** 1–2 mg t.i.d. (max 8 mg/d).

PHARMACOKINETICS **Absorption:** rapidly absorbed. Peak: 1–2 h. **Distribution:** crosses placenta. **Metabolism:** oxidized in liver to inactive metabolites. **Elimination:** half-life: 12–15 h; renal elimination.

CONTRAINDICATIONS & PRECAUTIONS **Contraindicated in:** sensitivity to benzodiazepines; acute narrow angle glaucoma; pulmonary disease; use alone in primary depression or psychotic disorders; during pregnancy (category D), in nursing mothers and children <18 y. **Cautious use in:** impaired renal or hepatic function; history of alcoholism; geriatric and debilitated patients. Effectiveness for long-term treatment (>4 mo) not established.

ADVERSE/SIDE EFFECTS **CNS:** *drowsiness, sedation,* light-headedness, dizziness, syncope, depression, headache, confusion, insomnia, nervousness, fatigue, clumsiness, unsteadiness, rigidity, tremor, restlessness, paradoxical excitement, hallucinations. **CV:** tachycardia, hypotension, ECG changes. **Other:** blurred vision, dyspnea.

DRUG INTERACTIONS **Alcohol** and other CNS DEPRESSANTS, ANTICONVULSANTS, ANTIHISTAMINES, BARBITURATES, NARCOTIC ANALGESICS, BENZODIAZEPINES compound CNS depressant effects; **cimetidine, disulfiram** increase alprazolam effects (decreased metabolism); ORAL CONTRACEPTIVES MAY INCREASE OR DECREASE ALPRAZOLAM EFFECTS.

NURSING IMPLICATIONS

Administration

- Alprazolam may be administered without regard to meals.
- Store in light-resistant containers at 15–30C (59–86F), unless otherwise directed.

Assessment & Drug Effects

- Patients receiving continuing therapy should have periodic blood counts, urinalyses, and blood chemistry studies.

- Drowsiness and sedation are the most common side effects. Monitor especially the elderly or debilitated, who may require supervised ambulation or side rails.

Patient & Family Education

- Adverse reactions, which may occur during early high-dose therapy, usually disappear with continuing therapy. Advise patient to keep physician informed; dosage adjustments may be indicated. Instruct patient to make position changes slowly and in stages.
- Alprazolam potentiates effects of alcoholic beverages and other CNS depressants; caution patient not to use them or OTC medications containing antihistamines (sleep aids, cold, hay fever, or allergy remedies) without consulting physician.
- Advise patient to avoid driving and other potentially hazardous activities until reaction to drug is determined.
- Following continuous use, dosage should be tapered off before drug is stopped. Abrupt discontinuation of drug may cause withdrawal symptoms: nausea, vomiting, abdominal and muscle cramps, sweating, confusion, tremors, convulsions.

ALPROSTADIL (PGE$_1$)

(al-pross′ta-dil)

Trade names: Prostin VR Pediatric, Caverject, Muse, Edex

Classification: PROSTAGLANDIN

Prototype: Dinoprostone

Pregnancy category: C

ACTIONS/PHARMACODYNAMICS Actions include vasodilation, inhibition of platelet aggregation, and stimulation of intestinal and uterine smooth muscles. Preserves ductal patency by relaxing smooth muscle of ductus arteriosus. Alprostadil induces penile erection by relaxing the smooth muscles of the corpus cavernosum and dilating the cavernosal arteries and their penile arterioles. Sufficient rigidity of the penis also requires increased venous outflow resistance, thus resulting in penile blood engorgement and erection.

USES Temporary measure to maintain patency of ductus arteriosus in infants with ductal-dependent congenital heart defects until corrective surgery can be performed. Also used in erectile dysfunction.

ROUTE & DOSAGE

To Maintain Patency of Ductus Arteriosus

Neonate: **IV/Intraarterial/Intraaortic** 0.05–0.1 μg/kg/min; may increase gradually to max of 0.4 μg/kg/min if necessary.

Erectile Dysfunction of Vasculogenic, Psychogenic, or Mixed Etiology

Adult: **Intracavernosal** Initiate with 2.5 μg; if inadequate response, increase dose by 2.5 μg. May then increase dose in 5- to 10-μg increments until a suitable erection occurs, not exceeding 1 h in duration. Doses > 60 μg not recommended.

Erectile Dysfunction of Pure Neurogenic Etiology

Adult: **Intracavernosal** Initiate with 1.25 μg; if inadequate response, increase dose by 1.25 μg, then increase by 2.5 μg, may then increase dose in 5 μg increments until a suitable erection occurs, not exceeding 1 h in duration. Doses > 60 μg not recommended.

PHARMACOKINETICS Onset: 15 min to 3 h. **Metabolism:** rapidly metabolized in lungs. **Elimination:** half-life: 5–10 min; metabolites excreted through kidneys.

CONTRAINDICATIONS & PRECAUTIONS Contraindicated in: ductus arteriosus respiratory distress syndrome (hyaline membrane disease); hypersensitivity to alprostadil; patients with penile implants. Muse, Edex: women, children, and newborns. Muse: patients with urethral stricture, inflammation/infection of glans of penis, severe hypospadias, acute or chronic urethritis; sickle cell anemia or trait, thrombocytopenia, polycethemia, multiple myeloma. **Cautious use in:** ductus arteriosus: bleeding tendencies; erectile dysfunction: hypersensitivity to alprostadil; sickle cell anemia or trait; multiple myeloma or leukemia; penile anatomic deformations or penile implants; patients on anticoagulants, vasoactive or antihypertensive drugs.

ADVERSE/SIDE EFFECTS CNS: *fever,* seizures; lethargy. **CV:** *flushing,* bradycardia, hypotension, syncope, tachycardia; CHF, <u>ventricular fibrillation</u>, <u>shock</u>. **GI:** diarrhea, gastric regurgitation. **Hematologic:** disseminated intravascular coagulation (DIC), thrombocytopenia. **Renal (infrequent):** oliguria, anuria. **Respiratory:** apnea. **Urogenital:** *penile pain,* prolonged erection, priapism, penile fibrosis, injection site hematoma/ecchymosis, penile rash and edema, prostatitis, perineal pain. **Other:** rash on face and arms, alopecia, leg pain.

DRUG INTERACTIONS May increase anticoagulant properties of **warfarin;** ANTIHYPERTENSIVE AGENTS increase risk of hypotension.

NURSING IMPLICATIONS

Administration

Parenteral (IV)

- Infusion solution is prepared by diluting 500 μg alprostadil with NaCl or dextrose injection to volume appropriate for pump delivery system. Prepare fresh solution q24h. Discard unused portions.
- A 500 μg ampule diluted in 250 ml yields a concentration of 2 μg/ml.
- May be infused at rate of 0.05–0.1 μg/kg/min up to a maximum of 0.4 μg/kg/min.
- Infusion rate should be reduced immediately if arterial pressure drops significantly or if fever occurs. If apnea or bradycardia occurs, infusion should be discontinued promptly.
- Store at 2–8C (36–46F) unless otherwise directed by manufacturer. Protect from freezing.

Intracavernosal Injection

- Proper training in the penile injection technique is required prior to administration. Refer to patient information on administration provided by the manufacturer.
- Reconstituted solutions should be used immediately.
- Store dry powder at or below 25C (77F) for up to 3 mo. Do not freeze.

Assessment & Drug Effects

Ductus Arteriosus

- Monitor intermittently throughout the infusion (1) arterial pressure, (2) arterial blood gases Po_2 and Pco_2, (3) arterial blood pH, (4) ECG, (5) heart rate, (6) BP, (7) respiratory rate, and (8) rectal temperature.

- With aortic arch abnormalities, also monitor for systemic BP, pulmonary artery and descending aorta pressures, return of palpable femoral pulse, and urinary output.
- Therapeutic response in infants with cyanotic heart disease (restricted pulmonary blood flow) is indicated by increase in blood oxygenation (Po_2), usually evident within 30 min. Normal Po_2 for neonates is 60–70 mm Hg.
- Therapeutic response in infants with restricted systemic blood flow is indicated by increased pH in those with acidosis, increased systemic BP and urinary output, return of palpable pulses, and decreased ratio of pulmonary artery to aortic pressure.

Patient & Family Education
Erectile Dysfunction

- The dose should not be changed without consulting the physician.
- Advise to use the drug no more often than 3 times a week with at least 24 h between uses.
- Instruct to report any of the following to the physician as soon as possible: nodules or hard tissue in penis; penile pain, redness, swelling, tenderness; or curvature of the erect penis.
- Instruct to seek immediate medical attention if an erection persists longer than 6 h.

ALTEPLASE RECOMBINANT

(al′te-plase)

Trade names: Actilyse, Activase

Classifications: BLOOD FORMERS AND COAGULATORS; THROMBOLYTIC ENZYME

Prototype: Streptokinase

Pregnancy category: C

ACTIONS/PHARMACODYNAMICS This recombinant DNA-derived form of human tissue-type plasminogen activator (t-PA) is a thrombolytic agent. t-PA promotes thrombolysis by forming the active proteolytic enzyme plasmin. Plasmin is capable of degrading fibrin, fibrinogen, and factors V, VIII, and XII.

USES Indicated in selective cases of acute MI, preferably within 6 h of attack for recanalization of the coronary artery; lysis of acute pulmonary emboli; acute ischemic stroke or thrombotic stroke (within 3 h of onset). **Unlabeled use:** lysis of arterial occlusions in peripheral vessels and bypass vessels.

ROUTE & DOSAGE

Acute MI

Adult: **IV** 60 mg over first hour, with 6–10 mg infused over first 1–2 min; then 20 mg/h over next 2 h (100 mg over 3 h).
Accelerated schedule: 15-mg bolus, then 0.75 mg/kg (up to 50 mg) over 30 min, then 0.5 mg/kg (up to 35 mg) over 60 min.

Acute Ischemic Stroke/Thrombotic Stroke

Adult: **IV** See accelerated schedule.

Pulmonary Embolism

Adult: **IV** 100 mg infused over 2 h.

PHARMACOKINETICS **Peak:** 5–10 min after infusion completed. **Duration:** baseline values restored in 3 h. **Metabolism:** metabolized in liver. **Elimination:** half-life: 26.5 min; excreted in urine.

CONTRAINDICATIONS & PRECAUTIONS **Contraindicated in:** active internal bleeding, history of cerebrovascular accident, recent (within 2 mo) intracranial or interspinal surgery or trauma, intercranial neoplasm, arteriovenous malformation, bleeding disorders, severe uncontrolled hypertension, likelihood of left heart thrombus, acute pericarditis, bacterial endocarditis, severe liver dysfunction, age >75, pregnancy (category C), septic thrombophlebitis, current use of oral anticoagulants. **Cautious use in:** recent major surgery (within 10 d), cerebral vascular disease, recent GI or GU bleeding, recent trauma, hypertension, hemorrhagic ophthalmic conditions. Safety and effectiveness in children have not been established.

ADVERSE/SIDE EFFECTS **Hematologic:** internal and superficial bleeding (cerebral, retroperitoneal, GU, GI).

NURSING IMPLICATIONS

Administration

- IV infusion of alteplase should be started as soon as possible after the thrombolytic event, preferably within 6 h.
- Reconstitution: Do not use the 20- or 50-mg vial if vacuum has been broken. Dilute contents of vial with sterile water for injection supplied by manufacturer. Use a large-bore needle (e.g., 18 gauge). Slight foaming is usual. Resulting concentration is 1 mg/ml.
- The 100-mg vial does not contain a vacuum. Follow manufacturer's directions and use supplied transfer device for reconstitution.
- Drug may be administered as reconstituted (1 mg/ml) or further diluted with an equal volume of NS or D5W to yield 0.5 mg/ml.
- For acute MI: Administer 60% of total dose in the first hour with 6–10 mg given as a bolus dose over 1–2 min and remainder of first dose infused over hour 1. Follow with second dose (20% of total) over hour 2, and third dose (20% of total) over hour 3. For patients weighing <65 kg: Calculate dose using 1.25 mg/kg over 3 h. See accelerated schedule in Route & Dosage table.
- For pulmonary embolism: Administer entire dose over a 2 h period.
- Do not exceed a total dose of 100 mg. Higher doses have been associated with intracranial bleeding.
- Follow infusion of drug by flushing IV tubing with 30–50 ml of NS or D5W.
- Reconstituted drug is stable for 8 h in above solutions at room temperature (2–30C; 36–86F). Since there are no preservatives, discard any unused solution after that time.
- While patient is receiving this medication, do not allow patient out of bed.

Assessment & Drug Effects

- Before administration, coagulation tests need to be done including APTT, bleeding time, PT, TT.
- Blood for Hct, Hgb, and platelet count should be drawn before administration for baseline values in case of bleeding.
- Check vital signs frequently. Be alert to changes in cardiac rhythm. Dysrhythmias signal need to stop therapy at once.
- Monitor for excess bleeding q15min for the first hour of therapy, q30min for second to eighth hour, then q8h.
- Monitor neurological checks throughout drug infusion q30min and qh for the first 8 h after infusion.
- Spontaneous bleeding occurs twice as often with alteplase as with heparin. Protect patient from invasive procedures: IM injections are contraindicated. Also prevent

physical manipulation of patient during thrombolytic therapy to prevent bruising.

- Report signs of bleeding: gum bleeding, epistaxis, hematoma, spontaneous ecchymoses, oozing at catheter site, increased pain from internal bleeding. The alteplase infusion should be interrupted, then resumed when bleeding stops.
- If blood gas determination is needed, select the radial rather than the femoral artery because of greater ease in applying a pressure dressing to control oozing. Pressure to puncture sites, if necessary, should be maintained for up to 30 min.
- Inquire about pregnancy, recent delivery, recent surgery of any type, as these increase the risk of bleeding.
- Patient is at risk for postthrombolytic bleeding for 2–4 d after intracoronary alteplase treatment. Continue monitoring vital signs until laboratory reports confirm anticoagulant control.
- Hct should be drawn following drug administration to detect possible blood loss.

Patient & Family Education

- Patient should report immediately a sudden severe headache.
- Patient should report blood in urine and bloody or tarry stools.
- Patient should report if there is any sign of bleeding or oozing from cuts or places of injection.
- While receiving this medicine, patient should move around as little as possible and not get out of bed when alone.
- To help prevent serious bleeding, advise patient to follow instructions given by physician very carefully.
- Instruct patient to report any unusual or allergic reactions to alteplase, anistreplase, streptokinase, or urokinase. Also report allergy to any other substances such as food, preservatives, or dyes.

ALTRETAMINE, HEXAMETHYLMELAMINE

(al-tre′-ta-meen)

Trade name: Hexalen

Classifications: ANTINEOPLASTIC; IMMUNOSUPPRESSANT

Prototype: Cyclophosphamide

Pregnancy category: D

ACTIONS/PHARMACODYNAMICS Altretamine, formally hexamethylmelamine, is a synthetic cytotoxic antineoplastic drug. The mechanism of action is not clearly understood. Altretamine probably requires the liver enzyme system for activation of its cytotoxic properties. Altretamine has demonstrated neoplastic activity in patients resistant to alkylating agents.

USE Ovarian cancer. **Unlabeled uses:** breast, cervical, colon, endometrial, head, and neck cancer; small-cell lung cancers and lymphomas.

ROUTE & DOSAGE

Ovarian Cancer

Adult: **PO** 260 mg/m^2/d for 14 or 21 consecutive d in a 28-day cycle. Give in 4 divided doses after meals and at bedtime.

PHARMACOKINETICS Absorption: rapidly absorbed from GI tract. Approximately 25% reaches systemic circulation due to extensive hepatic first-pass metabolism. **Metabolism:** rapidly demethylated in the liver to 5 minor and 4 major metabolites. **Elimination:** half-life: 13 h; 62% of the dose is excreted in the urine in 24 h. A small amount of altretamine is excreted through the lungs.

CONTRAINDICATIONS & PRECAUTIONS **Contraindicated in:** hypersensitivity to altretamine, severe bone marrow depression, neurologic toxicity, nursing mothers. **Cautious use in:** pregnancy (category D). Safety and efficacy in children not established.

ADVERSE/SIDE EFFECTS **CNS:** *paresthesias, hyporeflexia, muscle weakness, peripheral numbness, ataxia, parkinson-like tremors.* **GI:** *nausea, vomiting.* **Hematologic:** *leukopenia, thrombocytopenia.* **Renal:** slight increase in serum creatinine. **Other:** alopecia and eczema.

DRUG INTERACTIONS Concomitant administration of altretamine and tricyclic antidepressants (imipramine, amitriptyline), monoamine oxidase inhibitors, or selegiline have been reported to result in incapacitating dizziness and syncopal episodes during the first week of altretamine treatment. Patients became asymptomatic 24–96 h after discontinuing antidepressant.

NURSING IMPLICATIONS

Administration

- Administer only under supervision of a qualified physician experienced in the use of antineoplastics.
- Altretamine should be discontinued for 14 d or longer and restarted at 200 $mg/m^2/d$ if any of the following occur: severe GI intolerance; WBC count less than $2000/m^3$, granulocyte count less than $1000/m^3$; or progressive neurotoxicity.
- When neurotoxicity develops, concurrent administration of vitamin B_6, 100 mg b.i.d. may allow altretamine therapy to continue.
- Store at room temperature, 15–30C (59–86F).

Assessment & Drug Effects

- Peripheral blood counts should be monitored at least monthly and prior to each course of therapy.
- Neurologic examination should be performed regularly and patient questioned about the presence of any of the following: paresthesias, hypoesthesias, muscle weakness, peripheral numbness, ataxia, decreased sensations, and alterations in mood or consciousness.
- If neurologic symptoms fail to resolve with dose reduction, the medication should be discontinued.
- Monitor for nausea and vomiting, which are related to the cumulative dose of altretamine. After several weeks some patients develop tolerance to the GI effects. Antiemetics may be required to control GI distress.

Patient & Family Education

- Advise patient that taking altretamine after meals or with food or milk may decrease nausea.
- Inform patient of the symptoms indicative of neurotoxicity and advise to report these to the physician.
- Inform patient that GI, hematologic, and neurologic adverse effects are the major dose-limiting adverse effects associated with altretamine.

ALUMINUM HYDROXIDE

Trade names: ALternaGEL, Alu-Cap, Alugel, Alu-Tab, Amphojel, Dialume

ALUMINUM CARBONATE, BASIC

Trade name: Basaljel

ALUMINUM PHOSPHATE

Trade name: Phosphaljel

Prototype for classifications: GI AGENT; ANTACID; ADSORBENT

Pregnancy category: C

ACTIONS/PHARMACODYNAMICS Nonsystemic antacid with moderate neutralizing action. Decreases rate of gastric emptying and has demulcent, adsorbent, and mild astringent properties. Reduces acid concentration and pepsin activity by raising pH of gastric and intraesophageal secretions. Does not reduce gastric acid output. Lowers serum phosphate by binding dietary phosphorus to form insoluble aluminum phosphate, which is excreted in feces. This prevents formation of urinary phosphatic calculi by decreasing excretion of phosphates in urine. Its phosphate-binding capacity is not as great as that of aluminum carbonate.

USES Symptomatic relief of gastric hyperacidity associated with gastritis, esophageal reflux, and hiatal hernia; adjunct in treatment of gastric and duodenal ulcer. Also has been used in management of hyperphosphatemia of renal failure and in treatment of phosphatic urinary calculi. More commonly used in combination with other antacids. Aluminum carbonate is used primarily in conjunction with a low phosphate diet to reduce hyperphosphatemia in patients with renal insufficiency and for prophylaxis and treatment of phosphatic renal calculi. Also used as an antacid.

ROUTE & DOSAGE

Antacid (hydroxide & phosphate)
Adult: **PO** 600 mg t.i.d. or q.i.d.

Antacid (carbonate)
Adult: **PO** 10–30 ml of regular suspension, *or* 5–15 ml of extra strength suspension, *or* 2 capsules or tablets q2h.

Phosphate Lowering (carbonate)
Adult: **PO** 10–30 ml of regular suspension, *or* 5–15 ml of extra strength suspension, *or* 2–6 capsules or tablets 1 h p.c. and h.s.

PHARMACOKINETICS **Absorption:** minimal absorption. **Peak:** slow onset. **Duration:** 2 h when taken with food; 3 h when taken 1 h after food. **Elimination:** excreted in feces as insoluble phosphates.

CONTRAINDICATIONS & PRECAUTIONS **Contraindicated in:** prolonged use of high doses in presence of low serum phosphate; pregnancy (category C). **Cautious use in:** renal impairment; gastric outlet obstruction; elderly patients; decreased bowel activity (e.g., patients receiving anticholinergic, antidiarrheal, or antispasmodic agents); patients who are dehydrated or on fluid restriction.

ADVERSE/SIDE EFFECTS *Constipation*, fecal impaction, intestinal obstruction, hypophosphatemia, dialysis dementia (thought to be due to aluminum intoxication), hypomagnesemia.

DRUG INTERACTIONS Aluminum will decrease absorption of **chloroquine, cimetidine, ciprofloxacin, digoxin, isoniazid,** IRON SALTS, NSAIDS, **norfloxacin, ofloxacin, phenytoin, phenothiazines, quinidine, tetracycline, thyroxine. Sodium polystyrene sulfonate** may cause systemic alkalosis.

NURSING IMPLICATIONS

Administration

- Instruct patient to chew tablet until it is thoroughly wetted before swallowing it (undissolved particles increase risk of developing intestinal concretions). For antacid use: follow well-chewed tablet with one-half glass of water or milk; follow liquid preparation (suspension) with sip of water to ensure passage into stomach. For phosphate lowering, follow tablet, capsule, or suspension with full glass of water or fruit juice.

- For healing an active peptic ulcer, some physicians prescribe antacid 1 and 3 h after meals and at bedtime. Others alternate antacid and meals on a 2-h schedule and advise patients to take an extra antacid dose when discomfort is felt.
- Store between 15 and 30C (59 and 86F) in tightly closed container.

Assessment & Drug Effects

- Note number and consistency of stools. Constipation occurs commonly and is dose related. Intestinal obstruction from fecal concretions has been reported.
- Serum calcium and phosphorus levels should be determined at periodic intervals with prolonged high-dose therapy or impaired renal function.

Patient & Family Education

- Patients receiving large doses of antacids for prolonged periods and who eat a diet low in phosphorus can develop hypophosphatemia within 2 wk of continuous antacid use. The elderly patient in a poor nutritional state is at high risk.
- Since frequency of meals may vary in the elderly particularly, help patient design a diet-antacid regimen that will protect the gastric mucosa.
- Antacid may cause stools to appear speckled or whitish.
- Pain is used as a clinical guide for adjusting dosage. Keep physician informed. Pain that persists beyond 72 h may signify serious complications.
- Length of antacid therapy for patients with duodenal ulcer is usually 4–6 wk, and for gastric ulcers until healing has taken place.
- Caution individuals who self-medicate with antacids to seek medical help if indigestion is accompanied by shortness of breath, sweating, or chest pain, if stools are dark or tarry, or if symptoms are recurrent.
- A person should seek medical advice and supervision if self-prescribed antacid use exceeds 2 wk.

AMANTADINE HYDROCHLORIDE

(a-man'ta-deen)

Trade name: Symmetrel

Classifications: ANTIINFECTIVE; ANTIVIRAL; AUTONOMIC NERVOUS SYSTEM AGENT; ANTICHOLINERGIC (PARASYMPATHOLYTIC); ANTIPARKINSONISM AGENT

Prototype: Acyclovir

Pregnancy category: C

ACTIONS/PHARMACODYNAMICS

Because it does not suppress antibody formation, it can be administered for interim protection in combination with influenza A virus vaccine until antibody titer is adequate or to augment prophylaxis in a previously vaccinated individual. Active against several strains of influenza A virus; not effective against influenza B infections. Mechanism of action in parkinsonism not understood, but may be related to release of dopamine and other catecholamines from neuronal storage sites and also to anticholinergic effects.

USES In initial therapy or as adjunct with anticholinergic drugs or levodopa in treatment of all forms of parkinsonism (arteriosclerotic, idiopathic, postencephalitic) and for relief of drug-induced extrapyramidal reactions and symptomatic parkinsonism caused by carbon monoxide poisoning. Also used for prophylaxis and symptomatic treatment of influenza A infections. **Unlabeled uses:** primary enuresis, pseudosclerosis, neuroleptic malignant syndrome (NMS), management of cocaine dependency and withdrawal.

ROUTE & DOSAGE

Influenza A

Adult: **PO** 200 mg once/d *or* 100 mg q12h.
Child: **PO** 1–9 y, 4.4–8.8 mg/kg in 2–3 equal doses (max 150 mg/d).

Parkinsonism

Adult: **PO** 100 mg 1–2 times/d; start with 100 mg/d if patient is on other antiparkinsonism medications.

Drug-induced Extrapyramidal Symptoms

Adult: **PO** 100 mg b.i.d., up to 400 mg/d if needed.

Adjustment for Renal Impairment

Cl_{cr} 40–60 ml/min: 100 mg/d; 30–40 ml/min: 200 mg 2 times/wk; 10–20 ml/min: 100 mg 3 times/wk.

PHARMACOKINETICS **Absorption:** readily and almost completely absorbed from GI tract. **Onset:** within 48 h. **Peak:** 1–4 h. **Distribution:** distributed to saliva, nasal secretions, breast milk, placenta, CSF. **Metabolism:** not metabolized. **Elimination:** half-life: 9–37 h (prolonged in renal insufficiency); 90% excreted unchanged in urine.

CONTRAINDICATIONS & PRECAUTIONS **Contraindicated in:** safe use during pregnancy (category C), in nursing mothers, and in children <1 y not established. **Cautious use in:** history of epilepsy or other types of seizures; CHF, peripheral edema, orthostatic hypotension; recurrent eczematoid dermatitis; psychoses, severe psychoneuroses; hepatic disease; renal impairment; elderly patients with cerebral arteriosclerosis.

ADVERSE/SIDE EFFECTS Usually dose related. **CNS:** *dizziness, lightheadedness,* headache, ataxia, irritability, anxiety, *nervousness, difficulty in concentrating,* mood or other mental changes, confusion, visual and auditory hallucinations, *insomnia,* nightmares, convulsions. **CV:** orthostatic hypotension, peripheral edema, dyspnea. **Eye:** blurring or loss of vision. **GI:** anorexia, *nausea,* vomiting, dry mouth. **Hematologic:** leukopenia.

DRUG INTERACTIONS **Alcohol** enhances CNS effects; may potentiate effects of ANTICHOLINERGICS.

NURSING IMPLICATIONS

Administration

- Influenza prophylaxis: Drug is begun as soon as exposure to infected persons is anticipated and continued for at least 10 d.
- If insomnia is a problem, medication should be scheduled several hours before bedtime. Suggest that patient limit number of daytime naps.
- Amantadine may be swallowed with water, milk, or taken with food.

- Use supplied calibrated device for measuring syrup formulation.
- Amantadine may be used in conjunction with influenza A vaccine (generally in high-risk patients who have not been vaccinated previously) until protective antibodies develop (10–21 d) after vaccine administration.
- Store in tightly closed container preferably at 15–30C (59–86F) unless otherwise directed by manufacturer. Avoid freezing.

Assessment & Drug Effects

- Since drug may cause dizziness and light-headedness, supervision of ambulation and side rails may be indicated.
- Monitor for mental status changes; nervousness, difficulty concentrating, or insomnia may indicate need for dosage adjustment.
- Patients with history of seizures should be monitored closely for loss of seizure control.
- Establish a baseline profile of the patient's disabilities for accurate differentiation between disease symptoms (e.g., dementia) and drug-induced neuropsychiatric adverse reactions.
- Closely observe for toxicity with doses above 200 mg/d. Monitor vital signs for at least 3 or 4 d after increases in dosage.
- Patients with cerebrovascular disease or impaired renal function are more prone to develop symptoms of toxicity. Monitor particularly when dosage adjustments are made.
- Monitor urinary output and pH, serum electrolytes, vital signs.
- Livedo reticularis occurs most frequently in women receiving drug for 1 mo or longer for parkinsonism. It is a diffuse, rose-colored mottling of skin, usually confined to lower extremities, but it may also appear on arms and is preceded by or accompanied by ankle edema. Condition may be more noticeable when patient stands or is exposed to cold; color fades when legs are elevated. Appears within 1 mo–1 y after initiation of drug therapy and may subside with continued therapy, but disappears gradually 2–12 wk after drug is discontinued.
- Patients with parkinsonism may show reduction of salivation, akinesia, and rigidity within 4–48 h after initiation of therapy. Generally, drug has little effect on tremors. If significant improvement is not noted within 1–2 wk, drug is usually discontinued.
- Parkinsonism, extrapyramidal reactions: CNS and psychic disturbances are most likely to appear within 1 d to a few days after initiation of drug therapy or after dosage has been increased. Symptoms tend to subside when drug is given in two divided doses.

Patient & Family Education

- To be effective in treatment of influenza, must be administered preferably within 24 h but no later than 48 h after onset of symptoms and should be continued for 24–48 h after symptoms disappear. Advise patient to report to physician if there is no improvement within this time.
- Because orthostatic hypotension may be a problem, caution patient not to go to sleep in a sitting position, and advise elderly male patients particularly to sit down to urinate, especially at night.
- Advise patient to make all position changes slowly, particularly from recumbent to upright position, and to dangle legs a few minutes before standing. Caution patient to lie down immediately if faint or dizzy.

- Onset of shortness of breath, peripheral edema, significant weight gain, dizziness, inability to concentrate, and other changes in mental status, dysuria, and eye symptoms should be reported to physician.
- Activities requiring mental alertness such as driving a car should be avoided until patient's response to the drug has been evaluated.
- Maximum therapeutic response generally occurs within 2 wk–3 mo. Effectiveness sometimes wanes after 6–8 wk of treatment. Report to physician.
- Abrupt discontinuation of therapy for parkinsonism may precipitate within 1–3 d a parkinsonian crisis: severe akinesia, rigidity, tremor. Warn patient to adhere to established dosage regimen.
- In other patients, abrupt withdrawal can result in neuroleptic malignant syndrome: low-grade fever and symptoms similar to parkinsonian crisis.

AMBENONIUM CHLORIDE

(am-be-noe'nee-um)

Trade name: Mytelase

Classifications: AUTONOMIC NERVOUS SYSTEM AGENT; CHOLINERGIC (PARASYMPATHOMIMETIC); CHOLINESTERASE INHIBITOR

Prototype: Neostigmine

Pregnancy category: C

ACTIONS/PHARMACODYNAMICS Indirect-acting and a slowly reversible cholinesterase inhibitor approximately six times more potent than neostigmine. Inhibits destruction of acetylcholine (ACh) by cholinesterase, thereby prolonging effects of ACh (neurotransmitter) at postsynaptic receptor sites. Has direct stimulant effect on striated muscles.

USES Symptomatic treatment of myasthenia gravis for patients who cannot tolerate neostigmine bromide or pyridostigmine bromide because of bromide sensitivity. Has been used in conjunction with corticosteroids, ephedrine sulfate, and potassium chloride to increase muscle strength.

ROUTE & DOSAGE

Myasthenia Gravis

Adult: **PO** 2.5–5 mg t.i.d. or q.i.d.; may increase q1–2d to 50–75 mg t.i.d. or q.i.d. if necessary.

Child: **PO** 0.3 mg/kg/d in 3–4 divided doses; may need up to 1.5 mg/kg/d in 3–4 divided doses.

PHARMACOKINETICS Absorption: poorly absorbed from GI tract. **Onset:** 20–30 min. **Duration:** 3–8 h. **Metabolism:** unknown. **Elimination:** unknown.

CONTRAINDICATIONS & PRECAUTIONS Contraindicated in: intestinal or urinary tract obstruction; patients receiving mecamylamine. Safe use during pregnancy (category C) and in nursing women not established. **Cautious use in:** epilepsy, bradycardia, cardiac arrhythmias, recent coronary occlusion; bronchial asthma; hyperthyroidism; vagotonia; peptic ulcer, megacolon.

ADVERSE/SIDE EFFECTS Exaggerated cholinergic (muscarinic) effects. **CNS:** muscle cramps, headache, confusion, dizziness, incoordination, fasciculations, agitation, restlessness, muscle weakness, <u>paralysis</u>, slurred speech, convulsions, <u>respiratory depression</u>. **CV:** bradycardia. **GI:** nausea, vomiting, diarrhea, abdominal cramps, excessive salivation. **Eye:** blurred vision, lacrimation. **Respiratory:** bronchospasm, increased bronchial secretions, dyspnea. **Other:** diaphoresis.

DRUG INTERACTIONS **Demecarium** and other CHOLINESTERASE INHIBITORS possibly compound toxicity; **mecamylamine, succinylcholine, procainamide, quinidine,** AMINOGLYCOSIDES increase neuromuscular blocking effects with possibility of respiratory depression; **atropine** antagonizes effects of ambenonium.

NURSING IMPLICATIONS

Administration

- Administration with food or milk may minimize muscarinic side effects.
- In general, medication schedule is planned so that larger doses are given when patient experiences the most fatigue or muscle weakness. Patients who have difficulty in eating may benefit by taking drug 30 to 45 min before meals.
- Store preferably at 15–30C (59–86F) unless otherwise directed.

Assessment & Drug Effects

- Hazards of cumulative effects and overdosage are high; therefore, atropine sulfate should always be immediately available to treat severe cholinergic reactions.
- Monitor vital signs during dosage adjustment periods.
- Monitor for manifestations of inadequate ventilation: unusual apprehension, restlessness, rapid pulse and respirations, rising BP.
- Dosage requirements may vary according to disease exacerbations and remissions and stress-provoking factors. The effects of a given dosage change may not appear for several days because of cumulative action. If a dosage increase produces no effect, physician may reduce dose to previous level. Record drug effect and duration of drug action. Keep physician informed.
- It is important to record time that adverse symptoms appear. When muscle weakness occurs within 1 h after drug administration, suspect overdosage. Other signs of overdosage: headache, weakness of muscles of neck, chewing, and swallowing, increased salivation. Weakness that begins 3 h or more after drug administration is probably due to underdosage or drug resistance.

Patient & Family Education

- Patients and responsible family members should be taught to recognize adverse effects, how to modify the doses accordingly, and when and how atropine should be taken.
- Patients on long-term therapy may become refractory to drug. Responsiveness usually returns when dosage is reduced or drug is withdrawn for several days.
- Advise patient to carry card or jewelry indicating medical diagnosis and medication(s) being taken.

AMCINONIDE

(am-sin′oh-nide)

Trade name: Cyclocort

Classifications: SKIN AND MUCOUS MEMBRANE AGENT; ANTIINFLAMMATORY; GLUCOCORTICOID

Prototype: Hydrocortisone

Pregnancy category: C

See Appendix A.

AMIFOSTINE (WR-2721)

(am-i-fos′teen)

Trade name: Ethyol

Classification: CYTOPROTECTIVE AGENT
Pregnancy category: C

ACTIONS/PHARMACODYNAMICS Amifostine reduces cytotoxic damage induced by radiation or alkylating agents in well-oxygenated cells. Protective effects appear to be mediated by the formation of a thiol metabolite of amifostine (WR-1065), which removes free radicals from normal cells, and by promotion of the repair of macromolecules. The higher concentration of WR-1065, the metabolite, in normal tissues is available to bind to metabolites produced by cisplatin and also to remove free radicals that are generated in tissues exposed to cisplatin. Amifostine is cytoprotective in the kidney, bone marrow, and GI mucosa, but not in the brain or spinal cord. The cytoprotection results in decreased myelosuppression and peripheral neuropathy.

USE Reduction of the cumulative renal toxicity associated with cisplatin.

ROUTE & DOSAGE

Adult: **IV** 910 mg/m^2 once daily.

PHARMACOKINETICS Onset: 5–8 min. **Metabolism:** rapidly metabolized in liver to active free thiol metabolite. **Elimination:** half-life: 8 min; renally excreted.

CONTRAINDICATIONS & PRECAUTIONS Contraindicated in: sensitivity to aminothiol compounds or mannitol, patients with potentially curable malignancies, hypotensive patients or those who are dehydrated, pregnancy (category C), nursing mothers. **Cautious use in:** patients at risk for hypocalcemia, cardiovascular disease (i.e., arrhythmias, CHF, TIA, CVA).

ADVERSE/SIDE EFFECTS CV: *transient reduction in blood pressure.* **GI:** *nausea, vomiting.* **Other:** infusion reactions (flushing, feeling of warmth or coldness, chills, dizziness, somnolence, hiccups, sneezing), hypocalcemia, hypersensitivity reactions.

INCOMPATIBILITY Do not mix with any solutions other than normal saline.

NURSING IMPLICATIONS

Administration
- Prior to administration, patient should receive antiemetics, be adequately hydrated, and be off of antihypertensives for 24 h.
- Reconstituion of IV solution: Add 9.5 ml of 0.9% NaCl Injection to a single-dose vial.
- Administer IV infusion to supine patient over no more than 15 min, beginning 30 min before chemotherapy.
- Reconstituted solution is stable for 5 h at room temp or up to 24 h refrigerated.

Assessment & Drug Effects
- Monitor BP every 5 min during infusion. Stop infusion if systolic BP drops significantly from baseline (e.g., baseline[drop]: <100[20], 100–119[25], 120–139[30], 140–179[40], >80[50]) and place in Trendelenburg position. If BP returns to normal in 5 min, infusion may be restarted.
- Monitor for hypocalcemia, and monitor fluid balance if significant vomiting occurs.

Patient & Family Education
- Advise regarding potential adverse effects.

AMIKACIN SULFATE

(am-i-kay′sin)

Trade name: Amikin

Classifications: ANTIINFECTIVE; AMINOGLYCOSIDE ANTIBIOTIC

Prototype: Gentamicin

Pregnancy category: C

ACTIONS/PHARMACODYNAMICS Semisynthetic derivative of kanamycin with broad range of antimicrobial activity that includes many strains resistant to other aminoglycosides. Pharmacologic properties essentially the same as those of gentamicin. Appears to inhibit protein synthesis in bacterial cell and is usually bactericidal. Effective against a wide variety of gram-negative bacteria including *Escherichia coli, Enterobacter, Klebsiella pneumoniae,* most strains of *Pseudomonas aeruginosa,* and many strains of *Proteus* species, *Serratia, Providencia stuartii, Citrobacter freundii, Acinetobacter.* Also effective against penicillinase and non-penicillinase-producing *Staphylococcus* species, and against *Mycobacterium tuberculosis* and atypical mycobacteria.

USES Primarily for short-term treatment of serious infections of respiratory tract, bones, joints, skin, and soft tissue, CNS (including meningitis), peritonitis burns, recurrent urinary tract infections (UTIs). **Unlabeled use:** intrathecal or intraventricular administration, in conjunction with IM or IV dosage.

ROUTE & DOSAGE

Moderate to Severe Infections (all doses based on ideal body weight)

Adult: **IV/IM** 5–7.5 mg/kg loading dose; then 7.5 mg/kg q12h.

Child: **IV/IM** 5–7.5 mg/kg loading dose; then 5 mg/kg q8h or 7.5 mg/kg q12h.

Neonate: **IV/IM** 10 mg/kg loading dose; then 7.5 mg/kg q12–24h.

Uncomplicated UTI

Adult: **IV/IM** 250 mg q12h.

PHARMACOKINETICS **Peak:** 30 min IV; 45 min to 2 h IM. **Distribution:** does not cross blood–brain barrier; crosses placenta; accumulates in renal cortex. **Elimination:** half-life: 2–3 h in adults, 4–8 h in neonates; 94–98% excreted renally in 24 h, remainder in 10–30 d.

CONTRAINDICATIONS & PRECAUTIONS **Contraindicated in:** history of hypersensitivity or toxic reaction with an aminoglycoside antibiotic. Safe use during pregnancy (category C), in nursing mothers, neonates and infants, or use for period exceeding 14 d not determined. **Cautious use in:** impaired renal function; eighth cranial (auditory) nerve impairment; preexisting vertigo or dizziness, tinnitus, or dehydration, fever; the elderly, prematures, neonates and infants; myasthenia gravis; parkinsonism; hypocalcemia.

ADVERSE/SIDE EFFECTS **CNS:** neurotoxicity: drowsiness, unsteady gait, weakness, clumsiness, paresthesias, tremors, convulsions. **ENT:** ***ototoxicity:*** *auditory:* high-frequency hearing loss, complete hearing loss (occasionally permanent), tinnitus; ringing or buzzing in ears; *vestibular:* dizziness, ataxia. **GI:** nausea, vomiting. **Hypersensitivity:** skin rash, urticaria, pruritus, redness. **Renal:** oliguria, urinary frequency, hematuria, <u>tubular necrosis,</u> <u>azotemia</u>. **Other:** superinfections, peripheral neuritis, hepatotoxicity, hypokalemia, hypomagnesemia.

DRUG INTERACTIONS ANESTHETICS, SKELETAL MUSCLE RELAXANTS have additive neuromuscular blocking effects; **acyclovir, amphotericin B, bacitracin, capreomycin, cephalosporins, colistin, cisplatin, carboplatin, methoxyflurane, polymyxin B, vancomycin, furosemide, ethacrynic acid** increase risk of ototoxicity and nephrotoxicity.

INCOMPATIBILITIES **Solution/additive: aminophylline, amphotericin B,** CEPHALOSPORINS, **chlorothiazide, erythromycin, heparin, oxytetracycline,** PENICILLINS, **phenytoin, thiopental, vitamin B complex with C, warfarin. Y-site: amphotericin B, heparin, phenytoin, thiopental.**

NURSING IMPLICATIONS

Administration

- To prepare IV solution, add contents of 500 mg vial to 100 or 200 ml 5% dextrose or 0.9% NaCl injection or other diluent recommended by manufacturer. For pediatric patients, volume of diluent depends on patient need.
- Administer a single adult dose over at least 30–60 min by IV infusion. Increase infusion time to 1–2 h for infants.
- IV administration to neonates, infants, and children: Verify correct IV concentration and rate of infusion with physician.
- Monitor drip rate carefully. A rapid rise in serum amikacin level can cause respiratory depression (neuromuscular blockade) and other signs of toxicity.
- Color of solution may vary from colorless to light straw color or very pale yellow. Discard solutions that appear discolored or that contain particulate matter.
- Store at 15–30C (59–86F) unless otherwise directed.

Assessment & Drug Effects

- Culture and susceptibility tests should be performed before initial dose.
- Tests of renal function and vestibulocochlear nerve function should be performed before therapy and at regular intervals during therapy; should be closely monitored in the elderly, in patients with history of ear problems, patients with renal impairment, or during high dose or prolonged therapy.
- Blood for peak amikacin levels is drawn about 1 h after IM administration. If drug is administrated by IV infusion, time for drawing blood depends on IV infusion rate. In general, blood is drawn immediately after completion of a 1 h infusion or 30 min following completion of a 30 min infusion. Trough levels are drawn immediately before the next IM or IV dose.
- Periodic measurements of peak and trough serum amikacin levels in addition to serum creatinine or creatinine clearance (generally preferred) are advised, especially in the presence of impaired renal function, in neonates, and in the elderly.
- Peak serum amikacin concentrations above 30–35 μg/ml are not recommended; trough levels should not exceed 8 μg/ml. Prolonged high trough or peak levels are associated with toxicity.
- Amikacin serum levels are reportedly lower in patients with fever.
- Ototoxicity primarly involves the cochlear (auditory) branch. High-frequency deafness usually appears first and can be detected only by audiometer.

- Observe for and question about auditory symptoms (tinnitus, roaring noises, sensation of fullness in ears, hearing loss) and vestibular disturbances (dizziness or vertigo, nystagmus, ataxia).
- Monitor and report any changes in I&O, oliguria, hematuria, or cloudy urine. Keeping patient well hydrated reduces risk of nephrotoxicity. Consult physician regarding optimum fluid intake.
- Increasing serum creatinine and BUN, decreasing urine specific gravity and creatinine clearance, and presence of albumin and casts, WBC, and RBC in urine are indicators of declining renal function.
- If treatment is more than 10 d, daily tests of renal function and weekly audiograms and vestibular tests are strongly advised.
- Be on the alert for symptoms of respiratory tract infections and other symptoms indicative of superinfections. Notify physician should they occur.

AMILORIDE HYDROCHLORIDE

(a-mill′oh-ride)

Trade name: Midamor

Classifications: WATER BALANCE AGENT; POTASSIUM-SPARING DIURETIC

Prototype: Spironolactone

Pregnancy category: B

ACTIONS/PHARMACODYNAMICS Potassium-sparing diuretic with mild diuretic and antihypertensive actions. Induces urinary excretion of sodium and reduces excretion of potassium and hydrogen ions by direct action on distal renal tubules. Diuretic action is independent of aldosterone and carbonic anhydrase.

USES Potassium-sparing effect in prevention or treatment of diuretic-induced hypokalemia in patients with CHF, hepatic cirrhosis, or hypertension. Also used in management of primary hyperaldosteronism. Usually combined with a potassium-wasting (kaliuretic) diuretic such as a thiazide or loop diuretic. **Unlabeled uses:** with hydrochlorothiazide for recurrent calcium nephrolithiasis, lithium-induced polyuria.

ROUTE & DOSAGE

Diuretic

Adult: **PO** 5 mg/d; may increase up to 20 mg/d in 1–2 divided doses.

PHARMACOKINETICS **Absorption:** 50% absorbed from GI tract. **Onset:** 2 h. **Peak:** 6–10 h. **Duration:** 24 h. **Elimination:** half-life: 6–9 h; 20–50% excreted unchanged in urine, 40% in feces.

CONTRAINDICATIONS & PRECAUTIONS **Contraindicated in:** elevated serum potassium (>5.5 mEq/L), concomitant use of other potassium-sparing diuretics; anuria, acute or chronic renal insufficiency; evidence of diabetic nephropathy; type I (insulin-dependent) diabetes mellitus; metabolic or respiratory acidosis; hepatic function impairment. Safe use in pregnancy (category B), nursing mothers, and children not established. **Cautious use in:** debilitated patients; diet-controlled or uncontrolled diabetes mellitus; cardiopulmonary disease; the elderly.

ADVERSE/SIDE EFFECTS Generally well tolerated. **CNS:** *headache,* dizziness, nervousness, confusion, paresthesias, drowsiness. **CV:** cardiac arrhythmias. **Electrolyte imbalance/hematologic:** <u>hyperkalemia</u>, hyponatremia, positive Coombs' test, <u>aplastic anemia</u>. **ENT:** tinnitus, nasal congestion. **Eye:** visual disturbances, increased intraocular pressure. **GI:** *diarrhea* or constipation, anorexia, *nausea,* vomiting, abdominal cramps, dry mouth, thirst. **GU:** polyuria, dysuria, bladder spasms, urinary frequency. **Gynecologic:** impotence, decreased libido. **Respiratory:** dyspnea, shortness of breath. **Skin:** rash, pruritus, photosensitivity reactions. **Other:** weakness, fatigue, muscle cramps, photosensitivity.

DIAGNOSTIC TEST INTERFERENCE Manufacturer advises discontinuing amiloride in patients with diabetes mellitus at least 3 d before glucose tolerance tests.

DRUG INTERACTIONS Blood from blood banks, ACE INHIBITORS (e.g., **captopril**), **spironolactone, triamterene,** POTASSIUM SUPPLEMENTS may cause hyperkalemia with cardiac arrhythmias; possibility of increased **lithium** toxicity (decreased renal elimination); possibility of altered **digoxin** response; NSAIDS may attenuate antihypertensive effects. **Drug–food interactions:** POTASSIUM-CONTAINING SALT SUBSTITUTES increase risk of hyperkalemia.

NURSING IMPLICATIONS

Administration

- Once-a-day dose should be given in the morning.
- Administer with food to reduce possibility of gastric distress.
- Store at 15–30C (59–86F) in a tightly closed container unless otherwise directed.

Assessment & Drug Effects

- Serum potassium levels should be monitored for all patients, particularly when therapy is initiated, whenever dosage adjustments are made, and during any illness that may affect kidney function.
- Monitor for signs and symptoms of hyperkalemia and hyponatremia (see Appendix G).
- Hyperkalemia occurs in about 10% of patients receiving amiloride. Serum potassium can rise suddenly and without warning.
- Hyperkalemia is more common in the elderly and in patients with diabetes or renal disease.
- Intermittent evaluations of BUN, creatinine, and ECG are advised for patients with renal or hepatic dysfunction, diabetes mellitus, or who are elderly or debilitated.

Patient & Family Education

- Amiloride is generally taken in the morning to avoid interrupting nighttime sleep. Advise patient to take amiloride at the same time each day.
- Teach patients signs and symptoms of hyperkalemia and hyponatremia (see Appendix G) and instruct them to report any immediately.
- Potassium supplements, salt substitutes, high intake of dietary potassium are contraindicated. Exception: these measures may be prescribed for patients with severe or refractory hypokalemia.
- Because amiloride can cause visual disturbances and dizziness, particularly during early therapy, advise patient to be cautious when driving or performing other potentially hazardous tasks.

AMINOCAPROIC ACID

(a-mee-noe-ka-proe′ik)

Trade names: Amicar, EACA (epsilon-aminocaproic acid)

Prototype for classifications: BLOOD FORMER AND COAGULATOR; HEMOSTATIC

Pregnancy category: C

ACTIONS/PHARMACODYNAMICS Synthetic hemostatic with specific antifibrinolysis action. Acts principally by inhibiting plasminogen activator substance; to a lesser degree slightly inhibits activity of plasmin (fibrinolysin), which is concerned with destruction of clots. Does not control bleeding caused by loss of vascular integrity.

USES To control excessive bleeding resulting from systemic hyperfibrinolysis, a pathologic condition that may accompany heart surgery, portocaval shunt, abruptio placentae, aplastic anemia, and carcinoma of lung, prostate, cervix, and stomach. Also used in urinary fibrinolysis associated with severe trauma, anoxia, shock, urologic surgery, and neoplastic diseases of GU tract. **Unlabeled uses:** to prevent hemorrhage in hemophiliacs undergoing dental extraction; as a specific antidote for streptokinase or urokinase toxicity; to prevent recurrence of subarachnoid hemorrhage, especially when surgery is delayed; for management of amegakaryocytic thrombocytopenia; and to prevent or abort hereditary angioedema episodes.

ROUTE & DOSAGE

Hemostatic

Adult: **PO/IV** 4–5 g during first hour; then 1–1.25 g q.h. for 8 h or until bleeding is controlled (max 30 g/24h).
Child: **PO/IV** 100 mg/kg during first hour; then 33.3 mg/kg q.h. (max 18 g/m^2/24 h).

PHARMACOKINETICS Absorption: rapidly absorbed from GI tract. **Peak:** 2 h. **Distribution:** readily penetrates RBCs and other body cells. **Elimination:** 80% excreted as unmetabolized drug in 12 h.

CONTRAINDICATIONS & PRECAUTIONS Contraindicated in: severe renal impairment; active disseminated intravascular clotting (DIC); upper urinary tract bleeding. Safe use during pregnancy (category C) not established. **Cautious use in:** cardiac, renal, or hepatic disease; history of pulmonary embolus, or other thrombotic diseases.

ADVERSE/SIDE EFFECTS CNS: dizziness, malaise, headache, seizures. **CV:** faintness, orthostatic hypotension; dysrhythmias; thrombophlebitis, thromboses. **ENT:** tinnitus, nasal congestion. **Eye:** conjunctival erythema. **GI:** nausea, vomiting, cramps, diarrhea, anorexia. **GU:** diuresis, dysuria, urinary frequency, oliguria, reddish-brown urine (myoglobinuria), acute renal failure. **Gynecologic:** prolonged menstruation with cramping. **Skin:** rash.

DIAGNOSTIC TEST INTERFERENCE ***Serum potassium*** may be elevated (especially in patients with impaired renal function).

DRUG INTERACTIONS ESTROGENS, ORAL CONTRACEPTIVES may cause hypercoagulation.

NURSING IMPLICATIONS

Administration

- If oral therapy is prescribed, note that patient may have to take as many as 10 tablets or 4 tsp for a 5 g dose during the first hour of treatment. (Each tablet contains 500 mg; syrup contains 250 mg/ml.)
- IV preparation: Parenteral aminocaproic acid should always be diluted before use. Each 4 ml (1 g) of prepared solution is diluted with 50 ml of NS, 5% dextrose in water or saline, or Ringer's.
- IV administration: Physician will order specific IV flow rate. Usual

rate of administration is 5 g or a fraction thereof over first hour (5 g/250 ml); each additional gram over 1 h.

- Rapid IV administration should be avoided to prevent hypotension, faintness, and bradycardia or other arrhythmias.
- Check IV site at frequent intervals for extravasation. Observe for signs of thrombophlebitis (see Signs & Symptoms, Appendix G).
- Store in tightly closed containers at 15–30C (59–86F) unless otherwise directed. Avoid freezing.

Assessment & Drug Effects

- Monitor vital signs and I&O. Record response to aminocaproic therapy and keep physician informed.
- Report possible signs of myopathy: muscle weakness, myalgia, diaphoresis, fever, reddish-brown urine (myoglobinuria), oliguria. Drug should be discontinued promptly.
- Patients receiving prolonged therapy should have routine laboratory measurements of creatine phosphokinase activity and urinalyses for early detection of myopathy.
- Be alert to and report signs of thrombotic complications: arm or leg pain, tenderness or swelling, Homan's sign, prominence of superficial veins, chest pain, breathlessness, dyspnea.

Patient & Family Education

- Instruct patient to report difficulty urinating or reddish-brown urine.
- Report arm or leg pain, chest pain, or difficulty breathing.

AMINOGLUTETHIMIDE

(a-mee-noe-gloo-teth′i-mide)

Trade name: Cytadren

Classifications: ANTINEOPLASTIC; HORMONE ANTAGONIST

Pregnancy category: D

ACTIONS/PHARMACODYNAMICS

Blocks adrenal corticosteroid biosynthesis by inhibiting enzymatic conversion of cholesterol to precursors of cortisol and aldosterone. Also blocks aromatase, thereby preventing conversion of androgens to estrogens in peripheral tissues. Because estrogens are supplied principally by the adrenals in postmenopausal and oophorectomized women, aminoglutethimide-induced lowering of plasma estrogen levels (by adrenal suppression) is reportedly as effective as that produced by surgical adrenalectomy.

USES Temporary treatment of selected patients with Cushing's syndrome associated with adrenal carcinoma, ectopic ACTH-producing tumors, or adrenal hyperplasia. **Unlabeled uses:** to produce medical adrenalectomy in postmenopausal women with positive estrogen receptor test, metastatic breast cancer, or who fail or relapse with tamoxifen (Nolvadex), and for patients with prostatic carcinoma. Former use as an anticonvulsant supplement has been abandoned because of its adrenal suppressant activity.

ROUTE & DOSAGE

Cushing's Disease

Adult: **PO** 250 mg q6h; may be increased 250 mg/d q1–2wk if needed (max 2 g/d).

Breast Cancer

Adult: **PO** 250 mg b.i.d. and hydrocortisone 60 mg h.s., 20 mg in AM, and 20 mg at 2 PM daily for 2 wk; then 250 mg q.i.d. and hydrocortisone 20 mg h.s., 10 mg in AM, and 10 mg at 2 PM thereafter.

PHARMACOKINETICS Onset: 3–5 d. **Distribution:** crosses placenta. **Metabolism:** hepatic metabolism. **Elimination:** half-life: 13 h (7 h with long-term use); excreted by kidneys; recovery of adrenal responsiveness to stress occurs 36–72 h after discontinuation.

CONTRAINDICATIONS & PRECAUTIONS Contraindicated in: hypothyroidism; infection. Safe use in pregnancy (category D), nursing mothers, and in children not established. **Cautious use in:** elderly.

ADVERSE/SIDE EFFECTS CNS: lethargy, drowsiness, *dizziness*, uncontrolled eye movements (dose related); clumsiness, *headache*. **CV:** *hypotension, tachycardia*. **Endocrine:** masculinization. **GI:** nausea, vomiting, anorexia. **Hematologic (rare):** neutropenia, leukopenia, thrombocytopenia, pancytopenia, agranulocytosis, decreased Hgb and Hct, anemia, Coombs' negative hemolytic anemia. **Skin:** *measles-like (morbilliform) rash*, pruritus. **Other:** hepatotoxicity.

DRUG INTERACTIONS Dexamethasone decreases pharmacologic effects of aminoglutethimide; decreases anticoagulant response to **warfarin.**

NURSING IMPLICATIONS

Administration

- Treatment with aminoglutethimide normally is administered in the hospital until a stable dosage regimen is achieved.
- If glucocorticoid replacement is needed, 20–30 mg of hydrocortisone PO each morning may be ordered.
- Store at 15–30C (59–86F) in tightly closed containers unless otherwise directed.

Assessment & Drug Effects

- Baseline and periodic determinations should be made: 8 AM fasting plasma cortisol levels (normal: 5–30 μg/dl; excessively low levels indicate adrenal insufficiency); CBC; serum alkaline phosphatase (clue for early bone recurrence); AST (SGOT); bilirubin; thyroid function tests; urinary aldosterone (normal: 2–26 μg/24 h); serum electrolytes; CO_2.
- Baseline and regularly scheduled BP readings in the recumbent and upright positions indicate the effect of reduced aldosterone levels on BP. Orthostatic and persistent hypotension (subjectively experienced as dizziness, lightheadedness, weakness) result from reduced aldosterone production.
- Dose reduction or temporary discontinuation may be indicated if any of the following occur: extreme drowsiness, severe skin rash, extremely low cortisol levels.
- The elderly are particularly sensitive to the CNS effects of aminoglutethimide (e.g., lethargy, ataxia, orthostatic dizziness, light-headedness). Note implications for ambulation.
- Patients with Cushing's syndrome may show reduced effect with continuing therapy. These patients are generally not treated beyond 3 mo with aminoglutethimide.
- Adrenal insufficiency (hypoadrenalism) symptoms include anorexia, nausea, vomiting, weight loss, weakness, hypotension, dizziness, hypoglycemia, oliguria, low serum sodium, elevated potassium and BUN, arthralgia, myalgia, hyperpigmentation.

- Development of adrenal insufficiency is an indication for discontinuation of the drug.
- Report symptoms of hypothyroidism (see Signs & Symptoms, Appendix G) should they appear.

Patient & Family Education

- Make position changes gradually, pausing between each change. Do not stand still for prolonged periods. Support hose may be helpful. Consult physician.
- Drowsiness, nausea, and anorexia often disappear spontaneously within 1–2 wk of continuing therapy. Caution patient not to stop taking drug but to inform physician if symptoms persist or become pronounced.
- Report skin rash that persists beyond 5–8 d. Physician may discontinue drug.
- Tolerance to lethargy and ataxia usually develops after 4 wk of therapy. If symptoms are severe, however, drug discontinuation may be necessary. Keep physician informed.
- Contact physician immediately in times of stress such as surgery, dental work, acute illness, acute emotional situations. Steroid supplements may be indicated or physician may temporarily stop aminoglutethimide.
- Notify physician immediately if pregnancy is suspected.
- Because of the possibility of drowsiness and dizziness, warn patient to avoid driving and other potentially hazardous activities until the reaction to drug is known.
- Advise patient to carry card or jewelry (e.g., Medic Alert) indicating medical diagnosis, medication(s), physician's name, address, and telephone number.

AMINOPHYLLINE (THEOPHYLLINE ETHYLENEDIAMIDE)

(am-in-off'i-lin)

Trade names: Corophyllin ♣, Paladron ♣, Phyllocontin, Somophyllin, Somophyllin-DF, Truphylline

Classification: BRONCHODILATOR (RESPIRATORY SMOOTH MUSCLE RELAXANT); XANTHINE

Prototype: Theophylline

Pregnancy category: C

ACTIONS/PHARMACODYNAMICS

Aminophylline is a salt of theophylline with effects similar to those of other xanthines, e.g., caffeine and theobromine. Action is dependent on theophylline content (approximately 80%) and is measured as theophylline in the serum.

USES To prevent and relieve symptoms of acute bronchial asthma and treatment of bronchospasm associated with chronic bronchitis and emphysema. **Unlabeled uses:** as a respiratory stimulant in Cheyne-Stokes respiration; for treatment of apnea and bradycardia in prematures; as cardiac stimulant and diuretic in treatment of CHF. Use as antispasmodic for acute biliary attack has largely been replaced by more effective drugs.

ROUTE & DOSAGE

Bronchospasm (all doses based on ideal body weight)

Adult: **Loading dose** 6 mg/kg IV over 30 min. **Maintenance dose** IV by continuous infusion; PO divided q6h. *Nonsmoker:* **PO/IV** 0.5 mg/kg/h. *Smoker:* **PO/IV** 0.75 mg/kg/h. *With CHF or cirrhosis:* **PO/IV** 0.25 mg/kg/h.

Child: **Loading dose** 6 mg/kg IV over 30 min. **Maintenance dose** IV by continuous infusion; PO divided q6h; >9 y, 0.75 mg/kg/h; 1–9 y, 1 mg/kg/h. *Infant:* **PO/IV** 6–11 mo, 0.87 g/kg/h. 2–6 mo, 0.5 mg/kg/h. *Neonate:* **PO/IV** 0.16 mg/kg/h.

Neonatal Apnea

Neonate: **IV/PO** Loading dose 5 mg/kg; maintenance 5 mg/kg/d divided q12h.

PHARMACOKINETICS Absorption: most products are 100% absorbed from GI tract. **Peak:** IV 30 min; uncoated tablet 1 h; sustained release 4–6 h. **Duration:** 4–8 h; varies with age, smoking, and liver function. **Distribution:** crosses placenta. **Metabolism:** extensively metabolized in liver. **Elimination:** parent drug and metabolites excreted by kidneys; excreted in breast milk.

CONTRAINDICATIONS & PRECAUTIONS Contraindicated in: hypersensitivity to xanthine derivatives or to ethylenediamine component; cardiac arrhythmias. Safe use during pregnancy (category C) and in nursing mothers not established. **Cautious use in:** severe hypertension, cardiac disease, arrhythmias; impaired hepatic function; diabetes mellitus; hyperthyroidism; glaucoma; prostatic hypertrophy; fibrocystic breast disease; history of peptic ulcer; neonates and young children, patients over 55 y; COPD, acute influenza or patients receiving influenza immunization.

ADVERSE/SIDE EFFECTS CNS: *nervousness,* restlessness, depression, insomnia, irritability, headache, dizziness, muscle hyperactivity, convulsions. **CV:** cardiac arrhythmias, tachycardia, with rapid IV: hyperventilation; chest pain, severe hypotension, cardiac arrest. **GI:** *nausea, vomiting, anorexia,* hematemesis, diarrhea, epigastric pain.

DRUG INTERACTIONS Increases **lithium** excretion, lowering lithium levels; **cimetidine,** high-dose **allopurinol** (600 mg/d), **ciprofloxacin, erythromycin, troleandomycin** can significantly increase **theophylline** levels.

INCOMPATIBILITIES Solution/additive: amikacin, bleomycin, CEPHALOSPORINS, **chlorpromazine, ciprofloxacin, clindamycin, codeine phosphate, dimenhydrinate, dobutamine, dopamine, doxapram, doxorubicin, epinephrine, hydralazine, hydroyzine, insulin, isoproterenol, levorphanol, meperidine, methadone, methylprednisolone, morphine, nafcillin, norepinephrine, oxytetracycline, papaverine, penicillin G, pentazocine, procaine, prochlorperazine, promazine, promethazine, tetracycline, verapamil, vitamin B complex with C. Y-site: amiodarone, codeine phosphate, ciprofloxacin, clindamycin,** PHENOTHIAZINES (**chlorpromazine, prochlorperazine,** etc), **epinephrine, dobutamine, dopamine, levorphanol, morphine, meperidine, methadone, norepinephrine, verapamil.**

NURSING IMPLICATIONS

Administration

- Oral drug is absorbed faster if taken with a full glass of water on an empty stomach (1/2–1 h before or 2 h after meals).
- Absorption may be delayed but is not reduced by presence of food in stomach.
- GI symptoms may be minimized by taking immediately after a meal or with food.

- Extended (controlled) release preparations should not be chewed or crushed before swallowing; however, if tablet is scored, it can be broken in half, then swallowed.
- The contents of extended release capsules may be mixed with soft, moist food and swallowed without chewing.
- Rectal preparations are generally ordered when the patient must fast or cannot tolerate the drug orally. Drug absorption is enhanced if rectum is empty.

Parenteral (IV)

- Rapid infusion of IV aminophylline may cause cardiac arrest. Monitor infusion rate carefully.
- IV aminophylline, 25 mg/ml, may be given by direct IV undiluted at a rate of 25 mg/min.
- IV aminophylline, 25 mg/ml, may be further diluted in 100–200 ml of D5W or NS and infused at a rate not to exceed 25 mg/min.
- IV administration to neonates, infants, and children: Verify correct IV concentration and rate of infusion with physician.
- Do not use aminophylline solutions if discolored or if crystals are present.
- Store at 15–30C (59–86F) in tightly closed containers unless otherwise directed. Follow manufacturer's directions regarding storage of suppositories. Some are stored at room temperature; others must be refrigerated.

Assessment & Drug Effects

- Toxic effects are generally related to theophylline serum levels over 20 μg/ml (therapeutic range 10–20 μg/ml).
- High incidence of toxicity is associated with rectal suppository use because of erratic rate of absorption.
- Patients receiving parenteral aminophylline should be closely observed for signs of hypotension, arrhythmias, and convulsions until serum theophylline stabilizes within the therapeutic range.
- Monitor vital signs; measure and record I&O. Improvements in quality and rate of pulse and respiration, as well as diuresis, are expected clinical effects. A sudden, sharp, unexplained rise in heart rate is a useful clinical indicator of toxicity.
- The elderly, acutely ill, and patients with severe respiratory problems, liver dysfunction, or pulmonary edema are at greater risk of toxicity because of reduced drug clearance.
- Children appear to be more susceptible than adults to the CNS stimulating effects of xanthines (nervousness, restlessness, insomnia, hyperactive reflexes, twitching, convulsions). Dosage reduction may be indicated.

Patient & Family Education

- Smoking (tobacco or marijuana) tends to increase aminophylline elimination (prolongs half-life) and therefore dosage requirements may be higher and dosage intervals shorter than in nonsmokers.
- Advise patient to report excessive nervousness or insomnia. Dosage reduction may be indicated.
- Dizziness is a relatively common side effect, particularly in the elderly. Advise patient to take necessary safety precautions.
- Many popular OTC remedies for treatment of asthma or cough contain ephedrine in combination with various salts of theophylline. Caution patient to take only those medications approved by physician.

AMINOSALICYLATE SODIUM (PARA-AMINOSALICYLATE SODIUM)

(a-mee-noe-sal-i′si-late)

Trade names: Parasal Sodium ♣, P.A.S. Sodium

Prototype: Isoniazid

AMINOSALICYLIC ACID (PARA-AMINOSALICYLIC ACID)

(a-mee-noe-sal-i-sil′ik)

Trade name: P.A.S.

Classifications: ANTIINFECTIVE; ANTITUBERCULOSIS AGENT

Pregnancy category: C

ACTIONS/PHARMACODYNAMICS Mechanism of action resembles that of sulfonamides. Aminosalicylic acid and salts are highly specific bacteriostatic agents that suppress growth and multiplication of *Mycobacterium tuberculosis* by preventing folic acid synthesis. Aminosalicylates reportedly have potent hypolipemic action and reduce serum cholesterol and triglycerides by lowering LDL and VLDL. Mechanism of this effect has not been established.

USES In combination with streptomycin or isoniazid or both in treatment of pulmonary and extrapulmonary tuberculosis to delay emergence of strains resistant to these drugs. **Unlabeled use:** has been used for its lipid-lowering effect.

ROUTE & DOSAGE

Tuberculosis

Aminosalicylic Acid

Adult: **PO** 10–12 g/d in 2–3 divided doses.
Child: **PO** 150–300 mg/kg/d in 3–4 divided doses.

Aminosalicylate Sodium

Adult: **PO** 12–15 g/d in 2–4 divided doses.
Child: **PO** 240–360 mg/kg/d in 2–4 divided doses.

PHARMACOKINETICS Absorption: readily and almost completely absorbed from GI tract; aminosalicylate sodium is more rapidly and completely absorbed than the acid. **Peak effect:** 1.5–2 h. **Duration:** 4 h. **Distribution:** well distributed to most tissue and body fluids except CSF unless meninges are inflamed. **Metabolism:** metabolized in liver. **Elimination:** half-life: 1 h; >80% excreted in urine in 7–10 h.

CONTRAINDICATIONS & PRECAUTIONS Contraindicated in: hypersensitivity to aminosalicylates, salicylates, or to compounds containing *para*-aminophenyl groups (e.g., sulfonamides, certain hair dyes), G6PD deficiency, use of the sodium salt in patients on sodium restriction or CHF. Safe use during pregnancy (category C) not established. **Cautious use in:** impaired renal and hepatic function; blood dyscrasias; goiter; gastric ulcer.

ADVERSE/SIDE EFFECTS CNS: psychotic reactions. **GI:** *anorexia, nausea, vomiting, abdominal distress, diarrhea,* peptic ulceration. **Hematologic:** leukopenia, agranulocytosis, eosinophilia, lymphocytosis, thrombocytopenia, hemolytic anemia; (G6PD deficiency). **Hypersensitivity:** fever, chills, generalized malaise, joint pain, rash, fixed-drug eruptions, pruritus; vasculitis; Loeffler's syndrome. **Metabolic:** acute hepatitis, prothrombinemia. **Renal:** renal irritation, crystalluria. **Other:** malabsorption. With long-term administration, goiter.

DIAGNOSTIC TEST INTERFERENCE Aminosalicylates (PAS) may interfere with urine ***urobilinogen*** determinations (using ***Ehrlich's reagent***), and may cause false-positive ***urinary protein*** and ***VMA*** determinations (with ***diazoreagent***); false-positive ***urine glucose*** may result with ***cupric sulfate tests,*** e.g., ***Benedict's solution,*** but reportedly not with glucose oxidase reagents, e.g., TesTape, Clinistix. Reduces ***serum cholesterol,*** and possibly ***serum potassium, serum PBI,*** and 24-hour ***I-131 thyroidal uptake*** (effect may last almost 14 days).

DRUG INTERACTIONS Increases hypoprothrombinemic effects of ORAL ANTIACOAGULANTS; increased risk of crystalluria with **ammonium chloride, ascorbic acid;** decreased intestinal absorption of **cyanocobalamin, folic acid;** may decrease absorption of **digoxin;** ANTIHISTAMINES may inhibit PAS absorption; may increase or decrease **phenytoin** levels; **probenecid, sulfinpyrazone** decrease PAS elimination; SALICYLATES may enhance PAS toxicity.

NURSING IMPLICATIONS

Administration

- Administer with or immediately following meals to reduce irritative gastric effects. Physician may order an antacid to be given concomitantly. Generally, GI side effects disappear after a few days of therapy.
- Crystalluria may be minimized by keeping urine neutral or alkaline with adjunctive drugs, such as antacids or with diet.
- Aminosalicylic acid is an unstable drug that deteriorates rapidly on contact with heat, air, and moisture. Store in tight, light-resistant containers in a cool, dry place, preferably at 15–30C (59–86F), unless otherwise directed.

Assessment & Drug Effects

- I&O should be monitored and fluids encouraged. High concentrations are excreted in urine, and this can cause crystalluria and hematuria.
- Abrupt onset of fever, particularly during the early weeks of therapy, and clinical picture resembling that of infectious mononucleosis (malaise, fatigue, generalized lymphadenopathy, splenomegaly, sore throat), as well as minor complaints of pruritus, joint pains, and headache, are strongly suggestive of hypersensitivity; these symptoms should be reported promptly.

Patient & Family Education

- Aminosalicylic acid is mildly sour to the taste, and it sometimes leaves a bitter aftertaste that may be relieved by rinsing mouth with clear water or by chewing sugar-free gum or candy.
- Inform patient that urine may turn red on contact with hypochlorite bleach used in commercial toilet bowl cleaners.
- Hypersensitivity reactions may occur after a few days, but most commonly in the fourth or fifth week. Advise patient to report them promptly.
- Instruct patient to notify physician if sore throat or mouth, malaise, unusual fatigue, bleeding or bruising occur (symptoms of blood dyscrasia).
- Generally, chemotherapy is continued about 2 y. Patient and responsible family members must understand signs and symptoms of drug toxicity, importance of maintaining an established drug regimen, and need for remaining under close medical supervision to

detect covert adverse drug effects. Point out that resistant strains develop more rapidly when drug regimen is interrupted or is sporadic.

- Caution patient not to take aspirin or other OTC drugs without physician's approval.
- A brownish or purplish discoloration of the drug signifies decomposition; should this occur, discard drug.

AMIODARONE HYDROCHLORIDE

(a-mee'oh-da-rone)

Trade names: Cordarone, Amio-Aqueous, Pacerone

Classifications: CARDIOVASCULAR AGENT; ANTIARRHYTHMIC

Prototype: Procainamide

Pregnancy category: D

ACTIONS/PHARMACODYNAMICS Structurally related to thyroxine. Class III antiarrhythmic; also has antianginal and antiadrenergic properties. Totally unrelated to other antiarrhythmics. Acts directly on all cardiac tissues. Prolongs duration of action potential and refractory period without significantly affecting resting membrane potential. By direct action on smooth muscle, decreases peripheral resistance and increases coronary blood flow. Blocks effects of sympathetic stimulation.

USES Prophylaxis and treatment of life-threatening ventricular arrhythmias and supraventricular arrhythmias, particularly with atrial fibrillation. **Unlabeled use:** treatment of nonexertional angina.

ROUTE & DOSAGE

Arrhythmias

Adult: **PO** *Loading dose:* 800–1600 mg/d in 1–2 doses for 1–3 wk. *Maintenance dose:* 400–600 mg/d in 1–2 doses.
IV *Loading dose:* 150 mg over 10 min followed by 360 mg over next 6 h. *Maintenance dose:* 540 mg over 18 h (0.5 mg/min); may continue at 0.5 mg/min. *To convert from IV to PO:* If duration of infusion: < 1 wk, 800–1600 mg PO; 1–3 wk, 600–800 mg PO; > 3 wk, 400 mg PO.
Child: **PO** *Loading dose:* 10–15 mg/kg/d or 600–800 mg/1.73 m^2/d in 1–2 divided doses × 4–14 d or until adequate control of arrhythmia. *Maintenance dose:* 5 mg/kg/d or 200–400 mg/1.73 m^2/d once daily; may be able to reduce to 2–5 mg/kg/d 5 d per week.

PHARMACOKINETICS Absorption: approximately 50% absorbed (22–86%). **Onset:** 2–3 d to 1–3 wk. **Peak:** 3–7 h. **Distribution:** concentrates in adipose tissue, lungs, kidneys, spleen; crosses placenta. **Metabolism:** extensively hepatically metabolized; undergoes some enterohepatic cycling. **Elimination:** half-life: biphasic—initial 2.5–10 d, terminal 40–55 d; excreted chiefly in bile and feces; also excreted in breast milk.

CONTRAINDICATIONS & PRECAUTIONS Contraindicated in: hypersensitivity to amiodarone, cardiogenic shock, severe sinus bradycardia, advanced AV block unless a pacemaker is available; severe liver disease. Safe use during pregnancy (category D), in nursing women, and in children not established; it should not be used in children. **Cautious use in:** Hashimoto's thyroiditis, goiter, or history of other thyroid dysfunction; CHF; electrolyte imbalance; preexisting lung disease; open heart surgery; history of hypersensitivity to iodine.

ADVERSE/SIDE EFFECTS CNS: peripheral neuropathy (*muscle weakness,* wasting numbness, tingling), *fatigue,* abnormal gait, dyskinesias, *dizziness,* paresthesia, headache. **CV:** bradycardia, *hypotension* (IV), sinus arrest, cardiogenic shock, CHF, arrhythmias; AV block. **Eye:** *corneal microdeposits,* blurred vision, optic neuritis, optic neuropathy, permanent blindness, corneal degeneration, macular degeneration, photosensitivity. **GI:** *anorexia, nausea, vomiting, constipation.* **Respiratory (pulmonary toxicity):** alveolitis, pneumonitis (fever, dry cough, dyspnea), interstitial pulmonary fibrosis. **Skin:** slate-blue pigmentation, *photosensitivity,* rash. **Other (with chronic use):** angioedema, hyperthyroidism or hypothyroidism, hepatotoxicity; may cause neonatal hypo- or hyperthyroidism if taken during pregnancy.

DIAGNOSTIC TEST INTERFERENCE ***Thyroid function*** test abnormalities (in the absence of thyroid function impairment).

DRUG INTERACTIONS Significantly increases **digoxin** levels; enhances pharmacologic effects and toxicities of **disopyramide, procainamide, quinidine, flecainide, lidocaine;** anticoagulant effects of ORAL ANTICOAGULANTS enhanced; **verapamil, diltiazem**, BETA-ADRENERGIC BLOCKING AGENTS may potentiate sinus bradycardia, sinus arrest, or AV block; may increase **phenytoin** levels 2- to 3-fold; **cholestyramine** may decrease amiodarone levels; **fentanyl** may cause bradycardia, hypotension, or decreased output; may increase **cyclosporine** levels and toxicity; **cimetidine** may increase amiodarone levels; **ritonavir** may increase risk of amiodarone toxicity, including cardiotoxicity.

INCOMPATIBILITIES Solution/additive: sodium bicarbonate. Y-site: aminophylline, cefamandole, cefazolin, heparin; mezlocillin, sodium bicarbonate.

NURSING IMPLICATIONS

Administration

- With the oral drug GI symptoms occur commonly during high-dose therapy, especially with loading doses. Symptoms usually respond to dose reduction or to administration in divided dose and with food, including milk.
- IV dose for first 24 h: Prepare loading dose by adding 150 mg amiodarone to 100 ml D5W to yield 1.5 mg/ml; rapidly infuse at 15 mg/min over 10 min. Prepare the dose for the next 24 h by adding 900 mg amiodarone to 500 ml D5W to yield 1.8 mg/ml; infuse at 1 mg/min over 6 h, then decrease the rate to 0.5 mg/min for the remaining 18 h.
- IV dose after first 24 h: Use a concentration of 1–6 mg/ml (use central line for >2 mg/ml) and infuse at 0.5 mg/min (720 mg/24 h). Infusion rate may be increased to achieve needed effect.
- Store at 15–30C (59–86F) protected from light, unless otherwise directed.

Assessment & Drug Effects

- During IV infusion, carefully monitor blood pressure and slow the infusion if significant hypotension occurs. Bradycardia should be treated by slowing the infusion or discontinuing it if necessary.
- Sustained monitoring is essential because drug has an unusually long half-life (see Pharmacokinetics).
- Baseline and periodic assessments

should be made of liver, lung, thyroid, neurologic, and GI function.

- Regular ophthalmic exams, including fundoscopy and slit-lamp exam, are recommended throughout therapy.
- Report adverse reactions promptly. Bear in mind that long elimination half-life means that drug effects will persist long after dosage adjustments are made or drug is discontinued.
- Be alert to signs of pulmonary toxicity: progressive dyspnea, fatigue, cough, pleuritic pain, fever.
- Auscultate chest periodically or when patient complains of respiratory symptoms. Check for diminished breath sounds, rales, pleuritic friction rub; observe breathing pattern. Drug-induced pulmonary function problems must be distinguished from CHF or pneumonia. Keep physician informed.
- Monitor heart rate and rhythm and BP until drug response has stabilized. Report promptly symptomatic bradycardia (see Signs & Symptoms, Appendix G).
- Significant elevations of liver enzymes AST (SGOT) and ALT (SGPT) transaminases occur frequently without producing symptoms. If elevations persist or if they are 2–3 times above normal baseline readings, dosage should be reduced or drug promptly withdrawn, to prevent hepatotoxicity and liver damage.
- CNS symptoms generally develop within a week after amiodarone therapy begins. Proximal muscle weakness, a common side effect, intensified by tremors presents a great hazard to the ambulating patient. Assess severity of symptoms. Supervision of ambulation may be indicated.
- During early treatment period, especially, watch for and report symptoms of drug-induced hypothyroidism or hyperthyroidism (see Signs & Symptoms, Appendix G).
- Noncardiac side effects of amiodarone (especially lipofuscinosis, photophobia, insomnia) are major factors in noncompliance. Reinforce importance of adhering to established drug regimen.
- Patients already receiving antiarrhythmic therapy when amiodarone is started must be closely observed for adverse effects, particularly conduction disturbances and exacerbation of arrhythmias. Dosage of previous agent should be reduced by 30–50% several days after amiodarone therapy is started (anticipating onset of amiodarone antiarrhythmic effect).

Patient & Family Education

- Once stabilized, pulse should be checked daily (or as prescribed) by patient or primary caregiver. Instruct patient to report a pulse <60.
- Skin and corneal pigmentation (lipofuscinosis), seen in most patients who receive the drug for >2 mo, is reportedly reversible but may take 1–7 mo to fade completely because of amiodarone's long half-life. Generally, corneal deposits do not interfere with vision.
- Blue-gray skin pigmentation (associated with use >1 y) disappears slowly after amiodarone is discontinued. Occasionally, reversal is not complete.
- Photophobia may be eased by dark glasses, but some patients may not be unable to go outdoors at all in the daytime even with such protection.
- Alert patient to the possibility of a photosensitivity reaction (ery-

thema, pruritus). For maximum protection, patient should wear protective clothing and a barrier-type sunscreen that physically blocks penetration of skin by ultraviolet light (e.g., titanium oxide or zinc formulations) and should avoid exposure to sun and sunlamps.

AMITRIPTYLINE HYDROCHLORIDE

(a-mee-trip'ti-leen)

Trade names: Amitril, Apo-Amitriptyline ♣, Elavil, Emitrip, Endep, Enovil, Levate ♣, Meravil, Novotriptyn ♣, SK-Amitriptyline

Classifications: CNS AGENT; PSYCHOTHERAPEUTIC; TRICYCLIC ANTIDEPRESSANT

Prototype: Imipramine

Pregnancy category: C

ACTIONS/PHARMACODYNAMICS Among the most active of the tricyclic antidepressants (TCAs) in inhibition of serotonin uptake from synaptic gap; also inhibits norepinephrine reuptake to a moderate degree. Restoration of the levels of these neurotransmitters is a proposed mechanism of antidepressant action. Has H_2-receptor blocking activity (inhibits gastric acid secretion) and prominent anticholinergic and sedative actions.

USE Endogenous depression. **Unlabeled uses:** prophylaxis for cluster, migraine, and chronic tension headaches; intractable pain, peptic ulcer disease, to increase muscle strength in myotonic dystrophy, to treat pathologic weeping and laughing secondary to forebrain disease, for eating disorders associated with depression (anorexia or bulimia), and as sedative for nondepressed patients.

ROUTE & DOSAGE

Antidepressant

Adult: **PO** 75–100 mg/d; may gradually increase to 150–300 mg/d (use lower doses in outpatients). **IM** 20–30 mg q.i.d. until patient can take PO.
Adolescent: **PO** 25–50 mg/d in divided doses, may gradually increase to 100 mg/d (max 200 mg/d)
Geriatric: **PO** 10–25 mg h.s., may gradually increase to 25–150 mg/d. *Adolescent:* **PO** 10 mg t.i.d. and 20 mg h.s.

PHARMACOKINETICS Absorption: rapidly absorbed from GI and injection sites. **Peak levels:** 2–12 h. **Distribution:** crosses placenta. **Metabolism:** metabolized in liver to active metabolite. **Elimination:** half-life: 10–50 h; primarily excreted in urine; enters breast milk.

CONTRAINDICATIONS & PRECAUTIONS Contraindicated in: acute recovery period after MI, history of seizure disorders, pregnancy (category C), nursing mothers, children under 12 y. **Cautious use in:** prostatic hypertrophy, history of urinary retention or obstruction; angle-closure glaucoma; diabetes mellitus; hyperthyroidism; patient with cardiovascular, hepatic, or renal dysfunction; patient with suicidal tendency, electroshock therapy; elective surgery; schizophrenia; respiratory disorders; elderly, adolescents.

ADVERSE/SIDE EFFECTS CNS: *drowsiness, sedation, dizziness,* nervousness, restlessness, fatigue, headache, insomnia, abnormal movements (extrapyramidal symptoms), seizures. **CV:** *orthostatic hypotension,* tachycardia, palpitation, ECG changes. **Eye:** blurred vision, mydriasis. **GI:** *dry mouth,* increased appetite especially for sweets, *constipation,* weight gain, sour or metallic taste, nausea, vomiting. **Other:** *urinary retention,* bone marrow depression (rare).

DRUG INTERACTIONS ANTIHYPERTENSIVES may decrease some antihypertensive response; CNS DEPRESSANTS, **alcohol,** HYPNOTICS, BARBITURATES, SEDATIVES potentiate CNS depression; ANTICOAGULANTS, ORAL, may increase hypoprothombinemic effect; **ethchlorvynol,** transient delirium; **levodopa,** SYMPATHOMIMETICS (e.g., **epinephrine, norepinephrine),** possibility of sympathetic hyperactivity with hypertension and hyperpyrexia; MAO INHIBITORS, possibility of severe reactions, toxic psychosis, cardiovascular instability; **methylphenidate** increases plasma TCA levels; THYROID DRUGS may increase possibility of arrhythmias; **cimetidine** may increase plasma TCA levels.

NURSING IMPLICATIONS

Administration

- Oral drug may be taken with or immediately after food to reduce possibility of GI irritation. Tablet may be crushed if patient is unwilling to take it whole; administer with food or fluid.
- Dose increases by 25–50 mg are preferably made in late afternoon or at bedtime because sedative action precedes antidepressant effect.
- A single dose at bedtime is useful to promote sleep or for patients who complain of dizziness or when daytime sedation interferes with work productivity. Drug effect on depression is not affected by time of day dose is taken.
- Maintenance regimen is usually continued for at least 3 mo to prevent relapse. Typical length of therapy for depression is 6 mo–1 y.
- Abrupt discontinuation of therapy can precipitate withdrawal symptoms (headache, nausea, malaise, musculoskeletal pain, panic attack, weakness). This reaction can be avoided by tapering dosage over 2 wk.
- Store drug at 15–30C (59–86F) unless otherwise directed by manufacturer. Protect from light.

Assessment & Drug Effects

- Baseline and periodic leukocyte and differential counts, BP, cardiac, renal, and hepatic function tests, and eye examinations (including glaucoma testing) are recommended particularly for the elderly, adolescents, and for patients receiving high doses or prolonged therapy.
- Monitor BP and pulse rate in patients with preexisting cardiovascular disease. Withhold drug if there is a rise or fall in systolic BP (by 10–20 mm Hg), or a sudden increase or a significant change in pulse rate or rhythm. Notify physician.
- Monitor I&O, including bowel elimination pattern.
- During initial therapy, be alert to drowsiness and dizziness. Institute measures to prevent falling.
- If a patient uses excessive amounts of alcohol, it should be borne in mind that the potentiation of amitriptyline effects may increase the dangers of overdosage or suicide attempt.
- When used for migraine prophylaxis, therapeutic effect may occur in 1–6 wk. Drug is usually discontinued after patient has been headache-free for 1–2 mo. If headache recurs, physician may prescribe another course of treatment.

Patient & Family Education

- Monitor weight. Amitriptyline may increase the appetite and cause weight gain; some patients develop a craving for sweets.
- Tolerance or adaptation to distressing anticholinergic actions (see Appendix G) usually develops after patient goes on maintenance regimen. Keep physician informed.
- Advise patient that dry mouth can be relieved by taking frequent sips of water and by increasing total fluid intake.
- Instruct patient to change from recumbency to upright position slowly and in stages. Support stockings may help. Consult physician.
- Avoid potentially hazardous activities, such as driving, until response to the drug is known.
- Desired therapeutic effects for depression may not be evident until after 3–4 wk of therapy, because of long serum half-life.
- Advise patient not to use OTC drugs while he or she is on TCA therapy. Many preparations contain sympathomimetic amines.
- Inform patient that amitriptyline may make urine blue-green.

AMLEXANOX

(am-lex′-a-nox)

Trade name: Aphthasol

Classifications: SKIN AND MUCOUS MEMBRANE AGENT

Pregnancy category: B

ACTIONS/PHARMACODYNAMICS Mechanism of action by which healing of aphthous ulcers occurs is unknown. Amlexanox reduces healing time and pain related to aphthous ulcers or canker sores.

USE Treatment of aphthous ulcers in patients with normal immune systems.

ROUTE & DOSAGE

Aphthous Ulcers

Adult: **Topical** Apply 1/4 in. (0.5 cm) to finger and dab onto each mouth ulcer q.i.d. (after oral hygeine p.c. and h.s.) × 10 d.

PHARMACOKINETICS **Absorption:** minimally absorbed through ulcer. **Onset:** approximately 3 d. **Elimination:** half-life: 3.5 h; 17% of orally absorbed dose excreted in urine.

CONTRAINDICATIONS & PRECAUTIONS **Contraindicated in:** sensitivity to amlexanox. **Cautious use in:** pregnancy (category B), nursing mothers. Safety and efficacy in children have not been established.

ADVERSE/SIDE EFFECTS **Body as whole:** transient pain, stinging and/or burning at application site.

NURSING IMPLICATIONS

Administration

- Apply after oral hygiene following each meal and before bedtime.
- Avoid prolonged contact with skin and wash off skin if contact occurs.
- Store at 15–30C (59–86F) away from heat and moisture. Do not freeze.

Assessment & Drug Effects

- Therapeutic effectiveness is indicated by disappearance of oral ulcer.

Patient & Family Education

- Use at first sign of canker sore. Wash hands before and immediately after application.

- Flush eyes immediately with large amount of cold water if they accidentally contact paste.
- Discontinue use if rash or inflamed membranes develop.
- Contact physician if healing does not result after 10 d of therapy.

AMLODIPINE

(am-lo′-di-peen)

Trade name: Norvasc

Classifications: CARDIOVASCULAR AGENT; CALCIUM CHANNEL BLOCKER; NONNITRATE VASODILATOR

Prototype: Nifedipine (calcium channel blocker)

Pregnancy category: C

ACTIONS/PHARMACODYNAMICS Amlodipine is a calcium channel blocking agent that selectively blocks calcium ion reflux across cell membranes of cardiac and vascular smooth muscle without changing serum calcium concentrations. It predominantly acts on the peripheral circulation, decreasing peripheral vascular resistance, and increases cardiac output. It reduces systemic systolic, diastolic, and mean arterial blood pressure.

USE Treatment of mild to moderate hypertension and angina.

ROUTE & DOSAGE

Hypertension

Adult: **PO** 5–10 mg once daily; geriatric patients or patients with hepatic dysfunction should start with 2.5 mg; adjust dose at intervals of not less than 2 wk.

PHARMACOKINETICS **Absorption:** > 90% absorbed from GI tract. ***Onset:*** gradual. **Peak:** 6–9 h. Duration: 24 h. **Distribution:** > 95% protein bound. **Metabolism:** extensively metabolized in the liver to inactive metabolites. **Elimination:** half-life: < 45 y: 28–69 h; > 60 y: 40–120 h; inactive metabolites primarily excreted in urine (< 5–10% excreted unchanged), 20–25% excreted in feces.

CONTRAINDICATIONS & PRECAUTIONS **Contraindicated in:** hypersensitivity to amlodipine. **Cautious use in:** liver disease; concomitant use with hypotension; CHF; pregnancy (category C); nursing mothers; elderly.

ADVERSE/SIDE EFFECTS **CV:** palpitations, flushing tachycardia, *peripheral or facial edema,* bradycardia, chest pain, syncope, postural hypotension. **CNS:** light-headedness, fatigue, *headache.* **GI:** abdominal pain, nausea, anorexia, constipation, dyspepsia, dysphagia, diarrhea, flatulence, vomiting. **GU:** sexual dysfunction, frequency, nocturia. **Skin:** flushing, rash. **Other:** dyspnea, arthralgia, cramps, myalgia.

DRUG INTERACTIONS **Adenosine** may increase the risk of bradycardia **Drug–food:** grapefruit juice may increase amlodipine levels.

NURSING IMPLICATIONS

Administration

- Drug may be given without regard to meals.
- With frail elderly or those with hepatic dysfunction, dosage reductions to 2.5 mg daily may be warranted.
- Initial dosages of 2.5 mg daily are common with amlodipine if added to a regimen including other antihypertensive drugs.
- Dosage is generally titrated up over a period of 7–14 d or more rapidly if warranted.
- Store at room temperature (15–30C/59–86F).

Assessment & Drug Effects

- Monitor BP and postural changes. Report postural hypotension.
- Peak levels of amlodipine are achieved 6–9 h following oral doses with corresponding BP reduction.
- Monitor heart rate; dose-related palpitations (more common in women) may occur.
- Assess for dose-related peripheral or facial edema that may not be accompanied by weight gain. Rarely, edema may be severe enough to cause discontinuation of drug.

Patient & Family Education

- Instruct patient to report significant swelling of face or extremities.
- Warn of the possibility of dose-related light-headedness or dizziness. Advise of necessary precautions especially with frail or elderly patients.
- Advise patients to report shortness of breath, palpitations, irregular heartbeat, nausea, or constipation.

AMMONIUM CHLORIDE

(ah-mo'nium)

Classification: ELECTROLYTIC BALANCE AGENT

Pregnancy category: B

ACTIONS/PHARMACODYNAMICS Acidifying property is due to conversion of ammonium ion (NH_4^+) to urea in liver with liberation of H^+ and Cl^-. Potassium excretion also increases, but to a lesser extent. Tolerance to diuretic effect occurs within 2–3 d.

USES Systemic acidifier in patients with metabolic alkalosis; to correct chloride depletion after diuretic therapy; as adjunct to lower urinary pH in treatment of UTI; and as an aid in excretion of certain alkalinizing drugs, e.g., amphetamines. Limited use as a primary diuretic. Has been used to increase solubility of calcium and phosphate ions in urinary phosphatic calculi, and in treatment of bromism and lead poisoning, and for diuretic effect in premenstrual tension and Ménière's syndrome. Common ingredient in OTC cough mixtures for its expectorant action.

ROUTE & DOSAGE

Urine Acidifier, Diuretic

Adult: **PO** 4–12 g/d divided q4–6h.
Child: **PO** 75 mg/kg/d in 4 divided doses.

Metabolic Acidosis

Adult: **IM/IV** Dose calculated on basis of CO_2 combining power or serum Cl deficit; 50% of calculated deficit is administered slowly.
Child: **IM/IV** Same as for adult.

PHARMACOKINETICS **Absorption:** completely absorbed in 3–6 h. **Metabolism:** metabolized in liver to HCl and urea. **Elimination:** primarily excreted in urine.

CONTRAINDICATIONS & PRECAUTIONS **Contraindicated in:** severe renal or hepatic insufficiency; primary respiratory acidosis. Safe use during pregnancy (category B) not established. **Cautious use in:** cardiac edema, pulmonary insufficiency.

ADVERSE/SIDE EFFECTS Most are secondary to ammonia toxicity. **CNS:** headache, depression, drowsiness, twitching, excitability. **CV:** bradycardia and other arrhythmias. **GI:** gastric irritation, nausea, vomiting, anorexia. **Metabolic/electrolytes:** metabolic acidosis, hyperammonia. **Other:** skin rash, glycosuria, hyperventilation, EEG abnormalities; pain and irritation at IV site.

DIAGNOSTIC TEST INTERFERENCE Ammonium chloride may increase ***blood ammonia*** and ***SGOT (AST),*** decrease ***serum magnesium*** (by increasing urinary magnesium excretion), and decrease urine ***urobilinogen.***

DRUG INTERACTIONS **Aminosalicylic acid** may cause crystalluria; increases urinary excretion of AMPHETAMINES, **flecainide, mexiletine, methadone, ephedrine, pseudoephedrine;** decreased urinary excretion of SULFONYLUREAS, SALICYLATES.

INCOMPATIBILITIES **Solution/additive: codeine phosphate, levorphanol, methadone, nitrofurantoin, warfarin.**

NURSING IMPLICATIONS

Administration

- GI side effects may be minimized by giving oral drug immediately after meals or by use of enteric-coated tablets. Tablets should be swallowed whole.
- Note that ammonium chloride for injection is available in two strengths: 2.14% (0.4 mEq/ml) in 500 ml containers may be given without further dilution. The 26.75% (5 mEq/ml) concentrate in 20-ml vials must be diluted before administration. The concentrate may be prepared by diluting each 20 ml of ammonium chloride with 500 ml of 0.9% NaCl injection.
- Parenteral preparations of ammonium chloride should be administered slowly by IV infusion to avoid serious side effects (ammonia toxicity) and local irritation and pain.
- Administer diluted solution at a rate not to exceed 5 ml/min. Rate is much slower for infants (check with physician).
- Store in airtight container. Avoid freezing. Concentrated solutions of ammonium chloride tend to crystallize at low temperatures. Crystals can be dissolved by placing intact container in a warm water bath and warming to room temperature.

Assessment & Drug Effects

- Baseline and periodic determinations of CO_2 combining power, serum electrolytes, and urinary and arterial pH should be made during therapy to avoid serious acidosis. For some patients, dosage may be monitored by repeated serum chloride and CO_2 content (bicarbonate) determinations and urinary pH.
- Monitor rate and depth of respirations. Shortness of breath on exertion and increased ventilation at rest are signs of acidosis and should be reported promptly.
- Monitor I&O ratio and pattern. Because of compensatory mechanisms the diuretic effect of ammonium chloride lasts only 1 or 2 d.
- In the elderly, vigorous diuresis may precipitate renal insufficiency, urinary retention in men with prostatic hypertrophy, incontinence in both sexes, and acute Na^+ and K^+ depletion. Report signs of weakness and confusion and changes in voiding pattern and comfort.
- Check urine specific gravity of elderly patients on diuretic therapy. Elevation accompanying even mild diuresis is suggestive of renal insufficiency.

Patient & Family Education

- Unless contraindicated, diet of patients on diuretic therapy should include foods high in potassium,

e.g., bananas, oranges, dried fruits, cantaloupe, honeydew melon, milk (all types), tomatoes, potatoes, winter squash.
- Hyperglycemia and glycosuria are potential side effects. Note implications for the diabetic patient and instruct him or her accordingly.

AMOBARBITAL
(am-oh-bar′bi-tal)

Trade names: Amytal, Isobec, Novamobarb

AMOBARBITAL SODIUM
Trade name: Amytal Sodium

Classifications: CNS AGENT; BARBITURATE ANTICONVULSANT; SEDATIVE-HYPNOTIC

Prototype: Phenobarbital

Pregnancy category: D

Controlled substance: Schedule II

ACTIONS/PHARMACODYNAMICS Intermediate-acting barbiturate similar to phenobarbital. CNS depressant action appears to be related to ability to interfere with ascending impulse transmission from reticular activating system (concerned with body and behavioral alertness) to cerebral cortex. Does not impair pain perception.

USES Sedative, to relieve anxiety, and as short-term hypnotic to treat insomnia. Also used parenterally to control status epilepticus or acute convulsive episodes, agitated behavior, and for narcoanalysis and narcotherapy.

ROUTE & DOSAGE

Sedative

Adult: **PO** 30–50 mg b.i.d. or t.i.d.
Child: **PO** 2 mg/kg or 70 mg/m^2/d in 4 divided doses.

Preoperative Sedation

Adult: **PO/IM** 200 mg 1 h before surgery.

Labor

Adult: **PO** 200–400 mg repeated at 1–3 h intervals (max 1 g).

Hypnotic

Adult: **PO/IM** 65–200 mg (max 500 mg).
Child: **IM** 2–3 mg/kg.

Anticonvulsant, Agitated Behavior, Hypnotic

Adult: **IV** 65–500 mg, not to exceed 1 g.
Child: **IV** Same as for adult.

PHARMACOKINETICS **Onset:** 1 h PO; 5 min IV. **Duration:** 6–8 h PO; 3–6 h IV. **Distribution:** crosses placenta; appears in breast milk. **Metabolism:** metabolized primarily in liver. **Elimination:** half-life: 20–25 h; 40–50% of dose excreted in urine.

CONTRAINDICATIONS & PRECAUTIONS **Contraindicated in:** hypersensitivity to barbiturates; history of addiction; family or patient history of porphyria; severe respiratory, hepatic, or renal disease. Safe use during pregnancy (category D), in nursing women, and in children <6 y not established. **Cautious use in:** hypotension, hypertension, cardiac disease; acute or chronic pain; elderly patients.

ADVERSE/SIDE EFFECTS **CNS:** *drowsiness,* dizziness, hangover, unsteadiness, lethargy, paradoxical excitement. **Hematologic** (rare): agranulocytosis, thrombocytopenia. **Hypersensitivity:** rash, angioedema. **Other:** pain at IM injection site,

Stevens-Johnson syndrome, hypotension, respiratory depression.

DRUG INTERACTIONS Antagonizes effects of **phenmetrazine;** CNS DEPRESSANTS, **alcohol,** SEDATIVES compound CNS depression; MAO INHIBITORS cause excessive CNS depression; **methoxyflurane** presents risk of nephrotoxicity.

INCOMPATIBILITIES Solution/additive: codeine phosphate, dimenhydrinate, phenytoin, hydrocortisone, hydroxyzine, insulin, levophanol, meperidine, methadone, morphine, norepinephrine, pentazocine, procaine, streptomycin, tetracycline, vancomycin, penicillin G, PHENOTHIAZINES, **cimetidine, pancuronium.**

NURSING IMPLICATIONS

Administration

- Rate of absorption is increased if oral drug is taken on an empty stomach.
- For insomnia (hypnotic), dose is generally administered 30–60 min before bedtime. Hypnotic use should be limited to 2 wk. Amobarbital effectiveness appears to decrease by second week of continued use.
- Drug should be injected within 30 min after vial is opened.
- Parenteral solution is reconstituted with sterile water for injection. Add diluent slowly and rotate vial. Do not shake vial. If solution does not clear within 5 min or contains a precipitate, do not use. Consult manufacturer's package insert for reconstitution direction to prepare specific concentrations.
- IM injection should be deep in a large muscle mass, e.g., upper outer quadrant of gluteus maximus. Superficial injections are painful and can cause sterile abscess or sloughing. No more than 5 ml should be injected IM into any one site.
- IV administration rate should not exceed 100 mg/min for adults or 60 $mg/m^2/min$ for children.
- Reactions occur most frequently with rapid IV administration.
- Store at 15–30C (59–86F) unless otherwise directed. Avoid freezing.

Assessment & Drug Effects

- Vital signs should be monitored during IV infusion and for several hours after drug administration. Caution patient not to get out of bed without assistance. Side rails are indicated.
- Personnel and equipment for management of respiratory depression and hypotension should be immediately available when drug is administered IV.
- Observe IV injection site during and after administration. Extravasation can cause thrombophlebitis and tissue necrosis.
- Barbiturates may produce paradoxical restlessness, excitement, confusion, and depression in the elderly and in some children. Note implications for safety. Dosage adjustments may be required.

Patient & Family Education

- Caution patient not to take alcoholic beverages or other CNS depressants.
- Paradoxical excitement may also occur with onset of pain. Instruct patient to report this occurrence.
- Advise patient not to drive or engage in potentially hazardous activities until reaction to drug is known.
- Prolonged use may lead to tolerance and dependence. Advise patient to take drug only as ordered.

AMOXAPINE

(a-mox'a-peen)

Trade name: Asendin

Classifications: CNS AGENT; PSYCHOTHERAPEUTIC; TRICYCLIC ANTIDEPRESSANT

Prototype: Imipramine

Pregnancy category: C

ACTIONS/PHARMACODYNAMICS

Tricyclic antidepressant (TCA) and secondary amine with mixed antidepressant and neuroleptic properties. Action mechanism not clear. Appears to reduce reuptake of norepinephrine and serotonin and also blocks response to dopamine by dopaminergic receptors. Unlike other TCAs, not associated with severe cardiotoxicity, has mild sedative action, and causes slight orthostatic hypotension.

USE Neurotic and endogenous depression accompanied by anxiety or agitation.

ROUTE & DOSAGE

Antidepressant

Adult: **PO** Start at 50 mg b.i.d. or t.i.d.; may increase on third day to 100 mg t.i.d. *Maintenance doses* ≤300 mg/d may be given as a single dose at bedtime.
Geriatric: **PO** 25 mg h.s.; may increase q3–7d to 50–150 mg/d in divided doses (max 300 mg/d).

PHARMACOKINETICS Absorption: rapidly absorbed. **Peak:** 1–2 h. **Distribution:** probably crosses placenta; distributed into breast milk. **Metabolism:** metabolized active metabolite. **Elimination:** half-life: 8 h parent drug, 30 h metabolite; 60% excreted in urine in 6 d; 7–18% excreted in feces.

CONTRAINDICATIONS & PRECAUTIONS Contraindicated in: hypersensitivity to other tricyclic compounds; acute recovery period after MI; children <16 y of age; pregnancy (category C), nursing mothers. **Cautious use in:** history of convulsive disorders, schizophrenia, manic depression, electroshock therapy; alcohol abuse; history of urinary retention, benign prostatic hypertrophy; angle-closure glaucoma or increased intraocular pressure; cardiovascular disorders; impaired renal or hepatic function; elective surgery.

ADVERSE/SIDE EFFECTS CNS: *drowsiness,* dizziness, headache, fatigue, *sedation,* lethargy; extrapyramidal effects (acute dystonic reactions, panic attacks, parkinsonism, tardive dyskinesia), seizures (overdosage). **CV:** orthostatic hypotension; arrhythmias. **GI:** constipation, diarrhea, flatulence, *dry mouth,* peculiar taste, nausea, heartburn. **Other:** blurred vision, nephrotoxicity (overdosage), dry eyes.

DRUG INTERACTIONS May decrease response to ANTIHYPERTENSIVES; CNS DEPRESSANTS, **alcohol,** HYPNOTICS, BARBITURATES, SEDATIVES potentiate CNS depression; may increase hypoprothombinemic effect of ORAL ANTICOAGULANTS; **ethchlorvynol,** transient delirium; with **levodopa,** SYMPATHOMIMETICS (e.g., **epinephrine, norepinephrine**), possibility of sympathetic hyperactivity with hypertension and hyperpyrexia; with MAO INHIBITORS, possibility of severe reactions: toxic psychosis, cardiovascular instability; **methylphenidate** increases plasma TCA levels; thyroid drugs may increase possibility of arrhythmias; **cimetidine** may increase plasma TCA levels.

NURSING IMPLICATIONS

Administration

- Amoxapine may be taken with or after food to reduce GI irritation. Tablet may be crushed and taken with food or fluid of choice.
- Maintenance dose is generally taken as a single dose at bedtime to minimize daytime sedation and other annoying drug side effects.
- Store at 15–30C (59–86F) in tightly closed container unless otherwise directed.

Assessment & Drug Effects

- Initial antidepressant effect (mild euphoria, increased energy) may occur within 4–7 d; however, in most patients minimal clinical response does not occur until after 2 or 3 wk of drug therapy.
- Suicide risk may remain even when there is significant improvement. Supervise patient closely during therapy.
- Monitor I&O ratio and bowel elimination pattern. Report continuing constipation.
- Patient may experience sedation during early therapy, mostly when dosage increases are made. Note implications for ambulation, particularly in the elderly.
- Extrapyramidal reactions including parkinsonism, symptoms related to the reproductive system, and neuroleptic malignant syndrome reportedly occur more frequently with amoxapine than with other TCAs.
- Report immediately the onset of signs suggestive of tardive dyskinesia (see Signs & Symptoms, Appendix G). Careful observations and prompt reporting may prevent irreversibility.
- Immediately report signs of neuroleptic malignant syndrome: fever, sweating, rigidity (catatonia), unstable BP, rapid, irregular pulse; changes in level of consciousness, coma. Although rare, it can be life-threatening if drug is not stopped immediately. Death can result from acute respiratory, renal, or cardiovascular failure.
- Tolerance to amoxapine antidepressant effects develops in some patients after 1–3 mo of drug therapy. Close medical follow-up is essential.

Patient & Family Education

- Excessive alcohol may potentiate drug effects, thus increasing the dangers of overdosage or suicide.
- Drinking at least 2000 ml fluid daily and eating foods with high fiber content (if allowed) will provide needed roughage.
- Amoxapine may increase the appetite and cause weight gain. Some patients develop a craving for sweets.
- Alertness and skill in performing hazardous tasks, such as driving, may be impaired, particularly during early therapy.
- Xerostomia may be relieved by frequent sips of water, increasing total fluid intake, if allowed, and by use of sugarless gum or sourballs.
- Withdrawal symptoms (headache, nausea, musculoskeletal pain, weakness) can be avoided by tapering dosage over 2 wk.
- Impress on patient the necessity of maintaining established dosage regimen. Tell patient not to skip, reduce, or double doses or change dose intervals.
- OTC drug use should be approved by the physician.
- Smoking reportedly increases metabolism of tricyclic compounds. Higher doses may be required in some smokers.

AMOXICILLIN

(a-mox-i-sill'in)

Trade names: Amoxil, Apo-Amoxi ♣, Larotid, Novamoxin, Polymox, Sumox, Trimox, Utimox, Wymox

Classifications: ANTIINFECTIVE; BETA-LACTAM ANTIBIOTIC; AMINOPENICILLIN

Prototype: Ampicillin

Pregnancy category: B

ACTIONS/PHARMACODYNAMICS Broad-spectrum, acid-stable, semisynthetic aminopenicillin and analogue of ampicillin. Acts by inhibiting mucoprotein synthesis in cell wall of rapidly multiplying bacteria. It is bactericidal and is inactivated by penicillinase.

USES Infections of ear, nose, throat, GU tract, skin, and soft tissue caused by susceptible bacteria. Also used in uncomplicated gonorrhea. Available in combination with potassium clavulanate, which extends antibacterial spectrum of amoxicillin to include beta-lactamase-producing strains.

ROUTE & DOSAGE

Mild to Moderate Infections

Adult: **PO** 250–500 mg q8h.
Child: **PO** 25–50 mg/kg/d (max 60–80 mg/kg/d) divided q8h.

Gonorrhea

Adult: **PO** 3 g as single dose with 1 g probenecid.
Child ≥ 2 y: **PO** 50 mg/kg as single dose with probenecid 25 mg/kg.

PHARMACOKINETICS **Absorption:** rapid and nearly complete absorption. **Peak:** 1–2 h. **Distribution:** diffuses into most tissues and body fluids, except synovial fluid and CSF (unless meninges are inflamed); crosses placenta; distributed into breast milk in small amounts. **Metabolism:** metabolized in liver. **Elimination:** half-life: 1–1.3 h; 60% of dose excreted in urine in 6–8 h.

CONTRAINDICATIONS & PRECAUTIONS **Contraindicated in:** hypersensitivity to penicillins; infectious mononucleosis. Safe use during pregnancy (category B) not established. **Cautious use in:** history of or suspected atopy or allergy (hives, eczema, hay fever, asthma); severely impaired renal function; history of cephalosporin allergy.

ADVERSE/SIDE EFFECTS As with other penicillins. **GI:** diarrhea, nausea, vomiting, <u>pseudomembranous colitis</u> (rare). **Hematologic:** hemolytic anemia, eosinophilia, <u>agranulocytosis</u> (rare). **Hypersensitivity:** rash, <u>anaphylaxis</u>. **Skin:** pruritus, urticaria, or other skin eruptions. **Other:** superinfections, conjunctival ecchymosis.

DRUG INTERACTIONS TETRACYCLINES may inhibit activity of amoxicillin; **probenecid** prolongs the activity of amoxicillin.

NURSING IMPLICATIONS

Administration

- Chewable tablet should be chewed or crushed before being swallowed with a liquid.
- Amoxicillin may be given without regard to meals.
- For children, reconstituted pediatric drops may be placed directly on child's tongue for swallowing or added to formula, milk, fruit juice, water, ginger ale, or other soft drink. Have child drink all the prepared dose promptly.
- Store in tightly covered containers at 15–30C (59–86F) unless otherwise directed.

Assessment & Drug Effects

- Before therapy determine previous hypersensitivity reactions to penicillins, cephalosporins, and other allergens.
- Culture and sensitivity tests are done prior to initiation of therapy. Drug may be started pending results.
- Periodic assessments of renal, hepatic, and hematologic functions should be made during prolonged therapy.
- Diarrhea warrants appropriate diagnostic measures to rule out pseudomembranous colitis.
- Generalized, erythematous, maculopapular rash (ampicillin rash) is not due to hypersensitivity. It is usually mild, but can be severe. Report onset of rash to physician; hypersensitivity should be ruled out.
- An urticarial rash that occurs within a few days after start of amoxicillin is suggestive of a hypersensitivity reaction. If it occurs, look for other signs of hypersensitivity (fever, wheezing, generalized itching, dyspnea), and report to physician immediately.

Patient & Family Education

- Oral suspension and pediatric drops are reconstituted when they are dispensed from pharmacy. Date and time of reconstitution and discard date should appear on container. Stable for 7 d at room temperature, i.e., around 25C (77F) or 14 d if refrigerated, depending on manufacturer. Shake well before pouring.
- Instruct patient to take medication around the clock, not to miss a dose, and to continue therapy until all medication is taken, unless otherwise directed by physician.
- For most infections, treatment is continued for a minimum of 48–72 h beyond the time that patient is asymptomatic or cultures are negative.
- Patients with hemolytic streptococcal infections should receive at least 10 d of treatment to prevent occurrence of acute rheumatic fever.
- Advise patient to report to physician the onset of diarrhea and other possible symptoms of superinfection (see Signs & Symptoms, Appendix G).

AMOXICILLIN AND CLAVULANATE POTASSIUM

(a-mox-i-sill′in)

Trade names: Augmentin, Clavulin ♣

Classifications: ANTIINFECTIVE; BETA-LACTAM ANTIBIOTIC; AMINOPENICILLIN

Prototype: Ampicillin

Pregnancy category: B

ACTIONS/PHARMACODYNAMICS

Semisynthetic broad-spectrum antibiotic. Fixed combination of amoxicillin, an aminopenicillin, and the potassium salt to clavulanic acid, a competitive beta-lactamase inhibitor. Used alone, clavulanic acid antibacterial activity is weak. In combination, it inhibits enzyme (beta-lactamase) degradation of amoxicillin and by synergism extends both spectrum of activity and bactericidal effect of amoxicillin against many strains of beta-lactamase-producing bacteria resistant to amoxicillin alone. Active against gram-positive bacteria including *Staphylococcus aureus, Streptococcus pneumoniae, Clostridium, Peptococcus, Bacteroides fragilis* group, and many gram-negative organisms including *Branhamella catarrhalis* (formerly *Neisseria catarrhalis*), *Hemophilus influenzae, Proteus mirabilis; Salmonella, Shigella,* and *Klebsiella* sp. Generally inactive against *Pseudomonas*.

USES Infections caused by susceptible beta-lactamase-producing organisms: lower respiratory tract infections, otitis media, sinusitis, skin and skin structure infections, and UTI.

ROUTE & DOSAGE

Mild to Moderate Infections
Adult: **PO** 250 or 500 mg tablet (each with 125 mg clavulanic acid) q8–12h.
Child <40 kg: **PO** 20–40 mg/kg/d (based on amoxicillin component) divided q8–12h.
Neonates/Infants < 3 mo: **PO** 30 mg/kg/d (amoxicillin) divided q12h.

PHARMACOKINETICS Absorption: rapid and nearly complete absorption. **Peak:** 1–2 h. **Distribution:** diffuses into most tissues and body fluids, except synovial fluid and CSF (unless meninges are inflamed); crosses placenta; distributed into breast milk in very small amounts. **Metabolism:** metabolized in liver. **Elimination:** half-life: amoxicillin 1–1.3 h, clavulanate 0.78–1.2 h; 50–73% of the amoxicillin and 25–45% of the clavulanate dose excreted in urine in 2 h.

CONTRAINDICATIONS & PRECAUTIONS Contraindicated in: combination shares toxic potentials of ampicillin. Hypersensitivity to penicillins; infectious mononucleosis. **Cautious use in:** lactation, pregnancy (category B).

ADVERSE/SIDE EFFECTS GI: *diarrhea*, nausea, vomiting. **Skin:** rash, urticaria. **Other:** candidal vaginitis; moderate increases in serum ALT, AST; glomerulonephritis; agranulocytosis (rare).

DIAGNOSTIC TEST INTERFERENCE May interfere with ***urinary glucose*** determinations using ***cupric sulfate, Benedict's solution, Clinitest;*** does not affect glucose oxidase methods, e.g., Clinistix, TesTape. Positive direct ***antiglobulin (Coombs')*** test results may be reported, a reaction that could interfere with ***hematologic studies*** or with ***transfusion cross-matching*** procedures.

DRUG INTERACTIONS TETRACYCLINES may inhibit activity of amoxicillin; **probenecid prolongs the activity of amoxicillin**.

NURSING IMPLICATIONS

Administration

- Both 250- and 500-mg tablets contain the exact amount of clavulanic acid (125 mg and potassium salt); therefore, two 250-mg tablets are not equivalent to one 500-mg tablet.
- Drug may be given without regard to meals.
- Oral probenecid administered before or with amoxicillin–clavulanate potassium competitively inhibits tubular secretion of amoxicillin, thereby increasing its concentration and prolonging its effects.
- Reconstitute oral suspension by adding amount of water specified to provide suspension containing 125 mg amoxicillin per 31.25 mg clavulanic acid, or 250 mg amoxicillin per 62.5 mg clavulanic acid per 5 ml. Tap bottle before adding water to loosen powder, then add water in 2 portions, agitating suspension well before each addition. Discard reconstituted suspension after 10 d.

- Suspension should be agitated well just before administration of each dose.
- Patient compliance may be aided by using the chewable formulation with its lemon-lime flavor.
- A suggested schedule for the dialysis period is a 500 mg tablet (500 mg amoxicillin/125 mg clavulanate potassium) halfway through period and an additional 500 mg tablet at its conclusion.
- Store tablets in tight containers at <24C (71F). Reconstituted oral suspension should be refrigerated at 2–8C (36–46F).

Assessment & Drug Effects

- Before therapy is initiated, determine previous hypersensitivity to penicillins, cephalosporins, and other drugs.
- Before establishing a therapeutic regimen, culture and susceptibility tests are run. Drug may be started pending results.
- Generalized, erythematous, maculopapular rash (ampicillin rash) is not due to hypersensitivity. It is usually mild but can be severe. Report onset of rash to physician.
- An urticarial rash that occurs within a few days after start of amoxicillin is suggestive of a hypersensitivity reaction. Assess for other signs of hypersensitivity (see Appendix G).

Patient & Family Education

- Advise female patient to report onset of symptoms of candidal vaginitis. Therapy may have to be discontinued. Candidal vaginitis symptoms include moderate amount of white, cheesy, nonodorous vaginal discharge; vaginal inflammation and itching; vulvar excoriation, inflammation, burning, itching. Miconazole (topical) and oral nystatin are effective treatment agents.
- Caution patient with diabetes mellitus to use Clinistix or TesTape for monitoring urinary glucose to avoid false readings.

AMPHETAMINE SULFATE

(am-fet′a-meen)

Trade name: Racemic Amphetamine Sulfate, Adderall

Prototype for Classifications: CNS AGENT; RESPIRATORY AND CEREBRAL STIMULANT; AMPHETAMINE; ANOREXIANT

Pregnancy category: C

Controlled substance: Schedule II

ACTIONS/PHARMACODYNAMICS

Indirect-acting synthetic sympathomimetic amine with peripheral alpha- and beta-adrenergic activity. Marked stimulant effect on CNS thought to be due to action on cerebral cortex and possibly the reticular activating system. Acts indirectly on adrenergic receptors by increasing synaptic release of norepinephrine and dopamine in brain and by blocking reuptake at presynaptic membranes. CNS stimulation results in increased motor activity, diminished sense of fatigue, alertness, wakefulness, and mood elevation. In hyperkinetic children, it exerts a paradoxic sedative effect by unclear mechanism. Anorexigenic effect thought to result from direct inhibition of lateral hypothalamic appetite center, as well as mood elevation.

USES Narcolepsy, attention deficit disorder in children (hyperkinetic behavioral syndrome, minimal brain dysfunction). Use as short-term adjunct to control exogenous obesity not generally recommended because of its potential for abuse. **Unlabeled use:** in combination with other drugs for treatment-resistant depression.

ROUTE & DOSAGE

Narcolepsy

Adult: **PO** 5–60 mg/d divided q4–6h in 2–3 doses.
Child: **PO** >12 y, 10 mg/d; may increase by 10 mg at weekly intervals; 6–12 y, 5 mg/d; may increase by 5 mg at weekly intervals.

Attention Deficit Disorder

Child: **PO** 6 y, 5 mg 1–2 times/d; may increase by 5 mg at weekly intervals (max 40 mg/d); 3–5 y, 2.5 mg 1–2 times/d; may increase by 2.5 mg at weekly intervals.

Obesity

Adult: **PO** 5–10 mg 1 h before meals.

PHARMACOKINETICS **Absorption:** rapid. **Peak effect:** 1–5 h. **Duration:** up to 10 h. **Distribution:** all tissues, especially CNS. **Metabolism:** metabolized in liver. **Elimination:** half-life: 10–30 h; renal elimination; excreted in breast milk.

CONTRAINDICATIONS & PRECAUTIONS **Contraindicated in:** hypersensitivity to sympathomimetic amines; history of drug abuse; severe agitation; hyperthyroidism; diabetes mellitus; moderate to severe hypertension, advanced arteriosclerosis, angina pectoris or other cardiovascular disorders; Gilles de la Tourette disorder; glaucoma; during or within 14 d after treatment with MAOIs. Safe use during pregnancy (category C) and in nursing mothers not established. **Cautious use in:** mild hypertension.

ADVERSE/SIDE EFFECTS **Allergy:** urticaria. **CNS:** *irritability,* psychosis, *restlessness,* nervousness, headache, *insomnia,* weakness, *euphoria,* dysphoria, drowsiness, trembling hyperactive reflexes. **CV:** *palpitation,* elevated BP; *tachycardia,* vasculitis. Endocrine (with high doses): impotence, change in libido. **GI:** dry mouth, anorexia, unusual weight loss, nausea, vomiting, diarrhea, or constipation.

DIAGNOSTIC TEST INTERFERENCE Elevations in ***serum thyroxine*** (T_4) levels with high amphetamine doses.

DRUG INTERACTIONS **Acetazolamide, sodium bicarbonate** decrease amphetamine elimination; **ammonium chloride, ascorbic acid** increase amphetamine elimination; effects of both amphetamine and BARBITURATE may be antagonized if given together; **furazolidone** may increase BP effects of amphetamines, and interaction may persist for several weeks after furazolidone is discontinued; **guanethidine, guanadryl** antagonize antihypertensive effects; because MAO INHIBITORS, **selegiline** can precipitate hypertensive crisis (fatalities reported), do not administer amphetamines during or within 14 d of these drugs; PHENOTHIAZINES may inhibit mood elevating effects of amphetamines; TRICYCLIC ANTIDEPRESSANTS enhance amphetamine effects through increased norepinephrine release; BETA AGONISTS increase cardiovascular adverse effects.

NURSING IMPLICATIONS

Administration

- Give first dose on awakening.
- The last dose should be administered no later than 6 h before patient retires to avoid insomnia.
- As an anorexigenic, drug is administered on an empty stomach 30–60 min before meal.

- Store at 15–30C (59–86F) unless otherwise directed.

Assessment & Drug Effects

- Monitor for and report complaints of insomnia or anorexia. Dosage reduction may be required.
- Tolerance to the mood-elevating effects commonly occurs within a few weeks. When clinical effectiveness appears to be waning, evaluation is indicated, not a dose increase.
- Insulin dose in diabetes may require adjustment. Monitor closely.
- Effect of amphetamines on growth in children is not known. Close monitoring is advised.
- Response to the drug is more variable in children than in adults. Acute toxicity has occurred over a wide range of dosage.

Patient & Family Education

- Keep physician informed of clinical response and persistent or bothersome side effects. Amphetamine exerts a stimulating effect that masks fatigue. After the exhilaration has disappeared, fatigue and depression are usually greater than before, and a longer period of rest is needed.
- Report insomnia or undesired weight loss.
- Drug may impair ability to engage in hazardous activities such as operating an automobile or machinery.
- To relieve mouth dryness: Rinse frequently with clear water, especially after eating; increase fluid intake, if allowed; chew sugarless gum.
- Meticulous oral hygiene is required, as decreased saliva encourages demineralization of tooth surfaces and mucosal erosion. Gentle brushing of tongue surface helps to reduce halitosis. Use of a commercially avilable oral lubricant, such as Moi-Stir or Xero-Lube, can relieve soft tissue problems and reduce the potential of caries.
- Tolerance to the anorexiant effect usually occurs within a few weeks. As effect lessens (appetite increases), dose increase is not indicated.
- Caffeine-containing beverages should be avoided, as caffeine increases amphetamine-like and related amine effects.
- Following prolonged administration of high doses, amphetamine should gradually be withdrawn. Abrupt withdrawal may result in lethargy, profound depression, or other psychotic manifestations that may persist for several weeks.
- Tolerance almost invariably develops to the euphoric and anorexigenic effects of amphetamines. Drug should be discontinued when tolerance develops. Generally, tolerance does not occur when amphetamine is used for attention deficit disorders or narcolepsy.
- Amphetamines have a high abuse potential because of their excitatory and euphoric effects.

AMPHOTERICIN B

(am-foe-ter′i-sin)

Trade name: Fungizone

AMPHOTERICIN B LIPOSOMAL COMPLEX

Trade name: ABELCET, Ambisome

AMPHOTERICIN B CHOLESTERYL SULFATE COMPLEX

Trade name: Amphotec

Classifications: ANTIINFECTIVE; ANTIFUNGAL ANTIBIOTIC

Pregnancy category: B

ACTIONS/PHARMACODYNAMICS
Fungistatic antibiotic produced by *Streptomyces nodosus*. Fungicidal at higher concentrations, depending on sensitivity of fungus. Exerts antifungal action on both resting and growing cells at least in part by selectively binding to sterols in fungus cell membrane. Because it may also bind somewhat to human cytoplasmic sterols, it can have severe adverse effects.

USES Used intravenously for a wide spectrum of potentially fatal systemic fungal (mycotic) infections including aspergillosis, blastomycosis, coccidioidomycosis, cryptococcosis, disseminated candidiasis, histoplasmosis, paracoccidioidomycosis, sporotrichosis, and others. Has been used to potentiate antifungal effects of flucytosine (Ancobon) and to provide anticandidal prophylaxis in certain susceptible patients receiving immunosuppressive therapy. Used topically for cutaneous and mucocutaneous infections caused by *Candida* (monilia). ABELCET: aspergillosis. **Unlabeled uses:** treatment of candiduria, fungal endocarditis, meningitis, septicemia; fungal infections of urinary bladder and urinary tract; amebic meningoencephalitis, and paracoccidioidomycosis.

ROUTE & DOSAGE

All Systemic Indications

Adult: **IV** An IV test dose of 1 mg dissolved in 20 ml of D5W by slow infusion (over 10–30 min) is recommended to lessen the risk of an anaphylactic reaction. *Initial dose:* 250 µg/kg/d IV infused over 4–6 h in a single dose, adjusted daily in increments of 250 µg/kg/d, or faster if tolerated, up to 1.0 mg/kg/d or 1.5 mg/kg/d q.o.d.; a total daily dosage of 1.5 mg/kg should not be exceeded; usual daily dose is about 50 mg/d except in severe infections.
Child: **IV** Test dose: 0.1 mg/kg up to 1 mg; if tolerated, may give 0.4 mg/kg; may increase by 0.25 mg/kg/d to target dose of 0.25–1 mg/kg/d infused over 2–6 h.
The *minimum dilution* of amphotericin B in pediatric patients (≤17 y) is 0.1 mg/ml in D5W administered over 2–6 h.

ABELCET

Adult: **IV** 5 mg/kg/d infused at 2.5 mg/kg/h.
Child: **IV** Same as adult.

Amphotec

Adult: **IV** 3–4 mg/kg/d (max 7.5 mg/kg/d). Infuse a test dose (10 ml of total first dose) over 15–30 min; if no reaction after 30 min, infuse rest of dose at rate of 1 mg/kg/h (min 2 h)
Child: **IV** Same as adult.

Ambisome

Adult: **IV** 3–5 mg/kg/d infused over 1–2 h.

Candiduria (bladder irrigation)

Adult: 5–50 mg/1000 ml sterile water instilled continuously into the bladder via a 3-way closed drainage catheter system at a rate of 1000 ml/24 h.

PHARMACOKINETICS **Peak effect:** 1–2 h after IV infusion. **Duration:** 20 h. **Distribution:** minimal amounts enter CNS, eye, bile, pleural, pericardial, synovial, or amniotic fluids; similar plasma and urine concentrations. **Elimination:** half-life: 24–48 h; excreted renally; can be detected in blood up to 4 wk and in urine for 4–8 wk after discontinuing therapy.

CONTRAINDICATIONS & PRECAUTIONS **Contraindicated in:** hypersensitivity to amphotericin. **Cautious use in:** severe bone marrow depression or renal function impairment. Safe use during pregnancy (category B) and in nursing mothers not established.

ADVERSE/SIDE EFFECTS **CNS:** headache, sedation, muscle pain, arthralgia, weakness, **CV:** hypotension, cardiac arrest. **ENT (ototoxicity):** tinnitus, vertigo, loss of hearing. **GI:** nausea, vomiting, diarrhea, epigastric cramps, anorexia, weight loss. **Hematologic:** anemia, thrombocytopenia. **Metabolic:** *hypokalemia, hypomagnesemia.* **Hypersensitivity:** pruritus, urticaria, skin rashes, fever, dyspnea, anaphylaxis. **Renal:** nephrotoxicity, urine with low specific gravity. **Topical:** dry skin, erythema, pruritus, burning sensation; allergic contact dermatitis, exacerbation of lesions. **Other:** *fever, chills,* pain; arthralgias, thrombophlebitis (IV site), superinfections.

DRUG INTERACTIONS AMINOGLYCOSIDES, **capreomycin, cisplatin, carboplatin, colistin, cyclosporine, mechlorethamine, furosemide, vancomycin** increase the possibility of nephrotoxicity; CORTICOSTEROIDS potentiate hypokalemia; with DIGITALIS GLYCOSIDES, hypokalemia increases the risk of digitalis toxicity.

INCOMPATIBILITIES **Solution/additive:** any **saline**-containing solution (precipitate will form), PARENTERAL NUTRITION SOLUTIONS, **calcium chloride, calcium gluconate, cimetidine, edetate calcium disodium, metaraminol, methyldopa, polymyxin, potassium chloride, ranitidine, verapamil.** **Y-site:** AMINOGLYCOSIDES, PENICILLINS, PHENOTHIAZINES, **clindamycin, co-trimoxazole, diphenhydramine, dopamine, dobutamine, heparin** (flush lines with D5W, not NS), **lidocaine, procaine, tetracycline, fluconazole, vitamins, TPN.** Do not mix ABELCET or Amphotec with any other drugs.

NURSING IMPLICATIONS

Administration

- ABELCET: Shake vial gently to suspend all of drug before withdrawing dose. Inject through 5-μm filter needle into bag of D5W. Shake bag thoroughly before infusing. If infusion takes longer than 2 h, reshake bag to mix. Do not use in-line filter.
- IV preparation: Directions for IV preparation vary according to manufacturer. Refer to specific manufacturer's guidelines.
- IV administration: Directions for IV administration vary according to manufacturer. Refer to specific manufacturer's guidelines for type of in-line filter and rate of administration.
- Check with physician regarding IV flow rate. Rapid infusion can cause cardiovascular collapse. If a reaction occurs, interrupt therapy and report promptly to physician.
- Amphotericin B commonly causes local inflammatory reaction or thrombosis at injection site, particularly if extravasation occurs. Risk of thrombophlebitis associated with IV infusion may be reduced by using scalp vein needle in the most distal vein possible, by alternating veins, by addition of heparin or hydrocortisone (as prescribed) to the infusion, and by alternate day dosage schedule.
- Frequently check IV site for leakage. It is more likely to occur in the

elderly patient because loss of tissue elasticity with aging may promote extravasation around the needle.

- Intensity of adverse reactions may be reduced by reduction of dosage or by administering drug on alternate days. Some physicians prescribe prophylactic use (e.g., 1 h before infusion) of aspirin or acetaminophen, antiemetics, antihistamines, and corticosteroids.
- Check each manufacturer's directions for storage of reconstituted and unopened vials.

Topical Application

- Do not cover with plastic wrap, plastic cloth, rubber, or other occlusive dressings. Ask physician to specify when and how lesions are to be washed.
- Topical treatment should be discontinued promptly if signs of hypersensitivity, irritation, or worsening of lesions occurs.
- Store topical forms in well-closed containers at room temperature, 15–30C (59–86F), unless otherwise directed.

Assessment & Drug Effects

- Prior to systemic therapy, diagnosis is confirmed by positive cultures or histologic studies.
- During initial IV therapy, monitor TPR and BP and observe patient closely for adverse effects. If a test dose (1 mg over 20–30 min) is given, monitor vital signs every 30 min for at least 4 h. Febrile reactions (fever, chills, headache, nausea) occur in 20–90% of patients, usually 1–2 h after beginning infusion, and subside within 4 h after drug is discontinued. The severity of this reaction usually decreases with continued therapy. Keep physician informed.
- The appearance of mild erythema surrounding skin lesions may be an indication to reduce frequency of topical application. Consult with physician.
- Renal and hematologic status should be determined before therapy. During dosage regulation period, CBC, serum electrolytes (especially K, Mg, Na, Ca), and renal function tests (e.g., BUN, serum creatinine, creatinine clearance) including urinalysis are performed 2 or 3 times weekly, then at least weekly during therapy. Liver function tests are also done periodically throughout therapy.
- Adequate hydration and adjustment of daily dose reportedly are possible means of avoiding or minimizing nephrotoxicity. Consult physician for guidelines.
- Monitor I&O and weight. Report immediately oliguria, any change in I&O ratio and pattern, or appearance of urine, e.g., sediment, pink or cloudy urine (hematuria), abnormal renal function tests, unusual weight gain or loss. Generally, renal damage is reversible if drug is discontinued when first signs of renal dysfunction appear.
- If BUN exceeds 40 mg/dl or serum creatinine rises above 3 mg/dl, withhold drug and report to physician. Dosage should be reduced or drug discontinued until renal function improves.
- Hypokalemia occurs commonly and occasionally can be life threatening. Potassium supplementation is usually necessary. Monitor laboratory reports and observe for and report immediately the onset of possible signs of hypokalemia (see Appendix G).
- The drug is potentially ototoxic. Report promptly any evidence of hearing loss or complaints of tinnitus, vertigo, or unsteady gait. Tinnitus may not be a complaint in the

elderly or in the very young. Other signs of ototoxicity (i.e., vertigo or hearing loss) are more reliably reported in these age groups.

Patient & Family Education

- Notify physician if improvement does not occur within 1–2 wk or if lesions appear to worsen.
- Nail infections (onychomycoses) usually require several months or longer.
- Towels and clothing in contact with affected areas should be washed after each treatment.
- Topical cream slightly discolors the skin. Generally, lotion and ointment do not stain skin when rubbed in, but nail lesions may be stained.
- To remove cream or lotion from fabric, wash with soap and water. Ointment can be removed from fabric with a standard cleaning fluid.

AMPICILLIN

(am-pi-sill'in)

Trade names: Amcill, Ampicin, Novo-Ampicillin ♣, Omnipen, Penbritin ♣, Pfizerpen-A, Polycillin, Principen, SK-Ampicillin, Totacillin

AMPICILLIN SODIUM

Trade names: Ampicin ♣, Omnipen-N, Penbritin ♣, Polycillin-N, SK-Ampicillin-N, Totacillin-N

Prototype for Classifications: ANTIINFECTIVE; BETA-LACTAM ANTIBIOTIC; AMINOPENICILLIN

Pregnancy category: B

ACTIONS/PHARMACODYNAMICS

A broad-spectrum semisynthetic aminopenicillin, ampicillin is relatively stable in gastric acid, is highly bactericidal even at low concentrations, but is inactivated by penicillinase (beta-lactamase). Resembles penicillin G in its activity against gram-positive microorganisms such as alpha- and beta-hemolytic streptococci, *Diplococcus pneumoniae*, non-penicillinase-producing staphylococci, and *Listeria*. Major advantage over penicillin G is enhanced action against most strains of enterococci and several gram-negative strains including *Escherichia coli, Neisseria gonorrhoeae, N. meningitidis, Hemophilus influenzae, Proteus mirabilis, Salmonella* (including *typhosa*), and *Shigella*. Inactive against *Mycoplasma*, rickettsiae, fungi, and viruses.

USES Infections of GU, respiratory, and GI tracts and skin and soft tissues; also gonococcal infections, bacterial meningitis, otitis media, sinusitis, and septicemia and for prophylaxis of bacterial endocarditis. Used parenterally only for moderately severe to severe infections.

ROUTE & DOSAGE

Systemic Infections

Adult: **PO** 250–500 mg q6h. **IM/IV** 250 mg–2 g q6h.
Child: **PO** 25–50 mg/kg/d divided q6h. **IM/IV** 25–100 mg/kg/d divided q6h.
Neonates: **IM/IV** ≤7 d, ≤2000 g: 50 mg/kg/d divided q12h; >2000 g: 75 mg/kg/d divided q8h. >7 d, 50–100 mg/kg/d divided q6–12h.

Meningitis

Adult: **IV** 150–200 mg/kg/d divided q4–6h.
Child: **IV** Same as for adult.
Neonates: **IM/IV** ≤7 d, ≤2000 g: 100 mg/kg/d divided q12h; >2000 g: 150 mg/kg/d divided q8h. >7 d, 100–200 mg/kg/d divided q6–12h.

Gonorrhea
Adult: **PO** 3.5 g with 1 g probenecid × 1. **IM/IV** 500 mg q8–12h.

PHARMACOKINETICS Absorption: oral dose is 50% absorbed. **Peak effect:** 5 min IV, 1 h IM, 2 h PO. **Duration:** 6–8 h. **Distribution:** most body tissues; high CNS concentrations only with inflamed meninges; crosses the placenta. **Metabolism:** minimal hepatic metabolism. **Elimination:** half-life: 1–1.8 h; 90% excreted in urine; excreted into breast milk.

CONTRAINDICATIONS & PRECAUTIONS Contraindicated in: hypersensitivity to penicillin derivatives. Safe use during pregnancy (category B) not established. **Cautious use in:** history of severe reactions to cephalosporins, infectious mononucleosis.

ADVERSE/SIDE EFFECTS Similar to those for penicillin G. **CNS (with high doses):** convulsive seizures. **GI:** *diarrhea,* nausea, vomiting, pseudomembranous colitis. **Hypersensitivity:** pruritus, urticaria, eosinophilia, hemolytic anemia, interstitial nephritis, anaphylactoid reaction. **Other:** severe pain (following IM); phlebitis (following IV); *rash;* superinfections.

DIAGNOSTIC TEST INTERFERENCE Elevated ***CPK*** levels may result from local skeletal muscle injury following IM injection. ***Urine glucose:*** high urine drug concentrations can result in false-positive test results with Clinitest or Benedict's (enzymatic glucose oxidase methods, e.g., Clinistix, Diastix, TesTape are not affected). ***SGOT (AST)*** may be elevated (significance not known).

DRUG INTERACTIONS Allopurinol increases incidence of rash. Effectiveness of the AMINOGLYCOSIDES may be impaired in patients with severe end-stage renal disease. **Chloramphenicol, erythromycin**, and **tetracycline** may reduce bactericidal effects of ampicillin; this interaction is primarily significant when low doses of ampicillin are used. Ampicillin may interfere with the contraceptive action of ORAL CONTRACEPTIVES. Female patients should be advised to consider nonhormonal contraception while on antibiotics. **Drug–food:** food may decrease absorption of ampicillin, so it should be taken 1 h before or 2 h after meals.

INCOMPATIBILITIES Solution/additive: any dextrose-containing solution, including parenteral nutrition solutions. **Y-site: clindamycin, erythromycin**, AMINOGLYCOSIDES, **lidocaine, verapamil.**

NURSING IMPLICATIONS

Administration

- Food hampers rate and extent of oral absorption. Maximum absorption is achieved if it is taken with a full glass of water on an empty stomach (at least 1 h before or 2 h after meals).
- IV preparation: Ampicillin may be reconstituted with sterile or bacteriostatic water for injection. Follow manufacturer's directions for amount of diluent to use. Solutions for IM or direct IV should be administered within 1 h after preparation.
- For IV infusion, the reconstituted solution must be added to suitable IV fluid, such as 0.9% NaCl, 5% dextrose, 5% dextrose in 0.45% NaCl, or lactated Ringer's.
- IV administration: Administration of drug by direct IV should be done slowly, over at least 10–15 min. Drug may be further diluted

and given over 15–30 min. Rapid administration can result in seizures.

- IV administration to neonates, infants, and children: Verify correct IV concentration and rate of infusion with physician.
- Contact dermatitis occurs frequently in sensitized individuals. Those who must handle ampicillin repeatedly are advised to wear disposable gloves.
- Capsules and unopened vials are stored between 15 and 30C (59 and 86F) unless otherwise directed. Keep oral preparations tightly covered.

Assessment & Drug Effects

- Before therapy begins, determine previous hypersensitivity reactions to penicillins, cephalosporins, and other allergens.
- Culture and sensitivity tests should be done initially and periodically during therapy. Therapy may be initiated before results are known.
- Note that the sodium content must be taken into consideration in patients on sodium restriction.
- Inspect skin daily and instruct patient to do the same. The appearance of a rash should be carefully evaluated to differentiate an ampicillin rash (nonallergenic) from a hypersensitivity reaction. Report promptly to physician if it appears.
- Ampicillin rash characteristically is dull red, macular or maculopapular, and mildly pruritic. It generally begins on light-exposed or pressure areas such as knees, elbows, palms, and soles and may spread in a symmetric pattern over most of body. The rash usually develops after 5–14 d of treatment, but occasionally appears on first day of therapy or after therapy has stopped. It disappears within 1 wk after discontinuation of drug therapy.
- The incidence of ampicillin rash is higher in patients with infectious mononucleosis or other viral infections, *Salmonella* infections, lymphocytic leukemia, or hyperuricemia or in patients taking allopurinol.
- Baseline and periodic assessments of renal, hepatic, and hematologic functions are advised, particularly during prolonged or high-dose therapy.

Patient & Family Education

- Because ampicillin rash is believed to be nonallergenic, its appearance is not an absolute contraindication to future therapy.
- Advise patient to report diarrhea and not to self-medicate. A detailed report should be given to the physician regarding onset, duration, character of stools, associated symptoms, and patient's temperature and weight to help rule out the possibility of drug-induced, potentially fatal pseudomembranous colitis (see Appendix G).
- Superinfections (see Appendix G) are more likely to occur with broad-spectrum derivatives of penicillin, such as ampicillin. Instruct patient to report the onset of black, hairy tongue; oral lesions (stomatitis, glossitis); rectal or vaginal itching; vaginal discharge; loose, foul-smelling stools; or unusual odor to urine.
- Instruct patient to take medication around the clock, not to miss a dose, and to continue taking medication until it is all gone (usually 10 d) unless otherwise directed by physician or pharmacist.
- If no improvement is noted within a few days after therapy is started, physician should be notified.
- Treatment for most infections is

continued 48–72 h beyond the time that patient becomes asymptomatic or negative cultures are obtained.

Child ≥ 1 y: **IV** 300 mg/kg/d (200 mg/kg ampicillin and 100 mg/kg sulbactam) divided q6h. If child weighs ≥ 40 kg, give adult dose.

AMPICILLIN SODIUM AND SULBACTAM SODIUM

(am-pi-sill'in/sul-bak'tam)

Trade name: Unasyn

Classifications: ANTIINFECTIVE; BETA-LACTAM ANTIBIOTIC; AMINOPENICILLIN

Prototype: Ampicillin

Pregnancy category: B

ACTIONS/PHARMACODYNAMICS Antibiotic agent with broad spectrum of activity resulting from beta-lactamase inhibition. Sulbactam inhibits beta-lactamases most frequently responsible for transferred drug resistance. Because of this action, a wide range of beta-lactamases found in organisms resistant to penicillins and cephalosporins are irreversibily inhibited.

USES Treatment of infections due to susceptible organisms in skin and skin structures (e.g., *Klebsiella pneumoniae, Staphylococcus aureus)* and intraabdominal infections (e.g., *Escherichia coli*) and for gynecologic infections (e.g., *Bacteroides* sp. including *B. fragilis*). Also used for infections caused by ampicillin-susceptible organisms.

ROUTE & DOSAGE

Systemic Infections

Adult: **IM/IV** 1.5 (1 g ampicillin, 0.5 g sulbactam) to 3 g (2 g ampicillin, 1 g sulbactam) q6h (max 4 g sulbactam/d).

PHARMACOKINETICS **Peak:** immediate after IV. **Duration:** 6–8 h. **Distribution:** most body tissues; high CNS concentrations only with inflamed meninges; crosses placenta; appears in breast milk. **Metabolism:** minimal hepatic metabolism. **Elimination:** half-life: 1 h; excreted in urine.

CONTRAINDICATIONS & PRECAUTIONS **Contraindicated in:** hypersensitivity to penicillins; mononucleosis. Safe use during pregnancy (category B), by nursing mothers. **Cautious use in:** hypersensitivity to cephalosporins.

ADVERSE/SIDE EFFECTS **GI:** *diarrhea, nausea,* vomiting, abdominal distension, candidiasis. **Hematologic:** neutropenia, thrombocytopenia. **Hypersensitivity:** rash, itching, <u>anaphylactoid reaction</u>. **Renal:** dysuria. **Other:** fatigue, malaise, headache, chills, seizures, edema. **Local:** pain at injection sites; thrombophlebitis.

DRUG INTERACTIONS **Allopurinol** increases incidence of rash; effectiveness of the AMINOGLYCOSIDES may be impaired in patients with severe endstage renal disease; **chloramphenicol, erythromycin, tetracycline** may reduce bactericidal effects of ampicillin—this interaction is primarily significant when low doses are used; ampicillin may interfere with the contraceptive action of ORAL CONTRACEPTIVES—female patients should be advised to consider nonhormonal contraception while on antibiotics.

INCOMPATIBILITIES **Solution/additive:** incompatible in any dextrose-containing solution, including parenteral nutrition solutions. **Y-site: clindamycin, erythromycin,** AMINOGLYCOSIDES, **lidocaine, verapamil.**

NURSING IMPLICATIONS

Administration

- IM solution: Reconstitute with sterile water for injection. Consult manufacturer's directions. IM injections should be made deeply into a large muscle such as the gluteus maximus. Rotate injection sites.
- IV preparation: Reconstitute each 1.5 g with 4 ml of sterile water for injection to yield solutions of 375 mg/ml (250 mg ampicillin/125 mg sulbactam); then with suitable diluent, immediately add sufficient volume to yield solutions of 3–45 mg/ml (2–30 mg ampicillin/1–11 mg sulbactam/ml).
- IV administration: Administer properly diluted IV solution slowly over at least 10–15 min. Convulsions may be induced by too rapid administration.
- Use only freshly prepared solution; administer within 1 h after preparation.
- Store powder for injection at 15–30C (59–86F) before reconstitution. Storage times and temperatures vary for different concentrations of reconstituted solutions. Consult manufacturer's directions.

Assessment & Drug Effects

- Culture and sensitivity studies should be done before therapy is begun. Therapy may be started before results of susceptibility testing are known.
- Before therapy is begun, inquiry should be made regarding past hypersensitivity reactions to penicillin, cephalosporins, and other allergens.
- Report promptly unexplained bleeding (e.g., epistaxis, purpura, ecchymoses). These may be hypersensitivity phenomena and are usually reversible when drug is withdrawn.
- Monitor patient carefully during the first 30 min after initiation of IV therapy for signs of hypersensitivity and anaphylactoid reaction (see Appendix G).
- Serious anaphylactoid reactions require immediate use of epinephrine, oxygen, IV steroids, and airway management.
- Observe for and report symptoms of superinfections (see Signs & Symptoms, Appendix G). Ampicillin-sulbactam should be withdrawn.
- Monitor renal function: I&O ratio and pattern. Report dysuria, urine retention, and hematuria (adverse effects of ampicillin).

Patient & Family Education

- Instruct patient to immediately report chills, wheezing, pruritus, respiratory distress, or palpitations.

AMRINONE LACTATE

(am′ri-none)

Trade name: Inocor

Classifications: CARDIAC INOTROPIC AGENT; ENZYME INHIBITOR; VASODILATOR

Pregnancy category: C

ACTIONS/PHARMACODYNAMICS

A new chemical class of cardiac inotropic agents with vasodilator activity. Mode of action appears to differ from that of the digitalis glycosides and beta-adrenergic stimulants. In patients with depressed myocardial function, it enhances myocardial contractility, increases cardiac output and stroke volume, and reduces right and left ventricular filling pressure, pulmonary capillary wedge pressure (PCWP), and systemic vascular resistance.

USES Short-term management of CHF in patients not adequately controlled by traditional therapy, such as digitalis, diuretics, and vasodilators, and may be used in conjunction with these agents.

ROUTE & DOSAGE

Congestive Heart Failure

Adult: **IV** 0.75 mg/kg bolus given slowly over 2–3 min; then start infusion at 5–10 μg/kg/min; may repeat bolus in 30 min; should not exceed 10 mg/kg/d.

PHARMACOKINETICS **Onset:** 2–5 min. **Peak:** 10 min. **Duration:** about 2 h. **Distribution:** unknown if it crosses placenta or into breast milk. **Metabolism:** metabolized in liver. **Elimination:** half-life: 3.6–7.5 h; excreted primarily in urine.

CONTRAINDICATIONS & PRECAUTIONS **Contraindicated in:** hypersensitivity to amrinone or to bisulfites; severe aortic or pulmonic valvular disease in lieu of appropriate surgery, acute MI; uncorrected hypokalemia or dehydration. Safe use during pregnancy (category C), in nursing women, and in children not established. **Cautious use in:** compromised renal or hepatic function, hypertrophic subaortic stenosis. Concomitant cardiac glycoside therapy recommended in patients with atrial flutter or fibrillation.

ADVERSE/SIDE EFFECTS **CV:** hypotension, arrhythmias. **Endocrine:** nephrogenic diabetes insipidus. **GI:** nausea, vomiting, anorexia, abdominal cramps, hepatotoxicity. **Hematologic:** asymptomatic thrombocytopenia. **Hypersensitivity:** pericarditis, pleuritis; myositis with interstitial shadows on chest x-ray and elevated sedimentation rate; vasculitis with nodular pulmonary densities, hypoxemia, ascites, jaundice.

DRUG INTERACTION Possibility of excessive hypotension with **disopyramide.**

INCOMPATIBILITIES **Solution/additive:** sodium bicarbonate, dextrose-containing solutions. **Y-site:** furosemide.

NURSING IMPLICATIONS

Administration

- Do not dilute IV amrinone with dextrose solutions. However, manufacturer states that amrinone may be injected into a running dextrose infusion through Y-connector or directly into tubing.
- Amrinone is reportedly compatible with 0.45 and 0.9% NaCl injection. IV amrinone may be diluted by adding 1 ml of NS or 0.45% saline to each 5 mg (1 ml) of medication.
- IV amrinone may be administered undiluted by direct IV in a single dose over 2–3 min. The diluted solution may be infused at a rate of 5 μg/kg/min.
- Natural color of IV amrinone is clear yellow. Discard discolored solutions and those that contain a precipitate.
- All diluted solutions should be used within 24 h. Store at 15–30C (59–86F) unless otherwise directed. Protect ampuls from light.

Assessment & Drug Effects

- During IV administration, monitor BP, heart rate, and respirations and keep physician informed. Rate of administration and duration of therapy are prescribed according to clinical response and adverse effects.
- Consult physician for guidelines. In general, rate of infusion should

be slowed or stopped with excessive drop in BP or arrhythmias.

- Monitor infusion site to prevent extravasation.
- Monitor I&O ratio and pattern and daily weights. Improvement in cardiac output enhances diuresis with consequent danger of hypokalemia and arrhythmias, particularly in digitalized patients. Hypokalemia should be corrected before and during amrinone therapy.
- Principal hemodynamic parameters indicating clinical improvement include: increased cardiac output, decreased PCWP. Central venous pressure may be used to assess hypotension and blood volume (hydration state).
- The following laboratory values should also be closely monitored throughout therapy to detect adverse effects of amrinone: platelet counts, liver enzymes, fluid and electrolyte balances, renal function studies.
- Another measurement used to evaluate patient response is relief of symptoms of CHF.
- Thrombocytopenia may occur during prolonged therapy or with high dosages. Platelet counts should be taken before treatment begins and frequently during therapy. Close monitoring of platelet counts, appropriate dosage reduction or drug discontinuation should prevent symptoms of thrombocytopenia and allow reversibility. If platelet count falls below 150,000/mm^3, report immediately to physician.
- Amrinone IV preparation contains sodium metabisulfite, a reducing agent to which certain susceptible individuals are allergic. Drug should be discontinued immediately if patient manifests clinical symptoms suggestive of hypersensitivity reactions.
- Patient must be closely observed when drug is withdrawn after prolonged therapy because clinical deterioration may occur within hours.

AMYL NITRITE

(am'il)

Classifications: CARDIOVASCULAR AGENT; NITRATE VASODILATOR; ANTIDOTE

Prototype: Nitroglycerin

Pregnancy category: C

ACTIONS/PHARMACODYNAMICS

Short-acting vasodilator and smooth muscle relaxant with actions, contraindications, and adverse reactions similar to those of nitroglycerin. Action in treatment of cyanide poisoning based on ability of amyl nitrite to convert hemoglobin to methemoglobin, which forms a nontoxic complex with cyanide ion.

USES To relieve pain of renal and gallbladder colic. Also used as an adjunct antidote in the immediate treatment of cyanide poisoning. (Because of adverse effects, unpleasant odor, and expense, infrequently used to treat angina pectoris.) **Unlabeled use:** change intensity of heart murmurs.

ROUTE & DOSAGE

Acute Angina

Adult: **Inhalation** 0.18–0.3 ml prn.

Cyanide Poisoning

Adult: **Inhalation** 0.3-ml perle crushed every minute and inhaled for 15–30 s until sodium nitrite infusion is ready.
Child: **Inhalation** Same as for adult.

PHARMACOKINETICS **Absorption:** rapidly absorbed from mucous membranes. **Onset:** 10–30 s. **Duration:** 3–5 min.

CONTRAINDICATIONS & PRECAUTIONS **Contraindicated in:** hypersensitivity to nitrites or nitrates; cerebral hemorrhage, head trauma; hypotension; glaucoma; severe anemia; hyperthyroidism; recent MI; acute alcoholism. Safe use during pregnancy (category C) and in nursing women not established.

ADVERSE/SIDE EFFECTS *Headache,* transient flushing, orthostatic hypotension, dizziness, weakness, syncope, palpitation, respiratory depression, nausea, vomiting, cardiovascular collapse, tachycardia, methemoglobinemia (large doses).

NURSING IMPLICATIONS

Administration

- Amyl nitrite is available in 0.18 ml and 0.3 ml perles (thin, friable glass ampuls enveloped with woven fabric cover). To prepare for administration, wrap ampul in gauze or cloth and crush between fingers.
- Syncope, due to a sudden drop in systolic BP, sometimes follows amyl nitrite inhalation, particularly in the elderly. Patient should be sitting while and immediately after drug is administered.
- Amyl nitrite is volatile and highly flammable. When mixed with air or oxygen, it forms a mixture that can explode if ignited.
- Store at 8–15C (46–59F), unless otherwise directed. Protect from light.

Assessment & Drug Effects

- After administration of drug, note length of time required for pain to subside; monitor vital signs until they are stable. Rapid pulse, which usually lasts for a brief period, is an expected baroreceptor response to the fall in BP produced by the nitrite ion.
- When amyl nitrite is used to change the intensity of heart murmur, those resulting from stenotic valves become louder; those associated with aortic or mitral regurgitation become softer.
- Tolerance may develop with repeated use over prolonged periods.

Patient & Family Education

- Inform patient that drug has a strongly fruity odor.
- Patients taking amyl nitrite for angina pectoris should be advised to consult physician or go to the hospital emergency room immediately if no relief is experienced after 3 doses 5 min apart.

ANAGRELIDE HYDROCHLORIDE

(a-na′gre-lyde)

Trade name: Agrylin

Classifications: BLOOD FORMER; ANTIPLATELET AGENT

Pregnancy category: C

ACTIONS/PHARMACODYNAMICS Anagrelide is associated with significant decreases in platelet counts, which appear to be related to a selective inhibition of platelet production. It inhibits platelet aggregation by affecting several aggregating agents (thrombin and arachidonic acid, ADP, and collagen). Anagrelide is thought to prevent early changes in shape of platelets.

USE Essential thrombocythemia. **Unlabeled use:** polycythemia vera.

ROUTE & DOSAGE

Essential Thrombocythemia

Adult age ≥ 16 y: **PO** start with 0.5 mg q.i.d. or 1 mg b.i.d. × 1 wk. May be increased by 0.5 mg/d qwk until platelet count is <600,000/µl (max 10 mg/d).

Common side effect in *italic,* life-threatening effects underlined: generic names in **bold;** drug class in SMALL CAPS

PHARMACOKINETICS **Absorption:** 70% absorbed from GI tract. Food reduces bioavailability. **Onset:** 7–14 d at appropriate dose. **Duration:** increased platelet counts were observed 4 d after discontinuing drug. **Metabolism:** Extensively metabolized. **Elimination:** half-life: 1.3–1.8 h; primarily excreted in urine as metabolites.

CONTRAINDICATIONS & PRECAUTIONS **Contraindicated in:** pregnancy (category C), nursing mothers, hypotension. **Cautious use in:** cardiovascular disease, renal function impairment, hepatic function impairment. Safety and efficacy in patients < 16 y have not been established.

ADVERSE/SIDE EFFECTS **Body as whole:** *asthenia, pain, edema (general)*, paresthesia, back pain, malaise, fever, chills, photosensitivity. **CNS:** *headache, dizziness,* CVA, syncope, seizures. **CV:** *palpitations,* chest pain, tachycardia, peripheral edema, CHF, MI, cardiomyopathy, heart block, atrial fibrillation, pericarditis, arrhythmia, hemorrhage. **GI:** *diarrhea, abdominal pain, nausea,* flatulence, vomiting, dyspepsia, anorexia, pancreatitis, constipation, GI hemorrhage, and ulceration. **Respiratory:** *dyspnea,* pulmonary infiltrates, pulmonary fibrosis, pulmonary hypertension. **Skin:** rash, urticaria. **Other:** anemia, thrombocytopenia, ecchymoses, lymphedema, dysuria.

NURSING IMPLICATIONS

Administration

- Dosage increments should not exceed 0.5 mg/d in any 1 wk.
- Store at 15–25C (59–77F) in a light-resistant container.

Assessment & Drug Effects

- Therapeutic effectiveness is indicated by reduction of platelets for at least 4 wk to ≤ 600,000/μl or 50% from baseline.
- Lab tests: monitor platelet count q2d for first wk, weekly thereafter until maintenance dose reached; closely monitor Hgb, WBC count, liver function tests, and BUN and creatinine while platelet count is being lowered.
- Monitor cardiovascular status closely assessing especially for S&S of CHF or ischemia.
- Monitor patients with renal insufficiency (creatinine ≥ 2 mg/dl) for S&S of renal toxicity.
- Monitor patients with liver functions > 1.5 times upper limit of normal for S&S of hepatic toxicity.

Patient & Family Education

- Contact physician if palpitations, fluid retention, breathing difficulty, or any other distressful symptoms develop.
- Avoid excessive exposure to sunlight or UV light.

ANASTROZOLE

(a-nas'tro-zole)

Trade name: Armidex

Prototype for classifications: ANTINEOPLASTIC; HORMONES AND SYNTHETIC SUBSTITUTES; AROMATASE INHIBITOR

Pregnancy category: D

ACTIONS/PHARMACODYNAMICS Anastrozole is an aromatase potent and selective nonsteroidal aromatase inhibitor. Aromatase converts estrone to estradiol. Anastrozole lowers estrogen levels in postmenopausal women by inhibiting adrenally generated androstenedione to estrone and estrone to estradiol. The mechanism occurs in peripheral tissues. Anastrozole does not affect cortisol or aldosterone secretion.

USE Advanced breast cancer in postmenopausal women with disease progression following tamoxifen therapy.

ROUTE & DOSAGE

Breast cancer
Adult: **PO** 1 mg once daily.

PHARMACOKINETICS Absorption: rapidly absorbed from GI tract. **Distribution:** 40% protein bound. **Metabolism:** 85% metabolized in liver to inactive metabolites. **Elimination:** half-life: 50 h; 10% excreted unchanged and 60% as metabolites in urine.

CONTRAINDICATIONS & PRECAUTIONS Contraindicated in: pregnancy (category D), children. Safety and efficacy in children not established. **Cautious use in:** nursing mothers, severe hepatic disease.

ADVERSE/SIDE EFFECTS CNS: asthenia, headache, hot flushes, pain, dizziness, depression, paresthesia, malaise, insomnia, confusion, anxiety, nervousness. **CV:** chest pain, hypertension, thrombophlebitis, edema. **GI:** *diarrhea*, nausea, vomiting, constipation, abdominal pain, anorexia, dry mouth, increased liver function tests (ALT, AST, GGT). **Respiratory:** dyspnea, cough, pharyngitis, bronchitis, rhinitis, sinusitis. **Other:** rash, peripheral edema, pelvic pain, flu-like syndrome.

NURSING IMPLICATIONS

Administration
- Best given on an empty stomach either 1 h before or 2 h after meals, as food affects extent of absorption.
- Store at 20–25C (68–77F).

Assessment & Drug Effects
- Periodically monitor liver enzymes, CBC with differential, alkaline phosphatases, total cholesterol, and lipid profile.
- Assess for hypertension, complications of edema, thrombotic events, and signs of liver toxicity.

Patient & Family Education
- Advise regarding common adverse effects and provide information on measures to control those that cause discomfort.
- Instruct to seek medical attention if S&S of thromboembolism or liver toxicity occur.

ANISTREPLASE (APSAC)

(a-ni'strep-lase)
Trade name: Eminase
Classifications: BLOOD FORMERS AND COAGULATORS; THROMBOLYTIC ENZYME
Prototype: Streptokinase
Pregnancy category: C

ACTIONS/PHARMACODYNAMICS
A derivative of plasminogen streptokinase activator complex (APSAC). Activation of anistreplase occurs with deacylation of the drug. The production of plasmin from plasminogen by deacylated anistreplase can take place in the bloodstream or within the thrombus. The latter process is more efficient, but both may contribute to thrombolysis.

USE Management of acute MI in adults by lysis of thrombi obstructing coronary arteries and reduction of infarct size. Initiation of treatment occurs immediately after the onset of acute MI.

ROUTE & DOSAGE

Acute MI
Adult: **IV** 30 U IV push over 2–5 min.

PHARMACOKINETICS Onset: immediate. **Peak:** 45 min after end of injection. **Duration:** 4–6 h. **Metabolism:** metabolized in plasma. **Elimination:** half-life: 105–120 min.

CONTRAINDICATIONS & PRECAUTIONS Contraindicated in: active internal bleeding, history of CVA, recent (within 2 mo) intracranial or intraspinal surgery or trauma, intracranial neoplasms, uncontrolled hypertension; severe allergic reactions to either anistreplase or streptokinase. **Cautious use in:** pregnancy (category C), major surgery within preceding 10 d, cerebral vascular disease, recent GI or GU bleeding, recent trauma, hypertension, age >75 y, hemorrhagic ophthalmic conditions, current use of oral anticoagulants.

ADVERSE/SIDE EFFECTS CV: hemorrhage, *reperfusion arrhythmias, hypotension*. **Hypersensitivity:** anaphylactic and anaphylactoid reactions in <1% of patients.

NURSING IMPLICATIONS

Administration
- The drug should be instituted as soon as possible following the onset of clinical symptoms of acute MI.
- Dilute each dose with 5 ml sterile water for injection. Slowly add diluent, rolling vial to mix; do not shake. Do not further dilute reconstituted solution and discard if it is not used within 30 min.
- Inject over 2–5 min directly into vein or IV line through the most proximal port.
- During administration, only essential handling or moving of the patient should be done.
- Diluted solution may be clear to pale yellow. Do not administer if particulate matter is present.

Assessment & Drug Effects
- Prior to administration, coagulation tests need to be done including APTT, bleeding time, PT, TT.
- Blood for Hct, Hgb, and platelet counts should be drawn before administration for baseline values in case of bleeding.
- Monitor vital signs q15min for first 6 h, including BP, pulse, respirations, and temperature. Watch for bradycardia and allergic reaction.
- Monitor neurological checks q30min for 6 h.
- Spontaneous bleeding occurs twice as often with anistreplase as with heparin. Protect patient from invasive procedures: IM injections are contraindicated. Also prevent manipulation during thrombolytic therapy to prevent bruising.
- Monitor for excess external or internal bleeding q15min for the first hour of therapy, every 30 min for second to eighth hour, then every 8 h.
- Report signs of bleeding: gum bleeding, epistaxis, hematoma, spontaneous ecchymoses, oozing at catheter site, increased pain from internal bleeding. The anistreplase infusion should be interrupted, then resumed when bleeding stops.
- If a blood gas determination is needed, select the radial rather than the femoral artery because a pressure dressing can more easily be applied to it to control oozing. It may be necessary to apply pressure to puncture sites for as long as 30 min.

- Patient is at risk for postthrombolytic bleeding for 2–4 d after intracoronary anistreplase treatment. Continue monitoring vital signs until laboratory reports confirm anticoagulant control.
- Following administration, coagulation tests, coronary angiography, and myocardial scanning should be done to determine effectiveness of treatment.
- Hct should be drawn to detect possible blood loss following administration.

Patient & Family Education

- Incidents of bleeding need to be reported to the nurse or doctor. Report blood in urine and bloody or tarry stools.
- Bed rest is essential during therapy to prevent bleeding.

ANTIHEMOPHILIC FACTOR, HUMAN (FACTOR VIII)

(an-tee-hee-moe-fill′ik)

Trade names: H.T. Factorate, H.T. Factorate Generation II, Hemofil CT, Humate, Koate-HS, Koate HT, Monoclate, Profilate

Classifications: BLOOD FORMER AND COAGULATOR; HEMOSTATIC

Pregnancy category: C

ACTIONS/PHARMACODYNAMICS Stable lyophilized concentrate of human antihemophilic factor (AHF) obtained from large pools of fresh normal human plasma. Commercial factor VIII preparations are now subjected to heat treatment to reduce potential for transmitting HIV and viral hepatitis. Factor VIII is essential in the body for conversion of prothrombin to thrombin by the intrinsic pathway and for maintaining effective hemostasis. Administration of AHF corrects or prevents bleeding episodes by replacing the missing clotting factor and obviates the need of administering large volumes of plasma, thus avoiding risk of hypervolemia and hyperproteinemia. Contains relatively small amounts of fibrinogen and other plasma proteins.

USES Hemophilia A (genetic deficiency of factor VIII) and in patients with acquired circulating factor VIII inhibitors.

ROUTE & DOSAGE

Acute Bleeding Episode

Adult: **IV** 8–30 U/kg q8–12h.
Child: **IV** 20–50 U/kg q12–24h.

Prophylaxis

Adult: **IV** >50 kg: 500 U/d in AM; <50 kg: 250 U/d in AM.
Child: **IV** >50 kg: 500 U/d in AM; <50 kg: 250 U/d in AM.

PHARMACOKINETICS **Distribution:** does not readily cross placenta. **Metabolism:** rapidly cleared from body. **Elimination:** half-life: 12 h (4–24 h).

CONTRAINDICATIONS & PRECAUTIONS **Contraindicated in:** von Willebrand's disease since it is not effective for controlling bleeding. Safe use during pregnancy (category C) not established. **Cautious use in:** hepatic disease, large or frequently repeated doses to patients with blood types A, B, and AB.

ADVERSE/SIDE EFFECTS Generally related to rate of administration. **CNS:** headache, paresthesias, somnolence, lethargy. **CV:** hypotension, tachycardia. **Hypersensitivity:** <u>anaphylactic</u> or febrile reaction; hemolysis. **Other:** dizziness, nausea, vomiting, transient chest discomfort and cough, bronchospasm; disturbed vision; <u>viral hepatitis</u>; <u>AIDS</u>; thrombosis.

NURSING IMPLICATIONS

Administration

- Reconstitute according to manufacturer's directions and with diluent supplied. Before reconstitution, the dried concentrate and diluent should be warmed to room temperature 20–30C (68–86F). Temperature should not exceed 37C (98.6F).
- After the addition of diluent to vial, rotate or agitate gently until concentrate is completely dissolved. Administer within 3 h to avoid microbial contamination. Do not refrigerate or keep at less than room temperature after reconstitution, as precipitation may occur.
- Physician will prescribe IV flow rate. Preparations containing 34 or more AHF U/ml should be administered at a carefully controlled rate, not exceeding 2 ml/min. Preparations containing less than 34 AHF U/ml are administered at rate of 10–20 ml over 3 min, as prescribed.
- Cryoprecipitated factor VIII must be kept frozen until ready to use. Then it should be thawed to room temperature by placing it in a warm water bath at no higher than 37C (98.6F). Higher temperatures may destroy factor VIII activity. Bag should be gently agitated to assure dissolution. Once thawed, it should be used within 3 h. It is administered through a filter.
- Store dried concentrate preparations in refrigerator at 2–8C (35–46F) unless otherwise directed. Avoid freezing.

Assessment & Drug Effects

- Observe for vasomotor and hypersensitivity reactions. Take vital signs before and during therapy. If there is a significant increase in pulse rate, IV flow rate should be reduced or administration stopped.
- Some patients manifest an acute, transient allergic reaction (erythema, urticaria, backache, fever) during or after administration of certain preparations. The reaction generally subsides within 20 min. Notify physician.
- Factor VIII activity is determined before therapy and daily during therapy. Normal value is 100% (range 50–200%).
- Tests for factor VIII inhibitor also should be done before initiation of therapy. Patients with inhibitor levels greater than 5–10 Bethesda U/ml may not respond to AHF or may require larger doses.
- Hct and direct Coombs' test should be monitored in patients with blood types A, B, or AB who are receiving large or frequently repeated doses to detect signs of intravascular hemolysis: fever, chills, tachycardia, rapid breathing, backache, hematuria, increased serum bilirubin, LDH, and reticulocytes. (AHF preparations contain small amounts of group A and B isohemagglutinins.) Reaction is life threatening and must be recognized and treated promptly.

Patient & Family Education

- Instruct patient to immediately report any subjective symptoms of a hypersensitivity reaction (see Appendix G).

APOMORPHINE HYDROCHLORIDE

(a-poe-mor′feen)

Classification: EMETIC

Pregnancy category: C

Controlled substance: Schedule II

ACTIONS/PHARMACODYNAMICS Centrally acting emetic prepared by treating morphine with dilute hydrochloric acid; results in marked reduction of analgesic activity but enhanced emetic action. Produces CNS excitation and depression; induces vomiting by direct stimulant action on chemoreceptor trigger zone (CTZ) and possibly by excitation of vestibular centers. Depresses medullary center that controls respiration and vasomotor tone and stimulates salivation. Used in subemetic doses to reduce tremor and rigidity in parkinsonism as well as levodopa-induced tremor, choreiform movements, and dyskinesia, and in alcoholism to reduce anxiety and craving for alcohol. Has sedative and hypnotic action in small nonemetic doses.

USES To produce emesis, particularly in acute oral drug overdosage or after oral ingestion of certain poisons. **Unlabeled uses:** for parkinsonism and in conditioned aversion techniques for alcoholism.

ROUTE & DOSAGE

Emesis
Adult: **SC** 2–10 mg as a single dose (average 5–6 mg).
Child: **SC** 0.07–0.1 mg/kg as a single dose.

PHARMACOKINETICS **Onset:** 10–15 min in adults; 1–2 min in children. **Duration:** sedative effects may last 2 h. **Metabolism:** metabolized in liver. **Elimination:** excreted in urine.

CONTRAINDICATIONS & PRECAUTIONS **Contraindicated in:** hypersensitivity to morphine and related opiates; after ingestion of caustics or corrosives (e.g., lye, acids) or volatile oils. Use for petroleum distillates or liquid hydrocarbons (gasoline, kerosene, and the like) depends on amount ingested and relative toxicity of substance. **Other contraindications:** strychnine poisoning, unconsciousness, during seizures; absent gag reflex, severely inebriated patients, shock; narcosis due to alcohol, barbiturates, opiates, and other CNS or respiratory depressants. Safe use during pregnancy (category C) and in nursing mothers not established. **Cautious use in:** children, elderly, and debilitated patients; impaired cardiac function; epilepsy; predisposition to nausea and vomiting; acute overdosage of digitalis glycosides (may potentiate heart block) or convulsant drugs (may precipitate convulsions).

ADVERSE/SIDE EFFECTS Nausea, weakness, drowsiness, orthostatic hypotension, syncope; CNS stimulation (restlessness, tremors, tachycardia). **With large doses:** violent and persistent vomiting, retching; <u>CNS depression</u> (<u>depressed respirations, coma</u>, bradycardia, <u>acute circulatory failure</u>).

NURSING IMPLICATIONS

Administration

- For the adult patient, administration of 200–300 ml of water or preferably evaporated milk immediately before injection induces more efficient emesis. Smaller amounts of liquid are recommended for the small child.
- Emesis may be enhanced by gently bouncing the child. Emetic effect is reportedly potentiated by motion and reduced by recumbency.
- Position patient on side to prevent aspiration of vomitus.
- If apomorphine fails to induce vomiting, dose is not repeated because it is not likely to work and

would increase the risk of CNS or respiratory depression.

- If patient has ingested an absorbable poison, activated charcoal may be given immediately after apomorphine-induced vomiting is completed. If delay in giving the emetic is anticipated, activated charcoal is administered before the injection to reduce absorption of poisons in stomach.
- Apomorphine deteriorates with age and on exposure to light and air. Solutions that are green or brown or otherwise discolored or that contain a precipitate should not be used. Note expiration date of prepared solutions of apomorphine.
- Solution is stable for 48 h when protected from light and air and stored in refrigerator at 2–8C (36–46F). Solution should be labeled and dated.
- Store tablets in tight, light-resistant container, preferably at 15–30C (59–86F), unless otherwise directed.

Assessment & Drug Effects

- Vomiting occurs in about 5 min and may be preceded by salivation and nausea. Save all emesis unless otherwise directed by physician. When vomiting ceases, patient usually falls into a profound sleep. Sedative effects persist for about 2 h. Side rails are indicated. Caution patient not to get out of bed without assistance.
- Monitor vital signs closely for at least 2 h after drug administration. As apomorphine may not evacuate all of the toxic substance ingested, patient should be observed closely for signs of poisoning after vomiting is complete.
- Have on hand equipment for gastric lavage, suction, seizure precautions, and respiratory assistance; naloxone (opiate antagonist) to combat respiratory depression and sedation, and atropine (for treatment of cardiac depression).

APRACLONIDINE

(a-pra-clo′ni-deen)

Trade name: Iopidine

Classifications: EYE PREPARATION; MIOTIC (ANTIGLAUCOMA AGENT)

Prototype: Pilocarpine

Pregnancy category: C

See Appendix A.

APROBARBITAL

(a-pro-bar′bi-tol)

Trade name: Alurate

Classifications: CNS AGENT; BARBITURATE ANXIOLYTIC, SEDATIVE-HYPNOTIC

Prototype: Secobarbital

Pregnancy category: D

ACTIONS/PHARMACODYNAMICS

Intermediate-acting barbiturate. Barbiturates can produce all levels of CNS mood alteration, from excitation to mild sedation, hypnosis, and deep coma. These agents depress the sensory cortex, decrease motor activity, alter cerebellar function, and produce drowsiness, sedation, and hypnosis. Barbiturates have little analgesic action at subanesthetic doses and may increase the reaction to painful stimuli. All barbiturates exhibit anticonvulsant activity in anesthetic doses. Barbiturates are respiratory depressants; the degree of respiratory depression is dose dependent. With hypnotic doses, respiratory depression is similar to that which occurs during physiologic sleep.

USE Indicated for routine sedation and as a hypnotic in the short-term treatment of insomnia for up to 2 wk.

Barbiturates seem to lose their efficacy for sleep induction and maintenance after this period of time.

ROUTE & DOSAGE

Sedative

Adult: **PO** 40 mg t.i.d.

Hypnotic

Adult: **PO** 40–160 mg.

PHARMACOKINETICS Absorption: well absorbed from GI tract. **Onset:** 45–60 min. **Duration:** 3 h. **Distribution:** crosses placenta; distributed into breast milk. **Metabolism:** metabolized in the liver. **Elimination:** half-life: 14–40 h; excreted in urine.

CONTRAINDICATIONS & PRECAUTIONS Contraindicated in: barbiturate hypersensitivity; history of manifest or latent porphyria; impaired liver function; impaired renal function; severe respiratory distress, respiratory disease where dyspnea, obstruction, or cor pulmonale is present; previous addiction to the sedative-hypnotic group; acute or chronic pain; pregnancy (category D), and lactation; children. **Cautious use in:** elderly or debilitated patients, presence of fever, hyperthyroidism, diabetes mellitus, severe anemia, debility, severely impaired liver function, pulmonary or cardiac disease, status asthmaticus, shock, uremia, borderline hypoadrenal function.

ADVERSE/SIDE EFFECTS CNS: *Somnolence,* agitation, confusion, hyperkinesia, ataxia, vertigo, CNS depression, nightmares, lethargy, *residual sedation (hangover effect),* paradoxical excitement, nervousness, psychiatric disturbance, hallucinations, insomnia, anxiety, dizziness, thinking abnormalities, delirium and stupor with excessive amounts. **Respiratory:** hypoventilation, apnea, respiratory depression, laryngospasm, bronchospasm. **CV:** bradycardia, circulatory collapse, hypotension, syncope. **GI:** nausea, vomiting, constipation, diarrhea, epigastric pain. **Hematologic:** agranulocytosis (rare).

DIAGNOSTIC TEST INTERFERENCE BARBITURATES may cause a false-positive ***phentolamine test*** and decrease serum bilirubin concentrations.

DRUG INTERACTIONS CNS DEPRESSANTS, **alcohol,** SEDATIVES compound CNS depression; MAO INHIBITORS cause excessive CNS depression; ANTICONVULSANTS, **rifampin, phenmetrazine** may decrease effects of aprobarbital.

NURSING IMPLICATIONS

Administration

- In patients with impaired renal or hepatic function, lower doses should be used initially.
- Patients on dialysis may require an increase in dosage.
- Prolonged administration is not recommended because drug has not been shown to be effective for a period of more than 2 wk.
- Store away from heat and direct light in airtight container at 15–30C (59–86F).

Assessment & Drug Effects

- Monitor for severe drowsiness, severe confusion, severe weakness, shortness of breath, slow or troubled breathing, slurred speech, staggering, and bradycardia.
- Monitor hematologic studies for blood dyscrasia.
- Monitor liver function studies with continuous or prolonged use.
- Monitor elderly patients for paradoxical response (i.e., irritability,

marked excitement, depression, and confusion).

- Monitor phenytoin and barbiturate blood levels frequently if these drugs are given concurrently, as the effect of barbiturates on metabolism is unpredictable.

Patient & Family Education

- Do not increase the dose of the drug without consulting a physician.
- Do not drive, operate machinery, or perform other tasks until response to drug is known.
- Avoid use of alcohol or other CNS depressants.
- Notify physician if any of the following occur: fever, sore throat, mouth sores, easy bruising or bleeding, nosebleed, or petechiae.
- Make regular visits to physician to check progress during prolonged use.
- Do not discontinue use of medication abruptly, as physician may want to gradually decrease dosage to avoid possibility of withdrawal symptoms.
- Check with physician for suspected psychological or physical dependence.
- Get emergency help at once for suspected overdose.
- Increase vitamin D-fortified foods (e.g., milk products), as drug increases vitamin D metabolism, leading to subtherapeutic levels and possible onset of osteomalacia or rickets.

APROTININ

(a-pro-ti′-nin)

Trade name: Trasylol

Classifications: BLOOD FORMER AND COAGULATOR; HEMOSTATIC

Prototype: Aminocaproic acid

Pregnancy category: B

ACTIONS/PHARMACODYNAMICS Polypeptide of bovine origin that inhibits protease. By interaction with certain proteases, aprotinin has antifibrinolytic effect, hemostatic stabilizing effect, and weak anticoagulant effect. Aprotinin reduces postoperative bleeding in coronary bypass surgery patients by inhibiting fibrinolytic activity while preserving platelet adhesive function and prolonging postoperative bleeding time.

USES Prophylactically to reduce perioperative blood loss and need for blood transfusions during cardiopulmonary bypass in the course of repeat coronary artery bypass surgery. May also be used in selected cases of primary coronary artery bypass graft surgery where the risk of bleeding is especially high (i.e., impaired hemostasis, coagulopathy).

ROUTE & DOSAGE

Cardiac Surgery

Adult: **IV** 1-ml (10,000 kallikrein inactivator units [KIU]) test dose given at least 10 min prior to loading dose (observe for signs of an allergic reaction). Give a loading dose of 2 million KIU over 20–30 min after induction of anesthesia but prior to sternotomy. An additional 2 million KIU dose is added to the priming fluid of the cardiopulmonary priming pump. Then start a constant infusion of 500,000 KIU/h. Continue until the patient leaves the OR.

PHARMACOKINETICS **Distribution:** rapidly distributes into the extracellular fluid, then accumulates in proximal renal tubular epithelial cells;

crosses placenta; distributed into breast milk. **Metabolism:** metabolized primarily in kidneys to small peptides or amino acids. **Elimination:** half-life: initial 0.7 h, terminal 7 h; excreted by kidneys.

CONTRAINDICATIONS & PRECAUTIONS **Contraindicated in:** hypersensitivity to aprotinin and bovine products. **Cautious use in:** patients with heparinized blood, patients previously treated with aprotinin, pregnancy (category B). Safety and efficacy in children not established.

ADVERSE/SIDE EFFECTS **CV:** tachycardia. **Hematologic:** thromboembolism. **Renal:** nephrotoxicity (elevated serum creatinine). **Skin:** rash, urticaria. **Other:** hypersensitivity reactions (rash, urticaria anaphylaxis), bronchospasm.

DRUG INTERACTIONS **Heparin** results in further prolongation of the whole blood activated clotting time (ACT).

INCOMPATIBILITIES **Solution/additive:** AMINO ACIDS, CORTICOSTEROIDS, fat emulsion, **heparin,** TETRACYCLINES.

NURSING IMPLICATIONS

Administration

- Aprotinin is supplied in concentrations of 10,000 KIU/ml (1.4 mg/ml). *Note:* One KIU is equal to 0.14 μg of aprotinin.
- Administer all IV doses through a central venous catheter used exclusively for aprotinin.
- With patient supine, slowly administer loading dose over 20–30 min.

Assessment & Drug Effects

- Patients with a history of hypersensitivity to any allergens or who have previously received aprotinin are at special risk for hypersensitivity.
- During administration, carefully monitor for signs of hypersensitivity (see Appendix G). If hypersensitivity occurs, immediately discontinue aprotinin and begin emergency treatment to prevent anaphylaxis.
- During infusion, carefully monitor cardiac status and pulmonary function. After surgery, monitor PTT, ACT, and cardiac, pulmonary, renal, and liver functions.

ARDEPARIN SODIUM

(ar-de′-pa-rin)

Trade name: Normiflo

Classifications: BLOOD FORMER AND COAGULATOR; ANTICOAGULANT

Prototype: Heparin

Pregnancy category: C

See Appendix A.

ASCORBIC ACID (VITAMIN C)

Trade names: Apo-C ♣, Ascorbicap, Cebid, Cecon, Cenolate, Cemill, C-Span, Cetane, Cevalin, Cevi-Bid, Ce-Vi-Sol ♣, Cevita, Flavorcee, Redoxon ♣, Schiff Effervescent Vitamin C, Vita-C.

ASCORBATE, SODIUM

(a-skor′bate)

Trade names: Cenolate, Cevita

Classification: VITAMIN

Pregnancy category: C

ACTIONS/PHARMACODYNAMICS Water-soluble vitamin essential for synthesis and maintenance of collagen and intercellular ground substance of body tissue cells, blood vessels, cartilage, bones, teeth, skin, and tendons. Increases protection mechanism of the immune system, thus supporting wound healing.

Necessary for wound healing and resistance to infection. Unlike most mammals, humans are unable to synthesize ascorbic acid in the body; therefore it must be consumed daily.

USES Prophylaxis and treatment of scurvy and as a dietary supplement. **Unlabeled uses:** to acidify urine; to prevent and treat cancer; to treat idiopathic methemoglobinemia; as adjuvant during deferoxamine therapy for iron toxicity; in megadoses will possibly reduce severity and duration of common cold. Widely used as an antioxidant in formulations of parenteral tetracycline and other drugs.

ROUTE & DOSAGE

Therapeutic

Adult: **PO/IM/IV/SC** 150–500 mg in 1–2 doses.
Child: **PO/IM/IV/SC** 100–300 mg/d in divided doses.

Prophylactic

Adult: **PO/IM/IV/SC** 45–60 mg/d.
Child: **PO/IM/IV/SC** 30–60 mg/d.

Urinary Acidifier

Adult: **PO/IM/IV/SC** 4–12 g/d in divided doses.
Child: **PO/IM/IV/SC** 500 mg q6–8 h.

PHARMACOKINETICS Absorption: readily absorbed PO; however, absorption may be limited with large doses. **Distribution:** widely distributed to body tissues; crosses placenta; distributed into breast milk. **Metabolism:** metabolized in liver. **Elimination:** rapidly excreted from body in urine when plasma level exceeds renal threshold of 1.4 mg/dl.

CONTRAINDICATIONS & PRECAUTIONS Contraindicated in: use of sodium ascorbate in patients on sodium restriction; use of calcium ascorbate in patients receiving digitalis. Safe use during pregnancy (category C) and in nursing mothers not established. **Cautious use in:** excessive doses in patients with G6PD deficiency; hemochromatosis, thalassemia, sideroblastic anemia, sickle cell anemia; patients prone to gout or renal calculi.

ADVERSE/SIDE EFFECTS Acute hemolytic anemia (patients with deficiency of G6PD); sickle cell crisis. **With high doses:** nausea, vomiting, heartburn, diarrhea, abdominal cramps, headache; insomnia, urethritis, dysuria, crystalluria, hyperoxaluria, hyperuricemia. **Parenteral:** mild soreness at injection site; dizziness and temporary faintness with rapid IV administration.

DIAGNOSTIC TEST INTERFERENCE High doses of absorbic acid can produce false-negative results for ***urine glucose*** with ***glucose oxidase methods*** (e.g., Clinitest, TesTape, Diastix); false-positive results with ***copper reduction methods*** (e.g., Benedict's solution, Clinitest); and false increases in ***serum uric acid*** determinations (by ***enzymatic methods***). Interferes with ***urinary steroid*** (17-OHCS) determinations (by ***modified Reddy, Jenkins, Thorn procedure***), decreases in ***serum bilirubin,*** and may cause increases in ***serum cholesterol, creatinine,*** and ***uric acid*** (methodologic inferences). May produce false-negative tests for ***occult blood*** in stools if taken with 48–72 h of test.

DRUG INTERACTIONS Large doses may attenuate hypoprothombinemic effects of ORAL ANTICOAGULANTS; SALICYLATES may inhibit ascorbic acid uptake by leukocytes and tissues, and ascorbic acid may decrease elimination of salicylates; chronic high doses of ascorbic acid may diminish the effects of **disulfiram.**

INCOMPATIBILITIES Solution/additive: aminophylline, bleomycin, cephapirin, erythromycin, nafcillin, sodium bicarbonate, warfarin. Y-site: cefazolin, doxapram, sodium bicarbonate.

NURSING IMPLICATIONS

Administration

- Oral solutions may be mixed with food.
- Effervescent tablet form should be dissolved in a glass of water immediately before ingestion.
- Open ampuls with caution. After prolonged storage, decomposition may occur with release of carbon dioxide and resulting increase in pressure within ampul.
- Ascorbic acid injection may gradually darken on exposure to light. Slight coloration reportedly does not affect its therapeutic action.
- Parenteral vitamin C is incompatible with many drugs. Consult pharmacist for compatibility information.
- IV ascorbic acid may be given undiluted at a rate of 100 mg or a fraction thereof over 1 min.
- IV ascorbic acid may be diluted in IV solutions and given as a continuous infusion.
- IV administration to children: Verify correct IV concentration and rate of infusion with physician.
- Store in airtight, light-resistant, nonmetallic containers, away from heat and sunlight, preferably at 15–30C (59–86F), unless otherwise specified by manufacturer.

Patient & Family Education

- High doses of vitamin C are not recommended during pregnancy. It has been suggested that the fetus may adapt to high levels of the vitamin by developing the capacity to inactivate it, leading to rebound scurvy in the offspring when vitamin C intake is reduced to normal.
- The nonprescription use of megadoses (more than 10 times the RDA) is not warranted and can be toxic for some individuals.
- Large doses of vitamin C should be prescribed in divided amounts because the body uses only what is needed at a particular time and excretes the rest in urine.
- Megadoses can increase pH of the small intestine, leading to interference with absorption of vitamin B_{12}. Rebound scurvy has been reported when treatment with high doses is abruptly stopped.
- Reportedly, patients taking oral contraceptives also require vitamin C supplements.
- Smokers appear to have increased requirements for ascorbic acid because the vitamin is oxidized and excreted more rapidly than in nonsmokers. Advise patient with vitamin C deficiency to modify or stop smoking. Replacement dosages will be higher for the smoker.
- Review the importance of foods as primary sources of vitamin C.
- Vitamin C is rapidly oxidized when exposed to air (deterioration is accelerated by light and heat). Slight darkening of tablets may occur without loss of potency.
- Vitamin C increases the absorption of iron when taken at the same time as iron-rich foods.

ASPARAGINASE

(a-spar′a-gi-nase)

Trade names: Colaspase, Elspar, Kidrolase♣, L-asparaginase

Classification: ANTINEOPLASTIC ENZYME
Pregnancy category: C

ACTIONS/PHARMACODYNAMICS A highly toxic drug with a low therapeutic index. Catalyzes hydrolysis of asparagine to aspartic acid and ammonia, thus depleting extracellular supply of an amino acid essential to synthesis of DNA and other nucleoproteins. Reduced availability of asparagine causes death of tumor cells, since unlike normal cells, tumor cells are unable to synthesize their own supply. Resistance to cytotoxic action develops rapidly; therefore asparaginase is not effective in treatment of solid tumors and is not recommended for maintenance therapy.

USES Primarily in combination regimens with other antineoplastic agents to treat acute lymphocytic leukemia (ALL). **Unlabeled uses:** other leukemias, lymphosarcoma, and (intraarterially) treatment of hypoglycemia due to pancreatic islet cell tumor.

ROUTE & DOSAGE

Induction Agent
Adult: **IV** 200 IU/kg/d for 28 d; inject over at least 30 min into running IV.
Child: **IV** Same as for adult.

PHARMACOKINETICS Distribution: distributed primarily into intravascular space (80%) and lymph; low levels in CSF, pleural and peritoneal fluids. **Metabolism:** unknown. **Elimination:** half-life: 8–30 h; small amounts found in urine.

CONTRAINDICATIONS & PRECAUTIONS Contraindicated in: history of or existing pancreatitis; chickenpox (existing or recent illness or exposure), herpetic infection. Safe use during pregnancy (category C) and in nursing mothers not established. **Cautious use in:** liver impairment; diabetes mellitus; infections; history of urate calculi or gout; antineoplastic or radiation therapy.

ADVERSE/SIDE EFFECTS CNS: depression, fatigue, lethargy, drowsiness, confusion, agitation, hallucinations, dizziness, Parkinson-like syndrome with tremor and progressive increase in muscle tone. **GI:** *severe vomiting, nausea,* anorexia, abdominal cramps, diarrhea, acute pancreatitis. **GU:** uric acid nephropathy, azotemia, proteinuria, renal failure. **Hematologic:** *reduced clotting factors* (especially V, VII, VIII, IX), *decreased circulating platelets and fibrinogen,* leukopenia. **Hepatotoxicity:** liver function abnormalities. **Hypersensitivity:** *skin rashes, urticaria,* respiratory distress, <u>anaphylaxis</u>. **Other:** chills, fever, fatal hyperthermia, perspiration, weight loss, hyperglycemia, glycosuria, polyuria, hypoalbuminemia, hypocalcemia, hyperuricemia; flank pain, infections.

DIAGNOSTIC TEST INTERFERENCE Asparaginase may interfere with ***thyroid function*** tests: decreased total ***serum thyroxine*** and increased ***thyroxine-binding globulin index;*** pretreatment values return within 4 wk after drug is discontinued.

DRUG INTERACTIONS Decreased hypoglycemic effects of SULFONYLUREAS, **insulin;** increased potential for toxicity if asparaginase is given concurrently or immediately before CORTICOSTEROIDS, **vincristine; methotrexate's** antitumor effect blocked if asparaginase is given concurrently or immediately before it.

NURSING IMPLICATIONS

Administration

- Because of the possibility of unpredictable allergic reactions, an intradermal skin test is performed before the initial dose and when the drug is readministered after an interval of a week or more.
- Observe test site for at least 1 h for evidence of positive reaction (wheal, erythema). A negative skin test, however, does not preclude possibility of an allergic reaction.
- Administered under constant supervision by clinician experienced in cancer chemotherapy.
- IV preparation: Reconstitute with sterile water for injection for IV administration or with 0.9% NaCl for injection for IV and IM administration. Each 10,000 IU vial is diluted with 5 ml of diluent to yield 2000 IU/ml. Shake vial well to promote dissolution of powder. Avoid vigorous shaking. Ordinary shaking does not inactivate the enzyme or cause foaming of content.
- IV administration: For IV infusion the reconstituted solution should be further diluted with 0.9% NaCl injection or 5% dextrose injection by administration into tubing of an already free flowing infusion of one of these solutions; administer over a period of not less than 30 min.
- Gelatinous fiberlike particles can develop in asparaginase solutions on standing. Use of a 5-µm filter will remove particles without affecting potency.
- Unless otherwise directed by manufacturer, store sealed vial of lyophilized powder below 8C (46F). Store reconstituted solutions and solutions diluted for IV infusion at 2–8C (36–46F) for up to 8 h; then discard. Use only clear solutions.

Assessment & Drug Effects

- Have immediately available personnel, drugs (epinephrine, antihistamine, diphenhydramine, IV corticosteroid), oxygen, and equipment for treating allergic reaction (which may range from urticaria to anaphylactic shock) whenever drug is administered, including skin testing.
- During administration, monitor vital signs and be alert to evidence of hypersensitivity or anaphylactoid reaction (see Signs & Symptoms, Appendix G). Anaphylaxis usually occurs within 30–60 min after dose has been given. It is more apt to happen with intermittent administrations, particularly when interval between doses is 7 d or more and when IM route is used.
- When asparaginase is given with or immediately before a course of prednisone and vincristine, toxicity potential is increased. When administered after these drugs, reportedly toxicity appears to be less pronounced.
- Monitor I&O and maintain adequate fluid intake.
- Because asparaginase may interfere with the synthesis of insulin, tests for glycosuria should be done regularly. Report polyuria, polydipsia, or positive urine test to the physician.
- Serum amylase, calcium blood glucose, coagulation factor determinations, ammonia and uric acid levels, hepatic and renal function tests, peripheral blood counts, and bone marrow function are monitored regularly during treatment. Liver function tests are done at least twice weekly during therapy.
- Circulating lymphoblasts decrease markedly in the first several days of treatment, and leukocyte counts may fall below normal. Protection from infection during this period is crucial. Protective isolation may

be indicated. Signs of infection (chill, fever, aches, sore throat) should be reported promptly.

- Report sudden severe abdominal pain with nausea and vomiting, particularly if these symptoms occur after medication is discontinued (possible indicators of pancreatitis).
- Elevations of BUN and serum ammonia are expected findings because of enzymatic action. In most patients, blood ammonia levels are as high as 700–900 μg/dl (normal 80–110 μg/dl). Watch for signs of hyperammonemia: anorexia, vomiting, lethargy, weak pulse, depressed temperature, irritability, asterixis, seizures, coma. Generally, the treatment consists of low-protein diet with ample amounts of simple carbohydrates.
- Because of potential serious hepatic dysfunction the enzymatic detoxification of other drugs may be reduced. Therefore, anticipate the possibility of prolonged or exaggerated effects of concurrently given drugs or their toxicity; report incidence promptly.
- CNS function (general behavior, emotional status, level of consciousness, thought content, motor function) should be evaluated before and during therapy.
- Neurotoxic reaction usually appears within the first few days of therapy. It is manifested by tiredness and changing levels of consciousness (ranging from confusion to coma). Neurotoxic reaction occurs in approximately 25% of patients.

Patient & Family Education

- Inform patient before initiation of treatment of the positive and negative effects of drug therapy. A therapeutic response will most likely be accompanied by some toxicity in all patients; toxicity is reportedly greater in adults than in children.
- Instruct patient to notify physician of continued loss of weight or onset of foot and ankle swelling.
- Nausea, vomiting, or anorexia can interrupt scheduled doses at first, but these symptoms lessen with continued treatment. Instruct patient to try to continue all prescribed medications if at all possible; if not possible, physician should be notified without delay.
- Advise patient to report the onset of unusual bleeding, bruising, petechiae, melena, skin rash or itching, yellowed skin and sclera, joint pain, puffy face, or dyspnea.
- Drowsiness, decreased alertness, and shakiness are symptoms that can accompany treatment with this drug. Driving or operating equipment that requires alertness and skill can be hazardous. Urge caution and inform patient that these effects can continue several weeks after last dose of the drug.
- Reinforce necessity to keep scheduled appointments for evaluation of therapy.

ASPIRIN (ACETYLSALICYLIC ACID)

Trade names: Alka-Seltzer, A.S.A., Aspergum, Astrin♣, Bayer, Bayer Children's, Cosprin, Easprin, Ecotrin, Empirin, Entrophen♣, Halfprin, Measurin, Novasen♣, St Joseph Children's, Supasa♣, Triaphen-10♣, ZORprin

Prototype for classifications: CNS AGENT; ANALGESIC, ANTIPYRETIC; SALICYLATE

Pregnancy category: D

ACTIONS/PHARMACODYNAMICS Major actions appear to be associated primarily with inhibiting the formation of prostaglandins involved in the production of inflammation, pain, and fever. **Antiinflammatory action:** inhibits prostaglandin synthesis. As an antiinflammatory agent, aspirin appears to be involved in enhancing antigen removal and in reducing the spread of inflammation in ground substances. These antiinflammatory actions also contribute to analgesic effects. **Analgesic action:** principally peripheral with limited action in the CNS, possibly on the hypothalamus; results in relief of mild to moderate pain. **Antipyretic action:** in addition to inhibiting prostaglandin synthesis, aspirin lowers body temperature in fever by indirectly causing centrally mediated peripheral vasodilation and sweating. **Antiplatelet action:** aspirin (but not other salicylates) powerfully inhibits platelet aggregation. High serum salicylate concentrations can impair hepatic synthesis of blood coagulation factors VII, IX, and X, possibly by inhibiting action of vitamin K.

USES To relieve pain of low to moderate intensity. Also for various inflammatory conditions, such as acute rheumatic fever, systemic LE, rheumatoid arthritis, osteoarthritis, bursitis, and calcific tendonitis, and to reduce fever in selected febrile conditions. Used to reduce recurrence of TIA due to fibrin platelet emboli and risk of stroke in men; to prevent recurrence of MI; as prophylaxis against MI in men with unstable angina. **Unlabeled uses:** as prophylactic against thromboembolism; to prevent cataract and progression of diabetic retinopathy; and to control symptoms related to gluten sensitivity.

ROUTE & DOSAGE

Analgesic/Antipyretic

Adult: **PO/PR** 350–650 mg q4h; max 4 g/d.
Child: **PO/PR** 10–15 mg/kg in 4–6 h (max 3.6 g/d).

Arthritic Conditions

Adult: **PO** 3.6–5.4 g/d in 4–6 divided doses.
Child: **PO** 80–100 mg/kg/d in 4–6 divided doses; max 130 mg/kg/d.

Thromboembolic Disorders

Adult: **PO** 325–650 mg 1 or 2 times/d.

TIA Prophylaxis

Adult: **PO** 650 mg b.i.d.

MI Prophylaxis

Adult: **PO** 80–325 mg/d.

PHARMACOKINETICS **Absorption:** 80–100% absorbed (depending on formulation), primarily in stomach and upper small intestine. **Peak levels:** 15 min to 2 h. **Distribution:** widely distributed in most body tissues; crosses placenta. **Metabolism:** asprin is hydrolyzed to salicylate in GI mucosa, plasma, and erythrocytes; salicylate is metabolized in liver. **Elimination:** half-life: aspirin 15–20 min; salicylate 2–18 h (dose dependent); 50% of dose is eliminated in the urine in 2–4 h (low doses) or 15–30 h (high doses). Excreted in breast milk.

CONTRAINDICATIONS & PRECAUTIONS **Contraindicated in:** history of hypersensitivity to salicylates including methyl salicylate (oil of wintergreen); sensitivity to other NSAIDS; patients with "aspirin triad" (aspirin sensitivity, nasal polyps, asthma); chronic rhinitis; chronic urticaria;

history of GI ulceration, bleeding, or other problems; hypoprothrombinemia, vitamin K deficiency, hemophilia, or other bleeding disorders; CHF. Do not use aspirin during pregnancy (category D), especially in third trimester, in nursing mothers, and in prematures, neonates, and children under 2 y, except under advice and supervision of physician; do not use in children and teenagers with chickenpox or influenza-like illnesses (because of possible association with Reye's syndrome). **Cautious use in:** otic diseases; gout; children with fever accompanied by dehydration; hyperthyroidism; cardiac disease; renal or hepatic impairment; G6PD deficiency; anemia; preoperatively; Hodgkin's disease.

ADVERSE/SIDE EFFECTS CNS: dizziness, confusion, drowsiness. **ENT:** tinnitus, hearing loss. **GI:** *nausea*, vomiting, diarrhea, anorexia, *heartburn, stomach pains*, ulceration, occult bleeding, GI bleeding. **Hematologic:** thrombocytopenia, hemolytic anemia. **Hypersensitivity:** urticaria, bronchospasm, <u>anaphylactic shock</u>, laryngeal edema. **Skin:** petechiae, easy bruising, rash. **Other:** impaired renal function, prolonged bleeding time, prolonged pregnancy and labor with increased bleeding.

DIAGNOSTIC TEST INTERFERENCE ***Bleeding time*** is prolonged 3–8 d (life of exposed platelets) following a single 325-mg (5 grains) dose of aspirin. Large doses of salicylates equivalent to 5 g or more of aspirin per day may cause prolonged ***prothrombin time*** by decreasing prothrombin production; interference with ***pregnancy tests*** (using mouse or rabbit); decreases in ***serum cholesterol, potassium, PBI,*** T_3 and T_4 ***concentrations,*** and an increase in T_3 ***resin uptake. Serum uric acid*** may increase when plasma salicylate levels are below 10 and decrease when above 15 mg/dl using colorimetric methods. ***Urine 5-HIAA:*** aspirin may interfere with tests using fluorescent methods. ***Urine ketones:*** salicylates interfere with Gerhardt test (reaction with ferric chloride produces a reddish color that persists after boiling). ***Urine glucose:*** moderate to large doses of salicylates equivalent to an aspirin dosage ≥ 2.4 g/d may produce false-negative results with glucose oxidase methods (e.g., Clinistix, Tes-Tape) and false-positive results with copper reduction methods (Benedict's solution, Clinitest). Urinary ***PSP excretion*** may be reduced by salicylates. Salicylates may cause ***urine VMA*** to be falsely elevated (by most tests), or reduced (by Pisano method). Salicylates may interfere with or cause false decreases in plasma theophylline levels using Schack and Waxler method. High plasma salicylate levels may cause abnormalities in ***liver function tests.***

DRUG INTERACTIONS **Aminosalicylic acid** increases risk of salicylate toxicity. **Ammonium chloride** and other ACIDIFYING AGENTS decrease renal elimination and increase risk of salicylate toxicity. ANTICOAGULANTS increase risk of bleeding. ORAL HYPOGLYCEMIC AGENTS increase hypoglycemic activity with aspirin doses >2 g/d. CARBONIC ANHYDRASE INHIBITORS enhance salicylate toxicity. CORTICOSTEROIDS add to ulcerogenic effects. **Methotrexate** toxicity is increased. Low doses of salicylates may antagonize uricosuric effects of **probenecid** and **sulfinpyrazone.**

NURSING IMPLICATIONS

Administration

- Gastric irritation may be minimized by administering with a full glass of water (240 ml), milk, food, or antacid. Enteric-coated tablets dissolve too quickly if administered with milk; also they should not be crushed or chewed.
- Schedule aspirin administration at least 30 min before physical therapy or other planned exercise to keep discomfort at a minimum.
- For treatment of rheumatic diseases, physician may prescribe daily dose increase of 1 or 2 tablets per day on basis of serum salicylate concentrations or until therapeutic response occurs (usually within 3–5 d after beginning regular dosing) or symptoms of toxicity (salicylism) intervene. Symptoms of toxicity are often eliminated after dosage reduction of as little as 325 mg (5 grains or 1 tablet).
- Store preferably between 15 and 30C (59 and 86F) in airtight container and a dry environment unless otherwise directed by manufacturer. Store suppositories in a cool place or refrigerate but do not freeze.

Assessment & Drug Effects

- Serum salicylate concentration associated with analgesia and antipyresis is 30–100 μg/ml. Therapeutic range for rheumatic disease is 250–300 μg/ml; for antiinflammatory action: 150–300 μg/ml; for antiplatelet action: 100 μg/ml. Symptoms of toxicity generally occur with serum salicylate levels over 300 μg/ml.
- Previous nonreaction to salicylates does not guarantee future safety. Some individuals develop an acute and specific intolerance to aspirin, although they may have taken it for years without incident. The reaction is nonimmunologic; symptoms usually occur 15 min to 3 h after ingestion: profuse rhinorrhea, erythema, nausea, vomiting, intestinal cramps, diarrhea.
- Patients with asthma, nasal polyps, perennial vasomotor rhinitis, hay fever, or chronic urticaria demonstrate a high frequency of salicylate hypersensitivity.
- In adults, a sensation of fullness in the ears, tinnitus, and decreased or muffled hearing are the most frequent symptoms associated with chronic salicylate overdosage.
- Potential for toxicity is high in elderly chronic aspirin users because they have less serum protein to bind salicylate and also are less able to excrete it.
- Children tend to manifest salicylate toxicity by hyperventilation, agitation, mental confusion, or other behavioral changes, drowsiness, lethargy, sweating, and constipation.
- In children, and infants particularly, salicylate toxicity is enhanced by the dehydration that frequently accompanies fever or illness. Monitor these patients closely.
- Children on high doses of aspirin are particularly prone to develop hypoglycemia (see Appendix G). Monitor the diabetic child carefully for indicated need of insulin adjustment. See also Diagnostic Test Interferences.
- Because of the possible association of aspirin usage with Reye's syndrome, do not give aspirin to children or teenagers with symptoms of varicella (chickenpox) or influenza-like illnesses before consulting a physician.

Patient & Family Education

- GI disturbances may be reduced

by use of enteric-coated tablets or extended release tablets.

- Buffered aspirin preparations in an effervescent vehicle, e.g., Alka-Seltzer, are more rapidly absorbed than plain aspirin and reportedly cause less GI irritation and bleeding. Alka-Seltzer, however, has a high sodium content (approximately 24 mEq of sodium per 32-mg tablet).
- Buffered aspirin or aspirin administered with an antacid may be better tolerated than conventional tablets.
- When aspirin is prescribed for dysmenorrhea, explain that for best results aspirin should be taken 1 or 2 d before menses (to reduce prostaglandin-induced uterine contractions). Patients having heavy menstrual blood loss should be advised to take another analgesic, such as acetaminophen, instead of aspirin.
- To reduce risk of bleeding, aspirin therapy is usually discontinued about 1 wk before surgery. Patients undergoing oral surgery should be advised not to take aspirin-containing gum or gargles and not to chew aspirin products for at least 1 wk following surgery. Prolonged contact with aspirin can cause hemorrhage and injury to oral tissues.
- Chronic administration of high-dose aspirin during the last 3 mo of pregnancy can prolong pregnancy and labor, increase maternal bleeding before and after delivery, and cause weight increase and hemorrhage in the neonate.
- Discontinue use with onset of ringing or buzzing in the ears, impaired hearing, dizziness, or GI discomfort or bleeding and report to physician. Hearing impairment resulting from salicylate overdosage can generally be reversed within 24 h by reducing the dose.
- In general, adults should not use aspirin for self-medication of pain beyond 5 d without consulting a physician. In adults or children, aspirin should not be used longer than 3 d for fever and never for fever over 39.5C (103F) or 38.9C (102F) if patient is over 60 or for recurrent fever without medical direction. Consult physician before using aspirin for any fever accompanied by rash, severe headache, stiff neck, marked irritability, or confusion (all possible symptoms of meningitis).
- Caution patient on large doses of aspirin to avoid alcohol. See Drug Interactions.
- Prolonged use of high salicylate doses can lead to iron-deficiency anemia, especially in women. Average blood loss with daily use of several aspirin tablets is reportedly 2–6 ml; 10% of patients on chronic high doses may lose as much as 80 ml/d.
- Observe and report signs of bleeding (e.g., petechiae, ecchymoses, bleeding gums, bloody or black stools, cloudy or bloody urine) and symptoms of salicylism.
- Maintain adequate fluid intake (consult physician for guidelines) to prevent salicylate crystalluria.
- Avoid other medications containing aspirin unless directed by physician, because of danger of overdosing. (There are more than 500 OTC aspirin-containing compounds.)
- Most aspirin tablets develop a hard shell with age, a change that lengthens disintegration time, increases risk of GI irritation, and delays onset of therapeutic action. Advise patient not to buy aspirin in large quantities.

- Aspirin tablets rapidly hydrolyze on exposure to heat, moisture, and air. Instruct patient to smell tablet before taking it. If a vinegarlike (acetic acid) odor is detected, discard all tablets.

ASTEMIZOLE

(ah-stem′me-zole)

Trade name: Hismanal

Classification: ANTIHISTAMINE (H_1-RECEPTOR ANTAGONIST)

Prototype: Diphenhydramine

Pregnancy category: C

ACTIONS/PHARMACODYNAMICS A long-acting selective histamine H_1-receptor antagonist. Binds preferentially to peripheral rather than central H_1 receptors. Does not block histamine release, antibody production, or antigen–antibody interactions. Has little or no anticholinergic and sedative effects as compared to diphenhydramine.

USES Indicated for relief of symptoms associated with seasonal allergic rhinitis and chronic idiopathic urticaria.

ROUTE & DOSAGE

Allergic Rhinitis

Adult: **PO** 10 mg once daily; to reduce time to steady-state concentrations may give 30 mg on day 1, 20 mg on day 2, then 10 mg/d thereafter.
Child: **PO** <6 y, 0.2 mg/kg/d once daily; 6–12 y, 5 mg/d.

PHARMACOKINETICS **Absorption:** readily absorbed from GI tract; absorption decreased by food. **Peak:** 1–4 h. **Duration:** up to 24 h. **Distribution:** crosses placenta; distributed into breast milk. **Metabolism:** extensively metabolized in liver (including first-pass metabolism) to an active metabolite. **Elimination:** half-life: 20–24 h, metabolities 12–20 d; 54–73% excreted in feces; 25–50% excreted in urine.

CONTRAINDICATIONS & PRECAUTIONS **Contraindicated in:** hypersensitivity to antihistamines of similar structure, narrow-angle glaucoma, stenosing peptic ulcer, symptomatic prostatic hypertrophy, asthmatic attack, bladder neck obstruction, pyloroduodenal obstruction, children less than age 12, lactation, pregnancy (category C). **Cautious use in:** history of asthma, increased intraocular pressure, renal or hepatic impairment, elderly patients, young children.

ADVERSE/SIDE EFFECTS **CNS:** headache, appetite increase, weight gain, nervousness, dizziness, depression. **GI:** nausea, diarrhea, abdominal pain. **ENT:** pharyngitis, conjunctivitis, epistaxis. **Respiratory:** bronchospasm. **CV:** angioedema, arrhythmias, palpitation. **Skin:** photosensitivity, pruritus, rash, edema.

DRUG INTERACTIONS **Erythromycin, ketoconazole, itraconazole,** other MACROLIDE ANTIBIOTICS, **indinavir, ritonavir, saquinavir,** elfinavir, **fluoxetine, fluvoxamine, sertraline, nefazodone, paroxetine, zileuton** may increase risk of arrhythmias.

NURSING IMPLICATIONS

Administration

- Take at least 2 h after a meal. Have no food for 1 h after taking the drug.
- Do not drink grapefruit juice with astemizole. It is best if taken with water. Grapefruit juice may alter metabolism of astemizole.
- Store in tightly closed containers at

15–30C (59–86F) unless otherwise directed by manufacturer.

Assessment & Drug Effects

- If taken for allergic manifestations, obtain careful history including change from usual pattern of recently ingested foods and drugs and social or emotional stress.

Patient & Family Education

- Avoid use of alcohol or other CNS depressants.
- Observe caution while driving or performing other tasks requiring alertness.
- Inform physician of a history of glaucoma, peptic ulcer, urinary retention, or pregnancy before antihistamine therapy is begun.
- Carry medical information card or jewelry indicating type of allergy, medication, and physician's name, address, and telephone number.
- Advise patient that antihistamines have no therapeutic effect on the common cold.

ATENOLOL

(a-ten′oh-lole)

Trade names: Apo-Atenolol ♣, Tenormin

Classifications: AUTONOMIC NERVOUS SYSTEM AGENT; BETA-ADRENERGIC ANTAGONIST (SYMPATHOLYTIC, BLOCKING AGENT); ANTIHYPERTENSIVE

Prototype: Propranolol

Pregnancy category: C

ACTIONS/PHARMACODYNAMICS

In therapeutic doses, atenolol selectively blocks $beta_1$-adrenergic receptors located chiefly in cardiac muscle. With large doses, preferential effect is lost and inhibition of $beta_2$-adrenergic receptors may lead to increased airway resistance, especially in patients with asthma or COPD. Mechanisms for antihypertensive action include central effect leading to decreased sympathetic outflow to periphery, reduction in renin activity with consequent suppression of the renin-angiotensin-aldosterone system, and competitive inhibition of catecholamine binding at beta-adrenergic receptor sites. Reduces rate and force of cardiac contractions (negative inotropic action); cardiac output is reduced, as well as systolic and diastolic BP. Atenolol increases peripheral vascular resistance both at rest and with exercise.

USES Management of hypertension as a single agent or concomitantly with other antihypertensive agents, especially a diuretic, and in treatment of stable angina pectoris, MI. **Unlabeled uses:** antiarrhythmic, mitral valve prolapse, adjunct in treatment of pheochromocytoma and of thyrotoxicosis; and for vascular headache prophylaxis.

ROUTE & DOSAGE

Hypertension, Angina

Adult: **PO** 25–50 mg/d; may increase to 100 mg/d.
Child: **PO** 0.8–1.5 mg/kg/d (max 2 mg/kg/d).

MI

Adult: **PO** 10 min after second IV dose, start 50 mg/d. **IV** 5 mg q5min × 2 doses; then switch to PO.

PHARMACOKINETICS **Absorption:** 50% of PO dose absorbed. **Peak:** 2–4 h PO; 5 min IV. **Duration:** 24 h. **Distribution:** does not readily cross blood–brain barrier. **Metabolism:** no hepatic metabolism. **Elimination:** half-life: 6–7 h; 40–50% excreted in urine; 50–60% excreted in feces.

CONTRAINDICATIONS & PRECAUTIONS **Contraindicated in:** sinus bradycardia, greater than first-degree heart block, overt cardiac failure, cardiogenic shock. Safe use during pregnancy (category C), in nursing women, and in children not established. **Cautious use in:** hypertensive patients with CHF controlled by digitalis and diuretics, asthma and COPD; diabetes mellitus; impaired renal function; hyperthyroidism.

ADVERSE/SIDE EFFECTS Usually well tolerated. **CNS:** dizziness, vertigo, light-headedness, syncope, fatigue or weakness, lethargy, drowsiness, insomnia, mental changes, depression. **CV:** *bradycardia, hypotension, CHF,* cold extremities, leg pains, dysrhythmias. **GI:** nausea, vomiting, diarrhea. **Respiratory:** pulmonary edema, dyspnea, bronchospasm. **Other:** may mask symptoms of hypoglycemia; decreased sexual ability.

DRUG INTERACTIONS **Atropine** and other ANTICHOLINERGICS may increase atenolol absorption from GI tract; NSAIDS may decrease hypotensive effects; may mask symptoms of a hypoglycemic reaction induced by **insulin,** SULFONYLUREAS; may increase **lidocaine** levels and toxicity; pharmacologic and toxic effects of both atenolol and **verapamil** are increased. **Prazosin, terazocin** may increase severe hypotensive response to first dose of atenolol.

NURSING IMPLICATIONS

Administration

- If necessary, tablet may be crushed before administration and taken with fluid of patient's choice.
- IV atenolol may be given undiluted by direct IV at a rate of one dose per 5 min.
- IV atenolol may be diluted in up to 50 ml of D5W, 0.45% NS, or NS and given as an infusion over 15–30 min.
- Store in tightly closed, light-resistant container at 15–30C (59–86F) unless otherwise directed.

Assessment & Drug Effects

- Check apical pulse before administration of drug, especially in patients receiving digitalis (both drugs slow AV conduction). If below 60 bpm, withhold dose and consult physician.
- Monitor apical pulse, BP, respirations, and peripheral circulation throughout dosage adjustment period. Consult physician for acceptable parameters.

Patient & Family Education

- Advise patients to adhere rigidly to dose regimen. Sudden discontinuation of drug can exacerbate angina and precipitate tachycardia or MI in patients with coronary artery disease, and thyroid storm in patients with hyperthyroidism.
- Caution patients to make position changes slowly and in stages, particularly from recumbent to upright posture.

ATORVASTATIN CALCIUM

(a-tor-va′sta-tin)

Trade name: Lipitor

Classifications: CARDIOVASCULAR AGENT; ANTILIPEMIC AGENT; HMG-COA REDUCTASE INHIBITOR (STATIN)

Prototype: Lovastatin

Pregnancy category: X

ACTIONS/PHARMACODYNAMICS Atorvastatin is an inhibitor of reductase 3-hydroxy-3-methyl-glutaryl coenzyme A (HMG-CoA), which is essential to hepatic production of cholesterol. Lipitor increases the number of hepatic low-density-lipid

(LDL) receptors, thus increasing LDL uptake and catabolism of LDL. Lipitor also reduces LDL and total triglyceride (TG) production as well as increases the plasma level of high-density lipids (HDL).

USES Adjunct to diet for the reduction of LDL cholesterol and triglycerides in patients with primary hypercholesterolemia and mixed dyslipidemia.

ROUTE & DOSAGE

Hypercholesterolemia
Adult: **PO** Start with 10 mg q.d., can titrate up to 80 mg/d.

PHARMACOKINETICS **Absorption:** rapidly absorbed from GI tract. 30% of active component reaches the systemic circulation. **Onset:** cholesterol reduction—2 wk. **Peak:** plasma concentration, 1–2 h; effect 2–4 wk. **Distribution:** ≥98% protein bound. Crosses placenta, distributed into breast milk of animals. **Metabolism:** metabolized in the liver by CYP3A4 to active metabolites. **Elimination:** half-life: 14 h, 20–30 h for active metabolites; excreted primarily in bile. <2% excreted in urine.

CONTRAINDICATIONS & PRECAUTIONS **Contraindicated in:** hypersensitivity to atorvastatin, myopathy, active liver disease, unexplained persistent transaminase elevations, pregnancy (category X), lactation. **Cautious use in:** hypersensitivity to other HMG-CoA reductase inhibitors, history of liver disease, patients who consume substantial quantities of alcohol. Safety and efficacy in children < 9 y have not been established.

ADVERSE/SIDE EFFECTS **Body as whole:** back pain, asthenia, hypersensitivity reaction, myalgia, rhabdomyolysis. **CNS:** headache. **GI:** abdominal pain, constipation, diarrhea, dyspepsia, flatulence, increased liver function tests. **Respiratory:** sinusitis, pharyngitis. **Skin:** rash.

DRUG INTERACTIONS May increase digoxin levels 20%, increases levels of norethindrone and ethinyl estradiol oral contraceptives; erythromycin may increase atorvastatin levels 40%; macrolide antibiotics, cyclosporine, niacin, clofibrate, azole antifungals (ketoconazole, itraconazole) may increase risk of rhabdomyolysis.

NURSING IMPLICATIONS

Administration

- May be given without regard to food.
- Store at 20–25C (68–77F).

Assessment & Drug Effects

- Therapeutic effectiveness is indicated by reduction in the level of LDL-C.
- Lab tests: monitor lipid levels within 2–4 wk after initiation of therapy or upon change in dosage; monitor liver functions at 6 and 12 wk after initiation or elevation of dose, and periodically thereafter.
- Assess for muscle pain, tenderness, or weakness; and, if present, monitor CPK level. Atorvastatin should be discontinued with marked elevations of CPK or if myopathy is suspected.
- With concurrent digoxin use, monitor carefully for digoxin toxicity.

Patient & Family Education

- Promptly report any of the following: unexplained muscle pain, tenderness, or weakness, especially with fever or malaise; yellowing of skin or eyes; stomach pain with nausea, vomiting, or loss of appetite; skin rash or hives.
- Atorvastatin taken during preg-

nancy may cause birth defects. Immediately inform physician of a suspected or known pregnancy.

- Inform the physician regarding concurrent use of any of the following drugs: erythromycin, niacin, antifungals, or birth control pills.
- Alcohol intake should be minimized while taking atorvastatin.

ATOVAQUONE

(a-to′-va-quone)

Trade names: Mepron, Mepron Suspension

Classifications: ANTIINFECTIVE; ANTIPROTOZOAL

Prototype: Metronidazole

Pregnancy category: C

ACTIONS/PHARMACODYNAMICS Atovaquone is an antiprotozoal with antipneumocystic activity, including *Pneumocystis carinii* and the *Plasmodium* species. Mechanism of action against *P. carinii* is unknown. In the *Plasmodium* species, the site of action is linked to inhibition of the electron transport system in the mitochondria. This results in the inhibition of nucleic acid and ATP synthesis.

USE Second-line oral therapy of mild to moderate *P. carinii* pneumonia (PCP) in immunocompromised patients intolerant of cotrimoxazole. **Unlabeled use:** may be effective in the treatment of cerebral toxoplasmosis.

ROUTE & DOSAGE

Mild to Moderate *Pneumocystis carinii* Pneumonia

Adult: **PO** 750 mg (5 ml) suspension b.i.d. for 21 d.

PHARMACOKINETICS Absorption: poorly absorbed from GI tract. Absorption is improved when taken with a fatty meal. **Duration:** 6–23 wk after a 3-wk course of therapy. **Distribution:** penetrates poorly into cerebrospinal fluid; >99.9% protein bound. **Metabolism:** not metabolized. **Elimination:** half-life: 2–3 d; >94% excreted in feces over 21 d (enterohepatically cycled).

CONTRAINDICATIONS & PRECAUTIONS Contraindicated in: history of potential life-threatening allergies to atovaquone. **Cautious use in:** severe PCP, concurrent pulmonary diseases, elderly patients, pregnancy (category C), and nursing women. Safe use in children not established.

ADVERSE/SIDE EFFECTS CV: hypotension. **CNS:** *headache, insomnia, dizziness.* **Hematologic:** anemia, neutropenia. **Metabolic:** *fever,* hyponatremia, hypoglycemia. **GI:** *nausea, diarrhea, vomiting,* abdominal pain, anorexia, dyspepsia, oral candidiasis. **Other:** cough, sinusitis, *rash,* pruritus, erythema multiforme.

DRUG INTERACTIONS Oral absorption is increased 3- to 4-fold when administered with food, especially with fatty foods. **Zidovudine** may increase risk of bone marrow toxicity.

DIAGNOSTIC TEST INTERFERENCE May cause increase in **amylase** and other **liver function tests.**

NURSING IMPLICATIONS

Administration

- Administer with meals, because food significantly enhances the absorption of the atovaquone.
- Store at room temperature 15– 30C (59–86F) unless otherwise directed by the manufacturer.

Assessment & Drug Effects

- Because atovaquone is highly protein bound (99.9%), it may compete with other protein-bound drugs for plasma-binding sites. Therefore, assess for toxicity of either drug when used concurrently with another highly plasma-protein-bound drug.

- Assess for therapeutic failure in patients with GI disorders that may limit absorption of atovaquone.
- Monitor creatinine, BUN, and serum amylase periodically. Report abnormal elevations in these values, because the drug may need to be discontinued.

Patient & Family Education

- Because atovaquone has a long half-life, stress the necessity of taking the drug exactly as prescribed.
- Be certain patient understands that the drug must be taken with meals.

ATRACURIUM BESYLATE

(a-tra-kyoor'ee-um)

Trade name: Tracrium

Classifications: AUTONOMIC NERVOUS SYSTEM AGENT; SKELETAL MUSCLE RELAXANT, NONDEPOLARIZING; NEUROMUSCULAR BLOCKER

Prototype: Tubocurarine

Pregnancy category: C

ACTIONS/PHARMACODYNAMICS Synthetic skeletal muscle relaxant pharmacologically similar to tubocurarine that produces shorter duration of neuromuscular blockade, exhibits minimal direct effects on cardiovascular system, and has less histamine-releasing action. Has minimal cumulative tendency with subsequent doses if recovery from the drug begins before dose is repeated. Inhibits neuromuscular transmission by binding competitively with acetylcholine to muscle end plate receptors. Lacks analgesic action and has no apparent effect on pain threshold, consciousness, or cerebration. Given in general anesthesia only after unconsciousness has been induced by other drugs.

USES Adjunct for general anesthesia to produce skeletal muscle relaxation during surgery; to facilitate endotracheal intubation. Especially useful for patients with severe renal or hepatic disease, limited cardiac reserve, and in patients with low or atypical pseudocholinesterase levels.

ROUTE & DOSAGE

Skeletal Muscle Relaxation

Adult: **IV** 0.4–0.5 mg/kg initial dose; then 0.08–0.1 mg/kg 20–45 min after the first dose if necessary; reduce doses if used with general anesthetics.
Child: **IV** *1 mo–2 y:* 0.3–0.4 mg/kg; *≥2 y:* same as for adult.

Mechanical Ventilation

Adult: **IV** 5–9 μg/kg/min by continuous infusion.

PHARMACOKINETICS Onset: 2 min. **Peak:** 3–5 min. **Duration:** 60–70 min. **Distribution:** well distributed to tissues and extracellular fluids; crosses placenta; distribution into breast milk unknown. **Metabolism:** rapid nonenzymatic degradation in bloodstream. **Elimination:** half-life: 20 min; 70–90% excreted in urine in 5–7 h.

CONTRAINDICATIONS & PRECAUTIONS Contraindicated in: myasthenia gravis; safe use during pregnancy (category C), lactation, in children <2 y not established. **Cautious use in:** when appreciable histamine release would be hazardous (as in asthma or anaphylactoid reactions, significant cardiovascular disease), neuromuscular disease (e.g., Eaton-Lambert syndrome), carcinomatosis, electrolyte or acid–base imbalances, dehydration, impaired pulmonary function.

ADVERSE/SIDE EFFECTS **CV:** bradycardia, tachycardia. **Respiratory:** respiratory depression. **Other:** increased salivation, anaphylaxis.

DRUG INTERACTIONS GENERAL ANESTHETICS increase magnitude and duration of neuromuscular blocking action; AMINOGLYCOSIDES, **bacitracin, polymyxin B, clindamycin, lidocaine, parenteral magnesium, quinidine, quinine, trimethaphan, verapamil** increase neuromuscular blockade; DIURETICS may increase or decrease neuromuscular blockade; **lithium** prolongs duration of neuromuscular blockade; NARCOTIC ANALGESICS present possibility of additive respiratory depression; **succinylcholine** increases onset and depth of neuromuscular blockade; **phenytoin** may cause resistance to or reversal of neuromuscular blockade.

NURSING IMPLICATIONS

Administration

- Initial IV bolus dose may be given undiluted over 30–60 s.
- Maintenance dose is further diluted with NS or D5W and is given as a continuous infusion.
- IV administration to infants, children: Verify correct IV concentration and rate of infusion/injection with physician.
- Atracurium is incompatible with alkaline solutions (e.g., barbiturates). Do not mix in same syringe or administer through same needle as used for alkaline solutions. Reportedly compatible with 5% dextrose and 0.9% NaCl.
- To preserve potency, store at 2–8C (36–46F) unless otherwise directed. Avoid freezing.

Assessment & Drug Effects

- Baseline determinations of serum electrolytes, acid–base balance, and renal function are generally done as part of preanesthetic assessment.
- Personnel and equipment required for endotracheal intubation, administration of oxygen under positive pressure, artificial respiration, and assisted or controlled ventilation should be immediately available.
- Use of peripheral nerve stimulator by qualified individual is recommended to evaluate degree of neuromuscular blockade and muscle paralysis and thus avoid risk of overdosage. Nerve stimulator is also used to identify residual paralysis during recovery period. It is especially indicated when cautious use of atracurium is specified.
- Monitor BP, pulse, and respirations and evaluate patient's recovery from neuromuscular blocking (curare-like) effect as evidenced by ability to breathe naturally or to take deep breaths and cough, keep eyes open, lift head keeping mouth closed, adequacy of handgrip strength. Notify physician if recovery is delayed.
- Patient may find oral communication difficult until head and neck muscles recover from blockade effects.
- Recovery from neuromuscular blockade usually begins 35–45 min after drug administration and is almost complete in about 1 h. Note that recovery time may be delayed in patients with cardiovascular disease, edematous states, and in the elderly.

ATROPINE SULFATE

(a'troe-peen)

Trade names: Atropair ♣, Atropisol, Isopto Atropine

Prototype for Classifications: AUTONOMIC NERVOUS SYSTEM AGENT; ANTICHOLINERGIC (PARASYMPATHOLYTIC); ANTIMUSCARINIC
Pregnancy category: C

ACTIONS/PHARMACODYNAMICS

Selectively blocks all muscarinic responses to acetylcholine (ACh), whether excitatory or inhibitory. Blocks vagal impulses to heart with resulting decrease in AV conduction time, increase in heart rate and cardiac output, and shortened PR interval. Selective depression of CNS relieves rigidity and tremor of Parkinson's syndrome. Antisecretory action (vagolytic effect) suppresses sweating, lacrimation, salivation, and secretions from nose, mouth, pharynx, and bronchi. Atropine is a potent bronchodilator when bronchoconstriction has been induced by parasympathomimetics. Produces mydriasis (dilation of pupils) and cycloplegia (paralysis of accommodation) by blocking responses of iris sphincter muscle and ciliary muscle of lens to cholinergic stimulation.

USES Adjunct in symptomatic treatment of GI disorders (e.g., peptic ulcer, pylorospasm, GI hypermotility, irritable bowel syndrome) and spastic disorders of biliary tract. Relaxes upper GI tract and colon during hypotonic radiography. **Ophthalmic use:** to produce mydriasis and cycloplegia before refraction and for treatment of anterior uveitis and iritis. **Preoperative use:** to suppress salivation, perspiration, and respiratory tract secretions; to reduce incidence of laryngospasm, reflex bradycardia arrhythmia, and hypotension during general anesthesia. **Cardiac uses:** for sinus bradycardia or asystole during CPR or that is induced by drugs or toxic substances (e.g., pilocarpine, beta-adrenergic blockers, organophosphate pesticides, and *Amanita* mushroom poisoning); for management of selected patients with symptomatic sinus bradycardia and associated hypotension and ventricular irritability; for diagnosis of sinus node dysfunction and in evaluation of coronary artery disease during atrial pacing; for management of chronic symptomatic sinus node dysfunction. **Other uses:** oral inhalation for short-term treatment and prevention of bronchospasms associated with asthma, bronchitis, and COPD and as drying agent in upper respiratory infection. Adjunctive therapy for hypermotility of GI tract.

ROUTE & DOSAGE

Preanesthesia

Adult: **IV/IM/SC** 0.2–1 mg 30–60 min before surgery.
Child: **IM/IV/SC** <5 kg: 0.02 mg/kg; >5 kg: 0.01–0.02 mg/kg 30–60 min before surgery.

Arrhythmias

Adult: **IV/IM** 0.5–1 mg q1–2h prn to a max of 2 mg.
Child: **IV/IM** 0.01–0.03 mg/kg for 1–2 doses.

Organophosphate Antidote

Adult: **IV/IM** 1–2 mg q5–60min until muscarinic signs and symptoms subside (may need up to 50 mg).
Child: **IV/IM** 0.05 mg/kg q10–30 min until muscarinic signs and symptoms subside.

COPD

Adult: **Nebulizer** 0.025 mg/kg diluted with 3–5 ml saline, administered via nebulizer 3–4 times daily (max 2.5 mg/d).

Child: **Nebulizer** 0.03–0.05 mg/kg diluted with 3–5 ml saline, administered via nebulizer 3–4 times daily.

Uveitis

Adult: **Ophthalmic** 1–2 drops of solution or small amount of ointment in eye up to t.i.d.
Child: **Ophthalmic** Same as for adult.

Cycloplegia

Adult: **Ophthalmic** 1 drop of solution or small amount of ointment in eye 1 h before the procedure.
Child: **Ophthalmic** 1–2 drops in eye b.i.d. for 1–3 d prior to procedure or a small amount of ointment in conjunctival sac t.i.d. for 1–3 d prior to procedure with last dose applied several hours before the procedure.

PHARMACOKINETICS Absorption: well absorbed from all administration sites. **Peak effect:** 30 min IM, 2–4 min IV, 1–2 h SC, 1.5–4 h inhalation, 30–40 min topical. **Duration:** inhibition of salivation 4 h; mydriasis 7–14 d. **Distribution:** distributed in most body tissues; crosses blood–brain barrier and placenta. **Metabolism:** metabolized in liver. **Elimination:** half-life: 2–3 h; 77–94% excreted in urine in 24 h.

CONTRAINDICATIONS & PRECAUTIONS Contraindicated in: hypersensitivity to belladonna alkaloids; synechiae; angle-closure glaucoma; parotitis; obstructive uropathy, e.g., bladder neck obstruction caused by prostatic hypertrophy; intestinal atony, paralytic ileus, obstructive diseases of GI tract, severe ulcerative colitis, toxic megacolon; tachycardia secondary to cardiac insufficiency or thyrotoxicosis; acute hemorrhage; myasthenia gravis. Safe use during pregnancy (category C) and in nursing women not established. **Cautious use in:** myocardial infarction, hypertension, hypotension; coronary artery disease, CHF, tachyarrhythmias; gastric ulcer, GI infections, hiatal hernia with reflux esophagitis; hyperthyroidism; chronic lung disease; hepatic or renal disease; the elderly; debilitated patients; children under 6 y of age; Down syndrome; autonomic neuropathy, spastic paralysis, brain damage in children; patients exposed to high environmental temperatures; patients with fever.

ADVERSE/SIDE EFFECTS CNS: headache, ataxia, dizziness, excitement, irritability, convulsions, drowsiness, fatigue, weakness; mental depression, confusion, disorientation, hallucinations. **CV:** hypertension or hypotension, ventricular tachycardia, palpitation, paradoxical bradycardia, AV dissociation, atrial or ventricular fibrillation. **Eye:** mydriasis, blurred vision, photophobia, increased intraocular pressure, cycloplegia, eye dryness, local redness. **GI:** dry mouth with thirst, dysphagia, loss of taste; nausea, vomiting, constipation, delayed gastric emptying, antral stasis, paralytic ileus. **GU:** urinary hesitancy and retention, dysuria, impotence. **Skin:** flushed, dry skin; anhidrosis, rash, urticaria, contact dermatitis, allergic conjunctivitis, fixed-drug eruption.

DIAGNOSTIC TEST INTERFERENCE ***Upper GI series:*** findings may require qualification because of anticholinergic effects of atropine (reduced gastric motility and delayed gastric emptying). ***PSP excretion test:*** atropine may decrease urinary excretion of PSP (phenolsulfonphthalein).

DRUG INTERACTIONS **Amantadine,** ANTIHISTAMINES, TRICYCLIC ANTIDEPRESSANTS, **quinidine, disopyramide, procainamide** add to anticholinergic effects. **Levodopa** effects decreased. **Methotrimeprazine** may precipitate extrapyramidal effects. PHENOTHIAZINES' antipsychotic effects decreased (decreased absorption).

NURSING IMPLICATIONS

Administration

- Smaller doses of atropine are indicated for the elderly.
- IV administration: IV atropine is given by direct IV undiluted or diluted in up to 10 ml of sterile water. Administer 1 mg or fraction thereof over 1 min.
- Protect in airtight, light-resistant containers at room temperature, preferably 15–30C (59–86F) unless otherwise directed by manufacturer.

Assessment & Drug Effects

- Monitor vital signs. Pulse is a sensitive indicator of patient's response to atropine. Be alert to changes in quality, rate, and rhythm of pulse and respiration and to changes in blood pressure and temperature.
- Initial paradoxic bradycardia following IV atropine usually lasts only 1–2 min; it most likely occurs when IV is administered slowly (more than 1 min) or when small doses (less than 0.5 mg) are used. Postural hypotension occurs when patient ambulates too soon after parenteral administration.
- Atropine may contribute to the problem of urinary retention. Palpate lower abdomen for distention. Monitor I&O, especially in older patients and in patients who have had surgery. Have patient void before giving atropine.
- If constipation is a problem, check for abdominal distention and auscultate for bowel sounds.
- Geriatric and debilitated patients sometimes manifest drowsiness or CNS stimulation (excitement, agitation, confusion) with usual doses of atropine or other belladonna alkaloids. In addition to dosage adjustment, side rails and supervision of ambulation may be indicated.
- Infants, small children, and the elderly are especially prone to developing "atropine fever" (hyperpyrexia due to suppression of perspiration and heat loss), which increases the risk of heatstroke.
- Intraocular tension and depth of anterior chamber should be determined before and during therapy with ophthalmic preparations to avoid glaucoma attacks. Note that ophthalmic solutions and ointments are available in various strengths.
- Frequent and continued use of eye preparations, as well as overdosage, can have systemic effects. Studies reveal that over one half of atropine deaths have resulted from systemic absorption following ocular administration in infants and children.
- Onset of mydriatic action may be slower and duration longer in persons with dark eyes.
- Infants, children with spastic paralysis, brain damage, or Down syndrome (mongolism), and blonde, blue-eyed individuals appear to be highly sensitive to the effects of atropine and related drugs.
- Patients receiving atropine via inhalation sometimes manifest mild CNS stimulation with doses in excess of 5 mg and mental depression and other mental disturbances with larger doses.

Patient & Family Education

- Urge patient to keep dentist appointments. Since saliva is a natural mouthwash, teeth are much more vulnerable to decay when salivation is suppressed.
- The following measures may help to relieve dry mouth: maintain adequate hydration; small, frequent mouth rinses with tepid water; meticulous mouth and dental hygiene; gum chewing or sucking hard, sour candy (sugarless).
- Prepare for visual acuity to be impaired for several days and to protect eyes from bright light by wearing dark glasses while pupils are dilated.
- In addition to causing drowsiness, sensitivity to light and blurring of near vision, atropine will temporarily impair ability to judge distance. Avoid driving and other activities requiring visual acuity and mental alertness.
- Ophthalmic preparations should be discontinued if eye pain, conjunctivitis, palpitation, rapid pulse, or dizziness occurs. Report symptoms promptly to physician.

AURANOFIN

(au-rane′eh-fin)

Trade name: Ridaura

Classifications: GOLD COMPOUND; ANTIRHEUMATIC; ANTIINFLAMMATORY

Prototype: Aurothioglucose

Pregnancy category: C

ACTIONS/PHARMACODYNAMICS Strongly lipophilic and almost neutral in solution, properties that may facilitate transport of agent across cell membranes. Action appears to be immunomodulatory: serum immunoglobulin concentrations and rheumatoid factor titers are decreased; and antiinflammatory: gold is taken up by macrophages with resulting inhibition of phagocytosis and lysosomal enzyme release.

USES Management of active stage of classic or definite rheumatoid arthritis in adults who do not respond to or tolerate other antiarthritis agents (e.g., NSAIDS, other gold compounds). **Unlabeled uses:** juvenile rheumatoid arthritis, active SLE, psoriatic arthritis.

ROUTE & DOSAGE

Rheumatoid Arthritis

Adult: **PO** 6 mg/d in 1–2 divided doses; may increase to 6–9 mg/d in 3 divided doses after 6 mo if tolerated and needed (max 9 mg/d).
Child: **PO** Initially 0.1 mg/kg/d; may increase to 0.15 mg/kg/d in 1–2 divided doses (max 0.2 mg/kg/d).

PHARMACOKINETICS Absorption: 20% absorbed from small intestine. **Peak:** 2 h. **Distribution:** highest concentrations in kidneys, spleen, lungs, adrenals, and liver; not known if crosses placenta; small amounts distributed into breast milk. **Elimination:** half-life: 11–23 d; 60% of absorbed gold eliminated in urine, remainder in feces.

CONTRAINDICATIONS & PRECAUTIONS Contraindicated in: history of gold-induced necrotizing enterocolitis, renal disease, exfoliative dermatitis or bone marrow aplasia; patient who has recently received radiation therapy, history of severe toxicity from previous exposure to gold or other heavy metals. Safe use during pregnancy (category C), lactation, or by children not established. **Cautious use in:** inflammatory bowel disease, rash, liver disease, history of bone marrow depression; elderly patients; diabetes mellitus, CHF.

ADVERSE/SIDE EFFECTS **GI:** *diarrhea, abdominal cramping* and pain; *nausea,* vomiting, anorexia, dysphagia; *stomatitis,* glossitis, metallic taste; flatulence, constipation, GI bleeding, melena. **Hematologic:** thrombocytopenia, leukopenia, eosinophilia, agranulocytosis, aplastic anemia. **Renal:** proteinuria, hematuria, renal failure. **Skin:** *rash, pruritus,* dermatitis, urticaria.

DIAGNOSTIC TEST INTERFERENCE Auranofin may enhance response to a ***tuberculin skin test.***

NURSING IMPLICATIONS

Administration

- Administer capsule with food or fluid of patient's choice.
- Store at 15–30C (59–86F); protect from light and moisture. Expiration date: 4 y after date of manufacture.

Assessment & Drug Effects

- Auranofin has many adverse side effects, but they appear to be less toxic and better tolerated than those of other gold compounds. They occur frequently in the first 6 mo of treatment but can occur at any time.
- The following symptoms should be reported promptly: unexplained bleeding or bruising, metallic taste, sore mouth; pruritus, rash; diarrhea and melena; yellow skin and sclera; unexplained cough or dyspnea.
- Therapeutic effects from auranofin treatment develop slowly and are not usually apparent for 3–4 mo.
- Drug-induced thrombocytopenia (mechanism not clear) is usually spontaneously reversible several weeks after drug is withdrawn; however, platelet transfusions or corticosteroids or both may be required if condition is severe.
- Laboratory signs of possible impending gold toxicity are decreased Hgb; leukocytes <4000/mm^3; granulocytes <1500/mm^3; platelets <150,000/mm^3; proteinuria >500 mg/d.
- If drug is discontinued, adverse effects may persist for many months requiring continued medical surveillance and supportive therapy: difficulty in breathing, diarrhea and abdominal pain, fatigue, weakness, unexplained bleeding and bruising, metallic taste.

Patient & Family Education

- Instruct patient to report adverse effects of therapy.
- Do not change dosage (dose or dose interval) by omission, increase, or decrease without first consulting physician.
- Drug-induced diarrhea may respond well to treatment with an antidiarrheal drug and high-fiber diet.
- Abdominal cramping and pain should be reported; discontinuance of therapy may be necessary.
- Exposure to sunlight (especially between 10 AM and 4 PM) or to artificial ultraviolet light should be kept to a minimum to prevent photosensitivity reaction.
- Among earliest subjective symptoms of impending gold toxicity are metallic taste and pruritus with or without rash. Report promptly to physician.
- Urge patient to maintain contact with physician at appointed times (usually monthly) for assessment of disease status and monitoring of the following: urinary protein, CBC with differential and platelet count; hepatic function.
- For symptomatic treatment of mild stomatitis, the manufacturer suggests rinsing mouth with a hypo-

tonic NaCl solution. Avoid commercial mouth rinses; clean teeth with soft tooth brush and gentle brushing to avoid gingival trauma. Floss at least once daily.

AUROTHIOGLUCOSE

(aur-oh-thye-oh-gloo′kose)

Trade names: Gold thioglucose, Solganal

Prototype for classifications: GOLD COMPOUND; ANTIINFLAMMATORY

Pregnancy category: C

ACTIONS/PHARMACODYNAMICS Major clinical effect is suppression of joint inflammation in early arthritic disease. Has no effect on reparative process, but studies suggest that it may significantly slow or arrest disease progression. Mechanism of antiinflammatory action not clearly understood. Gold uptake by macrophages with subsequent inhibition of migration and phagocytic action, thereby suppressing immune responsiveness, may be principal mechanism.

USES Adjunctive treatment of both adult and juvenile active rheumatoid arthritis. Generally used when adequate trial with salicylates or other NSAIDS has not been satisfactory. **Unlabeled uses:** psoriatic arthritis, Felty's syndrome, pemphigus, nondisseminated LE.

ROUTE & DOSAGE

Rheumatoid Arthritis

Adult: **IM** 10 mg 1st wk, 25 mg 2nd and 3rd wk, then 50 mg/wk to a cumulative dose of 1 g; if improvement occurs, continue at 25–50 mg q2–3wk, then q3–4wk indefinitely or until side effects occur.

Child 6–12 y: **IM** 0.25–1 mg/kg/wk (max 25 mg) for 20 wk; if improvement, continue at 1 mg/kg (max 25 mg) q2–4wk.

PHARMACOKINETICS Absorption: slowly and irregularly absorbed from IM site. **Peak:** 4–6 h. **Distribution:** widely distributed, especially to synovial fluid; does not cross blood–brain barrier; crosses placenta. **Metabolism:** unknown. **Elimination:** half-life: 3–27 d; 50–90% of dose ultimately excreted in urine; 10–50% in feces; excreted in breast milk.

CONTRAINDICATIONS & PRECAUTIONS Contraindicated in: Gold allergy or history of severe toxicity from previous therapy with gold or other heavy metals; severe debilitation; uncontrolled diabetes mellitus; renal or hepatic insufficiency, history of hepatitis; uncontrolled CHF; marked hypertension; tuberculosis; severe anemia, hemorrhagic diathesis, agranulocytosis or other blood dyscrasias; disseminated LE, Sjögren's syndrome, recent radiation therapy; colitis; urticaria, eczema, history of exfoliative dermatitis. Safe use during pregnancy (category C), in nursing women, and in children under 6 y not established. **Cautious use in:** elderly patients; history of drug allergy or hypersensitivity; history of blood dyscrasias; history of renal or hepatic disease; compromised cerebral or cardiovascular circulation; presence of skin rash.

ADVERSE/SIDE EFFECTS GI: nausea, vomiting, abdominal cramps, anorexia, metallic taste, diarrhea. **Hematologic:** eosinophilia, agranulocytosis, thrombocytopenia, leukopenia, granulocytopenia, aplastic anemia. **Hypersensitivity:** anaphylactic shock, syncope, bradycardia, thickening of tongue, dysphagia, dyspnea. **Renal:** nephrotic syndrome, proteinuria, hematuria. **Skin:** *pruritus, urticaria, erythema,* "gold dermatitis," fixed-drug eruptions, exfoliative dermatitis with alopecia and nail shedding; gingivitis, glossitis, Stevens-Johnson syndrome, photosensitivity reactions. **Other:** hepatitis, immunologic destruction of synovial fluid, exacerbation of arthralgia (temporary), fever, local irritation at injection site, vaginitis, proteinuria, nephrotic syndrome, pulmonary fibrosis, interstitial pneumonitis.

DIAGNOSTIC TEST INTERFERENCE

Low ***PBI*** (by ***chloric acid method***); test interference may persist for several weeks after gold therapy is discontinued.

DRUG INTERACTIONS

ANTIMALARIALS, IMMUNOSUPPRESSANTS, **penicillamine, phenylbutazone** increase risk of blood dyscrasias.

NURSING IMPLICATIONS

Administration

- Hold vial horizontally and shake vigorously to ensure uniform suspension. Heating vial to body temperature (by placing in a warm-water bath) facilitates drug withdrawal.
- Administer drug by deep IM injection (preferably intragluteally). An 18- or 20-gauge, 1 1/2-inch needle is recommended (for obese patients a 2-inch needle may be preferable). Patient should be lying down when drug is administered.
- Patient should remain recumbent for 10 min after injection to overcome possible nitritoid reaction. Observe patient for 20–30 min after injection for hypersensitivity reactions.
- Gold therapy is contraindicated following a severe reaction but may be attempted at reduced initial dosage schedule and careful monitoring after a mild reaction.
- Store in light-resistant containers at 15–30C (59–86F) unless otherwise directed. Protect from freezing and light.

Assessment & Drug Effects

- Baseline renal and hepatic function tests, CBC, and urinalysis should be done before initiation of therapy. Thereafter, urinalysis (for protein and sediment) should be performed before each injection. CBC (including Hgb, RBC, WBC and differential, platelet counts) should be determined before every second injection throughout therapy.
- Pregnancy should be ruled out before gold treatment begins. Women of childbearing age should be warned about the potential hazards of becoming pregnant during therapy and counseled about the use of birth control.
- Therapeutic effectiveness may not be apparent before 6–8 wk of gold therapy.
- During early treatment, some patients complain of exacerbation of joint pain after injection. It usually subsides after the first few injections.
- Interview and examine patient before each injection to detect early signs and symptoms suggestive of gold toxicity. Beginning toxicity generally involves skin and mucous membranes anywhere in body. Inspect skin carefully and use tongue blade and flashlight to examine mouth and throat. The following are suggestive of gold reaction and should be reported

promptly: itching (often precedes dermatitis and eosinophilia), bruising or bleeding, tenderness, metallic taste (frequently precedes sore mouth, tongue, or throat), gray-blue discoloration of skin and mucous membranes, diarrhea or loose stools, indigestion, unexplained malaise; signs of hepatotoxicity (yellow sclerae and skin, clay-colored stools, dark urine, pruritus).

- A rapid improvement in joint pain and mobility also may signify that patient is approaching toxic tissue levels. Interruption of therapy, at least temporarily, is indicated.
- Precipitous decline in platelets or counts <100,000/mm^3, or leukocytes <4000/mm^3, granulocytes <1500/mm^3, eosinophils >5%, rapid fall in Hgb value, and presence of proteinuria or hematuria are all indications to withhold therapy pending further studies.

Patient & Family Education

- Before initiation of treatment, patient should be well informed regarding dangers associated with gold therapy and requirements for compliance in receiving scheduled doses, keeping laboratory appointments, and prompt reporting of adverse effects.
- Provide patient with a list of possible adverse effects that should be reported. If therapy is interrupted at the onset of gold toxicity, serious reactions can be avoided. Note that elderly patients are particularly sensitive to the effects of gold therapy, and some patients appear to have a genetic predisposition to gold toxicity.
- Adverse reactions are most likely to occur during second and third month of therapy or when cumulative aurothioglucose dose is 300–500 mg. However, they may appear at any time during therapy or several months after treatment has been discontinued (gold is slowly eliminated from body).
- Instruct patient to report any unusual color or odor to urine, or change in I&O ratio and pattern.
- Advise patient to report early signs of infection that may indicate onset of agranulocytosis (unusual fatigue or weakness, malaise, chills, fever, sore throat); possible signs of reduced platelets (thrombocytopenia): unexplained bleeding, e.g., bleeding gums, nosebleeds, dark urine (hematuria), black stools, petechiae, purpura, easy bruising. Also instruct patient to report signs of hepatotoxicity (see Signs & Symptoms, Appendix G).
- Be alert to vulnerability of patient to secondary infection because of the possible immunosuppressive effect of gold. Caution patient to avoid contact with persons who have colds or recent vaccination or who have been exposed recently to communicable disease.
- Inform patient that the necessity to increase the amount of aspirin or other prescribed NSAID for analgesia is a significant indication of diminishing response to gold therapy and therefore should be reported to physician.
- Since gray to blue pigmentation (chrysiasis) may occur on light-exposed skin areas, caution patient to minimize exposure to sunlight and artificial ultraviolet light.
- Symptomatic treatment of stomatitis: advise careful oral hygiene. Use a soft toothbrush or finger covered with moistened cotton or moistened gauze. Rub gently. Floss carefully with waxed dental floss once daily. Rinse mouth frequently with warm water, tea, or saline (if allowed). Caution against

overuse of commercial mouthwashes especially those that are bactericidal. Many contain alcohol, which enhances drying and irritation and can change mouth flora.

AZATADINE MALEATE

(a-za'ta-deen)

Trade names: Optimine, Trinalin

Classification: ANTIHISTAMINE (H_1-RECEPTOR ANTAGONIST)

Prototype: Diphenhydramine

Pregnancy category: B

ACTIONS/PHARMACODYNAMICS Long-acting antihistamine that acts by competitively antagonizing the stimulating effects of histamine at H_1-receptor sites on smooth muscle of blood vessels and respiratory and GI tract. This action blocks or reduces intensity of allergic responses associated with histamine release, such as vasodilation, capillary permeability and tissue edema, and itching.

USES Symptomatic relief of hay fever (seasonal allergic rhinitis), perennial (or nonseasonal) allergic rhinitis, and chronic urticaria.

ROUTE & DOSAGE

Allergic Rhinitis

Adult: **PO** 1–2 mg b.i.d.

PHARMACOKINETICS Absorption: readily absorbed from GI tract. **Peak:** 4 h. **Distribution:** probably crosses blood–brain barrier; crosses placenta; distribution into breast milk unknown. **Metabolism:** partially metabolized in liver. **Elimination:** half-life: 9–12 h; 50% excreted in urine in 5 d.

CONTRAINDICATIONS & PRECAUTIONS Contraindicated in: hypersensitivity to azatadine or to other H_1-receptor antagonists; MAO INHIBITOR therapy. Safe use during pregnancy (category B), in nursing women, and in children <12 y not established. **Cautious use in:** increased intraocular pressure, narrow-angle glaucoma; pyloroduodenal obstruction, stenosing peptic ulcer; prostatic hypertrophy, bladder neck obstruction; hyperthyroidism; hypertension, cardiovascular disease; convulsive disorders; history of asthma or COPD.

ADVERSE/SIDE EFFECTS CNS: *drowsiness,* sedation, dizziness, disturbed coordination, fatigue, confusion, euphoria, excitation, nervousness, restlessness, insomnia, tremor, irritability. **CV:** hypotension, palpitation, tachycardia, extrasystoles. **ENT:** nasal stuffiness; dryness of nose and throat; tinnitus. **Eye:** blurred vision. **GI:** *dry mouth,* epigastric distress, nausea, vomiting, anorexia, diarrhea, or constipation. **GU:** urinary retention, early menses. **Hematologic:** hemolytic anemia, thrombocytopenia, agranulocytosis. **Respiratory:** thickening of bronchial secretions.

DIAGNOSTIC TEST INTERFERENCE As a general rule, H_1-receptor antagonists are discontinued about 4 d before ***skin testing*** procedures are to be performed since they may produce false-negative results.

DRUG INTERACTIONS Alcohol, CNS DEPRESSANTS add to sedation, drowsiness; MAO INHIBITORS may prolong anticholinergic effects of azatadine; TRICYCLIC ANTIDEPRESSANTS augment anticholinergic effects.

NURSING IMPLICATIONS

Administration

- GI side effects may be minimized

by administering drug with food or milk.
- Store in tightly closed container at 2–30C (36–86F), unless otherwise directed.

Assessment & Drug Effects
- Azatadine is most likely to cause sedation, dizziness, hypotension, and confusion in the elderly. Advise patient to report these effects. Reduction in dosage may be indicated.
- There may be additive CNS depression with alcohol and other CNS depressants (e.g., sedatives, tranquilizers, sleep medications).

Patient & Family Education
- Azatadine commonly causes drowsiness, sedation, and dizziness; caution patient not to drive a car or engage in other potentially hazardous activities until reaction to drug is known.
- Instruct patient to avoid concurrent use of alcohol because of potential for additive CNS depression.
- Advise patient to avoid prolonged exposure to sunlight or to artificial ultraviolet light. Photosensitivity is a possible adverse effect.
- Dry mouth (xerostomia) may be relieved by the following measures: (1) frequent rinses with tepid water, preferred to commercial mouthwashes, overuse of which can change oral flora; also, many contain alcohol, which enhances drying; (2) increase fluid intake (if allowed) or at least maintain normal intake; (3) brush with soft toothbrush after every meal; (4) floss teeth daily with waxed floss (before brushing); (5) sugarless gum or sugarless sourballs; (6) use of artificial saliva, e.g., Xero-Lube, Moi-Stir.

AZATHIOPRINE
(ay-za-thye'oh-preen)
Trade name: Imuran
Classification: IMMUNOSUPPRESSANT
Prototype: Cyclosporine
Pregnancy category: D

ACTIONS/PHARMACODYNAMICS
Precise mechanism of immunosuppressant and antiinflammatory actions not determined. Antagonizes purine metabolism and appears to inhibit DNA, RNA, and normal protein synthesis in rapidly growing cells. Suppresses T cell effects before transplant rejection.

USES Adjunctive agent to prevent rejection of kidney allografts, usually with other immunosuppressants. Also used in selective adult patients with severe, active rheumatoid arthritis; unresponsive to conventional therapy. **Unlabeled uses:** SLE, ulcerative colitis, pemphigus, nephrotic syndrome, and other inflammatory and immunologic diseases.

ROUTE & DOSAGE

Renal Transplantation
Adult: **PO** 3–5 mg/kg/d initially; may be able to reduce to 1–3 mg/kg/d. **IV** 3–5 mg/kg/d initially; may be able to reduce to 1–3 mg/kg/d.

Rheumatoid Arthritis
Adult: **PO** 1 mg/kg/d initially; may be increased by 0.5 mg/kg/d at 4–6 wk intervals if needed up to 2.5 mg/kg/d.

Renal Impairment
Cl_{cr} 10–50 ml/min: 75% of usual dose; **<10 ml/min:** 50% of usual dose.

Common side effect in *italic,* life-threatening effects underlined: generic names in **bold;** drug class in SMALL CAPS

PHARMACOKINETICS Absorption: readily absorbed from GI tract. **Distribution:** crosses placenta. **Metabolism:** extensively metabolized in liver to active metabolite mercaptopurine. **Elimination:** half-life: 3 h; eliminated in urine.

CONTRAINDICATIONS & PRECAUTIONS Contraindicated in: hypersensitivity to azathioprine or mercaptopurine; clinically active infection, immunization of patient or close family members with live virus vaccines; anuria; pancreatitis; patients receiving alkylating agents (increased risk of neoplasms), concurrent radiation therapy. Safe use during pregnancy (category D) and lactation not established. **Cautious use in:** impaired kidney and liver function; patients receiving cadaver kidney; myasthenia gravis.

ADVERSE/SIDE EFFECTS GI: nausea, vomiting, anorexia, esophagitis, diarrhea, steatorrhea. **Hematologic:** <u>bone marrow depression</u>, thrombocytopenia, leukopenia, anemia, <u>agranulocytosis</u>, pancytopenia. **Hepatic:** hepatitis with elevations in bilirubin, alkaline phosphatase, AST, ALT, biliary stasis, toxic hepatitis. **Hypersensitivity:** skin eruptions, rash, arthralgia. **Other:** *secondary infection (immunosuppression);* dysarthria, alopecia. Carcinogenic and teratogenic potential reported.

DIAGNOSTIC TEST INTERFERENCE Azathioprine may decrease plasma and urinary ***uric acid*** in patients with gout.

DRUG INTERACTIONS Allopurinol increases effects and toxicity of azathioprine by reducing metabolism of the active metabolite—allopurinol doses should be decreased by one third or one fourth; **tubocurarine** and other NONDEPOLARIZING SKELETAL MUSCLE RELAXANTS may reverse or inhibit neuromuscular blocking effects.

NURSING IMPLICATIONS

Administration

- Azathioprine therapy is usually started 1–5 d before kidney transplantation and restarted within 24 h after transplantation.
- Gastric disturbances may be minimized by administering oral drug in divided doses (prescribed), or with food or immediately after meals, or by dosage reduction.
- IV preparation: reconstitute azathioprine sodium for IV injection by adding 10 ml sterile water for injection into vial. Swirl vial until drug is dissolved. For IV infusion, reconstituted solution may be further diluted with 50 ml NaCl injection or 5% dextrose in NaCl injection.
- IV administration: IV azathioprine properly diluted may be administered by infusion over 30–60 min. Note: the final volume of the IV solution depends on time for infusion, which may range from 5 min to 8 h. Check with physician.
- Reconstituted IV solution may be stored at room temperature; but use within 24 h after reconstitution (contains no preservatives).
- Preserve in tightly closed, light-resistant containers at 15–30C (59–86F) unless otherwise directed.

Assessment & Drug Effects

- Monitor vital signs. Report signs of infection.
- CBC, including Hgb and platelet counts, should be performed before and at least weekly during first month of therapy, twice monthly during second and third months, and monthly, or more frequently

therafter if indicated (e.g., by dosage or therapy changes).

- Kidney function is monitored to prevent drug accumulation (urine protein, urine electrolytes, creatinine clearance, serum creatinine, BUN).
- Surveillance of I&O ratio is crucial. Up to a twofold increase in toxicity is possible in anephric or anuric patients. Note color, character, and specific gravity of urine. Report an abrupt decrease in urinary output or any change in I&O ratio.
- Azathioprine has a high toxic potential. Because it may have delayed action, dosage should be reduced or drug withdrawn at the first indication of an abnormally large or persistent decrease in leukocyte or platelet count to avoid irreversible bone marrow depression.
- Thrombocytopenia occurs less commonly than leukopenia; however, be alert to signs of abnormal bleeding (easy bruising, bleeding gums, petechiae, purpura, melena, epistaxis, dark urine [hematuria], hemoptysis, hematemesis). If thrombocytopenia occurs, invasive procedures should be withheld, if possible.
- Liver function tests (alkaline phosphatase, AST, ALT, serum bilirubin) should be repeated at least every 3 mo or more frequently if indicated. If hepatic toxicity (see Signs & Symptoms, Appendix G) develops, therapy may have to be withdrawn.
- Protective isolation may be indicated for the hospitalized patient to reduce risk of infections.

Patient & Family Education

- Therapeutic effectiveness in patients with rheumatoid arthritis usually occurs in 6–8 wk of therapy (improvement in morning stiffness and grip strength). If no improvement has occurred after 12-wk trial period, drug is generally discontinued.
- Intercurrent infection is a constant hazard of immunosuppressive therapy. Warn patient to avoid contact with persons who have colds or other infections and to report signs of impending infection, which are also possible symptoms of agranulocytosis. Personal hygiene should be scrupulous.
- Pregnancy should be ruled out before azathioprine therapy begins. Women of childbearing age should be warned about potential hazards and advised to practice birth control during therapy and for 4 mo after drug is discontinued.
- Vaccinations or other immunity-conferring agents are contraindicated because they may precipitate unusually severe reactions due to the immunosuppressive effects of azathioprine.

AZELAIC ACID

(a′-ze-laic)

Trade name: Azelex

Classifications: SKIN AND MUCOUS MEMBRANE AGENT; ANTIACNE

Prototype: Isotretinoin

Pregnancy category: B

ACTIONS/PHARMACODYNAMICS

Azelaic acid is a naturally occurring dicarboxylic acid. Topical 20% azelaic acid possesses antimicrobial activity against *Propionibacterium acnes* and *Staphylococcus epidermidis.* The antimicrobial action may be attributable to inhibition of the microbial cellular protein synthesis. A normalization of keratinization may also contribute to its clinical effectiveness.

Common side effect in *italic,* life-threatening effects underlined: generic names in **bold;** drug class in SMALL CAPS

USE Mild to moderate inflammatory acne vulgaris.

ROUTE & DOSAGE

Acne Vulgaris
Adult: **Topical** Apply thin film to clean and dry area b.i.d.
Child > 12 y: **Topical** Same as adult

PHARMACOKINETICS Absorption: approximately 4% is absorbed through the skin. **Onset:** 4–8 wk. **Distribution:** distributes into all tissues. **Metabolism:** partially metabolized by beta oxidation in liver. **Elimination:** half-life: 12 h; excreted primarily in urine.

CONTRAINDICATIONS & PRECAUTIONS Contraindicated in: hypersensitivity to any component in the drug. **Cautious use in:** dark complexion, pregnancy (category B), lactation. Safety and efficacy in children < 12 y have not been established.

ADVERSE/SIDE EFFECTS Skin: pruritus, burning, stinging, tingling, erythema, dryness, rash, peeling, irritation, contact dermatitis, vitiligo depigmentation, hypertrichosis. **Other:** worsening of asthma.

NURSING IMPLICATIONS

Administration
- Skin should be thoroughly washed and dried prior to application of azelaic acid cream.
- Apply by thoroughly massaging a thin film of the cream into the affected area. Avoid occlusive dressing.
- Wash hands before and after application of cream.
- Store at 15–30C (59–86F).

Assessment & Drug Effects
- Assess for signs of hypopigmentation and report immediately.
- Monitor for sensitivity or severe irritation, which may warrant drug dosage reduction or discontinuation.

Patient & Family Education
- Inform patient that transient pruritus, burning, and stinging are common; however, severe skin irritation or hypopigmentation should be reported.
- Instruct about proper application of cream and advise to avoid contact with eyes or mucous membranes.
- Advise to wash eyes with copious amounts of water if contact with medication occurs.

AZITHROMYCIN
(a-zi-thro-mye′sin)
Trade name: Zithromax
Classifications: ANTIINFECTIVE; MACROLIDE ANTIBIOTIC
Prototype: Erythromycin
Pregnancy category: B

ACTIONS/PHARMACODYNAMICS A macrolide antibiotic that reversibly binds to the 50S ribosomal subunit of susceptible organisms and consequently inhibits protein synthesis. Effective for treatment of mild to moderate infections caused by pyogenic streptococci, *Streptococcus pneumoniae, Hemophilus influenzae,* and *Staphylococcus aureus.*

USES Pneumonia, lower respiratory tract infections, pharyngitis/tonsillitis, gonorrhea, nongonococcal urethritis, skin and skin structure infections due to susceptible organisms, otitis media, *Mycobacterium avium–intracellulare* complex infections. **Unlabeled uses:** bronchitis, *Helicobacter* gastritis.

ROUTE & DOSAGE

Bacterial Infections

Adult: **PO** 500 mg on day 1; then 250 mg q24h for 4 more d. **IV** 500 mg q.d. × at least 2 d. Administer 1 mg/ml over 3 h or 2 mg/ml over 1 h.
Child ≥*6 mo:* **PO** 10 mg/kg on day 1, then 5 mg/kg for 4 more d (max 250 mg/d).

Gonorrhea

Adult: **PO** 2 g as a single dose.

Chancroid

Adult: **PO** 1 g as a single dose.
Child: **PO** 20 mg/kg as single dose (max 1 g).

PHARMACOKINETICS **Absorption:** 37% of dose reaches the systemic circulation. **Onset:** 48 h. **Peak:** 2.5–4 h. **Distribution:** extensively distributed to most tissues including sputum, blister, and vaginal secretions; tissue concentrations are often higher than serum concentrations. **Metabolism:** metabolized in liver. **Elimination:** half-life: the elimination half-life of azithromycin increases with time after the dose because of slow elimination from tissue sites and ranges from 9.6–40 h; 5–12% of dose is excreted in urine.

CONTRAINDICATIONS & PRECAUTIONS **Contraindicated in:** hypersensitivity to azithromycin, erythromycin, or any of the macrolide antibiotics. **Cautious use in:** elderly or debilitated persons, hepatic or renal impairment, ventricular arrhythmias, pregnancy (category B), lactation, and children <6 years of age.

ADVERSE/SIDE EFFECTS **CNS:** headache, dizziness. **GI:** nausea, vomiting, diarrhea, abdominal pain. **Hepatotoxicity:** mild elevations in liver function tests.

DRUG INTERACTIONS ANTACIDS may decrease peak level of azithromycin. **Drug–food:** food will decrease the amount of azithromycin absorbed by 50%.

DIAGNOSTIC TEST INTERFERENCE Liver function tests: reversible, asymptomatic elevations in ***liver enzymes (AST, ALT, gamma glutamyl transferase, alkaline phosphatase)*** have been reported in some patients treated with azithromycin.

NURSING IMPLICATIONS

Administration

- Give capsule at least 1 h before or 2 h after a meal. Tablets may be taken without regard to food.
- IV preparation: reconstitue 500-mg vial with 4.8 ml of sterile water for injection and shake until dissolved. Final concentration is 100 mg/ml. Solution must be further diluted to 1.0 or 2.0 mg/ml by adding 5 ml of the 100-mg/ml solution to 500 ml or 250 ml, respectively, of D5W, 0.9% NaCl, D5W + 0.45% NaCl, or other compatible solution.
- IV administration: administer diluted solution over at least 60 min. Do not give a bolus dose.
- When diluted as directed, IV solutions are stable for 24 h at or below 30C (86F) or for 7 d under 5C (41F).

Assessment & Drug Effects

- Monitor for and report loose stools or diarrhea, since pseudomembranous colitis must be ruled out.
- Since simultaneous use with warfarin may increase coagulation time, carefully monitor prothrombin times.

Patient & Family Education

- Instruct patient to take drug on an empty stomach 1 h before or 2 h after eating.
- Instruct patient to take aluminum or magnesium antacids 2 h before or after azithromycin.

AZTREONAM

(az-tree′oh-nam)

Trade name: Azactam

Classifications: ANTIINFECTIVE; BETA-LACTAM ANTIBIOTIC

Prototype: Imipenem-cilastatin

Pregnancy category: B

ACTIONS/PHARMACODYNAMICS Differs structurally from other beta-lactam antibiotics (penicillins and cephalosporins) in having a monocyclic rather than a bicyclic nucleus. Acts by inhibiting synthesis of bacterial cell wall, primarily in aerobic, gram-negative bacteria. Highly resistant to beta-lactamases and does not readily induce their formation. Spectrum of activity limited to aerobic, gram-negative bacteria. Active against *Hemophilus influenzae, Pseudomonas aeruginosa, Neisseria gonorrhoeae,* and against Enterobacteriaceae including most strains of *E. coli, Enterobacter, Klebsiella, Proteus, Providencia, Shigella, Salmonella,* and *Serratia*. There appears to be little cross-allergenicity with penicillins and cephalosporins.

USES Gram-negative infections of urinary tract, lower respiratory tract, skin and skin structures; and for intraabdominal and gynecologic infections, septicemia, and as adjunctive therapy for surgical infections. Often used in combination with other antibiotics active against gram-positive and anaerobic bacteria in mixed infections.

ROUTE & DOSAGE

Urinary Tract Infection

Adult: **IM/IV** 0.5–1 g q8–12h.

Moderate to Severe Infections

Adult: **IM/IV** 1–2 g q6–8h (max 8 g/24h).
Neonate: **IM/IV** *≤7 d:* 60–90 mg/kg/d divided q8–12h; *>7 d:* 60–120 mg/kg/d divided q6–12 h.
Child >1 mo: **IM/IV** 90–120 mg/kg/d divided q6–8h.

Cystic Fibrosis

Child: **IM/IV** 50 mg/kg q6–8h (max 8 g/d).

PHARMACOKINETICS Peak: 1 h IM. **Distribution:** widely distributed including synovial and blister fluid, bile, bronchial secretions, prostate, bone, and CSF; crosses placenta; distributed into breast milk in small amounts. **Metabolism:** not extensively metabolized. **Elimination:** half-life: 1.6–2.1 h; 60–70% excreted in urine within 24 h.

CONTRAINDICATIONS & PRECAUTIONS Contraindicated in: safe use during pregnancy (category B), in nursing women, infants, and children not established. **Cautious use in:** history of hypersensitivity reaction to penicillin, cephalosporins, or to other drugs; impaired renal or hepatic function.

ADVERSE/SIDE EFFECTS CNS: headache, dizziness, confusion, paresthesias, insomnia, seizures. **ENT:** tinnitus, nasal congestion, sneezing. **Eye:** diplopia. **GI:** nausea, *diarrhea,* vomiting. **Hematologic:** eosinophilia. **Hepatic:** elevations of liver function tests. **Hypersensitivity:** urticaria, eosinophilia, anaphylaxis. **Local reactions:** phlebitis, thrombophle-

B

bitis (following IV), pain at injection sites. **Skin:** rash, purpura, erythema multiforme, exfoliative dermatitis, diaphoresis; petechiae, pruritus. **Other:** superinfections (gram-positive cocci), vaginal candidiasis.

DIAGNOSTIC TEST INTERFERENCE
Aztreonam may cause transient elevations of ***liver function tests,*** increases in ***PT*** and ***PTT,*** minor changes in ***Hgb,*** and positive ***Coombs' test.***

DRUG INTERACTIONS **Imipenem-cilastatin, cefoxitin** may be antagonistic; **probenecid** slows renal elimination of aztreonam.

INCOMPATIBILITIES **Solution/additive: ampicillin, metronidazole, nafcillin.**

NURSING IMPLICATIONS

Administration

- For IM injection, reconstitute 15- or 30-ml vial with at least 3 ml of diluent per gram of aztreonam. Immediately and vigorously shake vial to dissolve. Suitable diluents include sterile water for injection; bacteriostatic water for injection (with benzyl alcohol and propyl parabens); NaCl 0.9% for injection.
- IM injections should be made deeply into large muscle mass such as the upper outer quadrant of the gluteus maximus or lateral thigh. Rotate injections sites.
- IV administration: IV aztreonam may be given direct IV with a single dose diluted in 6–10 ml of sterile water for injection. Immediately shake vial until solution is dissolved. Give over 3–5 min.
- IV administration to neonates, infants, and children: Verify correct IV concentration and rate of infusion/injection with physician.
- Refer to manufacturer's package insert for complete details of solution preparation for IV infusion and stability information.
- Reconstituted solutions are colorless to light straw yellow and turn slightly pink on standing. Reportedly, this does not affect potency.

Assessment & Drug Effects

- Culture and susceptibility tests should be performed before initiation of therapy.
- Before treatment is initiated, a detailed history should be obtained of drug allergies so that necessary precautions may be observed.
- Renal function should be monitored, particularly in the elderly and in those with history of renal impairment. Estimates of creatinine clearance should be made initially and at regular intervals during therapy and used as a guide to dosage.
- Be watchful for signs of opportunistic infections (diarrhea, rectal or vaginal itching or discharge, fever, cough), and promptly report this onset to physician. Overgrowth of nonsusceptible organisms, particularly staphylococci, streptococci, and fungi, is a threat, especially in patients receiving prolonged or repeated therapy.
- Inspect IV injection sites daily for signs of inflammation. Reportedly, pain and phlebitis occur in over 2% of patients.

BACAMPICILLIN HYDROCHLORIDE

(ba-kam-pi-sill'in)

Trade names: Penglobe ♣, Spectrobid

Classifications: ANTIINFECTIVE; ANTIBIOTIC; AMINOPENICILLIN

Prototype: Ampicillin

Pregnancy category: B

ACTIONS/PHARMACODYNAMICS Acid-stable, penicillinase-sensitive aminopenicillin that is rapidly hydrolyzed to ampicillin in body. Has broad spectrum of antimicrobial activity and exerts antibacterial action by inhibiting bacterial cell wall biosynthesis. More rapidly and completely absorbed from GI tract than ampicillin is, and serum concentrations attained are higher.

USES Infections caused by susceptible microorganisms of upper and lower respiratory tract, urinary tract, skin and skin structures; acute uncomplicated gonorrhea.

ROUTE & DOSAGE

Moderate to Severe Infections

Adult: **PO** 400–800 mg q12h.
Child: **PO** 12.5–25 mg/kg q12h.

Gonorrhea

Adult: **PO** 1.6 g with 1 g probenecid x 1.

PHARMACOKINETICS **Absorption:** rapidly and almost completely absorbed; hydrolyzed to ampicillin. **Distribution:** most body tissues; crosses placenta; appears in breast milk. **Metabolism:** metabolized in liver. **Elimination:** half-life: 0.7–1.1 h; 75% eliminated as ampicillin in urine within 8 h.

CONTRAINDICATIONS & PRECAUTIONS **Contraindicated in:** hypersensitivity to penicillins; pregnancy (category B); infectious mononucleosis or other viral diseases; children <25 kg. **Cautious use in:** history of allergy to cephalosporins; nursing mothers.

ADVERSE/SIDE EFFECTS **GI:** *nausea,* vomiting, anorexia, *diarrhea.* **Hematologic:** thrombocytopenia, eosinophilia, anemia. **Hypersensitivity:** erythematous rash; anaphylaxis (rare). **Other:** superinfections, fixed drug eruption.

DIAGNOSTIC TEST INTERFERENCE High urine bacampicillin concentrations can result in false positive ***urine glucose determinations with copper sulfate tests*** (Benedict's, Clinitest, Fehling's); glucose oxidase methods (Clinistix, Tes-Tape) are not affected. ***Serum ALT*** (SGPT) and ***AST*** (SGOT) may increase.

DRUG INTERACTIONS **Allopurinol** increases incidence of rash; since ampicillin may interfere with ORAL CONTRACEPTIVE action, female patients should be advised to consider nonhormonal contraception while on antibiotics. **Drug–food:** food may decrease absorption of bacampicillin; give 1 h before or 2 h after meals.

NURSING IMPLICATIONS

Administration

- Food does not retard or reduce absorption of bacampicillin in tablet form.
- Oral suspension is affected by food and therefore should be taken on an empty stomach. Administer preferably with a full glass (240 ml) of water either 1 h before or 2 h after meals.
- The oral suspension is intended for use in children and infants weighing <25 kg, or in children who are unable to swallow tablets.
- When dispensed, oral suspension should include a calibrated liquid measuring device.
- Store in tight container at 15–30C (59–86F) unless otherwise directed.

Assessment & Drug Effects

- Careful inquiry should be made

B

before initiation of therapy concerning previous hypersensitivity reactions to penicillins, cephalosporins, and other allergens.

- Culture and susceptibility tests should be performed before therapy is begun.
- Baseline and periodic checks of renal, hepatic, and hematopoietic status are advised during prolonged therapy, particularly in patients with history of impaired function of these systems, and in prematures and neonates.

Patient & Family Education

- Instruct patient to report symptoms of an allergic hypersensitivity reaction immediately (see Appendix G).
- Advise patient to report signs of superinfection (see Appendix G).
- Emphasize need to take medication for the full course of therapy as prescribed.
- Stubborn infections may require several months of clinical or bacteriologic follow-up, or both, after therapy has stopped. Urge patient to keep follow-up appointments.

BACITRACIN

(bass-i-tray′sin)

Trade names: Baciguent, Baciguent Ophthalmic, Bacitin, Bacitracin Ophthalmic

Classifications: ANTIINFECTIVE; ANTIBIOTIC

Pregnancy category: C

ACTIONS/PHARMACODYNAMICS Polypeptide antibiotic derived from cultures of *Bacillus subtilis*. Precise mechanism of action not known. Appears to interfere with function of bacterial cell membrane by inhibiting cell wall synthesis. Spectrum of antibacterial activity similar to that of penicillin. Bactericidal or bacteriostatic depending on concentration and susceptibility of organism. Active against many gram-positive organisms including streptococci, staphylococci, pneumococci, corynebacteria, *Clostridia, Neisseria, Hemophilus influenzae,* and *Treponema pallidum*. Also active against gonococci and meningococci; ineffective against most other gram-negative organisms. Has neuromuscular blocking action.

USES Parenteral therapy restricted to infants with staphylococcal pneumonia and empyema due to susceptible organisms where adequate laboratory facilities and constant supervision are available. Used topically in treatment of superficial infections of skin and eye. **Unlabeled uses:** orally for treatment of antibiotic-associated colitis. Has been used investigationally by various routes (intrathecal, intrapleural, intrasynovial) for serious infections.

ROUTE & DOSAGE

Systemic Infections

Child: **IM** <2.5 kg: up to 900 U/kg/24h divided q8–12h; >2.5 kg: up to 1000 U/kg/24h divided q8–12h.

Skin Infections

Adult: **Topical** Apply thin layer of ointment b.i.d. or t.i.d. or use a solution of 250–1000 U/ml as a wet dressing. **Ophthalmic ointment:** applied to conjunctival sac 1 or more times/d.

PHARMACOKINETICS Absorption: poorly absorbed from intact or denuded skin or mucous membranes. **Peak:** 1–2 h IM. **Duration:** 6–8 h. **Distribution:** widely distributed including peritoneal and ascitic fluids. **Elimination:** slow renal excretion (10–40% in 24 h).

CONTRAINDICATIONS & PRECAUTIONS **Contraindicated in:** toxic reaction or renal dysfunction associated with bacitracin; impaired renal function; atopic individuals; pregnancy (category C). **Cautious use in:** myasthenia gravis or other neuromuscular disease. Patients allergic to neomycin may be sensitive to bacitracin.

ADVERSE/SIDE EFFECTS **Eye:** delayed corneal healing. **GI:** anorexia, nausea, vomiting, diarrhea, rectal itching and burning. **Hematologic** (systemic use): bone marrow depression, blood dyscrasias; eosinophilia. **Hypersensitivity** (associated with both systemic and topical use): erythema, <u>anaphylaxis</u>. **GU:** <u>Nephrotoxicity</u> (dose related): increased BUN, uremia, renal tubular and <u>glomerular necrosis</u>. **Other:** pain and inflammation at injection site, fever, superinfection, neuromuscular blockade with <u>respiratory depression</u>; tinnitus.

DRUG INTERACTIONS With AMINOGLYCOSIDES, possibility of additive nephrotoxic and neuromuscular blocking effects; with **tubocurarine** and other NONDEPOLARIZING SKELETAL MUSCLE RELAXANTS, possibility of additive neuromuscular blocking effects.

NURSING IMPLICATIONS

Administration

- Bacitracin should not be reconstituted with diluents containing parabens because solution may precipitate or become cloudy.
- Parenteral solution (for IM use only) should be dissolved in 0.9% NaCl injection containing 2% procaine hydrochloride (prescribed). Alternate injection sites since injections are painful.
- Administration of parenteral bacitracin for longer than 12 d is not advised.
- Intramuscular bacitracin solution is stable for 1 wk if refrigerated; inactivation occurs at room temperature. Dry bacitracin should be stored in refrigerator at 2–8C (36–46F). Topical ointments should be stored in tightly closed containers at 15–30C (59–86F) unless otherwise directed.

Assessment & Drug Effects

- Culture and susceptibility tests should be performed before therapy begins and periodically during therapy.
- Before systemic therapy is begun, determinations should be made of BUN and nonprotein nitrogen (NPN), and urine should be examined for albumin, casts, and cellular elements. Renal function should be monitored daily throughout therapy.
- Be alert to signs of local allergic manifestations (itching, burning, redness) with topical skin applications. Local reactions have preceded life-threatening anaphylactic episodes.
- Monitor I&O during parenteral therapy. Adequate urinary output should be maintained to reduce possibility of renal toxicity. If fluid intake is inadequate or urinary output decreases, report to physician.
- Inspect urine for turbidity and hematuria, and be on the alert for other signs and symptoms of urinary tract dysfunction. Note and report any changes in urination pattern, e.g., oliguria, urinary frequency, nocturia.
- Prolonged use may result in overgrowth of nonsusceptible organisms, especially *Candida albicans.*

Patient & Family Education

- Instruct patient taking ophthalmic preparation to stop drug and notify physician if signs of hypersen-

B

sitivity appear: itching, burning, swelling of eyelids.

- Instruct patient to report local allergic manifestations with topical applications, e.g., itching, burning, redness.

BACLOFEN

(bak'loe-fen)

Trade names: Lioresal, Lioresal DS

Classifications: AUTONOMIC NERVOUS SYSTEM AGENT; CENTRAL-ACTING SKELETAL MUSCLE RELAXANT

Prototype: Cyclobenzaprine

Pregnancy category: C

ACTIONS/PHARMACODYNAMICS

Centrally acting skeletal muscle relaxant. Precise mechanism of action not determined. Depresses monosynaptic and polysynaptic afferent reflex activity at spinal cord level thereby reducing skeletal muscle spasm caused by upper motor neuron lesions.

USES To provide symptomatic relief of painful spasms in multiple sclerosis and in the management of detrusor sphincter dyssynergia in spinal cord injury or disease. **Unlabeled uses:** treatment of trigeminal neuralgia and of tardive dystonia associated with antipsychotic medications.

ROUTE & DOSAGE

Muscle Spasm

Adult: **PO** 5 mg t.i.d.; may increase by 5 mg/dose q3d prn (max 80 mg/d).
Child: **PO** 2–7 y: 10–15 mg/d divided q8h; may increase by 5–15 mg/d q3d to max of 40 mg/d; ≥8 y: as for 2–7 y to max of 60 mg/d.

Adult: **Intrathecal** Used with implantable intrathecal infusion pump. Prior to pump implantation, give patient a trial dose using an initial bolus of 50 μg/ml administered in intrathecal space by barbotage over a period not less than 1 min. Observe patient over next 4–8 h for significant decrease in muscle spasm. If response is less than desired, administer second bolus of 75 μg/1.5 ml and observe 4–8 h. May repeat in 24 h with a 100 μg/2-ml bolus if necessary. ***Postimplant titration:*** Use screening dose if response lasted >12 h or double screening dose if response lasted <12 h and administer over 24 h. After first 24 h, decrease dose by 10–30% q24h until desired response achieved. Maintenance doses range from 12–1500 μg/d, with most patients maintained on 300–800 μg/d.

PHARMACOKINETICS **Absorption:** readily absorbed from GI tract. **Peak:** 2–3 h. **Duration:** 8 h. **Distribution:** minimal amounts cross blood–brain barrier; crosses placenta; distribution into breast milk unknown. **Metabolism:** 15% of dose metabolized in liver. **Elimination:** half-life: 3–4 h; 70–85% excreted in urine within 72 h; some elimination in feces.

CONTRAINDICATIONS & PRECAUTIONS **Contraindicated in:** safe use during pregnancy (category C), in nursing mothers, and in children <12 yr not established. **Cautious use in:** impaired renal and hepatic function; epilepsy; diabetes mellitus; stroke; psychiatric or brain disorders; elderly patients.

B

ADVERSE/SIDE EFFECTS **CNS:** *transient drowsiness,* vertigo, dizziness, weakness, fatigue, headache, confusion, insomnia; ataxia, loss of seizure control in epileptic patients. **CV:** hypotension. **ENT:** tinnitus, nasal congestion. **Eye:** blurred vision, mydriasis, nystagmus, diplopia, strabismus, miosis. **GI:** nausea, constipation, vomiting. **GU:** urinary frequency. **Hepatic:** mild increases in AST (SGOT), and alkaline phosphatase, jaundice.

DIAGNOSTIC TEST INTERFERENCE Possibility of increases in ***blood glucose,*** serum ***alkaline phosphatase,*** and ***AST*** levels.

DRUG INTERACTIONS **Alcohol,** CNS DEPRESSANTS, MAO INHIBITORS, ANTIHISTAMINES compound CNS depression; baclofen may increase blood glucose levels, making it necessary to increase dosage of SULFONYLUREAS, **insulin.**

NURSING IMPLICATIONS

Administration

- For intrathecal use, give by direct intrathecal injection (via lumbar puncture or catheter) over at least 1 min or longer.
- For intrathecal use, dilute *only* with sterile, preservative-free 0.9% NaCl injection. Baclofen must be diluted to a concentration of 50 μg/ml when preparing test doses.
- If patient complains of GI distress, oral drug may be administered with food or milk.
- Store at 15–30C (59–86F) in tightly closed container unless otherwise directed.

Assessment & Drug Effects

- Supervise ambulation. Initially, the loss of spasticity induced by baclofen may affect patient's ability to stand or walk.
- Baseline and periodic checks should be made of BP, weight, blood sugar, hepatic function tests, and urine.
- Advise patient to report adverse reactions to physician. Most can be reduced by decreasing dosage. Incidence of CNS symptoms (drowsiness, dizziness, ataxia) are reportedly high in patients >40 y of age.
- Many of the adverse neuropsychiatric or genitourinary symptoms resemble those of the underlying disease. Carefully assess them and report them to the physician.
- The elderly are especially sensitive to this drug. Observe carefully for side effects: mental confusion, depression, hallucinations.
- Patients with epilepsy should be closely monitored by EEG, clinical observation, and interview at regular intervals for possible loss of seizure control.
- Observe for and record response to drug. Therapeutic effectiveness may be noted in a few hours to weeks.

Patient & Family Education

- Warn patient that CNS depressant effects will be additive to other CNS depressants, including alcohol.
- Inform diabetics that baclofen may raise blood glucose levels. Urge patient to report promptly changes in urine or blood tests to the physician. Dose adjustment of insulin and hypoglycemic agents may be indicated.
- Warn patient to avoid driving and other potentially hazardous activities until the reaction to baclofen is determined.
- Caution patient not to self-dose with OTC drugs without physician's approval.

B

- Inform patient that drug withdrawal should be accomplished gradually over a period of 2 wk or more. Abrupt withdrawal following prolonged administration may cause anxiety, agitated behavior, auditory and visual hallucinations, severe tachycardia, acute exacerbation of spasticity, and seizures.

BASILIXIMAB

(bas-i-lix'i-mab)

Trade name: Simulect

Prototype for classifications:
IMMUNOSUPPRESSANT; MONOCLONAL ANTIBODY; INTERLEUKIN-2 RECEPTOR ANTIBODY

Pregnancy category: B

ACTIONS/PHARMACODYNAMICS Immunosuppressant agent that is an interleukin-2 receptor monoclonal antibody produced by recombinant DNA technology. Binds to and blocks interleukin-2R-alpha chain (CD-25 antibody) on surface of activated T lymphocytes. This binding inhibits a critical pathway in the immune response of the lymphocytes involved in allograft rejection.

USE Prophylaxis of acute renal transplant rejection.

ROUTE & DOSAGE

Prophylaxis for transplant rejection

Adult: **IV** 20 mg × 2 doses, first dose given 2 h before transplant surgery and second dose 4 days after transplant.
Child 2–15 y: **IV** 12 mg/m^2 (max 20 mg/dose) × 2 doses, first dose given 2 h before transplant surgery and second dose 4 days after transplant.

PHARMACOKINETICS **Duration:** 36 days. **Distribution:** binds to interleukin-2R-alpha sites on lymphocytes. **Elimination:** half-life: 7.2 ± 3.2 d in adults, 11.5 ± 6.3 d in children.

CONTRAINDICATIONS & PRECAUTIONS **Contraindicated in:** hypersensitivity to basiliximab, serious infection, or exposure to viral infections, e.g., chickenpox, herpes zoster, nursing mothers. **Cautious use in:** history of untoward reactions to dacliximab or other monoclonal antibodies, pregnancy (category B).

ADVERSE/SIDE EFFECTS **Body as whole:** pain, peripheral edema, edema, fever, viral infection, asthenia, arthralgia. **CNS:** headache, tremor, dizziness, insomnia, paresthesias, agitation, depression. **CV:** hypertension, chest pain, hypotension, arrhythmias. **GI:** constipation, nausea, diarrhea, abdominal pain, vomiting, dyspepsia, moniliasis, flatulence, GI hemorrhage, melena, esophagitis, erosive stomatitis. **Hematologic:** anemia, thrombocytopenia, thrombosis, polycythemia. **Respiratory:** dyspnea, URI, cough, rhinitis, pharyngitis, bronchospasm. **Skin:** poor wound healing, acne. **Urinary:** dysuria, UTI, albuminuria, hematuria, oliguria, frequency, renal tubular necrosis, urinary retention. **Other:** hyperkalemia, hypokalemia, hyperglycemia, hyperuricemia, hypophosphatemia, hypocalcemia, increased weight, hypercholesterolemia, acidosis, cataract, conjunctivitis.

NURSING IMPLICATIONS

Administration

- IV preparation: Add 5 ml sterile water for injection, then rock vial gently to dissolve; further dilute with 50 ml 0.9% NaCl or D5W; in-

B

vert infusion bag to dissolve; do not shake. Discard if diluted solution is colored or has particulate matter.

- IV infusion for adults and children: Infuse diluted drug over 20–30 min.
- Reconstituted solution should be used immediately but may be stored at room temperature for 4 h or at 2–8C (36–46F) for 24 h. Discard after 24 h.
- Store undiluted drug at 2–8C (36–46F).

Assessment & Drug Effects

- Therapeutic effectiveness is indicated by prevention of renal transplant rejection.
- Carefully monitor for and immediately report S&S of opportunistic infection or anaphylactoid reaction (see Appendix G).

Patient & Family Education

- Report any distressing adverse effects.
- If possible avoid vaccination for 2 wk following last dose of drug.

BCG (BACILLUS CALMETTE-GUÉRIN) VACCINE

(ba-cil′lus cal′met-te guer′in)

Trade names: Tice, Theracys

Classifications: VACCINE; IMMUNOMODULATOR; ANTINEOPLASTIC; BIOLOGICAL RESPONSE MODIFIER

Pregnancy category: C

ACTIONS/PHARMACODYNAMICS

BCG vaccine is an immunization agent for tuberculosis (TB). It is an attenuated strain of the bacillus Calmette and Guérin strain of *Mycobacterium bovis*. BCG vaccine stimulates the reticuloendothelial system (RES) to produce macrophages that do not allow mycobacteria to multiply. BCG live is used intravesically as a biological response modifier for bladder cancer in situ. It is thought to cause a local, chronic inflammatory response involving macrophage and leukocyte infiltration of the bladder. This local inflammatory response leads to destruction of superficial tumor cells. BCG is active immunotherapy, which stimulates the immune mechanism to reject the tumor. It enhances the cytotoxicity of macrophages.

USES To protect tuberculin skin test-negative infants and children, and groups with an excessive rate of new TB infections; carcinoma in situ of the bladder. **Unlabeled use:** malignant melanoma.

ROUTE & DOSAGE

Prevention of Tuberculosis (Tice only)

Adult: **Intradermal** 0.1 ml
Adult: **Percutaneous** After reconstitution, the vaccine, 0.2–0.3 ml, is dropped onto the cleansed surface of the skin and administered using a multiple-puncture disk applied through the vaccine.
Child: **Intradermal** <3 mo, 0.05 ml; >3 mo, 0.1 ml.
Child: **Percutaneous** >1 mo, same as adult; <1 mo, reduce adult dose by half (reconstitute with 2 ml rather than 1 ml). May need to redose with full dose at 1 y.

Carcinoma of the Bladder

Adult: **Intravesical** *Theracys*: 3 vials (27 mg each, or 81 mg total) of BCG reconstituted with accompanying diluent, diluted in 50 ml of sterile, preservative-free 0.9% NaCl and instilled into bladder slowly by gravity flow via urethral catheter; suspension is retained for 2 h after which time the patient voids; treatments are begun 7 to 14 d after any biopsies or transurethral resections, and are administered once a week for total of 6 wk, followed by one treatment at 3, 6, 12, 18, and 24 mo. *Tice*: 1 vial per intravesical instillation; usually repeated weekly for 6 wk followed by monthly instillation for 6–12 mo.

CONTRAINDICATIONS & PRECAUTIONS **Contraindicated in:** Impaired immune responses, immunosuppressive corticosteroid therapy, asymptomatic carriers with positive HIV serology, fever, UTI, lactation. **Cautious use in:** hypersensitivity to BCG, pregnancy (category C).

ADVERSE/SIDE EFFECTS **CNS:** intravesical administration: *malaise,* dizziness, headache, weakness. **Endocrine:** hyperpyrexia. **GI:** abdominal pain, anorexia, constipation, nausea, vomiting, diarrhea. **GU:** intravesical administration: bladder spasms, clot retention, decreased bladder capacity, decreased urine flow, *dysuria, hematuria,* incontinence, nocturia, UTI, cystitis, hemorrhagic cystitis, penile pain, prostatism. **Hematologic:** thrombocytopenia, eosinophilia, *anemia,* leukopenia, disseminated intravascular coagulation. **Hepatic:** hepatic dysfunction following intratumor injection, granulomatous hepatitis. **Respiratory:** cough (rare), pulmonary granulomas, pulmonary infection. **Skin:** abscess with recurrent discharge, red papule that scales or ulcerates in about 5–6 wk, dermatomyositis, granulomas at injection site 4–6 wk after inoculation, keloid formation, lupus vulgaris. **Other:** systemic BCG infection, *chills, flu-like syndrome,* anaphylaxis (rare), allergic reactions, lymphadenitis.

DIAGNOSTIC TEST INTERFERENCE Prior BCG vaccination may result in false-positive tuberculin skin test (PPD). Following BCG vaccination, tuberculin sensitivity may persist for months to years.

DRUG INTERACTIONS Concurrent antimycobacterial therapy (**aminosalicylic acid, capreomycin, cycloserine, ethambutol, ethionamide, isoniazid, pyrazinamide, rifabutin, rifampin, streptomycin**) that inhibits multiplication of BCG bacilli has the potential to antagonize or altogether negate the BCG vaccine-mediated immune response. *Cyclosporine* may reduce the immunologic response to BCG vaccine. *Cytomegalovirus immune globulin* and other live vaccines (measles/mumps/rubella, oral polio) may interfere with immune response to BCG. Previous vaccination with or other exposure to BCG may induce variable sensitivity to tuberculin. A greater booster effect following repeat tuberculin testing has been reported in individuals with prior BCG vaccination when compared with individuals without prior vaccination.

NURSING IMPLICATIONS

Administration

- Warning: Do not inject intravenously, subcutaneously, or intradermally.
- To prepare solution, add 1 ml sterile water for injection to 1 ampul of vaccine. Draw into syringe and expel back into ampul 3 times to mix.
- To administer the drug, drop an immunizing dose of 0.2–0.3 ml onto clean surface of skin; then

use a sterile multiple-puncture disk to create percutaneous skin punctures.

- Keep vaccination site dry for 24 h; no dressing is needed.
- During preparation and administration, avoid contact with the vaccine.
- Store reconstituted vaccine and dry BCG powder and diluent refrigerated, 2–8C (35–46F). Use reconstituted solution within 2 h.
- Important: Care should be taken by those handling BCG vaccine to avoid contact with the product. Discarded containers, syringes, and other equipment used for handling the vaccine should be sterilized before disposal.

Assessment & Drug Effects

- Monitor for signs of systemic BCG infection: fever, chills, severe malaise, or cough.
- If systemic infection is suspected, blood and urine cultures should be done.
- Assess for regional lymph node enlargement and report fistula formation.

Patient & Family Education

- Inform patient of potential adverse effects of vaccination.
- Advise patient to keep vaccination site clean until local reaction has subsided.

BECAPLERMIN

(be-cap′ler-min)

Trade name: Regranex

Classifications: HORMONES AND SYNTHETIC SUBSTITUTES; GROWTH FACTOR

Pregnancy category: C

ACTIONS/PHARMACODYNAMICS Recombinant human platelet-derived growth factor B in a topical gel. It enhances formation of new granulation tissue. Becaplemin also induces fibroblast proliferation. It is effective against diabetic neuropathic ulcers that involve subcutaneous or deeper tissue and also have an adequate blood supply.

USE Lower-extremity diabetic neuropathic ulcers.

ROUTE & DOSAGE

Diabetic Neuropathic Ulcers

Adult: **Topical** Calculate the length of gel based on ulcer size (see Administration below), apply to ulcer area, and cover with saline-moistened dressing. After 12 h, remove dressing, clean ulcer, and apply new saline-moistened dressing (without becaplermin). Apply gel once daily until ulcer is healed.

PHARMACOKINETICS Absorption: <3% absorbed into systemic circulation.

CONTRAINDICATIONS & PRECAUTIONS Contraindicated in: hypersensitivity to bacaplemin or any component in formulation; neoplasms at site of application; wounds that close by primary intention; breastfeeding. **Cautious use in:** concurrent use of corticosteroids, cancer chemotherapy, or other immunosuppressive agents; ulcer wounds related to arterial or venous insufficiency; thermal, electrical, or radiation burns at wound site; malignancy; pregnancy (category C).

ADVERSE/SIDE EFFECTS Skin: erythematous rash.

NURSING IMPLICATIONS

Administration

- Apply to only ulcers with good blood supply.
- Dosage calculation: Measure

B

greatest length (L) and greatest width (W) of ulcer in inches or centimeters; using 15- or 7.5-g tube multiply $(L \times W) \times 0.6$ for dose in inches or $(L \times W)/4$ for dose in cm; using 2-g tube multiply $(L \times W) \times 1.3$ for dose in inches or $(L \times W)/2$ for dose in cm.

- Amount of drug needed should be recalculated weekly/biweekly by wound care provider.
- Application: Squeeze calculated length of gel onto clean, firm, nonabsorbable surface; with clean tongue depressor or cotton swab apply even layer over ulcer; cover for 12 h with gauze moistened with saline; remove gauze, rinse with water or saline to remove residual gel; recover only with moist gauze for next 12 h; repeat cycle.
- Store at 2–8C (36–46F). Do not freeze and do not use beyond expiration date.

Assessment & Drug Effects

- Therapeutic effectiveness is indicated by approximately 30% decrease in ulcer size after 10 wk or complete healing after 20 wk.
- Monitor for and report appearance of erythematous rash.

Patient & Family Education

- Dose should be recalculated weekly/biweekly by wound care provider.
- Carefully follow directions for application. Gel may be measured out on waxed paper.
- Wash hands prior to application and do not allow tip of tube to contact ulcer or any surface.
- Report worsening ulceration or development of skin rash.

BECLOMETHASONE DIPROPIONATE

(be-kloe-meth′a-sone)

Trade names: Beclovent, Beconase Nasal Inhaler, Vancenase Nasal Inhaler, Vanceril, Vanceril D, Vancenas AQ

Classifications: SYNTHETIC HORMONE; ADRENAL CORTICOSTEROID

Prototype: Hydrocortisone

Pregnancy category: C

See Appendix A.

BELLADONNA EXTRACT

BELLADONNA TINCTURE

(bell-a-don′a)

Classifications: AUTONOMIC NERVOUS SYSTEM AGENT; ANTICHOLINERGIC (PARASYMPATHOLYTIC); ANTIMUSCARINIC, ANTISPASMODIC

Prototype: Atropine

Pregnancy category: C

ACTIONS/PHARMACODYNAMICS

Reversibly blocks action of acetylcholine at parasympathetic neuroeffector sites, thereby inhibiting smooth muscle contractions and suppressing secretions of secretory glands.

USES Adjunct in treatment of peptic ulcer disease, irritable bowel syndrome, and neurogenic bowel disturbances. Also has been used for dysmenorrhea, nocturnal enuresis, spasms of urinary tract, nausea and vomiting of pregnancy, vertigo, and for symptomatic relief of parkinsonism.

ROUTE & DOSAGE

Antispasmodic

Adult: **PO** 15–30 mg of extract t.i.d. or q.i.d.; 0.6–1 ml of tincture t.i.d. or q.i.d.
Child: **PO** 0.1 ml/kg/d of tincture in 3–4 divided doses (max 3.5 ml/d).

PHARMACOKINETICS Absorption: readily absorbed from GI tract. **Onset:** 1–2 h. **Distribution:** well distributed in body; crosses blood–brain barrier. **Elimination:** excreted unchanged in urine.

CONTRAINDICATIONS & PRECAUTIONS Contraindicated in: hypersensitivity to anticholinergic drugs; obstructive uropathy, atony of urinary bladder; esophageal reflux, obstructive disease of GI tract, intestinal atony, paralytic ileus, severe ulcerative colitis, toxic megacolon; myasthenia gravis; narrow-angle glaucoma; unstable cardiovascular status in acute hemorrhages. Safe use during pregnancy (category C), in nursing women, and of belladonna extract tablets in children not established. **Cautious use in:** autonomic neuropathy; heart disease, hypertension; patients >40 y (higher incidence of glaucoma).

ADVERSE/SIDE EFFECTS Dose related. **CNS:** excitement (young children and the elderly), confusion, delirium. **CV:** rapid heart beat, tachycardia, palpitation. **Eye:** blurred vision, mydriasis, photophobia. **GI:** *dry mouth, constipation*. **GU:** urinary retention, urgency.

DRUG INTERACTIONS Amantadine, ANTIHISTAMINES, TRICYCLIC ANTIDEPRESSANTS, **quinidine, disopyramide, procainamide** have additive anticholinergic effects; **levodopa** effects decreased; **methotrimeprazine** may precipitate extrapyramidal effects; antipsychotic effects of phenothiazines decreased (decreased absorption).

NURSING IMPLICATIONS

Administration

- Usually administered 30–60 min before meals and at bedtime.
- If patient is receiving antacid therapy, the antacid is given after meals. Space administration of antacid and belladonna preparations at least 1 h apart.
- Store at 15–30C (59–86F) in tightly covered, light-resistant containers, unless otherwise directed.

Assessment & Drug Effects

- Assess patient for therapeutic drug effects.
- Since drug may cause drowsiness and confusion, carefully monitor ambulation of elderly or debilitated patient.
- Monitor I&O and assess for urinary retention.

Patient & Family Education

- Instruct patient to be aware of I&O. Increase in fluid intake and bulk in diet may be allowed to prevent or relieve constipation. If it persists, notify physician.
- Caution patient to avoid hot baths, saunas, and strenuous work or exercise during hot and humid weather.
- Advise patient to refrain from driving and other potentially hazardous activities until reaction to drug is determined.
- If mouth dryness is a problem, instruct patient to practice meticulous oral hygiene. Sugarless gum or lemon drops and frequent sips of water may help.

BENAZEPRIL HYDROCHLORIDE

(ben-a′ze-pril)

Trade name: Lotensin

Classifications: CARDIOVASCULAR AGENT; ANGIOTENSIN-CONVERTING ENZYME (ACE) INHIBITOR

Prototype: Captopril

Pregnancy category: D

ACTIONS/PHARMACODYNAMICS Lowers blood pressure by specific

B

inhibition of the angiotensin-converting enzyme (ACE) and by decreasing angiotensin II (a potent vasoconstrictor) and aldosterone secretion. Both actions achieve an antihypertensive effect by suppression of the renin-angiotensin-aldosterone system.

USE Treatment of mild to moderate hypertension. **Unlabeled use:** CHF.

ROUTE & DOSAGE

Hypertension

Adult: **PO** 10–40 mg/d in 1–2 divided doses.

PHARMACOKINETICS Absorption: readily absorbed from GI tract with 37% reaching the systemic circulation. **Peak:** 2–6 h. **Duration:** 20–24 h. **Distribution:** small amounts cross the blood-brain barrier; crosses placenta; small amount excreted in breast milk. **Metabolism:** metabolized in liver to active metabolite, benazeprilat. **Elimination:** half-life: benazepril 0.6 h; benazeprilat 22 h; benazeprilat is primarily excreted in urine.

CONTRAINDICATIONS & PRECAUTIONS Contraindicated in: hypersensitivity to benazepril or another ACE inhibitor. Safe use during pregnancy (category D), in nursing mothers, or in children not established. **Cautious use in:** renal impairment, renal-artery stenosis; patients with hypovolemia, receiving diuretics, undergoing dialysis; patients in whom excessive hypotension would present a hazard (e.g., cerebrovascular insufficiency); CHF; hepatic impairment; diabetes mellitus.

ADVERSE/SIDE EFFECTS CV: hypotension. **CNS:** *headache,* dizziness, fatigue, weakness. **Endocrine:** hyperkalemia (at higher doses). **GI:** nausea, diarrhea or constipation, gastritis. **GU:** azotemia, oliguria, renal failure in patients with CHF. **Other:** cough, rhinitis, bronchitis, back pain.

DRUG INTERACTIONS POTASSIUM-SPARING DIURETICS may increase the risk of hyperkalemia. Benazepril may increase **lithium** levels, resulting in lithium toxicity.

DIAGNOSTIC TEST INTERFERENCE Elevations in ***serum bilirubin*** have been observed after benazepril administration. Benazepril inhibits aldosterone secretion, which causes an increase in ***serum potassium.***

NURSING IMPLICATIONS

Administration

- To avoid hypotension, the initial dose usually is given 2–3 d after discontinuation of diuretic therapy.
- In the presence of concomitant diuretic therapy, the initial dose usually is limited to 5 mg.
- Drug may be administered without regard to meals.
- Drug may be stored at room temperature but not above 30C (86F).

Assessment & Drug Effects

- Assess for hypotension, especially in patients who may be volume depleted (eg, prolonged diuretic therapy, recent vomiting or diarrhea, salt restriction).
- Monitor for excessive hypotension in patients with CHF.
- Monitor serum potassium levels for hyperkalemia (see Appendix G).

Patient & Family Education

- Advise against salt substitutes unless they are recommended by physician.
- Instruct patient to immediately re-

port swelling of face, eyes, lips, or tongue or difficulty breathing.

BENDROFLUMETHIAZIDE

(ben-droe-floo-meth-eye′a-zide)
Trade name: Naturetin
Classifications: WATER BALANCE AGENT; THIAZIDE DIURETIC
Prototype: Hydrochlorothiazide
Pregnancy category: C

ACTIONS/PHARMACODYNAMICS Thiazide diuretic chemically related to the sulfonamides. Similar to hydrochlorothiazide in pharmacologic actions, uses, contraindications, precautions, adverse effects, and interactions. Reportedly does not alter serum electrolyte concentrations appreciably at recommended doses.

USES Management of edema associated with CHF, mild hypertension. **Unlabeled use:** lithium-associated diabetes insipidus.

ROUTE & DOSAGE

Hypertension
Adult: **PO** 2.5–20 mg/d in 1–2 divided doses.
Child: **PO** 0.05–0.4 mg/kg/d in 1–2 divided doses.

PHARMACOKINETICS **Absorption:** readily absorbed from GI tract. **Onset:** 1–2 h. **Peak:** 6–12 h. **Duration:** 18–24 h. **Elimination:** excreted unchanged in urine within 24 h.

CONTRAINDICATIONS & PRECAUTIONS **Contraindicated in:** anuria, hypersensitivity to thiazides, sulfonamides; pregnancy (category C), lactation. **Cautious use in:** renal and hepatic disease; gout; diabetes mellitus.

ADVERSE/SIDE EFFECTS Orthostatic hypotension, electrolyte imbalance, hypokalemia, hyperglycemia, impaired glucose tolerance, hyperuricemia, exacerbation of gout.

DRUG INTERACTIONS **Cholestyramine, colestipol** decrease absorption of the diuretic; **diazoxide** has additive effects; with **digoxin,** the hypokalemia may increase risk of digitalis toxicity; increases **lithium** levels and toxicity; may increase blood glucose levels, necessitating adjustment of hypoglycemic therapy, i.e., SULFONYLUREAS, **insulin.**

NURSING IMPLICATIONS

Administration
- Administer drug early in AM after patient has eaten to reduce gastric irritation and to prevent possibility of interrupted sleep because of diuresis. If 2 doses are ordered, administer second dose no later than 3 PM.
- Store tablets in tightly closed container at 15–30C (59–86F) unless otherwise specified.

Assessment & Drug Effects
- Antihypertensive effects are generally noted in 3–4 d; maximal effects may require 3–4 wk.
- Monitor BP, I&O ratio and pattern, and weight, particularly during first phase of antihypertensive therapy. Report a sudden fall in BP, which may initiate severe postural hypotension and potentially dangerous perfusion problems of the extremities, especially in older patients.
- Orthostatic hypotension can be a distressing side effect in the elderly.
- Monitor for hypokalemia (see Signs & Symptoms, Appendix G). Report promptly.
- Hyperuricemia can be asymptomatic because thiazides interfere

B

with uric acid excretion, although rarely precipitate acute gout. Report onset of joint pain and limitation of motion.

- The prediabetic or diabetes mellitus patient should be watched carefully for loss of control of diabetes or early signs of hyperglycemia (see Signs & Symptoms, Appendix G). These symptoms are slow to develop and difficult to recognize. Notify physician, and question need to adjust insulin dosage.

Patient & Family Education

- Hypokalemia is rarely severe with thiazides. However, to prevent onset, urge patient to eat potassium-rich foods such as fruit juices, potatoes, cereals, skim milk, and bananas.
- Counsel patient to avoid OTC drugs unless they are approved by physician. Many preparations contain both potassium and sodium and if misused, or if patient overdoses, could induce electrolyte imbalance side effects.

BENZALKONIUM CHLORIDE

(benz-al-koe′nee-um)

Trade names: Benza, Benzalchlor-50, Germicin, Pharmatex♣, Sabol, Zephiran

Classifications: SKIN AND MUCOUS MEMBRANE AGENT; TOPICAL ANTIINFECTIVE; ANTIBIOTIC

Pregnancy category: C

ACTIONS/PHARMACODYNAMICS Bactericidal or bacteriostatic action (depending on concentration), probably due to inactivation of bacterial enzyme. Effective against bacteria, some fungi (including yeasts) and certain protozoa, e.g., *Trichomonas vaginalis*. Generally not effective against spore-forming organisms.

USES Antisepsis of intact skin, mucous membranes, superficial injuries, and infected wounds; also for irrigations of the eye and body cavities and for vaginal douching. A component of several contact lens wetting and cushioning solutions, and a preservative for ophthalmic solutions.

ROUTE & DOSAGE

Minor Wounds or Preoperative Disinfection

Adult: **Topical** 1:750 tincture or spray.

Preoperative Disinfection of Denuded Skin and Mucous Membranes

Adult: **Topical** 1:10,000–1:2000 solution.

Wet Dressings

Adult: **Topical** 1:5000 solution.

Urinary Bladder Irrigation

Adult: **Topical** 1:20,000–1:5000 solution.

Urinary Bladder Instillation

Adult: **Topical** 1:40,000–1:20,000 solution.

Irrigation of Deep Infected Wounds

Adult: **Topical** 1:20,000–1:3000 solution.

Vaginal Irrigation

Adult: **Topical** 1:5000–1:2000 solution.

Sterile Storage of Instruments, Thermometers, Ampuls

Adult: **Topical** 1:750 solution.

CONTRAINDICATIONS & PRECAUTIONS **Contraindicated in:** casts, occlusive dressings, anal or vaginal packs, pregnancy (category C). **Cautious use in:** irrigation of body cavities.

ADVERSE/SIDE EFFECTS Few or no toxic effects in recommended dilutions. Erythema, local burning, hypersensitivity reactions.

NURSING IMPLICATIONS

Administration

- Detergent action is antagonized by pus and other organic matter, and by soap substitutes (e.g., pHisoHex, pHisoderm). If these agents have been used, rinse skin thoroughly with water, dry, and then apply benzalkonium.
- For preoperative skin preparation, follow use of soap with thorough rinsing, first with water, then with 70% alcohol, before applying benzalkonium. Avoid pooling or prolonged contact of solution with skin.
- Use sterile water for injection as diluent for aqueous solutions to be instilled in wounds or body cavities. For other uses, fresh sterile distilled water is used. Tap water (especially hard water) should not be used because it may contain metallic ions and organic matter that reduce antibacterial potency of benzalkonium chloride.
- If solution stronger than 1:5000 enters the eyes, irrigate immediately and repeatedly with water; see a physician promptly.
- Solutions used on denuded skin or inflamed or irritated tissues should be more dilute than those used on normal tissue.
- Store at room temperature in airtight container, protected from light.

BENZOCAINE

(ben'zoe-caine)

Trade names: Americaine, Americaine Anesthetic Lubricant, Americaine-Otic, Anbesol, Benzocol, Chigger-Tox, Dermoplast, Foille, Hurricaine, Orabase with Benzocaine, Oracin, Orajel, Rhulicaine, Solarcaine, T-caine, Unguentine

Classifications: CNS AGENT; LOCAL ANESTHETIC (ESTER TYPE); ANTIPRURITIC

Prototype: Procaine

Pregnancy category: C

ACTIONS/PHARMACODYNAMICS Produces surface anesthesia by inhibiting conduction of nerve impulses from sensory nerve endings. Probable action in certain OTC appetite suppressants is dulling taste for foods. Almost identical to procaine in chemical structure but has lower solubility; therefore it is slowly absorbed and has prolonged duration of anesthetic action.

USES Temporary relief of pain and discomfort in pruritic skin problems, minor burns and sunburn, minor wounds, and insect bites. Otic preparations are used to relieve pain and itching in acute congestive and serous otitis media, swimmer's ear, and otitis externa. Preparations are also available for toothache, minor sore throat pain, canker sores, hemorrhoids, rectal fissures, pruritus ani or vulvae, as male genital desensitizer to slow onset of ejaculation, and for use as anesthetic-lubricant for passage of catheters and endoscopic tubes.

B

ROUTE & DOSAGE

Anesthetic

Adult: **Topical** Lowest effective dose.
Child: **Topical** Lower strengths.

PHARMACOKINETICS **Absorption:** poorly absorbed through intact skin; readily absorbed from mucous membranes. **Peak:** 1 min. **Duration:** 15–30 min. **Metabolism:** metabolized by plasma cholinesterases and to a lesser extent by hepatic cholinesterases. **Elimination:** metabolites excreted in urine.

CONTRAINDICATIONS & PRECAUTIONS **Contraindicated in:** hypersensitivity to benzocaine or other PABA derivatives (e.g., sunscreen preparations), or to any of the components in the formulation; use of ear preparation in patients with perforated eardrum or ear discharge; applications to large areas; use in children <2 y. Safe use during pregnancy (category C) not established. **Cautious use in:** history of drug sensitivity; denuded skin or severely traumatized mucosa; children <6 y.

ADVERSE/SIDE EFFECTS Low toxicity. Sensitization in susceptible individuals; allergic reactions, anaphylaxis. Methemoglobinemia reported in infants.

DRUG INTERACTION Benzocaine may antagonize antibacterial activity of SULFONAMIDES.

NURSING IMPLICATIONS

Administration

- Avoid contact of all preparations with eyes and be careful not to inhale mist when spray form is used. Do not use spray near open flame or cautery and do not expose to high temperatures. Hold can at least 12 inches (30 cm) away from affected area when spraying.
- Chemical burns should be washed and neutralized before benzocaine is applied.
- Before administration of hemorrhoidal preparation, rectal area should be thoroughly cleaned and dried. Usually administered morning and evening and after each bowel movement.
- Store at 15–30C (59–86F) in tight, light-resistant containers unless otherwise specified.

Patient & Family Education

- Bear in mind that when used on oral mucosa, benzocaine may interfere with second (pharyngeal) stage of swallowing. If possible, liquids and foods should not be taken for about 1 h following administration to prevent possible aspiration and mouth injury (biting tongue or buccal mucosa).
- Use specific benzocaine preparation only for problem for which prescribed or recommended by manufacturer.
- Most local anesthetics are potentially sensitizing to susceptible individuals when applied repeatedly or over extensive areas. Instruct patient to discontinue medication if the condition being treated persists, worsens, or if signs of sensitivity, irritation, or infection occur.

BENZONATATE

(ben-zoe′na-tate)
Trade name: Tessalon
Prototype for classification: ANTITUSSIVE
Pregnancy category: C

ACTIONS/PHARMACODYNAMICS Nonnarcotic antitussive chemically related to **tetracaine.** Antitussive activity reported to be somewhat less effective than that of **codeine.** Does not inhibit respiratory center at recommended doses.

USES Decreases frequency and intensity of nonproductive cough in acute and chronic respiratory conditions. Also used in bronchoscopy, thoracentesis, and other procedures when coughing must be avoided.

ROUTE & DOSAGE

Antitussive

Adult: **PO** 100 mg t.i.d. prn up to 600 mg/d.
Child: **PO** <10 y: 8 mg/kg/d in 3–6 divided doses.

PHARMACOKINETICS **Onset:** 15–20 min. **Duration:** 3–8 h.

CONTRAINDICATIONS & PRECAUTIONS **Contraindicated in:** safe use during pregnancy (category C) and lactation not established.

ADVERSE/SIDE EFFECTS Low incidence. **CNS:** drowsiness, sedation headache, mild dizziness. **GI:** constipation, nausea. **Skin:** skin rash, pruritus.

NURSING IMPLICATIONS

Administration

- Oral medication is supplied in soft capsules called Perles.
- Perles must be swallowed whole.
- Store in airtight containers protected from light.

Assessment & Drug Effects

- Auscultate lungs anteriorly and posteriorly at scheduled intervals.
- Observe character and frequency of coughing and volume and quality of sputum. Keep physician informed.

Patient & Family Education

- Instruct patient not to chew oral preparation (Perle) and not to allow it to dissolve in mouth. It should be swallowed whole. If it dissolves, mouth, tongue, and pharynx will be anesthetized. Also it is unpleasant to taste.
- Objective of treatment with an antitussive agent is to reduce overactive nonproductive coughing but not to suppress the cough completely.

BENZPHETAMINE HYDROCHLORIDE

(benz-fet'a-meen)

Trade name: Didrex

Classifications: CNS AGENT; RESPIRATORY AND CEREBRAL STIMULANT; ANOREXIANT

Prototype: Amphetamine

Pregnancy category: X

Controlled substance: Schedule III

ACTIONS/PHARMACODYNAMICS Indirect acting sympathomimetic amine with amphetamine-like actions but with fewer side effects than amphetamine. Anorexiant effect thought to be secondary to stimulation of hypothalamus to release stored catecholamines in the CNS.

USE Short-term adjunct in management of exogenous obesity.

ROUTE & DOSAGE

Obesity

Adult: **PO** 25–50 mg 1–3 times/d.

PHARMACOKINETICS **Absorption:** readily absorbed from GI tract. **Duration:** 4 h. **Elimination:** renal elimination.

CONTRAINDICATIONS & PRECAUTIONS **Contraindicated in:** known hypersensitivity to sympathomimetic amines; angle-closure glau-

B

coma; advanced arteriosclerosis, angina pectoris, severe cardiovascular disease, moderate to severe hypertension; hyperthyroidism, agitated states; history of drug abuse; children <12 y. Safe use during pregnancy (category X) not established. **Cautious use in:** diabetes mellitus; the elderly; psychosis.

ADVERSE/SIDE EFFECTS **CNS:** euphoria, irritability, hyperactivity, nervousness, *restlessness, insomnia,* tremor, headache, light-headedness, dizziness, depression following stimulant effects. **CV:** *palpitation,* tachycardia, elevated BP, irregular heart beat. **GI:** xerostomia, nausea, vomiting, diarrhea or constipation, abdominal cramps. **Chronic intoxication:** marked insomnia, irritability, hyperactivity, personality changes, psychosis, severe dermatoses.

DRUG INTERACTIONS **Acetazolamide, sodium bicarbonate** decrease amphetamine elimination; **ammonium chloride, ascorbic acid** increase amphetamine elimination; BARBITURATES may antagonize the effects of both drugs; **furazolidone** may increase BP effects of amphetamines, and interaction may persist for several weeks after discontinuation of furazolidone; **guanethidine, guanadryl** antagonize antihypertensive effects; because MAO INHIBITORS, **selegiline** can cause hypertensive crisis (fatalities reported), do not administer amphetamines during or within 14 d of these drugs; PHENOTHIAZINES may inhibit mood-elevating effects of amphetamines; TRICYCLIC ANTIDEPRESSANTS enhance amphetamine effects because they increase norepinephrine release; BETA AGONISTS increase amphetamines' adverse cardiovascular effects.

NURSING IMPLICATIONS

Administration

- A single daily dose is taken, preferably midmorning or midafternoon, according to patient's eating habits.
- To avoid insomnia, the daily dose should be scheduled no later than 6 h before patient retires.
- Preserved in tight, light-resistant containers at 15–30C (59–86F) unless otherwise directed.

Assessment & Drug Effects

- Assess for signs of excessive CNS stimulation: insomnia, restlessness, tremor, palpitations. These may indicate need for dosage adjustment.
- Monitor vital signs; report elevated BP, tachycardia, and irregular heart rhythm.

Patient & Family Education

- Anorexiant effects are temporary, seldom lasting more than a few weeks; tolerance may occur. Therefore, long-term use is not indicated.
- Dosage of antidiabetic drug may require adjustment in diabetic patients because their food intake may change.
- Because dizziness and light-headedness are possible side effects, caution patient against driving a car or performing any other potentially hazardous activities until reaction to drug is determined.
- Abrupt termination of therapy following prolonged high dosages can result in GI distress, stomach cramps, trembling, unusual tiredness, weakness, and mental depression.
- The possibility of psychic dependence should be noted.

BENZQUINAMIDE HYDROCHLORIDE

(benz-kwin′a-mide)

Trade name: Emete-Con

Classifications: GI AGENT; ANTIEMETIC

Prototype: Prochlorperazine

Pregnancy category: C

ACTIONS/PHARMACODYNAMICS Antiemetic activity similar to that of phenothiazines and antihistamine antiemetics but chemically unrelated to both. Mechanism of antiemetic action unknown but is believed to be by depression of chemoreceptor trigger zone (CTZ). Also exhibits antihistaminic, antiserotonin, anticholinergic, and sedative properties.

USES Prevention and treatment of nausea and vomiting associated with anesthesia and surgery. **Unlabeled uses:** management of nausea and vomiting secondary to antineoplastic therapy; as an antipsychotic agent; and as a cardiovascular stimulant.

ROUTE & DOSAGE

Antiemetic

Adult: **IM** 50 mg (0.5–1 mg/kg); may repeat q3–4h if necessary. **IV** 25 mg (0.2–0.4 mg/kg) administered slowly at no more than 1 ml/min.

PHARMACOKINETICS **Absorption:** readily absorbed from IM injection site. **Onset:** 15 min. **Peak:** 30 min IM. **Duration:** 3–4 h. **Distribution:** distributed throughout body tissues, with highest concentrations in liver and kidneys; distribution to placenta and breast milk unknown. **Metabolism:** metabolized in liver. **Elimination:** half-life: 40 min; 95% of dose excreted in urine and feces within 72 h.

CONTRAINDICATIONS & PRECAUTIONS **Contraindicated in:** IV administration to patients with cardiovascular disease, moderate to severe hypertension, or to those who have received preanesthetic or concomitant cardiovascular drugs. Safe use during pregnancy (category C), in nursing women, and in children <12 y not established. **Cautious use in:** elderly and debilitated patients.

ADVERSE/SIDE EFFECTS **CNS:** *drowsiness,* insomnia, headache, dizziness, excitement, restlessness, nervousness; extrapyramidal symptoms (in large doses). **CV:** (particularly following IV): flushing, sudden increase in BP and respiration; hypotension, dizziness, tachycardia, atrial fibrillation, premature atrial and ventricular contractions. **GI:** dry mouth, salivation, anorexia, nausea, vomiting, abdominal cramps. **Other:** blurred vision, sweating, shivering, chills, hiccups.

INCOMPATIBILITIES **Solution/additive: chlordiazepoxide, diazepam, pentobarbital, phenobarbital, secobarbital, thiopental.**

NURSING IMPLICATIONS

Administration

- For IV administration, reconstitute with 2.2 ml sterile water for injection; for IM administration, reconstitute with bacteriostatic water for injection (with benzyl alcohol or parabens). Do not reconstitute with NaCl because precipitation may result.
- IM injection should be made well into mass of a large muscle. Aspirate carefully to avoid inadvertent intravascular injection.

B

- Deltoid area may be used only if well developed.
- When given for prophylaxis of nausea and vomiting, should be administered IM at least 15 min prior to expected emergence from anesthesia.
- IV benzquinamide may be given direct IV over 30–60 seconds.
- Reconstituted solutions maintain potency for 14 d at room temperature. Do not refrigerate.
- Preserve in light-resistant containers.

Assessment & Drug Effects

- Monitor patient for cardiovascular effects such as hypertension or hypotension and arrhythmias, particularly when drug is administered IV.
- Drowsiness is a common side effect. Be aware of implications for the postoperative patient and particularly the elderly.

BENZTHIAZIDE

(bens-thye′a-zide)

Trade names: Aquatag, Exna, Hydrex, Marazide, Proaqua

Classifications: WATER BALANCE AGENT; THIAZIDE DIURETIC; ANTIHYPERTENSIVE

Prototype: Hydrochlorothiazide

Pregnancy category: D

ACTIONS/PHARMACODYNAMICS Thiazide diuretic chemically related to sulfonamides. Similar to hydrochlorothiazide. Inhibits renal tubular reabsorption of sodium and chloride, resulting in excretion of sodium and water, accompanied by some loss of bicarbonate and potassium.

USES Edema and adjunctively with other agents for treatment of mild hypertension.

ROUTE & DOSAGE

Edema

Adult: **PO** 25–200 mg/d or q.o.d.
Child: **PO** 1–4 mg/kg/d in 3 divided doses.

Hypertension

Adult: **PO** 25–100 mg/d after breakfast, up to 200 mg/d in 2–4 divided doses.

PHARMACOKINETICS Absorption: readily absorbed from GI tract. **Onset:** 2 h. **Peak:** 4–6 h. **Duration:** 12–18 h. **Distribution:** crosses placenta; distributed into breast milk. **Elimination:** excreted in urine within 24 h.

CONTRAINDICATIONS & PRECAUTIONS Contraindicated in: hypersensitivity to thiazides or sulfonamides; anuria; pregnancy (category D), lactation. **Cautious use in:** history of renal, hepatic, or pancreatic disease; history of gout; diabetes mellitus; hypercalcemia, hypokalemia.

ADVERSE/SIDE EFFECTS CNS: headache, unusual fatigue. **CV:** irregular heartbeat, vasculitis, orthostatic hypotension, volume depletion. **GI:** nausea, vomiting, anorexia, constipation, cramps. **Electrolytes:** hyperglycemia, hypokalemia; hyperuricemia. **Hematologic** (rare): thrombocytopenia, agranulocytosis. **Hypersensitivity:** dermatitis, photosensitivity, urticaria. **Other:** jaundice, increased thirst.

DIAGNOSTIC TEST INTERFERENCE ***Serum PBI*** levels may be decreased. Thiazides should be discontinued before ***parathyroid function*** tests because they tend to reduce calcium excretion.

DRUG INTERACTIONS Cholestyramine, colestipol decrease absorption of the diuretic; **diazoxide** has additive effects; with **digoxin,** hypokalemia may increase risk of digitalis toxicity; increases **lithium** levels and toxicity; may increase blood glucose levels, necessitating adjustment of dosage of SULFONYLUREAS, **insulin.**

NURSING IMPLICATIONS

Administration

- Benzthiazide may be taken with food or milk to minimize gastric irritation unless otherwise directed by physician.
- When benzthiazide is used to promote diuresis, a single daily dose is administered, preferably early in the morning to prevent interrupted sleep because of diuresis.
- Store tablets in tightly closed container at 15–30C (59–86F) unless otherwise directed.

Assessment & Drug Effects

- Antihypertensive dosage regimens are highly individualized. Effects may be noted in 3 or 4 d; maximal effects usually require 3–4 wk.
- The elderly are more sensitive to the average adult dose. Monitor serum potassium levels and observe patient carefully for signs of hypokalemia (see Signs & Symptoms, Appendix G).
- Baseline and periodic determinations should be made of blood counts, serum electrolytes, uric acid, blood sugar, NPN, BUN, and serum creatinine.
- Monitor I&O ratio and pattern.
- The prediabetic or diabetes mellitus patient should be watched for loss of control of diabetes or early signs of hyperglycemia (see Appendix G). These signs are slow to develop and difficult to recognize. Notify physician of their appearance, since an adjustment of insulin dosage may be needed.

Patient & Family Education

- To prevent onset of hypokalemia (rarely severe in most patients even on long-term therapy with thiazides), urge patient to eat potassium-rich foods such as fruit juices and bananas.
- Instruct patient to weigh daily and report sudden weight gain.
- To prevent dehydration, caution patient to notify doctor if severe nausea, vomiting, or diarrhea occurs.
- Counsel patient to avoid use of OTC drugs unless approved by the physician. Many preparations contain potassium and sodium.
- Warn patient about the possibility of photosensitivity reaction (like an exaggerated sunburn). Notify physician if it occurs. Thiazide-related photosensitivity is considered a photoallergy. It occurs 1 1/2–2 wk after initial sun exposure.

BENZTROPINE MESYLATE

(benz′troe-peen)

Trade names: Apo-Benzotro-pine ♣, Bensylate ♣, Cogentin, PMS Benzotropine ♣

Classifications: AUTONOMIC NERVOUS SYSTEM AGENT; ANTICHOLINERGIC (PARASYMPATHOLYTIC); ANTIPARKINSONISM AGENT

Prototype: Levodopa

Pregnancy category: C

ACTIONS/PHARMACODYNAMICS

Synthetic centrally acting anticholinergic (antimuscarinic) agent. Also exhibits antihistaminic and local anesthetic activity. Acts by diminishing excess cholinergic effect associated with dopamine deficiency. Suppresses tremor and rigidity; does not alleviate tardive dyskinesia.

B

USES Symptomatic treatment of all forms of parkinsonism (arteriosclerotic, idiopathic, postencephalitic) and to relieve extrapyramidal symptoms associated with neuroleptic drugs, e.g., haloperidol (Haldol), phenothiazines, thiothixene (Navane). Commonly used as supplement with trihexyphenidyl, carbidopa, or levodopa therapy.

ROUTE & DOSAGE

Parkinsonism

Adult: **PO** 0.5–1 mg/d; gradually increased as needed up to 6 mg/d.

Extrapyramidal Reactions

Adult: **PO** 1–2 mg b.i.d. **IM/IV** 1–2 mg as needed.
Child >3 y: **PO/IM/IV** 0.02–0.05 mg/kg 1–2 times/d.

PHARMACOKINETICS **Onset:** 15 min IM/IV; 1 h PO. **Duration:** 6–10 h.

CONTRAINDICATIONS & PRECAUTIONS **Contraindicated in:** narrow angle glaucoma; myasthenia gravis; obstructive diseases of GU and GI tracts; tendency to tachycardia; tardive dyskinesia, children <3 y. Safe use during pregnancy (category C) and in nursing women not established. **Cautious use in:** older children, elderly or debilitated patients, patients with poor mental outlook, mental disorders; enlarged prostate; hypertension; history of renal or hepatic disease.

ADVERSE/SIDE EFFECTS **CNS:** *sedation,* drowsiness, dizziness, paresthesias; agitation, irritability, restlessness, nervousness, insomnia, hallucinations, delirium, mental confusion, toxic psychosis, muscular weakness, ataxia, inability to move certain muscle groups. **CV:** palpitation, tachycardia, flushing. **Eye:** blurred vision, mydriasis, photophobia. **GI:** nausea, vomiting, *constipation, dry mouth,* distention, paralytic ileus. **GU:** dysuria.

DRUG INTERACTIONS **Alcohol,** CNS DEPRESSANTS have additive sedation and depressant effects; **amantidine,** TRICYCLIC ANTIDEPRESSANTS, MAO INHIBITORS, PHENOTHIAZINES, **procainamide, quinidine** have additive anticholinergic effects and cause confusion, hallucinations, paralytic ileus.

NURSING IMPLICATIONS

Administration

- Administration of oral drug immediately after meals or with food may help to prevent gastric irritation. Tablet can be crushed prior to administration and sprinkled on or mixed with food.
- Patients with arteriosclerotic or idiopathic parkinsonism generally experience greatest relief by taking benztropine at bedtime.
- IV benztropine mesylate may be given undiluted by direct IV at a rate of 1 mg or a fraction thereof over 1 min.
- IV administration to infants and children: Verify correct IV concentration of injection with physician.
- Drug therapy should be initiated and withdrawn gradually. Effects of benztropine are cumulative.
- Preserve in tightly covered, light-resistant container at 15–30C (59–86F) unless otherwise directed.

Assessment & Drug Effects

- Clinical improvement may not be evident until 2 or 3 d after oral drug is started.
- The elderly and patients with mental illness should be closely observed for intensification of mental symptoms, particularly during

early therapy or whenever dosage increases are made.

- Acute extrapyramidal symptoms associated with initiation of antipsychotic therapy are generally transient. Report even minor symptoms to physician. Most adverse/side effects respond to dosage reduction or temporary withdrawal of drug.
- Monitor I&O ratio and pattern. Advise patient to report difficulty in urination or infrequent voiding. Dosage reduction may be indicated.
- Appearance of intermittent constipation, abdominal pain, diminution of bowel sounds on auscultation, and distension may herald onset of paralytic ileus. Patients receiving combination drugs with anticholinergic action should be closely monitored for these symptoms.
- Muscle weakness or inability to move certain muscle groups are adverse side effects and require dosage reduction.
- Most of the atropinelike side effects of benztropine are controlled by adjustment of dosage. However, severe reactions, such as signs and symptoms of CNS depression or stimulation (see Appendix G), usually require interruption of drug therapy.

Patient & Family Education

- Caution patient about possibility of drowsiness and blurred vision and advise against operating vehicles or machinery or other activities requiring alertness until reaction to the drug is known. Supervision of ambulation and side rails may be indicated.
- Alcohol and other CNS depressants may cause additive drowsiness and therefore should be avoided. Also advise patient not to take OTC cold, cough, or hay fever remedies unless approved by physician.
- Mouth dryness may be relieved by frequent rinsing of mouth with tepid water or by sugarless gum or hard candy.
- Anhidrosis (diminished sweating), especially in hot weather, may require dose adjustments because of possibility of heat stroke. This condition is most apt to occur in the elderly patient. Caution patient to avoid doing manual labor or strenuous exercise in a hot environment.

BEPRIDIL HYDROCHLORIDE

(be-pri′-dil)

Trade name: Vascor

Classifications: CARDIOVASCULAR AGENT; CALCIUM CHANNEL BLOCKER

Prototype: Nifedipine

Pregnancy category: C

ACTIONS/PHARMACODYNAMICS

Selectively blocks calcium ion influx across the cell membranes of cardiac muscle and vascular smooth muscle without changing serum calcium concentrations. Unlike other calcium channel blockers, it also blocks the sodium channel and possibly the potassium channel, resulting in quinidine-like effects. Bepridil reduces myocardial oxygen use and supply, and relaxes and prevents coronary artery spasm.

USE Chronic stable angina.

ROUTE & DOSAGE

Adult: **PO** start with 200 mg once daily; may be adjusted every 7 d to max of 400 mg/d.

B

PHARMACOKINETICS Absorption: completely absorbed from GI tract; approximately 60% reaches systemic circulation. **Onset:** 60 min. **Peak:** 2–3 h. **Duration:** 24 h. **Distribution:** distributed into breast milk. **Metabolism:** metabolized in liver, presumably by hepatic oxidative processes; 17 metabolites have been isolated. **Elimination:** half-life: 42 h; approximately 65% excreted in urine in 10 d, 23% excreted in feces.

CONTRAINDICATIONS & PRECAUTIONS Contraindicated in: Hypersensitivity to bepridil HCl or any other calcium channel blocker, sick sinus syndrome or second- or third-degree block, ventricular arrhythmias, hypotension, uncompensated cardiac insufficiency, congenital QT interval prolongation, and with concomitant use of drugs that prolong QT interval. **Cautious use in:** elderly, CHF, recent MI (≤ 3 months), serious hepatic or renal dysfunction, pregnancy (category C).

ADVERSE/SIDE EFFECTS CNS: nervousness, *dizziness,* asthenia, *headache.* **CV:** negative inotropic effect, <u>proarrhythmic effects (ventricular tachycardia or fibrillation, torsade de pointes)</u>, CHF. **GI:** *nausea, vomiting, diarrhea,* dyspepsia. **Hematologic (rare):** leukopenia, neutropenia, agranulocytosis. **Other:** <u>death</u> has been reported in arrhythmia trials.

DRUG INTERACTIONS Adenosine and BETA BLOCKERS may increase risk of bradycardia. **Amiodarone** may lead to heart block; may increase **digoxin** levels and digoxin toxicity. May cause significant hypotension with **fentanyl.** Use with diuretics may increase risk of arrhythmias. TRICYCLIC ANTIDEPRESSANTS may exaggerate prolongation of QT interval associated with bepridil. May enhance neuromuscular blockade induced by nondepolarizing agents such as **succinylcholine** and **tubocurarine; warfarin** may increase free bepridil levels.

NURSING IMPLICATIONS

Administration

- Bepredil may be given without respect to meals. If nausea occurs, administer with food.
- Store away from light and moisture in tightly closed containers at 15–30C (59–86F).

Assessment & Drug Effects

- Monitor cardiac status, as bepridil can induce new arrhythmias, including ventricular tachycardia and fibrillation, and congestive heart failure.
- Females over age 60 with hypokalemia and sinus bradycardia are at high risk for drug-induced torsade de pointes (a type of ventricular tachycardia). Monitor closely.
- As dizziness is a common adverse effect, assess safety and determine need for assistance with ambulation or other activities.
- Adverse gastrointestinal effects (nausea, vomiting, diarrhea) are common. Assess to determine need for intervention.
- Monitor serum transaminase levels periodically.
- When bepridil is given concomitantly with digoxin, monitor for significant increases in serum digoxin levels.
- When bepridil is given concomitantly with a diuretic, monitor potassium levels and correct hypokalemia immediately.
- Monitor for hyperglycemia in patients taking oral hypoglycemic agents.

Patient & Family Education

- Instruct patient to take drug with

food if gastrointestinal upset occurs.

- Advise patient to report ringing sounds, as tinnitus has been reported with bepridil.
- Inform patient of potential adverse drug effects and advise to report those that are bothersome to the physician.

BERACTANT

(ber-ac'tant)

Trade name: Survanta

Prototype for classification: LUNG SURFACTANT

ACTIONS/PHARMACODYNAMICS Beractant is a sterile nonpyrogenic pulmonary surfactant. Endogenous pulmonary surfactant lowers surface tension on alveolar surfaces during respiration and stabilizes the alveoli against collapse at resting pressures. Deficiency of surfactant causes respiratory distress syndrome (RDS) in premature infants. Beractant lowers minimum surface tension and restores pulmonary compliance and oxygenation in premature infants.

USES Prevention and treatment of RDS in premature infants, especially those weighing <1250 g. **Unlabeled uses:** infants weighing <600 g or >1750 g; treatment of RDS in adults.

ROUTE & DOSAGE

Neonate: **Endotracheal** Instill 100 mg/kg (4 ml/kg) birth weight through endotracheal tube; may be repeated no more frequently than q6h up to 4 doses in the first 48 h of life.

PHARMACOKINETICS Absorption: absorbed from the alveolus into lung tissue, where it can be extensively catabolized and reutilized for further phospholipid synthesis and secretion. **Onset:** 0.5–4 h. **Peak:** 2 h. **Duration:** 48–72 h; may need multiple doses to sustain improvement. **Distribution:** not distributed to the systemic circulation. **Metabolism:** surfactant is recycled and metabolized exclusively in the lungs. **Elimination:** half-life: 20–30 h; recycling may be a dominant metabolic pathway by which surfactant is taken up by type II pneumocytes and reused.

CONTRAINDICATIONS & PRECAUTIONS Cautious use in: nosocomial infections.

ADVERSE/SIDE EFFECTS CV: *transient bradycardia.* **Respiratory:** *oxygen desaturation.* **Other:** increased probability of posttreatment nosocomial sepsis in surfactant-treated infants was observed in the controlled clinical trials but was not associated with increased mortality.

DRUG INTERACTIONS None reported to date.

NURSING IMPLICATIONS

Administration

- Before administration, refrigerated beractant should be allowed to stand at room temperature for at least 20 min or warmed in the hand for at least 8 min. Do not use artificial warming methods.
- For premature infants weighing less than 1250 g, or who have a surfactant deficiency, beractant should be given preferably within 15 min of birth.
- In infants requiring mechanical ventilation and with RDS confirmed by x-ray examination, beractant should be given within 8 h of birth.
- The infant should be suctioned before administration of beractant. Do not suction for 1 h after drug is

B

administered unless signs of significant airway obstruction occur.
- Drug is white to light brown. If drug has settled, swirl vial gently to suspend.
- Drug is administered intratracheally through a 5 French endhole catheter inserted into the endotracheal tube. A specific dosing procedure is recommended by the manufacturer. Carefully read accompanying drug administration literature and follow it exactly.
- Unopened vials that have been warmed to room temperature will not lose potency if refrigerated within 8 h of warming. Drug should not be warmed and returned to refrigerator more than once.
- Refrigerate unopened vials at 2–8C (36–46F). Protect from light. Store vials in carton until ready to use. Vials are for single use only. Discard unused drug in opened vials.

Assessment & Drug Effects
- During administration, monitor heart rate, color, chest expansion, facial expressions, oximeter, and endotracheal tube patency and position. Most adverse side effects occur during dosing.
- Infants receiving beractant should be monitored frequently with arterial or transcutaneous measurement of systemic oxygen and CO_2.
- Note that rales and moist breath sounds may occur transiently following drug administration. These do not necessarily indicate a need for suctioning.

BETAMETHASONE
(bay-ta-meth'a-sone)
Trade names: Betnelan ♣, Celestone

BETAMETHASONE ACETATE AND BETAMETHASONE SODIUM PHOSPHATE
Trade name: Celestone Soluspan

BETAMETHASONE BENZOATE
Trade names: Beben ♣, Benisone, Uticort

BETAMETHASONE DIPROPIONATE
Trade names: Alphatrex, Diprogen, Diprolene, Diprosalic, Diprosone

BETAMETHASONE SODIUM PHOSPHATE (PH 8.5)
Trade names: Betameth, Betnesol ♣, Celestone Phosphate, Celestone S, Cel-U-Jec, Selestoject

BETAMETHASONE VALERATE
Trade names: Betacort, Betaderm ♣, Betatrex, Beta-Val, Betnovate ♣, Celestoderm ♣, Ectosone Lotion ♣, Metaderm ♣, Novobetamet ♣, Valisone, Valisone Scalp Lotion, Valnac
Classifications: HORMONE; ADRENAL CORTICOSTEROID; GLUCOCORTICOID; ANTIINFLAMMATORY
Prototype: Hydrocortisone
Pregnancy category: C

ACTIONS/PHARMACODYNAMICS
Synthetic, long-acting glucocorticoid with minor mineralocorticoid properties but strong immunosuppressive, antiinflammatory, and metabolic actions. For contraindications and precautions and adverse/side effects, see hydrocortisone.

USES Topical use provides relief of inflammatory manifestations of corticosteroid-responsive dermatoses. With exception of use as replacement therapy in adrenocortical insufficiency and salt-losing forms of adrenogenital syndromes, beta-

Common side effect in *italic*, life-threatening effects underlined; generic names in **bold**; drug class in SMALL CAPS

methasone has the same indications for use, limitations, and adverse/side effects as hydrocortisone. **Unlabeled use:** prevention of neonatal respiratory distress syndrome (hyaline membrane disease).

ROUTE & DOSAGE

Antiinflammatory Agent

Adult: **PO** 0.6–7.2 mg/d. **IM/IV** 0.5–9 mg/d as sodium phosphate. **Topical** See Appendix A.

Child: **PO** 0.0175–0.25 mg/kg/d or 0.5–0.75 mg/m^2/d divided q6–8h. **IM** 0.0175–0.125 mg/kg/d or 0.5–0.75 mg/m^2/d divided q6–8h.

Respiratory Distress Syndrome

Adult: **IM** 2 ml of sodium phosphate to mother once daily 2–3 d before delivery.

PHARMACOKINETICS Unknown.

DRUG INTERACTIONS Barbiturates, phenytoin, rifampin may reduce pharmacologic effect of betamethasone by increasing its metabolism.

NURSING IMPLICATIONS

Administration

- Administer oral betamethasone with food or milk to lessen stomach irritation.
- Celestone Soluspan is used for intraarticular, IM, and intralesional injection. The preparation is not intended for IV use. Do not mix with diluents containing preservatives, e.g., parabens, phenol. If prescribed, 1% or 2% lidocaine hydrochloride may be used. (Withdraw betamethasone mixture first, then lidocaine; shake syringe briefly.)
- IV administration: IV betamethasone sodium phosphate may be given by direct IV undiluted at a rate of 1 dose/min. Medication may be further diluted in dextrose or saline solution and infused at a prescribed rate.

Assessment & Drug Effects

- Response following intraarticular, intralesional, or intrasynovial administration occurs within a few hours and persists for 1–4 wk. Following IM administration response occurs in 2–3 h and persists for 3–7 d.

Patient & Family Education

- Betamethasone appears to cause weight gain. Advise patient to monitor weight at least weekly.
- Steroids should be discontinued slowly after systemic use of ≥1 wk. Abrupt withdrawal, especially following high doses or prolonged use, can cause dizziness, nausea, vomiting, fever, muscle and joint pain, weakness.

BETAXOLOL HYDROCHLORIDE

(be-tax′oh-lol)

Trade names: Betoptic, Betoptic-S, Kerlone

Classifications: EYE PREPARATION; MIOTIC (ANTIGLAUCOMA AGENT); AUTONOMIC NERVOUS SYSTEM AGENT; BETA-ADRENERGIC BLOCKER

Prototype: Propranolol

Pregnancy category: C

See Appendix A.

BETHANECHOL CHLORIDE

(be-than′e-kole)

Trade names: Duvoid, Urabeth, Urecholine

B

Prototype for classifications: AUTONOMIC NERVOUS SYSTEM AGENT; DIRECT-ACTING CHOLINERGIC (PARASYMPATHOMIMETIC)
Pregnancy category: C

ACTIONS/PHARMACODYNAMICS
Synthetic choline ester with effects similar to those of acetylcholine (ACh). Acts directly on postsynaptic receptors, and since it is not hydrolyzed by cholinesterase, its actions are more prolonged than those of ACh. Produces muscarinic effects primarily on GI tract and urinary bladder. Increases tone and peristaltic activity of esophagus, stomach, and intestines; contracts detrusor muscle of urinary bladder, usually enough to initiate micturition.

USES Acute postoperative and postpartum nonobstructive (functional) urinary retention, and for neurogenic atony of urinary bladder with retention. **Unlabeled uses:** in selected cases of adynamic ileus, gastric atony and retention, reflux esophagitis, congenital megacolon, familial dysautonomia; for prevention and treatment of bladder and salivary gland inhibition induced by tricyclic antidepressants, and for prophylaxis and treatment of phenothiazine-induced bladder dysfunction.

ROUTE & DOSAGE

Urinary Retention
Adult: **PO** 10–50 mg b.i.d. to q.i.d. (max 120 mg/d). **SC** 2.5–5 mg t.i.d. or q.i.d. prn. *Child:* **PO** 0.2 mg/kg or 0.6 mg/m^2 t.i.d.

PHARMACOKINETICS **Absorption:** well absorbed PO. **Onset:** 30 min PO; 5–15 min SC. **Peak:** 60–90 min PO; 15–30 min SC. **Duration:** 1–6 h PO; 2 h SC. **Distribution:** does not cross blood–brain barrier. **Metabolism:** unknown. **Elimination:** unknown.

CONTRAINDICATIONS & PRECAUTIONS **Contraindicated in:** COPD, history of or active bronchial asthma; hyperthyroidism; recent urinary bladder surgery, cystitis, bacteriuria, urinary bladder neck or intestinal obstruction, peptic ulcer, recent GI surgery, peritonitis, marked vagotonia, pronounced vasomotor instability, AV conduction defects, severe bradycardia, hypotension or hypertension, coronary artery disease, recent MI, epilepsy, parkinsonism. Safe use during pregnancy (category C), in nursing women, and in children <8 y not established. Do not give IM or IV.

ADVERSE/SIDE EFFECTS Dose-related. **CV:** hypotension with dizziness, faintness, flushing, orthostatic hypotension (large doses); mild reflex tachycardia, atrial fibrillation (hyperthyroid patients), transient complete heart block. **Eye:** blurred vision, miosis, lacrimation. **GI:** nausea, vomiting, abdominal cramps, diarrhea, borborygmi, belching, salivation, fecal incontinence (large doses), urge to defecate (or urinate). **Respiratory:** acute asthmatic attack, dyspnea (large doses). **Other:** increased sweating, malaise, headache, substernal pain or pressure, hypothermia.

DIAGNOSTIC TEST INTERFERENCE
Bethanechol may cause increases in ***serum amylase*** and ***serum lipase,*** by stimulating pancreatic secretions, and may increase ***AST, serum bilirubin,*** and ***BSP retention*** by causing spasms in sphincter of Oddi.

B

DRUG INTERACTIONS **Ambenonium, neostigmine,** other CHOLINESTERASE INHIBITORS compound cholinergic effects and toxicity; **mecamylamine** may cause abdominal symptoms and hypotension; **procainamide, quinidine, atropine, epinephrine** antagonize effects of bethanechol.

NURSING IMPLICATIONS

Administration

- Bethanechol (PO) should be given on an empty stomach (1 h before or at least 2 h after meals) to lessen possibility of nausea and vomiting, unless otherwise advised by physician.
- Bethanechol may be prescribed with meals following bilateral vagotomy in patients with gastric atony. The drug is given orally in incomplete gastric retention, and SC if retention is complete.
- To determine minimum effective PO dose, physician may prescribe initial test dose of 5–10 mg repeated at hourly intervals to a maximum of 30 mg, unless satisfactory response or disturbing side effects intervene. Alternatively, 10 mg followed at 6 h intervals by 25 mg then 50 mg, until desired response obtained.
- To determine minimum effective SC dose: physician may prescribe initial test dose of 2.5 mg repeated at 15 to 30 min intervals to a maximum of 4 doses, unless satisfactory response or disturbing side effects intervene.
- Sterile solution of bethanechol is intended for subcutaneous use only. After inserting needle, aspirate carefully before injecting drug to avoid inadvertent entry into a blood vessel. Life-threatening symptoms of cholinergic stimulation can occur if it is given IM or IV.
- Antidote: Syringe containing atropine sulfate (specific antidote) should be ready for instantaneous use to abolish severe side effects, 0.6–1.2 mg for adults administered IM, slow IV, or SC; and 0.01 mg/kg for infants and children repeated every 2 h, if necessary. Specific directions for administering antidote should be prescribed by physician.
- Store at 15–30C (59–86F), unless otherwise directed.

Assessment & Drug Effects

- Adverse effects are most commonly associated with subcutaneous administration, and high PO doses. Monitor BP and pulse in these patients. Observe patient for at least 1 h following SC administration. Report early signs of overdosage: salivation, sweating, flushing, abdominal cramps, nausea.
- Monitor I&O. Observe and record patient's response to bethanechol, and report any failure of the drug to relieve the particular condition for which it was prescribed.
- Monitor respiratory status. Promptly report dyspnea or any other indication of respiratory distress.
- Since drug may cause dizziness and blurred vision, supervision of ambulation may be indicated.

Patient & Family Education

- Orthostatic hypotension is a possible side effect. Therefore, caution patient to make position changes slowly and in stages, particularly from recumbent to upright posture, not to stand still for prolonged periods, to avoid hot baths or showers, and to sit or lie down at first indication of faintness.
- Because bethanechol may cause dizziness and faintness, caution patient to avoid driving or other potentially hazardous activities until reaction to drug has been determined.

B

- Inform patient that drug may cause blurred vision. Advise appropriate caution.

BICALUTAMIDE

(bi-ca-lu′ta-mide)

Trade name: Casodex

Classifications: HORMONE; ANTIANDROGEN

Prototype: Leuprolide

Pregnancy category: X

ACTIONS/PHARMACODYNAMICS Bicalutamide is a nonsteroidal antiandrogen. It inhibits the pharmacologic effects of androgen by binding to the androgen receptors in the target tissue. Prostatic carcinoma is androgen sensitive; it responds to removal of the source of androgen or treatment that counteracts the effect of androgen.

USE In combination with a luteinizing hormone-releasing hormone (LHRH) analog for advanced prostate cancer.

ROUTE & DOSAGE

Advanced Prostate Cancer

Adult: **PO** 50 mg once/d.

PHARMACOKINETICS Absorption: readily absorbed from GI tract. **Metabolism:** metabolized in liver. **Elimination:** half-life: 5.8 d; excreted in urine and feces.

CONTRAINDICATIONS & PRECAUTIONS Contraindicated in: hypersensitivity to bicalutamide, pregnancy (category X). **Cautious use in:** moderate to severe hepatic impairment, nursing mothers. Safety and efficacy in children have not been established.

ADVERSE/SIDE EFFECTS CNS: dizziness, paresthesia, insomnia, anxiety, decreased libido, confusion, neuropathy, somnolence, nervousness, headache. **CV:** *hot flashes,* hypertension, chest pain, CHF. **GI:** *constipation, nausea, diarrhea,* vomiting, increased liver function tests, abdominal pain, anorexia, dyspepsia, dry mouth, melena. **GU:** nocturia, hematuria, UTI, impotence, gynecomastia, incontinence, frequency, dysuria, urinary retention, urgency. **Metabolic:** peripheral edema, hyperglycemia, weight loss, weight gain, gout. **Musculoskeletal:** myasthenia, arthritis, myalgia, leg cramps, pathologic fractures. **Skin:** rash, sweating, dry skin, pruritus, alopecia. **Other:** flu syndrome, bone pain, infection, anemia.

DRUG INTERACTION May increase effects of ORAL ANTICOAGULANTS.

NURSING IMPLICATIONS

Administration

- Drug should be given at the same time each day.
- Treatment with bicalutamide should be started at the same time as treatment with a luteinizing hormone-releasing hormone (LHRH) analog.
- Store at 15–30C (59–86F).

Assessment & Drug Effects

- With long-term therapy, periodically monitor hepatic and renal function and CBC. Carefully monitor patients with moderate-to-severe hepatic impairment.
- With concurrent coumadin therapy, closely monitor PT and INR values.
- Monitor for signs and symptoms of disease progression with regular assessment of PSA level.

Patient & Family Education

- Advise to take bicalutamide at the same time each day.
- Inform patient of potential adverse effects, especially gynecomastia and breast pain.
- Advise to report immediately jaundice or any other troubling adverse effect.

BIPERIDEN HYDROCHLORIDE

(bye-per′i-den)

Trade name: Akineton

BIPERIDEN LACTATE

Trade name: Akineton

Classifications: AUTONOMIC NERVOUS SYSTEM AGENT; ANTICHOLINERGIC (PARASYMPATHOLYTIC); ANTIPARKINSONISM AGENT

Prototype: Levodopa

Pregnancy category: C

ACTIONS/PHARMACODYNAMICS Synthetic tertiary amine, antimuscarinic. In common with other antiparkinsonism drugs has atropinelike (anticholinergic) actions. Antiparkinsonism activity is thought to be by reducing central excitatory action of acetylcholine on cholinergic receptors in the extrapyramidal system. This action helps to establish some balance between cholinergic (excitatory) and dopaminergic (inhibitory) activity in the basal ganglia.

USES Adjunct in all forms of parkinsonism, particularly postencephalitic and idiopathic parkinsonism (appears to be less effective in arteriosclerotic type). Also used to control drug-induced parkinsonism (extrapyramidal symptoms) associated with reserpine and phenothiazine therapy.

ROUTE & DOSAGE

Parkinsonism

Adult: **PO** 2 mg 1–4 times/d. **IM/IV** 2 mg injected slowly; may repeat q30min up to 8 mg/24h.
Geriatric: **PO** 2 mg 1–2 times/d.
Child: **IM/IV** 0.04 mg/kg or 1.2 mg/m^2; may repeat q30min up to 8 mg/24h.

PHARMACOKINETICS Unknown.

CONTRAINDICATIONS & PRECAUTIONS **Contraindicated in:** narrow-angle glaucoma; GI or GU obstruction, megacolon; tardive dyskinesia. Safe use during pregnancy (category C), in nursing women, and in children not established. **Cautious use in:** elderly or debilitated patients; prostatic hypertrophy; glaucoma; cardiac arrhythmias; epilepsy.

ADVERSE/SIDE EFFECTS (dose-related): **CNS:** drowsiness, dizziness, muscle weakness, lack of coordination, disorientation, euphoria, agitation, confusion. **CV:** mild, transient postural hypotension (following IM), tachycardia. **Eye:** *blurred vision,* photophobia. **GI:** *dry mouth,* nausea, vomiting, constipation.

DRUG INTERACTIONS **Alcohol** and other CNS DEPRESSANTS increase sedation; **haloperidol,** PHENOTHIAZINES, OPIATES, TRICYCLIC ANTIDEPRESSANTS, **quinidine** increase risk of anticholinergic side effects.

NURSING IMPLICATIONS

Administration

- GI disturbances may be relieved by administering PO doses with or after meals.
- IV biperiden lactate may be given by direct IV undiluted at a rate of 2 mg or a fraction thereof over 1 min.
- Patient should be recumbent

B

when receiving parenteral biperiden. Postural hypotension, disturbances of coordination, and temporary euphoria can occur following IV administration.

- Preserve in tightly closed, light-resistant containers at 15–30C (59–86F) unless otherwise directed.

Assessment & Drug Effects

- Monitor BP and pulse after IV administration. Advise patient to make position changes slowly and in stages, particularly from recumbent to upright position.
- It is reported that certain susceptible patients may manifest mental confusion, drowsiness, dizziness, agitation, hematuria, and decrease in urinary flow. Report these symptoms immediately.
- Slight dryness of mouth and blurred vision are common dose-related side effects and may be relieved or eliminated by dosage reduction.
- Monitor I&O ratio and pattern. If constipation is a problem, increase in dietary fiber and fluid intake may help.
- Biperiden usually reduces sweating, drooling, excessive oiliness of skin, and muscle rigidity. In patients with severe parkinsonism, tremors may increase as spasticity is relieved.

Patient & Family Education

- Caution patient to avoid driving and other potentially hazardous activities until reaction to drug is determined.
- Patients on prolonged therapy can develop tolerance; an increase in dosage may be required.

BISACODYL

(bis-a-koe′dill)

Trade names: Apo-Bisacodyl ♣, Bisacolax, Bisco-Lax ♣, Dacodyl, Deficol, Dulcolax, Fleet Bisacodyl, Laxit ♣, Theralax

Prototype for classifications: GI AGENT; STIMULANT LAXATIVE

Pregnancy category: C

ACTIONS/PHARMACODYNAMICS Induces peristaltic contractions by direct stimulation of sensory nerve endings in the colonic wall. Bisacodyl also expands intestinal fluid volume by increasing epithelial permeability.

USES Temporary relief of acute constipation and for evacuation of colon before surgery, proctoscopic, sigmoidoscopic, and radiologic examinations. Also used to cleanse colon before delivery and to relieve constipation in patients with spinal cord damage.

ROUTE & DOSAGE

Laxative

Adult: **PO** 5–15 mg prn up to 30 mg for special procedures. **PR** 10 mg prn. *Child:* **PO** ≥ 6 y: 5–10 mg prn. **PR** ≥ 2 y: 10 mg; < 2 y: 5 mg.

PHARMACOKINETICS **Absorption:** 5–15% absorbed from GI tract. **Onset:** 6–8 h PO; 15–60 min PR. **Metabolism:** metabolized in liver. **Elimination:** excreted in urine, bile, and breast milk.

CONTRAINDICATIONS & PRECAUTIONS **Contraindicated in:** acute surgical abdomen, nausea, vomiting, abdominal cramps, intestinal obstruction, fecal impaction; use of rectal suppository in presence of anal or rectal fissures, ulcerated hemorrhoids, proctitis. **Cautious use in:** pregnancy (category C).

ADVERSE/SIDE EFFECTS Systemic effects not reported. Mild cramping, nausea, diarrhea, fluid and electrolyte disturbances (especially potassium and calcium).

DRUG INTERACTIONS ANTACIDS will cause early dissolution of enteric coated tablets, resulting in abdominal cramping.

NURSING IMPLICATIONS

Administration

- In view of action time, administer PO drug in the evening or before breakfast. Suppository may be inserted at time bowel movement is desired.
- Tablets are enteric coated; therefore, to avoid gastric irritation, they should be swallowed whole and not cut, crushed, or chewed. Preferably taken with a full glass (240 ml) of water or other liquid.
- Tablets should not be taken within 1 h of antacids or milk. These substances may cause premature dissolution of enteric coating, with release of drug in stomach resulting in gastric irritation and loss of cathartic action.
- Bisacodyl tablets and suppositories are preserved in tightly closed containers at temperatures not exceeding 30C (86F).

Assessment & Drug Effects

- Bisacodyl usually produces 1 or 2 soft formed stools. Periodically evaluate patient's need for continued use of bisacodyl.
- Because of OTC availability, laxative abuse, especially among the elderly, is widespread.
- Indiscriminate use of laxatives or dietary fiber can lead to changes in intestinal bacterial flora and to decreased absorption of vitamin K, drugs, and nutrients, because of decreased transit time in the intestine.

Patient & Family Education

- Instruct patient not to take bisacodyl within 1 h of taking antacids or milk.
- Inform the habitual laxative user that a normal pattern for elimination varies from 3 bowel movements a day to 3 a week, depending on a self-established functionally effective schedule.
- High-fiber diet is frequently prescribed as a supplement and eventual substitute for laxative use. Examples of high-fiber foods are fruits, vegetables, bran.
- High-fiber foods should be added slowly to regular diet to avoid gas and diarrhea, and fluid intake should be adequate (at least 6–8 glasses/d).

BISMUTH SUBSALICYLATE

Trade name: Pepto-Bismol
Classifications: GI AGENT; ANTIDIARRHEAL; SALICYLATE
Prototype: Diphenoxylate with atropine

ACTIONS/PHARMACODYNAMICS
Hydrolyzed in GI tract to salicylate, which is believed to inhibit synthesis of prostaglandins responsible for GI hypermotility and inflammation. Effectiveness as an antidiarrheal also appears to be due to direct antimicrobial action and to an antisecretory effect on intestinal secretions exposed to toxins particularly of *Escherichia coli* and *Vibrio cholerae*.

USES Prophylaxis and treatment of traveler's diarrhea (turista) and for temporary relief of indigestion. **Unlabeled use:** *Helicobacter pylori* associated with peptic ulcer disease.

ROUTE & DOSAGE

Diarrhea
Adult: **PO** 30 ml or 2 tab q30–60min prn up to 8 doses/d.

B

Child: **PO** *9–12 y,* 15 ml or 1 tab q30–60min prn up to 8 doses/d; *6–9 y,* 2/3 tab or 10 ml q30–60 min prn; *3–6 y,* 5 ml or 1/2 tab q30–60min prn up to 8 doses/d.

Traveler's Diarrhea

Adult: **PO** 2–4 tab or 15–30 ml q.i.d. for 3 wk.

Peptic Ulcer Disease

Adult: **PO** 2 tablets q.i.d. with 2 additional antibiotics for 10–14 d. *Child < 10 y:* **PO** 15 ml q.i.d. × 6 wk.

PHARMACOKINETICS **Absorption:** undergoes chemical dissociation in GI tract to bismuth subcarbonate and sodium salicylate; bismuth is minimally absorbed, but the salicylate is readily absorbed.

CONTRAINDICATIONS & PRECAUTIONS **Contraindicated in:** hypersensitivity to aspirin or other salicylates; use for more than 2 d in presence of high fever or in children <3 y unless prescribed by physician. **Cautious use in:** patient taking salicylates, pregnancy, and nursing mothers.

ADVERSE/SIDE EFFECTS Temporary *darkening of stool* and tongue. With high doses: fecal impaction, bismuth toxicity: encephalopathy (disorientation, muscle twitching), incontinence, metallic taste, bluish gum line; salicylism: tinnitus, hearing loss, bleeding tendencies.

DIAGNOSTIC TEST INTERFERENCE Because bismuth subsalicylate is radiopaque, it may interfere with radiographic studies of GI tract.

DRUG INTERACTIONS Bismuth may decrease the absorption of TETRACYCLINES, QUINOLONES **(ciprofloxacin, norfloxacin, ofloxacin).**

NURSING IMPLICATIONS

Patient & Family Education

- Chew chewable tablet or allow it to dissolve in mouth.
- Drug contains salicylate and therefore must be used with caution with aspirin and other salicylates. (Many OTC medications for colds, fever, and pain contain salicylates.)
- Consult physician if diarrhea is accompanied by fever or continues for more than 2 d.
- Prophylactic use should be limited to 3 wk or less. (Normal bismuth level should be less than 5 μg/L.)
- Temporary grayish black discoloration of tongue and stool may occur. (Note that this side effect may mask GI bleeding.)
- Store at room temperature and protect drug from light unless otherwise directed.

BISOPROLOL FUMARATE

(bis-o-pro′-lol fum′-a-rate)

Trade name: Zebeta

Classifications: AUTONOMIC NERVOUS SYSTEM AGENT; BETA-ADRENERGIC ANTAGONIST (BLOCKING AGENT); ANTIHYPERTENSIVE

Prototype: Propranolol

Pregnancy category: C

ACTIONS/PHARMACODYNAMICS Long-acting cardioselective ($beta_1$) adrenoreceptor blocking agent without membrane-stabilizing activity or intrinsic sympathomimetic activity. To maintain $beta_1$ cardioselectivity, the lowest effective dose is necessary. The mechanism of antihypertensive activity has not been completely established. Factors affecting hypertension may include decreased cardiac output, suppressed renin activity, and decreased sympathetic stimulation from vasomotor centers in the brain. Bisoprolol decreases heart rate, blood pressure, contractile force, and cardiac workload, which reduces myocardial oxygen consumption and increases blood flow to myocardium. Consequently, bisoprolol has antiangianl properties, especially improving exercise tolerance.

USE Hypertension. **Unlabeled use:** angina.

ROUTE & DOSAGE

Hypertension, Angina
Adult: **PO** 2.5–5 mg once daily; may increase to 20 mg/d if necessary.

PHARMACOKINETICS Absorption: Readily absorbed from GI tract; 82–94% reaches systemic circulation. **Peak:** therapeutic effect 2–4 wk. **Duration:** 24 h. **Distribution:** some CNS penetration. **Metabolism:** 50% metabolized in liver to inactive metabolites. **Elimination:** half-life: 10–12.4 h; 50–60% excreted unchanged in urine.

CONTRAINDICATIONS & PRECAUTIONS Contraindicated in: history of hypersensitivity to bisoprolol, severe sinus bradycardia, second- and third-degree AV block, overt cardiac failure, cardiogenic shock. **Cautious use in:** asthma or COPD, peripheral vascular disease, diabetes mellitus, hyperthyroidism, renal or hepatic insufficiency, pregnancy (category C), with anesthetic use.

ADVERSE/SIDE EFFECTS CNS dizziness, fatigue, tiredness, vertigo, anxiety, headache, sleep disturbances. **CV:** bradycardia, orthostatic hypotension, rebound/withdrawal angina or hypertension following abrupt discontinuation, may exacerbate intermittent claudication. **Endocrine:** increases serum levels of VLDL-C and decreases levels of HDL-C lipoproteins, may cause slight rise in serum potassium. **GI:** abdominal pain, dyspepsia, nausea, vomiting, constipation, diarrhea. **Respiratory:** asthma, bronchospasm, cough, dyspnea, pharyngitis, sinusitis. **Skin:** rash, acne, pruritus, eczema. **Other:** arthralgia.

DRUG INTERACTIONS Amiodarone may cause significant bradycardia; BETA BLOCKERS may reduce glucose tolerance, inhibit insulin secretion, alter rate of recovery from hypoglycemia, produce hypertension, reduce peripheral circulation, and suppress hypoglycemic symptoms; **rifampin** decreases bisoprolol blood levels.

NURSING IMPLICATIONS

Administration

- Bisoprolol may be given without regard to meals.
- When it is used for hypertension, dosage is individualized, with usual initial dose of 5 mg increased gradually until target BP level is reached.
- In patients with renal or liver dysfunction, usual initial dose is 2.5 mg, and frequent monitoring is needed if dose is titrated upward.
- To avoid rebound or withdrawal angina and/or hypertension, drug discontinuation should be gradual, over a period of 1–2 wk.
- Store at room temperature, 15–30C (59–86F).

Assessment & Drug Effects

- Time required to achieve optimum antihypertensive effect varies from a few days to several weeks.
- Monitor BP frequently during periods of dose adjustment or drug withdrawal.
- Monitor for activity-induced an-

B

gina both during therapy and following discontinuation of drug.

- Monitor for and report severe hypotension and bradycardia. Dosage adjustment may be required.
- Monitor for bronchospasms in patients with a history of asthma and/or COPD.
- With Type I diabetics, monitor for hypoglycemia as the drug may potentiate insulin-induced hypoglycemia.
- With Type II diabetics, monitor for hyperglycemia, which occurs more often than hypoglcemia.
- Monitor periodically for adverse changes in the lipid profile.

Patient & Family Education

- Inform patient that orthostatic hypotension and dizziness may occur and should be reported.
- Advise patient not to discontinue drug abruptly unless specifically instructed to do so.
- Inform patient of the potential for drug-induced nightmares and unpleasant dreams.
- Discuss potential for loss of glycemic control with diabetics.
- Advise patient to report cold extremities and development of symptoms of intermittent claudication.

BITOLTEROL MESYLATE

(bye-tole′ter-ole)

Trade name: Tornalate

Classifications: AUTONOMIC NERVOUS SYSTEM AGENT; BETA-ADRENERGIC AGONIST (SYMPATHOMIMETIC); BRONCHODILATOR

Prototype: Isoproterenol

Pregnancy category: C

ACTIONS/PHARMACODYNAMICS Produces prolonged bronchodilation as a beta-adrenergic agent. Relaxes bronchial smooth muscle and inhibits the release of mediators of immediate hypersensitivity (e.g., histamine) from lung tissue cells. Decreases airway resistance and increases vital capacity; bronchodilation is greater and longer in duration than that produced by isoproterenol. Cardiovascular effects appear to be similar to or less than those produced by isoproterenol.

USES Prophylaxis and treatment of bronchial asthma and reversible bronchospasm in monotherapy, or concomitantly with theophylline or corticosteroids or both.

ROUTE & DOSAGE

Bronchospasm

Adult: **Inhalation** 2 inhalations spaced 1–3 min apart q6–8h; max of 12 inhalations/d.

PHARMACOKINETICS Absorption: absorption from lungs not fully described. **Onset:** 3–5 min. **Peak:** 0.5–2 h. **Duration:** up to 8 h. **Distribution:** not known if crosses placenta or is distributed into breast milk. **Elimination:** half-life: 3 h.

CONTRAINDICATIONS & PRECAUTIONS Contraindicated in: safe use during pregnancy (category C), in nursing mothers, or in children <12 y not established. **Cautious use in:** cardiovascular disease, hypertension, hyperthyroidism, diabetes mellitus, convulsive disorders, unusual sensitivity to catecholamines; elderly patients, psychoneurosis; patient with longstanding bronchial asthma, and emphysema with degenerative heart disease.

ADVERSE/SIDE EFFECTS CNS (mild, transient): *tremors,* nervousness, headache, dizziness, light-headedness, insomnia; hyperkinesia. **CV:** palpitations, chest discomfort; tachycardia, flushing, PVCs. **Respiratory:** *throat irritation,* cough, paradoxical bronchoconstriction, dyspnea, chest tightness. **Other:** nausea, dyspepsia.

DRUG INTERACTIONS Effects of BETA-ADRENERGIC BLOCKERS (e.g., **propranolol**) and bitolterol may be antagonized.

NURSING IMPLICATIONS

Administration

- Follow manufacturer's directions for administration of drug by aerosol metered dose inhaler. Supervise patient a few times to be certain drug delivery is accomplished.
- Manufacturer recommends that the bottle containing the drug be removed from the inhaler and that the plastic mouthpiece be cleansed in warm tap water and thoroughly dried once daily.
- Avoid contacting eyes with bitolterol. If it should happen, flush out with copious amounts of water.
- If an adrenocorticoid inhalation is also being used, the two drugs should be administered 15 min apart unless otherwise directed by physician. This is to diminish the risk of fluorocarbon (propellant) toxicity.
- Store at 15–30C (59–86F); protect from freezing.

Assessment & Drug Effects

- Tremors, a common adverse effect and one due to skeletal muscle stimulation, tends to diminish with continued use of bitolterol. Some find the effect intolerable.
- Immediate hypersensitivity reactions (see Signs & Symptoms, Appendix G) can occur with this drug. Epinephrine 1:1000 should be readily available until reaction to drug is known.
- Overdosage leads to exaggerated drug effects listed in Adverse/Side Effects.

Patient & Family Education

- Caution patient not to change dose or dose intervals, i.e., not to omit, increase, or decrease number of inhalations. Patient should notify physician immediately if condition worsens or if patient fails to respond to the usual dose.
- Warn patient not to use any other inhaler medication (OTC or leftover medication) unless the physician approves.
- Contents of the inhaler are under pressure; therefore, caution patient not to puncture the canister, use or store it near heat or an open flame, and not to place it in a fire or incinerator for disposal.

BLEOMYCIN SULFATE

(blee-oh-mye′sin)

Trade name: Blenoxane

Classifications: ANTINEOPLASTIC; ANTIBIOTIC

Prototype: Doxorubicin

Pregnancy category: D

ACTIONS/PHARMACODYNAMICS

Mixture of cytotoxic antibiotics from a strain of *Streptomyces verticillus.* A toxic drug with low therapeutic index; intensely cytotoxic. By unclear mechanism, blocks DNA, RNA, and protein synthesis. A cell cycle–phase nonspecific agent. Weak antibiotic activity is overshadowed by potent cytotoxic effects. Has strong affinity for skin and lung tumor cells, in contrast to its low affinity for cells in hematopoietic tissue. Widely used in combination with other chemotherapeutic agents because it lacks

B

significant myelosuppressive activity.

USES As single agent or in combination with other chemotherapeutic agents, as adjunct to surgery and radiation therapy. Squamous cell carcinomas of head, neck, penis, cervix, and vulva; lymphomas (including reticular cell sarcoma, lymphosarcoma, Hodgkin's); testicular carcinoma; malignant pleural effusions. **Unlabeled uses:** mycosis fungoides and *verucca vulgaris* (common warts).

ROUTE & DOSAGE

Squamous Cell Carcinoma, Testicular Carcinoma

Adult/Child: **SC, IM, IV** 10–20 U/m^2 or 0.25–0.5 U/kg 1–2 times/wk up to a total dose of 300–400 U.

Lymphomas

Adult/Child: **SC, IM, IV** 10–20 U/m^2 1–2 times/wk after a 1–2 U test dose x 2 doses.

Hodgkin's Disease, Maintenance

Adult/Child: **SC, IM, IV** 1 U IM or IV/ d or 5 U/wk.

PHARMACOKINETICS Distribution: concentrates mainly in skin, lungs, kidneys, lymphocytes, and peritoneum. **Metabolism:** unknown. **Elimination:** half-life: 2 h; 60–70% recovered in urine as parent compound.

CONTRAINDICATIONS & PRECAUTIONS Contraindicated in: history of hypersensitivity or idiosyncrasy to bleomycin, pregnancy (category D), women of childbearing age. **Cautious use in:** compromised hepatic, renal, or pulmonary function; previous cytotoxic drug or radiation therapy.

ADVERSE/SIDE EFFECTS CNS: headache, mental confusion. **GI:** stomatitis, ulcerations of tongue and lips, anorexia, nausea, vomiting, diarrhea, weight loss. **Hematologic** (rare): thrombocytopenia, leukopenia. **Respiratory:** pulmonary toxicity (dose- and age-related): interstitial pneumonitis, pneumonia, or fibrosis. **Skin:** diffuse alopecia (reversible), *hyperpigmentation, pruritic erythema,* vesiculation, acne, thickening of skin and nail beds, *patchy hyperkeratosis,* striae, peeling, bleeding. **Other:** *mild febrile reaction,* anaphylactoid reaction, pain at tumor site, phlebitis; necrosis at injection site.

DRUG INTERACTIONS Other ANTINEOPLASTIC AGENTS increase bone marrow toxicity; decreases effects of **digoxin, phenytoin.**

INCOMPATIBILITIES Solution/additive: aminophylline, ascorbic acid, carbenicillin, CEPHALOSPORINS, **diazepam, hydrocortisone, methotrexate, mitomycin, nafcillin, penicillin G, terbutaline.**

NURSING IMPLICATIONS

Administration

- Used only under constant supervision by medical personnel experienced in cancer chemotherapy.
- For IV administration, dilute each 15 U with at least 5 ml of sterile water for injection, D5W, or NaCl for injection. May be further diluted in 50–100 ml of chosen diluent.
- Administer properly diluted IV solution at a rate of 15 U/10 min through Y-tube of free-flowing IV.
- IV administration to infants and children: Verify correct IV concentration and rate of infusion with physician.
- Inject IM bleomycin deeply into

upper outer quadrant of buttock; change sites with each injection.

- Reconstituted solutions are stable at room temperature for 2 wk or for 4 wk if refrigerated. Discard unused solutions.
- Store unopened ampuls at 15–30C (59–86F) unless otherwise specified by manufacturer.

Assessment & Drug Effects

- Anaphylactoid reaction (see Signs & Symptoms, Appendix G) can be fatal. It may occur immediately or several hours after first or second dose, especially in lymphoma patients (10%). Usually, a test dose of 2 U or less of bleomycin is given to these patients for the first 2 doses. Patient is closely monitored (vital signs, auscultation of chest, careful observations) for at least 24 h. If there is no acute reaction (hypotension, hyperpyrexia, chills, confusion, wheezing, cardiopulmonary collapse), regular dosage schedule is resumed.
- Favorable response, if any is to occur, is expected within 2 wk for treatment of Hodgkin's or testicular tumor, and within 3 wk for squamous cell cancers.
- Monitor vital signs. Febrile reaction (mild chills and fever) is relatively common in patients receiving bleomycin therapy. It usually occurs within the first few hours after administration of a large single dose and lasts about 4–12 h. Reaction tends to become less frequent with continued drug administration but can recur at any time.
- Although bone marrow toxicity is rare, unexplained bleeding or bruising should be promptly reported to the physician.
- Monitor patient for evidence of deterioration of renal function, i.e., changed I&O ratio and pattern, weight gain (edema), decreasing creatinine clearance.
- Pulmonary toxicity occurs in about 10% of all patients and most frequently in patients >70 y or when the total of all doses approaches 400 U. It may also occur in young people, however, and with lower doses.
- Monitor for nonproductive cough, chest pain, dyspnea; by auscultation for fine rales.
- Be alert to evidence of radiation recall, i.e., erythema that develops in a previously irradiated field. This most frequently occurs when chemotherapy is started during or shortly after radiation therapy, but it also may be observed several years after the treatment.
- Stomatitis can be a dose-limiting factor because oral ulcerations may interfere with adequate nutrient intake, leading to severe debilitation. Consult physician if an oral local anesthetic is indicated. It may help patient to eat if applied about 10 min before meals.
- Check weight at regular intervals under standard conditions. Weight loss and anorexia may persist a long time after therapy has been discontinued.

Patient & Family Education

- Counsel patient to avoid using OTC drugs during antineoplastic treatment period unless such drugs are approved by physician.
- Skin toxicity usually develops in second or third week of treatment and after 150–200 U of bleomycin have been administered. Report symptoms (hypoesthesias, urticaria, tender swollen hands) promptly; therapy may be discontinued.
- Hyperpigmentation may occur in areas subject to friction and pres-

B

sure, skin folds, nail cuticles, scars, and intramuscular sites.

- Raynaud's phenomenon has been reported in a few patients receiving bleomycin for testicular carcinoma. Advise patient to observe and report early signs: hands and feet constantly cold especially when exposed; intermittent blanching and cyanosis in finger and toe tips; swelling of fingers and toes. Signs can occur during or after therapy has been discontinued.

BRETYLIUM TOSYLATE

(bre-til′ee-um)

Trade names: Bretylate♣, Bretylol

Classifications: CARDIOVASCULAR AGENT; ANTIARRHYTHMIC; AUTONOMIC NERVOUS SYSTEM AGENT; ADRENERGIC ANTAGONIST (SYMPATHOLYTIC, BLOCKING AGENT)

Prototype: Procainamide

Pregnancy category: C

ACTIONS/PHARMACODYNAMICS Mechanism of action is complex and not fully understood. Suppresses ventricular fibrillation by direct action on the myocardium and ventricular tachycardia by adrenergic blockade. Shortly after administration, norepinephrine is released from adrenergic postganglionic nerve terminals, resulting in a moderate increase in BP, heart rate, and ventricular irritability. Subsequently, (1–2 h) drug-induced release and reuptake of norepinephrine are blocked, leading to a state resembling surgical sympathectomy. Suppresses arrhythmias with a reentry mechanism and decrease dispersion of ectopic foci. PR, QT, and QRS intervals are unchanged. Orthostatic hypotension occurs commonly as a result of peripheral adrenergic blockade; some degree of hypotension may occur even while patient is supine. Tolerance to this effect develops after several days in most patients as adrenergic receptors become more responsive to circulating catecholamines. Because onset of desired action is delayed, bretylium is not a first-line antiarrhythmic agent.

USES Short-term prophylaxis and treatment of ventricular fibrillation; life-threatening arrhythmias such as ventricular fibrillation not responsive to conventional therapy, e.g., lidocaine, procainamide, direct current (cardioversion).

ROUTE & DOSAGE

Ventricular Fibrillation

Adult: **IV** 5 mg/kg rapid IV injection; may increase to 10 mg/kg and repeat q15–30min up to 30 mg/kg/d; may also give by continuous infusion at 1–2 mg/min. **IM** 5–10 mg/kg; may repeat in 1–2 h if arrhythmia persists, then 5–10 mg/kg q6–8h for maintenance.

Child: **IV** 5 mg/kg; may repeat q10–20min to total of 30 mg/kg. **IM** 2–5 mg/kg as single dose.

PHARMACOKINETICS **Onset:** minutes after IV; up to 6 h IM. **Peak:** 6–9 h. **Duration:** 6–24 h. **Distribution:** does not cross blood–brain barrier; not known if crosses placenta or distributed into breast milk. **Metabolism:** not metabolized. **Elimination:** half-life: 4–17 h; 70–80% excreted in urine in 24 h.

CONTRAINDICATIONS & PRECAUTIONS No contraindications for use in life-threatening refractory ventricular arrhythmias. Safe use during

Common side effect in *italic*, life-threatening effects underlined: generic names in **bold**; drug class in SMALL CAPS

pregnancy (category C), in nursing mothers, and in children not established. **Cautious use in:** digitalis-induced arrhythmias, patients with fixed cardiac output, e.g., severe aortic stenosis or severe pulmonary hypertension (profound hypotension can result without compensatory increase in cardiac output); sinus bradycardia, patients on digitalis maintenance, angina pectoris; impaired renal function.

ADVERSE/SIDE EFFECTS **CV:** both supine and postural *hypotension* with dizziness, vertigo, light-headedness, faintness, syncope, transitory hypertension, bradycardia, increased frequency of PVCs, exacerbation of digitalis-induced arrhythmias. **GI:** *nausea, vomiting* (particularly with rapid IV). **Other:** respiratory depression.

DIAGNOSTIC TEST INTERFERENCE ***Urinary VMA, epinephrine,*** and ***norepinephrine*** levels may be decreased during bretylium therapy.

DRUG INTERACTIONS **Lidocaine, procainamide, quinidine, propranolol** may antagonize antiarrhythmic effects and compound hypotension; ANTIHYPERTENSIVE AGENTS will add to hypotensive effects; DIGITALIS GLYCOSIDES may worsen arrhythmias through digitalis toxicity.

INCOMPATIBILITIES **Solution/additive: dobutamine, nitroglycerin, phenytoin. Y-site: phenytoin.**

NURSING IMPLICATIONS

Administration

- Use of bretylium should be limited to patients in facilities adequately equipped and staffed for constant monitoring of ECG and BP and for cardiopulmonary resuscitation and cardioversion if necessary.
- Administer no more than 5 ml in any one IM site. Avoid injecting into or near a major nerve. Keep a record of injection sites. Injection into same site can cause muscle atrophy, necrosis, and fibrosis.
- In ventricular fibrillation, IV bretylium may be given by direct IV undiluted at a rate of 1 dose/15 seconds.
- IV bretylium may be diluted in 50 ml or more of NS or D5W and infused at a rate of 1–2 mg/min.
- IV administration to infants and children: Verify correct IV concentration and rate of infusion/injection with physician.
- Store at 15–30C (59–86F) unless otherwise directed.

Assessment & Drug Effects

- Anticipate vomiting. IV administration is associated with a high incidence of nausea and vomiting. These side effects can be minimized by slow administration of drug (≥10 min).
- Establish baseline readings and monitor BP and ECG when drug is administered. Observe for initial transient rise in BP, increased heart rate, PVCs and other arrhythmias, or worsening of existing arrhythmias, which may occur within a few minutes to 1 h after drug administration. Keep physician informed. Usually, patients eventually adjust to these effects and stabilize.
- Initial effect of hypertension is usually followed within 1 h by a fall in supine BP and by orthostatic hypotension.
- The supine position is recommended until patient develops tolerance to the hypotensive effect of bretylium (generally in several days). Hypotension can occur in the supine position, particularly in patients with severely compromised cardiac function. It may not

B

readily respond to therapy (e.g., vasopressors, fluids); early reporting is essential.

- To prevent orthostatic hypotension, raise or lower head of bed slowly and advise patient to make position changes slowly. If patient is allowed to be out of bed, caution to dangle legs for a few minutes before standing and not to stand still for prolonged periods. Advise men to sit on toilet to urinate.
- Monitor I&O, particularly in patients with impaired renal function. Usually, these patients are given lower dosages or longer dosage intervals.

BRIMONIDINE TARTRATE

(bry-mon′-i-deen)

Trade name: Alphagan

Classifications: EYE PREPARATION; MIOTIC (ANTIGLAUCOMA AGENT)

Prototype: Pilocarpine

Pregnancy category: B

See Appendix A.

BRINZOLAMIDE

(brin-zol′a-mide)

Trade name: Azopt

Classifications: EYE PREPARATION; MIOTIC (ANTIGLAUCOMA AGENT); AUTONOMIC NERVOUS SYSTEM AGENT; DIRECT-ACTING CHOLINERGIC (PARASYMPATHOMIMETIC)

Prototype: Pilocarpine Hydrochloride

Pregnancy category: C

See Appendix A.

BROMOCRIPTINE MESYLATE

(broe-moe-krip′teen)

Trade name: Parlodel

Classifications: AUTONOMIC NERVOUS SYSTEM AGENT; ERGOT ALKALOID; ANTIPARKINSONISM AGENT

Prototype: Ergotamine

Pregnancy category: C

ACTIONS/PHARMACODYNAMICS

Semisynthetic ergot alkaloid derivative, but devoid of oxytocic activity generally attributed to drugs of this class. Reduces elevated serum prolactin levels in men and women by activating postsynaptic dopaminergic receptors in hypothalamus to stimulate release of prolactin-inhibiting factor and possibly luteinizing hormone release factor. Ovulation and ovarian function in amenorrheic women are restored, thus correcting female infertility secondary to elevated prolactin levels. Activates dopaminergic receptors in neostriatum of CNS, which may explain action in parkinsonism. Also reduces BP in the hypertensive and normotensive individual and may cause peripheral vasoconstriction (large doses) and increased sodium excretion.

USES Short-term management of amenorrhea/galactorrhea or female infertility associated with hyperprolactemia (when there is no indication of pituitary tumor). Also used as adjunctive to levodopa or levodopa/carbidopa therapy to relieve symptoms of Parkinson's disease and to lower plasma growth hormone in patients with acromegaly. **Unlabeled uses:** to prevent postpartum lactation, to relieve premenstrual symptoms, to treat hypogonadism and galactorrhea in hyperprolactinemic men; for management of hepatic encephalopathy,

B

Cushing's syndrome, drug-induced neuroleptic malignant syndrome, and cocaine withdrawal.

ROUTE & DOSAGE

Amenorrhea or Galactorrhea, Female Infertility

Adult: **PO** 1.25–2.5 mg/d up to 2.5 mg 2–3 times/d.

Suppression of Postpartum Lactation

Adult: **PO** 2.5 mg b.i.d. starting at least 4 h after delivery for 14–21 d.

Parkinson's Disease

Adult: **PO** 1.25–2.5 mg/d up to 100 mg/d in divided doses.

Acromegaly

Adult: **PO** 1.25–2.5 mg/d for 3 d; then increase by 1.25–2.5 mg q3–7d until desired effect achieved; usually 30–60 mg/d in divided doses.

PHARMACOKINETICS **Absorption:** approximately 28% absorbed from GI tract. **Peak:** 1–2 h. **Duration:** 4– 8 h. **Metabolism:** metabolized in liver. **Elimination:** half-life: 50 h; 85% excreted in feces in 5 d; 3–6% eliminated in urine.

CONTRAINDICATIONS & PRECAUTIONS **Contraindicated in:** hypersensitivity to ergot alkaloids; uncontrolled hypertension; severe ischemic heart disease or peripheral vascular disease; pituitary tumor; normal prolactin levels, nursing women. Safe use during pregnancy (category C) and in children <15 y not established. **Cautious use in:** hepatic and renal dysfunction; history of psychiatric disorder; history of MI with residual arrhythmia.

ADVERSE/SIDE EFFECTS Mostly dose related. **CNS:** headache, dizziness, vertigo, light-headedness, fainting, sedation, nightmares, insomnia, dyskinesia, ataxia; mania, nervousness, anxiety, depression. **CV:** *orthostatic hypotension*, shock, postpartum hypertension, palpitation, extrasystoles, Raynaud's phenomenon, red, tender, hot, edematous extremities (erythromelalgia), exacerbation of angina, arrhythmias, acute MI. **Eye:** blurred vision, burning sensation in eyes, blepharospasm, diplopia. **GI:** *nausea,* vomiting, abdominal cramps, epigastric pain, constipation (long-term use) or diarrhea; metallic taste, dry mouth, dysphagia, anorexia, peptic ulcers. **Skin:** urticaria, rash, mottling, livedo reticularis. **Other:** fatigue, nasal congestion, asthenia.

DRUG INTERACTIONS Possibility of decreased tolerance to **alcohol;** ANTIHYPERTENSIVE AGENTS add to hypotensive effects; ORAL CONTRACEPTIVES, **estrogen, progestins** may interfere with effect of bromocriptine by causing amenorrhea and galactorrhea; PHENOTHIAZINES, TRICYCLIC ANTIDEPRESSANTS, **methyldopa, reserpine** can cause an increase in prolactin, which may interfere with bromocriptine activity.

NURSING IMPLICATIONS

Administration

- Administer with meals, milk, or other food to reduce incidence of GI side effects.
- Hypotension with dizziness and fainting may occur, particularly following first dose in sensitive patients. For this reason, initial dose is usually prescribed for evening administration.
- Suppression of puerperal lactation: Because hypotension occurs

most commonly in the postpartum patient, it is recommended that therapy not be started any sooner than 4 h after delivery and then only if vital signs have stabilized.

- Store in tightly closed, light-resistant containers, preferably at 15–30C (59–86F) unless otherwise directed.

Assessment & Drug Effects

- Establish data regarding baseline vital signs. Therapy should not be initiated until vital signs are stable.
- BP should be monitored closely during the first few days of therapy and periodically throughout therapy for all patients. Compare readings with baseline data.
- Side effects are common, but they are usually mild to moderate in degree and respond to dosage reduction or discontinuation of drug.
- Periodic evaluations should be made of hepatic, hematologic, cardiovascular, and renal function in patients on prolonged therapy.
- Note that dosages for Parkinson's disease may be almost 10 times larger than those for galactorrhea and amenorrhea. Therefore, psychotic symptoms and other adverse reactions occur most frequently in Parkinson's patients.
- Improvement in Parkinson's disease may be noted in 30–90 min following administration of bromocriptine, with maximum effect in 2 h.
- Recurrence rates of amenorrhea and galactorrhea are high (70–80%) following withdrawal of bromocriptine. Amenorrhea usually returns within 4–24 wk; galactorrhea within 2–12 wk; serum prolactin increases to pretreatment levels within 1–6 wk.

Patient & Family Education

- Instruct patient to make position changes slowly and in stages, especially from recumbent to upright posture, and to dangle legs over bed for a few minutes before ambulating. Caution patient to lie down immediately if light-headedness or dizziness occurs.
- Inform patient that a mild diuresis may occur because of vasodilating action of bromocriptine on renal arteries.
- Since bromocriptine is associated with dose-related light-headedness, dizziness, and syncope, caution patient to avoid driving and other potentially hazardous activities until reaction to drug has been determined.
- Bromocriptine can cause digital vasospasm, particularly in patients with acromegaly and patients receiving high dosages. Advise patient to avoid exposure to cold and to report the onset of pallor of fingers or toes.
- Advise patient that bromocriptine may increase sensitivity to the effects of alcohol.
- Patients receiving bromocriptine to suppress postpartum lactation may have temporary rebound breast enlargement and pain following drug withdrawal.
- Patients being treated for amenorrhea or galactorrhea should be informed that restoration of regular menses usually occurs in 6– 8 wk (range: a few days to 24 wk). (If patient has been amenorrheic more than 4 y, restoration of menses may require considerable time.) Galactorrhea suppression is usually seen after 7–12 wk of therapy but may not occur for more than 24 wk. Because long-term drug effects are not known, it is recommended that duration of therapy for amenorrhea and galactorrhea not exceed 6 mo.
- Since restoration of fertility may result during therapy, patients being

treated for amenorrhea and galactorrhea should be advised to use barrier-type contraceptive measures until normal ovulating cycle is restored. Oral contraceptives are contraindicated because they may cause amenorrhea and galactorrhea.

- Inform physician immediately if pregnancy occurs during therapy. Bromocriptine should be discontinued without delay. These patients should be carefully observed throughout pregnancy.

BROMPHENIRAMINE MALEATE

(brome-fen-ir′a-meen)

Trade names: Bromphen, Codimal-A, Conjec-B, Cophene-B, Dehist, Dimetane, Dimetane Extentabs, Nasahist B, Sinusol-B

Classification: ANTIHISTAMINE (H_1-RECEPTOR ANTAGONIST)

Prototype: Diphenhydramine

Pregnancy category: C

ACTIONS/PHARMACODYNAMICS

Antihistamine similar to diphenhydramine; shares properties of other antihistamines. Competes with histamine for H_1-receptor sites on effector cells, thus blocking histamine-mediated responses. Has less sedative effect than diphenhydramine.

USES Symptomatic treatment of allergic manifestations. Also used in various cough mixtures and antihistamine-decongestant cold formulations.

ROUTE & DOSAGE

Allergy

Adult: **PO** 4–8 mg t.i.d. or q.i.d. *or* 8–12 mg of sustained release b.i.d. or t.i.d. **IM/IV** 5–20 mg q6–12h (max 40 mg/24 h).
Geriatric: **PO** 4 mg 1–2 times/d.
Child: **PO** >6 y, 2–4 mg t.i.d. or q.i.d. *or* 8–12 mg of sustained release b.i.d. (max 12 mg/24 h); <6 y, 0.5 mg/kg in 3–4 divided doses.

PHARMACOKINETICS **Peak:** 3–9 h. **Duration:** up to 48 h. **Distribution:** crosses placenta. **Elimination:** half-life: 12–34 h; 40% excreted in urine within 72 h; 2% in feces.

CONTRAINDICATIONS & PRECAUTIONS **Contraindicated in:** hypersensitivity to antihistamines; newborns, nursing mothers; acute asthma; pregnancy (category C). **Cautious use in:** the elderly; prostatic hypertrophy; narrow-angle glaucoma; cardiovascular or renal disease; hyperthyroidism.

ADVERSE/SIDE EFFECTS *Sedation,* drowsiness, dry mouth, throat, and nose, ringing or buzzing in ears, hypotension, dizziness, headache, disturbed coordination, urticaria, rash, increased sweating, stomach upset, constipation, photosensitivity, hypersensitivity reaction, <u>agranulocytosis</u>.

DIAGNOSTIC TEST INTERFERENCE May cause false-negative ***allergy skin tests.***

DRUG INTERACTIONS **Alcohol** and other CNS DEPRESSANTS add to sedation.

INCOMPATIBILITIES **Solution/additive: Radio-contrast media (diatrizoate, iothalomalate).**

NURSING IMPLICATIONS

Administration

- If gastric distress occurs, advise patient to take medication with meals or a snack.

- IV brompheniramine maleate may be given undiluted or diluted with 10 ml 0.9% NaCl injection unless otherwise specified by manufacturer. Administer one dose direct IV over 1 min.
- Initially diluted IV solution may be further diluted with NS for injection or D5W and infused at the ordered rate.
- Read labels carefully. Note that the 100 mg/ml concentration is not recommended for IV use. It is intended for IM administration and is given either without further dilution or diluted 1:10 with sterile saline for injection.
- Store in tightly covered container at 15–30C (59–86F) unless otherwise directed. Elixir and parenteral form should be protected from light. Avoid freezing.

Assessment & Drug Effects

- Acute hypersensitivity reaction with sudden severe agranulocytosis reportedly can occur within minutes to hours after drug ingestion. The reaction is manifested by high fever, chills, and possible development of gangrenous ulcerations of mouth and throat, pneumonia, and prostration. Patient should seek medical attention immediately.
- Drowsiness, sweating, transient hypotension, and syncope may follow IV administration. Patient should be recumbent while receiving injection, and reaction to drug should be evaluated. Keep physician informed.
- Elderly patients tend to be particularly susceptible to sedative effect, dizziness, and hypotension. Most symptoms respond to reduction in dosage.
- Bear in mind that brompheniramine has an atropinelike effect (thickens bronchial secretions) that may make expectoration difficult.
- Blood counts should be performed in patients receiving long-term therapy to reduce possibility of blood dyscrasias.

Patient & Family Education

- Thickened bronchial secretions and dry mouth, nose, and throat may be relieved by increasing fluid intake (check with physician). Advise patient that relief of dry mouth may be provided by sugarless gum or lemon drops, frequent rinses with warm water, diligent mouth care.
- Caution patient to avoid driving a car or other potentially hazardous activities until reaction to drug is known.
- Advise patient not to take alcoholic beverages and other CNS depressants, e.g., tranquilizers, sedatives, pain or sleeping medicines, without consulting physician.
- May cause false-negative allergy skin tests. The drug should be discontinued about 4 d before such tests are done.

BUCLIZINE HYDROCHLORIDE

(byoo-cli'zeen)

Trade name: Bucladin-S Softab

Classifications: ANTIHISTAMINE; ANTIVERTIGO

Prototype: Meclizine

Pregnancy category: C

ACTIONS/PHARMACODYNAMICS

Buclizine is a piperazine derivative structurally and pharmacologically related to meclizine and cyclizine. Mechanism of action not precisely known but may be related to its central anticholinergic actions. It diminishes vestibular stimulation and depresses labyrinthine function. An action on the medullary chemoreceptive trigger zone (CTZ) may also be involved in its antiemetic effect. Exhibits antihistaminic, anticholinergic, antivertigo, CNS depressant, and local anesthetic effects.

USES Prevention and treatment of motion sickness and the symptomatic treatment of vertigo.

ROUTE & DOSAGE

Motion Sickness

Adult: **PO** 50 mg 30 min before travel; may repeat in 4–6 h if needed.

Vertigo

Adult: **PO** 50 mg 1–3 times/d.

PHARMACOKINETICS **Absorption:** readily absorbed from GI tract. **Onset:** 1 h. **Duration:** 4–6 h.

CONTRAINDICATIONS & PRECAUTIONS **Contraindicated in:** hypersensitivity to buclizine hydrochloride, pediatric patients, elderly, lactation, pregnancy (category C). **Cautious use in:** patients receiving other CNS depressants or depressant drugs, angle-closure glaucoma, prostatic hypertrophy, bladder neck obstruction, pyloroduodenal obstruction.

ADVERSE/SIDE EFFECTS *Drowsiness,* dry mouth, headache, nausea, jitteriness.

DIAGNOSTIC TEST INTERFERENCE May interfere with ***allergy skin tests.***

DRUG INTERACTIONS **Alcohol** and other CNS DEPRESSANTS compound CNS depression.

NURSING IMPLICATIONS

Administration

- Administer with food, water, or milk to minimize gastric irritation.
- Tablet may be swallowed whole, chewed, or allowed to dissolve in mouth without water.
- Store away from heat, light, or moist areas at 15–30C in a tightly closed container.

Assessment & Drug Effects

- Inquire about history of aspirin allergy. Withhold buclizine if aspirin hypersensitivity reported.
- Buclizine may suppress dizziness, nausea, and vomiting associated with drug toxicity and serious disease conditions.
- Buclizine may mask ototoxic effects of large doses of salicylates.

Patient & Family Education

- Advise patient to take at least 30 min before traveling for motion sickness.
- Do not take more medication than recommended.
- Observe caution while driving or performing other tasks requiring alertness until reaction to drug is known.
- Avoid alcohol and other CNS depressants.
- This drug may interfere with skin tests using allergens; inform physician of use.

BUDESONIDE

(bu-des′-o-nide)

Trade names: Pulmicort Turbuhaler, Rhinocort, Rhinocort Turbuhaler

Classifications: HORMONE; ADRENAL CORTICOSTEROID; GLUCOCORTICOID; MINERALOCORTICOID

Prototype: Hydrocortisone

Pregnancy category: C

See Appendix A.

B

BUMETANIDE

(byoo-met′a-nide)
Trade name: Bumex
Classifications: WATER BALANCE AGENT; LOOP DIURETIC
Prototype: Furosemide
Pregnancy category: C

ACTIONS/PHARMACODYNAMICS Sulfonamide derivative structurally related to furosemide and with similar pharmacologic effects. Diuretic activity is 40 times greater, however, and duration of action is shorter than that of furosemide. Inhibits sodium and chloride reabsorption by direct action on proximal ascending limb of the loop of Henle. Also appears to inhibit phosphate and bicarbonate reabsorption. Produces only mild hypotensive effects at usual diuretic doses. Causes both potassium and magnesium wastage.

USES Edema associated with CHF; hepatic or renal disease, including nephrotic syndrome. Has been used in management of postoperative and premenstrual edema, edema accompanying disseminated carcinoma, and mild hypertension. May be used concomitantly with a potassium-sparing diuretic.

ROUTE & DOSAGE

Edema

Adult: **PO** 0.5–2 mg once/d; may repeat at 4–5 h intervals if needed (max 10 mg/d). **IM/IV** 0.5–1 mg over 1–2 min; repeated q2–3h prn (max 10 mg/d).
Neonates: **PO/IM/IV** 0.01–0.05 mg/kg q24–48h.
Infant/child: **PO/IM/IV** 0.015–0.1 mg/kg q6–24h (max 10 mg/d).

PHARMACOKINETICS Absorption: readily absorbed from GI tract. **Onset:** 30–60 min PO; 40 min IV. **Peak:** 0.5–2 h. **Duration:** 4–6 h. **Distribution:** distributed into breast milk. **Metabolism:** partially metabolized in liver. **Elimination:** half-life: 60–90 min; 80% excreted in urine in 48 h, 10–20% excreted in feces.

CONTRAINDICATIONS & PRECAUTIONS Contraindicated in: hypersensitivity to bumetanide or to other sulfonamides; anuria, markedly elevated BUN; hepatic coma; severe electrolyte deficiency. Safe use during pregnancy (category C), in nursing mothers, and in children <18 y not established. **Cautious use in:** hepatic cirrhosis, ascites; history of gout; history of hypersensitivity to furosemide.

ADVERSE/SIDE EFFECTS CNS: dizziness, headache, weakness, fatigue. **CV:** hypotension, ECG changes, chest pain, *hypovolemia*. **GI:** nausea, vomiting, abdominal or stomach pain, GI distress, diarrhea, dry mouth. **Electrolytes:** *hypokalemia*, hyponatremia, hyperuricemia, hyperglycemia; *hypomagnesemia;* decreased calcium, chloride. **Musculoskeletal:** muscle cramps, muscle pain, stiffness or tenderness; arthritic pain. **Ototoxicity:** ear discomfort, ringing or buzzing in ears, impaired hearing. **Other:** sweating, hyperventilation, glycosuria.

DRUG INTERACTIONS AMINOGLYCOSIDES, **cisplatin** increase risk of ototoxicity; bumetanide increases risk of hypokalemia-induced **digoxin** toxicity; NONSTEROIDAL ANTIINFLAMMATORY DRUGS may attenuate diuretic and hypotensive response; **probenecid** may antagonize diuretic activity; bumetanide may decrease renal elimination of **lithium.**

INCOMPATIBILITIES Solution/additive: dobutamine.

NURSING IMPLICATIONS

Administration

- Oral drug may be taken with food or milk to reduce risk of gastrointestinal irritation.
- Drug is usually administered in the morning as a single dose, either daily or by intermittent schedule. For some patients, diuresis is reportedly more effective when administered in two divided doses, morning and evening.
- IV bumetanide may be given direct IV undiluted at a rate of a single dose over 1–2 min.
- For IV infusion, parenteral bumetanide is compatible with 5% dextrose, 0.9% NaCl, and lactated Ringer's. Infusion should be used within 24 h after preparation.
- IV administration to neonates, infants and children: Verify correct IV concentration and rate of infusion/injection with physician.
- Drug will discolor on exposure to light. Inspect parenteral bumetanide before administration. Discard if it contains particles or is discolored.
- Store in tight, light-resistant container at 15–30C (59–86F) unless otherwise directed.

Assessment & Drug Effects

- Monitor I&O, BUN, and serum creatinine. Report promptly the onset of oliguria or other changes in I&O ratio and pattern and significant increases in BUN or serum creatinine.
- Monitor weight, BP, and pulse rate. Assess for hypovolemia by assessing BP and pulse rate while patient is lying, sitting, and standing.
- High doses or frequent administration, particularly in the elderly, can cause profound diuresis, hypovolemia, and resulting circulatory collapse with development of thrombi and emboli. Careful monitoring is essential.
- Both hypomagnesemia and hypokalemia (see Signs & Symptoms, Appendix G) pose a constant threat to all patients and particularly those receiving digitalis or who have CHF, hepatic cirrhosis, ascites, diarrhea, or potassium-depleting nephropathy. Careful monitoring and hospitalization during initial therapy and dosage adjustment periods are advised in these patients.
- Patients with hepatic disease should be carefully observed. Alterations in fluid and electrolyte balance can precipitate encephalopathy (inappropriate behavior, altered mood, impaired judgment, confusion, drowsiness, coma).
- Be alert to complaints about hearing difficulty or ear discomfort. Patients at risk of ototoxic effects (see Signs & Symptoms, Appendix G) include those receiving the drug IV, especially at high doses, those with severely impaired renal function, and those receiving other potentially ototoxic or nephrotoxic drugs. Hearing tests at periodic intervals are indicated for these patients.
- Serum electrolytes, blood studies, liver and kidney function tests, uric acid (particularly patients with history of gout), and blood sugar (particularly diabetics) values should be determined initially and at regular intervals. These determinations are especially important in patients receiving prolonged treatment, high doses, or who are on sodium restriction.

Patient & Family Education

- Advise patient to report symptoms

B

of electrolyte imbalance promptly to physician: weakness, dizziness, fatigue, faintness, confusion, muscle cramps, headache, paresthesias.

- Inform patient that serum magnesium, potassium, and sodium should be monitored during therapy.
- It is important for patient to maintain an adequate daily intake of potassium while taking bumetanide.
- Advise patient to promptly report signs and symptoms of ototoxicity.
- Advise diabetics that drug may cause loss of glycemic control and that they should inform physician of their diabetes, since adjustment in insulin dose may be required.

BUPIVACAINE HYDROCHLORIDE

(byoo-piv'a-kane)

Trade names: Marcaine, Sensorcaine

Classifications: CNS AGENT; LOCAL ANESTHETIC (AMIDE-TYPE)

Prototype: Procaine

Pregnancy category: C

ACTIONS/PHARMACODYNAMICS

Anesthetic of the amide type. Decreases sodium flux into nerve cell, inhibiting initial depolarization, and prevents propagation and conduction of the nerve impulse. Progression of anesthesia, related to diameter, myelination, and conduction velocity of affected fibers manifests clinically as sequential loss of nerve function: pain, temperature, touch, proprioception, and skeletal muscle tone. CV system effects are minimal; toxic blood concentrations depress cardiac condition and excitability and myocardial contractility and cause vasodilation. Bupivacaine may stimulate or depress the CNS or do both. Primary depressant effect is in medulla and higher centers.

USES Infiltration anesthesia; peripheral, sympathetic nerve, and epidural (including caudal) block anesthesia; 0.75% bupivacaine solution in dextrose is used for spinal anesthesia.

ROUTE & DOSAGE

Infiltration Anesthesia

Adult: **IM Local infiltration, sympathetic block:** 0.25% solution; **Lumbar epidural:** 0.25%, 0.5%, 0.75% solutions; **Caudal block, peripheral nerve block:** 0.25%, 0.5% solutions; **Retrobulbar block:** 0.75% solution.

Child: **IM** 1–3.7 mg/kg.

PHARMACOKINETICS **Onset:** 4–17 min for epidural, caudal, peripheral, or sympathetic block; within 1 min for spinal block. **Duration:** 3–5 h for epidural, caudal, peripheral, or sympathetic block; 1.25–2.5 h for spinal block. **Distribution:** crosses placenta. **Metabolism:** metabolized in liver. **Elimination:** half-life: 1.5–5.5 h in adults, 8.1 h in neonates; 6% excreted unchanged in urine.

CONTRAINDICATIONS & PRECAUTIONS **Contraindicated in:** known sensitivity to bupivacaine or to other amide-type anesthetics or to parabens or metabisulfites; acidosis; heart block; severe hemorrhage; hypotension and shock; hypertension, cerebrospinal diseases; obstetrical paracervical anesthesia or spinal anesthesia in septicemia; topical or IV regional anesthesia; intercurrent use with chloroprocaine; history of malignant hyperthermia. Safe use during pregnancy (category C) other than during labor and lactation or in children <12 y not established. **Cautious use in:** the elderly or debilitated patient; hepatic or renal disease; known drug allergies and sensitivities, dysrhythmias, children >12 y, obstetrical delivery.

ADVERSE/SIDE EFFECTS **CNS:** nervousness, unusual anxiety, excitement, dizziness, drowsiness, tremors, convulsions, unconsciousness, respiratory arrest. Associated with epidural anesthesia: total spinal block, urinary retention, fecal incontinence, loss of perineal sensation and sexual function; persistent analgesia, paresthesia, slowing of labor, increased incidence of forceps delivery, cranial nerve palsies (with inadvertent intrathecal injection). **CV:** hypotension, ventricular arrhythmias, myocardial depression, decreased cardiac output, bradycardia (fatal bradycardia during delivery), maternal hypotension, cardiac arrest. **Eye:** pupillary constriction; blurred or double vision. **GI:** nausea, vomiting. **Hypersensitivity:** cutaneous lesions, urticaria, sneezing, diaphoresis, syncope, hyperthermia, angioneurotic edema (including laryngeal edema), anaphylaxis, anaphylactoid reactions. **Ototoxicity:** tinnitus. **Other:** inflammation or sepsis at injection site, chills, pupillary constriction.

DRUG INTERACTIONS CNS DEPRESSANTS augment CNS depression; with **isoproterenol, ergonovine** there is persistent hypertension and a risk of CVA if bupivacaine used with **epinephrine:** MAO INHIBITORS, TRICYCLIC ANTIDEPRESSANTS, PHENOTHIAZINES cause severe or prolonged hypotension or hypertension if bupivacaine used with epinephrine.

INCOMPATIBILITIES **Solution/additive: sodium bicarbonate.**

NURSING IMPLICATIONS

Administration

- Preparations containing preservatives should not be used for epidural or spinal anesthesia.
- Bupivacaine with dextrose may be autoclaved once (repeated autoclaving or prolonged storage discolors solution because of caramelizing of dextrose).
- Do not use multiple-dose vial for lumbar or caudal epidural block; it is not known whether intrathecal administration of the preservatives in this vial is safe.
- The addition of a vasoconstrictor (epinephrine) to decrease rate of absorption also reduces risk of systemic toxic reaction, prolongs anesthetic effect, and permits administration of a larger maximum single dose of anesthetic.
- Store ampuls at 15–30C (59–85F); protect from freezing. Solutions with epinephrine should be protected from light.

Assessment & Drug Effects

- Observe for clinical response to an inadvertent intravascular injection, which can produce within 45 seconds a transient "epinephrine response" (increased heart rate or systolic BP or both, circumoral pallor, palpitations, nervousness) in the unsedated patient and an increase by 20 bpm or more in heart rate for at least 15 seconds in sedated patient.
- Risk of toxicity and degree of motor block increase with repeated doses (e.g., 2 doses of 0.5% solution can produce complete motor block).
- Vasoconstrictor-containing solution should be administered cautiously, if at all, to areas with end arteries (e.g., digits, penis) or to areas that have a compromised blood supply; ischemia and gan-

grene can result. Inspect areas for evidence of reduced perfusion because of vasospasm: pale, cold, sensitive skin.

- Systemic reactions (toxicity) are more apt to occur in children or the elderly and may develop rapidly or be delayed for as long as 30 min after administration.
- CNS stimulation (unusual anxiety, excitement, restlessness) usually occurs first, followed by CNS depression (drowsiness, unconsciousness, respiratory arrest). However, because stimulation is apt to be transient or absent, drowsiness may be the first sign of toxicity in some patients (especially children, elderly).
- Maternal hypotension may accompany regional anesthesia. Place mother on left side with legs elevated; monitor BP and fetal heart rate continuously.
- Monitor fetal heart rate during paracervical anesthesia. The risk of fetal bradycardia is high in prematurity, postmaturity, preeclampsia, uteroplacental insufficiency, and fetal distress.
- Patients receiving retrobulbar and dental blocks should have continuous monitoring of cardiac and respiratory status.
- During preparation for retrobulbar or dental anesthesia, inadvertent intraarterial injection of bupivacaine with subsequent retrograde flow into cerebral circulation may cause confusion, respiratory depression or arrest, convulsions, and CV stimulation or depression.

Patient & Family Education

- Tell patient who is given spinal anesthesia that sensation to lower extremities may not return for 2.5–3.5 h.

BUPRENORPHINE HYDROCHLORIDE

(byoo-pre-nor′feen)

Trade name: Buprenex

Classifications: CNS AGENT; ANALGESIC; NARCOTIC (OPIATE) AGONIST-ANTAGONIST

Prototype: Pentazocine

Pregnancy category: C

Controlled substance: Schedule V

ACTIONS/PHARMACODYNAMICS

Opiate agonist-antagonist with agonist activity approximately 30 times that of morphine and antagonist activity equal to or up to 3 times greater than that of naloxone. Dose-related analgesia results from a high affinity of buprenorphine for mu- and possibly kappa-opiate receptors in the CNS. Respiratory depression occurs infrequently and is of limited clinical significance to most patients. General absence of dose-related respiratory depression at higher than usual doses may be due to drug's opiate antagonist activity. Psychologic and limited physical dependence develops infrequently. Tolerance to drug rarely develops.

USES Principally for moderate to severe postoperative pain. Also for pain associated with cancer and trigeminal neuralgia, accidental trauma, ureteral calculi, MI. **Unlabeled uses:** to reverse fentanyl-induced anesthesia, to reduce opiate consumption in physical dependence on opiates (e.g., heroin).

ROUTE & DOSAGE

Postoperative Pain

Adult: **IM/IV** 0.3 mg q6h up to 0.6 mg q4h *or* 25–50 μg/h by IV infusion, *or* 60–180 μg over 48 h by epidural injection.

PHARMACOKINETICS **Onset:** 10–30 min. **Peak:** 1 h. **Duration:** 6–10 h. **Metabolism:** metabolized extensively in liver. **Elimination:** half-life: 2.2 h; 70% eliminated in feces and 20% in urine in 7 d.

CONTRAINDICATIONS & PRECAUTIONS **Contraindicated in:** known hypersensitivity to buprenorphine. Safe use in children <13 y and during pregnancy (category C) and lactation not established. **Cautious use in:** patient with history of opiate use, compromised respiratory function, concomitant use of other respiratory depressants; hypothyroidism, myxedema, Addison's disease; severe renal or hepatic impairment; geriatric or debilitated patients; acute alcoholism, delirium tremens; prostatic hypertrophy, urethral stricture; comatose patient; patients with CNS depression, head injury or intracranial lesion; biliary tract dysfunction.

ADVERSE/SIDE EFFECTS **CNS:** *sedation, drowsiness,* dizziness, vertigo, headache, amnesia, euphoria. **CV:** hypotension. **Eye:** miosis. **GI:** *nausea,* vomiting. **Respiratory:** respiratory depression, hyperventilation. **Skin:** pruritus, injection site reactions. **Other:** diaphoresis.

DRUG INTERACTIONS **Alcohol,** OPIATES, other CNS DEPRESSANTS, BENZODIAZEPINES augment CNS depression; **diazepam** may cause respiratory or cardiovascular collapse.

NURSING IMPLICATIONS

Administration

- Inspect buprenorphine solution visually for particulate matter and discoloration before administration.
- IV buprenorphine HCl may be given undiluted by direct IV at a rate of 0.3 mg over 2 min.
- IV administration precautions include patient in recumbent position during infusion and for short period afterward and immediately available emergency equipment and drugs.
- Gradual dose reduction may be necessary to avoid withdrawal symptoms.
- Store at 15–30C (59–86F); avoid freezing.

Assessment & Drug Effects

- Monitor respiratory status during therapy. Buprenorphine-induced respiratory depression is about equal to that produced by 10 mg morphine, but onset is slower, and if it occurs, it lasts longer.
- It may be difficult to identify respiratory depression because compensatory increases in depth of respiration prevent changes in arterial blood gas values. Also reduced pain intensity can reduce rate of respirations.
- Respiratory depression in the healthy adult plateaus or may even decrease in severity with doses more than 1.2 mg because of antagonist activity of the drug.
- Additive analgesic effect with a concurrent NSAID or other nonnarcotic analgesic permits lower dosing of buprenorphine.
- Treatment of chronic pain is thought to be more effective if scheduled rather than on an as-needed basis. This regimen is more likely to prevent peaks and troughs of pain and to provide sustained freedom from pain.
- Monitor I&O ratio and pattern during buprenorphine therapy; urinary retention is a potential adverse effect.
- Drowsiness occurs in about 66% of patients on this drug. Dizziness and vertigo are experienced by about 10% of patients.

Patient & Family Education

- Supervise ambulation. Also warn

patient that the drug may impair ability to perform hazardous activities requiring mental alertness or physical coordination (e.g., driving a car).

- Instruct patient on measures to relieve dry mouth.
- Inform patient of additive effect of other CNS depressants including alcohol.
- Warn patient not to take diazepam without medical supervision.

BUPROPION HYDROCHLORIDE

(byoo-pro′pi-on)

Trade names: Wellbutrin, Wellbutrin SR, Zyban

Classification: ANTIDEPRESSANT

Pregnancy category: B

ACTIONS/PHARMACODYNAMICS The neurochemical mechanism of bupropion is unknown. It does not inhibit monamine oxidase. Compared to tricyclic antidepressants it is a weak blocker of neural uptake of serotonin and norepinephrine.

USES Indicated for mental depression; since it has been associated with increased risk of seizures, it is not the agent of first choice; adjunct for smoking cessation. **Unlabeled uses:** cyclic mood disorders, schizoaffective disorders.

ROUTE & DOSAGE

Depression

Adult: **PO** 75–100 mg t.i.d.; doses >450 mg/d are associated with an increased risk of adverse reactions (including seizures); max 150 mg/dose; start with 75 mg t.i.d. or 100 mg b.i.d. and increase dose q3d to 300 mg/d.
Geriatric: **PO** 50–100 mg/d, may increase by 50–100 mg q3–4d.

Smoking Cessation

Adult: **PO** Start with 150 mg q.d. × 3 d, then increase to 150 mg b.i.d. (max 300 mg/d) for 7–12 wk.

PHARMACOKINETICS Absorption: readily absorbed from GI tract. **Onset:** 3–4 wk. **Peak:** 1–3 h. **Metabolism:** metabolized in liver (including first pass metabolism) to active metabolites. **Elimination:** half-life: 8–24 h; 80% excreted in urine as inactive metabolites.

CONTRAINDICATIONS & PRECAUTIONS Contraindicated in: hypersensitivity to drug, history of seizure disorder, current or prior diagnosis of bulimia or anorexia nervosa, concurrent administration of MAO inhibitor, head trauma, CNS tumor, recent MI, nursing mothers. **Cautious use in:** renal or hepatic function impairment, drug abuse or dependence, pregnancy (category B).

ADVERSE/SIDE EFFECTS CNS: <u>seizures</u>. The risk of seizure appears to be strongly associated with dose (especially >450 mg/d) and may be increased by predisposing factors (e.g., head trauma, CNS tumor) or a history of prior seizure; *agitation, insomnia, dry mouth, blurred vision, headache, dizziness, tremor*. **GI:** *nausea, vomiting, constipation*. **CV:** tachycardia. **Other:** weight loss, weight gain, rash.

DRUG INTERACTIONS Bupropion may increase metabolism of **carbamazepine, cimetidine, phenytoin, phenobarbital,** decreasing their effect; may increase incidence of adverse effects of **levodopa,** MAO INHIBITORS.

B

NURSING IMPLICATIONS

Administration

- Bupropion may be administered with meals to decrease the incidence of nausea and vomiting.
- Increases in dosage should not exceed 100 mg/d over a 3 d period. Greater increments increase the seizure potential.
- Store away from heat and direct light as well as moist areas.

Assessment & Drug Effects

- Use extreme caution when administering drug to patient with history of seizures, cranial trauma, or other factors predisposing to seizures.
- During sudden and large increments in dose, seizure potential is increased.
- A substantial proportion of patients experience some degree of increased restlessness, agitation, anxiety, and insomnia. Symptoms may require treatment or discontinuation of drug.
- Monitor for delusions, hallucinations, psychotic episodes, confusion, and paranoia.
- Bupropion may cause ECG changes such as premature beats and nonspecific ST-T changes with long-term use.
- Hepatic and renal function tests should be monitored while patient is on this drug.
- The full antidepressant effect of drug may not be realized for 4 or more weeks.

Patient & Family Education

- Drug should be taken at same times each day.
- Weight gain of ≥2 kg (5 lb) may occur.
- Alcohol increases the risk of seizures. Therefore, its consumption should be minimized or preferably avoided.
- Ability to perform tasks requiring judgment or motor and cognitive skills may be impaired. Patient should refrain from driving or other hazardous activities until reaction to drug is known.
- Patient should check with physician before discontinuing this medication. Gradual dosage reduction may be necessary to prevent adverse effects.
- Advise patient not to take any OTC drugs without informing physician.

BUSPIRONE HYDROCHLORIDE

(byoo-spye′rone)

Trade name: BuSpar

Classifications: CNS AGENT; ANXIOLYTIC

Prototype: Lorazepam

Pregnancy category: B

ACTIONS/PHARMACODYNAMICS

First generation agent in a new class of anxiolytics. Has chemical and pharmacologic properties unrelated to those of the benzodiazepines or other psychotherapeutic agents. Action is unclear but appears to be focused mainly on the brain dopamine system. Buspirone has agonist effects on presynaptic dopamine receptors and also a high affinity for serotonin receptors. Lacks the anticonvulsant, sedative, muscle relaxant properties of the benzodiazepines, and its abuse potential appears to be minimal. Identifiable abstinence syndrome with withdrawal after long-term use has not been reported. Unlike other anxiolytics, it seems to cause less clinically significant impairment of cognitive and motor performance and produces minimal if any interaction with other brain depressants, including alcohol.

B

USES Management of anxiety disorders and for short-term treatment of generalized anxiety. **Unlabeled use:** adjuvant for nicotine withdrawal.

ROUTE & DOSAGE

Anxiety

Adult: **PO** 7.5–15 mg/d in divided doses; may increase by 5 mg/d q2–3d as needed (max 60 mg/d).
Geriatric: **PO** 5 mg bid, may increase to max 60 mg/d.

PHARMACOKINETICS Absorption: readily absorbed from GI tract but undergoes first pass metabolism. **Onset:** 5–7 d. **Peak:** 1 h. **Metabolism:** metabolized in liver. **Elimination:** half-life: 2–4 h; 30–63% excreted in urine as metabolites within 24 h.

CONTRAINDICATIONS & PRECAUTIONS Contraindicated in: safe use during pregnancy (category B), lactation, or in children <18 y not established. **Cautious use in:** renal or hepatic impairment.

ADVERSE/SIDE EFFECTS CNS: numbness, paresthesia, tremors, *dizziness, headache,* nervousness, *drowsiness,* light-headedness, dream disturbances, decreased concentration, excitement, mood changes. **CV:** tachycardia, palpitation. **Eye:** blurred vision. **GI:** *nausea,* vomiting, dry mouth, abdominal/gastric distress, diarrhea, constipation. **GU:** urinary frequency, hesitancy. **Musculoskeletal:** arthralgias. **Respiratory:** hyperventilation, shortness of breath. **Skin:** rash, edema, pruritus, flushing, easy bruising, hair loss, dry skin. **Other:** headache, fatigue, weakness.

DIAGNOSTIC TEST INTERFERENCE Buspirone may increase serum concentrations of ***hepatic aminotransferases*** (ALT, AST).

DRUG INTERACTIONS MAO INHIBITORS, hypertension; **trazadone,** possible increase in liver transaminases; increased **haloperidol** serum levels.

NURSING IMPLICATIONS

Administration

- Administer with food to decrease first-pass metabolism. Rate of absorption may be delayed, but administration with food increases bioavailability of drug.
- Store at 15–30C (59–86F) in tightly closed container unless otherwise directed.

Assessment & Drug Effects

- Buspirone may displace digoxin from its serum binding. This could increase the potential for toxic serum levels of digoxin. If the two drugs must be given concomitantly, monitor cardiovascular parameters (BP, pulse) until dosage has been stabilized.
- Benzodiazepines or sedative-hypnotic drugs are withdrawn gradually before buspirone therapy is started. Observe patient for rebound symptoms, which may occur over varying time periods during first phase of treatment.
- Involuntary movements may manifest in a small number of patients during early therapy. Symptoms include dystonia, motor restlessness, and involuntary repetitious movement of facial or cervical muscle and should be reported.
- Observe for swollen ankles, decreased urinary output, changes in voiding pattern. These symptoms as well as symptoms of hepatic impairment (jaundice, itching, nausea, vomiting) should be reported promptly.

Patient & Family Education

- Buspirone should be taken exactly as prescribed: specifically patient should not omit, skip, increase or decrease doses without advice of the physician.

- Concomitant self-medication with OTC drugs without advice of the physician should be discouraged.
- Desired therapeutic response may begin within 7–10 d; however, optimal results are not achieved for 3–4 wk. Inform patient of this expected lag in effects and reinforce the importance of continuing treatment.
- Compliance during the initial therapy period requires reinforcement because adverse/side effects usually appear early in therapy. Assure patient that these effects subside during continued therapy with or without dosage adjustment.
- Buspirone's CNS effects are not always predictable. Caution patient about driving or working with dangerous equipment until reaction to the drug is known.
- Drug will be discontinued during pregnancy.
- Any changes that persist such as decreased acuity of smell, roaring noises in head, blurred vision, nightmares, weakness, should be reported.
- Patient should discuss limits of alcohol intake with physician. Cautious use is generally advised.
- Incidence of withdrawal or rebound symptoms when buspirone therapy is completed is low; when drug use is to be discontinued, be certain patient understands the planned schedule for changes in doses and intervals.

BUSULFAN

(byoo-sul′fan)

Trade name: Myleran

Classifications: ANTINEOPLASTIC; ALKYLATING AGENT

Prototype: Cyclophosphamide

Pregnancy category: D

ACTIONS/PHARMACODYNAMICS

Potent cytotoxic alkylating agent that may be a carcinogen in itself. Cell cycle nonspecific. Acts predominantly on slowly proliferating stem cells by inducing cross linkage in DNA, thus blocking replication and causing cell death. Reduces total granulocyte mass but has little effect on lymphocytes and platelets except in large doses. May cause widespread epithelial cellular dysplasia severe enough to make it difficult to interpret exfoliative cytologic examinations from lung, breast, bladder, and uterine cervix. May be mutagenic and carcinogenic. Acquired resistance may develop and is thought to be due to intracellular inactivation of busulfan before it reaches nuclear DNA.

USES Palliative treatment of chronic myelogenous (myeloid, granulocytic, myelocytic) leukemia for patients no longer responsive to radiation therapy or to previously tried antineoplastics. Does not appreciably extend survival time. **Unlabeled uses:** polycythemia vera, severe thrombocytosis, as adjunct in treatment of myelofibrosis, allogenic bone transplantation in patients with acute nonlymphocytic leukemia.

ROUTE & DOSAGE

Chronic Myelogenous Leukemia

Adult: **PO** 4–8 mg/d until maximal clinical and hematologic improvement; may use 1–4 mg/d if remission is shorter than 3 mo.
Child: **PO** 0.06–0.12 mg/kg/d or 1.8–4.6 mg/m^2.

B

PHARMACOKINETICS **Absorption:** readily absorbed from GI tract. **Peak:** 4 h. **Duration:** 4 h. **Metabolism:** metabolized in liver. **Elimination:** half-life: unknown; 10–50% excreted in urine within 48 h.

CONTRAINDICATIONS & PRECAUTIONS **Contraindicated in:** therapy-resistant chronic lymphocytic leukemia; **blastic** crisis of chronic myelogenous leukemia; bone marrow depression, immunizations (patient and household members), chickenpox (including recent exposure), herpetic infections. Safe use during pregnancy (category D) and in nursing mothers not established. **Cautious use in:** men and women in childbearing years; history of gout or urate renal stones; prior irradiation or chemotherapy.

ADVERSE/SIDE EFFECTS Major toxic effects are related to bone marrow failure. **GU:** flank pain, renal calculi, uric acid nephropathy, acute renal failure, gynecomastia, testicular atrophy, azoospermia, impotence, sterility in males, ovarian suppression, menstrual changes, amenorrhea (potentially irreversible), menopausal symptoms. **Hematologic:** agranulocytosis (rare), pancytopenia, thrombocytopenia, leukopenia, *anemia*. **Respiratory:** irreversible pulmonary fibrosis ("busulfan lung"). **Skin:** alopecia, hyperpigmentation. **Other:** endocardial fibrosis, dizziness, cholestatic jaundice, infections.

DIAGNOSTIC TEST INTERFERENCE Busulfan may decrease ***urinary 17-OHCS excretion,*** and may increase ***blood and urine uric acid*** levels. Drug-induced cellular dysplasia may interfere with interpretation of ***cytologic studies.***

DRUG INTERACTIONS **Probenecid, sulfinpyrazone** may increase uric acid levels.

NURSING IMPLICATIONS

Administration

- Medication should be taken at same time each day.
- Taking drug on an empty stomach may minimize nausea and vomiting.
- Store drug in tightly capped, light-resistant container at 15–30C (59–86F), unless otherwise specified.

Assessment & Drug Effects

- Establish data base with flow chart, recording initial vital signs and weight.
- Hgb, Hct, total and differential WBC counts, platelet counts, liver and kidney function tests, serum uric acid are obtained initially and at least weekly during therapy with busulfan.
- During remission, patient is examined at monthly intervals at least. When total leukocyte count increases to approximately 50,000/mm^3, induction dosage is resumed.
- With recommended dosage of busulfan, the normal leukocyte count is usually achieved in about 2 mo.
- There may be abrupt onset of hematotoxicity. Recovery from busulfan-induced pancytopenia may take 1 mo–2 y. It can be irreversible in some patients.
- Usually, the WBC count does not start to decrease for about 10–15 d after therapy begins; it may actually increase during this period. Since the count continues to fall for more than 1 mo after busulfan is withdrawn, usually therapy will be discontinued when the total leukocyte count reaches approxi-

mately 15,000/mm^3 (i.e., before the count reaches normal range).

- Be alert to symptoms suggestive of superinfection (see Signs & Symptoms, Appendix G), particularly when patient develops leukopenia.
- Remissions are characterized by increased appetite and sense of well-being within a few days after therapy begins.
- Weigh patient at least weekly. A slow but steady change in weight should be communicated to physician.
- Monitor I&O ratio and pattern. Urge patient to increase fluid intake to 10–12 (240 ml [8 oz]) glasses daily (if allowed) to assure adequate urinary output.
- Inspect skin and oral membranes daily and carefully examine urine and stools for abnormal bleeding due to thrombocytopenia. Ecchymotic or petechial bleeding, epistaxis, bleeding gums, cloudy or pink urine, and dark or black stools should be reported promptly.
- Auscultate lungs on a regular basis and monitor temperature. Advise patient to report immediately the onset of cough, low-grade fever, dyspnea, possible symptoms of pulmonary fibrosis (busulfan lung).
- Ovarian suppression and amenorrhea with menopausal symptoms commonly occur in premenopausal women. Effects are not apparent for 4–6 mo. Amenorrhea may be irreversible.

Patient & Family Education

- Busulfan should be taken as directed, at the same time each day.
- If possible, intrusive procedures should be avoided or at least limited during period of decreased platelet count. Caution patient to avoid trauma, floss teeth gently, use a soft toothbrush, and shave with a safety razor. Occult blood tests of urine, stool, and emesis may be indicated.
- Because of hyperpigmentation, signs of jaundice may be overlooked. Patient should report yellow sclera, dark urine, light-colored stools, abdominal discomfort, or pruritus.
- Instruct patient to report easy bruising or bleeding, sore mouth or throat, unusual fatigue (agranulocytosis), blurred vision (cataract), flank or joint pain, swelling of lower legs and feet (hyperuricemia).
- Contraceptive measures should be used during busulfan therapy and for at least 3 mo after drug is withdrawn.
- Discuss possibility of alopecia. Advise patient to brush hair gently and not more than is necessary.
- Busulfan is a highly toxic drug, and some patients eventually develop resistance to it. Keep follow-up appointments.

BUTABARBITAL SODIUM

(byoo-ta-bar′bi-tal)

Trade names: Barbased, Butalan, Butisol Sodium, Sarisol No. 2

Classifications: CNS AGENT; BARBITURATE ANXIOLYTIC, SEDATIVE-HYPNOTIC

Prototype: Phenobarbital

Pregnancy category: D

Controlled substance: Schedule III

ACTIONS/PHARMACODYNAMICS

Intermediate-acting barbiturate, similar to phenobarbital. Appears to act at thalamus level, where it interferes with transmission of impulses to the cerebral cortex.

USES Hypnotic in short-term treatment of simple insomnia, as sedative

B

for relief of anxiety, and to provide sedation preoperatively.

ROUTE & DOSAGE

Daytime Sedation

Adult: **PO** 15–30 mg t.i.d. or q.i.d. *Child:* **PO** 7.5–30 mg t.i.d.

Preoperative Sedation

Adult: **PO** 50–100 mg 60–90 min before surgery. *Child:* **PO** 2–6 mg/kg in 3 equally divided doses (max 100 mg).

Hypnotic

Adult: **PO** 50–100 mg h.s.

PHARMACOKINETICS **Absorption:** readily absorbed from GI tract. **Onset:** 40–60 min. **Peak:** 3–4 h. **Duration:** 6–8 h. **Distribution:** crosses placenta; distributed into breast milk. **Metabolism:** metabolized in liver. **Elimination:** half-life: average 100 h; excreted in urine primarily as metabolites.

CONTRAINDICATIONS & PRECAUTIONS **Contraindicated in:** porphyria; uncontrolled pain; severe respiratory disease; history of addiction; pregnancy (category D). **Cautious use in:** renal or hepatic impairment.

ADVERSE/SIDE EFFECTS Drowsiness, *residual sedation* ("hangover"), headache, nausea, vomiting, constipation, diarrhea, urticaria, skin rash, muscle or joint pain.

DRUG INTERACTIONS **Alcohol** and other CNS DEPRESSANTS add to CNS and respiratory depression; butabarbital increases the metabolism of ORAL ANTICOAGULANTS, BETA BLOCKERS, CORTICOSTEROIDS, **doxycycline, griseofulvin, quinidine,** THEOPHYLLINES, ORAL CONTRACEPTIVES, decreasing their effectiveness.

NURSING IMPLICATIONS

Administration

- Prolonged administration is not recommended because tolerance to butabarbital occurs in about 14 d.
- Physical and psychological dependence may develop with prolonged use. Following long-term use, drug should be withdrawn slowly to avoid precipitating withdrawal symptoms.
- Store in tightly covered containers, preferably at 15–30C (59–86F), unless otherwise directed by manufacturer.

Assessment & Drug Effects

- Elderly and debilitated patients sometimes manifest morbid excitement, confusion, or depression. Some children also react with paradoxical excitement. Side rails may be advisable. Report these reactions to physician.

Patient & Family Education

- Drug may cause drowsiness; caution patient not to drive and to avoid other potentially hazardous activities until reaction to drug is known.
- Advise patient not to drink alcoholic beverages while taking this drug. Other CNS depressants may produce additive drowsiness and should not be taken without approval of physician.

BUTENAFINE HYDROCHLORIDE

(bu-ten′a-feen)

Trade name: Mentax

Classifications: ANTIINFECTIVE; ANTIFUNGAL ANTIBIOTIC

Prototype: Fluconazole

Pregnancy category: B

ACTIONS/PHARMACODYNAMICS Exerts antifungal action by inhibiting sterol synthesis, which may enhance susceptibility of the fungal membrane to damage by butenafine.

USE Treatment of tinea pedis due to *Epidermophyton floccosum, Trichophyton mentagraphytes, Trichophyton rubium.*

ROUTE & DOSAGE

Tinea Pedis
Adult: **Topical** Apply to affected area and surrounding skin q.d. × 4 wk.
Child 12–16 y: **Topical** Same as adult.

CONTRAINDICATIONS & PRECAUTIONS **Contraindicated in:** hypersensitivity to butenafine. **Cautious use in:** hypersensitivity to naftinine or tolnaftate; pregnancy (category B); nursing mothers. Safety and efficacy in children < 12 y have not been established.

ADVERSE/SIDE EFFECTS **Skin:** burning/stinging at application site, contact dermatitis, erythema, irritation, itching.

NURSING IMPLICATIONS

Administration
- Apply sufficient cream to cover affected skin and surrounding areas.
- Do not use occlusive dressing unless specifically directed to do so.
- Store at 5–30C (41– 86F).

Assessment & Drug Effects
- Therapeutic effectiveness is indicated by resolution of fungal infection.
- Usually 2–4 wk of therapy are required for effective treatment.

Patient & Family Education
- Discontinue medication and notify physician if irritation or sensitivity develops.
- Contact with mucous membranes should be avoided.
- Wash hands thoroughly before and after application of cream.

BUTOCONAZOLE NITRATE

(byoo-toe-koe′na-zole)
Trade names: Femstat 3, Femstat-One
Classifications: ANTIINFECTIVE; ANTIFUNGAL ANTIBIOTIC
Prototype: Fluconazole
Pregnancy category: C

ACTIONS/PHARMACODYNAMICS Imidazole derivative with antifungal activity. Alters fungal cell membrane permeability, permitting loss of phosphorous compounds, potassium, and other essential intracellular constituents with consequent loss of ability to replicate. Action takes place primarily on medicated infected surface tissues. Has fungicidal activity against *Candida, Trichophyton, Microsporum,* and *Epidermophyton* as well as some gram-positive bacteria.

USE Local treatment of vulvovaginal candidiasis.

ROUTE & DOSAGE

Vulvovaginal Candidiasis
Adult: **Topical** 1 applicatorful intravaginally h.s. for 3 d; may be extended another 3 d if needed.
Pregnant women: **Topical** 1 applicatorful intravaginally h.s. for 6 d.

PHARMACOKINETICS **Absorption:** small amount absorbed systemically from intravaginal administration. **Distribution:** crosses placenta in animals. **Metabolism:** metabolized in liver. **Elimination:** half-life: 21–24 h;

B

excreted in equal amounts in urine and feces within 4–7 d.

CONTRAINDICATIONS & PRECAUTIONS **Contraindicated in:** first trimester of pregnancy (category C). Safe use in nursing mothers and in children not established. **Cautious use in:** second and third trimester of pregnancy.

ADVERSE/SIDE EFFECTS Vulvar or vaginal burning, vulvar itching, discharge, soreness, swelling; itching of fingers; urinary frequency and burning; headache.

NURSING IMPLICATIONS

Administration

- The usual course of treatment is 3 d. Vulvovaginal candidiasis may be more difficult to control during pregnancy; consequently a 6 d regimen is commonly prescribed.
- Treatment should be continued even during menstruation.
- Store medication at 15–30C (59–86F); avoid extreme temperature and freezing.

Assessment & Drug Effects

- Candidiasis in nonpregnant women is usually controlled in 3 d.

Patient & Family Education

- Butoconazole can be used with oral contraceptives and antibiotic therapy.
- Caution patient to take medication exactly as prescribed; she should not increase or decrease dosage or discontinue or extend the treatment period. If symptoms (vaginal burning, discharge, or itching) persist, she should contact the physician. Drug should be discontinued if irritation occurs.
- Patient's sexual partner should wear a condom during intercourse.

BUTORPHANOL TARTRATE

(byoo-tor'fa-nole)

Trade names: Stadol, Stadol NS

Classifications: CNS AGENT; ANALGESIC; NARCOTIC (OPIATE) AGONIST-ANTAGONIST

Prototype: Pentazocine

Pregnancy category: C

ACTIONS/PHARMACODYNAMICS Synthetic, centrally acting analgesic with mixed narcotic agonist and antagonist actions. Acts as agonist on one type of opioid receptor and as a competitive antagonist at others. Site of analgesic action believed to be subcortical, possibly in the limbic system. On a weight basis, analgesic potency appears to be about 5 times that of morphine, 40 times that of merperidine, and 15–30 times that of pentazocine. Narcotic antagonist potential is approximately 30 times that of pentazocine and 1/40 that of naloxone. Two milligrams of butorphanol produce about the same degree of respiratory depression as 10 mg morphine. Respiratory depression does not increase appreciably with higher doses, as it does with morphine, but duration of action increases. Like pentazocine, analgesic doses may increase pulmonary arterial pressure and cardiac work load. Appears to have low potential for dependence. Tends to inhibit release of antidiuretic hormone (ADH) from hypothalamus.

USES Relief of moderate to severe pain, preoperative or preanesthetic sedation and analgesia, obstetrical analgesia during labor, cancer pain, renal colic, burns. **Unlabeled uses:** musculoskeletal and postepesiotomy pain.

ROUTE & DOSAGE

Pain Relief

Adult: **IM** 1–4 mg q3–4h as needed (max 4 mg/dose). **IV** 0.5–2 mg q3–4h as needed.
Geriatric: **IM/IV** 0.5–2 mg q6–8 h.
Intranasal 1 mg (1 spray) in one nostril; may repeat in 90 s; may repeat these 2 doses q3– 4h prn.

PHARMACOKINETICS **Onset:** 10–30 min IM; 1 min IV. **Peak:** 0.5–1 h IM; 4–5 min IV. **Duration:** 3–4 h IM; 2– 4 h IV. **Distribution:** crosses placenta; distributed into breast milk. **Metabolism:** metabolized in liver in inactive metabolites. **Elimination:** half-life: 3–4 h; excreted primarily in urine.

CONTRAINDICATIONS & PRECAUTIONS **Contraindicated in:** narcotic-dependent patients. Safe use during pregnancy prior to labor (category C), in nursing women, and in children <18 y not established. **Cautious use in:** history of drug abuse or dependence, emotionally unstable individuals; head injury, increased intracranial pressure; acute MI, ventricular dysfunction, coronary insufficiency, hypertension; patients undergoing biliary tract surgery; respiratory depression, bronchial asthma, obstructive respiratory disease; and renal or hepatic dysfunction.

ADVERSE/SIDE EFFECTS **CNS:** drowsiness, *sedation,* headache, vertigo, dizziness, floating feeling, weakness, lethargy, confusion, lightheadedness, insomnia, nervousness, respiratory depression. **CV:** palpitation, bradycardia. **GI:** nausea. **Skin:** clammy skin, tingling sensation, flushing and warmth, cyanosis of extremities, diaphoresis, sensitivity to cold, urticaria, pruritus. **Other:** difficulty in urinating; biliary spasm.

DRUG INTERACTIONS **Alcohol** and other CNS DEPRESSANTS augment CNS and respiratory depression.

INCOMPATIBILITIES **Solution/additive: dimenhydrinate, pentobarbital. Y-site: pentobarbital.**

NURSING IMPLICATIONS

Administration

- IV butorphanol tartrate may be given undilted at a rate of 2 mg over 3–5 min.
- Store at 15–30C (59–86F) unless otherwise directed. Protect from light.

Assessment & Drug Effects

- Monitor for respiratory depression. Do not administer drug if respiratory rate is <12 breaths/min.
- Monitor vital signs. Report marked changes in BP or bradycardia.
- If butorphanol is used during labor or delivery, observe neonate for signs of respiratory depression.
- Butorphanol has habit-forming potential.
- Because butorphanol has agonist as well as antagonist actions, it can induce acute withdrawal symptoms in opiate-dependent patients.
- Abrupt withdrawal following chronic administration may produce vomiting, loss of appetite, restlessness, abdominal cramps, increase in BP and temperature, mydriasis, faintness. Withdrawal symptoms peak 48 h after discontinuation of drug.

Patient & Family Education

- Drug-induced nausea may be controlled by lying down.
- Warn patient not to take alcohol or other CNS depressant without consulting physician because of possible additive effects.
- Butorphanol causes sedation and

dizziness; therefore, observe safety precautions.

CABERGOLINE

(ka-ber'go-leen)
Trade name: Dostinex
Classifications: AUTONOMIC NERVOUS SYSTEM AGENT; ERGOT ALKALOID
Prototype: Ergotamine
Pregnancy category: B

ACTIONS/PHARMACODYNAMICS Cabergoline is a synthetic ergot derivative long-acting dopamine receptor agonist with a high affinity for D_2 receptors. Cabergoline inhibits both puerperal lactation and pathologic hyperprolactinemia.

USES Treatment of hyperprolactinemia (idiopathic or secondary to pituitary adenomas). **Unlabeled use:** treatment of Parkinson's disease.

ROUTE & DOSAGE

Hyperprolactinemia
Adult: **PO** Start with 0.25 mg 2 times/wk; may increase by 0.25 mg 2 times/wk to a max of 1 mg 2 times/wk.

Parkinson's Disease
Adult: **PO** Start with 0.5 mg q.d.; may increase up to 2.5 mg q.d. (max 5 mg/d).

PHARMACOKINETICS Absorption: rapidly absorbed from GI tract, undergoes first-pass metabolism. **Peak:** 2–3 h. **Distribution:** 40–42% protein bound. Crosses placenta, will interfere with ability to lactate. **Metabolism:** extensively metabolized. **Elimination:** half-life: 63–69 h; approx 22% excreted in urine, 60% in feces.

CONTRAINDICATIONS & PRECAUTIONS Contraindicated in: Uncontrolled hypertension and hypersensitivity to ergot derivatives; pregnancy (category B), pregnancy-induced hyertension, nursing mothers. **Cautious use in:** hepatic function impairment. Safety and efficacy in pediatric patients are unknown.

ADVERSE/SIDE EFFECTS Body as Whole: asthenia, fatigue, hot flashes. **CNS:** *headache, dizziness,* paresthesia, somnolence, depression, nervousness. **CV:** postural hypotension. **GI:** *nausea, constipation,* abdominal pain, dyspepsia, vomiting, dry mouth, diarrhea, flatulence. **Other:** breast pain, dysmenorrhea.

NURSING IMPLICATIONS

Administration
- Allow 4 wk intervals between dosage increases.
- Store at 20–25C (68–77F).

Assessment & Drug Effects
- Therapeutic effectiveness is indicated by return of serum prolactin levels to normal.
- Lab tests: serum prolactin levels are monitored to assess response to each dosing level.
- Monitor for hypotension, especially when given with other drugs known to lower BP.

Patient & Family Education
- Drug is usually discontinued after normal serum prolactin level has been maintained for 6 mo.
- Drug should not be taken by women who are breast-feeding or intend to do so.

CAFFEINE

(kaf-een')
Trade names: Caffedrine, Dexitac, NoDoz, Quick Pep, S-250, Tirend, Vivarin

C

CAFFEINE AND SODIUM BENZOATE

CITRATED CAFFEINE

Prototype for classifications: CNS AGENT; RESPIRATORY AND CEREBRAL STIMULANT; XANTHINE

Pregnancy category: C

ACTIONS/PHARMACODYNAMICS Chief action is thought to be related to inhibition of the enzyme phosphodiesterase, which results in higher concentrations of cyclic AMP. Releases epinephrine and norepinephrine from adrenal medulla, producing CNS stimulation. Small doses improve psychic and sensory awareness and reduce drowsiness and fatigue by stimulating cerebral cortex. Higher doses stimulate medullary, respiratory, vasomotor, and vagal centers. Produces smooth muscle relaxation (especially bronchi) and dilation of coronary, pulmonary, and systemic blood vessels by direct action on vascular musculature. Mild diuretic action may result from increase in renal blood flow and glomerular filtration rate and decrease in renal tubular reabsorption of sodium and water. Increases contractile force of heart and cardiac output by direct stimulation of myocardium. Also stimulates secretion of gastric acid and digestive enzymes. Relief of headache is perhaps due to mild cerebral vasoconstriction action and increased vascular tone.

USES Orally as a mild CNS stimulant to aid in staying awake and restoring mental alertness, and as an adjunct in narcotic and nonnarcotic analgesia. Used parenterally as an emergency stimulant in acute circulatory failure, as a diuretic, and to relieve spinal puncture headache. **Unlabeled uses:** topical treatment of atopic dermatitis, neonatal apnea.

ROUTE & DOSAGE

Mental Stimulant

Adult: **PO** 100–200 mg q3–4h prn.

Circulatory Stimulant

Adult: **IM** 200–500 mg prn.

Spinal Puncture Headaches

Adult: **IV** 500 mg over 1 h; may repeat × 1 dose

Neonatal Apnea

Child: **PO/IV** 10–20 mg/kg as a loading dose, followed by a maintenance dose 2–3 d later of 5–10 mg/kg 1–2 times/d.

PHARMACOKINETICS Absorption: rapidly absorbed. **Peak:** 15–45 min. **Distribution:** widely distributed throughout body; crosses blood-brain barrier and placenta. **Metabolism:** metabolized in liver. **Elimination:** half-life: 3–5 h in adults, 36–144 h in neonates; excreted in urine as metabolites; excreted in breast milk in small amounts.

CONTRAINDICATIONS & PRECAUTIONS Contraindicated in: acute MI, symptomatic cardiac arrhythmias, palpitations; peptic ulcer; insomnia, panic attacks. Safe use during pregnancy (category C), in nursing women, and in children not established. **Cautious use in:** diabetes mellitus; hiatal hernia; hypertension with heart disease.

ADVERSE/SIDE EFFECTS CNS: *nervousness, insomnia,* restlessness, irritability, confusion, agitation, fasciculations, delirium, twitching, tremors, clonic convulsions. **CV:** tingling of face, flushing, palpitation,

C

tachycardia or bradycardia, ventricular ectopic beats. **GI:** nausea, vomiting; epigastric discomfort, gastric irritation (oral form), diarrhea, hematemesis, kernicterus (neonates). **Other:** scintillating scotomas, tinnitus, increased urination, diuresis, tachypnea.

DIAGNOSTIC TEST INTERFERENCE Caffeine reportedly may interfere with diagnosis of pheochromocytoma or neuroblastoma by increasing urinary excretion of ***catecholamines, VMA,*** and ***5-HIAA*** and may cause false positive increases in ***serum urate*** (by ***Bittner method***).

DRUG INTERACTIONS Caffeine may increase effects of **cimetidine** by inhibiting its metabolism; caffeine increases cardiovascular stimulating effects of BETA-ADRENERGIC AGONISTS; possibly increases **theophylline** toxicity.

NURSING IMPLICATIONS

Administration

- Timed-release oral preparations should be administered not less than 6 h before bedtime.
- IV caffeine may be administered undiluted by direct IV at a rate of 250 mg or a fraction thereof over 1 min when used in an emergency situation.
- With neonates, caffeine without sodium benzoate is ordinarily used.
- Caffeine should be administered slowly by IV route to neonates. Check with physician regarding preferred rate.
- IV caffeine given to adults for spinal puncture headache is administered at a rate of 500 mg over 1 h by infusion.

Assessment & Drug Effects

- Large doses may cause intensification rather than reversal of severe drug-induced depressions. Monitor vital signs closely.
- Children are more susceptible than adults to the CNS effects of caffeine and therefore should be closely observed following administration.
- Monitor blood glucose levels in diabetics, as caffeine may elevate serum level.

Patient & Family Education

- Caffeine usually restricted with ulcers because caffeine stimulates gastric secretions. Patients who insist on drinking coffee should be advised to drink it with meals, well diluted, and with milk.
- Patients with diabetes should be advised that caffeine in large amounts may impair glucose tolerance.
- Advise patients who consume large amounts of caffeine that headache, dizziness, anxiety, irritability, nervousness, and muscle tension may result from excessive use, as well as from abrupt withdrawal of coffee (or oral caffeine) in heavy users. Withdrawal symptoms usually occur 12–18 h following last coffee intake.

CALCIFEDIOL

(kal-si-fe-dye′ole)

Trade name: Calderol

Classifications: HORMONE; VITAMIN D ANALOG

Pregnancy category: C

ACTIONS/PHARMACODYNAMICS

Vitamin D analog and major transport form of cholecalciferol (D_3); fat soluble. Because it is activated in the body and has regulatory effects, it is considered a hormone. Primary action leads to regulation of serum calcium, which is affected also by the activity of other vitamin D analogs (e.g., ergocalciferol), parathyroid hormone, and calcitonin. Pharmacologic effects of calcifediol are related to its intrinsic vitamin D activity as well as to the properties of active metabolites (e.g., calcitriol), which result from renal metabolism.

USES Management of metabolic bone disease and hypocalcemia associated with chronic renal failure in patients undergoing renal dialysis. **Unlabeled uses:** osteopenia caused by prolonged glucocorticoid therapy and osteomalacia secondary to hepatic disease.

ROUTE & DOSAGE

Metabolic Bone Disease in Patients with Chronic Renal Failure

Adult: **PO** Initially 300–350 µg/wk administered on a daily or alternate day schedule; may increase at 4-wk intervals if necessary; patients with normal calcium may only need 20 µg q.o.d. (usual range 50–100 µg/d *or* 100–200 µg q.o.d.).

PHARMACOKINETICS **Absorption:** readily absorbed from small intestines. **Peak:** 4 h. **Duration:** 15–20 d. **Distribution:** stored chiefly in liver and fat deposits. **Metabolism:** activated in kidneys. **Elimination:** half-life: 12–22 d; excreted primarily in bile and feces.

CONTRAINDICATIONS & PRECAUTIONS **Contraindicated in:** hypersensitivity to vitamin D, vitamin D toxicity, hypercalcemia. Safe use of doses in excess of RDA during pregnancy (category C), in nursing women, and in children not established. **Cautious use in:** patients receiving digitalis glycosides.

ADVERSE/SIDE EFFECTS Vitamin D intoxication and hypercalcemia. **CNS:** lethargy, headache, weakness, vertigo. **GI:** anorexia, nausea, vomiting, dry mouth, thirst, constipation, diarrhea, abdominal cramps, metallic taste. **Other:** muscle or bone pain, polyuria, hypercalciuria, hyperphosphatemia; idiosyncratic reaction (headache, nausea, vomiting, diarrhea, fever).

DRUG INTERACTIONS THIAZIDE DIURETICS may cause hypercalcemia; calcifediol-induced hypercalcemia may precipitate digitalis arrhythmias in patients taking DIGITALIS GLYCOSIDES.

NURSING IMPLICATIONS

Administration

- Calcifediol can be taken without regard to food.
- Patients undergoing dialysis may require aluminum carbonate or hydroxide gels to bind intestinal phosphate and thus lower serum phosphate levels.
- Since calcitriol is a metabolite of vitamin D_3, all sources of vitamin D are usually withheld during therapy or at least must be considered when calculating dosage.
- Store at 15–30C (59–86F) in tightly covered, light-resistant container unless otherwise directed.

Assessment & Drug Effects

- Baseline and periodic determinations should be made of serum calcium, phosphorus, magnesium, and alkaline phosphatase, and urinary calcium and phosphorus levels should be measured q24h.
- Effectiveness of therapy depends on an adequate daily intake of calcium. Since dietary calcium and phosphate are difficult to control, the physician may prescribe a calcium supplement as needed.
- Serum calcium levels particularly

should be monitored at least once weekly, or whenever dosage adjustments are made, and at periodic intervals thereafter.

- Monitor for manifestations of hypercalcemia (see Appendix G). If hypercalcemia occurs, calcifediol should be discontinued until serum calcium returns to normal (9–10.6 mg/dl).
- A fall in serum alkaline phosphatase usually signals the onset of hypercalcemia.

Patient & Family Education

- Instruct patient to withhold drug and report immediately signs and symptoms of hypercalcemia (see Appendix G).
- Advise patient to consult physician before taking an OTC medication. Calcium, phosphate, or magnesium-containing laxatives and antacids, mineral oil, and vitamin D preparations may increase side effects of calcifediol and therefore should be avoided.

CALCIPOTRIENE

(cal-ci′-po-tri-een)

Trade name: Dovonex

Classifications: SKIN AND MUCOUS MEMBRANE AGENT; ANTIINFLAMMATORY; IMMUNOSUPPRESSANT

Pregnancy category: C

ACTIONS/PHARMACODYNAMICS

Calcipotriene is a synthetic vitamin D_3 analog for the treatment of moderate plaque psoriasis. The scaly red patches of psoriasis are caused by abnormal growth and production of skin cells known as keratinocytes. Calcipotriene affects psoriasis by inhibiting proliferation of keratinocytes, reducing the number of polymorphonuclear leukocytes (PMNs) in the skin cells, and decreasing the number of epithelial cells.

USE Treatment of moderate plaque psoriasis.

ROUTE & DOSAGE

Adult: **Topical** Apply a thin layer to affected area once or twice daily.

PHARMACOKINETICS **Absorption:** approximately 6% absorbed systemically. **Onset:** 1 wk. **Peak:** 8 wk. **Duration:** 4 wk. **Metabolism:** recycled via liver. **Elimination:** excreted in bile.

CONTRAINDICATIONS & PRECAUTIONS **Contraindicated in:** hypersensitivity to calcipotriene, hypercalcemia or vitamin D toxicity. **Cautious use in:** dermatoses other than psoriasis, patients > 65 y old, pregnancy (category C), nursing mothers. Safety and efficacy in children not established.

ADVERSE/SIDE EFFECTS **Skin:** facial dermatitis, burning, stinging, erythema, folliculitis, mild transient itching.

NURSING IMPLICATIONS

Administration

- A thin layer should be applied to the affected skin and rubbed in gently and completely.
- Calcipotriene should not be applied to the face.
- Wash hands before and after application of medication.
- Store at room temperature, 15–30C (59–86F).

Assessment & Drug Effects

- A reduction in scaling, erythema, and lesion thickness indicates a positive therapeutic response.
- Significant reduction in psoriatic lesions usually occurs following 1 wk of treatment. Marked im-

provement is generally noted by the 8th wk of treatment.

- During long-term therapy, periodically monitor serum calcium, phosphate, and calcitriol levels.

Patient & Family Education

- Inform patient that treatment with calcipotriene may be indefinite, as reappearance of psoriatic lesions is common following discontinuation of the drug.
- Inform patient that burning and stinging may occur with drug application; these side effects are usually transient.
- Advise patient not to mix calcipotriene with any other topical medicine.
- Instruct patient to report appearance of facial dermatitis (erythema and scaling around mouth and nose).

CALCITONIN (HUMAN)

(kal-si-toe′nin)

Trade name: Cibacalcin

CALCITONIN (SALMON)

Trade names: Calcimar, Miacalcin

Classifications: HORMONE; BONE METABOLISM REGULATOR

Pregnancy category: C

ACTIONS/PHARMACODYNAMICS Calcitonin human and calcitonin salmon are synthetic polypeptides. Pharmacologic actions are the same, but calcitonin salmon is considerably more potent and has a longer duration of action. Antibody formation occurs commonly with calcitonin salmon and only rarely with calcitonin human. Calcitonin opposes the effects of parathyroid hormone on bone and kidneys, reduces serum calcium by binding to specific receptor site on osteoclast cell membrane, and alters transmembrane passage of calcium and phosphorus. Promotes renal excretion of calcium and phosphorus and causes transient sodium and water loss. In Paget's disease, slows rate of bone turnover, with resultant decreases in serum alkaline phosphatase and urinary hydroxyproline, biochemical changes that seem to correspond to more normal bone formation. In some patients, long-term use initiates drug resistance through formation of neutralizing antibodies.

USES Symptomatic Paget's disease of bone (osteitis deformans), postmenopausal osteoporosis. **Orphan drug approval (calcitonin human):** short-term adjunctive treatment of severe hypercalcemic emergencies. **Unlabeled uses:** diagnosis and management of medullary carcinoma of thyroid; treatment of osteogenesis imperfecta.

ROUTE & DOSAGE

Paget's Disease

Adult: **SC** Human 0.5 mg/d *or* 2–3 times/wk *or* 0.25 mg/d up to 0.5 mg b.i.d. **SC/IM** Salmon 100 IU/d; may decrease to 50–100 IU/d or q.o.d.

Hypercalcemia

Adult: **SC/IM** Salmon 4 IU/kg q12h; may increase to 8 U/kg q6h if needed.

Postmenopausal Osteoporosis

Adult: **SC/IM** Salmon 100 IU/d. ***Intranasal:*** Miacalcin 1 spray (200 IU) daily, alternate nostrils.

PHARMACOKINETICS (salmon calcitonin). **Onset:** 15 min. **Peak:** 4 h. **Duration:** 8–24 h. **Distribution:** does not cross placenta; distribution into breast milk unknown. **Metabolism:** metabolized in kidneys. **Elimination:**

half-life: 1.25 h (1 h for human calcitonin); excreted in urine.

C

CONTRAINDICATIONS & PRECAUTIONS **Contraindicated in:** hypersensitivity to fish proteins or to synthetic calcitonins; history of allergy. Safe use in children, pregnancy (category C), nursing mothers not established. **Cautious use in:** renal impairment; osteoporosis; pernicious anemia; Zollinger-Ellison syndrome.

ADVERSE/SIDE EFFECTS **GI:** *transient nausea,* vomiting, anorexia, unusual taste sensation, abdominal pain, diarrhea. **Skin:** inflammatory reactions at injection site, flushing of face or hands, pruritus of ear lobes, edema of feet, skin rashes. **Other:** headache, eye pain, nocturia, diuresis, feverish sensation, hypersensitivity reactions, <u>anaphylaxis</u>, abnormal urine sediment. Reported for calcitonin human only: urinary frequency, chills, chest pressure, weakness, paresthesias, tender palms and soles, dizziness, nasal congestion, shortness of breath.

NURSING IMPLICATIONS

Administration

- Note that calcitonin human is administered only by SC injection; dosages are smaller than those of calcitonin salmon and are expressed in milligrams. Calcitonin salmon may be administered by SC or IM injection.
- When the volume of calcitonin salmon to be injected is more than 2 ml, the IM route is employed. Rotate injection sites.
- The transient flushing that commonly occurs following injection of calcitonin, particularly during early therapy, may be minimized by administrating the drug at bedtime. Consult physician.
- The nasal spray is administered in one nostril daily; alternate nostrils.
- Store calcitonin (human) at 25C (77F) or less, protected from light, unless otherwise specified by manufacturer.
- Store calcitonin (salmon) in refrigerator, preferably at 2–8C (36–46F) unless otherwise directed.
- Once the nasal pump is activated, it may be stored at room temperature for 2 wk.

Assessment & Drug Effects

- An allergy skin test is usually done prior to initiation of therapy. The appearance of more than mild erythema or wheal 15 min after intracutaneous injection indicates that the drug should not be given.
- Have on hand epinephrine 1:1000, antihistamines, oxygen in the event of a reaction. Also have readily available parenteral calcium, particularly during early therapy. Hypocalcemic tetany is a theoretical possibility.
- Periodic laboratory examination of urine specimens for sediment is recommended with long-term therapy.
- Monitor for hypocalcemia (see Signs & Symptoms, Appendix G). Theoretically, calcitonin can lead to hypocalcemic tetany. Latent tetany may be demonstrated by Chvostek's or Trousseau's signs and by serum calcium values: 7–8 mg/dl (latent tetany); below 7 mg/dl (manifest tetany).
- Nasal exams should be performed prior to treatment with the nasal spray and anytime nasal irritation occurs.
- Nasal ulceration or heavy bleeding are indications for drug discontinuation.

Patient & Family Education

- SC route is preferred for self-administration.

- Teach patient to recognize and seek advice about local inflammatory reaction at site of injection.
- Teach patient the importance of maintaining drug regimen even though symptoms have been ameliorated, to prevent early relapses.
- Instruct patient on proper use of nasal pump. Advise patient to notify physician if significant nasal irritation occurs.
- Advise patient to consult physician before using OTC preparations. Some supervitamins, hematinics, and antacids contain calcium and vitamin D (vitamin may antagonize calcitonin effects).

CALCITRIOL

(kal-si-trye'ole)

Trade names: Calcijex, Rocaltrol

Prototype for classifications: HORMONE; VITAMIN D ANALOG

Pregnancy category: C

ACTIONS/PHARMACODYNAMICS Synthetic form of an active metabolite of ergocalciferol (vitamin D_2). In the liver, cholecalciferol (vitamin D_3) and ergocalciferol (vitamin D_2) are enzymatically metabolized to calcifediol, an activated form of vitamin D_3. Calcifediol is biodegraded in the kidney to calcitriol, the most potent form of vitamin D_3. Patients with nonfunctioning kidneys are unable to synthesize sufficient calcitriol and therefore must receive it pharmacologically. By promoting intestinal absorption and renal retention of calcium, calcitriol elevates serum calcium levels, decreases elevated blood levels of phosphatase and parathyroid hormone, and decreases subperiosteal bone resorption and mineralization defects in some patients.

USES Management of hypocalcemia in patients undergoing chronic renal dialysis and in patients with hypoparathyroidism or pseudohypoparathyroidism. **Unlabeled uses:** in selected patients with vitamin D-dependent rickets, familial hypophosphatemia (vitamin D-resistant rickets), and in management of hypocalcemia in premature infants.

ROUTE & DOSAGE

Hypocalcemia

Adult: **PO** 0.25 μg/d; may be increased by 0.25 μg/d q4– 8wk for dialysis patients or q2– 4wk for hypoparathyroid patients if necessary. **IV** 0.5 μg 3 times/wk at the end of dialysis; may need up to 3 μg 3 times/wk.
Child: **PO** On hemodialysis: 0.25–2 μg/d. **IV** 0.01–0.05 μg/kg 3 times/wk. Renal failure without dialysis: **PO** 0.014–0.041 μg/kg/d.

PHARMACOKINETICS **Absorption:** readily absorbed from GI tract. **Onset:** 2–6 h. **Peak:** 10–12 h. **Duration:** 3–5 d. **Metabolism:** metabolized in liver. **Elimination:** half-life: 3–6 h; excreted mainly in feces.

CONTRAINDICATIONS & PRECAUTIONS **Contraindicated in:** hypercalcemia or vitamin D toxicity. Safe use during pregnancy (category C), in nursing women, and in children not established. **Cautious use in:** hyperphosphatemia, patients receiving digitalis glycosides.

ADVERSE/SIDE EFFECTS Vitamin D intoxication and hypercalcemia. **CNS:** headache, weakness. **Eye:** blurred vision, photophobia. **GI:** anorexia, nausea, vomiting, dry mouth, thirst, constipation, abdominal cramps, metallic taste. **Other:**

palpitation, increased urination, muscle or bone pain, hypercalciuria, hyperphosphatemia.

DRUG INTERACTIONS THIAZIDE DIURETICS may cause hypercalcemia; calcifediol-induced hypercalcemia may precipitate digitalis arrhythmias in patients receiving DIGITALIS GLYCOSIDES.

NURSING IMPLICATIONS

Administration

- Oral dose can be taken either with food or milk or on an empty stomach. Discuss with physician.
- When given for hypoparathyroidism, the dose is given in the morning.
- IV administration: Calcitriol is given direct IV over 30–60 s.
- Effectiveness of therapy depends on an adequate daily intake of calcium and phosphate. The physician may prescribe a calcium supplement on an as-needed basis.
- Capsules should be protected from heat, light, and moisture. Store in tightly closed container, preferably at 15–30C (59–86F) unless otherwise directed.

Assessment & Drug Effects

- Baseline and periodic determinations should be made of serum calcium, phosphorus, magnesium, alkaline phosphatase, creatinine; urinary calcium and phosphorus levels should be measured q24h.
- Monitor for hypercalcemia (see Signs & Symptoms, Appendix G). During dosage adjustment period, serum calcium levels particularly should be monitored twice weekly to avoid hypercalcemia.
- Excessive intake of calcium and phosphate can cause hypercalcemia, hypercalciuria, and hyperphosphatemia.
- If hypercalcemia develops, calcitriol and calcium supplements should be discontinued until serum calcium returns to normal. Reduction of dietary calcium intake should also be considered.

Patient & Family Education

- Review symptoms of hypercalcemia (see Appendix G) and advise patient to withhold drug and contact physician if they occur.
- Since calcitriol is the most potent form of vitamin D_3, all sources of vitamin D should be withheld during therapy to avoid possibility of hypercalcemia.
- Advise patient to consult physician before taking an OTC medication. (Many products contain calcium, vitamin D, phosphates, or magnesium, which can increase adverse effects of calcitriol.)
- Patients with normal renal function should maintain an adequate fluid intake.

CALCIUM CARBONATE

Trade names: Apo-Cal ♣, BioCal, Calcite-500, Calsan ♣, Cal-Sup, Caltrate ♣, Chooz, Dicarbosil, Equilet, Mallamint, Mega-Cal, Nu-Cal, Os-Cal, Oystercal, Titralac, Tums

CALCIUM ACETATE

Trade names: Phos-Ex, PhosLo

CALCIUM CITRATE

Trade name: Citracal

CALCIUM PHOSPHATE TRIBASIC (TRICALCIUM PHOSPHATE)

Trade name: Posture

Classifications: ELECTROLYTIC BALANCE AGENT; REPLACEMENT SOLUTION; ANTACID

Prototype: Calcium gluconate

Pregnancy category: C for calcium acetate; other salts not rated

ACTIONS/PHARMACODYNAMICS Rapid-acting antacid with high neutralizing capacity and relatively prolonged duration of action. Decreases gastric acidity, thereby inhibiting proteolytic action of pepsin on gastric mucosa. Also increases lower esophageal sphincter tone. Although classified as a nonsystemic antacid, a slight to moderate alkalosis usually develops with prolonged therapy. Acid rebound, which may follow even low doses, is thought to be caused by release of gastrin triggered by action of calcium in small intestines.

USES Relief of transient symptoms of hyperacidity as in acid indigestion, heartburn, peptic esophagitis, and hiatal hernia. Also used as calcium supplement when calcium intake may be inadequate and in treatment of mild calcium deficiency states. Control of hyperphosphatemia in chronic renal failure (calcium acetate). **Unlabeled uses:** for treatment of hyperphosphatemia in patients with chronic renal failure and to lower BP in selected patients with hypertension.

ROUTE & DOSAGE

All doses are in terms of *elemental calcium:* 1 g calcium carbonate = 400 mg (20 mEq) elemental calcium; 1 g calcium acetate = 250 mg (12.6 mEq) elemental calcium; 1 g calcium citrate = 210 mg (12 mEq) elemental calcium; 1 g tricalcium phosphate = 390 mg (19.3 mEq) elemental calcium

Supplement for Osteoporosis

Adult: **PO** 1–2 g b.i.d. or t.i.d.

Antacid

Adult: **PO** 0.5–2 g 4–6 times/d.

Hyperphosphatemia

Adult: **PO** calcium acetate 2–4 tablets with each meal.

PHARMACOKINETICS Absorption: approximately 1/3 of dose absorbed from small intestine. **Distribution:** crosses placenta. **Elimination:** primarily excreted in feces; small amounts excreted in urine, pancreatic juice, saliva, breast milk.

CONTRAINDICATIONS & PRECAUTIONS Contraindicated in: hypercalcemia and hypercalciuria (e.g., hyperparathyroidism, vitamin D overdosage, decalcifying tumors, bone metastases), calcium loss due to immobilization, severe renal disease, renal calculi, GI hemorrhage or obstruction, dehydration, hypochloremic alkalosis, ventricular fibrillation, cardiac disease, pregnancy (category C). **Cautious use in:** decreased bowel motility (e.g., with anticholinergics, antidiarrheals, antispasmodics), the elderly.

ADVERSE/SIDE EFFECTS *Constipation* or laxative effect, acid rebound, nausea, eructation, *flatulence.* With prolonged use of high doses: hypercalcemia with alkalosis, metastatic calcinosis, hypercalciuria, hypomagnesemia, hypophosphatemia (when phosphate intake is low), mood and mental changes, polyuria, renal calculi, vomiting, fecal concretions.

DRUG INTERACTIONS May enhance inotropic and toxic effects of **digoxin; magnesium** may compete for GI absorption; decreases absorption of TETRACYCLINES, QUINOLONES **(ciprofloxacin).**

NURSING IMPLICATIONS

Administration

- When used as antacid, it is taken 1 h after meals and at bedtime.

C

When used as calcium supplement, it is taken 1–1 1/2 h after meals, unless otherwise directed by physician.

- Chewable tablet should be chewed well before swallowing or allowed to dissolve completely in mouth, followed with water. Powder form may be mixed with water.
- Store at 15–30C (59–86F) in tightly closed container unless otherwise directed.

Assessment & Drug Effects

- Note number and consistency of stools. If constipation is a problem, physician may prescribe alternate or combination therapy with a magnesium antacid or advise patient to take a laxative or stool softener as necessary.
- Weekly serum and urine calcium determinations are recommended in patients receiving prolonged therapy and in patients with renal dysfunction.
- Record amelioration of symptoms of hypocalcemia (see Signs & Symptoms, Appendix G).
- Observe for signs and symptoms of hypercalcemia in patients receiving frequent or high doses, or who have impaired renal function (see Appendix G).

Patient & Family Education

- Because of acid rebound, which generally occurs after repeated use for 1 or 2 wk, one can quickly become a chronic user of calcium carbonate. Explain to patient the potential dangers of self-medication. Caution not to take antacids longer than 2 wk without medical supervision.
- Avoid taking calcium carbonate with cereals or other foods high in oxylates. Oxalates combine with calcium carbonate to form insoluble, nonabsorbable compounds.
- Chronic use of calcium carbonate taken together with foods high in vitamin D (such as milk) or sodium bicarbonate can cause milk-alkali syndrome: hypercalcemia, distaste for food, headache, confusion, nausea, vomiting, abdominal pain, metabolic alkalosis, hypercalciuria, polyuria, soft tissue calcification (calcinosis), hyperphosphatemia and renal insufficiency. Predisposing factors include renal dysfunction, dehydration, electrolyte imbalance, and hypertension.

CALCIUM CHLORIDE

Classifications: ELECTROLYTIC BALANCE AGENT; REPLACEMENT SOLUTION

Prototype: Calcium gluconate

Pregnancy category: C

ACTIONS/PHARMACODYNAMICS

Actions similar to those of calcium gluconate. Ionizes more readily and thus is more potent than calcium gluconate and more irritating to tissues. Provides excess chloride ions that promote acidosis and temporary (1–2 d) diuresis secondary to excretion of sodium.

USES Treatment of cardiac resuscitation when epinephrine fails to improve myocardial contractions; for treatment of acute hypocalcemia (as in tetany due to parathyroid deficiency, vitamin D deficiency, alkalosis, insect bites or stings, and during exchange transfusions), for treatment of hypermagnesemia, and for cardiac disturbances of hyperkalemia.

ROUTE & DOSAGE

All doses are in terms of *elemental calcium:* 1 g calcium

chloride = 272 mg (13.6 mEq) elemental calcium

Hypocalcemia

Adult: **IV** 0.5–1 g (7–14 mEq) at 1–3 d intervals as determined by patient response and serum calcium levels.
Child: **IV** 25 mg/kg (1–7 mEq) administered slowly.
Neonate: **IV** <1 mEq/d.

Hypocalcemic Tetany

Adult: **IV** 4.5–16 mEq prn.
Child: **IV** 0.5–0.7 mEq/kg t.i.d. or q.i.d.
Neonate: **IV** 2.4 mEq/kg/d in divided doses.

CPR

Adult: **IV** 2.7–3.7 mEq x 1.
Child: **IV** 20 mg/kg; may repeat in 10 min.

PHARMACOKINETICS Distribution: crosses placenta. **Elimination:** primarily excreted in feces; small amounts excreted in urine, pancreatic juice, saliva, and breast milk.

CONTRAINDICATIONS & PRECAUTIONS Contraindicated in: ventricular fibrillation, hypercalcemia, digitalis toxicity, injection into myocardium or other tissue. Safe use during pregnancy (category C), in nursing women, and in children not established. **Cautious use in:** digitalized patients; sarcoidosis, renal insufficiency, history of renal stone formation; cor pulmonale, respiratory acidosis, respiratory failure.

ADVERSE/SIDE EFFECTS Tingling sensation. With rapid IV, sensations of heat waves (peripheral vasodilation), fainting, hypotension, bradycardia, cardiac arrhythmias, <u>cardiac arrest</u>, pain and burning at IV site, severe venous thrombosis, necrosis and sloughing (with extravasation).

DRUG INTERACTIONS May enhance inotropic and toxic effects of **digoxin;** antagonizes the effects of **verapamil** and possibly other CALCIUM CHANNEL BLOCKERS.

NURSING IMPLICATIONS

Administration

- Solution should be warmed to body temperature before administration.
- IV preparation: May be given undiluted or diluted (preferred) with an equal volume of NS for injection.
- IV administration: Give at 0.5–1 ml/min or more slowly if irritation develops. Use a small-bore needle and inject into a large vein to minimize venous irritation and undesirable reactions.
- IV administration to neonates, infants and children: Verify correct IV concentration and rate of infusion/injection with physician.
- Extravasation must be avoided during IV injection, since cellulitis, necrosis, and sloughing can result. Local necrosis can occur with leakage from vein. If given IV to children, scalp veins should be avoided.
- Calcium chloride should never be given subcutaneously or IM or by gavage, as it is a tissue irritant.
- Calcium chloride is incompatible with bicarbonates, carbonates, phosphates, sulfates, and tartrates. Consult pharmacist for compatible admixtures.
- Store at 15–30C (59–86F) unless otherwise directed.

Assessment & Drug Effects

- Monitor ECG, BP, and flow rate and observe patient closely during administration.
- IV injection may be accompanied by cutaneous burning sensation

C

and peripheral vasodilation, with moderate fall in BP. Following injection, advise ambulatory patient to remain in bed for 15–30 min or more depending on response.

- Digitalized patients must be closely observed since an increase in serum calcium increases risk of digitalis toxicity.
- Frequent determinations of serum pH, calcium, and other electrolytes should be performed as guides to dosage adjustments.

CALCIUM GLUCEPTATE

(gloo-sep′tate)

Classifications: ELECTROLYTIC BALANCE AGENT; REPLACEMENT SOLUTION
Prototype: Calcium gluconate
Pregnancy category: C

ACTIONS/PHARMACODYNAMICS

Similar to calcium gluconate in actions, uses, and contraindications and precautions but reportedly is less irritating. Preferred for use when IM administration is required as in neonatal tetany.

USES To correct hypocalcemia and following each 100 ml of exchange transfusion in newborns.

ROUTE & DOSAGE

All doses are in terms of ***elemental calcium:*** **1 g calcium gluceptate = 82 mg (4.1 mEq) elemental calcium**

Hypocalcemia

Adult: **IV** 1.1–4.4 g/d. **IM** 0.5–1.1 g.d.
Child: **IV** 200–500 mg/kg/d divided q6h.

Exchange Transfusions with Citrated Blood

Neonate: **IV** 0.5 ml after each 100 ml of blood exchanged.

PHARMACOKINETICS **Duration:** 2–3 h IV; 1–4 h IM. **Distribution:** crosses placenta. **Elimination:** primarily excreted in feces; small amounts excreted in urine, pancreatic juice, saliva, and breast milk.

ADVERSE/SIDE EFFECTS See calcium gluconate.

DRUG INTERACTIONS May enhance inotropic and toxic effects of **digoxin;** antagonizes the effects of **verapamil** and possibly other CALCIUM CHANNEL BLOCKERS.

NURSING IMPLICATIONS

Administration

- Calcium gluceptate may be given undiluted by direct IV at a rate not to exceed 1 ml/min or slower if irritation develops.
- Patient may complain of a transient tingling sensation and metallic taste following IV administration.
- IM injection may produce mild local reactions. Generally, this route is used only in adults when IV administration is not feasible.
- Recommended IM site for adults is the upper outer quadrant of the buttock and in infants (if prescribed) the midlateral thigh.

See calcium gluconate for additonal nursing implications, contraindications & precautions, and adverse/side effects.

CALCIUM GLUCONATE

(gloo′koe-nate)

Trade name: Kalcinate
Prototype for classifications: ELECTROLYTIC AND WATER BALANCE AGENT; REPLACEMENT SOLUTION

C

ACTIONS/PHARMACODYNAMICS Calcium is an essential element for regulating the excitation threshold of nerves and muscles, for blood clotting mechanisms, cardiac function (rhythm, tonicity, contractility), maintenance of renal function, for body skeleton and teeth. Also plays a role in regulating storage and release of neurotransmitters and hormones; regulating amino acid uptake and absorption of vitamin B_{12}; gastrin secretion, and in maintaining structural and functional integrity of cell membranes and capillaries. Calcium gluconate acts like digitalis on heart, increasing cardiac muscle tone and force of systolic contractions (positive inotropic effect).

USES Negative calcium balance (as in neonatal tetany, hypoparathyroidism, vitamin D deficiency, alkalosis). Also to overcome cardiac toxicity of hyperkalemia, for cardiopulmonary resuscitation, to prevent hypocalcemia during transfusion of citrated blood. Also as antidote for magnesium sulfate, for acute symptoms of lead colic, to decrease capillary permeability in sensitivity reactions, and to relieve muscle cramps from insect bites or stings. Oral calcium may be used to maintain normal calcium balance during pregnancy, lactation, and childhood growth and to prevent primary osteoporosis. Also in osteoporosis, osteomalacia, chronic hypoparathyroidism, rickets, and as adjunct in treatment of myasthenia gravis and Eaton-Lambert syndrome. **Unlabeled uses:** to antagonize aminoglycoside-induced neuromuscular blockage, and as "calcium challenge" to diagnose Zollinger-Ellison syndrome and medullary thyroid carcinoma.

ROUTE & DOSAGE

All doses are in terms of ***elemental calcium:*** **1 g calcium gluconate = 90 mg (4.5 mEq) elemental calcium**

Supplement for Osteoporosis

Adult: **PO** 1–2 g b.i.d. to q.i.d. **IV** 7 mEq q1–3d.
Child: **PO** 45–65 mg/kg/d in divided doses. **IV** 1–7 mEq q1–3d.
Neonate: **PO** 50–150 mg/kg/d (max 1 g). **IV** 1 mEq q1–3d.

Hypocalcemic Tetany

Adult: **IV** 4.5–16 mEq prn.
Child: **IV** 0.5–0.7 mEq/kg t.i.d. or q.i.d.
Neonate: **IV** 2.4 mEq/kg/d in divided doses.

CPR

Adult: **IV** 2.3–3.7 mEq × 1.

Hyperkalemia with Cardiac Toxicity

Adult: **IV** 2.25–14 mEq q1– 2min.

Exchange Transfusions with Citrated Blood

Adult: **IV** 1.35 mEq for each 100 ml of blood.
Neonate: **IV** 0.45 mEq for each 100 ml of blood.

PHARMACOKINETICS **Absorption:** approximately 1/3 of dose absorbed from small intestine. **Onset:** immediately after IV. **Distribution:** crosses placenta. **Elimination:** primarily excreted in feces; small amounts excreted in urine, pancreatic juice, saliva, and breast milk.

CONTRAINDICATIONS & PRECAUTIONS **Contraindicated in:** ventricular fibrillation, metastatic bone disease, injection into myocardium; administration by SC or IM routes; renal calculi, hypercalcemia, predisposition to hypercalcemia (hyper-

C

parathyroidism, certain malignancies). **Cautious use in:** digitalized patients, renal or cardiac insufficiency, sarcoidosis, history of lithiasis, immobilized patients.

ADVERSE/SIDE EFFECTS *Hypercalcemia.* **IV injection:** tingling sensations. **Rapid IV:** sense of oppression or "heat waves" (vasodilation), hypotension, bradycardia and other arrhythmias, syncope, <u>cardiac arrest</u>. **Local reactions:** tissue irritation, burning, cellulitis, soft tissue calcification, necrosis and sloughing (following IV extravasation). **PO preparation:** constipation, increased gastric acid secretion.

DIAGNOSTIC TEST INTERFERENCE IV calcium may cause false decreases in ***serum and urine magnesium*** (by Titan yellow method) and transient elevations of ***plasma 11-OHCS*** levels by Glenn-Nelson technique. Values usually return to control levels after 60 min; ***urinary steroid*** values (17-OHCS) may be decreased.

DRUG INTERACTIONS May enhance inotropic and toxic effects of **digoxin; magnesium** may compete for GI absorption; decreases absorption of TETRACYCLINES, QUINOLONES **(ciprofloxacin)**; antagonizes the effects of verapamil and possibly other CALCIUM CHANNEL BLOCKERS (IV administration).

NURSING IMPLICATIONS

Administration

- Oral calcium preparations are best utilized when administered 2–3 h after meals.
- IV calcium should be administered slowly through a small-bore needle into a large vein to avoid possibility of extravasation and resultant necrosis. If calcium is administered to children, scalp veins should be avoided.
- Most often, physician will prescribe a specific IV flow rate. High concentrations of calcium suddenly reaching the heart can cause fatal cardiac arrest.
- IV injection: IV solution may be given undiluted direct IV at a rate of 0.5 ml or a fraction thereof over 1 min.
- IV infusion: IV solution may be diluted in 1 L of NS and given over 12–24 h.

Assessment & Drug Effects

- Direct IV injection may be accompanied by cutaneous burning sensations and peripheral vasodilation, with moderate fall in BP. Injection should be stopped if patient complains of any discomfort. Patient should be advised to remain in bed for 15–30 min or more following injection, depending on response.
- During IV administration, ECG is monitored to detect evidence of hypercalcemia: decreased QT interval associated with inverted T wave.
- Observe IV site closely. Extravasation may result in tissue irritation and necrosis.
- Monitor for hypocalcemia and hypercalcemia (see Signs & Symptoms, Appendix G).
- In sustained therapy, frequent determinations should be made of calcium and phosphorus (tend to vary inversely) and magnesium. Deficiencies in other ions, particularly magnesium, frequently coexist with calcium ion depletion.

Patient & Family Education

- Instruct patients regarding signs and symptoms of hypercalcemia (see Appendix G) and advise them to report any promptly.
- Inform patient that milk and milk products are best sources of calcium (and phosphorus). Other good sources include dark green

vegetables, soy beans, tofu, and canned fish with bones.

- Advise patient that calcium absorption can also be inhibited by zinc-rich foods: nuts, seeds, sprouts, legumes, soy products (tofu).
- Advise patient to check with physician before self-medicating with a calcium supplement.

CALCIUM LACTATE

(lak′tate)

Classifications: ELECTROLYTIC BALANCE AGENT; REPLACEMENT SOLUTION

Prototype: Calcium gluconate

ACTIONS/PHARMACODYNAMICS Oral calcium preparation reportedly well tolerated. Similar to calcium gluconate in actions, contraindications, and adverse reactions.

USES Mild hypocalcemia and maintenance calcium therapy.

ROUTE & DOSAGE

All doses are in terms of *elemental calcium:* 1 g calcium lactate = 130 mg (6.5 mEq) elemental calcium

Supplement for Mild Hypocalcemia

Adult: **PO** 325 mg–1.3 g t.i.d. with meals.
Child: **PO** 500 mg/kg/d in divided doses.

PHARMACOKINETICS Absorption: approximately 1/3 of dose absorbed from small intestine. **Distribution:** crosses placenta. **Elimination:** primarily excreted in feces; small amounts excreted in urine, pancreatic juice, saliva, and breast milk.

ADVERSE/SIDE EFFECTS See calcium carbonate.

DRUG INTERACTIONS May enhance inotropic and toxic effects of **digoxin; magnesium** may compete for GI absorption; decreases absorption of TETRACYCLINES, QUINOLONES **(ciprofloxacin).**

NURSING IMPLICATIONS

Administration

- Tablets or powder can be dissolved in hot water; then add cool water to patient's taste.
- Calcium lactate may be administered with lactose (amount prescribed) to increase solubility.
- Store in airtight containers.

Assessment & Drug Effects

- Monitor for hypercalcemia (see Signs & Symptoms, Appendix G).
- Blood calcium levels should be checked periodically. Hypercalcemia can occur during prolonged administration particularly if patient is also taking vitamin D.
- Bear in mind that an increase in serum calcium in digitalized patients increases risk of digitalis toxicity.

Patient & Family Education

- Advise patient to confer with physician regarding need for vitamin D supplementation.
- Advise patient that calcium absorption can be inhibited by zinc-rich foods such as nuts, sprouts, legumes, and soy products.

CALCIUM POLYCARBOPHIL

(pol-ee-kar′boe-fil)

Trade names: FiberCon, Mitrolan

Classifications: GI AGENT; BULK LAXATIVE; ANTIDIARRHEAL

Prototype: Psyllium hydrophilic muciloid

Pregnancy category: C

C

ACTIONS/PHARMACODYNAMICS Hydrophilic, bulk-producing laxative that restores normal moisture level and bulk content of intestinal tract. In constipation, retains free water in intestinal lumen, thereby indirectly opposing dehydrating forces of the bowel; in diarrhea, when intestinal mucosa is incapable of absorbing fluid, drug absorbs fecal fluid to form a gel. In both conditions, peristalsis is encouraged and a well-formed stool is produced.

USES Constipation or diarrhea associated with diverticulitis or irritable bowel syndrome; acute nonspecific diarrhea.

ROUTE & DOSAGE

Constipation or Diarrhea
Adult: **PO** 1 g q.i.d. as needed (max 6 g/24 h).
Child: **PO** 6–12 y, 500 mg 1–3 times/d (max 3 g/24 h); < 6 y, 500 mg 1–2 times/d (max 1.5 g/24 h).

CONTRAINDICATIONS & PRECAUTIONS **Contraindicated in:** GI obstruction; children <6 y. **Cautious use in:** pregnancy (category C); nursing mothers.

ADVERSE/SIDE EFFECTS *Flatulence,* abdominal fullness, intestinal obstruction; laxative dependence (long-term use).

NURSING IMPLICATIONS

Administration
- Tablets should be chewed before swallowing them. Administer with at least 180–240 ml (6–8 oz) water or other fluid of patient's choice when used as a laxative and with at least 60–90 ml (2–3 oz) of fluid when used as an antidiarrheal. Chewed tablets should not be swallowed dry.
- If diarrhea is severe, dose can be repeated every half hour up to maximum daily dose.
- Store at 15–30C (59–86F).

Assessment & Drug Effects
- Evaluate effectiveness of medication. If it is ineffective as an antidiarrheal, report to physician.
- Rectal bleeding, very dark stools, or abdominal pain should be reported promptly.

Patient & Family Education
- Drug generally produces a bowel movement within 12–72 h.
- This is an OTC product. Discuss with patient the importance of taking the drug exactly as ordered. Patient should be cautioned not to increase the dose if response is inadequate. Consult physician. Advise patients not to use another laxative while they are taking calcium polycarbophil.

CALFACTANT

(cal-fac'tant)
Trade name: Infasurf
Classifications: LUNG SURFACTANT
Prototype: Beractant

ACTIONS/PHARMACODYNAMICS Pulmonary surfactant. Lowers the surface tension on alveolar surfaces during respiration and stabilizes the alveoli against collapse at resting pressure. Deficiency of surfactant causes respiratory disease syndrome (RDS) in premature infants.

USE Prevention and treatment of RDS in infants at high risk for RDS.

ROUTE & DOSAGE

Prevention & Treatment of RDS
Infant: **Intrathecal** 3 ml/kg of birth

weight administered through an endotracheal tube q12h × 3 doses.

PHARMACOKINETICS Absorption: Absorbs rapidly to air:liquid interface of lung surface. No other human pharmacokinetic information available.

CONTRAINDICATIONS & PRECAUTIONS Contraindicated in: nosocomial infections.

ADVERSE/SIDE EFFECTS CV: *bradycardia.* **Respiratory:** *cyanosis, airway obstruction.* **Other:** *reflux of surfactant into endotracheal tube.*

NURSING IMPLICATIONS

Administration

- Swirl vial to disperse suspension; DO NOT SHAKE. Withdraw with 20-gauge or larger needle. Avoid excess foaming.
- Stop administration of calfactant if reflux into endotracheal tube occurs as indicated by cyanosis, bradycardia, or other signs of airway obstruction.
- Store at 2–8C (36–46F) in a tightly closed container and protect from light.

Assessment & Drug Effects

- Close clinical monitoring is required during and after administration; adjustments in oxygen therapy and ventilator pressures are usually needed.

CANDESARTAN CILEXETIL

(can-de-sar′tan ci-lex′e-til)

Trade name: Atacand

Classifications: CARDIOVASCULAR AGENT; ANTIHYPERTENSIVE AGENT; ANGIOTENSIN II RECEPTOR ANTAGONIST

Prototype: Losartan

Pregnancy category: C (first trimester); D (second and third trimesters)

ACTIONS/PHARMACODYNAMICS Angiotensin II receptor (type AT_1) antagonist. Angiotensin II is a potent vasoconstrictor and primary vasoactive hormone of the renin–angiotensin–aldosterone system. Candesartan selectively blocks binding of angiotensin II to the AT_1 receptors found in many tissues (e.g., vascular smooth muscle, adrenal glands). This results in blocking the vasoconstricting and the aldosterone-secreting effects of angiotensin II, resulting in an antihypertensive effect.

USE Hypertension.

ROUTE & DOSAGE

Hypertension

Adult: **PO** Start at 16 mg q.d. (range 8–32 mg divided once or twice daily).

PHARMACOKINETICS Absorption: rapidly absorbed from GI tract; activated by ester hydrolysis during absorption; 15% reaches systemic circulation. **Peak:** serum concentration, 3–4 h; therapeutic effect, 2–4 wk. **Duration:** 24 h. **Distribution:** >99% protein bound; crosses placenta; distributed into breast milk. **Metabolism:** minimally metabolized in liver. **Elimination:** half-life: 9 h; excreted primarily unchanged in bile (67%) and urine (33%).

CONTRAINDICATIONS & PRECAUTIONS Contraindicated in: known sensitivity to candesartan or any other angiotensin II (AT_1) receptor antagonist (e.g., losartan, valsartan); primary hyperaldosteronism; bilateral renal artery stenosis; pregnancy (category C, first trimester; category D, second and third trimesters); lactation. **Cautious use in:** concurrent administration with high-dose diuretics, potassium-sparing diuretics, or potassium salt substitutes; unilateral renal artery stenosis; aortic or mitral valve stenosis; hypertrophic cardiomyopathy; CHF; diabetes; breastfeeding; significant renal failure.

ADVERSE/SIDE EFFECTS **Body as whole:** fatigue, peripheral edema. **CNS:** headache, dizziness. **CV:** chest pain. **GI:** nausea, abdominal pain, diarrhea, vomiting. **Respiratory:** cough, sinusitis, upper respiratory infection, pharyngitis, rhinitis. **Other:** back pain, arthralgia, albuminuria.

NURSING IMPLICATIONS

Administration

- To prevent hypotension, volume depletion should be corrected prior to initiation of therapy.
- Dose is individualized and may be given once or twice daily. The daily dose may be titrated up to 32 mg; larger doses are not likely to provide additional benefit.
- Store at 15–30C (59–86F).

Assessment & Drug Effects

- Therapeutic effectiveness is indicated by decreases in systolic and diastolic BP within 2 wk with maximal effect at 4–6 wk.
- Monitor for transient hypotension in volume/salt-depleted patients; if hypotension occurs, place in supine position and notify physician.
- Monitor BP periodically; trough readings, just prior to the next scheduled dose, should be made when possible.
- Lab tests: Periodically monitor BUN and creatinine, serum potassium, liver enzymes, and CBC with differential.

Patient & Family Education

- Women who become pregnant should immediately inform their physicians.
- Nursing mothers should discuss continuing drug use with their physicians.
- Maximum pressure-lowering effect may not be evident for 6 wk.
- Report episodes of dizziness especially when making position changes.

CAPECITABINE

(cap-e-si′ta-been)

Trade name: Xeloda

Classifications: ANTINEOPLASTIC; ANTIMETABOLITE

Prototype: Fluorouracil (5-FU)

Pregnancy category: D

ACTIONS/PHARMACODYNAMICS Pyrimidine antagonist and cell cycle-specific antimetabolite. Prodrug of 5-FU. Blocks actions of enzymes essential to normal DNA and RNA synthesis. May become incorporated into RNA molecules thereby interfering with RNA processing and protein synthesis.

USE Metastatic breast cancer refractory to other treatments.

ROUTE & DOSAGE

Breast Cancer

Adult: **PO** 2500 mg/m^2/d in 2 divided doses × 2 wk, then 1 wk off. Repeat.

PHARMACOKINETICS **Absorption:** absorption significantly reduced by food. **Peak:** 1.5–2 h. **Distribution:** approx 35% protein bound. **Metabolism:** extensively metabolized to 5-FU. **Elimination:** half-life: 45 min; excreted in urine.

C

CONTRAINDICATIONS & PRECAUTIONS **Contraindicated in:** hypersensitivity to capecitabine, doxifluridine, 5-FU; myelosuppression; pregnancy (category D); use with lactation is not known. **Cautious use in:** renal or hepatic dysfunction; bacterial or viral infection.

ADVERSE/SIDE EFFECTS **Body as whole:** *fatigue,* pyrexia, pain, myalgia. **CNS:** paresthesias, headache, dizziness, insomnia. **CV:** edema. **GI:** *severe diarrhea, nausea, vomiting, stomatitis,* abdominal pain, constipation, dyspepsia, *anorexia.* **Hematologic:** *neutropenia, thrombocytopenia, anemia, lymphopenia.* **Skin:** *hand-and-foot syndrome, dermatitis,* nail disorder. **Other:** dehydration, eye irritation, *hyperbilirubinemia.*

DRUG INTERACTIONS **Leucovorin** increases concentration and toxicity of 5-FU.

NURSING IMPLICATIONS

Administration

- Morning and evening doses (about 12 h apart) should be given at the end of a meal.
- Store at room temperature (or at 15–30C/59–86F) and keep tightly closed.

Assessment & Drug Effects

- Lab tests: Periodically monitor CBC with differential and liver functions including bilirubin, transaminases, alkaline phosphatase.
- Carefully monitor for S&S of grade 2 or greater toxicity: diarrhea > 4 BMs/day or at night; vomiting >1 time/24 h; significant loss of appetite or anorexia; stomatitis; hand-and-foot syndrome (pain, swelling, erythema, desquamation, blistering); temperature ≥ 100.5F; and S&S of infection.
- Withhold drug and immediately report S&S of grade 2 or greater toxicity.
- Monitor for dehydration and replace fluids as needed.
- Carefully monitor patients with coronary artery disease for S&S of cardiotoxicity (e.g., increasing angina).

Patient & Family Education

- Take tablets with adequate water within 30 min of a meal.
- Immediately report significant nausea, loss of appetite, diarrhea, soreness of tongue, fever of 100.5F or more, or signs of infection. Carefully review patient drug package insert for more detail.
- Women who become pregnant should immediately inform their physicians.
- Mothers should discuss advisability of nursing their infants with their physicians.

CAPREOMYCIN SULFATE

(kap-ree-oh-mye′sin)

Trade name: Capastat Sulfate

Classifications: ANTIINFECTIVE; ANTITUBERCULOSIS AGENT

Prototype: Isoniazid

Pregnancy category: C

ACTIONS/PHARMACODYNAMICS Polypeptide antibiotic derived from *Streptomyces capreolus.* Action mechanism not clear. Bacteriostatic against human strains of *Mycobacterium tuberculosis* and other species of *Mycobacterium.* Cross-resistance between capreomycin and both kanamycin and neomycin has been reported. Bacterial resistance can develop rapidly when used alone.

USES Only in conjunction with other appropriate antitubercular drugs in treatment of pulmonary tu-

C

berculosis when bactericidal agents, e.g., isoniazid and rifampin, cannot be tolerated or when causative organism has become resistant.

ROUTE & DOSAGE

Tuberculosis

Adult: **IM** 1 g/d (not to exceed 20 mg/kg/d) for 60–120 d; then 1 g 2–3 times/wk. See prescribing information for dose adjustments for renal insufficiency.

PHARMACOKINETICS **Peak:** 1–2 h. **Distribution:** does not cross blood–brain barrier; crosses placenta; distribution into breast milk unknown. **Elimination:** half-life: 4–6 h; 52% excreted in urine unchanged in 12 h; small amount excreted in bile.

CONTRAINDICATIONS & PRECAUTIONS **Contraindicated in:** safe use during pregnancy (category C), in nursing women, infants, and children not established. **Cautious use in:** renal insufficiency (extreme caution); acoustic nerve impairment; history of allergies (especially to drugs); preexisting liver disease; myasthenia gravis; parkinsonism.

ADVERSE/SIDE EFFECTS **CNS:** neuromuscular blockage (large doses): skeletal muscle weakness, <u>respiratory depression or arrest</u>. **Hematologic:** leukocytosis, leukopenia, *eosinophilia*. **Hypersensitivity:** urticaria, maculopapular rash, photosensitivity. **Renal:** <u>nephrotoxicity</u> (long-term therapy), <u>tubular necrosis</u>. **Ear:** ***ototoxicity:*** eighth nerve (auditory and vestibular) damage. **Other:** hypokalemia, and other electrolyte imbalances; impaired hepatic function (decreased BSP excretion); IM site reactions: pain, induration, excessive bleeding, sterile abscesses.

DIAGNOSTIC TEST INTERFERENCE ***BSP*** and ***PSP*** excretion tests may be decreased.

DRUG INTERACTIONS Increased risk of nephrotoxicity and ototoxicity with AMINOGLYCOSIDES, **amphotericin B, colistin, polymyxin B, cisplatin, vancomycin.**

NURSING IMPLICATIONS

Administration

- Reconstitute by adding 2 ml of 0.9% isotonic NaCl injection or sterile water for injection to each 1 g vial. Allow 2–3 min for drug to dissolve completely.
- IM injections should be made deep into large muscle mass. Superficial injections are more painful and are associated with sterile abscess. Rotate injection sites.
- Solution may become pale straw color and darken with time, but this does not indicate loss of potency.
- After reconstitution, solution may be stored 48 h at room temperature and up to 14 d under refrigeration unless otherwise directed.
- Store at 15–30C (59–86F) unless otherwise directed.

Assessment & Drug Effects

- Observe injection sites for signs of excessive bleeding and inflammation.
- The following determinations are used as guidelines for therapy and should be performed before drug is started and at regular intervals during therapy: (1) appropriate bacterial susceptibility tests; (2) audiometric measurements (twice weekly or weekly) and tests of vestibular function (periodically); (3) CBC; SMA-12 screening weekly; (4) weekly renal function studies (BUN, NPN, creatinine clearance, sediment); (5) liver function tests

(periodically); (6) serum potassium levels (monthly).

- Capreomycin is cumulative in patients with impaired renal function. Dosage should be reduced in these patients and renal function tests closely followed.
- Monitor I&O. Report immediately any change in output or I&O ratio, any unusual appearance of urine, or elevation of BUN above 30 mg/dl. (Normal BUN: 10–20 mg/dl.)

Patient & Family Education

- Instruct patient to report any change in hearing or disturbance of balance. These effects are sometimes reversible if drug is withdrawn promptly when first symptoms appear.
- Patient and responsible family members should be completely informed about adverse reactions. They should be urged to report immediately the appearance of any unusual symptom, regardless of how vague it may seem.

CAPSAICIN

(cap-say′i-sin)

Trade names: Axsain, Capsacin-P, Zostrix, Zostrix-HP

Classifications: SKIN AND MUCOUS MEMBRANE AGENT: TOPICAL ANALGESIC

ACTIONS/PHARMACODYNAMICS Capsaicin is an alkaloid derived from plants and is the active ingredient in hot peppers. It is used as a topical analgesic. Capsaicin's precise mechanism is not fully understood; however, it is thought that the drug renders skin and joints insensitive to pain by preventing the reaccumulation of substance P in peripheral sensory neurons. Substance P is thought to act as a principal neurotransmitter of pain sensations from the peripheral neurons to the CNS.

USES Temporary relief of pain from arthritis, neuralgias, diabetic neuropathy, and herpes zoster. **Unlabeled uses:** phantom limb pain, psoriasis, intractable pruritus.

ROUTE & DOSAGE

Analgesia

Adult: **Topical** Apply to affected area not more than 3–4 times/d
Child ≥2*y:* **Topical** Apply to affected area not more than 3–4 times/d.

PHARMACOKINETICS **Onset:** postherpetic neuralgia: 2–6 wk.

CONTRAINDICATIONS & PRECAUTIONS **Contraindicated in:** hypersensitivity to capsaicin or any ingredient in the cream. **Cautious use in:** patients on ACE inhibitors. Safety and efficacy in children < 2 y have not been established.

ADVERSE/SIDE EFFECTS **CNS:** concentration >1%: neurotoxicity, hyperalgesia. **Skin:** *burning, stinging, redness,* itching. **Other:** cough.

DRUG INTERACTION May increase incidence of cough with ACE INHIBITORS.

NURSING IMPLICATIONS

Administration

- Apply to affected areas only and avoid contact with eyes or broken or irritated skin.
- If applied with bare hand, wash immediately following application. An applicator or gloved hand may be used to apply cream.
- Avoid tight bandages over areas of application of the cream.
- Store at 15–30C (59–86F).

C

Assessment & Drug Effects

- Monitor for significant pain relief, which may require 4–6 wk of application three or four times daily.
- Monitor for and report signs of skin breakdown as these generally indicate need for drug discontinuation.

Patient & Family Education

- Instruct to report local discomfort at site of application if discomfort is distressing or persists beyond the first 3–4 d of use.
- Instruct to use caution in handling contact lenses following application of cream. Hands should be thoroughly washed before touching lenses.
- Advise to notify physician if symptoms do not improve or condition worsens within 14–28 d.
- Therapeutic effectiveness is maximized by frequent applications three or four times daily.

CAPTOPRIL

(kap′toe-pril)

Trade name: Capoten

Prototype for classifications: CARDIOVASCULAR AGENT; ANGIOTENSIN-CONVERTING ENZYME INHIBITOR; ANTIHYPERTENSIVE

Pregnancy category: D

ACTIONS/PHARMACODYNAMICS Lowers blood pressure by specific inhibition of the angiotensin-converting enzyme (ACE). This interrupts conversion sequences initiated by renin that lead to formation of angiotensin II, a potent endogenous vasoconstrictor. ACE inhibition alters hemodynamics without compensatory reflex tachycardia or changes in cardiac output (except in patient with CHF). Peripheral vascular resistance is lowered by vasodilation. Inhibition of ACE also leads to decreased circulating aldosterone. Reduced circulating aldosterone is associated with a potassium-sparing effect. In heart failure, captopril administration is followed by a fall in CVP and pulmonary wedge pressure; hypotensive action appears to be unrelated to plasma renin levels.

USES Hypertension; in conjunction with digitalis and diuretics in CHF, diabetic nephropathy. **Unlabeled use:** idiopathic edema.

ROUTE & DOSAGE

Hypertension

Adult: **PO** 6.25–25 mg t.i.d.; may increase to 50 mg t.i.d. (max 450 mg/d).
Premature infant: **PO** 0.01 mg/kg q8–12h.
Neonate: **PO** 0.05–0.1 mg/kg q8–24 h; may titrate up to 0.5 mg/kg q6–24 h.
Infant: **PO** 0.15–0.3 mg/kg; titrate up to 6 mg/kg/d in 1–4 divided doses;
Child: **PO** 0.3–12.5 mg/kg q12–24h; titrated up to max of 6 mg/kg/d in 2–4 divided doses.

Congestive Heart Failure

Adult: **PO** 6.25–12.5 mg t.i.d.; may increase to 50 mg t.i.d. (max 450 mg/d).

PHARMACOKINETICS Absorption: 60–75% absorbed; food may decrease absorption 25–40%. **Onset:** 15 min. **Peak:** 1–2 h. **Duration:** 6– 12 h. **Distribution:** distributed to all tissues except CNS; crosses placenta. **Metabolism:** some liver metabolism. **Elimination:** excreted primarily in urine; excreted in breast milk.

CONTRAINDICATIONS & PRECAUTIONS Contraindicated in: pregnancy (category D); safe use in nursing mothers and children not established. **Cautious use in:** impaired renal function, patient with solitary kidney; collagen-vascular diseases (scleroderma, SLE); patients receiving IMMUNOSUPPRESSANTS or other drugs that cause leukopenia or agranulocytosis; coronary or cerebrovascular disease; severe salt/volume depletion.

ADVERSE/SIDE EFFECTS **CV:** slight increase in heart rate, first dose hypotension, dizziness, fainting. **GI:** altered taste sensation (loss of taste perception, persistent salt or metallic taste); weight loss. **Hematologic:** hyperkalemia, neutropenia, agranulocytosis (rare). **Hypersensitivity:** serum sickness-like reaction, arthralgia, skin eruptions. **Renal:** azotemia, impaired renal function, nephrotic syndrome, membranous glomerulonephritis. **Skin:** *maculopapular rash*, urticaria, pruritus, angioedema, photosensitivity. **Other:** positive antinuclear antibody (ANA) titers, *cough*.

DIAGNOSTIC TEST INTERFERENCE In some patients, elevated ***urine protein levels*** may persist even after captopril has been discontinued. Possibility of transient elevations of ***BUN*** and ***serum creatinine,*** slight increase in ***serum potassium,*** and ***serum prolactin,*** increases in ***liver enzymes,*** and false-positive ***urine acetone*** (using sodium nitroprusside reagent). Captopril may decrease ***fasting blood sugar*** in the nondiabetic and cause hypoglycemia in the diabetic patient controlled with antidiabetic drug therapy.

DRUG INTERACTIONS NITRATES, DIURETICS, and ANTIHYPERTENSIVES enhance hypotensive effects. **Aspirin** and other NSAIDS may antagonize hypotensive effects. POTASSIUM-SPARING DIURETICS (**spironolactone, amiloride**) increase potassium levels. **Probenecid** decreases elimination and increases effects. **Drug–food:** Food decreases absorption; take 30–60 min before meals.

NURSING IMPLICATIONS

Administration

- Captopril is best administered 1 h before meals. Food reduces absorption by 30–40%. Tablet may have a slight sulfurous odor.
- Store in light-resistant containers at no more than 30C (86F) unless otherwise directed.

Assessment & Drug Effects

- A sudden exaggerated hypotensive response may occur within 1–3 h of first dose, especially in those with high BP or on a diuretic and restricted salt intake.
- Bed rest and BP monitoring are advised for the first 3 h after the initial dose.
- At least 2 wk of therapy may be required before full therapeutic effects are achieved.
- Baseline urinary protein levels should be established before initiation of therapy and checked at monthly intervals for the first 8 mo of treatment and then periodically thereafter.
- Proteinuria occurs in 1–2% of patients and may reach levels as high as 1 g/d. (Normal value: <150 mg/24 h.)
- WBC and differential counts are recommended before therapy is begun and at approximately 2-wk intervals for the first 3 mo of therapy and then periodically thereafter.

Patient & Family Education

- Report to physician without delay the onset of unexplained fever, unusual fatigue, sore mouth or

C

throat, easy bruising or bleeding (pathognomonic of agranulocytosis).

- Mild skin eruptions are most likely to appear during the first 4 wk of therapy and may be accompanied by fever and eosinophilia.
- Patient should consult physician promptly if vomiting or diarrhea occur.
- Darkening or crumbling of nail-beds may occur but is reversible with dosage reduction.
- Taste impairment occurs in 5–10% of patients and generally reverses in 2–3 mo even with continued therapy.
- Use OTC medications only with approval of the physician. Inform surgeon or dentist that captopril is being taken. Alert diabetic patient that captopril may produce hypoglycemia. Monitor blood glucose closely during first few weeks of therapy.

CARBACHOL INTRAOCULAR

(kar'ba-kole)

Trade name: Miostat

CARBACHOL TOPICAL

Trade name: Isopto Carbachol

Classifications: EYE PREPARATION; MIOTIC; AUTONOMIC NERVOUS SYSTEM AGENT; DIRECT-ACTING CHOLINERGIC (PARASYMPATHOMIMETIC)

Prototype: Pilocarpine

Pregnancy category: C

See Appendix A.

CARBAMAZEPINE

(kar-ba-maz'e-peen)

Trade names: Apo-Carbamazepine ♣, Carbatrol, Epitol, Mazepine ♣, PMS-Carbamazepine ♣, Tegretol, Tegretol XR

Classifications: CNS AGENT; ANTICONVULSANT

Prototype: Phenytoin

Pregnancy category: C

ACTIONS/PHARMACODYNAMICS

Structurally related to tricyclic antidepressants (TCAs) but lacks antidepressant properties. Anticonvulsant actions appear qualitatively similar to those of phenytoin (Dilantin). Like phenytoin, provides relief in trigeminal neuralgia by reducing synaptic transmission within trigeminal nucleus. Also has sedative, anticholinergic, antidepressant, and muscle relaxant (by inhibition of neuromuscular transmission) and slight analgesic actions.

USES Alone or concomitantly with other anticonvulsants in treatment of grand mal and psychomotor or temporal lobe epilepsy and mixed seizures in patients who have not responded satisfactorily to other agents. Also used for symptomatic treatment of trigeminal (tic douloureux) and glossopharyngeal neuralgias and for pain and paroxysmal symptoms associated with multiple sclerosis and other neurologic disorders. **Unlabeled uses:** certain psychiatric disorders including prophylaxis and treatment of manic-depressive illness, treatment of schizoaffective illness, resistant schizophrenia, dyscontrol syndrome; for management of alcohol withdrawal, rage outbursts, and for antidiuretic effect in diabetes insipidus.

ROUTE & DOSAGE

Epilepsy

Adult: **PO** 200 mg b.i.d., gradually increased to 800–1200 mg/d in 3–4 divided doses. Tegretol XR dosed b.i.d.

Child: **PO** *<6 y:* 10–20 mg/kg/d, may gradually increase weekly, recommended max 35 mg/kg/d in 3–4 divided doses; *6–12 y:* 100 mg b.i.d., gradually increased to 400–800 mg/d in 3–4 divided doses (max 1 g/d); *<6 y:* 20–30 mg/kg/d in 3–4 divided doses.

Trigeminal Neuralgia

Adult: **PO** 100 mg b.i.d., gradually increased by 100 mg increments q12h until relief; usual dose 200–800 mg/d in 3–4 divided doses (max 1.2 g/d). Tegretol XR dosed b.i.d.

PHARMACOKINETICS Absorption: slowly absorbed from GI tract. **Peak:** 2–8 h. **Distribution:** widely distributed; high concentrations in CSF; crosses placenta; distributed into breast milk. **Metabolism:** metabolized in liver; can induce liver microsomal enzymes. **Elimination:** half-life: 14–16 h (decreases with long-term use); excreted in urine and feces.

CONTRAINDICATIONS & PRECAUTIONS Contraindicated in: hypersensitivity to carbamazepine and to TCAs; history of myelosuppression or hematologic reaction to other drugs; increased IOP; SLE; cardiac, hepatic, or renal disease; coronary artery disease; hypertension. Safe use during pregnancy (category C), in nursing women, and in children <6 y not established. **Cautious use in:** the elderly; history of cardiac disease.

ADVERSE/SIDE EFFECTS CNS: dizziness, vertigo, drowsiness, disturbances of coordination, ataxia, confusion, headache, fatigue, listlessness, speech difficulty, development of minor motor seizures, hyperreflexia, akathisia, involuntary movements, tremors, visual hallucinations, activation of latent psychosis, aggression; agitation, <u>respiratory depression</u>. **CV:** edema, syncope, arrhythmias, <u>heart block</u>. **ENT:** abnormal hearing acuity. **Eye:** scotomas, conjunctivitis, blurred vision, transient diplopia, oculomotor disturbances, oscillopsia, nystagmus. **GI:** nausea, vomiting, anorexia, abdominal pain, diarrhea, constipation, dry mouth and pharynx. **GU:** urinary frequency or retention, oliguria, impotence. **Hematologic:** <u>aplastic anemia</u>, *leukopenia* (transient), leukocytosis, <u>agranulocytosis</u>, eosinophilia, thrombocytopenia. **Hepatic:** abnormal liver function tests, hepatitis, cholestatic and hepatocellular jaundice. **Skin:** skin rashes, urticaria, petechiae, extreme multiforme, Stevens-Johnson syndrome, photosensitivity reactions, altered skin pigmentation, <u>exfoliative dermatitis</u>, alopecia. **Other:** myalgia, arthralgia, leg cramps, carbamazepine-induced SLE, pancreatitis, hypothyroidism, SIADH.

DIAGNOSTIC TEST INTERFERENCE False-negative ***pregnancy test*** results with tests involving human chorionic gonadotropin.

DRUG INTERACTIONS Serum concentrations of other ANTICONVULSANTS may decrease because of increased metabolism; **verapamil, erythromycin, ketoconazole, nefazadone** may increase carbamazepine levels; decreases hypoprothrombinemic effects of ORAL ANTICOAGULANTS; increases metabolism of estrogens, thus decreasing effectiveness of ORAL CONTRACEPTIVES.

NURSING IMPLICATIONS

Administration

- Absorption of drug is enhanced by administration with meals.

C

- Do not administer carbamazepine suspension simultaneously with other liquid medications: a precipitate may form in the stomach.
- Store at 15–30C (59–86F) unless otherwise directed.

Assessment & Drug Effects

- Before initiation of carbamazepine therapy, the following procedures for eliciting baseline data are recommended: ophthalmoscopy, ECG, and laboratory studies: CBCs including platelets, reticulocytes, serum electrolytes and serum iron, liver function tests, BUN, and complete urinalysis.
- At least 3 mo into therapy, it is recommended that physician attempt dosage reduction or termination of drug therapy, if possible, in patients with trigeminal neuralgia. Some patients develop tolerance to the effects of carbamazepine.
- The following reactions commonly occur during early therapy: drowsiness, dizziness, light-headedness, ataxia, gastric upset. If these symptoms do not subside within a few days, dosage adjustments may be indicated.
- In general, therapy should be discontinued if any of the following signs of myelosuppression occur: RBC <4 million/mm^3, Hct <32%, Hgb <11 g/dl, WBC <4000/mm^3, platelet count <100,000/mm^3, reticulocyte count <20,000/mm^3, serum iron > 150 μg/dl.
- Toxicity can develop when serum concentrations are even slightly above the therapeutic range.
- The pain of tic douloureux is so excruciating that it has driven some patients to suicide. Common triggering stimuli include drafts, shaving, washing face, talking, chewing, hot or cold fluids or foods, jarring the bed, sudden noises. Carbamazepine relieves pain for 24–72 h in these patients.
- Monitor I&O ratio and vital signs during period of dosage adjustment. Report oliguria, signs of fluid retention, changes in I&O ratio, and changes in BP or pulse patterns.
- Cardiac syncope may resemble epileptic seizures. Therefore, it is recommended that patients who experience an apparent increase in frequency of seizures or a change in their character should be checked by continuous ECG monitoring for 24 h.
- Doses higher than 600 mg/d may precipitate arrhythmias in patients with heart disease.
- Confusion and agitation may be aggravated in the elderly; therefore, side rails and supervision of ambulation may be indicated.

Patient & Family Education

- Home patients and responsible family members should be instructed to withhold drug and notify physician immediately if early signs of toxicity or a possible hematologic problem appear, (e.g., anorexia, fever, sore throat or mouth, malaise, unusual fatigue, tendency to bruise or bleed, petechiae, ecchymoses, bleeding gums, nose bleeds).
- Because dizziness, drowsiness, and ataxia are common side effects, warn patient to avoid hazardous tasks requiring mental alertness and physical coordination until reaction to drug is known.
- Impress on the patient and family the importance of remaining under close medical supervision throughout therapy.
- Photosensitivity reactions have been reported; therefore caution patient to avoid excessive sunlight. Suggest application of a sunscreen (if allowed) with SPF of 12 or above.

- Patients taking oral contraceptives should be informed that carbamazepine may cause breakthrough bleeding and may also affect the reliability of oral contraceptives.
- In patients with epilepsy, abrupt withdrawal of any anticonvulsant drug may precipitate seizures or even status epilepticus.

CARBENICILLIN INDANYL SODIUM

(kar-ben-i-sill′in)

Trade names: Geocillin, Geopen Oral ♣

Classifications: ANTIINFECTIVE; ANTIBIOTIC; ANTIPSEUDOMONAL PENICILLIN

Prototype: Mezlocillin

Pregnancy category: B

ACTIONS/PHARMACODYNAMICS Broad-spectrum, semisynthetic penicillin and acid stable ester of carbenicillin prepared for oral use. Rapidly hydrolyzed to carbenicillin in body. Like carbenicillin disodium, it is bactericidal and penicillinase sensitive and has similar antimicrobial activity but achieves lower blood concentrations than parent compound.

USES Mainly in the treatment of prostatitis and acute and chronic infections of upper and lower urinary tract caused by susceptible strains of *Escherichia coli, Enterobacter, Enterococcus, Proteus,* and *Pseudomonas* species.

ROUTE & DOSAGE

Urinary Tract Infections

Adult: **PO** 382–764 mg q6h for 10 d; continue for 2–4 wk for prostatitis.

PHARMACOKINETICS Absorption: incompletely absorbed from GI tract. **Peak:** 0.5–1 h. **Distribution:** very low systemic concentrations; crosses placenta; distributed into breast milk. **Elimination:** half-life: 67 min; 80–99% excreted unchanged in urine within 24 h.

CONTRAINDICATIONS & PRECAUTIONS Contraindicated in: hypersensitivity to penicillins. Safe use in children and during pregnancy (category B) not established. **Cautious use in:** history of or suspected atopy or allergies; history of allergy to cephalosporins; impaired renal and hepatic function; patients on sodium restriction.

ADVERSE/SIDE EFFECTS Dose-related. **GI:** *nausea,* vomiting, heartburn; *diarrhea,* abdominal cramps, flatulence, unpleasant aftertaste, dry mouth. **Hematologic:** neutropenia, leukopenia, thrombocytopenia, <u>hemolytic anemia</u>, increased AST. **Hypersensitivity:** rash, fever, urticaria, eosinophilia, pruritus, <u>anaphylaxis</u>. **Other:** superinfections, especially of vagina.

NURSING IMPLICATIONS

Administration

- This drug is best taken with a full glass (240 ml) of water on an empty stomach (either 1 h before or 2 h after meals) to attain maximum therapeutic drug levels in urine. Consult physician.
- Protect tablets from moisture. Unless otherwise specified, store at 15–30C (59–86F).

Assessment & Drug Effects

- Culture and susceptibility test should be performed prior to and at regular intervals throughout therapy. Therapy may be initiated pending test results.
- Before treatment is initiated, a

C

careful inquiry should be made concerning patient's previous exposure and sensitivity to penicillin and cephalosporins and other allergic reactions of any kind.

- Drug-induced nausea, unpleasant aftertaste and smell, dry mouth, and furry tongue may be so objectionable as to necessitate drug withdrawal. Report to physician if symptoms persist.
- During prolonged therapy, evaluations of renal, hepatic, and hematopoietic systems are advised at regular intervals. Patients with creatinine clearance of less than 10 ml/min (normal: 105–130 ml/min) will not attain therapeutic urine levels.
- Check with physician regarding optimum daily fluid intake. Report any change in quality or quantity of urine or in I&O ratio.
- Observe patient for signs of electrolyte imbalance. Each 1 g of drug contains approximately 1 mEq of sodium.

Patient & Family Education

- Instruct patient to take with a full glass of water on an empty stomach.
- Instruct patient to take medication around the clock, not to miss any doses, and to continue taking medication until it is all gone unless otherwise directed by physician.

CARBIDOPA-LEVODOPA

(kar-bi-doe'pa)

Trade names: Sinemet, Sinemet-CR

CARBIDOPA

Trade name: Lodosyn

Classifications: AUTONOMIC NERVOUS SYSTEM AGENT; ANTICHOLINERGIC (PARASYMPATHOLYTIC); ANTIPARKINSONISM AGENT

Prototype: Levodopa

Pregnancy category: C

ACTIONS/PHARMACODYNAMICS

When levodopa is given alone, large doses must be administered. Carbidopa prevents peripheral metabolism (decarboxylation) of levodopa and thereby makes more levodopa available for transport to the brain. Carbidopa does not cross blood-brain barrier and therefore does not affect metabolism of levodopa within the brain. Carbidopa also prevents the inhibitory effect of pyridoxine (vitamin B_6) on levodopa.

USES Symptomatic treatment of idiopathic Parkinson's disease (paralysis agitans), postencephalitic parkinsonism, and parkinsonism following carbon dioxide and manganese intoxication. Carbidopa is available alone from manufacturer, on request by physician, for use with levodopa when separate titration of each agent is indicated and for investigational purposes.

ROUTE & DOSAGE

Parkinson's Disease in Patients Not Currently Receiving Levodopa

Adult: **PO** 1 tablet containing 10 mg carbidopa/100 mg levodopa *or* 25 mg carbidopa/100 mg levodopa t.i.d., increased by 1 tablet q.d. or q.o.d. up to 6 tablets/d.

Patients Receiving Levodopa

Adult: **PO** 1 tablet of the 25/250 mixture t.i.d. or q.i.d., adjusted by 1/2–1 tablet as needed up to 8 tablets/d (start at 20–25% of initial dose of levodopa).

PHARMACOKINETICS Absorption: 40–70% of carbidopa absorbed after PO dose; carbidopa may enhance absorption of levodopa. **Distribution:**

widely distributed in most body tissues except CNS; crosses placenta; excreted in breast milk. **Elimination:** half-life: 2 h; excreted in urine.

CONTRAINDICATIONS & PRECAUTIONS **Contraindicated in:** hypersensitivity to carbidopa or levodopa; narrow-angle glaucoma; history of or suspected melanoma. Safe use in women of childbearing potential, during pregnancy (category C), in nursing mothers, and in children <18 y not established. **Cautious use in:** cardiovascular, hepatic, pulmonary, or renal disorders; urinary retention; history of peptic ulcer; psychiatric states; endocrine disease; chronic wide-angle glaucoma; seizure disorders.

ADVERSE/SIDE EFFECTS No reactions reported for carbidopa alone. Adverse reactions are those of enhanced levodopa effects: **CNS:** *involuntary movements (dyskinetic, dystonic, choreiform),* ataxia, muscle twitching, increase in hand tremor, numbness, headache, dizziness, euphoria, fatigue, confusion, insomnia, nightmares, mental disturbances, anxiety, <u>depression with suicidal tendencies</u>, delirium, seizures. **CV:** orthostatic hypotension, irregular heart beat, palpitation, arrhythmias, phlebitis, edema. **Eye:** blepharospasm, mydriasis, miosis, blurred vision, diplopia, oculogyric crisis. **GI:** nausea, anorexia, dry mouth, bruxism, vomiting, excess salivation. **GU:** dark urine, priapism, urinary frequency, retention, incontinence. **Hematologic:** hemolytic and nonhemolytic anemia, thrombocytopenia, <u>agranulocytosis</u>. **Skin:** body odor, skin rash, dark sweat, loss of hair. **Other:** hoarseness, unusual breathing patterns, <u>neuroleptic malignant syndrome</u>, abnormal liver function tests, abnormal BUN.

DIAGNOSTIC TEST INTERFERENCE ***Urine glucose:*** false-negative tests may result with use of ***glucose oxidase methods*** (e.g., ***Clinistix, Tes-Tape***) and false-positive results with ***copper reduction methods*** (e.g., ***Benedict's, Clinitest***), especially in patients receiving large doses. It is reported that Clinistix and TesTape may be used if reading is taken at margin of wet and dry tape. There is also the possibility of false-positive tests for ***urinary ketones*** by ***dipstick tests,*** e.g., ***Acetest*** (equivocal), ***Ketostix, Labstix;*** false elevation of ***serum*** and ***urinary uric acid*** levels by colorimetric methods (not with uricase); and interference with ***urine PKU test*** results.

DRUG INTERACTIONS MAO INHIBITORS may precipitate hypertensive crisis; TRICYCLIC ANTIDEPRESSANTS potentiate postural hypotension; PHENOTHIAZINES, **haloperidol** may antagonize effects of levodopa; ANTICHOLINERGIC AGENTS may enhance levodopa effects but can exacerbate involuntary movements; **methyldopa, guanethidine** increase hypotensive and CNS effects; **phenytoin, papaverine** may interfere with levodopa effects.

NURSING IMPLICATIONS

Administration

- Administer with meals or food, unless otherwise directed by physician.
- Food–drug relationship: Ingestion of levodopa with meals high in protein appears to interfere with plasma-to-CNS transport of the drug.
- When patient has been taking levodopa alone, carbidopa-levodopa is usually initiated with a morning dose after patient has been without levodopa for at least 8 h.
- Store in tight, light-resistant con-

tainers at 15–30C (59–86F) unless otherwise directed.

C

Assessment & Drug Effects

- Rate of dosage increase is determined primarily by patient's tolerance and response to levodopa. Make accurate observations and report promptly adverse reactions and therapeutic effects.
- Monitor vital signs, particularly during period of dosage adjustment. Report alterations in BP, pulse, and respiratory rate and rhythm.
- All patients should be closely monitored for behavior changes. Patients in depression should be closely observed for suicidal tendencies.
- Patients with chronic wide-angle glaucoma should be monitored during therapy for changes in intraocular pressure.
- Monitor patients with diabetes carefully for alterations in diabetes control. Frequent monitoring of blood sugar is advised.
- All patients on extended therapy should be checked periodically for symptoms of diabetes and acromegaly and for functioning of hematopoietic, hepatic, and renal systems.
- About 50% of patients on full therapeutic doses for 1 y or longer develop abnormal involuntary movement such as facial grimacing, exaggerated chewing, protrusion of tongue, rhythmic opening and closing of mouth, bobbing of head, jerky arm and leg movements, and exaggerated respiration. Report immediately to physician.
- Chronic management may be accompanied by the "on-off" phenomenon: sudden, unpredictable loss of drug effectiveness ("off" effect), which lasts 1 min–1 h. This is followed by an equally abrupt return of function ("on" effect). Sometimes symptoms can be controlled by increasing number of doses per day.
- Some patients manifest increase in bradykinesia ("leg freezing" or slow body movement). The patient is unable to start walking and frequently falls. Reduction of dosage may be indicated in these patients.
- Patients who require more frequent drug administration are most likely to manifest gradual return of parkinsonian symptoms toward the end of a dose period.

Patient & Family Education

- Patients who have been taking levodopa must be carefully instructed regarding continuation or discontinuation of levodopa as prescribed by physician. Both adverse reactions and therapeutic effects occur more rapidly with carbidopa-levodopa combination than with levodopa alone.
- Orthostatic hypotension is usually asymptomatic, but some patients experience weakness, dizziness, and faintness. Advise patient to make positional changes slowly and in stages, particularly from recumbent to upright position, to dangle legs a few minutes before standing, and to walk in place before ambulating. Tolerance to this effect usually develops within a few months of therapy. Support stockings may help. Consult physician.
- Muscle twitching and spasmodic winking are early signs of overdosage; report them promptly.
- Elevation of mood and sense of well-being may precede objective improvement. Stress the importance of resuming activities gradually and observing safety precautions to avoid injury.

- Urge patient to maintain prescribed drug regimen. Abrupt withdrawal can lead to parkinsonian crisis with return of marked muscle rigidity, akinesia, tremor, hyperpyrexia, mental changes.
- Caution patient to avoid driving or other hazardous activities until reaction to drug is determined.
- Levodopa may cause urine to darken on standing and may also cause sweat to be dark-colored. This effect is not clinically significant.
- Advise patient to wear medical identification. All health care providers should be informed that patient is taking carbidopa-levodopa.

CARBOPLATIN

(car-bo-pla′-tin)

Trade name: Paraplatin

Classifications: ANTINEOPLASTIC; ALKYLATING AGENT

Prototype: Cyclophosphamide

Pregnancy category: D

ACTIONS/PHARMACODYNAMICS Carboplatin is a platinum compound that is a chemotherapeutic agent. It produces interstrand DNA cross-linkages, thus interfering with DNA, RNA, and protein synthesis. Carboplatin is cell-cycle nonspecific, i.e., effective throughout the entire cell life cycle.

USES Monotherapy or combination therapy for ovarian cancer. **Unlabeled uses:** combination therapy for breast, cervical, colon, endometrial, head and neck, and lung cancer; leukemia, lymphoma, and melanoma.

ROUTE & DOSAGE

Ovarian Cancer

Adult: **IV** 360 mg/m^2 once q4wk. May be repeated when neutrophil count is at least 2000 mm^3 and platelet count is at least 100,000 mm^3. If neutrophil and platelet counts are lower, dose of carboplatin should be reduced by 50–75% of initial dose. Alternatively, 400 mg/m^2 as a 24-h infusion for 2 consecutive d can be used.

Head and Neck and Small Cell Lung Cancer

Adult: **IV** 300–400 mg/m^2 q4wk
Child: **IV** Up to 560 mg/m^2 once q4wk or up to 175 mg/m^2 q2wk.

Other dosage regimens have been used for specific dosing protocols.

Important Note

Aluminum reacts with carboplatin to form an inactive precipitate; therefore, intravenous infusion sets and needles containing aluminum should not be used.

PHARMACOKINETICS Onset: 8 wk (2 cycles). **Duration:** 2–16 mo. **Distribution:** highest concentration is seen in the liver, lung, kidney, skin, and tumors. Not bound to plasma proteins. **Metabolism:** hydrolyzed in the serum. **Elimination:** Half-life: 3 h; primarily eliminated by the kidneys; 60–80% excreted in urine within 24 h.

CONTRAINDICATIONS & PRECAUTIONS Contraindicated in: history of severe reactions to carboplatin or other platinum compounds, severe bone marrow depression; significant bleeding; impaired renal function and nursing mothers. **Cautious use in:** pregnancy (category D), and use with other nephrotoxic drugs. Safety and efficacy in children not established.

C

ADVERSE/SIDE EFFECTS **CNS:** peripheral neuropathy. **GI:** *mild to moderate nausea and vomiting,* anorexia, hypogeusia, dysgeusia, mucositis, diarrhea, and constipation. **GU:** nephrotoxicity. **Hematologic:** <u>thrombocytopenia, leukopenia, neutropenia, anemia</u>. **Metabolic:** *mild hyponatremia, hypomagnesemia, hypocalcemia, and hypokalemia.* **Other:** elevated liver enzymes, rash, alopecia, tinnitus, hypersensitivity reactions.

DRUG INTERACTIONS AMINOGLYCOSIDES may increase the risk of ototoxicity and nephrotoxicity. May decrease phenytoin levels.

DIAGNOSTIC TEST INTERFERENCE Decreased **calcium levels;** mild increases in **liver function tests;** decreased levels of **magnesium, potassium,** and **sodium.**

INCOMPATIBILITY **Solution/additive: dextrose solutions.**

NURSING IMPLICATIONS

Administration

- Carboplatin should be given only under the supervision of a physician specifically trained in the use of antineoplastic drugs.
- Needles or IV sets containing aluminum parts that may come in contact with the carboplatin must not be used.
- Immediately before use, reconstitute with either sterile water for injection or 5% dextrose in water or NaCl injection, as follows: 50-mg vial plus 5 ml diluent; 150-mg vial plus 15 ml diluent; 450-mg vial plus 45 ml diluent. All dilutions yield 10 mg/ml. May be further diluted to 0.5 mg/ml with 5% dextrose in water or NaCl injection.
- Rate of administration of the IV solution must be over 15 min or longer, as determined by physician. Lengthening duration of administration may decrease nausea and vomiting.
- Premedication with a parenteral antiemetic 1/2 h before and on a scheduled basis thereafter is normally used.
- Do not repeat doses until the neutrophil count is at least 2000/ mm^3 and platelet count at least 100,000/ mm^3.
- Store unopened vials at room temperature, 15–30C (59–86F). Protect from light. Reconstituted solutions are stable for 8 h at room temperature; discard solutions 8 h after dilution.

Assessment & Drug Effects

- Allergic reactions have occurred within minutes of carboplatin administration. Monitor closely during first 15 min of infusion.
- Frequently monitor peripheral blood counts. Median nadir occurs at day 21. Leukopenia, neutropenia, and thrombocytopenia are dose related and may produce dose-limiting toxicity.
- Periodically monitor kidney function with creatinine clearance tests.
- Monitor for peripheral neuropathy (e.g., paresthesias), ototoxicity, and visual disturbances.
- Periodically monitor serum electrolytes, because carboplatin has been associated with decreases in sodium, potassium, calcium, and magnesium. Special precautions may be warranted for patients on diuretic therapy.

Patient & Family Education

- Discuss with patient the range of potential adverse effects. Strategies for nausea prevention should receive special attention.
- Inform the patient about the po-

tential for infection and hemorrhagic complications related to bone marrow suppression. Advise to avoid unnecessary exposure during the nadir period.
- Instruct patient to report paresthesias, visual disturbances, or symptoms of ototoxicity (hearing loss and/or tinnitus).

CARBOPROST TROMETHAMINE

(kar′boe-prost)

Trade names: Hemabate, Prostin/15 M

Classifications: OXYTOCIC; PROSTAGLANDIN; ABORTIFACIENT

Prototype: Dinosprostone

Pregnancy category: C

ACTIONS/PHARMACODYNAMICS

Synthetic analog of naturally occurring prostaglandin F_2 alpha with longer duration of biologic activity. Stimulates myometrial contractions of gravid uterus; contractions are qualitatively similar to those occurring at term labor. Mean time to abortion 16 h; mean dose required 2.6 ml. Length of time to abortion and total dose of carboprost required decrease with greater parity but increase with greater gestational age. Can be employed as abortifacient even if membranes are ruptured.

USES To induce abortion between 13th and 20th week of pregnancy, as calculated from first day of last menstrual period. Also for refractory postpartum bleeding. **Unlabeled uses:** to reduce blood loss secondary to uterine atony; to induce labor in intrauterine fetal death and hydatidiform mole.

ROUTE & DOSAGE

Adult: **IM** Initial: 250 μg (1 ml) repeated at 1 1/2 – 3 1/2-h intervals if indicated by uterine response; dosage may be increased to 500 μg (2 ml) if uterine contractility is inadequate after several doses of 250 μg (1 ml); not to exceed total dose of 12 mg or continuous administration for more than 2 d.

CONTRAINDICATIONS & PRECAUTIONS **Contraindicated in:** acute pelvic inflammatory disease; active cardiac, pulmonary, renal, or hepatic disease; pregnancy (category C). **Cautious use in:** history of asthma; adrenal disease; anemia; hypotension; hypertension; diabetes mellitus; epilepsy; history of uterine surgery; cervical stenosis; fibroids.

ADVERSE/SIDE EFFECTS Generally transient and reversible with discontinuation of drug. *Nausea,* diarrhea, vomiting, fever, flushing, chills, cough, headache, pain (muscles, joints, lower abdomen, eyes), hiccups, breast tenderness.

NURSING IMPLICATIONS

Administration

- Because nausea and diarrhea occur in about 60% of patients, an antiemetic and an antidiarrheal agent may be prescribed before and during carboprost administration.
- Administer deeply into muscle. Aspirate carefully before injecting drug to avoid inadvertent entry into blood vessel which can result in bronchospasm, tetanic contractions, and shock. Do not use same site for subsequent doses.
- Store drug in refrigerator at 2–4C (36–39F) unless otherwise specified.

C

Assessment & Drug Effects

- Complete medical history and baseline physical examination should be performed before drug is administered. Patient should be completely informed of the potential risks associated with carboprost-induced abortions.
- Patient should not be left unattended during induced labor. Monitor uterine contractions and observe and report excessive vaginal bleeding and cramping pain. Save all clots and tissue for physician inspection and laboratory analysis.
- Check vital signs at regular intervals. Carboprost-induced febrile reaction occurs in more than 10% of patients and must be differentiated from endometritis, which occurs around third day after abortion.

Patient & Family Education

- Report promptly onset of bleeding, foul-smelling lochia, abdominal pain, or fever.
- In some women, ovulation may be reinstated as early as 2 wk postabortion. Patient should be informed so that appropriate contraception may be started if desired.

CARISOPRODOL

(kar-eye-soe-proe′dole)

Trade names: Rela, Soma, Soprodol

Classifications: AUTONOMIC NERVOUS SYSTEM AGENT; CENTRAL-ACTING SKELETAL MUSCLE RELAXANT

Prototype: Cyclobenzaprine

Pregnancy category: C

ACTIONS/PHARMACODYNAMICS Propanediol derivative carbamate with central depressant action pharmacologically related to meprobamate. CNS depressant precise action mechanism is not clear. Skeletal muscle relaxant effect, unlike that of neuromuscular blocking agents, appears to be due to sedative action. Voluntary motor function is not lost, but there may be slight reduction in muscle tone leading to relief of pain and discomfort of muscle spasm.

USES Skeletal muscle spasm, stiffness, and pain in a variety of musculoskeletal disorders and to relieve spasticity and rigidity in cerebral palsy.

ROUTE & DOSAGE

Adult: **PO** 350 mg t.i.d.
Child: **PO** >5 y, 25 mg/kg/d in 4 divided doses.

PHARMACOKINETICS Onset: 30 min. **Duration:** 4–6 h. **Distribution:** crosses placenta. **Metabolism:** metabolized in liver. **Elimination:** half-life: 8 h; excreted by kidneys; excreted in breast milk (2–4 times the plasma concentrations).

CONTRAINDICATIONS & PRECAUTIONS Contraindicated in: hypersensitivity to carisoprodol and related compounds (e.g., meprobamate, tybamate); acute intermittent porphyria; children <12 y. Safe use during pregnancy (category C) and in nursing women not established. **Cautious use in:** impaired liver or kidney function, addiction-prone individuals.

ADVERSE/SIDE EFFECTS Low incidence of toxicity. **CNS:** *drowsiness, dizziness,* vertigo, ataxia, tremor, headache, irritability, depressive reactions, syncope, insomnia. **CV:** tachycardia, postural hypotension, facial flushing. **GI:** nausea, vomiting, hiccups. **Hypersensitivity:** skin rash, erythema multiforme, pruritus, eosinophilia, asthma, fever, anaphylactic shock.

DRUG INTERACTIONS **Alcohol,** CNS DEPRESSANTS potentiate CNS effects.

NURSING IMPLICATIONS

Administration

- Carisoprodol may be taken with food to reduce GI symptoms. Last dose should be taken at bedtime.
- Store in tightly closed container at 15–30C (59–86F) unless otherwise directed.

Assessment & Drug Effects

- Allergic or idiosyncratic reactions generally occur within the period from the first to the fourth dose in patients taking the drug for the first time. Symptoms usually subside after several hours; they are treated by supportive and symptomatic measures.
- There are some indications that psychologic dependence may occur with long-term use.

Patient & Family Education

- Drowsiness is a common side effect and may require reduction in dosage. Driving and other potentially hazardous activities should be avoided until response to the drug has been evaluated.
- Carisoprodol may cause dizziness and faintness. Symptoms may be controlled by making position changes slowly and in stages. Patient should report to physician if symptoms persist.
- Caution patient not to take alcohol or other CNS depressants (effects may be additive) unless otherwise directed by physician.
- Advise patient to discontinue drug and notify physician if skin rash, diplopia, dizziness, or other unusual signs or symptoms appear.

CARMUSTINE

(kar-mus′teen)

Trade names: BCNU, BiCNU, Gliadel

Classifications: ANTINEOPLASTIC; ALKYLATING AGENT

Prototype: Cyclophosphamide

Pregnancy category: D

ACTIONS/PHARMACODYNAMICS

Highly lipid-soluble nitrosourea derivative with cell-cycle-nonspecific activity against rapidly proliferating cell populations. Produces cross-linkage of DNA strands, thereby blocking DNA, RNA, and protein synthesis. Drug metabolites thought to be responsible for antineoplastic and toxic activities. Major toxic effect is bone marrow suppression.

USES As single agent or in combination with other antineoplastics in treatment of Hodgkin's disease and other lymphomas, melanoma, primary and metastatic tumors of brain, and GI tract malignancies. **Unlabeled uses:** treatment of carcinomas of breast and lungs, Ewing's sarcoma, Burkitt's tumor, malignant melanoma, and topically for mycosis fungoides.

ROUTE & DOSAGE

Previously Untreated Patients—Carcinoma

Adult: **IV** 150–200 mg/m^2 q6wk in one dose *or* given over 2 d.
Child: **IV** 200–250 mg/m^2 q4–6wk as single dose.
Doses adjusted based on hematologic parameters.

Mycosis Fungoides

Adult: **Topical** 0.05–0.4% solution or ointment 1–2 times/ d for 6–8 wk (10 mg/d).

PHARMACOKINETICS **Distribution:** readily crosses blood–brain barrier; CSF concentrations 15–70% of plasma concentrations. **Metabolism:** rapidly metabolized; metabolic fate not completely known. **Elimination:** 60–70% excreted in urine in 96 h; 6% excreted through lungs, 1% in feces; excreted in breast milk.

CONTRAINDICATIONS & PRECAUTIONS **Contraindicated in:** history of pulmonary function impairment; recent illness with or exposure to chickenpox or herpes zoster; infection, decreased circulating platelets, leukocytes, or erythrocytes. Safe use during pregnancy (category D) and in nursing women not established. **Cautious use in:** hepatic and renal insufficiency; patient with previous cytotoxic medication, or radiation therapy.

ADVERSE/SIDE EFFECTS **CNS:** dizziness, ataxia. **Eye (with high doses):** infarctions, retinal hemorrhage, suffusion of conjunctiva. **GI:** stomatitis, *nausea, vomiting*. **Hematologic:** delayed myelosuppression (dose-related); thrombocytopenia. **Respiratory:** pulmonary infiltration or fibrosis. **Other:** skin flushing and burning pain at injection site, hyperpigmentation of skin (from contact).

DRUG INTERACTIONS **Cimetidine** may potentiate neutropenia and thrombocytopenia.

NURSING IMPLICATIONS

Administration

- Use only when a physician experienced in cancer chemotherapy can provide constant supervision.
- Wear disposable gloves when preparing carmustine. Contact of drug with skin can cause burning, dermatitis, and hyperpigmentation.
- To prepare for IV administration, add supplied diluent to the 100 mg vial. Further dilute with 27 ml of sterile water for injection to yield a concentration of 3.3 mg/ml. Each dose is then added to 100–500 ml of D5W or NS and infused over at least 1 h.
- If possible avoid starting infusion into dorsum of hand, wrist, or the antecubital veins; extravasation in these areas can damage underlying tendons and nerves leading to loss of mobility of entire limb.
- Slow infusion over 1–2 h (by IV drip) and adequate dilution will reduce pain of administration. Frequently check rate of flow and blood return; palpate injection site for extravasation. If there is any question about patency, line should be restarted.
- IV administration to infants and children: Verify correct IV concentration and rate of infusion with physician.
- Reconstituted solutions of carmustine are clear and colorless and may be stored at 2–8C (36–46F) for 24 h protected from light.
- Store unopened vials at 2–8C (36–46F), protected from light, unless otherwise directed by manufacturer.
- Signs of decomposition of carmustine in unopened vial: liquefaction and appearance of oil film at bottom of vial. Discard drug in this condition.

Assessment & Drug Effects

- Nausea and vomiting (dose related) may occur within 2 h after drug administration and persist for up to 6 h. Prior administration of an antiemetic may help to decrease or prevent these side effects.
- Platelet nadir usually occurs within 4–5 wk, and leukocyte nadir within 5–6 wk after therapy is terminated. Thrombocytopenia may

be more severe than leukopenia; anemia is less severe. Blood studies are continued following infusion, at weekly intervals, for at least 6 wk.

- Check temperature daily. Avoid use of rectal thermometer to prevent injury to mucosa. An elevation of 0.6F or more above usual temperature warrants reporting.
- Baseline and periodic tests of hepatic, pulmonary, and renal function are recommended throughout therapy. Most patients receiving carmustine inevitably show some signs of toxicity.
- Symptoms of lung toxicity (cough, shortness of breath, fever) should be reported to the physician immediately.
- Be alert to signs of hepatic toxicity (jaundice, dark urine, pruritus, light-colored stools) and renal insufficiency (dysuria, oliguria, hematuria, swelling of lower legs and feet).

Patient & Family Education

- Carmustine can cause burning discomfort even in the absence of extravasation. Report burning sensation immediately. Infusion will be discontinued and restarted in another site. Ice application over the area may decrease the discomfort.
- Intense flushing of skin may occur during IV infusion. This usually disappears in 2–4 h.
- Patient will be highly susceptible to infection and to hemorrhagic disorders. Be alert to hazardous periods that occur 4–6 wk after a dose of carmustine. If possible, invasive procedures (e.g., IM injections, enemas, rectal temperatures) should be avoided during this period.
- Report promptly the onset of sore throat, weakness, fever, chills, infection of any kind, or abnormal bleeding (ecchymosis, petechiae, epistaxis, bleeding gums, hematemesis, melena).

CARTEOLOL HYDROCHLORIDE

(car'tee-oh-lole)

Trade names: Cartrol, Ocupress

Classifications: AUTONOMIC NERVOUS SYSTEM AGENT; BETA-ADRENERGIC ANTAGONIST (BLOCKING AGENT, SYMPATHOLYTIC); ANTIHYPERTENSIVE

Prototype: Propranolol

Pregnancy category: C

ACTIONS/PHARMACODYNAMICS

Carteolol is a beta-adrenergic blocking agent that competes for available beta receptor sites. It inhibits both $beta_1$ receptors (chiefly in cardiac muscle) and $beta_2$ receptors (chiefly in the bronchial and vascular musculature). It decreases standing and supine hypertension.

USES For hypertension, either alone or in combination with other drugs, particularly a thiazide diuretic (not indicated for hypertensive crisis); chronic open-angle glaucoma. **Unlabeled use:** to reduce the frequency of anginal attacks.

ROUTE & DOSAGE

Hypertension

Adult: **PO** 2.5 mg once/d; may increase to 5–10 mg if needed (max 10 mg/d).

Open-angle Glaucoma

Ophthalmic: 1 drop in affected eye b.i.d.

PHARMACOKINETICS **Absorption:** readily absorbed from GI tract; 85% reaches systemic circulation. **Peak:**

1–3 h. **Duration:** 24–48 h. **Distribution:** crosses placenta; distributed into breast milk. **Metabolism:** metabolized in liver to active metabolite. **Elimination:** half-life: 4–6 h; excreted primarily in urine.

CONTRAINDICATIONS & PRECAUTIONS Contraindicated in: sinus bradycardia, greater than first-degree heart block, cardiogenic shock, CHF secondary to tachycardia treatable with beta-blockers, overt cardiac failure, hypersensitivity to beta-blocking agents, persistent severe bradycardia, bronchial asthma or bronchospasm, and severe COPD. **Cautious use in:** CHF patients treated with digitalis and diuretics, peripheral vascular disease; diabetes, hypoglycemia, thyrotoxicosis; pregnancy (category C) and nursing mothers.

ADVERSE/SIDE EFFECTS CV: increased angina, hypotension, CHF, bradycardia. **CNS:** *headache, dizziness,* drowsiness, insomnia, anxiety, tremor, paresthesia, weakness. **Endocrine:** hyperglycemia. **GI:** abdominal pain, diarrhea, nausea. **Other:** rash, muscle cramps, bronchospasm.

DRUG INTERACTIONS DIURETICS and other HYPOTENSIVE AGENTS increase hypotensive effect; carteolol and **albuterol, metoproterenol, terbutaline, pirbuterol** are mutually antagonistic; NSAIDS may blunt hypotensive effect; decreases hypoglycemic effect of **glyburide**; may increase bradycardia and sinus arrest with **amiodarone.**

NURSING IMPLICATIONS

Administration

- For patients with renal impairment, dose is lowered according to creatinine clearance.
- Since rate of absorption is not appreciably slowed by food, it may be given without regard to meals.
- Administer capsule or tablet whole. Do not crush or break and instruct patient not to chew before swallowing.
- Store away from heat, light, or moisture.

Assessment & Drug Effects

- Before administration, assess heart rate. If pulse is less than 50 bpm, withhold drug and notify physician.
- Do not administer to patients with asthma or severe COPD.
- Monitor BP and pulse frequently during period of adjustment and periodically throughout therapy.
- If hypotension (systolic BP ≤ 90 mm Hg) occurs, discontinue the drug and carefully assess the hemodynamic status of the patient.
- Monitor daily weight and assess for evidence of fluid overload since drug may precipitate CHF (see Signs & Symptoms, Appendix G).
- Mental depression may be increased by use of this drug.
- If the patient has history of bronchitis or emphysema, assess for respiratory difficulty.
- Drug may prevent the appearance of early signs and symptoms of acute hypoglycemia (see Appendix G).
- Monitor diabetic for signs and symptoms of loss of diabetic control.
- Drug may reduce tolerance to cold temperatures in elderly patients or in those who have circulatory problems.

Patient & Family Education

- Advise patient to report the first sign or symptom of impending CHF (see Signs & Symptoms, Appendix G) or unexplained respiratory symptoms.
- Advise patient not to discontinue medication abruptly, since sudden withdrawal may precipitate or exacerbate angina.

- Advise patient not to use any OTC products such as nasal decongestants and cold preparations without consultation.
- Instruct patient to report slow pulse rate, confusion or depression, dizziness or light-headedness, skin rash, fever, sore throat, or unusual bleeding or bruising.
- Advise patient to be cautious while driving or performing other hazardous activities until response to drug is known.
- Stress the importance of compliance no matter how well the patient feels.
- Instruct patient to take BP at least twice a week and to report significant changes.
- Instruct patient to take pulse before and after taking the medication. If it is much slower than normal rate (or less than 50 bpm), check with the physician.

CARVEDILOL

(car-ve-di′ lol)

Trade name: Coreg, Kredex♣

Classifications: AUTONOMIC NERVOUS SYSTEM AGENT; ALPHA- AND BETA-ADRENERGIC ANTAGONIST; ANTIHYPERTENSIVE

Prototype: Propanolol HCl

Pregnancy category: C

ACTIONS/PHARMACODYNAMICS Adrenergic receptor blocking agent that combines selective alpha activity and nonselective beta-adrenergic blocking actions. Both activities contribute to blood pressure reduction. Peripheral vasodilatation and, therefore, decreased peripheral resistance results from $alpha_1$-blocking activity of Coreg. It is 3–5 times more potent than labetalol in lowering blood pressure.

USES Management of essential hypertension, mild to moderate CHF, in conjunction with other heart failure medications.

ROUTE & DOSAGE

CHF

Adult: **PO** Start with 3.125 mg b.i.d. × 2 wk; may double dose q2wk as tolerated up to 25 mg b.i.d. if <85 kg *or* 50 mg b.i.d. if >85 kg.

Hypertension

Adult: **PO** Start with 6.25 mg b.i.d.: may increase by 6.25 mg b.i.d. to max of 50 mg/d.

PHARMOCOKINETICS Absorption: rapidly absorbed from GI tract, 25–35% reaches the systemic circulation. **Peak:** antihypertensive effect 7–14 d. **Distribution:** >98% protein bound. **Metabolism:** metabolized in the liver by CYP2D6 and CYP2C9 enzymes. **Elimination:** half-life 7–10 h; primarily eliminated via the bile through the feces.

CONTRAINDICATIONS & PRECAUTIONS Contraindicated in: patients with class IV decompensated cardiac failure, bronchial asthma, or related bronchospastic conditions (e.g., chronic bronchitis and emphysema), second- and third-degree AV block, cardiogenic shock or severe bradycardia, lactation. **Cautious use in:** patients on MAOI agents, diabetes, hypoglycemia; patients at high risk for anaphylactic reaction, peripheral vascular disease, hepatic impairment. Safety and efficacy in patients < 18 y of age have not been established.

ADVERSE/SIDE EFFECTS Body as whole: increased sweating, fatigue, chest pain, pain. **CNS:** *dizziness,*

C

headache, paresthesias. **CV:** bradycardia, hypotension, syncope, hypertension, AV block, angina. **GI:** diarrhea, nausea, abdominal pain, vomiting. **Respiratory:** sinusitis, bronchitis. **Other:** thrombocytopenia, hyperglycemia, weight increase, gout, arthralgia.

DRUG INTERACTIONS Rifampin significantly decreases carvedilol levels; cimetidine may increase carvedilol levels; clonidine, reserpine, MAO inhibitors may cause hypotension or bradycardia; carvedilol may increase digoxin levels and may enhance hypoglycemic effects of insulin and oral hypoglycemic agents.

NURSING IMPLICATIONS

Administration

- Give with food to slow absorption and minimize risk of orthostatic hypotension.
- Dose increments should be made at 7- to 14-day intervals. The maximum total daily dose should not exceed 50 mg.
- Store at 15–30C (59–86F).

Assessment & Drug Effects

- Therapeutic effectiveness is indicated by lessening of S&S of CHF and improved BP control.
- Lab tests: periodically monitor liver function tests; at first sign of hepatic toxicity (see Appendix G) stop drug and notify physician.
- In patients with PVD, monitor for worsening of symptoms.
- Monitor digoxin levels with concurrent use; plasma digoxin concentration may increase.

Patient & Family Education

- This drug should not be abruptly discontinued.
- Patients should be aware of the risk of orthostatic hypotension.
- Do not engage in hazardous activities while experiencing dizziness.
- In diabetics, the drug may increase effects of hypoglycemic drugs and mask S&S of hypoglycemia.

CASCARA SAGRADA

(kas-kar'a)

Trade names: Cascara Sagrada Aromatic Fluid-extract, Cascara Sagrada Fluidextract

Classifications: GI AGENT; STIMULANT LAXATIVE

Prototype: Bisacodyl

Pregnancy category: C

ACTIONS/PHARMACODYNAMICS

Anthraquinone derivative obtained from bark of buckhorn tree (*Rhamnus purshiana*). Acts principally in large intestine by stimulating propulsive movements of colon through direct chemical irritation. Casanthrol, which is present in a variety of OTC mixtures, is a derivative of cascara sagrada.

USES Temporary relief of constipation and to prevent straining at stool in various disease conditions. Sometimes used with milk of magnesia.

ROUTE & DOSAGE

Laxative

Adult: **PO** Tablet: 325–1000 mg/d; fluid extract: 0.5–1.5 ml/d; aromatic fluid extract: 2–6 ml/d.
Child: **PO** *2–12 y:* 1/2 of adult dose; *<2 y:* 1/4 of adult dose.
Infant: **PO** Aromatic fluid extract: 1.25 ml/d as single dose.

PHARMOCOKINETICS **Absorption:** minimal absorption from GI tract. **Onset:** 6–12 h. **Metabolism:** metabolized in liver. **Elimination:** eliminated in feces and urine; excreted in breast milk.

CONTRAINDICATIONS & PRECAUTIONS **Contraindicated in:** abdominal pain, fecal impaction; GI bleeding, ulcerations; appendicitis, gastroenteritis, intestinal obstruction, nursing mothers, CHF.

ADVERSE/SIDE EFFECTS **Large doses:** anorexia, nausea, gripping, abnormally loose stools, hypokalemia, impaired glucose tolerance, calcium deficiency, discoloration of urine. **Chronic use:** constipation rebound, melanosis of colon.

DIAGNOSTIC TEST INTERFERENCE Possibility of interference with ***PSP excretion test*** because of urine discoloration.

NURSING IMPLICATIONS

Administration

- For best results administer with a full glass of water on an empty stomach. Results may be delayed somewhat by food.
- Store preferably between 15 and 30C (59 and 86F), in tightly covered, light-resistant containers, unless otherwise directed by manufacturer.

Patient & Family Education

- A single dose taken before retiring usually results in evacuation of soft stool 6–12 h later.
- Frequent or prolonged use of irritant cathartics disrupts normal reflex activity of colon and rectum and can lead to drug dependence for evacuation.

See bisacodyl for other patient teaching points.

CEFACLOR

(sef′a-klor)

Trade names: Ceclor, Ceclor CD

Classifications: ANTIINFECTIVE; ANTIBIOTIC; SECOND-GENERATION CEPHALOSPORIN

Prototype: Cefonicid

Pregnancy category: B

ACTIONS/PHARMACODYNAMICS
Semisynthetic, second-generation oral cephalosporin antibiotic similar to cefonicid. Possibly more active than other oral cephalosporins against gram-negative bacilli, especially beta-lactamase-producing *Hemophilus influenzae,* including ampicillin-resistant strains. Also active against *Escherichia coli, Proteus mirabilis, Klebsiella* sp and certain gram-positive strains, e.g., *Streptococcus pneumoniae, S. pyogenes,* and *Staphylococcus aureus.* Preferentially binds to one or more of the penicillin-binding proteins (PBPs) located on cell walls of susceptible organisms. This inhibits third and final stage of bacterial cell wall synthesis, thus killing the bacterium. Partial cross-allergenicity between penicillins and cephalosporins has been reported.

USES Treatment of otitis media and infections of upper and lower respiratory tract, urinary tract, and skin and skin structures caused by ampicillin-resistant *H. influenzae;* acute uncomplicated UTI.

ROUTE & DOSAGE

Mild to Moderate Infections

Adult: **PO** 250–500 mg q8h, or Ceclor CD 250–500 mg/q12h.
Child >1 mo: **PO** 20–40 mg/kg/d divided q8h (max 2 g/d).

PHARMACOKINETICS **Absorption:** well absorbed; acid stable. **Peak:** 30–60 min. **Elimination:** half-life 0.5–1 h; 60% of dose eliminated renally in

8 h; crosses placenta; excreted in breast milk.

C

CONTRAINDICATIONS & PRECAUTIONS **Contraindicated in:** hypersensitivity to cephalosporins and related antibiotics. Safe use during pregnancy (category B), in nursing mothers, and infants < 1 mo not established. **Cautious use in:** history of sensitivity to penicillins or other drug allergies; markedly impaired renal function.

ADVERSE/SIDE EFFECTS **GI:** *diarrhea;* nausea, vomiting, anorexia, pseudomembranous colitis (rare). **Hypersensitivity:** serum sickness-like reaction: urticaria, pruritus, morbilliform eruptions, eosinophilia, joint pain or swelling, fever. **Other:** superinfections.

DIAGNOSTIC TEST INTERFERENCE Cefaclor may produce positive direct Coombs' test, which can complicate ***cross-matching procedures*** and ***hematologic studies.*** False-positive ***urine glucose*** determinations may result with use of copper sulfate reduction methods, e.g., Clinitest or Benedict's reagent, but not with glucose oxidase (enzymatic) tests such as Clinistix, Diastix, TesTape.

DRUG INTERACTIONS **Probenecid** decreases renal excretion of cefaclor.

NURSING IMPLICATIONS

Administration

- Administer with food if nausea and vomiting appear to be associated with gastric irritation. Although food in the intestinal tract delays absorption and reduces blood level totals, amount absorbed is unchanged.
- After stock oral suspension is prepared, it should be kept refrigerated. Expiration date should appear on label. Discard unused portion after 14 d. Shake well before pouring.
- Store pulvules at 15–30C (59–86F) in tightly closed container unless otherwise directed.

Assessment & Drug Effects

- Culture and susceptibility tests recommended prior to and periodically during therapy.
- Before therapy is initiated, a careful inquiry should be made concerning previous hypersensitivity to cephalosporins, penicillins, and other drug allergies.
- Diarrhea, the most frequent adverse effect, may be due to a pharmacologic effect or to associated change in intestinal flora. If it persists, interruption of therapy may be necessary.
- Monitor for manifestations of drug hypersensitivity (see Appendix G). Discontinue drug and promptly report them if they appear.
- Monitor for manifestations of superinfection (see Appendix G). Promptly report their appearance.

Patient & Family Education

- Urge patient to report promptly signs and symptoms of superinfection (see Appendix G).
- Yogurt or buttermilk (if allowed) may serve as a prophylactic against intestinal superinfections by helping to maintain normal intestinal flora.
- Instruct patient to take medication for the full course of therapy as directed by physician.

CEFADROXIL

(sef-a-drox′ill)

Trade names: Duricef, Ultracef

Classifications: ANTIINFECTIVE; ANTIBIOTIC; FIRST-GENERATION CEPHALOSPORIN

Prototype: Cephalothin
Pregnancy category: B

ACTIONS/PHARMACODYNAMICS Semisynthetic, first-generation cephalosporin antibiotic with antibacterial spectrum similar to that of cephalothin. Bactericidal action (similar to that of penicillins): drug penetrates bacterial cell wall, resists beta-lactamases and inactivates enzymes essential to cell wall synthesis. At equivalent doses, reportedly attains greater concentrations in serum and urine than other oral cephalosporins. Active against organisms that liberate cephalosporinase and penicillinase (beta-lactamases). According to clinical and laboratory evidence, partial cross-allergenicity exists between penicillins and cephalosporins.

USES Primarily in treatment of urinary tract infections caused by *Escherichia coli, Proteus mirabilis,* and *Klebsiella* sp; infections of skin and skin structures caused by staphylococci and streptococci; and for treatment of group A beta-hemolytic streptococcal pharyngitis and tonsillitis.

ROUTE & DOSAGE

Uncomplicated Urinary Tract Infection
Adult: **PO** 1–2 g/d in 1–2 divided doses.
Child: **PO** 30 mg/kg/d in 2 divided doses.

Skin and Skin Structure Infections, Streptococcal Pharyngitis, or Tonsillitis
Adult: **PO** 1 g/d in 1–2 divided doses.
Child: **PO** 30 mg/kg/d in 2 divided doses.

Adjustment for Renal Impairment (Cl_{cr} <25 ml/min)
Adult: **PO** 1 g q24h.
Child: **PO** 15 mg/kg q24h.

PHARMACOKINETICS Absorption: acid stable; rapidly absorbed from GI tract. **Peak:** 1 h. **Elimination:** half-life: 1–12 h; 90% excreted unchanged in urine within 8 h; bacterial inhibitory levels persist 20–22 h; crosses placenta; excreted in breast milk.

CONTRAINDICATIONS & PRECAUTIONS Contraindicated in: hypersensitivity to cephalosporins and related antibiotics. Safe use during pregnancy (category B), in nursing mothers, and in children not established. **Cautious use in:** sensitivity to penicillins or other drug allergies; impaired renal function, history of colitis.

ADVERSE/SIDE EFFECTS GI: nausea, *diarrhea,* vomiting, heartburn, gastritis, bloating, abdominal cramps. **Hypersensitivity:** rash, swollen eyelids (<u>angioedema</u>), pruritus, chills. **Other:** superinfections.

DIAGNOSTIC TEST INTERFERENCE False-positive ***urine glucose*** determinations using copper sulfate reduction reagents, such as Clinitest or Benedict's reagent, but not with glucose oxidase tests, e.g., Clinistix, Diastix, TesTape. Cefadroxil-induced positive direct Coombs' test may interfere with ***cross-matching procedures*** and ***hematologic studies.***

DRUG INTERACTION Probenecid decreases renal excretion of cefadroxil.

NURSING IMPLICATIONS

Administration

- Nausea may be reduced by administration of drug with food or

C

milk. If nausea persists, termination of therapy may be necessary.

- Directions for mixing the oral suspension are on the label. Reconstituted solution contains 125 mg or 250 mg cefadroxil per 5 ml suspension. Shake well before use; discard after 14 d.
- Store in tight container at 15–30C (59–86F) unless otherwise directed. Oral suspensions are stable for 14 d under refrigeration at 2–8C (36–46F). Avoid freezing. Note expiration date on label.

Assessment & Drug Effects

- Culture and susceptibility testing are recommended prior to and periodically during therapy.
- Before therapy is initiated, a careful inquiry should be made concerning previous hypersensitivity to cephalosporins, penicillins, and other drug allergies.
- Baseline and periodic renal function studies should be performed in patients with renal function impairment, and I&O ratio and pattern should be monitored.
- Monitor for manifestations of drug hypersensitivity (see Signs & Symptoms, Appendix G). Discontinue drug and promptly report them if they appear.
- Monitor for manifestations of superinfection (see Signs & Symptoms, Appendix G). Promptly report their appearance.

Patient & Family Education

- If patient is allergic to penicillin, the possibility of an allergic reaction is high. Report promptly the onset of rash, urticaria, pruritus, fever.
- Instruct patient to take medication for the full course of therapy as directed by the physician.
- Report promptly signs and symptoms of superinfections (see Appendix G).

CEFAMANDOLE NAFATE

(sef-a-man'dole)

Trade name: Mandol

Classifications: ANTIINFECTIVE; ANTIBIOTIC; SECOND-GENERATION CEPHALOSPORIN

Prototype: Cefonicid

Pregnancy category: B

ACTIONS/PHARMACODYNAMICS

Semisynthetic, second-generation cephalosporin antibiotic similar to other drugs of this class. Preferentially binds to one or more of the penicillin-binding proteins (PBP) located on cell walls of susceptible organisms. This inhibits third and final stage of bacterial wall synthesis, thus killing the bacterium. Usually active against organisms susceptible to first generation cephalosporins. In addition, it is active against the anaerobes *Clostridium* sp, *Peptococcus* sp, *Fusobacterium* sp; and against some strains of *Providencia* sp, *Enterobacter, Serratia, Proteus, E. coli,* and *Klebsiella* resistant to first generation cephalosporins. Inactive against enterococci, methicillin-resistant staphylococci, *Listeria monocytogenes* and *Pseudomonas*. Partial cross-allergenicity between penicillins and cephalosporins has been reported.

USES Serious infections of respiratory, genitourinary, and biliary tracts, skin and soft tissue, bones and joints, and in septicemia and peritonitis (caused by *E. coli* and other coliform microbes); also perioperative prophylaxis to reduce infections in patient undergoing potentially contaminated procedure.

ROUTE & DOSAGE

Moderate to Severe Infections

Adult: **IV/IM** 500 mg–1 g q4–8h, up to 2 g q4h.

Child: **IV/IM** 50–100 mg/kg/d in 3–6 divided doses, up to 150 mg/kg/d (not to exceed adult doses).

Surgical Prophylaxis

Adult: **IV/IM** 1–2 g 30–60 min before surgery, then q6h for 24 h. *Child:* **IV/IM** 50–100 mg/kg 30–60 min before surgery, then q6h for 24 h.

PHARMACOKINETICS Peak levels: 0.5–2 h after IM; 10 min after IV. **Distribution:** poor CNS penetration even with inflamed meninges; extensive enterohepatic circulation; high concentrations in bile. **Metabolism:** rapidly hydrolyzed in plasma to active metabolite. **Elimination:** half-life: 30–120 min; 68–85% excreted unchanged in urine in 6–8 h.

CONTRAINDICATIONS & PRECAUTIONS Contraindicated in: hypersensitivity to cephalosporins and related antibiotics. Safe use during pregnancy (category B), in nursing mothers, and in children between 1 and 6 mo not established. **Cautious use in:** history of sensitivity to penicillins or other drug allergies; renal function impairment; history of GI disease, particularly colitis.

ADVERSE/SIDE EFFECTS GI: abdominal cramps, *diarrhea,* pseudomembranous colitis. **Hematologic:** hypoprothrombinemia (vitamin K deficiency). **Hypersensitivity:** rash, urticaria, drug fever, eosinophilia. **Other:** pain, redness and induration, sterile abscess at injection site, superinfections.

DIAGNOSTIC TEST INTERFERENCE False-positive ***urine glucose*** determinations using copper sulfate reduction methods, e.g., Clinitest or Benedict's reagent, but not with glucose oxidase (enzymatic) tests such as Clinistix, Diastix, TesTape. Cefamandole-induced positive direct Coombs' test may interfere with ***cross-matching procedures*** and ***hematologic studies.***

DRUG INTERACTIONS Probenecid decreases renal elimination of cefamandole; **alcohol** causes disulfiram reaction.

INCOMPATIBILITIES Solution/additive: Ringer's lactate, calcium gluconate, calcium gluceptate, cimetidine, AMINOGLYCOSIDES, **metronidazole, magnesium. Y-site:** AMINOGLYCOSIDES.

NURSING IMPLICATIONS

Administration

- For IM administration: to each gram of cefamandole add 3 ml of sterile water for injection or bacteriostatic water for injection, 0.9% NaCl injection or 0.9% bacteriostatic NaCl injection. Resulting solution will contain 285 mg cefamandole per milliliter.
- Administer IM deep into a large muscle mass such as gluteus maximus or lateral thigh.
- For direct IV administration: each gram of cefamandole should be reconstituted with 10 ml sterile water for injection, 5% dextrose injection, or 0.9% NaCl injection. Appropriate dose is administered slowly over 3–5 min.
- Cefamandole may be further diluted in 100–1000 ml of D5W or NS and given by IV intermittent or continuous infusion. The rate of infusion is determined by the amount of solution.
- Prolonged exposure to light causes cefamandole powder to discolor. Once reconstituted, cefamandole is no longer light sensitive. Solutions appear light yellow to amber. Do not use if otherwise

C

colored or if a precipitate is present.

- Because cefamandole is formulated with sodium carbonate, it is incompatible with fluids containing magnesium or calcium ions. Consult package insert for compatible IV infusion fluids and stability and storage times.
- After reconstitution, cefamandole may liberate CO_2. Do not store medication in syringes, as pressure build-up from CO_2 may force plunger out of barrel.
- Store cefamandole powder at 15–30C (59–86F). Protect from light. Reconstituted drug remains stable at 15–30C (59–86F) for 24 h and when refrigerated at 5C (41F), for 96 h.

Assessment & Drug Effects

- Culture and susceptibility testing recommended prior to and periodically during therapy. Cefamandole therapy may be instituted pending test results.
- Before therapy is initiated, determine previous hypersensitivity to cephalosporins, penicillins, and other drugs.
- Baseline and periodic studies of renal function and PT determinations should be performed.
- Monitor I&O ratio and pattern, particularly in patients with impaired renal function, patients > 50 y, or patients who are receiving high doses.
- Antibiotic-associated pseudomembranous enterocolitis (life-threatening) is a superinfection caused by *Clostridia difficile* (spore- and toxin-forming bacteria) and may occur in 4–9 d or as long as 6 wk after cefamandole is discontinued (see Signs & Symptoms, Appendix G). Most likely to occur in the chronically ill or debilitated elderly patient especially if undergoing abdominal surgery or if in an ICU.
- At onset of diarrhea, patient should check for fever and report fever and diarrhea to physician.
- Monitor for manifestations of hypersensitivity (see Appendix G). If they appear, discontinue drug and report them promptly.

Patient & Family Education

- Advise patient to avoid use of alcohol during and for 48–72 h after taking cefamandole. A drug-induced disulfiram-like reaction (see Appendix G) may follow alcohol intake.
- Drug therapy for beta-hemolytic streptococcal infections should continue for at least 10 d to guard against risk of rheumatic fever and glomerulonephritis.
- Superinfections may occur, particularly during prolonged use of cephalosporins. Report promptly signs and symptoms of superinfection (see Appendix G).
- Patient should report loose stools or diarrhea.
- Yogurt or buttermilk, 120 ml (4 oz) of either (if allowed), may serve as a prophylactic against intestinal superinfection by helping to maintain normal intestinal flora.

CEFAZOLIN SODIUM

(sef-a'zoe-lin)

Trade names: Ancef, Kefzol, Zolicef

Classifications: ANTIINFECTIVE; ANTIBIOTIC; FIRST-GENERATION CEPHALOSPORIN

Prototype: Cephalothin

Pregnancy category: B

ACTIONS/PHARMACODYNAMICS

Semisynthetic, first-generation derivative of cephalosporin C; antibiotic activity similar to that of cephalothin. Activity against gram-negative organisms is limited. Bactericidal action: preferentially binds to one or more of the penicillin-binding proteins (PBP) located on cell walls of susceptible organisms. This inhibits third and final stage of bacterial cell wall synthesis, thus killing the bacterium.

USES Severe infections of urinary and biliary tracts, skin, soft tissue, and bone, and for bacteremia and endocarditis caused by susceptible organisms; also perioperative prophylaxis in patients undergoing procedures associated with high risk of infection, e.g., open heart surgery.

ROUTE & DOSAGE

Moderate to Severe Infections

Adult: **IV/IM** 250 mg–2 g q8h, up to 2 g q4h (max 12 g/d).
Child: **IV/IM** 25–100 mg/kg/d in 3–4 divided doses, up to 100 mg/kg/d (not to exceed adult doses).
Neonate: **IV** ≤7 d: 40 mg/kg/d divided q12h; >7 d: 40–60 mg/kg/d divided q8–12h.

Adjustment for Renal Impairment

Cl_{cr} <35 ml/min: dose q12h.

Surgical Prophylaxis

Adult: **IV/IM** 1–2 g 30–60 min before surgery, then q8h for 24 h.
Child: **IV/IM** 25–50 mg/kg 30–60 min before surgery, then q8h for 24 h.

PHARMACOKINETICS **Peak:** 1–2 h after IM; 5 min after IV. **Distribution:** poor CNS penetration even with inflamed meninges; high concentrations in bile and in diseased bone; crosses placenta. **Elimination:** half-life: 90–130 min; 70% excreted unchanged in urine in 6 h; small amount excreted in breast milk.

CONTRAINDICATIONS & PRECAUTIONS **Contraindicated in:** hypersensitivity to any cephalosporin and related antibiotics. Safe use during pregnancy (category B), in nursing mothers, and in infants < 1 mo not established. **Cautious use in:** history of penicillin sensitivity, impaired renal function, patients on sodium restriction.

ADVERSE/SIDE EFFECTS **GI:** *diarrhea,* anorexia, abdominal cramps. **Hypersensitivity:** anaphylaxis, maculopapular rash, urticaria, fever, eosinophilia. **Other:** superinfections, seizure (high doses in patients with renal insufficiency).

DIAGNOSTIC TEST INTERFERENCE Because of cefazolin effect on the direct Coombs' test, transfusion ***cross-matching procedures*** and ***hematologic studies*** may be complicated. False-positive ***urine glucose*** determinations are possible with use of copper sulfate tests (e.g., Clinitest or Benedict's reagent) but not with glucose oxidase tests such as TesTape, Diastix, or Clinistix.

DRUG INTERACTION **Probenecid** decreases renal elimination of cefazolin.

INCOMPATIBILITIES **Solution/additive:** AMINOGLYCOSIDES, **bleomycin, ascorbic acid, cimetidine, lidocaine, vitamin B complex with C, amobarbital, calcium chloride, calcium gluceptate, calcium gluconate, colistin, erythromycin,** TETRACYCLINES, **pentobarbital, polymyxin B.** **Y-site:** AMINOGLYCOSIDES, **pentamidine.**

C

NURSING IMPLICATIONS

Administration

- Preparation of IM solution: Reconstitute with sterile water for injection, bacteriostatic water for injection, or 0.9% sodium chloride injection. Reconstituted solutions are stable for 24 hr at room temperature and for 96 hr refrigerated.
- IM injections should be made deep into large muscle mass. Pain on injection is usually minimal. Rotate injection sites.
- IV administration: Dilute each 1 g with 10 ml of sterile water for injection. May be further diluted with 50–100 ml of NS or D5W. Infuse 1 g over 5 min or longer as determined by the amount of solution.
- IV administration to neonates, infants, and children: Verify correct IV concentration and rate of infusion with physician.
- The risk of IV site reactions may be reduced by proper dilution of IV solution, use of small bore IV needle in a large vein, and by rotating injection sites.
- Store vials preferably between 15 and 30C (59 and 86F), unless otherwise directed by manufacturer.

Assessment & Drug Effects

- Before therapy is initiated, determine history of hypersensitivity to cephalosporins, penicillins, and other drugs.
- Culture and susceptibility testing is recommended prior to and during therapy. Therapy may be initiated pending results.
- Monitor intake and output ratio and pattern. Be alert to changes in BUN, serum creatinine.
- If patient has had a reaction to penicillin, be alert to signs of hypersensitivity with use of cefazolin. Cross-allergenicity between cephalosporins and penicillin has been reported. Prompt attention should be given to onset of signs of hypersensitivity (see Appendix G).
- Promptly report the onset of diarrhea, which may or may not be dose related. It is seen especially in patients with history of drug-related GI disturbances. Pseudomembranous colitis, a potentially life-threatening condition, starts with diarrhea.

Patient & Family Education

- Report promptly signs and symptoms of superinfection (see Appendix G).
- Report signs of hemostatic defects: ecchymoses, petechiae, nosebleed.

CEFDINIR

(cef′di-nir)

Trade name: Omnicef

Classifications: ANTIINFECTIVE; THIRD-GENERATION CEPHALOSPORIN

Prototype: Cefonicid sodium

Pregnancy category: B

ACTIONS/PHARMACODYNAMICS

Broad-spectrum semisynthetic third-generation cephalosporin antibiotic. Generally active against a wide variety of gram-positive and gram-negative bacteria, including most *Enterobacteriaceae* and *Pseudomonas.* Effective against most strains of staphylococci and streptococci including methicillin-resistant strains (MRSA).

USES Community-acquired pneumonia, acute exacerbations of chronic bronchitis, acute maxillary sinusitis, pharyngitis, tonsillitis, uncomplicated skin infections, bacterial otitis media.

C

ROUTE & DOSAGE

Community-Acquired Pneumonia, Skin Infections

Adult: **PO** 300 mg q12h × 10 d.
Child 6 mo–12 y: **PO** 7 mg/kg q12h × 10 d.

Chronic Bronchitis, Maxillary Sinusitis, Pharyngitis, Tonsillitis

Adult: **PO** 600 mg q24h or 300 mg q12h × 10 d.
Child 6 mo–12 y: **PO** 14 mg/kg q24h or 7 mg/kg q12h × 10 d.

PHARMACOKINETICS **Absorption:** 16–25% bioavailability. **Peak:** 2–4 h. **Distribution:** 60–70% protein bound; penetrates sinus tissue, blister fluid, lung tissue, middle ear fluid. **Metabolism:** not metabolized. **Elimination:** half-life: 1.6 h; excreted in urine.

CONTRAINDICATIONS & PRECAUTIONS **Contraindicated in:** hypersensitivity to cefdinir and other cephalosporins. Safe use in pregnancy (category B) and nursing mothers not established. **Cautious use in:** hypersensitivity to penicillins, penicillin derivatives; renal impairment; ulcerative colitis or antibiotic-induced colitis; bleeding disorders; GI disorders; liver or kidney disease. Safety and efficacy in neonates and infants <6 mo old not established.

ADVERSE/SIDE EFFECTS **CNS:** headache. **GI:** *diarrhea,* nausea, abdominal pain. **Metabolic:** increased GGT, increased urine protein, hematuria. **Skin:** rash, cutaneous moniliasis. **Other:** vaginal moniliasis, vaginitis.

DIAGNOSTIC TEST INTERFERENCE false positive for ketones or glucose in urine using nitroprusside or Clinitest.

DRUG INTERACTIONS Antacids should be taken at least 2 h before or after cefdinir; probenecid prolongs cefdinir elimination; iron decreases absorption.

NURSING IMPLICATIONS

Administration

- Do not give within 2 h of aluminum- or magnesium-containing antacids or iron supplements.
- Reconstitute oral suspension to 125 mg/ml by adding water (38-ml to 60-ml bottle and 63-ml to 100-ml bottle). Shake well before each use.
- Dosage adjustment is recommended if creatinine clearance <30 ml/min and for patients on hemodialysis.
- Store at 15–30C (59–86F) in tightly closed container. Discard after 10 days.

Assessment & Drug Effects

- Before therapy is initiated, determine previous hypersensitivity to cephalosporins, penicillins, and other drug allergies.
- Carefully monitor for and immediately report S&S of: hypersensitivity, superinfection, or pseudomembranous colitis (see Appendix G).
- Discontinue drug and notify physician if seizures associated with drug therapy occur.

Patient & Family Education

- Allow a minimum of 2 h between cefdinir and antacids containing aluminum or magnesium, or drugs containing iron.
- Immediately contact physician if a rash, diarrhea, or new infection (e.g., yeast infection) develops.
- Drug may cause false positive for urine ketones or glucose. Consult package insert.

C

CEFEPIME HYDROCHLORIDE

(cef′e-peem)

Trade name: Maxipime

Classifications: ANTIINFECTIVE; ANTIBIOTIC; FOURTH-GENERATION CEPHALOSPORIN

Prototype: Cefotaxime

Pregnancy category: B

ACTIONS/PHARMACODYNAMICS Cefepime, considered to be a fourth-generation cephalosporin antibiotic, is similar to third-generation cephalosporins with respect to broad gram-negative coverage; however, cefepime has broader gram-positive coverage than third-generation cephalosporins. It is highly resistant to hydrolysis by most β-lactamase bacteria. Cefepime preferentially binds to one or more of the penicillin-binding proteins located on cell walls of susceptible organisms. This inhibits the third and final stage of bacterial cell wall synthesis, thus killing the bacteria (bactericidal).

USES Uncomplicated and complicated UTI, skin and skin structure infections, pneumonia caused by susceptible organisms (*Escherichia coli, Klebsiella pneumoniae, Proteus mirabilis, Staphylococcus aureus* [methicillin-sensitive], *Streptococcus pyogenes, Streptococcus pneumoniae, Pseudomonas aeruginosa, Enterobacter* sp). Empiric monotherapy for febrile neutropenic patients.

ROUTE & DOSAGE

Mild to Moderate Infections

Adult: **IV/IM** 0.5–1g q12h × 7–10 d.

Moderate to Severe Infections

Adult: **IV** 1–2g q12h × 10 d.

Febrile Neutropenia

Adult: **IV** 2 g q8h for 7 d or until resolution of neutropenia.

Adjustment for Renal Impairment

Cl_{cr} 30–60 ml/min: dose q24h; 11–29 ml/min: give 50% of normal dose q24h; <10 ml/min: 250–500 mg q24h.

PHARMACOKINETICS Absorption: well absorbed after IM administration; serum levels significantly lower than after equivalent IV dose. **Distribution:** 20% protein bound, widely distributed, may cross inflamed meninges; crosses placenta, secreted into breast milk. **Metabolism:** metabolized in liver. **Elimination:** half-life: 2 h; excreted in urine.

CONTRAINDICATIONS & PRECAUTIONS Contraindicated in: hypersensitivity to cefepime, other cephalosporins, penicillins, or other β-lactam antibiotics. **Cautious use in:** patients with history of GI disease, particularly colitis, renal insufficiency, pregnancy (category B), nursing mothers. Safety and efficacy of cefepime in children <12 y not known.

ADVERSE/SIDE EFFECTS CNS: headache, fever. **GI:** antibiotic-associated colitis, diarrhea, nausea, oral moniliasis, vomiting, elevated liver function tests (ALT, AST). **Local injection reactions:** phlebitis, pain, inflammation, rash. **Other:** pruritus, urticaria, vaginitis, eosinophilia.

DIAGNOSTIC TEST INTERFERENCE Positive Coombs' test without hemolysis. May cause false-positive urine glucose test with Clinitest.

INCOMPATIBILITIES Solution/additive: AMINOGLYCOSIDES, **ampicillin,**

aminophylline, metronidazole, vancomycin.

NURSING IMPLICATIONS

Administration

- IM reconstitution: Reconstitute 500-mg vial and 1-g vial, respectively, with 1.3 or 2.4 ml of one of the following: Sterile Water for Injection, 0.9% NaCl Injection, Bacteriostatic Water for Injection with Parabens or benzyl alcohol, or other compatible solution.
- IV reconstitution: Dilute with 50–100 ml of one of the following: 0.9% NaCl Injection, 5% Dextrose Injection, or other compatible solution.
- IV administration: Infuse over 30 min; with Y-type administration set, discontinue other compatible solutions while infusing cefepime.
- Store reconstituted solution at 20–25C (68–77F) for 24 h or in refrigerator at 2–8C (36–46F) for 7 days. Protect from light.

Assessment & Drug Effects

- Culture and sensitivity tests should be performed before initiation of therapy. Dosage may be started pending test results.
- Before therapy is initiated, determine history of hypersensitivity reactions to cephalosporins, penicillins, or other drugs.
- Monitor for S&S of hypersensitivity (see Appendix G). Report their appearance promptly and discontinue drug.
- Monitor for S&S of superinfection or pseudomembranous colitis (see Appendix G); immediately report either to physician.
- With concurrent high-dose aminoglycoside therapy, closely monitor for nephrotoxicity and ototoxicity.

Patient & Family Education

- Teach S&S of hypersensitivity, superinfection, and pseudomembranous colitis; instruct to promptly report any of these.

CEFIXIME

(ce-fix′ime)

Trade name: Suprax

Classifications: ANTIINFECTIVE; ANTIBIOTIC; THIRD-GENERATION CEPHALOSPORIN

Prototype: Cefotaxime

Pregnancy category: B

ACTIONS/PHARMACODYNAMICS

A third-generation cephalosporin that is highly stable in the presence of beta-lactamases (penicillinases and cephalosporinases) and therefore has excellent activity against a wide range of gram-negative bacteria. It is bactericidal against susceptible bacteria. Cephalosporins inhibit mucopeptide synthesis in the bacterial cell wall.

USES Effective against *Streptococcus pyogenes, Streptococcus pneumoniae,* and gram-negative bacilli, including *Hemophilus influenzae, Branhamella catarrhalis,* and *Neisseria gonorrhoeae.* Little activity against staphylococci, and no activity against *Pseudomonas aeruginosa;* also uncomplicated UTI, otitis media, pharyngitis, tonsillitis, and bronchitis.

ROUTE & DOSAGE

Infection

Adult: **PO** 400 mg/d in 1–2 divided doses.
Child: **PO** 8 mg/kg/d in 1–2 divided doses.

C

PHARMACOKINETICS **Absorption:** 40–50% absorbed from GI tract. **Peak:** 2–6 h. **Distribution:** distributed into breast milk. **Elimination:** half-life: 3–4 h; 50% excreted in urine, 50% in bile.

CONTRAINDICATIONS & PRECAUTIONS **Contraindicated in:** patients with known allergy to the cephalosporin group of antibiotics. **Cautious use in:** allergy to penicillin, history of colitis, renal insufficiency, pregnancy (category B), lactation. Safety and effectiveness in infants < 6 mo have not been established.

ADVERSE/SIDE EFFECTS **GI:** *diarrhea,* loose stools, nausea, vomiting, dyspepsia, flatulence. **CNS:** drug fever, headache, dizziness. **Other:** rash, pruritus, vaginitis, genital pruritus.

NURSING IMPLICATIONS

Administration

- Oral drug may be administered without regard to meals.
- Because of lack of bioequivalence, tablets should not be substituted for liquid in treatment of otitis media.
- After reconstitution, suspension may be kept for 14 d at room temperature or refrigerated. Store away from heat and light. Keep tightly closed and shake well before using.

Assessment & Drug Effects

- Culture and susceptibility tests should be performed prior to initiation of therapy and periodically during therapy. Therapy may be implemented pending test results.
- Before therapy is initiated, a careful inquiry should be made to determine previous hypersensitivity reactions to cephalosporins, penicillins, and history of other allergies, particularly to drugs.
- If seizures associated with the drug therapy occur, the drug should be discontinued.
- Superinfections (see Appendix G) caused by overgrowth of nonsusceptible organisms may occur, particularly during prolonged use.
- Monitor I&O ratio and pattern. Nephrotoxicity occurs more frequently in patients > 50 y, with impaired renal function, in the debilitated, and in patients receiving high doses or other nephrotoxic drugs.
- Carefully monitor anyone with a history of allergies, especially to drugs. Report manifestations of hypersensitivity (see Appendix G).
- Promptly report loose stools or diarrhea, which may indicate pseudomembranous colitis (see Appendix G). Discontinuation of drug may be necessary.

Patient & Family Education

- Instruct patient to report loose stools or diarrhea during drug therapy and for several weeks after. Elderly patients are especially susceptible to pseudomembranous colitis.
- Instruct patient to take antibiotic for the full course of treatment.
- Instruct patient not to miss any doses and to take the doses at evenly spaced times, day and night.

CEFMETAZOLE

(sef-met′a-zol)

Trade name: Zefazone

Classifications: ANTIINFECTIVE; ANTIBIOTIC; THIRD-GENERATION CEPHALOSPORIN

Prototype: Cefotaxime

Pregnancy category: B

ACTIONS/PHARMACODYNAMICS Cefmetazole is a synthetic cephalosporin antibiotic. Its bactericidal action results from inhibition of cell wall synthesis. It is active against a wide range of aerobic and anaerobic gram-positive and gram-negative bacteria.

USES UTI infections caused by *Escherichia coli,* lower respiratory tract infections, namely pneumonia and bronchitis caused by *Streptococcus pneumoniae, Staphylococcus aureus, E. coli, Hemophilus influenzae.* In addition, it is effective against *Staphylococcus epidermidis, Streptococcus pyogenes, Streptococcus agalactiae, Proteus vulgaris,* and *Bacteroides fragilis;* preoperative prophylaxis of cesarean section, hysterectomy, cholecystectomy, and colorectal surgery.

ROUTE & DOSAGE

Systemic Infections
Adult: **IV** 1–2 g q6–12h.

Adjustment for Renal Impairment
Cl_{cr} <30 ml/min: 1–2 g q24h.

Surgical Prophylaxis
Adult: **IV** 1–2 g 30–90 min before surgery; then q8h for 2 more doses.

PHARMACOKINETICS Elimination: half-life: 1.2 h; excreted unchanged in urine.

CONTRAINDICATIONS & PRECAUTIONS Contraindicated in: patients with known allergy to cefmetazole or to any other cephalosporin antibiotic. **Cautious use in:** allergy to penicillin, history of colitis, renal insufficiency, pregnancy (category B), lactation.

ADVERSE/SIDE EFFECTS GI: *diarrhea,* loose stools, nausea, vomiting, dyspepsia, flatulence. **CNS:** drug fever, headache, dizziness. **Other:** rash, pruritus, vaginitis, genital pruritus, hypersensitivity reactions.

DRUG INTERACTION Probenecid decreases renal elimination of cefmetazole.

INCOMPATIBILITIES Solution/additive: AMINOGLYCOSIDES. **Y-site:** AMINOGLYCOSIDES.

NURSING IMPLICATIONS

Administration

- Reconstitute with sterile water for injection, bacteriostatic water for injection, or 0.9% NaCl injection. Dilute 1 g with 3.7 ml to yield 250 mg/ml or with 10 ml to yield 100 mg/ml. Dilute 2 g with 7 ml to yield 250 mg/ml or with 15 ml to yield 125 mg/ml.
- Solution may be further diluted to concentrations ranging from 1–20 mg/ml by adding it to 0.9% NaCl, 5% dextrose, or lactate Ringer's injection.
- Drug can be given direct IV over 3–5 min or infused over 10–60 min.
- Observe IV sites for evidence of inflammatory reaction. Risk of phlebitis may be reduced by use of a small needle in a large vein.
- Potency is retained for 24 h after reconstitution at room temperature, 7 d under refrigeration, and for 6 wk if frozen. Store away from heat, light, and moisture; do not refreeze.

Assessment & Drug Effects

- Culture and susceptibility tests should be performed before initiation of therapy and periodically during therapy. Therapy may be implemented pending test results.
- Before therapy is initiated, a careful inquiry should be made to determine previous hypersensitivity

C

to cephalosporins, penicillins, and history of other allergies, particularly to drugs.

- Assess for signs and symptoms of superinfections (see Appendix G) caused by overgrowth of nonsusceptible organisms, particularly with prolonged use.
- Monitor PT in patients with renal or hepatic disease or those receiving a long course of antibiotic therapy.
- Promptly report loose stools or diarrhea because of risk of pseudomembranous colitis (see Appendix G). Elderly are especially susceptible. Drug may be discontinued.

Patient & Family Education

- Patient should report onset of loose stools or diarrhea even for several weeks after drug is discontinued.
- Advise patient that ingestion of alcohol within 24 h of drug may cause a disulfiram-like reaction (see Appendix G).

CEFONICID SODIUM

(se-fon'i-sid)

Trade name: Monocid

Prototype for classifications: ANTIINFECTIVE; BETA-LACTAM ANTIBIOTIC; SECOND-GENERATION CEPHALOSPORIN

Pregnancy category: B

ACTIONS/PHARMACODYNAMICS Semisynthetic, second-generation cephalosporin antibiotic with drug structure characterized by a β-lactam ring (like the penicillin structure); generally resistant to hydrolysis by β-lactamases. Preferentially binds to one or more of the penicillin-binding proteins (PBP) located on cell walls of susceptible organisms. This inhibits third and final stage of bacterial wall synthesis, thus killing the bacterium. Second generation cephalosporins are usually active against the organisms susceptible to first generation cephalosporins. In addition they are active against *Hemophilus influenzae, Providencia* sp, *Clostridium* sp, *Peptococcus* sp, and against some strains of *Citrobacter, Enterobacter, Serratia, Neisseria, Proteus, Escherichia coli,* and *Klebsiella* that are resistant to first generation cephalosporins. Second generation agents are generally inactive against enterococci, methicillin-resistant staphylococci, *Acinetobacter, Listeria monocytogenes,* and *Pseudomonas.*

USES Moderate to severe infections such as septicemia, infections of lower respiratory tract, bones and joints, skin and skin structures, and urinary tract (UTI). Also used for perioperative prophylaxis. **Unlabeled use:** uncomplicated gonorrhea.

ROUTE & DOSAGE

Moderate to Severe Infections

Adult: **IV/IM** 1 g q24h, up to 2 g/24 h.

Surgical Prophylaxis

Adult: **IV/IM** 1 g 60 min before surgery.

PHARMACOKINETICS **Peak levels:** 1 h after IM; 5 min after IV. **Distribution:** poor CNS penetration even with inflamed meninges; crosses placenta. **Metabolism:** not metabolized. **Elimination:** half-life: 3.5– 5.8 h; 90–99% excreted unchanged in urine within 24 h; small amount excreted in breast milk.

CONTRAINDICATIONS & PRECAUTIONS **Contraindicated in:** hypersensitivity to cephalosporins and related antibiotics; severely impaired renal or hepatic function. Safe use during pregnancy (category B) and in children not established. **Cautious use in:** nursing mothers, patient with history of delayed-type reaction to penicillins or other drugs; GI disease, especially colitis.

ADVERSE/SIDE EFFECTS **GI:** Nausea, vomiting, *diarrhea*, pseudomembranous enterocolitis. **Hypersensitivity:** fever, rash, pruritus, erythema, myalgia, anaphylactoid reaction. **Other:** pain with IM injection; burning sensation, phlebitis (IV administration), flu-like syndrome, superinfections (by *Candida, Pseudomonas, Enterobacter* sp). Neutropenia (rare).

DIAGNOSTIC TEST INTERFERENCE A false-positive reaction for ***urine glucose*** may occur with copper sulfate reduction reagents, e.g., Benedict's or Clinitest; tests based on glucose oxidase reactions are apparently not affected, e.g., TesTape, Clinistix, Diastix.

DRUG INTERACTIONS **Probenecid** decreases renal elimination.

INCOMPATIBILITIES **Solution/additive:** AMINOGLYCOSIDES. **Y-site:** AMINOGLYCOSIDES.

NURSING IMPLICATIONS

Administration

- When cefonicid is given for prophylaxis during cesarean section, it is administered only after umbilical cord has been clamped.
- IM injections should be made deeply into large muscle mass. Pain and discomfort at IM site occurs commonly. If dose is 2 g, give 1/2 dose in different large muscle masses. Rotate injection sites.
- Single dose IM or direct (bolus) IV preparation: Reconstitute with sterile water for injection and shake well to assure complete dissolution of drug; 500 mg of drug to 2 ml diluent gives about 220 mg/ml; 1 g drug to 2.5 ml diluent gives about 325 mg/ml. After reconstitution, inspect for particulate matter; if present, discard solution.
- IV infusion preparation: Dilute reconstituted cefonicid in 50–100 ml 0.9% NaCl injection, Ringer's injection, or other diluent suggested by manufacturer.
- Direct (bolus) IV injections of reconstituted solution should be made slowly over 3–5 min. Injection may be made directly or through IV tubing if patient is receiving a compatible parenteral fluid recommended by manufacturer. Examine IV site daily for evidence of inflammation.
- After reconstitution or dilution, solutions are stable for 24 h at room temperature or 72 h if refrigerated 5C (41F). Slight yellowing does not indicate loss of potency.

Assessment & Drug Effects

- Culture and susceptibility tests should be performed before and periodically during therapy, if indicated. Therapy may be initiated before test results are available.
- Before therapy begins, determine history of hypersensitivity to cephalosporins, penicillins, or other drugs.
- Although cephalosporins may be used in individuals with history of hypersensitivity to penicillin, they should not be used if individual has experienced an immediate reaction to penicillin, such as bronchospasm, urticaria, angioedema.
- Monitor I&O ratio and pattern, particularly in patients with impaired renal function, patients > 50 y, or who are receiving high doses.

C

- Monitor temperature. Report temperature alterations and the onset of flu-like symptoms (chills, malaise).
- Superinfections caused by overgrowth of nonsusceptible organisms may occur, particularly during prolonged use of cephalosporins.
- Antibiotic-associated pseudomembranous enterocolitis is a life-threatening superinfection caused by *Clostridium difficile;* may occur in 4–9 d or as long as 6 wk after cephalothin is discontinued. Most apt to occur in the chronically ill or debilitated elderly patient, especially if undergoing abdominal surgery or if in an intensive care unit.
- If diarrhea occurs, check for fever. Report diarrhea and fever promptly.
- Periodic hematologic studies including PT and PTT and evaluations of renal and hepatic functions are recommended in patients receiving high doses and during prolonged therapy.

Patient & Family Education

- Superinfections caused by overgrowth of nonsusceptible organisms may occur, particularly during prolonged use of cephalosporins. Report early signs and symptoms (see Appendix G) promptly.
- Instruct patient to report loose stools or diarrhea.
- Yogurt or buttermilk, 120 ml (4 oz) of either (if allowed), may serve as a prophylactic against intestinal superinfection by helping to maintain normal intestinal flora.

CEFOPERAZONE SODIUM

(sef-oh-per'a-zone)

Trade name: Cefobid

Classifications: ANTIINFECTIVE; ANTIBIOTIC; THIRD-GENERATION CEPHALOSPORIN

Prototype: Cefotaxime

Pregnancy category: B

ACTIONS/PHARMACODYNAMICS

Semisynthetic third-generation cephalosporin antibiotic. Preferentially binds to one or more of the penicillin-binding proteins (PBP) located on cell walls of susceptible organisms. This inhibits third and final stage of bacterial cell wall synthesis, thus killing the bacterium. Spectrum of activity is similar to that of cefotaxime. Generally active against a wide variety of gram-negative bacteria, including some strains of *Pseudomonas aeruginosa.* Also active against some organisms resistant to first and second generation cephalosporins and currently available aminoglycoside antibiotics and penicillins: e.g., *Escherichia coli, Klebsiella pneumoniae,* and *Serratia marcescens.* Other susceptible organisms include *Proteus mirabilis, Salmonella, Shigella, Hemophilus influenzae, Neisseria gonorrhoeae,* groups A and B streptococci, *Staphylococcus aureus,* and some strains of *Pseudomonas* sp. Cefoperazone inhibits some strains of *Clostridium,* but *C. difficile* is resistant to the drug, as is *Listeria monocytogenes.*

USES Infections of skin and skin structures, urinary tract, respiratory tract; and peritonitis and other intraabdominal infections, pelvic inflammatory disease, endometritis and other infections of the female genital tract; and bacterial septicemia. **Unlabeled use:** children <12 y.

ROUTE & DOSAGE

Moderate to Severe Infections

Adult: **IV/IM** 1–2 g q12h; 16 g/d in 2–4 divided doses.

Child <12 y: **IV/IM** 100–150 mg/kg/d divided q8–12h (max 12 g/d).

PHARMACOKINETICS **Peak levels:** 1–2 h after IM; 15–20 min after IV. **Distribution:** low CNS penetration except with inflamed meninges; highest concentrations in bile; crosses placenta. **Elimination:** half-life: 2 h, 70–75% excreted unchanged in bile in 6–12 h, small amount excreted in breast milk.

CONTRAINDICATIONS & PRECAUTIONS **Contraindicated in:** hypersensitivity to cephalosporins and related beta-lactam antibiotics. Safe use during pregnancy (category B) and in children <12 y not established. **Cautious use in:** history of hypersensitivity to penicillins, history of allergy, particularly to drugs; hepatic disease, history of colitis or other GI disease, history of bleeding disorders; nursing mothers.

ADVERSE/SIDE EFFECTS **GI:** abdominal cramps, bloating, loose stools or *diarrhea*, *pseudomembranous colitis*. **Hematologic:** abnormal PT and PTT; hypoprothrombinemia. **Hypersensitivity:** skin rash, urticaria, pruritus, fever, eosinophilia. **Hepatic:** elevated liver function tests (AST, ALT, alkaline phosphatase). **Renal:** transient increases in serum creatinine and BUN, oliguria. **Other:** phlebitis (IV site), transient pain (IM site), superinfections.

DIAGNOSTIC TEST INTERFERENCE Cefoperazone can cause positive direct ***Coombs' test,*** which may result in interferences with ***hematologic studies*** and ***cross-matching*** procedures. False-positive results for ***urine glucose*** using copper sulfate tests (Benedict's, Clinitest), but not with glucose enzymatic tests, e.g., Clinistix, TesTape, Diastix. Also causes prolonged prothrombin twice during therapy.

DRUG INTERACTIONS **Probenecid** decreases renal elimination of cefoperazone; **alcohol** produces disulfiram reaction.

INCOMPATIBILITIES **Solution/additive:** AMINOGLYCOSIDES, **doxapram.** **Y-site:** AMINOGLYCOSIDES, **LABETALOL, MEPERIDINE, PERPHENAZINE.**

NURSING IMPLICATIONS

Administration

- To prepare IM injections, appropriate diluents include sterile water for injection, bacteriostatic water for injection, and 0.5% lidocaine. See package insert for reconstitution procedure.
- IV preparation: Dilute each 1 g with 5 ml sterile water. Shake vigorously to dissolve. May be further diluted in 50–100 ml of D5W or NS for intermittent infusion or 500–1000 ml for continuous infusion. See manufacturer's directions for reconstitution and dilution and for compatible diluents.
- Rapid, direct (bolus) IV injections are not recommended. Cefoperazone may be administered by intermittent IV over a 15–30 min period or by continuous IV infusion, as prescribed.
- IV administration to infants, children: Verify correct IV concentration and rate of infusion with physician.
- Protect sterile powder and piggyback units from light and store at or below 25C (77F). Reconstituted solutions may be stored in original containers for 24 h at 15–25C (59–77F); for 5 d under refrigeration at 5C (41F) or less, or for at least 3 wk in freezer.

Assessment & Drug Effects

- Culture and susceptibility studies

C

should be performed before initiation of therapy and during therapy, as indicated. Therapy may begin pending test results.
- Before therapy begins, determine hypersensitivity to cephalosporins, penicillins, and other drug allergies.
- PTT and PT should be performed before and during therapy.
- Observe for and question patient about signs of hemostatic defects: wound bleeding (e.g., surgical patient), nose bleeds, bleeding gums, bloody sputum, hematuria. Hypoprothrombinemia and vitamin K deficiency are possible complications of therapy and can result in significant blood loss in some patients. Reversible with vitamin K and plasma if necessary.
- Drug-induced vitamin K deficiency develops in conditions that reduce vitamin K-producing bacteria in GI tract. Patients at risk are those with poor nutritional states, malabsorption problems, patients on hyperalimentation regimens, and alcoholism. Vitamin K supplements may be prescribed for these patients, if indicated.
- Report the onset of loose stools or diarrhea. Most patients respond to replacement of fluids, electrolytes, and proteins. Discontinuation of drug may be required for some patients.
- Cefoperazone serum levels (at steady state: 150 μg/ml) should be monitored in patients with hepatic disease or biliary obstruction who are receiving over 4 g/d, patients with both hepatic and renal disease receiving over 1–2 g/d, and patients with renal impairment on high dose therapy.

Patient & Family Education

- Warn patient that ingestion of alcohol within 72 h after drug administration will cause a disulfiram-like reaction (see Signs & Symptoms, Appendix G). Effects generally appear within 15–30 min after alcohol is taken and disappear spontaneously 1–2 h later.
- Instruct patient to report promptly signs and symptoms of superinfection (see Appendix G).

CEFORANIDE

(se-for′a-nide)

Trade name: Precef

Classifications: ANTIINFECTIVE; ANTIBIOTIC; SECOND-GENERATION CEPHALOSPORIN

Prototype: Cefonicid

Pregnancy category: B

ACTIONS/PHARMACODYNAMICS Semisynthetic, second-generation cephalosporin antibiotic; generally resistant to hydrolysis by beta-lactamases. Bactericidal action: preferentially binds to one or more of the penicillin-binding proteins (PBP) located on cell wall of susceptible organisms. This inhibits third and final stage of bacterial cell walls synthesis, thus killing the bacterium. Ceforanide is usually active against the organisms susceptible to first generation cephalosporins. In addition, it is bactericidal against *Providencia* sp, *Clostridium* sp, *Peptococcus* sp, and against strains of *Citrobacter, Enterobacter, Serratia, Neisseria, Proteus, Escherichia coli,* and *Klebsiella* that are resistant to first generation cephalosporins; generally inactive against enterococci, methicillin-resistant staphylococci, *Acinetobacter, Listeria monocytogenes,* and *Pseudomonas.*

USES To treat infections caused by susceptible organisms in the lower respiratory tract, urinary tract, skin and skin structures, bones and joints, endocarditis, and septicemia and for perioperative prophylaxis in patient undergoing prosthetic arthroplasty or cardiovascular surgery. **Unlabeled use:** prophylaxis during biliary tract or gastric bypass surgery.

ROUTE & DOSAGE

Moderate to Severe Infections

Adult: **IV/IM** 500 mg–1 g q12h.
Child: **IV/IM** 20–40 mg/kg/d in 2 divided doses.

Surgical Prophylaxis

Adult: **IV/IM** 500 mg–1 g 60 min before surgery, then q12h for 24 h.
Child: **IV/IM** 20–40 mg/kg 60 min before surgery, then q12h for 24 h.

PHARMACOKINETICS Peak: 1 h after IM; 30 min after IV. **Distribution:** poor CNS penetration even with inflamed meninges; crosses placenta. **Metabolism:** not metabolized. **Elimination:** half-life: 2.3–3.3 h; 78–95% excreted unchanged in urine; small amount excreted in breast milk.

CONTRAINDICATIONS & PRECAUTIONS Contraindicated in: hypersensitivity to cephalosporins and related antibiotics; severely impaired renal or hepatic function. Safe use during pregnancy (category B) and in children not established. **Cautious use in:** nursing mothers.

ADVERSE/SIDE EFFECTS GI: nausea, vomiting, *diarrhea,* abdominal cramps, <u>pseudomembranous colitis</u>. **Hematologic:** *transient thrombocytosis* (20% of patients). **Other:** superinfections; infection site reactions; hypersensitivity reactions.

DIAGNOSTIC TEST INTERFERENCE Ceforanide causes false-positive direct Coombs' test (may interfere with ***cross-matching procedures*** and ***hematologic studies***).

DRUG INTERACTIONS Probenecid decreases renal elimination of ceforanide.

INCOMPATIBILITIES Solution/additive: AMINOGLYCOSIDES. **Y-site:** AMINOGLYCOSIDES.

NURSING IMPLICATIONS

Administration

- IM injections should be made deeply into large muscle mass. Pain and discomfort at IM site occurs commonly. Rotate injection sites.
- IM reconstitution: Dilute contents of 500 mg vial with 1.7 ml diluent to make 250 mg/ml solution (see manufacturer's directions).
- IV administration: Dilute contents of 500 mg vial in 5 ml of sterile water or NS for injection; administer slowly by direct IV administration over 3–5 min or further dilute in 50–100 ml D5W or NS and infuse over 30 min.
- Reconstituted solution may become discolored (usually light yellow to amber) if exposed to high temperatures; however, potency is not affected. Solution may be cloudy immediately after reconstitution; let stand and it will clear.
- A supplemental dose (1 g) is generally given immediately following hemodialysis.
- After reconstitution, solution is stable for 48 h at 25C (77F); 14 d when refrigerated at 4C (39F), or 90 d when frozen at –15C (5F). Do not refreeze.

Assessment & Drug Effects

- Before therapy begins determine history of hypersensitivity to

C

cephalosporins, penicillins, or other beta-lactam antibiotics.

- Report onset of diarrhea (may be dose related). If severe, pseudomembranous colitis (see Appendix G) must be ruled out. Elderly patients are especially susceptible.
- Ceforanide serum concentrations should be monitored when drug is used for patient with renal impairment.
- Monitor for manifestations of hypersensitivity (see Appendix G).

Patient & Family Education

- Report promptly signs and symptoms of superinfection (see Appendix G). Discontinue drug and promptly report this to physician.

CEFOTAXIME SODIUM

(sef-oh-taks′eem)

Trade name: Claforan

Prototype for classifications: ANTIINFECTIVE; BETA-LACTAM ANTIBIOTIC; THIRD-GENERATION CEPHALOSPORIN

Pregnancy category: B

ACTIONS/PHARMACODYNAMICS Broad-spectrum semisynthetic third-generation cephalosporin antibiotic. Preferentially binds to one or more of the penicillin-binding proteins (PBP) located on cell walls of susceptible organisms. This inhibits third and final stage of bacterial cell wall synthesis, thus killing the bacterium. Generally active against a wide variety of gram-negative bacteria including most of the Enterobacteriaceae. Also active against some organisms resistant to first and second generation cephalosporins and currently available aminoglycoside antibiotics and penicillins, e.g., *Escherichia coli, Klebsiella pneumoniae,* and *Serratia marcescens.* Other susceptible organisms: *Bacteroides fragilis, Morganella morganii, Proteus mirabilis, Salmonella, Shigella, Hemophilus influenzae, Neisseria gonorrhoeae,* groups A and B streptococci, *Staphylococcus aureus, Bacteroides, Eubacterium, Peptostreptococcus,* and *Peptococcus.* Inhibits some strains of *Clostridium,* but *C. difficile* is resistant to the drug, as is *Listeria monocytogenes.*

USES Serious infections of lower respiratory tract, skin and skin structures, bones and joints, CNS (including meningitis and ventriculitis), gynecologic and GU tract infections, including uncomplicated gonococcal infections caused by penicillinase-producing *Neisseria gonorrhoeae* (PPNG). Also used to treat bacteremia or septicemia, intraabdominal infections, and for perioperative prophylaxis. **Unlabeled uses:** currently recommended by CDC for treatment of disseminated gonococcal infections (gonococcal arthritis-dermatitis syndrome) and as drug of choice for gonococcal ophthalmia caused by PPNG in adults, children, and neonates.

ROUTE & DOSAGE

Moderate to Severe Infections

Adult: **IV/IM** 1–2 g q8–12h, up to 2 g q4h (max 12 g/d).
Child: **IV/IM** ≤ 1 wk: 50 mg/ kg q12h; 1–4 wk: 50 mg/kg q8h; 1 mo–12 y: 100–200 mg/kg/d divided q4–8h.

Surgical Prophylaxis

Adult: **IV/IM** 1 g 30–90 min before surgery.

PHARMACOKINETICS **Peak levels:** 30 min after IM; 5 min after IV. **Dis-**

tribution: CNS penetration except with inflamed meninges; also penetrates aqueous humor, ascitic and prostatic fluids; crosses placenta. **Metabolism:** partially metabolized in liver to active metabolites. **Elimination:** half-life: 1 h; 50–60% excreted unchanged in urine in 24 h; small amount excreted in breast milk.

CONTRAINDICATIONS & PRECAUTIONS **Contraindicated in:** hypersensitivity to cephalosporins and other β-lactam antibiotics. Safe use during pregnancy (category B) not established. **Cautious use in:** history of type I hypersensitivity reactions to penicillins; history of allergy to other β-lactams; renal impairment; history of colitis or other GI disease; nursing mothers. Safety and effectiveness in children < 12 y have not been established.

ADVERSE/SIDE EFFECTS **GI:** nausea, vomiting, *diarrhea*, abdominal pain, colitis, pseudomembranous colitis, anorexia. **Hypersensitivity:** rash, pruritus, fever. **Other:** nocturnal perspiration; ***IV site reactions:*** inflammatory reaction, phlebitis, thrombophlebitis; ***IM site:*** pain, induration, and tenderness. Also, superinfections, transient increases in serum AST, ALT, LDH, bilirubin, alkaline phosphatase concentrations.

DIAGNOSTIC TEST INTERFERENCE May cause falsely elevated ***serum*** or ***urine creatinine*** values (Jaffe reaction). False-positive reactions for ***urine glucose*** have not been reported using copper sulfate reduction methods, e.g., Benedict's, Clinitest; however, since it has occurred with other cephalosporins, it may be advisable to use glucose oxidase tests (Clinistix, TesTape, Diastix). Positive direct antiglobulin (Coombs') test results may interfere with ***hematologic studies*** and ***cross-matching*** procedures.

DRUG INTERACTIONS **Probenecid** decreases renal elimination; **alcohol** produces disulfiram reaction.

INCOMPATIBILITIES **Solution/additive:** AMINOGLYCOSIDES, **aminophylline, sodium bicarbonate, vancomycin. Y-site:** AMINOGLYCOSIDES, **doxapram, aminophylline, sodium bicarbonate; pentamidine.**

NURSING IMPLICATIONS

Administration

- Follow manufacturer's suggestions concerning appropriate diluents.
- IM injections: Add 3 ml diluent to vial containing 1 g drug providing a solution of approximately 300 mg cefotaxime/ml. Administer IM injection deeply into large muscle mass (e.g., upper outer quadrant of gluteus maximus). Aspirate to avoid inadvertent injection into blood vessel. If IM dose is 2 g, divide dose and administer into 2 different sites.
- IV infusion: Add 50 or 100 ml diluent to 1 or 2 g drug. Generally, intermittent IV infusion is infused over 20–30 min, preferably via butterfly or scalp vein–type needles.
- IV injection: Add 10 ml diluent to vial with 1 or 2 g drug providing a solution containing 95 or 180 mg cefotaxime/ml, respectively. Inject directly into vein over 3–5 min period or slowly into tubing of freely flowing compatible IV solution.
- IV administration to infants and children: Verify correct IV concentration and rate of infusion with physician.
- Do not admix cefotaxime with sodium bicarbonate or any fluid with a pH > 7.5 or with an aminoglycoside.

C

- Risk of phlebitis may be reduced by use of a small needle in a large vein.
- Cefotaxime therapy should continue for at least 48–72 h after patient becomes afebrile or other signs of infection have disappeared. Therapy for group A beta-hemolytic streptococci should be continued for a minimum of 10 d to reduce risk of glomerulonephritis and rheumatic fever.
- Store dry powder preferably at 15–30C (59–86F), unless otherwise directed by manufacturer. Protect from excessive light. Reconstituted solutions may be stored in original containers for 24 h at room temperature at 15–30C (59–86F); for 10 days under refrigeration at 5C (41F) or less; or for at least 13 wk in frozen state.

Assessment & Drug Effects

- Culture and susceptibility tests should be performed before initiation of therapy and periodically during therapy, if indicated. Therapy may be instituted pending test results.
- Before therapy is initiated, determine previous hypersensitivity reactions to cephalosporins and penicillins, and history of other allergies, particularly to drugs.
- Report change in I&O ratio and pattern in patients with impaired renal function or with chronic UTI or who are receiving high dosages or an aminoglycoside concomitantly. Renal status (serum creatinine, creatinine clearance, BUN) should be evaluated at regular intervals during therapy and for several months after drug has been discontinued.
- Superinfection due to overgrowth of nonsusceptible organisms may occur, particularly with prolonged therapy.
- Report onset of diarrhea promptly. Check for fever. If diarrhea is mild, discontinuation of cefotaxime may be sufficient.
- If diarrhea is severe, suspect antibiotic-associated pseudomembranous colitis, a life-threatening superinfection (may occur in 4–9 d or as long as 6 wk after cephalosporin therapy is discontinued). Chronically ill or debilitated elderly patients undergoing abdominal surgery or those in an intensive care unit are most vulnerable.
- Periodic hematologic studies (including PT and PTT) and evaluation of renal and hepatic functions are recommended with high doses or prolonged therapy.

Patient & Family Education

- Superinfections caused by overgrowth of nonsusceptible organisms may occur, particularly during prolonged use. Report early signs and symptoms promptly.
- Yogurt or buttermilk, 120 ml (4 oz) of either (if allowed), may serve as a prophylactic against intestinal superinfection by helping to maintain normal intestinal flora.
- Report loose stools or diarrhea.

CEFOTETAN DISODIUM

(sef′oh-tee-tan)

Trade name: Cefotan

Classifications: ANTIINFECTIVE; ANTIBIOTIC; THIRD-GENERATION CEPHALOSPORIN

Prototype: Cefotaxime

Pregnancy category: B

ACTIONS/PHARMACODYNAMICS

Semisynthetic beta-lactam antibiotic, classified as a third-generation cephalosporin. Preferentially binds to one or more of the penicillin-binding proteins (PBP) located on cell walls of susceptible organisms. This inhibits third and final stage of bacterial cell wall synthesis, thus killing the bacterium. Generally less active against susceptible staphylococci than first generation cephalosporins are but has broad spectrum of activity against gram-negative bacteria when compared to first and second generation cephalosporins. Spectrum of activity is like that of cefotaxime including *Escherichia coli, Klebsiella* sp, *Enterobacter* sp, *Proteus* sp, *Streptococcus pneumoniae, Staphylococcus aureus,* penicillinase- and nonpenicillinase-producing *Hemophilus influenzae, Salmonella, Shigella, Neisseria gonorrhoeae,* and many anaerobes. Generally inactive against *Pseudomonas aeruginosa*.

USES Infections caused by susceptible organisms in urinary tract, lower respiratory tract, skin and skin structures, bones and joints, gynecologic tract; also intraabdominal infections, bacteremia, and perioperative prophylaxis.

ROUTE & DOSAGE

Moderate to Severe Infections

Adult: **IV/IM** 1–2 g q12h.
Child: **IV/IM** 40–80 mg/kg/d divided q12h (max 6 g/d).

Surgical Prophylaxis

Adult: **IV/IM** 1–2 g 30–60 min before surgery.

PHARMACOKINETICS **Peak:** 1.5–3 h after IM. **Distribution:** poor CNS penetration; widely distributed to body tissues and fluids, including bile, sputum, prostatic and peritoneal fluids; crosses placenta. **Elimination:** half-life: 180–270 min; 51–81% excreted unchanged in urine; 20% excreted in bile; small amount excreted in breast milk.

CONTRAINDICATIONS & PRECAUTIONS **Contraindicated in:** hypersensitivity to cephalosporins and related beta-lactam antibiotics. Safe use in pregnancy (category B) and children not established. **Cautious use in:** nursing mothers.

ADVERSE/SIDE EFFECTS **GI:** nausea, vomiting, *diarrhea,* abdominal pain. **Hematologic:** antibiotic-associated colitis, thrombocytopenia, prolongation of bleeding time or prothrombin time. **Hypersensitivity:** rash, pruritus, fever, chills. **Other:** injection site pain, inflammation, disulfiram-like reaction.

DIAGNOSTIC TEST INTERFERENCE May cause falsely elevated ***serum*** or ***urine creatinine*** values (Jaffe reaction). False-positive reactions for ***urine glucose*** have not been reported using copper sulfate reduction methods, e.g., Benedict's, Clinitest; however, since it has occurred with other cephalosporins, it may be advisable to use glucose oxidase tests (Clinistix, TesTape, Diastix). Positive direct antiglobulin (Coombs') test results may interfere with ***hematologic studies*** and ***cross-matching*** procedures.

DRUG INTERACTIONS **Probenecid** decreases renal elimination of cefotetan; **alcohol** produces disulfiram reaction.

INCOMPATIBILITIES **Solution/additive:** AMINOGLYCOSIDES, **doxapram,** HEPARIN, **promethazine,** TETRACYCLINES. **Y-site:** AMINOGLYCOSIDES, **promethazine.**

NURSING IMPLICATIONS

Administration

- For direct IV administration, dilute each 1 g with 10 ml of sterile water for injection. May be given by direct IV over 3–5 min.

- For IM reconstitution (follow manufacturer's directions for selection of diluent), add 2 ml diluent to 1 g vial; withdraw approximately 2.4 ml to yield 375 mg drug/ml.
- For IM administration, inject well into body of large muscle such as upper outer quadrant of buttock (gluteus maximus).
- For intermittent IV infusion, dilute each 1 g with 50–100 ml of D5W or NS and administer a single dose over 30 min.
- For IV infusion, solution may be given for longer period of time through tubing system through which other IV solutions are being given. Butterfly or scalp vein-type needles are preferred. During infusion, temporarily discontinue administration of other solutions at same site.
- IV administration to infants and children: Verify correct IV concentration and rate of infusion with physician.
- Protect sterile powder from light; store at 22C (71.6F) or less; remains stable 24 mo after date of manufacture. May darken with age, but potency is unaffected. Reconstituted solutions: stable for 24 h at 25C (77F); 96 h when refrigerated at 5C (41F); or at least 1 wk when frozen at –20C (–4F). Piggyback reconstituted solutions: stable for 24 h at 25C (77F) or for 96 h at 5C (41F). Reconstituted solutions transferred to plastic syringes: stable for 24 h at room temperature, or 96 h when refrigerated. Thaw frozen solutions at room temperature. Do not refreeze.

Assessment & Drug Effects

- Culture and susceptibility studies should be performed before initiation of therapy and during therapy, as indicated. Therapy may begin pending test results.
- Before therapy begins, determine history of hypersensitivity to cephalosporins and penicillins, and other drug allergies.
- Monitor renal function, especially if cefotetan dose is high or if therapy is prolonged in order to recognize symptoms of nephrotoxicity and ototoxicity (see Appendix G).
- Report onset of loose stools or diarrhea. If diarrhea is severe, suspect pseudomembranous colitis (see Appendix G) caused by *Clostridium difficile*. Check temperature. Report fever and severe diarrhea to physician; drug should be discontinued.

Patient & Family Education

- Report promptly signs and symptoms of superinfection (see Appendix G).
- Report loose stools or diarrhea.

CEFOXITIN SODIUM

(se-fox'i-tin)

Trade name: Mefoxin

Classifications: ANTIINFECTIVE; ANTIBIOTIC; SECOND-GENERATION CEPHALOSPORIN

Prototype: Cefonicid

Pregnancy category: B

ACTIONS/PHARMACODYNAMICS

Semisynthetic, broad-spectrum betalactam antibiotic derivative of cephamycin C (produced by *Streptomyces lactamdurans*). Classified as second generation cephalosporin; structurally and pharmacologically related to cephalosporins and penicillins. Antimicrobial spectrum of activity resembles that of cefonicid. Considerably less active than most cephalosporins against staphylococci. Preferentially binds to one or more of the penicillin-binding proteins (PBP) located on cell walls of susceptible organisms.

USES Infections caused by susceptible organisms in the lower respiratory tract, urinary tract, skin and skin structures, bones and joints; also intraabdominal endocarditis, gynecological infections, septicemia, uncomplicated gonorrhea, and periooperative prophylaxis in prosthetic arthroplasty or cardiovascular surgery. May be cephalosporin of choice for mixed aerobic-anaerobic infections (e.g., *Bacteroides fragilis*).

ROUTE & DOSAGE

Moderate to Severe Infections

Adult: **IV/IM** 1–2 g q6–8 h; up to 12 g/d.
Child >3 mo: **IV/IM** 80–160 mg/kg/d in 4–6 divided doses (max 12 g/d).
Neonate: **IV/IM** 90–100 mg/kg/d divided q8h.

Surgical Prophylaxis

Adult: **IV/IM** 2 g 30–60 min before surgery; then 2 g q6h for 24 h.
Child: **IV/IM** 30–40 mg/kg 30–60 min before surgery; then 2 g q6h for 24 h.

Uncomplicated Gonorrhea

Adult: **IV/IM** 2 g given concurrently with 1 g probenecid PO.

PHARMACOKINETICS **Peak:** 20–30 min after IM; 5 min after IV. **Distribution:** poor CNS penetration even with inflamed meninges; widely distributed in body tissues including pleural, synovial, and ascitic fluid and bile; crosses placenta. **Elimination:** half-life: 45–60 min, 85% excreted unchanged in urine in 6 h, small amount excreted in breast milk.

CONTRAINDICATIONS & PRECAUTIONS **Contraindicated in:** hypersensitivity to cephalosporins and related antibiotics. Safe use during pregnancy (category B), in nursing mothers, and in children <3 mo not established. **Cautious use in:** history of sensitivity to penicillin or other allergies, particularly to drugs, impaired renal function.

ADVERSE/SIDE EFFECTS **GI:** *diarrhea,* <u>pseudomembranous colitis</u>. **Hypersensitivity:** rash, <u>exfoliative dermatitis</u>, pruritus, urticaria, drug fever, eosinophilia. **Other:** superinfections, local reactions: pain, tenderness, and induration (IM site), thrombophlebitis (IV site); nephrotoxicity, interstitial nephritis.

DIAGNOSTIC TEST INTERFERENCE Cefoxitin causes false-positive (black-brown or green-brown color) ***urine glucose*** reaction with copper reduction reagents such as Benedict's or Clinitest, but not with enzymatic glucose oxidase reagents (Clinistix, TesTape). With high doses, falsely elevated ***serum and urine creatinine*** (with Jaffee reaction) reported. False-positive direct Coombs' test (may interfere with ***cross-matching procedures*** and ***hematologic studies***) has also been reported.

DRUG INTERACTIONS **Probenecid** decreases renal elimination of cefoxitin.

INCOMPATIBILITIES **Solution/additive:** AMINOGLYCOSIDES. **Y-site:** AMINOGLYCOSIDES.

NURSING IMPLICATIONS

Administration

- Recommended diluents for IM solution include sterile water for

C

injection or 0.5 or 1% lidocaine hydrochloride (without epinephrine), used to reduce discomfort of IM injection. Consult physician before using lidocaine.

- After reconstitution for IM use, shake vial and allow solution to stand until it becomes clear. Solutions retain potency for 24 h at room temperature, for 7 d if refrigerated, and for at least 26 wk if frozen.
- Administer IM injections deep into large muscle mass such as upper outer quadrant of gluteus maximus. Aspirate before injecting drug. Rotate injection sites.
- For direct IV administration, dilute each 1 g with 10 ml sterile water, D5W, or NS. May be given by direct IV over 3–5 min.
- For IV infusion, dilute one dose (1–2 g) in 50–1000 ml of compatible solution and give at a rate determined by the volume of solution.
- IV administration to neonates, infants and children: Verify correct IV concentration and rate of infusion/injection with physician.
- Drug therapy for beta-hemolytic streptococcal infections should continue for at least 10 d to guard against risk of rheumatic fever.
- Reconstituted solution may become discolored (usually light yellow to amber) if exposed to high temperatures; however, potency is not affected. Solution may be cloudy immediately after reconstitution; let stand and it will clear.
- After reconstitution, solution is stable for 24 h at room temperature 25C (77F); 7 d when refrigerated at 4C (39F), or 30 wk when frozen at −20C (−4F).

Assessment & Drug Effects

- Before therapy is initiated, determine previous hypersensitivity to cephalosporins, penicillins, and other drug allergies.
- Culture and susceptibility testing is advised prior to and periodically during therapy.
- Inspect injection sites regularly. Report evidence of inflammation and patient's complaint of pain.
- Monitor I&O ratio and pattern. Nephrotoxicity occurs most frequently in patients >50 y, in patients with impaired renal function, the debilitated, and in patients receiving high doses or other nephrotoxic drugs.
- Be alert to signs and symptoms of superinfections (see Appendix G). This condition is most apt to occur in elderly patients, especially when drug has been used for prolonged period.
- Report onset of diarrhea (may be dose related). If severe, pseudomembranous colitis (see Signs & Symptoms, Appendix G) must be ruled out. Elderly patients are especially susceptible.

CEFPODOXIME

(cef-po-dox′-eem)

Trade name: Vantin

Classifications: ANTIINFECTIVE; ANTIBIOTIC; THIRD-GENERATION CEPHALOSPORIN

Prototype: Cefotaxime

Pregnancy category: B

ACTIONS/PHARMACODYNAMICS

Semisynthetic cephalosporin antibiotic with antibacterial activity resembling that of other third-generation cephalosporins. Stable in the presence of beta-lactamases. Highly active against gram-negative bacteria.

USES Gonorrhea, otitis media, lower and upper respiratory tract infections, urinary tract infections. **Unlabeled uses:** skin and soft tissue infections.

ROUTE & DOSAGE

Respiratory Tract, Skin, and Soft Tissue Infections

Adult: **PO** 200 mg q12h for 10 d.
Child: **PO** 10 mg/kg/d divided q12h.

Urinary Tract Infections

Adult: **PO** 100 mg q12h.

Gonorrhea

Adult: **PO** 200 mg as single dose.

Otitis Media

Child 5 mo–12 y: **PO** 10 mg/kg/d divided q12–24h.

PHARMACOKINETICS Absorption 40–50% absorbed from GI tract—increased with food. **Onset:** therapeutic effect in 3 d. **Distribution:** distributes well into inflammatory, pulmonary, and pleural fluid, and tonsils. Some distribution into prostate. 40% bound to plasma proteins. Distributed into breast milk. **Elimination:** half-life: 2–3 h; 80% excreted in urine.

CONTRAINDICATIONS & PRECAUTIONS Contraindicated in: hypersensitivity to cephalosporins and other beta-lactam antibiotics. Safe use during pregnancy (category B) not established. **Cautious use in:** renal impairment, history of type I hypersensitivity reactions to penicillins; history of colitis or other GI disease; nursing mothers.

ADVERSE/SIDE EFFECTS CNS: rare: headache, asthenia, dizziness, fatigue, anxiety, insomnia, flushing, nightmares, weakness. **GI:** diarrhea, nausea, vomiting, abdominal pain, soft stools, flatulance, <u>pseudomembranous colitis</u> (rare). **GU:** vaginal candidiasis. **Skin:** urticaria, rash, scaling, peeling. **Other:** eye itching, cough, epistaxis, fever, decreased appetite, malaise.

DRUG INTERACTIONS ANTACIDS, **ranitidine** may decrease absorption. **Drug–food:** food may increase the absorption.

NURSING IMPLICATIONS

Administration

- Drug should be administered with food to enhance absorption.
- Drug should be given 1 h before or 2 h after an antacid.
- In patients with renal impairment (i.e., creatinine clearance less than 30 ml/min), dosage intervals should be every 12 h.
- Patients on hemodialysis should be given usual dose 3 times weekly after hemodialysis.
- To either the 50 mg/5 ml strength or the 100 mg/5 ml strength, add 25 ml of distilled water, then shake vigorously for 15 seconds. Next, to the 50 mg/5 ml strength add 33 ml, or to the 100 mg/5 ml strength add 32 ml, of distilled water, and shake for at least 3 minutes.
- Store suspension for up to 14 d in a refrigerator (2–8C/36–46F). Shake well before using.

Assessment & Drug Effects

- Culture and susceptibility tests should be performed before initiation of therapy and periodically during therapy, if indicated. Therapy may be instituted pending test results.
- Before therapy is initiated, determine history of hypersensitivity reactions to cephalosporins and penicillins, and history of allergies, particularly to drugs.

- Report onset of loose stools or diarrhea. Although pseudomembranous enterocolitis (see Appendix G) rarely occurs, this potentially life-threatening complication should be ruled out as the cause of diarrhea during and after antibiotic therapy.
- Monitor for manifestations of hypersensitivity (see Appendix G). Discontinue drug and report signs and symptoms of hypersensitivity promptly.
- Monitor I&O ratio and pattern, especially with high doses. Report any significant changes.

Patient & Family Education

- Advise to immediately report signs and symptoms of hypersensitivity.
- Advise to report loose stools, or diarrhea, especially if containing blood, mucus, or pus.
- Stress the importance of completing the full course of drug therapy even if symptoms improve.

CEFPROZIL

(cef'pro-zil)

Trade name: Cefzil

Classifications: ANTIBIOTIC; ANTI-INFECTIVE; SECOND-GENERATION CEPHALOSPORIN

Prototype: Cefonicid

Pregnancy category: B

ACTIONS/PHARMACODYNAMICS Semisynthetic, second-generation cephalosporin antibiotic with drug structure characterized by a beta-lactam ring; generally resistant to hydrolysis by beta-lactamases. Preferentially binds to proteins in cell walls of susceptible organisms, thus killing the bacteria. Also active against organisms susceptible to first generation cephalosporin. Active against *Streptococcus pyogenes, Streptococcus pneumoniae, Hemophilus influenzae, Moraxella catarrhalis,* and *Staphylococcus aureus.*

USES Upper and lower respiratory tract infections, otitis media, skin infections.

ROUTE & DOSAGE

Mild to Moderate Infections

Adult: **PO** 250–500 mg q12–24h for 10–14 d.
Child >6 mo: **PO** 15 mg/kg q12h.

PHARMACOKINETICS **Absorption:** readily absorbed from GI tract. **Peak:** 1-2 h. **Distribution:** distributes into blister fluid at 50% of the serum level. **Elimination:** half-life: 1-2 h; primarily excreted by the kidneys.

CONTRAINDICATIONS & PRECAUTIONS Hypersensitivity to cephalosporin and related antibiotics; severely impaired renal or hepatic function. Safe use during pregnancy (category B) and in children not established. **Cautious use in:** nursing mothers, patients with delayed reaction to penicillin or other drugs, GI disease, especially colitis.

ADVERSE/SIDE EFFECTS **CNS:** headache. **GI:** nausea, vomiting, diarrhea, abdominal pain. **GU:** genital pruritus, vaginal candidiasis. **Hematologic:** eosinophilia. **Other:** hypersensitivity reactions, rash, diaper rash, superinfections.

DRUG INTERACTIONS **Probenecid** prolongs the elimination of cefprozil.

DIAGNOSTIC TEST INTERFERENCE May cause a positive direct ***Coombs' test;*** false-negative results in the ferricyanide assay for ***blood glucose;*** false-positive reactions for ***urine glucose*** with copper reduction tests

C

such as Benedict's or Fehling's solution or Clinitest tablets; increased ***partial thromboplastin time,*** indicating thrombocytosis, eosinophilia; minor elevations in ***serum alanine aminotransferase (ALT), aspartate aminotransferase (AST),*** and ***bilirubin.***

NURSING IMPLICATIONS

Administration

- Drug may be given without regard to meals.
- With impaired renal function, dose is reduced by 50% when creatinine clearance is 0–30 ml/min.
- Administer after hemodialysis since drug is partially removed by dialysis.
- After reconstitution, oral suspension is refrigerated. Discard unused portion after 14 days.
- Store at 15–30C (59–86F).

Assessment & Drug Effects

- Before treatment, inquire about previous hypersensitivity to cephalosporins or penicillins.
- If hypersensitivity occurs (e.g., rash, urticaria) discontinue drug and notify physician.
- Culture and sensitivity tests should be done before and periodically during therapy. Therapy may be initiated while results are pending.
- Monitor for and report diarrhea, as pseudomembranous colitis is a potential adverse effect.
- Monitor for and report signs of superinfection (see Appendix G).
- When given concurrently with other cephalosporins or aminoglycosides, monitor for signs of nephrotoxicity.

Patient & Family Education

- Stress importance of completing prescribed course of therapy.
- Advise patient to immediately report rash or other signs of hypersensitivity.
- Advise patient to report signs of superinfection (see Appendix G).
- Instruct patient to report loose stools and diarrhea even after completion of drug therapy.

CEFTAZIDIME

(sef'tay-zi-deem)

Trade names: Fortaz, Tazicef, Tazidime

Classifications: ANTIINFECTIVE; ANTIBIOTIC; THIRD-GENERATION CEPHALOSPORIN

Prototype: Ceftazidime

Pregnancy category: B

ACTIONS/PHARMACODYNAMICS

Semisynthetic, third-generation broad-spectrum cephalosporin similar to cefotaxime but more active against *Pseudomonas aeruginosa* and less active against staphylococci and *Bacteroides fragilis*. Preferentially binds to one or more of the penicillin-binding proteins (PBP) located on cell walls of susceptible microbes; this inhibits third and final stage of bacterial cell wall synthesis, leading to cell death. Most strains of gonococci, meningococci, and *Hemophilus influenzae* are highly susceptible to ceftazidime; *Listeria monocytogenes* organisms are resistant. Emergence of resistance during treatment has been reported. May be used concomitantly with other antibiotics (e.g., aminoglycosides, vancomycin, clindamycin).

USES To treat infections of lower respiratory tract, skin and skin structures, urinary tract, bones and joints; also used to treat bacteremia, gynecological, intraabdominal and CNS infections (including meningitis). **Unlabeled use:** surgical prophylaxis.

C

ROUTE & DOSAGE

Moderate to Severe Infections

Adult: **IV/IM** 1–2 g q8–12h; up to 2 g q6h. *Geriatric:* 1–2 g q 12h.
Child: **IV/IM** <4 wk, 30 mg/kg q12h; 1 mo–12 y, 30–50 mg/kg/d in 3 divided doses (max 6 g/d).

PHARMACOKINETICS **Peak:** 1 h after IM or IV. **Distribution:** CNS penetration with inflamed meninges; also penetrates bone, gallbladder, bile, endometrium, heart, skin, and ascitic and pleural fluids; crosses placenta. **Metabolism:** not metabolized. **Elimination:** half-life: 25–60 min; 80–90% excreted unchanged in urine in 24 h; small amount excreted in breast milk.

CONTRAINDICATIONS & PRECAUTIONS **Contraindicated in:** hypersensitivity to cephalosporins and related beta-lactam antibiotics. Safe use in pregnancy (category B) and children not established. **Cautious use in:** nursing mothers.

ADVERSE/SIDE EFFECTS **GI:** nausea, vomiting, *diarrhea,* abdominal pain, metallic taste, drug-associated <u>pseudomembranous colitis</u>. **GU:** vaginitis, candidiasis. **Hypersensitivity:** (1– 3%): pruritus, rash, urticaria, fever. **Other:** phlebitis, pain or inflammation at injection site, superinfections.

DIAGNOSTIC TEST INTERFERENCE False-positive reactions for ***urine glucose*** have been reported using copper sulfate (e.g., Benedict's solution, Clinitest). Glucose oxidase tests (Clinistix, TesTape) are unaffected. May cause positive direct antiglobulin (Coombs') test results which can interfere with ***hematologic studies*** and ***transfusion cross-matching procedures.***

DRUG INTERACTIONS **Probenecid** decreases renal elimination of ceftazidime.

INCOMPATIBILITIES **Solution/additive:** AMINOGLYCOSIDES. **Y-site:** AMINOGLYCOSIDES, **fluconazole; pentamidine.**

NURSING IMPLICATIONS

Administration

- IM reconstitution: Refer to manufacturer's directions regarding diluent and method. IM: add 3 ml diluent to 1 g-size vial to yield 280 mg/ml.
- IM administration: Inject into large muscle mass (e.g., upper outer quadrant of gluteus maximus or lateral part of thigh).
- IV administration: Add 10 ml of sterile water for injection to 1 g to yield 280 mg/ml. May be given direct IV over 3–5 min or may be further diluted with 50–100 ml of D5W or NS and infused over 30 min.
- Infuse IV solution through tubing or administration set while patient is also receiving one of the compatible IV fluids. Intermittent administration with Y-type set: during infusion of ceftazidime solution, discontinue other solutions.
- Protect sterile powder from light; store at 15–30C (59–86F). Store commercially available frozen ceftazidime at temperature no greater than –20C (–4F). Reconstituted solution is stable 7 d when refrigerated at 4–5C (39–41F); for 18–24 h when stored at 15–30C (59–86F).

Assessment & Drug Effects

- Culture and susceptibility studies should be performed before initiation of therapy and during therapy as indicated. Therapy may begin pending test results.

Common side effect in *italic,* life-threatening effects <u>underlined</u>; generic names in **bold;** drug class in SMALL CAPS

- Before therapy begins, determine history of hypersensitivity to cephalosporins and penicillins, and other drug allergies.
- If administered concomitantly with another antibiotic, monitor renal function and report if dysfunction symptoms appear (e.g., changes in I&O ratio and pattern, dysuria).
- Be alert to onset of rash, itching, and dyspnea. Check patient's temperature. If it is elevated, suspect onset of hypersensitivity reaction (see Signs & Symptoms, Appendix G).
- Superinfections have occurred and are usually caused by *Enterobacter, Pseudomonas* or *Candida* (see Signs & Symptoms, Appendix G).
- If diarrhea occurs and is severe, suspect pseudomembranous colitis (caused by *Clostridium difficile*). Check temperature: Report fever and severe diarrhea to physician; drug should be discontinued.

Patient & Family Education

- Instruct patient to report loose stools or diarrhea promptly.
- Advise patient to report signs and symptoms of superinfection promptly (see Appendix G).

CEFTIBUTEN

(sef-ti-bu′ten)

Trade name: Cedax

Classifications: ANTIINFECTIVE; BETA-LACTAM ANTIBIOTIC; THIRD-GENERATION CEPHALOSPORIN

Prototype: Cefotaxime

Pregnancy category: B

ACTIONS/PHARMACODYNAMICS Ceftibuten is a broad-spectrum, third-generation β-lactam antibiotic. Preferentially binds to one or more of the penicillin-binding proteins located in the cell wall of susceptible organisms. This inhibits third and final stage of bacterial cell wall synthesis, thus killing the bacterium. It is highly resistant to hydrolysis by most β-lactamase bacteria. It has antibacterial activity against both gram-negative and gram-positive bacteria, including *Hemophilus influenzae* (β-lactamase-producing strains also), *Streptococcus pneumoniae,* and *Streptococcus pyogenes.*

USES Acute bacterial exacerbations of chronic bronchitis caused by *H. influenzae, Moraxella catarrhalis,* or *S. pneumoniae;* acute bacterial otitis media caused by *H. influenzae, M. catarrhalis,* or *S. pyogenes;* pharyngitis or tonsillitis caused by *S. pyogenes.*

ROUTE & DOSAGE

Mild to Moderate Infections

Adult: **PO** 400 mg once daily for 10 d. **Adjustment for renal insufficiency:** Cl_{cr} 30–49: 200 mg q24h; Cl_{cr} <30: 100 mg q24h.
Child (6 mo–12 y): **PO** 9 mg/kg once daily (max 400 mg) for 10 d.

Adjustment for Renal Impairment

Cl_{cr} 30–49 ml/min: 4.5 mg/kg q24h; <30 ml/min: 2.25 mg/kg q24h.

PHARMACOKINETICS Absorption: rapidly absorbed from GI tract. **Peak:** approx 2–3 h. **Distribution:** bronchial mucosa levels are approx 37% of plasma levels, middle ear levels approx 50% of plasma levels. **Elimination:** half-life: 1.5–2.5 h; excreted primarily in urine.

CONTRAINDICATIONS & PRECAUTIONS Contraindicated in: hypersensitivity to ceftibuten or cephalosporins. **Cautious use in:** renal

C

dysfunction, penicillin hypersensitivity, history of colitis or diabetes, pregnancy (category B), nursing mothers. Safety and efficacy in infants <6 mo not established.

ADVERSE/SIDE EFFECTS CNS: headache, dizziness, nasal congestion, somnolence. **GI:** nausea, vomiting, diarrhea, dyspepsia, abdominal pain, anorexia, constipation, dry mouth, eructation, flatulence. **Other:** dyspnea, dysuria, fatigue, vaginitis, moniliasis, urticaria, pruritus, rash, paresthesia, taste perversion.

NURSING IMPLICATIONS

Administration

- Oral suspension must be given 1 h before or 2 h after a meal.
- Children weighing more than 45 kg may receive maximum daily dose.
- Doses should be reduced if Cl_{cr} >50 ml/min.
- Hemodialysis patients should receive drug at the end of dialysis.
- Store capsules at 2–25C (36–77F); keep container tightly closed. Reconstituted oral suspension is stable for 14 d under refrigeration at 2–8C (36–46F).

Assessment & Drug Effects

- Culture and sensitivity tests should be performed before initiation of therapy. Dosage may be started pending test results.
- Before therapy is initiated, determine history of hypersensitivity reactions to cephalosporins, penicillins, or other drugs. Monitor for S&S of hypersensitivity (see Appendix G); report their appearance promptly and discontinue drug.
- Monitor for S&S of superinfection or pseudomembranous colitis (see Appendix G); immediately report either to physician.
- Closely monitor patients with renal impairment; if seizures develop discontinue drug and notify physician.

Patient & Family Education

- Instruct patient on hemodialysis to take drug after dialysis.
- Teach S&S of hypersensitivity, superinfection, and pseudomembranous colitis; instruct to promptly report any of these.

CEFTIZOXIME SODIUM

(sef-ti-zox′eem)

Trade name: Cefizox

Classifications: ANTIINFECTIVE; ANTIBIOTIC; THIRD-GENERATION CEPHALOSPORIN

Prototype: Cefotaxime

Pregnancy category: B

ACTIONS/PHARMACODYNAMICS

Semisynthetic third-generation cephalosporin antibiotic. Preferentially binds to one or more of the penicillin-binding proteins (PBP) located on cell walls of susceptible organisms. This inhibits third and final stage of bacterial cell wall synthesis, thus killing the bacterium. Spectrum of activity similar to that of cefotaxime. Generally resistant to inactivation by beta-lactamases that act principally as cephalosporinases and penicillinases. *Clostridium difficile,* enterococci including *Streptococcus faecalis,* and most strains of *Listeria monocytogenes* are resistant to ceftizoxime. Incompatible with the aminoglycoside antibiotics. Evidence of partial cross-allergenicity among cephalosporins and other betalactamase antibiotics has been reported.

USES Infections caused by susceptible organisms in lower respiratory tract, skin and skin structures, urinary tract, bones and joints; also used to treat intraabdominal infections, pelvic inflammatory disease, uncomplicated gonorrhea, meningitis *(Hemophilus influenzae, Streptococcus pneumoniae),* and for surgical prophylaxis. **Unlabeled use:** meningitis caused by *Neisseria meningitidis* and *Escherichia coli.*

ROUTE & DOSAGE

Moderate to Severe Infections
Adult: **IV/IM** 1–2 g q8–12h, up to 2 g q4h.
Child: **IV/IM** ≥ 6 mo, 50 mg/ kg q6–8h, up to 200 mg/kg/d.

PHARMACOKINETICS **Peak:** 1 h after IM or IV. **Distribution:** crosses placenta. **Metabolism:** not metabolized. **Elimination:** half-life: 25–60 min; 80–90% excreted unchanged in urine in 24 h; small amount excreted in breast milk.

CONTRAINDICATIONS & PRECAUTIONS **Contraindicated in:** hypersensitivity to cephalosporins and other beta-lactam antibiotics. Safe use during pregnancy (category B) and for infants and children not established. **Cautious use in:** nursing mothers.

ADVERSE/SIDE EFFECTS **GI:** nausea, vomiting, diarrhea, pseudomembranous colitis. **Hypersensitivity:** rash, pruritus, fever. **Other:** phlebitis. ***Vaginitis (local):*** burning, cellulitis. ***Injection sites:*** pain, induration, paresthesia.

DIAGNOSTIC TEST INTERFERENCE Ceftizoxime causes false-positive direct Coombs' test (may interfere with ***cross-matching procedures*** and ***hematologic studies***).

DRUG INTERACTIONS **Probenecid** decreases renal elimination of ceftizoxime.

INCOMPATIBILITIES **Solution/additive:** AMINOGLYCOSIDES. **Y-site:** AMINOGLYCOSIDES.

NURSING IMPLICATIONS

Administration
- For IV administration, dilute each 1 g with 10 ml sterile water. May be given by direct IV over 3–5 min or further diluted in 50–100 ml of D5W or NS and infused over 30 min.
- Store sterile powder at 15–30C (59–86F); protect from light. Consult manufacturer's directions concerning storage of reconstituted solutions.

Assessment & Drug Effects
- Before therapy is instituted, determine history of hypersensitivity reactions to cephalosporins, penicillin, or other drugs. Report to physician history of allergy, particularly to drugs.
- Culture and sensitivity tests should be performed before initiation of therapy and periodically during therapy if indicated. Therapy may be instituted pending test results.
- Be alert to symptoms of hypersensitivity reaction (see Appendix G). Serious reactions may require emergency measures.
- It is not known whether this cephalosporin causes false-positive results with urine glucose determination using cupric sulfate solution (Benedict's reagent, or Clinitest).

Patient & Family Education
- Instruct patient to report loose stools or diarrhea promptly.
- Advise patient to report symptoms of hypersensitivity (see Appendix G) promptly.

CEFTRIAXONE SODIUM

(sef-try-ax′one)

Trade name: Rocephin

Classifications: ANTIINFECTIVE; AN-

TIBIOTIC; THIRD-GENERATION CEPHALOSPORIN
Prototype: Cefotaxime
Pregnancy category: B

C

ACTIONS/PHARMACODYNAMICS Semisynthetic third-generation cephalosporin antibiotic. Preferentially binds to one or more of the penicillin-binding proteins (PBP) located on cell walls of susceptible organisms. This inhibits third and final stage of bacterial cell wall synthesis, thus killing the bacterium. Spectrum of activity similar to that of cefotaxime including most Enterobacteriaceae, most gram-positive aerobic cocci, *Neisseria meningitidis,* and most strains of penicillinase-producing and nonpenicillinase-producing *Neisseria gonorrhoeae*. Has some activity against *Treponema pallidum* but none against most strains of clostridia.

USES Infections caused by susceptible organisms in lower respiratory tract, skin and skin structures, urinary tract, bones and joints; also intraabdominal infections, pelvic inflammatory disease, uncomplicated gonorrhea, meningitis, and surgical prophylaxis.

ROUTE & DOSAGE

Moderate to Severe Infections

Adult: **IV/IM** 1–2 g q12–24h (max 4 g/d).
Child: **IV/IM** 50–75 mg/kg/d in 2 divided doses (max 2 g/d).

Meningitis

Adult: **IV/IM** 2 g q12h.
Child: **IV/IM** 75 mg/kg loading dose, then 100 mg/kg/d in 2 divided doses (max 4 g/d).

Surgical Prophylaxis

Adult: **IV/IM** 1 g 30–120 min before surgery.

Uncomplicated Gonorrhea

Adult: **IM** 250 mg as single dose.
Child: **IM** 125 mg as single dose.

PHARMACOKINETICS Peak: 1.5–4 h after IM; immediately after IV infusion. **Distribution:** widely distributed in body tissues and fluids; good CNS penetration, especially with inflamed meninges; crosses placenta. **Metabolism:** not metabolized. **Elimination:** half-life: 5–10 h; 33–65% excreted unchanged in urine; also excreted in bile; small amount excreted in breast milk.

CONTRAINDICATIONS & PRECAUTIONS Contraindicated in: hypersensitivity to cephalosporins and related antibiotics. Safe use during pregnancy (category B) not established. **Cautious use in:** nursing mothers.

ADVERSE/SIDE EFFECTS GI: *diarrhea,* abdominal cramps, pseudomembranous colitis. **Gynecologic:** genital pruritus; moniliasis. **Hypersensitivity:** pruritus, fever, chills. **Other:** pain, induration at IM injection site; phlebitis (IV site); biliary sludge.

DIAGNOSTIC TEST INTERFERENCE Causes prolonged PT during therapy.

DRUG INTERACTIONS Probenecid decreases renal elimination of ceftriaxone; **alcohol** produces disulfiram reaction.

INCOMPATIBILITIES Solution/additive: aminophylline, theophylline, AMINOGLYCOSIDES, **clindamycin. Y-site:** AMINOGLYCOSIDES, **pentamidine**.

NURSING IMPLICATIONS

Administration

- For IV administration, dilute each 250 mg with 2.4 ml of sterile water, D5W, or NS to yield 100 mg/ml. Further dilute with 50–100 ml D5W or NS and infuse over 30 min.
- IV administration to infants and children: Verify correct IV concentration and rate of infusion with physician.
- Reconstituted solutions should be light yellow to amber.
- Because of its long elimination half-life, ceftriaxone can be given in a single daily dose instead of multiple doses.
- Protect sterile powder from light. Store at 15–25C (59–77F). Reconstituted solutions: diluent, concentration of solutions are determinants of stability. See manufacturer's instructions.

Assessment & Drug Effects

- Culture and sensitivity tests should be performed before initiation of therapy and periodically during therapy. Dosage may be started pending test results.
- Before therapy is initiated, determine history of hypersensitivity reactions to cephalosporins and penicillins and history of other allergies, particularly to drugs.
- Inspect injection sites for induration and inflammation. Rotate sites. Note IV injection sites for signs of phlebitis (redness, swelling, pain).
- No dosage adjustment is necessary if patient has hepatic or renal impairment; however, if impairment is severe, blood levels are carefully monitored.
- Monitor for manifestations of hypersensitivity (see Signs & Symptoms, Appendix G). Report their appearance promptly and discontinue drug.
- Ceftriaxone appears to alter vitamin K-producing gut bacteria; therefore, hypoprothrombinemic bleeding may occur. Watch for and report signs: petechiae, ecchymotic areas, epistaxis, or any unexplained bleeding.
- The incidence of antibiotic-produced pseudomembranous colitis (see Appendix G) is higher than with most cephalosporins. Most vulnerable patients: chronically ill or debilitated elderly patients undergoing abdominal surgery and those who may be in intensive care. If diarrhea occurs, check for fever. Report both promptly.

Patient & Family Education

- Report any signs of bleeding.
- Report loose stools or diarrhea promptly.

CEFUROXIME SODIUM

(se-fyoor-ox′eem)

Trade names: Kefurox, Zinacef

CEFUROXIME AXETIL

Trade name: Ceftin

Classifications: ANTIINFECTIVE; ANTIBIOTIC; SECOND-GENERATION CEPHALOSPORIN

Prototype: Cefonicid

Pregnancy category: B

ACTIONS/PHARMACODYNAMICS

Semisynthetic second-generation cephalosporin antibiotic with structure similar to that of the penicillins. Resistance against beta-lactamase-producing strains exceeds that of first generation cephalosporins. Antimicrobial spectrum of activity resembles that of cefonicid. Preferentially binds to one or more of the penicillin-binding proteins (PBP) located on cell walls of susceptible or-

C

ganisms. This inhibits third and final stage of bacterial cell wall synthesis, thus killing the bacterium. Partial cross-allergenicity between other beta-lactam antibiotics and cephalosporins has been reported.

USES Infections caused by susceptible organisms in the lower respiratory tract, urinary tract, skin, and skin structures; also used for treatment of meningitis, gonorrhea, and otitis media and for perioperative prophylaxis (e.g., open-heart surgery), early Lyme disease.

ROUTE & DOSAGE

Moderate to Severe Infections

Adult: **PO** 250–500 mg q12h. **IV/IM** 750 mg–1.5 g q6–8h.
Child (3 mo–12 y): **PO** 10–15 mg/kg (125–250 mg) q12h. **IV/IM** 75–100 mg/kg/d divided q8h (max 6 g/d).
Neonate: **IM/IV** 20–100 mg/kg/d divided q12h.

Bacterial Meningitis

Adult: **IV/IM** 3 g q8h.
Child: **IV/IM** 200–240 mg/kg/d divided q6–8h; reduced to 100 mg/kg/d upon improvement.

Surgical Prophylaxis

Adult: **IV/IM** 1.5 g 30–60 min before surgery, then 750 mg q8h for 24 h.
Child: **IV/IM** Same as for adult.

PHARMACOKINETICS **Absorption:** axetil salt well absorbed from GI tract; hydrolyzed to active drug in GI mucosa. **Peak effect:** PO 2 h; IM 30 min. **Distribution:** widely distributed in body tissues and fluids; adequate CNS penetration with inflamed meninges; crosses placenta. **Elimination:** half-life: 1–2 h; 66–100% excreted in urine in 24 h; excreted in breast milk.

CONTRAINDICATIONS & PRECAUTIONS **Contraindicated in:** hypersensitivity to cephalosporins and related antibiotics. Safe use during pregnancy (category B), in nursing women, and in children <3 mo not established. **Cautious use in:** history of allergy, particularly to drugs; penicillin sensitivity; renal insufficiency; history of colitis or other GI disease; potent diuretics.

ADVERSE/SIDE EFFECTS **GI:** *diarrhea,* nausea, antibiotic-associated colitis. **Hypersensitivity:** rash, pruritus, urticaria, positive Coombs' test. **Renal:** increased serum creatinine and BUN, decreased creatinine clearance. **Other:** local reactions: thrombophlebitis (IV site); pain, burning, cellulitis (IM site); superinfections.

DIAGNOSTIC TEST INTERFERENCE Cefuroxime causes false-positive (black-brown or green-brown color) ***urine glucose*** reaction with copper reduction reagents, e.g., Benedict's or Clinitest, but not with enzymatic glucose oxidase reagents, e.g., Clinistix, TesTape. False-positive direct Coombs' test (may interfere with ***cross-matching procedures*** and ***hematologic studies***) has been reported.

DRUG INTERACTIONS **Probenecid** decreases renal elimination of cefuroxime, thus prolonging its action.

INCOMPATIBILITIES **Solution/additive:** AMINOGLYCOSIDES, **doxapram, sodium bicarbonate.** **Y-site:** AMINOGLYCOSIDES, **sodium bicarbonate.**

NURSING IMPLICATIONS

Administration

- Cefuroxime tablets and oral suspension are not substitutable on a mg/mg basis.

- The oral suspension is for infants and children 3 mo to 12 y. Each teaspoon (5 ml) contains the equivalent of 125 mg cefuroxime. Shake oral suspension well before each use.
- Shake IM suspension gently before administration. IM injections should be made deeply into large muscle mass. Rotate injection sites.
- For IV administration, dilute each 750 mg with 9 ml sterile water, D5W, or NS. May be given by direct IV or further diluted in 50–100 ml of compatible solution. May also be added to 1000 ml of IV solution for continuous infusion.
- For direct intermittent IV, solution is injected slowly into a vein over 3–5 min, or injection may be made slowly through tubing system of a freely running compatible IV solution.
- For intermittent infusion, administer over 30 min. Rate of continuous infusion should be ordered by physician.
- IV administration to neonates, infants and children: Verify correct IV concentration and rate of infusion/injection with physician.
- Cefuroxime powder and solutions of the drug may range in color from light yellow to amber without adversely affecting product potency.
- When reconstituted as directed with sterile water for injection, solutions retain potency 24 h at room temperature and 48 h under refrigeration (5C); then they should be discarded.
- Store powder at 15–30C (59–86F) protected from light unless otherwise directed.
- After reconstitution, store suspension at 2–30C (36–86F). Discard after 10 d.

Assessment & Drug Effects

- Culture and susceptibility tests should be performed before initiation of therapy and periodically during therapy, if indicated. Therapy may be instituted pending test results.
- Before therapy is initiated, determine history of hypersensitivity reactions to cephalosporins, penicillins, and history of allergies, particularly to drugs.
- Inspect IM and IV injection sites frequently for signs of phlebitis.
- Report onset of loose stools or diarrhea. Although pseudomembranous colitis (see Signs & Symptoms, Appendix G) rarely occurs, this potentially life-threatening complication should be ruled out as the cause of diarrhea during and after antibiotic therapy.
- Monitor for manifestations of hypersensitivity (see Appendix G). Discontinue drug and report their appearance promptly.
- Monitor I&O ratio and pattern, especially in severely ill patients receiving high doses. Report any significant changes.

Patient & Family Education

- Advise patient to report loose stools or diarrhea promptly.
- Advise patient to report signs and symptoms of hypersensitivity (see Appendix G).

CELECOXIB

(cel-e-cox′ib)

Trade name: Celebrex

Classifications: CNS AGENT, ANALGESIC, NSAID, CYCLOOXYGENASE-2 INHIBITOR, ANTIPYRETIC

Prototype: Ibuprofen

Pregnancy category: C (first and second trimesters), D (third trimester)

ACTIONS/PHARMACODYNAMICS NSAID that exhibits antiinflammatory, analgesic, and antipyretic activities. Unlike ibuprofen, inhibits prostaglandin synthesis by inhibiting cyclooxygenase-2 (COX-2), but does not inhibit cyclooxygenase-1 (COX-1).

USE Relief of signs and symptoms of osteoarthritis and rheumatoid arthritis.

ROUTE & DOSAGE

Arthritis

Adult: **PO** 100–200 mg b.i.d. or 200 mg q.d.

PHARMACOKINETICS **Peak:** 3 h. **Distribution:** 97% protein bound; crosses placenta. **Metabolism:** metabolized in liver by cytochrome P450 2C9 enzymes. **Elimination:** half-life: 11.2 h; excreted primarily in feces (57%), 27% excreted in urine.

CONTRAINDICATIONS & PRECAUTIONS **Contraindicated in:** severe hepatic impairment; hypersensitivity to celecoxib; asthmatic patients with aspirin triad; advanced renal disease; concurrent use of diuretics and ACE inhibitors; anemia; pregnancy (category D) in third trimester. **Cautious use in:** patients who are P450 2C9 poor metabolizers; patients who weigh < 50 kg; moderate hepatic impairment; renal insufficiency; aspirin use; prior history of GI bleeding or peptic ulcer disease; asthmatics; pregnancy (category C) in first and second trimesters, and category D in third trimester; elevated liver function tests; heart failure; kidney disease; hypertension; fluid retention.

ADVERSE/SIDE EFFECTS **Body as whole:** back pain, peripheral edema. **CNS:** dizziness, headache, insomnia. **GI:** abdominal pain, diarrhea, dyspepsia, flatulence, nausea. **Respiratory:** pharyngitis, rhinitis, sinusitis, URI. **Skin:** rash.

DRUG INTERACTIONS May diminish effectiveness of ACE inhibitors; **fluconazole** increases celecoxib concentrations; may increase **lithium** concentrations.

NURSING IMPLICATIONS

Administration

- Celecoxib may be more effective if given 2 h before/after magnesium or aluminum-containing antacids.
- Store at 15–30C (59–86F) in tightly closed container and protect from light.

Assessment & Drug Effects

- Therapeutic effectiveness is indicated by relief of joint pain.
- Lab tests: Periodically monitor Hct and Hgb, liver functions, BUN and creatinine, and serum electrolytes.
- Periodically monitor lithium levels when the two drugs are given concurrently.
- Monitor for fluid retention and edema especially in those with a history of hypertension or CHF.

Patient & Family Education

- Pregnant women should avoid using celecoxib during the third trimester of pregnancy.
- Promptly report any of the following: unexplained weight gain, edema, skin rash.
- Stop taking celecoxib and promptly report to physician if any of the following occur: S&S of liver dysfunction including nausea, fatigue, lethargy, itching, jaundice, abdominal pain, and flulike symptoms; S&S of GI ulceration including black, tarry stools and upper GI distress.

C

CELLULOSE SODIUM PHOSPHATE (CSP)

Trade name: Calcibind
Classifications: RESIN EXCHANGE AGENT, CATION; ANTILITHIC
Pregnancy category: C

ACTIONS/PHARMACODYNAMICS When taken with meals, releases sodium in exchange for bivalent cations (e.g., dietary and secreted calcium and magnesium) in intestines to form a nonabsorbable complex. Binding of these bivalent ions renders them unavailable for complexing with oxalate; thus formation of renal calculi is inhibited. Does not generally cause significant alterations in serum phosphate or calcium in most patients. Serum magnesium is predictably reduced, however, and therefore supplemention is necessary.

USES Adjunct to dietary restriction to reduce renal calculi formation in absorptive hypercalciuria type I with recurrent calcium oxalate and calcium phosphate nephrolithiasis. **Unlabeled uses:** adjunct in treatment of hypercalcemia (e.g., associated with parathyroid carcinoma or sarcoidosis) and in management of calcinosis cutis.

ROUTE & DOSAGE

Urinary Calcium Exceeding 300 mg/d

Adult: **PO** Initial: 5 g t.i.d. with each meal; decrease to 5 g with the main meal and 2.5 g with the other 2 meals when urinary calcium is <150 mg/d.

PHARMACOKINETICS Absorption: not absorbed from GI tract. **Metabolism:** partially hydrolyzed in intestines, causing release of phosphorous ions, which are absorbed by the intestines. **Elimination:** nonabsorbable complex of calcium and cellulose phosphate excreted in feces along with unchanged resin.

CONTRAINDICATIONS & PRECAUTIONS Contraindicated in: bone disease, hypocalcemia, hypomagnesemia, hyperoxaluria; primary and secondary hyperparathyroidism, including renal hypercalciuria; high fasting urinary calcium or hypophosphatemia; conditions associated with high skeletal mobilization of calcium. Safe use during pregnancy (category C), in nursing mothers, and in children <16 y not established. **Cautious use in:** sodium restriction, CHF, ascites, nephrotic syndrome.

ADVERSE/SIDE EFFECTS GI: loose stools, diarrhea, GI discomfort, dyspepsia, anorexia, nausea, vomiting. **With long-term use:** <u>hypomagnesemia</u>, hypomagnesuria, hyperoxaluria, acute arthritis, arthralgia, hyperparathyroid bone disease, symptoms related to electrolyte imbalances, or depletion of trace elements copper, zinc, and iron.

DRUG INTERACTIONS CALCIUM SUPPLEMENTS counteract calcium-lowering effects of CSP; CSP also binds **magnesium,** decreasing its absorption—separate administration by at least 1 h; THIAZIDE DIURETICS may have additive effects; **ascorbic acid** is metabolized to oxalate and can counteract oxalate-lowering effects of CSP.

NURSING IMPLICATIONS

Administration

- Powder can be mixed with full glass (240 ml) of water, soft drink, or fruit juice and taken with meals. CSP is not palatable.

C

- Oral magnesium supplement (e.g., magnesium gluconate) should be administered to prevent hypomagnesemia. It can be given at any time as long as it is at least 1 h before or after CSP to avoid binding of magnesium.
- Doses of oral magnesium supplement depend on dose of CSP. Patients receiving 15 g/d of CSP should take 1.5 g magnesium gluconate before breakfast and again at bedtime (separately from CSP). Patients taking 10 g/d of CSP should take 1 g magnesium gluconate twice a day.
- Store in tightly closed container at 15–30C (59–86F), protected from moisture, unless otherwise directed.

Assessment & Drug Effects

- Monitor I&O ratio and pattern. Fluid intake should be encouraged to maintain a urinary output of at least 2 L/d (approximately 240 ml/h while awake).
- Serum parathyroid hormone (PTH) levels should be evaluated at least once between first 2 wk– 3 mo of therapy, and then every 3–6 mo during therapy. Serum and urinary calcium and oxalate, serum magnesium, copper, iron, and zinc, and CBC should be monitored every 3–6 mo throughout therapy.
- Observe urinary calcium levels. A reduction of less than 30 mg/5 g in urinary calcium in patients on moderate calcium and sodium restriction indicates treatment failure. Drug is usually discontinued.
- Discontinuation of therapy is also indicated in patients on moderate oxalate restriction with urinary oxalate levels in excess of 55 mg/d. A rise in serum PTH above normal also points to the need to adjust dosage or stop the drug.
- To increase therapeutic effectiveness of CSP, dietary restriction of sodium, calcium, oxalate, and ascorbic acid is essential. Collaborate with physician and dietitian.
- With long-term use, monitor for manifestations of hypomagnesemia (see Signs & Symptoms, Appendix G).

Patient & Family Education

- Be sure that patient understands drug will not work unless it is taken with meals or at least within 30 min of a meal.
- Instruct patients on long-term therapy to report signs and symptoms of hypomagnesemia (see Appendix G).

CEPHALEXIN

(sef-a-lex′in)

Trade names: Cefanex, Ceporex♣, Keflet, Keflex, Keftab, Novolexin♣

Classifications: ANTIINFECTIVE; ANTIBIOTIC; FIRST-GENERATION CEPHALOSPORIN

Prototype: Cephalothin

Pregnancy category: B

ACTIONS/PHARMACODYNAMICS

Semisynthetic derivative of cephalosporin C. Broad-spectrum, first-generation cephalosporin antibiotic with antiinfective activity similar to that of cephalothin but reportedly less potent. Preferentially binds to one or more of the penicillin-binding proteins (PBP) located on cell walls of susceptible organisms. This inhibits third and final stage of bacterial cell wall synthesis, thus killing the bacterium. Ineffective against many gram-negative or anaerobic organisms. Cross-allergenicity between cephalosporins and penicillins has been reported.

C

USES To treat infections caused by susceptible pathogens in respiratory and urinary tracts, middle ear, skin, soft tissue, and bone.

ROUTE & DOSAGE

Mild to Moderate Infection

Adult: **PO** 250–500 mg q6h.
Child: **PO** 25–100 mg/kg/d in 4 divided doses.

Skin and Skin Structure Infections

Adult: **PO** 500 mg q12h.

Otitis Media

Child: **PO** 75–100 mg/kg/d in 4 divided doses.

PHARMACOKINETICS Absorption: rapidly absorbed from GI tract; stable in stomach acid. **Peak:** 1 h. **Distribution:** widely distributed in body fluids with highest concentration in kidney; crosses placenta. **Elimination:** half-life: 38–70 min; 80–100% eliminated unchanged in urine in 8 h; excreted in breast milk.

CONTRAINDICATIONS & PRECAUTIONS Contraindicated in: hypersensitivity to cephalosporins and related antibiotics. Safe use during pregnancy (category B), by nursing mothers, and infants <1 mo not established. **Cautious use in:** history of hypersensitivity to penicillin or other drug allergy; severely impaired renal function.

ADVERSE/SIDE EFFECTS CNS: dizziness, headache, fatigue. **GI:** *diarrhea* (generally mild), nausea, vomiting, anorexia, abdominal pain. **Hypersensitivity:** angioedema, rash, urticaria, anaphylaxis. **Other:** superinfections.

DIAGNOSTIC TEST INTERFERENCE False-positive ***urine glucose*** determinations using copper sulfate reagents, e.g., Clinitest, Benedict's reagent, but not with glucose oxidase (enzymatic) tests, e.g., Tes-Tape, Diastix, Clinistix. Positive direct Coombs' test may complicate transfusion ***cross-matching procedures*** and ***hematologic studies.***

DRUG INTERACTIONS Probenecid decreases renal elimination of cephalexin.

NURSING IMPLICATIONS

Administration

- Cephalexin is not destroyed by gastric acid, but peak blood levels are slightly lower and delayed when cephalexin is administered with food. Total amount absorbed, however, is unchanged.
- Cephalexin oral suspension should be refrigerated; discard unused portions 14 d after preparation. Label should indicate expiration date. Keep tightly covered. Shake suspension well before pouring.
- Store capsules and tablets at 15–30C (59–86F) unless otherwise specified.

Assessment & Drug Effects

- Periodic evaluations of renal and hepatic function should be made in patients receiving prolonged therapy.
- Monitor for manifestations of hypersensitivity (see Signs & Symptoms, Appendix G). Discontinue drug and report their appearance promptly.

Patient & Family Education

- Take medication for the full course of therapy as directed by physician.
- Drug therapy for beta-hemolytic streptococcal infections should continue for at least 10 d to guard

against risk of rheumatic fever and glomerulonephritis.

- Keep physician informed if adverse reactions appear.
- Be alert to signs and symptoms of superinfections (see Appendix G). These symptoms should be reported promptly and appropriate therapy instituted.

CEPHALOTHIN SODIUM

(sef-a'loe-thin)

Trade names: Ceporacin✤, Keflin, Seffin

Prototype for classifications: ANTIINFECTIVE; BETA-LACTAM ANTIBIOTIC; FIRST-GENERATION CEPHALOSPORIN

Pregnancy category: B

ACTIONS/PHARMACODYNAMICS Semisynthetic first generation cephalosporin is derived from cephalosporin C. Drug structure characterized by a beta-lactam ring (like the penicillin structure). First-generation cephalosporins are characterized by the most narrow gram-negative antibacterial spectrum and by the greatest antibacterial activity against gram-positive bacteria when compared to second and third generation agents. Preferentially binds to one or more of the penicillin-binding proteins (PBP) located on cell walls of susceptible organisms. This inhibits third and final stage of bacterial wall synthesis, thus killing the bacterium. Active against gram-positive organisms including staphylococci, *Streptococcus pneumoniae,* beta-hemolytic streptococci, *Streptococcus faecalis;* and against gram-negative microbes including *Escherichia coli, Klebsiella* sp, *Proteus mirabilis;* variable activity on *Salmonella* sp, *Hemophilus influenzae, Shigella* sp, *Bacteroides fragilis,* and anaerobes.

USES Severe infections of respiratory, GI, and GU tracts; bone and joint infections, skin and soft tissue infections; and for septicemia, endocarditis, meningitis. Also used for perioperative prophylaxis in patients with high risk of infection. Used in intraperitoneal dialysis procedures. **Unlabeled use:** treatment of ventriculitis in hydrocephalic children.

ROUTE & DOSAGE

Moderate to Severe Infections

Adult: **IV/IM** 250 mg–2 g q4–6h, up to 2 g q4h (max 12 g/d).
Child: **IV/IM** 80–160 mg/kg/d in 4–6 divided doses.
Neonate: **IV** ≤7 d: 40–60 mg/kg/d divided q8–12h; >7 d: 40–80 mg/kg/d divided q6–12h.

Surgical Prophylaxis

Adult: **IV/IM** 1–2 g 30–60 min before surgery, then q6h for 24 h.
Child: **IV/IM** 20–30 mg/kg 30–60 min before surgery, then q6h for 24 h.

PHARMACOKINETICS **Peak levels:** 30 min after IM; 15 min after IV. **Distribution:** poor CNS penetration except with inflamed meninges; penetrates aqueous humor and other body fluids; crosses placenta. **Elimination:** half-life: 30–60 min; 52–75% excreted unchanged in urine in 24 h; small amount excreted in breast milk.

CONTRAINDICATIONS & PRECAUTIONS **Contraindicated in:** hypersensitivity to cephalosporin. Safety for use during pregnancy (category B) not determined. **Cautious use in:** history of allergies to other beta-lactams; impaired renal or hepatic function, patient on sodium restriction; nursing mothers; concomitant use of high doses of heparin; GI disease, especially colitis.

ADVERSE/SIDE EFFECTS **CNS:** dizziness, vertigo, headache, fatigue, malaise. **GI:** dysgeusia, glossitis, *nausea, vomiting,* anorexia, abdominal cramps, *diarrhea,* flatulence, pseudomembranous enterocolitis. **Hematologic:** agranulocytosis (rare). **Hypersensitivity:** morbilliform rash, pruritus, urticaria, serum sickness-like reactions, anaphylactic shock, eosinophilia, drug fever. **Other:** superinfections, especially *Pseudomonas* or *Candida;* local reactions: pain, induration, slough, abscess (IM site); thrombophlebitis (IV site).

DIAGNOSTIC TEST INTERFERENCE Most cephalosporins cause false-positive (black-brown or green-brown color) ***urine glucose*** reaction with copper reduction reagents, e.g., Benedict's or Clinitest, but not with enzymatic glucose oxidase reagents, e.g., Clinistix, TesTape. With high doses, falsely elevated ***serum and urine creatinine*** (with Jaffe reaction) reported. False-positive direct Coombs' test (may interfere with ***cross-matching procedures*** and ***hematologic studies***), false-positive ***urinary protein*** (sulfosalicylic acid method), and falsely elevated ***urinary 17-ketosteroids*** (Zimmerman reaction) have also been reported.

DRUG INTERACTION **Probenecid** decreases renal elimination.

INCOMPATIBILITIES **Solution/additive:** AMINOGLYCOSIDES, **aminophylline, bleomycin, cimetidine, colistimethate, cytarabine, diphenhydramine, dopamine, methylprednisolone, calcium chloride, calcium gluceptate, calcium gluconate, erythromycin,** TETRACYCLINES, **penicillin G, phenobarbital, polymyxin B, metoclopramide. Y-site:** AMINOGLYCOSIDES, **cytarabine, erythromycin, tetracyclines, polymyxin B,** METOCLOPRAMIDE.

NURSING IMPLICATIONS

Administration

- IM injection is prepared by adding 4 ml sterile water for injection to each gram of cephalothin (resultant solution: 500 mg/2.2 ml). If vial contents do not completely dissolve, add more diluent (0.2–0.4 ml), and warm vial slightly.
- IM injection causes intense pain and induration. If cephalothin IM is prescribed, administer injection deep into large muscle mass such as gluteus maximus or lateral aspect of thigh. Rotate injection sites.
- IV preparation: Dilute each 1 g with at least 10 ml sterile water for injection. Reconstituted solution may be further diluted with IV solution recommended by manufacturer.
- IV administration: IV cephalothin may be given by direct IV at a rate of 1 g over 3–5 min or by intermittent infusion.
- IV administration to neonates, infants and children: Verify correct IV concentration and rate of infusion with physician.
- Risk of phlebitis may be reduced by use of a small needle in a large vein for IV administration.
- Solutions for IM and intermittent IV infusion (may be stored at room temperature) should be administered within 12 h after reconstitution. Replace freshly prepared solution every 24 h in prolonged treatment with IV infusion.
- Slight discoloration of solution may occur, especially when stored

at room temperature; however, this does not affect potency.

- Refrigeration protects potency for 96 h after reconstitution.

Assessment & Drug Effects

- Culture and sensitivity tests should be performed before and during therapy. Therapy may be started pending test results.
- Before therapy is initiated, determine history of hypersensitivity to cephalosporins or penicillins, other allergies, particularly to drugs.
- Observe IV sites for evidence of inflammatory reaction. IV infusions of doses larger than 6 g/d for > 3 d can result in thrombophlebitis.
- Report falling urinary output or change in I&O ratio. Patients with renal dysfunction and those receiving high doses in the presence of dehydration are particularly susceptible to nephrotoxic reactions.
- Superinfections caused by overgrowth of nonsusceptible organisms may occur, particularly during prolonged use of cephalosporins.
- Antibiotic-associated pseudomembranous enterocolitis is a life-threatening superinfection caused by *Clostridium difficile;* may occur in 4–9 d or as long as 6 wk after cephalothin is discontinued. Most apt to occur in the chronically ill or debilitated elderly patient, especially if undergoing abdominal surgery or if in an intensive care unit.
- If diarrhea occurs, check for fever. Report diarrhea and fever promptly.
- Periodic hematologic studies including PT and PTT and evaluations of renal and hepatic functions are recommended in patients receiving high doses and during prolonged therapy.
- If an unexplained fever develops, check temperature twice daily. If temperature remains high, suspect drug-induced fever. Discuss with physician.

Patient & Family Education

- Report early signs of superinfections (see Appendix G).
- Report loose stools or diarrhea promptly.
- Yogurt or buttermilk, 120 ml (4 oz) of either (if allowed), may serve as a prophylactic against intestinal superinfection by helping to maintain normal intestinal flora.
- Signs and symptoms of hypersensitivity reaction (see Appendix G) should be reported promptly. Drug should be discontinued.
- Advise patient to report signs of hemostatic defects (ecchymoses, petechiae, nose bleeds).

CEPHAPIRIN SODIUM

(sef-a-pye′rin)

Trade name: Cefadyl

Classifications: ANTIINFECTIVE; ANTIBIOTIC; FIRST-GENERATION CEPHALOSPORIN

Prototype: Cephalothin

Pregnancy category: B

ACTIONS/PHARMACODYNAMICS

Semisynthetic, first-generation, broad-spectrum cephalosporin antibiotic similar to cephalothin. Reported to cause less tissue irritation and to be less nephrotoxic than cephalothin. Preferentially binds to one or more of the penicillin-binding proteins (PBP) located on cell walls of susceptible organisms. This inhibits third and final stage of bacterial cell wall synthesis, thus killing the bacterium. Cross-allergenicity between cephalosporins and penicillins has been reported.

USES Serious infections of respiratory and urinary tracts, skin and soft tissue, and for osteomyelitis, septicemia, and endocarditis caused by susceptible pathogens, e.g., group A beta-hemolytic streptococci, penicillinase- and nonpenicillinase-producing *Staphylococcus aureus, Streptococcus pneumoniae, viridans streptococci, Hemophilus influenzae, Escherichia coli, Proteus mirabilis,* and *Klebsiella* sp; also to prevent postoperative infection when infection at operative site is a risk.

ROUTE & DOSAGE

Mild to Moderate Infection

Adult: **IM/IV** 500 mg–1 g q4–6h up to 12 g/d.
Child: **IM/IV** 40–80 mg/kg/d in 4 divided doses.

Perioperative Prophylaxis

Adult: **IM/IV** 1–2 g 30–60 min before surgery; 1–2 g during surgery; then 1–2 g q6h for 24 h.

Adjustment for Renal Impairment

Cl_{cr} < 5 mg/dl: IM/IV 7.5–15 mg/kg q12h.

PHARMACOKINETICS **Peak:** 30 min after IM; 5 min after IV. **Distribution:** widely distributed in body fluids with highest concentration in kidney; crosses placenta. **Metabolism:** partially metabolized in liver and kidneys. **Elimination:** half-life: 36–54 min; 60–85% eliminated unchanged in urine in 6 h; excreted in breast milk.

CONTRAINDICATIONS & PRECAUTIONS **Contraindicated in:** hypersensitivity to cephalosporins and related antibiotics. Safe use during pregnancy (category B), in nursing mothers, and in children <3 mo not established. **Cautious use in:** history of sensitivity to penicillins and other allergies, particularly to drugs; sodium restriction, impaired renal function.

ADVERSE/SIDE EFFECTS **GI:** nausea, vomiting, *diarrhea,* abdominal cramps. **Hypersensitivity:** rash, urticaria, drug fever, eosinophilia, serum sickness–like reactions, <u>anaphylaxis</u>. **Other:** needle site reactions (infrequent).

DIAGNOSTIC TEST INTERFERENCE False-positive ***urine glucose*** determinations, using copper sulfate reduction methods, e.g., Clinitest or Benedict's reagent, but not with glucose oxidase (enzymatic) tests, e.g., Clinistix, Diastix, TesTape. Positive Coombs' test may complicate ***cross-matching procedures*** and ***hematologic studies.***

DRUG INTERACTIONS **Probenecid** decreases renal elimination of cephapirin.

INCOMPATIBILITIES **Solution/additive:** AMINOGLYCOSIDES, **aminophylline, ascorbic acid, epinephrine, norepinephrine, mannitol, phenytoin,** TETRACYCLINES, **thiopental.** **Y-site:** AMINOGLYCOSIDES, TETRACYCLINES, **thiopental, phenytoin.**

NURSING IMPLICATIONS

Administration

- IM injections should be made deep into large muscle mass. Rotate injection sites.
- For IM use, the 500 mg and 1 g vials are reconstituted with 1 or 2 ml sterile water for injection or bacteriostatic water for injection, respectively. Resulting solutions will contain 500 mg of cephapirin per 1.2 ml.

C

- For direct IV injection the 1 g or 2 g vial is reconstituted with 10 ml or more 0.9% NaCl injection, bacteriostatic water for injection, or dextrose injection. May be given by direct IV over 5 min or may be further diluted with 50–100 ml of D5W or NS and infused over 30 min.
- After reconstitution, depending on diluent and amount used, solutions retain potency for 12–48 h at room temperature or for 10 d if refrigerated at 4C. See package insert for specific information.
- Solutions may become slightly yellow, but this does not affect potency.

Assessment & Drug Effects

- Culture and susceptibility testing should be performed before treatment is begun. Therapy may be initiated before results are obtained.
- Before therapy begins, determine history of previous hypersensitivity to cephalosporins, penicillins, and other allergies, particularly to drugs.
- Periodic monitoring of renal function is important. Advise patient to report changes in I&O ratio and pattern or evidence of blood or pus in urine.
- Monitor for manifestations of hypersensitivity (see Signs & Symptoms, Appendix G). Discontinue drug and report their appearance promptly.

Patient & Family Education

- Advise patient to report promptly signs and symptoms of superinfections (see Appendix G).
- Advise patient to report signs and symptoms of hypersensitivity (see Appendix G).

CEPHRADINE

(sef′ra-deen)

Trade names: Anspor, Velosef

Classifications: ANTIINFECTIVE; ANTIBIOTIC; FIRST-GENERATION CEPHALOSPORIN

Prototype: Cephalothin

Pregnancy category: B

ACTIONS/PHARMACODYNAMICS

Semisynthetic acid-stable, first generation, broad-spectrum cephalosporin similar to cephalothin. Preferentially binds to one or more of the penicillin-binding proteins (PBP) located on cell walls of susceptible organisms. This inhibits third and final stage of bacterial cell wall synthesis, thus killing the bacterium. Cross-allergenicity between cephalosporins and penicillins has been reported.

USES Serious infections of respiratory and urinary tracts, skin and soft tissues, and for otitis media caused by susceptible pathogens; for perioperative prophylaxis, in cesarean section (intraoperative and postoperative); in septicemia (due to *Streptococcus pneumoniae, Staphylococcus aureus, Proteus mirabilis,* and *Escherichia coli*). Also used to treat urinary tract infections due to *Klebsiella* sp and enterococci *(Streptococcus faecalis)*.

ROUTE & DOSAGE

Mild to Moderate Infection

Adult: **PO** 250–500 mg q6h or 500 mg–1 g q12h up to 4 g/d. **IM/IV** 2–4 g/d in 4 divided doses (max 8 g/d).
Child: **PO** 25–50 mg/kg/d in 2–4 divided doses up to 4 g/d. **IM/IV** 50–100 mg/kg/d in 4 divided doses up to 8 g/d.

Perioperative Prophylaxis

Adult: **PO** 1 g 30–60 min before surgery; 1 g during surgery; then 1 g q4–6h for 24 h.

PHARMACOKINETICS **Absorption:** well absorbed from GI tract. **Peak:** 1 h after PO; 1–2 h after IM; 5 min after IV. **Distribution:** widely distributed in body fluids, with highest concentration in kidney; crosses placenta. **Elimination:** half-life: 1–2 h; 80–90% eliminated unchanged in urine in 6 h; excreted in breast milk.

CONTRAINDICATIONS & PRECAUTIONS **Contraindicated in:** hypersensitivity to cephalosporins and related antibiotics. Safe use during pregnancy (category B), in nursing mothers, and children <9 mo not established. **Cautious use in:** history of penicillin or other allergies, particularly to drugs; impaired renal function, sodium restriction (parenteral cephradine).

ADVERSE/SIDE EFFECTS **GI:** *diarrhea* or loose stools, abdominal pain, heartburn. **Hypersensitivity:** urticaria, rash, pruritus, joint pains, eosinophilia. **Other:** dizziness, tightness in chest, pain, induration and tissue sloughing (IM injection site); thrombophlebitis (IV site); paresthesias, superinfections.

DIAGNOSTIC TEST INTERFERENCE Cephradine causes false-positive (black-brown or green-brown color) ***urine glucose*** reaction with copper reduction reagents, e.g., as Benedict's or Clinitest, but not with enzymatic glucose oxidase reagents, e.g., Clinistix, TesTape. False-positive direct Coombs' test (may interfere with ***cross-matching procedures*** and ***hematologic studies***) has also been reported.

DRUG INTERACTIONS **Probenecid** decreases renal elimination of cephradine.

INCOMPATIBILITIES **Solution/additive:** AMINOGLYCOSIDES, TPN SOLUTIONS, other ANTIBIOTICS. **Y-site:** AMINOGLYCOSIDES, TPN SOLUTIONS, other ANTIBIOTICS.

NURSING IMPLICATIONS

Administration

- Oral cephradine may be given without regard to meals (acid stable); however, the presence of food may delay absorption.
- To minimize pain and induration of IM site, inject deep into large muscle mass such as gluteus maximus or lateral aspect of thigh.
- For IV administration, dilute each 500 mg with 5 ml sterile water for injection. May be further diluted (preferred) in 10–20 ml of D5W or NS.
- Give properly diluted solution by direct IV over 3–5 min. May be further diluted in 50–100 ml and infused over 30–60 min.
- The risk of thrombophlebitis may be reduced by proper dilution of IV fluid, use of small IV needles and large veins, and by alternating injection sites.
- Following reconstitution, oral suspension may be stored at room temperature up to 7 d or in refrigerator for up to 14 d. Shake well before pouring.
- After reconstitution, IM or IV solutions should be used within 2 h at room temperature. With refrigeration (5C), potency is retained 24 h. Reconstituted solutions may vary in color from light straw to yellow; this does not affect potency.
- All forms of cephradine are stored at 15–30C (59–86F) unless otherwise directed. Protect from concentrated light or direct sunlight.

Assessment & Drug Effects

- Before therapy is initiated, determine history of previous hypersensitivity to cephalosporins, penicillins, and other drug allergies.
- Culture and sensitivity tests and

renal function studies should be performed before and periodically during drug therapy.

- Recommended dosage schedule in patients with reduced renal function is lowered based on creatinine clearance determinations and severity of infection.
- Inspect IV insertion site frequently for thrombophlebitis (see Signs & Symptoms, Appendix G).
- Pseudomembranous enterocolitis, a potentially life-threatening superinfection caused by *Clostridium difficile,* may occur during or after cephalosporin therapy. If diarrhea occurs, check for fever. Report diarrhea and fever promptly.
- Monitor for signs of superinfection (see Appendix G). Report their appearance promptly.

Patient & Family Education

- Instruct patient to take medication for the full course of therapy as directed by physician. Therapy is usually continued for at least 48–72 h after patient becomes asymptomatic.
- Superinfections caused by overgrowth of nonsusceptible organisms may occur. Instruct patient to report early signs and symptoms (see Appendix G) promptly.
- Instruct patient to report loose stools or diarrhea promptly.

CERIVASTATIN SODIUM

(cer-i-va′sta-tin)

Trade name: Baychol

Classifications: CARDIOVASCULAR AGENT; ANTILIPEMIC; HMG-COA REDUCTASE INHIBITOR (STATIN)

Prototype: Lovastatin

Pregnancy category: X

ACTIONS/PHARMACODYNAMICS Competitively inhibits HMG-CoA reductase, the enzyme that catalyzes cholesterol biosynthesis. HMG-CoA reductase inhibitors increase serum HDL lipoprotein levels, and decrease serum LDL lipoprotein, VLDL lipoprotein, and plasma triglyceride levels. Effective in reducing total cholesterol and LDL lipoprotein in various forms of hypercholesterolemia.

USE Adjunct to diet for reduction of total and LDL cholesterol.

ROUTE & DOSAGE

Cholesterol Reduction

Adult: **PO** 0.3 mg q.d. in evening. **Renal impairment** (Cl_{cr} ≤60 ml/min) 0.2 mg q.d. in evening.

PHARMACOKINETICS Absorption: rapidly absorbed from GI tract; approx 60% reaches systemic circulation. **Distribution:** >99% protein bound; crosses placenta; distributed into breast milk. **Metabolism:** metabolized in liver to active metabolites. **Elimination:** half-life: 2–3 h; 24% excreted in urine, 70% excreted in feces primarily as metabolites.

CONTRAINDICATIONS & PRECAUTIONS Contraindicated in: hypersensitivity to cerivastatin; active hepatic disease or unexplained persistent transaminase elevation; pregnancy (category X); nursing mothers. Safety and efficacy in individuals <18 y not known. **Cautious use in:** history of alcohol abuse or liver disease; renal impairment; sepsis; hypotension; trauma.

ADVERSE/SIDE EFFECTS Body as whole: flulike syndrome, back pain, asthenia, arthralgia, myalgia. **CNS:** headache, dizziness, insomnia. **CV:** chest pain, peripheral edema. **GI:** abdominal pain, dyspepsia, diarrhea, flatulence, nausea constipation. **Respiratory:** rhinitis, pharyngitis, sinusitis, cough. **Skin:** rash.

DRUG INTERACTIONS cyclosporine, clofibrate, erythromycin, AZOLE ANTIFUNGALS, **niacin** may increase risk of rhabdomyolysis; **cholestryamine** (administered simultaneously) can decrease absorption of cerivastatin.

NURSING IMPLICATIONS

Administration
- Cerivastatin should be given in the evening (h.s.) for maximum effectiveness.
- Give at least 1 h before or 4 h after cholestyramine.
- Store at 20–25C (68–77F) in tightly closed container.

Assessment & Drug Effects
- Therapeutic effectiveness is indicated by reduction in level of LDL-C.
- Lab tests: Monitor lipid levels 4 wk after initiation of therapy or change in dosage; monitor liver functions 6 and 12 wk after initiation or elevation of dose and periodically thereafter.
- Assess for muscle pain, tenderness, or weakness and, if present, monitor CPK level. Cerivastatin should be discontinued with marked elevations of CPK or if myopathy is suspected.

Patient & Family Education
- Promptly report any of the following: unexplained muscle pain, tenderness, or weakness, especially with fever or malaise; yellowing of skin or eyes; nausea or loss of appetite; skin rash or hives.
- Cerivastatin taken during pregnancy may cause birth defects. Immediately inform physician of a suspected or known pregnancy.
- Inform the physician regarding concurrent use of cholestyramine, niacin, erythromycin, or antifungals.
- Alcohol intake should be minimized while taking cerivastatin.

CETIRIZINE

(ce-tir′i-zeen)

Trade names: Reactine ♣, Zyrtec

Classifications: ANTIHISTAMINE; H_1-RECEPTOR ANTAGONIST

Prototype: Diphenhydramine

Pregnancy category: B

ACTIONS/PHARMACODYNAMICS Cetirizine is a potent H_1-receptor antihistamine without significant anticholinergic or CNS activity. Low lipophilicity combined with its H_1-receptor selectivity probably accounts for its relative lack of anticholinergic and sedative properties.

USES Seasonal and perennial allergic rhinitis and chronic idiopathic urticaria.

ROUTE & DOSAGE

Allergic Rhinitis

Adult: **PO** 5–10 mg once/d.
Child: **PO** *2–5 y:* 2.5 mg q.d. (max 5 mg/d); *≥6 y:* 5–10 mg q.d.

Chronic Urticaria

Adult: **PO** 10 mg q.d. or b.i.d.

PHARMACOKINETICS Absorption: readily absorbed from GI tract. **Peak:** 1 h. **Distribution:** 93% protein bound; minimal CNS concentrations. **Metabolism:** minimal. **Elimination:** half-life: 7.4 h; 60% excreted unchanged in urine within 24 h, 5% excreted in feces.

C

CONTRAINDICATIONS & PRECAUTIONS **Contraindicated in:** hypersensitivity to H_1-receptor antihistamines. **Cautious use in:** renal impairment, pregnancy (category B), nursing mothers.

ADVERSE/SIDE EFFECTS **CNS:** *drowsiness, sedation, headache,* depression. **GI:** constipation, diarrhea, dry mouth.

NURSING IMPLICATIONS

Administration

- As elimination half-life is prolonged in the elderly, dosage adjustments may be warranted.
- Store at 15–30C (59–86F).

Assessment & Drug Effects

- As the drug is highly protein bound, the potential for interactions with other protein-bound drugs exists.
- Monitor for sedation, especially the elderly.

Patient & Family Education

- Advise not to use in combination with OTC antihistamines.
- Caution to determine response to drug before engaging in hazardous activities.

CHARCOAL, ACTIVATED (LIQUID ANTIDOTE)

Trade names: Actidose, Charcoaid, Charcocaps, Charcodote, Insta-Char

Classifications: ANTIDOTE; ADSORBENT

Pregnancy category: C

ACTIONS/PHARMACODYNAMICS Residue from destructive distillation of organic materials treated to reduce particle size, which increases surface area and adsorptive power. Activated charcoal (carbon) is a chemically inert, odorless, tasteless, fine black powder with wide spectrum of adsorptive activity. Acts by binding (adsorbing) toxic substances, thereby inhibiting their GI absorption, enterohepatic circulation, and thus bioavailability. Recent studies indicate that administration by "gastric dialysis" (repetitive doses) effectively increases clearance of drugs already absorbed into the systemic circulation. Action appears to result from increased rate of drug diffusion from plasma into GI tract where it is adsorbed by activated charcoal.

USES General purpose emergency antidote in the treatment of poisonings by most drugs and chemicals, e.g., acetaminophen, aspirin, atropine, barbiturates, digitalis glycosides, phenytoin, propoxyphene, strychnine, tricyclic antidepressants, among many others. Gastric dialysis (repetitive doses) in uremia to adsorb various waste products from GI tract; severe acute poisoning. Has been used to adsorb intestinal gases in treatment of dyspepsia, flatulence, and distension (value in these conditions not established). Sometimes used topically as a deodorant for foul-smelling wounds and ulcers.

ROUTE & DOSAGE

Acute Poisonings

Adult: **PO** 30–100 g in at least 180–240 ml (6–8 oz) of water or 1 g/kg.
Child 1–12 y: **PO** 1–2 g/kg or 15–30 g in at least 6–8 oz of water.
Infant <1 y: **PO** 1 g/kg.

Gastric Dialysis

Adult: **PO** 20–40 g q6h for 1 or 2 d.

GI Disturbances

Adult: **PO** 520–975 mg p.c. up to 5 g/d.

PHARMACOKINETICS **Absorption:** not absorbed. **Elimination:** excreted in feces.

CONTRAINDICATIONS & PRECAUTIONS **Contraindicated in:** reportedly not effective for poisonings by cyanide, mineral acids, caustic alkalis, organic solvents, iron, ethanol, methanol. Safe use as antiflatulent in children < 3 y not established. **Cautious use in:** pregnancy (category C).

ADVERSE/SIDE EFFECTS Vomiting (rapid ingestion of high doses), constipation, diarrhea (from sorbitol).

DRUG INTERACTIONS May decrease absorption of all other oral medications—administer at least 2 h apart.

NURSING IMPLICATIONS

Administration

- Before using charcoal as an antidote, call a poison control center, an emergency room, or a physician immediately for advice.
- Activated charcoal tablets or capsules are less adsorptive and thus less effective than powder or liquid form; therefore they are not recommended in treatment of acute poisoning.
- Drug is most effective when administered as soon as possible after acute poisoning (preferably within 30 min).
- In an emergency, dose may be approximated by stirring sufficient activated charcoal into tap water to make a slurry the consistency of soup (about 20–30 g in at least 240 ml of water).
- Activated charcoal can be swallowed or given through a nasogastric tube. If administered too rapidly, patient may vomit.
- If necessary, palatability may be improved by adding a small amount of concentrated fruit juice or chocolate powder to the slurry. Reportedly, these agents do not appreciably alter adsorptive activity.
- To prevent adsorption of gases from the air, store in tightly covered container at 15–30C (59–86F) unless otherwise directed.

Assessment & Drug Effects

- Record appearance, color, consistency, frequency, and relative amount of stools. Inform patient that activated charcoal will color feces black.

CHENODIOL (CHENODEOXYCHOLIC ACID)

(kee-noe-dye′ole)
Trade name: Chenix
Classification: GALLSTONE SOLUBILIZING AGENT
Pregnancy category: X

ACTIONS/PHARMACODYNAMICS Naturally occurring human bile acid synthesized by liver. After PO administration of chenodiol, biliary cholesterol saturation decreases, perhaps because of drug-induced suppression of hepatic synthesis of cholesterol and cholic acid and decreased biliary cholesterol secretion. By reducing cholesterol saturation in bile, chenodiol promotes dissolution of uncalcified cholesterol gallstones. Chenodiol has no effect on bile pigment stones. Inhibition of fluid absorption in colon by chenodiol and perhaps increase in fluid secretion may be the cause of loose stools or diarrhea. Increases in low-density lipoproteins (LDL) may pose a potential risk to patients with atherosclerosis. Prophylactic use of low doses in preventing stone recurrence is ineffective.

C

USES To dissolve small or floatable radiolucent cholesterol gallstones in carefully selected patients with radiographically well-visualized gallbladders and who are high surgical risks because of systemic disease or age.

ROUTE & DOSAGE

Cholesterol Gallstones

Adult: **PO** 250 mg b.i.d., AM and PM, for first 2 wk therapy; increase by 250 mg at weekly intervals to 13–16 mg/kg/d in 2 divided doses for up to 24 mo.

PHARMACOKINETICS Absorption: rapidly absorbed from small intestine. **Distribution:** distributed mainly into bile; crosses placenta. **Metabolism:** partially metabolized in intestines by anaerobic bacteria to lithocolic acid. **Elimination:** half-life (biphasic): 3.1 min and 16.4 min; 80% excreted in bile and feces; excreted in breast milk.

CONTRAINDICATIONS & PRECAUTIONS Contraindicated in: hepatocellular dysfunction, bile duct abnormalities, nonvisualized gallbladder after two consecutive single doses of PO cholecystographic agent; patients with radiopaque or radiolucent bile pigment stones, gallstone complications, compelling reasons for gallbladder surgery (e.g., unremitting acute cholecystitis, biliary obstruction, biliary GI fistula). Safe use during pregnancy (category X), in fertile women, nursing mothers, and children, and for longer than 6 mo not established. **Cautious use in:** atherosclerosis.

ADVERSE/SIDE EFFECTS GI: *mild diarrhea* (dose related), severe diarrhea (overdosage), fecal urgency, nausea, vomiting, dyspepsia, epigastric distress, anorexia, heartburn, flatulence, abdominal cramps. **Hepatic:** *transient elevations of serum transaminases,* particularly ALT or AST, *elevated serum total cholesterol, elevated LDL,* slight reduction of serum triglycerides, <u>hepatitis</u>.

DRUG INTERACTIONS Cholestyramine, colistipol, ANION EXCHANGE RESINS, ALUMINUM-CONTAINING ANTACIDS decrease absorption of chenodiol; ESTROGENS, ORAL CONTRACEPTIVES may counteract chenodiol effects by increasing biliary cholesterol secretion.

NURSING IMPLICATIONS

Administration

- Chenodiol should be taken with meals or milk. Food generally decreases rate but not extent of absorption.
- Store at 15–30C (59–86F) in tightly closed container unless otherwise directed.

Assessment & Drug Effects

- If partial stone dissolution does not occur by 9–12 mo, it is unlikely that further treatment will be effective. Therapy should be discontinued if no response has occurred by 16–18 mo following therapy initiation.
- Diarrhea is usually mild, transient, and dose related. It occurs in about 30–40% of patients, more frequently at beginning of therapy, but may occur at any time during therapy. Treatment generally consists of temporary dosage reduction (by about 1/2) until diarrhea is controlled; dosage is then gradually increased to original level. Antidiarrheal agents may also be prescribed.

Patient & Family Education

- Advise patient that the crampy abdominal pain that sometimes accompanies bouts of diarrhea is to be distinguished from the pain of biliary colic. The pain of biliary colic occurs in right upper quadrant or epigastric region, is frequently associated with nausea and vomiting, and should be reported to physician immediately.

- To reduce risk of stone recurrence, attain and maintain ideal body weight, include high-fiber foods in diet, and reduce cholesterol and carbohydrate intake.

CHLORAL HYDRATE

(klor′al hye′drate)

Trade names: Aquachloral Supprettes, Noctec, Novochlorhydrate♣

Classifications: CNS AGENT; ANXIOLYTIC, SEDATIVE-HYPNOTIC

Prototype: Secobarbital

Pregnancy category: C

Controlled substance: Schedule IV

ACTIONS/PHARMACODYNAMICS Produces "physiologic sleep" by mild cerebral depression with little effect on respirations or BP and little or no hangover. Does not affect sleep physiology (e.g., REM sleep) in low doses. It is the oldest chloral derivative and is still regarded as a relatively safe, effective, and inexpensive sedative-hypnotic. Has little or no analgesic action.

USES Short-term management of insomnia, for general sedation (especially in the young and the elderly), for sedation before and after surgery, to reduce anxiety associated with drug withdrawal, and alone or with paraldehyde to prevent or suppress alcohol withdrawal symptoms.

ROUTE & DOSAGE

Sedative

Adult: **PO/PR** 250 mg t.i.d. p.c.

Child: **PO/PR** 25–50 mg/kg/d divided q6–8h (max 500 mg/dose).

Hypnotic

Adult: **PO/PR** 500 mg–1 g 15–30 min before h.s. or 30 min before surgery.

Geriatric: **PO/PR** 250 mg h.s.

Child: **PO/PR** 50 mg/kg 15–30 min before h.s. or 30 min before surgery (max 1 g).

EEG Premedication

Child: **PO/PR** 20–25 mg/kg 30–60 min prior to procedure.

PHARMACOKINETICS Absorption: readily absorbed from oral or rectal administration. **Onset:** 30–60 min. **Peak:** 1–3 h. **Duration:** 4–8 h. **Distribution:** well distributed to all tissues; 70–80% protein bound; crosses placenta. **Metabolism:** metabolized in liver to the active metabolite trichloroethanol. **Elimination:** half-life: 8–11 h; excreted primarily by kidneys, with a small amount excreted in feces via bile.

CONTRAINDICATIONS & PRECAUTIONS Contraindicated in: known hypersensitivity to drug; severe hepatic, renal, or cardiac disease; rectal dosage form in patients with proctitis; oral use in patients with esophagitis, gastritis, gastric or duodenal ulcers. Safe use during pregnancy (category C) and in nursing women not established. **Cautious use in:** history of intermittent porphyria, asthma, history of or proneness to drug dependence, depression, suicidal tendencies.

ADVERSE/SIDE EFFECTS Generally well tolerated. **CNS:** dizziness, motor incoordination, headache. **CV (overdosage):** arrhythmias, <u>cardiac arrest</u>. **GI:** *nausea, vomiting, diar-*

C

rhea. **Hypersensitivity:** purpura, urticaria, erythematous rash, eczema, erythema multiforme, angioedema, eosinophilia. **Other:** breath odor, leukopenia, ketonuria, conjunctivitis. **Chronic use:** fixed drug eruptions, severe gastritis, renal, and hepatic damage, sudden death.

DIAGNOSTIC TEST INTERFERENCE False-positive results for ***urine glucose*** with Benedict's solutions, and possibly with Clinitest but not with glucose oxidase methods (e.g., Clinistix, Diastix, TesTape). Possible interference with fluorometric test for ***urine catecholamines*** (if chloral hydrate is administered within 48 h of test) and ***urinary 17-OHCS*** determinations (by modification of Reddy, Jenkins, Thorn procedure).

DRUG INTERACTIONS Alcohol, BARBITURATES, **paraldehyde,** other CNS DEPRESSANTS potentiate CNS depression; tachycardia may also occur with **alcohol;** increases anticoagulant effect of ORAL ANTICOAGULANTS; **furosemide** IV can produce flushing, diaphoresis, BP changes.

NURSING IMPLICATIONS

Administration

- Chloral hydrate is corrosive to skin and mucous membranes unless well diluted. It has an aromatic, pungent odor and bitter, pungent taste; these may be minimized by use of the capsule form or by dilution of liquid preparations in chilled fluids.
- Watch to see that drug is not cheeked and hoarded.
- Solutions are preserved in tightly covered, light-resistant containers. All forms preferably stored at 15–30C (59–86F) unless otherwise directed.

Assessment & Drug Effects

- Chloral hydrate is not intended for relief of pain. When used in the presence of pain, it may cause excitement and delirium.
- Remove matches, cigarettes, etc., if patient is a smoker. Side rails may be advisable for the elderly patient.
- Prolonged use can lead to tolerance, physical dependence, and addiction. Sudden withdrawal from dependent patients may produce delirium, mania, or convulsions.
- Allergic skin reactions may occur within several hours or as long as 10 d after drug administration.
- Evaluate patient's response to chloral hydrate and continued need for the drug.

Patient & Family Education

- Because hypnotic doses may cause dizziness, caution patient not to ambulate without assistance.
- Caution patient to avoid concomitant use of alcoholic beverages.
- Driving and other potentially hazardous activities should be avoided while patient is under the influence of chloral hydrate.

CHLORAMBUCIL

(klor-am'byoo-sil)

Trade name: Leukeran

Classifications: ANTINEOPLASTIC; ALKYLATING AGENT

Prototype: Cyclophosphamide

Pregnancy category: D

ACTIONS/PHARMACODYNAMICS Potent aromatic derivative of the alkylating agent nitrogen mustard and slowest acting and least toxic of the nitrogen mustards. A cell-cycle nonspecific (kills both resting and dividing cells), it causes cytotoxic cross linkage in DNA, thus preventing synthesis of DNA, RNA, and proteins. Myelosuppression in therapeutic doses is moderate and rapidly reversible. Lymphocytic effect is marked. Has mutagenic and embryotoxic properties.

USES As single agent or in combination with other antineoplastics in treatment of chronic lymphocytic leukemia, malignant lymphomas including lymphosarcoma, Hodgkin's disease, and giant follicular lymphoma, and in treatment of carcinoma of the ovary, breast, and testes. **Unlabeled uses:** nonneoplastic conditions: vasculitis complicating rheumatoid arthritis, autoimmune hemolytic anemias associated with cold agglutinins, lupus glomerulonephritis, idiopathic nephrotic syndrome, polycythemia vera, macroglobulinemia.

ROUTE & DOSAGE

Malignant Diseases (Lymphomas, Hodgkin's Disease, etc.)

Adult: **PO** 0.1–0.2 mg/kg/d (usual dose 4–10 mg/d).
Child: **PO** 0.1–0.2 mg/kg/d in single or divided doses.

PHARMACOKINETICS Absorption: rapidly and completely absorbed from GI tract. **Peak:** 1 h. **Distribution:** extensively bound to plasma and tissue proteins; crosses placenta. **Metabolism:** extensively metabolized in liver. **Elimination:** half-life: 1.5–2.5 h; 60% eliminated in urine as metabolites within 24 h.

CONTRAINDICATIONS & PRECAUTIONS Contraindicated in: hypersensitivity to chlorambucil or to other alkylating agents; administration within 4 wk of a full course of radiation or chemotherapy; full dosage if bone marrow is infiltrated with lymphomatous tissue or is hypoplastic; smallpox and other vaccines. Safe use during pregnancy (category D) and in nursing women not established. **Cautious use in:** excessive or prolonged dosage, pneumococcus vaccination, history of seizures or head trauma.

ADVERSE/SIDE EFFECTS Hematologic: bone marrow depression: *leukopenia,* thrombocytopenia, anemia. **Metabolic:** sterility, hyperuricemia. **GI:** low incidence of gastric discomfort. **Other:** drug fever, skin rashes, papilledema, alopecia, peripheral neuropathy, sterile cystitis, pulmonary complications, hepatotoxicity, seizures (high doses).

DRUG INTERACTIONS May have to adjust dose of **allopurinol, colchicine** because of chlorambucil-associated hyperuricemia.

NURSING IMPLICATIONS

Administration

- Nausea and vomiting may be controlled by giving entire daily dose at one time, 1 h before breakfast or 2 h after evening meal, or at bedtime. Consult physician.
- With confirmation of bone marrow depression (low platelet and neutrophil counts or peripheral lymphocytosis), it is recommended that dosage not exceed 0.1 mg/kg.
- Store at 15–30C (59–86F) in tightly closed, light-resistant container.

Assessment & Drug Effects

- CBC, hemoglobin, total and differential leukocyte counts, and serum uric acid should be checked initially and at least once weekly during treatment.
- Body weight, size of spleen, and temperature charted before initiation of therapy and at the time of blood counts provide a useful profile for determining degree of bone marrow suppression.
- Leukopenia usually develops after

C

the third week of treatment; it may continue for up to 10 d after last dose, then rapidly return to normal. About 25% of patients receiving a total dose of approximately 450 mg and 50% of those receiving this dosage for ≥ 8 wk may develop severe neutropenia.

- If possible, avoid or reduce to minimum injections and other invasive procedures (e.g., rectal temperatures, enemas) when platelet count is low because of danger of bleeding.

Patient & Family Education

- During treatment it is dangerous to go longer than 2 wk without a clinical examination and blood studies. Keeping appointments with the physician is imperative.
- Advise patient to notify physician if the following symptoms occur: unusual bleeding or bruising, sores on lips or in mouth; flank, stomach, or joint pain; fever, chills, or other signs of infection, sore throat, cough, dyspnea.
- Skin reactions are rare, but all appear to show a consistent pattern: pustular eruption on mouth, chin, cheeks; urticarial erythema on trunk that spreads to legs. The rash occurs early in treatment period and lasts about 10 d after last dose. Urge the patient to report immediately the onset of cutaneous reaction.
- If physician agrees, urge patient to drink at least 10–12 glasses (240 ml [8 oz] each) of fluid per day and to report to physician if urine output decreases below normal amounts.
- Advise patient to report to physician immediately if she becomes pregnant. She should be informed of the potential hazard to the fetus.
- Discuss possibility of gonadal suppression with patient (amenorrhea or azoospermia may be irreversible), which occurs especially with high doses.

CHLORAMPHENICOL

(klor-am-fen'i-kole)

Trade names: Chlorofair, Chloromycetin, Chloroptic, Chloroptic S.O.P., Fenicol, Isopto Fenicol, Novochlorocap ♣, Ophthochlor, Pentamycetin ♣

CHLORAMPHENICOL SODIUM SUCCINATE

Trade name: Chloromycetin Sodium Succinate

Classifications: ANTIINFECTIVE; ANTIBIOTIC

Pregnancy category: C

ACTIONS/PHARMACODYNAMICS Synthetic broad-spectrum antibiotic formerly derived from *Streptomyces venezuelae*. Principally bacteriostatic but may be bactericidal in certain species (e.g., *Hemophilus influenzae*) or when given in higher concentrations. Effective against a wide variety of gram-negative and gram-positive bacteria and most anaerobic microorganisms. Believed to act by binding to the 50S ribosome of bacteria and by interfering with protein synthesis.

USES Severe infections when other antibiotics are ineffective or are contraindicated. Particularly effective against *Salmonella typhi* and other *Salmonella* sp, *Streptococcus pneumoniae, Neisseria,* meningeal infections caused by *H. influenzae,* and infections involving *Bacteroides fragilis* and other anaerobic organisms, *Rickettsia rickettsii* (cause of Rocky Mountain spotted fever) and other rickettsiae, the lymphogranuloma-psittacosis group *(Chlamydia),* and *Mycoplasma*. Also used in cystic fibrosis antiinfective regimens and topically for infections of skin, eyes, and external auditory canal.

ROUTE & DOSAGE

Serious Infections

Adult: **PO/IV** 50 mg/kg/d in 4 divided doses. **Topical** 1–2 drops of ophthalmic solution q3–6h or small strip of ophthalmic ointment in lower conjunctival sac q3–6h or 2–3 drops of otic solution in ear t.i.d.
Neonate: **IV** 25–50 mg/kg/d divided q12–24h.
Infant/Child: **PO/IV** 50–75 mg/kg/d divided q6h (max 4 g/d).

Meningitis

Adult: **IV** 75–100 mg/kg/d divided q6h.
Child: **IV** Same as for adult.

PHARMACOKINETICS **Absorption:** rapidly absorbed from GI tract. **Peak:** PO: 1–3 h; IV: 1 h. **Distribution:** widely distributed to most body tissues including saliva and ascitic, pleural and synovial fluid; concentrates in liver and kidneys; penetrates CNS; crosses placenta. **Metabolism:** primarily inactivated in liver. **Elimination:** half-life: 1.5–4.1 h; much longer in neonates; metabolite and free drug excreted in urine; excreted in breast milk.

CONTRAINDICATIONS & PRECAUTIONS **Contraindicated in:** history of hypersensitivity or toxic reaction to chloramphenicol; treatment of minor infections, prophylactic use; typhoid carrier state, history or family history of drug-induced bone marrow depression, concomitant therapy with drugs that produce bone marrow depression. Safe use during pregnancy (category C) and in nursing mothers not established. **Cautious use in:** impaired hepatic or renal function, premature and full-term infants, children; intermittent porphyria; patients with G6PD deficiency; patient or family history of drug-induced bone marrow depression.

ADVERSE/SIDE EFFECTS **CNS:** Neurotoxicity: headache, mental depression, confusion, delirium, digital paresthesias, peripheral neuritis. **Eye (long-term, high-dose use):** visual disturbances, optic neuritis, optic nerve atrophy, contact conjunctivitis. **GI:** nausea, vomiting, diarrhea, perianal irritation, enterocolitis, glossitis, stomatitis, unpleasant taste, xerostomia. **Hematologic:** <u>bone marrow depression (dose-related and reversible):</u> reticulocytosis, leukopenia, granulocytopenia, thrombocytopenia, increased plasma iron, reduced Hgb, hypoplastic anemia. <u>Non-dose-related and irreversible pancytopenia, agranulocytosis, aplastic anemia,</u> paroxysmal nocturnal hemoglobinuria, leukemia. **Hypersensitivity:** <u>angioedema</u>, urticaria, contact dermatitis, maculopapular and vesicular rashes, dyspnea, fever, <u>anaphylaxis</u>. **Other:** hypoprothrombinemia, fixed-drug eruptions, superinfections, gray syndrome.

DIAGNOSTIC TEST INTERFERENCE Possibility of false-positive results for ***urine glucose*** by copper reduction methods (e.g., Benedict's solution, Clinitest). Chloramphenicol may interfere with ***17-OHCS*** (urinary steroid) determinations (modification of Reddy, Jenkins, Thorn procedure not affected), with ***urobilinogen excretion,*** and with responses to ***tetanus toxoid*** and possibly other active immunizing agents.

DRUG INTERACTIONS The metabolism of **chlorpropamide, di-**

cumarol, phenytoin, tolbutamide may be decreased, prolonging their activity. **Phenobarbital** decreases chloramphenicol levels. The response to iron preparations, folic acid, and vitamin B_{12} may be delayed.

INCOMPATIBILITIES Solutions/additives: chlorpromazine, polymyxin B, prochlorperazine, promethazine, TETRACYCLINES, **vancomycin, glycopyrrolate, metoclopramide.**

NURSING IMPLICATIONS

Administration

- Oral drug is taken preferably with a full glass of water on an empty stomach, at least 1 h before or 2 h after a meal, to achieve optimum blood levels.
- Instillation of eyedrops: after instillation apply light pressure to lacrimal duct for 1–2 min to prevent drainage into nasopharynx and systemic absorption. This is an extremely important step to decrease absorption. Several cases of aplastic anemia have been associated with use of ophthalmic preparations.
- Chloramphenicol sodium succinate is intended for IV administration only. Dilute each 1 g with 10 ml of sterile water or D5W. Give direct IV slowly over a period of at least 1 min.
- IV solution may be further diluted in 50–100 ml of 5% dextrose and infused over 30–60 min.
- Solution for injection may form crystals or a second layer when stored at low temperatures. Solution can be clarified by shaking vial. Do not use cloudy solutions.
- IV administration to neonates, infants, children: Verify correct IV concentration and rate of infusion with physician.
- Store topical ophthalmic, otic, and skin preparations, PO forms, and unopened ampuls preferably between 15–30C (59–86F) and protected from light unless otherwise directed by manufacturer.

Assessment & Drug Effects

- Bacterial culture and susceptibility tests are performed prior to first dose and periodically thereafter.
- Baseline CBC, platelets, serum iron, and reticulocyte cell counts are recommended before initiation of therapy, at 48 h intervals during therapy, and periodically during follow-up period. Chloramphenicol should be discontinued upon appearance of leukopenia, reticulocytopenia, thrombocytopenia, or anemia.
- Non-dose-related irreversible bone marrow depression may appear weeks or months after drug therapy is terminated. The potential for this side effect is greatest in patients with impaired hepatic or renal function, infants, children, and premenopausal women.
- Close observation of the patient is also crucial, because blood studies are not always reliable predictors of irreversible bone marrow depression.
- Chloramphenicol blood levels should be closely monitored weekly. More frequent determinations are made in patients with hepatic dysfunction and in patients receiving therapy for longer than 2 wk. Desired concentrations: peak 10–20 μg/ml; through 5–10 μg/ml.
- Check temperature at least q4h. Usually chloramphenicol is discontinued if temperature remains normal for 48 h.
- Report any appreciable change in I&O ratio or pattern.
- More frequent determinations of

serum glucose are recommended in patients receiving oral antidiabetic agents.

- Gray syndrome has occurred 2–9 d after initiation of high dose chloramphenicol therapy in premature infants and neonates and in children ≤ 2 y. It appears to be associated with initiation of therapy within the first 48 h of life and in children with preexisting liver dysfunction. Report early signs: abdominal distention, failure to feed, pallor, changes in vital signs. Early detection and prompt termination of therapy can interrupt a potentially fatal course.

Patient & Family Education

- Inform patient that bitter taste may occur 15–20 s after IV injection and that it usually lasts only 2–3 min.
- Report immediately sore throat, fever, fatigue, petechiae, nose bleeds, bleeding gums, or other unusual bleeding or bruising, or any other suspicious sign of symptom. Drug therapy should be discontinued if abnormal bleeding occurs.
- Watch for signs and symptoms of superinfection (see Appendix G).
- Advise patient to follow dosage and duration of therapy as prescribed by physician.
- Prolonged or frequent intermittent use of topical preparations should be avoided because systemic absorption and toxicity can occur.
- Withhold medication and check with physician immediately if signs of hypersensitivity reaction (see Appendix G), irritation, superinfection, or other adverse reactions appear.
- Applications to skin are generally preceded by a soap and water cleansing and thorough drying of part before reapplication of medication. Consult physician.

CHLORDIAZEPOXIDE HYDROCHLORIDE

(klor-dye-az-e-pox′ide)

Trade names: Libritabs, Librium, Lipoxide, Medilium♣, Novopoxide ♣, Sereen, Solium♣

Classifications: CNS AGENT; ANXIOLYTIC; SEDATIVE-HYPNOTIC; BENZODIAZEPINE

Prototype: Lorazepam

Pregnancy category: D

Controlled substance: Schedule IV

ACTIONS/PHARMACODYNAMICS

Benzodiazepine derivative. Acts on the limbic, thalamic, and hypothalamic areas of the CNS. Produces mild sedative, anticonvulsant, anxiolytic, and skeletal muscle relaxant effects. Has long-acting hypnotic properties. Causes mild suppression of REM sleep and of deeper phases, particularly stage 4, while increasing total sleep time.

USES Relief of various anxiety and tension states, preoperative apprehension and anxiety, and for management of alcohol withdrawal. **Unlabeled use:** essential, familial, and senile action tremors.

ROUTE & DOSAGE

Mild Anxiety, Preoperative Anxiety

Adult: **PO** 5–10 mg t.i.d. or q.i.d. **IM/IV** 50–100 mg 1 h before surgery.
Geriatric: **PO** 5 mg b.i.d. to q.i.d.
Child: **PO** 5 mg b.i.d. to q.i.d.; may be increased to 10 mg t.i.d.

Severe Anxiety and Tension

Adult: **PO** 20–25 mg t.i.d. or q.i.d. **IM/IV** 50–100 mg; then 25–50 mg t.i.d. or q.i.d.

C

Alcohol Withdrawal Syndrome

Adult: **PO** 50–100 mg prn up to 300 mg/d. **IM/IV** 50–100 mg; may repeat in 2–3 h if necessary.

PHARMACOKINETICS Absorption: well absorbed from GI tract; slow erratic absorption from IM. **Peak:** 1–4 h PO; 15–30 min IM; 3–30 min IV. **Distribution:** widely distributed throughout body; crosses placenta. **Metabolism:** metabolized in liver to long-acting active metabolite. **Elimination:** half-life: 5–30 h; slowly excreted in urine (may last several days); excreted in breast milk.

CONTRAINDICATIONS & PRECAUTIONS Contraindicated in: hypersensitivity to chlordiazepoxide and other benzodiazepines; narrow angle glaucoma, prostatic hypertrophy, shock, comatose states, primary depressive disorder or psychoses, pregnancy (category D), nursing mothers, lactation, oral use in children <6 y, parenteral use in children <12 y, acute alcohol intoxication. **Cautious use in:** anxiety states associated with impending depression, history of impaired hepatic or renal function; addiction-prone individuals, blood dyscrasias; in the elderly, debilitated patients, children; hyperkinesis, COPD.

ADVERSE/SIDE EFFECTS CNS: *drowsiness,* dizziness, *lethargy,* changes in EEG pattern; vivid dreams, nightmares, headache, vertigo, syncope, tinnitus, confusion, hallucinations, parodoxic rage, depression, delirium, ataxia. **CV:** orthostatic hypotension, tachycardia, changes in ECG patterns seen with rapid IV administration. **GI:** nausea, dry mouth, vomiting, constipation, increased appetite. **GU:** urinary frequency. **Other:** edema, pain in injection site, photosensitivity, skin rash, jaundice, hiccups, respiratory depression.

DIAGNOSTIC TEST INTERFERENCE Chlordiazepoxide increases ***serum bilirubin, AST*** and ***ALT;*** decreases ***radioactive iodine uptake;*** and may falsely increase readings for urinary ***17-OHCS*** (modified Glenn-Nelson technique).

DRUG INTERACTIONS Alcohol, CNS DEPRESSANTS, ANTICONVULSANTS potentiate CNS depression; **cimetidine** increases **chlordiazepoxide** plasma levels, thus increasing toxicity; may decrease antiparkinson effects of **levodopa;** may increase **phenytoin** levels; smoking decreases sedative and antianxiety effects.

NURSING IMPLICATIONS

Administration

- Patients who complain of gastric distress may obtain relief by taking the oral drug with or immediately after meals or with milk. If an antacid is prescribed, it should be taken at least 1 h before or after chlordiazepoxide to prevent delay in drug absorption.
- Supervise drug ingestion to prevent "cheeking" pills, a maneuver that leads to hoarding or omission of drug.
- Prepare parenteral solution immediately before use; discard unused portion. Drug is unstable in light and when in solution.
- Use special diluent provided by manufacturer to make the IM solution. Add diluent carefully to avoid bubble formation; gently agitate until solution is clear. Resulting solution: 50 mg/ml. Discard diluent if it is not clear.
- For IV injection, 5 ml of sterile water for injection or NaCl 0.9% is

added to each 100 mg ampul of dry powder and agitated gently until dissolved. Do not use IM diluent for the IV solution because it may contain air bubbles.

- Do not mix any other drug with chlordiazepoxide solution.
- IV chlordiazepoxide is administered by direct IV, properly diluted, at a rate of 100 mg or a fraction thereof over 1 min.
- Store in tight, light-resistant containers at 15–30C (59–86F) unless otherwise specified by manufacturer. The special diluent supplied by manufacturer for IM preparation should be kept refrigerated, preferably at 2–8C (36–46F) until ready for use.

Assessment & Drug Effects

- In early part of therapy, check BP and pulse before giving benzodiazepine. If blood pressure falls 20 mm Hg or more or if pulse rate is above 120 bpm, delay medication and consult physician.
- Orthostatic hypotension and tachycardia occur more frequently with parenteral administration. Patient should stay recumbent 2–3 h after IM or IV injection; observe closely and monitor vital signs.
- Until drug dosage is stabilized, monitor I&O. Report changes in I&O ratio and dysuria to physician. Cumulative (overdosage) effects can result with renal dysfunction. The elderly are especially vulnerable.
- Observe intake of patient who is seriously agitated or depressed; willful reduction of fluids can be hazardous.
- Paradoxic reactions—excitement, stimulation, disturbed sleep patterns, acute rage—may occur during first few weeks of therapy in psychiatric patients and in hyperactive and aggressive children receiving chlordiazepoxide. Withhold drug and report to physician.
- Observe patient's sleep pattern and quality. If dreams or nightmares interfere with rest, notify physician. A change in the dosing schedule, dose, or an alternate drug may be prescribed.
- If drug has been prescribed for anxiety-induced insomnia and is used every day, its effect begins in 2 or 3 nights; however, usefulness for this problem lasts only a few weeks.
- Periodic blood cell counts and liver function tests are recommended during prolonged therapy.
- Sore throat or mouth, upper respiratory infection, fever, and malaise should alert one to the possibility of agranulocytosis. Total and differential WBC counts should be ordered immediately, and protective isolation instituted.
- Adverse reactions are dose related but even at lower ranges may occur in elderly and debilitated patients. Supervision of ambulation is indicated, and possibly side rails.
- Some studies suggest that smoking increases clearance rate of chlordiazepoxide. The heavy smoker may require higher dosage of the drug for therapeutic effectiveness than the nonsmoker.
- Habituation and physical dependence can occur.
- Observe for signs of developing physical or psychologic dependency such as requests for change in drug regimen (dose and dose interval), diminishing favorable response (e.g., disturbed sleep pattern, increase in psychomotor activity), manipulative behavior, withdrawal symptoms. Investigate the symptoms of ataxia, vertigo, slurred speech; the patient may be taking more than the prescribed dose.

C

- Abrupt discontinuation of drug in patients receiving high doses for long periods (≥4 mo) has precipitated withdrawal symptoms, but not for at least 5–7 d because of slow elimination. Symptoms may include restlessness, headache, unreal or distant feelings, paresthesias, abdominal and muscle cramps, abnormal perceptions of motion, tremors, insomnia, vomiting, anorexia, profuse sweating, psychomotor activity including convulsions and delirium. In most cases, after usual doses there is no withdrawal syndrome.

Patient & Family Education

- Advise patient to take drug specifically as prescribed: not to skip, increase, or decrease doses, change intervals, or terminate therapy without physician's advice and not to lend or offer any of drug to another person.
- Advise patient that OTC drugs should not be taken unless prescribed.
- Long-term use of this drug may cause xerostomia. Inform patient that good oral hygiene can alleviate the discomfort.
- Sedation may occur during early therapy. Advise patient that activities requiring mental alertness and precision should be avoided until reaction to the drug has been evaluated.
- Caution against drinking alcoholic beverages. When combined with chlordiazepoxide, effects of both are potentiated.
- If patient becomes pregnant during therapy or intends to become pregnant, advise her to communicate with physician about continuing therapy.
- Caution patient to avoid excessive sunlight. Photosensitivity has been reported. A sun screen lotion (SPF 12 or above) should be used (if allowed).

CHLOROPROCAINE HYDROCHLORIDE

(klor-oh-proe'kane)

Trade names: Nesacaine, Nesacaine-CE ♣

Classifications: CNS AGENT; LOCAL ANESTHETIC (ESTER-TYPE)

Prototype: Procaine

Pregnancy category: C

ACTIONS/PHARMACODYNAMICS

Short-acting ester-type local anesthetic similar to procaine. Decreases sodium flux into nerve cells, thus preventing initial depolarization, propagation, and conduction of the nerve impulse. Not used for spinal, topical, or IV regional anesthesia.

USES Infiltration anesthesia and for peripheral, sympathetic, and epidural (including caudal) block anesthesia.

ROUTE & DOSAGE

Infiltration and Nerve Block

Adult: 1–2% solution: max 800 mg without epinephrine, 1 g with epinephrine.

Caudal and Epidural Block (Without Preservatives)

Adult: 2–3% solution: max 800 mg without epinephrine, 1 g with epinephrine.

PHARMACOKINETICS **Onset:** 6–12 min. **Duration:** 30–60 min without epinephrine; 60–90 min with epinephrine. **Metabolism:** hydrolyzed by plasma pseudocholinesterases. **Elimination:** excreted by kidneys.

CONTRAINDICATIONS & PRECAUTIONS **Contraindicated in:** known sensitivity to ester-type anesthetics, bisulfites, parabens (preservative) or PABA; intercurrent use of bupivacaine. Safe use during pregnancy (category C), by nursing mothers or children <12 y not established. **Cautious use in:** cardiac function impairment; history of drug hypersensitivity; debilitated, elderly, or acutely ill patients; dysrhythmias.

ADVERSE/SIDE EFFECTS **CNS:** anxiety, nervousness, tremors, sedation, circumoral paresthesia, convulsions followed by drowsiness, <u>respiratory arrest</u>. **CV:** myocardial depression, hypotension, arrhythmias, bradycardia, <u>cardiac arrest</u>. **Eye:** blurred or double vision. **Ear:** tinnitus. **GI:** nausea, vomiting. **Hypersensitivity:** cutaneous lesions of delayed onset; urticaria, sneezing, <u>anaphylactoid reactions</u>. **Other:** with caudal or epidural anesthesia: urinary retention, fecal or urinary incontinence, slowing of labor and increased incidence of forceps delivery, headache, backache, edema, status asthmaticus.

NURSING IMPLICATIONS

Administration

- A test dose (3 ml of 3% solution or 5 ml of 2% solution) is given before epidural use to check for intravascular or subarachnoid injection. Signs of intravascular injection: "epinephrine response" (tachycardia, circumoral pallor, palpitations, nervousness). Signs of subarachnoid injection: motor paralysis and extensive sensory anesthesia.
- If patient is moved with potential displacement of epidural catheter, test dose is repeated. At least 5 min should elapse between each test dose. Total dose for anesthesia is administered in fractional doses.
- Nesacaine formulation incorporates parabens (preservative) and sodium bisulfite; Nesacaine-CE is preservative-free but incorporates sodium bisulfite. Both parabens and bisulfites may initiate an allergic reaction in some individuals. Determine patient's sensitivity before administration of drug.
- Chloroprocaine is incompatible with alkali hydroxides and their carbonates: soaps, iodine, iodides, silver salts. Avoid use of any of these agents for skin or mucous membrane disinfection before chloroprocaine administration.
- Do not administer solution that is colored. Discard partially used solutions that are preservative-free.
- Store vials at 15–30C (59–86F); protect from freezing and from direct light.

Assessment & Drug Effects

- Monitor vital signs throughout period of drug use.
- Resuscitation equipment, oxygen, resuscitative drugs, and vasopressors should be immediately available when chloroprocaine is in use.

CHLOROQUINE HYDROCHLORIDE

(klor′oh-kwin)

Trade name: Aralen Hydrochloride

CHLOROQUINE PHOSPHATE

Trade name: Aralen Phosphate

Prototype for classifications: ANTIINFECTIVE; ANTIMALARIAL

Pregnancy category: C

ACTIONS/PHARMACODYNAMICS Antimalarial activity is believed to be based on ability to form complexes with DNA of parasite, thereby inhibiting replication and transcription to RNA and nucleic acid synthesis.

C

Highly active against asexual erythrocytic forms of the four species of *Plasmodium: P. vivax, P. malariae, P. ovale,* and most strains of *P. falciparum*. Action mechanism is unknown. Acts as a suppressive agent in patient with vivax or malariae malaria; terminates acute attacks and increases intervals between treatment and relapse of malaria. Abolishes the acute attack of *P. falciparum* malaria but does not prevent the infection. Chloroquine-resistant strains have been reported. Also acts as a tissue amebicide, has antiinflammatory action, antihistamine, and antiserotonic properties.

USES Suppression and treatment of malaria caused by *P. malariae, P. ovale, P. vivax,* and susceptible forms of *P. falciparum,* and in the treatment of extraintestinal amebiasis. Concomitant therapy with primaquine is necessary for radical cure of vivax and malariae malarias. **Unlabeled uses:** discoid and systemic lupus erythematosus, porphyria cutanea tarda, solar urticaria, polymorphous light eruptions, and in rheumatoid arthritis (as second-line therapy).

ROUTE & DOSAGE

Doses are expressed in terms of chloroquine base: 500 mg tablet = 300 mg base; 50 mg injection = 40 mg base

Acute Malaria

Adult: **PO** 600 mg base followed by 300 mg base at 6, 24, and 48 h. **IM** 200 mg base q6h prn; not to exceed 800 mg base/24 h.
Child: **PO** 10 mg base/kg; then 5 mg base/kg at 6, 24, and 48 h. **IM** 5 mg base/kg q12h.

Malaria Suppression

Adult: **PO** 300 mg base the same day each week starting 2 wk before exposure and continuing for 4–6 wk after leaving the area of exposure (max 300 mg base/wk).
Child: **PO** 5 mg base/kg the same day each week starting 2 wk before exposure and continuing for 4–6 wk after leaving the area of exposure (max 300 mg base/wk).

Extraintestinal Amebiasis

Adult: **PO** 600 mg base/d for 2 d; then 300 mg base/d for 2–3 wk.
Child: **PO** 10 mg base/kg/d for 2–3 wk.

Rheumatoid Arthritis, SLE

Adult: **PO** 150 mg base/d with evening meal.

PHARMACOKINETICS Absorption: rapidly and almost completely absorbed. **Peak:** 1–2 h. **Distribution:** widely distributed; concentrates in lungs, liver, erythrocytes, eyes, skin, and kidneys; crosses placenta. **Metabolism:** partially metabolized in liver to active metabolites. **Elimination:** half-life: 70–120 h; eliminated in urine; excreted in breast milk.

CONTRAINDICATIONS & PRECAUTIONS Contraindicated in: hypersensitivity to 4-aminoquinolines, psoriasis; porphyria, renal disease, 4-aminoquinoline-induced retinal or visual field changes; long-term therapy in children. Safe use during pregnancy (category C), in nursing women, and women of childbearing potential not established. **Cautious use in:** impaired hepatic function, alcoholism, eczema, patients with G6PD deficiency, infants and children, hematologic, GI, and neurologic disorders.

ADVERSE/SIDE EFFECTS CNS: mild transient headache, fatigue, irritability, confusion, nightmares, skeletal muscle weakness, paresthesias, reduced reflexes, vertigo. **CV:** hypotension; ECG changes. **Eye:** (usually reversible): blurred vision, disturbances of accommodation, night blindness, scotomas, visual field defects, photophobia, corneal edema, opacity or deposits. **GI:** *diarrhea,* abdominal cramps, *nausea,* vomiting, anorexia. **Hematologic:** hemolytic anemia in patients with G6PD deficiency. **Other:** bleaching of scalp, eyebrows, body hair, and freckles, pruritus, patchy alopecia (reversible), slight weight loss, myalgia, lymphedema of upper limbs, ototoxicity (rare).

DRUG INTERACTIONS Aluminum- and **magnesium**-containing ANTACIDS and LAXATIVES decrease chloroquine absorption, so separate administration by at least 4 h; chloroquine may interfere with response to **rabies vaccine.**

NURSING IMPLICATIONS

Administration

- GI side effects may be minimized by administering PO drug immediately before or after meals.
- Children are extremely susceptible to overdosage of chloroquine (especially the parenteral formulation) and other 4-aminoquinoline compounds. PO administration should begin as soon as possible. Long-term therapy is not recommended in children.
- Store in tightly closed container preferably between 15–30C (59–86F), unless otherwise directed by manufacturer.

Assessment & Drug Effects

- CBC and ECG are advised before initiation of therapy and periodically thereafter in patients on long-term therapy.
- A test for G6PD deficiency is recommended for American blacks and individuals of Mediterranean ancestry before therapy.
- Retinopathy (generally irreversible) can be progressive even after termination of therapy. Patient may be asymptomatic or complain of night blindness, scotomas, visual field changes, blurred vision, or difficulty in focusing. Chloroquine should be discontinued immediately.
- Patients on long-term therapy should be questioned regularly about skeletal muscle weakness, and periodic tests should be made of muscle strength and deep tendon reflexes. Positive signs are indications to terminate therapy.

Patient & Family Education

- Report promptly visual or hearing disturbances, muscle weakness, or loss of balance, symptoms of blood dyscrasia (fever, sore mouth or throat, unexplained fatigue, easy bruising or bleeding).
- Use of dark glasses in sunlight or bright light may provide comfort (because of photophobia) and reduce risk of ocular damage.
- Therapeutic effects in rheumatoid arthritis do not generally occur until after several weeks of therapy. Chloroquine can cause dizziness. Therefore, advise patient to avoid driving or other potentially hazardous activities until reaction to drug is known.
- May cause rusty yellow or brown discoloration of urine.

CHLOROTHIAZIDE

(klor-oh-thye'a-zide)

Trade names: Diachlor, Diuril, SK-Chlorothiazide

C

CHLOROTHIAZIDE SODIUM

Trade name: Sodium Diuril
Classifications: WATER BALANCE AGENT; THIAZIDE DIURETIC; ANTIHYPERTENSIVE
Prototype: Hydrochlorothiazide
Pregnancy category: B

ACTIONS/PHARMACODYNAMICS Thiazide diuretic chemically related to sulfonamides. Primary action is production of diuresis by direct action on the distal convoluted tubules. Inhibits reabsorption of sodium, potassium, and chloride ions. Promotes renal excretion of sodium (and water), bicarbonate, and potassium; decreases renal calcium excretion and supports uric acid retention. Antihypertensive mechanism is unclear but correlates with contraction of extracellular and intravascular fluid volumes and direct vasodilatory effect on vascular wall. This initially reduces cardiac output with subsequent decrease in peripheral resistance through autoregulatory mechanisms.

USES Adjunctively to manage edema associated with CHF, hepatic cirrhosis, renal dysfunction, corticosteroid, or estrogen therapy. Used alone as step 1 agent in stepped-care approach, or in combination with other agents for treatment of hypertension. **Unlabeled uses:** to reduce polyuria of central and nephrogenic diabetes insipidus, to prevent calcium-containing renal stones, and to treat renal tubular acidosis.

ROUTE & DOSAGE

Hypertension, Edema

Adult: **PO** 250 mg–1 g/d in 1–2 divided doses. **IV** 250 mg–1 g/d in 1–2 divided doses.

Geriatric: **PO** 500 mg qd or 1 g 3 times/wk.

Edema

Child: **PO** *<6 mo:* 20–40 mg/kg/d in 1–2 divided doses; *≥6 mo:* 20 mg/kg/d in 2 divided doses. **IV** *<6 mo:* 2–4 mg/kg/d in 2 divided doses; *≥6 mo:* 4 mg/kg/d.

PHARMACOKINETICS Absorption: incompletely absorbed PO. **Onset:** 2 h PO; 15 min IV. **Peak:** 3–6 h PO; 30 min IV. **Duration:** 6–12 h PO; 2 h IV. **Distribution:** distributed throughout extracellular tissue; concentrates in kidney; crosses placenta. **Metabolism:** does not appear to be metabolized. **Elimination:** half-life: 45–120 min; excreted in urine and breast milk.

CONTRAINDICATIONS & PRECAUTIONS Contraindicated in: hypersensitivity to thiazides or sulfonamides; anuria; hypokalemia; IV use in infants and children; during pregnancy (category B) and in nursing mothers. **Cautious use in:** history of sulfa allergy; impaired renal or hepatic function or gout; hypercalcemia, diabetes mellitus, elderly or debilitated patients, pancreatitis, sympathectomy, jaundiced children.

ADVERSE/SIDE EFFECTS CNS: unusual fatigue, dizziness, mental changes, vertigo, headache. **CV:** irregular heart beat, weak pulse, orthostatic hypotension. **GI:** vomiting, acute pancreatitis, diarrhea. **Hematologic:** agranulocytosis (rare), aplastic anemia (rare), asymptomatic hyperuricemia, hyperglycemia, glycosuria, SIADH secretion. **Hypersensitivity:** urticaria, photosensitivity, skin rash, fever, respiratory distress, anaphylactic reaction. **Other:** *hypokalemia*, hypercalcemia, hyponatremia, hypochloremic alkalosis, elevated cholesterol and triglyceride levels.

DIAGNOSTIC TEST INTERFERENCE Chlorothiazide (thiazides) may cause: marked increases in ***serum amylase*** values, decrease in ***PBI*** determinations; increase in excretion of ***PSP;*** increase in ***BSP retention;*** false-negative ***phentolamine*** and ***tyramine*** tests; interference with ***urine steroid*** determinations, and possibly the ***histamine test*** for pheochromocytoma. Thiazides should be discontinued at least 3 d before ***bentiromide test*** (thiazides can invalidate test) and before ***parathyroid function tests*** because they tend to decrease calcium excretion.

DRUG INTERACTIONS **Amphotericin B,** CORTICOSTEROIDS increase hypokalemic effects of chlorothiazide; the hypoglycemic effects of sulfonylureas and **insulin may be antagonized; cholestyramine, colestipol** decrease thiazide absorption; intensifies hypoglycemic and hypotensive effects of **diazoxide;** increased potassium and magnesium loss may cause **digoxin** toxicity; decreases **lithium** excretion, increasing its toxicity; increases risk of nsaid-induced renal failure and may attenuate diuresis.

INCOMPATIBILITIES **Y-site: chlorpromazine, amikacin, codeine phosphate, hydralazine, insulin, levorphanol, methadone, morphine, norepinephrine, polymyxin B, procaine, prochlorperazine, promazine, promethazine, streptomycin,** TETRACYCLINES, **trifluromazine, vancomycin,** MULTIVITAMINS.

NURSING IMPLICATIONS

Administration

- Oral drug may be administered with or after food to prevent gastric irritation. Extent of absorption appears to be increased by taking it with food.
- Schedule daily doses to avoid nocturia and interrupted sleep.
- IV administration: Reconstitute with no less than 18 ml sterile water for injection (500 mg/20 ml vial). Solution may be further diluted for IV administration with dextrose or NaCl injection. May be given by direct IV at a rate of 0.5 gram over 5 min.
- IV administration to infants and children: Verify corrrect IV concentration and rate of infusion with physician.
- Thiazide preparations are extremely irritating to the tissues, and great care must be taken to avoid extravasation. If infiltration occurs, stop medication, remove needle, and apply ice if area is small.
- Store tablets, PO solutions, and parenteral dosage forms at 15–30C (59–86F) unless otherwise directed by manufacturer. Unused reconstituted IV solutions may be stored at room temperature up to 24 h. Use only clear solutions.

Assessment & Drug Effects

- Baseline and periodic determinations are indicated for blood count, serum electrolytes, CO_2, BUN, creatinine, uric acid, and blood sugar.
- Thiazide therapy can cause hyperglycemia (see Signs & Symptoms, Appendix G) and glycosuria in diabetic and diabetic-prone individuals. Dosage adjustment of hypoglycemic drugs may be required.
- Asymptomatic hyperuricemia can be produced because of interference with uric acid excretion. Patient with history of gout may be continued on a thiazide with adjusted doses of uricosuric agent.

C

- Establish baseline weight before initiation of therapy. Weigh patient at the same time each AM under standard conditions. usually a gain of more than 1 kg (2 lb) within 2 or 3 d and a gradual weight gain over the week's period is reportable. Tell patient to check for signs of edema (hands, ankles, pretibial areas).
- BP should be closely monitored during early drug therapy. Physician may want initial measurements for patients with hypertension taken with patient standing, sitting, and to evaluate drug effects.
- Skin and mucous membranes should be inspected daily for evidence of petechiae in patients receiving large doses and those on prolonged therapy.
- In an attempt to relieve dry mouth, patient may significantly increase fluid intake. Consult physician about permissible intake volume.
- Patients on digitalis therapy should be observed closely for signs and symptoms of hypokalemia (see Appendix G). Even moderate reduction in serum potassium can precipitate digitalis intoxication in these patients.

Patient & Family Education

- Explain to patient that he or she will be urinating greater amounts and more frequently than usual and that there will be an unusual sense of tiredness. With continued therapy, diuretic action decreases; hypotensive effects usually are maintained, and sense of tiredness diminishes.
- Antihypertensive action of a thiazide diuretic requires several days before effects are observed; usually optimum therapeutic effect is not established for 3–4 wk.
- Monitor I&O ratio. Excessive diuresis or oliguria may cause electrolyte imbalance and necessitate prompt dosage adjustment. To prevent dehydration, urge patient to report GI illness accompanied by protracted vomiting or prolonged period of diarrhea.
- If orthostatic hypotension is a troublesome symptom (and it may be, especially in the elderly), inform patient of measures that may help him or her tolerate the effect and to prevent falling.
- Because of the possibility of dehydration, caution patient against drinking large quantities of coffee or other caffeine drinks. Caffeine is a CNS stimulant with diuretic effects.
- Advise patient to watch for and report signs and symptoms of hypokalemia, hypercalcemia, or hyperglycemia (see Appendix G).
- Hypokalemia may be prevented if the daily diet contains potassium-rich foods. Urge patient to eat a banana and drink at least 6 oz orange juice every day. Collaborate with dietitian and physician.
- Warn patient about the possibility of photosensitivity reaction and to notify physician if it occurs. Thiazide-related photosensitivity is considered a photoallergy (radiation changes drug structure and makes it allergenic for some individuals). It occurs 1 1/2–2 wk after initial sun exposure.

CHLOROTRIANISENE

(klor-oh-trye-an′i-seen)

Trade name: TACE

Classifications: HORMONE; SYNTHETIC ESTROGEN

Prototype: Estradiol

Pregnancy category: X

ACTIONS/PHARMACODYNAMICS

Nonesteroidal synthetic estrogen

derived from diethylstilbestrol. Properties similar to those of other estrogens. Has weak estrogenic properties until metabolized.

USES Inoperable progressing prostatic cancer; short-term treatment of symptoms of estrogen deficiency, e.g., atrophic vaginitis, female hypogonadism, kraurosis vulvae, vasomotor symptoms of menopause. Use for prevention of postpartum breast engorgement no longer recommended because large doses required increase risk of thrombophlebitis.

ROUTE & DOSAGE

Menopausal Symptoms
Adult: **PO** 12–25 mg/d x 30 d.

Prostatic Cancer
Adult: **PO** 12–25 mg/d.

Female Hypogonadism
Adult: **PO** 12–25 mg/d x 21 d followed by IM progesterone or PO progestin for 5 d.

PHARMACOKINETICS **Onset:** approximately day 14 of therapy. **Distribution:** stored in fat tissues, from where it is slowly released. **Metabolism:** converted in liver to active estrogen.

CONTRAINDICATIONS & PRECAUTIONS **Contraindicated in:** thrombophlebitis or thromboembolic disorders, breast cancer, undiagnosed abnormal vaginal bleeding, pregnancy (category X). Safe use during lactation not established. **Cautious use in:** history of jaundice, metabolic bone diseases, hypertension, impaired renal function, asthma, history of gallbladder disease, diabetes mellitus.

ADVERSE/SIDE EFFECTS **CNS:** headache, dizziness, sudden loss of coordination, slurred speech, mental depression, irritability. **CV:** thromboembolism, thrombophlebitis, edema. **GI:** abdominal cramps, anorexia, *nausea,* vomiting, diarrhea. **Gynecologic:** spotting, breakthrough bleeding, prolonged bleeding, amenorrhea, decrease in libido; testicular atrophy, gynecomastia (males); lumps in breast, breast tenderness, pigmentation of nipples and areola. **Other:** jaundice, loss of hair, shortness of breath, aggravation of migraine, photosensitivity, visual disturbances, intolerance to contact lenses.

NURSING IMPLICATIONS

Administration

- Instruct patient to swallow the capsule whole. It may be taken with or immediately after food to reduce nausea.
- When chlorotrianisene is administered for postpartum breast engorgement, first dose should be given within the first 8 h after delivery.
- Capsules should be stored in tightly closed container in a dry place, preferably at 15–30C (59–86F). Protect from extremes of temperature and humidity above 50%.

Assessment & Drug Effects

- Monitor for signs and symptoms of thrombophlebitis (see Appendix G) in the lower extremities.
- Monitor BP, especially in hypertensive patients, as drug may cause fluid retention.

Patient & Family Education

- May cause loss of diabetes control. Monitor blood and urine glucose closely.
- If pregnancy occurs during therapy, stop medication and report promptly to physician.

- Inform patient of the importance of keeping follow-up appointments.
- Instruct patient to report signs and symptoms of thrombophlebitis (see Appendix G).

CHLORPHENIRAMINE MALEATE

(klor-fen-eer'a-meen)

Trade names: Aller-Chlor, Chlo-Amine, Chlorate, Chlor-Pro, Chlor-span, Chlortab, Chlor-Trimeton, Chlor-Tripolon ♣, Novopheniram ♣, Pfeiffer Allergy, Phenetron, Tela-chlor, Teldrin, Trymegan

Classification: ANTIHISTAMINE (H_1-RECEPTOR ANTAGONIST)

Prototype: Diphenhydramine

Pregnancy category: B

ACTIONS/PHARMACODYNAMICS Antihistamine that generally produces less drowsiness than other antihistamines, but side effects involving CNS stimulation may be more common. Competes with histamine for H_1-receptor sites on effector cells, thus prevents histamine action that promotes capillary permeability and edema formation and constrictive action on respiratory, gastrointestinal, and vascular smooth muscles. Has antiemetic, antitussive, anticholinergic, and local anesthetic actions.

USES Symptomatic relief of various uncomplicated allergic conditions; to prevent transfusion and drug reactions in susceptible patients, and as adjunct to epinephrine and other standard measures in anaphylactic reactions.

ROUTE & DOSAGE

Symptomatic Allergy Relief

Adult: **PO** 2–4 mg t.i.d. or q.i.d.; 8–12 mg b.i.d. or t.i.d.; max 24 mg/d.

Geriatric: **PO** 4 mg q.d. or b.i.d. or 8 mg sustained-release h.s.

Child: **PO** 6–12 y: 2 mg q4–6h (max 12 mg/d); 2–6 y: 1 mg q4–6h.

Allergic Reactions to Blood

Adult: **SC/IV/IM** 10–20 mg (max 40 mg/d).

PHARMACOKINETICS Absorption: well absorbed from GI tract; about 45% of dose reaches systemic circulation intact. **Onset:** within 6 h. **Peak:** 2–6 h. **Distribution:** highest concentrations in lung, heart, kidney, brain, small intestine, and spleen. **Elimination:** half-life: 12–43 h.

CONTRAINDICATIONS & PRECAUTIONS Contraindicated in: Hypersensitivity to antihistamines of similar structure; lower respiratory tract symptoms, narrow-angle glaucoma, obstructive prostatic hypertrophy or other bladder neck obstruction, GI obstruction or stenosis, pregnancy (category B), nursing mothers, premature and newborn infants, during or within 14 days of MAO INHIBITOR therapy. **Cautious use in:** convulsive disorders, increased intraocular pressure, hyperthyroidism, cardiovascular disease, hypertension, diabetes mellitus, history of bronchial asthma, elderly patients, patients with G6PD deficiency.

ADVERSE/SIDE EFFECTS Low incidence of side effects. **CNS:** *drowsiness,* sedation, headache, dizziness, vertigo, fatigue, disturbed coordination, tremors, euphoria, nervousness, restlessness, insomnia. **CV:** palpitation, tachycardia, mild hypotension or hypertension. **ENT:** *dryness of mouth,* nose, and throat, tinnitus, vertigo, acute labyrinthitis, thickened bronchial secretions, sensation of chest tightness. **Eye:**

blurred vision, diplopia. **GI:** epigastric distress, anorexia, nausea, vomiting, constipation or diarrhea. **GU:** urinary frequency or retention, dysuria.

DIAGNOSTIC TEST INTERFERENCE Antihistamines should be discontinued 4 d before ***skin testing*** procedures for allergy because they may obscure otherwise positive reactions.

DRUG INTERACTIONS Alcohol (ethanol) and other CNS DEPRESSANTS produce additive sedation and CNS depression.

NURSING IMPLICATIONS

Administration

- Sustained-release tablets should be swallowed whole and not crushed or chewed.
- The 100 mg/ml preparation is intended for IM or SC use only. It should not be administered IV because it contains preservatives. The 10 mg/ml injection can be given IV, IM, or SC. It contains no preservatives.
- IV chlorpheniramine may be given by direct IV undiluted. Administer 10 mg or fraction thereof over at least 1 min.
- If patient manifests any reaction after parenteral administration, drug should be discontinued. (Exception: Patient may experience transitory stinging sensation that rarely lasts longer than a few minutes.)
- Store preferably between 15 and 30C (59 and 86F) unless otherwise directed by manufacturer. Syrup and injection forms should be protected from light to prevent discoloration.

Assessment & Drug Effects

- Monitor for CNS depression and sedation, especially when chlorpheniramine is given in combination with other CNS depressants.
- Monitor BP in hypertensive patients since chlorpheniramine may elevate BP.

Patient & Family Education

- Driving a car and other potentially hazardous activities should be avoided until drug response has been determined.
- Antihistamines have additive effects with alcohol. Therefore, advise cautious use.
- Patients on prolonged therapy should have periodic blood cell counts.
- Store antihistamines out of reach of children. Fatalities have been reported.
- Patients with allergies should be advised to carry at all times medical identification jewelry or card indicating specific allergy, name, and physician's name, address, and telephone number.

CHLORPROMAZINE
(klor-proe'ma-zeen)

CHLORPROMAZINE HYDROCHLORIDE

Trade names: Chlorpromanyl ♣, Largactil ♣, Novochlorpromazine ♣, Ormazine, Promapar, Promaz, Sonazine, Thorazine, Thor-Prom

Classifications: CNS AGENT; PSYCHOTHERAPEUTIC; ANTIPSYCHOTIC; PHENOTHIAZINE; ANTIEMETIC

Pregnancy category: C

ACTIONS/PHARMACODYNAMICS
Phenothiazine derivative with actions at all levels of CNS. Mechanism that produces strong antipsychotic effects is unclear, but thought to be related to blockade of postsynaptic dopamine receptors in the brain. Actions on hypothalamus and reticular

formation produce strong sedation, hypotension, and depressed temperature regulation. Has strong alpha-adrenergic blocking action and weak anticholinergic effects. Directly depresses the heart; may increase coronary blood flow. Exerts quinidinelike antiarrhythmic action. Antiemetic effect by suppression of the chemoreceptor trigger zone (CTZ). Inhibitory effect on dopamine reuptake, may be the basis for moderate extrapyramidal symptoms. Antipsychotic drugs are sometimes called neuroleptics (or tranquilizers) because they tend to reduce initiative and interest in environment, decrease displays of emotions or affect, suppress spontaneous movements and complex behavior, and decrease psychotic symptoms. Spinal reflexes and unconditioned nociceptive-avoidance behaviors remain intact.

USES To control manic phase of manic-depressive illness, for symptomatic management of psychotic disorders, including schizophrenia, in management of severe nausea and vomiting, to control excessive anxiety and agitation before surgery, and for treatment of severe behavior problems in children, e.g., attention deficit disorder. Also used for treatment of acute intermittent porphyria, intractable hiccups, and as adjunct in treatment of tetanus.

ROUTE & DOSAGE

Psychotic Disorders, Agitation

Adult: **PO** 25–100 mg t.i.d. or q.i.d.; may need up to 1000 mg/d. **IM/IV** 25–50 mg up to 600 mg q4–6h.
Child: **PO** *>6 mo,* 0.55 mg/kg q4–6h prn up to 500 mg/d. **PR** *>6 mo,* 1.1 mg/kg q6–8h. **IM/IV** *>6 mo,* 0.55 mg/kg q6–8h.

Nausea and Vomiting

Adult: **PO** 10–25 mg q4–6h prn. **PR** 50–100 mg q6–8h. **IM/IV** 25–50 mg q3–4h prn.
Child: **PO** *>6 mo,* 0.55 mg/kg q4–6h prn up to 500 mg/d. **PR** *>6 mo,* 1.1 mg/kg q6–8h. **IM/IV** *>6 mo,* 0.55 mg/kg q6–8h.

Dementia

Geriatric: **PO** Initial 10–25 mg 1–2 times/d, may increase q4–7d by 10–25 mg/d (max 800 mg/d).

Intractable Hiccups

Adult: **PO/IM/IV** 25–50 mg t.i.d. or q.i.d.

PHARMACOKINETICS Absorption: rapid absorption with considerable first pass metabolism in liver; rapid absorption after IM. **Onset:** 30–60 min. **Peak:** 2–4 h PO; 15–20 min IM. **Duration:** 4–6 h. **Distribution:** widely distributed; accumulates in brain; crosses placenta. **Metabolism:** metabolized in liver. **Elimination:** half-life: biphasic 2 and 30 h; excreted in urine as metabolites; excreted in breast milk.

CONTRAINDICATIONS & PRECAUTIONS Contraindicated in: hypersensitivity to phenothiazine derivatives; withdrawal states from alcohol; comatose states, brain damage, bone marrow depression, Reye's syndrome; children < 6 mo. Safe use during pregnancy (category C), and in nursing mothers not established. **Cautious use in:** agitated states accompanied by depression, seizure disorders, respiratory impairment due to infection or COPD; glaucoma, diabetes, hypertensive disease, peptic ulcer, prostatic hypertrophy; thyroid, cardiovascular, and hepatic disorders; patients exposed to extreme heat or organophosphate insecticides; previously detected breast cancer.

ADVERSE/SIDE EFFECTS Usually dose related. **CNS:** *sedation, drowsiness,* dizziness, restlessness, neuroleptic malignant syndrome, tardive dyskinesias, tumor, syncope, headache, weakness, insomnia, reduced REM sleep, bizarre dreams, cerebral edema, convulsive seizures, hypothermia, inability to sweat, depressed cough reflex, *extrapyramidal symptoms,* EEG changes. **CV:** orthostatic hypotension, palpitation, tachycardia, ECG changes (usually reversible): prolonged QT and PR intervals, blunting of T waves, ST depression. **Eye:** blurred vision, lenticular opacities, mydriasis, photophobia. **GI:** dry mouth; constipation, adynamic ileus, cholestatic jaundice, aggravation of peptic ulcer, dyspepsia, increased appetite. **GU:** anovulation, infertility, pseudopregnancy, menstrual irregularity, gynecomastia, galactorrhea, priapism, inhibition of ejaculation, reduced libido, urinary retention and frequency. **Hematologic:** agranulocytosis, thrombocytopenic purpura, pancytopenia (rare). **Respiratory:** laryngospasm. **Skin/hypersensitivity:** fixed-drug eruption, urticaria, reduced perspiration, contact dermatitis, exfoliative dermatitis, photosensitivity, eczema, anaphylactoid reactions, hypersensitivity vasculitis; hirsutism (long-term therapy). **Other:** weight gain, hypoglycemia, hyperglycemia, glycosuria (high doses), enlargement of parotid glands, idiopathic edema, muscle necrosis (following IM), SLE-like syndrome, sudden unexplained death.

DIAGNOSTIC TEST INTERFERENCE Chlorpromazine (phenothiazines) may increase ***cephalin flocculation,*** and possibly other ***liver function tests;*** also may increase ***PBI.*** False-positive result may occur for ***amylase, 5-hydroxyindole acetic acid, porphobilinogens, urobilinogen*** (Ehrlich's reagent), and ***urine bilirubin*** (Bili-Labstix). False-positive or false-negative ***pregnancy test*** results possibly caused by a metabolite of phenothiazines, which discolors urine depending on test used.

DRUG INTERACTIONS **Alcohol,** CNS DEPRESSANTS increase CNS depression; ANTACIDS, ANTIDIARRHEALS decrease absorption—space administration 2 h before or after administration of chlorpromazine; **phenobarbital** increases metabolism of phenothiazine; GENERAL ANESTHETICS increase excitation and hypotension; antagonizes antihypertensive action of **guanethidine; phenylpropanolamine** poses possibility of sudden death; TRICYCLIC ANTIDEPRESSANTS intensify hypotensive and anticholinergic effects; ANTICONVULSANTS decrease seizure threshold—may need to increase anticonvulsant dose.

INCOMPATIBILITIES **Solution/additive: aminophylline, amphotericin B, ampicillin, chloramphenicol, chlorothiazide, cimetidine, dimenhydrinate, heparin, methacillin, methohexital, penicillin G, pentobarbital, phenobarbital, ranitidine, thiopental. Y-site: aminophylline, amphotericin B, ampicillin, chloramphenicol, chlorothiazide, methacillin, methohexital, penicillin G, phenobarbital, thiopental.**

NURSING IMPLICATIONS

Administration

- Watch to see that oral drug is swallowed and not hoarded. Suicide attempt is a constant possibility in depressed patients, particularly when they are improving.

- Chlorpromazine concentrate should be mixed just before administration in at least 1/2 glass juice, milk, water, coffee, tea, carbonated beverage, or with semisolid food.
- Maintenance therapy is usually administered as a single dose at bedtime.
- Avoid parenteral drug contact with skin, eyes, and clothing because of its potential for causing contact dermatitis.
- Inject IM preparations slowly and deep into upper outer quadrant of buttock; massage site well. Avoid SC injection; it may cause tissue irritation and nodule formation. If irritation is a problem, consult physician about diluting medication with normal saline or 2% procaine. Rotate injection sites.
- The patient should remain recumbent for at least 1/2 h after parenteral administration. Observe closely. Hypotensive reactions may require head-low position and pressor drugs, e.g., phenylephrine (Neo-Synephrine), norepinephrine (Levophed). Epinephrine and other pressor agents are contraindicated since they may cause sudden paradoxical drop in BP.
- IV preparation: Avoid injecting undiluted chlorpromazine into a vein. Each 25 mg should be diluted with 24 ml of NS to produce a concentration of 1 mg/ml. May be further diluted in up to 1000 ml of NS for continuous infusion.
- IV administration: IV chlorpromazine may be given by direct IV diluted in 24 ml of NS. Administer 1 mg or fraction thereof over 2 min. A specific flow rate should be ordered for the IV infusion. Usual rate: 1–2 mg/min. Monitor BP.
- Lemon yellow color of parenteral preparation does not alter potency; if otherwise colored or markedly discolored, solution should be discarded.
- All forms are stored preferably between 15–30C (59–86F) protected from light, unless otherwise specified by the manufacturer. Avoid freezing.

Assessment & Drug Effects

- Before initiating treatment, establish baseline BP (in standing and recumbent positions), pulse, and respiratory capacity values.
- Hypotensive reactions, dizziness, and sedation are common during early therapy, particularly in patients on high doses and in the elderly receiving parenteral doses. Patients usually develop tolerance to these side effects; however, lower doses or longer intervals between doses may be required.
- Be alert for signs of neuroleptic malignant syndrome (see Appendix G). Report immediately.
- Smoking increases metabolism of phenothiazines, resulting in shortened half-life and more rapid clearance of drug. Higher dosage in smokers may be required. Advise patient to stop or at least reduce smoking, if possible.
- Monitor I&O ratio and pattern. Urinary retention due to mental depression and compromised renal function may occur. If serum creatinine becomes elevated, therapy should be discontinued.
- Note that chlorpromazine can suppress the cough reflex. Be alert to danger of bronchopneumonia, which may occur in the severely depressed patient, especially the elderly.
- Support hose and elevation of legs when sitting may minimize drug-induced hypotension (discuss with physician). Supervise ambulation.

- Chlorpromazine may affect temperature regulating mechanism.
- Antiemetic effect of chlorpromazine may obscure signs of overdosage of other drugs or other causes of nausea and vomiting.
- Be alert to complaints of diminished visual acuity, reduced night vision, photophobia, and a perceived brownish discoloration of objects. Patient may be more comfortable with dark glasses.
- Diabetics or prediabetics on long-term, high-dose therapy should be monitored for reduced glucose tolerance and loss of diabetes control. Urine and blood glucose should be checked regularly.
- Early manifestations of agranulocytosis (see Appendix G) are most likely to occur within first 4–10 wk of therapy, particularly in women and the elderly. Blood studies should be instituted promptly.
- CBC, liver function tests, urinalysis, ocular examinations, EEG (in patients > 50 y) are recommended before and periodically during prolonged therapy.

Patient & Family Education
- Take chlorpromazine with food or a full glass of water or milk (240 ml) to reduce possibility of gastric irritation.
- Some patients fail to experience improvement until 7 or 8 wk into therapy and therefore may not realize the importance of medication compliance. Stress necessity of keeping appointments for follow-up evaluation of dosage regimen.
- Urge patient on home therapy not to alter dosing regimen; tell patient not to give the drug to another person.
- May cause pink to red-brown discoloration of urine.
- Photosensitivity associated with chlorpromazine therapy is a phototoxic reaction. Severity of response depends on amount of exposure and drug dose. Exposed skin areas have appearance of an exaggerated sunburn. If reaction occurs, report to physician. Patient should wear protective clothing and sunscreen lotion with SPF above 12 when outdoors, even on dark days.
- Oral candidiasis occurs frequently in patients receiving phenothiazines. Emphasize meticulous oral hygiene.
- Extrapyramidal symptoms occur most often in patients on high dosage, the pediatric patient with severe dehydration and acute infection, the elderly, and women. These symptoms are frightening to the uninformed. Be sure patient and family members understand the importance of prompt reporting. Usually, symptoms disappear with dosage adjustment.
- Chlorpromazine may impair mental and physical abilities, especially during early therapy. Caution patient against driving a car or undertaking activities requiring precision and mental alertness until drug response is known.
- Abrupt withdrawal of drug or deliberate dose skipping, especially after prolonged therapy with large doses, can cause onset of extrapyramidal symptoms (see Appendix G) and severe GI disturbances. Urge patient to adhere to dosage regimen without changes. When treatment is to be discontinued, dosage must be tapered off gradually over a period of several weeks.

CHLORPROPAMIDE

(klor-proe'pa-mide)

Trade names: Apo-Chlorpropamide ♣, Chloronase, Diabinese, Glucamide, Novopropamide ♣

C

Classifications: HORMONE SYNTHETIC SUBSTITUTE; SULFONYLUREA ANTIDIABETIC
Prototype: Tolbutamide
Pregnancy category: C

ACTIONS/PHARMACODYNAMICS

Longest-acting first-generation sulfonylurea compound, structurally and pharmacologically related to tolbutamide. Although a sulfonamide derivative, it has no antiinfective activity. Lowers blood glucose by stimulating beta cells in pancreas to release endogenous insulin. May potentiate available antidiuretic hormone (ADH) secretion, a property not shared by other sulfonylureas.

USES Mild to moderately severe, stable non-insulin-dependent diabetes mellitus (type II, NIDDM) in patients who cannot be controlled by diet alone and who do not have complications of diabetes. **Unlabeled use:** neurogenic diabetes insipidus.

ROUTE & DOSAGE

Antidiabetic

Adult: **PO** Initial: 100–250 mg/d with breakfast; adjust by 50–125 mg/d q3–5d until glycemic control is achieved, up to 750 mg/d.

Antidiuretic

Adult: **PO** 100–250 mg/d; may adjust q2–3d up to 500 mg/d.

PHARMACOKINETICS **Absorption:** readily absorbed from GI tract. **Onset:** 1 h. **Peak:** 3–6 h. **Distribution:** highly protein bound; distributed into breast milk. **Metabolism:** metabolized in liver. **Elimination:** half-life: 36 h; 80–90% excreted in urine in 96 h.

CONTRAINDICATIONS & PRECAUTIONS **Contraindicated in:** known hypersensitivity to sulfonylureas and to sulfonamides; as sole therapy for type I (IDDM) diabetes; diabetes complicated by severe infection; acidosis; severe renal, hepatic, or thyroid insufficiency. Safe use during pregnancy (category C), in nursing mothers, and in children not established. **Cautious use in:** elderly patients, Addison's disease, CHF, and hepatic porphyria.

ADVERSE/SIDE EFFECTS **CNS:** drowsiness, muscle cramps, weakness, paresthesias. **GI:** GI distress, anorexia, nausea, diarrhea, constipation, cholestatic jaundice. **Hematologic:** leukopenia, thrombocytopenia, agranulocytosis. **Hypersensitivity:** rash, pruritus. **Other:** hypoglycemia, antidiuretic effect (SIADH): dilutional hyponatremia, water intoxication, hyposthenuria, flushing, photosensitivity, alcohol intolerance.

DRUG INTERACTIONS Adverse effects of ORAL ANTICOAGULANTS, **phenytoin,** SALICYLATES, NSAIDS may be increased along with those of chlorpropamide; THIAZIDE DIURETICS may increase blood sugar; **alcohol** produces disulfiram reaction; **probenecid,** mao inhibitors may increase hypoglycemic effects.

NURSING IMPLICATIONS

Administration

- Chlorpropamide is generally prescribed as a single morning dose with breakfast. Alternatively, it may be prescribed to be divided into 2 or 3 doses and taken with meals to minimize GI side effects and to achieve maximum diabetes control.
- Store below 40C (104F), preferably at 15–30C (59–86F) in a tightly

closed container, unless otherwise directed.

Assessment & Drug Effects

- Monitor blood and urine glucose to determine effectiveness of glycemic control.
- Glycosylated hemoglobin levels should be determined every 2–3 mo.
- Monitor for signs and symptoms of hypoglycemia (see Appendix G).
- Baseline and periodic hematologic and hepatic studies are advisable, particularly in patients receiving high doses. A CBC should be performed if symptoms of anemia appear; advise patient to report dizziness, shortness of breath, malaise, fatigue.
- In the treatment of diabetes insipidus, the expected therapeutic effect of chlorpropamide is the promotion of a significant decrease in urinary output. Monitor I&O ratio and check with physician regarding allowable parameters.

Patient & Family Education

- With long-acting hypoglycemic agents such as chlorpropamide, mild CNS symptoms of hypoglycemia predominate, whereas other symptoms may go unnoticed or simply may be tolerated.
- Because chlorpropamide has a long half-life, hypoglycemia can be severe, although onset is not as fast or as dramatic as with use of insulin.
- The more severe toxic effects, jaundice and agranulocytosis, are often preceded by skin eruptions, malaise, fever, or photosensitivity. Immediately report these symptoms to the physician. A change to another hypoglycemic agent may be indicated.
- Caution patient not to self-dose with OTC drugs unless approved or prescribed by the physician.
- Instruct the controlled diabetic patient to monitor weight and to be aware of I&O ratio and pattern. Infrequently, chlorpropamide produces an antidiuretic effect, with resulting severe hyponatremia, edema, and water intoxication. If fluid intake far exceeds output and edema develops (weight gain), the patient should report to the physician.

C

CHLORPROTHIXENE

(klor-proe-thix′een)

Trade names: Taractan, Tarasan ♣

Classifications: CNS AGENT; PSYCHOTHERAPEUTIC; PHENOTHIAZINE ANTIPSYCHOTIC (TRANQUILIZER)

Prototype: Chlorpromazine

Pregnancy category: C

ACTIONS/PHARMACODYNAMICS

Structurally and pharmacologically similar to the phenothiazines. Believed to act by blocking dopamine receptor sites in brain. Produces strong antiemetic effect by inhibiting medullary chemoreceptor trigger zone (CTZ). Also has prominent sedative effect but less hypotensive, anticholinergic, and antihistaminic activity than chlorpromazine, and incidence of extrapyramidal symptoms is less.

USE Management of manifestations of psychotic disorders.

ROUTE & DOSAGE

Antipsychotic

Adult: **PO** 25–50 mg t.i.d. or q.i.d. (max 600 mg/d). **IM** 25–50 mg; may repeat t.i.d. or q.i.d. if needed.

Child: **PO** 10–25 mg t.i.d. or q.i.d.

C

PHARMACOKINETICS Absorption: partially absorbed from GI tract. **Onset:** 10–30 min IM. **Metabolism:** metabolized in liver. **Elimination:** half-life: 30 h; excreted primarily in urine with some elimination in feces.

CONTRAINDICATIONS & PRECAUTIONS Contraindicated in: hypersensitivity to phenothiazine derivatives; bone marrow depression, circulatory collapse, coronary artery disease, cerebrovascular disorders, CHF, alcoholism, comatose states. Safe use during pregnancy (category C) or in nursing mothers or safe PO use in children <6 y or parenteral use in those <12 y not established. **Cautious use in:** persons exposed to extreme heat or organophosphate insecticides, persons with suicide tendency; history of drug abuse, peptic ulcer, cardiovascular or respiratory disease, breast cancer, persons receiving electroshock treatment.

ADVERSE/SIDE EFFECTS CNS: *sedation,* drowsiness, lethargy, dizziness, ataxia, convulsions, tardive dyskinesia, pseudoparkinsonism and other extrapyramidal symptoms. **CV:** orthostatic hypotension, Q and T wave distortions, tachycardia. **Eye:** blurred vision, ocular disturbances. **GI:** *dry mouth,* constipation. **GU:** difficult urination, urinary retention, galactorrhea, gynecomastia, increased libido, impotence, amenorrhea. **Hematologic:** transient leukopenia, agranulocytosis, thrombocytopenic purpura. **Skin:** inability to sweat, contact dermatitis, photosensitivity, urticaria. **Other:** uricosuria, increased appetite, excessive weight gain, thirst, nasal stuffiness, jaundice.

DIAGNOSTIC TEST INTERFERENCE ***Immunologic urine pregnancy tests*** may produce false-positive or false-negative results depending on test used. ***Urine bilinogen test*** results may be false-positive.

DRUG INTERACTIONS Alcohol, other CNS DEPRESSANTS increase sedation and CNS depression.

NURSING IMPLICATIONS

Administration

- May be taken with food or a full glass of water or milk to reduce risk of gastric irritation.
- Oral concentrate may be given alone or diluted in water, milk, fruit juice, coffee, or carbonated beverage just before administration. Warn patient not to spill oral liquid on skin or clothing because drug can cause contact dermatitis.
- Administer IM in upper outer quadrant of buttock or midlateral thigh. Rotate injection sites.
- Since postural hypotension may occur in some patients, IM injection should be given with patient recumbent. Patient should remain lying down for at least 1/2 h.
- Monitor patient closely when changeover from parenteral to oral dose is made. Oral dose is alternated with parenteral dose on same day, then oral dose only.
- When therapy is to be discontinued, doses should be reduced gradually over a several-day period. Abrupt withdrawal may produce nausea, vomiting, gastritis, dizziness, and tremulousness.
- Store in light-resistant, tightly covered container at 15–30C (59–86F) unless otherwise specified.

Assessment & Drug Effects

- Before treatment is initiated, establish baseline BP readings (standing and recumbent) and pulse and respiratory patterns.

- Geriatric and debilitated patients should be closely supervised particularly during ambulation. Lethargy and drowsiness are easily controlled by dosage adjustment.
- Monitor I&O ratio and bowel elimination pattern. Patient should know what laxative to use if necessary. Consult physician about prescribing a high-fiber diet.
- Patients on high dose or prolonged therapy should have the following follow-up checks at periodic intervals: blood cell counts and differential, liver function tests, urine tests for bile and bilirubin, ophthalmologic examinations.
- Hepatotoxicity (see Appendix G) generally occurs after 4–10 wk of continuous therapy. Agranulocytosis (see Signs & Symptoms, Appendix G) is most likely to occur after 2–4 wk of treatment.
- Therapy may be accompanied by inability to sweat, which can increase body temperature. Patient exposed to extremes in environmental temperature or to high fever due to illness may develop heat stroke. Inform physician and prepare to institute measures (evaporative cooling, and antipyretics) to rapidly lower body temperature.

Patient & Family Education

- Be certain patient understands dosing regimen and the importance of not changing or omitting doses.
- Patients for whom prolonged therapy is contemplated should be informed about the risk of developing tardive dyskinesia (see Appendix G). Early symptoms, such as wormlike movements of the tongue and bizarre, rhythmic movements of mouth and face, should be reported immediately.
- Alcohol and other CNS depressants should be avoided during treatment with chlorprothixene.
- Caution patient to avoid excessive exposure to sunlight. Use sunscreen lotion (SPF above 12) when outdoors, even if it is a cloudy day.
- Warn patient to avoid driving and other potentially hazardous activities until his or her reaction to drug is known.
- Urge patient to keep follow-up appointments. Periodic evaluations should be made to determine possibility of dosage reduction or termination of drug therapy.
- Drug may discolor urine pink to red or red brown.

CHLORTHALIDONE

(klor-thal'i-done)

Trade names: Hygroton, Hylidone, Novothalidone ♣, Thalitone, Uridon ♣

Classifications: WATER BALANCE AGENT; THIAZIDE DIURETIC; ANTIHYPERTENSIVE

Prototype: Hydrochlorothiazide

Pregnancy category: B

ACTIONS/PHARMACODYNAMICS
Sulfonamide derivative. Differs chemically from thiazides but shares similar actions, uses, contraindications, adverse reactions, and drug interactions. Increases excretion of sodium and chloride by inhibiting their reabsorption in the cortical diluting segment of the ascending loop of Henle. Reportedly causes elevations in total cholesterol, LDL cholesterol, and triglycerides, in some patients.

USES Edema associated with CHF, renal decompensation, hepatic cirrhosis, corticosteroid and estrogen therapy; as sole agent or with other antihypertensives to treat hypertension.

ROUTE & DOSAGE

Hypertension

Adult: **PO** 12.5–25 mg/d; may be increased to 100 mg/d if needed.
Child: **PO** 2 mg/kg 3 times/wk.

Edema

Adult: **PO** 50–100 mg/d; may be increased to 200 mg/d if needed.

PHARMACOKINETICS **Absorption:** readily absorbed from GI tract. **Onset:** 2 h. **Peak:** 3–6 h. **Duration:** 24–72 h. **Distribution:** crosses placenta; appears in breast milk. **Elimination:** half-life: 54 h; 30–60% excreted in urine in 24 h.

CONTRAINDICATIONS & PRECAUTIONS **Contraindicated in:** hypersensitivity to sulfonamide derivatives; anuria, hypokalemia. Safe use during pregnancy (category B), in nursing mothers, and children not established. **Cautious use in:** history of renal and hepatic disease, gout, SLE, diabetes mellitus.

ADVERSE/SIDE EFFECTS **CNS:** dizziness, vertigo, paresthesias, headache. **CV:** orthostatic hypotension. **GI:** anorexia, nausea, vomiting, diarrhea, constipation, cramping, jaundice. **Hematologic:** *hypokalemia,* hyponatremia, hypochloremia, hypercalcemia, <u>agranulocytosis</u>, thrombocytopenia, <u>aplastic anemia</u>. **Skin/Hypersensitivity:** rash, urticaria, photosensitivity, vasculitis. **Other:** glycosuria, hyperglycemia, impotence, exacerbation of gout.

DRUG INTERACTIONS Increased risk of **digoxin** toxicity because of hypokalemia; CORTICOSTEROIDS, **amphotericin B** increase hypokalemia; decreases **lithium** elimination; may antagonize the hypoglycemic effects of SULFONYLUREAS; NSAIDS may attenuate diuretic effects; **cholestyramine** decreases thiazide absorption.

NURSING IMPLICATIONS

Administration

- When chlorthalidone is used as a diuretic, an intermittent dose schedule may reduce incidence of adverse reactions.
- Administer as single dose in AM to reduce potential for interrupted sleep because of diuresis.
- Store tablets in tightly closed container at 15–30C (59–86F) unless otherwise advised.

Assessment & Drug Effects

- When chlorthalidone is used for hypertension, establish baseline BP measurements and check at regular intervals during period of dosage adjustment.
- Elderly patients are more sensitive to adverse effects of drug-induced diuresis because of age-related changes in the cardiovascular and renal systems. Be alert to signs of hypokalemia (see Appendix G).
- The following laboratory values should be obtained initially and periodically throughout therapy: serum electrolytes (particularly K, Mg, Ca), serum uric acid, creatinine, BUN, and uric acid and blood sugar (especially in patients with diabetes).

Patient & Family Education

- Advise patient to maintain adequate potassium intake, to monitor weight, and to make a daily estimate of I&O ratio.

CHLORZOXAZONE

(klor-zox'a-zone)

Trade names: Paraflex, Parafon Forte

Classifications: AUTONOMIC NERVOUS SYSTEM AGENT; CENTRAL-ACTING SKELETAL MUSCLE RELAXANT
Prototype: Cyclobenzaprine
Pregnancy category: C

ACTIONS/PHARMACODYNAMICS Centrally acting skeletal muscle relaxant. Acts indirectly by depressing nerve transmission through polysynaptic pathways in spinal cord, subcortical centers, and brainstem and possibly by sedative effect. Not effective for spastic or dyskinetic CNS disorders, e.g., cerebral palsy.

USE Symptomatic treatment of muscle spasm and pain associated with various musculoskeletal conditions.

ROUTE & DOSAGE

Skeletal Muscle Relaxant
Adult: **PO** 250–500 mg t.i.d. or q.i.d. (max 3 g/d).
Child: **PO** 20 mg/kg/d in 3–4 divided doses.

PHARMACOKINETICS Absorption: readily absorbed from GI tract. **Onset:** 1 h. **Peak:** 1–4 h. **Duration:** 3–4 h. **Distribution:** not known if crosses placenta or distributed into breast milk. **Metabolism:** metabolized in liver. **Elimination:** half-life: 66 min; excreted in urine.

CONTRAINDICATIONS & PRECAUTIONS Contraindicated in: impaired liver function. Safe use during pregnancy (category C) not established. **Cautious use in:** patients with known allergies or history of drug allergies; history of liver disease; elderly patients.

ADVERSE/SIDE EFFECTS CNS: *drowsiness, dizziness,* light-headedness, headache, malaise, overstimulation. **GI:** anorexia, heartburn, nausea, vomiting, constipation, diarrhea, abdominal pain. **Hypersensitivity:** erythema, rash, pruritus, urticaria, petechiae, ecchymoses. **Other:** hepatotoxicity: jaundice, liver damage.

DRUG INTERACTIONS Alcohol, CNS DEPRESSANTS add to CNS depression.

NURSING IMPLICATIONS

Administration

- Chlorzoxazone may be taken with food or meals to prevent gastric distress. If necessary, tablet may be crushed and mixed with food or liquid, e.g., milk, fruit juice.
- Store in tight container at 15–30C (59–86F) unless otherwise directed.

Assessment & Drug Effects

- Some patients may require supervision of ambulation during early drug therapy.
- Periodic liver function tests are advised in patients receiving long-term therapy even if sporadic.
- Since chlorzoxazone metabolite may discolor urine, dark urine cannot be a reliable sign of a hepatotoxic reaction.

Patient & Family Education

- Since sedation, drowsiness, and dizziness may occur, advise patient not to undertake activities requiring mental alertness, judgment, and physical coordination until reaction to drug is known.
- Drug may discolor urine orange to purplish red, but this is of no clinical significance.
- Drug should be discontinued if signs of hypersensitivity (see Appendix G) or of liver dysfunction appear (abdominal discomfort, yellow sclerae or skin, pruritus, malaise, nausea, vomiting).
- Advise patient to check with physician before taking an OTC

depressant (e.g., antihistamine, sedative, alcohol) since effects may be additive.

C

CHOLESTYRAMINE RESIN

(koe-less-tear'a-meen)

Trade names: Cholybar, Questran, Questran Light, Prevalyte

Prototype for classifications: CARDIOVASCULAR AGENT; ANTILIPEMIC; BILE ACID SEQUESTRANT; ANTIPRURITIC

Pregnancy category: C

ACTIONS/PHARMACODYNAMICS Anion-exchange resin used for its cholesterol-lowering effect. Adsorbs and combines with intestinal bile acids in exchange for chloride ions to form an insoluble, nonabsorbable complex that is excreted in the feces. As a result, bile salts are continually (but not entirely) prevented from reentry to the enterohepatic circulation. Increased fecal loss of bile acids leads to lowered serum total cholesterol by decrease in low-density lipoprotein (LDL) cholesterol and in reduction of bile acid deposit in dermal tissues. Serum triglyceride levels may increase or remain unchanged.

USES As adjunct to diet therapy in management of patients with primary hypercholesterolemia (type IIa hyperlipedemia) with a significant risk of atherosclerotic heart disease and MI; for relief of pruritus secondary to partial biliary stasis. **Unlabeled uses:** to control diarrhea caused by excess bile acids in colon; for hyperoxaluria.

ROUTE & DOSAGE

Hypercholesterolemia

Adult: **PO** 4 g b.i.d. to q.i.d. a.c. and h.s.; may need up to 24 g/d.

Child: **PO** 240 mg/kg/d in 3 divided doses.

Hyperlipoproteinemia

Adult: **PO** 4–8 g b.i.d. to q.i.d. a.c. and h.s. (≤ 32 g/d).

Pruritus

Adult: **PO** 4 g b.i.d. to q.i.d. a.c. and h.s. (≤ 16 g/d).

PHARMACOKINETICS Absorption: not absorbed from GI tract. **Elimination:** excreted in feces as insoluble complex.

CONTRAINDICATIONS & PRECAUTIONS Contraindicated in: complete biliary obstruction, hypersensitivity to bile acid sequestrants. Safe use by pregnant women (category C), nursing mothers, and children ≤ 6 y not established. **Cautious use in:** bleeding disorders; hemorrhoids; impaired GI function, peptic ulcer, malabsorption states (e.g., steatorrhea); phenylketonuria (Questran Light only).

ADVERSE/SIDE EFFECTS Eye: arcus juvenilis, uveitis. **GI:** *constipation,* fecal impaction, hemorrhoids, abdominal pain and distension, flatulence, bloating sensation, belching, nausea, vomiting, heartburn, anorexia, diarrhea, steatorrhea. **Other:** weight loss or gain, increased libido, iron, calcium, vitamin A, D, and K deficiencies (from poor absorption); hypoprothrombinemia, hyperchloremic acidosis, decreased erythrocyte folate levels, rash, irritations of skin, tongue, and perianal areas.

DIAGNOSTIC TEST INTERFERENCE Cholestyramine therapy may be accompanied by increased serum ***AST, phosphorus, chloride,*** and ***alkaline phosphatase*** levels; decreased ***serum calcium, sodium,*** and ***potassium*** levels.

DRUG INTERACTIONS Decreases the absorption of ORAL ANTICOAGULANTS, **digoxin,** TETRACYCLINES, **penicillins, phenobarbital,** THYROID HORMONES, THIAZIDE DIURETICS, IRON SALTS, FAT-SOLUBLE VITAMINS (A, D, E, K) from the GI tract—administer cholestyramine 4 h before or 2 h after these drugs.

NURSING IMPLICATIONS

Administration

- Place contents of one packet or one level scoopful on surface of at least 120 to 180 ml (4–6 oz) of water or other preferred liquid. Permit drug to hydrate by standing without stirring 1–2 min, twirling glass occasionally; then stir until suspension is uniform. Rinse glass with small amount of liquid and have patient drink remainder to ensure entire dose is taken. Administer before meals.
- Water, highly flavored liquids, or other noncarbonated drinks, thin soups, diluted pulpy fruit juices, or fruits with high moisture content such as applesauce or crushed pineapple disguise taste somewhat and may encourage compliance.
- Always dissolve cholestyramine before administration; it is irritating to mucous membranes and may cause esophageal impaction if administered dry.
- Color may vary with different batches, but this does not affect drug action. Has a slight aminelike odor and a disagreeable taste; in solution its consistency is sandy or gritty.
- Store in tightly closed container at 15–30C (59–86F) unless otherwise specified.

Assessment & Drug Effects

- Long-term use of cholestyramine resin can increase bleeding tendency. Be alert to early symptoms of hypoprothrombinemia (petechiae, ecchymoses, abnormal bleeding from mucous membranes, tarry stools) and report their occurrence promptly.
- Preexisting constipation may be worsened in the elderly, women, and in those taking >24 g/d.
- Supplemental vitamins A and D and folic acid may be required by patient on long-term therapy.
- Serum cholesterol levels are reduced within 24–48 h after treatment starts and may continue to decline for a year. After withdrawal of cholestyramine, cholesterol levels usually return to baseline level in about 2 to 4 wk.
- If response is unsatisfactory after 3 mo of treatment, drug is usually withdrawn.
- Periodic erythrocyte folate levels are recommended, particularly in children.

Patient & Family Education

- Report constipation immediately to physician.
- High-bulk diet with adequate fluid intake is an essential adjunct to cholestyramine treatment and generally resolves the problems of constipation and bloating sensation.
- Warn patient not to omit doses. Sudden withdrawal can promote uninhibited absorption of other drugs taken concomitantly, leading to toxicity or overdosage.
- Usually, GI side effects subside after the first month of drug therapy.
- The following symptoms may be drug-induced and should be reported promptly: severe gastric distress with nausea and vomiting,

unusual weight loss, black stools, severe hemorrhoids (GI bleeding), sudden back pain.

C

CHOLINE MAGNESIUM TRISALICYLATE

(cho′leen mag-ne′si-um tri-sal′i-cilate)

Trade name: Trilisate

Classifications: CNS AGENT; ANALGESIC, ANTIPYRETIC; SALICYLATE

Prototype: Aspirin

Pregnancy category: C

ACTIONS/PHARMACODYNAMICS Trilisate is a nonsteroidal, antiinflammatory preparation combining choline salicylate and magnesium salicylate. It also has analgesic and antipyretic action. Mode of action is by inhibiting prostaglandin synthesis. Platelet aggregation is not affected.

USES Osteoarthritis, rheumatoid arthritis, and other arthrides. Preferable to aspirin for patients with GI bleeding.

ROUTE & DOSAGE

Arthritis

Adult: **PO** 1.5–2.5 g/d in 1–3 divided doses (max 4.5 g/d).

Mild to Moderate Pain, Fever

Adult: **PO** 2–3 g/d in 2 divided doses.
Child: **PO** 30–60 mg/kg/d in 3–4 divided doses.

PHARMACOKINETICS **Absorption:** readily absorbed from small intestine. **Onset:** 30 min. **Peak:** 1–3 h. **Metabolism:** metabolized in liver. **Elimination:** half-life: 2–3 h; excreted in urine.

CONTRAINDICATIONS & PRECAUTIONS **Contraindicated in:** hypersensitivity to nonacetylated salicylates. **Cautious use in:** chronic renal and hepatic failure, peptic ulcer; patients on coumadin or heparin; pregnancy (category C); children and teenagers with chickenpox, influenza, or flu symptoms because of the potential for Reye's syndrome.

ADVERSE/SIDE EFFECTS **CNS:** headache, vertigo, confusion, drowsiness. **GI:** vomiting, diarrhea. **Ear:** tinnitus.

DRUG INTERACTIONS **Aminosalicylic acid** increases risk of salicylate toxicity; **ammonium chloride** and other **acidifying agents** decrease its renal elimination, increasing risk of salicylate toxicity; ANTICOAGULANTS increase risk of bleeding; CARBONIC ANHYDRASE INHIBITORS enhance salicylate toxicity; CORTICOSTEROIDS compound ulcerogenic effects; increases **methotrexate** toxicity; low doses of salicylates may antagonize uricosuric effects of **probenecid, sulfinpyrazone.**

NURSING IMPLICATIONS

Administration

- Drug may be given with food to reduce gastric upset. Do not give with antacids.
- Store at 59–86F (15–30C).

Assessment & Drug Effects

- As with other NSAIDS, the antipyretic and antiinflammatory effects may mask usual signs and symptoms of infection or other diseases.
- Assess for GI discomfort; nausea, gastric irritation, indigestion, diarrhea, and constipation are frequent complaints.
- If used concurrently with warfarin, monitor for signs and symptoms

of bleeding and closely monitor PT.

Patient & Family Education

- Avoid taking aspirin or acetaminophen concurrently with drug.
- Inform patient of possible CNS effects (e.g., vertigo, drowsiness) and caution to avoid dangerous activities until reaction to drug is determined.
- Instruct patient to report tinnitus to physician.
- Instruct patient to report persistent gastric irritation and epigastric pain.
- Instruct patients with type II diabetes who are taking an oral hypoglycemic agent (OHA) that hypoglycemic effects may be enhanced.
- Do not give to children or teenagers with chickenpox, influenza, or flu symptoms because of association with Reye's syndrome.

CHOLINE SALICYLATE

(koe'leen)

Trade name: Arthropan

Classifications: CNS AGENT; ANALGESIC, ANTIPYRETIC; SALICYLATE

Prototype: Aspirin

Pregnancy category: C

ACTIONS/PHARMACODYNAMICS Choline salt of salicylic acid available commercially as a liquid salicylate preparation. Reported to be less potent than aspirin as an analgesic, antiinflammatory, and antipyretic, and produces less gastric irritation and bleeding. Clinical significance of the claim that it is absorbed more rapidly than aspirin is unclear. Unlike aspirin, believed to have no appreciable effect on platelet function.

USES Analgesic and antiinflammatory in rheumatoid arthritis, rheumatic fever, osteoarthritis, and other conditions for which oral salicylates are usually recommended. May be indicated for patients who have difficulty swallowing tablets or capsules or as an alternative preparation for patients who show gastric intolerance to aspirin or who should avoid sodium-containing salicylates.

ROUTE & DOSAGE

Analgesic, Antipyretic

Adult: **PO** 435–870 mg (2.5–5 ml) q4h.
Child: **PO** 2–11 y: 2 g (115 ml)/m^2 in 4–6 divided doses.

Arthritis

Adult: **PO** 4.8–7.2 g (28–41 ml)/d in 4–6 divided doses.
Child: **PO** 107–134 mg (0.6–0.8 ml)/kg/d in 4–6 divided doses.

PHARMACOKINETICS Absorption: readily absorbed from GI tract. **Peak:** 10–30 min. **Distribution:** widely distributed in most body tissues; crosses placenta; distributed in breast milk. **Elimination:** half-life: 2–3 h; excreted in urine.

CONTRAINDICATIONS & PRECAUTIONS Contraindicated in: salicylate hypersensitivity. **Cautious use in:** history of peptic ulcer disease, pregnancy (category C).

ADVERSE/SIDE EFFECTS *Nausea,* vomiting. **High doses:** tinnitus, deafness, dizziness, sweating, mental confusion, hyperventilation; hepatotoxicity.

DIAGNOSTIC TEST INTERFERENCE As for aspirin with the exception of ***5-HIAA*** which is not affected by choline salicylate.

DRUG INTERACTIONS Aminosalicylate increases risk of salicylate toxicity; increases risk of bleeding with ORAL ANTICOAGULANTS; SULFONYLUREAS pose increased risk of hypo-

C

glycemia with large doses of salicylates; CARBONIC ANHYDRASE INHIBITORS cause metabolic acidosis that may increase salicylate toxicity; CORTICOSTEROIDS add to ulcerogenic effects; may increase **methotrexate** levels; small doses of salicylates may blunt uricosuric effects of **probenecid, sulfinpyrazone.**

NURSING IMPLICATIONS

Administration

- Choline salicylate may be mixed with or followed by fruit juice, a carbonated beverage, or water. Do not administer with an antacid.
- If patient requires an antacid, administer choline salicylate before meals and the antacid 2 h after meals.
- Store in tightly capped container at temperature between 15 and 30C (59 and 86F). Protect from freezing.

Assessment & Drug Effects

- Monitor effectiveness of drug in relieving pain in arthritic joints.
- Assess for signs of bleeding, especially in patients on anticoagulant therapy.

Patient & Family Education

- This drug is available OTC. Caution patient not to exceed recommended dosage and to keep medicine out of the reach of children.
- Avoid concurrent use of other drugs containing aspirin or salicylates unless otherwise advised by physician.

CHORIONIC GONADOTROPIN

(go-nad'oh-troe-pin)

Trade names: Antuitrin, A.P.L., Chorex, Chorigon, Choron 10, Corgonject-5, Follutein, Glukor, Gonic, HCG, Pregnyl, Profasi HP

Classification: HORMONE

Pregnancy category: C

ACTIONS/PHARMACODYNAMICS

Human chorionic gonadotropin (hCG) is a polypeptide hormone produced by the placenta and extracted from urine during first trimester of pregnancy. Actions nearly identical to those of pituitary luteinizing hormone (LH). Promotes production of gonadal steroid hormones by stimulating interstitial cells of the testes to produce androgen, and the corpus luteum of the ovary to produce progesterone. Administration of HCG to women of childbearing age with normal functioning ovaries causes maturation of the ovarian follicle and triggers ovulation. When given during normal pregnancy, it maintains corpus luteum after LH decreases, supports continuing secretion of estrogen and progesterone, and prevents ovulation.

USES Prepubertal cryptorchidism not due to anatomic obstruction and male hypogonadism secondary to pituitary deficiency. Also used in conjunction with menotropins to induce ovulation and pregnancy in infertile women in whom the cause of anovulation is secondary (ovulation usually occurs within 18 h). To stimulate spermatogenesis in males with hypogonadism. **Unlabeled use:** corpus luteum dysfunction.

ROUTE & DOSAGE

Prepubertal Cryptorchidism

Child: **IM** 4000 units 3 times/wk for 3 wk, *or* 5000 U q.o.d. for 4 doses, *or* 500–1000 U 3 times/wk for 4–6 wk.

Hypogonadotropic Hypogonadism

Adult: **IM** 500–1000 U 3 times/wk for 3 wk; then 2 times/wk for 3 wk *or* 4000 U 3

times/wk for 6–9 mo followed by 2000 U 3 times/wk for 3 mo.

Stimulation of Spermatogenesis

Adult: **IM** 5000 U 3 times/wk until normal testosterone levels are achieved (4–6 mo), then 2000 U 2 times/wk with menotropins for 4 mo.

Induction of Ovulation

Adult: **IM** 500–1000 U 1 d following last dose of menotropins.

PHARMACOKINETICS **Onset:** 2 h. **Peak:** 6 h. **Distribution:** testes in males, ovaries in females. **Elimination:** half-life: 23 h; 10–12% excreted in urine within 24 h.

CONTRAINDICATIONS & PRECAUTIONS **Contraindicated in:** known hypersensitivity to hCG, hypogonadism of testicular origin, hypertrophy or tumor of pituitary, prostatic carcinoma or other androgen-dependent neoplasms, precocious puberty. Safe use during pregnancy (category C) not established. **Cautious use in:** epilepsy, migraine, asthma, cardiac or renal disease.

ADVERSE/SIDE EFFECTS Headache, irritability, restlessness, depression, fatigue, gynecomastia, edema, precocious puberty, pain at injection site, increased urinary steroid excretion, ectopic pregnancy (incidence low). When used with menotropins (human menopausal gonadotropin): ovarian hyperstimulation (ascites with or without pain, pleural effusion, ruptured ovarian cysts with resultant hemoperitoneum, multiple births), arterial thromboembolism.

DIAGNOSTIC TEST INTERFERENCE ***Pregnancy tests:*** possibility of false results.

NURSING IMPLICATIONS

Administration

- Following reconstitution (diluent furnished by manufacturer), solution is stable for 30–90 d, depending on manufacturer, when refrigerated; thereafter potency decreases.
- Store powder for injection at 15–30C (59–86F) unless otherwise directed.

Patient & Family Education

- This hormone is given to the anovulatory patient after failure to respond to therapy with clomiphene citrate.
- Treatment for prepubertal cryptorchidism is usually started between 4 and 9 y. HCG can help predict whether orchidopexy will be needed in the future.
- When used for treatment of infertility, timing of coitus is important. Daily intercourse is encouraged from day before HCG is given until ovulation occurs.
- Instruct patient to report promptly onset of abdominal pain and distension (ovarian hyperstimulation syndrome).
- Induction of androgen secretion by HCG may induce precocious puberty in patient treated for cryptorchidism. Instruct parent to report to physician if the following appear: axillary, facial, pubic hair; penile growth; acne; deepening of voice.
- Observe for signs of fluid retention. A weight chart should be maintained for a biweekly record. Report to physician if weight gain is associated with edema.
- Vaginal bleeding during treatment of corpus luteum deficiency should be reported; drug will be discontinued.

C

CICLOPIROX OLAMINE

(sye-kloe-peer′ox)
Trade name: Loprox
Classifications: ANTIINFECTIVE; ANTIFUNGAL ANTIBIOTIC
Prototype: Fluconazole
Pregnancy category: B

ACTIONS/PHARMACODYNAMICS Synthetic broad-spectrum antifungal agent with activity against pathogenic fungi including dermatophytes, yeasts, and *Malassezia furfur,* some species of *Mycoplasma* and *Trichomonas vaginalis,* and certain strains of gram-positive and gram-negative bacteria. Inhibits transport of amino acids within fungal cell, thereby interfering with synthesis of protein, RNA, and DNA.

USES Topically for treatment of tinea cruris and tinea corporis (ringworm) due to *Trichophyton rubrum, Trichophyton mentagrophytes, Epidermophyton floccosum,* and *Microsporum canis,* and for tinea (pityriasis) versicolor due to *Malassezia furfur;* also cutaneous candidiasis (moniliasis) caused by *Candida albicans.*

ROUTE & DOSAGE

Tinea

Adult: **Topical** Massage cream into affected area and surrounding skin twice daily, morning and evening.

PHARMACOKINETICS Absorption: 1.3% absorbed through intact skin. **Distribution:** distributed to epidermis, corium (dermis), including hair and hair follicles and sebaceous glands; not known if crosses placenta or is distributed into breast milk. **Elimination:** half-life: 1.7 h; excreted primarily by kidneys.

CONTRAINDICATIONS & PRECAUTIONS Contraindicated in: hypersensitivity to ciclopirox olamine or to any excipients in the formulation. Safe use during pregnancy (category B), in nursing women, and in children <10 y not established.

ADVERSE/SIDE EFFECTS Irritation, pruritus, burning, worsening of clinical condition.

NURSING IMPLICATIONS

Administration

- Wash hands thoroughly before and after treatments.
- Consult with physician about specific procedure for cleansing the skin before medication is applied. Regardless of method used, dry skin thoroughly before drug application.
- Store at 15–30C (59–86F) unless otherwise directed.

Assessment & Drug Effects

- In general, tinea versicolor responds to drug treatment in about 2 wk. Tinea pedis ("athlete's foot"), tinea corporis (ringworm), tinea cruris ("jock itch"), and candidiasis (moniliasis) require about 4 wk of therapy.
- Recurrences are especially likely to occur in patients with diabetes or other predisposing illnesses.

Patient & Family Education

- Instruct patient to use medication for the prescribed time even though symptoms improve.
- Report skin irritation or other possible signs of sensitization. A reaction suggestive of sensitization warrants drug discontinuation.
- Caution patient not to use occlusive dressings or wrappings.
- Warn patient to avoid contact of drug in or near the eyes.
- Wear light clothing and footwear

that will allow ventilation. Loose-fitting cotton underwear or socks are ideal.

CIDOFOVIR

(cye-do′fo-ver)

Trade name: Vistide

Classifications: ANTIINFECTIVE; ANTIVIRAL

Prototype: Acyclovir

Pregnancy category: C

ACTIONS/PHARMACODYNAMICS Cidofovir, a nucleotide analog, suppresses cytomegalovirus (CMV) replication by inhibiting CMV DNA polymerase. This results in a reduction in the rate of viral DNA synthesis of CMV.

USE Treatment of CMV retinitis in patients with AIDS.

ROUTE & DOSAGE

CMV Retinitis: Induction

Adult: **IV** 5 mg/kg once weekly for 2 wk. Also give 2 g probenecid 3 h prior to infusion and 1 g 8 h after infusion (4 g total).

CMV Retinitis: Maintenance

Adult: **IV** 5 mg/kg once every 2 wk. Also give 2 g probenecid 3 h prior to infusion and 1 g 8 h after infusion (4 g total).

Adjustment for Renal Impairment

Cl_{cr} 41–55 ml/min: 2 mg/kg; 30–40: 1.5 mg/kg; 20–29 ml/min: 1 mg/kg; <20 ml/min: 0.5 mg/kg.

PHARMACOKINETICS Duration: probenecid increases serum levels and area under concentration–time curve. **Elimination:** 80–100% recovered in urine, probenecid delays urinary excretion.

CONTRAINDICATIONS & PRECAUTIONS Contraindicated in: hypersensitivity to cidofovir, history of severe hypersensitivity to probenecid or other sulfa-containing medications, nursing mothers. **Cautious use in:** renal function impairment, history of diabetes, myelosuppression, previous hypersensitivity to other nucleoside analogs, pregnancy (category C). Safety and effectiveness in children not established.

ADVERSE/SIDE EFFECTS CNS: *fever, headache,* asthenia. **GI:** nausea, vomiting, diarrhea. **Renal:** *nephrotoxicity, proteinuria.* **Respiratory:** dyspnea, pneumonia. **Other:** metabolic acidosis, neutropenia, infection, ocular hypotony, allergic reactions.

DRUG INTERACTIONS AMINOGLYCOSIDES, **amphotericin B, foscarnet, pentamidine** can increase risk of nephrotoxicity.

NURSING IMPLICATIONS

Administration

- Initiate treatment only in patients with serum creatinine ≤1.5 mg/dl, Cl_{cr} >55 ml/min, and urine protein <100 mg/dl.
- Pretreatment: Prehydrate with IV of 1 L NS infused over 1–2 h immediately before cidofovir infusion. If able to tolerate fluid load, infuse second liter over 1–3 h starting at beginning (or end) of cidofovir infusion.
- Preparation & administration of IV solution: Dilute in 100 ml of 0.9% NS and infuse over 1 h at constant rate.
- Do not coadminister with other agents with significant nephrotoxic potential.
- Ingestion of food and antiemetics prior to each dose of probenecid may reduce nausea.

C

- Store vials at 20–25C (68–77F); may store diluted IV solution at 2–8C (36–46F) for up to 24 h.

Assessment & Drug Effects

- Monitor serum creatinine, urine protein, and WBC count with differential prior to each dose. Dose adjustments or discontinuation may be required.
- In patients with proteinuria, administer IV hydration and repeat test.
- Periodically monitor visual acuity and intraocular pressure.
- Monitor for S&S of hypersensitivity (see Appendix G). Report their appearance promptly.

Patient & Family Education

- Advise those taking zidovudine to discontinue or decrease dose to 50% on days of cidofovir administration.
- Advise of importance of regular ophthalmologic exams.
- Warn patient of potential adverse reactions caused by probenecid (e.g., headache, nausea, vomiting, hypersensitivity reactions) and cidofovir.
- Emphasize need for closely monitoring renal function.
- Advise women to use effective contraception during and 1 mo after treatment.
- Advise men to use barrier contraception during and 3 mo after treatment.

CIMETIDINE

(sye-met′i-deen)

Trade names: Novocimetine ♣, Peptol ♣, Tagamet, Tagamet HB

Prototype for classifications: GI AGENT; ANTISECRETORY (H_2-RECEPTOR ANTAGONIST)

Pregnancy category: B

ACTIONS/PHARMACODYNAMICS

Enzyme inhibitor structurally similar to histamine. Belongs to the antihistamine group with high selectivity for histamine H_2-receptors on parietal cells (minimal effect on H_1-receptors). By reversible competitive inhibition of histamine at the H_2-receptor sites suppresses all phases of daytime and nocturnal basal gastric acid secretion. Indirectly reduces pepsin secretion. Is not a cholinergic. Has no effect on lower esophageal sphincter pressure, gastric motility or emptying, biliary or pancreatic secretion.

USES Short-term treatment of active duodenal ulcer and prevention of ulcer recurrence (at reduced dosage) after it is healed. Also used for short-term treatment of active benign gastric ulcer, pathologic hypersecretory conditions such as Zollinger-Ellison syndrome, and heartburn. **Unlabeled uses:** prophylaxis of stress-induced ulcers, upper GI bleeding, and aspiration pneumonitis; gastroesophageal reflux; chronic urticaria; acetaminophen toxicity.

ROUTE & DOSAGE

Duodenal Ulcer

Adult: **PO** 300 mg q.i.d. *or* 400 mg b.i.d. *or* 800 mg h.s. **IM/IV** 300 mg q6–8h.
Child: **PO/IM/IV** 20–40 mg/kg/d in 4 divided doses.
Neonate: **PO/IM/IV** 5–10 mg/kg/d divided q8–12h. *Infant:* **PO/IM/IV** 10–20 mg/kg/d divided q6–12h.

Duodenal Ulcer, Maintenance Therapy

Adult: **PO** 400 mg h.s.

Gastric Ulcer

Adult: **PO** 300 mg q.i.d. with meals and h.s. **IM/IV** 300 mg q6–8h.

Heartburn

Adult: **PO** 200 mg 2–4 times/d.

Pathologic Hypersecretory Disease

Adult: **PO** 300 mg q.i.d. with meals and h.s.; may increase up to 2400 mg/d. **IM/IV** 300 mg q6–8h; may increase up to 2400 mg/d.

Adjustment for Renal Impairment

Cl_{cr} 20–40 ml/min: dose q8h; Cl_{cr} <20 ml/min: dose q12h.

PHARMACOKINETICS **Absorption:** 70% of oral dose absorbed from GI tract. **Peak:** 1–1.5 h. **Distribution:** widely distributed; crosses blood-brain barrier and placenta. **Metabolism:** metabolized in liver. **Elimination:** half-life: 2 h; most of drug excreted in urine in 24 h; excreted in breast milk.

CONTRAINDICATIONS & PRECAUTIONS **Contraindicated in:** known hypersensitivity to cimetidine. Safe use in nursing mothers, during pregnancy (category B), or in children <16 y not established. **Cautious use in:** elderly or critically ill patients; impaired renal or hepatic function; organic brain syndrome.

ADVERSE/SIDE EFFECTS **CNS:** drowsiness, dizziness, light-headedness, depression, headache, reversible confusional states, paranoid psychosis. **CV (rare):** <u>cardiac arrhythmias and cardiac arrest after rapid IV bolus dose.</u> **GI:** mild transient diarrhea; severe diarrhea, constipation, abdominal discomfort. **Gynecologic:** gynecomastia and breast soreness, galactorrhea, reversible impotence. **Hematologic:** increased prothrombin time; neutropenia (rare), thrombocytopenia (rare), <u>aplastic anemia</u>. **Musculoskeletal:** exacerbation of joint symptoms in patients with preexisting arthritis. **Other:** rash, Stevens-Johnson syndrome, reversible alopecia, fever; slight increase in serum uric acid, BUN, creatinine; transient pain at IM site; hypospermia.

DIAGNOSTIC TEST INTERFERENCE Cimetidine may cause false-positive ***hemoccult test for gastric bleeding*** if test is performed within 15 min of oral cimetidine administration.

DRUG INTERACTIONS Cimetidine decreases the hepatic metabolism of **warfarin, phenobarbital, phenytoin, diazepam, propranolol, lidocaine, theophylline,** thus increasing their activity and toxicity; ANTACIDS may decrease absorption of cimetidine.

INCOMPATIBILITIES **Solution/additive: amphotericin B, cefamandole, cephalothin, atropine, cefazolin, chlorpromazine, pentobarbital, secobarbital.**

NURSING IMPLICATIONS

Administration

- Oral form may be taken with meals. Absorption may be decreased by antacids but is unaffected by food.
- Administration of antacid to control acute ulcer pain should be at least 1 h before or 2 h after food.
- Intermittent IV injection: Dilute 300 mg in at least 50 ml 5% dextrose injection or other compatible IV solution and infuse over 15–20 min.
- IV injection: Dilute in 0.9% NaCl injection or other compatible IV solution to a total volume of 20 ml

C

and inject within not less than 2 min.

- IV administration to neonates, infants and children: Verify correct IV concentration and rate of infusion/injection with physician.
- Parenteral solutions are stable for 48 h at room temperature when added to commonly used IV solutions for dilution. Follow manufacturer's directions.
- Store all forms of cimetidine at 15–30C (59–86F) protected from light unless otherwise directed by manufacturer.

Assessment & Drug Effects

- Ulcer healing may occur within the first 2 wk of therapy but generally requires at least 4 wk in most patients. Short-term (i.e., 8 wk) therapy of active duodenal ulcer does not prevent ulcer recurrence when drug is discontinued.
- Monitor pulse of patient during first few days of drug regimen. Bradycardia after PO as well as IV administration should be reported. Pulse usually returns to normal within 24 h after drug discontinuation.
- Monitor I&O ratio and pattern, particularly in the elderly, severely ill, and in patients with impaired renal function.
- Adynamic ileus has been reported in patients receiving cimetidine to prevent and treat stress ulcers. Report loss of bowel sounds, absence of bowel movement or flatus, vomiting, crampy pain, abdominal distention.
- Periodic evaluations of blood count and renal and hepatic function are advised during therapy.
- Be alert to onset of confusional states, particularly in the elderly or severely ill patient. Symptoms occur within 2–3 d after first dose. Report immediately: drug should be withdrawn. Symptoms usually resolve within 3–4 d after therapy is discontinued.
- If patient complains of severe headache, check BP and report an elevation to the physician.
- Ingestion of tyramine-rich foods (cheddar cheese, beef-extract, yogurt, aged meats, soy sauce, Chianti wine) can lead to transient hypertension and severe headache (MAOI-like reaction), especially if patient is elderly and has hepatic impairment. Cimetidine interference with liver metabolism can lead to excess in circulation of tyramine.
- Cimetidine impairs absorption of protein-bound vitamin B_{12}; therefore patient who takes cimetidine in divided doses to continuously suppress acid gastric secretion is at risk for vitamin B_{12} deficiency (no risk for patient who takes drug at bedtime to suppress nocturnal acid production).

Patient & Family Education

- Be certain that patient is aware of the importance of taking cimetidine exactly as prescribed. Sudden discontinuation of therapy reportedly has caused perforation of chronic peptic ulcer.
- Urge patient to seek advice about self-medication with any OTC drug.
- Mild bilateral gynecomastia and breast soreness may occur after ≥ 1 mo of therapy. It may disappear spontaneously or remain throughout therapy. Instruct patient to report this symptom to physician.
- Caution patient to promptly report recurrence of gastric pain or bleeding (black, tarry stools or "coffee ground" vomitus) and to notify physician if diarrhea continues more than 1 d.
- Caution patient to avoid driving

and other potentially hazardous activities until reaction to drug is known.

- Impress on patient and responsible family member(s) that duodenal or gastric ulcer is a chronic, recurrent condition that requires long-term maintenance drug therapy.
- Therapy for active duodenal ulcer is continued until healing is demonstrated by endoscopy (usually 4–6 wk, but not to exceed 8 wk).
- Maintenance therapy at reduced dosage after healing of active duodenal ulcer appears to limit recurrence, particularly if patient understands importance of other antiulcer therapeutic measures: no smoking, life-style that promotes reduced stress.

CINOXACIN

(sin-ox'a-sin)

Trade name: Cinobac

Classifications: URINARY TRACT ANTIINFECTIVE; QUINOLONE

Prototype: Trimethoprim

Pregnancy category: B

ACTIONS/PHARMACODYNAMICS Synthetic bactericidal agent with properties similar to those of nalidixic acid but with fewer side effects. Acts intracellularly to inhibit bacterial DNA replication and protein synthesis. Effective against a wide variety of gram-negative pathogens, particularly most strains of *Escherichia coli, Klebsiella* and *Enterobacter* species, *Proteus mirabilis,* and *Proteus vulgaris*. Not active against staphylococci, enterococci, or *Pseudomonas*.

USE Initial and recurrent UTIs in adults caused by susceptible microorganisms.

ROUTE & DOSAGE

UTI

Adult: **PO** 1 g/d in 2–4 divided doses.

PHARMACOKINETICS **Absorption:** readily absorbed from GI tract. **Peak:** 2–3 h. **Duration:** 12 h. **Distribution:** concentrates in renal and prostatic tissues; crosses placenta; distribution into breast milk unknown. **Elimination:** half-life: 1.5 h; 97% excreted in urine within 24 h.

CONTRAINDICATIONS & PRECAUTIONS **Contraindicated in:** hypersensitivity to cinoxacin or to other quinolones; anuria. Safe use during pregnancy (category B), in nursing mothers, and in prepubertal children not established. **Cautious use in:** impaired renal or hepatic function.

ADVERSE/SIDE EFFECTS **CNS:** *headache, dizziness,* insomnia, tingling sensations, agitation, anxiety. **Ear:** tinnitus. **Eye:** photophobia, blurred vision. **GI:** *nausea,* vomiting, anorexia, constipation, rectal itching, metallic taste, sore gums, abdominal cramps, diarrhea. **Hypersensitivity:** urticaria, pruritus, rash, edema. **Other:** swelling of extremities, arthropathy.

DRUG INTERACTION **Probenecid** decreases renal elimination of cinoxacin.

NURSING IMPLICATIONS

Administration

- Cinoxacin may be taken with food. Although presence of food in stomach may reduce peak serum concentrations, total amount absorbed is not affected.
- Therapeutic effectiveness is enhanced by taking the drug at evenly spaced intervals through-

out 24 h so that urinary drug concentration is maintained.

C

Assessment & Drug Effects

- Susceptibility tests should be performed before start of therapy and during therapy if response is not satisfactory.
- Since dizziness is a possible side effect, supervision of ambulation, especially with the elderly and debilitated, may be warranted.

Patient & Family Education

- Advise patient to take drug for the full course of therapy as prescribed.
- Instruct patient to report to physician if symptoms do not improve within a few days or if they become worse.
- Caution patient to avoid driving and other potentially hazardous tasks until reaction to drug is known.
- Photophobia may be relieved by wearing dark glasses.

CIPROFLOXACIN HYDROCHLORIDE

(ci-pro-flox'a-cin)

Trade names: Cipro, Cipro IV

CIPROFLOXACIN OPHTHALMIC

Trade name: Ciloxan

Prototype for classifications: ANTIINFECTIVE; QUINOLONE

Pregnancy Category: X

ACTIONS/PHARMACODYNAMICS Synthetic quinolone that is a broad spectrum bactericidal agent. Inhibits DNA-gyrase, an enzyme necessary for bacterial DNA replication and some aspects of transcription, repair, recombination, and transposition. Effective against many gram-positive and gram-negative organisms including *Citrobacter diversus, Enterobacter cloacae, Enterobacter aerogenes, Escherichia coli, Hemophilus influenzae, Klebsiella pneumoniae, Neisseria gonorrhoeae, Proteus mirabalis, Proteus vulgaris, Pseudomonas aeruginosa, Serratia marcescens, Staphylococcus aureus, Staphylococcus pyogenes, Shigella,* and *Salmonella*. Less active against gram-positive than gram-negative bacteria, although active against many gram-positive aerobic bacteria, including penicillinase-producing, non-penicillinase-producing, and methicillin-resistant staphylococci. However, many strains of streptococci are relatively resistant to the drug. Inactive against most anaerobic bacteria. Resistant to some strains of methicillin-resistant *S. aureus* (MRSA).

USES UTIs, lower respiratory tract infections, skin and skin structure infections, bone and joint infections, GI infection or infectious diarrhea, chronic bacterial prostatitis, nosocomial pneumonia, acute sinusitis. **Ophthalmic:** corneal ulcers, bacterial conjunctivitis caused by staphylococci, streptococci, and *P. aeruginosa.*

ROUTE & DOSAGE

UTI

Adult: **PO** 250 mg q12h. **IV** 200 mg q12h, infused over 60 min.

Moderate to Severe Systemic Infection

Adult: **PO** 500–750 mg q12h. **IV** 200–400 mg q12h, infused over 60 min.

Corneal Ulcers

Adult: **Ophthalmic** 2 drops q15min for 6 h, then 2 drops q30min for the next 18 h, then 2 drops q1h for 24 h, then 2 drops q4h for 14 d.

Bacterial Conjunctivitis

Adult: **Ophthalmic** 1–2 drops in conjunctival sac q2h while awake for 2 d, then 1–2 drops q4h while awake for the next 5 d.
Ointment: $\frac{1}{2}$-inch ribbon into conjunctival sac t.i.d. × 2 d, then b.i.d. × 5 d.

Acute Sinusitis

Adult: **PO** 500 mg b.i.d. × 10 d.

PHARMACOKINETICS Absorption: 60–80% absorbed from GI tract. **Ophthalmic:** minimal absorption through cornea or conjuctiva. **Onset:** topical 0.5–2 h. **Duration:** topical 12 h. **Peak:** 1–2 h. **Distribution:** widely distributed including prostate, lung, and bone; crosses placenta; distributed into breast milk. **Elimination:** half-life: 3.5–4 h; excreted primarily in urine with some biliary excretion.

CONTRAINDICATIONS & PRECAUTIONS Contraindicated in: known hypersensitivity to ciprofloxacin or other quinolones, pregnant women (category X), nursing mothers, and children. **Cautious use in:** known or suspected CNS disorders (i.e., severe cerebral arteriosclerosis or seizure disorders), patients receiving theophylline derivatives or caffeine, severe renal impairment and crystalluria during ciprofloxacin therapy, and patients on coumarin therapy.

ADVERSE/SIDE EFFECTS CNS: headache, vertigo, malaise, seizures (especially with rapid IV infusion). **GI:** nausea, vomiting, diarrhea, cramps, gas. **Ophthalmic:** *local burning and discomfort, crystalline precipitate on superficial portion of cornea,* lid margin crusting, scales, foreign body sensation, itching, and conjunctival hyperemia. **Skin:** rash, transient increases in liver transaminases, alkaline phosphatase, lactic dehydrogenase, and eosinophilia count, phlebitis, pain, burning, pruritus, and erythema at infusion site. **Other:** tendon rupture.

DIAGNOSTIC TEST INTERFERENCE Ciprofloxacin does not interfere with urinary glucose determinations using cupric sulfate solution or with glucose ovadase tests.

DRUG INTERACTIONS May increase **theophylline** levels 15–30%; ANTACIDS, **sulcralfate, iron** decrease absorption of ciprofloxacin; may increase PT for patients on warfarin.

INCOMPATABILITIES Solution/additive: aminophylline, clindamycin, dexamethasone, furosemide, heparin, hydrocortisone, magnesium sulfate, methylprednisolone, mezlocillin, phenytoin, sodium bicarbonate, theophylline. Y-site: aminophylline, clindamycin, furosemide, heparin, phenytoin, sodium bicarbonate, theophylline.

NURSING IMPLICATIONS

Administration

- Administration of an antacid should not be concomitant with or within 4 h of the oral ciprofloxacin dose.
- For patients with renal impairment, dose is lowered according to creatinine clearance.
- IV preparation: IV ciprofloxacin must be diluted before administration in NS or D5W to a final concentration of 1–2 mg/ml. Appropriate dilutions are 200 mg in 100 ml and 400 mg in 200 ml.
- IV administration: Properly diluted IV ciprofloxacin solution should be infused slowly over 60 min.
- Discontinue other IV infusion

while infusing ciprofloxacin or infuse through another site.
- Reconstituted IV solution is stable for 14 d refrigerated.

Assessment & Drug Effects
- Culture and sensitivity tests should be done prior to initial dose. Treatment may be implemented pending results.
- Urine pH should be less than 6.8, especially in the elderly and patients receiving high dosages of ciprofloxacin, to reduce the risk of crystalluria.
- Patients should be well hydrated; monitor I&O and assess for signs and symptoms of crystalluria.
- Monitor plasma theophylline concentrations, since drug may interfere with half-life.
- Administration with theophylline derivatives or caffeine can cause CNS stimulation.
- Assess for signs and symptoms of GI irritation (e.g., nausea, diarrhea, vomiting, abdominal discomfort) in clients receiving high dosages and in the elderly.
- Monitor PT in patients receiving coumarin therapy.
- Assess for signs and symptoms of superinfections (see Appendix G).

Patient & Family Education
- Advise fluid intake of 2–3 L/d if not contraindicated.
- Instruct patient not to exceed the recommended dosage.
- Instruct patient to restrict caffeine and advise of the effects (e.g., nervousness, insomnia, anxiety, tachycardia).
- Instruct patient of potential adverse effects of taking a theophylline derivative and of the need to report possible toxicity.
- Instruct patient to report nausea, diarrhea, vomiting, and abdominal pain or discomfort.
- Inform patient that drug may cause light-headedness and that caution should be taken with hazardous activities until reaction to drug is known.

CISAPRIDE

(cis′-a-pride)

Trade name: Propulsid

Classifications: AUTONOMIC NERVOUS SYSTEM AGENT; DIRECT-ACTING CHOLINERGIC (PARASYMPATHOMIMETIC); GI PROKINETIC AGENT

Prototype: Metoclopramide

Pregnancy category: C

ACTIONS/PHARMACODYNAMICS Cisapride's mechanism of action appears to enhance the release of acetylcholine at the myenteric plexus. It is a serotonin-4 ($5\text{-}HT_4$) receptor agonist. This may result in increased GI motility (prokinetic activity) and increased cardiac rate. Cisapride increases the lower esophagus sphincter pressure and lower esophagus peristalsis. It also accelerates gastric emptying time.

USE Indicated for second-line therapy for nocturnal heartburn due to reflux esophagitis. **Unlabeled uses:** gastroparesis, chronic constipation, postprandial epigastric distress, dyspepsia, postoperative GI atony, chronic intestinal pseudo-obstruction, anorexia nervosa.

ROUTE & DOSAGE

Gastroesophageal Reflux

Adult: **PO** 10 mg q.i.d. 15 min before meals and at bedtime.
Child: **PO** 0.2–0.3 mg/kg t.i.d.–q.i.d.

PHARMACOKINETICS **Absorption:** rapid; food increases rate and extent absorption, bioavailability averages

40–50%. **Onset:** 30–60 min. **Peak:** 1–1.5 h. Maximum effect occurs in 8–12 wk. **Distribution:** 98% protein bound. Does not readily cross blood–brain barrier. Excreted in breast milk. **Metabolism:** extensive hepatic metabolism. **Half-life:** 8–10 h. **Elimination:** found 50% in the urine and 50% in the feces.

CONTRAINDICATIONS & PRECAUTIONS **Contraindicated in:** GI hemorrhage; GI mechanical obstruction; GI perforation; hypersensitivity to cisapride; patients taking any medications that may increase cisapride levels (see Drug Interactions), patients with history of prolonged QT interval on ECG, renal failure, history of ventricular arrhythmias, ischemic heart disease, CHF; patients with hypokalemia, hypomagnesia, loss of K^+ ion due to diuretics or insulin; respiratory failure. **Cautious use in:** elderly, pregnancy (category C), and nursing mothers. Safety and efficacy in children has not been established.

ADVERSE/SIDE EFFECTS **GI:** diarrhea, abdominal pain, nausea, vomiting, epigastric pain. **Other (rare):** palpitations, tachycardia, elevated liver enzymes, dizziness.

DRUG INTERACTIONS Concurrent administration of ANTICHOLINERGIC COMPOUNDS (e.g., atropine) would compromise beneficial effects. Acceleration of gastric emptying could affect rate of absorption of drugs with narrow therapeutic range (e.g., **digoxin**). **Cimetidine** will increase plasma concentration of cisapride. Cisapride with **diazepam** will increase plasma concentrations of diazepam by 17%. Coagulation time may increase with concomitant ORAL ANTICOAGULANTS and cisapride. **Clarithromycin, erythromycin, fluconazole, itraconazole, ketoconazole, miconazole, indinavir, nefazodone, saquinavir, troleandomycin** may increase cisapride levels, resulting in prolonged QT interval and ventricular arrhythmias or torsade de pointes. **Quinidine, procainamide, sotalol,** TRICYCLIC ANTIDEPRESSANTS, PHENOTHIAZINES, **sertindole, astemizole, bepridil, sparfloxacin** may increase risk of arrhythmias.

NURSING IMPLICATIONS

Administration

- Cisapride should be given no sooner than 15 minutes before meals.
- If satisfactory results are not obtained with 10 mg q.i.d., the dose may be increased to 20 mg q.i.d.
- Patients with hepatic disease should be started on half the regular dose (5 mg q.i.d.).
- Store at room temperature 15–30C (59–86F) and protect from moisture.

Assessment & Drug Effects

- Because cisapride accelerates gastric emptying, it could affect the rate of absorption of other drugs. Closely monitor patients receiving narrow therapeutic ratio drugs or drugs requiring careful titration.
- For patients on concurrent oral anticoagulant therapy, check coagulation time approximately 1 wk after starting/stopping cisapride.
- Monitor for cisapride toxicity (e.g., dizziness, tachycardia, GI discomfort) when given concurrently with cimetidine. In patients on both drugs, the dose of cisapride may need to be reduced.

Patient & Family Education

- Advise patient that sedative effects of alcohol and benzodiazepine may be accelerated by cisapride.
- Stress need to take cisapride 15 min before meals.

C

- Inform patient that therapeutic effectiveness is indicated by decreased postprandial discomfort (e.g., fewer reflux symptoms such as nausea and heartburn).

CISATRACURIUM BESYLATE

(cis-a-tra-kyoo-ri′um)

Trade name: Nimbex

Classifications: AUTONOMIC NERVOUS SYSTEM AGENT; SKELETAL MUSCLE RELAXANT AGENT, NONDEPOLARIZING

Prototype: Tubocurarine chloride

Pregnancy category: B

ACTIONS/PHARMACODYNAMICS Cisatracurium is a neuromuscular blocking agent with intermediate onset and duration of action compared with similar agents. It binds competitively to cholinergic receptors on motor endplate of neurons, antagonizing the action of acetylcholine. This blocks neuromuscular transmission of impulses. This action can be reversed or antagonized by acetylcholinesterase inhibitors (e.g., neostigmine).

USES Adjunct to general anesthesia to facilitate tracheal intubation and provide skeletal muscle relaxation during surgery or mechanical ventilation.

ROUTE & DOSAGE

Intubation

Adult: **IV** 0.15 or 0.20 mg/kg.
Child ≥2 *y:* **IV** 0.1 mg/kg over 5–10 sec.

Maintenance

Adult: **IV** 0.03 mg/kg q20min prn or 1–2 μg/kg/min.
Child ≥ 2 *y:* **IV** 1–2 μg/kg/min.

Mechanical Ventilation in ICU

Adult: **IV** 3 μg/kg/min (can range from 0.5 to 10.2 μg/kg/min).

PHARMACOKINETICS **Onset:** varies with dose from 1.5 to 3.3 min (higher the dose, faster the onset). **Peak:** varies with dose from 1.5 to 3.3 min (higher the dose, faster to peak). **Duration:** varies with dose from 46 to 121 min (higher dose, longer recovery time). **Metabolism:** undergoes Hoffman elimination (pH- and temperature-dependent degradation) and hydrolysis by plasma esterases. **Elimination:** half-life: 22 min; excreted in urine.

CONTRAINDICATIONS & PRECAUTIONS **Contraindicated in:** hypersensitivity to cisatracurium or other related agents; rapid-sequence endotracheal intubation. **Cautious use in:** history of hemiparesis, electrolyte imbalances, burn patients, neuromuscular diseases (e.g., myasthenia gravis), elderly, renal function impairment, pregnancy (category B), nursing mothers. Not studied in children <2 y.

ADVERSE/SIDE EFFECTS **CV:** bradycardia, hypotension, flushing. **Respiratory:** bronchospasm. **Skin:** Rash.

INCOMPATIBILITIES **Solution/additive: ketorolac, propofol, sodium bicarbonate. Y-site: sodium bicarbonate.**

NURSING IMPLICATIONS

Administration

- Administer carefully adjusted, individualized doses using a peripheral nerve stimulator to evaluate neuromuscular function.
- Give only by or under supervision of expert clinician familiar with the drug's actions and potential complications.

- Have immediately available personnel and facilities for resuscitation and life support and an antagonist of cisatracurium.
- Refer to manufacturer's guidelines for preparation and administration. Note that 10-ml multiple-dose vials contain benzyl alcohol and should not be used with neonates.
- Refrigerate vials at 2–8C (36–46F). Protect from light. Diluted solutions may be stored refrigerated or at room temperature for 24 h.

Assessment & Drug Effects

- Perform neuromuscular monitoring only on nonparetic limbs.
- Time to maximum neuromuscular block is ≈ 1 min slower in the elderly.
- Monitor for bradycardia, hypotension, and bronchospasms; monitor ICU patients for spontaneous seizures.
- Antagonists should not be given when complete neuromuscular block is present.

CISPLATIN (cis-DDP, cis-PLATINUM II)

(sis'pla-tin)

Trade names: Abiplatin ♣, Platinol
Classifications: ANTINEOPLASTIC; ALKYLATING AGENT
Prototype: Cyclophosphamide
Pregnancy category: D

ACTIONS/PHARMACODYNAMICS

A heavy metal complex with platinum as central atom surrounded by 2 chloride atoms and 2 ammonia molecules in the *cis* position. Biochemical properties similar to those of bifunctional alkylating agents. Produces interstrand and intrastrand crosslinkage in DNA of rapidly dividing cells, thus preventing DNA, RNA, and protein synthesis. Cell-cycle nonspecific, i.e., effective throughout the entire cell life cycle. Carcinogenicity has not been fully studied, but other compounds with similar action mechanisms and mutogenicity have been reported to be carcinogenic.

USES Established combination therapy (cisplatin, vinblastine, bleomycin) in patient with metastatic testicular tumors and with doxorubicin for metastatic ovarian tumors following appropriate surgical or radiation therapy. **Unlabeled uses:** carcinoma of endometrium, bladder, head, and neck.

ROUTE & DOSAGE

Testicular Neoplasms

Adult: **IV** 20 mg/m^2/d for 5 d q3–4wk for 3 courses.

Ovarian Neoplasms

Adult: **IV** *Combination therapy:* 50 mg/m^2 once q3–4wk; *Single agent:* 100 mg/m^2 once q3–4wk.

PHARMACOKINETICS **Peak:** immediately after end of infusion. **Distribution:** widely distributed in body fluids and tissues; concentrated in kidneys, liver, and prostate; accumulated in tissues. **Metabolism:** not completely known. **Elimination:** half-life: 73–290 h; 15–50% of dose excreted in urine within 24–48 h.

CONTRAINDICATIONS & PRECAUTIONS **Contraindicated in:** history of hypersensitivity to cisplatin or other platinum-containing compounds; impaired renal function; myelosuppression; impaired hearing; history of gout and urate renal stones. Safe use during pregnancy (category D), in nursing women, and in children not established. **Cautious use in:** previous cytoxic drug or radiation therapy; with other ototoxic and nephrotoxic drugs.

ADVERSE/SIDE EFFECTS CNS: seizures, headache; peripheral neuropathies (may be irreversible): paresthesia, unsteady gait, clumsiness of hands and feet, exacerbation of neuropathy with exercise, loss of taste. **ENT:** ototoxicity (may be irreversible): tinnitus, hearing loss, deafness, vertigo. **Eye:** blurred vision, changes in ability to see colors (optic neuritis, papilledema). **GI:** *marked nausea, vomiting*, anorexia, stomatitis, xerostomia, diarrhea, constipation. **Hematologic:** myelosuppression (25–30% patients): leukopenia, thrombocytopenia; hemolytic anemia, hemolysis. **Hypersensitivity:** anaphylactic-like reactions. **Renal** (dose-related; cumulative): nephrotoxicity. **Other:** cardiac abnormalities, hypocalcemia, *hypomagnesemia*, hyperuricemia, elevated AST, SIADH.

DRUG INTERACTIONS AMINOGLYCOSIDES, **amphotericin B, vancomycin,** other **nephrotoxic drugs** increase nephrotoxicity and acute renal failure—try to separate by at least 1–2 wk; AMINOGLYCOSIDES, **furosemide** increase risk of ototoxicity.

INCOMPATIBILITIES Solution/additive: 5% dextrose, sodium bicarbonate, metoclopramide. Y-site: TPN.

NURSING IMPLICATIONS

Administration

- Administered only under supervision of a qualified physician experienced in the use of antineoplastics.
- Before the initial dose is given, hydration is started with 1–2 L IV infusion fluid to reduce risk of nephrotoxicity and ototoxicity. Drug is then diluted in 2 L 5% dextrose in 1/2 or 1/3 normal saline containing 37.5 g mannitol (an osmotic diuretic) and infused over 6–8 h. Hydration and forced diuresis are continued for at least 24 h after drug administration to ensure adequate urinary output.
- Usually a parenteral antiemetic agent is administered 1/2 h before cisplatin therapy is instituted and given on a scheduled basis throughout day and night as long as necessary.
- Use disposable gloves when preparing cisplatin solutions. If drug accidentally contacts skin or mucosa, wash immediately and thoroughly with soap and water.
- Reconstituted drug with sterile water for injection (1 mg/ml dilution) should be clear and colorless. Keep reconstituted solutions at room temperature; refrigeration will cause a precipitate to form. Since it lacks bacterial preservatives, it should be used within 20 h.
- Unless otherwise specified by manufacturer, store unopened vials in refrigerator at 2–8C (36–46F).

Assessment & Drug Effects

- A pretreatment ECG and cardiac monitoring during induction therapy are indicated because of possible myocarditis or focal irritability.
- Monitor urine output and specific gravity for 4 consecutive hours before treatment and for 24 h after therapy. Report if output is less than 100 ml/h or if specific gravity is more than 1.030. A urine output of less than 75 ml/h necessitates medical intervention to avert a renal emergency.
- Audiometric testing should be performed before the first dose and

before each subsequent dose. Ototoxicity (reported in 31% of patients) may occur after a single dose of 50 mg/m^2. Children who receive repeated doses are especially susceptible.

- Anaphylactoid reactions (particularly in patient previously exposed to cisplatin) may occur within minutes of drug administration.
- The following tests should be done *before* initiating every course of therapy and repeated each week during treatment period: serum uric acid, serum creatinine, BUN, urinary creatinine clearance.
- Patient should be closely monitored for dose-related adverse reactions. Drug action is cumulative; therefore severity of most adverse effects increases with repeated doses.
- A repeat course of therapy should not be given until (1) serum creatinine is below 1.5 mg/dl; (2) BUN is below 25 mg/dl; (3) platelets ≥ 100,000/mm^3; (4) WBC ≥ 4000/mm^3; (5) audiometric test is within normal limits.
- Nephrotoxicity (reported in 28–36% of patients receiving a single dose of 50 mg/m^2) usually occurs within 2 wk after drug administration and becomes more severe and prolonged with repeated courses of cisplatin.
- Suspect ototoxicity if patient manifests tinnitus or difficulty hearing in the high frequency range.
- Intractable nausea and vomiting severe enough to warrant discontinuation of drug usually begin 1–4 h after treatment and may last 24 h or persist for up to 1 wk after treatment is ended.
- Monitor and report abnormal electrolyte levels: sodium > 145 or < 135 mEq/L, and potassium > 5 or < 3.5 mEq/L.
- CBC and platelet counts are done weekly for 2 wk after each course of treatment. The nadirs in platelet and leukocyte counts occur between day 18 and 23 (range: 7.5–45) with most patients recovering in 13–62 d. A decrease in hemoglobin (more than 2 g/dl) occurs at approximately the same time and with the same frequency.
- Check BP, mental status, pupils, and fundi every hour during therapy. Hydration and mannitol may increase the danger of elevated intracranial pressure (ICP).
- Neurologic examinations at regular intervals should include tests of muscle strength, Romberg, vibratory and position sense, tests of sensation.
- Monitor and report abnormal bowel elimination pattern. Constipation and the possibility of fecal impaction may be caused by neurotoxicity; diarrhea is a possible response to GI irritation.
- Inspect oral membranes daily for xerostomia (white patches and ulcerations) and tongue for signs of fungal overgrowth (black, furry appearance).
- Infection precautions should be instituted promptly if a temperature increase of 0.6F over the previous reading is noted.
- The patient should be weighed under standard conditions (same time, clothing, scale) every day. A gradual ascending weight profile occurring over a period of several days should be reported.

Patient & Family Education

- Continue maintenance of adequate hydration (at least 3000 ml/24 h oral fluid if physician agrees) and report promptly the symptoms of nephrotoxicity: reduced urinary output, flank pain, anorexia, nausea, vomiting, dry mucosae, itching skin, urine odor

C

on breath, fluid retention, and weight gain.

- Keep vestibular stimulation to the minimum to avoid dizziness or falling: avoid unnecessary turning in bed, and change position gradually and slowly.
- Tingling, numbness, and tremors of extremities, loss of position sense and taste, and constipation are early signs of neurotoxicity. Report their occurrence promptly to prevent irreversibility. Pain with heel walking and difficulty in getting out of bed or chair are late indicators of nerve damage.
- If patient's oral discomfort interferes with eating, report to physician.
- Report promptly evidence of unexplained bleeding and easy bruising.
- Report unusual fatigue, fever, sore mouth and throat, abnormal body discharges.

CITALOPRAM HYDROBROMIDE

(cit-a-lo'pram)

Trade name: Celexa

Classifications: CNS AGENT; PSYCHOTHERAPEUTIC; SELECTIVE SEROTONIN-REUPTAKE INHIBITOR

Prototype: Fluoxetine

Pregnancy category: C

ACTIONS/PHARMACODYNAMICS Selective serotonin reuptake inhibitor (SSRI) in the CNS neurons which results in antidepressant activity. Does not produce any sympathomimetic response or anticholinergic activity. Does not inhibit MAOIs.

USE Depression.

ROUTE & DOSAGE

Depression

Adult: **PO** Start at 20 mg q.d.; may increase to 40 mg q.d. if needed.

Geriatric: **PO** 20 mg q.d.

PHARMACOKINETICS Absorption: rapidly absorbed from GI tract; approximately 80% reaches systemic circulation. **Peak:** steady-state serum concentrations in 1 wk; peak blood levels at 4 h. **Distribution:** 80% protein bound; crosses placenta; distributed into breast milk. **Metabolism:** metabolized in liver by cytochrome P450 3A4 and cytochrome P450 2C9 enzymes. **Elimination:** half-life:35 h; 20% excreted in urine, 80% in bile.

CONTRAINDICATIONS & PRECAUTIONS Contraindicated in: hypersensitivity to citalopram; concurrent use of MAOIs or use within 14 d of discontinuing MAOIs. **Cautious use in:** hypersensitivity to other SSRIs; renal or hepatic insufficiency; elderly patients; cardiovascular disease (e.g., dysrhythmias, conduction defects, myocardial ischemia); history of seizure disorders or suicidal tendencies; children and adolescents; pregnancy (category C); nursing mothers.

ADVERSE/SIDE EFFECTS Body as whole: asthenia, fatigue, fever, arthralgia, myalgia. **CNS:** dizziness, *insomnia, somnolence,* agitation, tremor, anxiety, paresthesia, migraine. **CV:** tachycardia, postural hypotension, hypotension. **GI:** *nausea,* vomiting, diarrhea, dyspepsia, abdominal pain, *dry mouth,* anorexia, flatulence. **Respiratory:** URI, rhinitis, sinusitis. **Skin:** increased sweating. **Other:** dysmenorrhea, decreased libido, ejaculation disorder, impotence.

DRUG INTERACTIONS Combination with MAOIs could result in hypertensive crisis, hyperthermia, rigidity, myoclonus, autonomic instability; **cimetidine** may increase citalopram levels.

NURSING IMPLICATIONS

Administration

- Do not begin this drug within 14 d of stopping an MAOI.
- Reduced doses are advised for the elderly and those with hepatic or renal impairment.
- Dose increments should be separated by at least 1 wk.
- Store at 15–30C (59–86F) in tightly closed container and protect from light.

Assessment & Drug Effects

- Therapeutic effectiveness is indicated by elevation of mood; 1–4 wk may be needed before improvement is noted.
- Lab tests: Periodically monitor hepatic functions, CBC, serum sodium, and lithium levels when the two drugs are given concurrently.
- Periodically monitor HR and BP, and carefully monitor complete cardiac status in person with known or suspected cardiac disease.
- Closely monitor elderly patients for adverse effects especially with doses >20 mg/d.

Patient & Family Education

- Do not engage in hazardous activities until reaction to this drug is known.
- Avoid using alcohol while taking citalopram.
- Inform physician of commonly used OTC drugs as there is potential for drug interactions.
- Report distressing side effects including any changes in sexual functioning or response.
- Periodic ophthalmology exams are advised with long-term treatment.

CLADRIBINE

(cla′dri-been)

Trade name: Leustatin

Classification: ANTINEOPLASTIC

Pregnancy category: D

ACTIONS/PHARMACODYNAMICS Cladribine is a synthetic antineoplastic agent with selective toxicity toward certain normal and malignant lymphocytes and monocytes. It accumulates intracellularly, preventing repair of single-stranded DNA breaks and ultimately interfering with cellular metabolism and DNA synthesis. Cladribine is cytotoxic to both actively dividing and quiescent lymphocytes and monocytes, inhibiting both DNA synthesis and repair.

USE Treatment of hairy cell leukemia. **Unlabeled uses:** advanced cutaneous T-cell lymphomas, chronic lymphocytic leukemia, non-Hodgkin's lymphomas, acute myeloid leukemia, autoimmune hemolytic anemia, mycosis fungoides.

ROUTE & DOSAGE

Hairy Cell Leukemia

Adult: **IV** 0.09 mg/kg/d by 7-d continuous infusion.

Chronic Lymphocytic Leukemia

Adult: **IV** 0.1 mg/kg/d by 7-d continuous infusion, or 0.028–0.14 mg/kg/d as 2-h bolus infusion for 5 consecutive d.

C

PHARMACOKINETICS Onset: therapeutic effect 10 d to 4 mo. **Duration:** 7–25+ mo. **Distribution:** crosses placenta; distributed into breast milk. **Metabolism:** In malignant leukocytes, cladribine is phosphorylated to form its monophosphate and triphosphate forms, presumably its active forms, which are subsequently incorporated into cellular DNA. **Elimination:** half-life: initial 35 min, terminal 6.7 h.

CONTRAINDICATIONS & PRECAUTIONS Contraindicated in: hypersensitivity to cladribine, pregnancy (category D). **Cautious use in:** hepatic or renal impairment. Safety and efficacy in children not established.

ADVERSE/SIDE EFFECTS CNS: headache, dizziness. **GI:** nausea, diarrhea. **Hematologic:** <u>*myelosuppression (neutropenia),*</u> *anemia,* thrombocytopenia. **Metabolic:** *fever*. **Renal:** elevated serum creatinine.

INCOMPATIBILITIES Solution/additive: do not mix with any other diluents or drugs.

NURSING IMPLICATIONS

Administration

- Refer to manufacturer's directions for preparation of the IV solution.
- Solutions for cladribine should not be mixed with any other IV drugs or additives, nor administered through an IV line used for other drugs or solutions.
- Use disposable gloves and protective clothing when handling the drug. Wash immediately if skin contact occurs.
- Diluted solutions of cladribine may be stored refrigerated for up to 8 h prior to administration.
- Store unopened vials in refrigerator (2–8C/36–46F) and protect from light.

Assessment & Drug Effects

- Monitor vital signs during and after drug infusion. Fever (>100F) is common during the 5th to 7th days in patients with hairy cell leukemia, and severe fever (>104F) may develop within the first month of therapy.
- Closely monitor hematologic status; myelosuppression is common during the first month after starting therapy.
- Monitor for and report signs and symptoms of infection. Note that within the first month, fever may occur in the absence of infection.
- Periodically assess serum creatinine and serum transaminase levels.
- With high doses of cladribine, monitor for neurologic toxicity (paraparesis/quadriparesis) and acute nephrotoxicity.

Patient & Family Education

- The patient should be fully informed regarding adverse responses to the drug.
- The patient should understand the need for close follow-up during and after treatment with the drug.

CLARITHROMYCIN

(clar'i-thro-my-sin)

Trade name: Biaxin Filmtabs

Classifications: ANTIINFECTIVE; MACROLIDE ANTIBIOTIC

Prototype: Erythromycin

Pregnancy category: C

ACTIONS/PHARMACODYNAMICS A semisynthetic macrolide antibiotic that binds to the 50S ribosomal subunit of susceptible bacterial organisms and thus inhibits protein synthesis. It is active against both aerobic and anaerobic gram-positive and gram-negative organisms including *Streptococcus pyogenes,*

C

Streptococcus pneumoniae, Hemophilus influenzae, Moraxella catarrhalis, Mycoplasma pneumoniae, and *Staphylococcus aureus.*

USES Treatment of upper-respiratory, lower-respiratory infections; acute maxillary sinusitis; otitis media; and skin and soft tissue infections caused by clinically significant aerobic and anaerobic gram-negative and gram-positive organisms, including *S. aureus, H. influenzae, S. pneumoniae, M. catarrhalis, S. pyogenes, M. pneumoniae.* Prevention and treatment of *Mycobacterium avium* complex (MAC) infections in patients with HIV. Used in combination for *H. pylori.*

ROUTE & DOSAGE

Mild to Moderate Infections

Adult: **PO** 250–500 mg b.i.d. for 10–14 d.
Child: **PO** 7.5 mg/kg q12h.

Mycobacterial Infections

Adult: **PO** 500 mg q12h.
Child: **PO** 7.5 mg/kg q12h.

***H. pylori* Infections**

Adult: **PO** 500 mg b.i.d. to t.i.d.

PHARMACOKINETICS Absorption: readily absorbed from GI tract; 50% reaches the systemic circulation. **Peak:** 2-4 h. **Distribution:** widely distributes into most body tissue (excluding CNS); high pulmonary tissue concentrations. **Metabolism:** partially metabolized in the liver; active 14-OH metabolite acts synergistically with the parent compound against *H. influenzae.* **Elimination:** half-life: 3-5 h; 20% excreted unchanged in urine; 10-15% of 14-OH metabolite excreted in urine.

CONTRAINDICATIONS & PRECAUTIONS Contraindicated in: hypersensitivity to clarithromycin, erythromycin, or any other macrolide antibiotics. **Cautious use in:** renal impairment, pregnancy (category C), and nursing mothers. Safety and efficacy in children < 12 y not established.

ADVERSE/SIDE EFFECTS CNS: headache. **GI:** diarrhea, abdominal discomfort, nausea, abnormal taste, dyspepsia. **Other:** rash, urticaria, eosinophilia.

DRUG INTERACTIONS 20% increase in **theophylline** levels; clinical significance of other drugs metabolized by cytochrome P450 has not been determined. Patients receiving other drugs known to interact with erythromycin (i.e., **digoxin, carbamazepine, triazolam, warfarin, ergotamine**) should be monitored carefully for increased levels and toxicity of these drugs until more data are available.

DIAGNOSTIC TEST INTERFERENCE May increase serum AST and ALT levels.

NURSING IMPLICATIONS

Administration

- Clarithromycin may be given without regard to meals.
- In the presence of severe renal impairment, a decreased dose or prolongation of the dosing interval are recommended.
- Store at 15–30C (59–86F).

Assessment & Drug Effects

- Before treatment, inquire about previous hypersensitivity to other macrolides (e.g., erythromycin).
- If hypersensitivity occurs (e.g., rash, urticaria), discontinue drug and notify physician.
- Monitor for and report loose stools or diarrhea, since pseudomembranous colitis must be ruled out.
- When clarithromycin is given concurrently with anticoagulants,

C

digoxin, or theophylline, blood levels of these drugs may be elevated. Monitor appropriate serum levels and assess for signs and symptoms of drug toxicity.

Patient & Family Education

- Stress importance of completing prescribed course of therapy.
- Advise patient to immediately report rash or other signs of hypersensitivity.
- Instruct patient to report loose stools or diarrhea even after completion of drug therapy.
- Advise lactating mothers that drug may be excreted in breast milk (not yet established).

CLEMASTINE FUMARATE

(klem'as-teen)

Trade names: Tavist, Tavist-1

Classification: ANTIHISTAMINE (H_1-RECEPTOR ANTAGONIST)

Prototype: Diphenhydramine

Pregnancy category: C

ACTIONS/PHARMACODYNAMICS An antihistamine (H_1-receptor antagonist) with prominent antipruritic activity and low incidence of unpleasant side effects. Anticholinergic effects are weak, and central sedative effects are generally mild.

USES Symptomatic relief of allergic rhinitis (sneezing, rhinorrhea, pruritus) and mild uncomplicated allergic skin manifestations such as urticaria and angioedema.

ROUTE & DOSAGE

Allergic Rhinitis

Adult: **PO** 1.34 mg b.i.d.; may increase up to 8.04 mg/d.
Child: **PO** >6 *y:* 0.67 mg b.i.d.; may increase up to 4.02 mg/d; <6 *y:* 0.335–0.67 mg/kg/d in 2 divided doses (max 1.34 mg/d).

Allergic Urticaria

Adult: **PO** 2.68 mg b.i.d. or t.i.d.; may increase up to 8.04 mg/d.
Child: **PO** 1.34 mg b.i.d.; may increase up to 4.02 mg/d.

PHARMACOKINETICS Absorption: readily absorbed from GI tract. **Peak:** 5–7 h. **Duration:** 10–12 h. **Distribution:** distributed into breast milk. **Metabolism:** metabolized in liver. **Elimination:** excreted chiefly in urine.

CONTRAINDICATIONS & PRECAUTIONS Contraindicated in: hypersensitivity to clemastine or to other antihistamines of similar chemical structure; lower respiratory tract symptoms, including acute asthma; concomitant MAO INHIBITOR therapy. Safe use during pregnancy (category C) and in nursing mothers not established. **Cautious use in:** history of bronchial asthma, increased intraocular pressure, GI or GU obstruction, hyperthyroidism, cardiovascular disease, hypertension, elderly patients.

ADVERSE/SIDE EFFECTS CNS: Sedation, *transient drowsiness,* dry nose and throat, headache, dizziness, weakness, fatigue, disturbed coordination; confusion, restlessness, nervousness, hysteria, convulsions, tremors, irritability, euphoria, insomnia, paresthesias, neuritis. **CV:** hypotension, palpitation, tachycardia, extrasystoles. **ENT:** vertigo, tinnitus, acute labyrinthitis. **Eye:** blurred vision, diplopia. **GI:** *dry mouth,* epigastric distress, anorexia, nausea, vomiting, diarrhea, constipation. **GU:** difficult urination, urinary retention, early menses. **Hematologic:** hemolytic anemia, thrombocytopenia, agranulocytosis. **Hypersensitivity:** urticaria, rash, photosensitivity, anaphylaxis. **Respiratory:** dry nose and throat, thickening of bronchial secretions, tightness of chest, wheezing, nasal stuffiness. **Other:** excess perspiration, chills.

DRUG INTERACTIONS **Alcohol** and other CNS DEPRESSANTS increase sedation; MAO INHIBITORS may prolong and intensify anticholinergic effects.

NURSING IMPLICATIONS

Administration

- Drug may be administered with food, water, or milk to reduce possibility of gastric irritation.
- Elderly patients usually require less than average adult dose.
- Store at 15–30C (59–86F) unless otherwise directed.

Assessment & Drug Effects

- Monitor for drowsiness, poor coordination, or dizziness, especially in the elderly or debilitated. Supervision of ambulation may be warranted.
- Assess for symptomatic relief with use of the medication.

Patient & Family Education

- Advise patient to check with physician before taking alcohol or other CNS depressants, since effects may be additive.
- Clemastine may cause lethargy and drowsiness; therefore necessary safety precautions should be taken.
- Advise elderly patients to make position changes slowly and in stages, particularly from recumbent to upright posture since they are more likely to experience dizziness and hypotension than younger patients.
- Caution patient not to drive and to avoid other potentially hazardous activities until response to the drug has been established.
- Discontinue about 4 d before skin testing procedures since it may prevent otherwise positive reactions.
- Advise frequent sips of water or sugarless hard candy to relieve dry mouth.

C

CLINDAMYCIN HYDROCHLORIDE

(klin-da-mye′sin)

Trade names: Cleocin, Dalacin C♣

CLINDAMYCIN PALMITATE HYDROCHLORIDE

Trade name: Cleocin Pediatric

CLINDAMYCIN PHOSPHATE

Trade names: Cleocin Phosphate, Cleocin T, Dalacin C

Prototype for classifications: ANTIINFECTIVE; ANTIBIOTIC; SKIN AGENT; ANTIACNE

Pregnancy category: B

ACTIONS/PHARMACODYNAMICS Semisynthetic derivative of lincomycin with which it shares neuromuscular blocking properties and other actions. Reported to have greater degree of antibacterial activity in vitro, better absorption, and lower incidence of GI side effects than lincomycin. Suppresses protein synthesis by binding to 50 S subunits of bacterial ribosomes, and therefore inhibits other antibiotics (e.g., erythromycin) that act at this site. Particularly effective against susceptible strains of anaerobic streptococci, *Bacteroides* (especially *B. fragilis*), *Fusobacterium, Actinomyces israelii, Peptococcus,* and *Clostridium* sp. Also effective against aerobic gram-positive cocci, including *Staphylococcus aureus, Staphylococcus epidermidis,* streptococci (except *S. faecalis*), and pneumococci.

USES Serious infections when less toxic alternatives are inappropriate. Topical applications are used in treatment of acne vulgaris. **Unlabeled**

C

uses: in combination with pyrimethamine for toxoplasmosis in patients with AIDS.

ROUTE & DOSAGE

Moderate to Severe Infections

Adult: **PO** 150–450 mg q6h. **IM/IV** 300–900 mg q6–8h (max 2700 mg/d).
Child: **PO** 10–30 mg/kg/d q6–8h. **IM/IV** 25–40 mg/kg/d q6–8h.
Neonate: **IM/IV** ≤7 d: 10–15 mg/kg/d divided q8–12h; >7 d: 10–20 mg/kg/d divided q6–12h.

Acne Vulgaris

Adult: **Topical** Apply to affected areas b.i.d.

PHARMACOKINETICS **Absorption:** approximately 90% absorbed from GI tract; 10% of topical application is absorbed through skin. **Peak:** 45–60 min PO; 3 h IM. **Duration:** 6 h PO; 8–12 h IM. **Distribution:** widely distributed except for CNS; crosses placenta; distributed into breast milk. **Metabolism:** metabolized in liver. **Elimination:** half-life: 2–3 h; excreted in urine and feces.

CONTRAINDICATIONS & PRECAUTIONS **Contraindicated in:** history of hypersensitivity to clindamycin or lincomycin; history of regional enteritis, ulcerative colitis, or antibiotic-associated colitis. Safe use during pregnancy (category B) and in nursing mothers not established. Not recommended for infants <1 mo. **Cautious use in:** history of GI disease, renal or hepatic disease; atopic individuals (history of eczema, asthma, hay fever); older patients.

ADVERSE/SIDE EFFECTS **GI:** *diarrhea,* abdominal pain, flatulence, bloating, *nausea, vomiting,* pseudomembranous colitis; esophageal irritation, loss of taste, medicinal taste (high IV doses). **Hematologic:** leukopenia, eosinophilia, agranulocytosis, thrombocytopenia. **Hepatic:** jaundice, abnormal liver function tests. **Hypersensitivity:** *skin rashes,* urticaria, pruritus, fever, serum sickness. **Skin:** dryness, contact dermatitis, gram-negative folliculitis, irritation, oily skin. **Other:** sensitization, swelling of face (following topical use); hypotension (following IM), cardiac arrest (rapid IV), generalized myalgia, superinfections, proctitis, vaginitis. **Local reactions:** pain, induration, sterile abscess (following IM injections); thrombophlebitis (IV infusion).

DIAGNOSTIC TEST INTERFERENCE Clindamycin may cause increases in ***serum alkaline phosphatase, bilirubin, creatine phosphokinase*** (CPK) from muscle irritation following IM injection; ***AST, ALT.***

DRUG INTERACTIONS **Chloramphenicol, erythromycin** possibly are mutually antagonistic to clindamycin; neuromuscular blocking action enhanced by NEUROMUSCULAR BLOCKING AGENTS **(atracurium, tubocurarine, pancuronium).**

INCOMPATIBILITIES **Solution/additive: ceftriaxone, ranitidine, tobramycin, fluconazole.**

NURSING IMPLICATIONS

Administration

- Determine history of any previous sensitivities to drugs or other allergens.
- Administer clindamycin capsules with a full (240 ml [8 oz]) glass of water to prevent esophagitis.
- Absorption of oral clindamycin is not significantly affected by food or gastric acid, although peak

serum levels may be somewhat delayed.

- Note expiration date of oral solution; retains potency for 14 d at room temperature. Do not refrigerate, as chilling causes thickening and thus makes pouring it difficult.
- Deep IM injection is recommended. Rotate injection sites and observe daily for evidence of inflammatory reaction. Single IM doses should not exceed 600 mg.
- IV preparation: Dilute to a concentration of not more than 18 mg/ml using 0.9% NaCl, 5% D5W, 0.45% NaCl + D5W, or other compatible solution.
- IV infusion: Do not give >1200 mg in a single 1-h infusion.
- IV clindamycin is never given as a bolus dose. The infusion should not exceed 1200 mg in 1 h. Prescribed continuous flow rate is slow to minimize risk of cardiac arrhythmias.
- Follow manufacturer's directions for reconstituting the parenteral drug, for storage time, compatible IV fluids, and IV infusion rates. Reportedly, local reactions following IV administration can be minimized by avoiding prolonged use of indwelling catheters.
- IV administration to neonates, infants and children: Verify correct IV concentration and rate of infusion with physician.
- Store in tight containers at 15–30C (59–86F) unless otherwise directed.

Assessment & Drug Effects

- Culture and susceptibility testing should be performed initially and periodically during therapy.
- Monitor BP and pulse in patients receiving drug parenterally. Hypotension has occurred following IM injection. Advise patient to remain recumbent following drug administration until BP has stabilized.
- Severe diarrhea and colitis, including pseudomembranous colitis, have been associated with oral (highest incidence), parenteral, and topical clindamycin. Report immediately the onset of watery diarrhea, with or without fever; passage of tarry or bloody stools, pus, intestinal tissue, or mucus; abdominal cramps, or ileus. Symptoms may appear within a few days to 2 wk after therapy is begun or up to several weeks following cessation of therapy.
- Elderly and bedridden patients are at a higher risk of developing severe colitis and therefore should be closely observed.
- Be alert to signs of superinfection (see Appendix G).
- Be alert for signs of anaphylactoid reactions (see Appendix G), that require immediate attention.

Patient & Family Education

- Instruct patient to take drug for the full course of therapy as prescribed.
- Instruct patient to report loose stools or diarrhea promptly.
- Drug therapy is stopped if patient develops significant diarrhea (more than 5 loose stools daily).
- Antiperistaltic agents may prolong and worsen diarrhea by delaying removal of toxins from colon. Advise patient not to self-medicate with antidiarrheal preparations.
- Patients using topical preparation for acne should be instructed to discontinue other acne preparations unless otherwise directed by physician. Advise patient to keep medication away from eyes.
- Since 10% absorption of topical medication is possible, instruct patient to report the onset of systemic reactions to physician.

C

CLIOQUINOL (IODOCHLORHYDROXYQUIN)

(klee-oh-kwee'nole)

Trade names: Torofor, Vioform

Classifications: ANTIINFECTIVE; ANTIBIOTIC; ANTIFUNGAL

Prototype: Fluconazole

Pregnancy category: C

ACTIONS/PHARMACODYNAMICS Halogenated hydroxyquinoline with broad spectrum of antifungal and antibacterial activity. Available OTC.

USES Topically for treatment of inflamed cutaneous conditions such as eczema, athlete's foot, and other fungal conditions.

ROUTE & DOSAGE

Inflamed Cutaneous Conditions

Adult: **Topical** Apply thin layer to affected area b.i.d. or t.i.d. for 1 wk only.

PHARMACOKINETICS Absorption: minimally absorbed through intact skin. **Elimination:** some is rapidly excreted in urine; the rest may persist in body 1 mo or more.

CONTRAINDICATIONS & PRECAUTIONS Contraindicated in: hypersensitivity to chloroxine, iodine, or iodine-containing preparations; tuberculosis; vaccinia, varicella, or other viral skin conditions; severe renal disease; hepatic damage; thyroid disorder. Safe use during pregnancy (category C) and in nursing mothers not established.

ADVERSE/SIDE EFFECTS Infrequent: local burning, irritation, redness, swelling, itching, rash, staining of hair and skin. **Systemic reactions (if used on large skin areas):** iodism, hypersensitivity reaction, slight enlargement of thyroid gland, hair loss, agranulocytosis, subacute myeloptic neuropathy.

DIAGNOSTIC TEST INTERFERENCE Possibility of elevated ***PBI,*** decreased ***iodine 131 thyroidal uptake,*** and elevation of butanol-extractable iodine ***(BEI).*** False-positive ferric chloride test for phenylketonuria ***(PKU)*** may result if clioquinol is present on diaper or in urine.

NURSING IMPLICATIONS

Administration

- Area to be treated is generally washed with soap and water and dried thoroughly before each application. Consult physician.
- Do not apply an occlusive dressing without a physician's order.
- Preserve in tightly covered, light-resistant containers at 15–30C (59–86F) unless otherwise directed.

Assessment & Drug Effects

- Monitor for signs of skin irritation. Notify physician if they appear. Drug may be discontinued.
- Monitor for signs of systemic absorption such as thyroid enlargement and hair loss. Notify physician if they occur. Drug may be discontinued.

Patient & Family Education

- Avoid contact of drug in or around eyes. Drug may stain fabric, skin, or hair yellow on contact.
- Clioquinol should be discontinued if skin irritation, rash, or other signs of sensitivity or systemic absorption develop. Report to physician.
- Treatment is usually continued 4 wk for athlete's foot or ringworm and 2 wk for jock itch.
- Notify physician if there is no improvement within 1–2 wk. Apply

the drug as directed and only for the period of time prescribed.

CLOBETASOL PROPIONATE

(cloe-bay'ta-sol)

Trade names: Dermovate, Temovate

Classifications: SKIN AND MUCOUS MEMBRANE AGENT; ANTIINFLAMMATORY; STEROID

Prototype: Hydrocortisone

Pregnancy category: C

See Appendix A.

CLOCORTOLONE PIVALATE

(kloe-kor'toe-lone)

Trade name: Cloderm

Classifications: SKIN AND MUCOUS MEMBRANE AGENT; ANTIINFLAMMATORY; STEROID

Prototype: Hydrocortisone

Pregnancy category: C

See Appendix A.

CLOFAZIMINE

(kloe-fa'zi-meen)

Trade name: Lamprene

Classifications: ANTIINFECTIVE; ANTILEPROSY AGENT

Prototype: Dapsone

Pregnancy category: C

ACTIONS/PHARMACODYNAMICS Exerts a slow bactericidal effect on *Mycobacterium leprae* (Hansen's bacillus) and has antiinflammatory activity. Binds preferentially to DNA of all mycobacteria and inhibits their growth. Its antiinflammatory action (precise mechanism unknown) controls erythema nodosum leprosum reactions. Bacterial killing is not detectable in biopsy tissue from leprosy patient until 50 d after start of therapy. Clofazimine is not effective against all forms of leprosy. Does not show cross-resistance with rifampin or dapsone. Has no clinically useful activity against microorganisms other than mycobacteria.

USES Chiefly in multiinfective therapy of multibacillary leprosy (with dapsone, rifampin, ethionamide) to prevent development of drug resistance. Also in lepromatous leprosy, including dapsone-resistant lepromatous leprosy and leprosy complicated by erythema nodosum leprosum (lepra) reaction. **Unlabeled use:** *Mycobacterium avium-intracellulare* complex infections in patients with AIDS.

ROUTE & DOSAGE

Dapsone-resistant Leprosy

Adult: **PO** 100 mg/d in combination with 1 or more antileprosy drugs for 3 y, then 100 mg/d as monotherapy.
Child: **PO** 1 mg/kg/d in combination with dapsone and rifampin.

Erythema Nodosum Leprosum

Adult: **PO** 100–300 mg/d for up to 3 mo; taper dose to 100 mg/d as soon as possible.

Mycobacterium avium-intracellulare

Adult: **PO** 100 mg 1–3 times/d.
Child: **PO** 1–2 mg/kg/d (max 100 mg/d).

PHARMACOKINETICS **Absorption:** slowly absorbed from GI tract; approximately 50% absorbed. **Peak:** 4–12 h. **Distribution:** distributed predominantly to fatty tissues and reticuloendothelial system; crosses placenta; distributed into breast milk. **Elimination:** half-life: 70 d; primarily eliminated in feces through bile.

CONTRAINDICATIONS & PRECAUTIONS **Contraindicated in:** safe use during pregnancy (category C) and by nursing mothers not established. **Cautious use in:** patient with GI problems, children.

ADVERSE/SIDE EFFECTS **CNS:** drowsiness, fatigue, headache, giddiness, dizziness, neuralgia, taste disorder. **Eye:** *conjunctival and corneal discoloration,* dryness, burning, itching, irritation. **GI:** *abdominal/epigastric pain* (dose-related), *nausea, vomiting, diarrhea,* bowel obstruction, hepatitis, jaundice, enlarged liver. **Skin:** *pink-brown skin discoloration, ichthyosis, dryness,* rash, pruritus, phototoxicity. **Other:** hypokalemia; elevated albumin, serum bilirubin, and AST; eosinophilia; erythema nodosum leprosum (lepra) reaction.

DRUG INTERACTION **Isoniazid** may decrease clofazimine concentrations in skin. **Food–drug:** food will increase absorption.

NURSING IMPLICATIONS

Administration

- Drug should be taken with meals or milk to reduce gastric irritation.
- Doses of more than 100 mg/d are given for as short a period of time as possible and should be administered under close medical supervision.
- Store capsules at 15–30C (59–86F); protect from moisture.

Assessment & Drug Effects

- Clofazimine is well tolerated in dosages no greater than 100 mg/d. Most adverse effects are dose related and reversible with discontinuation of drug.
- Abnormal crystalline deposits may result and cause serious side effects (e.g., pain in bones and joints, GI bleeding, diminished vision). Reactions are usually reversible but may require months or years to diminish.
- Severe abdominal symptoms (including splenic infarction, bowel obstruction, and GI bleeding) have occurred (although rarely), requiring explorative laparotomies. Deaths have been reported.
- Drug-induced reddish-brown discoloration of skin, cornea, conjunctiva, and body fluids (including tears, sweat, sputum, urine, and feces) occurs in 75–90% of patients within a few weeks of treatment. Skin discoloration may take months or years to disappear after drug is discontinued.
- The onset of tender, erythematous nodules with lymphadenopathy, joint swelling, epistaxis, iritis suggests a type 2 leprosy reactional state. Dosage may be increased to 200 mg/d. After reactive episode is controlled, dosage is tapered to 100 mg/d as soon as possible. Patient should remain under medical surveillance during the episode.

Patient & Family Education

- Caution patient to adhere strictly to established drug regimen. No drug dosage should be omitted, increased, or decreased without advice of physician.
- Advise patient to report promptly bone and joint pain; GI bleeding, colicky abdominal pain, nausea, vomiting, diarrhea; diminished vision.
- Skin dryness and ichthyosis (thickening and scaling of skin) may respond well to hydration and lubrication measures. Advise patient to minimize use of soap, avoid ap-

plying it directly to dry skin, and to thoroughly rinse it off.

- When dizziness, drowsiness, or visual impairment side effects are experienced, patient should not drive or work with hazardous equipment. These symptoms are generally dose related. Discuss with physician.

CLOFIBRATE

(kloe-fy′brate)

Trade names: Atromid-S, Claripex♣, Novofibrate♣

Classifications: CARDIOVASCULAR DRUG; ANTILIPEMIC; LIPID-LOWERING AGENT

Pregnancy category: C

ACTIONS/PHARMACODYNAMICS Structurally related to gemfibrozil. Reduces very low density lipoproteins (VLDL) to a greater extent than it reduces low density lipoproteins (LDL). Mechanism of action is unclear; it appears to inhibit cholesterol biosynthesis prior to mevalonate formation and transfer of triglycerides from liver to serum. Interferes with binding of free fatty acids to albumin and increases fecal excretion of neutral sterols. Its ability to cause regression of xanthomatous lesions is thought to be due to mobilization of cholesterol from tissue. Reduces platelet adhesiveness and increases release of ADH from posterior pituitary.

USES Adjunct for treatment of severe primary (type III) hyperlipidemia. **Unlabeled use:** management of diabetes insipidus.

ROUTE & DOSAGE

Hyperlipidemia
Adult: **PO** 2 g/d in 2–4 divided doses.

Diabetes Insipidus
Adult: **PO** 1.5–2 g/d in 2–4 divided doses.

PHARMACOKINETICS **Absorption:** readily absorbed from GI tract. **Peak:** 4–6 h. **Distribution:** distributed to extracellular space; crosses placenta; distribution into breast milk unknown. **Metabolism:** hydrolyzed in plasma to clofibric acid, which is further metabolized in liver. **Elimination:** half-life: 12–35 h; excreted in urine.

CONTRAINDICATIONS & PRECAUTIONS **Contraindicated in:** impaired renal or hepatic function, primary biliary cirrhosis. Safe use during pregnancy (category C), in nursing mothers, and in children <14 y not established. **Cautious use in:** history of jaundice or hepatic disease; gallstones; peptic ulcer; hypothyroidism; cardiovascular disease.

ADVERSE/SIDE EFFECTS **CNS:** drowsiness, dizziness, headache. **CV:** increase or decrease in angina, CHF, arrhythmias. **GI:** *nausea,* vomiting, loose stools, diarrhea, flatulence, abdominal distress, gastritis, stomatitis, cholelithiasis. **GU:** renal insufficiency. **Gynecologic:** impotence, decreased libido. **Hematologic:** neutropenia, leukopenia, anemia, eosinophilia, <u>agranulocytosis</u>, potentiation of anticoagulant effect. **Musculoskeletal:** flu-like symptoms. **Skin:** swelling and phlebitis at xanthoma sites, skin rash, allergy, urticaria, pruritus. **Other:** elevated AST and ALT.

DIAGNOSTIC TEST INTERFERENCE Clofibrate therapy may lead to increased ***BSP*** retention, ***thymol*** turbidity; increased ***serum creatine phosphokinase (CPK); proteinuria,*** parodoxical increase in ***LDL*** or ***cholesterol*** levels (if there is a large decrease in VLDL level). Lower fasting ***blood glucose*** and ***serum insulin*** levels in patients with diabetes mellitus.

DRUG INTERACTIONS ORAL ANTICOAGULANTS increase hypoprothrombinemia and increase risk of bleeding; **probenecid** increases effects of clofibrate; SULFONYLUREAS increase hypoglycemic effects.

NURSING IMPLICATIONS

Administration

- If gastric distress is a problem, administer drug with meals.
- Preserve in closed, light-resistant containers at 15–30C (59–86F) unless otherwise directed.

Assessment & Drug Effects

- Serum LDL and VLDL levels should be determined initially and evaluated every 2 wk during first few months of therapy, and then at monthly intervals. If tests show a steady rise or are otherwise abnormal, clofibrate should be withdrawn.
- Frequent serum transaminase and other liver tests are advocated, as well as periodic CBC, renal function tests, and determinations of plasma and urine steroid levels, serum electrolyte levels, and blood sugar.
- Therapeutic response generally occurs during the first or second month of therapy. Rebound may occur in second or third month, followed by a further decrease, and may also occur with sudden withdrawal of drug.
- Clofibrate therapy for increased serum cholesterol and triglycerides is generally withdrawn after 3 mo if the response is not adequate.

Patient & Family Education

- Flu-like symptoms (malaise, muscle soreness, aching, weakness) should be reported promptly to the physician. Other reportable conditions include leukopenia, pulmonary edema, and renal insufficiency (see Appendix G) and gastric pain, nausea, and vomiting.
- Women of childbearing years should be on birth control regimen. If pregnancy is desired, clofibrate therapy should be discontinued at least 2 mo before conception.
- Advise patient to adhere to drug regimen as established and not to stop taking the drug without consulting the physician.
- Caution patient about self-dosing with OTC drugs without the approval of the physician.

CLOMIPHENE CITRATE

(kloe′mi-feen)

Trade names: Clomid, Milophene, Serophene

Classifications: OVULATION STIMULANT; ANTIESTROGENIC

Pregnancy category: X

ACTIONS/PHARMACODYNAMICS Oral nonsteroidal estrogen agonist or antagonist. Induces ovulation in selected anovulatory women. Lacks androgenic, antiandrogenic, or progestational effects and does not appear to effect pituitary-adrenal or pituitary-thyroid functions. May act by binding to hypothalamic estrogen receptors, decreasing their numbers, and by inhibiting receptor replenishment. Resulting false hypoestrogenic state stimulates pituitary release of luteinizing hormone (LH), follicle-stimulating hormone (FSH), and gonadotropins, leading to ovarian stimulation. Normal ovulatory function does not usually resume after treatment or after pregnancy.

USES Infertility in appropriately selected women desiring pregnancy whose partners are fertile and potent. **Unlabeled uses:** male infertility, menstrual abnormalities, gynecomastia, fibrocystic breast disease, regulation of cycles in patients using rhythm method of contraception, endometrial hyperplasia, persistent lactation.

ROUTE & DOSAGE

Infertility

Adult: **PO *First course:*** 50 mg/d for 5 d; start on 5th day of cycle following start of spontaneous or induced bleeding (with progestin) or at any time in the patient who has had no recent uterine bleeding;
Second course if ovulation: repeat first course until conception or for 3 cycles;
Second course if no ovulation: 100 mg/d for 5 d as above (max 100 mg/d).

PHARMACOKINETICS Absorption: readily absorbed from GI tract. **Metabolism:** metabolized in liver. **Elimination:** half-life: 5 d; excreted primarily in feces in 5 d; the remainder is excreted slowly from enterohepatic pool or is stored in body fat for later release.

CONTRAINDICATIONS & PRECAUTIONS Contraindicated in: pregnancy (category X); neoplastic lesions, ovarian cyst; hepatic disease or dysfunction; abnormal bleeding; visual abnormalities; mental depression; thrombophlebitis. **Cautious use in:** polycystic ovarian enlargement, pelvic discomfort, sensitivity to pituitary gonadotropins.

ADVERSE/SIDE EFFECTS Dose related. **GI:** nausea, vomiting, increased appetite with weight gain, constipation, bloating. **GU:** urinary frequency, polyuria. **Eye (reversible and of short duration):** transient blurring, diplopia, scotomas, photophobia, floaters, prolonged after-images. **Reproductive:** spontaneous abortion, multiple ovulations, ovarian failure, *ovarian hyperstimulation syndrome, enlarged ovaries with multiple follicular cysts.* **Other:** *vasomotor flushes,* breast discomfort, abdominal pain, heavy menses, exacerbation of endometriosis; mental depression, headache, fatigue, insomnia, dizziness, vertigo.

DIAGNOSTIC TEST INTERFERENCE Clomiphene may increase BSP retention; ***plasma transcortin, thyroxine*** and ***sex hormone binding globulin*** levels. Also increases ***follicle-stimulating*** and ***luteinizing hormone*** secretion in most patients.

NURSING IMPLICATIONS

Administration

- Pretreatment with estrogen is indicated for the patient who has been hypoestrogenic for a long time. Estrogen therapy is stopped immediately before clomiphene therapy begins.
- Each course of therapy should start on or about the 5th cycle day once ovulation has been established.
- Store at 15–30C (59–86F) in tightly capped, light-resistant container.

Assessment & Drug Effects

- If abnormal bleeding occurs, full diagnostic measures are crucial. Report it immediately.

- If patient needs to wear dark glasses even inside or if she has blurred or decreased vision or scotomas (signs of ocular toxicity), she should promptly report for a complete ophthalmologic evaluation. Drug will be stopped until symptoms subside.
- If clomiphene is continued more than 1 y, patient should have an ophthalmologic examination at regular intervals.
- Pelvic pain indicates the need for immediate pelvic examination for diagnostic purposes.

Patient & Family Education

- Advise patient to take the medicine at same time every day to maintain drug levels and prevent forgetting a dose.
- Missed dose: Instruct patient to take drug as soon as possible. If not remembered until time for next dose, double the dose, then resume regular dosing schedule. If more than one dose is missed, patient should check with physician.
- Incidence of multiple births during clomiphene use is reportedly increased to 6 times normal and appears to increase with dose increases. Multiple births other than twins are rare.
- Patient who is going to respond usually ovulates 4–10 d after last day of treatment.
- The likelihood of conception diminishes with each succeeding course of therapy. If pregnancy is not achieved after 3 ovulatory responses, further treatment with clomiphene is not recommended.
- Usually, the couple is told to attempt conception 2 d before ovulation and to have intercourse every other day starting within 48 h after ovulation.
- Symptoms that should be reported: hot flushes resembling those associated with menopause; nausea, vomiting, headache. Appropriate drug therapy may be prescribed. Symptoms disappear after clomiphene is discontinued.
- Yellowing of eyes, light-colored stools, yellow, itchy skin, and fever symptomatic of jaundice should be reported promptly.
- Instruct patient to stop taking clomiphene if she suspects pregnancy and to contact physician for a confirmatory examination.
- Because of the possibility of lightheadedness, dizziness, and visual disturbances, caution the patient against performing hazardous tasks requiring skill and coordination in an environment with variable lighting.
- Warn patient to report promptly excessive weight gain, signs of edema, bloating, decreased urinary output.

CLOMIPRAMINE HYDROCHLORIDE

(clo-mi'pra-meen)

Trade name: Anafranil

Classifications: PSYCHOTHERAPEUTIC; CNS AGENT; TRICYCLIC ANTIDEPRESSANT

Prototype: Imipramine

Pregnancy category: C

ACTIONS/PHARMACODYNAMICS

Inhibits the reuptake of norepinephrine and serotonin at the presynaptic neuron. Elevated serum levels of these two amines are thought to be the basis of antidepressant effects. Exhibits anticholinergic, antihistaminic, hypotensive, sedative, mild analgesic, and peripheral vasodilator effects.

USES Obsessive-compulsive disorder (OCD). **Unlabeled uses:** panic disorder, anxiety, agoraphobia.

ROUTE & DOSAGE

Obsessive-compulsive Disorder
Adult: **PO** 75–300 mg/d in divided doses.
Child: **PO** 10–18 y: 100–200 mg/d in divided doses; start at 50 mg/d.

Depression
Adult: **PO** 50–150 mg/d in single or divided doses.

PHARMOCOKINETICS **Absorption:** rapidly absorbed from GI tract; 20–78% reaches systemic circulation. **Onset:** depression: approx 2 wk; OCD: approx 4–10 wk. **Peak** 2–6 h. **Distribution:** widely distributed including the CSF; crosses placenta. **Metabolism:** extensive first-pass metabolism in the liver; active metabolite is desmethylclomipramine. **Elimination:** half-life: 20–30 h; 50–60% excreted in urine, 24–32% in feces.

CONTRAINDICATIONS & PRECAUTIONS **Contraindicated in:** hypersensitivity to other tricyclic compounds; acute recovery period after MI, children < 10 y, pregnancy (category C), nursing mothers. **Cautious use in:** history of convulsive disorders, prostatic hypertrophy, urinary retention, cardiovascular, hepatic, GI, or blood disorders.

ADVERSE/SIDE EFFECTS **CNS:** mania, *tremor,* dizziness, hyperthermia, <u>neuroleptic malignant syndrome,</u> seizures (especially with abrupt withdrawal). **CV:** hypotension, tachycardia. **Endocrine:** galactorrhea, hyperprolactinemia, amenorrhea, *weight gain*. **Hematologic:** leukopenia, <u>agranulocytosis,</u> thrombocytopenia, anemia. **GI:** constipation, *dry mouth*. **GU:** delayed ejaculation, anorgasmia. **Other:** diaphoresis.

DRUG INTERACTION Clomipramine has the same drug interaction potential as other tricyclic antidepressants.

DIAGNOSTIC TEST INTERFERENCE Clomipramine appears to elevate serum ***prolactin*** levels. ***Serum AST and ALT*** are elevated. Serum levels of ***triiodothyronine (T_3) and free triiodothyronine (FT_3) have been significantly reduced from baseline. Thyroxine-binding globulin (TBG)*** levels were increased from baseline, whereas thyroxine (T_4), free thyroxine (FT_4), and reverse T_3 were unchanged.

NURSING IMPLICATIONS

Administration

- Drug should be initiated with a 25-mg/d dose, which is gradually increased to approximately 200 mg/d over a 2-wk period.
- Give in divided doses with meals to reduce GI side effects.
- Following titration to the full dose, drug may be given as a single dose at bedtime to reduce daytime sedation.
- Store at 15–30C (59–86F).

Assessment & Drug Effects

- Monitor for seizures, especially in those with predisposing factors such as alcoholism, brain injury, or concurrent therapy with other drugs that lower seizure threshold.
- Monitor liver functions, especially with long-term therapy.
- Monitor for and report signs of neuroleptic malignant syndrome (see Appendix G).
- Monitor for sedation and vertigo, especially at the beginning of therapy and following dosage increases. Supervision of ambulation may be indicated.
- Notify physician of fever and complaints of sore throat since WBC count with differential may be in-

dicated to rule out adverse hematologic changes.

C

Patient & Family Education

- Instruct patient not to take nonprescribed drugs or to discontinue therapy without consent of physician. Abrupt discontinuation may cause nausea, headache, malaise, or seizures.
- Men should understand that the drug may cause impotence or ejaculation failure. Advise them to report this problem to physician.
- Advise prompt reporting of sore throat accompanied by fever.
- Advise caution with ambulation until response to drug is known.
- Inform patient that excessive alcohol intake may potentiate adverse drug effects.

CLONAZEPAM

(kloe-na′zi-pam)

Trade names: Klonopin, Rivotril ♣

Classifications: CENTRAL NERVOUS SYSTEM AGENT; ANTICONVULSANT; BENZODIAZEPINE

Prototype: Diazepam

Pregnancy category: C

Controlled substance: Schedule IV

ACTIONS/PHARMACODYNAMICS BENZODIAZEPINE derivative with strong anticonvulsant activity and several other pharmacologic properties characteristic of the drug class. Suppresses spike and wave discharge in absence seizures (petit mal) and decreases amplitude, frequency, duration, and spread of discharge in minor motor seizures.

USES Alone or with other drugs in absence, myoclonic, and akinetic seizures, Lennox-Gastaut syndrome, absence seizures refractory to succinimides or valproic acid, and for infantile spasms and restless legs. **Unlabeled uses:** panic disorder, complex partial seizure pattern and generalized tonic-clonic convulsions.

ROUTE & DOSAGE

Seizures

Adult: **PO** 1.5 mg/d in 3 divided doses, increased by 0.5–1 mg q3d until seizures are controlled or until intolerable side effects (max recommended dose 20 mg/d).

Child: **PO** <10 y, 0.01–0.03 mg/kg/d (not to exceed 0.05 mg/kg/d) in 3 divided doses; may increase by 0.25–0.5 mg q3d until seizures are controlled or until intolerable side effects (max recommended dose 0.2 mg/kg/d).

Panic Disorders

Adult: **PO** 1–2 mg/d in divided doses (max 4 mg/d).

PHARMACOKINETICS **Absorption:** readily absorbed from GI tract. **Onset:** 60 min. **Peak:** 1–2 h. **Duration:** up to 12 h in adults; 6–8 h in children. **Distribution:** crosses placenta; distributed into breast milk. **Metabolism:** metabolized in liver. **Elimination:** half-life: 18–40 h; excreted in urine primarily as metabolites.

CONTRAINDICATIONS & PRECAUTIONS **Contraindicated in:** hypersensitivity to benzodiazepines; liver disease; acute narrow-angle glaucoma; breastfeeding. Safe use in pregnancy (category C) not established. **Cautious use in:** renal disease; COPD; drug-controlled open-angle glaucoma; addiction-prone individuals; children (because of unknown consequences of long-term use on growth and development); patient with mixed seizure disorders.

ADVERSE/SIDE EFFECTS CNS: *drowsiness, sedation, ataxia,* insomnia, aphonia, choreiform movements, coma, dysarthria, "glassy-eyed" appearance, headache, hemiparesis, hypotonia, slurred speech, tremor, vertigo. **CV:** palpitations. **Eye:** diplopia, nystagmus, abnormal eye movements. **GI:** dry mouth, sore gums, anorexia, coated tongue, increased salivation, increased appetite, nausea, constipation, diarrhea. **GU:** increased libido, dysuria, enuresis, nocturia, urinary retention. **Hematologic:** anemia, leukopenia, thrombocytopenia, eosinophilia. **Psychiatric:** confusion, depression, hallucinations, aggressive behavior problems, hysteria, suicide attempt. **Respiratory:** chest congestion, respiratory depression, rhinorrhea, dyspnea, hypersecretion in upper respiratory passages. **Skin:** hirsutism, hair loss, skin rash, ankle and facial edema.

DIAGNOSTIC TEST INTERFERENCE Clonazepam causes transient elevations of ***serum transaminase*** and ***alkaline phosphatase.***

DRUG INTERACTIONS Alcohol and other CNS DEPRESSANTS increase sedation and CNS depression; may increase **phenytoin** levels.

NURSING IMPLICATIONS

Administration

- If a new anticonvulsant is to be substituted, it is usually added to the drug regimen as the former medication is gradually withdrawn. Slow tapering of dose over several days' time is imperative. Abrupt withdrawal in patient on high doses or long-term therapy can precipitate status epilepticus. Other withdrawal symptoms include convulsion, tremor, abdominal and muscle cramps, vomiting, sweating.
- Store in tightly closed container protected from light at 15–30C (59–86F) unless otherwise specified.

Assessment & Drug Effects

- Monitor I&O ratio and other indicators of renal function. Excess accumulation of metabolites because of impaired excretion leads to toxicity.
- If multiple anticonvulsants are being given, watch patient carefully for signs of overdosage or drug interaction, i.e., increased depressant adverse effects.
- Liver function tests, platelet counts, blood counts, and clinical evaluation of drug efficacy should be a part of the follow-up care of the patient on clonazepam.
- Both psychological and physical dependence may occur in the patient on long-term, high-dose therapy. Watch patient to see that he or she does not cheek the tablet. Limit availability of large amounts of drug in the addiction-prone individual.
- Overdose symptoms are: somnolence, confusion, irritability, sweating, muscle and abdominal cramps, diminished reflexes, coma.

Patient & Family Education

- Anticonvulsant activity is often lost after 3 mo of therapy; dosage adjustment may reestablish efficacy. Patient should be aware of necessity to report loss of seizure control promptly.
- Counsel patient to take drug as prescribed and not to alter dosing regimen or stop medication without consulting physician.
- Caution patient not to self-medicate with OTC drugs before consulting the physician.
- Advise patient not to drive a car or engage in other activities requiring mental alertness and phys-

ical coordination until reaction to the drug is known. Drowsiness occurs in approximately 50% of patients.

- Patient should carry identification (e.g., Medic Alert) bearing information about medication in use and the diagnosis.

CLONIDINE HYDROCHLORIDE

(kloe′ni-deen)

Trade names: Catapres, Catapres-TTS, Dixaril ♣, Duraclon

Classifications: CARDIOVASCULAR AGENT; CENTRAL-ACTING ANTIHYPERTENSIVE; ANALGESIC

Prototype: Methyldopa

Pregnancy category: C

ACTIONS/PHARMACODYNAMICS Centrally acting antiadrenergic derivative. Stimulates $alpha_2$-adrenergic receptors in CNS to inhibit sympathetic vasomotor centers. Central actions reduce plasma concentrations of norepinephrine and decrease systolic and diastolic BP and heart rate. Orthostatic effects tend to be mild and occur infrequently. Also inhibits renin release from kidneys. Reportedly minimizes or eliminates many of the common clinical signs and symptoms associated with withdrawal of heroin, methadone, or other opiates.

USES Step 2 drug in stepped-care approach to treatment of hypertension, either alone or with diuretic or other antihypertensive agents. Epidural administration as adjunct therapy for severe pain. **Unlabeled uses:** prophylaxis for migraine; treatment of dysmenorrhea, menopausal flushing, diarrhea, paroxysmal localized hyperhidroses; alcohol, smoking, opiate, and benzodiazepine withdrawal; in the clonidine suppression test for diagnosis of pheochromocytoma; Gilles de la Tourette syndrome; attention deficit disorder with hyperactivity (ADDH) in children.

ROUTE & DOSAGE

Hypertension

Adult: **PO** 0.1 mg b.i.d. or t.i.d.; may increase by 0.1–0.2 mg/d until desired response is achieved (max 2.4 mg/d). **Transdermal** 0.1 mg patch once q7d; may increase by 0.1 mg q1–2wk.

Geriatric: **PO** Start with 0.1 mg once daily.

Child: **PO** 5–10 µg/kg/d divided q8–12h, may increase to 5–25 µg/kg/d divided q6h (max 0.9 mg/d).

Severe Pain

Adult: Epidural; start infusion at 30 µg/h and titrate to response. Use rates >40 µg/h with caution.

Child: Epidural; start infusion at 0.5 µg/kg/h and titrate to response.

ADDH

Child: **PO** 5 µg/kg/d in 4 divided doses (average dose, 0.15–0.2 mg/d). **Transdermal** 0.2–0.3 mg/d q5–7d.

PHARMACOKINETICS Absorption: readily absorbed from GI tract. **Onset:** 30–60 min PO; 1–3 d transdermal. **Peak:** 2–4 h PO; 2–3 d transdermal. **Duration:** 8 h PO; 7 d transdermal. **Distribution:** widely distributed; crosses blood–brain barrier; not known if crosses placenta or distributed into breast milk. **Metabolism:** metabolized in liver. **Elimination:** half-life: 6–20 h; 80% excreted in urine, 20% in feces.

CONTRAINDICATIONS & PRECAUTIONS Contraindicated in: pregnancy (category C), nursing women. Use of clonidine patch in polyarteritis nodosa, scleroderma, SLE. **Cautious use in:** severe coronary insufficiency, recent MI, sinus node dysfunction, cerebrovascular disease; chronic renal failure; Raynaud's disease, thromboangiitis obliterans; history of mental depression.

ADVERSE/SIDE EFFECTS CNS: *drowsiness, sedation,* dizziness, headache, fatigue, weakness, sluggishness, dyspnea, vivid dreams, nightmares, insomnia, behavior changes, agitation, hallucination, nervousness, restlessness, anxiety, mental depression. **CV:** *hypotension (epidural),* postural hypotension (mild), peripheral edema, ECG changes, tachycardia, bradycardia, flushing, rapid increase in BP with abrupt withdrawal. **Eye:** dry eyes. **GI/Metabolic:** *dry mouth, constipation,* abdominal pain, pseudo-obstruction of large bowel, altered taste, nausea, vomiting, hepatitis, hyperbilirubinemia, weight gain (sodium retention). **GU:** impotence, loss of libido. **Skin:** rash, pruritus, thinning of hair, exacerbation of psoriasis; with transdermal patch: hyperpigmentation, recurrent herpes simplex, skin irritation, contact dermatitis, mild erythema.

DIAGNOSTIC TEST INTERFERENCE Possibility of decreased urinary excretion of ***aldosterone, catecholamines,*** and ***VMA*** (however, sudden withdrawal of clonidine may cause increases in these values); transient increases in blood glucose; weakly positive direct antiglobulin (Coombs') tests.

DRUG INTERACTIONS Alcohol and other CNS DEPRESSANTS add to CNS depression; TRICYCLIC ANTIDEPRESSANTS may reduce antihypertensive effects. Opiate analgesics increase hypotension with epidural clonidine. Increased risk of bradycardia or AV block when epidural clonidine is used with digoxin, calcium channel blockers, or beta blockers.

NURSING IMPLICATIONS

Administration

- Last PO dose is commonly administered immediately before patient retires to ensure overnight BP control and to minimize daytime drowsiness.
- Oral dosage is increased gradually over a period of weeks so as not to lower BP abruptly (especially important in the elderly). Follow-up visits should be scheduled every 2–4 wk until BP stabilizes, then every 2–4 mo.
- Apply transdermal patch to dry skin, free of hair and rash. Avoid irritated, abraded, or scarred skin.
- Recommended areas for applying transdermal patch are upper outer arm and anterior chest. Less drug is absorbed from thighs. Rotate application sites and keep a record.
- During change from PO clonidine to transdermal system, PO clonidine should be maintained for at least 24 h after patch is applied. If patient is taking high PO doses, PO dosage may have to be tapered over several days. Directions should be written out and reviewed with patient so there is no misunderstanding.
- Epidural infusion rate is titrated up or down according to pain relief.
- If drug is to be discontinued, it is withdrawn over a period of 2–4 d. Abrupt withdrawal resembles sympathetic stimulation and may result in restlessness and headache 2–3 h after a missed dose and a hypertensive crisis within 8–18 h.
- Store in tightly closed container at 15–30C (59–86F) unless otherwise directed.

C

Assessment & Drug Effects

- Discuss with physician schedule for BP determinations: when to take readings, how often to take readings; position of patient (supine, sitting, standing; after exercise).
- With epidural administration, frequently monitor BP and HR. Hypotension is a common side effect that may require intervention.
- BP should be closely monitored whenever a drug is added to or withdrawn from therapeutic regimen.
- Tolerance sometimes develops in some patients. Physician may increase dosage or prescribe concomitant administration of a diuretic to enhance antihypertensive response.
- Monitor I&O during period of dosage adjustment. Report change in I&O ratio or change in voiding pattern.
- Determine weight daily. Patients not receiving a concomitant diuretic agent may gain weight, particularly during first 3 or 4 d of therapy, because of marked sodium and water retention.
- Patients with history of mental depression require close supervision, as they may be subject to further depressive episodes.

Patient & Family Education

- Although postural hypotension occurs infrequently, advise patient to make position changes slowly, and in stages, particularly from recumbent to upright position, and to dangle and move legs a few minutes before standing. Caution patient to lie down immediately if faintness or dizziness occurs.
- Inform patient of the possible sedative effect and caution against potentially hazardous activities until reaction to drug has been determined.
- Warn patient of the danger of omitting doses or of stopping the drug without consulting the physician.
- Advise patient to carry Medic Alert or other appropriate medical identification card.
- Caution patient not to take OTC medications, alcohol, or other CNS depressants without prior discussion with physician.
- Instruct patient to examine site when transdermal patch is removed and to report to physician if erythema, rash, irritation, or hyperpigmentation occurs.
- Advise patient that if transdermal patch loosens, it can be taped in place with adhesive. The patch should never be cut or trimmed.

CLOPIDROGREL BISULFATE

(clo-pi′dro-grel)

Trade name: Plavix

Classifications: BLOOD FORMER; ANTIPLATELET AGENT

Prototype: Ticlopidine

Pregnancy category: B

ACTIONS/PHARMACODYNAMICS

Inhibits platelet aggregation by selectively preventing the binding of ADP to its platelet receptor. An analog of ticlopidine. Its effect on the ADP receptor of a platelet is irreversible. Consequently, clopidrogrel prolongs bleeding time.

USE Secondary prevention of MI, stroke, and vascular death in patients with recent MI, stroke, or established peripheral arterial disease. **Unlabeled use:** reduction of restenosis after stent placement.

ROUTE & DOSAGE

Secondary Prevention

Adult: **PO** 75 mg q.d.

PHARMACOKINETICS **Absorption:** rapidly absorbed from GI tract. **Onset:** 2 h; reaches steady state in 3–7 d. **Distribution:** 94–98% protein bound. **Metabolism:** rapidly hydrolyzed in plasma to active metabolite. **Elimination:** half-life: 8 h; 50% excreted in urine and 50% in feces.

CONTRAINDICATIONS & PRECAUTIONS **Contraindicated in:** hypersensitivity to clopidogrel; intracranial hemorrhage, peptic ulcer, or any other active pathologic bleeding. Discontinue clopidogrel 7 days before surgery and during lactation. Safety and efficacy not established in children. **Cautious use in:** concurrent use with drugs that might induce gastrointestinal bleeding; GI bleeding; hepatic impairment (moderate to severe); patients at risk for increased bleeding; pregnancy (category B).

ADVERSE/SIDE EFFECTS **Body as whole:** flu-like syndrome, fatigue, pain, arthralgia, back pain. **CNS:** headache, dizziness, depression. **CV:** chest pain, edema, hypertension. **GI:** abdominal pain, dyspepsia, diarrhea, nausea, hypercholesterolemia. **Hematologic:** purpura, epistaxis. **Respiratory:** URI, dyspnea, rhinitis, bronchitis, cough. **Skin:** rash, pruritus. **Other:** UTI.

DRUG INTERACTIONS NSAIDS may increase risk of bleeding events.

NURSING IMPLICATIONS

Administration

- Do not administer to persons with active pathologic bleeding.
- Discontinue drug 7 d prior to surgery.
- Store at 15–30C (59–86F) in tightly closed container and protect from light.

Assessment & Drug Effects

- Therapeutic effectiveness is indicated by reduction in atherosclerotic events.
- Carefully monitor for and immediately report S&S of GI bleeding, especially when coadministered with NSAIDS, aspirin, heparin, or warfarin.
- Patients with unexplained fever or infection should be evaluated for myelotoxicity.

Patient & Family Education

- Promptly report any unusual bleeding (e.g., black, tarry stools).
- Avoid chronic aspirin or NSAID use unless approved by physician.

CLORAZEPATE DIPOTASSIUM

(klor-az′e-pate)

Trade names: Novoclopate ♣, Tranxene, Tranxene-SD

Classifications: CENTRAL NERVOUS SYSTEM AGENT; ANXIOLYTIC; SEDATIVE-HYPNOTIC; ANTICONVULSANT; BENZODIAZEPINE

Prototype: Lorazepam

Pregnancy category: C

Controlled substance: Schedule IV

ACTIONS/PHARMACODYNAMICS Anxiolytic with actions, uses, and interactions qualitatively similar to those of lorazepam but with fewer unwanted side effects, e.g., sedation.

USES Management of anxiety disorders, short-term relief of anxiety symptoms, as adjunct in management of partial seizures, and symptomatic relief of acute alcohol withdrawal.

ROUTE & DOSAGE

Anxiety

Adult: **PO** 15 mg/d h.s.; may increase to 15–60 mg/d in divided doses (max 60 mg/d).

C

Acute Alcohol Withdrawal

Adult: **PO** 30 mg followed by 30–60 mg in divided doses (max 90 mg/d); taper by 15 mg/d over 4 d to 7.5–15 mg/d until patient is stable.

Partial Seizures

Adult: **PO** 7.5 mg t.i.d.
Child 9–12 y: **PO** 3.75–7.5 mg b.i.d.; may increase by no more than 3.75 mg/wk (max 60 mg/d).

PHARMACOKINETICS **Absorption:** decarboxylated in stomach; absorbed as active metabolite, desmethyldiazepam. **Peak:** 1 h. **Duration:** 24 h. **Distribution:** crosses placenta; distributed into breast milk. **Metabolism:** metabolized in liver to oxazepam. **Elimination:** half-life: 30–200 h; excreted primarily in urine.

CONTRAINDICATIONS & PRECAUTIONS **Contraindicated in:** hypersensitivity to clorazepate and other benzodiazepines; patients <9 y; acute narrow-angle glaucoma; depressive neuroses, psychotic reactions, drug abusers. Safe use during pregnancy (category C), in nursing mothers, and in children <9 y not established. **Cautious use in:** elderly, debilitated patients; hepatic disease; kidney disease.

ADVERSE/SIDE EFFECTS *Drowsiness,* ataxia, GI disturbances, xerostomia, diplopia, blurred vision, dizziness, headache, paradoxical excitement, mental confusion, insomnia, hypotension; abnormal liver function tests, decreased Hct, blood dyscrasias; allergic reactions.

DRUG INTERACTIONS **Alcohol** and other CNS DEPRESSANTS compound CNS depression; clorazepate increases effects of **cimetidine, disulfiram,** causing excessive sedation.

NURSING IMPLICATIONS

Administration

- Antacids delay absorption of drug. If patient has gastric distress, advise taking drug with food or milk. If necessary to use an antacid (with approval), it should be taken no less than 1 h before or 1 h after drug ingestion.
- Drug dose should be tapered gradually over several day's time when regimen is to be discontinued. Abrupt termination may lead to memory impairment, severe GI symptoms, muscle pain, restlessness, irritability, fatigue, insomnia.
- Store in light-resistant container at 15–30C (59–86F) unless otherwise specified.

Assessment & Drug Effects

- Effectiveness of clorazepate for long-term use (more than 4 mo) has not been determined. Usefulness of drug should be periodically reassessed.
- Drowsiness, a common side effect, is more likely to occur at initiation of therapy and with dose increments on successive days.
- Periodic blood counts and tests of liver and kidney function should be performed throughout therapy.
- Patient with history of or actual cardiovascular disease should be monitored in early therapy for drug-induced responses. If systolic BP drops more than 20 mm Hg or if there is a sudden increase in pulse rate, withhold drug and notify physician.

Patient & Family Education

- Counsel patient to take drug as prescribed and not to change dose or abruptly stop taking the drug without physician's approval.

- Caution patient not to self-dose with OTC drugs (cold remedies, sleep medications, antacids) without consulting physician.
- Caution patient to avoid driving and other potentially hazardous activities until reaction to drug is known.
- Warn patient not to use alcohol and other CNS depressants while on clorazepate therapy.
- Patient should be advised that if she becomes pregnant during therapy or intends to become pregnant, she should communicate with her physician about the desirability of discontinuing the drug.
- Alert responsible family member(s) to report signs of possible drug abuse and dependency to physician: nervousness, insomnia, memory impairment, diarrhea.

CLOTRIMAZOLE

(kloe-trim′a-zole)

Trade names: Canesten ♣, Gyne-Lotrimin, Gyne-Lotrimin-3, Lotrimin, Mycelex, Mycelex-G

Classifications: ANTIINFECTIVE; ANTIBIOTIC; ANTIFUNGAL

Prototype: Fluconazole

Pregnancy category: B (topical); category C (oral)

ACTIONS/PHARMACODYNAMICS Has broad-spectrum fungicidal activity. Acts by altering fungal cell membrane permeability, permitting loss of phosphorous compounds, potassium, and other essential intracellular constituents with consequent loss of ability to replicate. Active against *Trichophyton rubrum, Trichophyton mentagrophytes, Epidermophyton floccosum, Microsporum canis, Malassezia furfur,* and *Candida* sp, including *Candida albicans.* Natural or acquired fungal resistance to clotrimazole is rare.

USES Dermal infections including tinea pedis, tinea cruris, tinea corporis, tinea versicolor; also vulvovaginal and oropharyngeal candidiasis. **Unlabeled use:** trichomoniasis.

ROUTE & DOSAGE

Dermal Infections
Adult: **Topical** Apply small amount onto affected areas b.i.d. AM and PM.

Vulvovaginal Infections
Adult: **Intravaginal** Insert 1 applicatorful or one 100 mg vaginal tablet into vagina at bedtime for 7 d, or one 500 mg vaginal tablet at bedtime for 1 dose.

Oropharyngeal Candidiasis
Adult/child: **PO** 1 troche (lozenge) 5 times/d q3h for 14 d.

PHARMACOKINETICS Absorption: minimal systemic absorption; minimally absorbed topically. **Peak:** high saliva concentrations <3h; high vaginal concentrations in 8–24 h. **Metabolism:** metabolized in liver. **Elimination:** eliminated as metabolite in bile.

CONTRAINDICATIONS & PRECAUTIONS Contraindicated in: ophthalmic uses; systemic mycoses. Safe use during pregnancy (category C for oral troches, category B for topical preparations), in nursing mothers, and in children <3 y not established. **Cautious use in:** hepatic impairment.

ADVERSE/SIDE EFFECTS Skin preparations: stinging, erythema, edema, vesication, desquamation, pruritus, urticaria, skin fissures. **Vaginal preparations:** mild burning sen-

C

sation, lower abdominal cramps, bloating, cystitis, urethritis, mild urinary frequency, vulval erythema and itching, pain and vaginal soreness during intercourse. **Other:** abnormal liver function tests; occasional nausea and vomiting (with oral troche).

NURSING IMPLICATIONS

Administration

- Instruct patient taking the oral lozenge to allow it to dissolve slowly in mouth over 15–30 min for maximum effectiveness.
- Vaginal preparations are effective only for candidiasis.
- Skin cream and solution preparations should be applied sparingly. Protect hands with latex gloves when applying medication.
- Avoid contact of clotrimazole preparations with the eyes.
- Occlusive dressings should not be applied unless otherwise directed by physician.
- Consult physician about skin cleansing procedure before applying medication. Regardless of procedure used, dry skin thoroughly.
- Store cream and solution formulations at 15–30C (59–86F); do not store troches or vaginal tablets above 35 (95F) unless otherwise directed.

Assessment & Drug Effects

- Evaluate effectiveness of treatment. Report any signs of skin irritation with dermal preparations.
- Anticipate signs of clinical improvement within the first week of drug use.

Patient & Family Education

- Advise patient to use clotrimazole as directed and for the length of time prescribed by physician.
- Generally, clinical improvement is apparent during first week of therapy. Advise patient to report to physician if condition worsens or if signs of irritation or sensitivity develop, or if no improvement is noted after 4 wk of therapy.
- Inform patient receiving the drug vaginally that sexual partner may experience burning and irritation of penis or urethritis and advise refraining from sexual intercourse during therapy or that sexual partner wear a condom.

CLOXACILLIN, SODIUM

(klox-a-sill′in)

Trade names: Apo-Cloxi ♣, Cloxapen, Cloxilean, Novocloxin ♣, Orbenin, Tegopen

Classifications: ANTIINFECTIVE; ANTIBIOTIC, NATURAL PENICILLIN; BETA-LACTAM

Prototype: Penicillin G

Pregnancy category: B

ACTIONS/PHARMACODYNAMICS

Semisynthetic, acid-stable, penicillinase-resistant, isoxazolyl penicillin. In common with other isoxazolyl penicillins (dicloxacillin, oxacillin), highly active against most penicillinase-producing staphylococci, less potent than penicillin G against penicillin-sensitive microorganisms, and generally ineffective against gram-negative bacteria and methicillin-resistant staphylococci.

USES Primarily in infections caused by penicillinase-producing staphylococci and penicillin-resistant staphylococci. May be used to initiate therapy in suspected staphylococcal infections pending culture and susceptibility test results. As with other penicillins, serum concentrations are enhanced by concurrent use of probenecid.

ROUTE & DOSAGE

Mild to Moderate Infections

Adult: **PO** 250–500 mg q6h.
Child: **PO** <20 kg: 12.5–25 mg/kg q6h (max 4 g/d).

PHARMACOKINETICS **Absorption:** 37–60% absorbed from GI tract. **Peak:** 0.5–2 h. **Duration:** 4–6 h. **Distribution:** distributed throughout body with highest concentrations in liver, kidney, spleen, bone, bile, and pleural fluid; low CSF penetration; crosses placenta; distributed into breast milk. **Metabolism:** metabolized in liver. **Elimination:** half-life: 30–60 min; excreted primarily in urine with some elimination through bile.

CONTRAINDICATIONS & PRECAUTIONS **Contraindicated in:** sensitivity to penicillins. Safe use during pregnancy (category B), in nursing mothers, and in neonates not established. **Cautious use in:** history of or suspected atopy or allergy (asthma, eczema, hives, hay fever), renal or hepatic function impairment, history of allergy to cephalosporins.

ADVERSE/SIDE EFFECTS **GI:** *nausea,* vomiting, flatulence, *diarrhea*. **Hematologic:** eosinophilia, leukopenia, agranulocytosis. **Hypersensitivity:** pruritus, urticaria, rash, wheezing, sneezing, chills, drug fever, anaphylaxis. **Other:** elevated AST, ALT; jaundice (possibly of allergic etiology); superinfections.

DRUG INTERACTION **Probenecid** decreases cloxacillin elimination.

NURSING IMPLICATIONS

Administration

- Cloxacillin is best taken on an empty stomach (at least 1 h before or 2 h after meals) unless otherwise advised by physician. Food reduces rate and extent of drug absorption.
- After reconstitution (by pharmacist), PO solution retains potency for 14 d if refrigerated (container should be so labeled and dated). Shake well before pouring.
- Unless otherwise advised, store capsules at 15–30C (59–86F).

Assessment & Drug Effects

- Before treatment is initiated, determine previous exposure and sensitivity to penicillins and cephalosporins and other allergic reactions of any kind.
- As with other penicillins, monitor for signs and symptoms of anaphylactoid reaction (see Appendix G) or other signs or symptoms of hypersensitivity reaction (see Appendix G).
- Periodic assessments of renal, hepatic, and hematopoietic function are advised in patients on long-term therapy.

Patient & Family Education

- Instruct patient to take medication around the clock, not to miss a dose, and to continue taking the medication until it is all gone, unless otherwise directed by physician.
- Inform patient to report to physician the onset of hypersensitivity reaction (see Appendix G) and superinfections.
- Advise patient to check with physician if GI side effects (nausea, vomiting, diarrhea) appear.

CLOZAPINE

(clo′za-pin)

Trade name: Clozaril

Prototype for classifications: CENTRAL NERVOUS SYSTEM (CNS) AGENT; PSYCHOTHERAPEUTIC; NEUROLEPTIC AGENT; DOPAMINE-REUPTAKE INHIBITOR

Pregnancy category: B

C

ACTIONS/PHARMACODYNAMICS Mechanism is not defined. Interferes with binding of dopamine to D_1 and D_2 receptors in the limbic region of brain. It binds primarily to nondopaminergic sites (e.g., alpha-adrenergic, serotonergic, and cholinergic receptors).

USE Indicated only in the management of severely ill schizophrenic patients who have failed to respond to other neuroleptic agents.

ROUTE & DOSAGE

Schizophrenia

Adult: **PO** >16 y: Initiate at 25–50 mg/d and titrate to a target dose of 350–450 mg/d in 3 divided doses at 2 wk intervals; further increases can be made if necessary; max 900 mg/d.

PHARMACOKINETICS Absorption: readily absorbed from GI tract. **Onset:** 2–4 wk. **Peak:** 2.5 h. **Distribution:** possibly distributed into breast milk. **Metabolism:** metabolized in liver. **Elimination:** half-life: 8–12 h; 50% excreted in urine, 30% in feces.

CONTRAINDICATIONS & PRECAUTIONS Contraindicated in: severe CNS depression, blood dyscrasia, history of bone marrow depression; patients with myeloproliferative disorders, uncontrolled epilepsy; clozapine-induced agranulocytosis, severe granulocytosis, concurrent administration of benzodiazepines or other psychotropic drugs; pregnancy (category B), lactation. **Cautious use in:** arrhythmias, GI disorders, narrow-angle glaucoma, hepatic and renal impairment, prostatic hypertrophy, history of seizures; patients with cardiovascular and/or pulmonary disease; previous history of agranulocytosis. Safety and efficiacy in children have not been established.

ADVERSE/SIDE EFFECTS CNS: seizures, *transient fever,* sedation. **CV:** orthostatic hypotension, *tachycardia,* ECG changes. **GI:** nausea, dry mouth, constipation, hypersalivation. **Other:** <u>agranulocytosis</u>, urinary retention.

DRUG INTERACTIONS Alcohol and other CNS DEPRESSANTS compound depressant effects; ANTICHOLINERGIC AGENTS potentiate anticholinergic effects; ANTIHYPERTENSIVE AGENTS may potentiate hypotension.

NURSING IMPLICATIONS

Administration

- If therapy must be discontinued, the drug is usually withdrawn gradually over 1–2 wk.
- Store the drug away from heat or light.

Assessment & Drug Effects

- Because of risk of agranulocytosis (see Appendix G) a baseline white blood count and differential count must be made before initial treatment, every week for first 6 mo, then every 2 wk for next 6 mo, and for 4 wk after the drug is discontinued.
- Monitor for seizure activity; seizure potential increases at the higher dose level.
- If the drug is being discontinued, closely monitor for recurrence of psychotic symptoms.
- Monitor for development of tachycardia or hypotension, which may pose a serious risk for patients with compromised cardiovascular function.
- Monitor daily temperature and report fever. Transient elevation above 38C (100.4F), with peak incidence during first 3 wk of drug therapy, may occur.

Patient & Family Education

- Advise patient not to engage in any hazardous activity until response to the drug is known. Drowsiness and sedation are common side effects.
- Warn patient about the risk of agranulocytosis (see Appendix G). Emphasize importance of complying with blood test regimen. Advise patient to report flulike symptoms, fever, sore throat, lethargy, malaise, or other signs of infection.
- Instruct patient to rise slowly to avoid orthostatic hypotension.
- Instruct patient that drug should be taken exactly as ordered.
- Instruct patient not to use OTC drugs or alcohol without permission of physician.
- Instruct patient to notify physician of pregnancy, as drug is not normally administered during pregnancy.
- Instruct patient not to breastfeed while she is taking clozapine.

COCAINE
(koe-kane′)

COCAINE HYDROCHLORIDE

Classifications: CENTRAL NERVOUS SYSTEM AGENT; ANESTHETIC, LOCAL
Prototype: Procaine
Pregnancy category: C
Controlled substance: Schedule II

ACTIONS/PHARMACODYNAMICS Alkaloid obtained from leaves of *Erythroxylon coca*. Topical application blocks nerve conduction and produces surface anesthesia accompanied by local vasoconstriction. Exerts adrenergic effect by potentiating action of endogenous (and injected) epinephrine and norepinephrine, possibly by inhibiting reuptake of catecholamines into sympathetic nerve terminals. Systemic absorption produces descending CNS stimulation, with intense, short-lived euphoria accompanied by indifference to pain or hunger and with illusions of great strength, endurance, and mental capacity, all the bases for drug abuse.

USES Surface anesthesia of ear, nose, throat, rectum, and vagina. Ophthalmic use largely abandoned because of its tendency to cause corneal sloughing. Sometimes used as ingredient in Brompton's cocktail.

ROUTE & DOSAGE

Surface Anesthesia
Adult: **Topical** 1–10% solution (use > 4% solution with caution); max single dose 1 mg/kg.

PHARMACOKINETICS Absorption: readily absorbed from mucous membranes; absorption limited by vasoconstriction. **Onset:** 1 min. **Peak:** 15–120 min. **Duration:** 30 min–2 h. **Distribution:** crosses placenta; distributed into breast milk. **Metabolism:** hydrolyzed in serum. **Elimination:** half-life: 1–2.5 h; excreted in urine; detectable for up to 30 h.

CONTRAINDICATIONS & PRECAUTIONS Contraindicated in: hypersensitivity to local anesthetics; sepsis in region of proposed application. Safe use during pregnancy (category C) and in nursing mothers not established. **Cautious use in:** history of drug sensitivities, history of drug abuse.

ADVERSE/SIDE EFFECTS CNS: *CNS stimulation* and CNS depression (respiratory and circulatory failure). **CV:** tachycardia, ventricular fibrillation, MI, angina pectoris. **ENT:** runny nose, perforated nasal septum. **Eye:** clouding, pitting, and ulceration of cornea. **GI:** nausea, vomiting,

C

anorexia, abdominal pain. **Other:** formication ("cocaine bugs"), hypersensitivity reactions; pneumonia, lung damage (chronic cocaine smoking).

DRUG INTERACTIONS **Epinephrine** entails risk of severe hypertension and arrhythmias; MAO INHIBITORS potentiate pharmacologic effects of cocaine.

NURSING IMPLICATIONS

Administration

- To discourage illegal use, cocaine solutions for topical application are often tinted with an antiseptic dye such as methylene blue. This dye also inhibits mold growth in the solution.
- Preserve in tightly closed, light-resistant containers.

Assessment & Drug Effects

- When used for anesthesia of throat, cocaine causes temporary paralysis of cilia of respiratory tract cells, reducing protection against aspiration. It also may interfere with pharyngeal stage of swallowing. Give nothing by mouth until sensation returns.
- Monitor cardiovascular status, especially in patients with known cardiac disease. Report promptly cardiac arrhythmias.

Patient & Family Education

- Instruct patients with a known history of cardiac disease to promptly report angina or other distress.

CODEINE

(koe′deen)

CODEINE PHOSPHATE

Trade name: Paveral♣

CODEINE SULFATE

Classifications: CNS AGENT; NARCOTIC (OPIATE) AGONIST ANALGESIC; ANTITUSSIVE

Prototype: Morphine

Pregnancy category: C

Controlled substance: Schedule II

ACTIONS/PHARMACODYNAMICS Opium derivative similar to morphine in actions, uses, contraindications, precautions, and adverse reactions. In equianalgesic doses, parenteral codeine produces degree of respiratory depression similar to that of morphine. In contrast to morphine, orally administered codeine is about 60% as potent as the parenteral form. Histamine-releasing action appears to be more potent than that of morphine and may result in hypotension, flushing, and rarely bronchoconstriction. Analgesic potency is about one-sixth that of morphine; antitussive activity is also a little less than that of morphine.

USES Symptomatic relief of mild to moderately severe pain when control cannot be obtained by nonnarcotic analgesics and to suppress hyperactive or nonproductive cough.

ROUTE & DOSAGE

Analgesic

Adult: **PO/IM/SC** 15–60 mg q.i.d.
Child: **PO/IM/SC** 0.5–1 mg/kg q4–6h prn (max 60 mg/dose).

Antitussive

Adult: **PO** 10–20 mg q4–6h prn (max 120 mg/24h).
Child: **PO** 6–12 y: 5–10 mg q4–6h (max 60 mg/24 h); 2–6 y: 2.5–5 mg q4–6h (max 30 mg/24 h).

Common side effect in *italic,* life-threatening effects underlined: generic names in **bold;** drug class in SMALL CAPS

PHARMACOKINETICS Absorption: readily absorbed from GI tract. **Onset:** 15–30 min. **Peak:** 1–1.5 h. **Duration:** 4–6 h. **Distribution:** crosses placenta; distributed into breast milk. **Metabolism:** metabolized in liver. **Elimination:** half-life: 2.5–4 h; excreted in urine.

CONTRAINDICATIONS & PRECAUTIONS Contraindicated in: hypersensitivity to codeine or other morphine derivatives; acute asthma, COPD; increased intracranial pressure, head injury, acute alcoholism, hepatic or renal dysfunction, hypothyroidism. Safe use during pregnancy (category C), in nursing mothers, and in neonates not established. **Cautious use in:** prostatic hypertrophy, debilitated patients, very young and very old patients; history of drug abuse.

ADVERSE/SIDE EFFECTS CNS: *dizziness,* light-headedness, *drowsiness,* sedation, lethargy, euphoria, agitation; restlessness, exhilaration, convulsions, narcosis, <u>respiratory depression</u>. **CV:** palpitation, hypotension, orthostatic hypotension, bradycardia, tachycardia, <u>circulatory collapse</u>. **GI:** *nausea,* vomiting, *constipation*. **GU:** urinary retention. **Hypersensitivity:** diffuse erythema, rash, urticaria, *pruritus,* excessive perspiration, facial flushing, shortness of breath, <u>anaphylactoid reaction</u>. **Other:** miosis, fixed-drug eruption.

DRUG INTERACTIONS Alcohol and other CNS DEPRESSANTS augment CNS depressant effects.

NURSING IMPLICATIONS

Administration

- Administer PO codeine with milk or other food to reduce possibility of GI distress.
- Patient's individual need for medication should be evaluated before each administration.
- Preserve in tight, light-resistant containers at 15–30C (59–86F) unless otherwise directed.

Assessment & Drug Effects

- Record relief of pain and duration of analgesia.
- Treatment of cough is directed toward decreasing frequency and intensity of cough without abolishing protective cough reflex, which serves the important function of removing bronchial secretions.
- Although codeine has less abuse liability than morphine, dependence is a major unwanted effect.
- Since drug may cause dizziness and light-headedness, supervision of ambulation and other safety precautions may be warranted.
- Nausea is a common side effect. Report nausea accompanied by vomiting. Change to another analgesic may be warranted.

Patient & Family Education

- Because orthostatic hypotension is a possible side effect, instruct patient to make position changes slowly and in stages particularly from recumbent to upright posture. Also advise patient to lie down immediately if light-headedness or dizziness occurs.
- Nausea appears to be aggravated by ambulation. Advise patient to lie down when feeling nauseated and to notify physician if this symptom persists.
- Inform patient that codeine may impair ability to perform tasks requiring mental alertness and therefore to avoid driving and other potentially hazardous activities until reaction to drug is known.
- Advise patient not to take alcohol or other CNS depressants unless approved by physician.
- Inform patient that hyperactive cough may be lessened by avoid-

ing irritants such as smoking, dust, fumes, and other air pollutants. Humidification of ambient air may provide some relief.

C

COLCHICINE

(kol′chi-seen)

Trade name: Novocolchine ♣

Prototype for classification: ANTIGOUT AGENT

Pregnancy category: C

ACTIONS/PHARMACODYNAMICS Alkaloid of the autumn crocus *Colchicum autumnale* with antimitotic and indirect antiinflammatory properties. Inhibition of inflammation and reduction of pain and swelling occurs in gouty arthritis. Colchicine is nonanalgesic and nonuricosuric. Tolerance to colchicine does not develop.

USES Prophylactically for recurrent gouty arthritis and for acute gout, either as single agent or in combination with a uricosuric such as probenecid, allopurinol, or sulfinpyrazone. **Unlabeled uses:** sarcoid arthritis, chondrocalcinosis (pseudogout), arthritis associated with erythema nodosum, leukemia, adenocarcinoma, acute calcific tendonitis, familial Mediterranean fever, multiple sclerosis, primary biliary cirrhosis, mycosis fungoides, and in experimental studies of normal and abnormal cell division.

ROUTE & DOSAGE

Acute Gouty Attack

Adult: **PO** 0.5–1.2 mg followed by 0.5–0.6 mg q1–2h until pain relief or intolerable GI symptoms (max 4 mg/attack). **IV** 2 mg followed by 0.5 mg q6h until relief or intolerable GI symptoms (max 4 mg/attack).

Prophylaxis

Adult: **PO** 0.5 or 0.6 mg every night or every other night as needed (up to 1.8 mg/d may be needed for severe cases). **IV** 0.5–1 mg 1–2 times/d.

Surgical Patients

Adult: **PO** 0.5 or 0.6 mg t.i.d. starting 3 d before surgery and continuing for 3 d after surgery.

PHARMACOKINETICS Absorption: rapidly absorbed from GI tract. **Peak:** 0.5–2 h; may have multiple peaks because of enterohepatic cycling. **Distribution:** widely distributed; concentrates in leukocytes, kidney, liver, spleen, and intestinal tract. **Metabolism:** partially metabolized in liver. **Elimination:** primarily excreted in feces; 10–20% excreted in urine in 24 h.

CONTRAINDICATIONS & PRECAUTIONS Contraindicated in: blood dyscrasias; severe GI, renal, hepatic, or cardiac disease; use of IV colchicine in patients with both renal and hepatic dysfunction. Severe local irritation can result from SC or IM use. Safe use during pregnancy (category C), in nursing mothers, and in children not established. **Cautious use in:** elderly and debilitated patients, early manifestations of GI, renal, hepatic, or cardiac disease.

ADVERSE/SIDE EFFECTS Dose-related. **CNS:** mental confusion, peripheral neuritis, syndrome of muscle weakness (accompanied by elevated serum creatine kinase). **GI:** *nausea, vomiting, diarrhea, abdominal pain,* anorexia, hemorrhagic gastroenteritis, steatorrhea, hepatotoxicity, pancreatitis. **Hematologic:** neutropenia, bone marrow depression, thrombocytopenia, agranulocytosis, aplastic anemia. **Renal:**

azotemia, proteinuria, hematuria, oliguria.

DIAGNOSTIC TEST INTERFERENCE Possible interference with ***urinary steroid (17-OHCS)*** determinations when done by modifications of Reddy, Jenkins, Thorn procedure. False-positive ***urine tests for RBCs and hemoglobin*** reported.

DRUG INTERACTION May decrease intestinal absorption of vitamin B_{12}.

NURSING IMPLICATIONS

Administration

- Administer oral drug with milk or food to reduce possibility of GI upset.
- To avoid cumulative toxicity, a given course of colchicine therapy for acute gout is generally not repeated within 3 d.
- IV preparation: Dilute with 0.9% NaCl injection that does not contain a bacteriostatic agent. Discard turbid solutions. Do not dilute colchicine with 5% dextrose injection or other fluids that may change pH of colchicine solution, since a precipitate may form.
- IV administration: Injection should be made over 2–5 min by direct IV or into tubing of free-flowing IV with compatible fluid.
- Care must be taken to prevent extravasation of IV colchicine because severe tissue irritation including nerve damage can result.
- Preserved in tight, light-resistant containers preferably between 15 and 30C (59 and 86F), unless otherwise directed by manufacturer.

Assessment & Drug Effects

- Baseline and periodic determinations of serum uric acid and creatinine are advised, as well as CBC, including Hgb, serum electrolytes, and urinalysis.
- Side effects (dose-related) are most likely to occur during the initial course of treatment. A latent period of several hours between drug administration and onset of toxic symptoms is usual.
- Early signs of colchicine toxicity include weakness, abdominal discomfort, anorexia, nausea, vomiting, and diarrhea, regardless of administration route. Report to physician. To avoid more serious toxicity, drug should be discontinued promptly until symptoms subside.
- Monitor I&O (during acute gouty attack). High fluid intake promotes excretion and reduces danger of crystal formation in kidneys and ureters.
- Keep physician informed of patient's progress. Drug should be stopped when pain of acute gout is relieved. Therapeutic response: articular pain and swelling generally subside within 8–12 h and usually disappear in 24–72 h after PO therapy, and 6–12 h after IV administration.

Patient & Family Education

- Patients taking colchicine at home should be advised to withhold drug and report to the physician the onset of GI symptoms or signs of bone marrow depression (nausea, sore throat, bleeding gums, sore mouth, fever, fatigue, malaise, unusual bleeding or bruising).
- Patients with gout should be instructed to keep colchicine at hand at all times so they can start therapy or increase dosage, as prescribed by physician, at the first suggestion of an acute attack.
- Physician may prescribe sodium bicarbonate, or sodium or potassium citrate, to maintain alkaline urine and thus prevent formation of urate stones.
- Fermented beverages such as beer, ale, and wine may precipi-

C

tate gouty attack and therefore should be avoided. The physician may allow distilled alcoholic beverages in moderation.

COLESTIPOL HYDROCHLORIDE

(koe-les′ti-pole)

Trade names: Cholestabyl ♣, Colestid, Lestid ♣

Classifications: CARDIOVASCULAR DRUG; ANTILIPEMIC; BILE ACID SEQUESTRANT

Prototype: Cholestyramine

Pregnancy category: C

ACTIONS/PHARMACODYNAMICS Insoluble chloride salt of a basic anion exchange resin, with high molecular weight. Binds with bile acids in intestinal tract to form an insoluble complex that is excreted in the feces, thus reducing circulating cholesterol and increasing serum LDL removal rate. Serum triglycerides are not affected or are minimally increased. Route and dosage, contraindications, adverse reactions, interactions are similar to those of cholestyramine.

USES Pruritus associated with partial biliary obstruction; also as adjunct to diet therapy of patient with primary hypercholesterolemia (type IIa hyperlipoproteinemia) or with coronary artery disease unresponsive to diet or other measures alone. **Unlabeled uses:** digitoxin overdose and hyperoxaluria and to control postoperative diarrhea caused by excess bile acids in colon.

ROUTE & DOSAGE

Hypercholesterolemia

Adult: **PO** 15–30 g/d in 2–4 doses a.c. and h.s., or 1–2 tabs 1–2 times/d.

Digitalis Toxicity

Adult: **PO** 10 g followed by 5 g q6–8h as needed.

PHARMACOKINETICS Absorption: not absorbed from GI tract. **Elimination:** excreted in feces as insoluble complex.

CONTRAINDICATIONS & PRECAUTIONS Contraindicated in: complete biliary obstruction, hypersensitivity to bile acid sequestrants. Safe use during pregnancy (category C), in nursing mothers, and in children not established. **Cautious use in:** hemorrhoids; bleeding disorders; malabsorption states; the elderly.

ADVERSE/SIDE EFFECTS GI: *constipation,* abdominal pain or distention, belching, flatulence, nausea, vomiting, diarrhea. **Other:** dermatitis, urticaria, joint and muscle pain, arthritis, shortness of breath, transient increases in liver enzyme tests, serum phosphorus and chloride; decreases in serum sodium and potassium.

DRUG INTERACTIONS Because it decreases the absorption from the GI tract of ORAL ANTICOAGULANTS, **digoxin,** TETRACYCLINES, PENICILLINS, **phenobarbital,** THYROID HORMONES, THIAZIDE DIURETICS, IRON SALTS, FAT-SOLUBLE VITAMINS (A, D, E, K), administer cholestyramine 4 h before or 2 h after these drugs.

NURSING IMPLICATIONS

Administration

- To prevent accidental inhalation or esophageal distress with the granule form, always mix with liquids, juices, soups, cereals, or pulpy fruits. Add powder to at least 90 ml fluid. When carbonated drink is used, slowly stir in a large glass because excess foaming may occur.

Rinse glass with small amount extra fluid to be sure all the drug is taken.
- Drugs given concomitantly should be scheduled at least 1 h before or 4 h after ingestion of colestipol to reduce interference with their absorption (see drug interactions).
- Store at 15–30C (59–86F) in tightly closed container unless otherwise instructed.

Assessment & Drug Effects
- Watch for changes in bowel elimination pattern. Constipation should not be allowed to persist without medical attention.
- Monitor serum sodium and potassium levels. Monitor for and report signs and symptoms of hyponatremia and hypokalemia (see Appendix G).

Patient & Family Education
- Be sure patient understands importance of established regimens for colestipol and other drugs that patient is taking. Patient should not change the times for taking each drug, nor omit or increase doses. Any change in established regimens should be approved by the physician.
- Patients receiving prolonged therapy should report unusual bleeding (vitamin K deficiency). Colestipol prevents absorption of FAT-SOLUBLE VITAMINS (A, D, E, K).
- Urge patient not to use OTC drugs unless physician has given approval.
- Check with physician regarding permitted amount of alcohol intake.

COLFOSCERIL PALMITATE
(col-fos′ce-ril)
Trade name: Exosurf Neonatal
Classification: LUNG SURFACTANT
Prototype: Beractant

C

ACTIONS/PHARMACODYNAMICS Synthetic lung surfactant. Endogenous pulmonary surfactant lowers surface tension on alveolar surfaces during respiration and stabilizes the alveoli against collapse at resting pressures. Deficiency of surfactant causes respiratory distress syndrome (RDS) in premature infants. Colfosceril lowers minimum surface tension and restores pulmonary compliance and oxygenation in premature infants.

USES Prophylactic treatment of infants with birth weights <1350 g who are at risk of developing RDS. Prophylactic therapy of infants with birth weights >1350 g who show evidence of pulmonary immaturity. **Unlabeled uses:** rescue treatment of infants with established RDS; RDS in adults.

ROUTE & DOSAGE

Prophylaxis
Infant: **Intratracheal** 3 doses of 5 ml/kg are recommended, with the first dose being given as soon as possible after birth and repeat doses 12 and 24 h later to infants who remain on mechanical ventilation.

Rescue Therapy
Infant: **Intratracheal** 2 doses of 5 ml/kg are recommended, the first dose being initiated as soon as the diagnosis of RDS is confirmed and the second 12 h later in infants remaining on mechanical ventilation.

PHARMACOKINETICS **Absorption:** absorbed fom the alveolus into lung tissue, where it can be extensively catabolized and reutilized for further phospholipid synthesis and secretion. **Duration:** improvements in the arterial:alveolar oxygen tension (a:A) ratio, A-a gradient, and oxygen and ventilator needs have persisted for at least 7 d. **Distribution:** uniformly to all lobes of the lung, distal airways, and alveolar spaces; gravitation to dependent areas of lung does not occur. **Metabolism:** sufactant is recycled and metabolized exclusively in the lungs of healthy infants and is not distributed to the systemic circulation; in infants with RDS, however, the disrupted integrity of the alveolar lining could result in escape of surfactant to systemic circulation. **Elimination:** half-life: 20-36 h; recycling may be a dominant metabolic pathway by which surfactant is taken up by type II pneumocytes and reused.

CONTRAINDICATIONS & PRECAUTIONS **Contraindicated in:** infants who have major congenital abnormalities or who are suspected of having congenital infections.

ADVERSE/SIDE EFFECTS **CV:** bradycardia, tachycardia. **Respiratory:** decreased oxygen saturation, mucous plugging, apnea, pulmonary hemorrhage.

NURSING IMPLICATIONS

Administration

- Reconstitute immediately before use if possible. Use only supplied diluent for reconstitution.
- Reconstitute as follows: (1) withdraw diluent with 18–19-gauge needle attached to 10–12-ml syringe; (2) inject into vial by allowing vacuum to draw diluent in; (3) do not withdraw needle and aspirate as much of solution as possible back into syringe; (4) maintain vacuum and quickly release plunger. Repeat steps 3 and 4 three or four times to ensure adequate mixing.
- Reconstituted drug is a milky white suspension. Gently shake if needed to resuspend it.
- Before administration of drug, ensure that endotracheal tube tip is in the trachea.
- Before administration of drug, the infant should be suctioned. If possible, avoid suctioning for 2 h after drug administration.
- Drug is administered without interrupting mechanical ventilation. Use side port on the endotracheal tube adaptor.
- Withdraw entire ordered dose into syringe while maintaining vacuum in vial.
- Administer dose in halves, each half over 1–2 min. Give first half dose with head in midline position; then turn head and torso to the right. Wait 30 s; then return to midline position for second half dose. Give each dose in short bursts timed with inspiration. After second half dose, turn head and torso to left for 30 s; then return to midline.
- Slow or stop drug administration and adjust ventilator rate or FIO_2 if any of the following occur: heart rate decreases, infant becomes dusky or agitated, or O_2 saturation drops.
- Store Exosurf at 15–30C (59–86F) in a dry place. Reconstituted solution is stable for 12 h.

Assessment & Drug Effects

- During administration of drug, continuous ECG and transcutaneous monitoring are required. Also monitor chest expansion and facial expression.
- Monitor pulmonary function during administration. Rapid changes may require immediate adjustment

of peak inspiratory pressure, ventilator rate, or FIO_2.
- Following administration, monitor continuously for 30 min. Frequent arterial blood gas sampling is required to prevent hyperoxia and hypocarbia.

C

COLISTIMETHATE SODIUM

(koe-lis-ti-meth′ate)

Trade name: Coly-Mycin M

Classification: URINARY TRACT ANTIINFECTIVE

Prototype: Trimethoprim

ACTIONS/PHARMACODYNAMICS Polymyxin antibiotic and parenteral form of colistin. Similar to polymyxin B in structure and actions but about one-third to one-fifth as potent. Antibacterial activity and overall toxicity are less, but nephrotoxic potential is almost identical with that of polymyxin B. Believed to act by affecting phospholipid component in bacterial cytoplasmic membranes with resulting damage and leakage of essential intracellular components. Bactericidal against most gram-negative organisms including *Pseudomonas aeruginosa, Escherichia coli, Enterobacter aerogenes, Hemophilus* sp, *Klebsiella pneumoniae, Brucella, Salmonella, Shigella, Bordetella, Pasteurella,* and *Vibrio.* Not effective against *Proteus* or *Neisseria* species. Complete cross-resistance and cross-sensitivity to polymyxin B reported but not to broad-spectrum antibiotics.

USES Particularly for severe, acute and chronic UTIs caused by susceptible strains of gram-negative organisms resistant to other antibiotics. Has been used with carbenicillin for *Pseudomonas* sepsis in children with acute leukopenia.

ROUTE & DOSAGE

Urinary Tract Infections

Adult: **IM/IV** 2.5–5 mg/kg/d divided in 2–4 doses; max 5 mg/kg/d.
Child: **IM/IV** Same as for adult.

PHARMACOKINETICS Peak: 1–2 h IM. **Duration:** 8–12 h. **Distribution:** widely distributed in most tissues except CNS; crosses placenta; distributed into breast milk. **Metabolism:** metabolized in liver. **Elimination:** half-life: 2–3 h; 66–75% excreted in urine within 24h.

CONTRAINDICATIONS & PRECAUTIONS Contraindicated in: hypersensitivity to polypeptide antibiotics; concomitant use of drugs that potentiate neuromuscular blocking effect (aminoglycoside antibiotics, other polymyxins, anticholinesterases, curariform muscle relaxants, ether, sodium citrate); nephrotoxic and ototoxic drugs. Safe use during pregnancy not established. **Cautious use in:** impaired renal function; myasthenia gravis; elderly patients, infants.

ADVERSE/SIDE EFFECTS Respiratory arrest after IM injection. **CNS:** circumoral, lingual, and peripheral paresthesias; visual and speech disturbances, neuromuscular blockade (generalized muscle weakness, dyspnea, respiratory depression or paralysis), seizures, psychosis. **Ear:** ototoxicity. **Hypersensitivity:** drug fever, pruritus, urticaria, dermatoses. **Renal:** nephrotoxicity. **Other:** GI disturbances, pain at IM site.

DRUG INTERACTIONS Tubocurarine, pancuronium, atracur-

C

ium, AMINOGLYCOSIDES may compound and prolong respiratory depression; AMINOGLYCOSIDES, **amphotericin B, vancomycin** augment nephrotoxicity.

INCOMPATIBILITIES Solution/additive: carbenicillin, cephalothin, erythromycin, hydrocortisone, kanamycin.

NURSING IMPLICATIONS

Administration

- Reconstitute each 150-mg vial with 2 ml of sterile water for injection to yield a concentration of 75 mg/ml. Swirl vial gently during reconstitution to avoid bubble formation. For IV use, further dilute with 20 ml sterile water for injection.
- IM injection should be made deep into upper outer quadrant of buttock. Patients commonly experience pain at injection site. Rotate sites.
- IV infusion solution should be freshly prepared and used within 24 h.
- A single initial dose properly diluted is given by direct IV at a rate of 75 mg over 5 min. Subsequent doses are usually further diluted in an additional 50 ml or more of compatible solution and infused over a period of hours.
- IV infusion rate is prescribed by physician. (Rate of 5–6 mg/h is recommended for patients with normal renal function.)
- Reconstituted solution may be stored in refrigerator at 2–8C (36–46F) or at controlled room temperature of 15–30C (59–86F). Use within 7 d. Store unopened vials at controlled room temperature.

Assessment & Drug Effects

- Culture and susceptibility tests should be performed initially and periodically during therapy to determine responsiveness of causative organisms.
- Respiratory arrest has been reported after IM administration. Report restlessness or dyspnea promptly.
- Baseline renal function tests should be performed prior to therapy; frequent monitoring of renal function and urine drug levels is advisable during therapy. Impaired renal function increases the possibility of nephrotoxicity, apnea, and neuromuscular blockade.
- Monitor I&O. Decrease in urine output or change in I&O ratio and rising BUN, serum creatinine, and serum drug levels (without dosage increase) are indications of renal toxicity. If they occur, withhold drug and report to physician.
- Elderly patients and infants are particularly prone to renal toxicity because they tend to have inadequate renal reserves. Close monitoring is essential.
- Be alert to neurologic symptoms: changes in speech and hearing, visual changes, drowsiness, dizziness, ataxia, and transient paresthesias, and keep physician informed.
- Postoperative patients who have received curariform muscle relaxants, ether, or sodium citrate should be closely monitored for signs of neuromuscular blockade (delayed recovery, muscle weakness, depressed respiration).

Patient & Family Education

- Because of the possibility of transient neurologic disturbances, caution ambulatory patient to avoid operating a vehicle or other potentially hazardous activities while on drug therapy.

C

CORTICOTROPIN

(kor-ti-koe-troe′pin)

Trade names: ACTH, Acthar

CORTICOTROPIN REPOSITORY

Trade names: ACTH Gel, Acthron, Cortigel, Cortrophin-Gel, Cotropic Gel, H.P. Acthar Gel

Classifications: HORMONE; ADRENAL CORTICOSTEROID

Prototype: Prednisone

Pregnancy category: C

ACTIONS/PHARMACODYNAMICS Adrenocorticotropic hormone (ACTH) extracted from pituitary of domestic animals (usually pigs). Stimulates functioning adrenal cortex to produce and secrete corticosterone, cortisol (hydrocortisone), several weak androgens, and limited amounts of aldosterone. Therapeutic effects appear more rapidly than do those of prednisone. Suppresses further release of corticotropin by negative feedback mechanism. Chronic administration of exogenous corticosteroids decreases ACTH store and causes structural changes in pituitary. Lack of ACTH stimulation can lead to adrenal cortex atrophy.

USES Diagnostic test of adrenocortical function and adjunctively to treat adrenal insufficiency secondary to inadequate corticotropin secretion. Effective in treatment of adrenocorticoid-responsive diseases, such as multiple sclerosis, but adrenocorticoid therapy is preferred.

ROUTE & DOSAGE

Diagnostic Test

Adult: **IV** 10–25 U in 500 ml D5W infused over 8 h.

Therapeutic

Adult: **IM/SC** 40–80 U/d; dose and frequency individualized; ***repository*** 40–80 U q24–72h. *Child:* **IM/IV/SC** 1.6 U/kg/d divided q6–8h; repository 0.8 U/kg/d divided q12h.

Acute Multiple Sclerosis

Adult: **IM/SC** 80–120 U/d for 2–3 wk; ***repository*** 80–120 U/d for 2–3 wk.

PHARMACOKINETICS Absorption: readily absorbed from IM site. **Onset:** 6 h. **Duration:** 2–4 h IV/IM; 12–24 h repository. **Distribution:** concentrated in many tissues; not known if crosses placenta or distributed into breast milk. **Metabolism:** metabolized in liver. **Elimination:** half-life: <20 min; excreted in urine.

CONTRAINDICATIONS & PRECAUTIONS Contraindicated in: ocular herpes simplex; recent surgery; CHF; scleroderma; osteoporosis; systemic fungoid infections; hypertension; sensitivity to porcine proteins; conditions accompanied by primary adrenocortical insufficiency or hyperfunction. Use during pregnancy (category C) or in lactating women requires evaluation of expected benefits against possible hazards to mother and child. **Cautious use in:** patients with latent tuberculosis or those reacting to tuberculin; hypothyroiditis, impaired hepatic function.

ADVERSE/SIDE EFFECTS CNS: euphoria, insomnia, headache, convulsions, papilledema, mood swings, depression. **Eye:** cataract, glaucoma. **GI:** nausea, vomiting, abdominal distention, peptic ulcer with perforation and hemorrhage. **Gynecologic:** hirsutism,

C

amenorrhea. **Metabolic:** sodium and water retention; potassium and calcium loss, negative nitrogen balance, hyperglycemia. **Skin:** acne, impaired wound healing, fragile skin, petechiae, ecchymosis. **Other:** osteoporosis, loss of muscle mass, hypersensitivity, cushingoid state, activation of latent diabetes mellitus or tuberculosis, vertebral compression fracture.

DRUG INTERACTIONS Aspirin, NSAIDS increase potential for hypoprothrombinemia; because of enzyme induction, BARBITURATES, **phenytoin, rifampin** decrease effects of corticotropin; ESTROGENS may increase corticotropin binding and effects; **amphotericin B,** diuretics increase potassium loss.

INCOMPATIBILITIES Solution/additive: aminophylline, sodium bicarbonate.

NURSING IMPLICATIONS

Administration

- Dosage is individualized. Changes in dosage regimen are gradual and only after full drug effects have become apparent.
- Corticotropin zinc hydroxide and corticotropin repository forms are not suitable for IV use.
- Shake corticotropin zinc hydroxide bottle well before injecting drug deep into gluteal muscle.
- For IV administration, dilute powder with 2 ml sterile water or NS for injection; desired dose is withdrawn from vial and further diluted with 500 ml of D5W and infused over 8 h.
- IV administration to infants and children: Verify correct IV concentration and rate of infusion with physician.
- Administration of the hormone at high dosage levels is tapered rather than withdrawn suddenly. A 2–5 d period of adrenocortical hypofunction follows discontinuation of corticotropin.
- Storage: Corticotropin for injection (reconstituted solution) is stable for 24 h or 7 d, depending on product, when stored at 2–8C (36–46F). Store corticotropin repository at 2–15C (36–59F). Store corticotropin zinc hydroxide at 15–30C (59–86F).

Assessment & Drug Effects

- Before giving corticotropin to patient with suspected sensitivity to porcine proteins, hypersensitivity skin testing should be performed.
- Observe patient closely for 15 min for hypersensitivity reactions during IV administration or immediately after SC or IM injections (urticaria, pruritus, dizziness, nausea, vomiting, anaphylactic shock). Epinephrine 1:1000 should be readily available for emergency treatment.
- Adrenal response to corticotropin is measured against a baseline plasma cortisol level 1 h before the 8 h test. Another plasma level is determined after at least 1 h of the infusion.
- Test results: Patient with normal adrenal reserves shows an increase in plasma cortisol levels of 15–40 μg/dl by the eighth hour of the 8-h corticotropin infusion (plasma cortisol levels more than 45 μg/dl by 8 h, urinary 17-OHCS increase to 12–25 mg/g creatinine; 17-KS increase by 1.5–2.5 times control level). Patient with complete primary adrenal suppression has no change from baseline plasma cortisol or urinary 17-OHCS or 17-KS excretion levels. In patient with hypopituitarism, plasma cortisol levels and urinary 17-OHCS increase in subnormal increments after the 8-h test daily for 5 d.
- Corticotropin may suppress signs and symptoms of chronic disease.
- New infections can appear during

treatment. Because of decreased resistance and inability to localize the infection, it may be severe. Report immediately.
- Prolonged use of corticotropin increases risk of hypersensitivity reaction (see Appendix G).
- Growth and development of a child receiving this drug should be carefully monitored.

Patient & Family Education
- Corticotropin administration increases requirements for insulin and oral antidiabetic agents. Make patient with diabetes mellitus aware of the need to monitor blood glucose closely until response to the drug is stabilized.
- Advise patient to monitor weight and report a steady gain, especially if accompanied by edema. Patient should also promptly report headache, muscle weakness, abdominal pain.
- Caution patient against self-medicating with OTC drugs without consulting physician.
- Eye examinations should be done before initiation of expected long-term therapy and periodically during treatment. Instruct patient to report to physician if blurred vision occurs.
- Dietary salt restriction and potassium supplementation may be necessary to minimize edema caused by overstimulation of the adrenal cortex by corticotropin.
- Patient should not be immunized with live vaccines while receiving corticotropin.

CORTISONE ACETATE

(kor′ti-sone)

Trade names: Cortistan, Cortone

Classifications: HORMONE; SYNTHETIC ADRENAL CORTICOSTEROID; GLUCOCORTICOID

Prototype: Prednisone

Pregnancy category: D

C

ACTIONS/PHARMACODYNAMICS

Short-acting synthetic steroid with prominent glucocorticoid activity and mineralocorticoid effects approximately equal to those of prednisone (cortisol). Because therapeutic activity of cortisone results from its conversion in body to cortisol, its effects simulate those of hydrocortisone. Has antiinflammatory and immunosuppressive actions. Metabolic effects include promotion of protein, carbohydrate, and fat metabolism and interference with linear growth in children. Mineralocorticoid actions include promotion of sodium retention and potassium excretion. May foster development of osteoporosis.

USES Replacement therapy for primary or secondary adrenocortical insufficiency and inflammatory and allergic disorders.

ROUTE & DOSAGE

Replacement or Inflammatory Disorders

Adult: **PO/IM** 20–300 mg/d in 1 or more divided doses; try to reduce periodically by 10–25 mg/d to lowest effective dose.
Child: **PO** 2.5–10 mg/kg/d divided q6–8h; **IM** 1–5 mg/kg/d divided q12–24h.

PHARMACOKINETICS **Absorption:** readily absorbed from GI tract. **Onset:** rapid PO; 24–48 h IM. **Peak:** 2 h PO; 24–48 h IM. **Duration:** 1.25–1.5 d. **Distribution:** concentrated in many tissues; crosses placenta; distributed into breast milk. **Metabolism:** metabolized in liver. **Elimination:** half-life: 0.5 h; HPA suppression: 8–12 h; excreted in urine.

C

CONTRAINDICATIONS & PRECAUTIONS **Contraindicated in:** hypersensitivity to glucocorticoids; psychoses; viral or bacterial diseases of skin; Cushing's syndrome, immunologic procedures. Safe use in pregnancy (category D), by nursing mothers, and children not established. **Cautious use in:** diabetes mellitus; hypertension, CHF; active or arrested tuberculosis; active or latent peptic ulcer.

ADVERSE/SIDE EFFECTS **CNS:** euphoria, insomnia, vertigo, nystagmus. **CV:** CHF, hypertension, *edema.* **Endocrine:** hyperglycemia. **Eye:** *cataracts,* glaucoma, blurred vision. **GI:** *nausea,* peptic ulcer, pancreatitis. **Hematologic:** thrombocytopenia. **Musculoskeletal:** *compression fracture,* osteoporosis, muscle weakness. **Skin:** impaired wound healing, petechiae, ecchymosis, acne.

DRUG INTERACTIONS BARBITURATES, **phenytoin, rifampin,** because of enzyme induction, decrease effects of cortisone.

NURSING IMPLICATIONS

Administration

- Administer cortisone (usually in AM) with food or fluid of patient's choice to reduce gastric irritation.
- Sodium chloride and a mineralocorticoid are usually given with cortisone as part of replacement therapy.
- Parenteral cortisone is a suspension (25 mg/ml) and therefore should not be used IV. Shake bottle well before withdrawing dose.
- Admixtures with other parenteral medications are not recommended because of state of suspension and altered absorption rate.
- Alternate-day therapy with an oral intermediate acting glucocorticoid may decrease growth retardation effect in children.
- Store at 15–30C (59–86F) in tightly closed container unless otherwise directed by manufacturer. Protect from heat and freezing.

Assessment & Drug Effects

- Monitor for signs and symptoms of Cushing's syndrome (see Appendix G), especially in patients on long-term therapy.
- Cortisone may mask some signs of infection, and new infections may appear.
- Be alert to clinical indications of infection: malaise, anorexia, depression, and evidence of delayed healing. (Classic signs of inflammation are suppressed by cortisone.)
- Ecchymotic areas, unexplained bleeding, and easy bruising are reportable signs.

Patient & Family Education

- Advise patient to take drug exactly as prescribed, and caution against altering dose intervals or stopping therapy abruptly.
- Patient should monitor weight and report a steady gain especially if it is accompanied by signs of fluid retention (e.g., edema of ankles or hands).
- Changes in visual acuity, including blurring, should be reported promptly.
- Inform physician or dentist that cortisone is being taken. Patient should carry identification card or jewelry that states drug being taken and physician's name.

COSYNTROPIN

(koe-sin-troe′pin)

Trade name: Cortrosyn

Classification: DIAGNOSTIC AGENT

Prototype: Prednisone

Pregnancy category: C

ACTIONS/PHARMACODYNAMICS Synthetic polypeptide resembling corticotropin (ACTH) in the first 24 of the 39 amino acids in naturally occurring ACTH. Has less immunologic activity and is associated with less risk of sensitivity than corticotropin. In patient with normal adrenocortical function, stimulates adrenal cortex to secrete corticosterone, cortisol (hydrocortisone), several weak androgenic substances, and limited amounts of aldosterone. Extra-adrenal actions, not used therapeutically, include melanotropic and adipokinetic effects and increased secretion of growth hormone.

USES Diagnostic tool to differentiate primary adrenal from secondary (pituitary) adrenocortical insufficiency. **Unlabeled use:** in patients with normal adrenocortical function for the long-term treatment of chronic inflammatory or degenerative disorders responsive to glucocorticoids.

ROUTE & DOSAGE

Rapid Screening Test
Adult: **IM/IV** 0.25 mg injected over 2 min
Child <2 y: **IM** 0.125 mg injected over 2 min; **IV** 0.125 mg at 0.04 mg/h over 6 h.
Child >2 y: same as adult.
Neonate: **IM/IV** 0.015 mg/kg.

PHARMACOKINETICS Absorption: plasma cortisol levels double in 15–30 min. **Peak:** 1 h. **Duration:** 2–4 h. **Distribution:** unknown; does not cross placenta. **Metabolism:** unknown.

CONTRAINDICATIONS & PRECAUTIONS Contraindicated in: history of allergic disorders. Safe use during pregnancy (category C) and in nursing women not established.

ADVERSE/SIDE EFFECTS Pruritus, mild fever, chronic pancreatitis.

DIAGNOSTIC TEST INTERFERENCE **Cortisone, hydrocortisone, estrogen, spironolactone,** elevated bilirubin, and presence of free Hgb in plasma may interfere with ***plasma cortisol*** determinations.

NURSING IMPLICATIONS

Administration

- Reconstitute cosyntropin powder by adding 1.1 ml 0.9% NaCl injection (diluent provided by manufacturer) to vial labeled 0.25 mg to provide solution containing 0.25 mg cosyntropin/ml.
- Reconstituted drug may be given by direct IV over 2 min or further diluted in D5W or NS and infused over 4–8 h.
- IV administration to neonates, infants and children: Verify correct IV concentration and rate of infusion/injection with physician.
- Reconstituted solutions remain stable 24 h at room temperature or 21 d at 2–8C.
- Cosyntropin should not be added to blood or to plasma infusions.

Assessment & Drug Effects

- Although plasma cortisol levels are better indicators of adrenal function, the response can also be measured by 24 h urinary 17-KS or 17-OHCS excretion before and at end of IV infusion.
- Normal 17-KS levels in men are 10–25 mg/24 h; in women <50 y, 5–15 mg/24 h; and in women >50 y, 4–8 mg/24 h.
- Normal 17-OHCS levels in men are 5–12 mg/24 h; in women, 3–10 mg/24 h; in children 8–12 y, <4.5 mg/24 h; in younger children, 1.5 mg/24 h. Levels may be slightly higher in obese or muscular individuals.
- Urine collection for study of 17-KS excretion may have to be postponed if female patient is menstruating.

C

- If patient is on prednisone, dexamethasone, or betamethasone, therapy can continue through the test period because these drugs do not interfere with analysis of serum cortisol.

CROMOLYN SODIUM

(kroe′moe-lin)

Trade names: Disodium Cromoglycate, DSCG, Fivent ♣, Intal, Nasalcrom, Rynacrom ♣, Vistacrom ♣

Prototype for classifications: ANTIASTHMATIC; MAST CELL STABILIZER; ANTIINFLAMMATORY

Pregnancy category: B

ACTIONS/PHARMACODYNAMICS Synthetic asthma-prophylactic agent with unique action. Inhibits release of bronchoconstrictors—histamine and SRS-A (slow-reacting substance of anaphylaxis)—from sensitized pulmonary mast cells, thereby suppressing an allergic response. Has no intrinsic bronchodilator, antihistaminic, or vasoconstrictor properties, thus only of value when taken prophylactically. Particularly effective for IgE-mediated or "extrinsic asthma" precipitated by exposure to specific allergen, e.g., pollens, dust, animal dander.

USES Primarily for prophylaxis of mild to moderate seasonal and perennial bronchial asthma and allergic rhinitis. Also used for prevention of exercise-related bronchospasm, prevention of acute bronchospasm induced by known pollutants or antigens, and for prevention and treatment of allergic rhinitis. **Ophthalmic use:** allergic ocular disorders. **Unlabeled uses:** orally for systemic mastocytosis and for prophylaxis of GI and systemic reactions to food allergy. **Orphan drug:** proposed use: mastocytosis; vernal keratoconjunctivitis.

ROUTE & DOSAGE

Allergies

Adult: **Inhalation** Metered dose inhaler or capsule: 1 spray or 1 capsule inhaled q.i.d.; nasal solution: 1 spray in each nostril 3–6 times/d at regular intervals.
Child: **Inhalation** >6 y: Metered dose inhaler or capsule: same as for adult; >6 y: nasal solution: same as for adult.

PHARMACOKINETICS **Absorption:** approximately 8% of dose absorbed from lungs. **Onset:** 1 wk with regular use. **Peak:** 15 min. **Duration:** 4–6 h; may last as long as 2–3 wk. **Elimination:** half-life: 80 min; excreted in bile and urine in equal amounts.

CONTRAINDICATIONS & PRECAUTIONS **Contraindicated in:** use of aerosol (because of fluorocarbon propellants) in patients with coronary artery disease or history of arrhythmias; dyspnea, acute asthma, status asthmaticus; patients unable to coordinate actions or follow instructions. Safe use in children <6 y not determined; use of capsule not recommended for children. Safe use during (category B) and in nursing women not established. **Cautious use in:** renal or hepatic dysfunction.

ADVERSE/SIDE EFFECTS Generally well tolerated. **CNS:** headache, dizziness, peripheral neuritis. **ENT:** *sneezing, nasal stinging and burning,* dryness and *irritation of throat and trachea; cough;* nasal congestion. **Eye:** itchy, puffy eyes, lacrimation, *transient burning, stinging.* **GI:** swelling of parotid glands, dry mouth, slightly bitter after-taste, *nausea,* vomiting, esophagitis. **Hypersensitivity:** erythema, urticaria, rash, contact dermatitis, peripheral eosinophilia, angioedema, bronchospasm, anaphylaxis (rare).

NURSING IMPLICATIONS

Administration

- Patients should receive detailed instructions for loading and administering the spinhaler or nasalmatic device. See manufacturer's instructions. Therapeutic effect is dependent on proper inhalation technique.
- Advise patient to clear as much mucus as possible before inhalation treatments.
- Instruct patient to exhale as completely as possible before placing inhaler mouthpiece between lips, tilt head backward and inhale rapidly and deeply with steady, even breaths. Remove inhaler from mouth, hold breath for a few seconds, then exhale into the air. Repeat until entire dose is taken.
- Caution patient not to exhale into inhaler because moisture from breath will interfere with its proper operation. Also inform patient that capsule is intended for inhalation only and is ineffective if swallowed.
- Protect cromolyn from moisture and heat. Store in tightly closed, light-resistant container at 15–30C (59–86F) unless otherwise directed.

Assessment & Drug Effects

- A drug history is advisable before treatment is initiated. Cromolyn capsules contain a lactose vehicle to which patients with lactose deficiency may react.
- Exacerbation of asthmatic symptoms including breathlessness and cough may occur in patients receiving cromolyn during corticosteroid withdrawal. The same is true of patients on maintenance steroid therapy when cromolyn is withdrawn.
- Cromolyn does not eliminate the continued need for therapy with bronchodilators, expectorants, antibiotics, or corticosteroids, but the amount and frequency of use of these medications may be appreciably reduced.
- Eosinophil count is a reliable indicator of developing allergy and therefore should be monitored.
- For patients with asthma, therapeutic effects may be noted within a few days but generally not until after 1–2 wk of therapy.

Patient & Family Education

- Inform patient that throat irritation, cough, and hoarseness can be minimized by gargling with water, drinking a few swallows of water, or by sucking on a lozenge after each treatment.
- Provide patient with specific instructions regarding what to do in the event of an acute asthmatic attack. Cromolyn is of no value in acute asthma.
- Advise patient to report any unusual signs or symptoms. Hypersensitivity reactions (see Signs & Symptoms, Appendix G) can be severe and life-threatening. Drug should be discontinued if an allergic reaction occurs.
- Treatment with cromolyn 15 min before doing protracted exercises reportedly blunts the effects of vigorous exercise as well as cold air.
- Ophthalmic use: Patient should be advised not to wear soft contact lenses during therapy with ophthalmic drug. They may be worn within a few hours after therapy is discontinued.
- Instruct patient in the proper technique for instillation of ophthalmic drops.

C

CROTAMITON

(kroe-tam′i-tonn)
Trade name: Eurax
Classifications: SKIN AND MUCOUS MEMBRANE AGENT; SCABICIDE; ANTIPRURITIC
Prototype: Lindane
Pregnancy category: C

ACTIONS/PHARMACODYNAMICS Scabicidal and antipruritic agent. Available in an emollient-lotion base or in a vanishing cream. By unknown mechanisms, drug eradicates *Sarcoptes scabiei* and effectively relieves itching. Carcinogenesis, mutagenesis, and impairment to fertility: data not available.

USES Treatment of scabies and for symptomatic treatment of pruritus.

ROUTE & DOSAGE

Scabies
Adult/child: **Topical** Apply a thin layer of cream from neck to toes; apply a second layer 24 h later; bathe 48 h after last application to remove drug.

CONTRAINDICATIONS & PRECAUTIONS **Contraindicated in:** application to acutely inflamed skin, raw or weeping surfaces, eyes, or mouth; history of previous sensitivity to crotamiton. Safe use during pregnancy (category C) or in children not established.

ADVERSE/SIDE EFFECTS Skin irritation (particularly with prolonged use), rash, erythema, sensation of warmth, allergic sensitization.

NURSING IMPLICATIONS

Administration

- Shake container well before use of solution.
- The skin must be thoroughly dry before applying medication.
- If drug accidentally contacts eyes, thoroughly flush out medication with water.
- Pruritus treatment: massage medication gently into affected areas until it is completely absorbed. Repeat as needed (usually effective for 6–10 h).
- Store in tightly closed containers at 15–30C (59–86F). Do not freeze.

Patient & Family Education

- Review package insert with patient before treatment begins.
- Instruct the patient to discontinue medication and report to physician if irritation or sensitization develops.

CYANOCOBALAMIN

(sye-an-oh-koe-bal′a-min)
Trade names: Anacobin ♣, Bedoz ♣, Betalin 12, Cobex, Crystamine, Crysti-12, Cyanabin, Cyanoject, Kaybovite, Redisol, Rubesol, Rubion ♣, Rubramin PC
Prototype for classification: VITAMIN B_{12}
Pregnancy category: A; C (parenteral)

ACTIONS/PHARMACODYNAMICS Vitamin B_{12} is a cobalt-containing B complex vitamin produced by *Streptomyces griseus*. Essential for normal growth, cell reproduction, maturation of RBCs, nucleoprotein synthesis, maintenance of nervous system (myelin synthesis), and believed to be involved in protein and carbohydrate metabolism. Also acts as coenzyme in various biologic reactions. Vitamin B_{12} deficiency results in megaloblastic anemia, dysfunction of spinal cord with paralysis, GI lesions.

C

USES Vitamin B_{12} deficiency due to malabsorption syndrome as in pernicious (Addison's) anemia, sprue; GI pathology, dysfunction, or surgery; fish tapeworm infestation, and gluten enteropathy. Also used in B_{12} deficiency caused by increased physiologic requirements or inadequate dietary intake, and in vitamin B_{12} absorption (Schilling) test. **Unlabeled use:** to prevent and treat toxicity associated with sodium nitroprusside.

ROUTE & DOSAGE

Vitamin B_{12} Deficiency

Adult: **IM/Deep SC** 30 μg/d for 5–10 d; then 100–200 μg/ mo.
Child: **IM/Deep SC** 100 μg doses to a total of 1–5 mg over 2 wk; then 60 μg/mo.

Pernicious Anemia

Adult: **IM/Deep SC** 100–1000 μg/d for 2–3 wk; then 100–1000 μg q2–4wk.
Child: **IM** 30–50 μg/d × 2 wk to total of 1000 μg, then 100 μg/mo.
Infant: **IM** 1000 μg/d × at least 2 wk, then 50 μg/mo.

Diagnosis of Megaloblastic Anemia

Adult: **IM/Deep SC** 1 μg/d for 10 d while maintaining a low folate and vitamin B_{12} diet.

Schilling Test

Adult: **IM/Deep SC** 1000 μg × 1 dose.

Nutritional Supplement

Adult: **PO** 1–25 μg/d.
Child: **PO** <1 y: 0.3 μg/d; ≥1 y: 1 μg/d.

PHARMACOKINETICS Absorption: intestinal absorption requires presence of intrinsic factor in terminal ileum. **Distribution:** widely distributed; principally stored in liver, kidneys, and adrenals; crosses placenta. **Metabolism:** converted in tissues to active co-enzymes; enterohepatically cycled. **Elimination:** 50–95% of doses ≥100 μg are excreted in urine in 48 h; excreted in breast milk.

CONTRAINDICATIONS & PRECAUTIONS Contraindicated in: history of sensitivity to vitamin B_{12}, other cobalamins, or cobalt; early Leber's disease (hereditary optic nerve atrophy), indiscriminate use in folic acid deficiency. Safe use during pregnancy [category A, category C (parenteral)], in nursing women, and in children not established. **Cautious use in:** heart disease, anemia, pulmonary disease.

ADVERSE/SIDE EFFECTS CV: feeling of swelling of body, peripheral vascular thrombosis, pulmonary edema, CHF. **GI:** mild transient diarrhea. **Skin:** itching, rash, flushing. **Other:** hypokalemia, sudden death; severe optic nerve atrophy (patients with Leber's disease), anaphylactic shock; unmasking of polycythemia vera (with correction of vitamin B_{12} deficiency).

DIAGNOSTIC TEST INTERFERENCE Most antibiotics, methotrexate, and pyrimethamine may produce invalid diagnostic ***blood assays for vitamin B_{12}. Possibility of false-positive test for intrinsic factor antibodies.***

DRUG INTERACTIONS Alcohol, aminosalicylic acid, neomycin, colchicine may decrease absorption of oral cyanocobalamin; **chloramphenicol** may interfere with therapeutic response to cyanocobalamin.

C

NURSING IMPLICATIONS

Administration

- PO preparations may be mixed with fruit juices. However, administer promptly since ascorbic acid affects the stability of vitamin B_{12}.
- Administration of oral vitamin B_{12} with meals increases its absorption, presumably by stimulating production of intrinsic factor.
- Parenteral therapy is the preferred treatment for patients with pernicious anemia, since oral administration may be unreliable. However, oral therapy may be used when the condition is mild and is without neurologic signs or in rare patients who are sensitive to the parenteral form or who refuse it.
- Preserved in light-resistant containers at room temperature preferably at 15–30C (59–86F) unless otherwise directed by manufacturer.

Assessment & Drug Effects

- Before initiation of therapy, reticulocyte and erythrocyte counts, Hgb, Hct, vitamin B_{12}, and serum folate levels should be determined; these studies should be repeated between 5 and 7 d after start of therapy and at regular intervals during therapy.
- A careful history of sensitivities should be obtained. Sensitization to cyanocobalamin can take as long as 8 y to develop.
- Potassium levels should be monitored during the first 48 h, particularly in patients with addisonian pernicious anemia or megaloblastic anemia. Conversion to normal erythropoiesis increases erythrocyte potassium requirement and can result in severe hypokalemia and sudden death.
- Monitor vital signs in patients with cardiac disease and in those receiving parenteral cyanocobalamin, and be alert to symptoms of pulmonary edema, which generally occur early in therapy.
- Therapeutic response to drug therapy is usually dramatic, occurring within 48 h. Effectiveness is measured by laboratory values and improvement in manifestations of vitamin B_{12} deficiency.
- Characteristically, reticulocyte concentration rises in 3–4 d, peaks in 5–8 d, and then gradually declines as erythrocyte count and hemoglobin rise to normal levels (in 4–6 wk).
- Usually, demonstrable neurologic damage is considered irreversible if there is no improvement after 1–1 1/2 y of adequate therapy.
- Bowel regularity is essential for consistent absorption of oral preparations.
- Smokers appear to have increased requirements for vitamin B_{12}.
- A complete diet and drug history and an inquiry into alcohol drinking patterns should be obtained on all patients receiving cyanocobalamin to identify and correct poor habits.

Patient & Family Education

- Advise patient to notify physician of any intercurrent disease or infection. Increased dosage may be required.
- It is imperative that the patient with pernicious anemia understand that parenteral drug therapy must be continued throughout life to prevent irreversible neurologic damage.
- Dietary deficiency of vitamin B_{12} has been observed in strict vegetarians (vegans) and their breastfed infants and in the elderly. Advise vegetarians of the relationship between vitamin B_{12} deficiency and their diet.
- Rich food sources are nutrient-

added breakfast cereals, vitamin B_{12}-fortified soy milk, organ meats, clams, oysters, egg yolk, crab, salmon, sardines, muscle meat, milk, and dairy products.

CYCLIZINE HYDROCHLORIDE

(sye'kli-zeen)

Trade names: Marezine, Marzine♣

CYCLIZINE LACTATE

Trade names: Marezine Lactate, Marzine

Classifications: ANTIHISTAMINE (H_1-RECEPTOR ANTAGONIST); ANTIVERTIGO AGENT; ANTIEMETIC

Prototype: Meclizine

Pregnancy category: B

ACTIONS/PHARMACODYNAMICS Piperazine antihistamine (H_1-receptor blocking agent) structurally and pharmacologically related to other cyclizine compounds (e.g., buclizine, hydroxyzine, meclizine). In common with these agents, it exhibits CNS depression and anticholinergic, antispasmodic, local anesthetic, and antihistaminic activity. Has prominent depressant action on labyrinthine excitability and on conduction in vestibular-cerebellar pathways, thus producing marked antimotion and antiemetic effects. Mechanism of action not known.

USES Chiefly for prevention and treatment of motion sickness and postoperative nausea and vomiting.

ROUTE & DOSAGE

Motion Sickness

Adult: **PO** 50 mg 30 min before travel; then q4–6h prn (max 200 mg/d). **IM** 50 mg q4–6h prn.
Child: **PO** 6–12 y, 25 mg q4–6h prn (max 75 mg/d). **IM** 6–12 y, 1 mg/kg t.i.d. prn (max 75 mg/d).

Postoperative Vomiting

Adult: **IM** 50 mg 15–30 min before end of operation; may repeat q4–6h (t.i.d.) prn during first few days after surgery.

PHARMACOKINETICS **Onset:** rapid. **Duration:** 4–6 h. **Metabolism:** unknown.

CONTRAINDICATIONS & PRECAUTIONS **Contraindicated in:** pregnancy (category B), nursing mothers, children <6 y. **Cautious use in:** narrow-angle glaucoma; prostatic hypertrophy; obstructive disease of GU or GI tracts; postoperative patients.

ADVERSE/SIDE EFFECTS Usually dose-related. **CNS:** *drowsiness,* excitement, euphoria, auditory and visual hallucinations, hyperexcitability alternating with drowsiness, convulsions, <u>respiratory paralysis</u> (rare). **CV:** hypotension, palpitation, tachycardia. **EENT:** *dry mouth,* nose, and throat; blurred vision, diplopia; tinnitus. **GI:** anorexia, nausea, vomiting, diarrhea, or constipation. **Hypersensitivity:** urticaria, rash, cholestatic jaundice. **Other:** pain at IM injection site.

DIAGNOSTIC TEST INTERFERENCE Because cyclizine is an antihistamine, inform patient that ***skin testing*** procedures should not be scheduled for about 4 d after drug is discontinued or false-negative reactions may result.

DRUG INTERACTIONS **Alcohol,** BARBITURATES, CNS DEPRESSANTS (e.g., HYPNOTICS, SEDATIVES, and ANXIOLYTICS) may compound effects of cyclizine.

NURSING IMPLICATIONS

Administration

- Aspirate needle carefully before injecting IM. Anaphylactic reactions following inadvertent IV injection have been reported.

- For prophylaxis of postoperative nausea and vomiting, drug usually prescribed with preoperative medication or is administered 20–30 min before expected termination of surgery.
- Store tablets in tight, light-resistant container at 15–30C (59–86F) unless otherwise directed. Store parenteral form in a cold place at 5–10C (41–50F). When parenteral solution is stored at room temperature for prolonged periods, it may become slightly yellow, but this does not indicate loss of potency.

Assessment & Drug Effects

- Because cyclizine can cause hypotension, the postoperative patient receiving the drug will require close monitoring of vital signs.
- Monitor for and report signs of CNS stimulation (e.g., hyperexcitability, euphoria). Dose reduction or discontinuation of drug may be indicated.

Patient & Family Education

- Advise patient to take cyclizine with food or a glass of milk or water to minimize GI irritation.
- Forewarn patient about side effects of drowsiness and dizziness and advise not to drive a car or engage in other potentially hazardous activities until reaction to the drug is known.
- Caution patient that alcohol, barbiturates, narcotic analgesic, and other CNS depressants may compound sedative action.

CYCLOBENZAPRINE HYDROCHLORIDE

(sye-kloe-ben′za-preen)

Trade names: Cycoflex, Flexeril

Prototype for classifications: AUTONOMIC NERVOUS SYSTEM AGENT; CENTRAL-ACTING SKELETAL MUSCLE RELAXANT

Pregnancy category: B

ACTIONS/PHARMACODYNAMICS

Structurally and pharmacologically related to tricyclic antidepressants. Relieves skeletal muscle spasm of local origin without interfering with muscle function. Believed to act primarily within CNS at brain stem; some action at spinal cord level is also probable. Depresses tonic somatic motor activity, although both gamma and alpha motoneurons are affected. In common with other tricyclic compounds, it increases circulating norepinephrine by blocking its synaptic reuptake. Also has sedative effects and potent central and peripheral anticholinergic activity.

USES Short-term adjunct to rest and physical therapy for relief of muscle spasm associated with acute musculoskeletal conditions. Not effective in treatment of spasticity associated with cerebral palsy or cerebral or cord disease.

ROUTE & DOSAGE

Muscle Spasm

Adult: **PO** 20–40 mg/d in 2–4 divided doses; max 60 mg/d.

PHARMACOKINETICS **Absorption:** well absorbed from GI tract with some first-pass elimination in liver. **Onset:** 1 h. **Peak:** 3–8 h. **Duration:** 12–24 h. **Distribution:** highly protein bound (93%). **Metabolism:** metabolized in liver to inactive metabolites. **Elimination:** half-life: 1–3 d; slowly excreted in urine with some elimination in feces; may be excreted in breast milk.

CONTRAINDICATIONS & PRECAUTIONS **Contraindicated in:** acute recovery phase of MI, patients with cardiac arrhythmias, heart block or conduction disturbances, CHF, hyperthyroidism. Use for periods longer than 2 or 3 wk not recommended by manufacturer. Safe use during pregnancy (category B), in nursing mothers, and children < 15 y not established. **Cautious use in:** patients receiving anticholinergic medications; prostatic hypertrophy, history of urinary retention, angle-closure glaucoma; increased IOP, seizures; cardiovascular disease; hepatic impairment; elderly, debilitated patients; history of psychiatric illness.

ADVERSE/SIDE EFFECTS **CNS:** *drowsiness, dizziness,* weakness, fatigue, asthenia, paresthesias, tremors, muscle twitching, insomnia, euphoria, disorientation, mania, ataxia. **CV:** tachycardia, syncope, palpitation, vasodilation, chest pain, orthostatic hypotension, dyspnea; with high doses, possibility of severe arrhythmias. **GI:** *dry mouth,* indigestion, unpleasant taste, coated tongue, tongue discoloration, vomiting, anorexia, abdominal pain, flatulence, diarrhea, paralytic ileus. **GU:** increased or decreased libido, impotence. **Hypersensitivity:** pruritus, urticaria, skin rash, edema of tongue and face. **Other:** sweating, myalgia, hepatitis, alopecia. Shares toxic potential of tricyclic antidepressants.

DRUG INTERACTIONS **Alcohol,** BARBITURATES, other CNS DEPRESSANTS enhance CNS depression; potentiates anticholinergic effects of **phenothiazine** and other ANTICHOLINERGICS; MAO INHIBITORS may precipitate hypertensive crisis — use with extreme caution.

NURSING IMPLICATIONS

Administration

- Do not administer drug if patient is receiving an MAO INHIBITOR (e.g., furazolidone, isocarboxazid, pargyline, tranylcypromine).
- Cyclobenzaprine is intended for short-term (2 or 3 wk) treatment because risk–benefit associated with prolonged use is not known.
- Store in tightly closed container, preferably at 15–30C (59–86F) unless otherwise directed by manufacturer.

Assessment & Drug Effects

- Because of risk of drowsiness and dizziness, supervision of ambulation may be indicated, especially in the elderly.
- Withhold drug and notify physician if signs of hypersensitivity, e.g., pruritus, urticaria, rash, appear.

Patient & Family Education

- Forewarn patient about side effects of drowsiness and dizziness. Advise patient to avoid driving and other potentially hazardous activities until reaction to drug is known.
- Caution patient to avoid alcohol and other CNS DEPRESSANTS (unless otherwise directed by physician) because cyclobenzaprine enhances their effects.
- Advise patient that dry mouth may be relieved by increasing total fluid intake (if not contraindicated).
- Keep physician informed of therapeutic effectiveness. Spasmolytic effect usually begins within 1 or 2 d and may be manifested by lessening of pain and tenderness, increase in range of motion, and ability to perform ADL.

C

CYCLOPENTOLATE HYDROCHLORIDE

(sye-kloe-pen'toe-late)

Trade names: Ak-Pentolate, Cyclogyl, Pentalair

Prototype for classifications: EYE PREPARATION; CYCLOPLEGIC; MYDRIATIC; AUTONOMIC NERVOUS SYSTEM AGENT; ANTICHOLINERGIC (PARASYMPATHOLYTIC)

Pregnancy category: C

See Appendix A.

CYCLOPHOSPHAMIDE

(sye-kloe-foss'fa-mide)

Trade names: Cytoxan, Neosar, Procytox ♣

Protype for classifications: ANTINEOPLASTIC; ALKYLATING AGENT; IMMUNOSUPPRESSANT

Pregnancy category: C

ACTIONS/PHARMACODYNAMICS Cell-cycle-nonspecific alkylating agent chemically related to the nitrogen mustards. Action mechanism unknown but thought to be the result of cross-linkage of DNA strands, thereby blocking synthesis of DNA, RNA, and protein. Has pronounced immunosuppressive activity and is a highly toxic drug; thus therapeutic effects are usually accompanied by some evidence of toxicity. Associated with increased risk of secondary malignancies that may be detected several years after cyclophosphamide has been discontinued.

USES As single agent or in combination with other chemotherapeutic agents in treatment of malignant lymphoma, multiple myeloma, leukemias, mycosis fungoides (advanced disease), neuroblastoma, adenocarcinoma of ovary, carcinoma of breast, or malignant neoplasms of lung. **Unlabeled uses:** to prevent rejection in homotransplantation; to treat severe rheumatoid arthritis, multiple sclerosis, systemic lupus erythematosus, Wegener's granulomatosis, nephrotic syndrome.

ROUTE & DOSAGE

Neoplasm

Adult: **PO** ***initial:*** 1–5 mg/kg/d; ***maintenance:*** 1–5 mg/kg q7–10d. **IV** ***initial:*** 40–50 mg/kg in divided doses over 2–5 d up to 100 mg/kg; ***maintenance:*** 10–15 mg/kg q7–10d *or* 3–5 mg twice weekly.

Child: **PO** ***initial:*** 2–8 mg/kg or 60–250 mg/m^2; ***maintenance:*** 2–5 mg/kg *or* 50–150 mg/m^2 twice weekly. **IV** ***initial:*** 2–8 mg/kg *or* 60–250 mg/m^2.

PHARMACOKINETICS Absorption: readily absorbed from GI tract. **Peak:** 1 h PO. **Distribution:** widely distributed, including brain, breast milk; crosses placenta. **Metabolism:** metabolized in liver. **Elimination:** half-life: 4–6 h; excreted in urine as active metabolites and unchanged drug.

CONTRAINDICATIONS & PRECAUTIONS Contraindicated in: men and women in childbearing years; serious infections (including chickenpox, herpes zoster); live virus vaccines; myelosuppression; pregnancy (category C), nursing mothers. **Cautious use in:** history of radiation or cytotoxic drug therapy; hepatic and renal impairment, recent history of steroid therapy; bone marrow infiltration with tumor cells; history of urate calculi and gout; patients with leukopenia, thrombocytopenia.

ADVERSE/SIDE EFFECTS **GI:** *nausea, vomiting,* mucositis, *anorexia,* hepatotoxicity, diarrhea. **GU:** sterile hemorrhagic and nonhemorrhagic cystitis, bladder fibrosis, nephrotoxicity. **Metabolic:** severe hyperkalemia, SIADH, hyponatremia, weight gain (but without edema) or weight loss, hyperuricemia. **Myelosuppression:** leukopenia, *neutropenia,* acute myeloid leukemia, anemia, thrombophlebitis, interference with normal healing. **Pulmonary:** pulmonary emboli and edema, pneumonitis, interstitial pulmonary fibrosis. **Skin:** *alopecia* (reversible), transverse ridging of nails, pigmentation of nail beds and skin (reversible), nonspecific dermatitis. **Other:** transient dizziness, fatigue, facial flushing, diaphoresis, drug fever, anaphylaxis, secondary neoplasia.

DIAGNOSTIC TEST INTERFERENCE Cyclophosphamide suppresses positive reactions to ***Candida, mumps, trichophytons,*** and ***tuberculin PPD skin tests. Papanicolaou (PAP)*** smear may be falsely positive.

DRUG INTERACTIONS **Succinylcholine,** prolonged neuromuscular blocking activity; **doxorubicin** may increase cardiac toxicity.

NURSING IMPLICATIONS

Administration

- Administer PO drug on empty stomach. If nausea and vomiting are severe, however, it may be taken with food. An antiemetic medication may be prescribed to be given before the drug.
- Store cyclophosphamide PO solution in refrigerator at 2–8C (36–46F), and use within 14 d.
- IV preparation: To reconstitute, add sterile water for injection or bacteriostatic water for injection (paraben-preserved only) to vial and shake vigorously to dissolve (5-ml to 100-mg vial). Solution should be used within 24 h if stored at room temperature, or within 6 d if refrigerated.
- IV administration: Administer each 100 mg or fraction thereof over 1 min or longer.
- Store at temperature between 2 and 30C (36 and 86F) unless otherwise recommended by the manufacturer.

Assessment & Drug Effects

- Total and differential leukocyte count, platelet count, and hematocrit are determined initially and at least 2 times per week during maintenance period. Baseline and periodic determinations of liver and kidney function and serum electrolytes also should be made. Microscopic urine examinations are recommended after large IV doses.
- Thrombocytopenia is rare, but if it occurs (count of 100,000/mm^3 or lower), watch for signs of unexplained bleeding or easy bruising. If count continues to descend, drug will be discontinued.
- Ordinarily a leukopenia of 3000–4000 mm^3 can be maintained without risk of serious complications.
- Marked leukopenia is the most serious side effect. It can be fatal. Nadir may occur in 2–8 d after first dose but may be as late as 1 mo after a series of several daily doses. Leukopenia usually reverses 7–10 d after therapy is discontinued.
- Check leukocyte count. During severe leukopenic period, protect patient from infection and trauma and from visitors and medical personnel who have colds or other infections.
- Report onset of unexplained chills, sore throat, tachycardia. Monitor

temperature carefully and report an elevation immediately. The development of fever in a neutropenic patient (granulocyte count < 1000) is a medical emergency because sepsis can develop quickly in these patients.

- During period of neutropenia, purulent drainage may become serosanguineous because there are not enough WBC to create pus. Because of suppressed immune mechanisms, wound healing may be prolonged or incomplete. Observe and report character of wound drainage.
- I&O ratio and pattern should be monitored. Since the drug is a chemical irritant, PO and IV fluid intake is generally increased to help prevent renal irritation and hemorrhagic cystitis. Have patient void frequently, especially after each dose and just before retiring to bed. Paradoxically, in patients with SIADH (a rare side effect) fluid intake may have to be restricted. Consult physician.
- Because patients are usually well hydrated as part of the therapy, watch for symptoms of water intoxication or dilutional hyponatremia. Should this condition occur, fluid intake will be reduced. Report to physician.
- Promptly report hematuria or dysuria. Drug schedule is usually interrupted and fluids are forced. Alert patient to the fact that hematuria may resolve spontaneously, or it may persist several months. In some cases, it has been serious enough to require transfusions.
- Record body weight at least twice weekly (basis for dose determination). Alert physician to sudden change or slow, steady weight gain or loss over a period of time that appears inconsistent with caloric intake.
- Diarrhea may signal onset of hyperkalemia, particularly if accompanied by colicky pain, nausea, bradycardia, and skeletal muscle weakness. These symptoms warrant prompt reporting to physician.
- Hyperuricemia occurs commonly during early treatment period in patients with leukemias or lymphoma. Report edema of lower legs and feet; joint, flank, or stomach pain.
- Before institution of cyclophosphamide therapy, observe and report the signs of hepatotoxicity (frothy dark urine, light-colored stools, jaundice, pruritus) that are most apt to appear in the patient with liver impairment.
- The immunosuppressive property of cyclophosphamide makes the patient particularly susceptible to varicella-zoster infections (chickenpox, herpes zoster). Particular care should be taken to screen young visitors.
- Report any sign of overgrowth with opportunistic organisms, especially in patient receiving corticosteroids or who has recently been on steroid therapy.
- Report fever, dyspnea, and nonproductive cough. Pulmonary toxicity is not common, but the already debilitated patient is particularly susceptible.

Patient & Family Education

- Urge patient to adhere to dosage regimen and not to omit, increase, decrease, or delay doses. If for any reason drug cannot be taken, notify physician.
- Alopecia occurs in about 33% of patients on cyclophosphamide therapy. Hair loss may be noted 3 wk after therapy begins; regrowth (often differs in texture and color) usually starts 5–6 wk after drug is

withdrawn and may occur while patient is on maintenance doses.

- Because of mutagenic potential, adequate means of contraception should be employed during and for at least 4 mo after termination of drug treatment. Breast-feeding should be discontinued before cyclophosphamide therapy is initiated.
- Amenorrhea may last up to 1 y after cessation of therapy in 10–30% of women.

CYCLOSERINE

(sye-kloe-ser′een)

Trade name: Seromycin

Classifications: ANTIINFECTIVE; ANTITUBERCULOSIS AGENT

Prototype: Isoniazid

Pregnancy category: C

ACTIONS/PHARMACODYNAMICS Broad-spectrum antiinfective derived from strains of *Streptomyces orchidaceus* or *S. garyphalus;* also produced synthetically. Structural analog of the amino acid D-alanine. Inhibits cell wall synthesis in susceptible strains of gram-positive and gram-negative bacteria and in *Mycobacterium tuberculosis* by competitively interfering with the incorporation of D-alanine into the bacterial cell wall. bacteriostatic or bactericidal depending on concentration and susceptibility of organism.

USES In conjunction with other tuberculostatic drugs in treatment of active pulmonary and extrapulmonary tuberculosis when primary agents isoniazid, rifampin, ethambutol, streptomycin have failed. Also used in treatment of acute UTI caused by *Enterobacter* sp and *Escherichia coli* that are unresponsive to conventional treatment. **Unlabeled use:** treatment of tuberculosis meningitis and nocardiosis.

ROUTE & DOSAGE

Tuberculosis

Adult: **PO** 250 mg q12h for 2 wk; may increase to 500 mg q12h (max 1g/d).

Urinary Tract Infection

Adult: **PO** 250 mg q12h for 2 wk.

PHARMACOKINETICS **Absorption:** 70–90% absorbed from GI tract. **Peak:** 3–4 h. **Distribution:** distributed to lung, ascitic, pleural and synovial fluids, and CSF; crosses placenta; distributed into breast milk. **Metabolism:** not metabolized. **Elimination:** half-life: 10 h; 60–70% excreted in urine within 72 h; small amount in feces.

CONTRAINDICATIONS & PRECAUTIONS **Contraindicated in:** epilepsy; depression, severe anxiety, history of psychoses; severe renal insufficiency; chronic alcoholism. Safe use during pregnancy (category C), in nursing women, and in children not established.

ADVERSE/SIDE EFFECTS **CNS:** *drowsiness,* anxiety, *headache,* tremors, myoclonic jerking, convulsions, vertigo, visual disturbances, speech difficulties (dysarthria), lethargy, depression, disorientation with loss of memory, confusion, nervousness, psychoses, tic episodes, character changes, hyperirritability, aggression, hyperreflexia, peripheral neuropathy, paresthesias, paresis, dyskinesias. **CV:** arrhythmias, CHF. **Eye:** eye pain (optic neuritis), photophobia. **Hematologic:** vitamin B_{12} and folic acid deficiency, megaloblastic or sideroblastic anemia. **Hypersensitivity:** dermatitis, photosensitivity.

C

DRUG INTERACTIONS **Alcohol** increases risk of seizures; **ethionamide, isoniazid** potentiate neurotoxic effects; may inhibit **phenytoin** metabolism, increasing its toxicity.

NURSING IMPLICATIONS

Administration

- Pyridoxine 200–300 mg/d may be ordered concurrently to prevent neurotoxic effects of cycloserine.
- Store in tightly closed container at 15–30C (59–86F) unless otherwise directed.

Assessment & Drug Effects

- Culture and susceptibility tests should be performed before initiation of therapy and periodically thereafter to detect possible bacterial resistance.
- Monitoring of blood-drug levels and hematologic, renal, and hepatic function at regular intervals is advised.
- Maintenance of blood-drug level below 30 μg/ml considerably reduces incidence of neurotoxicity. Possibility of neurotoxicity increases when dose is 500 mg or more or when renal clearance is inadequate. Blood-drug levels should be determined at least weekly in these patients.
- Observe patient carefully for signs of hypersensitivity and neurologic effects. Neurotoxicity generally appears within first 2 wk of therapy and disappears after drug is discontinued.
- Drug should be discontinued or dosage reduced if symptoms of CNS toxicity or hypersensitivity reaction (see Appendix G) develop.

Patient & Family Education

- Advise patient to take cycloserine after meals to prevent GI irritation.
- Advise patient or responsible family member to notify physician immediately of the onset of skin rash and early signs of CNS toxicity (see Appendix G).
- Advise patient to avoid potentially hazardous tasks such as driving until reaction to cycloserine has been determined.
- Instruct patient to take drug precisely as prescribed and to keep follow-up appointments. Continuous therapy may extend into months or years.

CYCLOSPORINE

(sye'kloe-spor-een)

Trade names: Neoral, Sandimmune

Prototype for classification: IMMUNOSUPPRESSANT

Pregnancy category: C

ACTIONS/PHARMACODYNAMICS Immunosuppressant agent derived from extract of a soil fungus. Action in reducing transplant rejection appears to be due to selective and reversible inhibition of helper T-lymphocytes (which normally stimulate antibody function). This creates an imbalance in favor of suppressor T-lymphocytes (which inhibit antibody production); thus immune response is subdued. Unlike other immunosuppressive agents, it does not cause clinically significant bone marrow suppression.

USES In conjunction with adrenal corticosteroids to prevent organ rejection after kidney, liver, and heart transplants (allografts). Has had limited use in pancreas, bone marrow, and heart/lung transplantations. Also used for treatment of chronic transplant rejection in patients previously treated with other immunosuppressants; rheumatoid arthritis, severe psoriasis. **Unlabeled use:** Sjögren's syndrome, to prevent rejection of heart–lung and pancreatic transplants, ulcerative colitis.

ROUTE & DOSAGE

Prevention of Organ Rejection

Adult: **PO** 14–18 mg/kg beginning 4–12 h before transplantation and continued for 1–2 wk after surgery; then gradual reduction by 5%/wk; max dose of microemulsion, 10 mg/kg/d; ***maintenance:*** 5–10 mg/kg/d. **IV** 5–6 mg/kg beginning 4–12 h before transplantation and continued after surgery until patient can take oral.
Child: **PO** Same as for adult. **IV** Same as for adult.

Rheumatoid Arthritis (Neoral)

Adult: **PO** 2.5 mg/kg/d divided into 2 doses. May increase by 0.5–0.75 mg/kg/d q4wk to a max of 4 mg/kg/d.

Severe Psoriasis (Neoral)

Adult: **PO** 1.25 mg/kg b.i.d. If significant improvement has not occurred after 4 wk, may increase dose by 0.5 mg/kg/d every 2 wk to max of 4 mg/kg/d.

PHARMACOKINETICS Absorption: variably and incompletely absorbed (30%). Microemulsion formulation (Neoral) has less variability in absorption and may produce significantly higher serum levels compared with the standard formulation. **Peak:** 3–4 h. **Distribution:** widely distributed; 33–47% distributed to plasma; 41–50% to RBCs; crosses placenta; distributed into breast milk. **Metabolism:** extensively metabolized in liver, including significant first pass metabolism; considerable enterohepatic circulation. **Elimination:** half-life: 19–27 h; primarily eliminated in bile and feces; 6% excreted in urine.

CONTRAINDICATIONS & PRECAUTIONS Contraindicated in: hypersensitivity to cyclosporine or to ingredients in commercially available formulations, e.g., Cremophor (polyoxyl 35 castor oil); recent contact with or bout of chickenpox, herpes zoster; administration of live virus vaccines, to patient or family members; RA patients with abnormal renal function, uncontrolled hypertension, or malignancies. Safe use during pregnancy (category C) and in nursing women. **Cautious use in:** renal, hepatic, pancreatic, or bowel dysfunction; hyperkalemia; hypertension; infection; malabsorption problems (e.g., liver transplant patients).

ADVERSE/SIDE EFFECTS CNS: *tremor,* convulsions, headache, paresthesias, hyperesthesia, flushing, night sweats, insomnia, visual hallucinations, confusion, anxiety, flat affect, depression, lethargy, weakness, paraparesis, ataxia, amnesia. **CV:** *hypertension,* MI (rare). **ENT:** sinusitis, tinnitus, hearing loss, sore throat. **GI:** gingival hyperplasia, diarrhea, nausea, *vomiting,* abdominal discomfort, anorexia, gastritis, constipation. **Hematologic:** leukopenia, anemia, thrombocytopenia, *hypermagnesemia, hyperkalemia,* hyperuricemia, *decreased serum bicarbonate,* hyperglycemia. **Renal:** urinary retention, frequency, *nephrotoxicity (oliguria).* **Skin:** *hirsutism,* acne, oily skin, flushing. **Other:** lymphoma, gynecomastia, chest pain, leg cramps, edema, fever, chills, weight loss, increased risk of skin malignancies in psoriasis patients previously treated with methotrexate, psoralens, or UV light therapy.

C

DIAGNOSTIC TEST INTERFERENCE ***Hyperlipidemia*** and abnormalities in ***electrophoresis*** reported; believed to be due to polyoxyl 35 castor oil (Cremophor) in IV cyclosporine.

DRUG INTERACTIONS AMINOGLYCOSIDES, **danazol, diltiazem, doxycycline, erythromycin, ketoconazole, methylprednisolone, metoclopramide, nicardipine,** NSAIDS, **prednisolone, verapamil** may increase cyclosporine levels; **carbamazepine, isoniazid, octreotide, phenobarbital, phenytoin, rifampin** may decrease cyclosporine levels; **acyclovir,** AMINOGLYCOSIDES, **amphotericin B, cimetidine, erythromycin, ketoconazole, melphalan, ranitidine, cotrimoxazole, trimethoprim** may increase risk of nephrotoxicity; POTASSIUM-SPARING DIURETICS, ACE INHIBITORS **(captopril, enalapril)** may potentiate hyperkalemia.

INCOMPATIBILITIES Y-site: TPN.

NURSING IMPLICATIONS

Administration

- Neoral (microemulsion) and Sandimmune are not bioequivalent and cannot be used interchangeably without physician supervision.
- Before use, inspect IV for particulate matter and discoloration. Cyclosporine parenteral concentrate must be diluted immediately before administration: dilute each ml in 20–100 ml of 0.9% NaCl or 5% dextrose injection.
- Administer IV solution by slow infusion over approximately 2–6 h, as prescribed by physician. Rapid IV can result in nephrotoxicity.
- Store preferably at 15–30C (59–86F) in well-closed containers. Do not refrigerate. Protect ampuls from light. Once opened, PO solution should be dated and contents used within 2 mo.

Assessment & Drug Effects

- Patients receiving the drug parenterally should be observed continuously for at least 30 min after start of IV infusion and at frequent intervals thereafter to detect allergic or other adverse reactions.
- Hypersensitivity reactions have been associated with Cremophor emulsifying agent in the parenteral formulation but not with the PO solution, which does not contain this ingredient.
- Monitor I&O ratio and pattern. Nephrotoxicity has been reported in about one third of transplant patients. It has occurred in mild forms as late as 2–3 mo after transplantation. In severe form, it can be irreversible, and therefore early recognition is critical.
- Report signs and symptoms suggestive of nephrotoxicity (see Appendix G). Laboratory values respond to dosage reduction.
- Monitor vital signs. Be alert to indicators of local or systemic infection that can be fungal, viral, or bacterial. Also report significant rise in BP.
- In psoriasis patients, BP, CBC, BUN, uric acid, potassium, lipids, and magnesium should be monitored biweekly during first 3 mo.
- Periodic tests should be made of neurologic function. Neurotoxic effects generally occur over 13–195 days after initiation of cyclosporine therapy. Signs and symptoms are reportedly fully reversible with dosage reduction or discontinuation of drug.
- Baseline and periodic tests are advised for (1) renal function (BUN, serum creatinine), (2) liver function (AST, ALT, serum amylase, biliru-

bin, and alkaline phosphatase), and (3) serum potassium.

- Blood or plasma drug concentrations should be monitored at regular intervals, particularly in patients receiving the drug orally for prolonged periods, as drug absorption is erratic.

Patient & Family Education

- Use the specially calibrated pipette provided to measure dose.
- Medication may be taken with meals to reduce nausea or GI irritation.
- Palatability of oral solution may be enhanced by mixing it with milk, chocolate milk, or orange juice, preferably at room temperature. Mix in a glass rather than a plastic container. Stir well, drink immediately, and rinse glass with small quantity of diluent to assure getting entire dose.
- Take medication at same time each day to maintain therapeutic blood levels.
- Keep scheduled follow-up appointments.
- If possible, patient should see a dentist before start of cyclosporine treatment. Advise patient to practice good oral hygiene. Inspect mouth daily for white patches, sores, swollen gums.
- Reassure patient that hirsutism is reversible with discontinuation of drug.

CYPROHEPTADINE HYDROCHLORIDE

(si-proe-hep′ta-deen)

Trade names: Periactin, Vimicon ♣

Classifications: ANTIHISTAMINE; ANTIPRURITIC

Prototype: Diphenhydramine

Pregnancy category: B

ACTIONS/PHARMACODYNAMICS Potent piperidine antihistamine with pharmacologic actions similar to those of azatadine. Acts by competing with histamine for H_1-receptor sites on effector cells, thus preventing histamine-mediated responses. Produces mild central depression and moderate anticholinergic effects; lacks antiemetic action. Has significant antipruritic, local anesthetic, and antiserotonin activity.

USES Symptomatic relief of various allergic conditions, including hay fever, vasomotor rhinitis, allergic conjunctivitis, urticaria caused by cold sensitivity, and pruritus of allergic dermatoses. Effective in treatment of anaphylactoid reactions as adjunct to epinephrine and other standard measures after acute symptoms have been controlled. **Unlabeled uses:** Cushing's disease, carcinoid syndrome, vascular headaches, appetite stimulant.

ROUTE & DOSAGE

Allergies

Adult: **PO** 4 mg t.i.d. or q.i.d. (4–20 mg/d); max 0.5 mg/kg/ d.
Geriatric: **PO** Start with 4 mg b.i.d.
Child: **PO** 0.25 mg/kg/d in 3–4 divided doses (max 12 mg/d for 2–6 y, 16 mg/d for 6–12 y).

PHARMACOKINETICS **Absorption:** readily absorbed from GI tract. **Duration:** 6–9 h. **Distribution:** distribution into breast milk not known. **Metabolism:** metabolized in liver. **Elimination:** excreted in urine.

CONTRAINDICATIONS & PRECAUTIONS **Contraindicated in:** hypersensitivity to cyproheptadine or other H_1-receptor antagonist antihistamines; acute asthma attack. Safe use during pregnancy (category B), in nursing mothers, and in children <2 y not established. **Cautious use in:** elderly and debilitated patients; patients predisposed to urinary retention; glaucoma; asthma; hyperthyroidism; cardiovascular disease, hypertension; GI or GU tract obstruction.

ADVERSE/SIDE EFFECTS CNS: *drowsiness,* dizziness, faintness, headache, tremulousness, fatigue, disturbed coordination. **ENT:** dry nose and throat. **GI:** *dry mouth,* nausea, vomiting, epigastric distress, appetite stimulation, weight gain, transient decrease in fasting blood sugar level, increased serum amylase level, cholestatic jaundice. **GU:** urinary frequency, retention, and difficult urination. **Other:** thickened bronchial secretions, skin rash.

DIAGNOSTIC TEST INTERFERENCE
As a general rule, antihistamines are discontinued about 4 d before ***skin testing procedures*** are to be performed because they may produce false-negative results.

NURSING IMPLICATIONS

Administration

- GI side effects may be minimized by administering drug with food or milk.
- Store in tightly covered container at 15–30C (59–86F) unless otherwise directed.

Assessment & Drug Effects

- In some patients, the sedative effect disappears spontaneously after 3–4 d of drug administration.
- Since drug may cause dizziness, supervision of ambulation and other safety precautions may be warranted.

Patient & Family Education

- Warn the patient to avoid activities requiring mental alertness and physical coordination, such as driving a car, until reaction to the drug is known.
- Drug causes sedation, dizziness, and hypotension in the elderly. Advise patient to report these symptoms. Children are more apt to manifest CNS stimulation, e.g., confusion, agitation, tremors, hallucinations. Reduction in dosage may be indicated.
- Cyproheptadine may increase and prolong the effects of alcohol, barbiturates, narcotic analgesics, anxiolytics, and other CNS depressants.
- Patient should monitor weight and keep physician informed of any significant weight gain.
- Maintaining sufficient fluid intake may help to relieve dry mouth and also may reduce risk of cholestatic jaundice.

CYTARABINE

(sye-tare'a-been)

Trade names: ARA-C, Cytosar-U, Cytosine Arabinoside

Classifications: ANTINEOPLASTIC; ANTIMETABOLITE; IMMUNOSUPPRESSANT

Prototype: Fluorouracil

Pregnancy category: D

ACTIONS/PHARMACODYNAMICS
Pyrimidine analog with cell phase specificity affecting rapidly dividing cells in S phase (DNA synthesis). In certain conditions prevents development of cell from G_1 to S phase. Interferes with DNA synthesis by blocking conversion of cytidine to deoxycytidine and may be incorporated into RNA molecule. Has strong myelosuppressant activity. Immunosuppressant properties are exhibited by obliterated cell-mediated

immune responses, such as delayed hypersensitivity skin reactions.

USES To induce and maintain remission in acute myelocytic leukemia, acute lymphocytic leukemia, and meningeal leukemia and for treatment of lymphomas. Used in combination with other antineoplastics in established chemotherapeutic protocols.

ROUTE & DOSAGE

Leukemias

Adult: **IV** 200 mg/m^2 by continuous infusion over 24 h. **SC** 1 mg/kg 1–2 times/wk. **Intrathecal** 5–75 mg once q4d or once/d for 4 d.
Child: **IV** Same as for adult. **SC** Same as for adult. **Intrathecal** Same as for adult.

PHARMACOKINETICS **Peak:** 20–60 min SC. **Distribution:** crosses blood-brain barrier in moderate amounts; crosses placenta. **Metabolism:** metabolized primarily in liver. **Elimination:** half-life: 1–3 h; 80% excreted in urine in 24 h.

CONTRAINDICATIONS & PRECAUTIONS **Contraindicated in:** history of drug-induced myelosuppression; immunization procedures. Safe use during pregnancy (category D) particularly during first trimester, nursing mothers, and infants not established. **Cautious use in:** impaired renal or hepatic function, gout, drug-induced myelosuppression.

ADVERSE/SIDE EFFECTS **CNS:** headache, neurotoxicity; peripheral neuropathy, brachial plexus neuropathy, personality change, neuritis, vertigo, lethargy, somnolence, confusion. **Eye:** conjunctivitis, keratitis, photophobia. **GI:** *nausea, vomiting,* diarrhea, stomatitis, oral or anal inflammation or ulceration, esophagitis, anorexia, hemorrhage. **Hematologic:** *leukopenia, thrombocytopenia,* anemia, megaloblastosis, myelosuppression (reversible); transient hyperuricemia. **Hepatic:** hepatotoxicity, jaundice. **Renal:** renal dysfunction, urinary retention. **Skin:** rash, erythema, freckling, cellulitis, skin ulcerations, pruritus, urticaria, bulla formation, desquamation. **Other:** weight loss, sore throat, fever, thrombophlebitis and pain at injection site; pericarditis, bleeding (any site), pneumonia. Potentially carcinogenic and mutagenic.

DRUG INTERACTIONS GI toxicity may decrease **digoxin** absorption; decreases AMINOGLYCOSIDES activity against *Klebsiella pneumoniae.*

INCOMPATIBILITIES **Solution/additive: cephalothin, fluorouracil, gentamicin, heparin, insulin, nafcillin, oxacillin, penicillin G. Y-site: TPN.**

NURSING IMPLICATIONS

Administration

- The 100-mg and 500-mg vials are reconstituted with 5 ml and 10 ml, respectively, of bacteriostatic water for injection. (Diluents containing benzyl alcohol must not be used for neonates. A fatal toxic syndrome could result.)
- Reconstituted drug may be given by direct IV at a rate of 100 mg or a fraction thereof over 3 min.
- For IV infusion the reconstituted solution may be further diluted with 5% dextrose or 0.9% NaCl injection and infused over 1–24 h.
- For intrathecal injection, reconstitute with an isotonic, buffered diluent without preservatives. Follow manufacturer's recommendations. Solution should be adminis-

tered as soon as possible after preparation.

- Store cytarabine in refrigerator until reconstituted. Reconstituted solutions may be stored at 15–30C (59–86F) for 48 h. Solutions with a slight haze should be discarded.

Assessment & Drug Effects

- Inspect patient's mouth before the administration of each dose. Toxicity necessitating dosage alterations almost always occurs. Report adverse reactions immediately.
- Hematocrit and platelet counts and total and differential leukocyte counts should be evaluated daily during initial therapy. Serum uric acid and hepatic function tests should be performed at regular intervals throughout treatment period.
- Hyperuricemia due to rapid destruction of neoplastic cells may accompany cytarabine therapy. A regimen that includes a uricosuric agent such as allopurinol, urine alkalinization, and adequate hydration may be started. To reduce potential for urate stone formation, fluids are forced in excess of 2 L, if tolerated. Consult physician.
- Monitor I&O ratio and pattern.
- During granulocytic periods, development of usual signs of inflammation may be inhibited. Monitor body temperature. Be alert to the most subtle signs of infection, especially low-grade fever, and report promptly.
- When platelet count falls below 50,000/mm^3 and polymorphonuclear leukocytes to below 1000/mm^3, therapy may be suspended. WBC nadir is usually reached in 5–7 d after therapy has been stopped. Therapy is restarted with appearance of bone marrow recovery and when preceding cell counts are reached.
- Provide good oral hygiene to diminish side effects and chance of superinfection. Stomatitis and cheilosis usually appear 5–10 d into the therapy.

Patient & Family Education

- Advise patient to report promptly protracted vomiting or signs of nephrotoxicity (see Appendix G).
- Flu-like syndrome occurs usually within 6–12 wk after drug administration and may recur with successive therapy. Instruct patient to report chills, fever, achy joints and muscles.
- Advise patient to report any signs and symptoms of superinfection (see Appendix G).

CYTOMEGALOVIRUS IMMUNE GLOBULIN (CMVIG, CMV-IVIG)

(cy-to-meg'a-lo-vi-rus)

Trade name: CytoGam

Classifications: IMMUNOMODULATOR; ANTIVIRAL

Prototype: Interferon Alfa-2a

Pregnancy category: C

ACTIONS/PHARMACODYNAMICS
Cytomegalovirus immune globulin (CMVIG) is a preparation of immunoglobulin G (IgG) antibodies derived from a large number of healthy donors with high concentrations of antibodies directed against cytomegalovirus (CMV). These antibodies attenuate or reduce the incidence of serious CMV disease, such as CMV-associated pneumonia, CMV-associated hepatitis, and concomitant fungi and parasitic superinfections.

USES Attenuation of primary cytomegalovirus (CMV) disease associated with kidney transplantation. **Unlabeled use:** prevention of CMV disease in other organ transplants (especially heart) when the recipient is seronegative for CMV and the donor is seropositive.

ROUTE & DOSAGE

Prevention of CMV Disease

Adult: **IV** 150 mg/kg within 72 h of transplantation, then 100 mg/kg 2, 4, 6, and 8 wk posttransplant, then 50 mg/kg 12 and 16 wk posttransplant.

CONTRAINDICATIONS & PRECAUTIONS **Contraindicated in:** history of previous severe reactions associated with CMVIG or other human immunoglobulin preparations, selective immunoglobulin A (IgA) deficiency. **Cautious use in:** myelosuppression, cardiac disease, pregnancy (category C).

ADVERSE/SIDE EFFECTS **CNS:** headache, anxiety. **CV:** hypotension, palpitations. **GI:** nausea, vomiting, metallic taste. **Respiratory:** *shortness* of breath, wheezing. **Skin:** flushing. **Other:** muscle aches, back pain, <u>anaphylaxis (rare)</u>, fever and chills during infusion.

DRUG INTERACTIONS Antibodies present in immune globulin preparations may interfere with the immune response to live virus vaccines (BCG, measles/mumps/rubella, live polio). Vaccination with live viral vaccines should be deferred for approximately 3 mo after administration of CMVIG; revaccination may be necessary if these vaccines were given shortly after CMVIG.

NURSING IMPLICATIONS

Administration

- CMVIG should be administered through a separate IV line using an infusion pump. See manufacturer's directions if this is not possible.
- IV preparation: Reconstitute with 50 ml sterile water. Gently rotate vial to dissolve; do not shake. Allow 30 min to dissolve powder. Reconstituted solution contains 50 mg/ml.
- Infusion of initial IV dose: Give at rate of 15, 30, 60 mg/kg/h over first 30 min, second 30 min, third 30 min, respectively.
- Monitor closely during and after each rate change. If flushing, nausea, back pain, fever, or chills develop, slow or temporarily discontinue infusion. If BP begins to decrease, stop infusion and institute emergency measures.
- Infusion of subsequent IV doses: The intervals for increasing the dose from 15 to 30 to 60 mg may be shortened from 30 to 15 min.
- Never infuse more than 75 ml/h CMVIG.
- Reconstituted solution should be started within 6 h and completed within 12 h of preparation. Discard solution if cloudy.

Assessment & Drug Effects

- Monitor vital signs preinfusion, before increases in infusion rate, periodically during infusion, and postinfusion.
- Notify physician immediately if any of the following occur: flushing, nausea, back pain, fall in BP, other signs of anaphylaxis.
- Emergency drugs should be available for treatment of acute anaphylactic reactions.
- Monitor for CMV-associated syndromes (e.g., leukopenia, thrombocytopenia, hepatitis, pneumonia) and for superinfections.

Patient & Family Education

- Inform patient of potential adverse effects of drug.
- Instruct patient on symptoms that

should be immediately reported during drug infusion.

- Advise patient to defer vaccination with live viral vaccines for 3 mo after administration of CMVIG.

D

DACARBAZINE

(da-kar'ba-zeen)

Trade names: DTIC, DTIC-Dome, Imidazole Carboxamide

Classifications: ANTINEOPLASTIC; ALKYLATING AGENT

Prototype: Cyclophosphamide

Pregnancy category: C

ACTIONS/PHARMACODYNAMICS Cytotoxic agent with alkylating properties. Cell-cycle nonspecific. Interferes with purine metabolism and with RNA and protein synthesis in rapidly proliferating cells. Has minimal immunosuppressive activity; reportedly carcinogenic, mutagenic, and teratogenic.

USES As single agent or in combination with other antineoplastics in treatment of metastatic malignant melanoma, refractory Hodgkin's disease, various sarcomas, and neuroblastoma. **Unlabeled uses:** soft tissue metastatic sarcoma and malignant glucagonoma.

ROUTE & DOSAGE

Neoplasms

Adult: **IV** 2–4.5 mg/kg/d for 10 d repeated at 4-wk intervals, *or* 250 $mg/m^2/d$ for 5 d repeated at 3-wk intervals.

Child: **IV** 200–470 $mg/m^2/d$ over 5 d q21–28d.

PHARMACOKINETICS **Distribution:** localizes primarily in liver. **Metabolism:** extensively metabolized in liver. **Elimination:** half-life: 5 h; 35–50% excreted in urine in 6 h.

CONTRAINDICATIONS & PRECAUTIONS **Contraindicated in:** safe use during pregnancy (category C) not established.

ADVERSE/SIDE EFFECTS **CNS:** confusion, headache, seizures, blurred vision. **GI:** *anorexia, nausea, vomiting*. **Hematologic:** <u>severe leukopenia and thrombocytopenia</u>, mild anemia. **Hypersensitivity:** erythematosus, urticarial rashes, hepatotoxicity, photosensitivity. **Other:** alopecia, facial paresthesia and flushing, flulike syndrome, myalgia, malaise, anaphylaxis, *pain along injected vein*.

INCOMPATIBILITIES **Solution/additive:** heparin.

NURSING IMPLICATIONS

Administration

- Dacarbazine should be administered to hospitalized patients because close observation and frequent laboratory studies are required during and after therapy.
- All handlers of dacarbazine should wear gloves. If solution gets into the eyes, wash them with soap and water immediately, then irrigate with water or isotonic saline.
- Reconstitute drug with sterile water for injection to make a solution containing 10 mg/ml dacarbazine (pH 3.0–4.0) by adding 9.9 ml to 100 mg or 19.8 ml to 200 mg. The reconstituted solution may be further diluted.
- Resulting solution is administered through a free-flowing IV with 5% dextrose injection or NaCl injection. Administered by direct IV over 1 min or by IV infusion over 30 min.
- IV administration to infants and children: Verify correct IV concentration and rate of infusion with physician.

- IV extravasation: Monitor injection site frequently (instruct patient to do so, if able). Give prompt attention to patient's complaint of swelling, stinging, and burning sensation around injection site. Extravasation can occur painlessly and without visual signs.
- Danger areas for extravasation are dorsum of hand or ankle (especially if peripheral arteriosclerosis is present), joint spaces, and previously irradiated areas. If possible, avoid using antecubital vein or veins on dorsum of hand or wrist where extravasation could lead to loss of mobility of entire limb. Avoid veins in extremity with compromised venous or lymphatic drainage and veins near joint spaces.
- If extravasation is suspected, infusion should be stopped immediately and restarted in another vein. Report to the physician. Prompt institution of local treatment is imperative.
- Store reconstituted solution up to 72 h at 4C (39F) or at room temperature for up to 8 h. Store diluted reconstituted solution for 24 h at 4C (39F) or at room temperature for up to 8 h. Protect from light.

Assessment & Drug Effects

- Check patient's mouth for ulcerative stomatitis prior to the administration of each dose.
- Skin damage by dacarbazine can lead to deep necrosis requiring surgical debridement, skin grafting, and even amputation. At risk are the elderly, very young, comatose, and debilitated patients. Other risk factors include establishing an IV line in a vein previously punctured several times and nonplastic catheters.
- Hematopoietic toxicity usually appears about 4 wk after first dose. Generally, a leukocyte count of $<3000/mm^3$ and a platelet count of $<100{,}000/mm^3$ require suspension or cessation of therapy. Leukopenia and thrombocytopenia can be severe enough to cause death.
- During platelet nadir, avoid if possible all tests and treatments (e.g., IM) requiring needle punctures. Observe carefully and report evidence of unexplained bleeding.
- Severe nausea and vomiting (>90% of patients) begin within 1 h after drug administration and may last for as long as 12 h.
- Monitor I&O ratio and pattern and daily temperature. Renal impairment extends the half-life and increases danger of toxicity. Report symptoms of renal dysfunction and even a slight elevation of temperature.

Patient & Family Education

- Fully advise patient of all potential adverse drug effects.
- Flu-like syndrome may occur during or even a week after treatment is terminated and last 7–21 d. Symptoms frequently recur with successive treatments. Advise patient to report them to physician.
- Caution patient to avoid prolonged exposure to sunlight or to ultraviolet light during treatment period and for at least 2 wk after last dose. Protect exposed skin with sunscreen lotion (≥SPF 15) and avoid exposure in midday.
- Warn patient to report promptly the onset of blurred vision or paresthesia.

DACLIZUMAB

(dac′li-zu-mab)

Trade name: Zenapax

Classifications: IMMUNOSUPPRESSANT; MONOCLONAL ANTIBODY; INTERLEUKIN-2 RECEPTOR ANTAGONIST
Prototype: Basiliximab
Pregnancy category: C

D

ACTIONS/PHARMACODYNAMICS

Immunosuppressant IgG-1 monoclonal antibody produced by recombinant DNA technology. Binds to interleukin-2 (IL-2) receptor complex of lymphocytes. Therefore, daclizumab inhibits IL-2–mediated activation of lymphocytes which is the major pathway for cellular immune rejection of allografts.

USES Prophylaxis of acute organ rejection in renal transplant.

ROUTE & DOSAGE

Renal Transplant
Adult: **IV** 1 mg/kg. Start first dose no more than 24 h prior to transplant, then repeat q14d for 4 more doses.

PHARMACOKINETICS **Duration:** 120 d. **Elimination:** half-life: 20 d (11–38 d).

CONTRAINDICATIONS & PRECAUTIONS **Contraindicated in:** hypersensitivity to daclizumab, nursing mothers, pregnancy (category C). **Cautious use in:** moderate-to-severe renal impairment; allergies, asthma, or history of allergic responses to medications. No adequate or well-controlled studies in children available.

ADVERSE/SIDE EFFECTS **Body as whole:** edema (general and in extremities), pain, fever, fatigue, shivering, generalized weakness, arthralgia, myalgia. **CNS:** tremor, headache, dizziness, insomnia, anxiety, depression. **CV:** chest pain, hypertension, hypotension, tachycardia, thrombosis, bleeding. **GI:** constipation, nausea, diarrhea, vomiting, abdominal pain, dyspepsia, abdominal distention, epigastric pain, flatulence, gastritis, hemorrhoids. **GU:** oliguria, dysuria, renal tubular necrosis, hydronephrosis, urinary tract bleeding, renal insufficiency. **Respiratory:** dyspnea, pulmonary edema, cough, atelectasis, congestion, pharyngitis, rhinitis, hypoxia, rales, abnormal breath sounds, pleural effusion. **Skin:** impaired wound healing, acne, pruritus, hirsutism, rash, night sweats. **Other:** diabetes mellitus, dehydration, blurred vision.

NURSING IMPLICATIONS

Administration

- IV preparation: Add calculated amount of drug (based on patient's body weight) to 50 ml of 0.9% NaCl. Invert infusion bag to dissolve but do not shake. Discard if diluted solution is colored or has particulate matter.
- IV infusion: Infuse diluted drug over 15 min.
- Diluted solution should be used immediately but may be stored at room temperature for 4 h or at 2–8C (36–46F) for 24 h. Discard after 24 h.
- Store unopened vials at 2–8C (36–46F) and protect from light.

Assessment & Drug Effects

- Therapeutic effectiveness is indicated by prevention of renal transplant rejection.
- Carefully monitor for and immediately report S&S of opportunistic infection or anaphylactoid reaction (see Appendix G).

Patient & Family Education

- Women of childbearing age should use effective contraception before beginning daclizumab therapy, during therapy, and for 4 mo after completion of therapy.

- Effectiveness of immune response to vaccinations or infections during daclizumab therapy has not been determined.

DACTINOMYCIN

(dak-ti-noe-mye′sin)
Trade names: Actinomycin-D, Cosmegen
Classifications: ANTINEOPLASTIC; ANTIBIOTIC
Prototype: Doxorubicin
Pregnancy category: C

ACTIONS/PHARMACODYNAMICS Potent cytotoxic antibiotic derived from mixture of actinomycins produced by *Streptomyces parvullus*. Toxic properties preclude its use as antibiotic. Complexes with DNA, thereby inhibiting DNA, RNA, and protein synthesis. Causes delayed myelosuppression; is strongly tissue corrosive and has a low therapeutic index. Potentiates effects of x-ray therapy; the converse also appears likely. Recent reports indicate increased potential for secondary primary tumors following treatment with x-ray and dactinomycin.

USES As single agent or in combination with other antineoplastics or radiation to treat Wilms' tumor, rhabdomyosarcoma, carcinoma of testes and uterus, Ewing's sarcoma, and sarcoma botryoides. **Unlabeled uses:** malignant melanoma, trophoblastic tumors, Kaposi's sarcoma, osteogenic sarcoma, among others.

ROUTE & DOSAGE

Neoplasms

Adult: **IV** 500 μg/d for a maximum of 5 d; may repeat at 2–4 wk intervals if tolerated.
Child: **IV** 15 μg/kg/d (max 500 μg) for 5 d *or* 2.5 mg/m^2 over 7 d; may repeat at 2–4 wk intervals if tolerated.

Isolation Perfusion

Adult: **IV** 50 μg/kg for lower extremity or pelvis; 35 μg/kg for upper extremity.

PHARMACOKINETICS **Distribution:** concentrated in liver, spleen, kidneys, and bone marrow; does not cross blood–brain barrier; crosses placenta; distribution into breast milk not known. **Elimination:** half-life: 36 h; 50% excreted unchanged in bile and 10% in urine; only 30% excreted in urine over 9 d.

CONTRAINDICATIONS & PRECAUTIONS **Contraindicated in:** chickenpox, herpes zoster, and other viral infections; pregnancy (category C), lactation, infants <6 mo. **Cautious use in:** previous therapy with antineoplastics or radiation within 3–6 wk, bone marrow depression; infections; history of gout; impairment of kidney or liver function; obesity.

ADVERSE/SIDE EFFECTS **GI:** *nausea, vomiting*, anorexia, abdominal pain, diarrhea, proctitis, GI ulceration, *stomatitis,* cheilitis, glossitis, dysphagia, hepatitis. **Hematologic:** anemia (including aplastic anemia), agranulocytosis, *leukopenia, thrombocytopenia,* pancytopenia, reticulopenia. **Skin:** acne, desquamation, hyperpigmentation and reactivation of erythema especially over previously irradiated areas, *alopecia* (reversible). **Other:** malaise, fatigue, lethargy, fever, myalgia, anaphylaxis, gonadal suppression, hypocalcemia, hyperuricemia, thrombophlebitis; *necrosis, sloughing, and contractures at site of extravasation;* hepatitis, hepatomegaly.

D

DRUG INTERACTIONS Elevated uric acid level produced by dactinomycin may necessitate dose adjustment of ANTIGOUT AGENTS; effects of both dactinomycin and other MYELOSUPPRESSANTS are potentiated; effects of both **radiation** and dactinomycin are potentiated, and dactinomycin may reactivate erythema from previous radiation therapy; **vitamin K** effects (antihemorrhagic) decreased, leading to prolonged clotting time and potential hemorrhage.

NURSING IMPLICATIONS

Administration

- Manufacturer advises use of gloves and eye shield to protect the person making the solution. If skin is contaminated, rinse with running water for 10 min; then rinse with buffered phosphate solution. If solution gets into the eyes, wash with water immediately; then irrigate with water or isotonic saline for 10 min.
- Reconstitute by adding 1.1 mg sterile water for injection (without preservative); the resulting solution will contain approximately 0.5 mg/ml.
- Once reconstituted, dactinomycin may be added directly to infusion solutions of 5% dextrose injection or NaCl injection, or into tubing or side arm of a running IV infusion, and administered over a 10–15 min period. Discard unused portion.
- Following IV injection, some clinicians recommend injecting 5–10 ml IV solution into the side arm or flushing the vein with running IV infusion for 2–5 min to remove any remaining drug from tubing.
- Observe injection site frequently; if extravasation occurs, stop infusion immediately. Infusion should be restarted in another vein. Report to physician. Prompt institution of local treatment to prevent thrombophlebitis and necrosis is imperative.
- The obese or edematous patient is given a lower dose of dactinomycin calculated at 400–600 μg/m^2 to relate dosage to lean body mass. Monitor for symptoms of toxicity from overdosage.
- Store drug at 15–30C (59–86F) unless otherwise advised. Protect from heat and light.

Assessment & Drug Effects

- Severe toxic effects occur with high frequency. Effects usually appear 2–4 d after a course of therapy is stopped and may reach maximal severity 1–2 wk following discontinuation of therapy.
- Nausea and vomiting usually occur a few hours after drug administration and are generally controlled by an antiemetic drug. Vomiting may be severe enough to require intermittent therapy. Observe patient daily for signs of drug toxicity.
- Frequent determinations of renal, hepatic, and bone marrow function are advised. WBC counts should be performed daily and platelet counts every 3 d to detect hematopoietic depression.
- Monitor temperature and inspect oral membranes daily for stomatitis.
- The combination of stomatitis, diarrhea, and severe hematopoietic depression usually requires prompt interruption of therapy until drug toxicity subsides.
- Report onset of unexplained bleeding, jaundice, and wheezing. Also, be alert to signs of agranulocytosis (see Appendix G). Report to physician. Antibiotic therapy, protective isolation, and discon-

tinuation of the antineoplastic are indicated.

- Observe and report symptoms of hyperuricemia (see Appendix G). Urge patient to increase fluid intake up to 3000 ml/d if allowed.

Patient & Family Education

- Discuss possibility of gonadal suppression (amenorrhea or azoospermia) with patient before therapy is instituted. This may be an irreversible side effect.
- Patient should be advised of the potential for nausea and vomiting and of what preventative measures will be taken to minimize these side effects.
- Patient should be informed that reversible alopecia is an anticipated side effect. Appropriate supportive guidance should be provided.

DALTEPARIN SODIUM

(dal-tep′a-rin)

Trade name: Fragmin

Classifications: BLOOD FORMER AND COAGULATOR; ANTICOAGULANT

Prototype: Heparin

Pregnancy category: B

See Appendix A.

DANAPAROID SODIUM

(dan-a′pa-roid)

Trade name: Orgaran

Classifications: BLOOD FORMER AND COAGULATOR; ANTICOAGULANT

Prototype: Heparin

Pregnancy category: B

See Appendix A.

DANAZOL

(da′na-zole)

Trade names: Cyclomen♣, Danocrine

Classifications: SYNTHETIC HORMONE; ANDROGEN/ANABOLIC STEROID

Prototype: Testosterone

Pregnancy category: C

ACTIONS/PHARMACODYNAMICS

Synthetic androgen steroid; derivative of testosterone with dose-related mild androgenic effects but no estrogenic or progestational activity. Suppresses pituitary output of FSH and LH, resulting in anovulation and associated amenorrhea. Interrupts progress and pain of endometriosis by causing atrophy and involution of both normal and ectopic endometrial tissue.

USES Palliative treatment of endometriosis when alternative hormonal therapy is ineffective, contraindicated, or intolerable. Also used to treat fibrocystic breast disease and hereditary angioedema. **Unlabeled uses:** to treat precocious puberty, gynecomastia, menorrhagia, premenstrual syndrome (PMS), chronic immune thrombocytopenic purpura (ITP), autoimmune hemolytic anemia, hemophilia A and B.

ROUTE & DOSAGE

Endometriosis

Adult: **PO** 400 mg b.i.d. for 3–6 mo; start during menstruation or if pregnancy test is negative; therapy may be extended to 9 mo if necessary; regimen cannot be repeated.

Fibrocystic Breast Disease

Adult: **PO** 100–400 mg in 2 divided doses; start during menstruation or if pregnancy test is negative.

Hereditary Angioedema

Adult: **PO** 200 mg b.i.d. or t.i.d.;

may decrease by 50% at intervals of 1–3 mo or longer; start during menstruation or if pregnancy test is negative.

D

PHARMACOKINETICS **Elimination:** half-life: 4.5 h; other pharmacokinetic information is not known.

CONTRAINDICATIONS & PRECAUTIONS **Contraindicated in:** pregnancy (category C), nursing mothers, children, undiagnosed abnormal genital bleeding; impaired renal, cardiac, or hepatic function. **Cautious use in:** migraine headache, epilepsy.

ADVERSE/SIDE EFFECTS **Androgenic (virilization):** acne, mild hirsutism, deepening of voice, oily skin and hair, hair loss, edema, weight gain, pitch breaks, voice weakness, decrease in breast size. **CNS:** dizziness, sleep disorders, fatigue, tremor, irritability. **Eye:** conjunctival edema. **GI:** gastroenteritis. **GU:** decreased libido. **Hypersensitivity:** skin rashes, nasal congestion. **Hypoestrogenic:** *hot flushes;* sweating; emotional lability; nervousness; vaginitis with itching, drying, burning, or bleeding; *amenorrhea, irregular menstrual patterns.* **Musculoskeletal:** joint lock-up, joint swelling. **Other:** elevated BP, hepatic damage (rare), increased LDL, decreased HDL, impairment in glucose tolerance.

NURSING IMPLICATIONS

Administration

- For patients with endometriosis or irregular periods or fibrocystic breast disease, therapy should start during menstruation, or a pregnancy test should be performed before treatment is initiated.
- Store capsules at 15–30C (59–86F) in tightly closed container.

Assessment & Drug Effects

- Routine breast examinations should be carried out during therapy. Carcinoma of the breast should be ruled out prior to start of therapy for fibrocystic breast disease. Advise patient to report to physician if any nodule enlarges or becomes tender or hard during therapy.
- Because danazol may cause fluid retention, patients with cardiac or renal dysfunction, epilepsy, or migraine should be observed closely during therapy, as these problems could worsen. Monitor weight.
- Drug-induced edema may compress the median nerve, producing symptoms of carpal tunnel syndrome. If patient complains of wrist pain that worsens at night, paresthesias in radial palmar aspect of the hand and fingers, consult physician.
- Baseline and periodic liver function tests should be performed in all patients. Patients with diabetes (or history of) should have blood glucose tests.

Patient & Family Education

- In fibrocystic breast disease, inform patient that pain and discomfort are usually relieved in 2 or 3 mo; the nodularity in 4–6 mo. Menses may be regular or irregular in pattern during therapy.
- Drug-induced amenorrhea is reversible. Ovulation and cyclic bleeding usually return within 60–90 d after therapeutic regimen is discontinued. Advise patient that potential for conception may also be restored at that time.
- A nonhormonal contraceptive should be used during danazol treatment (because ovulation may not be suppressed) until 6–8 wk of therapy. If pregnancy occurs while patient is receiving the drug, danazol should be discontinued, and the question of continuing the pregnancy considered.
- Advise patient to report voice

changes promptly. Drug should be stopped to avoid permanent damage to voice. Virilizing side effects may persist even after drug therapy is terminated.

DANTROLENE SODIUM

(dan'troe-leen)

Trade name: Dantrium

Classifications: AUTONOMIC NERVOUS SYSTEM AGENT; CENTRAL-ACTING SKELETAL MUSCLE RELAXANT

Prototype: Cyclobenzaprine

Pregnancy category: C

ACTIONS/PHARMACODYNAMICS Hydantoin derivative, structurally related to phenytoin, with peripheral skeletal muscle relaxant action. Directly relaxes the spastic muscle by interfering with calcium ion release from sarcoplasmic reticulum. Clinical doses produce about a 50% decrease in contractility of skeletal muscles but no effect on smooth or cardiac muscles. Relief of spasticity may be accompanied by muscle weakness sufficient to affect overall functional capacity of the patient.

USES Orally for the symptomatic treatment of skeletal muscle spasms secondary to spinal cord injury, stroke, cerebral palsy, multiple sclerosis. Used intravenously for the management of malignant hyperthermia. Oral dantrolene has been used prophylactically (2 or 3 d before anesthesia) for patients with a history of malignant hyperthermia or with a family history of the disorder. **Unlabeled uses:** neuroleptic malignant syndrome, exercise-induced muscle pain, and flexor spasms.

ROUTE & DOSAGE

Relief of Spasticity

Adult: **PO** 25 mg once/d; increase to 25 mg b.i.d. to q.i.d.; may increase q4–7d up to 100 mg b.i.d. to q.i.d.
Child: **PO** 0.5 mg/kg b.i.d.; increase to 0.5 mg/kg t.i.d. or q.i.d.; may increase by 0.5 mg/kg up to 3 mg/kg b.i.d. to q.i.d. (max 100 mg q.i.d.).

Malignant Hyperthermia

Adult: **IV** 1 mg/kg rapid IV push repeated prn up to a total of 10 mg/kg. **PO** May be necessary to continue orally with 1–2 mg/kg q.i.d. for 1–3 d to prevent recurrence.
Child: **IV** Same as for adult. **PO** Same as for adult.

PHARMACOKINETICS **Absorption:** about 35% slowly and incompletely absorbed from GI tract. **Peak:** 5 h. **Distribution:** crosses placenta. **Metabolism:** metabolized in liver. **Elimination:** half-life: 8.7 h; excreted in urine chiefly as metabolites.

CONTRAINDICATIONS & PRECAUTIONS **Contraindicated in:** active hepatic disease; when spasticity is necessary to sustain upright posture and balance in locomotion or to maintain increased body function; spasticity due to rheumatic disorders. Safe use during pregnancy (category C), in nursing mothers, and in children <5 y not established. **Cautious use in:** impaired cardiac or pulmonary function, patients >35 y, especially women.

ADVERSE/SIDE EFFECTS **CNS:** drowsiness, *muscle weakness,* dizziness, light-headedness, unusual fatigue, speech disturbances, headache, confusion, nervousness, men-

D

tal depression, insomnia, euphoria, seizures. **CV:** tachycardia, erratic BP. **Eye:** blurred vision, diplopia, photophobia. **GI:** *diarrhea,* constipation, nausea, vomiting, anorexia, swallowing difficulty, alterations of taste, gastric irritation, abdominal cramps, GI bleeding. **GU:** crystalluria with pain or burning with urination, urinary frequency, urinary retention, nocturia, enuresis, difficult erection. **Hepatic (prolonged use of high doses):** hepatitis, jaundice, hepatomegaly, <u>hepatic necrosis</u>. **Hypersensitivity:** pruritus, urticaria, eczematoid skin eruption, photosensitivity, eosinophilic pleural effusion.

DRUG INTERACTIONS **Alcohol** and other CNS DEPRESSANTS compound CNS depression; ESTROGENS increase risk of hepatotoxicity in women >35 y; **verapamil** and other CALCIUM CHANNEL BLOCKERS increase risk of ventricular fibrillation and cardiovascular collapse with IV dantrolene.

NURSING IMPLICATIONS

Administration

- If necessary, an oral suspension for a single dose may be made by emptying contents of capsule(s) into fruit juice or other liquid. Suspension should be shaken well before it is poured. Since it will not contain a preservative, avoid contamination, keep refrigerated, and use within several days.
- For IV administration, dilute each 20 mg with 60 ml sterile water without preservatives. Shake until clear; then give by rapid direct IV injection.
- IV extravasation should be avoided. Solution has a high pH and therefore is extremely irritating to tissue. Observe and palpate entry site frequently during therapy.
- Store capsules in tightly closed, light-resistant container. Contents of vial (for IV use) must be protected from direct light and used within 6 h after reconstitution, since it does not contain a preservative. Both PO and parenteral forms are stored at 15–30C (59–86F) unless otherwise directed.

Assessment & Drug Effects

- Improvement may not be apparent until 1 wk or more of drug therapy.
- During IV infusion, monitor vital signs. ECG, CVP, and serum potassium should also be monitored.
- Supervise ambulation until patient's reaction to drug is known. Relief of spasticity may be accompanied by some loss of strength.
- The most common side effects are generally transient, lasting up to 14 d after initiation of therapy. Keep physician informed.
- Patients with impaired cardiac or pulmonary function should be closely monitored for cardiovascular or respiratory symptoms such as tachycardia, BP changes, feeling of suffocation.
- Because of the possibility of hepatotoxicity (see Appendix G), it is recommended that drug be discontinued if improvement is not evident within 45 d.
- Baseline and regularly scheduled hepatic function tests (alkaline phosphatase, AST, ALT, total bilirubin), blood cell counts, and renal function tests should be performed.
- Monitor bowel function. Persistent diarrhea may necessitate drug withdrawal. Severe constipation with abdominal distention and signs of intestinal obstruction have been reported.

Patient & Family Education

- Instruct patient to report promptly

the onset of jaundice: yellow skin or sclerae; dark urine, clay-colored stools, itching, abdominal discomfort. Hepatotoxicity more frequently occurs between 3rd and 12th mo of therapy.

- Advise patient to report symptoms of allergy and of allergic pleural effusion: shortness of breath, pleuritic pain, dry cough.
- Forewarn patient of the possibility of dizziness and drowsiness and advise to avoid driving and other potentially hazardous activities until reaction to drug is known.
- Since hepatotoxicity occurs more commonly when other drugs are taken concurrently, advise patient not to take OTC medications, alcoholic beverages, or other CNS depressants unless otherwise advised by physician.

DAPSONE

(dap′sone)

Trade names: Avlosulfon ♣, DDS

Prototype for classifications: ANTIINFECTIVE; ANTILEPROSY (SULFONE) AGENT

Pregnancy category: C

ACTIONS/PHARMACODYNAMICS

Sulfone derivative chemically related to sulfonamides, with bacteriostatic and bactericidal activity similar to that group. Spectrum of activity includes *Mycobacterium leprae* (Hansen's bacillus), *Mycobacterium tuberculosis,* and limited activity against *Pneumocystis carinii* and *Plasmodium*. Interferes with bacterial cell growth by competitive inhibition of folic acid synthesis by susceptible organisms. Drug is effective against dapsone-sensitive multibacillary (borderline, borderline lepromatous, or lepromatous) leprosy, and dapsone-sensitive paucibacillary (indeterminate, tuberculoid, or borderline tuberculoid) leprosy. Resistant strains of initially susceptible *M. leprae* develop slowly in a stepwise fashion over periods of 5–24 y.

USES Drug of choice for treatment of all forms of leprosy (unless organism is shown to be dapsone resistant). Used in dapsone-sensitive multibacillary leprosy (with clofazimine and rifampin) and in dapsone-sensitive paucibacillary leprosy (with rifampin, clofazimine, or ethionamide). Also used prophylactically in contacts of patients with all forms of leprosy except tuberculoid and indeterminate leprosy. Used for treatment of dermatitis herpetiformis. **Unlabeled uses:** chemoprophylaxis of malaria (with pyrimethamine), systemic and discoid lupus erythematosus, pemphigus vulgaris, dermatosis (especially those associated with bullous eruptions, mucocutaneous lesion, inflammation or pustules); rheumatoid arthritis, allergic vasculitis; treatment of initial episodes of *P. carinii* pneumonia (with trimethoprim) in limited number of adults with AIDS.

ROUTE & DOSAGE

Tuberculoid and Indeterminate-type Leprosy

Adult: **PO** 100 mg/d (with 6 mo of rifampin 600 mg/d) for a minimum of 3 y.

Lepromatous and Borderline Lepromatous Leprosy

Adult: **PO** 100 mg/d for ≥ 10 y.
Child: **PO** 1–2 mg/kg/d once daily in combination therapy (max 100 mg/d).

D

Dermatitis Herpetiformis
Adult: **PO** 50 mg/d; may be increased to 300 mg/d if necessary (max 500 mg/d).

Prophylaxis for Close Contacts of Patient with Multibacillary Leprosy
Adult: **PO** 50 mg/d.
Child: **PO** *6–12 y:* 25 mg/d; *2–5 y:* 25 mg 3 times/wk; 6–23 12 mg 3 times/wk; *<6 mo:* 6 mg 3 times/wk.

***P. carinii* Pneumonia Prophylaxis**
Adult: **PO** 50 mg b.i.d. or 100 mg q.d.
Child: **PO** 2 mg/kg once daily (max 100 mg/d).

PHARMACOKINETICS **Absorption:** rapidly and nearly completely absorbed from GI tract. **Peak:** 2–8 h. **Distribution:** distributed to all body tissues; high concentrations in kidney, liver, muscle, and skin; crosses placenta; distributed into breast milk. **Metabolism:** metabolized in liver. **Elimination:** half-life: 20–30 h; 70–85% excreted in urine; remainder excreted in feces; traces of drug may be found in body for 3 wk after discontinuation of repeated doses.

CONTRAINDICATIONS & PRECAUTIONS **Contraindicated in:** hypersensitivity to sulfones or its derivatives; advanced renal amyloidosis, anemia, methemoglobin reductase deficiency. Safe use during pregnancy (category C) and by nursing mothers not established. **Cautious use in:** chronic renal, hepatic, pulmonary, or cardiovascular disease, refractory anemias, albuminuria, G6PD deficiency.

ADVERSE/SIDE EFFECTS **CNS:** headache, nervousness, insomnia, vertigo; paresthesia, *muscle weakness.* **GI:** anorexia, nausea, vomiting, abdominal pain; toxic hepatitis, cholestatic jaundice (reversible with discontinuation of drug therapy); increased ALT, AST, LDH; hyperbilirubinemia. **Hematologic:** in patient with or without G6PD deficiency; *dose-related hemolysis,* Heinz body formation, *methemoglobinemia with cyanosis,* hemolytic anemia; aplastic anemia (rare), agranulocytosis. **Hypersensitivity:** cutaneous reactions (especially bullous multibilliform and scarlatiniform reactions); erythema multiforme, exfoliative dermatitis, toxic epidermal necrolysis (rare), allergic rhinitis, urticaria. **Skin:** drug-induced lupus erythematosus, phototoxicity. **Other:** tachycardia, blurred vision, tinnitus, fever, male infertility, infectious mononucleosis–like syndrome; *reactional states.* Sulfone syndrome: fever, malaise, exfoliative dermatitis, hepatic necrosis with jaundice, lymphadenopathy, methemoglobinemia, anemia.

DRUG INTERACTIONS **Activated charcoal** decreases dapsone absorption and enterohepatic circulation; **pyrimethamine, trimethoprim** increase risk of adverse hematologic reactions; **rifampin** decreases dapsone levels 7–10 fold.

NURSING IMPLICATIONS

Administration

- Administer with food to reduce possibility of GI distress.
- Preserve in tightly covered, light-resistant containers at 15–30C (59–86F). Drug discoloration apparently does not indicate a chemical change.

Assessment & Drug Effects

- CBC is performed before initiation of therapy, weekly during the first month of therapy, at monthly intervals for at least 6 mo, and semiannually thereafter.

- Periodic determinations of dapsone blood levels are recommended.
- Nearly all patients demonstrate hemolysis. Manufacturer states that Hgb level is generally decreased by 1–2 g/dl; reticulocytes increase by 2–12%; RBC life span is shortened; and methemoglobinemia occurs in most patients receiving dapsone. Unless hemolysis or methemoglobinemia is severe, drug is not discontinued.
- Therapeutic effects in leprosy may not appear until after 3–6 mo of therapy. Skin lesions respond well; recovery from nerve involvement is usually limited.
- Monitor temperature during first few weeks of therapy. If fever is frequent or severe, leprosy reactional state should be ruled out. Reduction of or interruption of therapy may be sufficient.
- Suspect methemoglobinemia if patient appears cyanotic and mucous membranes have a brownish hue. Report to physician.
- Patients who complain of malaise, fever, chills, anorexia, nausea, and vomiting and have jaundice should have liver function tests performed. Dapsone therapy should be suspended until etiology is identified.

Patient & Family Education

- Report to physician if symptoms of leprosy do not improve within 3 mo or if they get worse.
- The appearance of a rash with bullous lesions around elbows and other joints should be reported promptly. Drug-induced or worsening of skin lesions require withdrawal of dapsone.
- Caution patient to report promptly if symptoms of peripheral neuropathy with motor loss (muscle weakness) develop.

D

DAUNORUBICIN HYDROCHLORIDE

(daw-noe-roo'bi-sin)

Trade name: Cerubidine

DAUNORUBICIN CITRATED LIPOSOMAL

Trade name: DaunoXome

Classifications: ANTINEOPLASTIC; ANTIBIOTIC

Prototype: Doxorubicin

Pregnancy category: D

ACTIONS/PHARMACODYNAMICS

Cytotoxic and antimitotic glycoside antibiotic; cell-cycle specific for S-phase of cell division. Toxic properties preclude its use as an antibiotic. Action mechanism unclear but may be due to rapid intercalating of DNA molecule resulting in inhibition of DNA, RNA, and protein synthesis. A potent bone marrow suppressant, with immunosuppressive properties. Induces cardiac toxicity and may be mutagenic and carcinogenic (development of secondary carcinomas).

USES To induce remission in acute nonlymphocytic leukemia (myelogenous, monocytic, erythroid) in adults. **Unlabeled use:** solid tumors of childhood and non-Hodgkin's lymphoma.

ROUTE & DOSAGE

Neoplasms

Adult: **IV** ***Single agent:*** 30–60 mg/m²/d for 3–5 d q3–4wk (maximum total cumulative dose 500–600 mg/m²); ***combination***

D

therapy: 30–45 $mg/m^2/d$ on days 1, 2, 3 of first course and days 1 and 2 of subsequent courses.
Child: **IV Combination therapy:** ≥2 y, 25–45 mg/m^2; <2 y, calculated on body weight (mg/kg) rather than body surface area.

Kaposi's Sarcoma (DaunoXome)

Adult: **IV** 40 mg/m^2 over 1 h. Repeat q2wk. Serum bilirubin >3 mg/dl or S_{cr} >3 mg/dl, administer half normal dose.

PHARMACOKINETICS Distribution: highest concentrations in spleen, kidneys, liver, lungs, and heart; does not cross blood–brain barrier; crosses placenta; distribution into breast milk not known. **Metabolism:** metabolized in liver to active metabolite. **Elimination:** half-life: 18.5–26.7 h; 25% excreted in urine, 40% in bile.

CONTRAINDICATIONS & PRECAUTIONS Contraindicated in: severe myelosuppression; immunizations (patient, family), and preexisting cardiac disease unless risk-benefit is evaluated; lactation; uncontrolled systemic infection. Safe use during pregnancy (category D) and in nursing women not established. **Cautious use in:** history of gout, urate calculi, hepatic or renal function impairment; elderly patients with inadequate bone reserve due to age or previous cytotoxic drug therapy, tumor cell infiltration of bone marrow, patient who has received potentially cardiotoxic drugs or related antineoplastics.

ADVERSE/SIDE EFFECTS CNS: amnesia, anxiety, ataxia, confusion, hallucinations, emotional lability, tremors. **CV:** pericarditis, myocarditis, arrhythmias, peripheral edema, <u>CHF</u>, hypertension, tachycardia. **GI:** *acute nausea and vomiting* (mild), anorexia, *stomatitis,* mucositis, diarrhea (occasionally) hemorrhage. **GU:** dysuria, nocturia, polyuria, dry skin. **Hematopoietic:** <u>*bone marrow depression,*</u> *thrombocytopenia, leukopenia,* anemia. **Skin:** generalized *alopecia* (reversible), transverse pigmentation of nails. **Other:** hyperuricemia, fever, gonadal suppression, severe cellulitis or tissue necrosis at site of drug extravasation.

INCOMPATIBILITIES Solution/additive: dexamethasone, heparin.

NURSING IMPLICATIONS

Administration

- Use of gloves during preparation of the solution for infusion is recommended to prevent skin contact with the drug. If this occurs, decontaminate with copious amounts of water with soap.
- Reconstitute 20-mg vial with 4 ml sterile water for injection. Concentrations of the solution will be 5 mg/ml. Withdraw dose into syringe containing 10–15 ml normal saline and inject over approximately 3 min into the tubing or side arm of a rapidly flowing IV infusion of 5% glucose or normal saline solution. Do not use a filter with DaunoXome.
- Extravasation can cause severe tissue necrosis and therefore must be avoided.
- Reconstituted solution is stable 24 h at room temperature and 48 h under refrigeration at 2–8C (36–46F) protected from light.

Assessment & Drug Effects

- Monitor serum bilirubin; drug dose is reduced when bilirubin is >1.2 mg/dl.
- Hct, platelet count, total and differential leukocyte count, serum uric acid, chest x-ray, and cardiac, hepatic, and renal function tests

should be performed prior to and periodically during therapy.

- Monitor BP, temperature, pulse, and respiratory function during treatment.
- Acute CHF can occur suddenly, especially when total dosage exceeds 550 mg/m^2, or in patients with compromised heart function because of previous radiation therapy to heart area.
- Report immediately breathlessness, orthopnea, change in pulse and BP parameters. Early clinical diagnosis of drug-induced CHF is essential for successful treatment.
- A profound suppression of bone marrow is required to induce a complete remission. Nadirs for thrombocytes and leukocytes are usually reached in 10–14 d.
- Myelosuppression imposes risk of superimposed infection. Promptly report elevation of temperature, chills, symptoms of upper respiratory tract infection, tachycardia, symptoms of overgrowth with opportunistic organisms—superinfection (see Appendix G).
- Protect patient from contact with persons with infections. The most hazardous period is during nadirs of thrombocytes and leukocytes.
- Monitor serum uric acid levels; normal serum uric acid: 3–7 mg/dl.
- Nausea and vomiting are usually mild and may be controlled by antiemetic therapy.
- Inspect oral membranes daily. Mucositis may occur 3–7 d after drug is administered.

Patient & Family Education

- Discuss probability of onset of alopecia but inform patient that recovery is usual in 6–10 wk.
- Advise against conception during treatment because of teratogenic properties of the drug. Advise patient to report to the physician should she become pregnant.
- Forewarn patient that daunorubicin may turn urine red (a transient effect) on the day of infusion.

D

DEFEROXAMINE MESYLATE

(de-fer-ox′a-meen)

Trade name: Desferal

Classifications: CHELATING AGENT; ANTIDOTE

Pregnancy category: C

ACTIONS/PHARMACODYNAMICS

Chelating agent isolated from *Streptomyces pilosus* with specific affinity for ferric ion and low affinity for calcium. Binds ferric ions to form a stable water-soluble chelate readily excreted by kidneys. Main effect is removal of iron from ferritin, hemosiderin, and transferrin. Does not affect hemoglobin or cytochromes or increase excretion of electrolytes and other trace elements.

USES Adjunct in treatment of acute iron intoxication. Has been used in management of hemochromatosis and hemosiderosis secondary to increased iron storage as from multiple transfusions used in treatment of congenital anemias, e.g., thalassemia (Cooley's or Mediterranean anemia), sickle cell anemia, and other chronic anemias. **Unlabeled uses:** to promote aluminum excretion in aluminum-associated dialysis encephalopathy and aluminum accumulation in bones of patients in renal failure.

ROUTE & DOSAGE

Acute Iron Intoxication

Adult: **IM/IV** 1 g followed by 500 mg at 4 h intervals for 2 doses;

subsequent doses of 500 mg q4–12h may be given if necessary (max 6 g/24 h); infuse at ≤15 mg/kg/h.
Child: **IM/IV** 20 mg/kg followed by 10 mg/kg at 4 h intervals for 2 doses; subsequent doses of 10 mg/kg q4–12h may be given if necessary (max 6 g/24 h); infuse at ≤ 15 mg/kg/h.

Chronic Iron Overload

Adult: **IM** 500 mg–1 g/d. **IV** 2 g with each unit of blood transfused; infuse at ≤ 15 mg/ kg/h.
Child: **IM** Same as for adult. **IV** Same as for adult (max 12 g/d).

PHARMACOKINETICS Distribution: widely distributed in body tissues. **Metabolism:** forms nontoxic complex with iron. **Elimination:** excreted primarily in urine; some excreted in feces.

CONTRAINDICATIONS & PRECAUTIONS Contraindicated in: severe renal disease, anuria, pyelonephritis; pregnancy (category C), and children <3 y of age. **Cautious use in:** history of pyelonephritis.

ADVERSE/SIDE EFFECTS CV: hypotension, tachycardia. **ENT:** decreased hearing. **Eye:** blurred vision, decreased visual acuity and visual fields, color vision abnormalities, night blindness, retinal pigmentary degeneration. **GI:** abdominal discomfort, diarrhea. **GU:** dysuria, exacerbation of pyelonephritis, orange-rose discoloration of urine. **Hypersensitivity:** generalized itching, cutaneous wheal formation, rash, fever, anaphylactoid reaction. **Local:** *pain and induration at injection site.*

NURSING IMPLICATIONS

Administration

- Reconstitute by adding 2 ml sterile water for injection to 500-mg vial. Make certain that drug is completely dissolved before withdrawing it from vial. For IM or SC administration, the reconstituted solution can be given without further dilution. Rotate injection sites.
- For IV administration, reconstitute as for IM or SC use. After drug is completely dissolved, withdraw prescribed amount from vial and add to 0.9% NaCl, D5W, or lactated Ringer's solution.
- Physician will prescribe specific infusion flow rate (should not exceed 15 mg/kg/h) and volume of solution. Monitor vital signs.
- IV administration to infants and children: Verify correct IV concentration and rate of infusion with physician.
- Solutions reconstituted with sterile water may be stored at room temperature for not longer than 1 wk. Protect from light.

Assessment & Drug Effects

- Baseline tests of kidney function should be performed prior to drug administration.
- Monitor injection site. If pain and induration occur, infusion should be moved to another site.
- Side effects occur more often with too rapid IV infusion.
- Monitor I&O ratio and pattern. Report any change. Observe stools for blood (iron intoxication frequently causes necrosis of GI tract).
- Periodic ophthalmoscopic (slit lamp) examinations and audiometry are advisable for patients on prolonged or high-dose therapy for chronic iron overload.

Patient & Family Education

- Deferoxamine chelate imparts a

characteristic reddish color to urine.

- Instruct patient to report blurred vision or any other visual abnormality.

DELAVIRDINE MESYLATE

(del-a-vir′deen)

Trade name: Rescriptor

Classifications: ANTIINFECTIVE; ANTIVIRAL; NONNUCLEOSIDE REVERSE TRANSCRIPTASE INHIBITOR

Prototype: Nevirapine

Pregnancy category: C

ACTIONS/PHARMACODYNAMICS Nonnucleoside reverse transcriptase inhibitor (NNRTI) of HIV-1 binds directly to reverse transcriptase (RT) and blocks RNA- and DNA-dependent DNA polymerase activities. Thus, it prevents replication of the HIV-1 virus. HIV-2 RT and human DNA polymerases such as polymerases alpha, gamma, and delta are not inhibited by delavirdine. Resistant strains appear rapidly.

USES Treatment of HIV infection in combination with other antiretroviral agents.

ROUTE & DOSAGE

HIV Infection

Adult: **PO** 400 mg t.i.d.
Child ≤ 16 y: **PO** 400 mg t.i.d.

PHARMACOKINETICS Absorption: rapidly absorbed from GI tract, 80% reaches systemic circulation. **Peak:** 1 h. **Distribution:** 98% protein bound. **Metabolism:** metabolized in the liver by the CYP3A enzymes. **Elimination:** half-life: 2–11 h; approx 51% excreted in urine, 44% in feces.

CONTRAINDICATIONS & PRECAUTIONS Contraindicated in: hypersensitivity to delavirdine; lactation. **Cautious use in:** impaired liver function, pregnancy (category C). Safety and efficiency in children ≤ 16 y have not been established.

ADVERSE/SIDE EFFECTS Body as whole: headache, fatigue, allergic reaction, chills, edema, arthralgia. **CNS:** abnormal coordination, agitation, amnesia, anxiety, confusion, dizziness. **CV:** chest pain, bradycardia, palpitations, postural hypotension, tachycardia. **GI:** nausea, vomiting, diarrhea, increased LFTs, abdominal cramps, anorexia, aphthous stomatitis. **Hematologic:** <u>neutropenia</u>. **Respiratory:** bronchitis, cough, dyspnea. **Skin:** *rash*, pruritus.

DRUG INTERACTIONS ANTACIDS, H_2-RECEPTOR ANTAGONISTS decrease absorption; **didanosine** and **delavirdine** should be taken 1 h apart to apart to avoid decreased delavirdine levels; **clarithromycin, fluoxetine, ketoconazole** may increase delavirdine levels; **carbamazepine, phenobarbital, phenytoin, rifabutin, rifampin** may decrease delavirdine levels; delavirdine may increase levels of **clarithromycin, astemizole, indinavir, saquinavir, dapsone, rifabutin, alprazolam, midazolam, triazolam,** DIHYDROPYRIDINE, CALCIUM CHANNEL BLOCKERS (e.g., **nifedipine, nicardipine,** etc.), cisapride, **quinidine, warfarin.**

NURSING IMPLICATIONS

Administration

- To disperse in water: add a single dose to at least 3 oz of water, let stand for a few minutes, then stir to create a uniform suspension just prior to administration.
- Patients with achlorhydria should take drug with an acid beverage such as orange or cranberry juice.

D

- Store at 20–25C (68–77F) and protect from high humidity in a tightly closed container.

Assessment & Drug Effects
- Therapeutic effectiveness is indicated by decreased viral load.
- Monitor for and immediately report appearance of a rash, generally within 1–3 wk of starting therapy; rash is usually diffuse, maculopapular, erythematous, and pruritic.

Patient & Family Education
- Drug must be taken exactly as prescribed. Missed doses increase risk of drug resistance.
- Separate antacids and delavirdine by at least 1 h.
- Because of multiple drug interactions, report all prescription and nonprescription drugs used to physician.
- Discontinue medication and notify physician if rash accompanied by any of the following appears: fever, blistering, oral lesions, conjunctivitis, swelling, muscle or joint pain.

DEMECARIUM BROMIDE
(dem-e-kare′ee-um)
Trade name: Humorsol
Classifications: EYE PREPARATION; MIOTIC (ANTIGLAUCOMA); AUTONOMIC NERVOUS SYSTEM AGENT; CHOLINERGIC; CHOLINESTERASE INHIBITOR
Prototype: Pilocarpine hydrochloride
Pregnancy category: C
See Appendix A.

DEMECLOCYCLINE HYDROCHLORIDE
(dem-e-kloe-sye′kleen)
Trade name: Declomycin
Classifications: ANTIINFECTIVE; ANTIBIOTIC; TETRACYCLINE
Prototype: Tetracycline
Pregnancy category: D

ACTIONS/PHARMACODYNAMICS Broad-spectrum, tetracycline antibiotic isolated from mutant strain of *Streptomyces aureofaciens*. Similar to tetracycline but is absorbed more readily, excreted much more slowly, and has longer duration of effective blood levels; therefore intervals between doses can be longer. Primarily bacteriostatic in action.

USES Similar to those of tetracycline. **Unlabeled use:** treatment of chronic SIADH (syndrome of inappropriate [excessive] antidiuretic hormone) secretion.

ROUTE & DOSAGE

Antiinfective
Adult: **PO** 150 mg q6h or 300 mg q12h (max 2.4 g/d).
Child >8 y: **PO** 8–12 mg/kg/d divided q8–12h.

Gonorrhea
Adult: **PO** 600 mg followed by 300 mg q12h for 4 d.

SIADH
Adult: **PO** 600–1200 mg/d in 3–4 divided doses.

PHARMACOKINETICS Absorption: 60–80% absorbed from GI tract. **Peak:** 3–4 h. **Distribution:** concentrated in liver; crosses placenta; distributed into breast milk. **Metabolism:** metabolized in liver; enterohepatic circulation. **Elimination:** half-life: 10–17 h; 40–50% excreted in urine and 31% in feces in 48 h.

CONTRAINDICATIONS & PRECAUTIONS Contraindicated in: hypersensitivity to any of the tetracyclines; cirrhosis, common bile duct obstruction; period of tooth development (last half of pregnancy; category D), nursing women, children <8 y (causes permanent yellow discoloration of teeth, enamel hypoplasia, and retarded bone growth). **Cautious use in:** impaired renal or hepatic function; nephrogenic diabetes insipidus; use of capsule or tablet formulations in patients with esophageal compression or obstruction.

ADVERSE/SIDE EFFECTS **GI:** *nausea,* vomiting, *diarrhea,* esophageal irritation or ulceration, enterocolitis, abdominal cramps, anorexia. **Hypersensitivity:** *photosensitivity,* <u>pericarditis,</u> <u>anaphylaxis</u> (rare). **Renal:** diabetes insipidus, azotemia, hyperphosphatemia. **Skin:** pruritus, erythematous eruptions, exfoliative dermatitis.

DIAGNOSTIC TEST INTERFERENCE Like other tetracyclines, demeclocycline may cause false increases in ***urine catecholamines*** (fluorometric methods); false decreases in ***urine urobilinogen;*** and false-negative ***urine glucose*** with glucose oxidase methods (e.g., Clinistix, TesTape).

DRUG INTERACTIONS **Antacids, iron preparation, calcium, magnesium, zinc, kaolin-pectin, sodium bicarbonate** can significantly decrease demeclocycline absorption; effects of **desmopressin** and demeclocycline antagonized; increases **digoxin** absorption, increasing risk of digoxin toxicity; **methoxyflurane** increases risk of renal failure. **Food–drug:** dairy products significantly decrease demeclocycline absorption; food may decrease drug absorption also.

NURSING IMPLICATIONS

Administration

- Check expiration date before administering drug. Renal damage and death have resulted from use of outdated tetracyclines.
- Absorption may be impaired by foods rich in iron such as red meat or dark green vegetables, milk, milk products, or other calcium-containing foods. Of all tetracyclines, demeclocycline has the greatest affinity for calcium ions. Administer not less than 1 h before or 2 h after meals.
- If gastric distress is a problem, physician may prescribe taking drug with a light meal even though absorption may be reduced. The meal should not contain dairy products.
- Preserve in tight, light-resistant containers, preferably at 15–30C (59–86F) unless otherwise directed. Tetracyclines form toxic products when outdated or when exposed to light, heat, or humidity.

Assessment & Drug Effects

- Culture and susceptibility testing is recommended prior to initiation of therapy and at periodic intervals during prolonged therapy.
- If drug therapy is prolonged, periodic evaluations of serum drug levels, electrolytes, and renal, hepatic, and hematopoietic systems are recommended.
- Monitor I&O ratio and pattern and record weights in patients with impaired kidney or liver function, or on prolonged or high dose therapy. Some patients develop diabetes insipidus–like syndrome (SIADH).

Patient & Family Education

- Drug should be taken on an empty stomach to enhance absorption. Because esophageal irritation and ulceration have been reported, advise patient to (1) take each dose with a full glass (240 ml) of water; (2) remain upright for at least 90 s after taking medication; and (3) avoid taking drug within 1 h of lying down or bedtime.

D

- Stress importance of reporting symptoms of superinfections (see Appendix G).
- Demeclocycline-induced phototoxic reaction can be unusually severe. Advise patient to avoid sunlight as much as possible and use sunscreen.

DESIPRAMINE HYDROCHLORIDE

(dess-ip′ra-meen)

Trade names: Norpramin, Pertofrane

Classifications: CNS AGENT; PSYCHOTHERAPEUTIC; TRICYCLIC ANTIDEPRESSANT

Prototype: Imipramine

Pregnancy category: C

ACTIONS/PHARMACODYNAMICS Dibenzoxazepine tricyclic antidepressant (TCA) and secondary amine. Desipramine is the active metabolite of imipramine and has similar pharmacologic actions. Unlike imipramine, onset of action is more rapid, and it has lower potential for producing sedative and anticholinergic effects and orthostatic hypotension. In common with other TCAs, antidepressant activity appears to be related to inhibition of reuptake of norepinephrine and serotonin in the CNS. Restoration of the levels of these neurotransmitters is a proposed mechanism of antidepressant action.

USES Endogenous depression and various depression syndromes. **Unlabeled uses:** attention deficit disorder in children >6 y and adolescents; to prevent depression in cocaine withdrawal.

ROUTE & DOSAGE

Antidepressant

Adult: **PO** 75–100 mg/d at bedtime or in divided doses; may gradually increase to 150–300 mg/d (use lower doses in elderly patients).
Adolescent: **PO** 25–50 mg/d (max 100 mg/d) in divided doses.
Child 6–12 y: **PO** 1–3 mg/kg/d in divided doses (max 5 mg/kg/d).

PHARMACOKINETICS **Absorption:** rapidly absorbed from GI tract and injection sites. **Peak:** 4–6 h. **Distribution:** crosses placenta. **Metabolism:** metabolized in liver. **Elimination:** half-life: 7–60 h; primarily excreted in urine.

CONTRAINDICATIONS & PRECAUTIONS **Contraindicated in:** hypersensitivity to tricyclic compounds; recent MI. Safe use during pregnancy (category C), in nursing mothers, and in children <12 y not established. **Cautious use in:** urinary retention, prostatic hypertrophy; narrow-angle glaucoma; epilepsy; alcoholism; adolescents, the elderly; thyroid; cardiovascular, renal, and hepatic disease; suicidal tendency; ECT; elective surgery.

ADVERSE/SIDE EFFECTS **CNS:** *drowsiness,* dizziness, weakness, fatigue, headache, insomnia, confusional states, depressive reaction, paresthesias, ataxia. **CV:** *postural hypotension,* hypotension, palpitation, tachycardia, ECG changes, flushing, <u>heart block</u>. **ENT:** tinnitus, parotid swelling. **Eye:** blurred vision, disturbances in accommodation, mydriasis, increased IOP. **GI:** *dry mouth, constipation,* bad taste, diarrhea, nausea. **GU:** *urinary retention,* frequency, delayed micturition, nocturia. **Hematologic (rare):** bone marrow depression, agranulocytosis. **Hypersensitivity:** rash, urticaria, photosensitivity. **Reproduction:** impaired sexual function, galactorrhea. **Other:** sweating, craving for sweets, weight gain or loss, SIADH secretion, hyperpyrexia, eosinophilic pneumonia.

DRUG INTERACTIONS May somewhat decrease response to ANTIHYPERTENSIVES; CNS DEPRESSANTS, **alcohol,** HYPNOTICS, BARBITURATES, SEDATIVES potentiate CNS depression; may increase hypoprothombinemic effect of ORAL ANTICOAGULANTS; **ethchlorvynol** may cause transient delirium; **levodopa,** SYMPATHOMIMETICS (e.g., **epinephrine, norepinephrine**) pose possibility of sympathetic hyperactivity with hypertension and hyperpyrexia; MAO INHIBITORS pose possibility of severe reactions, toxic psychosis, cardiovascular instability; **methylphenidate** increases plasma TCA levels; THYROID AGENTS may increase possibility of arrhythmias; **cimetidine** may increase plasma TCA levels.

NURSING IMPLICATIONS

Administration

- Drug may be taken with or immediately after food to reduce possibility of gastric irritation.
- Maintenance dose is generally prescribed at bedtime to minimize daytime sedation.
- Store drug in tightly closed container at 15–30C (59–86F) unless otherwise specified.

Assessment & Drug Effects

- Full therapeutic effect usually not realized until at least 2 wk of therapy.
- Monitor BP and pulse rate during early phase of therapy, particularly in the elderly, debilitated, and cardiovascular patients. If BP rises or falls more than 20 mm Hg or if there is a sudden increase in pulse rate or change in rhythm, withhold drug and inform physician.
- Drowsiness, dizziness, and orthostatic hypotension in patient on long-term, high dosage therapy are signs of impending toxicity. Prolonged QT or QRS intervals indicate possible toxicity. Report to physician.
- Observe patient with history of glaucoma. Symptoms that may signal acute attack (severe headache, eye pain, dilated pupils, halos of light, nausea, vomiting) should be reported promptly.
- Monitor bowel elimination pattern and I&O ratio. Severe constipation and urinary retention are potential problems of TCA therapy.
- Norpramin tablets may contain tartrazine, which can cause allergic-type reactions including bronchial asthma in susceptible individuals. Such individuals are frequently also sensitive to aspirin.

Patient & Family Education

- Instruct patient to make all position changes slowly and in stages, particularly from recumbent to standing position.
- Caution patient to avoid potentially hazardous activities such as driving until reaction to drug is known.
- Instruct patient to take medication exactly as ordered and not to change dose or dose intervals.
- Abrupt discontinuation of desipramine can precipitate withdrawal symptoms in patients who have received high dosages for prolonged periods: headache, nausea, musculoskeletal pain, weakness.
- OTC drugs should not be taken unless the physician has approved their use.
- Smoking may increase the metabolism of desipramine, thereby di-

minishing its therapeutic action. Advise patient to stop or at least limit smoking.

D

DESMOPRESSIN ACETATE

(des-moe-press'in)

Trade names: DDAVP, Stimate

Classifications: SYNTHETIC PITUITARY HORMONE (ANTIDIURETIC); VASOPRESSOR; OXYTOCIC

Prototype: Vasopressin

Pregnancy category: B

ACTIONS/PHARMACODYNAMICS Synthetic analog of the natural human posterior pituitary (antidiuretic) hormone, arginine vasopressin. Has more specific and longer duration of action than antidiuretic hormone and lower incidence of allergic reactions. Also, oxytocic and vasopressor actions are not apparent at therapeutic dosages. Unlike vasopressin, it does not stimulate release of adrenocorticotropic hormone nor does it increase plasma cortisol, growth hormone, prolactin, or luteinizing hormone levels. Reduces urine volume and osmolality in patients with central diabetes insipidus by increasing reabsorption of water by kidney collecting tubules. Produces a dose-related increase in factor VIII (antihemophilic factor) and von Willebrand's factor.

USES To control and prevent symptoms and complications of central (neurohypophyseal) diabetes insipidus, and to relieve temporary polyuria and polydipsia associated with trauma or surgery in the pituitary region. **Unlabeled uses:** to increase factor VIII activity in selected patients with mild to moderate hemophilia A and in type I von Willebrand's disease or uremia, and to control enuresis in children.

ROUTE & DOSAGE

(0.1 ml = 10 μg)

Diabetes Insipidus

Adult: **Intranasal** 0.1–0.4 ml (10–40 μg) in 1–3 divided doses. **IV/SC** 2–4 μg in 2 divided doses. **PO** 0.2–0.4 mg/d.
Child: **Intranasal** *3 mo–12 y,* 0.05–0.3 ml in 1–2 divided doses. **IV/SC** 0.3 μg/kg infused over 15–30 min. **PO** 0.05 mg titrated to response.

Enuresis

Adult: **Intranasal** 5–40 μg h.s.
Child: **Intranasal** *3–12 y,* Same as for adult. **PO** *≥6 y,* 0.2 mg h.s., may titrate up to 0.6 mg h.s.

Von Willebrand's Disease

Adult: **IV/SC** 0.3 μg/kg 30 min preop; may repeat in 48 h if needed.
Child >3 mo: **IV/SC** Same as for adult.

PHARMACOKINETICS Absorption: 10–20% absorbed through nasal mucosa. **Onset:** 15–60 min. **Peak:** 1–5 h. **Duration:** 5–21 h. **Distribution:** small amount crosses blood–brain barrier; distributed into breast milk. **Elimination:** half-life: 76 min.

CONTRAINDICATIONS & PRECAUTIONS Contraindicated in: nephrogenic diabetes insipidus, type II B von Willebrand's disease. Safe use during pregnancy (category B) and in nursing mothers not established. **Cautious use in:** coronary artery insufficiency, hypertensive cardiovascular disease.

ADVERSE/SIDE EFFECTS Dose-related. **CNS:** transient headache, drowsiness, listlessness. **ENT:** nasal congestion, rhinitis, nasal irritation. **GI:**

nausea, heartburn, mild abdominal cramps. **Other:** vulval pain, shortness of breath, slight rise in BP, facial flushing, pain and swelling at injection site.

DRUG INTERACTIONS **Demeclocycline, lithium,** other VASOPRESSORS may decrease antidiuretic response; **carbamazepine, chlorpropamide, clofibrate** may prolong antidiuretic response.

NURSING IMPLICATIONS

Administration

- Note that 0.2 mg PO = 10 μg (0.1 ml) intranasal.
- Follow manufacturer's instructions for proper technique with nasal spray.
- Initial dose is usually administered in the evening, and antidiuretic effect observed. Dose is increased each evening until uninterrupted sleep is obtained. If daily urine volume is more than 2 L after nocturia is controlled, morning dose is started and adjusted daily until urine volume does not exceed 1.5–2 L/24 h.
- IV administration for diabetes insipidus: Desmopressin may be given undiluted by direct IV over 30 s.
- IV administration for von Willebrand's disease (type I): Dilute 0.3 μg/kg in 10 ml of NS (children ≤ 10 kg) or 50 ml of NS (children > 10 kg and adults) and infuse over 15–30 min.
- IV administration to infants and children: Verify correct IV concentration and rate of infusion/injection with physician.
- Store parenteral and nasal solution in refrigerator preferably at 4C (39.2F) unless otherwise directed. Avoid freezing. Nasal spray can be stored at room temperature. Discard solutions that are discolored or contain particulate matter.

Assessment & Drug Effects

- Monitor I&O ratio and pattern (intervals). Fluid intake must be carefully controlled, particularly in the elderly and in the very young to avoid water retention and sodium depletion.
- Weigh patient daily and observe for edema. Severe water retention may require reduction in dosage and use of a diuretic.
- Monitor BP during dosage-regulating period and whenever drug is administered parenterally.
- Therapeutic effectiveness is judged by control of polyuria and nocturia and relief of polydipsia.
- Monitor urine osmolality and plasma osmolality. An increase in urine osmolality and a decrease in plasma osmolality indicate effectiveness of treatment in diabetes insipidus.

Patient & Family Education

- Report upper respiratory tract infection or nasal congestion.
- Demonstrate administration technique to patient. Follow manufacturer's instructions to ensure delivery of drug high into nasal cavity and not down throat. A flexible calibrated plastic tube is provided.

DESONIDE

(dess′oh-nide)

Trade names: DesOwen, Tridesilon

Classifications: SKIN AND MUCOUS MEMBRANE; ANTIINFLAMMATORY; STEROID

Prototype: Hydrocortisone

Pregnancy category: C

See Appendix A.

D

DESOXIMETASONE

(des-ox-i-met′a-sone)

Trade names: Topicort, Topicort-LP

Classifications: SKIN AND MUCOUS MEMBRANE; ANTIINFLAMMATORY; STEROID

Prototype: Hydrocortisone

Pregnancy category: C

See Appendix A.

DEXAMETHASONE

(dex-a-meth′a-sone)

Trade names: Aeroseb-Dex, Decaderm, Decadron, Decaspray, Deronil ✦, Dexameth, Dexamethasone Intensol, Dexasone, Dexone, Hexadrol, Maxidex, Mymethasone, Oradexon ✦

DEXAMETHASONE ACETATE

Trade names: Dalalone D.P., Dalalone-LA, Decadron-LA, Decaject-LA, Dexacen LA-8, Dexasone-LA, Dexo-LA, Dexon LA, Dexone LA, Solurex-LA

DEXAMETHASONE SODIUM PHOSPHATE

Trade names: Ak-Dex, Alba Dex, Dalalone, Decadrol, Decadron Phosphate, Decaject, Dex-4, Dexacen-4, Dexasone, Dexon, Dexone, Hexadrol Phosphate, Maxidex Ophthalmic, Savacort-D, Solurex

Classifications: HORMONE; SYNTHETIC ADRENAL CORTICOSTEROID; GLUCOCORTICOID; STEROID

Prototype: Prednisone

Pregnancy category: C

ACTIONS/PHARMACODYNAMICS

Long-acting synthetic adrenocorticoid with intense antiinflammatory (glucocorticoid) activity and minimal mineralocorticoid activity. ***Antiinflammatory action:*** prevents accumulation of inflammatory cells at sites of infection; inhibits phagocytosis, lysosomal enzyme release, and synthesis of selected chemical mediators of inflammation; reduces capillary dilation and permeability. ***Immunosuppression:*** not clearly understood, but may be due to prevention or suppression of delayed hypersensitivity immune reaction.

USES Adrenal insufficiency concomitantly with a mineralocorticoid; inflammatory conditions, allergic states, collagen diseases, hematologic disorders, cerebral edema, and addisonian shock. Also palliative treatment of neoplastic disease, as adjunctive short-term therapy in acute rheumatic disorders and GI diseases, and as a diagnostic test for Cushing's syndrome and for differential diagnosis of adrenal hyperplasia and adrenal adenoma. **Unlabeled uses:** as an antiemetic in cancer chemotherapy; as a diagnostic test for endogenous depression; and to prevent hyaline membrane disease in prematures.

ROUTE & DOSAGE

Allergies, Inflammation, Neoplasias

Adult: **PO** 0.25–4 mg b.i.d. to q.i.d. **IM** 8–16 mg q1–3 wk or 0.8–1.6 mg intralesional q1–3wk.
Child: **PO/IM/IV** 0.08–0.3 mg/kg/d divided q6–12h.

Cerebral Edema

Adult: **IV** 10 mg followed by 4 mg q4h; reduce dose after 2–4 d; then taper over 5–7 d.
Child: **PO/IM/IV** 1–2 mg/kg loading dose, then 1–1.5 mg/kg/d divided q4–6h (max 16 mg/d).

Shock

Adult: **IV** 1–6 mg/kg as a single dose *or* 40 mg repeated q2–6h if needed.

Dexamethasone Suppression Test

Adult: **PO** 0.5 mg q6h for 48 h.

Inflammation

Adult: **Ophthalmic/topical/oral inhalation/intranasal** See Appendix A.
Child: **Oral inhalation/intranasal** See Appendix A.

PHARMACOKINETICS **Absorption:** readily absorbed from GI tract. **Onset:** rapid onset. **Peak:** 1–2 h PO; 8 h IM. **Duration:** 2.75 d PO; 6 d IM; 1–3 wk intralesional, intraarticular. **Distribution:** crosses placenta; distributed into breast milk. **Elimination:** half-life: 3–4.5 h; hypothalamus-pituitary axis suppression: 36–54 h.

CONTRAINDICATIONS & PRECAUTIONS **Contraindicated in:** systemic fungal infection, acute infections, active or resting tuberculosis, vaccinia, varicella, administration of live virus vaccines (to patient, family members), latent or active amebiasis. ***Ophthalmic use:*** primary open-angle glaucoma, eye infections, superficial ocular herpes simplex, keratitis and tuberculosis of eye. Safe use during pregnancy (category C), in nursing mothers, and in children not established. **Cautious use in:** stromal herpes simplex, keratitis, GI ulceration, renal disease, diabetes mellitus, hypothyroidism, myasthenia gravis, CHF, cirrhosis, psychic disorders, seizures.

ADVERSE/SIDE EFFECTS ***Aerosol therapy:*** *nasal irritation,* dryness, epistaxis, rebound congestion, bronchial asthma, anosomia, perforation of nasal septum. ***Systemic absorption:*** **CNS:** euphoria, insomnia, convulsions, increased ICP, vertigo, headache, psychic disturbances. **CV:** CHF, hypertension, *edema.* **Endocrine:** menstrual irregularities, *hyperglycemia;* cushingoid state; growth suppression in children; hirsutism. **Eye:** *posterior subcapsular cataract,* increased IOP, glaucoma, exophthalmos. **GI:** peptic ulcer with possible perforation, abdominal distension, nausea, increased appetite, heartburn, dyspepsia, pancreatitis, <u>bowel perforation</u>, *oral candidiasis.* **Musculoskeletal:** muscle weakness, loss of muscle mass, <u>vertebral compression fracture</u>, pathologic fracture of long bones, tendon rupture. **Skin:** acne, *impaired wound healing,* petechiae, ecchymoses, diaphoresis, allergic dermatitis, hypo- or hyperpigmentation, SC and cutaneous atrophy, burning and tingling in perineal area (following IV injection).

DIAGNOSTIC TEST INTERFERENCE ***Dexamethasone suppression test for endogenous depression:*** false-positive results may be caused by **alcohol, glutethimide, meprobamate;** false-negative results may be caused by high doses of BENZODIAZEPINES (e.g., **chlordiazepoxide** and **cyproheptadine**), long-term GLUCOCORTICOID treatment, **indomethacin, ephedrine,** ESTROGENS or HEPATIC ENZYME–INDUCING AGENTS **(phenytoin)** may also cause false-positive results in ***test for Cushing's syndrome.***

DRUG INTERACTIONS BARBITURATES, **phenytoin, rifampin** increase steroid metabolism—dosage of dexamethasone may need to be increased; **amphotericin B,** DIURETICS compound potassium loss; **ambenonium, neostigmine, pyri-**

D

dostigmine may cause severe muscle weakness in patients with myasthenia gravis; may inhibit antibody response to VACCINES, TOXOIDS.

INCOMPATIBILITIES Solution/additive: daunorubicin, doxorubicin, doxapram, glycopyrrolate, metaraminol, vancomycin.

NURSING IMPLICATIONS

Administration

- Once-daily oral doses should be administered in the AM with food or liquid of patient's choice.
- Administer IM injection deep into a large muscle mass (e.g., gluteus maximus). Avoid SC injection: atrophy and sterile abscesses may occur.
- The repository form, dexamethasone acetate (for IM or local injection only), is a white suspension that settles on standing; mild shaking will resuspend the drug.
- IV administration: Dexamethasone may be given undiluted by direct IV over 30 seconds or less. Drug may be added to an infusion of D5W or NS and administered over a prescribed period.
- IV administration to infants and children: Verify correct IV concentration and rate of infusion/injection with physician.
- Because adrenal suppression can occur with prolonged use, dosage should be tapered over a period of time before it is discontinued.
- Do not store or expose aerosol to temperature above 48.9C (120F); do not puncture or discard into a fire or an incinerator.
- Store at 15–30C (59–86F) unless otherwise directed.

Assessment & Drug Effects

- Cushing's syndrome (see Appendix G) and other systemic effects can occur. Monitor and report signs and symptoms.
- Hiccups occurring for several hours following each drug dose constitute an annoying complication of high-dose oral dexamethasone (treatment regimen of the cancer patient).
- The neonate born to a mother who has been receiving a corticosteroid during pregnancy should be monitored for symptoms of hypoadrenocorticism.
- The acetate and sodium phosphate formulations may contain bisulfites or parabens or both. These inactive ingredients are allergenic to some individuals. Monitor for signs and symptoms of a hypersensitivity reaction (see Appendix G).

Patient & Family Education

- Make certain patient is aware of the importance of taking dexamethasone exactly as prescribed.
- Lack of response to the medication may signal hypoadrenocorticism and be evidenced by malaise, orthostatic hypotension, muscular weakness and pain, nausea, vomiting, anorexia, hypoglycemic reactions (see Appendix G), mental depression. Patient should be instructed to report these symptoms.
- Symptoms of early hyperadrenocorticism may be subtle: increased appetite and weight gain, increased facial hair (women), full-looking face (moon facies), abdominal distension, easy bruising, extreme weakness, amenorrhea. Alert patient (and family) to potential changes in appearance; physician should be contacted if they appear.
- Electrolytes and BP should be evaluated during therapy at regular intervals. Urge patient to keep appointments for check-ups.
- If patient is also receiving a potassium-depleting diuretic, dexa-

methasone-induced potassium loss may be enhanced. Encourage patient to add potassium-rich foods to diet and to report signs of hypokalemia (see Appendix G).

- The dexamethasone dose regimen may need to be altered if patient is subjected to stress; e.g., surgery, infections, emotional stress, illness, acute bronchial attacks, trauma. Consult physician if change in living or working environment is anticipated.
- Inform patient that discontinuation of dexamethasone should be accomplished gradually and under the guidance of the physician.
- Emphasize the implications of immunosuppression with regard to prevention of exposure to infection, trauma, and to sudden changes in environmental factors.

DEXCHLORPHENIRAMINE MALEATE

(dex-klor-fen-eer′a-meen)

Trade names: Dexchlor, Poladex T.D., Polaramine, Polargen

Classification: ANTIHISTAMINE (H_1-RECEPTOR ANTAGONIST)

Prototype: Diphenhydramine

Pregnancy category: B

ACTIONS/PHARMACODYNAMICS H_1-receptor antagonist and alkylamine antihistamine. In common with other antihistamines, has anticholinergic properties and produces mild to moderate drowsiness and sedation.

USES Perennial and seasonal allergic rhinitis, other manifestations of allergy, and vasomotor rhinitis. Also as adjunct to epinephrine in treatment of anaphylactic reactions.

ROUTE & DOSAGE

Allergic Rhinitis

Adult: **PO** 2 mg q4–6h *or* 4–6 mg of repeat-action tablets h.s. *or* q8–10h during the day.
Child: **PO** *6–11 y,* 1 mg q4–6h (not to exceed 6 mg/24 h) *or* 4 mg of repeat-action tablets h.s.; *2–5 y,* 0.5 mg q4–6h (not to exceed 3 mg/24 h).

PHARMACOKINETICS **Absorption:** readily absorbed from GI tract. **Onset:** 15–30 min. **Peak:** 3 h. **Distribution:** small amounts distributed into breast milk. **Metabolism:** metabolized in liver. **Elimination:** excreted in urine within 24 h.

CONTRAINDICATIONS & PRECAUTIONS **Contraindicated in:** hypersensitivity to antihistamines of similar class; acute asthmatic attack, lower respiratory tract symptoms, newborns, premature infants. Safe use during pregnancy (category B) and in nursing mothers not established. **Cautious use in:** increased intraocular pressure; prostatic hypertrophy; hyperthyroidism; renal and cardiovascular disease, elderly patients.

ADVERSE/SIDE EFFECTS **CNS:** *drowsiness,* dizziness, weakness, headache, excitation, neuritis, disturbed coordination, insomnia, euphoria, paresthesias. **ENT:** vertigo, tinnitus, acute labyrinthitis. **CV:** palpitation, tachycardia, hypotension, extrasystoles. **GI:** nausea, vomiting, anorexia, *dry mouth,* constipation, diarrhea. **GU:** difficulty in urinating, *urinary retention,* urinary frequency, early menses. **Hematologic:** agranulocytosis (rare), hemolytic or hypoplastic anemia. **Other:** blurred vision, skin eruptions, photosensitivity.

DIAGNOSTIC TEST INTERFERENCE In common with other antihistamines, dexchlorpheniramine may interfere with ***skin tests for allergy;*** discontinue dexchlorpheniramine at least 72 h before tests.

DRUG INTERACTIONS **Alcohol** and other CNS DEPRESSANTS, MAO INHIBITORS compound CNS depression.

NURSING IMPLICATIONS

Administration

- Advise patient to take medication with food, water, or milk to lessen GI distress.
- Regular tablet may be crushed and taken with fluid or mixed with food.
- Store at 15–30C (59–86F) unless otherwise directed.

Assessment & Drug Effects

- Supervise ambulation and take safety precautions.
- Monitor I&O and assess for difficulty voiding (e.g., frequency or retention).

Patient & Family Education

- Instruct patient to swallow timed-release tablet whole. It should not be broken, crushed, or chewed.
- Because of the possibility of drowsiness, dizziness, and blurred vision, caution patient to avoid driving and other potentially hazardous activities until reaction to drug is known.
- Advise patient to ask physician about the use of alcohol, tranquilizers, sedatives, or other CNS depressants because the effects of dexchlorpheniramine will be additive.
- Dexchlorpheniramine should be discontinued about 4 d before skin tests for allergies, since it can affect test results, making them inaccurate.

DEXPANTHENOL (PANTOTHENIC ACID)

(dex-pan′the-nole)

Trade names: Dexol, Ilopan, Panthoderm

Classifications: AUTONOMIC NERVOUS SYSTEM AGENT; CHOLINERGIC, DIRECT ACTING; VITAMIN B COMPLEX

Prototype: Bethanechol

Pregnancy category: C

ACTIONS/PHARMACODYNAMICS Alcohol analog of the coenzyme vitamin pantothenic acid, to which it is readily converted. A member of the B-complex group and precursor of coenzyme A, which is essential to normal epithelial function and biosynthesis of fatty acids, amino acids, and acetylcholine. Increases GI peristalsis and intestinal tone by stimulating acetylation of choline to acetylcholine. Topical application reportedly relieves itching and may aid healing of skin lesions by stimulating epithelialization and granulation. Also has antibacterial activity.

USES Prevention or treatment of postoperative abdominal distention, intestinal atony, and paralytic ileus. Topically to relieve itching and to promote healing in minor skin lesions.

ROUTE & DOSAGE

Postoperative Abdominal Distension, Intestinal Atony, Paralytic Ileus

Adult: **IM** 250–500 mg; repeat in 2 h; then repeat q4–12h prn. **IV** 500 mg by slow IV infusion.
Child: **IM** 11–12.5 mg/kg; repeat in 2 h; then repeat q4– 12h prn.

Itching
Adult: **Topical** Apply to affected area 1–2 times/d.

PHARMACOKINETICS Absorption: readily absorbed from IM site. **Distribution:** highest concentration in liver, adrenals, heart, and kidneys; small amount distributed into breast milk. **Metabolism:** rapidly converted to pantothenic acid, the active moiety. **Elimination:** 70% excreted in urine, 30% in feces.

CONTRAINDICATIONS & PRECAUTIONS Contraindicated in: hemophilia; ileus due to mechanical obstruction. Safe use during pregnancy (category C), in nursing women, and in children not established. **Cautious use in:** hypokalemia.

ADVERSE/SIDE EFFECTS Generally well tolerated.

DRUG INTERACTION Prolongs muscle relaxation effects of **succinylcholine.**

NURSING IMPLICATIONS

Administration

- Do not administer within 1 h of succinylcholine administration.
- IV dexpanthenol is not intended for direct IV adminstration.
- IV dexpanthenol is diluted in at least 500 ml of D5W or lactated Ringer's solution and infused slowly over 3–6 h.
- Store at 15–30C (59–86F); protect from freezing and excessive heat.

Assessment & Drug Effects

- Observe for and report bleeding tendency. Dexpanthenol may prolong bleeding time in some patients.
- Report immediately any evidence of a hypersensitivity reaction (see Appendix G); drug should be discontinued.
- Therapeutic results may not be obtained in patients with hypokalemia.

Patient & Family Education

- Instruct patient to report abdominal cramping or diarrhea.

DEXRAZOXANE

(dex-ra-zox′ane)
Trade name: Zinecard
Classification: CARDIOPROTECTIVE FOR DOXORUBICIN
Pregnancy category: C

ACTIONS/PHARMACODYNAMICS Dexrazoxane is a derivative of EDTA that readily penetrates cell membranes. The mechanism by which dexrazoxane exerts its cardioprotective activity is not fully understood. Dexrazoxane is converted intracellularly to a chelating agent that interferes with iron-mediated free radical generation thought to be partially responsible for one form of cardiomyopathy.

USES Reduction of the incidence and severity of cardiomyopathy associated with doxorubicin in women with metastatic breast cancer who have received a cumulative doxorubicin dose of 300 mg/m^2.

ROUTE & DOSAGE

Cardiomyopathy
Adult: **IV** 10 parts dexrazoxane to 1 part doxorubicin or 500 mg/m^2 for every 50 mg/m^2 of doxorubicin, repeated q3wk. Administer by slow IV push or rapid IV infusion in 0.9% NaCl or D5W (must use within 6 h of reconstitution). Doxorubicin should be started within 30 min of beginning dexrazoxane.

PHARMACOKINETICS Distribution: not bound to plasma proteins. **Metabolism:** metabolized in liver. **Elimination:** half-life: 2–2.5 h; 42% excreted in urine.

D

CONTRAINDICATIONS & PRECAUTIONS Contraindicated in: chemotherapy regimens that do not contain anthracycline, nursing mothers. **Cautious use in:** myelosuppresion, pregnancy (category C). Safety and efficacy in children have not been established.

ADVERSE/SIDE EFFECTS It is difficult to distinguish the adverse effects of dexrazoxane from those of the chemotherapeutic agents. Pain at injection site, leukopenia, granulocytopenia, and thrombocytopenia appear to occur more frequently with the addition of dexrazoxane than with placebo.

NURSING IMPLICATIONS

Administration

- Gloves are recommended when handling dexrazoxane. Immediately wash with soap and water if drug contacts skin or mucosa.
- IV preparation: Reconstitute by adding 25 or 50 ml of 0.167 M sodium lactate injection (provided by manufacturer) to the 250- or 500-mg vial, respectively, to produce a 10-mg/ml solution. This may be further diluted in 0.9% NaCl or D5W in an IV bag to a concentration of 1.3–5.0 mg/ml for infusion.
- IV injection: The 10 mg/ml solution may be administered by slow IV push.
- IV infusion: The 1.3–5 mg/ml solution may be administered by rapid IV infusion.

Assessment & Drug Effects

- Monitor cardiac function as drug does not eliminate risk of doxorubicin cardiotoxicity.
- Monitor hepatic, renal, and hematopoietic status throughout course of therapy.
- Adverse effects are likely due to concurrent cytotoxic drugs rather than dexrazoxane.

DEXTRAN 40

(dex′tran)

Trade names: Gentran 40, Hyskon, 10% LMD, Rheomacrodex

Classifications: BLOOD DERIVATIVE; PLASMA VOLUME EXPANDER; REPLACEMENT SOLUTION

Prototype: Albumin

Pregnancy category: C

ACTIONS/PHARMACODYNAMICS Low-molecular-weight polysaccharide. As a hypertonic colloidal solution, produces immediate and short-lived expansion of plasma volume by increasing colloidal osmotic pressure and drawing fluid from interstitial to intravascular spaces. Cardiovascular response to volume expansion includes increased BP, pulse pressure, CVP, cardiac output, venous return to heart, and urinary output. Reduces possibility of deep venous thrombosis and pulmonary embolism, primarily by inhibiting venous stasis and platelet adhesiveness.

USES Adjunctively to expand plasma volume and provide fluid replacement in treatment of shock or impending shock caused by hemorrhage, burns, surgery, or other trauma. Also used in prophylaxis and therapy of venous thrombosis and pulmonary embolism. Used as priming fluid or as additive to other primers during extracorporeal circulation.

ROUTE & DOSAGE

Shock

Adult: **IV** 500 ml administered rapidly (over 15–30 min); additional doses may be given more slowly up to 20 ml/kg in the first 24 h; doses up to 10 ml/kg/d may be given for an additional 4 d if needed.
Child: **IV** Total dose ≤20 ml/kg in first 24 h and ≤10 ml/kg/d for max of 5 d total.

Prophylaxis for Thromboembolic Complications

Adult: **IV** 500–1000 ml (10 ml/kg) on the day of operation followed by 500 ml/d for 2–3 d; may continue with 500 ml q2–3d for up to 2 wk if necessary.

Priming for Extracorporeal Circulation

Adult: **IV** 10–20 ml/kg added to perfusion circuit.

PHARMACOKINETICS **Onset:** volume expansion within minutes of infusion. **Duration:** 12 h. **Metabolism:** degraded to glucose and metabolized to CO_2 and water over a period of a few weeks. **Elimination:** 75% excreted in urine within 24 h; small amount excreted in feces.

CONTRAINDICATIONS & PRECAUTIONS **Contraindicated in:** hypersensitivity to dextrans, renal failure, hypervolemic conditions, severe CHF, thrombocytopenia, significant anemia, hypofibrinogenemia or other marked hemostatic defects including those caused by drugs, e.g., heparin, warfarin, pregnancy (category C). **Cautious use in:** active hemorrhage; severe dehydration; chronic liver disease; impaired renal function; patients susceptible to pulmonary edema or CHF.

ADVERSE/SIDE EFFECTS **Hypersensitivity:** mild to generalized urticaria, pruritus, anaphylactic shock (rare), angioedema, dyspnea. **Other:** renal tubular vacuolization (osmotic nephrosis), stasis, and blocking; oliguria, renal failure; increased AST and ALT, interference with platelet function, prolonged bleeding and coagulation times.

DIAGNOSTIC TEST INTERFERENCE When blood samples are drawn for study, notify laboratory that patient has received dextran. ***Blood glucose:*** false increases (utilizing ortho-toluidine methods or sulfuric or acetic acid hydrolysis). ***Urinary protein:*** false increases (utilizing Lowry method). ***Bilirubin assays:*** false increases when alcohol is used. ***Total protein assays:*** false increases using biuret reagent. ***Rh testing, blood typing*** and ***cross-matching*** procedures: dextran may interfere with results (by inducing rouleaux formation) when proteolytic enzyme techniques are used (saline agglutination and indirect antiglobulin methods reportedly not affected).

NURSING IMPLICATIONS

Administration

- Use only if seal is intact, vacuum is detectable, and solution is absolutely clear.
- If blood is to be administered, a cross-match specimen should be drawn before dextran infusion.
- Specific flow rate should be prescribed by physician. Usually administered at a rate of 500 ml over 15–30 min.
- Dextran should be stored at a constant temperature, preferably 25C (77F). Once opened, unused portion should be discarded because dextran contains no preservative.

D

Assessment & Drug Effects

- Patient's state of hydration should be evaluated before dextran therapy begins. Administration of dextran to severely dehydrated patients can result in renal failure.
- Baseline Hct should be taken prior to and after initiation of dextran (dextran usually lowers Hct). Notify physician if Hct is depressed below 30% by volume.
- Hypersensitivity reaction is most likely to occur during the first few minutes of administration. Monitor vital signs and observe patient closely for at least the first 30 min of infusion. Therapy should be terminated at the first sign of a hypersensitivity reaction (see Appendix G).
- Monitoring CVP is advised as an estimate of blood volume status and as a guide for determining dosage. Normal CVP: 5–10 cm H_2O.
- Observe patient for clinical signs of circulatory overload (see Appendix G).
- In patients for whom sodium restriction is indicated, it should be noted that 500 ml of dextran 40 in 0.9% normal saline contains 77 mEq of both sodium and chloride.
- Monitor I&O ratio and check urine specific gravity at regular intervals. Low urine specific gravity may signify failure of renal dextran clearance and is an indication for discontinuing therapy.
- In poorly hydrated patients, dextran may attract water from extravascular spaces and cause dehydration. Monitor for signs of dehydration (see Appendix G).
- Report oliguria, anuria, or lack of improvement in urinary output (dextran usually causes an increase in urinary output). Dextran should be discontinued at the first indication of renal dysfunction.
- Transient prolongation of bleeding time and interference with normal blood coagulation may occur with high doses.

DEXTRAN 70

(dex′tran)

Trade name: Macrodex

DEXTRAN 75

Trade name: Gentran 75

Classifications: BLOOD DERIVATIVE; PLASMA VOLUME EXPANDER; REPLACEMENT SOLUTION

Prototype: Albumin

Pregnancy category: C

ACTIONS/PHARMACODYNAMICS

High-molecular-weight polysaccharides. Dextran 70 has an average molecular weight of 70,000; that of dextran 75 is 75,000. Colloidal properties approximate those of serum albumin. Differs from dextran 40 in molecular weight and in having less effect on rouleaux formation and sludging of red blood cells and a higher incidence of severe allergic reactions.

USES Primarily for emergency treatment of hypovolemic shock or impending shock caused by hemorrhage, burns, surgery, or other trauma. Intended for emergency treatment only when whole blood or blood products are not available or when haste precludes cross-matching of blood. **Unlabeled uses:** nephrosis, toxemia of pregnancy, and prophylaxis of deep-vein thrombosis.

ROUTE & DOSAGE

Shock

Adult: **IV** 500 ml administered rapidly (over 15–30 min); additional doses may be given more slowly up to 20 ml/kg in the first 24 h; doses up to 10 ml/kg/d may be given for an additional 4 d if needed.

PHARMACOKINETICS **Onset:** volume expansion within minutes of infusion. **Duration:** 12 h. **Metabolism:** degraded to glucose and metabolized to carbon dioxide and water over a period of a few weeks. **Elimination:** 75% excreted in urine within 24 h; small amount excreted in feces.

CONTRAINDICATIONS & PRECAUTIONS **Contraindicated in:** known hypersensitivity to dextrans; severe bleeding disorders; severe CHF; renal failure; pregnancy (category C).

ADVERSE/SIDE EFFECTS *Allergic reactions*, urticaria, wheezing, mild hypotension, nausea, vomiting, fever, arthralgia, severe anaphylactoid reaction.

NURSING IMPLICATIONS

Administration

- Use only if seal is intact, vacuum is detectable, and solution is absolutely clear.
- Specific flow rate should be prescribed by physician. (For emergency treatment of shock, rate of administration for first 500 ml may be 20–40 ml/min. In normovolemic patients, flow rate should not exceed 4 ml/min.)
- Store at a constant temperature, preferably 25C (77F).

Assessment & Drug Effects

- Bleeding time may be temporarily prolonged in patients receiving more than 1000 ml of dextran 70 or 75.
- Patient should be observed closely for signs of anaphylaxis (see Appendix G) especially during first 30 min of infusion. Severe reactions occasionally have resulted in fatalities.
- Monitor I&O ratio and pattern. Monitor vital signs frequently as warranted by condition of patient.

D

DEXTROAMPHETAMINE SULFATE

(dex-troe-am-fet′a-meen)

Trade names: Dexampex, Dexedrine, Oxydess II ♣, Spancap No. 1

Classifications: CNS AGENT; RESPIRATORY AND CEREBRAL STIMULANT; AMPHETAMINE; ANOREXIANT

Prototype: Amphetamine

Controlled substance: Schedule II

ACTIONS/PHARMACODYNAMICS Dextrorotatory isomer of amphetamine, with which it shares actions, uses, contraindications, precautions, and adverse reactions. On a weight basis, has less pronounced action on cardiovascular and peripheral nervous systems and is a more potent appetite suppressant. CNS stimulating effect approximately twice that of racemic amphetamine. Anorexigenic effect is thought to result from CNS stimulation and possibly from loss of acuity of smell and taste. In hyperkinetic children, amphetamines reduce motor restlessness by an unknown mechanism.

USES Adjunct in short-term treatment of exogenous obesity, narcolepsy, and attention deficit disorder with hyperactivity in children (also called minimal brain dysfunction or hyperkinetic syndrome). **Unlabeled uses:** adjunct in epilepsy to control ataxia and drowsiness induced by barbiturates; to combat sedative effects of trimethadione in absence seizures.

D

ROUTE & DOSAGE

Narcolepsy

Adult: **PO** 5–20 mg 1–3 times/d at 4–6 h intervals.
Child: **PO** >12 y, 10 mg/d; may increase by 10 mg at weekly intervals; 6–12 y, 5 mg/d; may increase by 5 mg at weekly intervals.

Attention Deficit Disorder

Child: **PO** ≥ 6 y, 5 mg 1–2 times/d; may increase by 5 mg at weekly intervals (max 40 mg/d); 3–5 y, 2.5 mg 1–2 times/d; may increase by 2.5 mg at weekly intervals.

Obesity

Adult: **PO** 5–10 mg 1–3 times/d *or* 10–15 mg of sustained release once/d 30–60 min a.c.

PHARMACOKINETICS **Absorption:** rapid. **Peak:** 1–5 h. **Duration:** up to 10 h. **Distribution:** all tissues especially the CNS. **Metabolism:** metabolized in liver. **Elimination:** half-life: 10–30 h; renal elimination; excreted in breast milk.

CONTRAINDICATIONS & PRECAUTIONS **Contraindicated in:** hypersensitivity to sympathomimetic amines, glaucoma, agitated states, psychoses (especially in children), advanced arteriosclerosis, symptomatic heart disease, moderate to severe hypertension, hyperthyroidism, history of drug abuse, during or within 14 d of MAO INHIBITOR therapy, as anorexiant in children <12 y, for attention deficit disorder in children <3 y, lactation. **Cautious use in:** pregnancy (category C). Safety and efficacy in children < 3 y have not been established.

ADVERSE/SIDE EFFECTS **CNS:** nervousness, *restlessness,* hyperactivity, *insomnia,* euphoria, dizziness, headache; ***With prolonged use:*** severe depression, psychotic reactions. **CV:** palpitation, tachycardia, elevated BP. **GI:** dry mouth, unpleasant taste, anorexia, weight loss, diarrhea, constipation, abdominal pain. **Other:** impotence, changes in libido, unusual fatigue, increased intraocular pressure, marked dystonia of head, neck, and extremities; sweating.

DIAGNOSTIC TEST INTERFERENCE Dextroamphetamine may cause significant elevations in ***plasma corticosteroids*** (evening levels are highest) and increases in ***urinary epinephrine*** excretion (during first 3 h after drug administration).

DRUG INTERACTIONS **Acetazolamide, sodium bicarbonate** decrease dextroamphetamine elimination; **ammonium chloride, ascorbic acid** increase dextroamphetamine elimination; effects of both BARBITURATES and dextroamphetamine may be antagonized; **furazolidone** may increase BP effects of amphetamines—interaction may persist for several weeks after discontinuing furazolidone; antagonizes antihypertensive effects of **guanethidine, guanadryl;** MAO INHIBITORS, **selegiline** can cause hypertensive crisis (fatalities reported)—do not administer amphetamines during or within 14 d of these drugs; PHENOTHIAZINES may inhibit mood elevating effects of amphetamines; TRICYCLIC ANTIDEPRESSANTS enhance dextroamphetamine effects because of increased norepinephrine release; BETA-ADRENERGIC AGONISTS increase cardiovascular adverse effects.

NURSING IMPLICATIONS

Administration

- Administer 30–60 min before meals for treatment of obesity. Long-acting form is administered in the morning.
- To avoid insomnia, administer last dose no later than 6 h before patient retires (10–14 h before bedtime for sustained-release form).
- Store in tightly closed containers at 15–30C (59–86F) unless otherwise directed.

Assessment & Drug Effects

- Growth rate should be closely monitored in children.
- Periodic interruption of therapy or reduction in dosage is recommended to assess effectiveness of therapy in behavior disorders.
- Tolerance to anorexiant effects may develop after a few weeks; however, tolerance does not appear to develop when dextroamphetamine is used in treatment of narcolepsy.

Patient & Family Education

- Instruct patient to swallow sustained-release capsule whole with a liquid and not to chew or crush it.
- Inform patient that drug may impair ability to drive or perform other potentially hazardous activities.
- Discontinuation of drug following long-term use should be accomplished gradually to avoid extreme fatigue, mental depression, and prolonged sleep pattern that follows abrupt withdrawal.

DEXTROMETHORPHAN HYDROBROMIDE

(dex-troe-meth-or'fan)

Trade names: Balminil DM ♣, Benylin DM, Cremacoat 1, Delsym, DM Cough, Hold, Koffex ♣, Mediquell, Neo-DM ♣, Ornex DM ♣, Pedia Care, Pertussin 8 Hour Cough Formula, Robidex ♣, Robitussin DM, Romilar CF, Romilar Children's Cough, Sedatuss ♣, Sucrets Cough Control

Classification: ANTITUSSIVE

Prototype: Benzonatate

Pregnancy category: C

ACTIONS/PHARMACODYNAMICS Nonnarcotic derivative of levorphanol. Chemically related to morphine but without central hypnotic or analgesic effect or capacity to cause tolerance or addiction. Controls cough spasms by depressing cough center in medulla. Antitussive activity comparable to that of codeine but is less likely than codeine to cause constipation, drowsiness, or GI disturbances.

USE Temporary relief of cough spasms in nonproductive coughs due to colds, pertussis, and influenza.

ROUTE & DOSAGE

Cough

Adult: **PO** 10–20 mg q4h *or* 30 mg q6–8h (max 120 mg/d); *or* 60 mg of sustained-action liquid b.i.d.
Child: **PO** *6–12 y,* 5–10 mg q4h *or* 15 mg q6–8h (max 60 mg/d) *or* 30 mg sustained-action liquid b.i.d.; *2–6 y,* 2.5–5 mg q4h *or* 7.5 mg q6–8h (max 30 mg/d) *or* 15 mg sustained-action liquid b.i.d.

PHARMACOKINETICS **Absorption:** readily absorbed from GI tract. **Onset:** 15–30 min. **Duration:** 3–6 h. **Metabolism:** metabolized in liver. **Elimination:** excreted in urine.

CONTRAINDICATIONS & PRECAUTIONS **Contraindicated in:** children

<2 y, asthma, productive cough, persistent or chronic cough; hepatic function impairment; pregnancy (category C). **Cautious use in:** chronic pulmonary disease; enlarged prostate; patients on MAO INHIBITORS.

ADVERSE/SIDE EFFECTS Dizziness, drowsiness, CNS depression with very large doses; excitability, especially in children; GI upset, constipation, abdominal discomfort.

DRUG INTERACTIONS High risk of excitation, hypotension, and hyperpyrexia with MAO INHIBITORS.

NURSING IMPLICATIONS

Administration

- Although soothing local effect of the syrup may be enhanced if administered undiluted, depression of cough center depends only on systemic absorption of drug.

Patient & Family Education

- Unnecessary cough may be lessened by avoiding irritants such as smoking, dust, fumes, and other air pollutants. Humidification of ambient air may provide some relief.
- Treatment is directed toward decreasing the frequency and intensity of cough without completely eliminating protective cough reflex.
- Dextromethorphan can be purchased over the counter. Advise patient that any cough persisting longer than 1 wk or 10 d should be medically diagnosed.

DEXTROTHYROXINE SODIUM

(dex-troe-thye-rox'een)

Trade name: Choloxin

Classifications: CARDIOVASCULAR DRUG; ANTILIPEMIC; LIPID-LOWERING AGENT

Prototype: Lovastatin

Pregnancy category: C

ACTIONS/PHARMACODYNAMICS Sodium salt and dextrorotatory isomer of thyroxine. Reduces serum cholesterol and LDL levels in hyperlipidemia; triglycerides and beta lipoproteins may also be lowered from previously elevated levels, but effect is variable. By an unclear mechanism, liver is stimulated to increase catabolism and excretion of cholesterol and its degradation products via the biliary route into feces. Greatest decrease in serum cholesterol occurs in patients with highest baseline concentrations, with maximum therapeutic effects in 1 or 2 mo.

USES Adjunct to other medications in the treatment of primary hypercholesterolemia (type IIa hyperlipidemia), particularly euthyroid patients with significant risk but no evidence of coronary artery disease.

ROUTE & DOSAGE

Euthyroid Hyperlipidemia

Adult: **PO** 1–2 mg/d, increased by 1 or 2 mg every month if needed (max 8 mg/d). *Child:* **PO** 0.05 mg/kg/d, increased by not more than 0.05 mg/kg every month if needed (max 4 mg/d).

PHARMACOKINETICS Absorption: about 25% absorbed from GI tract. **Distribution:** crosses placenta; distribution into breast milk not known. **Metabolism:** metabolized in liver. **Elimination:** half-life: 18 h; excreted in urine and feces.

CONTRAINDICATIONS & PRECAUTIONS Contraindicated in: euthyroids: known organic heart disease including angina pectoris, arrhythmias, decompensated or borderline compensated cardiac states; history of MI or CHF; rheumatic heart disease; hypertension; advanced liver or kidney disease; history of iodism; pregnancy (category C), nursing mothers; 2 wk prior to elective surgery. **Cautious use in:** hypothyroid patients with concomitant coronary artery disease; women of childbearing age with familial hypercholesterolemia; diabetes mellitus; liver and kidney impairment; children, the elderly.

ADVERSE/SIDE EFFECTS Mainly due to increased metabolism. **CNS:** insomnia, nervousness, dizziness, psychic changes, paresthesias. **CV:** angina pectoris, palpitation, cardiac arrhythmia, ECG evidence of ischemic myocardial changes, increase in heart size; MI (relationship not conclusive), worsening of peripheral vascular disease. **ENT:** tinnitus, hoarseness. **Eye:** visual disturbances, exophthalmos, retinopathy, lid lag. **GI:** nausea, constipation, diarrhea, bitter taste, weight loss. **Iodism:** acneiform rash, pruritus, coryza, conjunctivitis, stomatitis, brassy taste, laryngitis, bronchitis.

DRUG INTERACTIONS **Cholestyramine, colestipol** decrease absorption of dextrothyroxine; compounds thyroid effects of other THYROID PREPARATIONS; increases risk of hypoprothrombinemia associated with **warfarin; digoxin** may enhance myocardial stimulation; may increase blood glucose, requiring adjustment of **insulin** and SULFONYLUREAS.

NURSING IMPLICATIONS

Administration

- Dextrothyroxine may be given at any time without respect to meals.
- Store medication in light- and moisture-proof container at 15–30C (59–86F) unless otherwise specified.

Assessment & Drug Effects

- Serum lipids should be determined initially and evaluated at periodic intervals during therapy. Patient should be on a normal diet for several days prior to the test.
- Initial decrease in cholesterol levels may not occur until 2 wk–1 mo after initiation of therapy. Maximum decrease usually occurs during second or third month of therapy.
- Patients with cardiac disease should be observed closely, particularly during early therapy, and checked at frequent intervals throughout the treatment period.
- Hypothyroid patients with organic heart disease have a high incidence of adverse/side effects.
- Report immediately new signs and symptoms of cardiac disease or increased decompensation in the borderline compensated patient. Dose adjustment may be indicated.
- Patients with diabetes should be closely monitored. Dosage adjustment of insulin or oral antidiabetic agent may be required. Advise patient to report diminishing control of diabetes.

Patient & Family Education

- Serum lipids generally return to pretreatment levels within 6 wk–3 mo after drug is withdrawn.
- Instruct patient to report chest pain, palpitations, sweating, diarrhea, headache, or skin rash.
- Advise patient to report promptly the onset of iodism (see adverse/side effects). If iodism is developing, the drug will be withdrawn.
- Instruct patient not to self-dose with OTC medications unless physician's approval is obtained.
- Patient should inform physician or dentist in an emergency situation that he or she is taking dextrothyroxine before any surgery is performed.

D

DEZOCINE

(de′zo-ceen)

Trade name: Dalgan

Classifications: CNS AGENT; NARCOTIC (OPIATE) AGONIST-ANTAGONIST; ANALGESIC

Prototype: Pentazocine

Pregnancy category: C

Controlled substance: Scedule IV

ACTIONS/PHARMACODYNAMICS

Dezocine is an agonist–antagonist opioid. It is comparable to morphine in analgesic potency, onset, and duration of action in the relief of postoperative pain. Because of its narcotic antagonist activity, dezocine may precipitate withdrawal symptoms in individuals with opiate dependence. Dezocine causes less respiratory depression and hypotension than morphine or pentazocine and no bronchoconstrictive or histamine-releasing activity following its administration.

USE Management of pain when the use of an opioid is appropriate.

ROUTE & DOSAGE

Adult: **IV** 2.5–10 mg; (usually 5 mg) q2–4h. **IM** 5–20 mg (usually 10 mg); may repeat q3–6h.

PHARMACOKINETICS Absorption: completely absorbed from IM site. **Onset:** 15–30 min. **Peak:** 10–90 min IM. **Duration:** 4–6 h. **Metabolism:** metabolized in liver. **Elimination:** half-life: 2.6 h; excreted in urine.

CONTRAINDICATIONS & PRECAUTIONS Contraindicated in: hypersensitivity to dezocine or structurally related drugs, concurrent use of CNS depressants. **Cautious use in:** COPD, chronic bronchitis, emphysema, head injury, increased intracranial pressure, pregnancy (category C).

ADVERSE/SIDE EFFECTS CNS: headache, dizziness, anxiety, euphoria, dysphoria, sedation. **CV:** bradycardia, hypotension. **GI:** *nausea, vomiting*. **Other:** miosis, pruritus, mild itching, drug dependence. **Respiratory:** respiratory depression.

DRUG INTERACTIONS BARBITURATES, other OPIATES, INHALATION GENERAL ANESTHETICS, and other CNS DEPRESSANTS may enhance the cardiovascular and CNS effects; MONOAMINE OXIDASE INHIBITORS should be avoided; increased respiratory depression when used with other OPIOIDS.

NURSING IMPLICATIONS

Administration

- Do not administer to persons with a known sulfite allergy.
- The maximum single IM dose is 20 mg, and the maximum daily IM dose is 120 mg.
- Doses should be reduced for elderly patients and those with renal or hepatic insufficiency.
- IV administration: Dezocine may be given by direct IV over 30–60 s.
- Store at room temperature, 15–30C (59–86F), and protect from light. Do not use if precipitate is visible.

Assessment & Drug Effects

- Assess for pain relief; onset occurs within 15–30 min, with peak effect at 60 min. Effective analgesia usually lasts 4–6 h.
- Monitor for respiratory depression (especially with preexisting pulmonary disease), changes in BP and heart rate (especially hypotension and bradycardia), and excess CNS depression.
- Assess for safety with ambulation, as dezocine may cause dizziness.

Patient & Family Education

- Inform patient of potential for hypotension and dizziness; advise caution with position changes and ambulation.

- Advise patient not to perform hazardous activities until response to drug is known.
- Advise patient to report adverse drug effects. A dosage reduction or change of drug may be warranted.

DIAZEPAM

(dye-az'e-pam)

Trade names: Apo-Diazepam♣, Diazemuls♣, E-Pam♣, Meval♣, Novodipam♣, Valium, Valrelease, Vivol♣

DIAZEPAM EMULSIFIED

Trade name: Dizac

Prototype for classifications: CNS AGENT; BENZODIAZEPINE ANTICONVULSANT; ANXIOLYTIC

Pregnancy category: D

ACTIONS/PHARMACODYNAMICS Psychotherapeutic agent related to chlordiazepoxide; reportedly superior in antianxiety and anticonvulsant activity, with somewhat shorter duration of action. Like chlordiazepoxide, appears to act at both limbic and subcortical levels of CNS. Shortens REM and stage 4 sleep but increases total sleep time. Causes transient analgesia after IV administration.

USES Drug of choice for status epilepticus. Management of anxiety disorders, for short-term relief of anxiety symptoms, to allay anxiety and tension prior to surgery, cardioversion and endoscopic procedures, as an amnesic, and treatment for restless legs. Also used to alleviate acute withdrawal symptoms of alcoholism, voiding problems in the elderly, and adjunctively for relief of skeletal muscle spasm associated with cerebral palsy, paraplegia, athetosis, stiff-man syndrome, tetanus.

ROUTE & DOSAGE

Note: emulsion is administered IV only.

Status Epilepticus

Adult: **IM/IV** 5–10 mg; repeat if needed at 10–15 min intervals up to 30 mg; repeat if needed q2–4h. Administer emulsion at 5 mg/min IVP.
Child: **IM/IV** *<5 y,* 0.2–0.5 mg slowly q2–5min up to 5 mg. *>5 y,* 1 mg slowly q2–5min up to 10 mg; repeat if needed q2–4 h. Administer emulsion at 5 mg/min IVP.

Anxiety, Muscle Spasm, Convulsions, Alcohol Withdrawal

Adult: **PO** 2–10 mg b.i.d. to q.i.d. *or* 15–30 mg/d sustained release. **IM/IV** 2–10 mg; repeat if needed in 3–4 h. Administer emulsion at 5 mg/min IVP.
Geriatric: **PO** 1–2 mg 1–2 times/d (max 10 mg/d).
Child >6 mo: **PO** 1–2.5 mg b.i.d. or t.i.d.

PHARMACOKINETICS **Absorption:** readily absorbed from GI tract; erratic IM absorption. **Onset:** 30–60 min PO; 15–30 min IM; 1–5 min IV. **Peak:** 1–2 h PO. **Duration:** 15 min– 1 h IV; up to 3 h PO. **Distribution:** crosses blood–brain barrier and placenta; distributed into breast milk. **Metabolism:** metabolized in liver to active metabolites. **Elimination:** half-life: 20–50 h; excreted primarily in urine.

CONTRAINDICATIONS & PRECAUTIONS **Contraindicated in:** ***Injectable form:*** shock, coma, acute alcohol intoxication, depressed vital signs, obstetrical patients, infants ≤30 d of age. ***Tablet form:*** children <6 mo of age, acute narrow-angle glaucoma, untreated open-angle glaucoma, during or within 14 d of MAO INHIBITOR therapy. Safe use during pregnancy (category D) and lactation not established. **Cautious use in:** epilepsy, psychoses, mental depression; myasthenia gravis; impaired hepatic or renal function; drug abuse, addiction-prone individuals. Injectable diazepam used with extreme caution in the elderly, the very ill, and patients with COPD.

ADVERSE/SIDE EFFECTS **CNS:** *drowsiness*, fatigue, ataxia, confusion, paradoxic rage, dizziness, vertigo, amnesia, vivid dreams, headache, slurred speech, tremor; EEG changes, tardive dyskinesia. **CV:** hypotension, tachycardia, edema, <u>cardiovascular collapse.</u> **Eye:** blurred vision, diplopia, nystagmus. **GI:** xerostomia, nausea, constipation. **GU:** incontinence, urinary retention, gynecomastia (prolonged use), menstrual irregularities. **Other:** hiccups, coughing, throat and chest pain, <u>laryngospasm</u>, ovulation failure, pain, venous thrombosis, phlebitis at injection site, hepatic dysfunction.

DRUG INTERACTIONS **Alcohol,** CNS DEPRESSANTS, ANTICONVULSANTS potentiate CNS depression; **cimetidine** increases diazepam plasma levels, increases toxicity; may decrease antiparkinson effects of **levodopa;** may increase **phenytoin** levels; smoking decreases sedative and antianxiety effects.

INCOMPATIBILITIES **Solution/additive: bleomycin, benzquinamide, dobutamine, doxapram, doxorubicin, fluorouracil, glycopyrrolate, heparin, nalbuphone, sufentanil.** Emulsion also incompatible with **morphine. Y-site: furosemide, heparin, potassium chloride, vitamin B complex with C.** Emulsion also incompatible with **morphine.** Do not mix emulsion with any other drugs. Do not administer through polyvinyl chloride (PVC) infusion sets.

NURSING IMPLICATIONS

Administration

- Tablet may be crushed before administration and taken with fluid or mixed with food.
- Supervise oral ingestion to ensure drug is swallowed.
- Abrupt discontinuation of diazepam should generally be avoided. Doses should be tapered to termination.
- IM administration should be made deep into large muscle mass. Inject slowly. Rotate injection sites.
- The emulsion form is for IV use only; do not give IM or SC.
- IV administration: To prevent swelling, irritation, venous thrombosis, phlebitis, give direct IV by injecting drug slowly, taking at least 1 min for each 5 mg (1 ml) given to adults and taking at least 3 min to inject 0.25 mg/kg body weight of children.
- If injection cannot be made directly into vein, manufacturer suggests making injection slowly through infusion tubing as close as possible to vein insertion. The emulsion form is incompatible with PVC infusion sets.
- Avoid small veins and extreme care should be taken to avoid intraarterial administration or extravasation.
- Preserve in tight, light-resistant containers at 15–30C (59–86F), unless otherwise specified by manufacturer. Store emulsion at 2–8C (36–46F). Do not freeze.

Assessment & Drug Effects

- Most adverse reactions are dose

related. Physician will rely on accurate observations and reporting of patient's response to the drug to determine lowest effective maintenance dose.

- Maximum effect may require 1–2 wk; patient tolerance to therapeutic effects may develop after 4 wk of treatment.
- Suicidal tendencies may be present in anxiety states accompanied by depression. Observe necessary preventive precautions.
- When diazepam is given parenterally, hypotension, muscular weakness, tachycardia, and respiratory depression may occur. Observe patient closely and monitor vital signs.
- Periodic blood cell counts and liver function tests are recommended during prolonged therapy.
- Adverse reactions such as drowsiness, ataxia, constipation, and urinary retention are more likely to occur in the elderly and debilitated or in those receiving larger doses. Dosage adjustment may be necessary. Supervise ambulation.
- Monitor I&O ratio, including bowel elimination.
- Smoking increases metabolism of diazepam; therefore clinical effectiveness is lowered. Heavy smokers may need a higher dose than the nonsmoker.
- Psychic and physical dependence may occur in patients on long-term high dosage therapy, in those with histories of alcohol or drug addiction, or in those who self-medicate.

Patient & Family Education

- Alcohol and other CNS depressants should be avoided during therapy with diazepam, unless otherwise advised by physician. Concomitant use of these agents can cause severe drowsiness, respiratory depression, and apnea.
- Because of possible sedation, activities requiring mental alertness and precision should be avoided until reaction to diazepam has been evaluated.
- The patient should be advised that if she becomes pregnant during therapy or intends to become pregnant she should communicate with her physician regarding desirability of discontinuing drug.
- Caution patient to take drug as prescribed and not to change dose or dose intervals.
- Patient should check with physician before taking any OTC drug while on diazepam therapy.

DIAZOXIDE

(dye-az-ox′ide)

Trade names: Hyperstat I.V., Proglycem

Classifications: CARDIOVASCULAR DRUG; ANTIHYPERTENSIVE; VASODILATOR; SULFONYLUREA

Prototype: Hydralazine

Pregnancy category: C

ACTIONS/PHARMACODYNAMICS

Rapid-acting thiazide (benzothiadiazine) nondiuretic hypotensive and hyperglycemic agent. In contrast to thiazide diuretics, causes sodium and water retention and decreases urinary output, probably because it increases proximal tubular reabsorption of sodium and decreases glomerular filtration rate. Reduces peripheral vascular resistance and BP by direct vasodilatory effect on peripheral arteriolar smooth muscles, perhaps by direct competition for calcium receptor sites. Hypotensive effect may be accompanied by marked reflex increase in heart rate, cardiac output, and stroke volume; thus cerebral and coronary blood flow are usually maintained.

D

USES Intravenously for emergency lowering of BP in hospitalized patients with malignant hypertension, particularly when associated with renal impairment. Not effective in pheochromocytoma. Commonly used with a diuretic such as furosemide (Lasix) to counteract diazoxide-induced sodium and water retention. Orally in treatment of various diagnosed hypoglycemic states due to hyperinsulinism when other medical treatment or surgical management has been unsuccessful or is not feasible.

ROUTE & DOSAGE

Severe Hypertension
Adult: **IV** 1–3 mg/kg up to 150 mg repeated at 5–15 min intervals if necessary.
Child: **IV** Same as for adult.

Hypoglycemia
Adult/Child: **PO** 3–8 mg/kg/d divided q8–12h.
Neonates/Infants: **PO** 8–15 mg/kg/d divided q8–12h.

PHARMACOKINETICS **Onset:** 30–60 s IV; 1 h PO. **Peak:** 5 min IV. **Duration:** 2–12 or more h IV; 8 h PO. **Distribution:** crosses blood–brain barrier and placenta. **Metabolism:** partially metabolized in the liver. **Elimination:** half-life: 21–45 h; excreted in urine.

CONTRAINDICATIONS & PRECAUTIONS **Contraindicated in:** hypersensitivity to diazoxide or to other thiazides; cerebral bleeding, eclampsia; aortic coarctation; AV shunt, significant coronary artery disease. Safe use during pregnancy (category C) and in nursing mothers not established. Use of oral diazoxide for functional hypoglycemia or in presence of increased bilirubin in newborns. **Cautious use in:** diabetes mellitus; impaired cerebral or cardiac circulation; impaired renal function; patients taking corticosteroids or estrogen–progestogen combinations; hyperuricemia, history of gout, uremia.

ADVERSE/SIDE EFFECTS **CNS:** tinnitus, momentary hearing loss, headache, weakness, malaise, *dizziness,* polyneuritis, sleepiness, insomnia, euphoria, anxiety, extrapyramidal signs. **CV:** palpitations, atrial and ventricular arrhythmias, flushing, shock; *orthostatic hypotension,* CHF, transient hypertension. **Eye:** blurred vision, transient cataracts, subconjunctival hemorrhage, ring scotoma, diplopia, lacrimation, papilledema. **GI:** *nausea, vomiting,* abdominal discomfort, diarrhea, constipation, ileus, anorexia, transient loss of taste. **Hematologic:** transient neutropenia, eosinophilia, decreased Hgb/Hct, decreased IgG. **Hypersensitivity:** rash, fever, leukopenia. **Renal:** decreased urinary output, nephrotic syndrome (reversible), hematuria, increased nocturia, proteinuria, azotemia. **Skin:** pruritus, flushing, monilial dermatitis, herpes, hirsutism; loss of scalp hair, sweating, sensation of warmth, burning, or itching. **Other:** impaired hepatic function, chest and back pain, muscle cramps; advance in bone age (children); *hyperglycemia, sodium and water retention, edema,* hyperuricemia, glycosuria, inhibition of labor, enlargement of breast lump, galactorrhea; decreased immunoglobinemia, hirsutism.

DIAGNOSTIC TEST INTERFERENCE Diazoxide can cause false-negative response to ***glucagon.***

DRUG INTERACTIONS SULFONYLUREAS antagonize effects; THIAZIDE

DIURETICS may intensify hyperglycemia and antihypertensive effects; **phenytoin** increases risk of hyperglycemia, and diazoxide may increase phenytoin metabolism, causing loss of seizure control.

NURSING IMPLICATIONS

Administration

- IV diazoxide is given undiluted by rapid direct IV injection over 10–30 s.
- Patient should be recumbent while receiving IV diazoxide and should remain in bed for at least 30 min following administration.
- Since diazoxide causes sodium and water retention, a diuretic is generally prescribed to avoid CHF and drug resistance and to maximize hypotensive effect.
- When a diuretic, e.g., furosemide (Lasix), is prescribed, it is generally given 30–60 min prior to IV diazoxide. Patient should remain recumbent 8–10 h because of possible additive hypotensive effect.
- Darkened solutions may have lost potency and should not be administered.
- Store capsules, oral suspension, and injection at 2–30C (35.6–86F) unless otherwise directed. Protect from light, heat, and freezing.

Assessment & Drug Effects

- Check IV injection sites daily. Solution is strongly alkaline. Extravasation of medication into SC or IV tissues can cause severe inflammatory reaction. Diazoxide is administered only by peripheral vein.
- Diazoxide is discontinued if not effective in 2 or 3 wk.
- Blood glucose, serum electrolytes, and CBC should be determined at start of IV therapy and regularly thereafter in patients receiving multiple doses.
- Monitor BP q5min for the first 15–30 min or until stabilized, then hourly for balance of drug effect.
- If BP continues to fall 30 min or more after IV drug administration, suspect cause other than drug effect. Notify physician immediately.
- Monitor pulse: Tachycardia has occurred immediately following IV; palpitation and bradycardia have also been reported.
- Report promptly any change in I&O ratio.
- Observe patient closely for signs and symptoms of CHF (see Appendix G).
- Serum electrolyte levels should be evaluated at regular intervals, particularly in patient with impaired renal function. (Hypokalemia potentiates hyperglycemic effect of diazoxide.)
- In contrast to IV diazoxide, oral administration usually does not produce marked effects on BP. However, periodic measurements of BP and vital signs should be made.
- Prolonged surveillance of symptoms for up to 7 d may be essential because of long half-life of diazoxide (for both oral and parenteral forms).

Patient & Family Education

- Diazoxide may cause hyperglycemia and glycosuria in diabetic and diabetic-prone individuals. Blood and urine glucose should be closely monitored; report any abnormalities to physician.
- Instruct patient to report palpitations, chest pain, dizziness, fainting, or severe headache.
- Lanugo-type hirsutism occurs frequently and is most common in children and women. Reassure patient that it is reversible with discontinuation of drug.

D

DIBUCAINE

(dye'byoo-kane)

Trade name: Nupercainal

Classifications: CNS AGENT; ANESTHETIC, LOCAL (AMIDE-TYPE)

Prototype: Procaine

Pregnancy category: C

ACTIONS/PHARMACODYNAMICS Long-acting anesthetic of the amide type and reportedly one of the most potent and most toxic. Appears to inhibit initiation and conduction of nerve impulses by reducing permeability of nerve cell membrane to sodium ions.

USES Fast, temporary relief of pain and itching due to hemorrhoids and other anorectal disorders, nonpoisonous insect bites, sunburn, minor burns, cuts, and scratches.

ROUTE & DOSAGE

Itching Due to Insect Bites or Hemorrhoids

Adult: **Topical** Apply skin cream or ointment to affected area as needed (max 1 oz [28 g]/24 h); insert rectal ointment morning and evening and after each bowel movement.

Child: **Topical** Apply skin cream or ointment to affected area as needed (max 1/4 oz [7 g]/24 h).

PHARMACOKINETICS **Absorption:** poorly absorbed from intact skin; readily absorbed from mucous membranes or abraded skin. **Onset:** 15 min. **Duration:** 2–4 h.

CONTRAINDICATIONS & PRECAUTIONS **Contraindicated in:** hypersensitivity to amide-type anesthetics, pregnancy (category C).

ADVERSE/SIDE EFFECTS Irritation, contact dermatitis; rectal bleeding (suppository).

NURSING IMPLICATIONS

Administration

- The cream preparation is water soluble and therefore should be applied after bathing or swimming.
- Dibucaine preparations are stored at 15–30C (59–86F) in tight, light-resistant containers.

Patient & Family Education

- Instruct patient to use OTC preparations as directed. Review package instructions with patient.
- Caution patient to discontinue medication if irritation or rectal bleeding (following use of rectal preparations) develops and to consult physician.
- Remind patient that hemorrhoids can be caused or worsened by constipation, excessive straining at stool, and excessive standing, sitting, and coughing.
- Physician may prescribe sitz baths 3 or 4 times daily to reduce the swelling and pain of hemorrhoids.
- Medication is intended only for temporary relief of mild to moderate itching or pain.
- Seek medical advice for continuing discomfort, pain or bleeding, or sensation of rectal pressure.

DICHLORPHENAMIDE

(dye-klor-fen'a-mide)

Trade names: Daranide, Oratrol

Classifications: EYE PREPARATION; CARBONIC ANHYDRASE INHIBITOR; ANTIGLAUCOMA

Prototype: Acetazolamide

Pregnancy category: C

ACTIONS/PHARMACODYNAMICS Nonbacteriostatic sulfonamide derivative similar to acetazolamide except that chloride excretion is increased, and thus potential for significant metabolic acidosis is less. Lowers IOP by decreasing production of aqueous humor. Produces diuresis but is not used as a diuretic because effect is lost with chronic use.

USES Adjunctive treatment of open-angle glaucoma and preoperatively in narrow-angle glaucoma when delay of surgery is desired to lower IOP. Commonly used in conjunction with a miotic; an osmotic agent may also be used to enhance reduction of IOP in acute angle-closure glaucoma.

ROUTE & DOSAGE

Glaucoma
Adult: **PO** 100–200 mg followed by 100 mg q12h until desired response is obtained; **Maintenance:** 25–50 mg 1–3 times/d.

PHARMACOKINETICS Absorption: well absorbed from GI tract. **Onset:** 0.5–1 h. **Peak:** 2–4 h. **Duration:** 6–12 h.

CONTRAINDICATIONS & PRECAUTIONS Contraindicated in: hypersensitivity to sulfonamides and sulfonamide derivative diuretics; depressed sodium and potassium levels, severe pulmonary obstruction, marked kidney or liver dysfunction, hyperchloremic acidosis, adrenocortical insufficiency, long-term use in noncongestive angle-closure glaucoma. Safe use during pregnancy (category C) and in nursing mothers not established. **Cautious use in:** respiratory acidosis, reduced respiratory capacity, diabetes mellitus.

ADVERSE/SIDE EFFECTS CNS: paresthesia, sedation, drowsiness, fatigue, dizziness, ataxia. **GI:** anorexia, nausea, vomiting, metallic taste, diarrhea, abdominal discomfort. **Hematologic:** leukopenia, <u>agranulocytosis</u>, thrombocytopenia, hemolytic anemia. **Renal:** urinary frequency, crystalluria, renal calculi. **Skin:** urticaria, pruritus, rash. **Other:** weight loss, fever, glycosuria, asymptomatic hyperuricemia.

DRUG INTERACTIONS Renal excretion of AMPHETAMINES, **ephedrine, flecainide, quinidine, procainamide,** TRICYCLIC ANTIDEPRESSANTS may be decreased, thereby enhancing or prolonging their effects; increases renal excretion of **lithium;** excretion of **phenobarbital** may be increased; **amphotericin B,** CORTICOSTEROIDS may increase potassium loss; dichlorphenamide-induced hypokalemia may predispose patients taking DIGITALIS GLYCOSIDES to digitalis toxicity; patients on high doses of SALICYLATES are at higher risk for salicylate toxicity.

NURSING IMPLICATIONS

Administration

- Dichlorphenamide may be taken with meals to reduce gastric irritation.

Assessment & Drug Effects

- Since drug may cause dizziness and ataxia, supervision of ambulation and other safety precautions may be warranted.
- Monitor for hematologic reactions common to sulfonamides. Obtain baseline CBC and platelet counts before initiating therapy and at regular intervals during therapy.

Patient & Family Education

- High fluid intake is generally rec-

D

ommended to reduce risk of renal calculi. Consult physician.

- Advise patient to report to physician the onset of sore throat, fever, unusual bleeding or bruising, tremors, flank or loin pain, skin rash.
- Caution patient to avoid driving and other potentially hazardous activities until reaction to drug is known.

D

DICLOFENAC SODIUM

(di-klo'fen-ak)

Trade name: Voltaren

DICLOFENAC POTASSIUM

Trade name: Cataflam

Classifications: CNS AGENT; NSAID; ANALGESIC, NONNARCOTIC; ANTIPYRETIC

Prototype: Ibuprofen

Pregnancy category: B

ACTIONS/PHARMACODYNAMICS

Nonsteroidal antiinflammatory drug (NSAID) with analgesic and antipyretic activity. Although its exact mechanism of action has not been fully elucidated, it appears to be a potent inhibitor of cyclooxygenase, thereby decreasing the synthesis of prostaglandins, prostacyclin, and thromboxane. At therapeutic doses, has little effect on platelet aggregation.

USES Analgesic and antipyretic effects in symptomatic treatment of rheumatoid arthritis, osteoarthritis, and ankylosing spondylitis. Also acute gout; juvenile rheumatoid arthritis; various rheumatic conditions including bursitis, myalgia, sciatica, and tendinitis; acute soft tissue injuries including sprains and strains; dysmenorrhea; headache, migraine, and dental, minor surgical, and postpartum pain; and renal or biliary colic. **Ophthalmic:** cataract surgery; photophobia associated with refractive surgery.

ROUTE & DOSAGE

Rheumatoid Arthritis

Adult: **PO** 150–200 mg/d in 3–4 divided doses.
Child: **PO** 25 mg b.i.d. or t.i.d.

Osteoarthritis

Adult: **PO** 100–150 mg/d in 3–4 divided doses.

Ankylosing Spondylitis

Adult: **PO** 25 mg q.i.d. and 25 mg h.s.

Cataract Surgery

Adult: **ophthalmic** 1 drop of 0.1% solution in affected eye q.i.d. beginning 24 h after surgery and continuing for 2 wk.

PHARMACOKINETICS **Absorption:** readily absorbed from GI tract; 50–60% reaches systemic circulation. **Peak:** 2–3 h. **Distribution:** widely distributed including synovial fluid and into breast milk. **Metabolism:** extensively metabolized in liver. **Elimination:** half-life: 1.2–2 h; 50–70% excreted in urine, 30–35% in feces.

CONTRAINDICATIONS & PRECAUTIONS **Contraindicated in:** hypersensitivity to diclofenac, patients in whom asthma, urticaria, angioedema, bronchospasm, severe rhinitis, shock, or other sensitivity reaction is precipitated by aspirin or other NSAIDS, pregnancy (category B), lactation. **Cautious use in:** geriatric patients and children; patients receiving anticoagulant therapy; history of GI disease; GU tract problems such as dysuria, cystitis, hematuria, nephritis, nephrotic syndrome, patients who must restrict their sodium intake; impaired hepatic function; SLE; heart failure; hypertension.

ADVERSE/SIDE EFFECTS CNS: dizziness, headache, drowsiness. **ENT:** tinnitus. **Skin:** rash, pruritus. **GI:** *dyspepsia,* nausea, vomiting, abdominal pain, cramps, constipation, diarrhea, indigestion, abdominal distension, flatulence, peptic ulcer. **CV:** fluid retention, hypertension, CHF. **Hepatic:** liver enzymes, transaminases increased. **Respiratory:** asthma. **Other:** liver test abnormalities, back, leg, or joint pain, hyperglycemia, prolonged bleeding time; inhibits platelet aggregation.

DIAGNOSTIC TEST INTERFERENCE Liver function test values may be increased. Liver function test abnormalities may return to normal despite continued use; however, if significant abnormalities occur, clinical signs and symptoms consistent with liver disease develop, or systemic manifestations such as eosinophilia or rash occur, the medication should be discontinued. Serum uric acid concentrations may be decreased because of increased renal clearance.

DRUG INTERACTIONS Increases **cyclosporine**-induced nephrotoxicity; increases **methotrexate** levels (increases toxicity); may decrease BP-lowering effects of DIURETICS; may increase levels and toxicity of **lithium;** may increase **digoxin** levels.

NURSING IMPLICATIONS

Administration

- Administer on an empty stomach, 1 h before or after a meal, as absorption is delayed markedly by food.
- Schedule administration 30 min before physical therapy or planned exercise to keep discomfort at a minimum.
- Gastric irritation may be minimized by administering it with a full glass of water.
- Do not crush tablets or dissolve in water. They should be swallowed whole.
- To reduce risk of bleeding, discontinue therapy about 1 wk before surgery.
- Use with caution in those who must restrict sodium intake.
- Store at 15–30C (59–86F) away from heat and direct light.

Assessment & Drug Effects

- Monitor liver function and serum uric acid concentrations.
- Observe and report signs of bleeding (e.g., petechiae, ecchymoses, bleeding gums, bloody or black stools, cloudy or bloody urine). Monitor Hct and PT.
- Monitor BP for hypertension and blood sugar for hyperglycemia.
- Monitor for increased serum sodium and potassium in patients receiving potassium-sparing diuretics.
- Monitor weight and report gains greater than 1 kg (2 lb)/24 h.
- Monitor for signs and symptoms of GI irritation and ulceration.

Patient & Family Education

- Instruct patient not to lie down for 15–30 min after taking the medicine to decrease esophageal irritation.
- Advise patient to discontinue use with onset of ringing or buzzing in the ears, impaired hearing, dizziness, GI discomfort, or bleeding.
- Advise patient not to take aspirin or other OTC analgesics without permission of the physician.
- Instruct patient to avoid alcohol or other CNS depressants.

- Advise caution while driving, operating machines, or other hazardous activities until reaction to drug is known.

D

DICLOXACILLIN SODIUM

(dye-klox-a-sill'in)

Trade names: Dycill, Dynapen, Pathocil

Classifications: ANTIINFECTIVE; BETA-LACTAM ANTIBIOTIC; SEMISYNTHETIC PENICILLIN; ANTISTAPHYLOCOCCAL PENICILLIN

Prototype: Penicillin G potassium

Pregnancy category: B

ACTIONS/PHARMACODYNAMICS Semisynthetic, acid-stable, penicillinase-resistant isoxazolyl penicillin. Mechanism of action similar to that of penicillin G; however, platelet dysfunction not reported for dicloxacillin. Action is bactericidal. Inhibits biosynthesis of bacterial cell wall during stage of active multiplication. Reportedly the most active of the isoxazolyl penicillins (cloxacillin, oxacillin) against penicillinase-producing staphylococci. Less potent than penicillin G against penicillin-sensitive microorganisms and generally ineffective against methicillin-resistant staphylococci and gram-negative bacteria.

USES Primarily in systemic infections caused by penicillinase-producing staphylococci and penicillin-resistant staphylococci.

ROUTE & DOSAGE

Mild to Moderate Infections

Adult: **PO** 125–500 mg q6h.
Child: **PO** <40 kg, 12.5–25 mg/kg q6h (max 4 g/d).

PHARMACOKINETICS Absorption: 35–76% absorbed from GI tract. **Peak:** 0.5–2 h. **Duration:** 4–6 h. **Distribution:** distributed throughout body with highest concentrations in liver and kidney; low CSF penetration; crosses placenta; distributed into breast milk. **Metabolism:** metabolized in liver. **Elimination:** half-life: 30–60 min; excreted primarily in urine with some elimination through bile.

CONTRAINDICATIONS & PRECAUTIONS Contraindicated in: hypersensitivity to penicillins. Safe use during pregnancy (category B) and in neonates not established. **Cautious use in:** history of or suspected atopy or allergy (asthma, eczema, hives, hay fever); history of hypersensitivity to cephalosporins.

ADVERSE/SIDE EFFECTS GI: nausea, vomiting, flatulence, *diarrhea,* abdominal pain. **Hypersensitivity:** pruritus, urticaria, rash, wheezing, sneezing, <u>anaphylaxis</u>; eosinophilia. **Other:** transient elevations of ALT, superinfections.

DRUG INTERACTION Probenecid decreases dicloxacillin elimination.

NURSING IMPLICATIONS

Administration

- Dicloxacillin is best taken on an empty stomach at least 1 h before or 2 h after meals. Food reduces drug absorption.
- Following reconstitution (by pharmacist), oral suspensions are stable for 7 d at room temperature or 14 d under refrigeration at 2–8C (35.6–46.4F). Container should be so labeled and dated. Shake well before pouring.
- Capsules are stored at 15–30C (59–86F) in tight containers unless otherwise directed.

Assessment & Drug Effects

- Before initiation of therapy a careful inquiry should be made concerning patient's previous exposure and sensitivity to penicillins and cephlosporins, and other allergic reactions of any kind.
- Bacteriologic studies should be done prior to initiation of therapy to determine susceptibility of causative organism. Therapy may begin pending test results.
- Blood cultures, WBC, and differential counts are recommended before therapy begins and at least weekly for patients on prolonged therapy. Periodic ALT and AST determinations, urinalysis, BUN, and creatinine are also advised for these patients.

Patient & Family Education

- Instruct patient to take medication around the clock, not to miss a dose, and to continue taking the medication until it is all gone, unless otherwise directed by physician.
- Advise patient to check with physician if GI side effects appear.
- Instruct patient to watch for and report the signs of hypersensitivity reactions and superinfections (see Appendix G).

DICUMAROL

(dye-koo'ma-role)

Trade name: Bishydroxycoumarin

Classifications: BLOOD FORMERS AND COAGULATORS; ORAL ANTICOAGULANT

Prototype: Warfarin

Pregnancy category: D

ACTIONS/PHARMACODYNAMICS Long-acting coumarin derivative. Interferes with blood clotting by depressing hepatic synthesis of vitamin K–dependent coagulation factors: II, VII, IX, X.

USE Prophylaxis and treatment of DVT.

ROUTE & DOSAGE

Anticoagulant

Adult: **PO** 200–300 mg on day 1, then 25–200 mg/d based on PTs.

PHARMACOKINETICS **Absorption:** slowly and incompletely absorbed from GI tract. **Peak:** 1–4 d. **Duration:** 2–10 d. **Distribution:** crosses placenta; distributed into breast milk. **Metabolism:** metabolized in liver. **Elimination:** half-life: 1–2 d; 70–85% excreted in urine, 15–30% in feces.

CONTRAINDICATIONS & PRECAUTIONS **Contraindicated in:** hemorrhagic tendencies: hemophilia, thrombocytopenia, leukemia; open wounds or ulcers; renal or hepatic impairment, vitamin C or K deficiency; severe hypertension; subacute bacterial endocarditis; visceral carcinoma. Safe use during pregnancy (category D), in nursing women, and in children not established. **Cautious use in:** active tuberculosis, major surgery, indwelling catheters.

ADVERSE/SIDE EFFECTS **GI:** diarrhea, flatulence, nausea, vomiting, anorexia, abdominal cramping. **GU:** hematuria, priapism. **Hematologic:** leukopenia, agranulocytosis, hemorrhage. **Skin:** unusual hair loss, urticaria, dermatitis. **Other:** hypersensitivity, fever.

DRUG INTERACTIONS See **warfarin.**

NURSING IMPLICATIONS

Administration

- Frequent dosage adjustment may

be necessary during first 1 or 2 wk of therapy because drug absorption is so variable. Administration with food enhances drug absorption.

- Store in tightly closed container at 15–30C (59–86F) unless otherwise directed.

Assessment & Drug Effects

- During period of dosage adjustment, PT and INR should be checked daily and dose order obtained.
- Blood for PT and INR should be drawn at least 5 h after an IV bolus dose of heparin or 24 h following a full therapeutic SC dose. Continuous IV infusion or low doses of heparin SC usually do not cause a significant increase in PT; therefore, blood can be drawn at any time.
- When patient is controlled on maintenance dose, PT and INR may be checked semiweekly, weekly for 3–4 wk, then at 1- to 4-wk intervals, depending on stability of patient's response.

Patient & Family Education

- Instruct patient to inform physician if any other medication is being taken, including OTC drugs.
- Caution patient not to add or discontinue any medication without approval of physician or pharmacist.
- Instruct patient to report immediately any unexplained bleeding, easy bruising, or prolonged bleeding time.
- Advise patient to tell all doctors and dentists who may administer care that he or she is on anticoagulant therapy.
- Stress importance of avoiding unusual changes in vitamin intake, diet or life-style without consulting physician. Also advise patient to notify physician of any changes in health status. Illness may increase anticoagulant requirement.

DICYCLOMINE HYDROCHLORIDE

(dye-sye′kloe-meen)

Trade names: Antispas, A-spas, Bentyl, Bentylol♣, Byclomine, Dibent, Di-Cyclonex, Dilomine, Di-Spaz, Formulex♣, Lomine♣, Neoquess, Nospaz, Or-Tyl, Protylol♣, Spasmoban♣, Spasmoject, Viscerol♣

Classifications: AUTONOMIC NERVOUS SYSTEM AGENT; ANTICHOLINERGIC (PARASYMPATHOLYTIC); ANTISPASMODIC

Prototype: Atropine

Pregnancy category: B

ACTIONS/PHARMACODYNAMICS

Synthetic tertiary amine with antispasmodic properties. Relieves smooth muscle spasm in GI and biliary tracts, uterus, and ureters by nonspecific direct relaxant action. Atropine-like (antimuscarinic) side effects on salivary and sweat glands, gastric secretions, eyes, and cardiovascular system are generally slight with average dosage.

USES Adjunctively in treatment of functional bowel disorders/irritable bowel syndrome. **Unlabeled uses:** acute enterocolitis, peptic ulcer, and infant colic.

ROUTE & DOSAGE

Irritable Bowel Disorders

Adult: **PO** 20–40 mg q.i.d. **IM** 20 mg q.i.d.
Child: **PO** 10 mg t.i.d. or q.i.d. (max 40 mg/d).
Infants: **PO** 5 mg t.i.d. or q.i.d.

PHARMACOKINETICS **Absorption:** readily absorbed from GI tract. **Onset:** 1–2 h. **Duration:** 4 h. **Metabolism:** metabolized in liver. **Elimina-**

tion: half-life: 9–10 h; 80% excreted in urine, 10% in feces.

CONTRAINDICATIONS & PRECAUTIONS **Contraindicated in:** hypersensitivity to anticholinergic drugs; obstructive diseases of GU and GI tracts, paralytic ileus, intestinal atony, biliary tract disease; unstable cardiovascular status; severe ulcerative colitis, toxic megacolon; myasthenia gravis; infants <6 mo. Safe use during pregnancy (category B), in nursing mothers, and in children not established. **Cautious use in:** glaucoma; prostatic hypertrophy; autonomic neuropathy; ulcerative colitis; hyperthyroidism; coronary heart disease, CHF, arrhythmias, hypertension; hepatic or renal disease; hiatal hernia associated with esophageal reflux; infants ≤6 mo.

ADVERSE/SIDE EFFECTS Dose related. **CNS:** light-headedness, drowsiness, headache, insomnia, brief euphoria, fever, restlessness, irritability, coma, seizures. **CV:** fluctuations in heart rate, palpitation, tachycardia. **GI:** *dry mouth,* nausea, *constipation,* paralytic ileus, vomiting, diminished sense of taste, bloated feeling. **GU:** urinary hesitancy, *urinary retention,* impotence. **Other:** blurred vision, decreased sweating, suppression of lactation, urticaria, allergic reactions; curare-like effect (cyanosis, apnea, respiratory arrest).

NURSING IMPLICATIONS

Administration

- Administer 30 min before meals and at bedtime.
- Store below 30C (86F) unless otherwise directed.

Assessment & Drug Effects

- Treatment of infant colic with dicyclomine is not without some risk, especially in infants <2 mo of age. Doubling the usual dose of 5 mg can produce serious toxic effects.
- Infants ≤6 wk have developed respiratory symptoms as well as seizures, fluctuations in heart rate, weakness, and coma within minutes after taking syrup formulation. Symptoms generally last 20–30 min and are believed to be due to local irritation.
- Monitor I&O.
- If drug produces drowsiness and light-headedness, supervision of ambulation and other safety precautions are warranted.

Patient & Family Education

- Dicyclomine may increase risk of heatstroke by decreasing sweating, especially in the elderly.
- Since dicyclomine may produce drowsiness and blurred vision, avoid activities requiring mental alertness until reaction to drug is known.
- Report changes in urine volume, voiding pattern.

DIDANOSINE (DDI)

(di-dan′o-sine)

Trade name: Videx

Classifications: ANTIINFECTIVE; ANTIRETROVIRAL AGENT; NUCLEOSIDE REVERSE TRANSCRIPTASE INHIBITOR

Prototype: Zidovudine

Pregnancy category: B

ACTIONS/PHARMACODYNAMICS Synthetic purine nucleotide that inhibits replication of HIV. DDI interferes with the HIV RNA-dependent DNA polymerase (reverse transcriptase), thus preventing replication of the virus.

USES Advanced HIV infection in patients who are intolerant to zidovudine (AZT) or who demonstrate significant clinical or immunological deterioration during zidovudine therapy.

ROUTE & DOSAGE

Adult: **PO** 35–49 kg, tablets, 125 mg b.i.d.; powder, 167 mg b.i.d.; 50–74 kg, tablets, 200 mg b.i.d.; powder, 250 mg b.i.d.; ≥75 kg, tablets, 300 mg b.i.d.; powder, 375 mg b.i.d.; 2 tablets should be taken at each dose to ensure adequate buffering.
Child: **PO** BSA 1.1–1.4 m^2, tablets, 100 mg b.i.d.; powder, 125 mg b.i.d. BSA 0.8–1.0 m^2, tablets, 75 mg b.i.d; powder, 94 mg b.i.d. BSA 0.5–0.7 m^2, tablets, 50 mg b.i.d.; powder, 72 mg b.i.d. BSA ≤0.4 m^2, tablets, 25 mg b.i.d.; powder, 31 mg b.i.d. >1 y, should receive a 2-tablet dose. <1 y, should receive a 1-tablet dose.

PHARMACOKINETICS Absorption: rapidly absorbed from GI tract when administerded to fasting patient with antacids; 23-40% reaches systemic circulation. **Peak:** 0.6–1 h. **Distribution:** distributed primarily to body water; 21% reaches CSF; crosses placenta. **Elimination:** half-life: 0.8–1.5 h; 36% excreted in urine.

CONTRAINDICATIONS & PRECAUTIONS Contraindicated in: hypersensitivity to any of the components in the formulation, pregnancy (category B), and nursing mothers. **Cautious use in:** individuals with peripheral vascular disease, history of neuropathy, chronic pancreatitis, renal impairment, or any liver impairment.

ADVERSE/SIDE EFFECTS CV: palpitations, thrombophlebitis, arrhythmias, *vasodilation*. **CNS:** *headache, dizziness, nervousness, insomnia, peripheral neuropathy,* lethargy, poor coordination, seizures. **Eye:** retinal depigmentation, photophobia, blurred vision, optic neuritis, diplopia, blindness. **GI:** *abdominal pain, nausea, vomiting, diarrhea,* constipation, stomatitis, dry mouth, pancreatitis, increased liver enzymes. **Hematologic:** increased WBC, neutrophil, lymphocyte, and platelet counts; increased Hgb, thrombocytopenia, ecchymosis, hemorrhage, petechiae. **Metabolic:** hypocalcemia, hypokalemia, hypomagnesemia, hyperuricemia (asymptomatic), *hypertriglyceridemia*. **Musculoskeletal:** muscle atrophy, myalgia, arthritis, decreased strength. **Respiratory:** *asthma, cough, dyspnea, epistaxis, rhinitis, rhinorrhea,* hypoventilation, pharyngitis, rhonchi or rales, sinusitis, congestion. **Skin:** rash, impetigo, eczema, *pruritus, sweating,* erythema.

DRUG INTERACTIONS ALUMINUM- and MAGNESIUM-CONTAINING ANTACIDS may increase the aluminum- and magnesium-associated adverse effects of tablets. The effectiveness of **dapsone** in prophylaxis of *Pneumocystis carinii* pneumonia may be reduced by concomitant didanosine. May cause additive neuropathy with **zalcitabine** (ddC). **Drug–food:** absorption is significantly decreased by food. Take on an empty stomach.

NURSING IMPLICATIONS

Administration

- Didanosine should be taken on an empty stomach. Food should not be consumed within 15–30 min of drug administration.
- Administer with water. Do not administer with fruit juice or any other acid-containing liquid.
- Chewable tablets must be thoroughly chewed or crushed and dispersed in at least 30 ml (1 oz) of water and immediately swallowed.
- Powder for oral solution (buf-

fered) should be mixed with at least 120 ml (4 oz) of water, stirred until dissolved (requires 2–3 min), and immediately swallowed.

- Powder for oral solution (pediatric) is prepared by pharmacist to yield a concentration of 10 mg/ml. This solution should be shaken thoroughly before administration.
- Dosage reduction may be indicated in those with renal or hepatic impairment.
- Store reconstituted liquid in a tightly closed container in refrigerator for up to 30 d.

Assessment & Drug Effects

- Monitor for signs and symptoms of pancreatitis (e.g., abdominal pain, nausea, vomiting, elevated serum amylase). Report them to physician immediately and withhold drug until pancreatitis is ruled out.
- Monitor for signs and symptoms of peripheral neuropathy (e.g., numbness, tingling, burning, pain in hands or feet). Report them to physician, as dose reduction may be indicated.
- Patients with renal impairment should be monitored for drug toxicity and for hypermagnesemia manifested by muscle weakness and confusion.

Patient & Family Education

- Instruct patient on proper method of drug administration.
- Stress the importance of taking drug on an empty stomach.
- Advise patient to immediately report to physician any of the following: abdominal pain, nausea, or vomiting.

DIENESTROL

(dye-en-ess'trole)

Trade names: DV, Estraguard, Ortho Dienestrol

Classifications: SYNTHETIC HORMONE; ESTROGEN

Prototype: Estradiol

Pregnancy category: X

ACTIONS/PHARMACODYNAMICS

Synthetic nonsteroidal estrogen structurally related to diethylstilbestrol. See estradiol for actions and contraindications.

USES Atrophic vaginitis and kraurosis vulvae associated with menopause.

ROUTE & DOSAGE

Atrophic Vaginitis

Adult: **Intravaginal** 1–2 applicatorsful/d for 1–2 wk; then decrease dose by half for another 1–2 wk; ***Maintenance:*** 1 applicatorful 1–3 times/wk.

ADVERSE/SIDE EFFECTS Increased risk of endometrial cancer and gallbladder disease; thromboembolism. **GU:** vaginal candidiasis, breakthrough bleeding. **GI:** nausea, vomiting, abdominal cramps, bloating. **Skin:** erythema multiforme, loss of scalp hair, hirsutism. **CNS:** mental depression, headache, migraine, dizziness.

NURSING IMPLICATIONS

Administration

- Administration at bedtime increases absorption and thus effectiveness.
- Insert cream applicator (or suppository inserter) approximately 2 in. (5 cm), directing it slightly back toward sacrum. Patient should remain in recumbent position about 30 min to prevent losing the medication.
- If patient is to administer medication to herself, instruct her to wash her hands well before and after

procedure; also advise her not to use tampons while on vaginal therapy.

- Protect cream from light. Store at 8–15C (46–59F) in a tight container unless otherwise directed.

D

Patient & Family Education

- Review package insert with patient.

DIETHYLPROPION HYDROCHLORIDE

(dye-eth-il-proe′pee-on)

Trade names: Nobesine ♣, Propion, Ten-Tab, Tenuate, Tenuate Dospan, Tepanil

Prototype for classifications: GASTROINTESTINAL AGENT; ANOREXIANT

Pregnancy category: B

Controlled substance: Schedule IV

ACTIONS/PHARMACODYNAMICS Sympathomimetic amine and amphetamine cogener. Has lower incidence of amphetamine-type adverse effects but reportedly is less effective as an appetite suppressant. Anorexigenic action probably secondary to direct (CNS) stimulation of appetite control center in hypothalamus and limbic regions. Also produces mild psychic stimulation and vasopressor effects.

USE Used solely in management of exogenous obesity as short-term (a few weeks) adjunct in a regimen of weight reduction based on caloric restriction.

ROUTE & DOSAGE

Obesity

Adult: **PO** 25 mg t.i.d. 30–60 min a.c. or 75 mg sustained release q.d. midmorning.

PHARMACOKINETICS **Absorption:** Readily absorbed from GI tract. **Duration:** 4 h, regular tablets; 10–14 h, sustained release. **Elimination:** half-life: 4–6 h; excreted in urine.

CONTRAINDICATIONS & PRECAUTIONS **Contraindicated in:** known hypersensitivity or idiosyncrasy to sympathomimetic amines; severe hypertension, advanced arteriosclerosis; hyperthyroidism; glaucoma; agitated states, history of drug abuse. Safe use during pregnancy (category B) and in children < 12 not established. **Cautious use in:** hypertension, arrhythmias, symptomatic cardiovascular disease; epilepsy; diabetes mellitus.

ADVERSE/SIDE EFFECTS **CNS:** mild euphoria, restlessness, *nervousness,* dizziness, headache, irritability, hyperactivity, insomnia, drowsiness, mood changes, lethargy. **CV:** palpitation, tachycardia, precordial pain, rise in BP. **GI:** nausea, vomiting, diarrhea, constipation, dry mouth, unpleasant taste. **Hypersensitivity:** urticaria, rash, erythema. **Other:** muscle pain, dyspnea, hair loss, blurred vision, severe dermatoses (chronic intoxication); polyuria, dysuria, increased sweating, impotence, changes in libido, gynecomastia, menstrual irregularities, increase in convulsive episodes in patients with epilepsy.

DRUG INTERACTIONS **Acetazolamide, sodium bicarbonate** decrease diethylpropion elimination; **ammonium chloride, ascorbic acid** increase diethylpropion elimination; a BARBITURATE and diethylpropion taken together may antagonize the effects of both drugs; **furazolidone** may increase blood pressure effects of amphetamines, and interaction may persist for several weeks after discontinuation of furazolidone; **guanethidine,**

guanadryl antagonize antihypertensive effects; MAO INHIBITORS, **selegiline** can cause hypertensive crisis (fatalities reported)—amphetamines should not be administered at the same time as or within 14 days of these drugs; PHENOTHIAZINES may inhibit mood elevating effects of amphetamines; TRICYCLIC ANTIDEPRESSANTS enhance amphetamine effects by increasing norepinephrine release; BETA AGONISTS increase cardiovascular adverse effects.

NURSING IMPLICATIONS

Administration

- Administer on an empty stomach, 1/2–1 h before meals.
- Additional dose sometimes prescribed in midevening to control nighttime hunger. Rarely causes insomnia except in high doses.
- Dosage should be carefully titrated in patients with diabetes.
- Store between 15 and 30C (59 and 86F) in well-closed container unless otherwise specified.

Assessment & Drug Effects

- Patients with epilepsy should be observed closely for reduction in seizure control.
- Anorexigenic effect seldom lasts more than a few weeks. If tolerance develops, drug should be discontinued.
- Varying degrees of psychologic and rarely physical dependence can occur. Drugs related to amphetamines are frequently misused by emotionally unstable individuals.

Patient & Family Education

- Sustained-release tablets should be swallowed whole and not chewed.
- Avoid driving a car or other hazardous activities until reaction to drug is determined.

DIETHYLSTILBESTROL (DES)

(dye-eth-il-stil-bess'trole)

Trade name: Stilbestrol

DIETHYLSTILBESTROL DIPHOSPHATE

Trade names: Honval♣, Stilphostrol

Classifications: SYNTHETIC HORMONE; ESTROGEN; ANTINEOPLASTIC

Prototype: Estradiol

Pregnancy category: X

ACTIONS/PHARMACODYNAMICS

Potent nonsteroidal synthetic estrogen compound with strong teratogenic potential: may cause vaginal or cervical cancer in offspring if mother is treated with diethylstilbestrol (DES) during pregnancy. Competes for androgen or estrogen receptors on tumor cells, thereby changing the hormonal environment essential for their survival. Also interferes with release of FSH and LH with resultant inhibition of lactation, ovulation, and androgen secretion.

USES Estrogen deficiency states, including female hypogonadism or castration, primary ovarian failure, menopausal symptoms, atrophic vaginitis, kraurosis vulvae, and for palliative treatment of advanced metastatic carcinoma of the breast in selected men and postmenopausal women and advanced inoperable carcinoma of prostate. **Unlabeled use:** emergency postcoital contraceptive ("morning after pill").

ROUTE & DOSAGE

Carcinoma Palliation

Adult: **PO** ***Breast:*** 15 mg/d. ***Prostate:*** 1–3 mg/d; may increase in advanced cases.

Postcoital Contraception

Adult: **PO** 25 mg b.i.d. for 5 d; must start within 72 h after coitus.

Prostate Carcinoma

Adult: **PO** 50 mg t.i.d.; may increase to 200 mg or more t.i.d. depending on tolerance of patient. **IV** 0.5 g followed by 1 g/d for 5 or more days; then may reduce to 0.25–0.5 g 1–2 times/wk.

PHARMACOKINETICS Absorption: readily absorbed from GI tract. **Metabolism:** metabolized in liver. **Elimination:** excreted in urine and feces.

CONTRAINDICATIONS & PRECAUTIONS Contraindicated in: use for birth control (except emergency postcoital contraception); malignancies or precarcinomatous lesions (vagina, vulva, or breasts); pregnancy (category X); blood clotting disorders; hepatic dysfunction; undiagnosed vaginal bleeding; long-term use during menopause. **Cautious use in:** hypertension; migraine; diabetes mellitus; asthma.

ADVERSE/SIDE EFFECTS CV: <u>thromboembolic disorders</u>, hypertension, edema, <u>MI</u>. **CNS:** headache, dizziness, chronic depression. **Eye:** intolerance to contact lenses, worsening of myopia. **GI:** *nausea,* vomiting, diarrhea, anorexia, constipation, cramps, bloating, cholestatic jaundice. **Metabolic:** reduced carbohydrate tolerance, hypercalcemia, folic acid deficiency. **Reproduction:** gynecomastia, mastodynia, breast secretions, breakthrough bleeding, changes in menstrual flow, dysmenorrhea, amenorrhea, vaginal candidiasis, changes in libido. **Skin:** melasma (discoloration), erythema multiforme or nodosum, loss of scalp hair, hirsutism. **Other:** weight changes, leg cramps.

DRUG INTERACTIONS Rifampin may increase DES metabolism; may antagonize anticoagulant effects of **warfarin.**

NURSING IMPLICATIONS

Administration

- Enteric-coated tablets should be swallowed whole.
- Diethylstilbestrol diphosphate IV solution: Dissolve dose in 300 ml 0.9% NaCl for injection or 5% dextrose for injection. Infusion: administer slowly (1–2 ml/min) during first 10–15 min and then flow rate is adjusted to permit remainder of solution to be given over a period of 1 h.
- Patient should be lying down during infusion to reduce incidence of dizziness.
- After reconstitution, solution may be stored at room temperature if protected from direct light. Under these conditions, solution is stable for about 5 d. Do not use if a precipitate or cloudiness is present.
- Store tablets and ampuls at 15–30C (59–86F) in a tightly closed container. Protect from light and freezing.

Assessment & Drug Effects

- Nausea and vomiting are common in the menopausal group of patients receiving ≥1 mg/d and relatively uncommon in men and nonpregnant women even when doses are 3–5 mg/d.
- Severe nausea and vomiting with contraceptive doses can lead to noncompliance. An antiemetic may be required.
- Risk of blood clot formation is high. Monitor for signs & symptoms of deep vein thrombosis or thrombophlebitis (see Appendix G).

Patient & Family Education

- Patients with intact uterus should be closely monitored for endometrial cancer. Advise patient to report the onset of vaginal bleeding or any other unusual sign or symptom.

- Women should have breasts and pelvic organs examined before treatment begins and at intervals throughout therapy. Teach the patient self-examination of breasts. Urge her to keep check-up appointments.
- A pregnancy test is advised before the patient is started on therapy with DES. Patient should be informed of the teratogenic potential of this drug.
- Reassure the male patient that drug-induced loss of libido and development of feminine characteristics will disappear with termination of therapy.

DIFLORASONE DIACETATE

(dye-flor'a-sone)

Trade names: Florone, Florone E, Maxiflor, Psorcon

Classifications: SKIN AGENT; ANTI-INFLAMMATORY; STEROID

Prototype: Hydrocortisone

Pregnancy category: C

See Appendix A.

DIFLUNISAL

(dye-floo'ni-sal)

Trade name: Dolobid

Classifications: CNS AGENT; ANALGESIC; NSAID

Prototype: Ibuprofen

Pregnancy category: C

ACTIONS/PHARMACODYNAMICS Long-acting nonsteroidal antiinflammatory drug (NSAID) with peripheral analgesic properties by inhibition of prostaglandin synthesis. More potent than aspirin and acetaminophen in equianalgesic doses and has longer duration of effect. Unlike aspirin, inhibition of platelet function and effect on bleeding time are dose related and reversible, lasting only about 24 h after drug is discontinued. Exerts mild antipyretic effect; therefore not used clinically for this purpose. Has some uricosuric activity at usual dosages.

USES Acute and long-term relief of mild to moderate pain and symptomatic treatment of osteoarthritis and rheumatoid arthritis.

ROUTE & DOSAGE

Analgesia

Adult: **PO** 1000 mg followed by 500 mg q8–12h.

Arthritis

Adult: **PO** 500–1000 mg/d in 2 divided doses (max 1500 mg/d).

PHARMACOKINETICS **Absorption:** readily absorbed from GI tract. **Onset:** 1 h. **Peak:** 2–3 h. **Duration:** 12 h. **Distribution:** probably crosses placenta; distributed into breast milk. **Metabolism:** metabolized in liver. **Elimination:** half-life: 8–12 h; excreted in urine.

CONTRAINDICATIONS & PRECAUTIONS **Contraindicated in:** patients in whom aspirin or other NSAIDS precipitate an acute asthmatic attack (bronchospasm), urticaria, angioedema, severe rhinitis, or shock; active peptic ulcer, GI bleeding. Safe use during pregnancy (category C), in nursing mothers, and in children <12 y not established. Use during third trimester of pregnancy specifically contraindicated because NSAIDS are known to cause premature closure on ductus arteriosus in fetus.

D

Cautious use in: history of upper GI disease; impaired renal or hepatic function; compromised cardiac function, and other conditions associated with fluid retention; patients receiving diuretics; geriatric patients; hypertension; patients who may be adversely affected by prolonged bleeding time.

ADVERSE/SIDE EFFECTS CNS: headache, drowsiness, insomnia, dizziness, vertigo, light-headedness, fatigue, weakness, nervousness, confusion, disorientation. **CV:** palpitation, tachycardia, *peripheral edema*. **ENT:** tinnitus, hearing loss. **Eye:** blurred vision, reduced visual acuity, changes in color vision, scotomas, corneal deposits, retinal disturbances. **GI:** *nausea,* GI pain, flatulence, GI bleeding, peptic ulcer, anorexia, eructation, cholestatic jaundice. **GU:** hematuria, proteinuria, interstitial nephritis, renal failure. **Hematologic:** prolonged PT, anemia, decreased serum uric acid, transient elevations of liver function tests. **Hypersensitivity syndrome:** fever, chills, rash, eosinophilia, changes in renal and hepatic function, <u>anaphylactic reactions with bronchospasm.</u> **Skin:** rash, toxic epidermal necrolysis, exfoliative dermatitis, urticaria. **Other:** weight gain, hyperventilation, dyspnea, photosensitivity.

DIAGNOSTIC TEST INTERFERENCE Diflunisal can lower ***serum uric acid*** concentrations by as much as 1.4 mg/dl and increased renal clearance of uric acid.

DRUG INTERACTIONS ANTACIDS decrease diflunisal absorption; **aspirin** and other NSAIDS increase risk of GI bleeding; increases risk of **warfarin**-induced hypoprothombinemia; increases **methotrexate** levels and toxicity.

NURSING IMPLICATIONS

Administration

- Diflunisal can be taken with water, milk, or food to reduce GI irritation. Food causes slight reduction in absorption rate but does not affect total amount absorbed.
- Store at 15–30C (59–86F) in tightly closed containers unless otherwise directed.

Assessment & Drug Effects

- Full antiinflammatory effect for arthritis may not occur until 8 d to several weeks into therapy in some patients.
- Diflunisal should be discontinued if patient presents signs of hepatic toxicity (see Appendix G).
- Although the antipyretic effect is mild, chronic or high doses may mask fever in some patients.

Patient & Family Education

- Instruct patient to swallow tablet whole. It should not be crushed or chewed.
- Caution patient to take drug as prescribed. Doubling the dosage can produce greater than doubling of drug accumulation, particularly in patients receiving repetitive doses.
- Advise patient to report the onset of visual or auditory problems immediately to physician.
- Patients with impaired renal function should be closely monitored. Instruct patient to be aware of I&O ratio and pattern and to check for and report peripheral edema and unusual weight gain.
- Advise all patients and particularly those with history of GI problems to report promptly to physician the onset of melena, hematemesis, or severe stomach pain.
- Caution patient about potentially hazardous activities until reaction to drug is known.

D

DIGOXIN
(di-jox′in)
Trade names: Lanoxicaps, Lanoxin
Prototype for classifications: CARDIOVASCULAR AGENT; CARDIAC GLYCOSIDE; ANTIARRHYTHMIC
Pregnancy category: A

ACTIONS/PHARMACODYNAMICS Widely used glycoside of *Digitalis lanata*. Acts by increasing the force and velocity of myocardial systolic contraction (positive inotropic effect). It also decreases conduction velocity through the atrioventricular node. Action is more prompt and less prolonged than that of digitalis and digitoxin. Also, it is less likely to give rise to cumulative effects because it is more readily absorbed and exchanged in the body and is rather rapidly excreted in urine.

USES Rapid digitalization and for maintenance therapy in CHF, atrial fibrillation, atrial flutter, paroxysmal atrial tachycardia.

ROUTE & DOSAGE

Digitalizing Dose

Adult: **PO** 10–15 μg/kg (1 mg) in divided doses over 24–48 h. **IV** 10–15 μg/kg (1 mg) in divided doses over 24 h.
Child: **PO/IV** >10 y, 10–15 μg/kg (1.5–2 mg); 2–10 y, 20–40 μg/kg; <2 y, 40–60 μg/kg.
Neonate, term: 30–50 μg/kg; *premature:* 20 μg/kg.

Maintenance Dose

Adult: **PO/IV** 0.1–0.375 mg/d.
Child: **PO/IV** >10 y, 0.125–0.25 mg/d; 2–10 y, 6–7.5 μg/kg/d; <2 y, 7.5–9 μg/kg/d.
Neonate, term: 6–7.5 μg/kg/d; *premature:* 3.75 μg/kg/d.

PHARMACOKINETICS Absorption: 70% PO tablets; 90% PO liquid and capsules. **Onset:** 1–2 h PO; 5–30 min IV. **Peak:** 6–8 h PO; 1–5 h IV. **Duration:** 3–4 d in fully digitalized patient. **Distribution:** widely distributed; tissue levels significantly higher than plasma levels; crosses placenta. **Metabolism:** approximately 14% in liver. **Elimination:** half-life: 34–44 h; 80–90% excreted by kidneys; may appear in breast milk.

CONTRAINDICATIONS & PRECAUTIONS Contraindicated in: digitalis hypersensitivity, ventricular fibrillation, ventricular tachycardia unless due to CHF. Full digitalizing dose not given if patient has received digoxin during previous week or if slowly excreted cardiotonic glycoside has been given during previous 2 wk. **Cautious use in:** renal insufficiency, hypokalemia, advanced heart disease, acute MI, incomplete AV block, cor pulmonale; hypothyroidism; lung disease; pregnancy (category A), nursing women, premature and immature infants, children, elderly or debilitated patients.

ADVERSE/SIDE EFFECTS CNS: fatigue, muscle weakness, headache, facial neuralgia, mental depression, paresthesias, hallucinations, confusion, drowsiness, agitation, dizziness. **CV:** arrhythmias, hypotension, AV block. **Eye:** visual disturbances. **GI:** anorexia, *nausea,* vomiting, diarrhea. **Other:** diaphoresis, recurrent malaise, dysphagia.

DRUG INTERACTIONS ANTACIDS, **cholestyramine, colestipol** decrease digoxin absorption; DIURETICS, CORTICOSTEROIDS, **amphotericin B,** LAXATIVES, **sodium polystyrene sulfonate** may cause hypokalemia, increasing the risk of digoxin toxicity; **calcium IV** may increase risk of arrhythmias if administered together

D

with digoxin; **quinidine, verapamil, amiodarone, flecainide** significantly increase digoxin levels, and digoxin dose should be decreased by 50%; **erythromycin** may increase digoxin levels; **succinylcholine** may potentiate arrhythmogenic effects; **nefazadone** may increase digoxin levels.

INCOMPATIBILITIES Solution/additive: dobutamine, doxapram.

NURSING IMPLICATIONS

Administration

- Digoxin may be given without regard to food. Administration after food may slightly delay rate of absorption but total amount absorbed is not affected.
- Tablet may be crushed and mixed with fluid or food if patient cannot swallow it whole.
- IV administration: Direct IV injection of digoxin may be administered undiluted or diluted in 4 ml of sterile water, D5W, or NaCl 0.9% (if prescribed). Administer each direct IV dose over at least 5 min.
- Infiltration of parenteral drug into subcutaneous tissue can cause local irritation and sloughing.

Assessment & Drug Effects

- Be familiar with patient's baseline data (e.g., quality of peripheral pulses, blood pressure, clinical symptoms, serum electrolytes, creatinine clearance) as a foundation for making assessments.
- Before administering digoxin, check laboratory reports for serum levels of digoxin, potassium, magnesium, and calcium. Notify physician of abnormal values.
- Before administering digoxin, take apical pulse for 1 full min noting rate, rhythm, and quality. If changes are noted, withhold digoxin, take rhythm strip if patient is on ECG monitor, notify physician promptly.
- Monitor for signs and symptoms of digoxin toxicity.
- Although a fall in ventricular rate to 60/min in adults (70/min in children) is one criterion for withholding medication, any change in pulse rate or rhythm should be interpreted as a sign of digitalis intoxication and should be reported promptly.
- In children, cardiac arrhythmias are usually reliable signs of early toxicity. Early indicators in adults (anorexia, nausea, vomiting, diarrhea, visual disturbances) are rarely initial signs in children.
- Therapeutic range of serum digoxin is 0.8–2 ng/ml; toxic levels are >2 ng/ml. Blood samples for determining plasma digoxin levels should be drawn at least 6 h after daily dose and preferably just before next scheduled daily dose.
- Monitor I&O ratio during digitalization, particularly in patients with impaired renal function, and for edema daily and auscultate chest for rales.
- Concurrent antibiotic–digoxin therapy could precipitate toxicity because of altered intestinal flora. Monitor serum digoxin levels closely.
- Patient should be closely observed when being transferred from one preparation (tablet, elixir, or parenteral) to another; e.g., when tablet is replaced by elixir potential for toxicity increases since ≥ 30% of drug is absorbed.

Patient & Family Education

- When digoxin is prescribed for atrial fibrillation, advise patient to report to physician if pulse falls below 60 or rises above 110 or if patient detects skipped beats or other changes in rhythm.

- Instruct patient to suspect toxicity and report to physician if any of the following occur: anorexia, nausea, vomiting, diarrhea, or visual disturbances.
- Instruct patient to weigh each day under standard conditions. Report weight gain > 1 kg (2 lb)/d.
- Instruct patient to take digoxin precisely as prescribed, not to skip or double a dose or change dose intervals, and to take it at same time each day.
- Caution patient not to take OTC medications, especially those for coughs, colds, allergy, GI upset, or obesity without prior approval of physician.
- Patient should continue with brand originally prescribed unless otherwise directed by physician.

DIGOXIN IMMUNE FAB (OVINE)

Trade name: Digibind
Classification: ANTIDOTE
Pregnancy category: C

ACTIONS/PHARMACODYNAMICS

Purified fragments of antibodies specific for digoxin (but also effective for digitoxin) produced in sheep immunized with digoxin–albumin conjugate. Use of fragments of antidigoxin antibodies (Fab) instead of whole antibody molecules permits more extensive and faster distribution to serum and toxic cellular sites. Acts by selectively complexing with circulating digoxin or digitoxin, thereby preventing drug from binding at receptor sites; the complex is then eliminated in urine.

USES Treatment of potentially life-threatening digoxin or digitoxin intoxication in carefully selected patients.

ROUTE & DOSAGE

Serious Digoxin Toxicity Secondary to Overdose

IV Dosages vary according to amount of digoxin to be neutralized; dosages are based on total body load or steady state serum digoxin concentrations (see package insert); some patients may require a second dose after several hours.

PHARMACOKINETICS **Onset:** <1 min after IV administration. **Elimination:** half-life: 14–20 h; excreted in urine over 5–7 d.

CONTRAINDICATIONS & PRECAUTIONS **Contraindicated in:** hypersensitivity to sheep products; renal or cardiac failure. Safe use during pregnancy (category C) or in nursing women not established. **Cautious use in:** prior treatment with sheep antibodies or ovine Fab fragments; history of allergies; impaired renal function.

ADVERSE/SIDE EFFECTS Adverse reactions associated with use of digoxin immune Fab are related primarily to the effects of digitalis withdrawal on the heart (see Nursing Implications). Allergic reactions have been reported rarely. Hypokalemia.

DIAGNOSTIC TEST INTERFERENCE Digoxin immune Fab may interfere with ***serum digoxin*** determinations by immunoassay tests.

DRUG INTERACTIONS Not established.

NURSING IMPLICATIONS

Administration

- Reconstitute by dissolving 38 mg (1 vial) in 4 ml of sterile water for injection; mix gently (solution will contain 9.5 mg/ml). For administration by IV infusion, reconstituted solution may be diluted further with sterile isotonic saline injection.

- After reconstitution, digoxin immune Fab is administered by IV infusion over 30 min, preferably through a 0.22-μm membrane filter, or as bolus injection if cardiac arrest is imminent.
- For infants, reconstitute as directed and administer with a tuberculin syringe. For small doses (e.g., 2 mg or less), dilute the reconstituted 40 mg vial with 36 ml of sterile isotonic saline injection to make a concentration of 1 mg/ml. Children must be closely monitored for fluid overload.
- Reconstituted solutions should be used promptly or refrigerated at 2–8C (36–46F) for up to 4 h.

Assessment & Drug Effects

- Skin testing for allergy is performed prior to administration of immune Fab, particularly in patients with history of allergy or who have had previous therapy with immune Fab.
- As a precaution, emergency equipment and drugs should be immediately available before skin testing is done or first dose is given and should be kept readily accessible until patient is out of danger.
- The following measurements should be determined before administration of digoxin immune Fab and repeated at frequent intervals during therapy: temperature; BP; ECG; serum potassium; serum digoxin or digitoxin concentration (this measurement will not be accurate for at least 5–7 d after therapy begins because of test interference by immune Fab).
- Effective treatment should be reflected in improvement in cardiac rhythm abnormalities, mental orientation and other neurologic symptoms, and GI and visual disturbances.
- Reversal of signs and symptoms of digitalis toxicity occurs in 15–60 min in adults and usually within minutes in children.
- Cardiac status may deteriorate as inotropic action of digitalis is withdrawn by action of immune Fab. Closely monitor for CHF, arrhythmias, increase in heart rate, and hypokalemia.
- Close monitoring of serum potassium is particularly critical during first several hours following administration of immune Fab.
- Follow-up serum digoxin levels and ECG readings are recommended for at least 2–3 wk.

DIHYDROERGOTAMINE MESYLATE

(dye-hye-droe-er-got'a-meen)

Trade name: D.H.E. 45, Migranal

Classifications: AUTONOMIC NERVOUS SYSTEM AGENT; ALPHA-ADRENERGIC ANTAGONIST; ERGOT ALKALOID

Prototype: Ergotamine

Pregnancy category: X

ACTIONS/PHARMACODYNAMICS

Alpha-adrenergic blocking agent and dihydrogenated ergot alkaloid with direct constricting effect on smooth muscle of peripheral and cranial blood vessels. Maintains elevated levels of circulating norepinephrine (vasoconstrictor action) by inhibiting its reuptake. Vasoconstrictor action is more prominent on capacitance vessels (veins, venules) than on resistance vessels (arteries, arterioles). Reduces rate of serotonin-induced platelet aggregation. Has somewhat weaker vasoconstrictor action than ergotamine but greater adrenergic blocking activity.

USES To prevent or abort vascular headache (e.g., migraine or histaminic cephalalgia) when rapid control is desired or other routes are not feasible. With low-dose heparin therapy to prevent postoperative deep-vein thrombosis and pulmonary embolism. **Other use:** to treat postural hypotension.

ROUTE & DOSAGE

Migraine Headache

Adult: **IM/IV** 1 mg; may be repeated at 1 h intervals to a total of 3 mg IM or 2 mg IV (max 6 mg/wk). **Intranasal** 1 spray (0.5 mg) in each nostril; may repeat with additional spray in 15 min if no relief; max 4 sprays per attack; should wait 6–8 h before treating another attack (max 8 sprays per 24 h, 24 sprays/wk).

PHARMACOKINETICS **Onset:** 15–30 min IM; <5 min IV. **Duration:** 3–4 h. **Distribution:** probably distributed into breast milk. **Metabolism:** metabolized in liver. **Elimination:** half-life: 21–32 h; excreted primarily in urine; some excreted in feces.

CONTRAINDICATIONS & PRECAUTIONS **Contraindicated in:** history of hypersensitivity to ergot preparations; peripheral vascular disease, coronary heart disease, hypertension; peptic ulcer; impaired hepatic or renal function; sepsis. Safe use during pregnancy (category X), in nursing women, and in children not established.

ADVERSE/SIDE EFFECTS **CV:** vasospasm: coldness, numbness and tingling in fingers and toes, muscle pains and weakness of legs, precordial distress and pain, transient tachycardia or bradycardia, hypertension (large doses). **GI:** *nausea, vomiting.* **Other:** dizziness, dysphoria, *localized edema and itching;* ergotism (excessive doses).

DRUG INTERACTIONS BETA BLOCKERS, **erythromycin** increase peripheral vasoconstriction with risk of ischemia.

NURSING IMPLICATIONS

Administration

- Drug should be given at first warning of migraine headache. Optimum results are obtained by titrating the doses required to give relief for several headaches to determine the minimal effective dose. This dose is used for subsequent attacks.
- Onset of action after IM injection is delayed about 20 min; therefore, when more rapid relief is required, the IV route is prescribed.
- IV dihydroergotamine may be given by direct IV undiluted at a rate of 1 mg/60 seconds.
- Protect ampuls from heat and light; do not freeze. Discard ampul if solution appears discolored.
- Store at 15–30C (59–86F) unless otherwise directed.

Patient & Family Education

- Advise patient to lie down in a quiet, darkened room for several hours after drug administration for best results.
- Report the onset of nausea, vomiting, change in heartbeat, numbness, tingling, pain or weakness of extremities.

DIHYDROTACHYSTEROL

(dye-hye-droe-tak-iss'ter-ole)

Trade names: DHT, DHT Intensol, Hytakerol

Classifications: VITAMIN D; REGULATOR, SERUM CALCIUM
Pregnancy category: A

D

ACTIONS/PHARMACODYNAMICS

Oil-soluble reduction product of ergocalciferol (vitamin D_2) with pharmacologic actions similar to those of both ergocalciferol and parathyroid hormone. In comparison with ergocalciferol, dihydrotachysterol has weak antirachitic activity, promotes less intestinal absorption of calcium but almost equal phosphate diuresis. Acts like parathyroid hormone in ability to raise serum calcium concentrations rapidly; also reported to increase intestinal absorption of sodium, potassium, and magnesium.

USES Hypocalcemia associated with hypoparathyroidism, both postoperative and idiopathic, and in pseudohypoparathyroidism. Also for prophylaxis of hypocalcemic tetany following thyroid surgery. **Unlabeled uses:** vitamin D-resistant rickets (familial hypophosphatemia), osteoporosis, and renal osteodystrophy.

ROUTE & DOSAGE

Hypoparathyroidism, Pseudohypoparathyroidism

Adult: **PO** 0.75–2.5 mg/d for several days; then 0.2–1 mg/d (may need 1.5 mg/d).
Child: **PO** 1–5 mg/d for 4 d; then 0.5–1.5 mg/d.
Neonate: **PO** 0.05–0.1 mg/d.

Thyroidectomy-induced Hypocalcemia

Adult: **PO** 0.25 mg/d.

Renal Osteodystrophy

Adult: **PO** 0.1–0.6 mg/d. *Child:* **PO** 0.1–0.5 mg/d.

PHARMACOKINETICS Absorption: readily absorbed from small intestines. **Peak:** 2 wk. **Duration:** 2 wk. **Distribution:** distributed in breast milk. **Metabolism:** metabolized in liver to active metabolite. **Elimination:** excreted primarily in bile and feces.

CONTRAINDICATIONS & PRECAUTIONS Contraindicated in: sensitivity to vitamin D; hypercalcemia and hypocalcemia associated with renal insufficiency and hyperphosphatemia; renal stones, hypervitaminosis D. Safe use during pregnancy (category A), in nursing mothers, and in children in amounts exceeding RDA not established.

ADVERSE/SIDE EFFECTS Hypercalcemia. **CNS:** drowsiness, headache, weakness, vertigo, ataxia, atonia, mental depression. **GI:** anorexia, nausea, vomiting, metallic taste, dry mouth, thirst, diarrhea, constipation, abdominal pain. **GU:** nocturia, polyuria, renal calculi. **Other:** tinnitus.

DRUG INTERACTIONS Not established.

NURSING IMPLICATIONS

Administration

- Withhold drug if signs and symptoms of hypercalcemia appear (see Appendix G) and report to physician.
- Store in tightly closed, light-resistant containers at 15–30C (59–86F) unless otherwise directed.

Assessment & Drug Effects

- Determine serum and urinary calcium levels at least weekly during first month of therapy until they are stabilized, then monthly thereafter.
- Adequate calcium intake is necessary for clinical response to therapy. Usually supplemented with

10–15 g of oral calcium lactate or gluconate daily.

- Patients with hyperphosphatemia will require dietary restriction of phosphate or administration of calcium carbonate supplements with meals, or both, to bind intestinal phosphates and improve calcium balance.
- Hypoparathyroid patients receiving thiazide diuretics are prone to develop hypercalcemia and therefore require close monitoring.

Patient & Family Education

- Inform patients of the signs and symptoms of hypercalcemia (see Appendix G).

DILTIAZEM

(dil-tye'a-zem)

Trade names: Cardizem, Cardizem CD, Cardizem SR, Cardizen Lyo-Ject, Dilacor XR, Tiamate, Tiazac

DILTIAZEM IV

Trade name: Cardizem IV

Classifications: CARDIOVASCULAR AGENT; CALCIUM CHANNEL BLOCKING AGENT; ANTIHYPERTENSIVE

Prototype: Verapamil

Pregnancy category: C

ACTIONS/PHARMACODYNAMICS Slow channel blocker with pharmacologic actions similar to those of verapamil. Inhibits calcium ion influx through slow channels into cell of myocardial and arterial smooth muscle (both coronary and peripheral blood vessels). As a result, intracellular calcium remains at subthreshold levels insufficient to stimulate cell excitation and contraction. Dilates coronary arteries and arterioles and inhibits coronary artery spasm; thus myocardial oxygen delivery is increased (antianginal effect). Slows SA and AV node conduction (antiarrhythmic effect) without affecting normal arterial action potential or intraventricular conduction. By vasodilation of peripheral arterioles drug decreases total peripheral vascular resistance and reduces arterial BP at rest (antihypertensive effect). May cause slight decrease in heart rate. Does not alter total serum calcium levels.

USES Vasospastic angina (Prinzmetal's variant or at rest angina), chronic stable (classic effort-associated) angina, essential hypertension. **IV form:** atrial fibrillation, atrial flutter, supraventricular tachycardia. **Unlabeled use:** prevention of reinfarction in non-Q-wave MI.

ROUTE & DOSAGE

Angina

Adult: **PO** 30 mg q.i.d.; may increase q1–2d as required; usual dose range 180–360 mg/d in divided doses.

Hypertension

Adult: **PO** 60–120 mg sustained release b.i.d. (usual range: 240–360 mg/d).

Atrial Fibrillation

Adult: **IV** 0.25 mg/kg IV bolus over 2 min; if inadequate response, may repeat in 15 min with 0.35 mg/kg, followed by a continuous infusion of 5–10 mg/h (recommended max dose: 15 mg/h for 24 h).

PHARMACOKINETICS **Absorption:** approximately 80% absorbed from GI tract, with 40% reaching systemic circulation. **Peak:** 2–3 h; 6–11 h sustained release. **Distribution:** distributed into breast milk. **Metabolism:**

D

metabolized in liver. **Elimination:** half-life: oral 3.5–9 h, IV 2 h; excreted primarily in urine with some elimination in feces.

CONTRAINDICATIONS & PRECAUTIONS **Contraindicated in:** known hypersensitivity to drug; sick sinus syndrome (unless pacemaker is in place and functioning); second- or third-degree AV block; severe hypotension (systolic <90 mm Hg or diastolic <60 mm Hg); patients undergoing intracranial surgery; bleeding aneurysms. Safe use during pregnancy (category C), in nursing mothers, and in children not established. **Cautious use in:** CHF (especially if patient is also receiving beta blocker), conduction abnormalities; renal or hepatic impairment; the elderly; nursing mothers.

ADVERSE/SIDE EFFECTS **CNS:** *headache,* fatigue, dizziness, asthenia, drowsiness, nervousness, insomnia, confusion, tremor, gait abnormality. **CV:** edema, arrhythmias, angina, second- or third-degree AV block, bradycardia, CHF, flushing, hypotension, syncope, palpitations. **GI:** nausea, constipation, anorexia, vomiting, diarrhea, impaired taste, weight increase. **Skin:** rash.

DRUG INTERACTIONS BETA BLOCKERS, **digoxin** may have additive effects on av node conduction prolongation; may increase **digoxin** or **quinidine** levels; **cimetidine** may increase diltiazem levels, thus increasing effects; may increase **cyclosporine** levels.

INCOMPATIBILITIES **Solution/additive: furosemide. Y-site: furosemide.**

NURSING IMPLICATIONS

Administration

- Administer oral drug before meals and at bedtime.
- IV diltiazem may be given by direct IV as a bolus dose over 2 min. A second bolus may be administered after 15 min.
- IV diltiazem may be given by coninuous IV infusion. The recommended rate is 5–15 mg/h. Infusion duration longer than 24 h and infusion rate >15 mg/h are not recommended.
- For continuous IV infusion, diltiazem may be added to any of the following: D5W, NS, D5W/0.45% NaCl. Refrigerate until used and use within 24 h of dilution.
- Withhold drug if systolic BP is < 90 mm Hg or diastolic is < 60 mm Hg.
- Store oral forms at 15–30C (59–86F).

Assessment & Drug Effects

- BP and ECG should be evaluated before initiation of therapy and monitored particularly during dosage adjustment period. Baseline and periodic tests of liver and renal function are also recommended.
- Monitor for headache. An analgesic may be required.
- Drug may induce hyperglycemia. Monitor diabetes closely.

Patient & Family Education

- Because of the possibility of lightheadedness, dizziness (hypotension), advise patient to make position changes slowly and in stages. Supervision of ambulation may be indicated.
- Caution patient to avoid driving and other potentially hazardous activities until reaction to drug is known.
- Stress importance of keeping follow-up appointments and of keeping physician informed.

DIMENHYDRINATE

(dye-men-hye′dri-nate)

Trade names: Apo-Dimenhydrinate♣, Calm-X, Dimenhydrinate Injection, Dimentabs, Dinate, Dommanate, Dramanate, Dramamine, Dramilin, Dramocen, Dramoject, Dymenate, Gravol♣, Hydrate, Marmine, Motion-Aid, Nauseatol♣, Novodimenate♣, PMS Dimenhydrinate♣, Travamine♣, Travel Aid, Travel Eze, Wehamine

Classifications: ANTIHISTAMINE (H_1-RECEPTOR ANTAGONIST); ANTIEMETIC; ANTIVERTIGO AGENT

Prototype: Diphenhydramine

Pregnancy category: B

ACTIONS/PHARMACODYNAMICS

H_1-receptor antagonist and chlorotheophylline salt of diphenhydramine, with which it shares similar properties. Precise mode of antinauseant action not known, but thought to involve ability to inhibit cholinergic stimulation in vestibular and associated neural pathways.

USES Chiefly in prevention and treatment of motion sickness. Also has been used in management of vertigo, nausea, and vomiting associated with radiation sickness, labyrinthitis, Ménière's syndrome, stapedectomy, anesthesia, and various medications.

ROUTE & DOSAGE

Motion Sickness

Adult: **PO** 50–100 mg q4–6h (max 400 mg/24h). **IM/IV** 50 mg as needed.

Child: **PO** *6–12 y,* 25–50 mg q6–8h (max 150 mg/24h); *2–6 y,* up to 25 mg q6–8h (max 75 mg/24h). **IM/IV** *6–12 y,* 1.25 mg/kg q.i.d. up to 300 mg/d; *2–6 y,* 1.25 mg/kg q.i.d. up to 300 mg/d.

PHARMACOKINETICS Absorption: readily absorbed from GI tract. **Onset:** 15–30 min PO; immediate IV; 20–30 min IM. **Duration:** 3–6 h. **Distribution:** distributed into breast milk. **Elimination:** excreted in urine.

CONTRAINDICATIONS & PRECAUTIONS Contraindicated in: narrow-angle glaucoma, prostatic hypertrophy. Safe use during pregnancy (category B), in nursing women, and in children <2 y not established. **Cautious use in:** convulsive disorders.

ADVERSE/SIDE EFFECTS CNS: *drowsiness,* headache, incoordination, dizziness, blurred vision, nervousness, restlessness, *insomnia (especially children).* **CV:** hypotension, palpitation. **Other:** dry mouth, nose, throat. Less frequently: anorexia, constipation or diarrhea, urinary frequency, dysuria.

DIAGNOSTIC TEST INTERFERENCE ***Skin testing*** procedures should not be performed within 72 h after use of an antihistamine.

DRUG INTERACTIONS Alcohol and other CNS DEPRESSANTS enhance CNS depression, drowsiness; TRICYCLIC ANTIDEPRESSANTS compound anticholinergic effects.

INCOMPATIBILITIES Solution/additive: aminophylline, amobarbital, butorphanol, chlorpromazine, glycopyrrolate, hydroxyzine, midazolam, pentobarbital, prochlorperazine, promazine, promethazine, thiopental.

NURSING IMPLICATIONS

Administration

- IV injection: IV dimenhydrinate may be given by direct IV. Dilute each 50 mg in 10 ml of NS. Administer 50 mg or fraction thereof over 2 min.
- To prevent radiation sickness,

drug is usually administered 30–60 min before treatment, then repeated 1 1/2 h after treatment, and again in 3 h.

- Store preferably at 15–30C (59–86F), unless otherwise directed by manufacturer. Examine parenteral preparation for particulate matter and discoloration. Do not use unless absolutely clear.

Assessment & Drug Effects

- High incidence of drowsiness. Side rails and supervision of ambulation may be indicated.
- Tolerance to CNS depressant effects usually occurs after a few days of drug therapy. Some decrease in antiemetic action may result with prolonged use.
- Antihistamines can obscure signs of dizziness, nausea, and vomiting, associated with drug toxicity and serious disease conditions.

Patient & Family Education

- Caution ambulatory patient not to drive or operate dangerous machinery until reaction to drug is known.
- To prevent motion sickness, dimenhydrinate should be taken 30 min before departure and should be repeated before meals and upon retiring.

DIMERCAPROL

(dye-mer-kap′role)

Trade names: BAL in Oil, British Anti-Lewisite

Classifications: CHELATING AGENT; ANTIDOTE

Pregnancy category: D

ACTIONS/PHARMACODYNAMICS Dithiol compound that combines with ions of various heavy metals to form relatively stable, nontoxic, soluble complexes called chelates, which can be excreted; inhibition of sulfhydryl enzymes by toxic metals is thus prevented. May also reactivate affected enzymes but is most effective when administered prior to enzyme damage.

USES Acute poisoning by arsenic, gold, and mercury; as adjunct to edetate calcium disodium (EDTA) in treatment of lead encephalopathy. **Unlabeled uses:** chromium dermatitis; ocular and dermatologic manifestations of arsenic poisoning, as adjunct to penicillamine to increase rate of copper excretion in Wilson's disease, and for poisoning with antimony, bismuth, chromium, copper, nickel, tungsten, zinc.

ROUTE & DOSAGE

Arsenic or Gold Poisoning

Adult: **IM** 2.5–3 mg/kg q4h for first 2 d; then q.i.d. on third day; then b.i.d. for 10 d.
Child: **IM** Same as for adult.

Mercury Poisoning

Adult: **IM** 5 mg/kg initially; followed by 2.5 mg/kg 1–2 times/d for 10 d.
Child: **IM** Same as for adult.

Acute Lead Encephalopathy

Adult: **IM** 4 mg/kg initially; then 3–4 mg/kg q4h with EDTA for 2–7 d depending on response.
Child: **IM** Same as for adult.

PHARMACOKINETICS **Peak:** 30–60 min. **Distribution:** distributed mainly in intracellular spaces, including brain; highest concentrations in liver and kidneys. **Elimination:** half-life: short; completely excreted in urine and bile within 4 h.

CONTRAINDICATIONS & PRECAUTIONS **Contraindicated in:** hepatic insufficiency (with exception of postarsenical jaundice); severe renal insufficiency; poisoning due to cadmium, iron, selenium, or uranium. Safe use during pregnancy (category D) and in nursing women not established. **Cautious use in:** hypertension, patients with G6PD deficiency.

ADVERSE/SIDE EFFECTS CNS: headache, anxiety, muscle pain or weakness, restlessness, paresthesias, tremors, *convulsions,* shock. **CV:** *elevated BP,* tachycardia. **ENT:** rhinorrhea; burning sensation, feeling of pain and constriction in throat. **GI:** nausea, *vomiting*; burning sensation in lips and mouth, halitosis, salivation; abdominal pain, metabolic acidosis. **GU:** burning sensation in penis, renal damage. **Other:** pains in chest or hands, pain and sterile abscess at injection site, sweating, reduction in polymorphonuclear leukocytes, dental pain.

DIAGNOSTIC TEST INTERFERENCE ***^{131}I thyroidal uptake*** values may be decreased if test is done during or immediately following dimercaprol therapy.

DRUG INTERACTIONS **Iron, cadmium, selenium, uranium** form toxic complexes with dimercaprol.

NURSING IMPLICATIONS

Administration

- Because irreversible tissue damage may occur quickly, particularly in mercury poisoning, dimercaprol therapy must be initiated as soon as possible (within 1–2 h) after ingestion of the poison.
- Administered by deep IM injection only. Local pain, gluteal abscess, and skin sensitization reported. Rotate injection sites and observe daily.
- Contact of drug with skin may produce erythema, edema, dermatitis. Handle with caution.
- Presence of sediment in ampul reportedly does not indicate drug deterioration.

Assessment & Drug Effects

- Monitor vital signs. Elevations of systolic and diastolic BPs accompanied by tachycardia frequently occur within a few minutes following injection and may remain elevated up to 2 h.
- Fever occurs in approximately 30% of children receiving treatment and may persist throughout therapy.
- I&O should be monitored. Drug is potentially nephrotoxic. Report oliguria or change in I&O ratio.
- Urine should be kept alkaline to reduce possibility of renal damage during elimination of dimercaprol chelate.
- Daily urine examinations should be made for albumin, blood, casts, and pH. Blood and urinary levels of the metal serve as guides for dosage adjustments.
- Minor adverse reactions usually reach maximum 15–20 min after drug administration and generally subside in 30–90 min. Ephedrine or an antihistamine is sometimes administered to prevent symptoms.

DIMETHYL SULFOXIDE

(dye-meth′il sul-fox′ide)

Trade names: DMSO, Rimso-50

Classifications: SKIN AND MUCOUS MEMBRANE AGENT; ANTIINFLAMMATORY, LOCAL

Pregnancy category: C

ACTIONS/PHARMACODYNAMICS Mechanism of action not known. Reported actions and effects include

D

antiinflammatory effects, membrane penetration, collagen dissolution, peripheral nerve blockade (local analgesia), vasodilation, muscle relaxation, diuresis, weak bacteriostatic and antifungal actions, initiation of histamine release at administration site, cholinesterase inhibition. Enhances percutaneous absorption of many drugs by increasing permeability of skin.

USE Symptomatic treatment of interstitial cystitis. **Unlabeled uses:** topical treatment of a variety of musculoskeletal disorders, arthritis, scleroderma, tendinitis, breast and prostate malignancies, retinitis pigmentosa, herpesvirus infections, head and spinal cord injuries, shock, and as a carrier to enhance penetration and absorption of other drugs. Also used to protect living cells and tissues during cold storage (cryoprotection). Widely used as an industrial solvent and in veterinary medicine for treatment of musculoskeletal injuries.

ROUTE & DOSAGE

Interstitial Cystitis

Adult: **Intravesicular Instillation:** 50 ml of 50% solution instilled slowly into urinary bladder and retained for 15 min; may repeat q2wk until maximum relief obtained; then increase intervals between treatments.

PHARMACOKINETICS Absorption: readily absorbed systemically. **Peak:** 4–8 h. **Distribution:** widely distributed in tissues and body fluids; penetrates blood–brain barrier; distributed into breast milk. **Metabolism:** metabolized to dimethyl sulfide (garlic breath) and dimethyl sulfone. **Elimination:** dimethyl sulfide excreted through lungs and skin; dimethyl sulfone may remain in serum > 2 wk and is excreted in urine and feces.

CONTRAINDICATIONS & PRECAUTIONS Contraindicated in: safe use during pregnancy (category C), in nursing mothers, and in children not established. **Cautious use in:** hepatic or renal dysfunction.

ADVERSE/SIDE EFFECTS Eye: transient disturbances in color vision, photophobia. **GI:** nausea, diarrhea. **Hypersensitivity:** local or generalized rash, erythema, pruritus, urticaria, swelling of face, dyspnea (anaphylactoid reaction). **Other:** nasal congestion, headache, sedation, drowsiness. **Following intravesicular instillation:** *garlic-like odor on breath and skin; garlic-like taste;* discomfort during administration; transient cystitis. **Following topical application:** vesicle formation.

DRUG INTERACTIONS Decreases effectiveness of **sulindac,** possibly causing severe peripheral neuropathy.

NURSING IMPLICATIONS

Administration

- Manufacturer suggests application of analgesic lubricant such as lidocaine jelly to urethra to facilitate insertion of catheter.
- Patient retains instillation for 15 min and then expels it by spontaneous voiding.
- Discomfort associated with instillation usually becomes less prominent with repeated administration. Physician may prescribe an oral analgesic or suppository containing belladonna and an opiate prior to instillation to reduce bladder spasm.
- Store at 15–30C (59–86F) unless otherwise directed by manufacturer. Protect from strong light and avoid contact with plastics.

Assessment & Drug Effects
- CBCs and liver and renal function tests are recommended, initially and at 6-mo intervals.
- Complete eye evaluation including slit-lamp examination is recommended prior to and at regular intervals during therapy.

Patient & Family Education
- Garliclike taste may be experienced within minutes after drug instillation and may last for several hours. Garliclike odor on breath and skin may last as long as 72 h.
- Caution patient not to use OTC topical medications without consulting physician.

DINOPROSTONE (PGE_2, PROSTAGLANDIN E_2)
(dye-noe-prost'one)
Trade names: Cervidil, Prostin E_2, Prepidil
Prototype for classifications: PROSTAGLANDIN; OXYTOCIC

ACTIONS/PHARMACODYNAMICS Synthetically prepared member of the prostaglandin E_2 series that appears to act directly on myometrium and on gastrointestinal, bronchial, and vascular smooth muscle. Stimulation of gravid uterus in early weeks of gestation is more potent than that of oxytocin. Contractions are qualitatively similar to those that occur during term labor. Has high success rate when used as abortifacient before twentieth week and for stimulation of labor in cases of intrauterine fetal death.

USES To terminate pregnancy from twelfth week through second trimester as calculated from first day of last regular menstrual period; to evacuate uterine contents in management of missed abortion or intrauterine fetal death up to 28 wk gestational age; to manage benign hydatidiform mole; cervical ripening prior to labor induction.

ROUTE & DOSAGE

Induction of Labor
Adult: **Endocervical *Prepidil:*** Place 0.5 mg endocervically. May repeat q6h to a max of 1.5 mg. ***Cervidil:*** Place 10-mg insert transversely in the posterior fornix of the vagina. Remove on onset of active labor or 12 h after insertion.

Evacuation of Uterus
Adult: **Intravaginal** Insert suppository high in vagina; repeat q2–5h until abortion occurs or membranes rupture; max total dose 240 mg.

PHARMACOKINETICS Absorption: slowly absorbed from vagina; Cervidil insert releases approximately 0.3 mg/h. **Onset:** 10 min. **Duration:** 2–3 h. **Distribution:** widely distributed in body. **Metabolism:** rapidly metabolized in lungs, kidneys, spleen, and other tissues. **Elimination:** excreted mainly in urine; some excreted in feces.

CONTRAINDICATIONS & PRECAUTIONS Contraindicated in: acute pelvic inflammatory disease, history of pelvic surgery, uterine fibroids, cervical stenosis, active cardiac, pulmonary, renal, or hepatic disease. **Cautious use in:** history of hypertension, hypotension, asthma, epilepsy, anemia, diabetes mellitus; jaundice, history of hepatic, renal, or cardiovascular disease; cervicitis, acute vaginitis, infected endocervical lesion.

ADVERSE/SIDE EFFECTS CNS: headache, tremor, tension. **CV:** transient

D

hypotension, flushing, cardiac arrhythmias. **GI:** *nausea, vomiting, diarrhea.* **Reproductive:** vaginal pain, endometritis, uterine rupture. **Respiratory:** dyspnea, cough, hiccups. **Other:** chills, *fever,* dehydration, diaphoresis, rash.

DRUG INTERACTION OXYTOCICS used with extreme caution.

NURSING IMPLICATIONS

Administration

- Antiemetic and antidiarrheal medication may be prescribed before dinoprostone to minimize GI side effects.
- The vaginal insert must be placed in the vagina immediately after removal from the foil package. *Do not* use without retrieval system.
- Patient should remain in supine position for 10 min after administration of dinoprostone suppository to prevent expulsion and enhance absorption.
- Store suppositories in freezer at temperature not exceeding –20C (–4F) unless otherwise specified by manufacturer.

Assessment & Drug Effects

- Although rupture of the membranes is not a contraindication to use of dinoprostone, be aware that profuse bleeding may result in expulsion of the suppository. Observe patient carefully, after insertion of the drug.
- Monitor uterine contractions and observe for and report excessive vaginal bleeding and cramping pain. Keep pad count. Save all clots and tissues for physician inspection and laboratory analysis.
- In most patients, abortion usually occurs within 30 h. (When used in conjunction with oxytocin, time may be shortened to 12–14 h.)
- Monitor vital signs. Fever is a physiologic response of the hypothalamus to use of dinoprostone and occurs within 15–45 min after insertion of suppository. Temperature returns to normal within 2–6 h after discontinuation of medication.
- Observe patient closely during entire period of drug action: report wheezing, chest pain, dyspnea, and significant changes in BP and pulse to the physician.

Patient & Family Education

- Advise patient to continue taking her temperature (late afternoon) for a few days after discharge. Advise her to contact physician with onset of fever, bleeding, abdominal cramps, abnormal or foul-smelling vaginal discharge.
- Douches, tampons, intercourse, and tub baths should be avoided for at least 2 wk. Clarify with physician.
- If patient has had a joint disorder, dinoprostone may exacerbate pain and limitation because of its effect on the inflammatory process.

DIPHENHYDRAMINE HYDROCHLORIDE

(dye-fen-hye′dra-meen)

Trade names: Allerdryl ♣, Banophen, Belix, Ben-Allergin, Bena-D, Benadryl, Benadryl Dye-Free, Benahist, Benoject, Benylin, Compoz, Diahist, Dihydrex, Diphen, Diphenacen, Fenylhist, Hyrexin, Insomnal, Nordryl, Nytol with DPH, Sleep-Eze 3, Sominex Formula 2, Tusstat, Twilite, Valdrene, Wehdryl

Prototype for classifications: ANTIHISTAMINE; H_1-RECEPTOR ANTAGONIST

Pregnancy category: C

ACTIONS/PHARMACODYNAMICS

Ethanolamine antihistamine with significant anticholinergic activity.

High incidence of drowsiness, but GI side effects are minor. Competes for H_1-receptor sites on effector cells, thus blocking histamine release. Effects in parkinsonism and drug-induced extrapyramidal symptoms are apparently related to its ability to suppress central cholinergic activity and to prolong action of dopamine by inhibiting its reuptake and storage. Does not inhibit gastric secretion but has strong antiemetic effect.

USES Temporary symptomatic relief of various allergic conditions and to treat or prevent motion sickness, vertigo, and reactions to blood or plasma in susceptible patients. Also used in anaphylaxis as adjunct to epinephrine and other standard measures after acute symptoms have been controlled; in treatment of parkinsonism and drug-induced extrapyramidal reactions; as a nonnarcotic cough suppressant; as a sedative-hypnotic; and for treatment of intractable insomnia.

ROUTE & DOSAGE

Allergy Symptoms, Antiparkinsonism, Motion Sickness, Nighttime Sedation

Adult: **PO** 25–50 mg t.i.d. or q.i.d. (max 300 mg/d). **IV/IM** 10–50 mg q4–6h (max 400 mg/d).
Child: **PO/IV/IM** 6–12 y, 12.5 –25 mg q4–6h (max 300 mg/24 h); 2–6 y, 6.25 mg q4–6h (max 300 mg/24 h).

Nonproductive Cough

Adult: **PO** 25 mg q4–6h (max 100 mg/d).
Child: **PO** 6–12 y, 12.5 mg q4–6h (max 50 mg/24 h); 2–6 y, 6.25 mg q4–6h (max 25 mg/24 h).

PHARMACOKINETICS Absorption: readily absorbed from GI tract but only 40–60% reaches systemic circulation. **Onset:** 15–30 min. **Peak:** 1–4 h. **Duration:** 4–7 h. **Distribution:** crosses placenta; distributed into breast milk. **Metabolism:** metabolized in liver; some degradation in lung and kidney. **Elimination:** mostly excreted in urine within 24 h.

CONTRAINDICATIONS & PRECAUTIONS Contraindicated in: hypersensitivity to antihistamines of similar structure; lower respiratory tract symptoms (including acute asthma); narrow-angle glaucoma; prostatic hypertrophy, bladder neck obstruction; GI obstruction or stenosis; pregnancy (category C), nursing mothers, prematures, and newborns; use as nighttime sleep aid in children < age 12. **Cautious use in:** history of asthma; convulsive disorders; increased IOP; hyperthyroidism; hypertension, cardiovascular disease; diabetes mellitus; elderly patients, infants, and young children.

ADVERSE/SIDE EFFECTS CNS: *drowsiness,* dizziness, headache, fatigue, disturbed coordination, tingling, heaviness and weakness of hands, tremors, euphoria, nervousness, restlessness, insomnia; confusion; (especially in children): excitement, fever. **CV:** palpitation, *tachycardia,* mild hypotension or hypertension, <u>cardiovascular collapse</u>. **ENT:** tinnitus, vertigo, dry nose, throat, nasal stuffiness. **Eye:** blurred vision, diplopia, photosensitivity, dry eyes. **GI:** *dry mouth,* nausea, epigastric distress, anorexia, vomiting, constipation, or diarrhea. **GU:** urinary frequency or retention, dysuria. **Hypersensitivity:** skin rash, urticaria, photosensitivity, <u>anaphylactic shock</u>. **Respiratory:** thickened

D

bronchial secretions, wheezing, sensation of chest tightness.

DIAGNOSTIC TEST INTERFERENCE In common with other antihistamines, diphenhydramine should be discontinued 4 d prior to ***skin testing*** procedures for allergy because it may obscure otherwise positive reactions.

DRUG INTERACTIONS **Alcohol** and other CNS DEPRESSANTS, MAO INHIBITORS compound CNS depression.

INCOMPATIBILITY **Y-site: furosemide.**

NURSING IMPLICATIONS

Administration

- GI side effects of oral drug may be lessened by administration of drug with food or milk.
- When diphenhydramine is used for motion sickness, the first dose is given 30 min before exposure to motion. For duration of exposure, it is given before meals and on retiring.
- Administer IM injection deep into large muscle mass; alternate injection sites. Avoid perivascular or SC injections of the drug because of its irritating effects. Hypersensitivity reactions (including anaphylactic shock) are more likely to occur with parenteral injections than with PO administration.
- IV administration: IV diphenhydramine may be given by direct IV undiluted at a rate of 25 mg or a fraction thereof over 1 min.
- Store in tightly covered containers at 15–30C (59–86F) unless otherwise directed by manufacturer. Store injection and elixir formulations in light-resistant containers protected from light.
- Elixir or syrup formulations are used for relief of cough.

Assessment & Drug Effects

- Patients with blood pressure problems who are receiving the drug parenterally should be closely monitored.
- Drowsiness is most prominent during the first few days of therapy and often disappears with continued therapy. Elderly patients are especially likely to manifest dizziness, sedation, and hypotension. Side rails and supervision of ambulation may be advisable for some patients.

Patient & Family Education

- Warn the patient about possible additive CNS depressant effects with concurrent use of alcohol and other CNS depressants.
- Caution the patient against activities requiring alertness and coordination until drug response has been evaluated.
- The drug has an atropine-like drying effect (thickens bronchial secretions) that may make expectoration difficult. Advise patient to increase fluid intake if not contraindicated.

DIPHENIDOL

(di-phen′i-dol)

Trade name: Vontrol

Classifications: GI AGENT; ANTIEMETIC; ANTIVERTIGO

Prototype: Prochlorperazine

Pregnancy category: C

ACTIONS/PHARMACODYNAMICS

Mechanism of action not precisely known but may exert a specific effect on the vestibular apparatus to control vertigo and inhibit the chemoreceptor trigger zone (CTZ) to control nausea and vomiting. Has a weak peripheral anticholinergic effect.

USES Peripheral (labyrinthine) vertigo and associated nausea and vomiting, in Ménière's syndrome and middle and inner ear surgery (labyrinthitis). Also control of nausea and vomiting in postoperative states, malignant neoplasms, and labyrinthine disturbances.

ROUTE & DOSAGE

Nausea, Vomiting, Vertigo
Adult: **PO** 25–50 mg q4h prn (max 300 mg/d).
Child: **PO** > 25 kg, 0.88 mg/kg; may repeat in 1 h if needed; then q4h prn (max 5.5 mg/kg/d).

PHARMACOKINETICS **Absorption:** readily absorbed form GI tract. **Peak:** 1.5–3 h. **Metabolism:** metabolized in liver. **Elimination:** half-life: 4 h; excreted primarily in urine, small amount of feces.

CONTRAINDICATIONS & PRECAUTIONS **Contraindicated in:** hypersensitivity to diphenidol, anuria, pregnancy (category C), lactation, children <25 kg (55 lb). **Cautious use in:** glaucoma, obstructive lesions of the GI and GU tracts such as stenosing peptic ulcer, prostatic hypertrophy, pyloric and duodenal obstruction, organic cardiospasm.

ADVERSE/SIDE EFFECTS **CNS:** Auditory and visual hallucinations, disorientation, confusion, drowsiness, overstimulation, depression, blurred vision. **GI:** dry mouth, nausea, indigestion.

DRUG INTERACTIONS None noted.

CLINICAL IMPLICATIONS

Administration

- Tablets may be swallowed whole, chewed, or allowed to dissolve in mouth.
- Administer with food, water, or milk to minimize gastric irritation.
- Should be administered under close medical supervision.
- Store at 15–30C (59–86F) in a tight, light resistant container unless otherwise specified.

Assessment & Drug Effects

- Inquire about history of anuria, hypotension, or renal function impairment before starting therapy.
- Monitor I&O; assess weight daily.
- Assess BP for hypotension.
- Observe for blurred vision, confusion, or hallucinations.
- Because of anticholinergic effect of drug, patients with glaucoma and obstructive lesions of the GI or GU tract should be closely monitored for worsening of the condition.

Patient & Family Education

- Instruct patient not to take more medication than prescribed.
- Instruct patient to take as soon as possible if dose is missed but not to take if almost time for next dose nor to double dose.
- Instruct patient to avoid use of alcohol or other CNS depressants.
- Advise against driving or performing other hazardous activities until response to drug is known.
- Instruct patient to report severe or persistent nausea and vomiting.

DIPHENOXYLATE HYDROCHLORIDE WITH ATROPINE SULFATE

(dye-fen-ox'i-late)

Trade names: Diphenatol, Lofene, Lomanate, Lomotil, Lonox, Lo-Trol, Low-Quel, Nor-Mil

Prototype for classifications: GI AGENT; ANTIDIARRHEAL

Pregnancy category: C

Controlled substance: Schedule V

D

ACTIONS/PHARMACODYNAMICS Diphenoxylate is a synthetic narcotic structurally related to meperidine. Commercially available only with atropine sulfate, added in subtherapeutic doses to discourage deliberate overdosage. Inhibits mucosal receptors responsible for peristaltic reflex, thereby reducing GI motility. Has little or no analgesic activity or risk of dependence, except in high doses.

USE Adjunct in symptomatic management of diarrhea.

ROUTE & DOSAGE

Diarrhea

Adult: **PO** 1–2 tablets or 1–2 teaspoonsful (5 ml) 3–4 times/d (each tablet or 5 ml contains 2.5 mg diphenoxylate HCl and 0.025 mg atropine sulfate). *Child 2–12 y:* **PO** 0.3–0.4 mg/kg/d of liquid in divided doses.

PHARMACOKINETICS **Absorption:** readily absorbed from GI tract. **Onset:** 45–60 min. **Peak:** 2 h. **Duration:** 3–4 h. **Distribution:** distributed into breast milk. **Metabolism:** rapidly metabolized to active and inactive metabolites in liver. **Elimination:** half-life: 4.4 h; excreted slowly through bile into feces; small amount excreted in urine.

CONTRAINDICATIONS & PRECAUTIONS **Contraindicated in:** hypersensitivity to diphenoxylate or atropine; severe dehydration or electrolyte imbalance, advanced liver disease, obstructive jaundice, diarrhea caused by pseudomembranous enterocolitis associated with use of broad-spectrum antibiotics; diarrhea associated with organisms that penetrate intestinal mucosa; diarrhea induced by poisons until toxic material is eliminated from GI tract; glaucoma; children < 2 y of age. Safe use during pregnancy (category C) or in nursing women not established. **Cautious use in:** advanced hepatic disease, abnormal liver function tests; renal function impairment, patients receiving addicting drugs, addiction-prone individuals or those whose history suggests drug abuse; ulcerative colitis; young children (particularly patients with Down syndrome).

ADVERSE/SIDE EFFECTS **CNS:** headache, sedation, drowsiness, dizziness, lethargy, numbness of extremities; restlessness, euphoria, mental depression, weakness, general malaise. **CV:** flushing, palpitation, tachycardia. **Eye:** nystagmus, mydriasis, blurred vision, miosis (toxicity). **GI:** nausea, vomiting, anorexia, dry mouth, abdominal discomfort or distension, paralytic ileus, toxic megacolon. **Hypersensitivity:** pruritus, angioneurotic edema, giant urticaria, rash. **Other:** urinary retention, swelling of gums.

DRUG INTERACTIONS MAO INHIBITORS may precipitate hypertensive crisis; **alcohol** and other CNS DEPRESSANTS may enhance CNS effects; also see **atropine.**

NURSING IMPLICATIONS

Administration

- If necessary, tablet may be crushed and taken with fluid of patient's choice.
- Dosage should be reduced as soon as initial control of symptoms occurs.
- Drug should be withheld in presence of severe dehydration or electrolyte imbalance until appropriate corrective therapy has been initiated.
- Treatment is generally continued

for 24–36 h before it is considered ineffective.
- Store in tightly covered, light-resistant container, preferably between 15 and 30C (59 and 86F), unless otherwise directed by manufacturer.

Assessment & Drug Effects
- Assess GI function; report abdominal distention and signs of decreased peristalsis.
- Dehydration occurs more rapidly in the younger child and may further influence variability of response to diphenoxylate and predispose patient to delayed toxic effects. Close monitoring is essential.
- Monitor for signs and symptoms of dehydration (see Appendix G).
- Monitor frequency and consistency of stools.

Patient & Family Education
- Counsel patient to take medication only as directed by physician.
- Instruct patient to notify physician if diarrhea persists or if fever, bloody stools, palpitation, or other adverse reactions occur.
- Since drug can cause dizziness and drowsiness, advise patient to use caution when driving or performing other activities requiring coordination and alertness.

DIPIVEFRIN HYDROCHLORIDE
(dye-pi′ve-frin)

Trade name: Propine

Classifications: EYE PREPARATION; MYDRIATIC; AUTONOMIC NERVOUS SYSTEM AGENT; ADRENERGIC AGONIST (SYMPATHOMIMETIC)

Prototype: Pilocarpine

Pregnancy category: B

See Appendix A.

DIPYRIDAMOLE
(dye-peer-id′a-mole)

Trade names: Apo-Dipyridamole ♣, Persantine, Pyridamole, IV Persantine

Classifications: BLOOD FORMER; ANTIPLATELET AGENT

Prototype: Ticlopidine

Pregnancy category: C

ACTIONS/PHARMACODYNAMICS
Nonnitrate coronary vasodilator with many properties similar to those of papaverine. Increases coronary blood flow by selectively dilating coronary arteries, thereby increasing myocardial oxygen supply. Exhibits mild inotropic action. Has little effect on BP and blood flow in peripheral arteries.

USES To prevent postoperative thromboembolic complications associated with prosthetic heart valves and as adjunct for thallium stress testing. **Unlabeled uses:** to reduce rate of reinfarction following MI; to prevent TIAs (transient ischemic attacks) and coronary bypass graft occlusion.

ROUTE & DOSAGE

Prevention of Thromboembolism in Cardiac Valve Replacement

Adult: **PO** 75–100 mg q.i.d.
Child: **PO** 1–2 mg t.i.d.

Thromboembolic Disorders

Adult: **PO** 150–400 mg/d in divided doses.

Thallium Stress Test

Adult: **IV** 0.142 mg/kg/min for 4 min.

PHARMACOKINETICS Absorption: readily absorbed from GI tract. **Peak:**

45–150 min. **Distribution:** small amount crosses placenta. **Metabolism:** metabolized in liver. **Elimination:** half-life: 10–12 h; mainly excreted in feces.

D

CONTRAINDICATIONS & PRECAUTIONS **Contraindicated in:** safe use in pregnancy (category C) and nursing mothers not established. **Cautious use in:** hypotension, anticoagulant therapy.

ADVERSE/SIDE EFFECTS Usually dose related, minimal, and transient. **CNS:** headache, dizziness, faintness, syncope, weakness. **CV:** peripheral vasodilation, flushing. **GI:** nausea, vomiting, diarrhea, abdominal distress. **Other:** skin rash, pruritus.

NURSING IMPLICATIONS

Administration

- It is preferable to take on an empty stomach at least 1 h before or 2 h after meals, with a full glass of water. Physician may prescribe it to be taken with food if gastric distress persists.
- Before IV administration, dilute to at least a 1:2 ratio with 0.5N NaCl injection, 1N NaCl injection, or 5% dextrose injection for a total volume of 20 to 50 ml.
- The recommended IV dose is 0.142 mg/kg/min infused over 4 min.
- Store in tightly closed container at 15–30C (59–86F) unless otherwise directed. Protect IV dypyridamole from direct light.

Assessment & Drug Effects

- Clinical response may not be evident before second or third month of continuous therapy.
- Expected therapeutic effects are reduced frequency or elimination of anginal episodes, improved exercise tolerance, reduced requirement for nitrates.

Patient & Family Education

- Counsel patient to notify physician of any side effects.
- If postural (orthostatic) hypotension is a problem, advise patient to make all position changes slowly and in stages, especially from recumbent to upright posture.

DIRITHROMYCIN

(dir-ith-roe-my'sin)

Trade name: Dynabac

Classifications: ANTIINFECTIVE; MACROLIDE ANTIBIOTIC

Prototype: Erythromycin

Pregnancy category: C

ACTIONS/PHARMACODYNAMICS Dirithromycin is an analog of erythromycin. It binds reversibly to the 235 component of the 50-S ribosomal subunit, thus inhibiting RNA-dependent protein synthesis in bacterial cells. It is more active against gram-positive organisms than gram-negative organisms, including *Legionella, Helicobacter pylori,* and *Chlamydia trachomatis*. It is not effective against *Pseudomonas* or methicillin-resistant *Staphylococcus aureus, S. epidermidis, Listeria monocytogenes, Legionella pneumophila, Hemophilus influenzae,* or *Neisseria gonorrhoeae*.

USES Acute bacterial exacerbations of chronic bronchitis, community-acquired pneumonia, pharyngitis/tonsillitis, uncomplicated skin/skin structure infections due to susceptible bacteria.

ROUTE & DOSAGE

Bacterial Infections

Adult: **PO** 500 mg once/d.
Child ≥12 y: **PO** Same as for adult.

PHARMACOKINETICS Absorption: readily absorbed from GI tract; 60–90% hydrolyzed to active metabolite, erythromycylamine, within 35 min. **Peak:** 1.5 h. **Distribution:** high tissue concentrations of active metabolite; slowly released back into the circulation. **Metabolism:** rapidly converted to active metabolite, erythromycylamine, in absorption and distribution phases. **Elimination:** half-life: 20–50 h; 81–97% excreted in bile and feces.

CONTRAINDICATIONS & PRECAUTIONS Contraindicated in: known hypersensitivity to dirithromycin, erythromycin, or any other macrolide antibiotic; known or suspected bacteremias. **Cautious use in:** concurrent administration of terfenadine, hepatic impairment, pregnancy (category C). Safety and effectiveness in lactation, or children < 12 y have not been established.

ADVERSE/SIDE EFFECTS CNS: headache, dizziness, asthenia. **CV:** chest pain. **GI:** *abdominal pain, nausea, diarrhea, vomiting, dyspepsia, flatulence.* **Liver:** elevated liver function tests (ALT, AST, GGT). **Skin:** rash, urticaria. **Respiratory:** dyspnea, asthmalike symptoms, rhinitis, pharyngitis, increased coughing.

DRUG INTERACTIONS May increase **theophylline** levels. May increase risk of arrhythmias with terfenadine.

NURSING IMPLICATIONS

Administration

- Administer with food or within 1 h of eating.
- Tablets should not be cut, crushed, or chewed.
- Store at 15–30C (59–86F).

Assessment & Drug Effects

- Before therapy begins, inquire about previous hypersensitivity to other macrolides (e.g., erythromycin).
- Withhold drug and notify physician if signs and symptoms of hypersensitivity occur (see Appendix G).
- Monitor liver and renal function in patients with mild liver or renal impairment.
- Monitor for signs and symptoms of superinfection (see Appendix G).
- Monitor theophylline levels if given concurrently with dirithromycin.
- Dirithromycin may increase the blood level of theophylline, necessitating theophylline dosage adjustment.

Patient & Family Education

- Stress importance of taking tablets whole and with meals.
- Advise to monitor for and report signs and symptoms of superinfection or pseudomembranous enterocolitis (see Appendix G).
- Immediately report any worsening of signs and symptoms of infection.

DISOPYRAMIDE PHOSPHATE

(dye-soe-peer'a-mide)

Trade names: Napamide, Norpace, Norpace CR, Rythmodan ♣, Rythmodan-LA ♣

Classifications: CARDIOVASCULAR AGENT; ANTIARRHYTHMIC

Prototype: Procainamide

Pregnancy category: C

ACTIONS/PHARMACODYNAMICS Class IA antiarrhythmic agent with pharmacologic actions similar to those of quinidine and procainamide, although chemically unrelated. Acts as myocardial depressant by reducing rate of spontaneous diastolic depolarization in pacemaker cells, thereby suppressing ectopic focal activity. Disopyramide shortens sinus node recovery time and increases atrial and ventricular effective refractory period but has minimal effect on refractoriness and conduction time of AV node or on conduction time of His-Purkinje system or QRS duration.

USES To suppress and prevent recurrence of premature ventricular contractions (unifocal, multifocal, paired) and ventricular tachycardia not severe enough to require cardioversion. **Unlabeled uses:** in combination with other antiarrhythmic drugs to treat or prevent serious refractory arrhythmias. To convert atrial fibrillation, atrial flutter, and paroxysmal atrial tachycardia to normal sinus rhythm.

ROUTE & DOSAGE

Arrhythmias

Adult: **PO** >50 kg, 100–200 mg q6h or 300 mg controlled release capsule q12h; <50 kg, 100 mg q6h or 200 mg controlled release q12h.
Child: **PO** *12–18 y,* 6–15 mg/kg/d in divided doses q6h; *4–12 y,* 10–15 mg/kg/d in divided doses q6h; *1–4 y,* 10–20 mg/kg/d in divided doses q6h; *<1y,* 10–30 mg/kg/d in divided doses q6h.

PHARMACOKINETICS Absorption: readily absorbed from GI tract; 60–83% reaches systemic circulation. **Onset:** 30 min–3.5 h. **Peak:** 1–2 h. **Duration:** 1.5–8.5 h. **Distribution:** distributed in extracellular fluid; crosses placenta; distributed into breast milk. **Metabolism:** metabolized in liver. **Elimination:** half-life: 4–10 h; 80% excreted in urine, 10% in feces.

CONTRAINDICATIONS & PRECAUTIONS Contraindicated in: cardiogenic shock, preexisting 2nd or 3rd degree AV block (if no pacemaker is present); uncompensated or inadequately compensated CHF, hypotension (unless secondary to cardiac arrhythmia), hypokalemia. Safe use during pregnancy (category C), in nursing women, and in children not established. **Cautious use in:** sick sinus syndrome (bradycardia-tachycardia); Wolff-Parkinson-White (WPW) syndrome or bundle branch block, myocarditis or other cardiomyopathy, underlying cardiac conduction abnormalities; hepatic or renal impairment; urinary tract disease (especially prostatic hypertrophy); myasthenia gravis; narrow-angle glaucoma, family history of glaucoma.

ADVERSE/SIDE EFFECTS CNS: dizziness, headache, fatigue, muscle weakness, convulsions, paresthesias, nervousness, acute psychosis, peripheral neuropathy. **CV:** *hypotension,* chest pain, edema, dyspnea, syncope, bradycardia, tachycardia; worsening of CHF or cardiac arrhythmia; <u>cardiogenic shock</u>, <u>heart block</u>; edema with weight gain. **Eye:** *blurred vision,* dry eyes, increased IOP, precipitation of acute angle-closure glaucoma. **GI:** *dry mouth, constipation,* epigastric or abdominal pain, cholestatic jaundice. **GU:** *hesitancy and retention,* urinary frequency, urgency, renal insufficiency. **Hypersensitivity:** pruritus, urticaria, rash, photosensitivity, <u>laryngospasm</u>. **Other:** dry nose and throat, drying of bronchial secretions, initiation of uterine contractions (pregnant patient); muscle aches, precipitation of myasthenia gravis, <u>agranulocytosis</u> (rare), thrombocytopenia.

DRUG INTERACTIONS ANTICHOLINERGIC DRUGS (e.g., TRICYCLIC ANTIDE-

PRESSANTS, ANTIHISTAMINES) compound anticholinergic effects; other ANTIARRHYTHMICS compound toxicities; **phenytoin, rifampin** may increase disopyramide metabolism and decrease levels; may increase **warfarin**-induced hypoprothrombinemia.

NURSING IMPLICATIONS

Administration

- For patients who have been receiving either quinidine or procainamide, manufacturer suggests starting disopyramide 6–12 h after last quinidine dose and 3–6 h after last procainamide dose.
- Controlled-release capsules are not appropriate for use in loading doses when rapid control is required or in patients with creatinine clearance of ≤ 40 ml/min.
- When patient is to be transferred from conventional capsule to controlled-release capsule, start the latter 6 h after last dose of conventional capsule.
- Store at 15–30C (59–86F) unless otherwise directed.

Assessment & Drug Effects

- Check apical pulse before administering drug. Withhold drug and notify physician if pulse rate is slower than 60 bpm, faster than 120 bpm, or if there is any unusual change in rate, rhythm, or quality.
- ECG should be closely monitored. The following signs are indications for drug withdrawal: prolongation of QT interval and worsening of arrhythmia interval, QRS widening (> 25%).
- Baseline and periodic determinations should be made of hepatic and renal function, blood glucose, and serum potassium. Hypokalemia or other imbalances are corrected before initiation of therapy.
- Closely monitor BP in all patients during periods of dosage adjustment and in those receiving high dosages.
- Monitor I&O, particularly in the elderly and patients with impaired renal function or prostatic hypertrophy. Persistent urinary hesitancy or retention may necessitate lower dosage or discontinuation of drug.
- Toxic effects are enhanced by hyperkalemia. Report signs and symptoms (see Appendix G).
- Patients with a family history of glaucoma should have IOP measured before treatment begins.
- Monitor for signs and symptoms of CHF (see Appendix G).
- Disopyramide should be discontinued promptly if signs and symptoms of agranulocytosis, or peripheral neuritis, or jaundice (see Appendix G) appear.

Patient & Family Education

- Instruct patient to weigh daily under standard conditions and to check ankles and tibiae daily for edema. Report to physician a weekly weight gain of ≥ 1–2 kg (2–4 lb).
- Because of the possibility of hypotension, advise patient to make position changes slowly, particularly from recumbent posture, to dangle legs for a few minutes before ambulating, and to not stand still for prolonged periods. Instruct patient to lie down or sit down if he or she feels light-headed.
- To maintain regularity of heartbeat, drug must be taken precisely as prescribed. Emphasize importance of not skipping or stopping medication or changing dose without consulting physician.
- Advise patient not to take OTC medications unless approved by physician.

- Disopyramide may cause photosensitivity; therefore exposure to sunlight or ultraviolet light should be avoided.
- Since drug may cause dizziness and blurring of vision, caution patient to avoid driving and other potentially hazardous activities until reaction to drug effects is known.
- Warn patient not to drink alcoholic beverages while taking disopyramide.

D

DISULFIRAM

(dye-sul'fi-ram)

Trade names: Antabuse, Cronetal, Ro-sulfiram

Classifications: ENZYME INHIBITOR; ANTIALCOHOL AGENT

Pregnancy category: X

ACTIONS/PHARMACODYNAMICS Acts as a deterrent to alcohol ingestion by inhibiting the enzyme acetaldehyde dehydrogenase, which normally metabolizes alcohol in the body. When a small amount of alcohol is ingested, a complex of highly unpleasant symptoms known as the disulfiram reaction occurs, which serves as a deterrent to further drinking. Does not produce tolerance and is not a cure for alcoholism.

USE Adjunct in treatment of the patient with chronic alcoholism who sincerely wants to maintain sobriety.

ROUTE & DOSAGE

Alcoholism

Adult: **PO** 500 mg/d for 1–2 wk; then 125–500 mg/d (max 500 mg/d).

PHARMACOKINETICS **Absorption:** readily absorbed from GI tract. **Onset:** up to 12 h. **Duration:** up to 2 wk. **Distribution:** initially deposited in fat. **Metabolism:** metabolized slowly in liver. **Elimination:** 5–20% excreted in feces; 20% remains in body for 1–2 wk; some may be excreted in breath as carbon disulfide.

CONTRAINDICATIONS & PRECAUTIONS **Contraindicated in:** severe myocardial disease; psychoses; pregnancy (category X); or patients who have recently received alcohol, metronidazole, paraldehyde; multiple drug dependence. **Cautious use in:** diabetes mellitus; epilepsy; hypothyroidism; coronary artery disease, cerebral damage; chronic and acute nephritis; hepatic cirrhosis or insufficiency; abnormal EEG.

ADVERSE/SIDE EFFECTS Disulfiram reaction (with alcohol ingestion): flushing of face, chest, arms, pulsating headache, nausea, violent vomiting, thirst, sweating, marked uneasiness, confusion, weakness, vertigo, blurred vision, pruritic skin rash, hyperventilation, abnormal gait, slurred speech, disorientation, confusion, personality changes, bizarre behavior, psychoses, tachycardia, palpitation, chest pain. Severe reactions: <u>hypotension to shock level, arrhythmias, acute congestive failure, marked respiratory depression, unconsciousness, convulsions, sudden death</u>. **CNS:** drowsiness, fatigue, restlessness, headache, tremor, psychoses (usually with high doses), polyneuritis, peripheral neuropathy, optic neuritis. **GI:** mild GI disturbances, garliclike or metallic taste, <u>hepatotoxicity</u>, hypersensitivity hepatitis. **Hypersensitivity:** allergic or acneiform dermatitis; urticaria, fixed-drug eruption.

DIAGNOSTIC TEST INTERFERENCE Disulfiram can reduce ***uptake of***

I-131; or decreases ***PBI*** test results (rare).

DRUG INTERACTIONS **Alcohol** (including in liquid OTC drugs, **IV nitroglycerin, IV cotrimoxazole**), **metronidazole, paraldehyde** will produce disulfiram reaction; **isoniazid** can produce neurological symptoms; may increase blood levels and toxicity of **warfarin, paraldehyde,** BARBITURATES, **phenytoin.**

NURSING IMPLICATIONS

Administration

- Daily dose should be taken in the morning when the resolve not to drink may be strongest.
- To minimize sedative effect the drug may be prescribed to be taken at bedtime. Decrease in dose may also reduce sedative effect.
- Therapy is not initiated until patient has abstained from alcohol and alcohol-containing preparations for at least 12 h and preferably 48 h.
- Maintenance therapy with disulfiram may be required for months or even years. Compliance should be determined periodically.
- Protect tablets from light. Store at 15–30C (59–86F) unless otherwise directed.

Assessment & Drug Effects

- Complete physical examination, and careful drug history are advised prior to therapy. Baseline and follow-up transaminase studies every 10–14 d are suggested to detect hepatic dysfunction. In addition, CBC and sequential multiple analysis (SMA-12) tests should be performed every 6 mo.
- Disulfiram reaction occurs within 5–10 min following ingestion of alcohol and may last 30 min to several hours.
- Intensity of reaction varies with each individual, but it is generally proportional to the amount of alcohol ingested.
- Treat patient with severe disulfiram reaction as though he or she were in shock. Monitor potassium levels, especially if patient has diabetes mellitus.

Patient & Family Education

- Patient should be completely aware of and should consent to therapy with disulfiram. Patient and family should be fully informed of possible dangers if alcohol is ingested during disulfiram treatment.
- Instruct patient to report promptly to physician the onset of nausea with right upper quadrant pain or discomfort, itching, jaundiced sclerae or skin, dark urine, clay-colored stools. Disulfiram should be withheld pending liver function studies.
- Ingestion of even small amounts of alcohol or use of external applications that contain alcohol may be sufficient to produce a reaction. Teach patient to read labels and to avoid use of anything containing alcohol.
- Patient should be informed that prolonged administration of disulfiram does not produce tolerance; the longer one remains on therapy, the more sensitive one becomes to alcohol.
- Warn patient that alcohol sensitivity may last as long as 2 wk after disulfiram has been discontinued.
- During first 2 wk of therapy, patient may experience side effects of disulfiram itself (See Adverse/ Side Effects). These symptoms usually disappear with continued therapy or with dose reduction.
- Advise patient to carry an identification card stating that patient is on disulfiram therapy and describing the symptoms of disulfiram reaction. The name of the physician

or institution to contact in an emergency should also be provided.

- During early therapy when drowsiness may be a problem, the patient should avoid driving or performing other tasks requiring alertness.

D

DOBUTAMINE HYDROCHLORIDE

(doe-byoo′ta-meen)

Trade name: Dobutrex

Classifications: AUTONOMIC NERVOUS SYSTEM AGENT; BETA-ADRENERGIC AGONIST; CATECHOLAMINE

Prototype: Isoproterenol

Pregnancy category: C

ACTIONS/PHARMACODYNAMICS Produces inotropic effect by acting on beta receptors and primarily on myocardial alpha adrenergic receptors. Increases cardiac output and decreases pulmonary wedge pressure and total systemic vascular resistance with comparatively little or no effect on BP. Also increases conduction through AV node. Has lower potential for precipitating arrhythmias than dopamine. In CHF, increase in cardiac output enhances renal perfusion and increases renal output and renal sodium excretion.

USES Inotropic support in short-term treatment of adults with cardiac decompensation due to depressed myocardial contractility (cardiogenic shock) resulting from either organic heart disease or from cardiac surgery. **Unlabeled uses:** to augment cardiovascular function in children undergoing cardiac catheterization, stress thallium testing.

ROUTE & DOSAGE

Cardiac Decompensation

Adult: **IV** 2.5–10 μg/kg/min (up to 40 μg/kg/min); has been given for up to 72 h without decrease in effectiveness.

Child: **IV** Same as for adult.

PHARMACOKINETICS Onset: 2–10 min. **Peak:** 10–20 min. **Metabolism:** metabolized in liver and other tissues by COMT. **Elimination:** half-life: 2 min; excreted in urine.

CONTRAINDICATIONS & PRECAUTIONS Contraindicated in: history of hypersensitivity to other sympathomimetic amines, ventricular tachycardia, idiopathic hypertrophic subaortic stenosis. Safe use during pregnancy (category C), in nursing mothers and children, or following acute MI not established. **Cautious use in:** preexisting hypertension, atrial fibrillation.

ADVERSE/SIDE EFFECTS Generally dose related. **CNS:** headache, tremors, paresthesias, mild leg cramps, nervousness, fatigue (with overdosage). **CV:** *increased heart rate and BP,* premature ventricular beats, palpitation, *anginal pain.* **GI:** nausea, vomiting. **Other:** nonspecific chest pain, shortness of breath.

DRUG INTERACTIONS GENERAL ANESTHETICS (especially **cyclopropane** and **halothane**) may sensitize myocardium to effects of CATECHOLAMINES such as dobutamine and lead to serious arrhythmias—used with extreme caution; BETA-ADRENERGIC BLOCKING AGENTS, e.g., **metoprolol, propranolol**, may make dobutamine ineffective in increasing cardiac output, but total peripheral resistance may increase—concomitant use generally avoided; MAO INHIBITORS, tricylic antidepressants potentiate pressor effects—used with extreme caution.

INCOMPATIBILITIES Solution/additive: sodium bicarbonate, aminophylline, bretylium, bumetanide, calcium chloride, calcium gluconate, diazepam, doxapram, digoxin, epinephrine, furosemide, heparin, insulin, magnesium sulfate, phenytoin, potassium chloride, potassium phosphate. Y-site: acyclovir, aminophylline, sodium bicarbonate.

NURSING IMPLICATIONS

Administration

- Hypovolemia should be corrected by administration of appropriate volume expanders prior to initiation of therapy.
- Since dobutamine enhances AV conduction, patients with atrial fibrillation are generally given a digitalis preparation prior to initiation of therapy to reduce risk of ventricular tachycardia.
- Dobutamine may be reconstituted by adding 10 ml sterile water for injection or 5% dextrose injection to 250-mg vial. If not completely dissolved, additional 10 ml of diluent may be added.
- For IV infusion, reconstituted solution must be further diluted before administration to at least 50 ml with 5% dextrose, 0.9% NaCl, or sodium lactate injection. IV solutions should be used within 24 h.
- Rate of infusion should be controlled by an infusion pump (preferred) or a microdrip IV infusion set.
- Solutions containing dobutamine may exhibit color changes because of slight oxidation of drug. This does not affect potency.
- Dobutamine is incompatible with sodium bicarbonate and other alkaline solutions.
- Reconstituted solution may be refrigerated at 2–15C (36–59F) for 48 h or for 6 h at room temperature.

Assessment & Drug Effects

- At any given dosage level, drug takes 10–20 min to produce peak effects.
- ECG and BP should be monitored continuously during administration of dobutamine.
- IV infusion rate and duration of therapy are determined by heart rate, blood pressure, ectopic activity, urine output, and whenever possible, by measurements of cardiac output and central venous or pulmonary wedge pressures.
- Marked increases in blood pressure (systolic pressure is the most likely to be affected) and heart rate, or the appearance of arrhythmias or other adverse cardiac effects are usually reversed promptly by reduction in dosage.
- Patients with preexisting hypertension must be closely observed for exaggerated pressor response.
- Tolerance has been observed with continuous or prolonged dobutamine infusions. However, adverse reactions are no different than those seen with shorter infusions.
- Monitor intake and output ratio and pattern. Urine output and sodium excretion generally increase because of improved cardiac output and renal perfusion.

Patient & Family Education

- Instruct patient to promptly report anginal pain.

DOCETAXEL

(doc-e-tax′ el)

Trade name: Taxotere

D

Classifications: ANTINEOPLASTIC AGENT; TAXANE AGENT
Prototype: Paclitaxel
Pregnancy category: D

ACTIONS/PHARMACODYNAMICS Docetaxel is a semisynthetic analog of paclitaxel. Potential advantages over paclitaxel are greater antitumor activity and lower toxicity potential. Docetaxel, like paclitaxel, binds to the microtubule network essential for interphase and mitosis of the cell cycle. Docetaxel stabilizes the microtubules and prevents their normal functioning, which results in inhibiting mitosis in cells.

USE Metastatic breast cancer.

ROUTE & DOSAGE

Breast Cancer

Adult: **IV** 60–100 mg/m^2 once every 3 wk. Patients should be premedicated with dexamethasone 8 mg b.i.d. × 5 d, starting 1 d prior to docetaxel.

PHARMACOKINETICS Distribution: 97% protein bound. **Metabolism:** metabolized in liver by cytochrome P4503A isoenzymes. **Elimination:** half-life: 11.1 h; 80% eliminated in feces, 20% renally excreted.

CONTRAINDICATIONS & PRECAUTIONS Contraindicated in: hypersensitivity to docetaxel or other drugs formulated with polysorbate 80, paclitaxel, neutrophil count <1500 cells/mm^3, lactation, pregnancy (category D), acute infection. **Cautious use in:** hepatic disease, bone marrow suppression, bone marrow transplant patients, CHF, pulmonary disorders. Safety and effectiveness in children not established.

ADVERSE/SIDE EFFECTS CNS: paresthesia, pain, burning sensation, weakness, confusion. **CV:** hypotension, *fluid retention (peripheral edema, weight gain),* pleural effusion. **GI:** *nausea, vomiting, diarrhea, stomatitis,* abdominal pain. **Hematologic:** <u>*neutropenia, leukopenia, thrombocytopenia, anemia,*</u> febrile neutropenia. **Hepatic:** increased liver function tests (AST or ALT) **Skin:** rash, localized eruptions desquamation, *alopecia,* nail changes (hyper/hypopigmentation, onycholysis). **Other:** *hypersensitivity reactions,* infusion site reactions (hyperpigmentation, inflammation, redness, dryness, phlebitis, extravasation).

DRUG INTERACTIONS Possibility of interacting with other drugs metabolized by the cytochrome P4503A system (cyclosporine, erythromycin, ketoconazole, terfenadine, troleandomycin).

NURSING IMPLICATIONS

Administration

- Administer only after premedication with corticosteroids to prevent hypersensitivity.
- Preparation of IV solution: Bring vials to room temperature for 5 min; add provided diluent, gently rotate for 15 s; let stand until surface foam dissipates. Inject required amount of diluted solution into a 250-ml, or larger, bag of 0.9% NaCl injection or 5% Dextrose Injection; the final concentration should not exceed 0.9 mg/ml. Completely mix by manual rotation.
- IV administration: Give at a constant rate over 1 h.
- If skin contacts drug during preparation, wash immediately with soap and water.
- A 25% dose reduction is recom-

mended following severe neutropenia (<500 cells/mm^3) for 7 d or longer or febrile neutropenia, severe cutaneous reactions, or severe peripheral neuropathy.
- Refrigerate vials at 2–8C (36–46F). Protect from light. Do not store in PVC bags. Diluted solutions may be stored refrigerated or at room temperature for 8 h.

Assessment & Drug Effects
- Monitor bilirubin, AST or ALT, and alkaline phosphatase prior to each drug cycle. Generally, docetaxel should not be given to patients with elevations of bilirubin or with significant elevations of transaminases concurrent with elevations of alkaline phosphatases.
- Frequently monitor complete blood cell counts with differential. Withhold drug if platelets <100,000 or neutrophils <1500 cells/mm^3.
- Monitor for signs of hypersensitivity (see Appendix G) which may develop within a few minutes of initiation of infusion. It is usually not necessary to discontinue infusion for minor reactions (i.e., flushing or local skin reaction).
- Throughout therapy, assess for and report cardiovascular dysfunction, respiratory distress; fluid retention; development of neurosensory symptoms; severe, cutaneous eruptions on feet, hands, arms, face, or thorax; and S&S of infection.

Patient & Family Education
- Advise regarding common adverse effects and provide information on measures to control or minimize when possible. Instruct to immediately report any distressing adverse effects.
- Stress importance of compliance with corticosteroid therapy and with monitoring of lab values.
- Advise women to avoid pregnancy during therapy; advise lactating women to discontinue nursing prior to taking the drug.

D

DOCUSATE CALCIUM (DIOCTYL CALCIUM SULFOSUCCINATE)
(dok′yoo-sate)

Trade names: DCS, PMS-Docusate Calcium, Pro-Cal-Sof, Surfak

DOCUSATE POTASSIUM
Trade names: Dialose, Diocto-k, Kasof

DOCUSATE SODIUM
Trade names: Colace, Colace Enema, Dio-Sul, Disonate, DGSS, D-S-S, Duosol, Lax-gel, Laxinate 100, Modane Soft, Pro-Sof, Regulax ♣, Regutol, Therevac-Plus, Therevac-SB

Prototype for classifications: GI AGENT; STOOL SOFTNER

Pregnancy category: C

ACTIONS/PHARMACODYNAMICS
Anionic surface-active agent with emulsifying and wetting properties. Detergent action lowers surface tension, permitting water and fats to penetrate and soften stools for easier passage.

USES Prophylactically in patients who should avoid straining during defecation and for treatment of constipation associated with hard, dry stools (e.g., following anorectal surgery, MI).

ROUTE & DOSAGE

Stool Softener
Adult: **PO** 50–500 mg/d. **PR**

50–100 mg added to enema fluid. *Child:* **PO** *6–12 y,* 40–120 mg/d; *3–6 y,* 20–60 mg/d; *<3 y,* 10–40 mg/d.

D

CONTRAINDICATIONS & PRECAUTIONS **Contraindicated in:** atonic constipation, nausea, vomiting, abdominal pain, fecal impaction, structural anomalies of colon and rectum, intestinal obstruction or perforation; use of docusate sodium in patients on sodium restriction; use of docusate potassium in patients with renal dysfunction; concomitant use of mineral oil; pregnancy (category C).

ADVERSE/SIDE EFFECTS Rare: occasional mild abdominal cramps, *diarrhea,* nausea, bitter taste, throat irritation (liquid preparation), rash.

DRUG INTERACTION Docusate will increase systemic absorption of **mineral oil.**

NURSING IMPLICATIONS

Administration

- Administer oral dose with a full glass of water if allowed.
- Microenema: insert full length of nozzle (half length for children) into the rectum. Squeeze entire contents of tube and remove completely before releasing grip on tube.
- Store in tightly covered containers. Syrup formulations should be stored in tight, light-resistant containers at 15–30C (59–86F) unless directed otherwise.

Assessment & Drug Effects

- If diarrhea develops, withhold drug and notify physician.
- Effect on stools is usually apparent 1–3 d after first dose.

Patient & Family Education

- Advise patient to take sufficient liquid with each dose and to increase fluid intake during the day, if allowed. Oral liquid (not syrup) may be administered in milk, fruit juice, or infant formula to mask bitter taste.
- Docusate enhances systemic absorption of mineral oil; therefore, concomitant use is not recommended.
- Docusate should not be administered for prolonged periods in lieu of proper dietary management or treatment of underlying causes of constipation.

DOLASETRON MESYLATE

(dol-a-se′tron)

Trade name: Anzemet

Classifications: GI AGENT; ANTIEMETIC; 5-HT_3 ANTAGONIST

Prototype: Ondansetron

Pregnancy category: B

ACTIONS/PHARMACODYNAMICS Dolasetron is a selective serotonin (5-HT_3) receptor antagonist used for control of nausea and vomiting associated with cancer chemotherapy. Serotonin receptors affected by dolasetron are located in the chemoreceptor trigger zone (CTZ) of the brain and peripherally on the vagal nerve terminal. Serotonin, released from the cells of the small intestine, activate 5-HT_3 receptors located on vagal efferents, thus initiating the vomiting reflex. Dolasetron causes ECG changes lasting from 6 to 24 h.

USES Prevention of nausea and vomiting from emetogenic chemotherapy, prevention and treatment of postoperative nausea and vomiting.

ROUTE & DOSAGE

Prevention of Chemotherapy-induced Nausea and Vomiting

Adult: **IV** 1.8 mg/kg or 100 mg administered over 30 s, 30 min prior to chemotherapy. **PO** 100 mg 1 h prior to chemotherapy.
Child >2 y: **IV** 1.8 mg/kg or 100 mg administered over 30 s, 30 min prior to chemotherapy. **PO** 1.8 mg/kg up to 100 mg 1 h before chemotherapy.

Pre/Postoperative Nausea and Vomiting

Adult: **IV** 12.5 mg 15 min before cessation of anesthesia or when post-op nausea and vomiting occurs. **PO** 100 mg within 2 h prior to surgery.
Child >2 y: **IV** 0.35 mg/kg up to 12.5 mg 15 min before cessation of anesthesia or when post-op nausea and vomiting occurs. **PO** 1.2 mg/kg up to 100 mg starting 2 h prior to surgery (may also mix IV formulation in apple or apple-grape juice and administer orally.

PHARMACOKINETICS **Absorption:** rapidly absorbed from GI tract, converted to hydrodolasetron, the active metabolite. **Peak:** 0.6 h IV, 1 h PO. **Distribution:** crosses placenta, distributed into breast milk. **Metabolism:** metabolized to hydrodolasetron by carbonyl reductase. Hydrodolasetron is metabolized in the liver by CYP2D6. **Elimination:** half-life: 10 min dolasetron, 7.3 h hydrodolasetron; primarily excreted in urine as unchanged hydrodolasetron.

CONTRAINDICATIONS & PRECAUTIONS **Contraindicated in:** hypersensitivity to dolasetron. **Cautious use in:** patients who have or may develop prolongation of cardiac conduction intervals, particularly QT_C (i.e., patients with hypokalemia, hypomagnesia, diuretics, congenital QT syndrome; patients taking antiarrhythmic drugs and high-dose anthracycline therapy, etc.), pregnancy (category B), and lactation. Safety and efficacy in children < 2 y are not known.

ADVERSE/SIDE EFFECTS **Body as Whole:** fever, fatigue, pain, chills/shivering. **CNS:** *headache,* dizziness, drowsiness. **CV:** hypertension. **GI:** *diarrhea,* increased LFTs, abdominal pain. **Other:** urinary retention.

NURSING IMPLICATIONS

Administration

- For pediatric patients IV formulation may be dissolved in apple or apple-grape juice and given 1 h before chemotherapy.
- When used for post-op nausea, dose should be given within 2 h before surgery.
- IV preparation: may be given undiluted or diluted in 50 ml of any of the following: 0.9% NaCl, D5W, D5W+0.45% NaCl, D5W + lactated Ringer's, lactated Ringer's.
- IV infusion: undiluted drug may be injected over 30 s; diluted drug may be infused over 15 min.
- Store at 20–25C (66–77F) and protect from light. Diluted IV solution may be stored refrigerated up to 48 h.

Assessment & Drug Effects

- Therapeutic effectiveness is indicated by prevention of nausea and vomiting.
- Prior to administering dolasetron, serum electrolytes should be determined, and hypokalemia and hypomagnesemia should be corrected.

- Cardiac status should be closely monitored especially with vomiting, excess diuresis, or other conditions that may result in electrolyte imbalances.
- Monitor ECG especially in those taking concurrent antiarrhythmic or other drugs that may cause QT prolongation.
- Monitor for and report signs of bleeding (e.g., hematuria, epistaxis, purpura, hematoma).
- Lab tests: with prolonged therapy, periodically monitor liver functions, PTT, CBC with platelet count.

Patient & Family Education

- Headache requiring analgesic for relief is a common adverse effect.

DONEPEZIL HYDROCHLORIDE

(don-e′pe-zil)

Trade names: Aricept

Classifications: AUTONOMIC NERVOUS SYSTEM AGENT; CHOLINERGIC (PARASYMPATHOMIMETIC); CHOLINESTERASE INHIBITOR

Pregnancy category: C

ACTIONS/PHARMACODYNAMICS In early stages of Alzheimer's disease, pathologic changes in neurons result in deficiency of acethycholine. Aricept, a cholesterase inhibitor, presumably elevates acethylcholine concentration in the cerebral cortex by slowing degradation of acethylcholine released by remaining intact neurons.

USE Mild to moderate dementia of Alzheimer's type.

ROUTE & DOSAGE

Alzheimer's Disease

Adult: **PO** 5–10 mg h.s.

PHARMACOKINETICS Absorption: rapidly absorbed from GI tract. **Peak plasma concentration:** 3–4 h. **Distribution:** 96% protein bound. **Metabolism:** metabolized in the liver by CYP2D6 and CYP3A4 to at least 2 active metabolites. **Elimination:** half-life: 70 h; primarily excreted in urine.

CONTRAINDICATIONS & PRECAUTIONS Contraindicated in: hypersensitivity to donepezil or tracine. **Cautious use in:** anesthesia, sick sinus rhythm, bradycardia, hypotension; hyperthyroidism, history of ulcers, GI bleeding, abnormal liver function; patients with asthma or obstructive pulmonary disease, history of seizures, urinary tract obstruction, intestinal obstruction; pregnancy (category C). Safety and efficacy in children and nursing mothers have not been established.

ADVERSE/SIDE EFFECTS Body as Whole: *headache,* fatigue. **CNS:** *insomnia,* dizziness, depression, tremor, irritability, vertigo, ataxia. **CV:** syncope, hypertension, atrial fibrillation, hot flashes, hypotension. **GI:** *nausea, diarrhea, vomiting, muscle cramps, anorexia,* <u>GI bleeding,</u> bloating, fecal incontinence, epigastric pain. **Respiratory:** dyspnea. **Skin:** pruritus, sweating, urticaria. **Other:** ecchymoses, muscle cramps, dehydration, blurred vision, urinary incontinence, nocturia.

DRUG INTERACTIONS Ketoconazole, quinidine may inhibit donepezil metabolism; **carbamazepine, dexamethasone, phenobarbital, phenytoin, rifampin** may increase donepezil elimination; donepezil may interfere with the action of ANTICHOLINERGIC AGENTS.

NURSING IMPLICATIONS

Administration

- Drug should be taken at h.s. just prior to going to bed.
- Dosage increase to 10 mg should only be made after 4–6 wk of therapy with the 5-mg dose.
- Store at 15–30C (59–86F).

Assessment & Drug Effects

- Therapeutic effectiveness is indicated by improvement as noted on the Alzheimer's Disease Assessment Scale.
- Monitor closely for S&S of GI ulceration and bleeding, especially with concurrent use of NSAIDS.
- Carefully monitor patients with a history of asthma or obstructive pulmonary disease.
- Monitor cardiovascular status; drug may have vagotonic effect on the heart, causing bradycardia, especially in presence of conduction abnormalities.

Patient & Family Education

- Fainting episodes related to slowing the heart rate may occur. Caution should be exercised.
- Immediately report any S&S of GI ulceration or bleeding (e.g., "coffee-grounds" emesis, tarry stools, epigastric pain).

DOPAMINE HYDROCHLORIDE

(doe'pa-meen)

Trade names: Dopastat, Intropin, Revimine ♣

Classifications: AUTONOMIC NERVOUS SYSTEM AGENT; ALPHA- AND BETA-ADRENERGIC AGONIST (SYMPATHOMIMETIC)

Prototype: Epinephrine

Pregnancy category: C

ACTIONS/PHARMACODYNAMICS Naturally occurring neurotransmitter and immediate precursor of norepinephrine. Major cardiovascular effects produced by direct action on alpha- and beta-adrenergic receptors and on specific dopaminergic receptors in mesenteric and renal vascular beds. Positive inotropic effect on myocardium increases cardiac output with increase in systolic and pulse pressure and little or no effect on diastolic pressure. Improves circulation to renal vascular bed by decreasing renal vascular resistance with resulting increase in glomerular filtration rate and urinary output.

USES To correct hemodynamic imbalance in shock syndrome due to MI (cardiogenic shock), trauma, endotoxic septicemia (septic shock), open heart surgery, and CHF. **Unlabeled uses:** acute renal failure; cirrhosis; hepatorenal syndrome; barbiturate intoxication.

ROUTE & DOSAGE

Shock

Adult: **IV** 2–5 μg/kg/min increased gradually up to 20–50 μg/kg/min if necessary.
Child: **IV** Same as for adult.

Renal Failure

Adult: **IV** 2–5 μg/kg/min.

PHARMACOKINETICS **Onset:** <5 min. **Duration:** <10 min. **Distribution:** Widely distributed; does not cross blood–brain barrier. **Metabolism:** Inactive in the liver, kidney, and plasma by monoamine oxidase and COMT. **Elimination:** half-life: 2 min; excreted in urine.

CONTRAINDICATIONS & PRECAUTIONS **Contraindicated in:** pheochromocytoma; tachyarrhythmias or ventricular fibrillation. Safe use during pregnancy (category C), in nurs-

D

ing women, and in children not established. **Cautious use in:** patients with history of occlusive vascular disease (e.g., Buerger's or Raynaud's disease); cold injury; diabetic endarteritis, arterial embolism.

ADVERSE/SIDE EFFECTS **CV:** *hypotension,* ectopic beats, *tachycardia,* anginal pain, palpitation, vasoconstriction (indicated by disproportionate rise in diastolic pressure), cold extremities; less frequent: aberrant conduction, bradycardia, widening of QRS complex, elevated blood pressure. **GI:** nausea, vomiting **Other:** headache necrosis, tissue sloughing with extravasation, gangrene, azotemia, piloerection, dyspnea, dilated pupils (high doses).

DIAGNOSTIC TEST INTERFERENCE Dopamine may modify test response when histamine is used as a control for ***intradermal skin tests***.

DRUG INTERACTIONS MAO INHIBITORS, ERGOT ALKALOIDS, **furazolidine** increase alpha-adrenergic effects (headache, hyperpyrexia, hypertension); **guanethidine, phenytoin** may decrease dopamine action; BETA BLOCKERS antagonize cardiac effects; ALPHA BLOCKERS antagonize peripheral vasoconstriction; **halothane, cyclopropane** increase risk of hypertension and ventricular arrhythmias.

INCOMPATIBILITIES **Solution/additive:** sodium bicarbonate, **aminophylline, amphotericin B, ampicillin, cephalothin, penicillin G. Y-site: acyclovir, aminophylline, amphotericin B,** sodium bicarbonate.

NURSING IMPLICATIONS

Administration

- Before initiation of dopamine therapy, hypovolemia should be corrected, if possible, with either whole blood or plasma.
- Dilution should be made just prior to administration, although reportedly the solution may remain stable for 24 h after dilution.
- IV infusion rate and guidelines for adjusting rate of flow in relation to changes in blood pressure will be prescribed by physician. Microdrip or other reliable metering device should be used for accuracy of flow rate.
- Infusion rate must be continuously monitored for free flow, and care must be taken to avoid extravasation, which can result in tissue sloughing and gangrene. For this reason, infusion is made preferably into a large vein of the antecubital fossa.
- Antidote for extravasation: stop infusion promptly and remove needle. Immediately infiltrate the ischemic area, using syringe and fine needle. Recommended dose is 5–10 mg phentolamine mesylate in 10–15 ml of normal saline, using syringe and fine needle.
- Protect dopamine from light. Discolored solutions should not be used. Reconstituted solution is stable for 48 h when stored at 2–15C (36–59F) or 6 h at room temperature 15–30C (59–86F).

Assessment & Drug Effects

- Monitor blood pressure, pulse, peripheral pulses, and urinary output at intervals prescribed by physician. Precise measurements are essential for accurate titration of dosage.
- Close observation is critical when patient is receiving dopamine. The following indicators are used for decreasing or temporarily suspending dose (report promptly to physician): reduced urine flow rate in absence of hypotension; as-

cending tachycardia; dysrhythmias; disproportionate rise in diastolic pressure (marked decrease in pulse pressure); signs of peripheral ischemia (pallor, cyanosis, mottling, coldness, complaints of tenderness, pain, numbness, or burning sensation). Presence of peripheral pulses is not always indicative of adequate circulation.

- In addition to improvement in vital signs and urine flow, other indices of adequate dosage and perfusion of vital organs include loss of pallor, increase in toe temperature, adequacy of nail bed capillary filling, and reversal of confusion or comatose state.

DORNASE ALFA

(dor′naze)

Trade name: Pulmozyme

Classifications: SKIN AND MUCOUS MEMBRANE AGENT; MUCOLYTIC

Prototype: Acetylcysteine

Pregnancy category: B

ACTIONS/PHARMACODYNAMICS Dornase is a solution of recombinant human deoxyribonuclease (DNase), an enzyme that selectively cleaves DNA. In cystic fibrosis (CF) patients, viscous, purulent secretions in the airway reduce pulmonary function and lead to exacerbations of infection. Purulent pulmonary secretions contain very high concentrations of DNA released by degenerating leukocytes that are present in response to infection. Dornase hydrolyzes the DNA in sputum of CF patients and reduces sputum viscosity. Use of dornase significiantly reduces number of upper respiratory infections acquired by patients with CF.

USES In combination with standard therapies to reduce the frequency of respiratory infections in patients with CF and to improve pulmonary function.

ROUTE & DOSAGE

Adult: **Inhaled** 2.5 mg (1 ampule) inhaled once daily using a recommended nebulizer; may increase to twice daily; do not mix with other agents in nebulizer.
Child: **Inhaled** Same as adult.

PHARMACOKINETICS **Absorption:** minimal systemic absorption. **Onset:** 3–8 d. **Duration:** benefit lasts up to 4 d after discontinuing treatment.

CONTRAINDICATIONS & PRECAUTIONS **Contraindicated in:** hypersensitivity to dornase. **Cautious use in:** pregnancy (category B), nursing mothers. Safety and efficacy in children <5 y of age not studied.

ADVERSE/SIDE EFFECTS **Respiratory:** hoarseness, sore throat, voice alterations, pharyngitis, laryngitis, cough, rhinitis. **Other:** conjunctivitis, chest pain, rash.

NURSING IMPLICATIONS

Administration

- Dornase alfa should not be diluted or mixed with any other drugs or solutions in the nebulizer.
- The drug should be used only with nebulizer systems recommended by the drug manufacturer.
- Do not shake ampuls; do not use ampuls that have been at room temperature longer than 24 h or have become cloudy or discolored.
- Store under refrigeration (2–8C/36–46F) in protective foil pouch.

Assessment & Drug Effects

- Monitor for improvement in dyspnea and sputum clearance.
- Monitor for signs and symptoms of

hypersensitivity (see Appendix G). Patients with a history of hypersensitivity to bovine pancreatic dornase are at high risk.
- Monitor for adverse effects; rarely, dosage adjustments may be required.

Patient & Family Education
- Instruct patient to report rash, hives, itching, or other signs and symptoms of hypersensitivity immediately.
- Inform patient of potential adverse effects and advise to report those that are bothersome or do not disappear.
- Advise patient to take a missed dose as soon as possible; if it is almost time for the next dose, advise to skip the missed dose.

DORZOLAMIDE HYDROCHLORIDE

(dor-zo′la-mide)

Trade name: Trusopt

Classifications: EYE PREPARATION; CARBONIC ANHYDRASE INHIBITOR

Prototype: Acetazolamide

Pregnancy category: C

ACTIONS/PHARMACODYNAMICS Dorzolamine is a sulfonamide and inhibits carbonic anhydrase in the eye, thus reducing the rate of aqueous humor formation with subsequent lowering of IOP. Elevated IOP is a major risk factor in the pathogenesis of optic nerve damage and visual field loss due to glaucoma.

USE Elevated intraocular pressure in patients with ocular hypertension or open-angle glaucoma.

ROUTE & DOSAGE

Adult: **Ophthalmic** 1 drop in affected eye t.i.d.

PHARMACOKINETICS Absorption: some systemic absorption from topical instillation. **Onset:** 2 h. **Duration:** 8–12 h. **Distribution:** distributes into red blood cells. **Elimination:** half-life: RBC elimination about 4 mo; excreted in urine.

CONTRAINDICATIONS & PRECAUTIONS Contraindicated in: previous hypersensitivity to dorzolamide. **Cautious use in:** history of hypersensitivity to other carbonic anhydrase inhibitors, sulfonamides, or thiazide diuretics; ocular infection or inflammation; recent ocular surgery; moderate-to-severe renal or hepatic insufficiency; angle-closure glaucoma; concomitant use of oral carbonic anhydrase inhibitors; pregnancy (category C). Safety and efficacy in children have not been established.

ADVERSE/SIDE EFFECTS CNS: headache. **GI:** bitter taste, nausea. **Ocular:** *transient burning or stinging, transient blurred vision,* superficial punctate keratitis, tearing, dryness, photophobia, ocular allergic reaction. **Other:** rash.

NURSING IMPLICATIONS

Administration
- Apply gentle pressure to lacrimal sac during and immediately following drug instillation for about 1 min to lessen degree of systemic absorption.
- If another ophthalmic drug is being used concurrently, administer at least 10 min apart.
- Store at 15–30C (59–86F).

Assessment & Drug Effects
- Before therapy begins inquire about previous hypersensitivity to sulfonamides.
- Withhold drug and notify physician if signs and symptoms of local or systemic hypersensitivity occur (see Appendix G).

- Withhold the drug and notify the physician if ocular irritation occurs.
- With long-term use, periodically monitor CBC, serum electrolytes, and renal and liver function tests.

Patient & Family Education

- Instruct in proper technique for applying eyedrops.
- Emphasize need to prevent contact of tip of drug dispenser with the eye.
- Instruct to discontinue drug and report to physician if ocular irritation, infection, or signs and symptoms of systemic hypersensitivity occur (see Appendix G).

DOXACURIUM CHLORIDE

(dox′-a-cur-i-um)

Trade name: Nuromax

Classifications: AUTONOMIC NERVOUS SYSTEM AGENT; SKELETAL MUSCLE RELAXANT, NONDEPOLARIZING

Prototype: Tubocurarine

Pregnancy category: C

ACTIONS/PHARMACODYNAMICS Long-acting neuromuscular blocking agent. Binds competively to cholinergic receptors on the motor end-plate, resulting in a block of neuromuscular transmission. Most patients require a pharmacologic reversal prior to full spontaneous recovery from neuromuscular block using anticholinesterase.

USE Skeletal muscle relaxation during surgery after general anesthesia. **Unlabeled use:** facilitates endotracheal intubation.

ROUTE & DOSAGE

Intubation or Induction

Adult: **IV** 0.05 mg/kg administered as rapid bolus injection over 5–10 s. Use lower doses in elderly patients or patients with renal or hepatic dysfunction. doses in elderly patients or
Child 2–12 y: **IV** 0.03–0.05 mg/kg with halothane general anesthesia.

Maintenance with General Anesthesia

Adult: **IV** 0.0005–0.01 mg/kg q60–100 min administered as rapid bolus injection over 5–10 s. Dosing interval adjusted for each individual patient. Use lower patients with renal or hepatic dysfunction.
Child 2–12 y: **IV** Same dose as adult, but may have to give more frequently.

PHARMACOKINETICS **Onset:** 5–10 min. **Peak:** 10 min. **Duration:** 60–160 min depending on dose. **Distribution:** 30% protein bound. **Metabolism:** minimal to no hepatic metabolism. **Elimination:** half-life: 1.5 h; 40–50% excreted in urine within 12 h. some excretion in bile.

CONTRAINDICATIONS & PRECAUTIONS **Contraindicated in:** hypersensitivity to doxacurium. **Cautious use in:** neuromuscular diseases (e.g., myasthenia gravis), burn patients, acid–base or serum electrolyte imbalances, newborn infants, elderly patients, pregnancy (category C), nursing mothers, and children <2 years of age.

ADVERSE/SIDE EFFECTS **CV:** bradycardia, hypotension, cutaneous flushing, histamine release.

DRUG INTERACTIONS VOLATILE ANESTHETICS **(isoflurane, enflurane, halothane)** potentiate the effects of doxacurium, requiring a reduced dose of doxacurium. Certain ANTIBIOTICS, including the AMINOGLYCOSIDES, **capre-**

D

omycin, tetracycline, bacitracin, polymyxins, lincomycin, clindamycin, and **colistin,** increase the neuromuscular blocking effect of doxacurium. **Carbamazepine** or **phenytoin** may increase the onset and decrease the duration of neuromuscular blockade. **Lithium, magnesium, procainamide,** or **quinidine** may enhance neuromuscular blockade.

NURSING IMPLICATIONS

Administration

- Doses of doxacurium are individualized according to age, body size, and presence of kidney, liver, and neuromuscular diseases.
- Doxacurium contains benzyl alcohol, which has been associated with fatal complications in newborns.
- Doxacurium should be administered under the supervision of expert clinicians. See manufacturer's guidelines for dilution, compatibility, and administration.
- Store undiluted at room temperature (15–25C/41–77F). Do not freeze. Diluted drug may be stored in polypropylene syringes for up to 24 h at 5–25C/41–77F.

Assessment & Drug Effects

- Evidence of prolonged neuromuscular block may range from skeletal muscle weakness to prolonged paralysis with respiratory insufficiency and apnea.
- Monitor for full recovery of skeletal muscle function. Ventilation should be supported until full recovery occurs.
- Duration of neuromuscular block may be longer in persons >60 years old and in obese patients whose doses have not been adjusted according to ideal body weight.
- Drugs used to antagonize doxacurium may wear off before the effects of doxacurium. Monitor accordingly.

DOXAPRAM HYDROCHLORIDE

(dox′a-pram)

Trade name: Dopram

Classifications: CNS AGENT; RESPIRATORY AND CEREBRAL STIMULANT

Prototype: Caffeine

Pregnancy category: B

ACTIONS/PHARMACODYNAMICS

Short-acting analeptic capable of stimulating all levels of the cerebrospinal axis. Has minor effect on cortex. Respiratory stimulation by direct medullary action or possibly by indirect activation of peripheral chemoreceptors increases tidal volume and slightly increases respiratory rate. Decreases Pco_2 and increases Po_2 by increasing alveolar ventilation; may elevate BP and pulse rate by stimulation of brainstem vasomotor areas.

USES Short-term adjunctive therapy to alleviate postanesthesia and drug-induced respiratory depression and to hasten arousal and return of pharyngeal and laryngeal reflexes. Also as a temporary measure (approximately 2 h) in hospitalized patients with COPD associated with acute respiratory insufficiency as an aid to prevent elevation of $Paco_2$ during administration of oxygen. (Not used with mechanical ventilation.) **Unlabeled use:** neonatal apnea refractory to xanthine therapy.

ROUTE & DOSAGE

Postanesthesia

Adult: **IV** 0.5–1 mg/kg single injection not to exceed 1.5 mg/kg or 2 mg/kg total dose when repeated at 5 min intervals, *or* 1–3 mg/min infusion (max 4 mg/kg or 300 mg, not to exceed 3 g/d).

Common side effect in *italic,* life-threatening effects underlined: generic names in **bold;** drug class in SMALL CAPS

Drug-induced CNS Depression

Adult: **IV** 1–2 mg/kg; repeat in 5 min; then q1–2h until patient awakens; if relapse occurs, resume q1–2h injections (max total dose 3 g); if no response after priming dose, may give 1–3 mg/min for up to 2 h until patient awakens.

Chronic Obstructive Pulmonary Disease

Adult: **IV** 1–2 mg/min for a max of 2 h (max rate 3 mg/min).

Neonatal Apnea

Neonate: **IV** 2.5–3 mg/kg followed by 1 mg/kg/h, may titrate to max 2.5 mg/kg/h.

PHARMACOKINETICS **Onset:** 20–40 s. **Peak:** 1–2 min. **Duration:** 5–12 min. **Metabolism:** rapidly metabolized. **Elimination:** excreted in urine as metabolites.

CONTRAINDICATIONS & PRECAUTIONS **Contraindicated in:** epilepsy and other convulsive disorders; incompetence of ventilatory mechanism due to muscle paresis, pulmonary fibrosis, flail chest, pneumothorax, airway obstruction, extreme dyspnea, or acute bronchial asthma; severe hypertension, coronary artery disease, uncompensated heart failure, CVA. Safe use during pregnancy (category B), in nursing mothers, and in children <12 y not established. **Cautious use in:** history of bronchial asthma, COPD; cardiac disease, severe tachycardia, arrhythmias, hypertension; hyperthyroidism; pheochromocytoma; head injury, cerebral edema, increased intracranial pressure; peptic ulcer, patients undergoing gastric surgery; acute agitation.

ADVERSE/SIDE EFFECTS **CNS:** dizziness, sneezing, apprehension, confusion, *involuntary movements,* hyperactivity, paresthesias; feeling of warmth and burning, especially of genitalia and perineum; flushing, sweating, hyperpyrexia, headache, pilomotor erection, pruritus, muscle tremor, rigidity, convulsions, *increased deep-tendon reflexes,* bilateral Babinski sign, *carpopedal spasm,* pupillary dilation, mild delayed narcosis. **CV:** *mild to moderate increase in BP, sinus tachycardia,* bradycardia, extrasystoles, lowered T waves, PVCs, chest pains, tightness in chest. **GI:** nausea, vomiting, diarrhea, salivation, sour taste. **GU:** urinary retention, frequency, incontinence. **Respiratory:** dyspnea, tachypnea, cough, laryngospasm, bronchospasm, hiccups, rebound hypoventilation, hypocapnia with tetany. **Other:** local skin irritation, thrombophlebitis with extravasation; decreased Hgb, Hct, and RBC count; elevated BUN; albuminuria.

DRUG INTERACTIONS MAO INHIBITORS, SYMPATHOMIMETIC AGENTS add to pressor effects.

INCOMPATIBILITIES **Solution/additive: aminophylline, ascorbic acid,** CEPHALOSPORINS, **carbenicillin, dexamethasone, diazepam, digoxin, dobutamine, folic acid, furosemide, hydrocortisone, ketamine, methylprednisolone, minocycline, thiopental, ticarcillin.**

NURSING IMPLICATIONS

Administration

- Doxapram contains benzyl alcohol; therefore, do not use in newborns.
- Adequacy of airway and oxygenation must be ensured before initiation of doxapram therapy.
- Drug is available prediluted. For undiluted ampuls, follow manu-

D

facturer's recommendations for dilution.

- IV flow rate is prescribed by physician. Infusion rate may start at 1 mg/min until satisfactory respiratory response is observed. It should then be maintained at 1–2 mg/min and be adjusted to maintain desired respiratory response.
- IV administration to neonates: Verify correct IV concentration and rate of infusion with physician.
- Store at 15–30C (59–86F) unless otherwise directed.

Assessment & Drug Effects

- Extravasation or use of same IV site for prolonged periods can cause thrombophlebitis (see Appendix G) or tissue irritation.
- Careful monitoring and accurate observations of BP, pulse, deep tendon reflexes, airway, and arterial blood gases are essential guides for determining minimum effective dosage and preventing overdosage. Baseline determinations should be made for comparison.
- In patients with COPD, arterial Po_2 and Pco_2 and O_2 saturation should be drawn prior to initiation of doxapram infusion and oxygen administration and then at least every 30 min during infusion. Infusion should not be administered for longer than 2 h.
- Doxapram should be discontinued if arterial blood gases show evidence of deterioration and when mechanical ventilation is initiated.
- Observe patient continuously during therapy and maintain vigilance until patient is fully alert (usually about 1 h) and protective pharyngeal and laryngeal reflexes are completely restored.
- Notify physician immediately of any side effects. Be alert for early signs of toxicity: tachycardia, muscle tremor, spasticity, hyperactive reflexes.
- A mild to moderate increase in BP commonly occurs.
- If sudden hypotension or dyspnea develops, doxapram should be discontinued.

DOXAZOSIN MESYLATE

(dox-a′zo-sin)

Trade name: Cardura

Classifications: AUTONOMIC NERVOUS SYSTEM AGENT; ALPHA-ADRENERGIC ANTAGONIST (SYMPATHOLYTIC, BLOCKING AGENT)

Prototype: Prazosin

Pregnancy category: B

ACTIONS/PHARMACODYNAMICS By selective competitive inhibition of $alpha_1$-adrenoceptors produces vasodilation in both resistance (arterioles) and capacitance (veins) vessels with the result that both peripheral vascular resistance and blood pressure are reduced. Lowers blood pressure in supine or standing individuals with most pronounced effect on diastolic pressure.

USES Mild to moderate hypertension, benign prostatic hypertrophy. **Unlabeled use:** CHF.

ROUTE & DOSAGE

Hypertension

Adult: **PO** Start with 1 mg h.s. and titrate up to a max of 16 mg/d in 1–2 divided doses.
Geriatric: **PO** Start with 0.5 mg h.s.

PHARMACOKINETICS Absorption: readily absorbed from GI tract; 62–69% of dose reaches systemic circulation. **Peak:** 2–6 h. **Duration:** up to 24 h. **Distribution:** highly protein bound (98–99%). **Metabolism:** approximately 35% of dose is metabolized in liver. **Elimination:** half-life: 9–12 h; 9% excreted in urine, 63% in feces.

CONTRAINDICATIONS & PRECAUTIONS **Contraindicated in:** hypersensitivity to doxazosin, prazosin, and terazosin; nursing mothers; safe use during pregnancy (category B) and children has not been established. **Cautious use in:** hepatic impairment.

ADVERSE/SIDE EFFECTS **CV:** *Orthostatic hypotension,* edema. **CNS:** vertigo, *headache,* dizziness, somnolence, fatigue, nervousness, anxiety. **GI:** nausea, abdominal pain. **Hematologic:** leukopenia. **Skin:** pruritus, eczema.

NURSING IMPLICATIONS

Administration

- Give initial dose at bedtime to minimize problems with postural hypotension and syncope.
- Maintenance dose is individualized according to the standing BP response.
- Store at 15–30C (59–86F).

Assessment & Drug Effects

- Monitor BP with patient lying down and standing. Note that doses above 4 mg increase the risk of postural hypotension.
- Postural hypotension is most likely to occur between 2 and 6 h after the initial dose or any dose increase. Therefore, monitor BP during this time.

Patient & Family Education

- Instruct patient to avoid driving and other hazardous tasks for 12–24 h after the first dose or an increase in dosage or when medication is restarted after an interruption in dosage.
- To avoid orthostatic hypotension and syncope, the patient should be cautious when rising from a sitting or supine position and should make position and directional changes slowly and in stages.
- Report to the physician episodes of dizziness or palpitations. These will require a dosage adjustment.
- Until reaction to doxazosin is known (i.e., potential development of side effects), patient should not undertake any activity that might become a hazard in the presence of dizziness, syncope, or weakness.

D

DOXEPIN HYDROCHLORIDE

(dox′e-pin)

Trade names: Adapin, Sinequan, Triadapin♣, Zonalon

Classifications: CNS AGENT; PSYCHOTHERAPEUTIC; TRICYCLIC ANTIDEPRESSANT

Prototype: Imipramine

Pregnancy category: C

ACTIONS/PHARMACODYNAMICS Dibenzoxepin tricyclic antidepressant (TCA). Actions, limitations, and interactions are similar to those of imipramine. Reportedly one of the most sedating of the TCAs.

USES Psychoneurotic anxiety or depressive reactions; mixed symptoms of anxiety and depression; anxiety or depression associated with alcoholism; organic disease; psychotic depressive disorders; topical for treatment of pruritus. **Unlabeled uses:** peptic ulcer disease, neuralgia.

ROUTE & DOSAGE

Antidepressant

Adult: **PO** 30–150 mg/d h.s. *or* in divided doses; may gradually increase to 300 mg/d (use lower doses in elderly patients).

Geriatric: **PO** 10–25 mg h.s., may gradually increase to 75 mg/d.
Child: **PO** 1–3 mg/kg/d in single or divided doses.

Pruritus

Adult: **Topical** apply a thin film q.i.d. with at least 3–4 h between applications; may use up to 8 d.

PHARMACOKINETICS **Absorption:** rapidly absorbed from GI sites through intact skin. **Peak:** 2 h. **Distribution:** crosses placenta; distributed into breast milk. **Metabolism:** metabolized in liver. **Elimination:** half-life: 6–8 h; primarily excreted in urine.

CONTRAINDICATIONS & PRECAUTIONS **Contraindicated in:** prior sensitivity to any TCA; during acute recovery phase following MI; glaucoma; prostatic hypertrophy; tendency to urinary retention; concurrent use of MAO INHIBITORS. Safe use during pregnancy (category C), in nursing women, and in children <12 y not established. **Cautious use in:** patients receiving ECT, patients with suicidal tendency; renal, cardiovascular or hepatic dysfunction.

ADVERSE/SIDE EFFECTS Anticholinergic. **CNS:** *drowsiness,* dizziness, weakness, fatigue, headache, hypomania, confusion, tremors, paresthesias. **CV:** *orthostatic hypotension,* palpitation, hypertension, tachycardia, ECG changes. **Eye:** mydriasis, blurred vision, photophobia. **GI:** *dry mouth,* sour or metallic taste, epigastric distress, constipation. **GU:** urinary retention, delayed micturition, urinary frequency. **Other:** increased perspiration, tinnitus, weight gain, photosensitivity reaction, skin rash, agranulocytosis, *burning or stinging at application site,* edema.

DRUG INTERACTIONS May decrease some antihypertensive response to ANTIHYPERTENSIVES; CNS DEPRESSANTS, **alcohol,** HYPNOTICS, BARBITURATES, SEDATIVES potentiate CNS depression; may increase hypoprothombinemic effect of ORAL ANTICOAGULANTS; **ethchlorvynol** may cause transient delirium; **levodopa,** SYMPATHOMIMETICS (e.g., **epinephrine, norepinephrine**) introduce possibility of sympathetic hyperactivity with hypertension and hyperpyrexia; MAO INHIBITORS introduce possibility of severe reactions, toxic psychosis, cardiovascular instability; **methylphenidate** increases plasma TCA levels; thyroid agents may increase possibility of arrhythmias; **cimetidine** may increase plasma TCA levels.

NURSING IMPLICATIONS

Administration

- Oral concentrate must be diluted with approximately 120 ml water, milk, or fruit juice just before administration.
- Capsule may be emptied and contents swallowed with fluid or mixed with food.
- If daytime sedation is pronounced, inform physician. Entire daily dose (up to 150 mg) may be prescribed for bedtime administration.
- Store at 15–30C (59–86F) in tightly closed, light-resistant container.

Assessment & Drug Effects

- If a patient uses excessive amounts of alcohol, potentiation of doxepin effects may increase the danger of overdosage or suicide attempt.
- Doxepin has moderate to strong anticholinergic effects. Be alert to changes in I&O ratio and check patient for constipation and abdominal distention.

Patient & Family Education

- Teach the necessity to maintain established dosage regimen and to avoid change of intervals, doubling, reducing, or skipping doses.

- The actions of both alcohol and doxepin are potentiated when used together during therapy and for up to 2 wk after doxepin is discontinued. Consult physician about safe amount of alcohol, if any, that can be taken.
- Caution patient to avoid driving and other potentially hazardous activities until reaction to drug is known. Doxepin has a pronounced sedative effect; symptom tends to disappear with continued therapy.

D

DOXORUBICIN HYDROCHLORIDE (ADR)

(dox-oh-roo'bi-sin)

Trade names: Adriamycin, Rubex

DOXORUBICIN LIPOSOME

Trade name: Doxil

Prototype for classifications: ANTINEOPLASTIC; ANTIBIOTIC

Pregnancy category: D

ACTIONS/PHARMACODYNAMICS Cytotoxic antibiotic with wide spectrum of antitumor activity and strong immunosuppressive properties. Intercalates with preformed DNA residues, blocking effective DNA and RNA transcription. Highly destructive to rapidly proliferating cells and slowly developing carcinomas; selectively toxic to cardiac tissue. A potent radiosensitizer capable of enhancing radiation reactions. No clinical cross-resistance to standard antineoplastics; therefore, it may be especially effective in patients with less advanced disease.

USES To produce regression in neoplastic conditions, including acute lymphoblastic and myeloblastic leukemias, Wilms' tumor, neuroblastoma, soft tissue and bone sarcomas, breast and ovary carcinomas, lymphomas, bronchogenic carcinoma. Generally used in combined modalities with surgery, radiation, and immunotherapy. Effective pretreatment to sensitize superficial tumors to local radiation therapy. Kaposi's sarcoma (Doxil). **Unlabeled use:** multiple myeloma.

ROUTE & DOSAGE

Neoplasm

Adult: **IV** 60–75 mg/m^2 as single dose at 21 d intervals *or* 30 mg/m^2 on each of 3 consecutive days repeated every 4 wk (max total cumulative dose 500–550 mg/m^2).
Child: **IV** 35–75 mg/m^2 as single dose, repeat at 21-d interval, or 20–30 mg/m^2 once weekly.

Kaposi's Sarcoma

Adult: **IV** (Doxil) 20 mg/m^2 every 3 wk. Infuse over 30 min (do not use in-line filters).

PHARMACOKINETICS Distribution: widely distributed; does not cross blood–brain barrier; crosses placenta; distribution into breast milk not known. **Metabolism:** metabolized in liver to active metabolite. **Elimination:** half-life: 16.7–31.7 h; excreted primarily in bile.

CONTRAINDICATIONS & PRECAUTIONS Contraindicated in: myelosuppression, impaired cardiac function, obstructive jaundice, previous treatment with complete cumulative doses of doxorubicin or daunorubicin. Safe use during pregnancy (category D) not established. **Cautious use in:** impaired hepatic or renal function; patients who have received cyclophosphamide or pelvic irradiation or radiotherapy to areas surrounding heart; history of atopic dermatitis.

ADVERSE/SIDE EFFECTS **CV:** serious, irreversible myocardial toxicity with delayed CHF, ventricular arrhythmias, acute left ventricular failure, hypertension, hypotension. **GI:** *stomatitis*, esophagitis with ulcerations; nausea, vomiting, anorexia, inanition, diarrhea. **Hematopoietic:** *severe myelosuppression* (60–85% of patients); leukopenia (principally granulocytes), thrombocytopenia, anemia. **Hypersensitivity:** red flare around injection site, erythema, skin rash, pruritus, angioedema, urticaria, eosinophilia, fever, chills, anaphylactoid reaction. **Skin:** hyperpigmentation of nail beds, tongue, and buccal mucosa (especially in blacks); *complete alopecia* (reversible), hyperpigmentation of dermal creases (especially in children), rash, *recall phenomenon (skin reaction due to prior radiotherapy)*. **Other:** lacrimation, drowsiness, fever, facial flush with too rapid IV infusion rate, microscopic hematuria, hyperuricemia. *With extravasation: severe cellulitis, vesication, tissue necrosis,* lymphangitis, phlebosclerosis.

DRUG INTERACTIONS BARBITURATES may decrease pharmacologic effects of doxorubicin by increasing its hepatic metabolism—increase in doxorubicin dosage may be needed; **streptozocin** (Zanosar) may prolong doxorubicin half-life—dosage reduction of doxorubicin may be indicated.

INCOMPATIBILITIES **Solution/additive: aminophylline, cephalothin, dexamethasone, diazepam, fluorouracil, furosemide, hydrocortisone, heparin, vinblastine. Y-site: furosemide, heparin,** TPN.

NURSING IMPLICATIONS

Administration

- Caution should be observed in preparing doxorubicin solution. Wear gloves. If powder or solution contacts skin or mucosa, wash copiously with soap and water.
- Personnel who handle or are exposed to doxorubicin during the first trimester of pregnancy are at high risk of losing the fetus.
- IV preparation: Dilute the powder with 0.9% NaCl to yield a final concentration of 2 mg/ml. Bacteriostatic diluents are not recommended.
- IV administration: administer slowly into side arm of freely running IV infusion of NaCl injection or 5% dextrose injection. Tubing should be attached to a butterfly needle inserted into a large vein.
- Infusion rate usually permits administration of the dose in a 3- to 5-min period. Rate will be specifically ordered.
- IV administration to infants and children: Verify correct IV concentration and rate of infusion with physician.
- Facial flushing and local red streaking along the vein may occur if drug is administered too rapidly. Urticaria around injection site is usually self-limiting.
- If possible, avoid using antecubital vein or veins on dorsum of hand or wrist where extravasation could damage underlying tendons and nerves. Also avoid veins in extremity with compromised venous or lymphatic drainage.
- Reconstituted solution is stable for 24 h at room temperature and for 48 h under refrigeration (4–10C) (39–50F). Protect from sunlight; discard unused solution.

Assessment & Drug Effects

- Give prompt attention to complaint of stinging or burning sensation at the injection site. Infusion should be stopped promptly and IV needle removed. Notify physician promptly.

- Monitor area of extravasation closely for 3–4 wk. If ulceration begins (usually 1–4 wk after extravasation), a plastic surgeon should be consulted.
- Begin a flow chart to establish baseline data. Include temperature, pulse, respiration, BP, body weight, laboratory values, and I&O ratio and pattern.
- Evaluation of hepatic, renal, hematopoietic, and cardiac function (ECG) should be performed prior to initiation of therapy, at regular intervals thereafter, and at end of therapy.
- Be alert to and report early signs of cardiotoxicity (see Appendix G). Monitor pulse and BP frequently. Acute life-threatening arrhythmias may occur within a few hours of drug administration.
- Objective signs of hepatic dysfunction (jaundice, dark urine, pruritus) or kidney dysfunction (altered I&O ratio and pattern, local discomfort with voiding) should be reported promptly.
- Stomatitis, generally maximal in second week of therapy, frequently begins with a burning sensation accompanied by erythema of oral mucosa that may progress to ulceration and dysphagia in 2 or 3 d. Fastidious oral hygiene is required, especially before and after meals.
- The nadir of leukopenia (an expected 1000/mm^3) typically occurs 10–14 d after single dose, with recovery occurring within 21 d.
- Superinfections may result from antibiotic therapy during leukopenic period. Report signs of superinfection (see Appendix G) promptly.
- Bloody diarrhea may result from an antiblastic effect on rapidly growing intestinal mucosal cells. Avoid rectal medications and use of rectal thermometer to prevent trauma.

Patient & Family Education

- Complete alopecia (reversible) is an expected side effect.
- Inform patient that alopecia may also involve eyelashes and eyebrows, beard and mustache, pubic and axillary hair. Regrowth of hair usually begins 2–3 mo after drug is discontinued.
- Advise patient that drug turns urine red for 1–2 d after administration.
- Increased lacrimation for 5–10 d after a single dose is a possibility. Caution patient to keep hands away from eyes to prevent conjunctivitis.

DOXYCYCLINE HYCLATE

(dox-i-sye′kleen)

Trade names: Apo-Doxy ♣, Doryx, Doxy, Doxy-Caps, Doxychel, Doxycin ♣, Doxy-Lemmon, Novo-doxylin ♣, SK-Doxycycline, Vibramycin, Vibra-Tabs, Vivox

Classifications: ANTIINFECTIVE; ANTIBIOTIC; TETRACYCLINE

Prototype: Tetracycline

Pregnancy category: D

ACTIONS/PHARMACODYNAMICS

Semisynthetic broad-spectrum tetracycline antibiotic derived from oxytetracycline. More completely absorbed, effective blood levels maintained for longer periods and excreted more slowly than most other tetracyclines, thus requiring smaller and less frequent dosing. Primarily bacteriostatic in action.

USES Similar to those of tetracycline, e.g., chlamydial and mycoplasmal infections; gonorrhea, syphilis in penicillin-allergic patients; rickettsial diseases; acute exacerbations of chronic bronchitis. **Unlabeled uses:** treatment of acute PID, leptospirosis, prophylaxis for rape victims, suppression and chemoprophylaxis of chloroquine-resistant *Plasmodium falciparum* malaria, short-term prophylaxis and treatment of travelers' diarrhea caused by enterotoxigenic strains of *Escherichia coli*. **Intrapleural:** malignant pleural effusions.

D

ROUTE & DOSAGE

Antiinfective

Adult: **PO/IV** 100 mg q12h on day 1; then 100 mg/d as single dose up to 100 mg q12h. *Child:* **PO/IV** > 8 y, 4.4 mg/kg in 1–2 doses on day 1; then 2.2–4.4 mg/kg/d in 1–2 divided doses.

Gonorrhea

Adult: **PO** 200 mg immediately, followed by 100 mg h.s.; then 100 mg b.i.d. for 3 d.

Primary and Secondary Syphilis

Adult: **PO** 300 mg/d in divided doses for at least 10 d.

Travelers' Diarrhea

Adult: **PO** 100 mg/d during risk period (up to 2 wk) beginning day 1 of travel.

PHARMACOKINETICS **Absorption:** completely absorbed from GI tract. **Peak:** 1.5–4 h. **Distribution:** penetrates eye, prostate, and CSF; crosses placenta; distributed into breast milk. **Metabolism:** not metabolized. **Elimination:** half-life: 14–24 h; 20–30% excreted in urine and 20–40% in feces in 48 h.

CONTRAINDICATIONS & PRECAUTIONS **Contraindicated in:** sensitivity to any of the tetracyclines; use during period of tooth development: last half of pregnancy (category D), nursing women, infants, and children <8 y (causes permanent yellow discoloration of teeth, enamel hypoplasia, and retardation of bone growth). **Cautious use in:** alcoholism.

ADVERSE/SIDE EFFECTS **Eye:** interference with color vision. **GI:** anorexia, *nausea*, vomiting, diarrhea, enterocolitis; esophageal irritation (oral capsule and tablet). **Skin:** rashes, photosensitivity reaction. **Other:** thrombophlebitis (IV use), superinfections.

DIAGNOSTIC TEST INTERFERENCE Like other tetracyclines, doxycycline may cause false increases in ***urinary catecholamines*** (fluorometric methods); false decreases in ***urinary urobilinogen;*** false-negative ***urine glucose*** with glucose oxidase methods (e.g., Clinistix, TesTape); parenteral doxycycline (containing ascorbic acid) may cause false-positive determinations using Benedict's reagent or Clinitest.

DRUG INTERACTIONS ANTACIDS, **iron** preparation, **calcium, magnesium, zinc, kaolin-pectin, sodium bicarbonate** can significantly decrease absorption; effects of both doxycycline and **desmopressin** antagonized; increases **digoxin** absorption, thus increasing risk of digoxin toxicity; **methoxy flurane** increases risk of renal failure.

NURSING IMPLICATIONS

Administration

- Check expiration date. Degradation products of tetracycline are nephrotoxic.
- Unlike most tetracyclines, oral doxycycline may be taken with food or milk to minimize nausea

without significantly affecting bioavailability of drug.

- Consult physician about ordering the oral suspension for patients who are bedridden or have difficulty swallowing.
- IV preparation: Reconstitute by adding 10 ml sterile water for injection, or other diluent recommended by manufacturer, to each 100 mg of drug. Before administration, the reconstituted solution must then be diluted further with 100–1000 ml (per 100 mg of drug) of compatible infusion solution to produce concentrations ranging from 0.1 to 1 mg/ml.
- Administer properly diluted doxycycline at a rate of 100 mg over 1–4 h. Infusion should be completed within 12 h of dilution.
- IV infusion rate will be prescribed by physician. Duration of infusion varies with dose but is usually 1–4 h. Recommended minimum infusion time for 100 mg of 0.5 mg/ml solution is 1 h.
- When diluted with lactated Ringer's or dextrose 5% in lactated Ringer's injection, infusion must be completed within 6 h to ensure adequate stability.
- During infusion, all solutions must be protected from direct sunlight.
- Reconstituted solutions are stable for 72 h if refrigerated. After this time, infusion must be completed within 12 h.
- Doxycycline, oral and parenteral forms (prior to reconstitution), should be stored in tightly covered, light-resistant containers at 15–30C (59–86F) unless otherwise directed.

Assessment & Drug Effects

- Doxycycline (capsule and tablet forms) is associated with a comparatively high incidence of esophagitis, especially in patients > 40 y. Sudden onset of painful or difficult swallowing should be reported promptly to physician.
- Be alert for and report evidence of superinfections (see Appendix G).

Patient & Family Education

- Instructions for patients taking capsule or tablet forms (to prevent esophageal ulceration): Take drug with a full glass (240 ml) of water to ensure passage into stomach. Remain standing for about 90 s after taking medication. Avoid taking capsule or tablet within 1 h of lying down or retiring.
- To reduce risk of phototoxic reaction, caution patient to avoid exposure to direct sunlight and ultraviolet light while taking doxycycline and for 4 or 5 d after therapy is terminated. Phototoxic reaction appears like an exaggerated sunburn. Sunscreens provide little protection.

DRONABINOL

(droe-nab′i-nol)

Trade names: Marinol, THC

Classifications: CNS AGENT; ANTIEMETIC; CANNABINOID

Pregnancy category: B

Controlled substance: Schedule II

ACTIONS/PHARMACODYNAMICS

Synthetic derivative of tetrahydrocannabinol (THC), the principal psychoactive constituent of marijuana *(Cannabis sativa)*. Mechanism unclear: Inhibits vomiting control mechanism in the medulla oblongata, producing potent antiemetic effect; nontherapeutic actions are exactly like those of marijuana. Has complex CNS effect that necessitates close supervision of the patient during drug use. Decreases REM sleep;

effect on BP is unpredictable; oral temperature may be decreased, and heart rate may be increased. Risk of drug abuse is high.

D

USES To treat chemotherapy-induced nausea and vomiting in cancer patients who fail to respond to conventional antiemetic therapy. Appetite stimulant for AIDS patients. **Unlabeled use:** glaucoma.

ROUTE & DOSAGE

Chemotherapy-induced Nausea

Adult: **PO** 5 mg/m^2 1–3 h before administration of chemotherapy; then q2–4h after chemotherapy for a total of 4–6 doses; dose may be increased by 2.5 mg/m^2 up to a max of 15 mg/m^2 if necessary. *Child*: **PO** Same as for adult.

Appetite Stimulant

Adult: **PO** 2.5 mg b.i.d., before lunch and dinner.

PHARMACOKINETICS Absorption: rapidly absorbed from GI tract, with bioavailability of 10–20%. **Peak:** 2–3 h. **Distribution:** fat soluble; distributed to many organs; distributed into breast milk. **Metabolism:** metabolized in liver; extensive first-pass metabolism. **Elimination:** half-life: 25–36 h; excreted principally in bile; 50% excreted in feces within 72 h; 10–15% excreted in urine.

CONTRAINDICATIONS & PRECAUTIONS Contraindicated in: nausea and vomiting caused by other than chemotherapeutic agents; hypersensitivity to dronabinol or sesame oil; used during pregnancy (category B) only if clearly necessary. **Cautious use in:** first exposure, especially in elderly or cardiac patient; hypertension, cardiovascular disorders; epilepsy; psychiatric illness, patient receiving other psychoactive drugs; severe hepatic dysfunction.

ADVERSE/SIDE EFFECTS CNS: *drowsiness,* psychologic high, dizziness, anxiety, confusion, euphoria, sensory or perceptual difficulties, impaired coordination, depression, irritability, headache, ataxia, memory lapse, paresthesias, paranoia, depersonalization, disorientation, tinnitus, nightmares, speech difficulty, facial flush, diaphoresis. **CV:** tachycardia, orthostatic hypotension, hypertension, syncope. **GI:** dry mouth, diarrhea, fecal incontinence. **Other:** muscular pains.

DRUG INTERACTIONS Alcohol and other CNS DEPRESSANTS may exaggerate psychoactive effects of dronabinol; TRICYCLIC ANTIDEPRESSANTS, **atropine** may cause tachycardia.

NURSING IMPLICATIONS

Administration

- Doses are not repeated following a reaction until patient's mental state has returned to normal and the circumstances have been evaluated.
- Store dronabinol at 8–15C (46–59F).

Assessment & Drug Effects

- Patients with hypertension or heart disease should have monitoring of BP and cardiac status.
- Response to dronabinol is varied, and previous uneventful use does not guarantee that adverse reactions will not occur. Effects of drug may persist an unpredictably long time (days). Extended use at therapeutic dosage may cause accumulation of toxic amounts of dronabinol and its metabolites.
- If dose is increased, watch for disturbing psychiatric symptoms such as altered mental state, loss of coordination, evidence of a psychologic high (easy laughing, elation

and heightened awareness), or depression.

- Withdrawal symptoms have been observed within 12 h after abrupt withdrawal of the drug: irritability, insomnia, restlessness. Peak intensity of symptoms occurs at about 24 h: hot flashes, diaphoresis, rhinorrhea, watery diarrhea, hiccups, anorexia. Usually, syndrome is over in 96 h.

Patient & Family Education

- Caution patient to avoid driving or other potentially hazardous activities that require alertness and judgment because of high incidence of dizziness and drowsiness.
- Alert and prepare patient and family for possible (reversible) drug-induced mood changes or behavior changes that may occur during dronabinol use.
- Caution against ingestion of alcohol during period of systemic dronabinol effect. Effect on blood ethanol levels are complex and unpredictable.

DROPERIDOL

(droe-per′i-dole)

Trade name: Inapsine

Classifications: CNS AGENT; BUTYROPHENONE; ANTIEMETIC

Prototype: Haloperidol

Pregnancy category: C

ACTIONS/PHARMACODYNAMICS Butyrophenone derivative structurally and pharmacologically related to haloperidol. Antagonizes emetic effects of morphine-like analgesics and other drugs that act on CTZ. Mild alpha-adrenergic blocking activity and direct vasodilator effect may cause hypotension. Acts primarily at subcortical level to produce sedation. Sedative property reduces anxiety and motor activity without necessarily inducing sleep; patient remains responsive. Potentiates other CNS depressants.

USES To produce tranquilizing effect and to reduce nausea and vomiting during surgical and diagnostic procedures. Also for premedication, during induction, and as adjunct in maintenance of general or regional anesthesia. Principally used in fixed combination with the potent narcotic analgesic fentanyl (Innovar) to produce neuroleptanalgesia (quiescence, reduced motor activity, and indifference to pain and environmental stimuli) to permit carrying out a variety of diagnostic and minor surgical procedures. **Unlabeled use:** IV antiemetic in cancer chemotherapy.

ROUTE & DOSAGE

Premedication

Adult: **IM/IV** 2.5–10 mg 30–60 min preoperatively.
Child 2–12 y: **IM/IV** 0.088–0.165 mg/kg 30–60 min preoperatively.

Maintenance of General Anesthesia

Adult: **IM/IV** *Induction:* 0.22–0.275 mg/kg; **maintenance:** 1.25–2.5 mg.
Child 2–12 y: **IM/IV** 0.088–0.165 mg/kg.

PHARMACOKINETICS **Onset:** 3–10 min. **Peak:** 30 min. **Duration:** 2–4 h; may persist up to 12 h. **Distribution:** crosses placenta. **Metabolism:** metabolized in liver. **Elimination:** excreted in urine and feces.

CONTRAINDICATIONS & PRECAUTIONS **Contraindicated in:** known intolerance to droperidol. Safe use during pregnancy (category C) and in children <2 y not established. **Cau-**

tious use in: elderly, debilitated, and other poor-risk patients; Parkinson's disease; hypotension; liver, kidney, cardiac disease; cardiac bradyarrhythmias.

D

ADVERSE/SIDE EFFECTS **CNS:** *postoperative drowsiness, extrapyramidal symptoms:* dystonia, akathisia, oculogyric crisis; dizziness, restlessness, anxiety, hallucinations, mental depression. **CV:** *hypotension, tachycardia.* **Other:** chills, shivering, laryngospasm, bronchospasm.

INCOMPATIBILITIES **Solution/additive: fluorouracil, furosemide, heparin, leucovorin, methotrexate, pentobarbital. Y-site: fluorouracil, furosemide, heparin, leucovorin, methotrexate, nafcillin.**

NURSING IMPLICATIONS

Administration

- When patient is under the effect of another CNS depressant, the required dose of droperidol may be less than usual. Postoperative narcotics or other CNS depressants are prescribed in reduced doses since they have additive or potentiating effects.
- IV droperidol may be given undiluted by direct IV at a rate of 10 mg or fraction thereof over 30–60 seconds.
- IV administration to infants and children: Verify correct rate of IV injection with physician.
- Protect from light. Store at 15–30C (59–86F), unless otherwise directed by manufacturer.

Assessment & Drug Effects

- Monitor vital signs closely. Hypotension and tachycardia are common side effects.
- Because of possibility of severe orthostatic hypotension, always exercise care in moving and positioning the medicated patient. Avoid abrupt changes in position.
- Patient who receives a narcotic analgesic concurrently should be observed carefully for signs of impending respiratory depression.
- Elevated BP has been reported following administration of droperidol with parenteral analgesics.
- During the postoperative period, EEG patterns are slow to return to normal.
- Extrapyramidal symptoms may occur within 24–48 h postoperatively. Observe patient carefully for early signs of acute dystonia: facial grimacing, restlessness, tremors, torticollis, oculogyric crisis. Report promptly.
- Droperidol may aggravate symptoms of acute depression.

DYCLONINE HYDROCHLORIDE

(dye-kloe-neen)

Trade name: Dyclone

Classifications: CNS AGENT; ANESTHETIC, LOCAL (MUCOSAL); ANTIPRURITIC

Prototype: Procaine

Pregnancy category: C

ACTIONS/PHARMACODYNAMICS Organic ketone, synthetic local topical anesthetic agent. Unrelated to amide derivatives. Produces local anesthesia by blocking impulses at peripheral nerve endings in skin and mucous membranes.

USES Topical anesthesia of mucous membranes preparatory for endoscopic examinations and gynecologic and proctologic procedures. Also to suppress gag reflex, to relieve pain of minor burns or trauma, and to alleviate itching of pruritus ani or vulvae. **Unlabeled use:** to provide relief from discomfort of fever blisters.

ROUTE & DOSAGE

Topical Anesthesia

Adult: **Topical** Apply 0.5–1% solution by swabbing, gargling, spray, instillation, wet compress, or rinse.

Before Urologic Endoscopy

Adult: **Topical** Instill 30–60 ml of 0.5–1% solution into urethra and retain 5–10 min before procedure.

PHARMACOKINETICS Absorption: absorbed through skin and mucous membranes. **Onset:** 2–10 min. **Duration:** up to 1 h.

CONTRAINDICATIONS & PRECAUTIONS Contraindicated in: cystoscopic procedures following IV pyelography (because contrast media containing iodine may precipitate and interfere with visualization); applications to extensive areas or to bleeding surfaces. Safe use during pregnancy (category C) not established. **Cautious use in:** debilitated or elderly patients, children, patients with drug sensitivities or family history of allergies; severe trauma or sepsis in region of application.

ADVERSE/SIDE EFFECTS Skin: urticaria, edema, contact dermatitis (local): burning, tenderness, swelling, irritation, urethritis. **Systemic absorption:** nervousness, dizziness, drowsiness, excitement or depression, tremors, *seizures,* blurred vision, hypotension, bradycardia, cardiac or respiratory arrest.

DIAGNOSTIC TEST INTERFERENCE Dyclonine may interfere with visualization in cystoscopic procedures by causing precipitation of iodine in ***contrast media.***

NURSING IMPLICATIONS

Administration

- To relieve pain of esophageal lesions, 5–15 ml of 0.5% dyclonine solution may be swallowed (prescribed).
- Avoid contact with eyes or eyelids. Applications to large areas should be avoided.
- Store at 15–30C (59–86F) in tight, light-resistant container unless otherwise directed.

Assessment & Drug Effects

- When applied orally, dyclonine may interfere with second stage of swallowing. Do not give patient anything by mouth within 60 min (until return of gag reflex) following drug administration.
- If necessary, gag reflex may be tested by gently stroking soft palate with a cotton swab (while holding tongue down with a depressor). If patient does not gag or swallow, give nothing by mouth. Suctioning of secretions may be necessary to prevent aspiration.
- A sip of clear water should be the first thing swallowed when gag reflex returns.

Patient & Family Education

- If patient is to self-administer medication orally, he or she should be instructed on suppression of gag reflex and appropriate safety precautions.

DYPHYLLINE

(dye'fi-lin)

Trade names: Dilor, Dyflex, Dylline, Lufyllin, Neothylline, Protophylline♣, Thylline

Classifications: BRONCHODILATOR; RESPIRATORY SMOOTH MUSCLE RELAXANT; XANTHINE

Prototype: Theophylline

Pregnancy category: C

D

ACTIONS/PHARMACODYNAMICS Xanthine and derivative of theophylline with which it shares similar pharmacologic effects: bronchodilation, myocardial stimulation, vasodilation, diuresis, and smooth muscle relaxation. Unlike other xanthines, dyphylline is not metabolized to theophylline in body; therefore serum theophylline levels are not useful.

USES Acute bronchial asthma and reversible bronchospasm associated with chronic bronchitis and emphysema.

ROUTE & DOSAGE

Asthma

Adult: **PO** 200–800 mg q6h up to 15 mg/kg q.i.d.; **IM** 250–500 mg q6h up to 15 mg/kg q.i.d.
Child ≥6 y: **PO/IM** 4.4–6.6 mg/kg/d in divided doses.

PHARMACOKINETICS Absorption: readily absorbed from GI tract. **Peak:** 1 h. **Metabolism:** metabolized in liver (but not to theophylline). **Elimination:** half-life: 2 h; excreted in urine.

CONTRAINDICATIONS & PRECAUTIONS Contraindicated in: hypersensitivity to xanthine compounds; apnea in newborns. Safe use during pregnancy (category C) and in nursing mothers not established. **Cautious use in:** severe cardiac disease, hypertension, acute myocardial injury, renal or hepatic dysfunction, glaucoma, hyperthyroidism, peptic ulcer, in the elderly and in children; concomitant administration of other xanthine formulations or other CNS-stimulating drugs.

ADVERSE/SIDE EFFECTS CNS: headache, irritability, restlessness, dizziness, insomnia, light-headedness, muscle twitching, <u>convulsions</u>. **CV:** palpitation, *tachycardia,* extrasystoles, flushing, hypotension. **GI:** *nausea*, vomiting, diarrhea, anorexia, epigastric distress. **Respiratory:** tachypnea. **Other:** albuminuria, fever, dehydration.

DRUG INTERACTIONS BETA BLOCKERS may antagonize bronchodilating effects of dyphylline; **halothane** increases risk of cardiac arrhythmias; **probenecid** may decrease dyphylline elimination.

NURSING IMPLICATIONS

Administration

- Absorption is enhanced by taking oral preparation with a full glass of water on an empty stomach, e.g., 1 h before or 2 h after meals. However, administration after meals may help to relieve gastric discomfort.
- Care should be exercised in the amount of elixir given to children because it has a high alcohol content (18–20%).
- For IM administration, aspirate carefully before injecting and inject slowly.
- Do not use parenteral form if a precipitate is present.
- Store at 15–30C (59–86F) unless otherwise directed. Protect dyphylline injection from light.

Assessment & Drug Effects

- Baseline and periodic pulmonary function tests may be done to assess therapeutic effectiveness of dyphylline.
- Minimal effective therapeutic dyphylline blood level is reported to be 12 μg/ml.
- Toxic dyphylline plasma levels, although rare with normal dosage, are a risk in patients with a diminished capacity for dyphylline clearance, e.g., those with CHF or hepatic impairment or who are >55 y or <1 y of age.

Patient & Family Education

- Instruct patient to consistently take

medication with or without food at the same time each day.

- Instruct patient to notify physician of adverse effects: nausea, vomiting, insomnia, jitteriness, headache, rash, severe GI pain, restlessness, convulsions, or irregular heartbeat.
- Caution patient to avoid alcohol and also large amounts of coffee and other xanthine-containing beverages (e.g., tea, cocoa, cola) during therapy.
- Many OTC drugs for coughs, colds, and allergies contain ephedrine or other sympathomimetics and xanthines (e.g., caffeine, theophylline, aminophylline). Advise patient to consult physician before taking OTC preparations.

ECHOTHIOPHATE IODIDE

(ek-oh-thye′oh-fate)

Trade name: Phospholine Iodide

Classifications: EYE PREPARATION; MIOTIC (ANTIGLAUCOMA AGENT)

Prototype: Pilocarpine hydrochloride

Pregnancy category: C

See Appendix A.

ECONAZOLE NITRATE

(e-kone′a-zole)

Trade names: Ecostatin♣, Spectazole

Classifications: ANTIINFECTIVE; ANTIBIOTIC; ANTIFUNGAL

Prototype: Amphotericin

Pregnancy category: C

ACTIONS/PHARMACODYNAMICS Synthetic imidazole derivative with broad antifungal spectrum of activity similar to that of miconazole. Exerts fungistatic action but may be fungicidal for certain microorganisms. Active against dermatophytes (including *Trichophyton mentagrophytes, T. rubrum, T. tonsurans, Epidermophyton floccosum, Microsporum audouini, M. canis*), yeasts, e.g., *Candida albicans, Pityrosporum obiculare* (tinea versicolor), and many other genera of fungi. Also appears to be active against some gram-positive bacteria (e.g., *Staphylococcus aureus, Streptococcus pyogenes,* and *Corynebacterium diphtheriae*).

USES Topically for treatment of tinea pedis (athlete's foot or ringworm of foot), tinea cruris ("jock itch" or ringworm of groin), tinea corporis (ringworm of body), tinea versicolor, and cutaneous candidiasis (moniliasis). **Unlabeled uses:** has been used for topical treatment of erythrasma and with corticosteroids for fungal or bacterial dermatoses associated with inflammation.

ROUTE & DOSAGE

Tinea Cruris, Tinea Corporis, Tinea Pedis, Cutaneous Candidiasis

Adult/Child: **Topical** Apply sufficient amount to affected areas twice daily, morning and evening.

Tinea Versicolor

Adult: **Topical** Apply sufficient amount to affected areas once daily.

PHARMACOKINETICS Absorption: minimal percutaneous absorption through intact skin; increased absorption from denuded skin. **Peak:** 0.5–5 h. **Elimination:** < 1% of applied dose is eliminated in urine and feces.

CONTRAINDICATIONS & PRECAUTIONS Contraindicated in: safe use during pregnancy (category C) and in nursing women not established.

ADVERSE/SIDE EFFECTS Burning, stinging sensation, pruritus, erythema.

NURSING IMPLICATIONS

Administration

- Cleanse skin with soap and water and dry thoroughly before applying medication (unless otherwise directed by physician). Wash hands thoroughly before and after treatments.
- Do not use occlusive dressings unless prescribed by physician.
- Store at temperature less than 30C (86F) unless otherwise directed.

Patient & Family Education

- Instruct patient to use medication for the prescribed time even if symptoms improve and to report to physician skin reactions suggestive of irritation or sensitization.
- Clinical improvement should occur within the first 1 or 2 wk of therapy. Advise patient to notify physician if full course of therapy does not result in improvement. Diagnosis should be reevaluated.
- Caution patient not to apply the topical cream in or near the eyes or intravaginally.

EDETATE CALCIUM DISODIUM

(ed′e-tate)

Trade names: Calcium Disodium Versenate, Calcium EDTA

Classification: CHELATING AGENT

Pregnancy category: C

ACTIONS/PHARMACODYNAMICS Chelating agent that combines with divalent and trivalent metals to form stable, nonionizing soluble complexes that can be readily excreted by kidneys. Action is dependent on ability of heavy metal to displace the less strongly bound calcium in the drug molecule.

USES Principally as adjunct in treatment of acute and chronic lead poisoning (plumbism). Generally used in combination with dimercaprol (BAL) in treatment of lead encephalopathy or when blood lead level exceeds 100 µg/dl. Also used to diagnose suspected lead poisoning. **Unlabeled uses:** treatment of poisoning from other heavy metals such as chromium, manganese, nickel, zinc, and possibly vanadium; removal of radioactive and nuclear fission products such as plutonium, yttrium, uranium. Not effective in poisoning from arsenic, gold, or mercury.

ROUTE & DOSAGE

Diagnosis of Lead Poisoning

Adult: **IM/IV** 500 mg/m^2 (max 1 g) over 1 h; then collect urine for 24 h; if µg lead:mg EDTA ratio in urine is > 1, the test is positive. *Child:* **IM** 50 mg/kg (max 1 g); then collect urine for 6–8 h; if µg lead:mg EDTA ratio in urine is > 0.5, the test is positive.

Treatment of Lead Poisoning

Adult: **IV** 1–1.5 g/m^2 in 250–500 ml D5W or NS over 1 h q12h for up to 5 d; if patient is symptomatic, infuse over 2 h; may give the second dose 6 h after the first dose; then q12h. *Child:* **IM/IV** 35 mg/kg b.i.d. (not to exceed 50 mg/kg/d in mild cases) for 3–5 d.

PHARMACOKINETICS **Absorption:** well absorbed IM. **Onset:** 1 h. **Peak:** peak chelation 24–48 h. **Distribution:** distributed to extracellular fluid; does not enter CSF. **Metabolism:** not metabolized. **Elimination:** half-life: 20–60 min IV, 90 min IM; chelated lead excreted in urine; 50% excreted in 1 h.

CONTRAINDICATIONS & PRECAUTIONS **Contraindicated in:** severe renal disease, anuria; IV use in patients with lead encephalopathy not generally recommended (because of possible increase in intracranial pressure); during pregnancy (category C). **Cautious use in:** renal dysfunction; active tubercular lesions; history of gout.

ADVERSE/SIDE EFFECTS **CV:** hypotension, thrombophlebitis. **GI:** anorexia, nausea, vomiting, diarrhea, abdominal cramps, cheilosis. **Hematologic:** transient bone marrow depression, depletion of blood metals. **Renal:** <u>nephrotoxicity</u> (renal tubular necrosis), proteinuria, hematuria. **Other:** ***Febrile reaction:*** excessive thirst, fever, chills, severe myalgia, arthralgia, GI distress, and accompanied by ***histamine-like reactions:*** flushing, throbbing headache, sweating, sneezing, nasal congestion, lacrimation, postural hypotension, tachycardia.

DIAGNOSTIC TEST INTERFERENCE Edetate calcium disodium may decrease ***serum cholesterol, plasma lipid*** levels (if elevated), and ***serum potassium*** values. ***Glycosuria*** may occur with toxic doses.

DRUG INTERACTIONS None established.

INCOMPATABILITIES **Solution/additive: amphotericin B, hydralazine.**

NURSING IMPLICATIONS

Administration

- The IM route is preferred for symptomatic children and is recommended for patients with incipient or overt lead-induced encephalopathy.
- Procaine hydrochloride should be added to minimize pain at IM injection site (usually 1 ml of procaine 1% to each 1 ml of concentrated drug). Consult physician.
- When dimercaprol (BAL) and Calcium EDTA are given concurrently, each should be injected into separate IM sites.
- For IV administration, dilute the 5 ml ampule with 250–500 ml of NS or D5W.
- Warning: Rapid IV infusion may be lethal by suddenly increasing intracranial pressure in patients who already have cerebral edema.
- Calcium disodium edetate can produce potentially fatal effects when higher than recommended doses are used or when it is continued after toxic effects appear.

Assessment & Drug Effects

- Adequacy of urinary output must be determined before therapy is initiated. This may be done by administering IV fluids before giving first dose.
- Fluid intake is generally increased to enhance urinary excretion of chelates. Excess fluid intake, however, should be avoided in patients with lead encephalopathy because of the danger of further increasing intracranial pressure. Consult physician regarding allowable intake.
- Monitor I&O. Since drug is excreted almost exclusively via kidneys, toxicity may develop if output is inadequate. Therapy should be stopped if urine flow is markedly diminished or absent. Report any change in output or I&O ratio to physician.
- Serum creatinine, calcium, and phosphorus determinations should be done before and during each course of therapy.
- Baseline and frequent determinations of BUN and ECG should be monitored during therapy.

- Patients on prolonged therapy should have periodic determinations of blood trace element metals (e.g., copper, zinc, magnesium).
- Be alert for occurrence of febrile reaction that may appear 4–8 h after drug infusion (see Adverse/Side Effects).

E

EDETATE DISODIUM

(ed′e-tate)

Trade names: Disotate, Disodium EDTA, Endrate

Classifications: CHELATING AGENT; REGULATOR, SERUM CALCIUM

Pregnancy category: C

ACTIONS/PHARMACODYNAMICS Structurally distinct from edetate calcium disodium. Forms chelates with many bivalent and trivalent metals, e.g., magnesium, zinc, and other trace metals, but has particular affinity for calcium. Forms a stable, nonionizing soluble complex that can be readily excreted via kidneys. Does not chelate potassium but promotes its urinary excretion and may reduce serum potassium levels.

USES In selected patients for emergency treatment of hypercalcemia and to control ventricular arrhythmias and heart block associated with digitalis toxicity when other drugs, e.g., phenytoin and potassium are contraindicated or ineffective. **Unlabeled use:** in ophthalmology to remove corneal calcium deposits (topically or by iontophoresis).

ROUTE & DOSAGE

Hypercalcemia

Adult: **IV** 50 mg/kg/d (up to 3 g/d) diluted in 500 ml of D5W or NS and infused over 3–4 h.
Child: **IV** 40 mg/kg/d (up to 70 mg/kg/d) diluted to at least 30 mg/ml in D5W or NS and infused over 3–4 h.

Digitalis-induced Ventricular Arrhythmia

Adult: **IV** 15 mg/kg/h up to 60 mg/kg/d by IV infusion in D5W.
Child: **IV** Same as for adult.

PHARMACOKINETICS **Metabolism:** not metabolized. **Elimination:** approximately 95% of dose excreted renally as calcium chelate.

CONTRAINDICATIONS & PRECAUTIONS **Contraindicated in:** significant renal disease, anuria, hypocalcemia, history of seizure disorders or intracranial lesions, active or healed calcified tubercular lesions, generalized arteriosclerosis associated with advancing age, coronary or peripheral vascular disease. Safe use during pregnancy (category C) not established. **Cautious use in:** limited cardiac reserve, incipient CHF, potassium deficiency states.

ADVERSE/SIDE EFFECTS **CNS:** transient numbness, circumoral paresthesias, muscle cramps, muscle weakness, back pain, lassitude, malaise, headache, fatigue, convulsions. **CV:** hypotension, hypertension, arrhythmias, thrombophlebitis. **GI:** *nausea, vomiting, anorexia, diarrhea, abdominal cramps.* **Renal:** (with excessive dosage): nephrotoxicity: urgency, dysuria, nocturia, oliguria, polyuria, proteinuria, tubular necrosis. **Skin:** exfoliative dermatitis and other skin and mucous membrane lesions resembling those of pyridoxine (vitamin B_6) deficiency. **Other:** fever, chills, anemia, glycosuria, hyperuricemia, severe hypocalcemia (rapid IV or high dosages), tetany, hypomagnesemia (prolonged therapy), calcium embolization, damage to reticuloendothelial system with hemorrhagic tendencies (excessive dosage). ***Local reactions:*** pain, *erythema, dermatitis at infusion site.*

DIAGNOSTIC TEST INTERFERENCE Colorimetric method of determining ***serum calcium*** levels will not be accurate; oxalate method may yield artificially low serum calcium values. Greater accuracy may be possible by performing test immediately before dose due is administered or by acidifying the sample (atomic absorption spectrometry reportedly not affected). ***Serum alkaline phosphatase*** may be decreased (thought to be induced by low ***serum magnesium*** levels).

DRUG INTERACTIONS Edetate disodium may lower blood glucose levels and thus reduce **insulin** requirements in (IDDM) diabetic patients; reaction is thought to be due to chelation of the zinc in insulin preparations.

NURSING IMPLICATIONS

Administration

- The commercially available injection must be diluted before administration. Drug is extremely irritating to tissue and therefore should be well diluted before infusion.
- Dilute a single dose in 500 ml of D5W or NS and infuse over 3 or more hours.
- Monitor IV infusion rate as prescribed by physician. Rapid IV infusion (or high serum drug levels) can produce hypocalcemic tetany, cardiac arrhythmias, seizures, and cardiac arrest.
- Extravasation must be prevented.

Assessment & Drug Effects

- Serum calcium levels should be determined after each administration. Observe for and report immediately early signs and symptoms of hypocalcemia (see Appendix G).
- Cardiac function should be monitored, particularly in patients with arrhythmias and those with history of seizure disorders or intracranial lesions.
- Determine BP and HR before patient ambulates. Be alert to the possibility of postural hypotension.
- Monitor and report any significant change in I&O ratio to physician.
- Urinalyses should be done daily throughout therapy, and renal function studies (BUN, serum creatinine) should be performed prior to initiation of therapy, every 48 h during therapy, and 48 h after therapy is discontinued. Nephrotoxicity is usually reversible if drug is stopped promptly at the first appearance of symptoms.
- Insulin-dependent diabetic (IDDM) patients may require reduction of insulin dosage while receiving edetate disodium therapy (see section on Drug Interactions).

Patient & Family Education

- Advise patient to remain in bed for about 20 to 30 min after infusion because of the possibility of postural hypotension.

EDROPHONIUM CHLORIDE

(ed-roe-foe′nee-um)

Trade names: Enlon, Reversol, Tensilon

Classifications: AUTONOMIC NERVOUS SYSTEM AGENT; CHOLINERGIC (PARASYMPATHOMIMETIC) CHOLINESTERASE INHIBITOR

Prototype: Neostigmine

Pregnancy category: C

ACTIONS/PHARMACODYNAMICS Rapidly reversible indirect-acting cholinesterase inhibitor similar to neostigmine. Acts as antidote to curariform drugs by displacing them from muscle cell receptor sites, thus permitting resumption of normal transmission of neuromuscular impulses. However, like neostigmine, it prolongs skeletal muscle relaxant action of succinylcholine chloride and decamethonium bromide.

E

USES Differential diagnosis and as adjunct in evaluation of treatment requirements of myasthenia gravis, for differentiating myasthenic from cholinergic crisis, and to reverse neuromuscular blockade produced by overdosage of nondepolarizing skeletal muscle relaxants, e.g., tubocurarine, gallamine. Not recommended for maintenance therapy in myasthenia gravis because of its short duration of action. **Unlabeled uses:** to terminate paroxysmal atrial tachycardia, as an aid in diagnosing supraventricular tachyarrhythmias, and to evaluate function of demand pacemakers.

ROUTE & DOSAGE

Edrophonium Test for Myasthenia Gravis

Adult: **IV** Prepare 10 mg in a syringe; inject 2 mg over 15–30 s; if no reaction after 45 s, inject the remaining 8 mg; may repeat test after 30 min. **IM** Inject 10 mg; if cholinergic reaction occurs, retest after 30 min with 2 mg to rule out false-negative reaction.
Child: **IV** ≤ 34 kg, 1 mg; if no response after 45 s, dose may be titrated up to 5 mg; **IM** 2 mg; **IV** > 34 kg, 2 mg; if no response after 45 s, dose may be titrated up to 10 mg; **IM** 5 mg.
Infants: 0.5–1 mg IM.

Evaluation of Myasthenia Treatment

Adult: **IV** 1–2 mg administered 1 h after last PO dose of anticholinesterase medication.

Curare Antagonist

Adult: **IV** 10 mg administered over 30–45 s; may repeat q5–10min as needed up to 40 mg.

PHARMACOKINETICS **Onset:** 30–60 s IV; 2–10 min IM. **Duration:** 5–10 min IV; 5–30 min IM.

CONTRAINDICATIONS & PRECAUTIONS **Contraindicated in:** hypersensitivity to anticholinesterase agents; intestinal and urinary obstruction. Safe use during pregnancy (category C) and in nursing mothers not established. **Cautious use in:** bronchial asthma; cardiac arrhythmias; patients receiving digitalis.

ADVERSE/SIDE EFFECTS Severe side effects uncommon with usual doses. **CNS:** weakness, muscle cramps, dysphoria, fasciculations, incoordination, dysarthria, dysphagia, convulsions, respiratory paralysis. **CV:** bradycardia, irregular pulse, hypotension, pulmonary edema. **Eye:** miosis, blurred vision, diplopia, lacrimation. **GI:** diarrhea, abdominal cramps, nausea, vomiting, excessive salivation. **Respiratory:** increased bronchial secretions, bronchospasm, laryngospasm, pulmonary edema. **Other:** excessive sweating, urinary frequency, incontinence.

DRUG INTERACTIONS **Procainamide, quinidine** may antagonize the effects of edrophonium; DIGITALIS GLYCOSIDES increase the sensitivity of the heart to edrophonium; **succinylcholine, decamethonium** may prolong neuromuscular blockade.

NURSING IMPLICATIONS

Administration

- Edrophonium usually is administered by a physician.

- Some clinicians recommend giving a 1–2 mg test dose of edrophonium to elderly patients, to those with history of heart disease or who take digitalis, and possibly to all patients.
- Antidote (atropine sulfate) and facilities for endotracheal intubation, tracheostomy, suction, assisted respiration, and cardiac monitoring should be immediately available for treatment of cholinergic reaction.

Assessment & Drug Effects

- Monitor vital signs. Observe for signs of respiratory distress. Patients > 50 y are particularly likely to develop bradycardia, hypotension, and cardiac arrest.
- Edrophonium test for myasthenia gravis: all cholinesterase inhibitors (anticholinesterases) should be discontinued for at least 8 h before test. Positive response to edrophonium test consists of brief improvement in muscle strength unaccompanied by lingual or skeletal muscle fasciculations.
- Evaluation of myasthenic treatment: *Myasthenic response:* immediate subjective improvement with increased muscle strength, absence of fasciculations; generally indicates that patient requires larger dose of anticholinesterase agent or longer-acting drug. *Cholinergic response* (muscarinic side effects): lacrimation, diaphoresis, salivation, abdominal cramps, diarrhea, nausea, vomiting; accompanied by decrease in muscle strength; usually indicates overtreatment with cholinesterase inhibitor. *Adequate response:* no change in muscle strength; fasciculations may be present or absent; minimal cholinergic side effects (observed in patients at or near optimal dosage level).

EFAVIRENZ

(e-fa′vi-renz)

Trade name: Sustiva

Classifications: ANTIINFECTIVE; ANTIVIRAL; NONNUCLEOSIDE REVERSE TRANSCRIPTASE INHIBITOR

Prototype: Nevirapine

Pregnancy category: C

ACTIONS/PHARMACODYNAMICS

Nonnucleoside reverse transcriptase inhibitor (NNRTI) of HIV-1. Binds directly to reverse trascriptase and blocks RNA polymerase activities; thus it prevents replication of the HIV-1 virus. HIV-2 reverse transcriptase and DNA polymerases alpha, beta, gamma, and delta are not inhibited by efavirenz. Resistant strains appear rapidly.

USE HIV-1 infection in combination with other antiretroviral agents.

ROUTE & DOSAGE

HIV Infection

Adult: **PO** 600 mg q.d.
Child ≥3 y: **PO** *10–15 kg:* 200 mg q.d.; *15–20 kg:* 250 mg q.d.; *20–25 kg:* 300 mg q.d.; *25–32.5 kg:* 350 mg q.d.; *32.5–40 kg:* 400 mg q.d.; *≥40 kg:* 600 mg q.d.

PHARMACOKINETICS **Peak:** 5 h; steady-state 6–10 d. **Distribution:** 99% protein bound. **Metabolism:** metabolized in liver by cytochrome P450 3A4 and 2B6; can induce (increase) its own metabolism. **Elimination:** half-life: 52–76 h after single dose, 40–55 h after multiple doses; 14–34% excreted in urine, 16–61% excreted in feces.

CONTRAINDICATIONS & PRECAUTIONS **Contraindicated in:** hypersensitivity to efavirenz, pregnancy (category C), lactation. **Cautious use in:** liver disease, CNS disorders. Safety and efficacy in children <3 y old or who weigh <13 kg (29 lb) is not known.

E

ADVERSE/SIDE EFFECTS **Body as whole:** fatigue, fever. **CNS:** dizziness, headache, hypoesthesia, impaired concentration, insomnia, abnormal dreams, somnolence, depression, nervousness. **CV:** hypercholesterolemia. **GI:** *nausea,* vomiting, *diarrhea,* dyspepsia, abdominal pain, flatulence, anorexia, increased liver function tests (ALT, AST). **Respiratory:** cough. **Skin:** *rash* (erythematous rash, pruritus, *maculopapular rash,* erythema multiforme. Stevens–Johnson syndrome, toxic epidermal necrolysis), increased sweating. **Other:** renal calculus, hematuria.

DRUG INTERACTIONS Decreased concentrations of **clarithromycin, indinavir, nelfinavir, saquinavir;** increased concentrations of **ritonavir, azithromycin, ethinyl estradiol.** Efavirenz levels are increased by **ritonavir, fluconazole** and decreased by **saquinavir, rifampin.** Additional drugs not recommended for administration with efavirenz include **astemizole, midazolam, triazolam, cisapride,** ERGOT DERIVATIVES, **warfarin.**

DIAGNOSTIC TEST INTERFERENCE False-positive urine tests for marijuana.

NURSING IMPLICATIONS

Administration

- Bedtime dosing is recommended to increase tolerability of CNS adverse effects.
- Efavirenz should not be taken following a high fat meal.
- Store at 15–30C (59–86F) in a tightly closed container and protect from light.

Assessment & Drug Effects

- Therapeutic effectiveness is indicated by reduction in viral load (plasma HIV RNA).
- Lab tests: Periodically monitor liver functions and lipid profile.

Patient & Family Education

- Take exactly as ordered. Do not skip a dose or discontinue therapy without consulting the physician.
- Contact physician promptly if any of the following occur: skin rash, delusions, inappropriate behavior, thoughts of suicide.
- Women should use barrier contraception as well as oral/hormonal contraception.
- Women who become pregnant should immediately notify the physician.
- Avoid engaging in hazardous activities until reaction to the drug is known. Dizziness, impaired concentration, and drowsiness usually improve with continued therapy.

EMEDASTINE DIFUMARATE

(em-e-das′teen di-foom′a-rate)

Trade name: Emadine

Classifications: ANTIHISTAMINE; H_1-RECEPTOR ANTAGONIST

Prototype: Diphenhydramine

Pregnancy category: C

See Appendix A.

EMETINE HYDROCHLORIDE

(em′e-teen)

Classifications: ANTIINFECTIVE; AMEBICIDE

Pregnancy category: X

ACTIONS/PHARMACODYNAMICS Natural or synthetic alkaloid of ipecac with direct lethal action on *Entamoeba histolytica* in tissues. More effective against motile forms (trophozoites) than cysts. Causes degeneration of nucleus and cytoplasm of amebae and eradicates parasites, possibly by interfering with multiplication of trophozoites. Also has adrenergic and neuromuscular blocking activities and expectorant, diaphoretic, and emetic actions but is not used clinically for these effects.

USES In combination with other amebicides in management of acute fulminating amebic dysentery (intestinal amebiasis) or for acute exacerbations of chronic amebic dysentery. Highly effective in treatment of extraintestinal amebiasis (amebic abscess, amebic hepatitis). **Unlabeled uses:** irrigation solution (emetine in NaCl injection) used at site of amebic abscess (after pus aspiration); malaria (caused by *Plasmodium falciparum*).

ROUTE & DOSAGE

Amebic Dysentery

Adult: **IM/Deep SC** 1 mg/kg b.i.d. (morning & evening) for 3–10 d (max 65 mg/kg or 650 mg in 10 d).
Child: **IM/Deep SC** <*8 y,* 1 mg/kg b.i.d. for 4;pl d (max 10 mg/d); >*8 y,* 1 mg/kg b.i.d. for 4+ d (max 20 mg/d).

Hepatic Amebiasis or Abscess

Adult: **IM/Deep SC** 1 mg/kg b.i.d. (morning & evening) for up to 10 d (max 65 mg/kg or 650 mg in 10 d); do not repeat in <6 wk.

PHARMACOKINETICS Absorption: erratic oral absorption; therefore is given IM. **Distribution:** highest concentrations in lung, kidney, and spleen. **Elimination:** appears in urine 20–40 min after injection; still present in urine 40–60 d after discontinued.

CONTRAINDICATIONS & PRECAUTIONS Contraindicated in: patients who have received a course of emetine 6–8 wk previously; treatment of mild symptoms or carriers of amebiasis; heart or kidney disease; pregnancy (category X); children except those with severe dysentery not controlled by other amebicides. Safe use in nursing mothers not established. **Cautious use in:** debilitated or elderly patients; hypotension; patients about to have surgery.

ADVERSE/SIDE EFFECTS CNS (overdose): skeletal muscle weakness, tenderness, stiffness, pain; tremors, peripheral neuropathy. **CV (cardiotoxicity):** hypotension, tachycardia, arrhythmias, myocarditis, *pericarditis,* <u>precordial pain,</u> dyspnea, ECG abnormalities, gallop rhythm, cardiac dilatation, CHF. **GI:** *diarrhea;* abdominal cramps; *nausea and vomiting associated with dizziness, faintness, headache,* epigastric burning and pain. **Other:** large doses: <u>acute lesions in heart,</u> *liver,* kidney, intestinal tract, skeletal muscle; *injection site reactions (frequent):* aching, tenderness, and local muscle weakness; eczematous, urticarial, or purpuric lesions; necrosis, cellulitis, abscess.

DRUG INTERACTIONS Not established.

NURSING IMPLICATIONS

Administration

- Emetine is administered by deep SC or IM injection. Aspirate carefully after needle is introduced. *IV injection is dangerous and is specifically contraindicated.*
- Emetine is very irritating to tissues. Wash hands thoroughly after handling drug.
- Protect drug from light.

Assessment & Drug Effects

- Make a record of injection sites and observe these sites daily. Muscle ache and tenderness at area of injection occur frequently.
- Emetine is potentially toxic to the heart. An ECG should be taken before emetine is initiated, as well as after the fifth dose, on completion of therapy, and 1 wk later. ECG changes usually appear about 7 d after drug is administered. Report their appearance immediately.
- Pulse (rate and quality) and BP should be recorded at least 3 times daily. Tachycardia frequently precedes appearance of ECG abnormalities.
- Withhold drug and report to physician if any of the following occur: tachycardia, a precipitous fall in BP, marked weakness or other neuromuscular symptoms, and severe GI effects.
- Monitor I&O. Report oliguria or change in I&O ratio.
- Record number, unusual odor, and consistency of stools. Suspect emetine-induced reaction if stools increase in number following improvement of diarrhea.

Patient & Family Education

- Advise patients to remain sedentary and to restrict activity for several weeks after completion of drug therapy to prevent development of tachycardia.
- Advise patients to immediately report weakness, fatigue, listlessness, muscle stiffness, tenderness, or pain or other distressing reactions.

EMLA (EUTECTIC MIXTURE OF LIDOCAINE AND PRILOCAINE)

Trade name: EMLA cream

Classifications: CNS AGENT; LOCAL ANESTHETIC

Prototype: Procaine

Pregnancy category: B

ACTIONS/PHARMACODYNAMICS EMLA cream is a mixture of lidocaine and prilocaine. The mixture forms a liquid at room temperature. Concentration of anesthetic in liquid versus an emulsifier is 80% versus 20%. EMLA is a topical analgesic.

USE Topical anesthetic on normal intact skin for local anesthesia. **Unlabeled uses:** topical anesthetic prior to leg ulcer debridement; treatment of postherpetic neuralgia.

ROUTE & DOSAGE

Topical Anesthetic

Adult: **Topical** Apply 2.5 g of cream (1/2 of 5-g tube) over 20–25 cm^2 of skin. Cover with occlusive dressing and wait at least 1 h. Then remove dressing and wipe off cream. Cleanse area with an antiseptic solution and prepare patient for the procedure.

Child >1 mo: **Topical** Same as adult.

PHARMACOKINETICS Absorption: penetrates intact skin. **Onset:** 15–60 min. **Peak:** 2–3 h. **Duration:** 1–2 h after removal of cream. **Distribution:** crosses blood–brain barrier and placenta, distributed into breast milk. **Metabolism:** metabolized in liver. **Elimination:** half-life: 60–150 min; 98% of absorbed dose is excreted in urine.

CONTRAINDICATIONS & PRECAUTIONS Contraindicated in: patients with known sensitivity to local anesthetics, patients with congenital or idiopathy methemoglobinemia. **Cautious use in:** acutely ill, debilitated, or elderly patients; severe hepatic disease, pregnancy (category B), and nursing mothers; children under 7 years of age.

ADVERSE/SIDE EFFECTS **Hematologic:** methemoglobinemia, especially in infants, small children, and patients with G6PD deficiency. **Skin:** *blanching and redness,* itching, heat sensation. **Other:** edema, soreness, aching, numbness, heaviness. The adverse effects of lidocaine could occur with large doses or if there is significant systemic absorption.

NURSING IMPLICATIONS

Administration

- Apply a thick layer to skin (approximately 1/2 of 5-g tube per 20–25 cm^2 or 2 × 2 in) at site of procedure. Apply an occlusive dressing. Do not spread out cream. Seal edges of dressing well to avoid leakage.
- Apply EMLA cream 1 h before routine procedure and 2 h before painful procedure.
- Prior to skin puncture, remove EMLA cream and clean area with an aseptic solution.
- Store at room temperature (15–30C/59–86F).

Assessment & Drug Effects

- Monitor for local skin reactions including erythema, edema, itching, abnormal temperature sensations, and rash. These reactions are very common and usually disappear in 1–2 h.
- Note that persons taking Class 1 antiarrhythmic drugs may experience toxic effects on the cardiovascular system. EMLA should be used with caution in these patients.
- If contact with the eye occurs, wash immediately with water or saline; protect the eye until sensation returns.

Patient & Family Education

- Inform patient that analgesia may be accompanied by temporary loss of all sensation in the treated skin. Advise caution until sensation returns.
- Inform patient that skin analgesia lasts for 1 h following removal of the occlusive dressing.

ENALAPRIL MALEATE

(e-nal′a-pril)

Trade name: Vasotec

ENALAPRILAT

Trade name: Vasotec I.V.

Classifications: CARDIOVASCULAR AGENT; ANGIOTENSIN-CONVERTING ENZYME (ACE) INHIBITOR; ANTIHYPERTENSIVE

Prototype: Captopril

Pregnancy category: D

ACTIONS/PHARMACODYNAMICS Vasotec is an angiotensin-converting enzyme (ACE) inhibitor. ACE catalyzes the conversion of angiotensin I to angiotensin II, a vasoconstrictor substance. Therefore, inhibition of ACE decreases angiotensin II levels, which decreases vasopressor activity and aldosterone secretion. Both actions achieve an antihypertensive effect by suppression of the renin–angiotensin–aldosterone system. ACE inhibitors also reduce peripheral arterial resistance (afterload), pulmonary capillary wedge pressure (PCWP), a measure of preload, and pulmonary vascular resistance and improve cardiac output as well as exercise tolerance.

USES Management of mild to moderate hypertension as monotherapy or with a diuretic. Malignant, refractory, accelerated, and renovascular hypertension (except in bilateral renal artery stenosis or renal artery stenosis in a solitary kidney), CHF. **Unlabeled use:** hypertension or renal crisis in scleroderma.

E

ROUTE & DOSAGE

Hypertension

Adult: **PO** 5 mg/d; may increase to 10–40 mg/d in 1–2 divided doses; **IV** 1.25 q6h; may give up to 5 mg q6h in hypertensive emergencies.
Neonate: **PO** 0.1 mg/kg q24h. **IV** 5–10 μg/kg q8–24h.
Child: **PO** 0.1 mg/kg/d in 1–2 divided doses, may increase to max of 0.5 mg/kg/d. **IV** 5–10 μg/kg q8–24h.

Congestive Heart Failure

Adult: **PO** 2.5 mg 1–2 times/d; may increase up to 5–20 mg/d in 1–2 divided doses (max 40 mg/d).

PHARMACOKINETICS **Absorption:** 70% absorbed from GI tract. **Onset:** 1 h PO; 15 min IV. **Peak:** 4–8 h PO; 4 h IV. **Duration:** 12–24 h PO; 6 h IV. **Distribution:** limited amount crosses blood–brain barrier; crosses placenta. **Metabolism:** oral dose undergoes first-pass metabolism in liver to active form, enalaprilat. **Elimination:** half-life: 2 h; 60% excreted in urine, 33% in feces within 24 h.

CONTRAINDICATIONS & PRECAUTIONS **Contraindicated in:** hypersensitivity to enalapril or captopril. There has been evidence of fetotoxicity and renal damage in newborns exposed to ACE inhibitors during pregnancy (category D). Safety in nursing mothers and in children not established. **Cautious use in:** renal impairment, renal-artery stenosis; patients with hypovolemia, receiving diuretics, undergoing dialysis; patients in whom excessive hypotension would present a hazard (e.g., cerebrovascular insufficiency); CHF; hepatic impairment; diabetes mellitus.

ADVERSE/SIDE EFFECTS **CNS:** *headache, dizziness,* fatigue, nervousness, paresthesias, asthenia, insomnia, somnolence. **CV:** *hypotension including postural hypotension;* syncope, palpitations, chest pain. **GI:** diarrhea, nausea, abdominal pain, loss of taste, dyspepsia. **Hematologic:** decreased Hgb and Hct. **Renal:** (patient with CHF): <u>acute renal failure</u>, deterioration in renal function. **Skin:** pruritus with and without *rash,* angioedema, erythema. **Other:** hyperkalemia, cough.

DRUG INTERACTIONS **Indomethacin** and other NSAIDS may decrease antihypertensive activity; POTASSIUM SUPPLEMENTS, POTASSIUM-SPARING DIURETICS may cause hyperkalemia; may increase **lithium** levels and toxicity.

NURSING IMPLICATIONS

Administration

- If possible, diuretics should be discontinued for 2–3 d prior to initial PO dose to reduce incidence of hypotension. If the diuretic cannot be discontinued, an initial dose of 2.5 mg is given PO. Keep patient under medical supervision for at least 2 h and until BP has stabilized for at least an additional hour.
- Oral enalapril may be administered with food or drink of patient's choice.
- IV administration: 1.25 mg/ml of enalaprilat is administered slowly IV over at least 5 min through a port of a free flowing infusion of D5W or NS. It may be used as provided or diluted with up to 50 ml

of a compatible diluent (i.e., D5W, NS) as indicated.

- IV administration to neonates, infants, children: Verify correct IV concentration and rate of infusion/injection with physician.
- For conversion from IV to oral therapy the recommended initial dose is 5 mg once a day with a creatinine clearance of (Cl_{cr}) >30 ml/min, and 2.5 mg once daily with a Cl_{cr} <30 ml/min.
- Store tablets at <30C (86F); protect from heat and light. Expiration date: 30 mo following date of manufacture if stored at <30C.

Assessment & Drug Effects

- The peak effects after the first IV dose may not occur for up to 4 h. The peak effects of subsequent doses may exceed those of the first.
- First-dose phenomenon (i.e., a sudden exaggerated hypotensive response) may occur within 1–3 h of first IV dose, especially in the patient with very high blood pressure or one on a diuretic and controlled salt intake regimen. An IV infusion of normal saline for volume expansion may be ordered to counteract the hypotensive response. (This initial response is not an indicator to stop therapy.)
- Bedrest and BP monitoring are advised for the first 3 h after the initial IV dose.
- Monitor BP for first several days of therapy. If antihypertensive effect is diminished before 24 h, the total dose may be given as 2 divided doses.
- Transient hypotension with lightheadedness should be reported to physician. The elderly are particularly sensitive to drug-induced hypotension. Until BP has stabilized, patient should be cautious about ambulation and should not engage in hazardous activities including driving a car.
- Patients who have diabetes, impaired renal function, or CHF are at risk of developing hyperkalemia during enalapril treatment. Monitor serum potassium and be alert to symptoms of hyperkalemia (K^+ > 5.7 mEq/L).
- Renal function should be monitored closely during first few weeks of therapy. Advise patient to be aware of I&O ratio and pattern and to report significant changes (e.g., hematuria, dysuria) to physician.

Patient & Family Education

- The full antihypertensive effect may not be experienced until several weeks after enalapril therapy starts.
- If drug has to be discontinued because of syncope or severe hypotension, patient should be informed that the hypotensive effect may persist a week or longer after termination of therapy because of long duration of drug action.
- Advise against a self-selected low-sodium diet (e.g., low-sodium foods or low-sodium milk) without approval from physician.
- Because of the potential for hyperkalemia, patient should avoid use of a salt substitute (principal ingredient: potassium salt) and potassium supplements.
- A persistent nonproductive cough, especially at night, may be a disturbing side effect. This problem sometimes accompanied by nasal congestion should not be tolerated. Advise patient to report symptoms to physician. Enalapril may be discontinued.
- Angioedema is a rare side effect and, if accompanied by laryngeal edema, may be fatal. Advise patient to report to physician promptly if swelling of face, eyelids, tongue, lips, or extremities occurs.

E

ENOXACIN

(e-nox'a-sin)

Trade name: Penetrex

Classifications: ANTIINFECTIVE; QUINOLONE

Prototype: Ciprofloxacin

Pregnancy category: X

ACTIONS/PHARMACODYNAMICS Synthetic quinolone broad-spectrum antibiotic that inhibits DNA-gyrase, an enzyme necessary for bacterial DNA replication and some aspects of transcription, repair, recombination, and transposition. Effective against *Neisseria gonorrhoeae, Escherichia coli, Staphylococcus epidermidis, Staphylococcus saprophyticus, Klebsiella pneumoniae, Proteus mirabilis, Pseudomonas aeruginosa,* and *Enterobacter cloacae.*

USES Uncomplicated urethral or cervical gonorrhea and uncomplicated and complicated urinary tract infections due to susceptible organisms. **Unlabeled uses:** ear, nose, and throat infections, lower respiratory tract infections, and skin infections.

ROUTE & DOSAGE

Urinary Tract Infections*

Adult: **PO** 200–400 mg q12h for 7–14 d.

Uncomplicated Gonorrhea*

Adult: **PO** 400 mg single dose.

*Reduce dose by 50% in patients with creatinine clearance ≤ 30 ml/min.

PHARMACOKINETICS Absorption: readily absorbed from GI tract; 90% of dose reaches systemic circulation. **Peak:** serum, 1–2 h; urine, 2.5–7 h. **Distribution:** widely distributed including blister fluid, middle ear fluid, and prostatic tissue; crosses placenta; distributed into breast milk. **Metabolism:** 15–20% of dose metabolized in liver. **Elimination:** half-life: 3–6 h; 26–72% excreted in urine within 72 h.

CONTRAINDICATIONS & PRECAUTIONS Contraindicated in: known hypersensitvity to enoxacin, ciprofloxacin, or other quinolones, pregnant women (category X), nursing mothers, and children. **Cautious use in:** severe renal impairment and known or suspected CNS disorders.

ADVERSE/SIDE EFFECTS CNS: headache, hallucinations, seizures. **GI:** nausea, vomiting, gastric pain. **Other:** rash, photosensitivity.

DRUG INTERACTIONS Ranitidine may decrease enoxacin levels by 40% when given 2 h before enoxacin. Enoxocin decreases **theophylline** clearance by at least 50%, thus inceasing theophylline levels and toxicity. ALUMINUM- AND MAGNESIUM-CONTAINING ANTACIDS may decrease the absorption of enoxacin.

NURSING IMPLICATIONS

Administration

- Enoxacin should be taken 1 h before or 2 h after meals.
- While taking enoxacin, the patient should be well hydrated.
- For patients with renal impairment, dose is lowered according to creatinine clearance.

Assessment & Drug Effects

- Culture and sensitivity tests should be done before initial dose is given. Treatment may be implemented pending results.
- Hypersensitivity reaction, including skin rash or other allergic response, may occur after just one dose. Discontinue the drug immediately and notify physician.
- With concurrent digoxin adminis-

tration, monitor for increased digoxin level and possible toxicity.
- Carefully monitor patients with seizure disorders, since enoxacin may lower the seizure threshold.

Patient Education
- Instruct patient to promptly discontinue drug and notify the physician at the first sign of an allergic response.
- Advise patient to restrict caffeine intake since enoxacin may reduce rate of caffeine clearance, producing insomnia, nervousness, tachycardia.
- Inform patient that phototoxicity may occur with excessive exposure to sunlight.

ENOXAPARIN
(e-nox′-a-pa-rin)
Trade name: Lovenox
Classifications: BLOOD FORMER; ANTICOAGULANT
Prototype: Heparin
Pregnancy category: B
See Appendix A.

EPHEDRINE HYDROCHLORIDE
(e-fed′rin)
Trade name: Efedron

EPHEDRINE SULFATE
Trade names: Ectasule, Ephedsol, Vatronol
Classifications: AUTONOMIC NERVOUS SYSTEM AGENT; ALPHA- AND BETA-ADRENERGIC AGONIST (SYMPATHOMIMETIC); BRONCHODILATOR
Prototype: Epinephrine
Pregnancy category: C

ACTIONS/PHARMACODYNAMICS Both indirect- and direct-acting sympathomimetic amine. Thought to act indirectly by releasing tissue stores of norepinephrine and directly by stimulation of alpha-, beta$_1$-, and beta$_2$-adrenergic receptors. Like epinephrine, it contracts dilated arterioles of nasal mucosa, thus reducing engorgement and edema and facilitating ventilation and drainage. Local application to eye produces mydriasis without loss of light reflexes or accommodation or change in intraocular pressure (IOP).

USES Temporary relief of congestion of hay fever, allergic rhinitis, and sinusitis; and in treatment and prophylaxis of mild cases of acute asthma and in patients with chronic asthma requiring continuing treatment. Also has been used for its CNS stimulant actions in treatment of narcolepsy, to improve respiration in narcotic and barbiturate poisoning, to combat hypotensive states, especially those associated with spinal anesthesia; in management of enuresis or impaired bladder control; as adjunct in treatment of myasthenia gravis; as mydriatic; to relieve dysmenorrhea; and for temporary support of ventricular rate in Adams-Stokes syndrome; for peripheral edema secondary to type I diabetic neuropathy.

ROUTE & DOSAGE

Bronchodilator, Nasal Decongestant
Adult: **PO** 25–50 mg q3–4h prn (max 150 mg/24 h); **IM/IV/SC** 12.5–25 mg.
Child: **PO** >2 *y*, 2–3 mg/kg/d in 4–6 divided doses; *6–12 y*, 6.25–12.5 mg q4h (max 75 mg/24 h).

Hypotension
Adult: **PO** 25 mg 1–4 times/d

E

(max 150 mg/24 h); **IM/SC/IV** 10–50 mg IM/SC or 10–25 mg slow IV; may repeat in 5–10 min if necessary (max 150 mg/24 h). *Child:* **PO/IM/SC/IV** 3 mg/kg/d in 4–6 divided doses (max 75 mg/24 h).

Myasthenia Gravis

Adult: **PO** 25 mg t.i.d. or q.i.d.

Enuresis

Adult: **PO** 25 mg h.s.

Urinary Incontinence

Geriatric: **PO** 25–50 mg q6h.

Nasal Decongestant

Adult: **Intranasal** 2–4 drops or a small amount of jelly in each nostril no more than q.i.d. for 3–4 consecutive days.

PHARMACOKINETICS Absorption: readily absorbed from GI tract. **Peak:** 15 min–1 h. **Duration:** bronchodilation 2–4 h; cardiac & pressor effects up to 4 h PO and 1 h IV. **Distribution:** widely distributed; crosses blood–brain barrier and placenta; distributed into breast milk. **Metabolism:** small amounts metabolized in liver. **Elimination:** half-life: 3–6 h; excreted in urine.

CONTRAINDICATIONS & PRECAUTIONS Contraindicated in: history of hypersensitivity to ephedrine or other sympathomimetics; narrow-angle glaucoma. Safe use during pregnancy (category C) and in nursing women not established. **Cautious use in:** use with extreme caution if at all in hypertension, arteriosclerosis, angina pectoris, coronary insufficiency, chronic heart disease; diabetes mellitus; hyperthyroidism; prostatic hypertrophy.

ADVERSE/SIDE EFFECTS Systemic (usually with large doses): CNS: headache, insomnia, *nervousness,* anxiety, tremulousness, giddiness. **CV:** palpitation, tachycardia, precordial pain, cardiac arrhythmias. **GU:** difficult or painful urination, acute urinary retention (especially older men with prostatism). **GI:** nausea, vomiting, anorexia. **Other:** sweating, thirst, fixed-drug eruption. **Topical use:** *burning, stinging,* dryness of nasal mucosa, sneezing, rebound congestion. **Overdosage:** euphoria, confusion, delirium, convulsions, pyrexia, hypertension, rebound hypotension, respiratory difficulty.

DIAGNOSTIC TEST INTERFERENCE Ephedrine is generally withdrawn at least 12 h before ***sensitivity tests*** are made to prevent false-positive reactions.

DRUG INTERACTIONS MAO INHIBITORS, TRICYCLIC ANTIDEPRESSANTS, **furazolidine, guanethidine** may increase alpha-adrenergic effects (headache, hyperpyrexia, hypertension); **sodium bicarbonate** decreases renal elimination of ephedrine, increasing its CNS effects; **epinephrine, norepinephrine** compound sympathomimetic effects; effects of ALPHA AND BETA BLOCKERS and ephedrine antagonized.

INCOMPATIBILITIES Solution/additive: hydrocortisone, pentobarbital, phenobarbital, secobarbital, thiopental.

NURSING IMPLICATIONS

Administration

- If possible, administer last dose a few hours before bedtime to minimize insomnia.
- Have patient clear nose before instilling drops. Instruct patient to blow gently with both nostrils open. Generally, nose drops are instilled with head in lateral, head-low position to avoid entry of drug into throat. Check with physician.

- IV ephedrine may be given undiluted by direct IV at a rate of 10 mg or fraction thereof over 30–60 seconds.
- Preserve in tightly closed, light-resistant containers at 15–30C (59–86F) unless otherwise directed by manufacturer. Do not administer liquid medication unless absolutely clear.

Assessment & Drug Effects

- Patients receiving ephedrine IV must be under constant supervision. Take baseline BP and other vital signs. Check BP repeatedly during first 5 min, then q3–5min until stabilized.
- Monitor I&O ratio and pattern, especially in older male patients. Encourage patient to void before taking medication (see Adverse/Side Effects).
- Systemic effects of nose drops can occur because of excessive dosage from rapid absorption of drug solution through nasal mucosa. This is most likely to occur in the elderly.

Patient & Family Education

- Ephedrine is a commonly abused drug. Patients should be advised of side effects and dangers and should be cautioned to take medication only as prescribed.
- Warn patient not to take OTC medications for coughs, colds, allergies, or asthma unless approved by physician. Ephedrine is a common ingredient in these preparations

EPINEPHRINE
(ep-i-nef′rin)

Trade names: Bronkaid Mist, Epi-E-Zpen, Epinephrine Pediatric, EpiPen Auto-Injector, Primatene Mist Suspension

EPINEPHRINE BITARTRATE
Trade names: AsthmaHaler, Bronkaid Mist Suspension, Bronitin Mist Suspension, Epitrate, Medihaler-Epi, Primatene Mist Suspension

EPINEPHRINE HYDROCHLORIDE
Trade names: Adrenalin Chloride, Bronkaid Mistometer, Dysne-Inhal, Epifrin, Glaucon, SusPhrine ♣

EPINEPHRINE, RACEMIC
Trade names: AsthmaNefrin, Dey-Dose Epinephrine, microNefrin, Vaponefrin ♣

EPINEPHRYL BORATE
(ep-i-nef′rill bor′ate)

Trade names: Epinal, Eppy/N

Prototype for classifications: AUTONOMIC NERVOUS SYSTEM AGENT; ALPHA- AND BETA-ADRENERGIC AGONIST; BRONCHODILATOR

Pregnancy category: C

ACTIONS/PHARMACODYNAMICS
Naturally occurring catecholamine obtained from animal adrenal glands; also prepared synthetically. Acts directly on both alpha and beta receptors; the most potent activator of alpha receptors. Imitates all actions of sympathetic nervous system except those on arteries of the face and sweat glands. Strengthens myocardial contraction; increases systolic but may decrease diastolic blood pressure; increases cardiac rate and cardiac output. Constricts bronchial arterioles and inhibits histamine release, thus reducing congestion and edema and increasing tidal volume and vital capacity. Constricts arterioles, particularly in skin, mucous membranes, and kidneys, but dilates skeletal muscle blood vessels. Relaxes uterine smooth musculature and inhibits uterine contrac-

tions. CNS stimulation believed to result from peripheral effects.

USES Temporary relief of bronchospasm, acute asthmatic attack, mucosal congestion, hypersensitivity and anaphylactic reactions, syncope due to heart block or carotid sinus hypersensitivity, and to restore cardiac rhythm in cardiac arrest. Ophthalmic preparation is used in management of simple (open-angle) glaucoma, generally as an adjunct to topical miotics and oral carbonic anhydrase inhibitors; also used as ophthalmic decongestant. Relaxes myometrium and inhibits uterine contractions; prolongs action and delays systemic absorption of local and intraspinal anesthetics. Used topically to control superficial bleeding.

ROUTE & DOSAGE

Anaphylaxis

Adult: **SC** 0.1–0.5 ml of 1:1000 q10–15min prn. **IV** 0.1–0.25 ml of 1:1000 q10–15min.
Child: **SC** 0.01 ml/kg of 1:1000 q10–15min prn. **IV** 0.01 ml/kg of 1:1000 q10–15min.
Neonate: **IV, intratracheal** 0.01–0.03 mg/kg (0.1–0.3 ml/kg of 1:10,000) q3–5min prn.

Cardiac Arrest

Adult: **IV** 0.1–1 mg (1–10 ml of 1:10,000) q5min as needed. **Intracardiac** 0.1–1 mg.
Child: **IV** 0.01 mg/kg (0.1 ml/kg of 1:10,000) q5min as needed. **Intracardiac** 0.05–0.1 mg/kg.

Asthma

Adult: **SC** 0.1–0.5 ml of 1:1000 q20min–4h. **Inhalation** 1 inhalation q4h prn.
Child: **SC** 0.01 ml/kg of 1:1000 q20min–4h. **Inhalation** 1 inhalation q4h prn.

Glaucoma

Adult: **Topical** 1–2 drops 0.25–2% solution 1/d *or* b.i.d.
Child: **Topical** Same as for adult.

Ocular Mydriasis

See Appendix A.

Nasal Hemostasis

Adult: **Topical** 1–2 drops 0.1% ophthalmic or 0.1% nasal solution.
Child: **Topical** Same as for adult.

Topical Hemostatic

Adult: **Topical** 1:50,000–1:1000 applied topically; *or* 1:500,000–1:50,000 mixed with a local anesthetic.
Child: **Topical** Same as for adult.

PHARMACOKINETICS Absorption: inactivated in GI tract. **Onset:** 3–5 min, 1 h on conjunctiva. **Peak:** 20 min, 4–8 h on conjunctiva. **Duration:** 12–24 h topically. **Distribution:** widely distributed; does not cross blood–brain barrier; crosses placenta. **Metabolism:** metabolized in tissue and liver by monoamine oxidase (MAO) and catecholamine-methyltransferase (COMT). **Elimination:** small amount excreted unchanged in urine; excreted in breast milk.

CONTRAINDICATIONS & PRECAUTIONS Contraindicated in: hypersensitivity to sympathomimetic amines; narrow-angle glaucoma; hemorrhagic, traumatic, or cardiogenic shock; cardiac dilatation, cerebral arteriosclerosis, coronary insufficiency, arrhythmias, organic heart or brain disease; during second stage of labor; for local anesthesia of fingers, toes, ears, nose, genitalia. Safe use during pregnancy (category C), in nursing women, and in children not established. **Cautious use in:**

elderly or debilitated patients; prostatic hypertrophy; hypertension; diabetes mellitus; hyperthyroidism; Parkinson's disease; tuberculosis; psychoneurosis; in patients with long-standing bronchial asthma and emphysema with degenerative heart disease; in children <6 y of age.

ADVERSE/SIDE EFFECTS **Nasal use:** *burning, stinging,* dryness of nasal mucosa, sneezing, rebound congestion. **Ophthalmic use:** *transient stinging or burning of eyes,* lacrimation, browache, headache, rebound conjunctival hyperemia, allergy, iritis; with prolonged use: melanin-like deposits on lids, conjunctiva, and cornea; corneal edema; loss of lashes (reversible); maculopathy with central scotoma in aphakic patients (reversible). **Systemic reactions:** *nervousness,* restlessness, sleeplessness, fear, anxiety, *tremors,* severe headache, cerebrovascular accident, weakness, dizziness, syncope, pallor, nausea, vomiting, sweating, dyspnea, precordial pain, *palpitations,* hypertension, MI, tachyarrhythmias including ventricular fibrillation; bronchial and pulmonary edema, urinary retention, tissue necrosis with repeated injections. Metabolic acidoses, elevated serum lactic acid, transient elevations of blood glucose, altered state of perception and thought, psychosis.

DRUG INTERACTIONS May increase hypotension in circulatory collapse or hypotension caused by PHENOTHIAZINES. Additive toxicities with other SYMPATHOMIMETICS **(phenylpropanolamine).** ALPHA- AND BETA-ADRENERGIC BLOCKING AGENTS (e.g., **ergotamine, propranolol**) antagonize effects of epinephrine. GENERAL ANESTHETICS increase cardiac irritability.

INCOMPATIBILITIES **Solution/additive: aminophylline, cephapirin, hyaluronidase, mephentermine, sodium bicarbonate, warfarin. Y-site: aminophylline, sodium bicarbonate.**

NURSING IMPLICATIONS

Administration

Parenteral (SC and IV)

- A tuberculin syringe may ensure greater accuracy in measurement of parenteral doses.
- Epinephrine injection should be protected from exposure to light at all times. Do not remove ampul or vial from carton until ready to use.
- Before withdrawing epinephrine suspension into syringe, shake vial or ampul thoroughly to disperse particles; then inject promptly.
- Carefully aspirate before injecting epinephrine. Inadvertent IV injection of usual SC doses can result in sudden hypertension and possibly cerebral hemorrhage.
- Vascular constriction from repeated injections may cause tissue necrosis. Rotate injection sites and observe for signs of blanching.
- IV preparation: For IV use in cardiac resuscitation, if the 1:1000 1-ml ampuls are used, the dose should be further diluted with 10 ml of sodium chloride injection.
- As a maintenance dose, dilute in 500 ml 5% dextrose.
- IV administration: Give each 1 mg over 1 min or longer; may give more rapidly in cardiac arrest.
- IV administration to neonates, infants, children: Verify correct rate of IV injection with physician.

Inhalation

- Patient should be in an upright position when aerosol preparation is used. The reclining position can result in overdosage by producing large droplets instead of fine spray.
- Instruct patient to rinse mouth and throat with water immediately after inhalation to avoid swallow-

ing residual drug (may cause epigastric pain and systemic effects from the propellant in the aerosol preparation) and to prevent dryness of oropharyngeal membranes.

- Isoproterenol should not be used concurrently with epinephrine. A 4-h interval should elapse before a change is made from one drug to the other.

E

Topical

- Nose drops should be instilled with head in lateral, head-low position to prevent entry of drug into throat. Discuss with physician.
- Instruct patient to rinse nose dropper or spray tip with hot water after each use to prevent contamination of solution with nasal secretions.

Ophthalmic

- It is generally advisable to remove soft contact lenses before instilling eye drops.
- To prevent excessive systemic absorption, instruct patient to apply gentle finger pressure against nasolacrimal duct immediately after drug is instilled for at least 1 or 2 min following instillation.
- When separate solutions of epinephrine and a topical miotic are used, the miotic should be instilled 2–10 min prior to epinephrine because of the conjunctival sac's limited capacity.

Assessment & Drug Effects

Parenteral

- Following IV administration, monitor BP, pulse, respirations, and urinary output and observe patient closely. Epinephrine may widen pulse pressure. If disturbances in cardiac rhythm occur, withhold epinephrine and notify physician immediately. Keep physician informed of any changes in intake-output ratio.
- Patients receiving epinephrine IV should be on cardiac monitor. Have full crash cart immediately available.
- When epinephrine is administered IV, blood pressure should be checked repeatedly during first 5 min, then checked q3–5min until stabilized.

Inhalation

- Advise patient to report to physician if symptoms are not relieved in 20 min or if they become worse following inhalation.
- Advise patient to report bronchial irritation, nervousness, or sleeplessness. Dosage should be reduced.

Patient & Family Education

- Forewarn patient that intranasal application may sting slightly.
- Ophthalmic preparation may cause mydriasis, with blurred vision and sensitivity to light in some patients being treated for glaucoma. Drug is usually administered at bedtime or following prescribed miotic to minimize these symptoms.
- Inform patient that transitory stinging may follow initial ophthalmic administration and that headache and browache occur frequently at first but usually subside with continued use. Advise patient to report to physician if symptoms persist.
- Patient should be instructed to discontinue epinephrine eye drops and to consult a physician if signs of hypersensitivity develop (edema of lids, itching, discharge, crusting eyelids).
- Patients and responsible family members should be taught how to administer epinephrine subcutaneously. Medication and equipment should be available for home emergency. Confer with physician.
- Inhalation epinephrine reduces bronchial secretions and thus may make mucous plugs more difficult to dislodge.

- Tolerance can occur with repeated or prolonged use. Caution the patient to report tolerance to physician; continued use of epinephrine in the presence of tolerance can be dangerous.
- Epinephrine may increase blood glucose levels. Patients with diabetes may experience loss of diabetes control.
- Instruct patient to take medication only as prescribed and to report the onset of systemic effects of epinephrine.
- Discard discolored or precipitated solutions.

EPOETIN ALFA (HUMAN RECOMBINANT ERYTHROPOIETIN)

(e-po-e-tin)

Trade names: Epogen, Eprex ♣, Procrit

Prototype for classifications: BLOOD FORMER; HEMATOPOIETIC GROWTH FACTOR

Pregnancy category: C

ACTIONS/PHARMACODYNAMICS
Erythropoietin is a glycoprotein that stimulates RBC production. It is produced in the kidney and stimulates bone marrow production of RBCs (erythropoiesis). Hypoxia and anemia generally increase the production of erythropoietin.

USES Elevates the hematocrit of patients with anemia secondary to chronic renal failure (CRF)—patients may or may not be on dialysis; other anemias related to malignancies and AIDS. Autologous blood donations for anticipated transfusions. Reduce need for blood in anemic surgical patients.

ROUTE & DOSAGE

Anemia
Adult: **SC/IV** 3–500 U/kg/dose 3 times/wk; usually start with 50–100 U/kg/dose until target Hct range of 30–33% (max 36%) is reached; Hct should not increase by more than 4 points in any 2-wk period; rapid increase in Hct increases the risk of serious adverse reactions (hypertension, seizures); may increase dose if Hct has not increased 5–6 points after 8 wk of therapy; reduce dose after target range is reached or the Hct increases by > 4 points in any 2-wk period; dose usually increased or decreased by 25 U/kg increments.
Child: **SC** 150 U/kg/dose 3 times/wk initially; when Hct increased to 35%, decrease dose by 25 U/kg/dose until Hct reaches 40%.

PHARMACOKINETICS Onset: 7–14 d. **Metabolism:** metabolized in serum. **Elimination:** half-life: 4–13 h; minimal recovery in urine.

CONTRAINDICATIONS & PRECAUTIONS Contraindicated in: uncontrolled hypertension and known hypersensitivity to mammalian cell–derived products and albumin (human). **Cautious use in:** pregnancy (category C) and nursing mothers. Safety and effectiveness in children has not been established.

ADVERSE/SIDE EFFECTS CNS: seizures, *headache*. **CV:** *hypertension*. **GI:** nausea, diarrhea. **Hematologic:** *iron deficiency*, thrombocytosis, *clotting of AV fistula*. **Other:** sweating, bone pain, arthralgias.

E

NURSING IMPLICATIONS

Administration

- Do not shake solution. Shaking may denature the glycoprotein, rendering it biologically inactive.
- Prior to use visually inspect solution for particulate matter. Do not use if solution is discolored or if it contains particulate matter.
- Use only one dose per vial, and do not reenter vial.
- Do not give with any other drug solution.
- IV administration: Epoetin alfa may be given undiluted by direct IV as a bolus dose.
- Discard any unused portion of the vial. It contains no preservatives.
- Store at 2–8C (36–46F). Do not freeze or shake.

Assessment & Drug Effects

- Prior to initiation of therapy the patient's iron stores, including transferrin and serum ferritin, should be evaluated.
- BP should be adequately controlled prior to initiation of therapy and must be closely monitored and controlled during therapy. Hypertension is a side effect that must be controlled.
- BP may rise during early therapy as the Hct increases. Notify physician of a rapid rise in Hct (> 4 points in 2 wk). Dosage will need to be reduced because of risk of serious hypertension.
- Monitor for hypertensive encephalopathy in patients with CRF during period of increasing Hct.
- The potential for seizures exists during periods of rapid Hct increase (> 4 points in 2 wk). Monitor for premonitory neurological symptoms, i.e., aura, and report their appearance promptly.
- The risk of thrombotic events, e.g., MI, CVA, TIA, is increased, especially for patients with CRF. Monitor for them closely.
- Patients may require additional heparin during dialysis to prevent clotting of the vascular access or artificial kidney. Monitor APTT closely.
- Hct should be determined twice weekly until it is stabilized in the target range (30–33%) and the maintenance dose of epoetin alfa has been determined. Hct should then be monitored at regular intervals.
- A CBC with differential and platelet count should be performed regularly.
- Monitor BUN, creatinine, phosphorus, and potassium regularly.
- Epoetin alfa has caused polycythemia in cases where the Hct was not carefully monitored with appropriate dosage adjustments.

Patient & Family Education

- Stress the importance of complying with antihypertensive medication and dietary restrictions.
- During the first 90 d of therapy, patients should not drive or be involved in other hazardous activity because of possible seizure activity.
- As Hct increases, there is an improved sense of well-being and quality of life. The importance of compliance with dietary and dialysis prescriptions should be reinforced.
- Inform patient that headache is a common adverse effect. It should be reported if it is severe or persistent, as it may indicate developing hypertension.
- Stress importance of keeping all follow-up appointments.

EPOPROSTENOL SODIUM

(e-po-pros′-te-nol)

Trade name: Flolan

Classifications: PROSTAGLANDIN; ANTIHYPERTENSIVE; ANTIPLATELET AGENT
Prototype: Dinoprostone
Pregnancy category: B

ACTIONS/PHARMACODYNAMICS Epoprostenol (PGI_2, PGX, Prostacyclin) is a naturally occurring prostaglandin. It is a potent vasodilator of pulmonary and systemic arterial vascular beds and an inhibitor of platelet aggregation. Epoprostenol, by its vasodilation effect, reduces right and left ventricular afterload, increases cardiac output, and increases stroke volume. Depending on the dose, it may also decrease pulmonary vascular resistance and mean systemic arterial pressure.

USE Long-term treatment of primary pulmonary hypertension in NYHA Class III and IV patients.

ROUTE & DOSAGE

Primary Pulmonary Hypertension

Adult: **IV Acute dose ranging:** Initiate with 2 ng/kg/min, increase by 2 ng/kg/min q15min until dose-limiting effects occur (e.g., nausea, vomiting, headache, hypotension, flushing). **Chronic administration:** Start infusion at 4 ng/kg/min less than the maximum tolerated infusion. If maximum tolerated infusion is ≤5 ng/kg/min, start maintenance infusion at 50% of maximum tolerated dose.

PHARMACOKINETICS **Peak:** approx 15 min. **Metabolism:** rapidly hydrolyzed at neutral pH in blood; also subject to enzyme degradation. **Elimination:** half-life: approx 6 min; 82% eliminated in urine.

CONTRAINDICATIONS & PRECAUTIONS **Contraindicated in:** chronic use with CHF patients, hypersensitivity to epoprostenol or related compounds. **Cautious use in:** elderly, pregnancy (category B), lactation. Safety and efficacy in children not established.

ADVERSE/SIDE EFFECTS **Dose-limiting effects (acute dose ranging):** *nausea, vomiting, headache, hypotension, flushing, chest pain, anxiety,* dizziness, bradycardia, dyspnea, abdominal pain, musculoskeletal pain, tachycardia. **During chronic administration: CNS:** *chills, fever, flu-like syndrome, dizziness,* syncope, *headache, anxiety/nervousness,* hyperesthesia, paresthesia. **CV:** *tachycardia, flushing.* **GI:** *diarrhea, nausea, vomiting.* **Musculoskeletal:** *jaw pain, myalgia, nonspecific musculoskeletal pain.*

DRUG INTERACTIONS Hypotension if administered with other vasodilators or antihypertensives.

INCOMPATIBILITY Should NOT be mixed or infused with any other drugs.

NURSING IMPLICATIONS

Administration

- Must be reconstituted using sterile diluent for epoprostenol; must not be mixed with any other medications or solution prior to or during administration.
- Carefully follow manufacturer's directions for reconstitution and administration.
- Avoid abrupt infusion interruption or large dosage reduction.
- Anticoagulation therapy is generally initiated along with epoprostenol.
- Store unopened vials at 15–25C (59–77F). Protect from light. See manufacturer's directions for sta-

bility and/or storage of reconstituted solutions.

Assessment & Drug Effects

- Carefully assess for development of pulmonary edema during dose ranging.
- Frequently monitor respiratory and cardiovascular status during entire period of chronic use of epoprostenol.
- Monitor for and report recurrence or worsening of symptoms associated with primary pulmonary hypertension (e.g., dyspnea, dizziness, exercise intolerance) or adverse effects of drug; dosage adjustments may be needed.

Patient & Family Education

- With ambulatory patients carefully teach correct techniques for storage, reconstitution, and administration of drug, and maintenance of catheter site.
- Advise to immediately report S&S of worsening primary pulmonary hypertension, adverse drug reactions, and S&S of infection at catheter site or sepsis.

EPTIFIBATIDE

(ep-ti-fib′a-tide)

Trade name: Integrilin

Classifications: CARDIOVASCULAR AGENT; ANTITHROMBOTIC AGENT; ANTIPLATELET ANTIBODY; GLYCOPROTEIN IIB/IIIA INHIBITOR

Prototype: Abciximab

Pregnancy category: B

ACTIONS/PHARMACODYNAMICS Binds to the glycoprotein IIb/IIIa (GPIIb/IIIa) receptor sites of platelets. Inhibits platelet aggregation by preventing fibrinogen, von Willebrand's factor, and other molecules from adhering to GPIIb/IIIa receptor sites on platelets.

USES Treatment of acute coronary syndromes (unstable angina, non–Q-wave MI) and patients undergoing percutaneous coronary interventions (PCIs).

ROUTE & DOSAGE

Acute Coronary Syndromes (ACS)

Adult: **IV** 180 μg/kg initial bolus followed by 2 μg/kg/min until hospital discharge or up to 72 h.

PCI in Patients with ACS

Adult: **IV** 180 μg/kg initial bolus followed by 0.5 μg/kg/min for 20–24 h after end of procedure.

PCI in Patients without ACS

Adult: **IV** 135 μg/kg initial bolus followed by 0.5 μg/kg/min for 20–24 h after end of procedure.

PHARMACOKINETICS **Duration:** 6–8 h after stopping infusion. **Distribution:** 25% protein bound. **Metabolism:** minimally metabolized **Elimination:** half-life: 2.5 h; 50% excreted in urine.

CONTRAINDICATIONS & PRECAUTIONS **Contraindicated in:** hypersensitivity to eptifibatide; active bleeding; GI or GU bleeding within 6 weeks; thrombocytopenia; recent major surgery or trauma; intracranial neoplasm, intracranial bleeding within 6 mo; concurrent administration of another GPIIb/IIIa receptor inhibitor (e.g., abciximab); renal dialysis; severe hypertension (systolic blood pressure >200 mm Hg or diastolic blood pressure >110 mm Hg), aneurysm. **Cautious use in:** hypersensitivity to related compounds (e.g., abciximab, tirofiban, lamifiban); concurrent administration of other anticoagulants; pregnancy (category B); lactation. Safety and effectiveness in children not known.

ADVERSE/SIDE EFFECTS **CNS:** intracranial bleed (rare). **GI:** GI bleeding. **Hematologic:** *bleeding* (major bleeding 4.4–11%), anemia, thrombocytopenia.

NURSING IMPLICATIONS

Administration

- Review contraindications to administration prior to giving this drug.
- IV bolus injection: Withdraw bolus dose undiluted from the 10-ml vial and give by IV push over 1–2 min.
- IV infusion: May give undiluted directly from the 100-ml vial (at a rate based on patient's weight) using a vented infusion set or infused through an IV line with 0.9% NaCl or 0.9% NaCl + D5W (either solution may contain up to 60 mEq KCl).
- Store unopened vials at 2–8C (36–46F) and protect from light. Discard any unused portion in opened vial.

Assessment & Drug Effects

- Lab tests before infusion: PT/aPTT, ACT for those undergoing percutaneous coronary intervention (PCI); Hct or Hgb; platelet count; and serum creatinine.
- Monitor lab values: Target aPTT is 50–70 s; during PCI, target ACT is 300–350 s.
- Minimize all vascular and other trauma during treatment. When obtaining IV access, avoid using a noncompressible site such as the subclavian vein.
- Carefully monitor for and immediately report S&S of bleeding (e.g., femoral artery access site bleeding, intracerebral hemorrhage, GI bleeding).
- Note: Immediately stop infusion of eptifibatide and heparin if bleeding at the arterial access site cannot be controlled by pressure.
- Following discontinuation of eptifibatide and heparin, hemostasis at the arterial access site must be achieved by standard compression for a minimum of 4 h prior to hospital discharge.

E

ERGOCALCIFEROL

(er-goe-kal-sif′e-role)

Trade names: Activated Ergosterol, Calciferol, Deltalin, Drisdol, D-ViSol, Ostoforte ♣, Radiostol ♣, Radiostol Forte ♣, Vitamin D_2

Classification: VITAMIN D

Pregnancy category: C

ACTIONS/PHARMACODYNAMICS The name vitamin D encompasses two related fat-soluble substances (sterols) that occur in nature or are synthetically prepared. Vitamin D acts like a hormone in that it is distributed through the circulation and plays a major regulatory role. Maintains normal blood calcium and phosphate ion levels by enhancing their intestinal absorption and by promoting mobilization of calcium from bone and renal tubular resorption of phosphate.

USES Familial hypophosphatemia (vitamin D-resistant rickets), osteomalacia (adult rickets), anticonvulsant-induced rickets and osteomalacia, osteoporosis, renal osteodystrophy, hypocalcemia associated with hypoparathyroidism; prophylaxis and treatment of nutritional rickets. Also hypophosphatemia in Fanconi's syndrome. **Unlabeled uses:** with varying clinical results in lupus vulgaris, psoriasis, and rheumatoid arthritis.

ROUTE & DOSAGE

40 U = 1 μg

Nutritional Rickets, Osteomalacia

Adult: **PO/IM** 25–125 μg/d for 6–12 wk; may need up to 7.5 mg/d in patients with malabsorption.
Child: **PO/IM** 50–125 μg/d; may need up to 250–625 μg/d in patients with malabsorption.

Vitamin D–dependent Rickets

Adult: **PO/IM** 250 μg–1.5 mg/d; may need up to 12.5 mg/d (prolonged therapy with > 2.5 mg/d increases risk of toxicity).
Child: **PO/IM** 75–125 μg/d; may need up to 1.5 mg/d.

Hypoparathyroidism, Pseudohypoparathyroidism

Adult: **PO/IM** 625 μg–5 mg/d; may need up to 10 mg/d (prolonged therapy with > 2.5 mg/d increases risk of toxicity).
Child: **PO/IM** 1.25–5 mg/d; (prolonged therapy with > 2.5 mg/d increases risk of toxicity).

PHARMACOKINETICS Absorption: readily absorbed from GI tract. **Peak activity:** after 4 wk. **Duration:** 2 mo or more. **Distribution:** most of drug first appears in lymph, then concentrates in liver; stored chiefly in liver and to a lesser extent in skin, brain, spleen, and bones. **Metabolism:** metabolized in liver and kidney to active metabolites. **Elimination:** half-life: 12–24 h; about 50% of oral dose excreted in bile; may be stored in tissues for months.

CONTRAINDICATIONS & PRECAUTIONS Contraindicated in: hypersensitivity to vitamin D, hypervitaminosis D, hypercalcemia, hyperphosphatemia, renal osteodystrophy with hyperphosphatemia, malabsorption syndrome, decreased renal function. Safe use of amounts in excess of 400 IU (10 μg) daily in pregnancy (category C) not established. **Cautious use in:** coronary disease; nursing women; arteriosclerosis (especially in the elderly); history of renal stones.

ADVERSE/SIDE EFFECTS Vitamin D toxicity (hypervitaminosis D): produces symptoms of hypercalcemia. ***Initial:*** fatigue, weakness, headache, drowsiness, metallic taste, dry mouth, anorexia, nausea, vomiting, diarrhea, constipation, abdominal cramps, vertigo, tinnitus, ataxia, muscle and joint pain, hypotonia (infants), exanthema. ***Later:*** anemia; calcification of soft tissues (kidneys, blood vessels, myocardium, lungs, skin); nephrotoxicity (polyuria, hyposthenuria, polydipsia, nocturia, casts, albuminuria, hematuria); hypertension; conjunctivitis (calcific); photophobia; rhinorrhea; pruritus; mild acidosis; convulsions; cardiac arrhythmias; osteoporosis (adults); weight loss; renal failure. **Chronic hypervitaminosis D in children:** <u>mental and physical retardation</u>, suppression of linear growth.

DIAGNOSTIC TEST INTERFERENCE Vitamin D may cause false increase in ***serum cholesterol*** measurements (Zlatkis-Zak reaction).

DRUG INTERACTIONS Cholestyramine, colestipol, mineral oil may decrease absorption of vitamin D.

NURSING IMPLICATIONS

Administration

- IM injection should be made deeply, preferably into gluteus maximus and injected slowly. Aspirate carefully. Rotate injection sites.
- Once symptoms of vitamin D de-

ficiency are relieved, dosage should be reduced to prevent hypercalcemia.

- Preserve in tightly covered, light-resistant containers at 15–30C (59–86F), unless otherwise directed. Decomposes on exposure to light and air.

Assessment & Drug Effects

- Patients receiving therapeutic doses of vitamin D must remain under close medical supervision.
- When high therapeutic doses are used, progress is followed by frequent determinations (q2wk or more often) of serum calcium, phosphorus, magnesium, alkaline phosphatase, BUN, and determinations of urine calcium, casts, albumin, and RBC. Blood calcium concentration is generally kept between 9 and 10 mg/dl.
- In patients with osteomalacia a decrease in serum alkaline phosphatase may signal the onset of hypercalcemia.

Patient & Family Education

- Magnesium-containing antacids and laxatives should be avoided in patients with chronic renal failure receiving vitamin D preparations since they are more prone to develop magnesium intoxication than other patients.
- Advise patient not to use OTC medications unless approved by physician.

ERGOLOID MESYLATE

(er′goe-loid mess′i-late)

Trade names: Gerimal, Hydergine, Hydroloid-G, Niloric

Classifications: AUTONOMIC NERVOUS SYSTEM AGENT; ALPHA-ADRENERGIC ANTAGONIST (BLOCKING AGENT, SYMPATHOLYTIC); ERGOT ALKALOID

Prototype: Ergotamine tartrate

Pregnancy category: C

ACTIONS/PHARMACODYNAMICS Combination of three hydrogenated derivatives of ergot alkaloids. Produces peripheral vasodilation primarily by central action and may cause slight reduction in BP and heart rate. Reportedly relieves symptoms of cerebral arteriosclerosis, possibly by increasing cerebral metabolism with consequent increase in blood flow.

USE Senile dementia of Alzheimer type.

ROUTE & DOSAGE

Senile Dementia of Alzheimer Type

Adult: **PO/SL** 1 mg t.i.d.; doses up to 4.5–12 mg/d have been used.

PHARMACOKINETICS **Absorption:** incompletely absorbed from GI tract; approximately 50% reaches systemic circulation. **Peak:** 1.5–3 h. **Metabolism:** undergoes rapid first-pass metabolism in liver. **Elimination:** half-life: 2–12 h; primarily excreted in feces.

CONTRAINDICATIONS & PRECAUTIONS **Contraindicated in:** acute or chronic psychosis. Safe use during pregnancy (category C), in nursing women, and in children not determined. **Cautious use in:** acute intermittent porphyria.

ADVERSE/SIDE EFFECTS Mostly dose related. **CV:** orthostatic hypotension, dizziness or light-headedness, flushing, sinus bradycardia. **EENT:** blurred vision, nasal stuffiness, increased nasopharyngeal secretions. **GI:** sublingual irritation, anorexia, stomach cramps, transient nausea and vomiting, heartburn. **Other:** skin rash, drowsiness, headache, precipitation of acute intermittent porphyria.

NURSING IMPLICATIONS

Administration

- Instruct patient to allow SL tablet to dissolve under tongue and not to drink, eat, or smoke while tablet is in place. SL tablets should not be crushed.
- Store at 15–30C (59–86F) in tightly closed container unless otherwise directed.

Assessment & Drug Effects

- Establish baseline values of BP and pulse; check at regular intervals throughout therapy.
- Sinus bradycardia (40 bpm) has been reported in patients receiving 1.5 mg doses. Report to physician. Pulse rate usually returns to normal within 2 d after drug is discontinued.
- Drug should be permanently withdrawn if marked bradycardia or hypotension occurs.
- Improvement may not be apparent until after 3–4 wk of therapy.

Patient & Family Education

- Advise patient to make position changes slowly, particularly from recumbent to upright posture, and to move ankles and feet for a few minutes before ambulating.

ERGOTAMINE TARTRATE

(er-got'a-meen)

Trade names: Ergostat, Gynergen ♣, Medihaler Ergotamine, Wigrettes

Prototype for classifications: AUTONOMIC NERVOUS SYSTEM AGENT; ALPHA-ADRENERGIC ANTAGONIST (SYMPATHOLYTIC); ERGOT ALKALOID

Pregnancy category: X

ACTIONS/PHARMACODYNAMICS

Natural amino acid alkaloid of ergot. Alpha-adrenergic blocking agent with direct stimulating action on cranial and peripheral vascular smooth muscles and depressant effect on central vasomotor centers. In vascular headache, exerts vasoconstrictive action on previously dilated cerebral vessels, reduces amplitude of arterial pulsations, and antagonizes effects of serotonin. Does not demonstrate intrinsic sedative or analgesic actions. By unknown mechanism, ergotamine activity can damage vascular endothelium, with subsequent occlusion, thrombosis, and gangrene.

USES As single agent or in combination with caffeine to prevent or abort migraine, cluster headache (histamine cephalalgia), and other vascular headaches. Not recommended for migraine prophylaxis because of the possibility of adverse effects.

ROUTE & DOSAGE

Vascular Headaches

Adult: **PO** 1–2 mg followed by 1–2 mg q30min until headache abates or until max of 6 mg/24h or 10 mg/wk. **Inhalation** 1 inhalation (360 µg) q5min to a max of 6 inhalations in 24h or 15/wk.
PR 2 mg q.h. to a max of 4 mg/24h or 10 mg/wk.

PHARMACOKINETICS **Absorption:** variable absorption orally. **Peak:** 0.5–3 h. **Distribution:** crosses blood–brain barrier. **Metabolism:** extensive first-pass metabolism in liver. **Elimination:** half-life: 2.7 h initial phase, 21 h terminal phase; 96% eliminated in feces; excreted in breast milk.

Common side effect in *italic*, life-threatening effects underlined; generic names in **bold**; drug class in SMALL CAPS

CONTRAINDICATIONS & PRECAUTIONS **Contraindicated in:** hypersensitivity, pregnancy (category X), use in children, sepsis, obliterative vascular disease, thromboembolic disease, prolonged use of excessive dosage, hepatic and renal disease, severe pruritus, marked arteriosclerosis, history of MI, coronary artery disease, hypertension, infectious states, anemia, and malnutrition. **Cautious use in:** lactation, elderly patients.

ADVERSE/SIDE EFFECTS **Acute ergotism:** *nausea; vomiting;* diarrhea; abdominal pain; unquenchable thirst; paresthesias; pain (spasms) of facial muscles, tongue, limbs, and lumbar region with difficulty in walking; delirium; convulsive seizures; rapid, weak, or irregular pulse; confusion; itching and cold skin; (occasionally) gangrene of nose, digits, ears. **Chronic ergotism:** intermittent claudication, muscle pains, *weakness,* numbness, coldness and cyanosis of digits (Raynaud's phenomenon). **Other:** complete absence of medium- and large-vessel pulsations in extremities; precordial distress and pain; angina pectoris, transient bradycardia or tachycardia; elevated or lowered BP; depression; drowsiness; kidney failure; fibrotic changes (long-term therapy), partial necrosis of tongue, disagreeable aftertaste.

DRUG INTERACTIONS With high doses of BETA-ADRENERGIC BLOCKERS, possibility of additive vasoconstrictor effects; **erythromycin, troleandomycin** may cause severe peripheral vasospasm.

NURSING IMPLICATIONS

Administration

- Sublingual tablets should not be chewed or swallowed. They should be allowed to completely dissolve.
- Metered-dose nebulizers administer an exact dose and are safe if used as directed. Review instructions with patient.
- Preserve in light-resistant container preferably between 15 and 30C (59 and 86F) unless otherwise directed by manufacturer.

Assessment & Drug Effects

- Nausea and vomiting are adverse reactions that occur in about 10% of patients after they take ergotamine. Patient may need an antiemetic. Consult with physician.
- Carefully monitor patients with PVD for development of peripheral ischemia.
- Patients receiving high ergotamine doses for prolonged periods may experience increased frequency of headaches, fatigue, and depression. Discontinuation of the drug in these patients results in severe withdrawal headache that may last a few days.
- Overdose symptoms: nausea, vomiting, weakness and pain in legs, numbness and tingling in fingers and toes, tachycardia or bradycardia, hypertension or hypotension, and localized edema.

Patient & Family Education

- Drug therapy should begin as soon after onset of migraine attack as possible, preferably during migraine prodrome (scintillating scotomas, visual field defects, nausea, paresthesias usually on side opposite to that of the migraine).
- If migraine attacks occur more frequently or are not relieved, advise patient to report this to physician.
- Advise patient to lie down in a quiet, dark room for 2–3 h after drug administration.
- Instruct patient to report claudication, muscle pain or weakness of extremities, cold or numb digits, ir-

regular heartbeat, nausea, or vomiting. Carefully protect extremities from exposure to cold temperatures; provide warmth, but not heat, to ischemic areas.

- Warn patients not to increase dosage without consulting physician; overdosage is the chief cause of untoward effects from the drug.

ERYTHROMYCIN

(er-ith-roe-mye′sin)

Trade names: Akne-Mycin Ery-Tab, Apo-Erythro Base♣, A/T/S, E-Mycin, Eryc, EryDerm, Erythrocin, Erythromid♣, Erythromycin Base, Ilotycin, Novorythro♣, PCE, Robimycin, Ro-Mycin♣, Staticin, T-Stat

ERYTHROMYCIN ESTOLATE

Trade names: Ilosone, Nororythro♣

ERYTHROMYCIN STEARATE

Trade names: Apo-Erythro-S♣ Eramycin, Erypar, Ethril, Erythrocin Stearate, SK-Erythromycin, Wyamicin S

Classifications: ANTIINFECTIVE; MACROLIDE ANTIBIOTIC

Pregnancy category: B

ACTIONS/PHARMACODYNAMICS

Macrolide antibiotic produced by a strain of *Streptomyces erythreus*. Bacteriostatic or bactericidal, depending on nature of organism and drug concentration used. Antibacterial spectrum is similar to but broader than that of penicillin; commonly used as penicillin substitute in hypersensitive patients for infections not requiring high antibiotic blood levels. More active against gram-positive than gram-negative bacteria. Effectiveness against *Chlamydia trachomatis* is basis for its topical use in prophylaxis of neonatal inclusion conjunctivitis.

USES Pneumococcal pneumonia, *Mycoplasma pneumoniae* (primary atypical pneumonia), acute pelvic inflammatory disease caused by *Neisseria gonorrhoeae* in females sensitive to penicillin, infections caused by susceptible strains of staphylococci, streptococci, and certain strains of *Hemophilus influenzae*. Also used in intestinal amebiasis, Legionnaires' disease, uncomplicated urethral, endocervical, and rectal infections caused by *Chlamydia trachomatis*, for prophylaxis of ophthalmia neonatorum caused by *N. gonorrhoeae, C. trachomatis*, and for chlamydial conjunctivitis in neonates. Considered an acceptable alternative to penicillin for treatment of streptococcal pharyngitis, for prophylaxis of rheumatic fever and bacterial endocarditis, for treatment of diphtheria as adjunct to antitoxin and for carrier state, and as alternate choice in treatment of primary syphilis in patients allergic to penicillins. **Topical applications:** pyodermas, acne vulgaris, and external ocular infections, including neonatal chlamydial conjunctivitis and gonococcal ophthalmia.

ROUTE & DOSAGE

Moderate to Severe Infections

Adult: **PO** 250–500 mg q6h; 333 mg q8h.
Child: **PO** 30–50 mg/kg/d divided q6h. **Topical** Apply ointment to infected eye 1 or more times/d.
Neonate: **PO** *≤7 d:* 10 mg/kg q12h; *>7 d:* 10 mg/kg q8–12h. **Topical** 0.5–1 cm in conjunctival sac once.

***Chlamydia trachomatis* Infections**

Adult: **PO** 500 mg q.i.d. *or* 666 mg q8h.

Child: **Topical** Apply 0.5–1 cm ribbon in lower conjunctival sacs shortly after birth.

PHARMACOKINETICS Absorption: erythromycin base is acid labile; most erythromycins are absorbed in small intestine. **Peak:** 1–4 h PO. **Distribution:** widely distributed to most body tissues; low concentrations in CSF; concentrates in liver and bile; crosses placenta. **Metabolism:** partially metabolized in liver. **Elimination:** half-life: 1.5–2 h; primarily excreted in bile; excreted in breast milk.

CONTRAINDICATIONS & PRECAUTIONS Contraindicated in: hypersensitivity to erythromycins, pregnancy (category B). **Estolate:** history of erthromycin-associated hepatitis; hepatic dysfunction; treatment of skin disorders such as acne or furunculosis, prophylaxis of rheumatic fever. **Cautious use in:** impaired hepatic function.

ADVERSE/SIDE EFFECTS GI: *nausea, vomiting, abdominal cramping*, diarrhea, heartburn, anorexia. **Hypersensitivity reactions:** fever, eosinophilia, urticaria, skin eruptions, fixed drug eruption, anaphylaxis. **CNS:** ototoxicity: reversible bilateral hearing loss, tinnitus, vertigo. **Other:** superinfections by nonsusceptible bacteria, yeasts, or fungi. **Estolate:** cholestatic hepatitis syndrome. **Topical:** erythema, desquamation, burning, tenderness, dryness or oiliness, pruritus.

DIAGNOSTIC TEST INTERFERENCE False elevations of ***urinary catecholamines, urinary steroids,*** and AST (SGOT), ALT (SGPT) (by colorimetric methods).

DRUG INTERACTIONS Serum levels and toxicities of **carbamazepine, cyclosporine, digoxin, theophylline, triazolam, warfarin** are increased. **Ergotamine** may increase peripheral vasospasm. May increase risk of arrhythmias with **terfenadine, astemizole.**

NURSING IMPLICATIONS

Administration

- Administered preferably on an empty stomach 1 h before or 3 h after meals. Do not give with, or immediately before or after, fruit juices, and advise patient not to crush or chew tablets.
- Enteric-coated tablets may be given without regard to meals.
- When switching from tablet to a PO liquid preparation, dosing may require adjustment.
- Prophylaxis for neonatal eye infection: Ribbon of ointment approximately 0.5–1 cm long is placed into lower conjunctival sac of neonate shortly after birth. Use a new tube of erythromycin for each neonate.
- For treatment of eye infections, use only preparations labeled for ophthalmic use.
- Store in tightly capped containers preferably between 15 and 30C (59 and 86F) unless otherwise directed by manufacturer.

Assessment & Drug Effects

- GI symptoms after PO administration are dose related. Report their onset to physician. If symptoms persist after dosage reduction, physician may prescribe drug to be given with meals in spite of impaired absorption.
- Pseudomembranous enterocolitis (see Appendix G), a potentially life-threatening condition, may occur during or after antibiotic therapy.
- Observe for symptoms of superinfection by overgrowth of nonsus-

E

ceptible bacteria or fungi. Emergence of resistant staphylococcal strains is highly predictable during prolonged therapy.

- Hepatic function tests should be performed periodically during prolonged drug regimens.
- Hepatotoxicity is believed to be a hypersensitivity reaction. Premonitory signs and symptoms may include abdominal pain, nausea, vomiting, fever, leukocytosis, and eosinophilia. Jaundice may or may not be present.
- Symptoms of hepatotoxicity may appear a few days after initiation of drug but usually occur after 1–2 wk of continuous therapy. Symptoms are reversible with prompt discontinuation of erythromycin.
- Ototoxicity appears to develop most frequently in patients receiving 4 g/d or more, the elderly, female patients, and patients with renal or hepatic dysfunction. It is reversible with prompt discontinuation of drug.

Patient & Family Education

- Watch for signs and symptoms of superinfection (see Appendix G). Report immediately.
- Observe for signs and symptoms of pseudomembranous enterocolitis (see Appendix G), which may occur even after the drug is discontinued. Report immediately.
- Advise patient to report any ototoxic effects including dizziness, vertigo, nausea, tinnitus, roaring noises, hearing impairment (see Appendix G).

ERYTHROMYCIN ETHYLSUCCINATE

Trade names: Apo-Erythro-ES ♣, E.E.S., EES-200, EES-400, EryPed, Pediamycin, Wyamycin E

Classifications: ANTIINFECTIVE; MACROLIDE ANTIBIOTIC
Prototype: Erythromycin
Pregnancy category: B

ACTIONS/PHARMACODYNAMICS
Acid-stable ester salt of erythromycin.

USES See erythromycin.

ROUTE & DOSAGE

400 mg erythromycin ethylsuccinate is approximately equal to 250 mg erythromycin base.

Infection

Adult: **PO** 400 mg q6h up to 4 g/d according to severity of infection.
Child: **PO** 30–50 mg/kg/d in 4 divided doses up to 100 mg/kg/d for severe infections.

PHARMACOKINETICS **Absorption:** readily absorbed from GI tract. **Peak:** 2 h. **Distribution:** concentrates in liver; crosses placenta; distributed into breast milk. **Metabolism:** metabolized in liver. **Elimination:** half-life: 2–5 h; excreted primarily in bile and feces.

CONTRAINDICATIONS & PRECAUTIONS **Contraindicated in:** hypersensitivity to erythromycins; history of erythromycin-associated hepatitis; preexisting liver disease. Safe use during pregnancy (category B) not established.

ADVERSE/SIDE EFFECTS **GI:** diarrhea, *nausea,* vomiting, stomatitis, *abdominal cramps,* anorexia. **Other:** skin eruptions, hepatotoxicity and ototoxicity potential, superinfections.

DRUG INTERACTIONS May increase **carbamazepine, cyclosporine, theophylline, digoxin, triazolam,** and **warfarin** serum levels and toxicity; **ergotamine** may induce ischemia and peripheral vasospasm; may increase risk of arrhythmias with **terfenadine.**

NURSING IMPLICATIONS

Administration

- PO formulations may be administered without regard to meals in patients ≥ 2 y.
- Chewable tablets should be chewed and not swallowed whole.
- PO suspensions are stable for 14 d at room temperature unless otherwise stated by manufacturer. Note expiration date.
- Store tablets in tight containers at 15–30C (59–86F) unless otherwise directed.

Assessment & Drug Effects

- Culture and susceptibility testing should be performed before initiation of treatment.
- Cholestatic hepatitis syndrome is most likely to occur in adults who have received erythromycin estolate for > 10 d or who have had repeated courses of therapy. The condition generally clears within 3–5 d after cessation of therapy.
- Hepatic function tests and blood cell counts should be conducted periodically if therapy is prolonged 10 d or more.

Patient & Family Education

- Advise patient to report immediately the onset of adverse reactions and to be on the alert for signs and symptoms associated with jaundice (see Appendix G).
- Ototoxicity is most likely to occur in patients receiving high dosage or who have impaired renal function. Report immediately the onset of tinnitus, vertigo, or hearing impairment.

ERYTHROMYCIN GLUCEPTATE

Trade name: Ilotycin Gluceptate

ERYTHROMYCIN LACTOBIONATE

Trade name: Erythrocin Lactobionate-I.V.

Classifications: ANTIINFECTIVE; MACROLIDE ANTIBIOTIC

Prototype: Erythromycin

Pregnancy category: B

E

ACTIONS/PHARMACODYNAMICS Soluble salt of erythromycin.

USES When oral administration is not possible or the severity of infection requires immediate high serum levels. See erythromycin.

ROUTE & DOSAGE

Infections

Adult: **IV** 250 mg–1 g q6h up to 4 g/d according to severity of infection.

Child: **IV** 15–20 mg/kg/d in 4 divided doses up to 100 mg/kg/d for severe infections.

PHARMACOKINETICS Peak: 1 h. **Distribution:** concentrates in liver; crosses placenta; distributed into breast milk. **Metabolism:** metabolized in liver. **Elimination:** half-life: 3–5 h; excreted primarily in bile and feces; 12–15% excreted in urine.

CONTRAINDICATIONS & PRECAUTIONS Contraindicated in: hypersensitivity to erythromycins. Safe use during pregnancy (category B) not established. **Cautious use in:** impaired hepatic function.

ADVERSE/SIDE EFFECTS *Pain and venous irritation after IV injection;* allergic reactions, anaphylaxis (rare); superinfections; variations in liver function tests following prolonged or repeated therapy. **GI:** *nausea,* vomiting, diarrhea, *abdominal cramps*. See also **erythromycin.**

DRUG INTERACTIONS May increase **carbamazepine, cyclosporine, theophylline, digoxin, triazolam,** and **warfarin** serum levels and toxicity; **ergotamine** may induce ischemia and peripheral vasospasm; may increase risk of arrhythmias with **terfenadine**.

INCOMPATIBILITIES Solution/additive: aminophylline, TETRACYCLINES, **pentobarbital, secobarbital, streptomycin, heparin, cephalothin, colistimethate, metaraminol, metoclopramide**, vitamin B complex with C, **ampicillin, amikacin**. **Y-site: aminophylline, heparin,** TETRACYCLINES.

NURSING IMPLICATIONS

Administration

- Initial solution is prepared by adding 10 ml sterile water for injection without preservatives to each 500 mg or fraction thereof (see manufacturer's directions for dilution). Shake vial until drug is completely dissolved.
- Before administration, initial solution is further diluted with 80–250 ml of NS, lactated Ringer's or Normosol-R and buffer to neutrality (see manufacturer's directions). Stability of solution is dependent on pH and is optimal at pH 6–8.
- Continuous infusion is administered slowly within 24 h after dilution to a volume of 500 ml.
- Physician will prescribe specific IV infusion rate. Rate should be slow to avoid pain along course of vein.
- Initially, reconstituted solution is stable up to 7 d if refrigerated at 2–8C (36–46F).
- Store sterile powder at 15–30C (59–86F) unless otherwise directed.

Assessment & Drug Effects

- Culture and susceptibility testing should be performed prior to initiation of therapy.
- Hearing impairment may occur with large doses of this drug. It may occur as early as the second day and as late as the third week of therapy.
- IV infusion of large doses reported to increase risk of thrombophlebitis. Assess for signs and symptoms (see Appendix G).
- Periodic hepatic function tests are advised in patients receiving daily high doses or prolonged or repeated therapy.

Patient & Family Education

- Instruct patient to report immediately tinnitus, dizziness, or hearing impairment.

ESMOLOL HYDROCHLORIDE

(ess'moe-lol)

Trade name: Brevibloc

Classifications: AUTONOMIC NERVOUS SYSTEM AGENT; BETA-ADRENERGIC ANTAGONIST (BLOCKING AGENT, SYMPATHOLYTIC)

Prototype: Propranolol

Pregnancy category: C

ACTIONS/PHARMACODYNAMICS Ultrashort-acting $beta_1$-adrenergic blocking agent with cardioselective properties but devoid of intrinsic sympathetic activity (ISA) or membrane-stabilizing (quinidine-like) activity. Its hemodynamic effects are mild, with potency as a beta blocker about 1/100th that of propranolol. By competitive binding at beta-adrenergic receptors, inhibits the agonist effect of catecholamines. Since it binds predominantly to $beta_1$-receptors in cardiac tissue, sympathetically mediated increases in cardiac rate and BP are blocked.

USES Supraventricular tachyarrhythmias (SVT) in perioperative and postoperative periods or in other critical situations. Also short-term treatment of noncompensating sinus tachycardia and in the control of heart rate for patients with MI. **Unlabeled uses:** moderate postoperative hypertension; treatment of intense transient adrenergic response to surgical stress in cardiac as well as noncardiac surgery.

ROUTE & DOSAGE

Supraventricular Tachyarrhythmias

Adult: **IV** 500 μg/kg loading dose followed by 50 μg/kg/min; may increase dose q5–10min prn (max 200 μg/kg/min).

PHARMACOKINETICS Onset: <5 min. **Peak:** 10–20 min. **Duration:** 10–30 min. **Metabolism:** rapidly hydrolyzed by RBC esterases. **Elimination:** half-life: 9 min; eliminated in urine.

CONTRAINDICATIONS & PRECAUTIONS Contraindicated in: cardiac failure, heart block greater than first degree, sinus bradycardia, cardiogenic shock. Safe use during pregnancy (category C), in nursing mothers, and in children not established. **Cautious use in:** history of allergy or bronchial asthma, bronchospasm, emphysema; CHF; diabetes mellitus; renal function impairment.

ADVERSE/SIDE EFFECTS CNS: headache, *dizziness,* somnolence, confusion, agitation. **CV:** *hypotension* (dose related), cold hands and feet, bradyarrhythmias, flushing, myocardial depression. **GI:** nausea, vomiting. **Respiratory:** dyspnea, chest pain, rhonchi, bronchospasm. **Skin:** *infusion site inflammation* (redness, swelling, induration).

DRUG INTERACTIONS May increase **digoxin** IV levels 10–20%; **morphine** IV may increase esmolol levels by 45%; **succinylcholine** may prolong neuromuscular blockade.

INCOMPATIBILITY Y-site: furosemide.

NURSING IMPLICATIONS

Administration

- Esmolol must be diluted before administration (available as a solution: 250 mg/ml in 10-ml ampuls).
- Preparation of infusion: Dilute each 5 g with 500 ml of D5W, NS, or other appropriate diluent (see manufacturer's directions). Resulting solution yields 10 mg/ml. Caution: A stronger solution (e.g., 20 mg/ml) may cause venous irritation and thrombophlebitis.
- Do not admix with other drugs before dilution in a suitable IV fluid.
- Esmolol infusion may be administered via a central vein; use of butterfly needles is not recommended.
- The diluted infusion solution is stable for at least 24 h at room temperature.
- Store ampuls at 15–30C (59–86F) unless otherwise directed.

Assessment & Drug Effects

- Monitor BP, pulse, ECG, during esmolol infusion.
- Hypotension may have its onset during the initial titration phase; thereafter the risk increases with increasing doses.
- Usually the hypotension experienced during esmolol infusion is resolved within 30 min after infusion is reduced or discontinued.
- IV site reactions (burning, erythema) or diaphoresis may develop during infusion. Both reactions are

temporary, but injection site should be changed if local reaction occurs. Blood chemistry abnormalities have not been reported.
- Overdose symptoms: Discontinue administration if the following symptoms occur: bradycardia, severe dizziness or drowsiness, dyspnea, bluish-colored fingernails or palms of hands, seizures.

E

ESTAZOLAM

(es-ta-zo′lam)

Trade name: Prosom

Classifications: CNS AGENT; ANXIOLYTIC; SEDATIVE-HYPNOTIC; BENZODIAZEPINE

Prototype: Lorazepam

Pregnancy category: X

Controlled substance: Schedule IV

ACTIONS/PHARMACODYNAMICS Estazolam is a benzodiazepine whose effects (anxiolytic, sedative, hypnotic, skeletal muscle relaxant) are mediated by the inhibitory neurotransmitter gamma-aminobutyric acid (GABA). GABA acts at the thalamic, hypothalamic, and limbic levels of CNS. Benzodiazepines decrease the number of awakenings from sleep. Stage 2 (unequivocal sleep) is increased with all benzodiazepines. Estazolam shortens stages 3 and 4 (slow-wave sleep), and REM sleep is shortened. The total sleep time, however, is increased with estazolam.

USE Short-term management of insomnia.

ROUTE & DOSAGE

Adult: **PO** 1 mg h.s. may increase up to 2 mg if necessary; some debilitated elderly patients should start with 0.5 mg h.s.

PHARMACOKINETICS Absorption: rapidly absorbed from GI tract. **Onset:** 20–30 min. **Peak:** 2 h. **Distribution:** crosses rapidly into brain; crosses placenta; distributed into breast milk. **Metabolism:** extensively metabolized in liver. **Elimination:** half-life: 10–24 h; excreted in urine.

CONTRAINDICATIONS & PRECAUTIONS Contraindicated in: Known sensitivity to BENZODIAZEPINES, acute narrow-angle glaucoma, primary depressive disorders or psychosis, children < 12 y old, coma, shock, acute alcohol intoxication, pregnancy (category X), nursing mothers. **Cautious use in:** renal and hepatic impairment, organic brain syndrome, myasthenia gravis, narrow-angle glaucoma, suicide tendency, GI disorders, elderly and debilitated patients, limited pulmonary reserve.

ADVERSE/SIDE EFFECTS CNS: headache, dizziness, impaired coordination, headache, hypokinesia, *somnolence,* hangover. **CV (rare):** palpitations, arrhythmias, syncope. **Hematologic:** leukopenia, <u>agranulocytosis</u>. **GI:** constipation, xerostomia, anorexia, flatulence, vomiting. **Other:** arthritis, arthralgia, myalgia, muscle spasm.

DRUG INTERACTIONS Cimetidine may decrease metabolism of estazolam and increase its effects; alcohol and other CNS DEPRESSANTS may increase drowsiness.

NURSING IMPLICATIONS

Administration

- For elderly patients in good health, a 1-mg dose is indicated; however, for debilitated or small elderly patients, initial dose should be reduced to 0.5 mg.
- Dosage reduction may be needed in the presence of hepatic impairment.

Common side effect in *italic,* life-threatening effects <u>underlined</u>: generic names in **bold;** drug class in SMALL CAPS

- Store at room temperature, 15–30C (59–86F).

Assessment & Drug Effects
- Monitor for improvement in signs and symptoms of insomnia.
- Assess for excess CNS depression or daytime sedation.
- Assess for safety, especially with elderly or debilitated patients, as dizziness and impaired coordination are known side effects.

Patient & Family Education
- Inform patient of adverse effects and advise to report these to the physician.
- Instruct patient to avoid using this drug in combination with other CNS depressant drugs or alcohol.
- Advise caution with hazardous activities until response to drug is known.

ESTRADIOL
(ess-tra-dye'ole)
Trade names: Alora, Climara, Estrace, Estraderm; Fempatch, Menorest, Vivelle, Estring

ESTRADIOL CYPIONATE
Trade names: Depo-Estradiol Cypionate, depGynogen, Depogen, Dura-Estrin, Estro-Cyp, Estroject-LA, and others

ESTRADIOL VALERATE
Trade names: Delestrogen, Dioval, Duragen-10, Estraval, Femogex♣, Gynogen LA, Valergen
Prototype for classifications: HORMONE; ESTROGEN
Pregnancy category: X

ACTIONS/PHARMACODYNAMICS Natural or synthetic steroid hormone secreted principally by the ovarian follicles, and also by the adrenals, corpus luteum, placenta, and testes. Estrogen binds to a specific intracellular receptor, forming a complex that stimulates synthesis of proteins responsible for estrogenic effects. In general, estradiol (estrogens) effects simulate those produced by the endogenous hormone. Promotes endometrial lining development, but prolonged exposure leads to abnormal endometrial hyperplasia, a condition usually associated with an abnormal bleeding pattern. Conversely, estrogen-stimulated endometrium suddenly deprived of estrogen may bleed within 48–72 h. Reduces pituitary release of gonadotropins (LH and FSH), resulting in inhibition of lactation and ovulation and reduction of sebaceous secretion. May mask onset of climacteric.

USES Natural or surgical menopausal symptoms, kraurosis vulvae, atrophic vaginitis, primary ovarian failure, female hypogonadism, castration. Used adjunctively with diet, calcium, and physical therapy to prevent and treat postmenopausal osteoporosis; also for palliation in advanced prostatic carcinoma and inoperable metastic breast cancer in women at least 5 y after menopause. Combined with progestins in many oral contraceptive formulations.

ROUTE & DOSAGE

Menopause, Atrophic Vaginitis, Kraurosis Vulvae, Female Hypogonadism, Female Castration, Primary Ovarian Failure

Adult: **PO** 1–2 mg/d in a cyclic regimen. **Topical** 2–4 g *vaginal cream* intravaginally once/d for 1–2 wk, then 1–2 g/d for 1–2 wk, then 1 g 1–3 times/wk; *transdermal patch* **Estraderm** twice weekly; ***Climara, Fempatch*** qwk in a cyclic regimen. **IM** 1–5 mg once q3–4wk (cypionate); 10–25 mg once q4wk (valerate).

Metastatic Breast Cancer

Adult: **PO** 10 mg t.i.d.

Prostatic Cancer

Adult: **PO** 1–2 mg t.i.d.
IM 30 mg once q1–2wk (valerate).

Postpartum Breast Engorgement

Adult: **IM** 10–25 mg at end of first stage of labor (valerate).

E

PHARMACOKINETICS Absorption: rapid absorption from GI tract; readily absorbed through skin and mucous membranes; slow absorption from IM injections. **Distribution:** distributed throughout body tissues, especially in adipose tissue; crosses placenta. **Metabolism:** metabolized primarily in liver. **Elimination:** excreted in urine; excreted in breast milk.

CONTRAINDICATIONS & PRECAUTIONS Contraindicated in: known or suspected pregnancy (category X), estrogenic-dependent neoplasms, breast cancer (except in selected patients being treated for metastatic disease). History of thromboembolic disorders; active arterial thrombosis or thrombophlebitis; undiagnosed abnormal genital bleeding; history of cholestatic disease; thyroid dysfunction; blood dyscrasias. **Cautious use in:** adolescents with incomplete bone growth; endometriosis, lactation; hypertension, cardiac insufficiency; diseases of calcium and phosphate metabolism (metabolic bone disease); cerebrovascular disease; mental depression; benign breast disease, family history of breast or genital tract neoplasm; diabetes mellitus; gallbladder disease; preexisting leiomyoma, abnormal mammogram, history of idiopathic jaundice of pregnancy; varicosities; asthma; epilepsy; migraine headaches; hepatic or renal dysfunction; jaundice, acute intermittent porphyria, pyridoxine deficiency.

ADVERSE/SIDE EFFECTS CNS: headache, migraine, dizziness, mental depression, chorea, convulsions. **CV:** <u>thromboembolic disorders</u>, hypertension. **Eye:** intolerance to contact lenses, worsening of myopia or astigmatism, scotomas. **GI:** *nausea,* vomiting, anorexia, increased appetite, diarrhea, abdominal cramps or pain, constipation, bloating, colitis, acute pancreatitis, cholestatic jaundice, benign hepatoadenoma. **GU:** mastodynia, breast secretion, spotting, changes in menstrual flow, dysmenorrhea, amenorrhea, cervical erosion, altered cervical secretions, premenstrual-like syndrome, vaginal candidiasis, endometrial cystic hyperplasia, reactivation of endometriosis, increased size of preexisting fibromyomats, cystitis-like syndrome, hemolytic uremic syndrome; in men: gynecomastia, testicular atrophy, feminization, impotence (reversible). **Metabolic:** reduced carbohydrate tolerance, hyperglycemia, hypercalcemia, folic acid deficiency, fluid retention. **Skin:** dermatitis, pruritus, seborrhea, oily skin, acne; photosensitivity, chloasma, loss of scalp hair, hirsutism. **Other:** pain and postinjection flare at injection site; sterile abscess; leg cramps, weight changes, acute intermittent porphyria, change in libido.

DIAGNOSTIC TEST INTERFERENCE Estradiol reduces response of ***metyrapone*** test and excretion of ***pregnanediol.*** **Increases:** ***BSP*** retention, norepinephrine-induced ***platelet aggregability, hydrocortisone, PBI, T_4, sodium, thyroxine-binding globulin*** (TBG), ***pro-***

thrombin and factors VII, VIII, IX and ***X; serum triglyceride,*** and ***phospholipid*** concentrations, ***renin*** substrate. **Decreases:** ***antithrombin III, pyridoxine*** and ***serum folate*** concentrations, serum ***cholesterol,*** values for the ***T_3 resin uptake*** test, ***glucose tolerance.*** May cause false-positive test for ***LE cells*** or ***antinuclear antibodies*** (ANA).

DRUG INTERACTIONS BARBITURATES, **phenytoin, rifampin** decrease estrogen effect by increasing its metabolism; ORAL ANTICOAGULANTS may decrease hypoprothrombinemic effects.

NURSING IMPLICATIONS

Administration

- Take PO medication with or immediately after solid food to reduce nausea.
- For administration of intravaginal or transdermal drug forms, see specific information under patient and family education.
- Protect tablets from light and moisture in well-closed container. Store at 15–30C (59–86F) and protect from freezing, unless otherwise directed by manufacturer.

Assessment & Drug Effects

- Nausea, frequently at breakfast time, usually disappears after 1 or 2 wk of drug use.
- Spotting or breakthrough bleeding occurring when a barbiturate and estradiol are taken concurrently indicates reduced availability of the estrogen.
- Patients with cardiac or renal dysfunction or hypertension should be monitored carefully. Check BP on a regular basis.
- Severe hypercalcemia (> 15 mg/dl) may be caused by estradiol therapy in patients with breast cancer and bone metastasis.
- Estrogen treatment is usually interrupted at least 4 wk before surgery that may be associated with a prolonged period of immobilization or with vascular complications.

Patient & Family Education

- Emphasize need for compliance with established dosage schedule. It should not be altered unless physician prescribes a change.
- Urge patient to read the patient package insert (PPI) carefully; then discuss it with patient to assure her complete understanding of estrogen therapy.
- Patient should promptly report intermittent bleeding or unexplained and sudden pain to physician.
- Advise patient to determine weight under standard conditions 1 or 2 times/wk and to report sudden weight gain or other signs of fluid retention.
- Instruct patient to report positive Homan's sign and the following symptoms of thromboembolic disorders immediately: tenderness, swelling, and redness in extremity; sudden, severe headache or chest pain; slurring of speech; change in vision; tenderness, pain, sudden shortness of breath.
- Advise diabetic users to report positive urine or blood glucose tests promptly.
- Urge decreased caffeine intake, since estrogen depresses caffeine metabolism.
- Teach self-examination of breasts, emphasizing a monthly schedule.
- Long-term or high-dosage therapy with estrogens is reduced or terminated gradually.
- Reassure male patients that estrogen-induced feminization and impotence are reversible with termination of therapy.
- Estrogen-primed or -stimulated endometrium may bleed 48–72 h after dose is discontinued. In cyclic therapy, estradiol is resumed on

schedule before drug-induced vaginal bleeding stops.
- Withdrawal bleeding may occur even after oophorectomy and after menopause.

Intravaginal Application
- Instruct patient to insert calibrated dosage applicator approximately 5 cm (2 in.), directing it slightly back toward sacrum. Instill medication by pushing plunger. Patient should remain in recumbent position about 30 min to prevent losing the medication. Observe perineal area before each administration: if mucosa is red, swollen, or excoriated or if there is a change in vaginal discharge, report to physician.
- Instruct patient to wash her hands well before and after the application. Also tell her not to use tampons while on vaginal cream therapy.

Transdermal Application
- Cleanse and dry selected skin area on trunk of body, preferably the abdomen. Avoid application to the breasts, to an irritated, abrased, oily area, or to the waistline.
- If system falls off, the same system may be reapplied, or if necessary, a new one can be applied. Return to original treatment schedule.
- Rotate application site with an interval of at least 1 wk between applications to a particular site.

ESTRAMUSTINE PHOSPHATE SODIUM

(ess-tra-muss'teen)

Trade name: Emcyt

Classifications: ANTINEOPLASTIC; ALKYLATING AGENT

Prototype: Cyclophosphamide

Pregnancy category: X

ACTIONS/PHARMACODYNAMICS Conjugate of estradiol and the carbamate of nitrogen mustard. Extent of antitumor activity contributed by each, as well as precise mechanisms of action, unknown. Appears to act as a relatively weak alkylating agent and estrogen. Major effectiveness reported to be in patients who have been refractory to estrogen therapy alone.

USES Palliative treatment of metabolic or progressive carcinoma of prostate.

ROUTE & DOSAGE

Neoplasm

Adult: **PO** 14 mg/kg/d in 3–4 divided doses.

PHARMACOKINETICS Absorption: readily absorbed from GI tract. **Peak:** 2–3 h. **Metabolism:** dephosphorylated in intestines to estramustine, estradiol, estrone, and nitrogen mustard; further metabolized in liver. **Elimination:** half-life: 20 h; excreted in feces via bile.

CONTRAINDICATIONS & PRECAUTIONS Contraindicated in: hypersensitivity to either estradiol or nitrogen mustard; active thrombophlebitis or thromboembolic disorders; pregnancy (category X). **Cautious use in:** history of thrombophlebitis, thromboses, or thromboembolic disorders; cerebrovascular or coronary artery disease; gallstones or peptic ulcer; impaired liver function; metabolic bone diseases associated with hypercalcemia; diabetes mellitus; hypertension, conditions that might be aggravated by fluid retention (e.g., epilepsy, migraine, renal dysfunction); elderly patients.

ADVERSE/SIDE EFFECTS CNS: lethargy, emotional lability, insomnia, headache, anxiety. **CV:** CVA, MI, *thrombophlebitis*, CHF, *peripheral* *edema*. **GI:** *nausea*, diarrhea, anorexia, flatulence, vomiting, thirst, GI bleeding. **Hematologic:** leukopenia, thrombocytopenia, *abnormalities in liver function tests*, hypercalcemia, bone marrow depression (rare). **Respiratory:** hoarseness, burning sensation in throat, dyspnea, upper respiratory discharge, pulmonary emboli. **Skin:** rash, pruritus, urticaria, dry skin, easy bruising, flushing, peeling skin and fingertips, thinning hair. **Other:** tearing of eyes, gynecomastia, breast tenderness, impotence, leg cramps, decrease in glucose tolerance.

DRUG-FOOD INTERACTIONS Milk, dairy products, calcium supplements, may decrease estramustine absorption.

NURSING IMPLICATIONS

Administration

- Drug can be taken with meals to reduce incidence of GI side effects. Some patients require drug withdrawal because of intolerable GI effects.
- Store in refrigerator at 2–8C (38–46F) in tight, light-resistant containers, unless otherwise directed by manufacturer.

Assessment & Drug Effects

- Keep track of weight and examine for peripheral edema. Be mindful that drug can cause CHF.
- Monitor I&O ratio and pattern to prevent dehydration and electrolyte imbalance, especially with vomiting or diarrhea.
- Patients with diabetes should be closely observed because of possibility of estramustine-induced reduction in glucose tolerance. Baseline and periodic glucose tolerance tests are advised.
- Baseline and periodic hepatic enzymes and bilirubin tests should be performed, then repeated after drug has been discontinued for 2 mo.

Patient & Family Education

- To reduce drug-induced nausea, instruct patient to eat small feedings at frequent intervals; eat slowly; and attempt cold food if food odors are offensive.
- Advise patient to drink liquids 1 h before or 1 h after rather than with meals; clear liquids may be more palatable.

E

ESTROGENS, CONJUGATED

(ess′tro-jenz)

Trade names: C.E.S. ♣, Premarin, Progens

Classifications: HORMONE; ESTROGEN

Prototype: Estradiol

Pregnancy category: X

ACTIONS/PHARMACODYNAMICS Short-acting estrogen mixture of conjugated estrogens including sodium estrone sulfate and sodium equilin sulfate. Binds to intracellular receptors that stimulate DNA and RNA to synthesize proteins responsible for effects of estrogen.

USES Atrophic vaginitis, kraurosis vulvae, and abnormal bleeding (hormonal imbalance); also female hypogonadism, primary ovarian failure, vasomotor symptoms associated with menopause; to retard progression of osteoporosis and as palliative therapy of breast and prostatic carcinomas. **Unlabeled use:** postcoital contraceptive.

ROUTE & DOSAGE

Menopause, Osteoporosis, Atrophic Vaginitis, Kraurosis Vulvae

Adult: **PO** 0.3–1.25 mg/d for 21 d each month; adjust to lowest level that gives symptom control (≤0.625 mg/d); **IM/IV** 25 mg; repeated in 6–12 h if needed; **Topical** 2–4 g of cream/d.

Female Hypogonadism

Adult: **PO** 2.5–7.5 mg/d in 1–3 divided doses for 20 d; followed by a 10-d rest period.

Postcoital Contraception

Adult: **PO** 30 mg/d in divided doses for 5 consecutive days beginning within 72 h of coitus.

Breast Cancer

Adult: **PO** 10 mg t.i.d. for at least 3 mo.

Prostatic Cancer (palliation)

Adult: **PO** 1.25–2.5 mg t.i.d.

CONTRAINDICATIONS & PRECAUTIONS **Contraindicated in:** breast cancer, known or suspected pregnancy (category X). **Cautious use in:** hypertension; gallbladder disease; diabetes mellitus; heart failure; hepatic or renal dysfunction, history of thromboembolic disease.

ADVERSE/SIDE EFFECTS **CNS:** headache, dizziness, depression, *libido changes*. **CV:** <u>thromboembolic disorders</u>, hypertension. **GI:** *nausea,* vomiting, diarrhea, bloating, cholestatic jaundice. **GU:** mastodynia, spotting, changes in menstrual flow, dysmenorrhea, amenorrhea. **Metabolic:** reduced carbohydrate tolerance, fluid retention. **Other:** leg cramps, intolerance to contact lenses.

DRUG INTERACTIONS **Carbamazepine, phenytoin, rifampin** decrease estrogen levels because they increase its metabolism; may enhance steroid effects of CORTICOSTEROIDS; may decrease anticoagulant effects of ORAL ANTICOAGULANTS.

NURSING IMPLICATIONS

See numerous additional implications under estradiol.

Administration

- Conjugated estrogens are given cyclically except when used for treatment of postpartum breast engorgement and for palliation of cancer. Cyclic regimen is to dose for 3 wk followed by 1 wk off.
- Before reconstitution for IV or IM, refrigerate ampul at 2–8C (36–46F). To reconstitute, add diluent to ampul and agitate gently; use within a few hours.
- Conjugated estrogen solution is compatible with D5W and NS and is incompatible with any solution with an acid pH (<7.0). Rapid IV injection may cause skin flushing.
- IV estrogen is given slowly by direct IV injection at a rate of 5 mg/min.
- If reconstituted solution is stored in refrigerator and protected from light, it will remain stable for 60 d. Discard precipitated or discolored solution.
- Store vaginal cream at 15–30C (59–86F); protect from light and from freezing.

Patient & Family Education

- Be certain patient is aware of importance of taking drug exactly as prescribed: specifically, doses should not be omitted, increased, or decreased without advice of physician.
- A calibrated dosage applicator should be dispensed with the vaginal cream. Inform the patient.
- Intravaginal administration: If patient is to administer medication to herself, instruct her to wash her hands well before and after the application, and to avoid contact of denuded areas with the cream. Also tell her not to use tam-

pons while on vaginal cream therapy.
- Caution patient to report adverse symptoms of estrogen therapy to the physician promptly.
- Risk of blood clot formation is high with morning after pill. Discuss signs of thrombophlebitis (see Appendix G).
- Review package insert with patient to ensure understanding of estrogen therapy.

ESTROGENS, ESTERIFIED

Trade names: Estratab, Menest, Menrium, Neo-Estrone ♣
Classifications: HORMONE; ESTROGEN
Prototype: Estradiol
Pregnancy category: X

ACTIONS/PHARMACODYNAMICS Combination of same estrogens as found in conjugated estrogens (but in different proportions): sodium estrone sulfate and sodium equilin sulfate. Binds to intracellular receptors that stimulate DNA and RNA to synthesize proteins responsible for effects of estrogen.

USES Atrophic vaginitis, kraurosis vulvae and abnormal bleeding (hormonal imbalance), female hypogonadism, castration, primary ovarian failure, vasomotor symptoms associated with menopause, palliative therapy of breast and prostatic carcinomas; prevention of osteoporosis.

ROUTE & DOSAGE

Menopause
Adult: **PO** 0.3–1.25 mg/d for 21 d each month; adjust to lowest level that gives symptom control (≤0.625 mg/d).

Female Hypogonadism, Primary Ovarian Failure, Female Castration
Adult: **PO** 2.5–7.5 mg/d in 1–3 divided doses for 20 d followed by a 10-d rest period; during last 5 d of estrogen, give a PO progestin.

Breast Cancer
Adult: **PO** 10 mg t.i.d. for 2–3 mo.

Prostatic Cancer (palliation)
Adult: **PO** 1.25–2.5 mg t.i.d. for several weeks.

Prevention of Osteoporosis
Adult: 0.3 mg q.d.

CONTRAINDICATIONS & PRECAUTIONS **Contraindicated in:** breast cancer; known or suspected pregnancy (category X). **Cautious use in:** hypertension; gallbladder disease; diabetes mellitus; heart failure; hepatic or renal dysfunction; history of thromboembolic disease.

ADVERSE/SIDE EFFECTS **CNS:** headache, dizziness, depression, *libido changes*. **CV:** <u>thromboembolic disorders</u>, hypertension. **GI:** *nausea*, vomiting, diarrhea, bloating, cholestatic jaundice. **GU:** mastodynia, spotting, changes in menstrual flow, dysmenorrhea, amenorrhea. **Metabolic:** reduced carbohydrate tolerance, fluid retention. **Other:** leg cramps, intolerance to contact lenses.

DRUG INTERACTIONS **Carbamazepine, phenytoin, rifampin** decrease estrogen levels because they increase its metabolism; may enhance steroid effects of CORTICOSTEROIDS; may decrease anticoagulant effects of ORAL ANTICOAGULANTS.

NURSING IMPLICATIONS

See numerous nursing implications under estradiol.

Administration

- Tablet can be taken with food or fluid of patient's choice.
- Esterified estrogens are given cyclically, except when used for palliation of cancer.
- Store tablets at 15–30C (59–86F) in a tightly closed container.

Patient & Family Education

- Be certain patient is aware of importance of taking drug exactly as prescribed: specifically, doses should not be omitted, increased, or decreased without advice of physician. Patient should also be made aware of what to do when a dose is missed.
- Review package insert with patient to ensure understanding of estrogen therapy.

ESTRONE

(ess'trone)

Trade name: Femogen ✱

ESTRONE AQUEOUS SUSPENSION

Trade names: Estronol, Femogen Forte✱, Kestrone-5, Theelin Aqueous

ESTROGENIC SUBSTANCE AQUEOUS SUSPENSION

Trade name: Estroject-2

Classifications: HORMONE; ESTROGEN

Prototype: Estradiol

Pregnancy category: X

ACTIONS/PHARMACODYNAMICS First sex hormone isolated in pure form; present in urine of pregnant mares along with other estrogens. Binds to intracellular receptors that stimulate DNA and RNA to synthesize proteins responsible for effects of estrogen.

USES Atrophic vaginitis, kraurosis vulvae, and abnormal bleeding (hormonal imbalance); also female hypogonadism, primary ovarian failure, vasomotor symptoms associated with menopause, and as palliative therapy of prostatic carcinoma.

ROUTE & DOSAGE

Menopause

Adult: **IM** 0.1–0.5 mg 2–3 times/wk.

Female Hypogonadism, Primary Ovarian Failure

Adult: **IM** 0.1–1 mg/wk in single or divided doses.

Inoperable Prostatic Cancer (palliation)

Adult: **IM** 2–4 mg/d 2–3 times/wk.

CONTRAINDICATIONS & PRECAUTIONS **Contraindicated in:** breast cancer; known or suspected pregnancy (category X). **Cautious use in:** hypertension; gallbladder disease; diabetes mellitus; heart failure; hepatic or renal dysfunction; history of thromboembolic disease.

ADVERSE/SIDE EFFECTS **CNS:** headache, dizziness, depression, *libido changes*. **CV:** <u>thromboembolic disorders</u>, hypertension. **GI:** *nausea*, vomiting, diarrhea, bloating, cholestatic jaundice. **GU:** mastodynia, spotting, changes in menstrual flow, dysmenorrhea, amenorrhea. **Metabolic:** reduced carbohydrate tolerance, fluid retention. **Other:** leg cramps, intolerance to contact lenses.

DRUG INTERACTIONS **Carbamazepine, phenytoin, rifampin** decrease estrogen levels because they increase its metabolism; may enhance steroid effects of CORTICOSTEROIDS; may decrease anticoagulant effects of ORAL ANTICOAGULANTS.

NURSING IMPLICATIONS

See numerous nursing implications under estradiol.

Administration
- Shake vial and syringe well to suspend medication before withdrawing and injecting medication.
- Store at 15–30C (59–86F) unless otherwise directed by manufacturer. Protect from light and from freezing.

Assessment & Drug Effects
- Patients with conditions that may be influenced by fluid retention (migraine, cardiac or renal dysfunction, asthma, epilepsy, hypertension) should be monitored carefully. Check BP on a regular basis.
- Spotting or breakthrough bleeding occurring when a barbiturate and estrone are taken concurrently indicates reduced availability of the estrogen.

Patient & Family Education
- Review package insert with patient to assure understanding of estrogen therapy.
- Advise patient to determine weight under standard conditions 1 or 2 times/wk and to report sudden weight gain or other signs of fluid retention.
- Instruct patient to report positive Homan's sign and the following symptoms of thromboembolic disorders immediately: tenderness, swelling, and redness in extremity; sudden, severe headache or chest pain; slurring of speech; change in vision; sudden shortness of breath.
- Symptoms of vaginal candidiasis (thick, white, curdlike secretions and inflamed, congested introitus) should be reported to permit appropriate treatment.
- Advise patient to report severe abdominal pain and tenderness or abdominal mass.

ESTROPIPATE

(es-troe-pi′pate)

Trade name: Ogen

Classifications: HORMONE; ESTROGEN

Prototype: Estradiol

Pregnancy category: X

ACTIONS/PHARMACODYNAMICS

Water-soluble preparation of pure crystalline estrone (responsible for therapeutic actions conjugated as the sulfate and stabilized with piperazine). Binds to intracellular receptors that stimulate DNA and RNA to synthesize proteins responsible for effects of estrogen.

USES Atrophic vaginitis, kraurosis vulvae, and abnormal bleeding (hormonal imbalance); also female hypogonadism, primary ovarian failure, vasomotor symptoms associated with menopause, and as palliative therapy of prostatic carcinoma.

ROUTE & DOSAGE

Menopause, Atrophic Vaginitis, Kraurosis Vulvae

Adult: **PO** 0.75–6 mg/d for 21 d each month; adjust to lowest level that gives symptom control. **Intravaginal** 2–4 g of cream once/d in a cyclic regimen.

Female Hypogonadism, Primary Ovarian Failure, Female Castration

Adult: **PO** 1.5–9 mg/d in 1–3 divided doses for 21 d, followed by an 8–10-d drug-free period.

CONTRAINDICATIONS & PRECAUTIONS **Contraindicated in:** estrogen hypersensitivity, breast cancer, known or suspected pregnancy (category X). **Cautious use in:** hypertension; gallbladder disease; diabetes mellitus; heart failure; hepatic or renal dysfunction; history of thromboembolic disease.

E

ADVERSE/SIDE EFFECTS **CNS:** headache, dizziness, depression, *libido changes*. **CV:** thromboembolic disorders, hypertension. **GI:** *nausea*, vomiting, diarrhea, bloating, cholestatic jaundice. **GU:** mastodynia, spotting, changes in menstrual flow, dysmenorrhea, amenorrhea. **Metabolic:** reduced carbohydrate tolerance, fluid retention. **Other:** leg cramps, intolerance to contact lenses.

DRUG INTERACTIONS **Carbamazepine, phenytoin, rifampin** decrease estrogen levels because they increase its metabolism; may enhance steroid effects of CORTICOSTEROIDS; may decrease anticoagulant effects of ORAL ANTICOAGULANTS.

NURSING IMPLICATIONS

See numerous nursing implications under estradiol.

Administration

- Tablet may be taken with food or fluid of patient's choice.
- Vaginal cream is dispensed with a calibrated dosage applicator. Squeeze tube of cream to force sufficient amount into applicator so that number on plunger indicating prescribed dose is level with top of barrel.
- Store in tightly closed containers at 15–30C (59–86F) unless otherwise directed.

Patient & Family Education

- Between uses, pull plunger out of barrel and wash applicator in warm soapy water. Do not place plunger in hot or boiling water.
- Warn patient not to use tampons while on vaginal cream therapy.
- If patient is to administer medication to herself, instruct her to wash her hands well before and after the procedure.
- Sudden discontinuation of vaginal cream after high dosage or prolonged use may evoke withdrawal bleeding.
- Review patient package insert (PPI) with patient.

ETANERCEPT

(e-tan'er-cept)

Trade name: Enbrel

Classifications: IMMUNOMODULATOR; TUMOR NECROSIS FACTOR (TNF) RECEPTOR ANTAGONIST

Pregnancy category: B

ACTIONS/PHARMACODYNAMICS Produced by recombinant DNA technology. Binds specifically to tumor necrosis factor (TNF) and blocks it from attaching to cell surface TNF receptors. TNF is a naturally occurring cytokine (e.g., IL-6) that is part of the normal immune and inflammatory response. TNF mediates inflammation and modulates cellular immune responses. Elevated levels of TNF are found in the synovial fluids of rheumatoid arthritis (RA) patients.

USES Reduction of the signs and symptoms of RA in patients with inadequate response to other disease-modifying antirheumatic drugs.

ROUTE & DOSAGE

Rheumatoid Arthritis

Adult: **SC** 25 mg twice weekly.
Child >4y: **SC** 0.4 mg/kg (max 25 mg/dose) twice weekly.

PHARMACOKINETICS Onset: 1–2 wk. **Peak:** 72 h. **Elimination:** half-life: 115 h.

CONTRAINDICATIONS & PRECAUTIONS Contraindicated in: patients with sepsis; hypersensitivity to etanercept; malignancy; lactation. **Cautious use in:** immunosuppression; pregnancy (category B). Safety and efficacy in children < 4 y of age have not been studied.

ADVERSE/SIDE EFFECTS Body as whole: asthenia. **CNS:** headache, dizziness, cerebral ischemia, depression. **CV:** heart failure, MI, myocardial ischemia, hypertension, hypotension. **GI:** abdominal pain, dyspepsia, cholecystitis, pancreatitis, GI hemorrhage. **Respiratory:** rhinitis, URI, pharyngitis, cough, respiratory disorder, sinusitus, dyspnea. **Skin:** rash. **Other:** *infection,* bursitis. **Injection site reactions:** *erythema, itching, pain, swelling.*

NURSING IMPLICATIONS

Administration

- Do not administer to a patient who has known or suspected sepsis.
- Reconstitute by slowly injecting the supplied diluent into the vial. Swirl gently to dissolve and do not shake. Reconstituted solution should be clear and colorless. Use within 6 h of reconstitution.
- Inject SC into thigh, abdomen, upper arm; rotate injection sites and never inject into an old injection site or where skin is tender, bruised, red, or hard.
- Reconstituted solution may be stored for up to 6 h refrigerated at 2–8C (36–46F). Unopened dose tray must be stored refrigerated at 2–8C (36–46F).

Assessment & Drug Effects

- Therapeutic effectiveness is indicated by improved RA symptomatology.
- Carefully monitor for and immediately report S&S of infection.

Patient & Family Education

- Women should not nurse their infants while on etanercept.
- Discard all needles and syringes after use; do not reuse.
- If you develop an infection or are exposed to varicella virus, withhold etanercept and notify your prescriber before resuming the drug.
- Vaccinations, in general, and live vaccines, in particular, should be avoided while on etanercept.
- Injection site reactions (e.g., redness, pain, swelling) are common in the first month of therapy but generally decrease over time.

ETHACRYNIC ACID

(eth-a-krin'ik)

Trade name: Edecrin

ETHACRYNATE SODIUM

Trade name: Sodium Edecrin

Classifications: ELECTROLYTIC AND WATER BALANCE AGENT; LOOP DIURETIC

Prototype: Furosemide

Pregnancy category: B

ACTIONS/PHARMACODYNAMICS Has rapid and potent diuretic action. Action mechanism is unclear. Inhibits sodium and chloride reabsorption in proximal tubule and most segments of loop of Henle, promotes potassium and hydrogen ion excretion, and decreases urinary ammonium ion concentration and pH. Promotes calcium elimination in hypercalcemia and nephrogenic diabetes insipidus. Fluid-electrolyte loss may exceed that caused by thiazides, but the effect on carbohydrate metabolism and blood glucose is less. Hypotensive effect may be due to hypovolemia secondary to diuresis and in part to decreased vascular resistance.

USES Severe edema associated with CHF, hepatic cirrhosis, ascites of malignancy, renal disease, nephrotic syndrome, lymphedema. **Unlabeled uses:** treatment of nephrogenic diabetes insipidus, hypercalcemia, mild to moderate hypertension, and as adjunct in therapy of hypertensive crisis complicated by pulmonary edema.

ROUTE & DOSAGE

Edema

Adult: **PO** 50–100 mg 1–2 times/d; may increase by 25–50 mg prn up to 400 mg/d; **IV** 0.5–1 mg/kg or 50 mg up to 100 mg; may repeat if necessary.
Child: **PO** 1 mg/kg q.d.; may increase to 3 mg/kg/d.

PHARMACOKINETICS **Absorption:** rapidly absorbed from GI tract. **Onset:** 30 min PO; 5 min IV. **Peak:** 2 h PO; 15–30 min IV. **Duration:** 6–8 h PO; 2 h IV. **Distribution:** does not cross CSF. **Metabolism:** metabolized to cysteine conjugate. **Elimination:** half-life: 30–70 min; 30–65% excreted in urine; 35–40% excreted in bile.

CONTRAINDICATIONS & PRECAUTIONS **Contraindicated in:** history of hypersensitivity to ethacrynic acid; increasing azotemia, anuria; hepatic coma; severe diarrhea, dehydration, electrolyte imbalance, hypotension; pregnancy (category B), nursing mothers, infants, parenteral use in pediatric patients. **Cautious use in:** hepatic cirrhosis; elderly cardiac patients; diabetes mellitus; history of gout; pulmonary edema associated with acute MI; hyperaldosteronism; nephrotic syndrome; history of pancreatitis.

ADVERSE/SIDE EFFECTS **CNS:** headache, fatigue, apprehension, confusion. **CV:** *postural hypotension* (dizziness, light-headedness). **Electrolyte imbalance:** hyponatremia, *hypokalemia,* hypochloremic alkalosis, hypomagnesemia, hypocalcemia, hypercalciuria, hyperuricemia, hypovolemia. **ENT:** vertigo, tinnitus, sense of fullness in ears, temporary or permanent deafness. **GI:** anorexia, diarrhea, nausea, vomiting, dysphagia, abdominal discomfort or pain, GI bleeding (IV use), abnormal liver function tests. **Hematologic:** <u>thrombocytopenia</u>, <u>agranulocytosis</u> (rare), <u>severe neutropenia</u> (rare). **Skin:** skin rash, pruritus. **Other:** hematuria, glycosuria, hyperglycemia, gynecomastia, fever, chills, acute gout; elevated BUN, creatinine, and urate levels; local irritation and thrombophlebitis with IV injection.

DRUG INTERACTIONS THIAZIDE DIURETICS increase potassium loss; increased risk of **digoxin** toxicity from hypokalemia; CORTICOSTEROIDS, **amphotericin B** increase risk of hypokalemia; decreased **lithium** clearance, so increased risk of lithium toxicity; SULFONYLUREA effect may be blunted, causing hyperglycemia; ANTIHYPERTENSIVE AGENTS increase risk of orthostatic hypotension; AMINOGLYCOSIDES may increase risk of ototoxicity; **warfarin** potentiates hypoprothrombinemia.

INCOMPATIBILITIES **Solution/additive: hydralazine, procainamide, tolazoline, triflupromazine.**

NURSING IMPLICATIONS

Administration

- Administer PO drug after a meal or food to prevent gastric irritation.

- Schedule doses to avoid nocturia and thus sleep interference. Avoid administration within at least 4 h of bedtime, if possible. This recommendation may not apply to the patient who accumulates fluid and develops respiratory symptoms during sleep.
- Reconstitute for IV administration by adding 50 ml of 5% dextrose injection or 0.9% of NaCl injection to vial. Solution should be used within 24 h. Discard cloudy solutions.
- Give IV dose slowly into tubing of a running infusion of compatible IV fluid or by direct IV injection over several minutes.
- If a second IV dose is required, a new site should be selected to prevent thrombophlebitis.
- Store oral tablet and parenteral dosage form at 15–30C (59–86F) unless otherwise directed.

Assessment & Drug Effects

- Patient should be observed closely when receiving the drug by IV infusion. Rapid, copious diuresis following IV administration can produce hypotension.
- Extravasation of IV drug causes local pain and tissue irritation from dehydration and blood volume depletion.
- Monitor BP during initial therapy. Because orthostatic hypotension can occur, supervision of ambulation is indicated.
- For patients with impaired cardiac function, monitor BP and pulse throughout therapy. Diuretic-induced hypovolemia may reduce cardiac output, and electrolyte loss promotes cardiotoxicity in those receiving digitalis (cardiac) glycosides.
- Establish baseline weight prior to start of therapy; weigh patient under standard conditions. Keep physician informed of weight loss or gain in excess of 1 kg (2 lb)/d.
- Monitor I&O ratio. Drug should be discontinued if excessive diuresis, oliguria, hematuria, or sudden profuse diarrhea occurs. Report signs to physician.
- Baseline and periodic determinations should be made of blood count, serum electrolytes, CO_2, BUN, creatinine, blood sugar, uric acid, and liver function.
- Observe for and report warning signs and symptoms of electrolyte imbalance: anorexia, nausea, vomiting, thirst, dry mouth, polyuria, oliguria, weakness, fatigue, dizziness, faintness, headache, muscle cramps, paresthesias, drowsiness, mental confusion. Instruct patient to report these symptoms promptly to physician.
- Report immediately possible signs of thromboembolic complications (see Appendix G).
- In patients receiving any other potentially ototoxic drug concurrently with ethacrynic acid, renal status, audiograms, and vestibular function tests are advised before initiation of therapy and regularly throughout therapy.
- Impaired glucose tolerance with hyperglycemia and glycosuria has occurred in patients receiving doses in excess of 200 mg/d.

Patient & Family Education

- Teach patient signs and symptoms of hypokalemia and hyponatremia (see Appendix G), and advise patient to report any of these promptly.
- Caution patient to make position changes slowly, particularly from recumbent to upright posture.
- GI side effects occur most frequently after 1–3 mo of PO therapy or in patients on high dosage. The onset of loose stools or other

GI symptoms at any time during therapy should be reported to permit dosage adjustment or discontinuation of drug if indicated.

- Report immediately any evidence of impaired hearing. Hearing loss may be preceded by vertigo, tinnitus, or fullness in ears; it may be transient, lasting 1–24 h, or it may be permanent.

E

ETHAMBUTOL HYDROCHLORIDE

(e-tham′byoo-tole)

Trade names: Etibi♣, Myambutol

Classifications: ANTIINFECTIVE; ANTITUBERCULOSIS AGENT

Prototype: Isoniazid

Pregnancy category: B

ACTIONS/PHARMACODYNAMICS Synthetic antituberculosis agent with bacteriostatic action. Mode of action not completely understood, but it appears to inhibit RNA synthesis and thus arrests multiplication of tubercle bacilli. Not recommended for use as sole agent. The emergence of resistant strains is delayed by administering ethambutol in combination with other antituberculosis drugs.

USE In conjunction with at least one other antituberculosis agent in treatment of pulmonary tuberculosis. **Unlabeled use:** atypical mycobacterial infections.

ROUTE & DOSAGE

Tuberculosis

Adult: **PO** 15 mg/kg q24h; for retreatment start with 25 mg/kg/d for 60 d; then decrease to 15 mg/kg/d.
Child 6–12 y: **PO** 10–15 mg/kg/d.

PHARMACOKINETICS Absorption: 70–80% absorbed from GI tract. **Peak:** 2–4 h. **Distribution:** distributes to most body tissues; highest concentrations in erythrocytes, kidney, lungs, saliva; crosses placenta; distributed into breast milk. **Metabolism:** metabolized in liver. **Elimination:** half-life: 3–4 h; 50% excreted in urine within 24 h; 20–22% excreted in feces.

CONTRAINDICATIONS & PRECAUTIONS Contraindicated in: optic neuritis; children <13 y. Safe use during pregnancy (category B) not established. **Cautious use in:** patients with renal impairment; gout; ocular defects (e.g., cataract, recurrent ocular inflammatory conditions, diabetic retinopathy).

ADVERSE/SIDE EFFECTS CNS: headache, dizziness, confusion, hallucinations, paresthesias, joint pains. **Eye:** ocular toxicity: *retrobulbar optic neuritis;* possibility of anterior optic neuritis with decrease in visual acuity, temporary loss of vision, constriction of visual fields, red–green color blindness, central and peripheral scotomas, eye pain, photophobia; retinal hemorrhage and edema. **GI:** anorexia, nausea, vomiting, abdominal pain. **Hypersensitivity:** pruritus, dermatitis, anaphylaxis.

NURSING IMPLICATIONS

Administration

- Ethambutol may be taken with food if GI irritation occurs.
- Protect ethambutol from light, moisture, and excessive heat. Store in tightly closed container at 15–30C (59–86F) unless otherwise directed.

Assessment & Drug Effects

- Culture and susceptibility tests should be performed before initiation of therapy and repeated periodically throughout therapy.

- Ocular toxicity generally appears within 1–7 mo after start of therapy. Symptoms usually disappear within several weeks to months after drug is discontinued, depending on degree of ocular damage.
- Ophthalmoscopic examination should be performed prior to start of therapy and at monthly intervals during therapy. Eyes should be tested separately as well as together.
- Monitor I&O ratio in patients with renal impairment. Report oliguria or any significant changes in ratio or in laboratory reports of renal function. Systemic accumulation with toxicity can result from delayed drug excretion.
- Hepatic and renal function tests, blood cell counts, and serum uric acid determinations should be performed at regular intervals throughout therapy.

Patient & Family Education

- Emphasize importance of adhering to drug regimen and of keeping follow-up appointments.
- In general, therapy may continue for 1–2 y or longer, although shorter treatment regimens have been used with success.
- Advise patient to report promptly to physician the onset of blurred vision, changes in color perception, constriction of visual fields, or any other visual symptoms. Patient should be questioned periodically about eyes.

ETHAVERINE HYDROCHLORIDE

(e′tha-ve-rine)

Trade names: Ethaquin, Ethatab, Ethavex-100, Isovex

Classifications: CARDIOVASCULAR AGENT; NONNITRATE VASODILATOR

Prototype: Hydralazine hydrochloride

Pregnancy category: C

ACTIONS/PHARMACODYNAMICS

Ethaverine is an alkaloid prepared synthetically from opium. It has no narcotic properties. It directly relaxes all smooth muscles, especially when they have been spasmodically contracted. When spasm is present, action is especially pronounced on coronary, cerebral, pulmonary, and peripheral arteries. Like quinidine, acts directly on myocardium, depresses conduction and irritability, and prolongs refractory period. Relaxes smooth muscles of bronchi, GI tract, ureters, and biliary system.

USES Primarily for peripheral and cerebral vascular insufficiency associated with arterial spasm; also a smooth muscle spasmolytic in spastic conditions of the GI and GU tracts.

ROUTE & DOSAGE

Peripheral and Cerebral Vascular Insufficiency

Adult: **PO** 100 mg t.i.d.; may increase up to 200 mg t.i.d.

PHARMACOKINETICS Absorption: readily absorbed from GI tract. **Peak:** 1–2 h. **Duration:** 6 h regular tablets. **Metabolism:** metabolized in liver. **Elimination:** excreted in urine chiefly as metabolites.

CONTRAINDICATIONS & PRECAUTIONS Contraindicated in: complete atrioventricular dissociation (AV heart block) and severe hepatic disease. **Cautious use in:** patients with glaucoma, pregnancy (category C), nursing mothers, and myocardial depression.

ADVERSE/SIDE EFFECTS CNS: vertigo, *headache, drowsiness.* **CV:** *hy-*

potension, arrhythmias. **GI:** nausea, anorexia, abdominal distress, dry throat. **Other:** malaise, *flushing,* sweating, lassitude, respiratory depression.

DRUG INTERACTIONS May decrease **levodopa** effectiveness; **morphine** may antagonize smooth muscle relaxation effect of ethaverine.

NURSING IMPLICATIONS

Administration

- Monitor heart rate (apical pulse for 1 full minute) and BP; if significant changes occur (e.g., hypotension, arrhythmias), withhold drug and notify physician.
- Preserve in a tightly covered, light-resistant container.

Assessment & Drug Effects

- Routinely monitor apical pulse for changes in rate and rhythm. Drug may cause cardiac arrhythmias.
- Monitor BP for hypotension, and respiration rate for respiratory depression. Promptly report marked changed to physician.
- Liver function and blood tests should be performed periodically. Hepatotoxicity (thought to be a hypersensitivity reaction) is reversible with prompt drug withdrawal.

Patient & Family Education

- Since drug may cause dizziness and drowsiness, advise patients to avoid driving and potentially hazardous tasks until reaction to drug is known.
- Warn patient that alcohol may increase drowsiness and dizziness.
- Instruct patient to notify physician if jaundice or skin rash appear. Hepatic function tests may be indicated.
- Inform patient that drug may cause flushing, headache, and diaphoresis; physician should be notified if symptoms are pronounced.
- Advise patient to notify physician if GI distress develops and persists.

ETHCHLORVYNOL

(eth-klor-vi′nole)

Trade name: Placidyl

Classifications: CNS AGENT; ANXIOLYTIC; SEDATIVE-HYPNOTIC; BARBITURATE

Prototype: Secobarbital

Pregnancy category: C

Controlled substance: Schedule IV

ACTIONS/PHARMACODYNAMICS CNS depressant effects similar to those of chloral hydrate and barbiturates. Mechanism of action not known. Hypnotic doses produce cerebral depression and quiet, deep sleep; sedative doses reduce anxiety and apprehension. Also exhibits anticonvulsant and muscle relaxant activity. Has no analgesic properties. Effect on REM sleep not known. Not commonly used as a sedative because of its short duration of action.

USE Short-term therapy of simple insomnia for periods up to 1 wk.

ROUTE & DOSAGE

Sedative

Adult: **PO** 200 mg b.i.d. or t.i.d.

Hypnotic

Adult: **PO** 500 mg–1 g h.s.; may give an additional 200 mg if patient awakens early.

PHARMACOKINETICS Absorption: readily absorbed from GI tract. **Onset:** 15–30 min. **Peak:** 1–2 h. **Duration:** 5 h. **Distribution:** localizes in adipose tissue, liver, kidney, spleen, brain, CSF, bile; crosses placenta; distribution into breast milk unknown. **Metabolism:** metabolized in liver with enterohepatic cycling and possibly in kidney. **Elimination:** half-life: 20–100 h; 10% excreted in urine within 24 h.

CONTRAINDICATIONS & PRECAUTIONS **Contraindicated in:** porphyria; patients with uncontrolled pain; first and second trimesters of pregnancy (category C). Safe use in nursing mothers and in children not established. **Cautious use in:** third trimester of pregnancy; patients with mental depression or suicidal tendencies, addiction-prone individuals; impaired hepatic or renal function; elderly or debilitated patients; patients who respond unpredictably to alcohol or barbiturates.

ADVERSE/SIDE EFFECTS **CNS:** dizziness, facial numbness, headache, mild hangover, nightmares, coma, respiratory failure. **Eye:** blurred vision. **GI:** nausea, vomiting, aftertaste. **Hypersensitivity:** urticaria. **Other:** muscle weakness, tremors.

DIAGNOSTIC TEST INTERFERENCE ***Phentolamine test:*** false-positive test results (ethchlorvynol should be withdrawn at least 24 h before the test).

DRUG INTERACTIONS **Alcohol** and other CNS DEPRESSANTS amplify CNS depression; decrease anticoagulation effect of ORAL ANTICOAGULANTS.

NURSING IMPLICATIONS

Administration

- Ethchlorvynol produces transient giddiness and ataxia in some patients who apparently absorb the drug rapidly. Symptoms may be minimized by administering the drug with milk or other food.
- Preserve in tight, light-resistant containers (darkens on exposure to light; slight darkening does not affect potency). Store at 15–30C (59–86F) unless otherwise directed.

Assessment & Drug Effects

- Report the appearance of mental confusion, hallucinations, or drowsiness in patients receiving daytime sedation; decrease in dosage or drug discontinuation is indicated.
- The elderly may not tolerate average adult doses. Observe intensity and duration of drug action.
- Severe withdrawal symptoms may occur if drug is discontinued abruptly in patients taking regular doses.

Patient & Family Education

- Caution patient to avoid driving or engaging in other activities requiring mental alertness and physical coordination for at least 5 h after taking drug.
- Psychological and physical dependence is possible; therefore, prolonged administration is not recommended. Urge patient to adhere to established drug regimen.

ETHINYL ESTRADIOL

(eth′in-il ess-tra-dye′ole)

Trade names: Estinyl, Feminone

Classifications: HORMONE; ESTROGEN

Prototype: Estradiol

Pregnancy category: X

ACTIONS/PHARMACODYNAMICS Oral estrogen with actions similar to those of estradiol. Given cyclically for short-term use. Binds to intracellular receptors that stimulate DNA and RNA to synthesize proteins responsible for effects of estrogen.

USES Moderate to severe vasomotor symptoms associated with menopause; also postmenopausal osteoporosis, female gonadism, and as palliation for inoperable, metastatic cancer of female breast (at least 5 y postmenopause) and of the prostate. **Unlabeled use:** postcoital contraceptive.

ROUTE & DOSAGE

Menopause, Postmenopausal Osteoporosis

Adult: **PO** 0.02–0.05 mg/d for 21 d each month; adjust to lowest level that gives symptom control.

Female Hypogonadism

Adult: **PO** 0.05 mg 1–3 times/d for 2 wk, followed by 2 wk of progestin; continue this regimen for 3–6 mo.

Breast Cancer

Adult: **PO** 1 mg t.i.d. for 2–3 mo.

Prostatic Cancer (palliation)

Adult: **PO** 0.15–2 mg/d.

Postcoital Contraceptive

Adult: **PO** 5 mg/d for 5 consecutive days beginning within 72 h of coitus.

CONTRAINDICATIONS & PRECAUTIONS **Contraindicated in:** breast cancer, known or suspected pregnancy (category X). **Cautious use in:** hypertension; gallbladder disease; diabetes mellitus; heart failure; hepatic or renal dysfunction, history of thromboembolic disease.

ADVERSE/SIDE EFFECTS **CNS:** headache, dizziness, depression, *libido changes*. **CV:** thromboembolic disorders, hypertension. **GI:** *nausea,* vomiting, diarrhea, anorexia, weight changes, bloating, cholestatic jaundice. **GU:** mastodynia, breakthrough bleeding, changes in menstrual flow, dysmenorrhea, amenorrhea; in men: impotence, gynecomastia, testicular atrophy. **Metabolic:** reduced carbohydrate tolerance, fluid retention. **Other:** leg cramps, edema, intolerance to contact lenses.

DRUG INTERACTIONS **Carbamazepine, phenytoin, rifampin** decrease estrogen levels because they increase its metabolism; may enhance steroid effects of CORTICOSTEROIDS; may decrease anticoagulant effects of ORAL ANTICOAGULANTS.

NURSING IMPLICATIONS

Administration

- Tablet may be taken with food or fluid of patient's choice.
- Morning-after pill: When used as an emergency postcoital contraceptive, as for rape or for incest, drug is started within 24 h and not later than 72 h after sexual exposure. A pregnancy test is performed before dosing.
- Store at 15–30C (59–86F) in tight, light-resistant container.

Assessment & Drug Effects

- Patients with conditions that may be influenced by fluid retention (migraine, cardiac or renal dysfunction, asthma, epilepsy, hypertension) should be monitored carefully. Check BP on a regular basis.
- Pyridoxine (vitamin B_6) levels are lowered by estrogens. A supplement may be ordered for the patient on long-term therapy, especially if undernourished.

Patient & Family Education

- Be certain patient understands dose schedule and regimen. She should understand what to do if a dose is missed.
- Risk of blood clot formation is

high. Instruct patient to report immediately positive Homan's sign and the following symptoms of thromboembolic disorders: tenderness, pain, swelling, and redness in extremity; sudden, severe headache or chest pain, slurring of speech; change in vision; sudden shortness of breath. If physician is not available, patient should go to the nearest hospital emergency room.

- Advise patient to report severe abdominal pain and tenderness, or abdominal mass.
- Advise patient to determine weight under standard conditions 1 or 2 times/wk and to report sudden weight gain or other signs of fluid retention.
- A low-salt diet and diuretic may be prescribed to reduce cyclic fluid retention.
- History of jaundice in pregnancy increases the possibility of estrogen-induced jaundice. Instruct patient to report yellow skin and sclera, pruritus, dark urine, and light-colored stools. Estrogen therapy is usually interrupted pending clinical investigation.
- High vitamin C intake (e.g., 1 g/d) may increase ethinyl estradiol levels. Abrupt withdrawal of vitamin C may lead to breakthrough bleeding.
- Symptoms of vaginal candidiasis (thick, white, curdlike secretions and inflamed congested introitus) should be reported to permit appropriate treatment.
- Reassure male patients that estrogen-induced feminization and impotence are reversible with termination of therapy.
- Estrogenic depression of caffeine metabolism may cause caffeinism. Urge patient to decrease caffeine intake from sources such as tea, coffee, and cola.

ETHIONAMIDE

(e-thye-on-am′ide)

Trade name: Trecator-SC

Classifications: ANTIINFECTIVE; ANTITUBERCULOSIS AGENT; ANTILEPROSY (SULFONE) AGENT

Prototype: Isoniazid

Pregnancy category: D

E

ACTIONS/PHARMACODYNAMICS

Bacteriostatic or bactericidal depending on concentration used and susceptibility of organism. Effective against human and bovine strains of *Mycobacterium tuberculosis* and against of *Mycobacterium kansasii* and some strains of *Mycobacterium avium-intracellulare* complex. Also active against *Mycobacterium leprae.* Emergence of resistant strains may be delayed or prevented when administered concurrently with other antituberculosis drugs.

USES Any form of active tuberculosis when treatment with primary antituberculosis drugs (e.g., isoniazid, streptomycin, ethambutol, rifampin) has failed. Must be given with at least one other effective antituberculosis agent. **Unlabeled use:** atypical mycobacterial infections and tuberculous meningitis.

ROUTE & DOSAGE

Tuberculosis

Adult: **PO** 0.5–1 g/d divided q8–12h.
Child: **PO** 15–20 mg/kg/d in 2–3 equally divided doses (max 1 g/d).

PHARMACOKINETICS **Absorption:** 80% absorbed from GI tract. **Peak:** 3 h. **Duration:** 9 h. **Distribution:** widely distributed including CSF; crosses placenta; distribution into breast milk unknown. **Metabolism:** metabolized in liver. **Elimination:** half-life: 3 h; excreted in urine.

CONTRAINDICATIONS & PRECAUTIONS **Contraindicated in:** hypersensitivity to ethionamide and chemically related drugs, e.g., isoniazid, niacin (nicotinamide); severe hepatic damage. Safe use during pregnancy (category D), by nursing mothers or by children, and in women of childbearing potential not established. **Cautious use in:** diabetes mellitus, hepatic dysfunction.

ADVERSE/SIDE EFFECTS **CNS:** headache, restlessness, mental depression, drowsiness, dizziness, ataxia, hallucinations, paresthesias, convulsions. **GI:** dose related and frequent; symptoms may be due to CNS stimulation rather than to GI irritation: anorexia, *epigastric distress, nausea, vomiting,* metallic taste, *diarrhea,* stomatitis, sialorrhea. **Hepatic:** elevated ALT, AST; hepatitis (with jaundice). **Other:** postural hypotension, menorrhagia, impotence, hypothyroidism.

DRUG INTERACTIONS **Cycloserine, isoniazid** may increase neurotoxic effects.

NURSING IMPLICATIONS

Administration

- GI side effects may be minimized by taking drug with or after meals. Some patients tolerate ethionamide best when it is taken as a single dose after the evening meal or as a single dose at bedtime. (GI symptoms appear to increase with divided doses, although serum concentrations may be higher.)
- About 50% of patients cannot tolerate a single dose larger than 500 mg because of GI side effects. An antiemetic is sometimes prescribed, but if symptoms persist, drug should be discontinued.
- Physician may prescribe pyridoxine (vitamin B_6) concurrently to prevent or relieve peripheral neuritis and other neurotoxic effects.
- Store in a cool, dry place at 8–15C (46–59F) in a tightly closed container unless otherwise directed.

Assessment & Drug Effects

- Culture and susceptibility tests should be made before start of therapy.
- Report onset of skin rash. Progression to exfoliative dermatitis can occur if drug is not promptly discontinued.
- Liver function tests (AST and ALT), CBC, and renal function tests including urinalysis should be done prior to and every 2–4 wk during therapy.
- This drug may make it difficult to manage blood glucose levels in the diabetic. Alert the patient to monitor blood glucose closely until response to the drug is established. These patients appear to be especially prone to hepatotoxicity (see Appendix G).

Patient & Family Education

- Because ethionamide may increase potential for hepatic dysfunction, physician may suggest moderation or elimination of alcohol ingestion.
- Hepatotoxicity is generally reversible if drug is promptly withdrawn. Instruct patient to report onset of signs or symptoms (see Appendix G).
- Caution patient who is experiencing postural hypotension to make position changes slowly and in stages, particularly from recumbent to upright posture.

ETHOSUXIMIDE

(eth-oh-sux'i-mide)

Trade name: Zarontin

Common side effect in *italic,* life-threatening effects underlined: generic names in **bold;** drug class in SMALL CAPS

Prototype for classifications: CNS AGENT; SUCCINIMIDE ANTICONVULSANT
Pregnancy category: C

ACTIONS/PHARMACODYNAMICS Succinimide anticonvulsant. Reduces frequency of epileptiform attacks, apparently by depressing motor cortex and elevating CNS threshold to stimuli. Usually ineffective in management of psychomotor or major motor seizures.

USES Management of absence (petit mal) seizures, myoclonic seizures, and akinetic epilepsy. May be administered with other anticonvulsants when other forms of epilepsy coexist with petit mal.

ROUTE & DOSAGE

Absence Seizures
Adult: **PO** 250 mg b.i.d.; may increase q4–7d prn (max 1.5 g/d).
Child: **PO** *6–12 y,* Same as for adult; *3–6 y,* 250 mg/d; may increase q4–7d prn (max 1.5 g/d).

PHARMACOKINETICS Absorption: readily absorbed from GI tract. **Peak:** 4 h; steady state: 4–7 d. **Metabolism:** metabolized in liver. **Elimination:** half-life: 30 h in children, 60 h in adults; excreted slowly in urine; small amounts excreted in bile and feces.

CONTRAINDICATIONS & PRECAUTIONS Contraindicated in: hypersensitivity to succinimides; severe liver or renal disease; use alone in mixed types of epilepsy (may increase frequency of grand mal seizures). Safe use during pregnancy (category C), in nursing mothers, and in children <3 y not established.

ADVERSE/SIDE EFFECTS CNS: drowsiness, hiccups, ataxia, dizziness, headache, euphoria, restlessness, irritability, anxiety, hyperactivity, aggressiveness, inability to concentrate, lethargy, confusion, sleep disturbances, night terrors, hypochondriacal behavior, muscle weakness, fatigue. **Eye:** myopia. **GI:** nausea, vomiting, *anorexia, epigastric distress,* abdominal pain, *weight loss,* diarrhea, constipation. **GU:** vaginal bleeding. **Hematologic:** eosinophilia, leukopenia, thrombocytopenia, <u>agranulocytosis</u>, <u>pancytopenia</u>, <u>aplastic anemia</u>, positive direct Coombs' test. **Skin:** hirsutism, pruritic erythematous skin eruptions, urticaria, alopecia, erythema multiforme, exfoliative dermatitis. **Other:** gingival hyperplasia.

DRUG INTERACTIONS Carbamazepine decreases ethosuximide levels; **isoniazid** significantly increases ethosuximide levels; levels of both **phenobarbital** and ethosuximide may be altered with increased seizure frequency.

NURSING IMPLICATIONS

Administration

- Ethosuximide may be taken with food if GI distress occurs.
- Store capsules in tight containers, and syrup in light-resistant containers at 15–30C (59–86F); avoid freezing.

Assessment & Drug Effects

- Baseline and periodic hematologic studies and tests of liver and renal function should be made.
- GI symptoms, drowsiness, ataxia, dizziness, and other neurologic side effects occur frequently and indicate the need for dosage adjustment.

- Close observation is required during the period of dosage adjustment and whenever other medications are added to or eliminated from the drug regimen. Therapeutic serum levels: 40–80 μg/ml.
- Behavioral changes are most likely to occur in the patient with a prior history of psychiatric disturbances. Close supervision is indicated. Drug should be withdrawn slowly if these symptoms appear.

Patient & Family Education

- Abrupt withdrawal of ethosuximide (whether used alone or in combination therapy) may precipitate seizures or petit mal status. Caution patient to discontinue drug only under physician supervision.
- Ethosuximide may impair mental and physical abilities; caution the patient to avoid driving a motor vehicle and other hazardous activities.
- Instruct patient to monitor weight on a weekly basis. Anorexia and weight loss should be reported to physician and may indicate need to reduce dosage.

ETIDOCAINE HYDROCHLORIDE

(e-ti′doe-kane)

Trade name: Duranest

Classifications: CNS AGENT; LOCAL ANESTHETIC (AMIDE-TYPE)

Prototype: Procaine hydrochloride

Pregnancy category: B

ACTIONS/PHARMACODYNAMICS Amide-type anesthetic similar to bupivacaine in action and uses. Inhibits sodium fluxes into nerve cell required for initial depolarization, propagation, and conduction of nerve impulse.

USES Infiltration anesthesia, peripheral nerve blocks (intercostal, ulnar, inferior alveolar, brachial plexus) and central neural block (lumbar or caudal epidural blocks).

ROUTE & DOSAGE

Percutaneous Infiltration

Adult: **IM** 0.5% solution; max 300 mg, 400 mg if given with epinephrine.

Peripheral Nerve Block, Caudal

Adult: **IM** 0.5% or 1% solution; max 300 mg (400 mg if given with epinephrine).

Central Neural Block

Adult: **IM** 0.5% or 1.5% solution; max 300 mg (400 mg if given with epinephrine).

PHARMACOKINETICS **Absorption:** readily absorbed from parenteral injection sites. **Onset:** 2–8 min. **Duration:** 4.5–13 h. **Distribution:** crosses blood-brain barrier and placenta. **Metabolism:** metabolized in liver. **Elimination:** half-life: 1–2 h; excreted in urine.

CONTRAINDICATIONS & PRECAUTIONS **Contraindicated in:** known sensitivity to amide-type anesthetics, parabens, bisulfites; acidosis, heart block, severe hemorrhage, severe hypotension, hypertension; cerebrospinal deformities or disease; spinal block, epidural anesthesia in vaginal delivery; injection into inflamed or infected area. Safe use during pregnancy (category B) (except during labor), in nursing mothers, or in children <14 y not established. **Cautious use in:** known drug sensitivities; impaired cardiac function; renal or hepatic disease; severe shock; elderly, debilitated or severely ill patients.

ADVERSE/SIDE EFFECTS CNS: nervousness, headache, anxiety, excitement, <u>convulsions followed by drowsiness, unconsciousness, respiratory arrest</u>. **CV:** myocardial depression, arrhythmias, <u>cardiac arrest, fetal bradycardia during delivery</u>, maternal hypotension. **Ear/eye:** blurred vision, tinnitus. **GI:** nausea, vomiting. **Other:** skin rash, <u>anaphylaxis, anaphylactoid reactions</u>, injection site inflammation and pain, edema, pupillary constriction, backache.

NURSING IMPLICATIONS

Administration

- Discard partially used vial of etidocaine, since it has no preservative.
- Store vials at 15–30C (59–86F); protect from freezing. Solutions with epinephrine should be protected from direct light.

Assessment & Drug Effects

- When used for peridural analgesia, drug produces a profound degree of motor blockade and abdominal relaxation.
- Monitor patient's CV and respiratory status continuously during administration.
- Early warnings of CNS toxicity are: restlessness, anxiety, tinnitus, dizziness, blurred vision, tremors, and drowsiness. At first sign, oxygen is administered.
- Etidocaine may trigger familial malignant hyperthermia. Early unexplained signs of tachycardia, tachypnea, labile BP, metabolic acidosis, and skeletal muscle rigidity may precede temperature elevation.

Patient & Family Education

- Use for dental anesthesia: caution patient not to chew solid foods or test the anesthetized region by biting or probing before anesthesia wears off to prevent traumatizing tongue, lip, and buccal mucosa.
- When appropriate, inform patient that he or she may experience temporary loss of sensation and motor activity, usually in the lower part of the body, after proper administration of epidural anesthesia.

E

ETIDRONATE DISODIUM

(e-ti-droe′nate)

Trade names: Didronel, Didronel I.V., EHDP

Prototype for classifications: REGULATOR, BONE METABOLISM, BIPHOSPHONATE

Pregnancy category: B (PO); C (parenteral)

ACTIONS/PHARMACODYNAMICS Diphosphate preparation with primary action on bone. Mechanism of action not fully understood. Slows rate of bone resorption and new bone formation in pagetic bone lesions and in normal remodeling process. Lowers serum alkaline phosphatase and urinary hydroxyproline levels and reduces elevated cardiac output associated with Paget's disease by decreasing vascularity of bone. Induces reversible hyperphosphatemia without adverse effects.

USES Symptomatic Paget's disease and heterotopic ossification due to spinal cord injury or after total hip replacement. **Unlabeled uses:** to prevent parathyroid hormone-induced bone resorption, management of malignancy-associated hypercalcemia, treatment of osteoporosis.

E

ROUTE & DOSAGE

Paget's Disease

Adult: **PO** 5–10 mg/kg/d for up to 6 mo *or* 11–20 mg/kg/d for up to 3 mo; may repeat after 3–6 mo off the drug if necessary.

Heterotopic Ossification Due to Spinal Cord Injury

Adult: **PO** 20 mg/kg/d for 2 wk; then 10 mg/kg/d for an additional 10 wk.

Heterotopic Ossification Due to Total Hip Arthroplasty

Adult: **PO** 20 mg/kg/d starting 1 mo before the procedure and continuing for 3 mo after.

Malignancy-associated Hypercalcemia

Adult: **IV** 7.5 mg/kg/d for 3–7 d diluted in at least 250 ml NS and infused over at least 2 h; may repeat after 7 d off the drug if necessary.

PHARMACOKINETICS **Absorption:** variably absorbed from GI tract. **Distribution:** 50% of absorbed drug is distributed to bone. **Metabolism:** not metabolized. **Elimination:** half-life: 6 h; 50% of absorbed dose is excreted in urine.

CONTRAINDICATIONS & PRECAUTIONS **Contraindicated in:** enterocolitis; children; pathologic fractures, pregnancy [(category B, PO), (category C, parenteral)]. Safe use in nursing women, and in children not established. **Cautious use in:** renal impairment; patients on restricted calcium and vitamin D intake.

ADVERSE/SIDE EFFECTS **GI:** nausea, diarrhea, *loose bowel movements,* metallic or altered taste. **Other:** increased or recurrent bone pain in pagetic sites, onset of bone pain in previously asymptomatic sites, increased risk of fractures in patient with Paget's disease, hypocalcemia, hyperphosphatemia, renal insufficiency (high IV doses), elevated serum phosphatase, suppressed mineralization of uninvolved skeleton (focal osteomalacia).

DRUG INTERACTIONS CALCIUM SUPPLEMENTS, ANTACIDS, IRON AND OTHER MINERAL SUPPLEMENTS may decrease absorption of etidronate—give etidronate 2 h before other drugs. **Drug–food:** food, especially milk and dairy products, will decrease absorption of etidronate—give 2 h before meals.

NURSING IMPLICATIONS

Administration

- Administer as single dose on empty stomach 2 h before meals with full glass of water or juice to reduce gastric irritation.
- GI side effects may be relieved by dividing total oral daily dose.
- IV etidronate is prepared by diluting a single dose in 25 ml of NS.
- After dilution, it is important to administer the IV slowly over a period of at least 2 h.
- Store at 15–30C (59–86F) in tightly closed container unless otherwise directed.

Assessment & Drug Effects

- GI side effects may interfere with adequate nutritional status and should be treated promptly. Persistent nausea or diarrhea should be reported.
- Monitor I&O ratio, serum creatinine, or BUN of patient with impaired renal function.
- Latent tetany (hypocalcemia) may be detected by Chvostek's and Trousseau's signs and a serum calcium value of 7–8 mg/dl.

- Serum phosphate levels generally return to normal 2–4 wk after medication is discontinued.

Patient & Family Education
- Instruct patient to avoid eating 2 h before or after taking PO etidronate. Drug absorption is decreased by food, especially milk, milk products, and other foods high in calcium, mineral supplements, and antacids.
- The risk of pathological fractures increases when daily dose of 20 mg/kg is taken longer than 3 mo. Instruct patient to report promptly the sudden onset of unexplained pain.
- Response of Paget's disease to etidronate therapy may be slow (1–3 mo) and may continue for months after treatment is discontinued.
- Instruct patient to report promptly if bone pain, restricted mobility, heat over involved bone site occur.

ETODOLAC

(e-to′do-lac)

Trade names: Lodine, Lodine XL

Classifications: CNS AGENT; ANALGESIC, ANTIPYRETIC; NONSTEROIDAL ANTIINFLAMMATORY AGENT

Prototype: Ibuprofen

Pregnancy category: C

ACTIONS/PHARMACODYNAMICS Exact mechanism of action is unknown but may inhibit cyclooxygenase activity and prostaglandin synthesis. NSAIDS may also suppress production of rheumatoid factor.

USES Osteoarthritis and acute pain, rheumatoid arthritis. **Unlabeled use:** temporal arteritis.

ROUTE & DOSAGE

Acute Pain

Adult: **PO** 200–400 mg q6–8h prn.

Osteoarthritis

Adult: **PO** 600–1200 mg/d in 2–4 divided doses; total daily dose should not exceed 1200 mg or 20 mg/kg for patients ≤60 kg. Lodine XL 400–1000 mg once daily.

Rheumatoid Arthritis

Adult: **PO** 500 mg b.i.d.

PHARMACOKINETICS Absorption: readily absorbed from GI tract. **Onset:** 30 min. **Peak:** 1–2 h. **Duration:** 4–12 h. **Distribution:** widely distributed; 99% protein bound; not known if crosses placenta or if distributed into breast milk. **Metabolism:** extensively metabolized in liver. **Elimination:** half-life: 6–7 h; 72% excreted in urine, 16% in feces.

ADVERSE/SIDE EFFECTS CV: fluid retention, edema. **CNS:** dizziness, headache, drowsiness, insomnia. **GI:** *dyspepsia, nausea, vomiting, diarrhea,* indigestion, heartburn, abdominal pain, constipation, flatulence, gastritis, melena, peptic ulcer, GI bleeding. **Hematologic:** thrombocytopenia, increased bleeding time. **Skin:** rash, pruritus. **Other:** urinary frequency, hepatotoxicity, blurred vision, asthma, tinnitus

DRUG INTERACTIONS May reduce the effects of DIURETICS and the antihypertensive effects of BETA BLOCKERS and other ANTIHYPERTENSIVE MEDICATIONS. May increase **digoxin** and **lithium** levels and nephrotoxicity due to **cyclosporine.**

DIAGNOSTIC TEST INTERFERENCE May cause a false-positive ***urinary***

bilirubin test and a false-positive ***ketone*** test done with the dipstick method. May cause a small decrease (1 to 2 mg/dL) in ***serum uric acid*** levels.

CONTRAINDICATIONS & PRECAUTIONS **Contraindicated in:** hypersensitivity to NSAIDS and in GI ulceration or inflammation. Safety and efficacy in children <14 y have not been established. **Cautious use in:** renal impairment, hepatic function impairment, patients over 65 y, and pregnancy (category C).

NURSING IMPLICATIONS

Administration

- Administer etodolac with food or antacid to reduce risk of GI ulceration.
- Store capsules in bottles at 15–30C (59–86F). Store capsules in unit-dose packages at 15–25C (59–77F). Protect both forms from moisture.

Assessment & Drug Effects

- Assess for signs of GI ulceration and bleeding. Risk factors include high doses of etodolac, history of peptic ulcer disease, alcohol use, smoking, and concomitant use of aspirin.
- In patients with a history of CHF, carefully assess for fluid retention by monitoring weight and observing for edema.
- In hypertensive patients, monitor for decreased BP control.
- When used concurrently with either digoxin or lithium, monitor for toxicity of these drugs.
- Monitor for rhinitis, urticaria, or other signs of allergic reactions. Discontinue drug and notify physician.
- Carefully monitor increases in etodolac dosage with elderly patients, as side effects are more pronounced in this population.
- Monitor for headaches, especially at high doses. Discontinuation of the drug may be indicated.
- CBC and renal and hepatic function tests should be performed periodically during therapy.

Patient & Family Education

- Alert patients to the signs and symptoms of GI ulceration and bleeding and to the need to stop the medication and contact the physician immediately if these occur.
- Advise patient not to take aspirin, which may potentiate ulcerogenic effects.

ETOPOSIDE

(e-toe-po′side)

Trade names: Etopophos, Toposar, VePesid, VP-16

Classifications: ANTINEOPLASTIC; MITOTIC INHIBITOR

Prototype: Vincristine

Pregnancy category: D

ACTIONS/PHARMACODYNAMICS
Semisynthetic derivative of May apple plant. Produces cytotoxic action by unclear mechanism. Primary action is by arresting G_2 (resting or premitotic) phase of cell cycle; also acts on S (DNA synthesis) phase. High doses cause lysis of cells entering mitotic phase, and lower doses inhibit cells from entering prophase.

USES Treatment of refractory testicular neoplasms, in patients who have already received appropriate surgical, chemotherapeutic, and radiation therapy; for treatment of choriosarcoma in women and small cell carcinoma of the lung. **Unlabeled uses:** Hodgkin's and non-Hodgkin's lymphomas, acute myelogenous (nonlymphocytic) leukemia.

ROUTE & DOSAGE

Testicular Carcinoma

Adult: **IV** 50–100 $mg/m^2/d$ for 5 consecutive days q3–4wk for 3–4 courses *or* 100 mg/m^2 on days 1, 3, and 5 q3–4wk for 3–4 courses; **PO** Twice the IV dose rounded to the nearest 50 mg.

Small Cell Lung Carcinoma

Adult: **IV** 35 $mg/m^2/d$ for 4 consecutive days to 50 $mg/m^2/d$ for 5 consecutive days q3–4wk; **PO** Twice the IV dose rounded to the nearest 50 mg.

PHARMACOKINETICS Absorption: approximately 50% absorbed from GI tract. **Peak:** 1–1.5 h. **Distribution:** variable penetration into CSF. **Metabolism:** probably metabolized in liver. **Elimination:** half-life: 5–10 h; 44–60% excreted in urine, 2–16% excreted in feces over 3 d.

CONTRAINDICATIONS & PRECAUTIONS Contraindicated in: severe bone marrow depression; severe hepatic or renal impairment; existing or recent viral infection, bacterial infection; intraperitoneal, intrapleural, or intrathecal administration. Safe use during pregnancy (category D), in nursing mothers, and in children not established. **Cautious use in:** impaired renal or hepatic function; gout.

ADVERSE/SIDE EFFECTS CNS: peripheral neuropathy, paresthesias, weakness, somnolence, unusual tiredness, transient confusion. **CV:** transient hypotension. **GI:** *nausea, vomiting,* dyspepsia, anorexia, diarrhea, constipation, stomatitis. **Hematologic:** *leukopenia (principally granulocytopenia), thrombocytopenia,* <u>severe myelosuppression</u>, *anemia, pancytopenia, neutropenia.* **Hypersensitivity:** sweating, chills, fever, coryza, tachycardia; throat, back and general body pain; abdominal cramps, flushing, substernal chest pain, dyspnea, <u>bronchospasm</u>, pulmonary edema, <u>anaphylactoid reaction</u>. **Respiratory:** pleural effusion, bronchospasm. **Skin:** *reversible alopecia* (can progress to total baldness); radiation recall dermatitis. **Other:** necrosis, thrombophlebitis with extravasation, *pain at IV site.*

E

NURSING IMPLICATIONS

Administration

- Wear disposable surgical gloves when preparing or disposing of etoposide.
- Each 100 mg must be diluted with 250–500 ml of D5W or NS to produce final concentrations of 0.2–0.4 mg/ml.
- Administer by slow IV infusion over 30–60 min to reduce risk of hypotension and bronchospasm.
- Before administration, inspect solution for particulate matter and discoloration. Solution should be clear and yellow. If crystals are present, discard.
- Diluted solutions with concentration of 0.2 mg/ml are stable for 96 h, and the 0.4 mg/ml solutions are stable for 48 h under normal room fluorescent light in glass or plastic (PVC) containers.
- Store unopened vials at 15–30C (59–86F) unless otherwise directed.
- Refrigerate capsules at 2–8C (36–46F) unless otherwise directed. Do not freeze.

Assessment & Drug Effects

- Check IV site during and after infusion. Extravasation can cause thrombophlebitis and necrosis.
- Be prepared to treat an anaphylactoid reaction (see Appendix G). If the reaction occurs, infusion should be stopped immediately.
- Monitor vital signs during and after

infusion. If hypotension occurs, infusion should be stopped immediately.

- The following laboratory tests are advised before therapy is begun, at regular intervals during therapy, and before each subsequent treatment course: CBC, WBC counts; hepatic and renal function tests (AST, ALT, serum bilirubin, LDH, BUN, serum creatinine).
- An absolute neutrophil count below 500/mm^3 or a platelet count below 50,000/mm^3 signifies need to withhold therapy.
- Be alert to evidence of patient complaints that might suggest development of leukopenia (see Appendix G), infection (immunosuppression), and bleeding.
- During period of platelet nadir particularly, protect patient from any trauma that might precipitate bleeding. If possible, invasive procedures should be withheld.

Patient & Family Education

- Before treatment begins, patient and responsible family members should be informed of the possible adverse effects of etoposide, such as blood dyscrasias, alopecia, carcinogenesis.
- Because transient hypotension after therapy is a possible side effect, caution patient to make position changes slowly, particularly from recumbent to upright position.
- Inspect mouth daily for ulcerations and bleeding. Patients with stomatitis should avoid obvious irritants such as hot or spicy foods, smoking, alcohol.

ETRETINATE

(e-tret'i-nate)

Trade name: Tegison

Classifications: SKIN AGENT; ANTIPSORIATIC; RETINOID

Prototype: Isotretinoin

Pregnancy category: X

ACTIONS/PHARMACODYNAMICS

A second-generation retinoid related to retinoic acid and retinol (vitamin A). Mechanism of action unknown. Reduces redness, scaling, and thickness of psoriasis lesions by normalizing epidermal differentiation; also decreases stratum corneum thickness and inflammation in epidermis and dermis.

USE Treatment of severe recalcitrant psoriasis in patients unresponsive to or intolerant of standard therapies.

ROUTE & DOSAGE

Psoriasis

Adult: **PO** 0.75–1 mg/kg/d in divided doses, not to exceed 1.5 mg/kg/d; may be able to decrease to 0.5–0.75 mg/kg/d after 8–10 wk of therapy.

PHARMACOKINETICS **Absorption:** readily absorbed from GI tract with significant first pass metabolism. **Peak:** 2.5–5 h. **Duration:** detectable serum levels for years after discontinuation. **Distribution:** accumulates in adipose tissue, liver, and subcutaneous fat; crosses placenta; distributed into breast milk. **Metabolism:** metabolized in liver. **Elimination:** half-life: 120 h; excreted primarily in feces; some excretion in urine.

CONTRAINDICATIONS & PRECAUTIONS **Contraindicated in:** intolerance to isotretinoin, tretinoin, vitamin A derivatives, or to parabens (preservative in etretinate formulation); pregnancy (category X), lactation, severe obesity. **Cautious use in:** cardiovascular disease or family history of; children (used only if all alternative therapies have been ineffective); hepatic impairment; diabetes mellitus, patients predisposed to hypertriglyceridemia.

ADVERSE/SIDE EFFECTS Nearly all resemble those of hypervitaminosis A syndrome. **CNS:** *fatigue, headache, fever,* dizziness, lethargy, amnesia, anxiety, depression, pseudotumor cerebri. **CV:** edema; cardiac thrombotic or obstructive events; postural hypotension, coagulation disorders, MI (rare). **ENT:** dry nose, *nose bleeds,* change in hearing, earache, otitis externa. **Eye:** *eye irritation,* decreased night vision, *eyelid abnormalities; double vision;* corneal erosion and abrasions; dry eyes, eye pain, blurred vision, excessive tearing, conjunctivitis, scotomas, photophobia. **GI:** abdominal pain, *appetite change,* stomatitis, *sore tongue,* thirst, *nausea,* constipation, diarrhea, flatulence, weight loss, *gingival bleeding, dry mouth.* **GU:** abnormal menses, atrophic vaginitis, dysuria, polyuria. **Hematologic:** anemia; increased or decreased serum potassium, calcium, sodium, *phosphorus, chloride, fasting blood sugars,* platelets, Hgb, Hct, *PTT, MCHC,* prothrombin time; increased BUN, creatinine. **Hepatic:** *hypertriglyceridemia,* hepatitis (hepatotoxicity), *hypercholesterolemia,* lowered HDL, increased AST, ALT, bilirubin. **Musculoskeletal:** *bone and joint pain,* muscle cramps, myalgia, gout, hyperkinesia, *hyperostosis.* **Respiratory:** dyspnea, coughing. **Skin:** nail disorders, *photosensitivity; skin fragility and peeling;* changes in perspiration, *hair loss,* dry skin, rash, itching, skin atrophy, fissures, ulcerations; hirsutism, herpes simplex. **Other:** *chapped lips,* cheilitis; malignant neoplasms.

DRUG INTERACTIONS Alcohol may increase plasma triglyceride levels; **isotretinoin,** VITAMIN A PREPARATIONS compound toxic effects; **methotrexate** may increase risk of hepatotoxicity; TETRACYCLINES may increase risk of pseudotumor cerebri. **Drug–food:** milk will increase absorption of etretinate.

NURSING IMPLICATIONS

Administration

- Consistent administration of etretinate with whole milk or other high-fat food increases drug absorption and allows smaller doses. It may thus be easier to titrate lowest effective dosage range. Discuss with physician.
- Store capsules at 15–30C (59–86F); protect from light and moisture.

Assessment & Drug Effects

- Transient exacerbation of psoriasis may occur during the initial treatment period.
- Hepatic function tests are performed before beginning treatment, then at 1- to 2-wk intervals for 1–2 mo. Periodic tests continue thereafter at intervals of 1–3 mo during the treatment period. Drug is discontinued in presence of hepatitis.
- Blood lipid determinations are performed before treatment starts and then repeated at 1- to 2-wk intervals until lipid response is established (usually 4–8 wk).
- Effective contraception should be used at least 1 mo before starting treatment, continued during treatment, and perhaps for as long as 4 y after treatment ends.

Patient & Family Education

- Complete clearing of the disease has been observed after 4–9 mo of therapy in most patients.
- The most common sites for drug-induced hyperostosis (abnormal growth of bone tissue) in adults are in the ankles, pelvis, and knees. Pain and limitation of motion should be reported immediately; drug will be discontinued.

F

- If drug is prescribed for children, caution parent to report promptly the onset of pain or limitation of motion in the child.
- Caution patient to report immediately signs and symptoms of hepatitis: jaundice (see Appendix G), flu-like symptoms.
- If any visual difficulties develop, drug should be discontinued and patient should have an ophthalmic examination.
- High-fat foods in diet should be controlled because this drug can cause hypertriglyceridemia and increased LDLs.
- Patient should be advised to avoid vitamin A supplements because of the possibility of additive toxic effects.
- Caution patient to report early symptoms of pseudotumor cerebri: headache, vomiting, nausea, blurred vision.
- Because of potential drug-induced photosensitivity and photophobia, caution patient to avoid excessive sun exposure and sunlamp treatments.
- Drug-induced effects on oral mucosa and gingiva because of decreased salivary flow should be reported and treated.
- Patient should be completely aware of the teratogenic danger. If patient becomes pregnant, urge her to talk with the physician about the risk of continuing pregnancy.
- Patient should be warned not to donate blood while taking etretinate and for several years after therapy.

FACTOR IX COMPLEX

Trade names: Konyne, Konyne-HT, Profilnine, Proplex, Proplex SX

Classifications: BLOOD COAGULATOR; HEMOSTATIC (SYSTEMIC)

Pregnancy category: C

ACTIONS/PHARMACODYNAMICS

Dried, purified concentrate of vitamin K-dependent blood coagulation factors II, VII, IX, and X derived from fresh pooled plasma of healthy donors. Factor IX complex contains only traces of blood group A and B isohemagglutins; however, when large doses are administered, the amount of isohemagglutins becomes significant and can cause intravascular hemolysis. Congenital deficiency of any one of the four blood coagulation factors present in factor IX complex can result in a hemorrhagic problem. Factor VII, factor IX, and factor X or Stuart-Prower factor are all essential for conversion of factor II prothrombin to thrombin.

USES Primarily to control bleeding in patients with factor IX deficiency, i.e., hemophilia B (Christmas disease). Also to reverse effects of coumarin anticoagulants. Proplex is used to control bleeding in patients with hemophilia A (who have factor VIII inhibitors).

ROUTE & DOSAGE

Bleeding in Patient With Hemophilia A Who Has Factor VIII Inhibitors

Adult: **IV** 75 U/kg ideal body weight; a second dose may be given if necessary after 8–12 h.

Prophylaxis for Spontaneous Bleeding Episodes

Adult: **IV** 500 U/wk.

Prompt Reversal of Anticoagulant Effect of Coumarins or Drug-induced Bleeding

Adult: **IV** 15 U/kg.

PHARMACOKINETICS **Metabolism:** rapidly cleared from plasma after IV administration. **Elimination:** half-life: 17–32 h.

CONTRAINDICATIONS & PRECAUTIONS **Contraindicated in:** liver disease or suspicious signs of disseminated intravascular coagulation (DIC) or fibrinolysis; patients with mild factor IX deficiency who could be treated effectively with fresh-frozen plasma; patients who have had little exposure to blood products (at high risk of developing viral hepatitis); patients undergoing elective surgery (risk of thromboses); pregnancy (category C).

ADVERSE/SIDE EFFECTS Generally well tolerated. **With large doses:** fever, chills, DIC, thromboses, MI. **With rapid infusion:** vasomotor reactions (flushing, changes in BP or pulse rate), transient fever, chills, headache, tingling, urticaria, nausea, vomiting, somnolence, lethargy. **Other:** viral hepatitis, anaphylactic shock (rare).

NURSING IMPLICATIONS

Administration

- Dilute with at least 1 ml of sterile water for injection for each 50 U (50 U/ml). A more dilute solution using 2 ml of sterile water for injection for each 50 U (25 U/ml) may be preferred. Diluent is usually provided by manufacturer.
- Before reconstitution, warm diluent (sterile water for injection) to room temperature. After diluent is added, vial should be gently agitated to ensure complete dissolution of powder.
- Rate of flow is prescribed (generally not to exceed 3 ml/min).
- After reconstitution, solution should be administered within 3 h to avoid possibility of microbial contamination. It should not be refrigerated because precipitation may occur.
- Refrigerate unopened vials at 2–8C (35–46F) until reconstituted unless otherwise directed. Do not freeze.

Assessment & Drug Effects

- Coagulation assays should be performed before initiation of therapy and at regular intervals during therapy to individualize dosage.
- Be alert to signs of DIC, e.g., oliguria, mucosal bleeding, ecchymoses, abnormal coagulation tests, and hypersensitivity reactions.
- Monitor vital signs and I&O.

Patient & Family Education

- Instruct patient to report bleeding gums and signs and symptoms of hypersensitivity (see Appendix G).
- Patients with hemophilia A (classic hemophilia) commonly have hemarthrosis (i.e., bleeding into joints causing swelling, pain, and immobility). Bleeding into soft tissues and muscle causes hematomas that compress nerves, blood vessels, and even the airway. Prompt treatment and physical therapy can prevent irreversible joint damage and muscle atrophy.

FAMCICLOVIR

(fam-ci′clo-vir)

Trade name: Famvir

Classifications: ANTIINFECTIVE; ANTIVIRAL

Prototype: Acyclovir

Pregnancy category: B

ACTIONS/PHARMACODYNAMICS Famciclovir is the prodrug to the antiviral agent penciclovir. Famciclovir may have an advantage over acyclovir because of its greater stability intracellularly in infected cells. It prevents viral replication by inhibition of DNA synthesis in herpesvirus-infected cells, and has longer-lasting antiviral activity than acyclovir. Famciclovir interferes with DNA synthesis of herpes simplex virus type 1 and 2 (HSV-1 and HSV-2) infections, varicella-zoster virus and cytomegalovirus.

F

USES Management of acute herpes zoster, genital herpes, recurrent episodes of genital herpes in immunocompromized adults. Suppression of recurrent episodes of genital herpes in immunocompetent adults.

ROUTE & DOSAGE

Herpes Zoster, Treatment

Adult: **PO** 500 mg q8h × 7 d, should be started within 48–72 h of onset of rash; dose should be reduced in patients with renal insufficiency: Cl_{cr} 40–59 ml/min, 500 mg q12h; Cl_{cr} 20–39 ml/min, 500 mg q24h.

Treatment of Recurrent Genital Herpes

Adult: **PO** 125 mg b.i.d. × 5 d.

Suppression of Recurrent Genital Herpes

Adult: **PO** 250 mg b.i.d. for up to 1 y.

PHARMACOKINETICS **Absorption:** readily absorbed from GI tract and rapidly converted to penciclovir in intestinal and liver tissue. **Onset:** median times to full crusting of lesions, loss of vesicles, loss of ulcers, and loss of crusts were 6, 5, 7, and 19 d, respectively; median time to loss of acute pain was 21 d. **Peak:** 1 h. **Distribution:** distributes into breast milk of animals. **Metabolism:** metabolized in liver and intestinal tissue to penciclovir, which is the active antiviral agent. **Elimination:** half-life: penciclovir 2–3 h; approximately 60% recovered in urine as penciclovir.

CONTRAINDICATIONS & PRECAUTIONS **Contraindicated in:** hypersensitivity to famciclovir, nursing mothers. **Cautious use in:** renal and hepatic impairment, carcinoma, elderly, pregnancy (category B). Safe use in children <18 y not established.

ADVERSE/SIDE EFFECTS **CNS:** *headache,* somnolence, dizziness, paresthesias, fatigue, fever, rigors. **Hematologic:** purpura. **GI:** nausea, diarrhea, vomiting, constipation, anorexia, abdominal pain. **Other:** pharyngitis, sinusitis, pruritus.

DRUG INTERACTIONS **Probenecid** may decrease elimination; famciclovir may increase **digoxin** levels.

NURSING IMPLICATIONS

Administration

- In patients with reduced renal function, dosage reduction is recommended.
- Store at room temperature, 15–30C (59–86F).

Assessment & Drug Effects

- A positive therapeutic response is indicated by decreasing pain and crusting of lesions followed by loss of vesicles, ulcers, and crusts.
- Prior to and after short courses of therapy and periodically during prolonged treatment, complete blood counts and routine blood chemistry studies should be done.
- If digoxin is used concurrently with famciclovir, monitor digoxin level and assess for signs and symptoms of digoxin toxicity.

Patient & Family Education

- Inform patient of potential adverse

effects and instruct to report those that are bothersome.

- Inform patient that a full therapeutic response may take several weeks.
- Advise patient to report signs and symptoms of hypersensitivity immediately.

FAMOTIDINE

(fa-moe′ti-deen)

Trade names: Pepcid, Pepcid AC

Classifications: GASTROINTESTINAL AGENT; ANTISECRETORY AGENT (H_2-RECEPTOR ANTAGONIST)

Prototype: Cimetidine

Pregnancy category: B

ACTIONS/PHARMACODYNAMICS A thiazole derivative, structurally similar to histamine and pharmacologically similar to cimetidine. A potent competitive inhibitor of histamine at histamine (H_2) receptor sites in gastric parietal cells. This action reduces parietal cell output of hydrochloric acid; thus, detrimental effects of acid on gastric mucosa are diminished. Inhibits basal, nocturnal, meal-stimulated, and pentogastrin-stimulated gastric secretion; also inhibits pepsin secretion. Is 20–160 times more potent than cimetidine and 3–20 times more potent than ranitidine. Does not affect gastric emptying or exocrine pancreatic function.

USES Short-term treatment of active duodenal ulcer. Maintenance therapy for duodenal ulcer patients on reduced dosage after healing of an active ulcer. Treatment of pathologic hypersecretory conditions (e.g., Zollinger-Ellison syndrome), benign gastric ulcer, gastroesophageal reflux disease (GERD), gastritis. **Unlabeled use:** stress ulcer prophylaxis.

ROUTE & DOSAGE

Duodenal Ulcer

Adult: **PO** 40 mg h.s. or 20 mg b.i.d. **IV** 20 mg q12h.
Child: **PO/IV** 0.5 mg/kg q8–12h (max 40 mg/d).

Duodenal Ulcer, Maintenance Therapy

Adult: **PO** 20 mg h.s.

Pathological Hypersecretory Conditions

Adult: **PO** 20–160 mg q6h.

GERD, Gastritis

Adult: **PO** 10 mg b.i.d.

PHARMACOKINETICS Absorption: incompletely absorbed from GI tract (40–50% reaches systemic circulation). **Onset:** 1 h. **Peak:** 1–3 h PO; 0.5–3 h IV. **Duration:** 10–12 h. **Metabolism:** metabolized in liver. **Elimination:** half-life: 2.5–4 h; excreted in urine.

CONTRAINDICATIONS & PRECAUTIONS Contraindicated in: safe use during pregnancy (category B), by nursing mothers, or in children not established. **Cautious use in:** renal insufficiency.

ADVERSE/SIDE EFFECTS CNS: dizziness, headache, confusion, depression. **GI:** constipation, diarrhea. **Skin:** rash, acne, pruritus, dry skin, flushing. **Other:** thrombocytopenia, increases in BUN and serum creatinine.

DRUG INTERACTIONS None identified.

NURSING IMPLICATIONS

Administration

- Administer oral drug with liquid or food of patient's choice; an antacid may be given with famotidine if patient is also on antacid therapy.

- IV push: Dilute 20 mg (2 ml) famotidine IV solution (containing 10 mg/ml) with D5W, NS, or other compatible IV diluent (see manufacturer's directions) to a total volume of 5 or 10 ml; administer direct IV over not less than 2 min.
- IV infusion: Dilute 2 ml famotidine IV with 100 ml compatible IV solution; infuse over 15–30 min.
- IV administration to infants, children: Verify correct IV concentration and rate of infusion/injection with physician.
- In the patient with severe renal insufficiency, dosage adjustment may be made on basis of creatinine clearance. High plasma concentrations of famotidine do not appear to produce drug-related toxicity.
- Famotidine IV reconstituted solutions are stable for 48 h at room temperature (15–30C) (59–86F).
- Store at 15–30C (59–86F). Protect from moisture and strong light; do not freeze. Store IV solution at 2–8C (36–46F).

Assessment & Drug Effects

- Monitor for improvement in GI distress.
- Monitor for signs of GI bleeding.

Patient & Family Education

- Inform patient that pain relief may not be experienced for several days after starting therapy.

FAT EMULSION, INTRAVENOUS

Trade names: Intralipid, Liposyn, Nutralipid, Soyacal, Travamulsion

Classification: CALORIC AGENT

Pregnancy category: B for Soyacal 10%; C for all others

ACTIONS/PHARMACODYNAMICS Intralipid is a soybean oil in water emulsion containing egg yolk phospholipids and glycerin. Liposyn 10% is a safflower oil in water emulsion containing egg phosphatides and glycerin. Caloric value per milliliter of Intralipid 10% and Liposyn 10% is 1.1, and for Intralipid 20% it is 2. Fat emulsions contain a mixture of neutral triglycerides, mostly unsaturated fatty acids.

USES Fatty acid deficiency. Also to supply fatty acids and calories in high-density form to patients receiving prolonged TPN therapy who cannot tolerate high dextrose concentrations or when fluid intake must be restricted as in renal failure, CHF, ascites.

ROUTE & DOSAGE

Prevention of Essential Fatty Acid Deficiency

Adult: **IV** 500 ml of 10% *or* 250 ml of 20% solution infused over 8–12 h twice/wk (max rate of 100 ml/h).
Child: **IV** 0.5–1 g/kg infused slowly over 8–12 h twice/wk (max 3–4 g/kg/d; max infusion 0.25 g/kg/h).

Calorie Source in Fluid-restricted Patients

Adult: **IV** up to 2.5 g/kg or 60% of nonprotein calories daily infused over at least 8–12 h (max rate of 100 ml/h).
Child: **IV** up to 4 g/kg or 60% of nonprotein calories daily infused over at least 8–12 h (max rate of 100 ml/h).
Premature infant: **IV** 0.25–0.5 g/kg/d; increase by 0.25–0.5 g/kg/d to max of 3–4 g/kg/d (max infusion 0.15 g/kg/h).

CONTRAINDICATIONS & PRECAUTIONS **Contraindicated in:** hyperlipemia; bone marrow dyscrasias; impaired fat metabolism as in pathological hyperlipemia, lipoid nephrosis, acute pancreatitis accompanied by hyperlipemia. **Cautious use in:** severe hepatic or pulmonary disease; coagulation disorders; anemia; newborns, prematures, infants with hyperbilirubinemia; when danger of fat embolism exists; diabetes mellitus; thrombocytopenia; history of gastric ulcer.

ADVERSE/SIDE EFFECTS Hypersensitivity reactions (to egg protein), *hyperlipemia,* hypercoagulability, *transient increases in liver function tests,* thrombocytopenia in neonates, irritation at infusion site. **Long-term administration:** sepsis, jaundice (cholestasis), hepatomegaly, kernicterus (infants with hyperbilirubinemia), shock (rare).

DIAGNOSTIC TEST INTERFERENCE Blood samples drawn during or shortly after fat emulsion infusion may produce abnormally high ***hemoglobin MCH and MCHC*** values. Fat emulsions may cause transient abnormalities in ***liver function tests*** and may interfere with estimations of ***serum bilirubin*** (especially in infants).

INCOMPATIBILITIES Solution/additive: aminophylline, ampicillin, calcium chloride, calcium gluconate, hetastarch, magnesium chloride, methicillin, penicillin G, phenytoin, ranitidine, tetracycline, vitamin B complex. Y-site: hetastarch, phenytoin, tetracycline.

NURSING IMPLICATIONS

Administration

- If possible, allow preparations that have been refrigerated to stand at room temperature for about 30 min before using.
- Do not use if oil appears to be separating out of the emulsion.
- Fat emulsions may be administered via a separate peripheral site or by piggyback into same vein receiving amino acid injection and dextrose mixtures. Administered by piggyback through a Y-connector near infusion site so that the two solutions mix only in short piece of tubing proximal to needle.
- Fat emulsion must be hung higher than hyperalimentation solution bottle to prevent backup of fat emulsion into primary line.
- An in-line filter is not recommended because size of fat particles is larger than pore size.
- Flow rate of each solution should be controlled by separate infusion pumps.
- Check with a pharmacist before mixing fat emulsions with electrolytes, vitamins, drugs, or other nutrient solutions.
- Because newborns and prematures tend to metabolize fat slowly, it is usually administered at a constant rate over 20–24 h to reduce risk of hyperlipemia.
- Unless otherwise directed by manufacturer, Intralipid 10% and Liposyn 10% may be stored at room temperature (25C [77F] or below). Intralipid 20% should be refrigerated. Do not freeze.
- Contents of partly used containers should be discarded.

Assessment & Drug Effects

- Acute reactions tend to occur within the first $2\frac{1}{2}$ h of therapy. Observe patient closely.
- The following baseline determinations are recommended: hemogram, platelet count, blood coagulation, liver function tests, plasma lipid profile (especially serum triglycerides and cholesterol, free fatty acids in plasma). These tests are usually repeated 1

or 2 times weekly during therapy in adults, and more frequently in children. Significant deviations should be reported promptly.

- Because newborns are prone to develop thrombocytopenia, daily platelet counts are advised during first week of therapy, then every other day during second week and 3 times weekly thereafter.
- Lipemia must clear after each daily infusion. Degree of lipemia is measured by serum triglycerides and cholesterol levels 4–6 h after infusion has ceased.

Patient & Family Education

- Instruct patient to report difficulty breathing, nausea, vomiting, or headache.

F

FELBAMATE

(fel′-ba-mate)

Trade name: Felbatol

Classifications: CNS AGENT; ANTICONVULSANT

Prototype: Phenytoin

Pregnancy category: C

ACTIONS/PHARMACODYNAMICS Felbamate's anticonvulsant mechanism has not been identified. It blocks repetitive firing of neurons. Felbamate increases seizure threshold and prevents seizure spread. Felbamate is less potent than phenytoin.

USES Treatment of Lennox–Gastaut syndrome and partial seizures. **Unlabeled use:** monotherapy or in combination with other anticonvulsants for the treatment of generalized tonic/clonic seizures.

ROUTE & DOSAGE

Partial Seizures

Adult: **PO** Initiate with 1200 mg/d in 3–4 divided doses. May increase by 600 mg/d q2wk to max of 3600 mg/d. If converting to monotherapy, reduce the dose of concomitant anticonvulsants by 1/3 when initiating felbamate. Continue to decrease other anticonvulsants by 1/3 with each increase in felbamate q2wk. If using as adjunctive therapy, decrease other anticonvulsants by 20% when initiating felbamate. Further reductions in other anticonvulsants may be required to minimize side effects and drug interactions.

Lennox–Gastaut Syndrome

Child: **PO** Start at 15 mg/kg/d in 3 or 4 divided doses. Concurrent antiepileptic drugs should be reduced by 20%; further reductions may be required to minimize side effects due to drug interactions. May increase felbamate by 15 mg/kg/d at weekly intervals to max of 45 mg/kg/d.

PHARMACOKINETICS Absorption: 90% absorbed from GI tract. Absorption of tablet not affected by food. **Onset:** therapeutic effect approximately 14 d. **Peak:** peak plasma levels at 1–6 h. **Distribution:** 20–25% protein bound, readily crosses the blood–brain barrier. **Metabolism:** metabolized in the liver via the cytochrome P-450 system. **Elimination:** half-life: 20–23 h; 40–50% excreted unchanged in urine, rest excreted in urine as metabolites.

CONTRAINDICATIONS & PRECAUTIONS Contraindicated in: hypersensitivity to felbamate or other carbamates, history of blood dyscrasia or hepatic dysfunction. **Cautious use in:** pregnancy (category C), nursing mothers, elderly. Safety and effectiveness of felbamate in children other than those with Lennox–Gastaut syndrome have not been established.

ADVERSE/SIDE EFFECTS CNS: mild tremors, headache, dizziness, ataxia, diplopia, blurred vision; agitation, aggression, hallucinations, fatigue, psychological disturbances. **Endocrine:** slight elevation of serum cholesterol, hyponatremia, hypokalemia, weight gain and loss. **GI:** *nausea and vomiting,* anorexia, constipation, hiccup, taste disturbance, indigestion, esophagitis, increased appetite, <u>acute liver failure</u>. **Hematologic:** <u>*aplastic anemia.*</u>

DRUG INTERACTIONS Felbamate reduces serum **carbamazepine** levels by a mean of 25%, but increases levels of its active metabolite, increases serum **phenytoin** levels approximately 20%, and increases **valproic acid** levels.

NURSING IMPLICATIONS

Administration

- Do not give this drug to anyone with a history of blood dyscrasia or hepatic dysfunction.
- Titrate dose under close clinical supervision.
- Shake suspension well before administering a dose.
- Store in airtight container at room temperature 15–30C (59–86F).

Assessment & Drug Effects

- Complete hematologic studies should be done before initiating therapy, frequently during therapy, and for a lengthy period after discontinuation of felbamate.
- Immediately report any hematologic abnormalities.
- Monitor hepatic function tests throughout therapy.
- When used in combination with either phenytoin or carbamazepine, carefully monitor serum levels of these drugs when felbamate is added, when adjustments in felbamate dosing are made, or when felbamate is discontinued.
- Usually, a reduction in phenytoin of 10–40% is needed when felbamate is added to the regimen.
- Periodically monitor serum sodium and potassium levels because hyponatremia and hypokalemia have been reported.
- Monitor weight, because both weight gain and loss have been reported.
- Monitor for signs and symptoms of drug toxicity including GI distress and CNS toxicity.

Patient & Family Education

- It is highly recommended that patients and physicians sign an informed consent form that reviews the indication for treatment, an explanation of the risks associated with the drug, and the importance of undergoing regular blood monitoring. A copy of the form can be found in the package insert.
- Advise patient to report unusual changes (e.g., blurred vision, dysplopia).
- Advise patient to report signs and symptoms of hypersensitivity including pruritus, urticaria, and (rarely) photosensitivity allergic reaction.
- Inform patient of adverse side effects and advise to report these to physician immediately.

FELODIPINE

(fel-o′di-peen)

Trade name: Plendil

Classifications: CARDIOVASCULAR AGENT; CALCIUM CHANNEL BLOCKER

Prototype: Nifedipine

Pregnancy category: C

ACTIONS/PHARMACODYNAMICS Calcium antagonist with high vascular selectivity that reduces systolic, diastolic, and mean arterial pressure at rest and during exercise. BP reduction is due to a reduction in peripheral vascular resistance (afterload) against which the heart works. This reduces oxygen demand by the heart and consequently may account for its effectiveness in chronic stable angina.

F

USE Mild to moderate hypertension. **Unlabeled uses:** severe hypertension, angina, CHF, pulmonary hypertension.

ROUTE & DOSAGE

Adult: **PO** 5–10 mg once/d (max 20 mg/d); elderly patients and patients with impaired hepatic function should be started at 2.5 mg q.d.

PHARMACOKINETICS **Absorption:** completely absorbed from GI tract; it undergoes extensive first-pass metabolism with only about 15% of dose reaching systemic circulation. **Onset:** <1 h. **Peak:** 2–4 h. **Duration:** 20–24 h (extended release formulation). **Distribution:** >99% bound to plasma proteins. **Metabolism:** metabolized via hepatic cytochrome P-450 mixed function oxidase system. **Elimination:** half-life: 10 h; 60–70% of metabolites are excreted in urine within 72 h.

CONTRAINDICATIONS & PRECAUTIONS **Containdicated in:** hypersensitivity to felodipine and sick sinus rhythm or second- or third-degree heart block except with the use of a pacemaker. Safety and efficacy in children not established. **Cautious use in:** hypotension, CHF, hepatic impairment, pregnancy (category C), nursing mothers.

ADVERSE/SIDE EFFECTS **CV:** tachycardia, *palpitations, flushing, peripheral edema.* **CNS:** *Dizziness, fatigue,* headache. **GI:** nausea, flatulence, diarrhea, dyspepsia. **Hematologic:** small but significant decreases in Hct, Hgb, and RBC count. Most adverse effects appear to be dose dependent.

DRUG INTERACTIONS **Adenosine** may cause prolonged bradycardia if it is used to treat patients with toxic concentrations of calcum channel blockers. **Carbamazepine, phenobarbital, phenytoin** may decrease felodipine bioavailability and serum concentrations. **Cimetidine** may increase felodipine bioavailability (competes for hepatic metabolism). Concomitant felodipine and **digoxin** administration produces only transient increases in plasma digoxin concentrations (35–40% increase), which are not sustained with continued administration. This interaction may be of clinical relevance in patients whose plama digoxin concentration is in the upper portion of the therapeutic range or in patients with preexisting renal insufficiency.

DIAGNOSTIC TEST INTERFERENCE Serum ***alkaline phosphatase*** may be slightly but significantly inceased. Plasma total and ionized ***Calcium*** levels rise significantly. Serum ***gamma-glutamyl transferase*** may increase.

NURSING IMPLICATIONS

Administration

- Administer tablet whole. It should not be crushed or chewed.
- When given concomitantly with cimetidine, the felodipine dose should be reduced.
- Store at or below 30C (86F) in a

tightly closed, light-resistant container.

Assessment & Drug Effects

- Carefully monitor BP, especially at initiation of drug therapy, in patients >64 y, and in those with impaired hepatic function.
- Anticipate BP reduction with possible reflux heart rate increase (5–10 bpm) 2–5 h after dosing.
- Promptly report sustained hypotension, which is more common with concurrent beta-blocker therapy.
- Assess for and report reflex tachycardia, which may precipitate angina.
- Patients on concurrent digoxin therapy should be monitored for possible digoxin toxicity.

Patient Education

- Instruct patient not to chew or crush tablet.
- Instruct patient to report peripheral edema, headache, or flushing. These may necessitate discontinuation of drug.
- Advise of the potential for dizziness and hypotension. Instruct patient to arise slowly and in stages.

FENOFIBRATE

(fen-o-fi′brate)

Trade name: Tricor

Classifications: CARDIOVASCULAR AGENT; ANTILIPEMIC; LIPID-LOWERING AGENT

Prototype: Clofibrate

Pregnancy category: C

ACTIONS/PHARMACODYNAMICS Fibric acid derivative with lipid-regulating properties. Lowers plasma triglycerides apparently by inhibiting triglyceride synthesis and, as a result, lowers VLDL production as well as stimulates the catabolism of triglyceride-rich lipoprotein (e.g., VLDL). Produces a moderate increase in HDL cholesterol levels in most patients.

USES Adjunctive therapy to diet for patients with high triglycerides.

ROUTE & DOSAGE

Hypertriglyceridemia

Adult: **PO** 67 mg q.d.; may increase to max of 3 capsules (201 mg)/d.

PHARMACOKINETICS **Absorption:** well absorbed from the GI tract; absorption increased with food. **Peak:** 6–8 h. **Distribution:** 99% protein bound; excreted in breast milk. **Metabolism:** rapidly hydrolyzed by esterases to active metabolite, fenofibric acid. **Elimination:** half-life: 20 h; 60% excreted in urine, 25% in feces.

CONTRAINDICATIONS & PRECAUTIONS **Contraindicated in:** hypersensitivity to fenofibrate or other fibric acid derivatives (e.g., clofibrate, benzofibrate); hepatic or severe renal dysfunction; unexplained liver function abnormality; primary biliary cirrhosis; preexisting gallbladder disease; pregnancy (category C); lactation; thrombocytopenia. Safety and efficacy in children not established. **Cautious use in:** concomitant therapy with HMG-CoA reductase inhibitors (e.g., lovastatin, pravastatin, simvastatin), oral anticoagulant medications; renal impairment, elderly; history of bleeding disorders; myelosuppression.

ADVERSE/SIDE EFFECTS **Body as whole:** asthenia, fatigue, infections, flu-like syndrome, localized pain, arthralgia. **CNS:** headache, paresthesia, dizziness, insomnia. **CV:** arrhythmia. **GI:** dyspepsia, eructation, flatulence, nausea, vomiting, abdominal pain, constipation, diarrhea, increased appetite. **Respiratory:** cough, rhinitis, sinusitis. **Skin:** pruritus, rash. **Other:** decreased libido, earache, eye floaters, blurred vision, conjunctivitis, eye irritation, polyuria, vaginitis.

DRUG INTERACTIONS May potentiate anticoagulant effects of **warfarin;** combination with an HMG-COA REDUCTASE INHIBITOR (STATIN) may result in rhabdomyolysis or acute renal failure; **cholestyramine, colestipol** may decrease absorption (give fenofibrate 1 h before or 4–6 h after BILE ACID SEQUESTRANTS); may increase risk of nephrotoxicity of **cyclosporine**.

NURSING IMPLICATIONS

Administration

- Fenofibrate should be given with meals.
- In the elderly or those with impaired renal function, dose is limited to 67 mg/d.
- Give at least 1 h before or 4–6 h after cholestyramine.
- Store at 15–30C (59–86F) in a tightly closed container and protect from light.

Assessment & Drug Effects

- Therapeutic effectiveness is indicated by reduction in the level of serum triglycerides.
- Lab tests: Periodically monitor lipid levels, liver functions, and CBC with differential.
- Therapy should be discontinued after 2 mo if adequate lipid reduction is not achieved with the maximum dose of 201 mg/d.
- Assess for muscle pain, tenderness, or weakness and, if present, monitor CPK level. Cerivastatin should be discontinued with marked elevations of CPK or if myopathy is suspected.
- Patients on coumarin-type drugs should be closely monitored for prolongation of PT.

Patient & Family Education

- Immediately contact physician if any of the following develop: unexplained muscle pain, tenderness, or weakness, especially with fever or malaise; yellowing of skin or eyes; nausea or loss of appetite; skin rash or hives.
- Inform the physician regarding concurrent use of cholestyramine, oral anticoagulants, or cyclosporine.
- Mothers should not nurse their infants while on fenofibrate.

FENOLDOPAM MESYLATE

(fen-ol′do-pam mes′y-late)

Trade name: Corlopam

Classifications: CARDIOVASCULAR AGENT; ANTIHYPERTENSIVE; NONNITRATE VASODILATOR; DOPAMINE AGONIST AGENT

Pregnancy category: B

ACTIONS/PHARMACODYNAMICS
Rapid-acting vasodilator that is a dopamine D_1-like receptor agonist. Exerts hypotensive effects by decreasing peripheral vascular resistance while increasing renal blood flow, diuresis, and natriuresis.

USE Short-term (up to 48 h) management of severe hypertension.

ROUTE & DOSAGE

Severe Hypertension

Adult: **IV** 0.025–0.3 µg/kg/min by continuous infusion for up to 48 h; may increase by 0.05–0.1 µg/kg/min q15min; dosage range: 0.01–1.6 µg/kg/min.

Common side effect in *italic,* life-threatening effects underlined: generic names in **bold;** drug class in SMALL CAPS

PHARMACOKINETICS **Onset:** 5 min. **Peak:** 15 min. **Duration:** 15–30 min. **Distribution:** crosses placenta. **Metabolism:** conjugated in liver. **Elimination:** half-life: 5 min; 90% excreted in urine, 10% in feces.

CONTRAINDICATIONS & PRECAUTIONS **Contraindicated in:** hypersensitivity to fenoldopam. Avoid concomitant use with beta blockers. **Cautious use in:** asthmatic patients; hepatic cirrhosis, portal hypertension, or variceal bleeding; arrhythmias, tachycardia, or angina, particularly unstable angina; elevated IOP; angular-closure glaucoma; hypotension; hypokalemia; acute cerebral infarct or hemorrhage; lactation; pregnancy (category B). Safety and efficacy in children not established.

ADVERSE/SIDE EFFECTS **Body as whole:** injection site reaction, pyrexia, nonspecific chest pain. **CNS:** headache, nervousness, anxiety, insomnia, dizziness. **CV:** *hypotension, tachycardia,* T-wave inversion, flushing, postural hypotension, extrasystoles, palpitations, bradycardia, heart failure, ischemic heart disease, MI, angina. **GI:** nausea, vomiting, abdominal pain or fullness, constipation, diarrhea. **Metabolic:** increased creatinine, BUN, glucose, transaminases, LDH; hypokalemia. **Respiratory:** nasal congestion, dyspnea, upper respiratory disorder. **Skin:** sweating. **Other:** UTI, leukocytosis, bleeding.

NURSING IMPLICATIONS

Administration

- IV preparation: Dilute to a final concentration of 40 μg/ml by adding 1 ml (10 mg), 2 ml (20 mg), or 3 ml (30 mg) of fenoldopam to 250, 500, or 1000 ml, respectively, of 0.9% NaCl or D5W.
- IV infusion: Give only by continuous infusion; never give a bolus dose.
- Initial dose should be titrated up or down no more frequently than q15min.
- Diluted solution is stable under normal room temperature and light for 24 h. Discard any unused solution after 24 h.
- Store at 15–30C (59–86F) in a tightly closed container and protect from light.

Assessment & Drug Effects

- Therapeutic effectiveness is indicated by rapid reduction in BP.
- Carefully monitor BP and HR at least q15min or more often as warranted; expect dose-related tachycardia.
- Lab tests: Carefully monitor serum electrolytes (especially serum potassium), BUN and creatinine, liver enzymes, and blood glucose.

F

FENOPROFEN CALCIUM

(fen-oh-proe′fen)

Trade name: Nalfon

Classifications: CNS AGENT; ANALGESIC; ANTIPYRETIC; NSAID

Prototype: Ibuprofen

Pregnancy category: B (D in third trimester)

ACTIONS/PHARMACODYNAMICS Exhibits antiinflammatory, analgesic, and antipyretic properties. Claimed to be comparable to aspirin in antiinflammatory activity and to be associated with lower incidence of adverse GI symptoms.

USES Antiinflammatory and analgesic effects in the symptomatic treatment of acute and chronic rheumatoid arthritis and osteoarthritis; relief of mild to moderate pain. **Unlabeled uses:** juvenile rheumatoid arthritis, acute gouty arthritis, ankylosing spondylitis; fever associated with pulmonary tuberculosis, type A influenza, colds; neoplasms.

ROUTE & DOSAGE

Inflammatory Disease

Adult: **PO** 300–600 mg t.i.d. or q.i.d. (max 3200 mg/d).
Child: **PO** 900 mg/m^2 in divided doses; may increase over 4 wk to 1.8 g/m^2.

Mild to Moderate Pain

Adult: **PO** 200 mg q4–6h prn.

PHARMACOKINETICS **Absorption:** 80% absorbed from GI tract. **Onset:** 2 h. **Peak:** 2 h. **Duration:** 4–6 h. **Distribution:** small amounts distributed into breast milk. **Metabolism:** metabolized in liver. **Elimination:** half-life: 3 h; excreted primarily in urine; some biliary excretion.

CONTRAINDICATIONS & PRECAUTIONS **Contraindicated in:** history of nephrotic syndrome associated with aspirin or other NSAIDS; patient in whom urticaria, severe rhinitis, bronchospasm, angioedema, nasal polyps are precipitated by aspirin or other NSAIDS; significant renal or hepatic dysfunction; pregnancy (category B, category D in third trimester). Safe use in nursing mothers and in children not established. **Cautious use in:** history of upper GI tract disorders; hemophilia or other bleeding tendencies; compromised cardiac function, hypertension; impaired hearing.

ADVERSE/SIDE EFFECTS **CNS:** *headache, drowsiness,* dizziness, fatigue, lassitude, tremor, confusion, insomnia, nervousness, depression. **Ear/eye:** tinnitus, decreased hearing, deafness; blurred vision. **GI:** *indigestion, nausea, vomiting,* anorexia, *constipation,* diarrhea, flatulence, abdominal pain, dry mouth; infrequent: gastritis, peptic ulcer, <u>GI bleeding</u>. **GU:** dysuria, cystitis, hematuria, oliguria, azotemia, anuria, allergic nephritis, papillary necrosis, nephrotoxicity (rare). **Hematologic (infrequent):** thrombocytopenia, <u>hemolytic anemia, agranulocytosis, pancytopenia</u>. **Skin:** (may or may not be hypersensitivity reaction): pruritus, rash, purpura, increased sweating, urticaria. **Other:** dyspnea, malaise, <u>anaphylaxis</u>, edema.

DRUG INTERACTIONS Fenoprofen may prolong bleeding time—should not be given with ORAL ANTICOAGULANTS, **heparin;** action and side effects of **phenytoin,** SULFONYLUREAS, SULFONAMIDES, and fenoprofen may be potentiated.

NURSING IMPLICATIONS

Administration

- Best taken on an empty stomach 30–60 min before or 2 h after meals. May be administered with meals, milk, or antacid (prescribed), however, if patient experiences GI disturbances.
- Tablet may be crushed or capsule emptied and contents swallowed with fluid or mixed with food.
- Store capsules and tablets in tightly closed containers at 15–30C (59–86F); avoid freezing.

Assessment & Drug Effects

- Baseline and periodic evaluations of hemoglobin, renal and hepatic function, and auditory and ophthalmic examinations are recommended in patients receiving prolonged or high dose therapy.
- Monitor for signs and symptoms of GI bleeding.
- When phenobarbital is added to or withdrawn from patient's drug reg-

imen, dosage adjustment of fenoprofen may be required.

Patient & Family Education

- Because fenoprofen may cause dizziness and drowsiness, advise patient to exercise caution when driving or performing other potentially hazardous activities.
- Instruct patient to report immediately the onset of unexplained fever, rash, arthralgia, oliguria, edema, weight gain. Possible symptoms of nephrotic syndrome are rapidly reversible if drug is promptly withdrawn.
- Therapeutic effectiveness of fenoprofen in patients with arthritis may be evidenced within a few days with peak effect in 2–3 wk.
- Inform patient that alcohol and aspirin may increase risk of GI ulceration and bleeding tendencies and should be avoided unless otherwise advised by physician.
- Fenoprofen may prolong bleeding time; therefore, advise patient to inform dentist or surgeon that he is taking this drug.

FENTANYL CITRATE

(fen′ta-nil)

Trade names: Duragesic, Actiq Oralet, Sublimaze

Classifications: CNS AGENT; ANALGESIC; NARCOTIC (OPIATE) AGONIST

Prototype: Morphine

Pregnancy category: C

Controlled substance: Schedule II

ACTIONS/PHARMACODYNAMICS

Synthetic, potent narcotic agonist analgesic with pharmacologic actions qualitatively similar to those of morphine and meperidine, but action is more prompt and less prolonged. Principal actions: analgesia and sedation. Drug-induced alterations in respiratory rate and alveolar ventilation may persist beyond the analgesic effect. Emetic effect is less than with either morphine or meperidine.

USES Short-acting analgesic during operative and perioperative periods, as a narcotic analgesic supplement in general and regional anesthesia, and with droperidol or with diazepam to produce neuroleptoanalgesia. Also given with oxygen and a skeletal muscle relaxant (neuroleptoanesthesia) to selected high-risk patients (e.g., those undergoing open heart surgery) when attenuation of the response to surgical stress without use of additional anesthesia agents is important.

ROUTE & DOSAGE

Premedication

Adult: **IM** 50–100 μg 30–60 min before surgery. **PO** Suck on 400-μg lozenge until sedated.
Child: **PO** Suck on lozenge until sedated. Dose based on weight as follows: *10–25 kg,* 200-μg lozenge; *25–35 kg,* 300-μg lozenge; *35–40 kg,* 400-μg lozenge.
Neonate: **IV** 1–4-μg/kg slow IV push q2–4h or 1–2-μg/kg bolus, then infuse at 0.5–1-μg/kg/h.
Child 1–12 y: **IV/IM** 1–2 μg/kg q30–60 min or 1–2 μg/kg followed by 1–3 μg/kg/h infusion (max 5 μg/kg/h).

Adjunct for Regional Anesthesia

Adult: **IM** 50–100 μg; **IV** 2–20 μg/kg over 1–2 min up to 50 μg/kg.

F

General Anesthesia

Adult: **IV** up to 150 μg/kg as required.

Postoperative Pain

Adult: **IM** 50–100 μg q1–2h prn.
Child: **IM** 1.7–3.3 μg/kg q1–2h prn.

Chronic Pain

Adult: **Transdermal** Doses of transdermal fentanyl must be individualized and should be regularly reassessed; for patient not already receiving an opioid, the initial dose should be a 25 μg/h patch q3d; for patients already on opioids, see package insert for conversions.

Stick lozenge (Actiq) Place in mouth between cheek and lower gum and suck on lozenge; should be consumed over 15-min period.

PHARMACOKINETICS **Absorption:** absorbed through the skin, leveling off between 12–24 h. **Onset:** immediate IV; 7–15 min IM; 12–24 h transdermal. **Peak:** 3–5 min IV;24–72 h transdermal. **Duration:** 30–60 min IV; 1–2 h IM; 72 h transdermal. **Metabolism:** metabolized in liver. **Elimination:** excreted in urine

CONTRAINDICATIONS & PRECAUTIONS **Contraindicated in:** patients who have received MAO INHIBITORS within 14 d; myasthenia gravis. Safe use during pregnancy (category C) and in children <2 y not established. **Cautious use in:** head injuries, increased intracranial pressure; elderly, debilitated, poor-risk patients; COPD, other respiratory problems; liver and kidney dysfunction; bradyarrhythmias, by nursing mothers.

ADVERSE/SIDE EFFECTS **CNS:** *sedation,* euphoria, dizziness, diaphoresis, delirium, convulsions with high doses. **CV:** hypotension, bradycardia, circulatory depression, cardiac arrest. **Eye:** miosis, blurred vision. **GI:** *nausea,* vomiting, constipation, ileus. **Respiratory:** laryngospasm, bronchoconstriction, respiratory depression or arrest. **Other:** muscle rigidity, especially muscles of respiration after rapid IV infusion, urinary retention, rash, contact dermatitis from patch.

DRUG INTERACTIONS **Alcohol** and other CNS DEPRESSANTS potentiate effects; MAO INHIBITORS may precipitate hypertensive crisis.

INCOMPATIBILITIES **Solution/additive: pentobarbital, thiopental.**

NURSING IMPLICATIONS

Administration

- Parenteral doses may be given undiluted or diluted in 5 ml sterile water or NS. Administer by direct IV over 1–2 min.
- Store at 15–30C (59–86F) unless otherwise directed. Protect drug from light.

Assessment & Drug Effects

- Monitor vital signs and observe patient for signs of skeletal and thoracic muscle (depressed respirations) rigidity and weakness.
- During postoperative period, watch carefully for respiratory depression and for movements of various groups of skeletal muscle in extremities, external eye, and neck. These movements may present patient management problems and should be reported promptly.
- Duration of respiratory depressant effect may be considerably longer than narcotic analgesic effect. Have immediately available oxygen, resuscitative and intubation

equipment, and an opioid antagonist such as naloxone.

FERROUS SULFATE

Trade names: Feosol, Fer-In-Sol, Fer-Iron, Fero-Gradumet, Ferospace, Ferralyn, Ferra-TD, Fesofor, Hematinic, Mol-Iron, Novoferrosulfa ♣, Slow-Fe

FERROUS FUMARATE

(foo′ma-rate)

Trade names: Feco-T, Femiron, Feostat, Fersamal, Fumasorb, Fumerin, Hemocyte, Ircon-FA, Neo-Fer-50 ♣, Novofumar ♣, Palafer ♣, Palmiron

FERROUS GLUCONATE

(gloo′koe-nate)

Trade names: Fergon, Fertinic ♣, Novoferrogluc ♣, Simron

Prototype for classifications: BLOOD FORMER; IRON PREPARATION

Pregnancy category: A

ACTIONS/PHARMACODYNAMICS Ferrous sulfate is the standard iron preparation against which other oral iron preparations are usually measured. They correct erythropoietic abnormalities induced by iron deficiency but do not stimulate erythropoiesis. May reverse gastric, esophageal, and other tissue changes caused by lack of iron. Ferrous gluconate is claimed to cause less gastric irritation and to be better tolerated than ferrous sulfate.

USES To correct simple iron deficiency and to treat iron deficiency (microcytic, hypochromic) anemias. Also may be used prophylactically during periods of increased iron needs, as in infancy, childhood, and pregnancy.

ROUTE & DOSAGE

Iron Deficiency

Sulfate (30% elemental iron)
Adult: **PO** 750–1500 mg/d in 1–3 divided doses.
Child: **PO** *6–12 y:* 600 mg/d in divided doses; *<6 y:* 75–225 mg/d in divided doses.

Fumarate (33% elemental iron)
Adult: **PO** 200 mg t.i.d. or q.i.d.
Child: **PO** 3 mg/kg t.i.d.

Gluconate (12% elemental iron)
Adult: **PO** 325–600 mg q.i.d.; may be gradually increased to 650 mg q.i.d. as needed and tolerated.
Child: **PO** *6–12 y:* 100–300 mg t.i.d.; *<6 y:* 100–300 mg/d in divided doses.

Iron Supplement

Sulfate
Pregnancy: **PO** 300–600 mg/d in divided doses. *Infants:* **PO** 1 mg/kg/d for 3 y up to 15 mg/d. *Low birth weight:* **PO** 2 mg/kg/d up to 15 mg/d.

Fumarate
Adult: **PO** 200 mg once/d.
Child: **PO** 3 mg/kg once/d.

Gluconate
Adult: **PO** 325–600 mg once/d.
Child: **PO** *6–12 y:* 100–300 mg once/d; *<6 y:* 100–300 mg/d in divided doses.

PHARMACOKINETICS **Absorption:** 5–10% absorbed in healthy individuals; 10–30% absorbed in iron-deficiency; food decreases amount absorbed. **Distribution:** transported by transferrin to bone marrow, where it is incorporated into hemoglobin; crosses placenta. **Elimina-**

tion: most of iron released from hemoglobin is reused in body; small amounts are lost in desquamation of skin, GI mucosa, nails, and hair; 12–30 mg/mo lost through menstruation.

CONTRAINDICATIONS & PRECAUTIONS **Contraindicated in:** peptic ulcer, regional enteritis, ulcerative colitis; hemolytic anemias (in absence of iron deficiency), hemochromatosis, hemosiderosis, patients receiving repeated transfusions, pyridoxine-responsive anemia; cirrhosis of liver; pregnancy (category A).

ADVERSE/SIDE EFFECTS Generally minimal: **GI:** *nausea, heartburn,* anorexia, *constipation,* diarrhea, epigastric pain, abdominal distress, *black stools.* **Other:** yellow-brown discoloration of eyes and teeth (liquid forms.) **Large chronic doses in infants:** rickets (due to interference with phosphorus absorption). **Massive overdosage:** lethargy, drowsiness, nausea, vomiting, abdominal pain, diarrhea, local corrosion of stomach and small intestines, pallor or cyanosis, metabolic acidosis, shock, cardiovascular collapse, convulsions, liver necrosis, coma, renal failure, death.

DIAGNOSTIC TEST INTERFERENCE By coloring feces black, large iron doses may cause false-positive tests for ***occult blood with ortho-toluidine*** (Hematest, Occultest, Labstix); ***guaiac reagent benzidine test*** is reportedly not affected.

DRUG INTERACTIONS ANTACIDS decrease iron absorption; iron decreases absorption of TETRACYCLINES, **ciprofloxacin, ofloxacin; chloramphenicol** may delay iron's effects; iron may decrease absorption of **penicillamine. Drug–food:** food decreases absorption of iron; ascorbic acid (vitamin C) may increase iron absorption.

NURSING IMPLICATIONS

Administration

- PO iron preparations are best absorbed when taken on an empty stomach (i.e., between meals). However, to minimize gastric distress it may be necessary to administer the drug with or immediately after meals.
- Tablets or capsules should not be taken within 1 h of bedtime, with adequate liquid.
- If the patient experiences difficulty in swallowing tablet or capsule, consult physician about prescribing a liquid formulation or a less corrosive form, such as ferrous gluconate.
- Liquid preparations should be well diluted and administered through a straw or placed on the back of tongue with a dropper to prevent staining of teeth and to mask taste. Instruct the patient to rinse mouth with clear water immediately after ingestion.
- Feosol elixir may be mixed with water, but it is not compatible with milk or fruit juice. Fer-In-Sol (drops) may be given in water or in fruit or vegetable juice, according to manufacturer.
- Preserve in tightly closed containers. Protect from moisture. Do not use discolored tablets. Store at 15–30C (59–86F).

Assessment & Drug Effects

- Hemoglobin and reticulocyte values should be monitored during therapy. In the absence of satisfactory response after 3 wk of drug treatment, possible reasons for failure warrant investigation.
- Therapeutic response may be experienced within 48 h as a sense of

well-being, increased vigor, improved appetite, and decreased irritability (in children). Reticulocyte response begins in about 4 d; it usually peaks in 7–10 d (reticulocytosis) and returns to normal after 2 or 3 wk. Hemoglobin generally increases by 2 g/dl and hematocrit by 6% in 3 wk.

- Iron therapy is usually continued for 2–3 mo after the hemoglobin level has returned to normal (roughly twice the period required to normalize hemoglobin concentration).
- As a general rule, iron should not be administered for longer than 6 mo except in repeated pregnancies, persistent bleeding, or menorrhagia.

Patient & Family Education

- Instruct patient not to crush tablet or empty contents of capsule before administration.
- Ascorbic acid increases absorption of iron. Consuming citrus fruit or tomato juice with iron preparation (except the elixir) may increase its availability.
- Iron absorption may be inhibited if the iron preparation is taken with milk, eggs, or caffeine beverages.
- Inform patient that iron preparations cause dark green or black stools. Advise patient to report constipation or diarrhea. These symptoms may be relieved by adjustments in dosage or diet or by change to another iron preparation.

FEXOFENADINE

(fex-o-fen′a-deen)

Trade name: Allegra

Classifications: ANTIHISTAMINE; H_1-RECEPTOR ANTAGONIST

Prototype: Diphenhydramine

Pregnancy category: C

ACTIONS/PHARMACODYNAMICS
Antihistamines competitively antagonize histamine at the H_1-receptor site but do not bind with histamine to inactivate it. Fexofenadine inhibits antigen-induced bronchospasm and histamine release from peritoneal mast cells. No anticholinergic or sedative properties are associated with fexofenadine.

USE Relief of symptoms associated with seasonal allergic rhinitis.

ROUTE & DOSAGE

Allergic Rhinitis
Adult: **PO** 60 mg b.i.d. Start with 60 mg once daily in patients with impaired renal function.
Child >12 y: **PO** Same as adult.

PHARMACOKINETICS **Absorption:** rapidly absorbed from GI tract, 33% reaches systemic circulation. **Onset:** 1 h. **Peak:** 2–3 h. **Duration:** at least 12 h. **Distribution:** 60–70% bound to plasma proteins. **Metabolism:** only 5% of dose metabolized in liver. **Elimination:** half-life: 14.4 h; 80% excreted in urine, 11% in feces.

CONTRAINDICATIONS & PRECAUTIONS **Contraindicated in:** hypersensitivity to fexofenadine. **Cautious use in:** pregnancy (category C), lactation, renal insufficiency, hepatic insufficiency. Safety and effectiveness in children <12 y not established.

ADVERSE/SIDE EFFECTS **CNS:** *headache,* drowsiness, fatigue. **GI:** nausea, dyspepsia, throat irritation.

NURSING IMPLICATIONS

Administration

- A reduced starting dose is recommended for those with decreased renal function.

- Store at 20–25C (68–77F). Protect from excess moisture.

Assessment & Drug Effects

- Efficacy is indicated by reduction of the following: nasal congestion and sneezing; watery or red eyes; itching nose, palate, or eyes.

Patient & Family Education

- Advise that drug is well tolerated and causes minimal side effects.
- Inform nursing mothers that safety of drug for breastfed infants is unknown.

FIBRINOLYSIN AND DESOXYRIBONUCLEASE

(fye-bri-noe-lye′sin)

Trade name: Elase

Classification: DEBRIDING ENZYME

Pregnancy category: C

ACTIONS/PHARMACODYNAMICS

Combination of two bovine proteolytic enzymes: fibrinolysin extracted from bovine plasma acts primarily on fibrin in blood clots and exudates, and desoxyribonuclease derived from beef pancreas attacks DNA in devitalized tissue and disintegrating cells. Enzymatic debridement is directed primarily against denatured proteins in dead tissue; normal tissue remains relatively unaffected.

USES Debriding agent in a variety of inflammatory and infected lesions such as general surgical wounds, abscesses, fistulas, and sinus tracts; ulcerative lesions; second- and third-degree burns; circumcision and episiotomy; cervicitis; and vaginitis.

ROUTE & DOSAGE

Vaginitis

Adult: **Intravaginal** 5 g ointment inserted at bedtime for 5 d, *or* 10 ml of solution instilled into vagina and held in place with a cotton tampon for 24 h followed by the ointment.

Infected Wounds, Empyema Cavities, Fistulas, Sinus Tracts, Subcutaneous Hematomas

Adult: **Topical** Irrigate with the solution; solution should be drained and replaced q6–8h.

CONTRAINDICATIONS & PRECAUTIONS **Contraindicated in:** hypersensitivity to bovine products or to mercury derivatives (e.g., thimerosal): not recommended for parenteral use; pregnancy (category C); hematomas adjacent to or within adipose tissue.

ADVERSE/SIDE EFFECTS With higher than recommended dosage: local hyperemia.

NURSING IMPLICATIONS

Administration

- Application of ointment: Flush away necrotic debris and exudates with hydrogen peroxide, sterile warm water, or normal saline (as prescribed), and gently dry area. Apply thin layer of ointment and cover with vaseline gauze or other nonocclusive dressing (as prescribed).
- Reconstitute contents of vial with 10 ml sterile isotonic NaCl solution.
- Solution must be freshly prepared before use. Loss of potency is delayed somewhat by refrigeration; however, solution must be used within 24 h.
- Application of solution (wet-to-dry dressing method): (1) Mix vial of powder with 10–50 ml of saline. (2) Saturate fine mesh gauze or unfolded sterile gauze sponge with

the solution. (3) Carefully pack ulcerated area with the saturated gauze.

- The dry powder is stable at room temperature (59–86F). Note expiration date printed on package.

FILGRASTIM

(fil-gras′tim)

Trade name: Neupogen

Classifications: BLOOD FORMATION; HEMATOPOIETIC GROWTH FACTOR

Prototype: Epoetin alfa

Pregnancy category: C

ACTIONS/PHARMACODYNAMICS Filgrastim is a human granulocyte colony-stimulating factor (G-CSF) produced by recombinant DNA technology. Endogenous G-CSF regulates the production of neutrophils within the bone marrow. It is not species specific and primarily affects neutrophil progenitor proliferation, differentiation and selected end-cell functional activity (including enhanced phagocytic activity, antibody-dependent killing, and the increased expression of some functions associated with cell-surface antigens).

USES To decrease the incidence of infection, as manifested by febrile neutropenia, in patients with nonmyeloid malignancies receiving myelosuppressive anticancer drugs associated with a significant incidence of severe neutropenia with fever; to decrease neutropenia associated with bone marrow transplant; to treat chronic neutropenia; to mobilize peripheral blood stem cells (PBSCs) for autologous transplantation.

ROUTE & DOSAGE

Neutropenia

Adult: **IV** 5 µg/kg/d by 30 min infusion; dose may be increased by 5 µg/kg/d (max 30 µg/kg/d). **SC** 5 µg/kg/d as single dose; dose may be increased by 5 µg/kg/d (max 20 µg/kg/d).
Child: **IV** Same as for adult. **SC** Same as for adult

PHARMACOKINETICS **Absorption:** readily absorbed from SC site. **Onset:** 4 h. **Peak:** 1 h. **Elimination:** half-life: 1.4–7.2 h; probably excreted in urine.

CONTRAINDICATIONS & PRECAUTIONS **Contraindicated in:** hypersensitivity to *Escherichia coli*–derived proteins, simultaneous administration with chemotherapy, and myeloid cancers. **Cautious use in:** pregnancy (category C) and nursing mothers.

ADVERSE/SIDE EFFECTS **CV:** abnormal ST segment depression. **Hematologic:** anemia. **GI:** nausea, anorexia. **Other:** *bone pain,* hyperuricemia, *fever.*

DIAGNOSTIC TEST INTERFERENCE Elevations in **leukocyte alkaline phosphatase, serum alkaline phosphatase, lactate dehydrogenase,** and **uric acid** have been reported. These elevations appear to be related to increased bone marrow activity.

INCOMPATIBILITIES **Y-site:** gentamicin, imipenem.

NURSING IMPLICATIONS

Administration

- Do not administer filgrastim 24 h before or after cytotoxic chemotherapy.

- Use only one dose per vial; do not reenter the vial.
- Prior to injection, filgrastim may be allowed to reach room temperature for a maximum of 6 h. Discard any vial left at room temperature for > 6 h.
- Refrigerate at 2–8C (36–46F). Do not freeze. Avoid shaking.

F

Assessment & Drug Effects

- A baseline CBC with differential and platelet count is obtained prior to administering drug.
- CBC should be done twice weekly during therapy to monitor neutrophil count and leukocytosis. WBC ≥ 100,000/mm^3 has been observed with no apparent adverse effect.
- Discontinue filgrastim if absolute neutrophil count surpasses 10,000/mm^3 after the chemotherapy-induced nadir.
- With the discontinuation of filgrastim therapy, neutrophil counts return to normal.
- Regular monitoring of hematocrit and platelet count is recommended.
- Closely monitor patients with preexisting cardiac conditions. MI and arrhythmias have been associated with a small percent of patients receiving filgrastim.
- Monitor temperature q4h. Incidence of infection should be reduced after administration of filgrastim.
- Assess degree of bone pain if present. Physician should be consulted if nonnarcotic analgesics do not provide relief.
- The safety and efficacy of chronic administration of filgrastim over a period of several years has yet to be established.

Patient & Family Education

- Instruct patient to report bone pain and, if necessary, to request analgesics to control pain.
- If home use is prescribed, instruct patient in the importance of proper drug administration and disposal. A puncture-resistant container for the disposal of used syringes and needles should be available to the patient.

FINASTERIDE

(fin-as′te-ride)

Trade name: Propecia, Proscar

Classification: ANDROGEN HORMONE INHIBITOR

Pregnancy category: X

ACTIONS/PHARMACODYNAMICS

Finasteride is a specific inhibitor of the steroid 5α-reductase, an enzyme necessary to convert testosterone into the potent androgen 5α-dihydrotestosterone (DHT) in the prostate gland.

USES Benign prostatic hypertrophy, male pattern hair loss (androgenetic alopecia).

ROUTE & DOSAGE

Benign Prostatic Hypertrophy

Adult: **PO** 5 mg/d.

Male Pattern Hair Loss

Adult: **PO** 1 mg q.d.

PHARMACOKINETICS **Absorption:** readily absorbed from GI tract. **Onset:** 3–6 mo. **Duration:** 5–7 d. **Elimination:** half-life: 5–7 h; 39% excreted in urine, 57% in feces.

CONTRAINDICATIONS & PRECAUTIONS **Contraindicated in:** hypersensitivity to finasteride, pregnancy (category X), lactation, and children. **Cautious use in:** hepatic impairment, obstructive uropathy.

Common side effect in *italic,* life-threatening effects underlined: generic names in **bold;** drug class in SMALL CAPS

ADVERSE/SIDE EFFECTS GU: impotence, decreased libido, decreased volume of ejaculate.

DIAGNOSTIC TEST INTERFERENCES Depresses levels of **DHT** and **prostate-specific antigen (PSA). Testosterone** levels usually are increased.

NURSING IMPLICATIONS

Administration

- Tablets may be crushed if necessary. However, pregnant women should avoid skin contact with the crushed drug.
- Store at 15–30C (59–86F) unless otherwise directed.

Assessment & Drug Effects

- Carefully evaluate any sustained increase in serum PSA levels while patients are taking finasteride. It may indicate the presence of prostate cancer or noncompliance with the therapy.
- Monitor patients with a large residual urinary volume or decreased urinary flow. These patients may not be candidates for this therapy.

Patient & Family Education

- Inform patient that crushed finasteride tablets should not be handled by pregnant women. The drug may become absorbed through the skin and may be harmful to a male fetus.
- Advise patient to avoid exposing a woman who is or may become pregnant to his semen.
- Inform patient that impotence and decreased libido may occur with treatment. Also volume of ejaculation may be decreased in some patients during treatment.

FLAVOXATE HYDROCHLORIDE

(fla-vox′ate)

Trade name: Urispas

Classifications: AUTONOMIC NERVOUS SYSTEM AGENT; ANTICHOLINERGIC (PARASYMPATHOLYTIC); ANTISPASMODIC

Prototype: Atropine

Pregnancy category: C

ACTIONS/PHARMACODYNAMICS Exerts spasmolytic (papaverinelike) action on smooth muscle. Reported to produce an increase in urinary bladder capacity in patients with spastic bladder, possibly by direct action on detrusor muscle. Also demonstrates local anesthetic and analgesic action.

USES Symptomatic relief of dysuria, frequency, urgency, nocturia, incontinence, and suprapubic pain associated with various urologic disorders.

ROUTE & DOSAGE

Dysuria, Nocturia, Incontinence

Adult: **PO** 100–200 mg t.i.d. or q.i.d.

PHARMACOKINETICS Elimination: 10–30% excreted in urine within 6 h.

CONTRAINDICATIONS & PRECAUTIONS Contraindicated in: pyloric or duodenal obstruction, obstructive intestinal lesions, ileus, achalasia, GI hemorrhage; obstructive uropathies of lower urinary tract. Safe use during pregnancy (category C) and in children <12 y not established. **Cautious use in:** suspected glaucoma.

ADVERSE/SIDE EFFECTS CNS: headache, vertigo, drowsiness, mental confusion (especially in the elderly). **CV:** palpitation, tachycardia. **Eye:** blurred vision, increased intraocular tension, disturbances of eye accommodation. **GI:** nausea, vomiting, dry mouth (and throat), constipation (with high doses). **Skin:** dermatosis, urticaria. **Other:** dysuria, hyperpyrexia, eosinophilia, leukopenia (rare).

NURSING IMPLICATIONS

Administration

- Flavoxate may be given without regard to meals.
- Store at 15–30C (59–86F) unless otherwise directed.

F

Assessment & Drug Effects

- Monitor heart rate. Take apical pulse for 1 full minute. Report tachycardia.
- Periodic evaluation of blood counts is advisable during therapy.

Patient & Family Education

- Advise patients to avoid driving or performing tasks that require mental alertness and physical coordination until reaction to drug is known.
- Advise patient to report to physician adverse reactions, clinical improvement, or the lack of a favorable response.

FLECAINIDE

(fle-kay'nide)

Trade name: Tambocor

Classifications: CARDIOVASCULAR AGENT; ANTIARRHYTHMIC

Prototype: Procainamide

Pregnancy category: C

ACTIONS/PHARMACODYNAMICS Local (membrane) anesthetic and antiarrhythmic with electrophysiologic properties similar to other class IC antiarrhythmic drugs. Slows conduction velocity throughout myocardial conduction system, increases ventricular refractoriness but has little effect on repolarization. Prolongs His-ventricular (HQ) and QRS intervals at therapeutic doses. Clinically, flecainide causes both hypotension and negative inotropy (in higher dose ranges) and is an effective suppressant of PVCs and a variety of atrial and ventricular arrhythmias.

USE Life-threatening ventricular arrhythmias. **Unlabeled uses:** atrial tachycardia and other arrhythmias unresponsive to standard agents (e.g., quinidine), Wolff-Parkinson-White syndrome, and recurrent ventricular tachycardias.

ROUTE & DOSAGE

Life-threatening Ventricular Arrhythmias

Adult: **PO** 100 mg q12h; may increase by 50 mg b.i.d. q4d to a max of 400 mg/d.
Child: **PO** 1–3 mg/kg/d in 3 divided doses (max 8 mg/kg/d).

PHARMACOKINETICS **Absorption:** readily absorbed from GI tract. **Peak:** 2–3 h. **Distribution:** crosses placenta; distributed into breast milk. **Metabolism:** metabolized in liver. **Elimination:** half-life: 7–22 h; excreted mainly in urine.

CONTRAINDICATIONS & PRECAUTIONS **Contraindicated in:** hypersensitivity to flecainide; preexisting second- or third-degree AV block, right bundle branch block when associated with a left hemiblock unless a pacemaker is present; cardiogenic shock, significant hepatic impairment. Safe use during pregnancy (category C), in nursing mothers, and in children <18 y not established. **Cautious use in:** CHF, sick sinus syndrome, renal impairment.

ADVERSE/SIDE EFFECTS Usually dose-related. **CNS:** *dizziness,* headache, light-headedness, unsteadiness, paresthesias, fatigue. **CV:** arrhythmias, chest pain, worsening of CHF. **Eye:** *blurred vision, difficulty in focusing,*

Common side effect in *italic,* life-threatening effects underlined; generic names in **bold;** drug class in SMALL CAPS

spots before eyes. **GI:** *nausea,* constipation, change in taste perception. **Other:** dyspnea, fever, edema.

DRUG INTERACTIONS **Cimetidine** may increase flecainide levels; may increase **digoxin** levels 15–25%; BETA BLOCKERS may have additive negative inotropic effects.

NURSING IMPLICATIONS

Administration

- Dosage increases more frequently than every 4 d are not recommended.
- Store in tightly covered, light-resistant containers at 15–30C (59–86F) unless otherwise directed.

Assessment & Drug Effects

- Preexisting hypokalemia or hyperkalemia should be corrected before treatment is initiated.
- ECG monitoring, including Holter monitor for ambulating patients, is essential because of the possibility of drug-induced arrhythmias.
- Patients with pacemakers should have pacing threshold determination before initiation of therapy, after 1 wk of therapy, and at regular intervals thereafter.
- Plasma level monitoring is recommended, especially in patients with severe CHF or renal failure because drug elimination may be delayed in these patients.
- Effective trough plasma levels are between 0.7–1 μg/ml. The probability of adverse reactions increases when trough levels exceed 1 μg/ml.
- Once arrhythmia is controlled, dosage reduction may be attempted with caution.

Patient & Family Education

- Impress on patient the importance of taking drug at the prescribed times.
- Instruct patient to report visual disturbances.

FLOXURIDINE

(flox-yoor'i-deen)

Trade name: FUDR

Classifications: ANTINEOPLASTIC; ANTIMETABOLITE

Prototype: Fluorouracil

Pregnancy category: D

ACTIONS/PHARMACODYNAMICS Pyrimidine antagonist and cell-cycle specific. Catabolized to fluorouracil in vivo, thus producing same systemic effects as fluorouracil.

USE Palliative agent in management of selected patients with GI metastasis to liver. **Unlabeled uses:** carcinoma of breast, ovary, cervix, urinary bladder, and prostate not responsive to other antimetabolites.

ROUTE & DOSAGE

Carcinoma

Adult: **Intraarterial** 0.1–0.6 mg/kg/d by continuous intraarterial infusion.

PHARMACOKINETICS **Distribution:** distributed to tumor, intestinal mucosa, bone marrow, liver, and CSF; probably crosses placenta. **Metabolism:** rapidly metabolized in liver to fluorouracil. **Elimination:** half-life: 16 min; 15% excreted in urine, 60-80% excreted through lungs as carbon dioxide.

CONTRAINDICATIONS & PRECAUTIONS **Contraindicated in:** existing or recent viral infections. Pregnancy (category D). **Cautious use in:** poor nutritional status, bone marrow depression, serious infections; high-risk patients: prior high-dose pelvic irradiation, use of alkylating agents; impaired renal or hepatic function.

ADVERSE/SIDE EFFECTS CNS: vertigo, convulsions, depression, hemiplegia. **CV:** myocardial ischemia, angina. **GI:** *nausea, vomiting, stomatitis,* diarrhea, cramps, anorexia, enteritis, gastritis, esophagopharyngitis. **Hematologic:** leukopenia, *thrombocytopenia.* **Skin:** dermatitis, alopecia (usually reversible), *erythema* or increased skin pigmentation (photosensitivity), dry skin, pruritic ulcerations, rash. **Other:** hiccups, fever, epistaxis, decreased resistance to disease, renal insufficiency.

F

NURSING IMPLICATIONS

Administration

- Drug is reconstituted with 5 ml sterile distilled water for injection. It is further diluted with 5% dextrose or 0.9% NaCl injection to a volume appropriate for the infusion apparatus to be used. It is administered by pump only to overcome pressure in large arteries and to ensure a uniform rate.
- Examine infusion site frequently for signs of extravasation. If this occurs, infusion should be stopped and restarted in another vessel.
- Reconstituted solutions are stable at 2–8C (36–46F) for no more than 2 wk.
- Store at 15–30C (59–86F) unless otherwise directed.

Assessment & Drug Effects

- Therapy should be discontinued promptly with onset of any of the following: stomatitis, esophagopharyngitis, intractable vomiting, diarrhea, leukopenia (WBC <3500/mm^3), or rapidly falling WBC count, thrombocytopenia (platelets 100,000/mm^3), GI bleeding, hemorrhage from any site.
- Baseline and periodic determinations should be made of total and differential leukocyte counts, Hct, platelet count, serum uric acid creatinine, and liver function tests.

Patient & Family Education

- Inform patient that floxuridine sometimes causes temporary thinning of hair.
- Inform patient of potential for nausea and vomiting and measures to alleviate them.

FLUCONAZOLE

(flu-con'a-zole)

Trade name: Diflucan

Prototype for classifications: ANTIINFECTIVE; ANTIBIOTIC; ANTIFUNGAL

Pregnancy category: C

ACTIONS/PHARMACODYNAMICS Fungistatic but may be fungicidal depending on concentration. It interferes with formation of ergosterol. Ergosterol, the principal sterol in the fungal cell membrane, becomes depleted and interferes with membrane function.

USES Cryptococcal meningitis and oropharyngeal and systemic candidiasis, both commonly found in AIDS and other immunocompromised patients; vaginal candidiasis.

ROUTE & DOSAGE

Oropharyngeal Candidiasis

Adult: **PO/IV** 200 mg day 1, then 100 mg q.d. x 2 wk.
Child: **PO/IV** 3–6 mg/kg/d.

Esophageal Candidiasis

Adult: **PO/IV** 200 mg day 1, then 100 mg q.d. x 3 wk.
Child: **PO/IV** 3–6 mg/kg/d.

Systemic Candidiasis

Adult: **PO/IV** 400 mg day 1, then

200 mg q.d. x 4 wk.
Child: **PO/IV** 3–6 mg/kg/d.

Vaginal Candidiasis
Adult: **PO** 150 mg × 1 dose.

Cryptococcal Meningitis
Adult: **PO/IV** 400 mg day 1, then 200 mg q.d. x 10–12 wk.
Child: **PO/IV** 3–6 mg/kg/d.

PHARMACOKINETICS **Absorption:** 90% absorbed from GI tract. **Peak:** 1–2 h. **Distribution:** widely distributed, including CSF. **Metabolism:** 11% of dose metabolized in liver. **Elimination:** half-life: 20–50 h; excreted in urine.

CONTRAINDICATIONS & PRECAUTIONS **Contraindicated in:** hypersensitivity to fluconazole or other azole antifungals. **Cautious use in:** pregnancy (category C).

ADVERSE/SIDE EFFECTS **CNS:** headache. **GI:** nausea, vomiting, abdominal pain, diarrhea. **Other:** rash, increase in AST in patients with cryptococcal meningitis and AIDS.

DRUG INTERACTIONS Increased PT in patients on **warfarin;** increased **phenytoin, cyclosporine** levels; hypoglycemic reactions with ORAL SULFONYLUREAS; decreased fluconazole levels with **rifampin, cimetidine.**

INCOMPATIBILITIES **Solution/additive: piperacillin. Y-site: amphotericin B, ceftazidime.**

NURSING IMPLICATIONS

Administration

- IV fluconazole should be administered at a maximum rate of approximately 200 mg/h if given as a continuous infusion.
- IV admixtures of fluconazole and other medications are not recommended.
- Administer the drug after hemodialysis is completed.

Assessment & Drug Effects

- Patients allergic to other azole antifungals may be allergic to fluconazole.
- The drug may cause elevations of the following laboratory serum values: ALT, AST, alkaline phosphatase, bilirubin.
- Monitor BUN and serum creatinine concentrations.
- Liver function tests should be monitored. Monitor for signs and symptoms of hepatotoxicity (see Appendix G).

Patient & Family Education

- It is important that the medication be taken for the full course of therapy, which may take weeks or months.
- If a dose is missed, it should be taken as soon as possible; however, it should not be taken if it is almost time for next dose.

FLUCYTOSINE

(floo-sye′toe-seen)

Trade names: Ancobon, Ancotil ♣, 5-FC, 5-Fluorocytosine
Classifications: ANTIINFECTIVE; ANTIBIOTIC; ANTIFUNGAL
Prototype: Fluconazole
Pregnancy category: C

ACTIONS/PHARMACODYNAMICS Fluorinated pyrimidine structurally related to fluorouracil. Ineffective for cancerous tumors possibly because it does not enter mammalian cells. Selectively penetrates fungal cell and is converted to fluorouracil, an antimetabolite believed to be responsible for antifungal activity.

USES Alone or in combination with amphotericin B for serious systemic infections caused by susceptible strains of *Cryptococcus* and *Candida* species. **Unlabeled use:** chromomycosis.

ROUTE & DOSAGE

Fungal Infection
Adult: **PO** 50–150 mg/kg/d divided q6h.
Child: **PO** > *50 kg,* 50–150 mg/kg/d divided q6h; *<50 kg,* 1.5–4.5 g/m²/d divided q6h.
Neonate: **PO** 50–100 mg/kg/d in 1–2 divided doses.

PHARMACOKINETICS Absorption: readily absorbed from GI tract. **Peak:** 2 h. **Distribution:** widely distributed in body tissues including aqueous humor and CSF; crosses placenta. **Metabolism:** minimally metabolized. **Elimination:** half-life: 3–6 h; 75–90% excreted in urine unchanged.

CONTRAINDICATIONS & PRECAUTIONS Contraindicated in: safe use during pregnancy (category C) and in nursing women not established. Extreme caution in impaired renal function; bone marrow depression, hematologic disorders, patients being treated with or having received radiation or bone marrow depressant drugs.

ADVERSE/SIDE EFFECTS CNS: confusion, hallucinations, headache, sedation, vertigo. **GI:** nausea, vomiting, diarrhea, abdominal bloating, enterocolitis. **Hematologic:** hypoplasia of bone marrow: anemia, leukopenia, thrombocytopenia, agranulocytosis, eosinophilia. **Other:** rash; elevated levels of serum alkaline phosphatase, AST, ALT, BUN, serum creatinine; hepatomegaly, hepatitis.

DIAGNOSTIC TEST INTERFERENCE False elevations of ***serum creatinine*** can occur with ***Ektachem analyzer.***

DRUG INTERACTIONS Amphotericin B produces additive or synergistic effects and can increase flucytosine toxicity by inhibiting its renal clearance.

NURSING IMPLICATIONS

Administration
- Lower dosages and longer dosage intervals are recommended in patients with serum creatinine of 1.7 mg/dl or higher.
- Incidence and severity of nausea and vomiting may be decreased by giving capsules a few at a time over 15 min.
- Preserve in light-resistant containers at 15–30C (59–86F).

Assessment & Drug Effects
- Culture and susceptibility tests should be performed before initiation of therapy and at weekly intervals during therapy. Organism resistance has been reported.
- Hematologic, renal, and hepatic function tests should be performed on all patients before and at frequent intervals during therapy. Twice weekly leukocyte and platelet counts are recommended.
- Frequent assays of blood drug level are recommended, especially in patients with impaired renal function to determine adequacy of drug excretion (therapeutic range: 25–120 μg/ml).
- Monitor I&O. Report change in I&O ratio or pattern. Because most of drug is eliminated unchanged by kidneys, compromised function can lead to drug accumulation.

Patient & Family Education
- Instruct patient to report fever, sore mouth or throat, and unusual bleeding or bruising tendency.
- Duration of therapy is generally 4–6 wk, but it may continue for several months.

FLUDROCORTISONE ACETATE
(floo-droe-kor′ti-sone)
Trade name: Florinef Acetate
Prototype for classifications: SYNTHETIC HORMONE; ADRENAL CORTICOSTEROID; MINERALOCORTICOID
Pregnancy category: C

ACTIONS/PHARMACODYNAMICS Long-acting synthetic steroid with potent mineralocorticoid and moderate glucocorticoid activity. Small doses produce marked sodium retention, increased urinary potassium excretion, and elevated BP. If protein intake is inadequate, fludrocortisone induces negative nitrogen balance.

USES Partial replacement therapy for adrenocortical insufficiency and for treatment of salt-losing forms of congenital adrenogenital syndrome. **Unlabeled use:** to increase systolic and diastolic blood pressure in patients with severe hypotension secondary to diabetes mellitus or to levodopa therapy.

ROUTE & DOSAGE

Adrenocortical Insufficiency
Adult: **PO** 0.1 mg/d; dose may range from 0.1 mg 3 times/wk to 0.2 mg/d.
Child: **PO** 0.05–0.1 mg/d.

Salt-losing Adrenogenital Syndrome
Adult: **PO** 0.1–0.2 mg/d.
Child: **PO** 0.05–0.1 mg/d.

PHARMACOKINETICS **Absorption:** readily absorbed from GI tract. **Peak:** 1.7 h. **Metabolism:** metabolized in liver. **Elimination:** half-life: 3.5 h.

CONTRAINDICATIONS & PRECAUTIONS **Contraindicated in:** hypersensitivity to glucocorticoids, idiopathic thrombocytopenic purpura, psychoses, acute glomerulonephritis, viral or bacterial diseases of skin, infections not controlled by antibiotics, active or latent amebiasis, hypercorticism (Cushing's syndrome), smallpox vaccination or other immunologic procedures. (Topical steroids contraindicated in presence of varicella, vaccinia, on surfaces with compromised circulation, and in children < 2 y.) Safe use in nursing mothers, during pregnancy (category C) not established. **Cautious use in:** children; diabetes mellitus; chronic, active hepatitis positive for hepatitis B surface antigen; hyperlipidemia; cirrhosis; stromal herpes simplex; glaucoma, tuberculosis of eye; osteoporosis; convulsive disorders; hypothyroidism; diverticulitis; nonspecific ulcerative colitis; fresh intestinal anastomoses; active or latent peptic ulcer; gastritis; esophagitis; thromboembolic disorders; CHF; metastatic carcinoma; hypertension; renal insufficiency; history of allergies; active or arrested tuberculosis; systemic fungal infection; myasthenia gravis.

ADVERSE/SIDE EFFECTS Dose and treatment duration dependent. **CNS:** vertigo, headache, nystagmus, increased intracranial pressure with papilledema (usually after discontinuation of medication), mental disturbances, aggravation of preexisting psychiatric conditions, insomnia, ataxia (rare). **CV:** CHF, hypertension. thromboembolism (rare), tachycardia. **Endocrine:** suppressed linear growth in children, decreased glucose tolerance; hyperglycemia, manifestations of latent diabetes mellitus; hypocorticism; amenorrhea and other menstrual difficulties. **Eye:** posterior subcapsular cataracts (especially in children), glaucoma, exophthalmos, increased intraocular pressure with optic nerve damage, perforation of the globe. **Fluid and electrolyte disturbances:** hypocalcemia; *sodium and fluid retention;* hypokalemia and hypokalemic alkalosis. **GI:** *nausea,* increased appetite, ulcerative esophagitis, pancreatitis, abdominal distension, peptic ulcer with perforation and hemorrhage, melena. **Hematologic:** thrombocytopenia. **Musculoskeletal (long-term use):** osteoporosis, compression fractures, muscle wasting and weakness, tendon rupture, aseptic necrosis of femoral and humeral heads. **Skin:** skin thinning and atrophy, *acne, impaired wound healing;* petechiae, ecchymosis, easy bruising; suppression of skin test reaction; hypopigmentation or hyperpigmentation, hirsutism, acneiform eruptions, subcutaneous fat atrophy; allergic dermatitis, urticaria, angioneurotic edema, increased sweating. **Other:** negative nitrogen balance, aggravation or masking of infections; malaise, weight gain, obesity; increased or decreased motility and number of sperm, decreased serum concentration of vitamins A and C; anaphylactoid reactions (rare).

DRUG INTERACTIONS The antidiabetic effects of **insulin** and SULFONYLUREAS may be diminished; **amphotericin B,** DIURETICS may increase potassium loss; **warfarin** may decrease prothrombin time; **indomethacin, ibuprofen** can potentiate the pressor effect of fludrocortisone; ANABOLIC STEROIDS increase risk of edema and acne; **rifampin** may increase the hepatic metabolism of fludrocortisone.

NURSING IMPLICATIONS

Administration

- Concomitant oral cortisone or hydrocortisone therapy may be advisable to provide substitute therapy approximating normal adrenal activity.
- Store in airtight containers at 15–30C (59–86F). Protect from light.

Assessment & Drug Effects

- Monitor for signs of hypokalemia and hyperkalemic metabolic alkalosis (see Appendix G).
- Monitor serum electrolyte levels during prolonged therapy.
- Monitor weight and I&O ratio to observe onset of fluid accumulation, especially if patient is on unrestricted salt intake and without potassium supplement. Report weight gain of 2 kg (5 lb)/wk.
- Monitor and record BP daily. If hypertension develops as a consequence of therapy, report to physician. Usually, the dose will be reduced to 0.05 mg/d.
- During period of dosage adjustment, BP should be checked q4–6h and weight at least every other day.
- Signs of overdosage (hypercorticism) are psychosis, excess weight gain, edema, congestive heart failure, ravenous appetite, severe insomnia, and increase in BP.
- Signs of insufficient dosage (hypocorticism) are loss of weight and appetite, nausea, vomiting, diarrhea, muscular weakness, increased fatigue, and hypotension.

Patient & Family Education

- Instruct patient to report signs of hypokalemia (see Appendix G).
- Alert patient to signs of potassium depletion associated with high sodium intake: muscle weakness, paresthesias, circumoral numbness; fatigue, anorexia, nausea,

mental depression, polyuria, delirium, diminished reflexes, arrhythmias, cardiac failure, ileus, ECG changes.

- Patient may be advised to eat foods with high potassium content.
- Sodium intake may or may not require regulation, depending on individual needs and clinical situation. Teach the patient that salt intake is a significant regulator of drug efficacy. Signs of edema should be reported immediately.
- Instruct patient to weigh daily under standard conditions and to report steady weight gain.
- Intercurrent infection, trauma, or unexpected stress of any kind should be reported promptly by patient on maintenance therapy.
- Advise patient to wear or carry medical identification card or jewelry stating drug being used and physician's identity.

FLUMAZENIL

(flu-ma'ze-nil)

Trade names: Mazicon♣, Romazicon

Prototype for classification: BENZODIAZEPINE ANTAGONIST

Pregnancy category: C

ACTIONS/PHARMACODYNAMICS Antagonizes the effects of benzodiazepine on the CNS: sedation, impairment of recall, and psychomotor impairment. Does not reverse the effects of opioids.

USES Complete or partial reversal of sedation induced by benzodiazepine for anesthesia or diagnostic or therapeutic procedures and through overdose. **Unlabeled uses:** seizure disorders, alcohol intoxication, hepatic encephalopathy, facilitation of weaning from mechanical ventilation.

ROUTE & DOSAGE

Reversal of Sedation

Adult: **IV** 0.2 mg over 15 s; may repeat 0.2 mg q60s for 4 additional doses or a cumulative dose of 1 mg.

Benzodiazepine Overdose

Adult: **IV** 0.2 mg over 30 s; if no response after 30 s, then 0.3 mg over 30 s; may repeat with 0.5 mg q60s for a maximum cumulative dose of 3 mg.

PHARMACOKINETICS **Onset:** 1–5 min. **Peak:** 6–10 min. **Duration:** 2–4 h. **Metabolism:** metabolized in the liver to inactive metabolites. **Elimination:** half-life: 54 min; 90–95% excreted in urine, 5-10% in feces within 72 h.

CONTRAINDICATIONS & PRECAUTIONS **Contraindicated in:** hypersensitivity to flumazenil or to benzodiazepines; patients given a benzodiazepine for control of a life-threatening condition; patients showing signs of cyclic antidepressant overdose; seizure-prone individuals during labor and delivery. Effects on children are unknown. **Cautious use in:** hepatic function impairment, the elderly, pregnancy (category C), nursing mothers, intensive care patients, head injury, drug- and alcohol-dependent patients, and physical dependence upon benzodiazepines.

ADVERSE/SIDE EFFECTS **CNS:** emotional lability, headache, *dizziness,* agitation, *resedation,* seizures, blurred vision. **GI:** *nausea, vomiting,* hiccups. **Other:** shivering, pain at injection site, hypoventilation.

NURSING IMPLICATIONS

Administration

- Repeat doses should be reduced in patients with hepatic function impairment.
- Ensure patency of IV before administration of flumazenil, since extravasation will cause local irritation.
- Flumazenil should be administered through an IV that is freely flowing into a large vein.
- IV preparation: Flumazenil may be administered undiluted or diluted with D5W, lactated Ringer's, or 0.9% NaCl. All diluted solutions of flumazenil should be used within 24 h of dilution.
- IV administration: Flumazenil should not be administered as a bolus dose, but rather each 0.2 mg dose should be given in small quantities over 15 s. Doses of flumazenil are given at 60 s intervals (see Route & Dosage).
- In high-risk patients, slow the rate of administration of flumazenil to intervals of 6–10 min to provide the smallest effective dose.
- If resedation occurs, repeat doses may be given at 20 min intervals. Maximum dose for repeat treatment is 1 mg given at a rate of 0.2 mg/min, not to exceed 3 mg in any 1-h period.

Assessment & Drug Effects

- Monitor patients for reversal of benzodiazepine for up to 120 min for respiratory depression and resedation.
- Benzodiazepine-induced ventilatory insufficiency may not be fully reversed by flumazenil; carefully monitor respiratory status until risk of resedation is unlikely.
- Monitor carefully for seizures and take appropriate precautions.

Patient & Family Education

- Instruct patient, preferably in writing, not to engage in activities requiring alertness, such as driving or operating machinery, until at least 18–24 h after discharge following a procedure.
- Alcohol or nonprescription drugs should not be taken for 18–24 h after flumazenil administration or if the effects of the benzodiazepine persist.

FLUNISOLIDE

(floo-niss'oh-lide)

Trade names: AeroBid, Nasalide, Nasarel

Classifications: SKIN AND MUCOUS MEMBRANE AGENT; ANTIINFLAMMATORY; ADRENAL CORTICOSTEROID

Prototype: Hydrocortisone

Pregnancy category: C

See Appendix A.

FLUOCINOLONE ACETONIDE

(floo-oh-sin'oh-lone)

Trade names: Fluoderm♣, Fluolar, Fluonid, Flurosyn, Synalar, Synalar-HP, Synemol

Classifications: SKIN AGENT; ANTI-INFLAMMATORY; ADRENAL CORTICOSTEROID

Prototype: Hydrocortisone

Pregnancy category: C

See Appendix A.

FLUOCINONIDE

(floo-oh-sin'oh-nide)

Trade names: Lidemol, Lidex, Lidex-E, Lyderm, Topsyn

Classifications: SKIN AGENT; ANTI-INFLAMMATORY; ADRENAL CORTICOSTEROID

Prototype: Hydrocortisone

Pregnancy category: C

See Appendix A.

FLUORESCEIN SODIUM

(flure′e-seen)

Trade names: Fluorescite, Fluor-I-Strip, Fluor-I-Ful-Glo, Funduscein

Classification: DIAGNOSTIC AGENT

Pregnancy category: C

ACTIONS/PHARMACODYNAMICS

Mildly antiseptic fluorescent dye related chemically to phenolphthalein.

USES An aid in fitting hard contact lenses, applanation tonometry, detecting corneal epithelial defects, and testing potency of lacrimal system. Used IV as a diagnostic aid in retinal angiography. Also used as an antidote for aniline dye.

ROUTE & DOSAGE

Diagnostic Aid

Adult: **Topical** Instill 1–2 drops and have patient keep eyelid closed for 60 s; *or* moisten strip with sterile water, touch conjunctiva or fornix with moistened tip, and have patient blink to distribute.

Retinal Angiography

Adult: **IV** 5 ml of 10% solution or 3 ml of 25% solution injected rapidly in antecubital vein.
Child: **IV** 7.5 mg/kg injected rapidly in antecubital vein.

CONTRAINDICATIONS & PRECAUTIONS **Contraindicated in:** topical use with soft contact lenses not recommended. **Cautious use in:** history of hypersensitivity, allergies, bronchial asthma, pregnancy (category C).

ADVERSE/SIDE EFFECTS **Topical use:** *temporary stinging, burning sensation,* conjunctival redness. IV administration: **CNS:** headache, paresthesias, pyrexia, convulsions. **CV:** hypotension, transient dyspnea, acute pulmonary edema, basilar artery ischemia, syncope, severe shock, cardiac arrest. **GI:** nausea, vomiting. **Hypersensitivity:** urticaria, pruritus, angioneurotic edema, anaphylactic reaction. **Other:** thrombophlebitis at injection site, temporary discoloration of skin and urine, strong metallic taste following high dosage.

NURSING IMPLICATIONS

Administration

- Avoid touching eyelids or surrounding area with eyedropper when instilling medication.
- To fit hard contact lenses: Fluorescein is instilled with contact lenses in place. Patient should be instructed to blink several times to distribute dye. Under blue light, areas that lack fluorescein will appear black, indicating that contact lens is touching cornea at these points.
- To test for potency of lacrimal system: One drop of 2% solution is instilled into conjunctival sac. Instruct patient to blink at least 4 times. After 6 min, nasal secretions are examined under blue light. Traces of dye in secretions indicate that nasolacrimal drainage system is open.
- As an antidote for aniline dye (in indelible pencils): After removal of pencil point, eye is irrigated with 2% solution every 10 min until visible precipitate is no longer present. Irrigations are repeated every 30 min for 12–24 h.
- Solution container should be kept tightly closed when not in use.
- Store below 27C (80F). Protect from light and freezing.

Assessment & Drug Effects

- Facilities for treatment of anaphylactic reaction should be immediately available, e.g., epinephrine 1:1000 for IV or IM use, an antihistamine, and oxygen.

- Fluorescein should be discontinued immediately if signs of sensitivity develop.

Patient & Family Education

- IV administration may impart a yellowish orange discoloration to skin and to urine. Skin discoloration usually fades in 6–12 h; urine clears in 24–36 h.

FLUOROMETHOLONE

(flure-oh-meth′oh-lone)

Trade names: Fluor-Op, FML Forte, FML Liquifilm Ophthalmic

Classifications: SKIN AND MUCOUS MEMBRANE AGENT; ANTIINFLAMMATORY; ADRENAL CORTICOSTEROID

Prototype: Hydrocortisone

Pregnancy category: C

See Appendix A.

FLUOROURACIL (5-FLUOROURACIL [5-FU])

(flure-oh-yoor′a-sil)

Trade names: Adrucil, Efudex, Fluoroplex

Prototype for classifications: ANTINEOPLASTIC; ANTIMETABOLITE

Pregnancy category: D

ACTIONS/PHARMACODYNAMICS Pyrimidine antagonist and cell-cycle specific. Blocks action of enzymes essential to normal DNA and RNA synthesis and may become incorporated in RNA to form a fraudulent molecule; unbalanced growth and death of cell follow. Has higher affinity for tumor tissue than healthy tissue. Highly toxic, especially to proliferative cells in neoplasms, bone marrow, and intestinal mucosa. Low therapeutic index with high potential for severe hematologic toxicity.

USES Systemically as single agent and in combination with other antineoplastics for palliative treatment of carefully selected patients with inoperable neoplasms of breast, colon or rectum, stomach, pancreas, urinary bladder, ovary, cervix, liver. Also topically for solar or actinic keratoses and superficial basal cell carcinoma. **Unlabeled uses:** to induce repigmentation in vitiligo; actinic cheilitis; malignant effusions; mucosal leukoplakia.

ROUTE & DOSAGE

Carcinoma

Adult: **IV** 12 mg/kg/d for 4 consecutive days up to 800 mg *or* until toxicity develops *or* 12 d therapy; may repeat at 1 mo intervals; if toxicity occurs, 15 mg/kg once weekly can be given until toxicity subsides

Actinic and Solar Keratosis

Adult: **Topical** Apply cream b.i.d. for 2–4 wk.

Superficial Basal Cell Carcinoma

Adult: **Topical** Apply 5% cream b.i.d. for 3–6 wk.

PHARMACOKINETICS Distribution: distributed to tumor, intestinal mucosa, bone marrow, liver, and CSF; probably crosses placenta. **Metabolism:** rapidly metabolized in liver. **Elimination:** half-life: 16 min; 15% excreted in urine, 60–80% excreted through lungs as carbon dioxide.

CONTRAINDICATIONS & PRECAUTIONS Contraindicated in: poor nutritional status; myelosuppression. Safe use during pregnancy (category D) and in nursing women not established. **Cautious use in:** major surgery during previous month; history of high-dose pelvic irradiation, metastatic cell infiltration of bone marrow, previous use of alkylating agents; men and women in childbearing ages; hepatic and renal impairment.

ADVERSE/SIDE EFFECTS CNS: euphoria, acute cerebellar syndrome (dysmetria, nystagmus, ataxia, severe mental deterioration); pustular contact hypersensitivity. **CV:** cardiotoxicity (rare), angina. **GI:** anorexia, *nausea, vomiting, stomatitis,* esophagopharyngitis, medicinal taste, *diarrhea*, proctitis. **Hematologic:** anemia, <u>leukopenia</u>, thrombocytopenia, eosinophilia. **Hypersensitivity:** pustular contact eruption, edema of face, eyes, tongue, legs. **Skin:** SLE-like dermatitis, *alopecia*, photosensitivity, erythema, increased pigmentation, skin dryness and fissuring, pruritic maculopapular rash. **Topical:** local pain, pruritus, hyperpigmentation, burning at site of application, dermatitis, suppuration, swelling, scarring, toxic granulation.

DIAGNOSTIC TEST INTERFERENCE Fluorouracil may increase excretion of ***5-hydroxyindoleacetic acid (5-HIAA)*** and decrease ***plasma albumin*** (because of drug-induced protein malabsorption).

INCOMPATIBILITIES Solution/additive: cytarabine, diazepam, doxorubicin, droperidol. Y-site: droperidol, TPN.

NURSING IMPLICATIONS

Administration

Parenteral IV

- Dose is determined by actual weight unless patient is obese, in which case ideal weight is used.
- Currently recommended procedure for safe handling: Double-glove with latex gloves, and change the double set after every 30 min of exposure. If a drug spill occurs, gloves should be changed immediately after it is cleaned up.
- This drug may be given without dilution by direct IV injection over 1–2 min.
- Inspect injection site frequently; avoid extravasation. If it occurs, stop infusion and restart in another vein. Ice compresses may reduce danger of local tissue damage from infiltrated solution.
- Fluorouracil solution is normally colorless to faint yellow. Slight discoloration during storage does not appear to affect potency or safety. Discard dark yellow solution. If a precipitate forms, redissolve drug by heating to 60C (140F) and shake vigorously. Allow to cool to body temperature before administration.

Topical Application

- Use gloved fingers to apply topical drug.
- Occlusive dressings with topical drug are not recommended. A porous gauze dressing used for cosmetic purposes does not cause inflammation.
- Second-degree burns from contact of plastic eyeglass frames with treated skin have been reported. Risk of burns or irritation may be reduced by (1) treating skin that contacts frames only at night when glasses are not worn, and (2) using the lowest effective strength of topical preparation.
- Store drugs at 15–30C (59–86F) unless otherwise directed. Protect from light and freezing.

Assessment & Drug Effects

- Total and differential leukocyte counts should be determined before each dose is administered. Drug should be discontinued if leukopenia occurs (WBC <3500/mm^3) or if patient develops thrombocytopenia (platelet count <100,000/mm^3). Baseline and periodic checks of hematocrit and liver and kidney function test are also advised.
- During leukopenic period (WBC <3500/mm^3) patient should be in protective isolation.
- During thrombocytopenic period (day 7–17), watch for and report signs of abnormal bleeding from any source; inspect skin for ecchymotic and petechial areas. Protect patient from trauma.
- Report disorientation or confusion; drug should be withdrawn immediately.
- Establish a reference data base for body weight, I&O ratio and pattern, food preferences and dietary habits, bowel habits, and condition of mouth.
- If vomiting is intractable report it to physician.
- Indications for drug discontinuation are severe stomatitis, leukopenia (WBC < 3500/mm^3 or rapidly decreasing count), intractable vomiting, diarrhea, thrombocytopenia (platelets < 100,000/mm^3), and hemorrhage from any site.
- Inspect patient's mouth daily. Promptly report cracked lips, xerostomia, white patches, and erythema of buccal membranes.
- Report development of maculopapular rash, which usually responds to symptomatic treatment and is reversible.
- Expected response of lesion to topical 5-FU: erythema followed in sequence by vesiculation, erosion, ulceration, necrosis, epithelialization. Applications of drug are continued until ulcerative stage is reached (2–6 wk after initial applications) and then discontinued.
- Systemic toxicity may follow use of topical drug on large ulcerated area. Report symptoms promptly.

Patient & Family Education

- Inform the patient of the importance of prompt reporting of the first signs of toxicity: anorexia, vomiting, nausea, stomatitis, diarrhea, GI bleeding.
- Periodic checks on liver and kidney function will be scheduled.
- Caution patient not to change dosage regimen, i.e., not to increase, or omit doses or change dosage intervals.
- Caution patient to avoid exposure to sunlight or to ultraviolet lamp treatments. Protect exposed skin. Photosensitivity usually subsides 2–3 mo after last dose.
- If patient manifests difficulty in maintaining balance while ambulating, report symptom to physician promptly.
- Prepare patient for alopecia; new hair growth usually begins within 6–8 wk.
- Contraception is advisable during 5-FU treatment. Advise patient to report to physican if she suspects pregnancy.

FLUOXETINE HYDROCHLORIDE

(flu′-ox-e-tine)

Trade name: Prozac

Prototype for classifications: CNS AGENT; PSYCHOTHERAPEUTIC; SEROTONIN-REUPTAKE INHIBITOR

Pregnancy category: B

ACTIONS/PHARMACODYNAMICS Oral antidepressant chemically unrelated to tricyclic, tetracyclic, or other available antidepressants. Antidepressant effect is presumed to be linked to its inhibition of CNS presynaptic neuronal uptake of serotonin.

USES Depression, obsessive compulsive disorders, bulimia nervosa. **Unlabeled use:** obesity.

ROUTE & DOSAGE

Depression
Adult: **PO** 20 mg/d in AM; may increase to max of 80 mg/d.
Geriatric: **PO** May need to start with 10 mg/d.

PHARMACOKINETICS **Absorption:** 60–80% absorbed from GI tract. **Onset:** 1–3 wk. **Peak:** 4–8 h. **Distribution:** widely distributed, including CNS. **Metabolism:** metabolized in liver to active metabolite, norfluoxetine. **Elimination:** half-life: fluoxetine 2–3 d, norfluoxetine 7–9 d; > 80% excreted in urine; 12% in feces.

CONTRAINDICATIONS & PRECAUTIONS **Contraindicated in:** hypersensitivity to fluoxetine. **Cautious use in:** hepatic and renal impairment, anorexia, hyponatremia, diabetes, and patients with history of suicidal ideations. Elderly may require dose adjustments. Safety in pregnancy (category B), lactation, and in children not established.

ADVERSE/SIDE EFFECTS **CNS:** *headache, nervousness, anxiety, insomnia,* drowsiness, fatigue, tremor, dizziness. **CV:** palpitations, hot flushes, chest pain. **GI:** *nausea, diarrhea,* anorexia, dyspepsia, increased appetite, dry mouth. **Skin:** rash, pruritus, sweating, hypersensitivity reactions. **Other:** blurred vision, myalgias, arthralgias, flu-like syndrome, hyponatremia, sexual dysfunction, menstrual irregularities.

DRUG INTERACTIONS Concurrent use of **tryptophan** may cause agitation, restlessness, and GI distress; MAO INHIBITORS, **selegiline** may increase risk of severe hypertensive reaction and death; increases half-life of **diazepam**; may increase toxicity of TRICYCLIC ANTIDEPRESSANTS.

F

NURSING IMPLICATIONS

Administration

- Administer single dose in AM. Any additional doses should be administered at noon.
- Provide suicidal or potentially suicidal patient with small quantities of prescription medication.

Assessment & Drug Effects

- Use with caution in elderly patient and patient with impaired renal or hepatic function (may need lower dose).
- Use with caution in anorexic patient, since weight loss is a possible side effect.
- Monitor for signs and symptoms of anaphylactoid reaction (see Appendix G).
- Monitor for signs of improved affect. Requires approximately 2–3 wk for therapeutic effects to be felt.
- Weigh weekly to monitor weight loss, particularly in the elderly or nutritionally compromised patient. Report significant weight loss to physician.
- Observe for and promptly report rash or urticaria and signs and symptoms of fever, leukocytosis, arthralgias, carpal tunnel syndrome, edema, respiratory distress, and proteinuria. Drug may have to be discontinued or adjunctive therapy instituted with steroids or antihistamines.
- Observe for dizziness and drowsi-

ness and employ safety measures (up with assistance, side rails, etc.) as indicated.

- Observe for and report increased anxiety, nervousness, or insomnia; modification of drug dose may be needed.
- Observe for seizures in patients with a history of seizures. Use appropriate safety precautions.
- Closely supervise patients who are high suicide risks, especially during initial therapy.
- Carefully monitor patients with hepatic or renal impairment for signs of toxicity (e.g., agitation, restlessness, nausea, vomiting, seizures).
- Monitor serum sodium level for development of hyponatremia, especially in patients who are taking diuretics or are otherwise hypovolemic.
- Monitor diabetics for loss of control; hypoglycemia has occurred during initiation of therapy, and hyperglycemia during drug withdrawal.

Patient & Family Education

- Instruct patient to take medication in AM for single dose or AM and noon for divided doses to prevent insomnia.
- Instruct patient that therapeutic effects may take from several days to 5 wk to develop fully.
- Advise patient to notify physician of intent to become pregnant or if breast feeding.
- Instruct patient that a rash could be one sign of a serious group of adverse effects and to notify physician if noted.
- Caution patients, particularly the elderly, to exercise safety precautions and to avoid hazardous tasks if dizziness noted.
- Advise diabetics of possible loss of diabetic control and need for careful monitoring.
- Advise those with history of seizures of possible increase in seizure activity.

FLUOXYMESTERONE

(floo-ox-ee-mess′te-rone)

Trade names: Halotestin, Ora Testryl ♣

Classifications: SYNTHETIC HORMONE; ANDROGEN/ANABOLIC STEROID

Prototype: Testosterone

Pregnancy category: X

Controlled substance: Schedule III

ACTIONS/PHARMACODYNAMICS

Short-acting, orally effective derivative of testosterone. Has hypercholesterolemic effect. Retention of sodium is minimal; thus hypertension and edema rarely complicate therapy. Reduces nitrogen, potassium, and calcium excretion and promotes recalcification of osseous metastases and regression of soft tissue lesions.

USES In men as replacement therapy in conditions associated with testicular hormone deficiency; in women to antagonize effects of estrogen in androgen-responsive inoperable breast cancer. Also in combination with estrogens for management of severe postmenopausal vasomotor symptoms.

ROUTE & DOSAGE

Male Hypogonadism

Adult: **PO** 2.5–20 mg/d.

Metastatic Carcinoma of Female Breast

Adult: **PO** 10–40 mg/d in divided doses.

Postpartum Breast Engorgement

Adult: **PO** 2.5 mg shortly after delivery; then 5–10 mg/d in divided doses for 4–5 d.

PHARMACOKINETICS Absorption: readily absorbed from GI tract. **Metabolism:** metabolized in liver. **Elimination:** half-life: 9.5 h.

CONTRAINDICATIONS & PRECAUTIONS Contraindicated in: breast cancer in men, prostatic cancer, benign obstructive prostatic hypertrophy; hypercalcemia; diabetes mellitus; severe cardiorenal disease or liver damage; nephrosis or nephrotic phase of nephritis; history of MI; athletes; infants; women with inoperable mammary cancer <1 y or >5 y after menopause; pregnancy (category X), nursing mothers.

ADVERSE/SIDE EFFECTS Virilization (women); priapism, impotence, gynecomastia (men); jaundice (reversible), hypoglycemia, hypercalcemia, hepatocellular carcinoma, peliosis hepatitis, nausea, vomiting, diarrhea, symptoms resembling peptic ulcer, anaphylactic reactions (rare), *edema, acne.*

DRUG INTERACTIONS ORAL ANTICOAGULANTS increase risk of bleeding. Possibly increases risk of **cyclosporine** toxicity. **Insulin** and ORAL HYPOGLYCEMIC AGENTS may decrease glucose level; dose will need to be adjusted.

NURSING IMPLICATIONS

Administration

- Administer drug immediately before or with meals to diminish GI distress.

Assessment & Drug Effects

- Baseline and periodic determinations of liver function and serum electrolytes are indicated. Serial determinations of serum cholesterol are advised in patients with history of MI or coronary artery disease.
- Monitor I&O ratio and pattern and weight, and check for edema; report significant changes.
- Monitor for signs of hypercalcemia (see Appendix G), which is particularly likely to occur in patients with metastatic breast carcinoma. Anabolic therapy will be stopped if it develops.
- Be alert for voice change in female patient, an early sign of virilism. Virilism may be irreversible even after prompt discontinuation of therapy.
- When used in pediatrics, therapy is preceded by x-ray of wrist bones to establish level of bone maturation. During treatment, bone maturation may proceed more rapidly than linear growth; therefore, intermittent dosage schedule and periodic x-rays are usual.
- Children <7 y are particularly sensitive to androgenic effects and therefore should be closely observed for precocious development of male sexual characteristics or masculinization.
- Anabolic treatment may reduce blood glucose in diabetic patients. Watch for symptoms of hypoglycemia (see Appendix G) and report to physician.
- Observe patient on concomitant anticoagulant therapy for ecchymotic areas, petechiae, or abnormal bleeding from any site. Close monitoring of PT is essential.
- When fluoxymesterone is used for palliation of mammary cancer, subjective effects of therapy may not be experienced for about 1 mo; objective symptoms may be delayed for as long as 3 mo.
- Anabolic response may be evidenced by euphoria and gain in weight and appetite, especially in emaciated and debilitated patient.
- Baseline and periodic determinations should be made of Hgb, Hct, hepatic function, and serum and urine calcium.

Patient & Family Education

- Reinforce adherence to scheduled appointments for laboratory tests. Stress importance of good personal hygiene, including meticulous skin care (females and prepubertal males are especially likely to develop acne).
- Teach patient to note and report symptoms of jaundice (see Appendix G) to physician. Dose adjustment may reverse the condition.
- Instruct female patient to report menstrual irregularities.
- Teach parents the importance of keeping child's appointments for bone maturation studies (usually every 3–6 mo) to prevent compromised adult height.
- Instruct to report priapism (symptom of overdosage) promptly; temporary interruption of regimen is indicated. Also advise to report persistent GI distress, diarrhea, or the onset of jaundice.
- Explain to female that virilization usually occurs. Urge early reporting of voice change (hoarseness or deepening), increased libido (associated with clitoral enlargement), hirsutism. Usually, stopping therapy will end further development of symptoms but will not reverse hirsutism or voice change.

FLUPHENAZINE DECANOATE

(floo-fen′a-zeen)

Trade names: Prolixin Decanoate, Modecate Decanoate ♣

FLUPHENAZINE ENANTHATE

Trade names: Moditen Enanthate ♣ Prolixin Enanthate

FLUPHENAZINE HYDROCHLORIDE

Trade names: Moditen Hydrochloride ♣, Permitil, Prolixin

Classifications: CNS AGENT; PSYCHOTHERAPEUTIC; ANTIPSYCHOTIC; PHENOTHIAZINE

Prototype: Chlorpromazine

Pregnancy category: C

ACTIONS/PHARMACODYNAMICS

Potent phenothiazine. Blocks postsynaptic dopamine receptors in the brain. Similar to other phenothiazines with the following exceptions: more potent per weight, higher incidence of extrapyramidal complications, and lower frequency of sedative and hypotensive effects.

USE Management of manifestations of psychotic disorders. **Unlabeled use:** as antineuralgia adjunct.

ROUTE & DOSAGE

Psychosis

Adult: **PO** 0.5–10 mg/d in 1–4 divided doses, up to a usual max of 20 mg/d. **IM/SC** ***HCl:*** 2.5–10 mg/d divided q6–8h up to usual max of 10 mg/d. ***Decanoate:*** 12.5–25 mg q1–4wk. ***Enanthate:*** 25 mg q2wk.

Dementia Behavior

Geriatric **PO** 1–2.5 mg/d, may increase every 4–7 d by 1–2.5 mg/d to max 20 mg/d in 2–3 divided doses.

PHARMACOKINETICS **Absorption:** HCl is readily absorbed PO and IM; decanoate, enanthate have delayed IM absorption. **Onset:** 1 h HCl; 24–72 h decanoate, enanthate. **Peak:** 0.5 h PO; 1.5–2 h IM HCl. **Duration:** 6–8 h HCl; 1–6 wk decanoate; 2–4 wk enanthate. **Distribution:** crosses blood–brain barrier and placenta. **Metabolism:** metabolized in liver. **Elimination:** half-life: 15 h HCl; 3.6 d enanthate; 7–10 d decanoate.

CONTRAINDICATIONS & PRECAUTIONS **Contraindicated in:** known hypersensitivity to phenothiazines; subcortical brain damage, comatose or severely depressed states, blood dyscrasias, renal or hepatic disease. Safe use during pregnancy (category C) or in nursing women not established. Parenteral form not recommended for children <12 y. **Cautious use in:** with anticholinergic agents, other CNS depressants; elderly patients, previously diagnosed breast cancer; cardiovascular diseases; pheochromocytoma; history of convulsive disorders; patients exposed to extreme heat or phosphorous insecticides; peptic ulcer; respiratory impairment.

ADVERSE/SIDE EFFECTS **CNS:** *extrapyramidal symptoms* (resembling Parkinson's disease), tardive dyskinesia, sedation, drowsiness, dizziness, headache, mental depression, catatonic-like state, impaired thermoregulation, grand mal seizures. **CV:** tachycardia, hypertension, hypotension. **GI:** dry mouth, nausea, epigastric pain, constipation, fecal impaction, cholecystic jaundice. **GU:** urinary retention, polyuria. **Gynecologic:** inhibition of ejaculation. **Hematologic:** transient leukopenia, agranulocytosis. **Other:** contact dermatitis, peripheral edema, nasal congestion, blurred vision, increased intraocular pressure, *photosensitivity,* hyperprolactinemia.

DRUG INTERACTIONS **Alcohol** and other CNS DEPRESSANTS may potentiate depressive effects; decreases seizure threshold—may need to adjust dosage of ANTICONVULSANTS.

NURSING IMPLICATIONS

Administration

- Extended-release tablet should be swallowed whole (not recommended for children).
- Dilute PO concentrate in fruit juice, water, carbonated beverage, milk, soup. Avoid caffeine-containing beverages (cola, coffee) as a diluent, also tannic acid (tea) or pectinates (apple juice).
- Persons preparing PO concentrate or liquid preparations for injection should be careful not to contact skin or clothing with drug. Warn patient to avoid spilling drug. If skin is contacted, it should be rinsed promptly with warm water.
- Antacids diminish absorption; therefore administer PO preparations at least 1 h before or 2 h after the antacid.
- Fluphenazine enanthate and decanoate are given IM or SC.
- All preparations of fluphenazine should be protected from light and from freezing. Solutions may safely vary in color from almost colorless to light amber. Discard dark or otherwise discolored solutions.
- Store in tightly closed container at 15–30C (59–86F) unless otherwise specified by manufacturer.

Assessment & Drug Effects

- Report immediately the onset of mental depression and extrapyramidal symptoms. They occur frequently, particularly with long-acting forms (decanoate and enanthate). Be alert for appearance of acute dystonia (see Appendix G). Symptoms can be controlled by reducing fluphenazine dosage or by adding an antiparkinsonism drug such as benztropine (Cogentin).
- Extended exposure to high environmental temperature, to sun's rays, or to a high fever associated with serious illness places this patient at risk for heat stroke. Be alert to red, dry, hot skin; full, bounding pulse, dilated pupils, dyspnea,

mental confusion, elevated BP, temperature over 40.6C (105F). Inform physician and institute measures to reduce body temperature rapidly.

- Renal function should be monitored in patients on long-term treatment. The drug should be discontinued if BUN is elevated (normal BUN: 10–20 mg/dl). WBC with differential, hepatic function tests, and ophthalmologic examinations should also be performed periodically.
- Monitor BP during early therapy. If systolic drop is more than 20 mm Hg, inform physician.
- Monitor I&O ratio and bowel elimination pattern. Check for abdominal distension and pain. Monitor for xerostomia and constipation.
- Patients on large doses who undergo surgery and those with cerebrovascular, cardiac, or renal insufficiency are especially prone to hypotensive effects.

Patient & Family Education

- Caution patient against driving motor vehicle or other hazardous activities until reaction to the drug is known.
- Advise patient not to alter dosage regimen or stop it abruptly. Caution patient not to give the drug to any other person.
- The physician should give approval before patient self-doses with OTC drugs.
- Because both decanoate and enanthate formulations have a long duration of action, early detection of adverse effects is critical. Patient should inform the physician promptly if the following symptoms appear: light-colored stools, changes in vision, sore throat, fever, cellulitis, rash, any interference with volitional movement.
- Encourage adequate food and fluid intake as prophylaxis for constipation and for xerostomia.
- Patient may be unable to adjust to extreme temperatures. Advise caution because of possible impaired thermoregulation.
- Warn patient to avoid exposure to sun, to wear protective clothing and cover exposed skin surfaces with sun screen lotion (SPF above 12).
- Alcohol should be avoided while patient is on fluphenazine therapy.
- Inform patient that fluphenazine may discolor urine pink to red or reddish brown.

FLURANDRENOLIDE

(flure-an-dren'oh-lide)

Trade names: Cordran, Cordran SP, Drenison ♣

Classifications: SKIN AGENT; ANTI-INFLAMMATORY; ADRENAL CORTICOSTEROID

Prototype: Hydrocortisone

Pregnancy category: C

See Appendix A.

FLURAZEPAM HYDROCHLORIDE

(flure-az'e-pam)

Trade names: Apo-Flurazepam ♣, Dalmane, Durapam, Novoflupam ♣

Classifications: CNS AGENT ANXIOLYTIC; SEDATIVE-HYPNOTIC; BENZODIAZEPINE

Prototype: Lorazepam

Pregnancy category: X

Controlled substance: Schedule IV

ACTIONS/PHARMACODYNAMICS

Benzodiazepine derivative, with hypnotic activity equal to or greater than that produced by barbiturates or chloral hydrate. Mode and site of action not known but appears to act at limbic and subcortical levels of CNS to produce sedation, skeletal muscle relaxation, and anticonvulsant effects. Reduces sleep induction time; produces marked reduction of stage 4 sleep (deepest sleep stage) while at the same time increasing duration of total sleep time.

USES Hypnotic in management of all kinds of insomnia (e.g., difficulty in falling asleep, frequent nocturnal awakening or early morning awakening or both). Also for treatment of poor sleeping habits.

ROUTE & DOSAGE

Sedative, Hypnotic
Adult ≥*15 y:* **PO** 15–30 mg h.s.
Geriatric: **PO** 15 mg h.s.

PHARMACOKINETICS Absorption: readily absorbed from GI tract. **Onset:** 15–45 min. **Duration:** 7–8 h. **Distribution:** crosses blood–brain barrier and placenta; distributed into breast milk. **Metabolism:** metabolized in liver to active metabolites. **Elimination:** half-life: 47–100 h; excreted primarily in urine.

CONTRAINDICATIONS & PRECAUTIONS Contraindicated in: prolonged administration; sleep apnea; intermittent porphyria; acute narrow-angle glaucoma; children <15 y; pregnancy (category X), nursing mothers. **Cautious use in:** impaired renal or hepatic function; mental depression, psychoses, history of suicidal tendencies, addiction-prone individuals; elderly or debilitated patients; COPD.

ADVERSE/SIDE EFFECTS CNS: *residual sedation, drowsiness,* light-headedness, dizziness, ataxia, headache, nervousness, apprehension, talkativeness, irritability, depression, hallucinations, nightmares, confusion, paradoxic reactions: excitement, euphoria, hyperactivity, disorientation, coma (overdosage). **Eye:** blurred vision, burning eyes. **GI:** heartburn, nausea, vomiting, diarrhea, abdominal pain. **Other:** immediate allergic reaction, hypotension, granulocytopenia (rare), jaundice (rare).

DIAGNOSTIC TEST INTERFERENCE Flurazepam may increase serum levels of ***total and direct bilirubin, alkaline phosphatase, AST,*** and ***ALT.*** False-negative ***urine glucose*** reactions may occur with ***Clinistix*** and ***Diastix;*** no effect with TesTape.

DRUG INTERACTIONS Alcohol, CNS DEPRESSANTS, ANTICONVULSANTS potentiate CNS depression; **cimetidine, disulfiram** may increase flurazepam levels, thus increasing its toxicity.

NURSING IMPLICATIONS

Administration

- Encourage patient to remain upright in bed (e.g., reading) for 20–30 min after taking the drug. This may help patient experience the onset of natural sleepiness.
- Store in light-resistant container with childproof cap at 15–30C (59–86F) unless otherwise specified.

Assessment & Drug Effects

- Hypnotic effect is apparent on second or third night of consecutive use and continues 1 or 2 nights after drug is stopped (drug has a long half-life).
- Residual sedation and drowsiness are relatively common. Excessive drowsiness, ataxia, vertigo, and falling occur more frequently in elderly or debilitated patients. Supervise ambulation.
- Prolonged use of large doses can

result in psychic and physical dependence. If patient has a history of drug abuse, monitor drug ingestion.

- With repeated use, blood counts and liver and kidney function tests are advised.
- Withdrawal symptoms have occurred 3 d after abrupt discontinuation of flurazepam after prolonged use: worsening of insomnia, dizziness, blurred vision, anorexia, GI upset, nasal congestion, paresthesias.

F

Patient & Family Education

- Warn patients to avoid potentially hazardous activities until reaction to drug is known.
- Caution patient to avoid alcohol. Concurrent ingestion with flurazepam intensifies CNS depressant effects. Symptoms may occur even when alcohol is ingested as long as 10 h after last flurazepam dose.
- Caution patients about the possibility of additive depressant effects if flurazepam is combined with barbiturates, tranquilizers, or other CNS depressants.
- Dose intervals or dosage should not be changed. Instruct patient not to use it for a self-diagnosed problem.
- Patient should be advised that if she becomes pregnant during therapy or intends to become pregnant, she should ask her physician about the desirability of discontinuing the drug.
- Because insomnia is usually transient, the prolonged use of this hypnotic is inadvisable.

FLURBIPROFEN SODIUM

(flure-bi′proe-fen)

Trade names: Ansaid, Ocufen

Classifications: CNS AGENT; ANALGESIC, ANTIPYRETIC; NSAID

Prototype: Ibuprofen

Pregnancy category: C

ACTIONS/PHARMACODYNAMICS

Inhibitor of prostaglandin synthesis including in the conjunctiva and uvea; structurally and pharmacologically related to ibuprofen. When administered prophylactically, ocular flurbiprofen reduces miosis, permitting maintenance of drug-induced mydriasis during surgical procedures. Also inhibits migration of leukocytes into inflamed tissues, depresses monocyte function, and may inhibit platelet aggregation. Has no significant effect on IOP.

USES Inhibition of intraoperative miosis; arthritis and other inflammatory diseases; mild to moderate pain. **Unlabeled uses:** management of postoperative ocular inflammation, prevention of postcystoid macular edema.

ROUTE & DOSAGE

Inflammatory Disease

Adult: **PO** 200–300 mg/d in 2–4 divided doses (max 300 mg/d).

Mild-to-Moderate Pain

Adult: **PO** 50–100 mg q6–8h.

Inhibition of Intraoperative Miosis

Adult: **Topical** 1 drop in eye approximately q30min beginning 2 h before surgery for a total of 4 drops per affected eye.

PHARMACOKINETICS Absorption: 80% absorbed from GI tract. **Onset:** 2 h. **Peak:** 2 h. **Duration:** 6–8 h. **Distribution:** small amounts distributed into breast milk. **Metabolism:** metabolized in liver. **Elimination:** half-life: 5 h; excreted primarily in urine; some biliary excretion.

CONTRAINDICATIONS & PRECAUTIONS **Contraindicated in:** epithelial herpes simplex keratitis. Safe use during pregnancy (category C), by nursing mothers, or children not established. **Cautious use in:** concomitant use with other NSAIDS; patient who may be adversely affected by prolonged bleeding time; patient in whom asthma, rhinitis, or urticaria is precipitated by aspirin or other NSAIDS. For contraindications to oral use, see ibuprofen.

ADVERSE/SIDE EFFECTS **Ocular:** (transient): *mild ocular stinging,* burning, itching, or foreign body sensation. **Other:** slowed corneal healing; increased bleeding time. For adverse/side effects to oral preparations, see ibuprofen.

DRUG INTERACTIONS ORAL ANTICOAGULANTS, **heparin** may prolong bleeding time; actions and side effects of both flurbiprofen and **phenytoin**, SULFONYLUREAS, or SULFONAMIDES may be potentiated.

NURSING IMPLICATIONS

For nursing implications for oral preparation, see ibuprofen.

Administration of Eye Preparation

- Administer ophthalmic preparation with great care to avoid contamination of solution. Do not touch eye surface with dropper.
- Store at 15–30C (59–86F) in tight, light-resistant container.

Patient & Family Education for Eye Preparation

- Ocular irritation that persists after flurbiprofen use during surgery (tearing, dry eye sensation, dull eye pain, photophobia) should be reported to physician.
- Advise patient with bleeding tendency to report unexplained bleeding, prolongation of bleeding time, or bruises. Minor systemic absorption of flurbiprofen may temporarily increase bleeding time.

F

FLUTAMIDE

(flu′ta-mide)

Trade name: Eulexin

Classifications: ANTINEOPLASTIC; ANTIANDROGEN

Pregnancy category: D

ACTIONS/PHARMACODYNAMICS Flutamide is a nonsteroidal, nonhormonal, antiandrogenic drug. It exerts its antiandrogenic effects in inhibiting androgen uptake and/or inhibiting binding of androgen to target tissues (i.e., prostatic cancer cells). It interferes with the binding of both testosterone and dihydrotestosterone to target tissue.

USES In combination with luteinizing hormone-releasing hormone agonists (i.e., luprolide) or castration for early stage and metastatic prostate cancer.

ROUTE & DOSAGE

Prostate Cancer

Adult: **PO** 250 mg (2 caps) q8h.

PHARMACOKINETICS **Absorption:** readily absorbed from GI tract. **Onset:** antiandrogenic activity 2.2 h; symptomatic relief 2–4 wk. **Duration:** 3 mo–2.5 y, with an average of 10.5 mo. **Metabolism:** metabolized in liver to at least 10 different metabolites; the major metabolite, 2-hydroxyflutamide (SCH-16423), is an alpha-hydroxylated derivative that is biologically active. **Elimination:** half-life: 5–6 h; 98% excreted in urine.

CONTRAINDICATIONS & PRECAUTIONS **Contraindicated in:** hypersensitivity to flutamide, pregnancy (category D). **Cautious use in:** severe liver impairment.

F

ADVERSE/SIDE EFFECTS **CNS:** drowsiness, confusion, depression, anxiety, nervousness. **GI:** diarrhea, nausea, vomiting, anorexia, hepatitis, cholestatic jaundice, encephalopathy, hepatic necrosis, may increase SGOT, SGPT, bilirubin. **GU:** *hot flashes, loss of libido, impotence.* **Hematologic:** anemia, leukopenia, thrombocytopenia. **Other:** rash, edema, gynecomastia, galactorrhea.

NURSING IMPLICATIONS

Administration

- Flutamide should be used with caution in patients with severe hepatic impairment.
- Store at temperatures between 2 and 30C (36 and 86F) in a tightly closed, light-resistant container.

Assessment & Drug Effects

- Therapeutic response should be monitored with acid and alkaline phosphatase tests, bone and liver scans, chest x-ray, and physical exam.
- Monitor for symptomatic relief of bone pain.
- Assess for development of gynecomastia and galactorrhea; if these become bothersome, dosage reduction may be warranted.
- Monitor liver functions and serum bilirubin periodically.
- Monitor for and report development of a lupus-like syndrome.

Patient & Family Education

- Inform the patient of potential adverse effects of flutamide therapy.
- Advise patients to notify physician immediately if any of the following occur: pain in upper abdomen, yellowing of skin and eyes, dark urine, respiratory problems, rashes on face, difficulty urinating, sore throat, fever, chills.

FLUTICASONE

(flu-ti-ca′sone)

Trade names: Flonase, Flovent

Classifications: SKIN AND MUCOUS MEMBRANE AGENT; ANTIINFLAMMATORY; HORMONE; ADRENAL CORTICOSTEROID

Prototype: Hydrocortisone

Pregnancy category: C

See Appendix A.

FLUVASTATIN

(flu-vah-stat′-in)

Trade name: Lescol

Classifications: CARDIOVASCULAR AGENT; ANTILIPEMIC; HMG-COA REDUCTASE INHIBITOR (STATIN)

Prototype: Lovastatin

Pregnancy category: X

ACTIONS/PHARMACODYNAMICS Fluvastatin is an inhibitor of therapeutic reductase 3-hydroxy-3-methylglutaryl coenzyme A (HMG-CoA), which is essential to hepatic production of cholesterol. This cholesterol-lowering effect triggers induction of LDL receptors, which promote removal of LDL and VLDL remnants (precursors of LDL) from plasma. Fluvastatin therapy also results in an increase in plasma HDL concentrations. (HDLs collect excess cholesterol from body cells and transport it to the liver for excretion.)

USES Adjunct to diet for the reduction of elevated total LDL cholesterol in patients with primary hypercholesterolemia (Types IIa and IIb). **Unlabeled use:** other types of hyperlipidemias.

ROUTE & DOSAGE

Adult: **PO** 20 mg h.s.; may increase up to 80 mg/d in 1–2 doses.

PHARMACOKINETICS Absorption: readily absorbed from GI tract; about 24% reaches systemic circulation after first-pass metabolism **Onset:** 3–6 wk. **Peak:** serum level 0.5–1 h. **Distribution:** 98% protein bound; distributed into breast milk. **Metabolism:** metabolized in liver. **Elimination:** half-life: 0.5–1 h; 95% excreted in bile; 5% excreted in urine.

CONTRAINDICATIONS & PRECAUTIONS Contraindicated in: hypersensitivity to fluvastatin, lovastatin, pravastatin, or simvastatin; active liver disease or unexplained persistent elevated liver function tests; pregnancy (category X); lactation. **Cautious use in:** patients who consume substantial quantities of alcohol; history of liver disease; renal impairment.

ADVERSE/SIDE EFFECTS CNS: headache. **GI:** dyspepsia. **Skin:** rash.

DRUG INTERACTION May increase risk of bleeding with **warfarin.**

NURSING IMPLICATIONS

Administration

- Fluvastatin should be given at bedtime.
- When given concomitantly with a bile-acid resin (such as cholestyramine), separate the doses of the two drugs by at least 2 h.
- Dosage adjustments may be required in patients with significant renal or hepatic impairment.
- Store at room temperature, 15–30C (59–86F).

Assessment & Drug Effects

- Monitor lipoprotein levels; maximal lipid-lowering effect occurs in 4–6 wk.
- Monitor serum transaminase and CPK levels every 3–4 mo for the first year and periodically thereafter.
- Monitor PT in patients on concurrent warfarin therapy, as PT may be prolonged.

Patient & Family Education

- Stress the importance of taking fluvastatin at bedtime.
- Alert patients on warfarin therapy to report signs of bleeding immediately.
- Instruct patient to notify physician immediately if any of the following occur: fever; rash; muscle pain, weakness, tenderness, or cramping.
- Advise patient to reduce or eliminate alcohol consumption while on fluvastatin.

F

FLUVOXAMINE

(flu-vox'a-meen)

Trade name: Luvox

Classifications: CNS AGENTS; PSYCHOTHERAPEUTIC; SELECTIVE SEROTONIN REUPTAKE INHIBITOR

Prototype: Fluoxetine

Pregnancy category: B

ACTIONS/PHARMACODYNAMICS Fluvoxamine is an antidepressant with potent, selective, inhibitory activity on neuronal (5-HT) serotonin reuptake (SSRI); it is structurally unrelated to TCAs. Compared with TCAs, fluvoxamine has fewer anticholinergic effects and no severe cardiovascular effects.

USES Treatment of depression and obsessive-compulsive disorders. **Unlabeled uses:** chronic tension-type headaches, panic attacks.

ROUTE & DOSAGE

Depression, Obsessive-Compulsive Disorder

Adult: **PO** Start with 50 mg q.d.; may increase slowly up to 300 mg/d given q.h.s. or divided b.i.d.

Child 8–11 y: **PO** Start with 25 mg q.h.s.; may increase by 25 mg q4–7d to a max of 200 mg/d in divided doses.

F

PHARMACOKINETICS Absorption: almost completely absorbed from GI tract. **Onset:** 4–7d. **Distribution:** approximately 77% bound to plasma proteins; excreted in human breast milk but in an amount that poses little risk to the nursing infant. **Metabolism:** metabolized in liver. **Elimination:** half-life: 16–24 h; completely excreted in urine.

CONTRAINDICATIONS & PRECAUTIONS Contraindicated in: hypersensitivity to fluvoxamine or fluoxetine. **Cautious use in:** pregnancy (category B), lactation, liver disease, renal impairment, history of seizures.

ADVERSE/SIDE EFFECTS CNS: *somnolence, headache, agitation, insomnia, dizziness,* seizures. **CV:** orthostatic hypotension, slight bradycardia. **GI:** *nausea, vomiting, dry mouth, constipation, anorexia.* **GU:** sexual dysfunction. **Skin (rare):** <u>Stevens-Johnson syndrome, toxic epidermal necrolysis</u>.

DIAGNOSTIC TEST INTERFERENCE ***Gamma-glutamyl transferase*** increased by more than 3-fold following 3 wk of therapy.

DRUG INTERACTIONS Fluvoxamine has been shown to significantly increase plasma levels of **amitriptyline, clomipramine**, and other TRICYCLIC ANTIDEPRESSANTS to mildly increase levels of their metabolites. May antagonize the blood pressure-lowering effects of **atenolol** and other BETA BLOCKERS. May increase levels and toxicity of **carbamazepine.** May increase **lithium** levels causing neurotoxicity, serotonin syndrome, somnolence, and mania. One report of increased **theophylline** levels with toxicity. Increases prothrombin time in patients on **warfarin.**

NURSING IMPLICATIONS

Administration

- In adults low starting doses of 50 mg/d and/or giving total daily dose at bedtime may improve tolerance to nausea and vomiting, which are common early in therapy.
- Store at room temperature, 15–30C (59–86F), away from moisture and light.

Assessment & Drug Effects

- Monitor for significant nausea and vomiting, especially when therapy is initiated.
- Assess safety, as drowsiness and dizziness are common adverse effects.
- With concurrent warfarin therapy, monitor PT carefully and adjust warfarin as needed.

Patient & Family Education

- Inform patient that nausea and vomiting may occur when therapy is initiated. The physician should be notified if these adverse effects last more than a few days.
- Advise patient to exercise caution with hazardous activity until response to the drug is known.
- Advise patient to adhere strictly to directions for taking fluvoxamine.

FOLIC ACID (VITAMIN B_9, PTEROYLGLUTAMIC ACID)

Trade names: Apo-Folic♣, Folacin, Folvite, Novofolacid♣

FOLATE SODIUM

Trade name: Folvite Sodium
Classification: VITAMIN B_9
Pregnancy category: A

ACTIONS/PHARMACODYNAMICS Member of vitamin B complex essential for nucleoprotein synthesis and maintenance of normal erythropoiesis. Stimulates production of RBCs, WBCs, and platelets in patients with megaloblastic anemias. In folic acid deficiency, impaired thymidylate synthesis results in production of defective DNA that leads to megaloblast formation and arrest of bone marrow maturation.

USES Folate deficiency, macrocytic anemia, and megaloblastic anemias associated with malabsorption syndromes, alcoholism, primary liver disease, inadequate dietary intake, pregnancy, infancy, and childhood.

ROUTE & DOSAGE

Therapeutic

Adult: **PO/IM/SC/IV** ≤ 1 mg/d.
Child: **PO/IM/SC/IV** ≤1 mg/d.

Maintenance

Adult: **PO/IM/SC/IV** ≤0.4 mg/d.
Child: **PO/IM/SC/IV** *>4 y,* ≤0.4 mg/d; *<4 y,* ≤0.3 mg/d
Infants: ≤0.1 mg/d.

PHARMACOKINETICS Absorption: readily absorbed from proximal small intestine. **Peak:** 30–60 min PO. **Distribution:** distributed to all body tissues; high concentrations in CSF; crosses placenta; distributed into breast milk. **Metabolism:** metabolized in liver to active metabolites. **Elimination:** small amounts eliminated in urine in folate-deficient patients; large amounts excreted in urine with high doses.

CONTRAINDICATIONS & PRECAUTIONS Contraindicated in: folic acid-alone for pernicious anemia or other vitamin B_{12} deficiency states; normocytic, refractory, aplastic, or undiagnosed anemia. **Cautious use in:** pregnancy (category A).

ADVERSE/SIDE EFFECTS Reportedly nontoxic. Slight flushing and feeling of warmth following IV administration.

DIAGNOSTIC TEST INTERFERENCE Falsely low serum ***folate levels*** may occur with ***Lactobacillus casei assay*** in patients receiving antibiotics such as tetracyclines.

DRUG INTERACTIONS Chloramphenicol may antagonize effects of folate therapy; **phenytoin** metabolism may be increased, thus decreasing its levels in folate-deficient patients.

INCOMPATIBILITY Solution/additive: doxapram.

NURSING IMPLICATIONS

Administration

- IV folic acid may be given by direct IV undiluted over 30–60 seconds. May also be added to a continuous infusion.
- Store at 15–30C (59–86F) in tightly closed containers protected from light, unless otherwise directed.

Assessment & Drug Effects

- A careful history of dietary intake and drug and alcohol usage should be obtained before start of therapy. Drugs reported to cause folate deficiency include oral contraceptives, alcohol, barbiturates, methotrexate, phenytoin, primidone, and trimethoprim. Folate deficiency may also result from renal dialysis.

- Therapeutic effects of folic acid therapy include improvement in blood picture and gradual reversal of symptoms of folic acid deficiency: glossitis, diarrhea, constipation, weight loss, irritability, fatigue, restless legs, diffuse muscular pain, insomnia, forgetfulness, mental depression, pallor. Keep physician informed of patient's response.

Patient & Family Education

- Emphasize the need for the patient to remain under close medical supervision while he or she is receiving folic acid therapy. Adjustment of maintenance dose should be made if there is threat of relapse.

F

FOSCARNET

(fos′car-net)

Trade name: Foscavir

Classifications: ANTIINFECTIVE; ANTIVIRAL

Prototype: Acyclovir

Pregnancy category: C

ACTIONS/PHARMACODYNAMICS Inhibits the replication of all known herpesviruses in vitro including cytomegalovirus (CMV), herpes simplex virus types 1 and 2 (HSV-1, HSV-2), human herpesvirus 6 (HHV-6), Epstein-Barr virus (EBV), and varicella-zoster virus (VZV).

USES CMV retinitis, mucocutaneous HSV, acyclovir-resistant HSV in immunocompromised patients. **Unlabeled uses:** other CMV infections, herpes zoster infections in AIDS patients.

ROUTE & DOSAGE

CMV Retinitis

Adult: **IV** ***Induction*** 60 mg/kg infused over 1 h q8h for 2–3 wk; induction may be repeated if relapse occurs during maintenance therapy. ***Alternate induction therapies*** 100 mg/kg q12h for 2–3 wk or 20–30 mg/kg infused over 30 min followed by a continuous infusion of 180–230 mg/kg/d for 2–3 wk. ***Maintenance*** 90–120 mg/kg/d infused over 2 h.

Herpes Simplex Infections in AIDS

Adult: **IV** 40–60 mg/kg q8h for 2–3 wk; may be followed by 50 mg/kg/d for 5–7 d/wk for up to 15 wk.

Acyclovir-resistant HSV in Immunocompromised Patients

Adult: **IV** 40 mg/kg q8–12h for up to 3 wk or until lesions heal.

Dose must be adjusted for renal insufficiency. See package insert for specific dosing adjustment.

PHARMACOKINETICS **Onset:** 3–7 d. **Duration:** relapse usually occurs 3–4 wk after end of therapy. **Distribution:** 3–28% of dose may be deposited in bone; variable penetration into CSF; crosses placenta; distributed into breast milk. **Metabolism:** does not appear to be metabolized. **Elimination:** half-life: 3–4 h; 73–94% excreted in urine.

CONTRAINDICATIONS & PRECAUTIONS **Contraindicated in:** hypersensitivity to foscarnet. **Cautious use in:** renal function impairment, mineral and electrolyte imbalances, seizures, elderly, pregnancy (category C), and nursing women. Safety and efficacy in children have not been established.

ADVERSE/SIDE EFFECTS CV: thrombophlebitis if infused through a peripheral vein. **CNS:** tremor, muscle twitching, headache, weakness, fatigue, confusion, anxiety. **Endocrine:** *hyperphosphatemia,* hypophosphatemia, hypocalcemia. **GI:** nausea, vomiting, diarrhea. **GU:** penile ulceration. **Hematologic:** *anemia,* leukopenia, thrombocytopenia. **Renal:** *nephrotoxicity* (acute renal failure, tubular necrosis). **Skin:** fixed drug eruption, rash.

DIAGNOSTIC TEST INTERFERENCE May cause increase or decrease in serum ***calcium, phosphorus,*** and ***magnesium.*** Decreases ***Hct*** and ***Hgb.*** Increased serum ***creatinine.***

DRUG INTERACTIONS AMINOGLYCOSIDES, **amphotericin B, vancomycin** may increase risk of nephrotoxicity. **Etidronate, pamidronate, pentamidine (IV)** may exacerbate hypocalcemia.

INCOMPATIBILITIES Solution/additive: lactated Ringer's, acyclovir, amphotericin B, calcium, cotrimoxazole, diazepam, digoxin, diphenhydramine, dobutamine, droperidol, ganciclovir, haloperidol, leucovorin, lorazepam, midazolam, pentamidine, phenytoin, prochlorperazine, promethazine, trimetrexate, vancomycin. Y-site: acyclovir, amphotericin B, calcium, cotrimoxazole, diazepam, digoxin, diphenhydramine, dobutamine, droperidol, ganciclovir, haloperidol, leucovorin, lorazepam, midazolam, pentamidine, phenytoin, prochlorperazine, promethazine, trimetrexate, vancomycin.

NURSING IMPLICATIONS

Administration

- Foscarnet may be given undiluted (24 mg/ml) through a central line. For peripheral infusion, dilute to 12 mg/ml with D5W or 0.9% NaCl. No other IV solution or drug may be given through the same catheter with foscarnet.
- Foscarnet must be administered at a constant rate not to exceed 1 mg/kg/min over the specified period of infusion with an infusion pump. Do not increase the rate of infusion or shorten the specified interval between doses.
- Prehydration and continued daily hydration with 2.5 L of 0.9% NaCl are recommended to reduce nephrotoxicity.
- Prepared IV solutions must be used within 24 h.
- Store according to manufacturer's directions.

Assessment & Drug Effects

- Monitor serum creatinine and creatinine clearance throughout therapy. Drug dose will be decreased in response to decreased clearance.
- Monitor for electrolyte imbalances including hypocalcemia, hyperphosphatemia, hypophosphatemia, hypomagnesemia, and hypokalemia.
- Monitor for cardiac arrhythmias, especially in presence of known cardiac abnormalities.
- Monitor for seizures and take appropriate precautions.
- Complete blood count should be periodically monitored, as anemia and other blood dyscrasias are common.
- Question patients regarding local irritation of the penile or vulvovaginal epithelium. If either occurs, increased hydration and better personal hygiene are indicated.

Patient & Family Education

- Advise patient to immediately re-

port perioral tingling, numbness, and paresthesia.
- Advise patient that foscarnet is not a cure for CMV retinitis and that regular ophthalmologic exams are necessary.
- Advise patient of the importance of good hydration to maintain adequate diuresis.

F

FOSFOMYCIN TROMETHAMINE

(fos-fo-my′sin)

Trade name: Monurol

Classifications: ANTIINFECTIVE; ANTIBIOTIC

Prototype: Nitrofurantoin

Pregnancy category: B

ACTIONS/PHARMOCODYNAMICS Fosfomycin is a synthetic, broad-spectrum, bactericidal antibiotic active against gram-negative and gram-positive aerobic organisms. It blocks the first steps in bacterial cell wall synthesis. Fosfomycin is bactericidal against *Enterococcus faecalis, E. fascium,* and *Escherichia coli.* In addition, it is effective against *Klebsiella, Proteus,* and *Serratia.*

USES Treatment of uncomplicated UTIs in women due to susceptible strains of *E. coli* and *E. faecalis.*

ROUTE & DOSAGE

UTI

Adult: **PO** 1 × 3 g sachet dissolved in 3–4 oz of water as a single dose.

PHARMACOKINETICS Absorption: rapidly absorbed from GI tract, 37% of dose reaches systemic circulation as free acid. **Peak urine concentration:** 2–4 h. **Distribution:** not protein bound, distributed to kidneys, bladder wall, prostate, and seminal vesicles. **Elimination:** half-life: 5.7 h; primarily excreted in urine.

CONTRAINDICATIONS & PRECAUTIONS Contraindicated in: hypersensitivity to fosfomycin, lactation. **Cautious use in:** pregnancy (category B). Safety and efficiency in children < 12 y have not been established.

ADVERSE/SIDE EFFECTS Body as whole: pain. **CNS:** *headache,* dizziness. **GI:** *diarrhea*, nausea, abdominal pain, dyspepsia. **Respiratory:** rhinitis. **Other:** vaginitis, dysmenorrhea, pharyngitis.

DRUG INTERACTION Metoclopramide may decrease urinary excretion of fosfomycin.

NURSING IMPLICATIONS

Administration
- Pour entire contents of a single dose into 3–4 oz water (not hot), stir to dissolve completely, and give immediately. Drug must not be taken in the dry form.
- Store at 15–30C (59–86F).

Assessment & Drug Effects
- Therapeutic effectiveness is indicated by improvement in cystitis symptoms within 2–3 d.
- Lab tests: urine C&S should be done before and after therapy.

Patient & Family Education
- Follow directions for preparation and administration.

FOSINOPRIL

(fos-in′o-pril)

Trade name: Monopril

Classifications: CARDIOVASCULAR AGENT; ANGIOTENSIN-CONVERTING ENZYME (ACE) INHIBITOR

Prototype: Captopril

Pregnancy category: C (first trimester); D (second and third trimesters)

ACTIONS/PHARMOCODYNAMICS Lowers BP by interrupting conversion sequences initiated by renin that lead to formation of angiotensin II, a potent vasoconstrictor. Inhibition of ACE also leads to decreased circulating aldosterone, a secretory response to angiotensin II stimulation. ACE inhibitors also reduce peripheral arterial resistance (afterload) and improve cardiac output as well as activity tolerance.

USES Mild to moderate hypertension, CHF.

ROUTE & DOSAGE

Hypertension, CHF
Adult: **PO** 5–40 mg once/d (max 80 mg/d).

PHARMOCOKINETICS **Absorption:** readily absorbed from GI tract; converted to its active form, fosinoprilat, in the liver. **Peak:** 3 h. **Duration:** 24 h. **Distribution:** approximately 90% protein bound; crosses placenta. **Metabolism:** hydrolyzed by intestinal and hepatic esterases to its active form, fosinoprilat. **Elimination:** half-life: 3-4 h (fosinoprilat); 44% excreted in urine, 46% in feces.

CONTRAINDICATIONS & PRECAUTIONS **Contraindicated in:** hypersensitivity to fosinopril or any other ACE inhibitor. **Cautious use in:** impaired renal function, pregnancy [category C (first trimester) or D (second or third trimester)], hyperkalemia, and surgery and anesthesia.

ADVERSE/SIDE EFFECTS **CV:** hypotension. **CNS:** headache, fatigue, dizziness. **Endocrine:** hyperkalemia. **GI:** nausea, vomiting, diarrhea. **GU:** proteinuria. **Other:** cough, rash.

DRUG INTERACTIONS NSAIDS may decrease antihypertensive effects of fosinopril. POTASSIUM SUPPLEMENTS, POTASSIUM-SPARING DIURETICS increase risk of hyperkalemia. ACE inhibitors may increase **lithium** levels and toxicity.

NURSING IMPLICATIONS

Administration

- If possible, diuretics should be discontinued 2–3 d before initiation of fosinopril. If diuretics cannot be discontinued, the initial dose should not exceed 10 mg.
- Store at 15–30C (59–86F) and protect from moisture.

Assessment & Drug Effects

- Monitor BP at the time of peak effectiveness, 2–6 h after dosing and at the end of the dosing interval just before next dose.
- Report diminished antihypertensive effect toward the end of the dosing interval. An inadequate trough response may be an indication for dividing the daily dose.
- Monitor for first-dose hypotension, especially in salt- or volume-depleted persons.
- BUN and serum creatinine should be periodically monitored. Increases may necessitate dose reduction or discontinuation of the drug.
- Monitor serum potassium values and observe for signs and symptoms of hyperkalemia (see Appendix G).

Patient & Family Education

- Advise patient to discontinue fosinopril and report to physician if any of the following occur: signs and symptoms of angioedema (e.g., swelling of face or extremities, difficulty breathing or swallowing); syncope; chronic, nonproductive cough.

- Instruct patient to maintain adequate fluid intake and to avoid potassium supplements or salt substitutes unless specifically prescribed by the physician.
- Advise patient to immediately report vomiting or diarrhea to physician.

FOSPHENYTOIN SODIUM

(fos-phen′i-toin)

Trade name: Cerebyx

Classifications: CNS AGENT; HYDANTOIN ANTICONVULSANT AGENT

Prototype: Phenytoin

Pregnancy category: D

ACTIONS/PHARMOCODYNAMICS Fosphenytoin is a prodrug of phenytoin. Following parenteral administration fosphenytoin is converted to the anticonvulsant, phenytoin. The cellular mechanisms of phenytoin are thought to be responsible for fosphenytoin's anticonvulsant activity. Fosphenytoin is thought to modulate the sodium channels of neurons, modulate calcium flux across neuronal membranes, and enhance the sodium–potassium ATPase activity of neurons and glial cells.

USES Control of generalized convulsive status epilepticus and the prevention and treatment of seizures during neurosurgery, or as a parenteral short-term substitute for oral phenytoin. **Unlabeled uses:** see **phenytoin**.

ROUTE & DOSAGE

Note: all dosing is expressed in phenytoin sodium equivalents (PE) to avoid the need to calculate molecular weight adjustments between fosphenytoin and phenytoin sodium doses. Fosphenytoin should always be prescribed in PE units.

Status Epilepticus

Adult: **IV** Loading dose of 15–20 mg PE/kg administered at 100–150 mg PE/min. Initial maintenance dose is 4–6 mg PE/kg/d.

Substitution for Oral Phenytoin Therapy

Adult: **IV/IM** Substitute fosphenytoin at the same total daily dose in mg PE as the oral dose at a rate of infusion not greater than 150 mg PE/min.

PHARMOCOKINETICS Absorption: completely absorbed after IM administration. **Peak:** 30 min IM. **Distribution:** 95–99% bound to plasma proteins, displaces phenytoin from protein binding sites; crosses placenta, small amount in breast milk. **Metabolism:** converted to phenytoin by phosphatases; phenytoin is oxidized in liver to inactive metabolites. **Elimination:** half-life: 15 min to convert fosphenytoin to phenytoin, 22 h phenytoin; phenytoin metabolites excreted in urine.

CONTRAINDICATIONS & PRECAUTIONS Contraindicated in: hypersensitivity to hydantoin products, rash, seizures due to hypoglycemia, sinus bradycardia, complete or incomplete heart block, Adams–Stokes syndrome, pregnancy (category D), lactation. **Cautious use in:** impaired hepatic or renal function, alcoholism, hypotension, heart block, bradycardia, severe CAD, diabetes mellitus, hyperglycemia, respiratory depression, acute intermittent porphyria.

ADVERSE/SIDE EFFECTS CNS: usually dose related: paresthesia, tinnitus, *nystagmus, dizziness, somnolence, drowsiness,* ataxia, mental confusion, tremors, insomnia, headache, seizures, increased reflexes, dysarthria, intracranial hypertension. **CV:** bradycardia, tachycardia, hypotension, hypertension, cardiovascular collapse, ventricular fibrillation, phlebitis. **Eye:** photophobia, conjunctivitis, diplopia, blurred vision. **GI:** *gingival hyperplasia,* nausea, vomiting, constipation, epigastric pain, dysphagia, loss of taste, weight loss, hepatitis, liver necrosis. **Hematologic:** thrombocytopenia, leukopenia, leukocytosis, agranulocytosis, pancytopenia, eosinophilia; megaloblastic, hemolytic, or aplastic anemias. **Metabolic:** fever, hyperglycemia, glycosuria, weight gain, edema, transient increase in serum thyrotropic (TSH) level, hyperkalemia. **Skin:** alopecia, hirsutism (especially in young female); rash: scarlatiniform, maculopapular, urticarial, morbilliform (may be fatal); bullous, exfoliative, or purpuric dermatitis; Stevens–Johnson syndrome, toxic epidermal necrolysis, keratosis, neonatal hemorrhage, *pruritus.* **Other:** acute renal failure, osteomalacia or rickets associated with hypocalcemia and elevated alkaline phosphatase activity, acute pneumonitis, pulmonary fibrosis, periarteritis nodosum, acute systemic lupus erythematosus, craniofacial abnormalities (with enlargement of lips), Peyronie's disease, lymphadenopathy, injection site pain, chills.

DIAGNOSTIC TEST INTERFERENCE Fosphenytoin may produce lower than normal values for ***dexamethasone*** or ***metyrapone*** tests; may increase serum levels of ***glucose, BSP,*** and ***alkaline phosphatase*** and may decrease ***PBI*** and ***urinary steroid*** levels.

DRUG INTERACTIONS **Alcohol** decreases fosphenytoin effects; OTHER ANTICONVULSANTS may increase or decrease fosphenytoin levels; fosphenytoin may decrease absorption and increase metabolism of ORAL ANTICOAGULANTS; fosphenytoin increases metabolism of CORTICOSTEROIDS and ORAL CONTRACEPTIVES, thus decreasing their effectiveness; **amiodarone, chloramphenicol, omeprazole** increase fosphenytoin levels; ANTITUBERCULOSIS AGENTS decrease fosphenytoin levels. **Drug–food:** folic acid, calcium, vitamin D absorption may be decreased by fosphenytoin; fosphenytoin absorption may be decreased by enteral nutrition supplements.

INCOMPATIBILITIES Compatibility studies have not been done.

NURSING IMPLICATIONS

- See **phenytoin** for additional nursing implications related to assessment, drug effects, and patient/family education.

Administration

- IM injection: Follow institutional policy regarding maximum volume to inject into one IM site.
- IV preparation and administration: Dilute in 5% dextrose or 0.9% NaCl to a concentration of 1.5–25 mg PE/ml. Do not administer at a rate >150 mg PE/min.
- Store at 2–8C (36–46F). May be stored at room temperature for ≤ 48 h.

Assessment & Drug Effects

- During and for 10–20 min after infusion, continuously monitor ECG, BP, and respiratory function.

- Discontinue infusion and notify physician if rash appears. Note that rapid substitution of alternative therapy may be needed to prevent withdrawal-precipitated seizures.
- Allow at least 2 h after IV infusion and 4 h after IM injection before monitoring total plasma phenytoin concentration.
- Monitor electrolyte balance and blood glucose for hyperglycemia.
- Carefully monitor for adverse effects, especially in those with renal or hepatic disease or hypoalbuminemia.

Patient & Family Education

- Advise regarding potential adverse effects and inform that itching, burning, tingling, and/or paresthesia are common during and for some time following IV infusion.

F

FURAZOLIDONE

(fur-a-zoe'li-done)

Trade name: Furoxone

Classifications: ANTIINFECTIVE; MAO INHIBITOR

Pregnancy category: C

ACTIONS/PHARMACODYNAMICS Synthetic nitrofuran with antibacterial and antiprotozoal properties. Acts by interfering with several bacterial enzyme systems. Bactericidal against majority of GI pathogens, including species of *Enterobacter aerogenes, Escherichia coli, Giardia lamblia, Proteus, Salmonella, Shigella, Staphylococcus,* and *Vibrio cholerae.* Also has MAO INHIBITOR action that is cumulative and dose related (occurring after 4 or 5 d of therapy).

USES Bacterial or protozoal diarrhea and enteritis caused by susceptible organisms.

ROUTE & DOSAGE

Diarrhea and Enteritis

Adult: **PO** 100 mg q.i.d.
Child: **PO** ≥ 5 y, 25–50 mg q.i.d. (max 8.8 mg/kg/d); 1–4 y, 17–25 mg q.i.d.; 1 mo–1 y, 8–17 mg q.i.d.

PHARMACOKINETICS Absorption: poorly absorbed from GI tract. **Metabolism:** metabolized in intestines. **Elimination:** excreted in urine.

CONTRAINDICATIONS & PRECAUTIONS Contraindicated in: hypersensitivity to furazolidone, concurrent use with alcohol, other MAO INHIBITORS, tyramine-containing foods, indirect-acting sympathomimetic amines; infants <1 mo. Safe use during pregnancy (category C) and in nursing mothers not established. **Cautious use in:** if at all, patients with glucose-6-phosphate dehydrogenase (G6PD) deficiency.

ADVERSE/SIDE EFFECTS GI: *nausea, vomiting,* abdominal pain, diarrhea. **Hypersensitivity:** fever, arthralgia, hypotension, urticaria, angioedema, vesicular or morbilliform rash. **Other:** headache, malaise, dizziness, hypoglycemia. Rare: intravascular hemolysis in patients with G6PD deficiency, agranulocytosis, partial deafness.

DIAGNOSTIC TEST INTERFERENCE Furazolidone metabolite reportedly may cause false-positive reactions for ***urine glucose*** with copper sulfate reduction methods, e.g., ***Benedict's reagent, Clinitest,*** and ***Fehling's solution.***

DRUG INTERACTIONS Alcohol may elicit disulfiram-type reaction up to 4 d after the drug is stopped; MAO INHIBITORS, NARCOTICS, SYMPATHOMIMETIC AMINES, **ephedrine,**

phenylpropanolamine may cause a hypertensive reaction; TRICYCLIC ANTIDEPRESSANTS may cause toxic psychosis. **Food–drug:** may interact with tyramine-containing foods, resulting in flushing, tachycardia, and hypertensive crisis. See phenelzine (MAO inhibitor prototype).

NURSING IMPLICATIONS

Administration

- Preserve in tight, light-resistant containers (drug darkens on exposure to light). Protect from excessive heat.

Assessment & Drug Effects

- Nausea and vomiting occur commonly but may be relieved by reducing dosage. If symptoms persist, drug discontinuation may be necessary.
- Bed rest and fluid and electrolyte replacement (as indicated) are important adjuncts to drug therapy. Consult physician regarding dietary allowances.
- Keep physician informed of signs of dehydration (see Appendix G) and electrolyte imbalance.
- Since drug may cause hypoglycemia (see Signs & Symptoms, Appendix G), diabetic patients will require close monitoring. Use glucose oxidase methods for urine testing (e.g., Clinistix, Diastix, TesTape).

Patient & Family Education

- Faintness, weakness, and lightheadedness may be symptoms of hypersensitivity reaction or hypoglycemia and should be reported.
- Foods high in tyramine (e.g., aged and fermented food and drinks) may produce hypertensive reaction. Provide patient with list of high-tyramine foods. Hypertensive crisis is most likely to occur when drug is continued beyond 5 d or when large doses are given.
- Warn patients not to drink alcohol during furazolidone therapy and for at least 4 d after drug is stopped. Ingestion of alcohol may cause disulfiram-type reaction (see Appendix G); symptoms may last up to 24 h.
- Inform patients that drug may impart a harmless brown color to urine.
- Advise the diabetic of potential for hypoglycemia.

F

FUROSEMIDE

(fur-oh′se-mide)

Trade names: Fumide ♣, Furomide ♣, Lasix, Luramide ♣

Prototype for classifications: ELECTROLYTIC AND WATER BALANCE AGENT; LOOP DIURETIC

Pregnancy category: C

ACTIONS/PHARMACODYNAMICS

Rapid-acting potent sulfonamide "loop" diuretic and antihypertensive with pharmacologic effects and uses almost identical to those of ethacrynic acid. Exact mode of action not clearly defined. Renal vascular resistance decreases, and renal blood flow may increase during drug administration. Inhibits reabsorption of sodium and chloride primarily in loop of Henle and also in proximal and distal renal tubules. Reportedly less ototoxic than ethacrynic acid.

USES Treatment of edema associated with CHF, cirrhosis of liver, and renal disease, including nephrotic syndrome. May be used for management of hypertension, alone or in combination with other antihypertensive agents, and for treatment of hypercalcemia. Has been used concomitantly with mannitol for

F

treatment of severe cerebral edema, particularly in meningitis.

ROUTE & DOSAGE

Edema

Adult: **PO** 20–80 mg in 1 or more divided doses up to 600 mg/d if needed. **IV/IM** 20–40 mg in 1 or more divided doses up to 600 mg/d.
Child: **PO** 2 mg/kg; may be increased by 1–2 mg/kg q6–8h up to a max of 6 mg/kg/dose. **IV/IM** 1 mg/kg; may be increased by 1mg/kg q2h if needed up to a max of 6 mg/kg/dose.
Neonate: **PO** 1–4 mg/kg q12–24h. **IV/IM** 1–2 mg/kg q12–24h.

Hypertension

Adult: **PO** 10–40 mg b.i.d. (max 480 mg/d).

PHARMACOKINETICS **Absorption:** 60 of oral dose absorbed from GI tract. **Peak:** 60–70 min PO; 20–60 min IV. **Onset:** 30–60 min PO; 5 min IV. **Duration:** 2 h. **Distribution:** crosses placenta. **Metabolism:** small amount metabolized in liver. **Elimination:** half-life: 30 min; rapidly excreted in urine; 50% of oral dose and 80% of IV dose excreted within 24 h; excreted in breastmilk.

CONTRAINDICATIONS & PRECAUTIONS **Contraindicated in:** history of hypersensitivity to furosemide or sulfonamides; increasing oliguria, anuria, fluid and electrolyte depletion states; hepatic coma; pregnancy (category C). **Cautious use in:** infants, elderly patients; hepatic cirrhosis, nephrotic syndrome; cardiogenic shock associated with acute MI; history of SLE, history of gout; patients receiving digitalis glycosides or potassium-depleting steroids.

ADVERSE/SIDE EFFECTS **CV:** postural hypotension, dizziness with excessive diuresis, acute hypotensive episodes, circulatory collapse. **Fluid and electrolyte imbalance:** hypovolemia, dehydration, hyponatremia, *hypokalemia*, hypochloremia metabolic alkalosis, hypomagnesemia, hypocalcemia (tetany). **GI:** nausea, vomiting, oral and gastric burning, anorexia, diarrhea, constipation, abdominal cramping, acute pancreatitis, jaundice. **GU:** allergic interstitial nephritis, irreversible renal failure, urinary frequency. **Hematologic:** anemia, leukopenia, thrombocytopenic purpura. Rare: aplastic anemia, agranulocytosis. **Ototoxicity:** tinnitus, vertigo, feeling of fullness in ears, hearing loss (rarely permanent). **Skin:** pruritus, urticaria, exfoliative dermatitis, purpura, photosensitivity, porphyria cutanea tarde, necrotizing angiitis (vasculitis). **Other:** hyperglycemia, glycosuria, elevated BUN, hyperuricemia; increased perspiration; paresthesias; blurred vision, activation of SLE, muscle spasms, weakness; thrombophlebitis, pain at IM injection site.

DIAGNOSTIC TEST INTERFERENCE Furosemide may cause elevations in ***BUN, serum amylase, cholesterol, triglycerides, uric acid*** and ***blood glucose*** levels, and may decrease ***serum calcium, magnesium, potassium,*** and ***sodium*** levels.

DRUG INTERACTIONS OTHER DIURETICS enhance diuretic effects; with **digoxin,** increased risk of toxicity because of hypokalemia; NONDEPOLARIZING NEUROMUSCULAR BLOCKING AGENTS (e.g., **tubocurarine**) prolong neuromuscular blockage; CORTICO-

STEROIDS, **amphotericin B** potentiate hypokalemia; decreased **lithium** elimination and increased toxicity; SULFONYLUREAS, **insulin** blunt hypoglycemic effects; NSAIDS may attenuate diuretic effects.

INCOMPATIBILITIES Solution/additive: ciprofloxacin, diphenhydramine, dobutamine, doxapram, doxorubicin, droperidol, gentamicin, labetalol, meperidine, metoclopramide, milrinone, netilmicin, pancuronium, quinidine, thiamine. Y-site: amrinone, ciprofloxacin, diazepam, diphenhydramine, doxorubicin, droperidol, esmolol, fluconazole, gentamicin, methocarbamol, metoclopramide, morphine, netilmicin, ondansetron, quinidine, tobramycin, vinblastine, vincristine, vitamin B complex with C, TPN.

NURSING IMPLICATIONS

Administration

- Oral furosemide may be taken with food or milk to reduce possibility of gastric irritation.
- Schedule doses to avoid nocturia and sleep disturbance (e.g., a single dose is generally administered in the morning; twice-a-day doses may be prescribed for 8 AM and 2 PM).
- Intermittent dosage schedule is frequently used to allow time for natural correction of electrolyte and acid-base imbalance (e.g., drug is given for 2–4 consecutive days each week).
- Slight discoloration of tablets reportedly does not alter potency; however, yellow or otherwise discolored injection solutions should be discarded.
- Protect syringes from light once they are removed from package.
- IV administration: IV furosemide may be given by direct IV undiluted at a rate of 20 mg or a fraction thereof over 1 min. With high doses a rate of 4 mg/min is recommended to decrease risk of ototoxicity.
- IV administration to neonates, infants, children: Verify correct IV concentration and rate of infusion/injection with physician.
- Infusion solutions in which furosemide has been mixed should be used within 24 h.
- Store tablets and parenteral solution at controlled room temperature, preferably at 15–30C (59–86F) unless otherwise directed. Protect from light.
- Store oral solution in refrigerator, preferably at 2–8C (36–46F). Protect from light and freezing.

Assessment & Drug Effects

- Patients receiving the drug parenterally should be observed carefully, and BP and vital signs closely monitored. Sudden death from cardiac arrest has been reported.
- Close observation of the elderly patient is particularly essential during period of brisk diuresis. Sudden alteration in fluid and electrolyte balance may precipitate significant adverse reactions. Report these symptoms to physician.
- Lab tests: Frequent determinations should be made of blood count, serum and urine electrolytes, CO_2, BUN, blood sugar, and uric acid during first few months of therapy and periodically thereafter.
- Monitor for signs and symptoms of hypokalemia (see Appendix G).
- Monitor I&O ratio and pattern. Report decrease or unusual increase in output. Excessive diuresis can result in dehydration and hypovolemia, circulatory collapse, and hypotension.
- During periods of brisk diuresis, weigh patient daily under standard conditions.

- Monitor BP during periods of diuresis and through period of dosage adjustment.
- Excessive dehydration is most likely to occur in the elderly, in those with chronic cardiac disease on prolonged salt restriction, or in those receiving sympatholytic agents.

F

Patient & Family Education

- Consult physician regarding allowable salt and fluid intake.
- To reduce or prevent potassium depletion, daily ingestion of potassium-rich foods (e.g., bananas, oranges, peaches, dried dates) may be prescribed.
- Instruct patient regarding signs and symptoms of hypokalemia (see Appendix G). Advise patient to report muscle cramps or weakness.
- Patients receiving high doses of antihypertensive drugs concurrently are subject to episodes of postural hypotension. Caution patient to make position changes slowly.
- Instruct patient to avoid replacing fluid losses with large amounts of free water.
- Advise against prolonged exposure to direct sun.
- Furosemide may cause hyperglycemia. Diabetics and patients with decompensated hepatic cirrhosis require careful urine and blood glucose monitoring.

GABAPENTIN

(gab-a-pen'tin)

Trade name: Neurotin

Classifications: CNS AGENT; ANTICONVULSANT

Prototype: Phenytoin

Pregnancy category: C

ACTIONS/PHARMACODYNAMICS Gabapentin is a GABA neurotransmitter analog; however, it does not interact with GABA receptors, and it does not inhibit GABA uptake or degradation. Gabapentin is used in conjunction with other anticonvulsants to control certain types of seizures in patients with epilepsy. Mechanism of action is unknown. An effect of gabapentin on central serotonin metabolism has been postulated.

USES Adjunctive therapy for partial seizures with or without secondary generalization in adults. **Unlabeled use:** add-on therapy for generalized seizures.

ROUTE & DOSAGE

Adjunctive Therapy for Seizure Disorder

Adult: **PO** Initiate with 300 mg on day 1, 300 mg b.i.d. on day 2, and 300 mg t.i.d. on day 3. Continue to increase over a week to an initial total dose of 400 mg t.i.d. (1200 mg/d). May increase to 1800–2400 mg/d depending on response (most patients received 600–1800 mg/d in 3 divided doses).
Child: **PO** >12 y, same as adult.

PHARMACOKINETICS **Absorption:** 50–60% absorbed from GI tract. **Peak:** peak level 1–3 h; peak effect 2–4 wk. **Distribution:** crosses the blood–brain barrier comparable to other anticonvulsants; readily passes into cerebrospinal fluid; is not bound to plasma proteins; highest concentrations (in animal studies) found in pancreas and kidneys. **Metabolism:** does not appear to be metabolized. **Elimination:** half-life: 5–6 h; 76–81% excreted unchanged in 96 h; 10–23% recovered in feces.

CONTRAINDICATIONS & PRECAUTIONS **Contraindicated in:** hypersensitivity to gabapentin. **Cautious use in:** status epilepticus, renal impairment, elderly, pregnancy (category C), nursing mothers. Safety and efficacy in children < 12 y not established.

ADVERSE/SIDE EFFECTS **CNS:** *drowsiness, fatigue,* dizziness, tremor, slurred speech, impaired concentration, headache, increased frequency of partial seizures. **Endocrine:** weight gain. **GI:** nausea, gastric upset, vomiting. **Other:** blurred vision, nystagmus, rash, eczema.

DRUG INTERACTIONS May cause increase in **phenytoin** levels at higher doses (300–600 mg/d gabapentin). Does not appear to affect serum levels of other ANTICONVULSANTS. ANTACIDS reduce absorption of gabapentin about 20%.

NURSING IMPLICATIONS

Administration

- Dosage adjustments are recommended for patients with creatinine clearance of 60 ml/min or less. See manufacturer's recommendations.
- Separate doses of gabapentin and antacids by 2 h.
- Drug should be withdrawn gradually over 1 wk, as discontinuation may cause status epilepticus.
- Store at room temperature (15–30C/59–86F); protect from heat, moisture, and direct light.

Assessment & Drug Effects

- Assess frequency of seizures; in rare cases, the drug has increased the frequency of partial seizures.
- Assess safety, as vision, concentration, and coordination may be impaired by gabapentin.
- Maximum therapeutic effectiveness may not occur until several weeks following initiation of therapy.

Patient & Family Education

- Inform patient about potential adverse effects of drug.
- Advise patient to notify physician immediately if any of the following occur: increased seizure frequency, visual changes, unusual bruising or bleeding.
- Advise not to perform hazardous activities until reaction to drug is known.
- Caution against taking drug within 2 h of an antacid or abruptly discontinuing use of drug.

GALLAMINE TRIETHIODIDE

(gal'a-meen)

Trade name: Flaxedil

Classifications: AUTONOMIC NERVOUS SYSTEM AGENT; NONDEPOLARIZING SKELETAL MUSCLE RELAXANT

Prototype: Tubocurarine

Pregnancy category: C

ACTIONS/PHARMACODYNAMICS Synthetic, nondepolarizing neuromuscular blocking agent (curariform drug). Similar to tubocurarine in actions, uses, contraindications, precautions, and adverse reactions. Has parasympatholytic effect on vagus and may cause tachycardia and occasionally hypertension.

USES Preanesthetic and intraanesthetic medication to induce skeletal muscle relaxation for treatment of GI disorders and to reverse neuromuscular blockade.

ROUTE & DOSAGE

Skeletal Muscle Relaxation

Adult: **IV** 1 mg/kg initial dose; then 0.5–1 mg/kg q30–40min prn (max single dose 100 mg).

G

PHARMACOKINETICS **Peak:** 3 min. **Duration:** 15–20 min. **Distribution:** crosses placenta. **Elimination:** excreted primarily unchanged in urine.

CONTRAINDICATIONS & PRECAUTIONS **Contraindicated in:** hypersensitivity to gallamine or iodides; myasthenia gravis; impaired pulmonary or renal function; shock; infants weighing less than 5 kg; hyperthyroidism; hypertension, tachycardia, cardiac insufficiency; hypoalbuminemia. **Cautious use in:** impaired liver function.

ADVERSE/SIDE EFFECTS Decreased respiratory minute volume, transient tachycardia, prolonged apnea, residual muscle weakness, hypersensitivity.

DRUG INTERACTION AMINOGLYCOSIDES may prolong neuromuscular blockade.

NURSING IMPLICATIONS

Administration

- Gallamine may be given undiluted by direct IV. Administer a single dose over 30 to 60 seconds.
- Store at 5–30C (59–86F) unless otherwise directed and protect from light and excessive heat.

Assessment & Drug Effects

- Tachycardia occurs almost immediately after administration, reaches maximum within 3 min, and declines gradually to premedication level.
- Patients with electrolyte imbalance, dehydration, or elevated temperature may be more sensitive to the effects of gallamine.

GALLIUM NITRATE

(gal'li-um)

Trade name: Ganite

Prototype for classification: BONE METABOLISM REGULATOR

Pregnancy category: C

ACTIONS/PHARMACODYNAMICS Induces hypocalcemia by inhibiting calcium resorption from bone. The precise mechanism is not known.

USES Hypercalcemia of malignancy. **Unlabeled uses:** Paget's disease, painful bone metastases, adjuvant therapy for bladder cancer and lymphomas.

ROUTE & DOSAGE

Hypercalcemia

Adult: **IV** 100–200 mg/m^2/d for 5–7 d; dilute in 1000 ml D5W or 0.9% NaCl and infuse continuously over 24 h.

Bone Metastases

Adult: **IV** 200 mg/m^2/d for 7 d; dilute in 1000 ml D5W or 0.9% NaCl and infuse continuously over 24 h.

PHARMACOKINETICS **Onset:** 48 h. **Duration:** 4–14 d after discontinuation of therapy. **Distribution:** concentrates in tumors; distributed to lung, skin, muscle, and heart with high concentrations in liver and kidney; not known if crosses placenta or is distributed into breast milk. **Metabolism:** not metabolized. **Elimination:** half-life: 25–111 h; 35–71% is excreted through kidneys within first 24 h after administration.

CONTRAINDICATIONS & PRECAUTIONS **Contraindicated in:** severe renal impairment (serum creatinine >2.5 mg/dl). **Cautious use in:** renal function impairment, pregnancy (category C), and nursing mothers. The safety and efficacy in children have not been established.

ADVERSE/SIDE EFFECTS CNS: *fatigue,* paresthesia, hyperthermia. **CV:** hypotension. **GI:** *nausea, vomiting, diarrhea,* anorexia, stomatitis, dysgeusia, mucositis, metallic taste. **Hematologic:** anemia, granulocytopenia, thrombocytopenia. **Metabolic:** hypocalcemia, hypophosphatemia, hypomagnesemia. **GU:** nephrotoxicity, acute renal failure. **Other:** optic neuritis, maculopapular rash.

DRUG INTERACTIONS AMINOGLYCOSIDES, **amphotericin B, vancomycin** increase the risk of nephrotoxicity.

NURSING IMPLICATIONS

Administration

- Before initiation of therapy with gallium nitrate, patient should be well hydrated with oral or IV 0.9% NaCl to produce a urine output of 2 L/d. Adequate hydration should be maintained throughout treatment.
- Dilute each daily dose with 1000 ml D5W or 0.9% NaCl and infuse over 24 h. Avoid rapid infusion.
- Gallium nitrate should not be administered concurrently with potentially nephrotoxic drugs.
- IV solutions may be stored at 15–30C (59–86F) for 48 h or refrigerated at 2–8C (36–46F) for 7 d. Discard unused portions of gallium nitrate.

Assessment & Drug Effects

- Monitor BUN and serum creatinine throughout therapy. Notify physician if serum creatinine exceeds 2–5 mg/dl, since gallium nitrate should be discontinued if this occurs.
- In addition to baseline determinations, serum calcium and serum phosphorus should be assessed daily and twice weekly, respectively.
- If hypocalcemia occurs, stop gallium nitrate and notify physician.

Patient & Family Education

- Instruct the patient on signs and symptoms of hypocalcemia (see Appendix G). Advise patient to report them immediately.

GANCICLOVIR (DHPG)

(gan-ci′clo-vir)
Trade name: Cytovene
Classifications: ANTIINFECTIVE; ANTIVIRAL AGENT
Prototype: Acyclovir
Pregnancy category: C

ACTIONS/PHARMACODYNAMICS Ganciclovir is an antiviral drug active against cytomegalovirus (CMV). Sensitive human viruses include CMV, herpes simplex virus-1 and -2 (HSV-1, HSV-2), Epstein-Barr virus, and varicella zoster virus.

USES CMV retinitis, prophylaxis and treatment of systemic CMV infections in immunocompromised patients including HIV-positive and transplant patients.

ROUTE & DOSAGE

Note: See prescribing information for dosing in patients with renal impairment.

Induction Therapy

Adult/child >3 mo: **IV** 5 mg/kg over 1 h q12h for 14–21 d; doses have ranged from 2.5–5.0 mg/kg over 1 h q8–12h for 10–35 d.

Maintenance Therapy

Adult: **IV** 5 mg/kg over 1 h qd *or* 6 mg/kg over 1 h qd 5 d/wk.

PO 1000 mg t.i.d. or 500 mg 6 times/d q3h while awake.

Prevention of CMV Disease in Transplant Recipients

Adult/child: **IV** 5 mg/kg q12h × 7–14 d, then 5 mg/kg q.d. or 6 mg/kg/d 5 d/wk.

CMV Infection after Bone Marrow Transplant

Child: **IV** 7.5–19.5 mg/kg/d divided q8h.

PHARMACOKINETICS **Onset:** 3–8 d. **Duration:** clinical relapse can occur 14 d to 3.5 mo after stopping therapy; positive blood and urine cultures recur 12–60 d after therapy. **Distribution:** distributes throughout body including CSF, eye, lungs, liver, and kidneys; crosses placenta in animals; not known if distributed into breast milk. **Metabolism:** not metabolized. **Elimination:** half-life: 2.5–4.2 h; 94–99% of dose is excreted unchanged in urine.

CONTRAINDICATIONS & PRECAUTIONS **Contraindicated in:** hypersensitivity to ganciclovir or acyclovir. **Cautious use in:** renal impairment, the elderly, pregnancy (category C), and nursing mothers. Safety and efficacy in children have not been established.

ADVERSE/SIDE EFFECTS **CNS:** *fever,* headache, disorientation, mental status changes, ataxia, <u>coma</u>, confusion, dizziness, paresthesia, nervousness, somnolence, tremor. **CV:** edema, phlebitis. **GI:** *nausea, diarrhea,* anorexia. **Hematologic:** *<u>bone marrow suppression</u>, thrombocytopenia, granulocytopenia,* eosinophilia, *leukopenia.* **Hepatic:** elevated liver enzymes, hyperbilirubinemia. **Metabolic:** hyperthermia, hypoglycemia. **GU:** infertility. **Other:** rash.

DRUG INTERACTIONS ANTINEOPLASTIC AGENTS, **amphotericin B, didanosine, trimethoprim-sulfamethoxazole (TMP-SMZ), dapsone, pentamidine, probenecid, zidovudine** may increase bone marrow suppression and other toxic effects of ganciclovir; may increase risk of nephrotoxicity from cyclosporine; may increase risk of seizures due to **imipenem-cilastatin.**

INCOMPATIBILITIES **Solution/additive:** amino acid solutions (TPN), bacteriostatic water for injection, fludarabine, foscarnet, ondansetron. **Y-site:** total parenteral nutrition.

NURSING IMPLICATIONS

Administration

- Do not administer if neutrophil count falls below 500/mm^3 or platelet count falls below 25,000/mm^3.
- Give PO form with food.
- IV preparation: Reconstitute only with 10 ml of sterile water for injection (supplied) immediately before use to yield 50 mg/ml. Withdraw the ordered amount and add to 100 ml of 0.9% NaCl, D5W, Ringer's injection, or Ringer's lactate.
- IV administration: Give at a constant rate over 1 h. Avoid rapid infusion or bolus injection.
- IV administration to infants, children: Verify correct IV concentration and rate of infusion with physician.
- An in-line filter is required when infusing ganciclovir sodium solution. A 0.22 micron filter is preferred, but if that is not available, a 5 micron filter can be substituted.
- Avoid direct contact of powder in capsules or solution with skin and mucous membranes. Wash thoroughly with soap and water if contact occurs.

- Reconstituted solution should be stored at 4C (refrigeration) and used within 12 h.
- The infusion solution should be used immediately but may be stored refrigerated if used within 24 h of preparation.

Assessment & Drug Effects

- Neutrophil and platelet counts should be made at least every other day during twice-daily dosing and weekly thereafter. More frequent monitoring may be indicated in certain patients.
- Monitor serum creatinine or creatinine clearance at least q2wk. Closely monitor renal function in the elderly.
- Inspect IV insertion site throughout infusion for signs and symptoms of phlebitis.

Patient & Family Education

- Advise patient that drug is not a cure for CMV retinitis and stress importance of regular ophthalmologic examinations.
- Instruct patient on importance of maintaining adequate hydration during therapy.
- Advise men to use barrier contraception throughout therapy and for at least 90 d thereafter.
- Stress importance of frequent hematologic monitoring.

GEMCITABINE HYDROCHLORIDE

(gem-ci′ta-been)

Trade name: Gemzar

Classifications: ANTINEOPLASTIC AGENT; ANTIMETABOLITE; IMMUNOSUPPRESSANT

Prototype: Fluorouracil

Pregnancy category: D

ACTIONS/PHARMACODYNAMICS Pyrimidine analog with cell phase specificity by affecting rapidly dividing cells in S phase (DNA synthesis). It also blocks the progression of cells from G_1 phase to S phase of cell cycle. Gemcitabine interferes with DNA synthesis by inhibiting ribonucleotide reductase, which results in a reduction in the concentration of deoxynucleotides. In addition, if gemcitabine is incorporated into the DNA strand, it inhibits further growth of the DNA strand.

G

USE Locally advanced or metastatic adenocarcinoma of the pancreas.

ROUTE & DOSAGE

Pancreatic Cancer

Adult: **IV** 1000 mg/m^2 once weekly for up to 7 wk, followed by 1 wk rest from treatment. May repeat once weekly for 3 of every 4 wk.

PHARMACOKINETICS **Peak:** peak concentrations reached by 30 min after infusion; lower clearance in women and elderly results in higher concentrations at any given dose. **Distribution:** crosses placenta, distributed into breast milk. **Metabolism:** metabolized intracellularly by nucleoside kinases to active diphosphate (dFdCDP) and triphosphate (dFdCTP) nucleosides. **Elimination:** half-life: 32–94 min; 92–98% recovered in urine within 1 wk.

CONTRAINDICATIONS & PRECAUTIONS **Contraindicated in:** hypersensitivity to gemcitabine, severe thrombocytopenia, acute infection, pregnancy (category D), lactation. **Cautious use in:** myelosuppression, renal or hepatic dysfunction, history of bleeding disorders, infection, previous cytotoxic or radiation treatment. Safety and effectiveness in children not established.

ADVERSE/SIDE EFFECTS CNS: *fever, flu-like syndrome (anorexia, headache, cough, chills, myalgia),* paresthesias. **GI:** *nausea, vomiting, diarrhea,* stomatitis, *transient elevations of liver transaminases.* **Hematologic:** myelosuppression (anemia, leukopenia, neutropenia, thrombocytopenia). **Renal:** mild proteinuria and hematuria. **Other:** *dyspnea, edema, peripheral edema, infection.*

G

NURSING IMPLICATIONS

Administration

- IV reconstitution: Dilute with 0.9% NaCl without preservatives; add 5 ml or 25 ml to the 200-mg or 1-g vial, respectively, to yield 40 mg/ml. May be further diluted with 0.9% NaCl to concentrations as low as 0.1 mg/ml.
- IV administration: Infuse over 30 min. Infusion time > 60 min is associated with increased toxicity.
- Store reconstituted solutions unrefrigerated at 20–25C (68–77F). Use within 24 h of reconstitution.

Assessment & Drug Effects

- Prior to each dose, monitor CBC with differential and platelet count.
- Prior to initiation of therapy and periodically thereafter, monitor renal and hepatic function.

Patient & Family Education

- Advise regarding common adverse effects and provide information on measures to control or minimize when possible. Instruct to immediately report any distressing adverse effects.
- Advise that fever with flu-like symptoms, rash, and GI distress are very common.

GEMFIBROZIL

(gem-fi′broe-zil)

Trade name: Lopid

Classifications: CARDIOVASCULAR AGENT; ANTILIPEMIC; LIPID-LOWERING AGENT

Prototype: Lovastatin

Pregnancy category: B

ACTIONS/PHARMACODYNAMICS
Fibric acid derivative with lipid regulating properties. Blocks lipolysis of stored triglycerides in adipose tissue and inhibits hepatic uptake of fatty acids. This decreases VLDL (triglyceride) synthesis and secretion. Produces a moderate increase in HDL cholesterol levels and reduces levels of total and LDL cholesterol and triglycerides.

USES Patients with very high serum triglyceride levels (above 750 mg/dl) (type IV and V hyperlipidemia) who have not responded favorably to intensive diet restriction and who are at risk of pancreatitis and abdominal pain. Also severe familial hypercholesterolemia (type IIa or IIb) that developed in childhood and has failed to respond to dietary control or to other cholesterol-lowering drugs.

ROUTE & DOSAGE

Hypertriglyceridemia
Adult: **PO** 600 mg b.i.d. 30 min before morning and evening meal; may increase up to 1500 mg/d.

PHARMACOKINETICS Absorption: readily absorbed from GI tract. **Peak:** 1–2 h. **Metabolism:** undergoes enterohepatic circulation. **Elimination:** half-life: 1.3–1.5 h; excreted primarily in urine; 6% excreted in feces.

CONTRAINDICATIONS & PRECAUTIONS Contraindicated in: gallbladder disease, hepatic or severe kidney dysfunction. Safe use during pregnancy (category B), in nursing mothers, and in children not established. **Cautious use in:** diabetes mellitus, hypothyroidism.

ADVERSE/SIDE EFFECTS CNS: headache, dizziness, blurred vision. **GI:** *abdominal* or *epigastric pain,* diarrhea, nausea, vomiting, flatulence. **Hematologic:** eosinophilia, mild decreases in Hct, Hgb. **Musculoskeletal:** painful extremities, back pain, muscle cramps, myalgia, arthralgia, swollen joints. **Skin:** rash, dermatitis, pruritus, urticaria. **Other:** hypokalemia, moderate hyperglycemia.

DRUG INTERACTIONS May potentiate hypoprothrombinemic effects of ORAL ANTICOAGULANTS; **lovastatin** increases risk of myopathy and rhabdomyolysis.

NURSING IMPLICATIONS

Administration

- Instruct patient to take drug 30 min before breakfast and evening meal.
- Store at 15–30C (59–86F) unless otherwise directed.

Assessment & Drug Effects

- The following laboratory tests should be monitored initially and at regular intervals during first year of therapy: serum LDL and VLDL, triglycerides, total cholesterol, CBC, blood glucose, liver function tests.
- Mild decreases in WBC, Hgb, Hct may occur during early stage of treatment but generally stabilize with continued therapy.
- Frequent PT determinations are advisable until the drug effect is known.
- Gemfibrozil should be discontinued if the lipid response is not adequate after 3 mo of therapy.
- Gallbladder studies are indicated if patient presents signs and symptoms suggestive of cholelithiasis or cholecystitis. Symptoms often occur during the night or early morning; jaundice may or may not be present.

Patient & Family Education

- Advise patient to report promptly if unexplained bleeding occurs (e.g., easy bruising, epistaxis, hematuria).
- Caution patient to avoid driving and other potentially hazardous activities until reaction to drug is known.
- Patients with high serum triglyceride levels are generally advised to lose excess weight and to restrict carbohydrate and alcohol intake (alcohol increases serum triglyceride levels).

GENTAMICIN SULFATE

(jen-ta-mye′sin)

Trade names: Garamycin, Garamycin Ophthalmic, Genoptic

Prototype for classifications: ANTIINFECTIVE; AMINOGLYCOSIDE ANTIBIOTIC

Pregnancy category: C

ACTIONS/PHARMACODYNAMICS Broad-spectrum aminoglycoside antibiotic derived from *Micromonospora purpurea*, an actinomycete. Action is usually bactericidal. Active against a wide variety of gram-negative bacteria, including *Citrobacter, Escherichia coli, Enterobacter, Klebsiella, Proteus* (including indole-positive and indole-negative strains), *Pseudomonas aeruginosa*, and *Serratia* sp. Also effective against certain gram-positive organisms, particularly penicillin-sensitive and some methicillin-resistant strains of *Staphylococcus aureus*.

USES Parenteral use restricted to treatment of serious infections of GI, respiratory, and urinary tracts, CNS, bone, skin, and soft tissue (including burns) when other less toxic antimicrobial agents are ineffective or are contraindicated. Has been used in combination with other antibiotics. Also used topically for primary and secondary skin infections and for superficial infections of external eye and its adnexa. **Unlabeled use:** prophylaxis of bacterial endocarditis in patients undergoing operative procedures or instrumentation.

G

ROUTE & DOSAGE

Moderate to Severe Infection

Adult: **IV/IM** 1.5–2 mg/kg loading dose followed by 3–5 mg/kg/d in 2–3 divided doses. **Topical** 1–2 drops of solution in eye q4h up to 2 drops q1h *or* small amount of ointment b.i.d. or t.i.d.
Child: **IV/IM** 6–7.5 mg/kg/d in 3–4 divided doses.
Neonate: **IV/IM** 2.5 mg/kg q12–24h.

Acute Pelvic Inflammatory Disease

Adult: **IV/IM** 2 mg/kg followed by 1.5 mg/kg q8h.

Prophylaxis of Bacterial Endocarditis

Adult: **IV/IM** 1.5 mg/kg 30 min before procedure; may repeat in 8 h.
Child <27 kg: **IV/IM** 2 mg/kg 30 min before procedure; may repeat in 8 h.

PHARMACOKINETICS Absorption: well absorbed from IM site. **Peak:** 30–90 min IM. **Distribution:** widely distributed in body fluids, including ascitic, peritoneal, pleural, synovial, and abscess fluids; poor CNS penetration; concentrates in kidney and inner ear; crosses placenta. **Metabolism:** not metabolized. **Elimination:** half-life: 2–4 h; excreted unchanged in urine; small amounts accumulate in kidney and are eliminated over 10–20 d; small amount excreted in breast milk.

CONTRAINDICATIONS & PRECAUTIONS Contraindicated in: history of hypersensitivity to or toxic reaction with any aminoglycoside antibiotic. Safe use during pregnancy (category C) and in nursing mothers not established. **Cautious use in:** impaired renal function; history of eighth cranial (acoustic) nerve impairment; preexisting vertigo or dizziness or tinnitus; dehydration, fever; use in the elderly, prematures, neonates, and infants; obesity, neuromuscular disorders: myasthenia gravis, parkinsonian syndrome; hypocalcemia, heart failure, topical applications to widespread areas.

ADVERSE/SIDE EFFECTS CNS: ototoxicity (vestibular disturbances, impaired hearing), optic neuritis, neuromuscular blockade: skeletal muscle weakness, apnea, respiratory paralysis (high doses); arachnoiditis (intrathecal use). **GI:** nausea, vomiting. **Hematologic:** increased or decreased reticulocyte counts; granulocytopenia, thrombocytopenia (fever, bleeding tendency), thrombocytopenic purpura, anemia. **Hypersensitivity:** rash, pruritus, urticaria, exfoliative dermatitis, eosinophilia, burning sensation of skin, drug fever, joint pains, laryngeal edema, anaphylaxis. **Renal:** <u>nephrotoxicity</u>: proteinuria, tubular necrosis, cells or casts in urine, hematuria, rising BUN, nonprotein nitrogen, serum creatinine; *decreased creatinine clearance*. **Topical and ophthalmic:** photosensitivity, sensitization, erythema, pruritus; burning, stinging, and lacrimation (ophthalmic formulation). **Other:** transient increase in AST (SGOT), ALT (SGPT), and serum LDH and bilirubin; hepatomegaly, splenomegaly; hypotension or hypertension; local irritation and pain following IM use; thrombophlebitis, abscess, superinfections, syndrome of hypocalcemia (tetany, weakness, hypokalemia, hypomagnesemia).

DRUG INTERACTIONS **Amphotericin B, capreomycin, cisplatin, methoxyflurane, polymyxin B, vancomycin,** increase risk of nephrotoxicity. **Ethacrynic acid** and **furosemide** may increase risk of ototoxicity. GENERAL ANESTHETICS and NEUROMUSCULAR BLOCKING AGENTS (e.g., **succinylcholine**) potentiate neuromuscular blockade. **Indomethacin** may increase gentamicin levels in neonates.

INCOMPATIBILITIES **Solution/additive:** fat emulsion, TPN, **amphotericin B, ampicillin, carbenicillin,** CEPHALOSPORINS, **cytarabine, heparin. Y-site: furosemide, iodipamide.**

NURSING IMPLICATIONS

Administration

Parenteral (IV)

- For administration by intermittent IV infusion to adults, a single dose of gentamicin is diluted with 50–200 ml of 0.9% NaCl or 5% dextrose injection and infused over 30 min–2 h.
- For pediatric patients, amount of infusion fluid may be proportionately smaller depending on patient's needs but should be sufficient to be infused over the same time period as for adults.
- Gentamicin is stable for 24 h at room temperature in 0.9% NaCl or 5% dextrose injection, or other IV fluids recommended by manufacturer.
- Note that commercial IV piggyback preparations and gentamicin for intrathecal use contain no preservatives and therefore must be used promptly once opened. Any unused portion should be discarded.
- Gentamicin for IV or IM administration is clear and colorless or slightly yellow. Gentamicin for intrathecal use is a clear and colorless solution. Do not use solutions that are discolored or that contain particulate matter.

Ophthalmic

- Immediately apply pressure to inner canthus for 1 min after instillation of drops.
- After administration of ophthalmic ointment, instruct patient to keep eyes closed for 1–2 min to assure medication contact. Caution patient that vision will be blurred for a few minutes.

Topical

- Wash affected area with mild soap and water, rinse, and dry thoroughly, unless otherwise prescribed by physician. Gently apply small amount of medication to lesions. Cover with sterile gauze if desired.
- Topical applications, particularly gentamicin cream preparations, should not be made to large denuded body surfaces because systemic absorption and toxicity are possible.
- Store gentamicin preparations between 2–30C (36–86F) unless otherwise directed by manufacturer.

G

Assessment & Drug Effects

Parenteral

- Culture and susceptibility tests should be performed initially (before first dose) and periodically during continued therapy. Therapy may begin pending test results.
- If improvement does not occur in 3–5 d, susceptibility tests should be repeated and therapy reevaluated.
- Baseline weight, vital signs, and tests of renal function and vestibular and auditory function should be determined before therapy and at regular intervals during treatment. Vestibular and auditory function should be checked again 3–4 wk after drug is discontinued (the time that deafness is most likely to occur).
- Creatinine clearance and serum drug concentrations should be determined at frequent intervals, particularly for patients with impaired renal function, infants (renal immaturity), the elderly, and patients receiving high doses or therapy beyond 10 d, patients with fever or extensive burns, edema, obesity.
- I&O should be monitored. Patient is kept well hydrated during therapy to prevent chemical irritation of renal tubules. Report oliguria, unusual appearance of urine, change in I&O ratio or pattern, and presence of edema (prolongs elimination time).
- Ototoxic effect (see Appendix G) is greatest on the vestibular branch of eighth cranial (acoustic) nerve (symptoms: headache, dizziness or vertigo, nausea and vomiting with motion, ataxia, nystagmus). However, damage to the auditory branch (tinnitus, roaring noises, sensation of fullness in ears, hearing impairment) may also occur. Prompt reporting is critical to prevent permanent damage.
- Generally, dosages are adjusted to maintain peak serum gentamicin concentrations of 4–10 μg/ml, and trough concentrations of 1–2 μg/ml. Peak concentrations above 12 μg/ml and trough concentrations above 2 μg/ml are associated with toxicity.
- Blood specimens for peak serum gentamicin concentrations are generally drawn 30 min–1 h after IM administration, and 30 min after completion of a 30–60 min IV infusion. For trough levels, blood specimens are drawn just before the next IM or IV dose. Blood should be collected in nonheparinized tubes.
- Be alert for signs of bacterial overgrowth (opportunistic infections) with resistant or nonsusceptible organisms (diarrhea, anogenital itching, vaginal discharge, stomatitis, glossitis).

Patient & Family Education

- Caution patients using topical applications to: (1) avoid excessive exposure to sunlight because of danger of photosensitivity; (2) withhold medication and notify physician if condition fails to improve within 1 wk, worsens, or signs of irritation or sensitivity occur; and (3) apply medication as directed and only for length of time prescribed (overuse can result in superinfections).

GLATIRAMER ACETATE

(gla-tir′a-mer)

Trade name: Copaxone, Copolymer-1

Classifications: IMMUNOMODULATOR

Pregnancy category: B

ACTIONS/PHARMACODYNAMICS Glatiramer (formerly Copolymer-1) is a random synthetic copolymer of L-alanine, L-glutamic acid, L-lysine, and L-tyrosine. Its mechanism of action is unknown, but its function is to reduce the relapse rate of muscular sclerosis (MS), a demyelinating disease of the CNS of unknown origin. During an autoimmune response, glatiramer is thought to divert immune cells away from their myelin target.

USE Reduction of the frequency of relapses in patients with relapsing–remitting multiple sclerosis.

ROUTE & DOSAGE

Multiple Sclerosis
Adult: **SC** 20 mg q.d.

PHARMACOKINETICS No data in humans.

CONTRAINDICATIONS & PRECAUTIONS **Contraindicated in:** hypersensitivity to glatiramer acetate or mannitol. **Cautious use in:** pregnancy (category B), children < 18 y of age, nursing mothers, history of asthma or other respiratory disorders.

ADVERSE/SIDE EFFECTS **Body as whole:** *asthenia, back pain,* chills, facial edema, fever, *flu-like syndrome, infection, pain, arthralgia.* **CNS:** migraine, agitation, *anxiety, hypotonia.* **CV:** *chest pain, palpitations,* syncope, tachycardia, *vasodilation.* **GI:** *diarrhea, nausea,* anorexia, gastroenteritis, vomiting. **Respiratory:** *dyspnea, rhinitis,* bronchitis. **Skin:** *rash, pruritus, sweating.* **Other:** *postinjection reaction (flushing, chest pain, palpitations, anxiety, dyspnea, constriction of throat, urticaria), injection site reactions (erythema, hemorrhage, pain, pruritus, urticaria, swelling),* ecchymoses, *lymphadenopathy,* ear pain, dysmenorrhea, urinary urgency.

NURSING IMPLICATIONS

Administration

- Recommended SC injection sites are arms, abdomen, hips, and thighs.
- Reconstitute with supplied diluent, swirl gently, let stand at room temperature until completely dissolved, then use immediately.
- Do not store reconstituted drug. Before reconstitution, store vials at −20 to −10C (−4 to 14F).

Assessment & Drug Effects

- Therapeutic effectiveness is indicated by longer remission periods and reduced frequency of attacks.
- Assess for systemic postinjection reactions (see Patient & Family Education). Assure patient that reaction is self-limiting. Assess for local reactions at injection sites including erythema, itching, induration, and soreness.
- Monitor for S&S of compromised immune response (e.g., increasing frequency of infections).

Patient & Family Education

- Some persons experience a systemic postinjection reaction with chest pain, palpitations, flushing, urticaria, anxiety, dyspnea, and laryngeal constriction immediately after injection. These symptoms are transient (lasting from 30 s–30 min), requires no treatment, and resolves spontaneously.
- The physician should be informed of a planned or suspected pregnancy.
- Report any distressing adverse drug effects.

GLIMEPIRIDE

(gli-me′pi-ride)

Trade name: Amaryl

Classifications: SYNTHETIC HOR-

MONE; ANTIDIABETIC; SECOND-GENERATION SULFONYLUREA
Prototype: Tolbutamide
Pregnancy category: C

ACTIONS/PHARMACODYNAMICS Second-generation sulfonylurea hypoglycemic agent used for once-a-day dosing. Directly stimulates functioning pancreatic beta cells to secrete insulin, leading to direct drop in blood glucose. Indirect action leads to increased sensitivity of peripheral insulin receptors, resulting in increased insulin binding in peripheral tissues. Glimepiride improves postprandial glycemic control.

USES Adjunct to diet and exercise in patients with NIDDM, may also be used in combination with insulin in NIDDM.

ROUTE & DOSAGE

NIDDM

Adult: **PO** Start with 1–2 mg once daily with breakfast or first main meal, dose may be increased to usual maintenance dose of 1–4 mg once daily (max 8 mg/d.)

PHARMACOKINETICS Absorption: completely absorbed from GI tract. **Onset:** 1 h. **Peak:** 2–3 h. **Distribution:** >99.5% protein bound; probably secreted into breast milk. **Metabolism:** metabolized in liver by cytochrome P4502C9 (CYP2C9). **Elimination:** half-life: 5–9 h; 60% excreted in urine, 40% in feces.

CONTRAINDICATIONS & PRECAUTIONS Contraindicated in: hypersensitivity to glimepiride, diabetic ketoacidosis, pregnancy (category C), lactation, nondiabetic patients with renal glycosuria. **Cautious use in:** previous hypersensitivity to other sulfonylureas, sulfonamides, or thiazide diuretics; hypoglycemia or conditions predisposing to hypoglycemia (e.g., prolonged nausea and vomiting, alcohol ingestion, renal or hepatic function impairment, severe infections, surgery). Safe use in children not established.

ADVERSE/SIDE EFFECTS CNS: dizziness, asthenia, headache, blurred vision, changes in accommodation. **GI:** nausea, vomiting, diarrhea, abdominal pain. **Hematologic:** leukopenia, agranulocytosis (rare), thrombocytopenia. **Metabolic:** hypoglycemia. **Skin:** rash, pruritus, erythema, urticaria, maculopapular eruptions.

DRUG INTERACTIONS Hypoglycemic effects may be potentiated by other highly protein-bound drugs (e.g., β-ADRENERGIC ANTAGONISTS, **chloramphenicol,** MAO INHIBITORS, NSAIDS, **probenecid,** SALICYLATES, SULFONAMIDES, **warfarin**). CORTICOSTEROIDS, **phenytoin, isoniazid, nicotinic acid,** SYMPATHOMIMETIC AMINES, THIAZIDE DIURETICS may attenuate effects of glimepiride.

NURSING IMPLICATIONS

Administration

- Give with breakfast or first main meal.
- Maximum starting dose is ≤ 2 mg. With renal or hepatic insufficiency, initial recommended dose is 1 mg. Dose may be increased by ≤ 2 mg at 1- to 2-wk intervals to maximum of 8 mg/d.
- Store in tightly closed container at 15–30C (59–86F).

Assessment & Drug Effects

- Frequently monitor blood glucose and urinary glucose.
- Monitor glycosylated hemoglobin every 3–6 mo.
- With long-term therapy, periodically monitor liver function tests,

serum osmolarity, serum sodium, and CBC with differential.

Patient & Family Education

- Provide administration directions. Advise to take a missed dose as soon as possible unless it is almost time for next dose, but never take two doses at the same time.
- Advise to avoid drinking alcohol or using OTC drugs without informing physician.
- Advise to use sunscreen and avoid sunlamps.
- Advise regarding adverse reactions and drug interactions.

GLIPIZIDE

(glip′i-zide)

Trade names: Glucotrol, Glucotrol XL

Classifications: SULFONYLUREA; ANTIDIABETIC AGENT

Prototype: Tolbutamide

Pregnancy category: C

ACTIONS/PHARMACODYNAMICS Second generation sulfonylurea hypoglycemic agent. Potency is enhanced by as much as 200-fold over first generation agents. Directly stimulates functioning pancreatic beta cells to secrete insulin, leading to an acute drop in blood glucose. Indirect action leads to altered numbers and sensitivity of peripheral insulin receptors, resulting in increased insulin binding. It also causes inhibition of hepatic glucose production and reduction in serum glucagon levels.

USES Adjunct to diet for control of hyperglycemia in patient with type II (non-insulin-dependent) diabetes mellitus after dietary control alone has failed; also used to treat transient loss of control in patient usually controlled well on diet.

ROUTE & DOSAGE

Control of Hyperglycemia

Adult: **PO** 2.5–5 mg/d, 30 min before breakfast; may increase by 2.5–5 mg q1–2wk; > 15 mg/d should be given in divided doses 30 min before morning and evening meal (max 40 mg/d). **Sustained release:** 5–10 mg once/d.

PHARMACOKINETICS Absorption: readily absorbed from GI tract. **Onset:** 15–30 min. **Peak:** 1–2 h. **Duration:** up to 24 h. **Metabolism:** metabolized extensively in liver. **Elimination:** half-life: 3–5 h; excreted mainly in urine with some excretion via bile in feces.

CONTRAINDICATIONS & PRECAUTIONS Contraindicated in: diabetic ketoacidosis. Safe use during pregnancy (category C), in nursing mothers, and in children not established. **Cautious use in:** impaired renal and hepatic function, the elderly, debilitated, malnourished patient; patient with adrenal or pituitary insufficiency.

ADVERSE/SIDE EFFECTS GI: nausea, diarrhea, constipation, gastralgia, cholestatic jaundice (rare). **Metabolic:** hepatic porphyria. **Skin:** erythema, morbilliform or maculopapular rash, pruritus, urticaria, eczema (transient). **Other:** transient: drowsiness, headache, hypersensitivity. **Overdosage:** hypoglycemia, ***mild:*** fatigue, drowsiness, hunger, GI distress (heartburn, abdominal pain, anorexia), headache, anxiety; ***severe:*** visual disturbances, ataxia, confusion, tachycardia, seizures, coma.

DRUG INTERACTIONS Alcohol produces disulfiram-like reaction in some patients; ORAL ANTICOAGULANTS,

chloramphenicol, clofibrate, phenylbutazone, MAO INHIBITORS, SALICYLATES, **probenecid,** SULFONAMIDES may potentiate hypoglycemic actions; THIAZIDES may antagonize hypoglycemic effects; **cimetidine** may increase glipizide levels, causing hypoglycemia.

NURSING IMPLICATIONS

G

Administration

- For once-daily dosing, take 30 min before the first meal of the day.
- Store in tightly closed, light-resistant container at 15–30C (59–86F).

Assessment & Drug Effects

- Response to the initial dose and establishment of a maintenance regimen in the elderly or debilitated patient is approached cautiously. Observe for early signs of hypoglycemia (easily overlooked).
- Severe drug-induced skin rashes and pruritus may necessitate discontinuation of drug use. Symptoms usually subside rapidly when drug is withdrawn.
- During insulin withdrawal and transfer to glipizide, urine tests for sugar and ketone bodies should be checked at least 3 times daily. Advise patient to contact the physician if tests are abnormal.
- The patient who is transferred from a sulfonylurea with a long half-life (e.g., chlorpropamide, half-life: 30–40 h) must be observed for hypoglycemic responses (see Appendix G) for 1–2 wk because of potential overlapping of drug effect.
- If the patient is also receiving a beta blocker or is elderly, the first signs of hypoglycemia may be hard to detect.
- Overdose treatment: Mild hypoglycemia (reaction without loss of consciousness of neurologic symptoms) is treated with PO glucose and adjustment of dosage and meal pattern. The patient should be closely monitored for at least 5–7 d to assure reestablishment of safe control. Severe hypoglycemia requires emergency hospitalization to permit treatment to maintain a blood glucose level above 100 mg/dl.

Patient & Family Education

- Emphasize to the patient that glipizide treatment accompanies (does not substitute for) continued control of diet and (if patient is obese) a weight-loss program.
- Blood glucose testing is encouraged for the patient on a sulfonylurea.
- Inform patient about the importance of exercise as a part of the total control program.
- When a drug that affects the hypoglycemic action of sulfonylureas (see Drug Interactions) is withdrawn or added to the glipizide regimen, the patient should be alerted to the added danger of loss of control. Urine and blood glucose tests and test for ketone bodies should be carefully monitored.

GLUCAGON

(gloo′ka-gon)

Trade name: GlucaGen

Classifications: HORMONE; ANTIDIABETIC AGENT

Pregnancy category: B

ACTIONS/PHARMACODYNAMICS

Polypeptide hormone produced by alpha cells of islets of Langerhans. Stimulates uptake of amino acids and their conversion to glucose precursors. Promotes lipolysis in liver and adipose tissue with release of free fatty acid and glycerol, which further stimulates ketogenesis and hepatic gluconeogenesis. Action in hypoglycemia relies on presence of adequate liver glycogen stores. Increases heart rate and myocardial contractility, and improves AV conduction in a manner similar to that produced by catecholamines. Actions are independent of beta blockade.

USES Emergency treatment of severe hypoglycemic reactions in diabetic patients who are unconscious or unable to swallow food or liquids and in psychiatric patients receiving insulin shock therapy. Also radiologic studies of GI tract to relax smooth muscle and thereby allow finer detail of mucosa; to diagnose insulinoma. **Unlabeled uses:** GI disturbances associated with spasm, cardiovascular emergencies, and to overcome cardiotoxic effects of beta blockers, quinidine, tricyclic antidepressants; as an aid in abdominal imaging.

ROUTE & DOSAGE

(Note: 1 mg = 1 unit)

Hypoglycemia

Adult: **IM/IV/SC** 0.5–1 mg; may repeat q5–20min if no response for 1–2 more doses.
Child: **IM/IV/SC** 0.025 mg/kg (max 1 mg/dose); may repeat q5–20min if no response for 1–2 more doses.
Neonate: **IM/IV/SC** 0.3 mg/kg (max 1 mg)

Insulin Shock Therapy

Adult: **IM/IV/SC** 0.5–1 mg usually 1 h after coma develops; if no response, may repeat in 25 min.

Diagnostic Aid to Relax Stomach or Upper GI Tract

Adult: **IM/IV/SC** 0.25–2 mg 10 min before the procedure.

Diagnostic Aid for Examination of Colon

Adult: **IM/IV/SC** 2 mg 10 min before the procedure.

PHARMACOKINETICS Onset: 5–20 min. **Peak:** 30 min. **Duration:** 1–1.5 h. **Metabolism:** metabolized in liver, plasma, and kidneys. **Elimination:** half-life: 3–10 min.

G

CONTRAINDICATIONS & PRECAUTIONS Contraindicated in: hypersensitivity to glucagon or protein compounds. Safe use during pregnancy (category B) and in nursing women not established. **Cautious use in:** insulinoma, pheochromocytoma.

ADVERSE/SIDE EFFECTS Nausea and vomiting; hypersensitivity reactions; Stevens-Johnson syndrome (erythema multiforme); hyperglycemia, hypokalemia.

INCOMPATIBILITY Solution/additive: sodium chloride.

NURSING IMPLICATIONS

Administration

- Dilute 1 unit (1 mg) of glucagon with 1 ml of diluent supplied by manufacturer. Administer by direct IV. Flush line with 5% dextrose instead of NaCl solution.
- IV administration to neonates, infants, children: Verify correct rate of IV injection with physician.
- After reconstitution of dry powder, use solution immediately.
- Glucagon will form a precipitate in saline solutions and solutions with pH of 3–9.5 (pH of glucagon is 2.5–3). Glucagon should be considered incompatible in syringe with any other drug.
- Reconstituted solution remains potent for up to 3 mo if kept refrigerated at 2–8C (36–46F). Use only

special vehicle supplied by manufacturer for dilution. Indicate date on label. Lyophilized (dry powder) form is stable at room temperature.

Assessment & Drug Effects

- IV glucose must be given if patient fails to respond to glucagon.
- Patient usually awakens from (diabetic) hypoglycemic coma 5–20 min after glucagon injection. As soon as possible after patient regains consciousness, PO carbohydrate should be given.
- After recovery from hypoglycemic reaction, symptoms such as headache, nausea, and weakness may persist.

Patient & Family Education

- For patients with frequent or severe hypoglycemic reactions, physician may request that a responsible family member be taught how to administer glucagon SC or IM. Stress importance of notifying physician promptly whenever a hypoglycemic reaction occurs so that reason for the reaction can be ascertained. Also review package insert with patient and family member.

G

GLUTETHIMIDE

(gloo-teth'i-mide)

Trade name: Doriglute

Classifications: CNS AGENT; ANXIOLYTIC; SEDATIVE-HYPNOTIC, BARBITURATE

Prototype: Secobarbital

Pregnancy category: C

Controlled substance: Schedule III

ACTIONS/PHARMACODYNAMICS Pharmacologic actions similar to those of barbiturates. Can induce hypnosis without producing reliable analgesic, antitussive, or anticonvulsant action. Causes less respiratory depression but greater degree of hypotension than barbiturates. Significantly suppresses REM sleep; but following drug withdrawal after chronic administration, REM rebound occurs, and patient may experience markedly increased dreaming, nightmares, insomnia. Addiction liability similar to that of barbiturates.

USES Short-term treatment of insomnia and for sedative effect preoperatively and during first stage of labor. Not indicated for routine sedation or persistent insomnia.

ROUTE & DOSAGE

Insomnia

Adult: **PO** 250–500 mg h.s.; may repeat prn but not <4 h before arising.

Preoperative Sedation

Adult: **PO** 500 mg the night before surgery and 500 mg–1 g 1 h before anesthesia.

PHARMACOKINETICS **Absorption:** erratic absorption from GI tract. **Onset:** 30 min. **Duration:** 4–8 h. **Distribution:** widely distributed; localizes in adipose tissue, liver, kidney, brain, and bile; crosses placenta; distributed into breast milk in small quantities. **Metabolism:** metabolized in liver. **Elimination:** half-life: 10–12 h; metabolites excreted in urine.

CONTRAINDICATIONS & PRECAUTIONS **Contraindicated in:** uncontrolled pain; intermittent porphyria; severe hepatic and renal impairment; prolonged administration; children <12 y. Safe use during pregnancy [(category C) except with caution during first stage of labor] not established. **Cautious use in:** elderly or debilitated patients; prostatic hypertrophy, bladder neck obstruction; pyloroduodenal obstruction, stenosing peptic ulcer; narrow-angle glaucoma; hypotension, cardiac arrhythmias; mental depression (particularly in patients with suicidal tendencies), history of alcoholism or drug abuse.

ADVERSE/SIDE EFFECTS CNS: CNS depression in fetus; paradoxic excitement, headache, vertigo. **GI:** gastric irritation, nausea, drug "hangover," dry mouth. **Hematologic:** blood dyscrasias; **Skin:** generalized skin rash (occasionally, purpuric or urticarial), exfoliative dermatitis (rare). **Other:** acute hypersensitivity reactions, hiccups, blurred vision. **Acute overdosage (CNS depression):** coma; depressed reflexes, including corneal reflex; dilated, fixed pupils; hypotension; hypothermia followed by hyperpyrexia; tachycardia; respiratory depression, cyanosis, sudden apnea; decreased intestinal motility, adynamic ileus; facial twitching; intermittent spasticity; flaccid paralysis; pulmonary and cerebral edema; renal tubular necrosis; severe infections. **Chronic toxicity (toxic psychosis):** slurred speech, impaired memory, inability to concentrate, mydriasis, dry mouth, nystagmus, ataxia, hyporeflexia, tremors, peripheral neuropathy.

DRUG INTERACTIONS Alcohol, BARBITURATES, other CNS DEPRESSANTS compound depressant effects; TRICYCLIC ANTIDEPRESSANTS add to anticholinergic effects; decreases anticoagulant effects of ORAL ANTICOAGULANTS.

NURSING IMPLICATIONS

Administration

- If administered for insomnia, glutethimide should be given 4 h or more before the usual time of arising to avoid residual daytime effects.
- Abrupt withdrawal following regular use may produce nausea, vomiting, nervousness, tremors, abdominal cramps, nightmares, insomnia, tachycardia, chills, fever, numbness of extremities, dysphagia, delirium, hallucinations, or convulsions. Withdrawal should be gradual, with stepwise dose reduction over a period of several days or weeks.

Assessment & Drug Effects

- Keep physician informed of patient's response to drug. Smallest effective dosage should be used for the shortest period of time compatible with patient's needs.
- Overdosage of glutethimide is difficult to treat. Patients tend to go in and out of toxicity, possibly because of delayed absorption of the drug.

Patient & Family Education

- Advise patient to report onset of rash or any other unusual symptoms. Discontinuation of drug is indicated if a rash occurs.
- Caution patient to avoid driving a motor vehicle or engaging in other activities requiring mental alertness for 7–8 h after drug ingestion.
- Warn patient about possible adverse reactions when glutethimide is combined with alcohol or other CNS depressants.
- Prolonged use of moderate to high doses of glutethimide can produce tolerance and psychologic and physical dependence.

GLYBURIDE

(glye'byoor-ide)

Trade names: DiaBeta, Euglucon♣, Glynase, Micronase

Classifications: SULFONYLUREA; ANTIDIABETIC AGENT

Prototype: Tolbutamide
Pregnancy category: B

ACTIONS/PHARMACODYNAMICS One of the most potent of the sulfonylurea hypoglycemic agents. Second-generation sulfonylurea closely related in actions, uses, and limitations to glipizide. Potency is enhanced by as much as 200-fold over first-generation agents. Appears to lower blood sugar concentration in both diabetic and nondiabetic individuals by sensitizing functioning pancreatic beta cells to release insulin in the presence of elevated serum glucose levels. Blood glucose-lowering effect persists during long-term glyburide treatment, but there is a gradual decline in meal-stimulated secretion of endogenous insulin toward pretreatment levels.

G

USE Adjunct to diet to lower blood glucose in patients with type II diabetes mellitus (NIDDM) after dietary control alone has failed.

ROUTE & DOSAGE

Control of Hyperglycemia
Adult: **PO** 1.25–5 mg/d with breakfast; may increase by 2.5–5 mg q1–2wk; > 15 mg/d should be given in divided doses with morning and evening meal (max 20 mg/d). ***Glynase:*** 1.5–3 mg/d (max 12 mg/d).

PHARMACOKINETICS Absorption: readily absorbed from GI tract. **Onset:** 15–60 min. **Peak:** 1–2 h. **Duration:** up to 24 h. **Distribution:** distributed in highest concentrations in liver, kidneys, and intestines; crosses placenta. **Metabolism:** metabolized extensively in liver. **Elimination:** half-life: 10 h; excreted equally in urine and feces.

CONTRAINDICATIONS & PRECAUTIONS Contraindicated in: diabetic ketoacidosis, as sole therapy for type II diabetes mellitus. Safe use during pregnancy (category B), in nursing mothers, and in children not established. **Cautious use in:** renal or hepatic insufficiency, elderly, debilitated, or malnourished patients; adrenal or pituitary insufficiency.

ADVERSE/SIDE EFFECTS <u>Hypoglycemia</u>, epigastric fullness, heartburn, nausea, pruritus, erythema, urticarial or morbilliform eruptions, cholestatic jaundice (rare).

DRUG INTERACTIONS Alcohol causes disulfiram-like reaction in some patients; ORAL ANTICOAGULANTS, **chloramphenicol, clofibrate, phenylbutazone,** MAO INHIBITORS, SALICYLATES, **probenecid,** SULFONAMIDES may potentiate hypoglycemic actions; THIAZIDES may antagonize hypoglycemic effects; **cimetidine** may increase glyburide levels, causing hypoglycemia.

NURSING IMPLICATIONS

Administration
- Glyburide is generally administered once daily in the morning with breakfast or with first main meal.
- Store in tightly closed, light-resistant container at 15–30C (59–86F).

Assessment & Drug Effects
- The elderly patient is especially vulnerable to glyburide-induced hypoglycemia (see Appendix G) because the antidiabetic agent is long-acting. Blood glucose levels should be monitored carefully during the dangerous early treatment period when dosage is being individualized.
- If the patient is also receiving a beta blocker or if the patient is el-

derly, the first signs of hypoglycemia may be hard to detect.

- The following indices of patient's response to therapy should be monitored at regular intervals: blood and urine glucose, glycosylated hemoglobin, urine ketones.
- Persistence of acetonuria with glycosuria indicates that the patient may require insulin therapy.

Patient & Family Education

- If symptoms of hypoglycemia occur, patient should eat or drink some form of sugar (e.g., corn syrup, orange juice with 2 or 3 tsp of table sugar). Reaction should be reported to physician promptly.
- Remind patient that loss of control of diabetes may result from stress such as fever, surgery, trauma, or infection. Blood and urine glucose and ketone body detection may need to be checked more frequently during these stress periods, and transfer from the sulfonylurea to insulin may be necessary.
- Emphasize importance of keeping follow-up medical appointments and of adhering to dietary instructions, regular exercise program, and scheduled urine and blood testing.

GLYCERIN

(gli'ser-in)

Trade names: Fleet Babylax, Glycerol, Glyrol, Osmoglyn

GLYCERIN ANHYDROUS

Trade name: Ophthalgan

Classifications: HYPEROSMOTIC LAXATIVE; ANTIGLAUCOMA

Pregnancy category: C

ACTIONS/PHARMACODYNAMICS

When administered orally, glycerin raises plasma osmotic pressure by withdrawing fluid from extravascular spaces; lowers ocular tension by decreasing volume of intraocular fluid. Also may decrease CSF pressure and produce slight diuresis. Topical application to eye reduces edema by hygroscopic effect. Glycerin suppositories apparently work by causing dehydration of exposed tissue, which produces an irritant effect, and by absorbing water from tissues, thus creating more mass. Both actions stimulate peristalsis.

USES Orally to reduce elevated intraocular pressure (IOP) before or after surgery in patients with acute narrow-angle glaucoma, retinal detachment, or cataract and to reduce elevated CSF pressure. Sterile glycerin (anhydrous) is used topically to reduce superficial corneal edema resulting from trauma, surgery, or disease and to facilitate ophthalmoscopic examination. Used rectally (suppository or enema) to relieve constipation. **Unlabeled use:** to reduce mortality due to strokes in the elderly.

ROUTE & DOSAGE

Decrease IOP

Adult/Child: **PO** 1–1.8 g/kg 1–1.5 h before ocular surgery; may repeat q5h.

Constipation

Adult/Child ≥6 y: **PR** Insert 1 suppository *or* 5–15 ml of enema high into rectum and retain for 15 min.
Child <6 y: **PR** Insert 1 infant suppository *or* 2–5 ml of enema high into rectum and retain for 15 min.

Neonate: **PR** 0.5 ml of rectal solution (enema).

Reduction of Corneal Edema

Adult: **Topical** 1–2 drops instilled into eye q3–4h.

PHARMACOKINETICS **Absorption:** readily absorbed from GI tract after oral administration; rectal preparations are poorly absorbed. **Onset:** 10 min PO. **Peak:** 30 min–2 h. **Duration:** 4–8 h. **Metabolism:** 80% metabolized in liver; 10–20% metabolized in kidneys to CO_2 and water or utilized in glucose or glycogen synthesis. **Elimination:** half-life: 30–40 min; 7–14% excreted unchanged in urine.

CONTRAINDICATIONS & PRECAUTIONS **Contraindicated in:** safe use during pregnancy (category C) and in nursing women not established. **Cautious use in:** cardiac, renal, or hepatic disease; diabetes mellitus; dehydrated or elderly patients.

ADVERSE/SIDE EFFECTS Headache, dizziness, nausea, vomiting, thirst, diarrhea, hyperglycemia, glycosuria, dehydration, hyperosmolar nonketotic coma, irregular heartbeat, disorientation. **Suppository form:** abdominal cramps, rectal discomfort, hyperemia of rectal mucosa.

NURSING IMPLICATIONS

Administration

- Commercially available flavored solution may be poured over crushed ice and sipped through a straw. Lemon or lime juice and 0.9% NaCl (if allowed) may be added to unflavored solution for palatability.
- Headache (from cerebral dehydration) may be prevented or relieved by having patient lie down during and after administration of PO drug.

Assessment & Drug Effects

- Consult physician regarding fluid intake in patients receiving drug for elevated IOP. Although hypotonic fluids will relieve thirst and headache caused by the dehydrating action of glycerin, these fluids may nullify its osmotic effect.
- Monitor glycemic control in diabetics. Drug may cause hyperglycemia (see Appendix G).

Patient & Family Education

- After administration of glycerin rectal suppository or enema, patient will usually have an evacuation within 15–30 min.
- Slight hyperglycemia and glycosuria may occur with PO use. Patients with diabetes may require adjustment in insulin dosage.

GLYCOPYRROLATE

(glye-koe-pye′roe-late)

Trade names: Robinul, Robinul Forte

Classifications: AUTONOMIC NERVOUS SYSTEM AGENT; ANTICHOLINERGIC (PARASYMPATHOLYTIC); ANTIMUSCARINIC, ANTISPASMODIC

Prototype: Atropine

Pregnancy category: B

ACTIONS/PHARMACODYNAMICS Synthetic anticholinergic (antimuscarinic) compound with pharmacologic effects similar to those of atropine. Inhibits muscarinic actions of acetylcholine or autonomic neuroeffector sites innervated by postganglionic cholinergic nerves. Inhibits motility of GI tract and genitourinary tract and decreases volume of gastric and pancreatic secretions, saliva, and perspiration.

USES Adjunctive management of peptic ulcer and other GI disorders associated with hyperacidity, hypermotility, and spasm. Also used parenterally as preanesthetic and intraoperative medication and to reverse neuromuscular blockade.

ROUTE & DOSAGE

Peptic Ulcer

Adult: **PO** 1 mg t.i.d or 2 mg b.i.d. or t.i.d. in equally divided intervals (max 8 mg/d); should then decrease to 1 mg b.i.d. **IM/IV** 0.1–0.2 mg as single dose t.i.d. or q.i.d.

Reversal of Neuromuscular Blockade

Adult/Child: **IV** 0.2 mg glycopyrrolate administered with 1 mg of neostigmine *or* 5 mg pyridostigmine.

Control of Secretions

Child: **PO** 40–100 µg/kg t.i.d.–q.i.d. **IM/IV** 4–10 µg/kg t.i.d.–q.i.d.

PHARMACOKINETICS **Absorption:** poorly and incompletely absorbed from GI tract. **Onset:** 1 min IV; 15–30 min IM/SC; 1 h PO. **Peak:** 30–45 min IM/SC; 1 h PO. **Duration:** 2–7 h IM/SC; 8–12 h PO. **Distribution:** crosses placenta. **Metabolism:** minimally metabolized in liver. **Elimination:** 85% excreted in urine.

CONTRAINDICATIONS & PRECAUTIONS **Contraindicated in:** glaucoma; asthma; prostatic hypertrophy, obstructive uropathy; obstructive lesions or atony of GI tract; severe ulcerative colitis; myasthenia gravis; tachycardia; during cyclopropane anesthesia; children <12 y (except parenteral use in conjunction with anesthesia). Safe use during pregnancy (category B) or in nursing mothers not established. **Cautious use in:** autonomic neuropathy, hepatic or renal disease.

ADVERSE/SIDE EFFECTS *Xerostomia, decreased sweating, urinary hesitancy or retention,* blurred vision, mydriasis, constipation, palpitation, tachycardia, drowsiness, weakness, dizziness. **Overdosage:** neuromuscular blockade (curare-like action) leading to muscle weakness and paralysis is possible.

DRUG INTERACTIONS **Amantadine,** ANTIHISTAMINES, TRICYCLIC ANTIDEPRESSANTS, **quinidine, disopyramide, procainamide** compound anticholinergic effects; decreases **levodopa** effects; **methotrimeptrazine** may precipitate extrapyramidal effects; decreases antipsychotic effects (decreased absorption) of PHENOTHIAZINES.

INCOMPATIBILITIES **Solution/additive: methylprednisolone, chloramphenicol, dexamethasone, diazepam, dimenhydrinate, methohexital, pentazocine, phenobarbital, secobarbital, sodium bicarbonate, thiopental. Y-site: diazepam, dimenhydrinate, methohexital, pentazocine, phenobarbital, secobarbital, thiopental.**

NURSING IMPLICATIONS

Administration

- Do not combine glycopyrrolate in same syringe with drugs capable of raising the pH above 6.0 (see Incompatibilities). A precipitate and gas will form.
- May be given undiluted by direct IV. Administer 0.2 mg or fraction thereof over 1–2 min.
- Inspect parenteral products for cloudiness and discoloration. Discard such solutions.

Assessment & Drug Effects

- Incidence and severity of side effects are generally dose related.
- Monitor I&O ratio and pattern particularly in the elderly. Watch for urinary hesitancy and retention.
- Monitor vital signs, especially when drug is given parenterally. Report any changes in heart rate or rhythm.

G

Patient & Family Education

- Caution patient to avoid high environmental temperatures. (Heat prostration can occur because of decreased sweating.)
- Because glycopyrrolate may produce dizziness and blurred vision, warn patient not to engage in activities requiring mental alertness, such as operating a motor vehicle or performing other hazardous tasks.
- Instruct patient to use good oral hygiene, frequent mouth rinses with water, and a saliva substitute to lessen effects of xerostomia (dry mouth).

GOLD SODIUM THIOMALATE

(thye-oh-mah'late)

Trade name: Myochrysine

Classifications: GOLD COMPOUND

Prototype: Aurothioglucose

Pregnancy category: C

ACTIONS/PHARMACODYNAMICS Water-soluble gold compound similar to aurothioglucose in actions and uses. Has immunomodulatory and antiinflammatory effects. Action mechanism unclear: drug appears to act by suppression of phagocytosis, altered immune responses, and possibly by inhibition of prostaglandin synthesis. See aurothioglucose.

USES Selected patients (adults and juveniles) with acute rheumatoid arthritis. **Unlabeled uses:** psoriatic arthritis, Felty's syndrome.

ROUTE & DOSAGE

Rheumatoid Arthritis

Adult: **IM** 10 mg wk 1, 25 mg wk 2; then 25–50 mg/wk to a cumulative dose of 1 g; if improvement occurs, continue at 25–50 mg q2wk for 2–20 wk, then q3–4wk indefinitely or until side effects occur.
Child: **IM** 10 mg test dose; then 1 mg/kg/wk or 2.5–5 mg for wk 1 and 2; then 1 mg/kg q1–4wk (max single dose 50 mg).

PHARMACOKINETICS Absorption: slowly and irregularly absorbed from IM site. **Peak:** 3–6 h. **Distribution:** widely distributed, especially to synovial fluid, kidney, liver, and spleen; does not cross blood–brain barrier; crosses placenta. **Metabolism:** unknown. **Elimination:** half-life: 3–168 d; 60–90% of dose ultimately excreted in urine; also eliminated in feces; traces may be found in urine for ≥ 6 mo.

CONTRAINDICATIONS & PRECAUTIONS Contraindicated in: history of severe toxicity from previous exposure to gold or other heavy metals; severe debilitation; SLE, Sjögren's syndrome in rheumatoid arthritis; renal disease; hepatic dysfunction, history of infectious hepatitis or hematologic disorders; uncontrolled diabetes or CHF. Safe use during pregnancy (category C) not established. **Cautious use in:** history of drug allergies or hypersensitivity, hypertension.

ADVERSE/SIDE EFFECTS CNS: dizziness, syncope, sweating, flushing.

CV: bradycardia. **GI:** hepatitis, metallic taste, *stomatitis,* nausea, vomiting. **Hematologic (rare):** agranulocytosis, aplastic anemia, eosinophilia. **Renal:** nephrotic syndrome, glomerulitis with hematuria, *proteinuria.* **Skin:** transient pruritus, *erythema, dermatitis,* fixed drug eruption, alopecia, shedding of nails, gray to blue pigmentation of skin (chrysiasis). **Other:** gold deposits in ocular tissues, *photosensitivity,* peripheral neuritis, angioneurotic edema, pulmonary fibrosis, interstitial pneumonitis, anaphylaxis (rare).

DRUG INTERACTIONS ANTIMALARIALS, IMMUNOSUPPRESSANTS, **penicillamine, phenylbutazone** increase risk of blood dyscrasias.

NURSING IMPLICATIONS

Administration

- Agitate vial before withdrawing dose to ensure uniform suspension.
- Drug is usually administered deep into upper outer quadrant of gluteus with patient lying down. Patient should remain recumbent for at least 30 min after injection because of the danger of "nitritoid reaction" (transient giddiness, vertigo, facial flushing, fainting). Observe for allergic reactions.
- Preserve in tight, light-resistant containers at 15–30C (59–86F). Drug should not be used if it is any darker than pale yellow.

Assessment & Drug Effects

- Prior to each injection, urine should be analyzed for protein, blood, and sediment. Drug should be discontinued promptly if proteinuria or hematuria develops.
- Patient should be interviewed and examined before each injection to detect occurrence of transient pruritus or dermatitis (both are common early indications of toxicity), stomatitis (sore tongue, palate, or throat), metallic taste, indigestion, or other signs and symptoms of possible toxicity. Treatment should be interrupted immediately if any of these reactions occurs.
- Allergic reaction may occur almost immediately after injection, 10 min after injection, or at any time during therapy. If it is observed, treatment should be discontinued. At time of injection have antidote dimercaprol (BAL) on hand.
- Baseline Hgb and RBC determinations, WBC count, differential count, platelet count, and urinalysis should be obtained before initiation of therapy and at regular intervals thereafter.
- Rapid reduction in hemoglobin level, WBC count below 4000/mm^3, eosinophil count above 5%, and platelet count below 100,000/mm^3 signify possible toxicity.

Patient & Family Education

- Therapeutic effects may not appear until after 2 mo of therapy.
- Rapid improvement in joint swelling usually indicates that patient is closely approaching drug tolerance level; report to physician.
- Patients who develop gold dermatitis should be warned that exposure to sunlight may aggravate the problem.
- The appearance of purpura or ecchymoses is always an indication for doing a platelet count; instruct patient to report them to physician.
- Patients should be informed about possible adverse reactions and warned to report any symptom suggestive of toxicity as soon as it appears.

GONADORELIN HYDROCHLORIDE

(goe-nad-oh-rell'in)
Trade name: Factrel
Classifications: SYNTHETIC HORMONE; DIAGNOSTIC AGENT
Pregnancy category: B

G

ACTIONS/PHARMACODYNAMICS Synthetic luteinizing hormone–releasing hormone (LHRH) with structure identical to the natural hormone; also referred to as gonadotropin-releasing hormone (GnRH). Stimulates anterior pituitary to release the gonadotropin LH.

USES To evaluate functional capacity and response of the gonadotropes of anterior pituitary and in suspected gonadotropic deficiency. Also used to evaluate residual gonadotropic function of the pituitary following surgical or radiologic removal of a pituitary tumor. **Unlabeled uses:** treatment of delayed puberty, amenorrhea, and infertility in males.

ROUTE & DOSAGE

Evaluation of Functional Capacity of Anterior Pituitary
Adult: **SC/IV** 100 μg administered in women during early phase of menstrual cycle (days 1 to 7) if it can be determined.

PHARMACOKINETICS Duration: 3–5 h. **Distribution:** distributed into breast milk. **Metabolism:** hydrolyzed in plasma. **Elimination:** half-life: 10–40 min; metabolites excreted in urine.

CONTRAINDICATIONS & PRECAUTIONS Contraindicated in: safe use in pregnancy (category B) not established; concurrent use of other drugs having effect on pituitary-gonadotropic function.

ADVERSE/SIDE EFFECTS CNS: headache, light-headedness. **GI:** nausea, abdominal discomfort. **Other:** flushing, local inflammation at injection site if given SC, hypersensitivity reaction (rare).

DRUG INTERACTIONS ANDROGENS, ESTROGENS, PROGESTINS, GLUCOCORTICOIDS may cause false test results; **digoxin** may suppress gonadotropin levels; DOPAMINE ANTAGONISTS, PHENOTHIAZINES increase prolactin and blunt response to gonadorelin; **spironolactone, levodopa** increase gonadotropin levels.

NURSING IMPLICATIONS

Administration
- Preparation of the solution: Reconstitute 100-μg vial with 1 ml sterile diluent (supplied by manufacturer), and the 500-μg vial with 2 ml. Solution should be used immediately after preparation.
- Administer a single dose by direct IV over 15–30 s.
- After reconstitution, store drug at room temperature and use within 24 h. Discard unused diluted solution and diluent. Store ampule at room temperature.
- Test procedure is according to established protocol (see manufacturer's information).

Assessment & Drug Effects
- Repetitive high doses of gonadorelin may inhibit spermatogenesis and cause luteolysis.

Interpretation of Test
- In menopausal and postmenopausal women, baseline LH levels are elevated.
- Patient clinically diagnosed or with suspected pituitary or hypothalamus dysfunction often demon-

strates subnormal or absent LH response after test dose.

GOSERELIN ACETATE

(gos-er′e-lin)
Trade name: Zoladex
Classifications: HORMONE; GONADOTROPIN-RELEASING HORMONE (GnRH) ANALOG
Prototype: Leuprolide
Pregnancy category: X

ACTIONS/PHARMACODYNAMICS
A synthetic form of luteinizing hormone-releasing hormone (LHRH or GnRH) that inhibits pituitary gonadotropin secretion. With chronic administration, serum testosterone levels fall into the range normally seen with surgically castrated men.

USES Prostate cancer, breast cancer. Endometrial thinning agent prior to endometrial ablation for dysfunctional uterine bleeding. **Unlabeled uses:** endometriosis, uterine leiomyomas.

ROUTE & DOSAGE

Prostate Cancer, Breast Cancer, Endometriosis, Uterine Leiomyomas

Adult: **SC** 3.6 mg once q28d. 10.8 mg depot q12wk.

Endometrial Thinning Prior to Endometrial Ablation

Adult: **SC** 3.6 mg once q28d.

PHARMACOKINETICS Absorption: rapidly absorbed following SC administration. **Duration:** 29 d. **Elimination:** half-life: 4.9 h; excreted by kidneys.

CONTRAINDICATIONS & PRECAUTIONS Contraindicated in: pregnancy (category X) and nursing mothers; known hypersensitivity to LHRH; endometriosis or endometrial thinning; hypercalcemia. **Cautious use in:** urinary tract obstruction and children; family history of osteoporosis; concurrent use with anticonvulsants or corticosteroids. Safety and efficacy in children <18 y not known.

ADVERSE/SIDE EFFECTS CNS: headache, tumor flare. **Endocrine:** gynecomastia, breast swelling and tenderness, *postmenopausal symptoms* (*hot flashes,* vaginal dryness). **GI:** nausea. **GU:** vaginal spotting, breakthrough bleeding, decreased libido, *impotence*. **Musculoskeletal:** bone pain, bone loss.

DIAGNOSTIC TEST INTERFERENCE
Increased levels of ***alkaline phosphatase*** and ***estradiol*** in the first 1–8 d; initial increase then decrease in ***FSH, LH,*** and ***testosterone.***

DRUG INTERACTIONS None established.

NURSING IMPLICATIONS

Administration
- Follow manufacturer's directions exactly for implanting the drug SC in the upper abdominal wall.
- Store at room temperature not to exceed 25C (77F).

Assessment & Drug Effects
- In patients with prostate cancer, monitor carefully during the first month of therapy for signs and symptoms of spinal cord compression or ureteral obstruction. Report immediately to physician.
- In patients with prostate cancer, anticipate a transient worsening of symptoms (e.g., bone pain) during the first weeks of therapy.

Patient & Family Education
- Inform men that sexual dysfunc-

tion and hot flashes may accompany drug use.
- Advise patients to immediately report symptoms of spinal cord compression or urinary obstruction.

GRANISETRON

(gran′i-se-tron)

Trade name: Kytril
Classifications: GI AGENT; ANTIEMETIC; 5-HT_3 ANTAGONIST
Prototype: Ondansetron
Pregnancy category: B

G

ACTIONS/PHARMACODYNAMICS Granisetron is a selective serotonin (5-HT_3) receptor antagonist used for the prevention of nausea and vomiting associated with cancer chemotherapy. Serotonin receptors of the 5-HT_3 type are located centrally in the chemoreceptor trigger zone, and peripherally on the vagal nerve terminals. Serotonin is released from the wall of the small intestine, stimulates the vagal afferents through the serotonin (5-HT_3) receptors, and initiates the vomiting reflex.

USES Prevention of nausea and vomiting associated with initial and repeat courses of emetogenic cancer therapy, including high-dose cisplatin.

ROUTE & DOSAGE

Nausea and Vomiting
Adult: **IV** 10 μg/kg infused over 30 s–5 min, beginning at least 30 min before initiation of chemotherapy; up to 40 μg/kg per dose has been used. **PO** 1 mg b.i.d.: start 1 mg up to 1 h prior to chemotherapy, then second tab 12 h later; or 2 mg q.d.
Child 2–16 y: **IV** same as adult.

PHARMACOKINETICS **Onset:** several minutes. **Duration:** approximately 24 h. **Distribution:** widely distributed in body tissues. **Metabolism:** appears to be metabolized in liver. **Elimination:** half-life: 10–11 h in cancer patients, 4–5 h in healthy volunteers; excreted in urine as metabolites.

CONTRAINDICATIONS & PRECAUTIONS **Contraindicated in:** hypersensitiviy to granisetron. **Cautious use in:** liver disease, pregnancy (category B), lactation.

ADVERSE/SIDE EFFECTS **CNS:** *headache,* dizziness, somnolence, insomnia, labile mood, anxiety, fatigue. **GI:** constipation, diarrhea, elevated liver function tests.

NURSING IMPLICATIONS

Administration
- Granisetron may be given undiluted over 30 s.
- Granisetron injection may be diluted in 0.9% sodium chloride or 5% dextrose to a total volume of 20–50 ml for IV infusion.
- Diluted granisetron may be infused over 5 min, with the infusion completed 20–30 min prior to initiation of chemotherapy.
- Granisetron infusion should be prepared at time of administration; it should not be mixed in solution with other drugs.
- Granisetron infusion is stable for 24 h after dilution when stored at room temperature (15–30C/59–86F) under normal lighting conditions.

Assessment & Drug Effects
- Monitor the frequency and severity of nausea and vomiting.
- Monitor liver function tests; elevated AST and ALT values usually normalize within 2 wk of last dose of granisetron.

- Assess for headache, which usually responds to nonnarcotic analgesics.

Patient & Family Education
- Inform patient that headache requiring an analgesic for relief is a common adverse effect.
- Discuss with patient ways to manage constipation.

GREPAFLOXACIN HYDROCHLORIDE
(gre-pa′flox-a-sin)
Trade name: Raxar
Classifications: ANTIINFECTIVE; QUINOLONE ANTIBIOTIC
Prototype: Ciprofloxacin
Pregnancy category: C

ACTIONS/PHARMACODYNAMICS Grepafloxacin is a quinolone that is a synthetic, broad-spectrum antibacterial agent. Grepafloxacin is bactericidal, interfering with the enzyme DNA-gyrase, necessary for bacterial DNA replication. Effective against many gram-positive and gram-negative organisms including *Streptococcus pneumoniae* and penicillin-resistant strains such as *Pseudomonas aeruginosa, Hemophilus influenzae,* and *Chlamydia trachomatis.*

USES Chronic bronchitis, community-acquired pneumonia, uncomplicated gonorrhea, nongonoccal urethritis, cervicitis.

ROUTE & DOSAGE

Chronic Bronchitis
Adult: **PO** 400–600 mg q.d. × 10 d.

Community-acquired Pneumonia
Adult: **PO** 600 mg q.d. × 10 d.

Nongonoccal Urethritis or Cervicitis
Adult: **PO** 400 mg q.d. × 7 d.

Uncomplicated Gonorrhea
Adult: **PO** 400 mg once.

PHARMACOKINETICS Absorption: rapidly absorbed from GI tract, bioavailability 70%. **Peak:** 2–3 h. **Distribution:** 50% protein bound. **Metabolism:** metabolized in liver by cytochromes P450 1A2 (primary) and 3A4 (minor). **Elimination:** half-life: 15.7 h; 50% excreted in feces, 38% in urine.

CONTRAINDICATIONS & PRECAUTIONS Contraindicated in: hypersensitivity to grepafloxacin or related antibiotics such as ciprofloxacin, levofloxacin, norfloxacin, nalidixic acid, sparfloxacin; hepatic failure; patients with known QT_C prolongation; concomitantly with medications known to increase the QT_C interval or torsades de pointes (e.g., terfenadine) unless the patient is on a cardiac monitor; lactation; pregnancy (category C). **Cautious use in:** children and adolescents due to potential arthropathies; concomitant administration with NSAIDs, antidiabetic agents, caffeine, theobromide, theophylline; concomitant administration with products containing aluminum, calcium, iron, magnesium, zinc.

ADVERSE/SIDE EFFECTS Body as whole: asthenia, infection, pain, photosensitivity reaction. **CNS:** headache, dizziness, insomnia, somnolence, nervousness. **GI:** *nausea, taste perversion,* diarrhea, abdominal pain, vomiting, dyspepsia, anorexia, dry mouth, constipation. **Skin:** pruritus, rash. **Other:** vaginitis, leukorrhea.

DRUG INTERACTIONS Absorption decreased by ANTACIDS, IRON SALTS, **calcium; theophylline** levels may be increased; NSAIDS may increase risk of CNS stimulation or convulsions.

NURSING IMPLICATIONS

Administration

- Do not give oral drug within 2 h of drugs containing aluminum, magnesium, iron, zinc, or sucralfate.
- Store at 15–30C (59–86F) in a tightly closed container.

Assessment & Drug Effects

- C&S test should be done prior to beginning therapy and periodically during therapy.
- Therapy should be discontinued and physician immediately notified if any of the following occur: skin rash or other signs of a hypersensitivity reaction (see Appendix G); CNS symptoms such as seizures, restlessness, confusion, hallucinations, depression; skin eruption following sun exposure; symptoms of colitis such as persistent diarrhea; joint pain, inflammation, or rupture of a tendon; hypoglycemic reaction in a diabetic on an oral hypoglycemic agent.

Patient & Family Education

- Note important indications for discontinuing drug and immediately notify physician.
- Fluids should be consumed liberally while taking grepafloxacin.
- Allow a minimum of 4 h between grepafloxacin and drugs containing any of the following: aluminum and/or magnesium antacids, iron supplements, multivitamins with zinc, sucralfate.
- Avoid exposure to excess sunlight or artificial UV light.
- If possible, NSAIDS should be avoided while taking grepafloxacin.

GRISEOFULVIN MICROSIZE

(gri-see-oh-ful'vin)

Trade names: Fulvicin-U/F, Grifulvin V, Grisactin, Grisovin-FP ♣

GRISEOFULVIN ULTRAMICROSIZE

Trade names: Fulvicin P/G, Grisactin Ultra, Gris-PEG

Classifications: ANTIINFECTIVE; ANTIBIOTIC; ANTIFUNGAL

Prototype: Fluconazole

Pregnancy category: C

ACTIONS/PHARMACODYNAMICS

Fungistatic antibiotic derived from species of *Penicillium*. Arrests metaphase of cell division by disrupting mitotic spindle structure in fungal cells. Deposits in keratin precursor cells and has special affinity for diseased tissue. Tightly bound to new keratin of skin, hair, and nails, which becomes highly resistant to fungal invasion. Effective against various species of *Epidermophyton, Microsporum,* and *Trichophyton* (has no effect on other fungi, including *Candida,* bacteria, and yeasts). Has some direct vasodilatory activity. Efficacy of GI absorption of ultramicrosize formulation reported to be twice that of microsize griseofulvin. Theoretically, cross-sensitivity with penicillin is a possibility.

USES Mycotic disease of skin, hair, and nails not amenable to conventional topical measures. Concomitant use of appropriate topical agent may be required, particularly for tinea pedis. **Unlabeled uses:** Raynaud's disease, angina pectoris, and gout.

ROUTE & DOSAGE

Tinea Corporis, Tinea Cruris, Tinea Capitis

Adult: **PO** 500 mg microsize or

330–375 mg ultramicrosize daily in single or divided doses.
Child: **PO** 10–20 mg/kg/d microsize or 5–10 mg/kg/d ultramicrosize in single or divided doses.

Tinea Pedis, Tinea Unguium

Adult: **PO** 0.75–1 g microsize or 660–750 mg ultramicrosize daily in single or divided doses; microsize dose should be decreased to 500 mg/d after response is noted.
Child: **PO** 10–20 mg/kg/d microsize or 5–10 mg/kg/d ultramicrosize in single or divided doses.

PHARMACOKINETICS Absorption: absorbed primarily from duodenum; microsize is variably and unpredictably absorbed; ultramicrosize is almost completely absorbed. **Peak:** 4–8 h. **Distribution:** concentrates in skin, hair, nails, fat, and skeletal muscle; crosses placenta. **Metabolism:** metabolized in liver. **Elimination:** half-life: 9–24 h; excreted mainly in urine; some excretion in perspiration.

CONTRAINDICATIONS & PRECAUTIONS Contraindicated in: porphyria; hepatic disease; SLE. Safe use during pregnancy (category C), for children ≤ 2 y, or for prophylaxis against fungal infections not established. **Cautious use in:** penicillin-sensitive patients (possibility of cross-sensitivity with penicillin exists; however, reportedly penicillin-sensitive patients have been treated without difficulty).

ADVERSE/SIDE EFFECTS Low incidence of side effects. **CNS:** *severe headache,* insomnia, fatigue, mental confusion, impaired performance of routine functions, psychotic symptoms, vertigo. **GI:** heartburn, nausea, vomiting, diarrhea, flatulence, dry mouth, thirst, decreased taste acuity, anorexia, unpleasant taste, furred tongue, oral thrush. **Hematologic:** leukopenia, neutropenia, granulocytopenia, punctate basophilia, monocytosis. **Hypersensitivity:** urticaria, photosensitivity, skin rashes, pruritus, fixed drug eruption, serum sickness syndromes, severe angioedema. **Renal (nephrotoxicity):** proteinuria. **Other:** hepatotoxicity, estrogenlike effects (in children), aggravation of SLE, overgrowth of nonsusceptible organisms, candidal intertrigo.

DRUG INTERACTIONS Alcohol may cause flushing and tachycardia; BARBITURATES may decrease activity of griseofulvin; may decrease hypoprothrombinemic effects of ORAL ANTICOAGULANTS; may increase **estrogen** metabolism, resulting in break through bleeding, and decrease contraceptive efficacy of ORAL CONTRACEPTIVES.

NURSING IMPLICATIONS

Administration

- Giving the drug with or after meals may allay GI disturbances.
- Serum levels may be enhanced by giving the microsize formulations with a high fat content meal (increases drug absorption rate). Consult physician.
- Store griseofulvin preparations at 15–30C (59–86F) in tightly covered containers unless otherwise directed.

Assessment & Drug Effects

- Before treatment is initiated, inquire about history of sensitivity to griseofulvin, penicillins, or other allergies.
- Monitor food intake. Griseofulvin may alter taste sensations, and this may cause appetite suppression and inadequate nutrient intake.
- Blood studies should be per-

formed at least once weekly during first month of therapy or longer. Periodic tests of renal and hepatic function are also advised.
- Treatment should be continued until there is clinical improvement or until 2 or 3 consecutive weekly cultures are negative.

Patient & Family Education
- Patient may experience symptomatic relief after 48–96 h of therapy. Stress the importance of continuing treatment as prescribed to prevent relapse.
- Duration of treatment depends on time required to replace infected skin, hair, or nails, and thus varies with infection site. Average duration of treatment for tinea capitis (scalp ringworm), 4–6 wk; tinea corporis (body ringworm), 2–4 wk; tinea pedis (athlete's foot), 4–8 wk; tinea unguium (nail fungus), at least 4 mo for fingernails, depending on rate of growth, and 6 mo or more for toenails.
- Caution patient to avoid exposure to intense natural or artificial sunlight, because photosensitivity-type reactions may occur.
- Headaches often occur during early therapy but frequently disappear with continued drug administration.
- Warn patient of possible disulfiram-type reaction (see Appendix G) on ingestion of alcohol during therapy.
- Patient should be informed that pharmacologic effects of oral contraceptives may be reduced. Breakthrough bleeding and pregnancy may occur. Alternative form of birth control may be advisable during griseofulvin therapy.

GUAIFENESIN
(gwye-fen'e-sin)
Trade names: Amonidrin, Anti-Tuss, Breonesin, Gee-Gee, GG-Cen, Glyceryl Guaiacolate, Glycotuss, Glytuss, Guaituss, Hytuss, Malotuss, Mytussin, Nortussin, Resyl ♣, Robitussin
Prototype for classification: EXPECTORANT
Pregnancy category: C

ACTIONS/PHARMACODYNAMICS Enhances reflex outflow of respiratory tract fluids by irritation of gastric mucosa and aids in expectoration by reducing adhesiveness and surface tension of secretions.

USE To combat dry, nonproductive cough associated with colds and bronchitis. A common ingredient in cough mixtures.

ROUTE & DOSAGE

Cough
Adult: **PO** 200–400 mg q4h up to 2.4 g/d.
Child: **PO** *6–11 y:* 100–200 mg q4h up to 1.2 g/d; *2–5 y:* 50–100 mg q4h up to 600 mg/d; *<2 y:* 12 mg/kg/d in 6 divided doses.

CONTRAINDICATIONS & PRECAUTIONS **Contraindicated in:** hypersensitivity to guaifenesin; pregnancy (category C), lactation.

ADVERSE/SIDE EFFECTS Low incidence: GI upset, nausea, drowsiness.

DIAGNOSTIC TEST INTERFERENCE Guaifenesin may produce color interferences with certain laboratory determinations of urinary 5-hydroxyindoleacetic acid ***(5-HIAA)*** and vanillylmandelic acid ***(VMA).***

DRUG INTERACTIONS By inhibiting platelet function, guaifenesin may increase risk of hemorrhage in patients receiving **heparin** therapy.

NURSING IMPLICATIONS

Administration

- Drug is most effective when taken q4h around the clock or during waking hours.
- Carefully observe maximum daily doses for adults and children.
- Follow dose with a full glass of water if not contraindicated.

Assessment & Drug Effects

- Persistent cough may indicate a serious condition requiring further diagnostic work.
- Monitor effectiveness of drug. If high fever, rash, or headaches develop, notify physician.

Patient & Family Education

- Increase in fluid intake will also help to loosen mucus. Encourage patient to drink at least 8 glasses of fluid daily.
- Instruct patient to contact physician if cough persists beyond 1 wk.
- Advise patient to contact physician if high fever, rash, or headache develops.

GUANABENZ ACETATE

(gwan′a-benz)

Trade name: Wytensin

Classifications: CARDIOVASCULAR AGENT; CENTRAL-ACTING ANTIHYPERTENSIVE

Prototype: Methyldopa

Pregnancy category: C

ACTIONS/PHARMACODYNAMICS Centrally acting alpha$_2$-adrenergic agonist. Pharmacologic actions closely resemble those of clonidine. Lowers BP, primarily by stimulating central alpha-adrenergic receptors, which leads to inhibition of sympathetic outflow from brain. Reduces both supine and standing BP, usually without producing postural hypotension, and slightly lowers pulse rate. Has no effect on exercise tolerance or on potassium levels. It does not cause sodium retention or excretion; however, it appears to enhance urinary dilution and free water diuresis. Given the fact that central adrenergic hyperactivity causes symptoms of narcotic withdrawal, guanabenz appears to help control abstinence symptoms by reducing norepinephrine output.

USES Used alone in treatment of hypertension or in combination with a thiazide diuretic (stepped-care approach: step 2.) **Unlabeled uses:** opiate detoxification, analgesic for chronic pain.

ROUTE & DOSAGE

Hypertension
Adult: **PO** 4 mg b.i.d.; may increase by 4–8 mg/d q1–2wk up to 32 mg b.i.d.
Geriatric **PO** 4 mg once daily, may increase every 1–2 wk.

Opiate Withdrawal
Adult: **PO** 4 mg b.i.d. to q.i.d.

PHARMACOKINETICS **Absorption:** 75% absorbed from GI tract. **Onset:** 60 min. **Peak:** 2–5 h. **Duration:** 6–12 h. **Distribution:** widely distributed; crosses blood–brain barrier; not known if crosses placenta or distributed into breast milk. **Metabolism:** extensively metabolized. **Elimination:** half-life: 4–14 h; 80% excreted in urine; 20% in feces.

CONTRAINDICATIONS & PRECAUTIONS **Contraindicated in:** safe use during pregnancy (category C), in nursing mothers, and in children not established. **Cautious use in:** severe coronary insufficiency, recent MI, cerebrovascular disease, severe hepatic or renal failure.

ADVERSE/SIDE EFFECTS CNS: *drowsiness or sedation,* dizziness, weakness, headache, anxiety, ataxia, depression, sleep disturbances. **CV:** chest pain, edema, arrhythmias, palpitation. **GI:** *dry mouth,* nausea, epigastric pain, diarrhea, vomiting, constipation, abdominal discomfort, taste disorders. **GU:** increased urination, urinary frequency, sexual dysfunction. **Other:** blurred vision, nasal congestion, dyspnea, muscle aches, aches in extremities, rash, pruritus. **Overdosage:** hypotension; somnolence, lethargy, irritability, miosis, bradycardia, unusual fatigue or weakness, nervousness.

DRUG INTERACTIONS **Alcohol** and other CNS DEPRESSANTS compound CNS depression; TRICYCLIC ANTIDEPRESSANTS may reduce antihypertensive effects of guanabenz.

NURSING IMPLICATIONS

Administration

- One dose is usually prescribed for bedtime administration to ensure overnight control and to reduce possibility of daytime drowsiness or sedation.
- Store at 15–30C (59–86F) in tightly closed containers unless otherwise directed.

Assessment & Drug Effects

- Baseline and periodic tests should include blood chemistry (serum potassium, CBC, creatinine, uric acid, cholesterol, glucose), urinalysis for protein and sugar, and ECG.
- Dry mouth requires early attention and specific treatment because (1) it can interfere with patient's food and fluid intake; (2) deprivation of normal salivary flow is a potential dental hazard since it favors demineralization of teeth; and (3) it can be a factor in noncompliance.

Patient & Family Education

- Elderly patients tend to be more sensitive to normal adult doses of antihypertensive drugs because of deficient baroreceptor reflexes. Therefore, although orthostatic hypotension is not an expected guanabenz effect, caution patient to make all position changes slowly and in stages.
- Warn patient not to omit dosage and not to stop drug therapy without consulting the physician. Abrupt discontinuation of guanabenz may cause sympathetic overactivity: anxiety, nervousness, palpitation, chest pain, fast or irregular heartbeat, trembling, flushing, headache, increased sweating and salivation, elevation of BP (usually above basal level).
- Advise patient to use caution when driving or performing other potentially hazardous activities until reaction to drug is determined. Also warn patient that tolerance to alcohol and other CNS depressants may be reduced by guanabenz.

GUANADREL SULFATE

(gwahn'a-drel)

Trade name: Hylorel

Classifications: CARDIOVASCULAR AGENT; CENTRALLY ACTING ANTIHYPERTENSIVE

Prototype: Methyldopa

Pregnancy category: B

ACTIONS/PHARMACODYNAMICS Adrenergic ganglionic blocking agent structurally and pharmacologically related to guanethidine. Acts as a false neurotransmitter without adrenergic activity because it blocks the release of norepinephrine from adrenal medulla and adrenergic nerve endings that normally follows sympathetic nerve stimulation. The net effect is catecholamine depletion with resulting relaxation of vascular smooth muscle, reduction of peripheral vascular resistance, lowering of systolic and diastolic BP, and a relative increase in parasympathetic tone. Decreases standing more than supine BP and is more effective in lowering systolic than diastolic BP.

USES Stepped-care approach: step 2 treatment of hypertension, usually with a diuretic.

ROUTE & DOSAGE

Hypertension
Adult: **PO** 5 mg b.i.d.; may increase up to 20–75 mg/d in 2–4 divided doses.
Geriatric: **PO** Start with 5 mg once daily.

PHARMACOKINETICS Absorption: readily absorbed from GI tract. **Onset:** 0.5–2 h. **Peak:** 4–6 h. **Duration:** 4–14 h. **Distribution:** widely distributed. **Elimination:** half-life: 10–12 h; 85% excreted in urine within 24 h.

CONTRAINDICATIONS & PRECAUTIONS Contraindicated in: pheochromocytoma, CHF, patients taking MAO INHIBITORS. Safe use during pregnancy (category B), in nursing women, and in children not established. **Cautious use in:** cerebrovascular, coronary artery, or peripheral vascular disease, bronchial asthma, history of peptic ulcer, diarrhea, elderly patients.

ADVERSE/SIDE EFFECTS Mostly dose related. **CNS:** *fatigue, headache, drowsiness,* paresthesias, tremors, confusion, depression or other psychologic problems, sleep disorders. **CV:** *morning orthostatic hypotension* (light-headedness, weakness), *orthostatic hypotension during the day,* palpitation, chest pain. **GI:** *diarrhea,* or increased number of stools, indigestion, constipation, dry mouth and thirst, anorexia, glossitis, nausea, vomiting, abdominal distress or pain. **GU:** nocturia, urine retention, urinary urgency or frequency, hematuria, *impaired ejaculation,* impotence. **Other:** visual disturbances; musculoskeletal aches, pains, or inflammation; excessive weight gain or loss, peripheral edema, nasal stuffiness, cough, *shortness of breath at rest or with exercise.*

DRUG INTERACTIONS Alcohol intensifies orthostatic hypotension and sedation; ALPHA- OR BETA-ADRENERGIC BLOCKERS, **reserpine** may intensify orthostatic hypotension and bradycardia; may enhance the action of **epinephrine, norepinephrine, methoxamine;** MAO INHIBITORS, PHENOTHIAZINES, TRICYCLIC ANTIDEPRESSANTS, **ephedrine, phenylpropanolamine** may antagonize hypotensive effects of guanadrel.

NURSING IMPLICATIONS

Administration

- Because serum half-life of guanadrel averages about 10 h, dosage adjustments are generally made weekly or monthly.
- Store at 15–30C (59–86F) unless otherwise directed.

Assessment & Drug Effects

- Dosage adjustments should be based on BP response in supine position and after standing 2–20 min. Record baseline measurements for future comparison purposes.
- The full effect of guanadrel on standing (orthostatic) BP should be carefully evaluated before the hospitalized patient is discharged. For ambulatory patient, BP measurements should also be taken following exercise for complete assessment.
- Patients with cerebrovascular, coronary artery, or peripheral vascular disease are particularly prone to orthostatic hypotension and therefore should be closely monitored.
- Guanadrel tends to enhance sodium and water retention, but these effects are generally controlled by concurrent diuretic therapy.

Patient & Family Education

- Inform patient about the possibility of orthostatic hypotension.
- Caution elderly patients particularly not to get out of bed without assistance during initial dosage adjustment period.
- Warn patient to make position changes slowly and in stages, especially from recumbent to upright posture. These precautions should be observed throughout drug therapy.
- Advise patient to lie down immediately at first hint of faintness, dizziness, weakness, or light-headedness. All are possible manifestations of orthostatic hypotension.
- Teach patient to monitor weight and to check legs and ankles for edema and in particular to note if rings or shoes suddenly seem too tight. Advise patient to notify physician of peripheral edema or unexpected weight gain of ≥ 1 kg (2 lb)/day.
- To encourage patient compliance in taking guanadrel at the same time(s) each day, suggest that it be taken in relation to a daily routine activity.
- Most side effects disappear or at least diminish in intensity after about 8 wk of therapy.
- Patient should be specifically cautioned not to use OTC drugs for treatment of colds, allergy, asthma, or appetite suppressants without consulting the physician or pharmacist. Many of these products contain adrenergic (sympathomimetic) amines, which may interfere with hypotensive action of guanadrel.

GUANETHIDINE SULFATE

(gwahn-eth′i-deen)

Trade names: Apo-Guanethidine ♣, Ismelin

Classifications: CARDIOVASCULAR AGENT; CENTRALLY ACTING ANTIHYPERTENSIVE

Prototype: Methyldopa

Pregnancy category: C

ACTIONS/PHARMACODYNAMICS

Potent, long-acting, adrenergic blocking agent. Competes with norepinephrine for reuptake into adrenergic neurons; displaces stored norepinephrine, thus exposing it to degradation by MAO. Produces gradual prolonged fall in BP, usually associated with bradycardia and decreased pulse pressure. Antihypertensive effect results from venous dilatation with peripheral pooling, decreased venous return, and decreased cardiac output. Drug-induced sodium retention and expansion of plasma volume, with resulting tolerance to antihypertensive effect, may occur unless concomitant diuretic therapy is administered. It is more effective in lowering orthostatic than supine BP. Local instillation in eye causes miosis and reduces intraocular pressure in glaucomatous eyes.

USES Stepped care approach to treatment of moderate to severe hypertension either alone or in conjunction with a thiazide diuretic or hydralazine. **Unlabeled uses:** chronic open-angle glaucoma, endocrine ophthalmopathy. **Orphan drug:** reflex sympathetic dystrophy syndrome; causalgia.

ROUTE & DOSAGE

Hypertension

Adult: **PO** 10 mg once/d; may be increased by 10 mg q5–7d up to 300 mg/d; may start with 25–50 mg/d in hospitalized patients; increase by 25–50 mg q1–3d.
Geriatric: **PO** Start with 5 mg once daily.
Child: **PO** 0.2 mg/kg/d; may increase by 0.2 mg/kg q1–3wk if needed (max 1–1.6 mg/kg/d).

PHARMACOKINETICS **Absorption:** completely absorbed, but undergoes significant first pass metabolism by liver; 3–50% of dose reaches systemic circulation. **Peak effect:** 1–3 wk. **Distribution:** rapidly distributed to adrenergic neuron storage sites; does not cross blood–brain barrier. **Metabolism:** metabolized in liver to inactive metabolites. **Elimination:** half-life: 5 d; excreted in urine.

CONTRAINDICATIONS & PRECAUTIONS **Contraindicated in:** pheochromocytoma, frank CHF (not due to hypertension). Safe use during pregnancy (category C) not established. **Cautious use in:** diabetes mellitus, impaired renal or hepatic function, sinus bradycardia, limited cardiac reserve, coronary disease with insufficiency, recent MI, cerebrovascular insufficiency, febrile illnesses, the elderly; history of peptic ulcer, colitis, or bronchial asthma.

ADVERSE/SIDE EFFECTS **CV:** *marked orthostatic and exertional hypotension* with dizziness, light-headedness; bradycardia, symptomatic sick sinus syndrome (weakness, dizziness, blurred vision); angina, *edema with weight gain,* CHF, complete heart block. **EENT:** blurred vision, ptosis of eyelids, parotid tenderness, nasal congestion. **GI:** *severe diarrhea,* nausea, vomiting, constipation, dry mouth. **GU:** nocturia, urinary retention, incontinence, inhibition of ejaculation, impotence. **Skin:** skin eruptions, loss of scalp hair. **Other:** dyspnea, psychic depression, weakness, fatigue, myalgia, tremor, chest paresthesias, asthma, rise in BUN, polyarteritis nodosa.

DRUG INTERACTIONS **Alcohol, levodopa,** DIURETICS and other HYPOTENSIVE AGENTS increase hypotensive effects; MAO INHIBITORS may antagonize hypotensive effects; **norepinephrine, pseudoephedrine,** OTHER DECONGESTANTS, TRICYCLIC ANTIDEPRESSANTS, PHENOTHIAZINES block hypotensive effects.

NURSING IMPLICATIONS

Administration

- Tablet may be crushed before administration and taken with fluid of patient's choice.
- Dosage should be increased slowly (at intervals of no less than 5–7 d for adults and 1–3 wk in children) and only if there has been no reduction in standing BP from previous levels. BP should be monitored during dosage adjustment period.

Assessment & Drug Effects

- Ideal dosage is that which reduces orthostatic BP to within normal range without faintness, dizziness, weakness, or fatigue.
- Take BP first in supine position and then again after patient has been standing for 10 min.
- I&O should be monitored, especially in the elderly and in patients with limited cardiac reserve or impaired renal function. Report changes in I&O ratio.
- Patients with limited cardiac reserve are particularly susceptible to guanethidine-induced sodium and water retention, with resulting edema, CHF, and drug resistance.
- Observe for evidence of edema and weight gain. Sudden weight gain of 1 kg (2 lb) in 24 h or more should be reported to physician.
- Patients on antidiabetic therapy should be observed closely for signs of hypoglycemia.

Patient & Family Education

- Stress importance of not stopping drug without advice of physician.
- Supervise ambulation, particularly in the elderly, since they are prone to develop orthostatic hypotension.
- Patients should be informed that orthostatic hypotension is most prominent shortly after arising from sleep and when too rapid changes are made to sitting or upright positions. Warn patients to move gradually to sitting position and to make all position changes slowly and in stages. Advise patient to flex arms and legs slowly before standing to augment venous return.
- Patients should be informed that orthostatic hypotension is intensified by prolonged standing, hot baths or showers, hot weather, alcohol ingestion, and strenuous physical exercise (particularly if followed by immobility).
- Warn patients to lie down or sit down (in head-low position) immediately at the onset of dizziness, weakness, or faintness.
- Advise patient to report character and frequency of stools. Diarrhea may be explosive and embarrassing to patient.
- Advise patient to consult physician regarding allowable salt intake.
- Dosage requirements may be reduced in presence of febrile illnesses. Advise patient to report fever to physician.
- Guanethidine may sensitize the patient to some sympathomimetic agents found in OTC cold remedies and cause hypertensive crisis. Caution patient to consult physician or pharmacist before taking any OTC drug.

GUANFACINE HYDROCHLORIDE

(gwahn'fa-seen)

Trade name: Tenex

Classifications: CARDIOVASCULAR AGENT; CENTRAL-ACTING ANTIHYPERTENSIVE

Prototype: Methyldopa

Pregnancy category: B

ACTIONS/PHARMACODYNAMICS

CENTRAL-ACTING ANTIHYPERTENSIVE with alpha$_2$-adrenergic agonist properties. In cerebral cortex, stimulation of alpha$_2$-adrenoceptors triggers inhibitory neurons to reduce central sympathetic outflow (i.e., impulses from vasomotor center to heart and blood vessels) with the result that peripheral vascular resistance is decreased and heart rate is slightly reduced (5 bpm). Cardiac output is not altered by this agent.

USE Management of mild to moderate hypertension. **Unlabeled use:** adjunct in heroin withdrawal.

ROUTE & DOSAGE

Hypertension

Adult: **PO** 1 mg/d h.s.; may be gradually increased to 3 mg/d if needed.

PHARMACOKINETICS Absorption: readily absorbed from GI tract. **Onset:** 2 h. **Peak:** 6 h. **Duration:** up to 24 h. **Distribution:** crosses placenta. **Metabolism:** metabolized in liver. **Elimination:** half-life: 17 h; 80% excreted in the urine in 24 h.

CONTRAINDICATIONS & PRECAUTIONS Contraindicated in: treatment of acute hypertension associated with toxemia of pregnancy; pregnancy (category B); children <12 y. **Cautious use in:** severe coronary insufficiency, recent MI, cerebrovascular disease; chronic renal or hepatic failure; nursing mothers.

ADVERSE/SIDE EFFECTS CNS: confusion, amnesia, mental depression, drowsiness, *dizziness, sedation,* headache, asthenia, *fatigue,* insomnia. **CV:** bradycardia, palpitation, substernal pain. **ENT:** rhinitis, tinnitus, taste change. **Eye:** vision disturbances, conjunctivitis, iritis. **GI:** *dry mouth, constipation,* abdominal pain, diarrhea, dysphagia, nausea. **GU:** *impotence,* testicular disorder, urinary incontinence. **Musculoskeletal:** leg cramps, hypokinesia. **Skin:** dermatitis, pruritus, purpura, sweating. **Other:** dyspnea.

DRUG INTERACTIONS Alcohol and other CNS DEPRESSANTS compound sedation and CNS depression.

NURSING IMPLICATIONS

Administration

- Single dose is best taken at bedtime to reduce effect of somnolence.
- Discontinuation of guanfacine treatment is gradual with planned tapering of schedule.
- Store tablets at 15–30C (59–86F) in tightly closed container; protect from light.

Assessment & Drug Effects

- Abrupt discontinuation may cause plasma and urinary catecholamine increases, leading to symptoms of tachycardia, insomnia, anxiety, nervousness. Rebound hypertension (i.e., increases in BP to levels significantly greater than those before therapy) may occur 2–7 d after abrupt drug withdrawal, but serious effects rarely develop.
- Monitor BP until it is stabilized. Report a rise in pressure that occurs toward end of dose interval; a divided dose schedule may be ordered.
- Side effects tend to be dose-dependent, increasing significantly with doses above 3 mg/d.

Patient & Family Education

- Urge patients to continue with drug even after they feel well. Advise maintenance of dosage regimen (dose and dose intervals). If 2 or more doses are missed, consult physician about how to reestablish dosage regimen.
- Urge patient to employ measures to keep mouth moist; suggest, if necessary, a saliva substitute, e.g., Moi-Stir, Xero-Lube (available OTC). If dry mouth persists > 2 wk, patient should check with dentist.
- Advise caution about driving or performing other tasks requiring alertness until reaction to drug is known.
- Advise patients to avoid alcohol and not to self-medicate with nonprescription drugs such as sleeping

medications, or cough medications without advice of physician.

HAEMOPHILUS b CONJUGATE VACCINE

(hee-mof'il-us)

Trade names: HibTITER, Pedvax-HIB, ProHIBiT

Classification: VACCINE

Pregnancy category: C

H

ACTIONS/PHARMACODYNAMICS A highly purified capsular polysaccharide extracted from *Hemophilus influenzae* type b (Hib). Hib capsular polysaccharide, principal antigen in the vaccine, promotes production of Hib anticapsular antibody, which mediates complement-dependent bacteriolyses and opsinization of *H. influenzae* type b organism. Serum antibody response is age dependent; i.e., response is poor in infants, increasing significantly between 12–24 mo. Immunization against *H. influenzae* type b disease may be considered in children 2–18 mo of age.

USES To provide active immunity to *H. influenzae* type b (Hib) infection in children 2 mo–5 y. **Unlabeled uses:** adults at risk of Hib infection who have Hodgkin's disease, before immunosuppressive chemotherapy.

ROUTE & DOSAGE

Immunoprophylaxis for *H. influenzae* Type b Infection

Child: **IM** *2–6 mo,* HibTITER: 0.5 ml, 3 doses 2 mo apart with booster at 15 mo; PedvaxHIB: 0.5 ml, 2 doses 2 mo apart with booster at 12 mo; *7–11 mo,* HibTITER: 0.5 ml, 2 doses 2 mo apart with booster at 15 mo; PedvaxHIB: 0.5 ml, 2 doses 2 mo apart with booster at 15 mo; *12–14 mo,* HibTITER: 0.5 ml, 1 dose with booster at 15 mo; PedvaxHIB: 0.5 ml, 1 dose with booster at 15 mo; *15 mo–5 y,* all vaccines: 0.5 ml as 1 dose.

PHARMACOKINETICS **Onset:** antibody levels detected within 2 wk. **Peak:** 3 wk. **Duration:** 1.5–3.5 y. **Distribution:** crosses placenta; distributed into breast milk.

CONTRAINDICATIONS & PRECAUTIONS **Contraindicated in:** hypersensitivity to any component of vaccine (e.g., thiomerosal); febrile illness (other than upper respiratory tract infection); active infection. Safe use during pregnancy (category C), and by nursing mothers not established.

ADVERSE/SIDE EFFECTS Irritation at injection site (4–9%). **Other:** acute febrile reactions (13%), irritability, anorexia, <u>anaphylactoid reaction</u> (rare).

DIAGNOSTIC TEST INTERFERENCE Hib polysaccharide vaccine may interfere with interpretation of ***antigen detection tests*** (e.g., latex agglutination) used in diagnosis of systemic Hib disease.

DRUG INTERACTIONS IMMUNOSUPPRESSANT DRUGS, STEROIDS may decrease antibody response.

NURSING IMPLICATIONS

Administration

- Reconstitute lyophilized powder with supplied diluent to yield 25 μg/0.5 ml.
- Hib polysaccharide vaccine and DPT (diphtheria, pertussis, tetanus) may be given at the same time but at different sites.
- Store at 2–8C (36–46F) but may be

frozen without loss of potency. The diluent should not be frozen.

Assessment & Drug Effects

- Be prepared for anaphylactoid reaction (see Appendix G) by having epinephrine 1:1000 available.

Patient & Family Education

- Local reactions to the vaccine at the injection site (erythema, tenderness, induration, swelling, pain) may appear within 6 h after administration; usually symptoms are mild and disappear in 24 h.
- Monitor temperature after injection. An acute febrile reaction with temperature above 38.3C (101F) may follow vaccination (less than 1% of recipients). Report to physician.

HALAZEPAM

(hal-az′e-pam)

Trade name: Paxipam

Classifications: CNS AGENT; ANXIOLYTIC; SEDATIVE-HYPNOTIC; BENZODIAZEPINE

Prototype: Lorazepam

Pregnancy category: D

Controlled substance: Schedule IV

ACTIONS/PHARMACODYNAMICS Psychotropic drug that shares antianxiety actions of other short-term benzodiazepine derivatives. Exact mechanism of action is unknown, but clinically it produces dose-related CNS depressant effect ranging from mild improvement of psychomotor activity to hypnosis. Clinical efficacy in long-term use (i.e., > 4 mo) has not been evaluated.

USE To manage anxiety disorders or for short-term relief of anxiety symptoms.

ROUTE & DOSAGE

Anxiety

Adult: **PO** 20–40 mg t.i.d. or q.i.d.
Geriatric: **PO** 20 mg 1–2 times daily.

PHARMACOKINETICS **Absorption:** readily absorbed from GI tract. **Peak:** 1–3 h. **Distribution:** crosses placenta; distributed into breast milk. **Metabolism:** metabolized in liver to active form. **Elimination:** half-life: 30–200 h (active metabolite); excreted in urine.

CONTRAINDICATIONS & PRECAUTIONS **Contraindicated in:** hypersensitivity to halazepam or other benzodiazepines; psychosis, anxiety-free psychiatric disorders, acute narrow-angle glaucoma. **Cautious use in:** abnormal kidney or liver function. Safe use during pregnancy (category D), in nursing mothers, and in children < 18 y not established.

ADVERSE/SIDE EFFECTS **CNS:** *drowsiness, sedation,* headache, confusion, ataxia, paresthesia. **CV:** hypotension, tachycardia, bradycardia. **GI:** dry mouth, increased salivation, nausea, vomiting, constipation. **Other:** motion sickness, visual disturbances, GU distress, respiratory disturbances, abnormal liver values.

DRUG INTERACTIONS **Cimetidine, disulfiram,** ORAL CONTRACEPTIVES may increase effects of halazepam; **alcohol,** other CNS DEPRESSANTS compound CNS depression.

NURSING IMPLICATIONS

Administration

- Patients with renal or hepatic impairment may require lower doses.
- Store at 2–30C (36–86F) unless directed otherwise.

Assessment & Drug Effects

- Ataxia, confusion, or oversedation may be symptoms of overdosage and can occur at relatively low dosage in the elderly or debilitated patient.
- Smoking decreases sedative effects of halazepam.
- Response to halazepam should be reassessed periodically.

Patient & Family Education

- If patient becomes pregnant or plans on pregnancy, she should discuss with physician desirability of discontinuing drug because of its potential hazard to the fetus.
- Warn not to stop taking drug suddenly. Barbiturate-like withdrawal symptoms may occur (dysphoria, insomnia, abdominal and muscle cramps, vomiting, sweating, tremors, convulsions).
- Caution to avoid driving and other potentially hazardous activities until reaction to drug is known.
- Warn that alcohol or other CNS depressants can produce additive effects.

HALCINONIDE

(hal-sin′oh-nide)

Trade name: Halog

Classifications: SKIN AGENT; ANTI-INFLAMMATORY; STEROID

Prototype: Hydrocortisone

Pregnancy category: C

ACTIONS/PHARMACODYNAMICS Fluorinated steroid with substituted 17-hydroxyl group, chemically similar to flurandrenolide (Cordran). Crosses cell membranes, complexes with nuclear DNA and stimulates synthesis of enzymes thought to be responsible for antiinflammatory effects. Systemic absorption leads to actions, limitations, and drug interactions observed with use of hydrocortisone.

USE Relief of pruritic and inflammatory manifestations of corticosteroid-responsive dermatoses.

ROUTE & DOSAGE

Inflammation

Adult: **Topical** Apply thin layer b.i.d. or t.i.d.

Child: **Topical** Apply thin layer once/d.

PHARMACOKINETICS Absorption: minimum absorption through intact skin; increased absorption from axilla, eyelid, face, scalp, scrotum, or with occlusive dressing.

NURSING IMPLICATIONS

Administration

- Generally, skin is gently washed and thoroughly dried before each application.
- Ointment is usually preferred for dry scaly lesions. Moist lesions are appropriately treated with solution.
- Halcinonide is not to be applied in or around the eyes.
- Occlusive dressings should not be applied over areas covered with halcinonide unless specifically prescribed.
- Store at 15–3C (59–86F).

Assessment & Drug Effects

- Medication should be discontinued if signs of infection or irritation occur.
- Systemic corticosteroid effects may occur with occlusive dressings or topical applications over large areas of skin.

HALOPERIDOL
(ha-loe-per'i-dole)
Trade names: Haldol, Peridol ♣

HALOPERIDOL DECANOATE
Trade name: Haldol LA
Prototype for classifications: CNS AGENT; PSYCHOTHERAPEUTIC; ANTIPSYCHOTIC; BUTYROPHENONE
Pregnancy category: C

ACTIONS/PHARMACODYNAMICS Potent, long-acting butyrophenone derivative with pharmacologic actions similar to those of piperazine phenothiazines but with higher incidence of extrapyramidal effects and less hypotensive and relatively low sedative activity. Exerts strong antiemetic effect and impairs central thermoregulation. Produces weak central anticholinergic effects and transient orthostatic hypotension.

USES Management of manifestations of psychotic disorders and for control of tics and vocal utterances of Gilles de la Tourette's syndrome; for treatment of agitated states in acute and chronic psychoses. Used for short-term treatment of hyperactive children and for severe behavior problems in children of combative, explosive hyperexcitability. **Unlabeled uses:** cancer chemotherapy as an antiemetic in doses smaller than those required for antipsychotic effects; treatment of autism; alcohol dependence; chorea.

ROUTE & DOSAGE

Psychosis

Adult: **PO** 0.2–5 mg b.i.d. or t.i.d. **IM** 2–5 mg repeated q4h prn; decanoate: 50–100 mg q4wk. *Child:* **PO** 0.5 mg/d in 2–3 divided doses; may be increased by 0.5 mg q5–7d to 0.05–0.15 mg/kg/d.

Severe Psychosis

Adult: **PO** 3–5 mg b.i.d. or t.i.d.; may need up to 100 mg/d. **IM** 2–5 mg; may repeat q.h. prn; decanoate: 50 – 100 mg q4wk. *Child:* **PO** 0.05–0.15 mg/kg/d in 2–3 divided doses.

Dementia

Geriatric: **PO** 0.25–0.5 mg 1–2 times daily, may increase every 4–7 d to max 4 mg/d in 2–3 divided doses.

Tourette's Disorder

Adult: **PO** 0.2–5 mg b.i.d. or t.i.d. *Child:* **PO** 0.05–0.075 mg/kg/d in 2–3 divided doses.

PHARMACOKINETICS Absorption: well absorbed from GI tract; 60% reaches systemic circulation. **Onset:** 30–45 min IM. **Peak:** 2–6 h PO; 10–20 min IM; 6–7 d decanoate. **Distribution:** distributes mainly to liver with lower concentration in brain, lung, kidney, spleen, heart. **Metabolism:** metabolized in liver. **Elimination:** half-life: 13–35 h; 40% excreted in urine within 5 d; 15% eliminated in feces; excreted in breast milk.

CONTRAINDICATIONS & PRECAUTIONS Contraindicated in: Parkinson's disease, parkinsonism, seizure disorders, coma; alcoholism; severe mental depression, CNS depression; thyrotoxicosis. Safe use during pregnancy (category C), in nursing mothers, and in children <3 y not established. **Cautious use in:** elderly or debilitated patients, urinary retention, glaucoma, severe cardiovascular disorders; patients receiving anticonvulsant, anticoagulant, or lithium therapy.

ADVERSE/SIDE EFFECTS CNS: *extrapyramidal reactions:* parkinsonian symptoms, dystonia, akathisia, tardive dyskinesia (after long-term use); insomnia, restlessness, anxiety, euphoria, agitation, drowsiness, mental depression, lethargy, fatigue, weakness, tremor, ataxia, headache, confusion, vertigo; neuroleptic malignant syndrome, hyperthermia, grand mal seizures, exacerbation of psychotic symptoms. **CV:** tachycardia, ECG changes, hypotension, hypertension (with overdosage). **Endocrine:** menstrual irregularities, galactorrhea, lactation, gynecomastia, impotence, increased libido, hyponatremia, hyperglycemia, hypoglycemia. **Eyes:** blurred vision. **Hematologic:** mild transient leukopenia, agranulocytosis (rare). **GI:** dry mouth, anorexia, nausea, vomiting, constipation, diarrhea, hypersalivation. **GU:** urinary retention, priapism. **Respiratory:** laryngospasm, bronchospasm, increased depth of respiration, bronchopneumonia, respiratory depression. **Skin:** diaphoresis, maculopapular and acneiform rash, photosensitivity. **Other:** cholestatic jaundice, variations in liver function tests, decreased serum cholesterol.

DRUG INTERACTIONS CNS DEPRESSANTS, OPIATES, **alcohol** increase CNS depression; may antagonize activity of ORAL ANTICOAGULANTS; ANTICHOLINERGICS may increase intraocular pressure; **methyldopa** may precipitate dementia.

NURSING IMPLICATIONS

Administration

- Give with a full glass (240 ml) of water or with food or milk.
- Concentrate may form a precipitate when mixed with coffee or tea. Avoid these as diluents.
- Haloperidol should be administered by deep IM injection into a large muscle. Do not exceed 3 ml per injection site.
- Have patient recumbent at time of parenteral administration and for about 1 h after injection. Assess for orthostatic hypotension.
- Dosing regimen should be tapered when therapy is to be discontinued. Abrupt termination can initiate extrapyramidal symptoms.
- Store in light-resistant container at 15–30C (59–86F), unless otherwise specified by manufacturer. Discard darkened solutions.

Assessment & Drug Effects

- Target symptoms expected to decrease with successful haloperidol treatment include hallucinations, insomnia, hostility, agitation, and delusions.
- Because of long half-life, therapeutic effects are slow to develop in early therapy or when established dosing regimen is changed.
- Monitor patient's mental status daily.
- "Therapeutic window" effect (point at which increased dose or concentration actually decreases therapeutic response) may occur after long period of high doses. Close observation is imperative when doses are changed.
- Monitor for NMS (see Appendix G), especially in those with hypertension or taking lithium. Immediately discontinue drug if NMS suspected.
- Symptoms of NMS can appear suddenly after initiation of therapy or after months or years of taking neuroleptic (antipsychotic) medication.
- Monitor for parkinsonism and tardive dyskinesia (see Appendix G).
- Risk of tardive dyskinesia appears to be greater in women receiving high doses and in the elderly. It can occur after long-term therapy and even after therapy is discontinued.

- Extrapyramidal (neuromuscular) reactions occur frequently during first few days of treatment. Symptoms are usually dose related and are controlled by dosage reduction or concomitant administration of antiparkinson drugs.
- Be alert for behavioral changes in patients who are concurrently receiving antiparkinson drugs.
- Monitor for exacerbation of seizure activity.
- When haloperidol is used to control mania or cyclic disorders, the patient should be closely observed for rapid mood shift to depression. Depression may represent a drug side effect or reversion from a manic state.
- Monitor WBC count with differential and liver function tests in patients on prolonged therapy.

Patient & Family Education

- Advise to avoid use of alcohol during therapy.
- Advise not to engage in potentially hazardous activities until drug response is known.
- Xerostomia may promote dental problems. Discuss oral hygiene with patient. Encourage adequate fluid intake.
- Caution that drug can cause a photosensitivity reaction; advise to avoid overexposure to sun or sunlamp and to use a suncreen.

HALOPROGIN

(ha-loe-proe′jin)

Trade name: Halotex

Classifications: ANTIINFECTIVE; ANTIBIOTIC; ANTIFUNGAL

Prototype: Fluconazole

Pregnancy category: B

ACTIONS/PHARMACODYNAMICS Synthetic iodinated phenolic ether. Fungicidal or fungistatic against various species of *Trichophyton, Epidermophyton, Microsporum, Malassezia,* and *Candida*. Also active in vitro against *Staphylococcus aureus* and *Streptococcus pyogenes*.

USES Superficial fungal infections such as tinea pedis, tinea cruris, tinea corporis, and tinea manus. Also tinea versicolor caused by *Malassezia furfur*. May be used in combination antiinfective therapy for mixed infections.

ROUTE & DOSAGE

Superficial Fungal Infections

Adult: **Topical** Apply liberally to affected area b.i.d. for 2–3 wk.

PHARMACOKINETICS Absorption: minimum absorption through intact skin.

CONTRAINDICATIONS & PRECAUTIONS Contraindicated in: safe use during pregnancy (category B) not established.

ADVERSE/SIDE EFFECTS Local irritation, burning sensation, vesiculation, increased maceration, exacerbation of preexisting lesions, sensitization, pruritus. Low incidence of systemic toxicity.

NURSING IMPLICATIONS

Administration

- Generally, skin is gently washed and thoroughly dried before each application.
- Avoid contact of medication with eyes.

Assessment & Drug Effects

- Medication should be discontinued if signs of infection or irritation occur.
- Therapy should be reevaluated

if no improvement is noted after 2–3 wk.

Patient & Family Education

- Advise to discontinue medication if condition worsens or if burning, irritation, or signs of sensitization occur, and consult physician.
- Advise patients with tinea pedis (athlete's foot) not to wear occlusive footwear because it promotes drug absorption and enhances fungal growth.

H

HEMIN

(hee′min)

Trade name: Panhematin

Classifications: ENZYME INHIBITOR; BLOOD DERIVATIVE

Pregnancy category: C

ACTIONS/PHARMACODYNAMICS Sterile, nonpyrogenic ferric iron complex of protoporphyrin IX; derived from processed red blood cells. Represses synthesis of porphyrin in liver or bone marrow by blocking production of delta-aminolevulinic acid (ALA) synthetase, an essential enzyme in the porphyrin-heme biosynthetic pathway.

USE Recurrent attacks of acute intermittent porphyria (AIP) only after an appropriate period of alternate therapy has been tried (i.e., glucose 400 g/d for 1–2 d).

ROUTE & DOSAGE

Acute Intermittent Porphyria

Adult: **IV** 1–4 mg/kg/d administered over 10–15 min for 3–14 d; dose should not be repeated earlier than q12h (max 6 mg/kg in 24 h).

PHARMACOKINETICS **Duration:** can be detected in plasma up to 5 d. **Elimination:** excess amounts eliminated in bile and urine.

CONTRAINDICATIONS & PRECAUTIONS **Contraindicated in:** history of hypersensitivity to hemin; porphyria cutanea tarda. Safe use during pregnancy (category C), in nursing women, and in children not established.

ADVERSE/SIDE EFFECTS *Phlebitis* (when administered into small veins); anticoagulant effect: prolonged PT, thromboplastin time, thrombocytopenia, hypofibrinogenemia; decreased Hct; reversible renal shutdown (with excessive doses).

DRUG INTERACTIONS Potentiates anticoagulant effects of ANTICOAGULANTS; BARBITURATES, ESTROGENS, SULFONAMIDES may antagonize hemin effect.

NURSING IMPLICATIONS

Administration

- Hemin should be administered via a large arm vein or central venous catheter to reduce risk of phlebitis. Terminal filtration through a sterile 0.45 μm or smaller filter is recommended.
- Reconstitute immediately before use by aseptically adding 43 ml sterile water for injection to vial. Shake well for 2–3 min to dissolve all particles. Discard unused portions.
- Freeze and store lyophilized powder until time of use.

Assessment & Drug Effects

- Monitor IV site for signs and symptoms of thrombophlebitis (see Appendix G).
- The following are monitored throughout hemin therapy (decrease in these values is an indication of a favorable clinical

response): ALA, UPG (uroporphyrinogen), PBG (porphobilinogen or coproporphyrin).

- To monitor clinical effect of drug therapy, be aware of the patient's symptoms and complaints associated with acute porphyria, which may include depression, insomnia, anxiety, disorientation, hallucinations, psychoses; dark urine, nausea, vomiting, abdominal pain, low back and leg pain, pareses (neuropathy), seizures.
- Monitor I&O and promptly report the onset of oliguria or anuria.

Patient & Family Education

- Instruct to report bruising, hematuria, tarry black stools, and nosebleeds.

HEPARIN CALCIUM

(hep′a-rin)

Trade names: Calcilean ♣, Calciparine

HEPARIN SODIUM

Trade names: Hepalean ♣, Heparin Sodium Lock Flush Solution, Hep-Lock, Lipo-Hepin, Liquaemin Sodium

Prototype for classifications: BLOOD FORMERS AND COAGULATORS; ANTICOAGULANT

Pregnancy category: C

ACTIONS/PHARMACODYNAMICS Strongly acidic, high molecular weight mucopolysaccharide with rapid anticoagulant effect, prepared from bovine lung tissue or porcine intestinal mucosa. Exerts direct effect on blood coagulation (clotting) by enhancing the inhibitory actions of antithrombin III (heparin cofactor) on several factors essential to normal blood clotting, thereby blocking the conversion of prothrombin to thrombin and fibrinogen to fibrin. Does not lyse already existing thrombi but may prevent their extension and propagation. Inhibits formation on new clots.

USES Prophylaxis and treatment of venous thrombosis and pulmonary embolism and to prevent thromboembolic complications arising from cardiac and vascular surgery, frostbite, and during acute stage of MI. Also used in treatment of disseminated intravascular coagulation (DIC), atrial fibrillation with embolization, and as anticoagulant in blood transfusions, extracorporeal circulation, and dialysis procedures. **Unlabeled uses:** prophylaxis in hip and knee surgery. Heparin Sodium Lock Flush Solution is used to maintain potency of indwelling IV catheters in intermittent IV therapy or blood sampling. It is not intended for anticoagulant therapy.

ROUTE & DOSAGE

Treatment of Thromboembolism

Adult: **IV** 5000-U bolus dose; then 20,000–40,000 U infused over 24 h; dose adjusted to maintain desired APTT; *or* 5000–10,000 U IV piggyback q4–6h. **SC** 10,000–20,000 U followed by 8000–20,000 U q8–12h.
Child: **IV** 50 U/kg bolus; then 20,000 U/m^2/24 h or 50–100 U/kg q4h *or* 15–25 U/kg/h.

Open Heart Surgery

Adult: **IV** 150–300 U/kg.

Prophylaxis of Embolism

Adult: **SC** 5000 U q8–12h.

PHARMACOKINETICS **Onset:** 20–60 min SC. **Peak:** within minutes. **Duration:** 2–6 h IV; 8–12 h SC. **Distribution:** does not cross placenta; not distributed into breast milk. **Metabolism:**

metabolized in liver and by reticuloendothelial system. **Elimination:** half-life: 90 min; excreted slowly in urine.

CONTRAINDICATIONS & PRECAUTIONS **Contraindicated in:** history of hypersensitivity to heparin (white clot syndrome); active bleeding, bleeding tendencies (hemophilia, purpura, thrombocytopenia); jaundice; ascorbic acid deficiency; inaccessible ulcerative lesions; visceral carcinoma; open wounds, extensive denudation of skin, suppurative thrombophlebitis; advanced kidney, liver, or biliary disease; active tuberculosis; bacterial endocarditis; continuous tube drainage of stomach or small intestines; threatened abortion; suspected intracranial hemorrhage, severe hypertension; recent surgery of eye, brain, or spinal cord; spinal tap; shock. Teratogenic potential not established. **Cautious use in:** alcoholism; history of atopy or allergy (asthma, hives, hay fever, eczema); during menstruation, pregnancy (category C) especially the last trimester, and immediate postpartum period; patients with indwelling catheters; the elderly; use of acid-citrate-dextrose (ACD)-converted blood (may contain heparin); patients in hazardous occupations; cerebral embolism.

H

ADVERSE/SIDE EFFECTS Spontaneous bleeding, injection site reactions: pain, itching, ecchymoses, tissue irritation and sloughing; cyanosis and pains in arms or legs (vasospasm); *transient thrombocytopenia,* hypofibrinogenemia, increased AST, ALT, "white clot syndrome"; priaprism (rare). **Hypersensitivity:** fever, chills, urticaria, pruritus, skin rashes, itching and burning sensations of feet, numbness and tingling of hands and feet, elevated BP, headache, reversible transient alopecia (usually around temporal area), nasal congestion, lacrimation, conjunctivitis, chest pains, arthralgia, bronchospasm, anaphylactoid reactions. **Large doses for prolonged periods:** osteoporosis, hypoaldosteronism, suppressed renal function, hyperkalemia; rebound hyperlipidemia (following termination of heparin therapy).

DIAGNOSTIC TEST INTERFERENCE Notify laboratory that patient is receiving heparin, when a test is to be performed. Possibility of false-positive rise in ***BSP*** test and in ***serum thyroxine;*** and increases in ***resin*** T_3 ***uptake;*** false-negative ^{125}I ***fibrinogen uptake.*** Heparin prolongs PT. Valid readings may be obtained by drawing blood samples at least 4–6 h after an IV dose (but at any time during heparin infusion) and 12–24 h after an SC heparin dose.

DRUG INTERACTIONS May prolong PT, which is used to monitor therapy with ORAL ANTICOAGULANTS; **aspirin,** NSAIDS increase risk of bleeding; **nitroglycerin** IV may decrease anticoagulant activity; **protamine** antagonizes effects of heparin.

INCOMPATIBILITIES **Solution/additive: amikacin, codeine, chlorpromazine, cytarabine, diazepam, dobutamine, doxorubicin, droperidol, erythromycin, gentamicin, haloperidol, hyaluronidase, hydrocortisone, kanamycin, levorphanol, meperidine, methadone, methicillin, methotrimeprazine, morphine, netilmicin, nitroglycerin, pentazocine, polymyxin B, promethazine, streptomycin, tetracycline, tobramycin, triflupromazine, vancomycin. Y-site: amikacin, decarbazine, diaze-**

pam, diphenhydramine, doxycycline, doxorubicin, droperidol, ergotamine, erythromycin, gentamicin, haloperidol, kanamycin, methotrimeprazine, netilmicin, nitroglycerin, phenytoin, polymyxin B, streptomycin, tobramycin, triflupromazine, vancomycin.

NURSING IMPLICATIONS

Administration

- Before administration, check coagulation test values; if results are not within therapeutic range, notify physician for dosage adjustment.
- Solutions of heparin or heparin lock-flush that contain benzyl alcohol preservative should not be used in neonates.

SC Administration

- More concentrated heparin solutions are recommended for SC injection.
- Preferably, SC injections are made into the fatty layer of the abdomen or just above the iliac crest. Avoid injecting within 5 cm (2 in) of umbilicus or bruise. Insert needle into tissue roll perpendicular to skin surface. Do not withdraw plunger to check entry into blood vessel. Systematically rotate injection sites and keep record.

IV Administration

- A single dose of IV heparin (adult 5000 U, child 50 U/kg) may be given undiluted by direct IV injection over 60 seconds.
- IV heparin may be added to NS, D5W, or Ringer's for injection and infused intermittently or continuously. When heparin is added to an infusion solution, invert container at least 6 times to ensure adequate mixing.
- Continuous IV infusion of heparin requires a constant infusion pump.
- Heparin is stable at 15–30C (59–86F). Protect from freezing.

Assessment & Drug Effects

- Baseline blood coagulation tests, Hct, Hgb, RBC, and platelet counts should be performed before therapy is initiated, at regular intervals throughout therapy.
- In general, dosage is adjusted to keep APTT between 1.5–2.5 times normal control level.
- During dosage adjustment period, blood is drawn for coagulation test 30 min before each scheduled SC or intermittent IV dose and approximately q4h for patients receiving continuous IV heparin. After dosage is established, tests may be done once daily.
- Patients vary widely in their reaction to heparin. The risk of hemorrhage appears to be greatest in women, all patients ≥ 60 y, and patients with liver disease or renal insufficiency.
- Monitor vital signs. Report fever, drop in BP, rapid pulse, and other S & S of hemorrhage.
- Observe all needle sites daily for hematoma and signs of inflammation (swelling, heat, redness, pain).
- Antidote: Have on hand protamine sulfate (1% solution), specific heparin antagonist.

Patient & Family Education

- Advise to protect from injury and report pink, red, dark brown, or cloudy urine; red or dark brown vomitus; red or black stools; bleeding gums or oral mucosa; ecchymoses, hematoma, epistaxis, bloody sputum; chest pain; abdominal or lumbar pain or swelling; unusual increase in menstrual flow; pelvic pain; severe or continuous headache, faintness, or dizziness.
- Inform women that menstruation may be somewhat increased and prolonged. Usually, this is not a

contraindication to continued therapy if bleeding is not excessive.

- If patient is to be discharged on heparin, teach the correct technique for SC administration.
- In the absence of a low platelet (thrombocyte) count, patient may carry out normal activities such as shaving with a safety razor. Usually, heparin does not affect bleeding time.
- Smoking and alcohol consumption may alter response to heparin and therefore are not advised. Caution not to take aspirin or any other OTC medication without physician's approval.

H

HEPATITIS A VACCINE

(hep'a-ti-tis)

Trade names: Havrix, Vaqta

Classifications: VACCINE; VIRAL, HEPATITIS A

Prototype: Hepatitis B vaccine

Pregnancy category: C

ACTIONS/PHARMACODYNAMICS Anti-hepatitis A virus antibody titers following administration of hepatitis A vaccine (inactivated) are comparable to those observed after natural hepatitis A virus infection. Antibody levels are 50- to 300-fold higher with inactivated vaccine than with passive immunity with human immune globulin.

USE Active immunization against hepatitis A.

ROUTE & DOSAGE

Hepatitis A Immunization

Adult: **IM** 1 ml in deltoid muscle; booster dose (1 ml) should be given 6–12 mo after primary dose. *Child 2–18 y:* **IM** 2 doses of 0.5 ml in deltoid muscle given 1 mo apart; booster dose (0.5 ml) should be given 6–12 mo after primary doses.

PHARMACOKINETICS **Onset:** 3 wk. **Duration:** 1–3 y with single dose, 5–10 y with booster.

CONTRAINDICATIONS & PRECAUTIONS **Contraindicated in:** hypersensitivity to any component in vaccine, pregnancy (category C), children < 2 y. **Cautious use in:** nursing mothers.

ADVERSE/SIDE EFFECTS **CNS:** *headache,* fatigue, fever, malaise, somnolence, vertigo, insomnia, photophobia, convulsions, neuropathy, paresthesia. **GI:** anorexia, nausea, abdominal pain, diarrhea, dysgeusia, vomiting. **Skin:** pruritus, rash, urticaria, erythema multiforme, hyperhydrosis, angioedema (rare). **Other:** *soreness at injection site, pain, swelling, redness at injection site,* pharyngitis, lymphadenopathy.

NURSING IMPLICATIONS

Administration

- Give IM only in deltoid for adults and children older than 2 y. Do not give IV, SC, or intradermally.
- Use vaccine as packaged without dilution.
- Shake vial and syringe well before withdrawal and injection, respectively. Vaccine should be an opaque white suspension; discard if it looks otherwise.
- Store at 2–8C (36–47F). Discard vaccine if it has been frozen.

Assessment & Drug Effects

- The vaccine is usually withheld during a febrile illness.
- Assess for signs and symptoms of anaphylaxis and have epinephrine available.

Patient & Family Education

- Inform that injection site soreness

is common and that most adverse reactions are mild and usually last less than 24 h.

- Advise to have a booster injection within 6–12 mo if risk of exposure is still present.

HEPATITIS B IMMUNE GLOBULIN

Trade names: H-BIG, Hep-B-Gammagee, HyperHep

Classifications: VACCINE; VIRAL, HEPATITIS B

Pregnancy category: C

ACTIONS/PHARMACODYNAMICS Sterile solution of immunoglobulins (not less than 80% immunoglobulin G [IgG]) prepared by a special process using pooled human plasma. Preparation contains a high antibody titer specific to hepatitis B surface antigen (anti-HBs); plasma does not show serologic evidence of hepatitis B surface antigen (HBsAg). Serum has also been tested for and found free of antibody to HIV. The possibility of transmission of hepatitis infection or AIDS from HBIG is remote.

USES Prophylactically to provide passive immunity to hepatitis B infection in individuals exposed to HBV or HBsAg-positive materials (blood plasma, serum). Also as postexposure prophylaxis after bite or percutaneous exposure, ingestion, direct mucous membrane contact, sexual or intimate contact, and in neonates born to HBsAg-positive women.

ROUTE & DOSAGE

Hepatitis B Prophylaxis

Adult: **IM** 0.06 ml/kg as soon as possible after exposure, preferably within 24 h, but no later than 7 d; repeat 28–30 d after exposure.
Child: **IM** Same as for adult.

Newborn Exposure

Child: **IM** 0.5 ml as soon as possible after birth but no later than 24 h; repeat dose 3 and 6 mo later.

PHARMACOKINETICS Absorption: slowly absorbed from IM site. **Onset:** 1–6 d. **Peak:** 3–11 d. **Duration:** 2–6 mo. **Elimination:** half-life: 21 d.

CONTRAINDICATIONS & PRECAUTIONS Cautious use in: history of systemic allergic reactions to immune globulin, thrombocytopenia or bleeding disorders, HBsAg-positive individuals, patients with specific immunoglobulin A (IgA) deficiency; pregnancy (category C).

ADVERSE/SIDE EFFECTS Usually infrequent and mild. **Skin/hypersensitivity:** urticaria, rash, angioedema, pruritus, erythema, sensitization (following large or repeated doses), anaphylaxis (rare). **Local:** muscle stiffness; pain, tenderness, swelling, erythema of injection site. **Other:** nausea, faintness, fever, dizziness, malaise, lassitude, body and joint pain, leg cramps.

DRUG INTERACTIONS May interfere with immune response to LIVE-VIRUS VACCINES (measles/mumps/rubella/poliovirus).

NURSING IMPLICATIONS

Administration

- Hepatitis B immune globulin may be administered at the same time or up to 1 mo preceding hepatitis B vaccination (hepatitis B vaccine) without impairing the active immune response from the vaccination.
- IM injections should be made preferably into deltoid muscle or anterolateral aspect of thigh.
- For neonates and small children the preferred IM injection site is

H

the anterolateral aspect of the thigh.

- Inadvertent IV administration can cause a precipitous fall in BP and an anaphylactic reaction.
- Store at 2–8C (36–46F) unless otherwise directed. Avoid freezing.

Assessment & Drug Effects

- Hypersensitivity reactions are most likely to occur in patients receiving large doses or repeated injections. Have epinephrine 1:1000 readily available.

Patient & Family Education

- Advise regarding potential adverse reactions.

HEPATITIS B VACCINE (RECOMBINANT)

Trade names: Engerix-B, Recombivax HB

Prototype for classifications: VACCINE; VIRAL, HEPATITIS B

Pregnancy category: C

ACTIONS/PHARMACODYNAMICS Suspension of inactivated and purified hepatitis B surface antigen (HBsAg) derived from human plasma of screened asymptomatic HBsAg-positive carriers of hepatitis B virus. Hepatitis B vaccine recombinant is the first vaccine produced by gene splicing. No human plasma is used in its production. The recommended 3-dose regimen produces active immunity against hepatitis B infection by inducing protective antibody (anti-HBs) formation.

USES To promote active immunity in individuals at high risk of potential exposure to hepatitis B virus or HBsAg-positive materials. Has been used simultaneously (into different sites) with hepatitis B immune globulin (HBIG) for postexposure prophylaxis in selected patients and in infants born to HBsAg-positive mothers.

ROUTE & DOSAGE

Hepatitis B Prophylaxis

Adult: **IM *Recombivax:*** 1 ml (10 µg) at 0, 1, and 6 mo. ***Engerix B:*** 1 ml (20 µg) at 0, 1, and 6 mo or 0, 1, 2, and 12 mo.
Child: **IM *Recombivax:*** 0.5 ml (5 µg) at 0, 1, and 6 mo. ***Engerix B:*** 0.5 ml (10 µg) at 0, 1, and 6 mo or 0, 1, 2, and 12 mo.

Dialysis and Immunodeficient Patients

Adult: **IM *Recombivax:*** 2 ml (20 µg) at 0, 1, and 6 mo. ***Engerix B:*** 2 ml (40 µg) at 0, 1, and 6 mo or 0, 1, 2, and 12 mo.

PHARMACOKINETICS **Absorption:** slowly absorbed from IM site. **Onset:** 2 wk. **Peak:** 6 mo. **Duration:** at least 3 y.

CONTRAINDICATIONS & PRECAUTIONS **Contraindicated in:** history of allergic reaction to hepatitis B vaccine or to any ingredient in the formulation; HBsAg carriers. Safe use during pregnancy (category C) and in nursing mothers not established. **Cautious use in:** compromised cardiopulmonary status, serious active infection or fever; thrombocytopenia or other bleeding disorders.

ADVERSE/SIDE EFFECTS *Mild local tenderness at injection site, local inflammatory reaction* (swelling, heat, redness, induration, pain); *fever, malaise, fatigue,* headache, dizziness, faintness, leg cramps, myalgia, arthralgia, nausea, vomiting, urticaria, diarrhea, rash, pruritus; possibility of subcutaneous nodules following SC injections; hypersensitivity.

NURSING IMPLICATIONS

Administration

- Preferably IM injection should be made into the deltoid and in neonates into the anterolateral thigh, avoiding blood vessels and nerves. Carefully aspirate to prevent inadvertent intravascular injection.
- Epinephrine should be immediately available to treat anaphylaxis.
- Shake vial well before withdrawing dose to assure uniform suspension.
- Store unopened and opened vials at 2–8C (36–46F) unless otherwise directed. Avoid freezing (freezing destroys potency).

Assessment & Drug Effects

- The ACIP recommends serologic confirmation of postvaccination immunity in patients undergoing dialysis and in immunodeficient patients.
- Monitor temperature. Some patients develop a temperature elevation of 38.3C (101F) following vaccination that may last 1 or 2 d.
- Advise regarding potential adverse reaction.

HETASTARCH

(het'a-starch)

Trade names: HES, Hespan, Hydroxyethyl Starch

Classification: PLASMA VOLUME EXPANDER

Prototype: Albumin

Pregnancy category: C

ACTIONS/PHARMACODYNAMICS Synthetic starch closely resembling human glycogen. Colloidal osmotic properties are approximately equal to those of human serum albumin. Acts much like albumin and dextran but is claimed to be less likely to produce anaphylaxis or to interfere with cross matching or blood typing procedures. Causes no significant alterations in fibrinogen or clotting time but may prolong the PPT and PT. In hypovolemic patients, it increases arterial and venous pressures, heart rate, cardiac output, urine output, and colloidal osmotic pressure. Not a substitute for blood or plasma.

USES Early fluid replacement and plasma volume expansion when whole blood is not available or when there is no time for necessary cross matching. Used to expand plasma volume during cardiopulmonary bypass and in adjunctive treatment of shock caused by hemorrhage, burns, surgery, sepsis, or other trauma. Also used as sedimenting agent in preparation of granulocytes by leukopheresis. **Unlabeled uses:** as a priming fluid in pump oxygenators for perfusion during extracorporeal circulation and as a cryoprotective agent for long-term storage of whole blood.

ROUTE & DOSAGE

Plasma Volume Expansion

Adult: **IV** 500–1000 ml at a max rate of 20 ml/kg/h (max 1500 ml/d).
Child: **IV** 10 ml/kg/dose (max 20 ml/kg/24 h).

Leukapheresis

Adult: **IV** 250–750 ml infused at a constant fixed ratio of 8:1 to venous whole blood.

PHARMACOKINETICS **Duration:** 24–36 h. **Distribution:** remains in intravascular space. **Metabolism:** metabolized in reticuloendothelial system. **Elimination:** excreted in urine with some biliary excretion.

CONTRAINDICATIONS & PRECAUTIONS **Contraindicated in:** severe bleeding disorders, CHF, renal failure with oliguria and anuria, treatment of shock not accompanied by hypovolemia, pregnancy (category C). Safe use in children not established. **Cautious use in:** hepatic or renal insufficiency, pulmonary edema in the very young or the elderly, patients on sodium restriction.

H

ADVERSE/SIDE EFFECTS **CV:** peripheral edema, circulatory overload, heart failure. **Hematologic:** (with large volumes) prolongation of PT, PPT, clotting time, and bleeding time; decreased Hct, Hgb, platelets, calcium, and fibrinogen; dilution of plasma proteins, hyperbilirubinemia, increased sedimentation rate. **Hypersensitivity:** pruritus, anaphylactoid reactions (periorbital edema, urticaria, wheezing). **Other:** vomiting, mild fever, chills, influenza-like symptoms, headache, muscle pains, submaxillary and parotid glandular swelling.

DRUG INTERACTIONS None established.

NURSING IMPLICATIONS

Administration

- Hetastarch is administered undiluted by IV infusion.
- Specific flow rate is prescribed by physician. Rate may be as high as 20 ml/kg/h in acute hemorrhagic shock.
- Store at room temperature. Avoid extremes of heat or cold. Partially used bags should be discarded.

Assessment & Drug Effects

- Monitor for signs and symptoms of hypersensitivity reaction (see Appendix G).
- Measure and record I&O. Report oliguria or significant changes in I&O ratio.
- Monitor BP and vital signs and observe patient for unusual bruising or bleeding.
- Observe for signs of circulatory overload (see Appendix G).
- Check laboratory reports of Hct values. Notify physician if there is an appreciable drop in Hct or if value approaches 30% by volume. Hct should not be allowed to drop below 30%.

HOMATROPINE HYDROBROMIDE

(hoe-ma'troe-peen)

Trade names: AK-Homatropine, Homatrine, Isopto Homatropine

Prototype for classifications: EYE PREPARATION; MYDRIATIC; AUTONOMIC NERVOUS SYSTEM AGENT; ANTICHOLINERGIC (PARASYMPATHOLYTIC)

Pregnancy category: C

See Appendix A.

HYALURONIDASE

(hye-al-yoor-on'i dase)

Trade name: Wydase

Classification: ENZYME

Pregnancy category: C

ACTIONS/PHARMACODYNAMICS Mucolytic enzyme prepared from purified bovine testicular hyaluronidase. Hydrolyzes hyaluronidase, thereby modifying connective tissue permeability, permitting diffusion and spreading of substances injected subcutaneously and the absorption of transudates and exudates. Hastens disappearance of swelling after clysis and reduces pain related to distention.

USES To increase rate of absorption of parenteral fluids given by hypodermoclysis, to enhance diffusion of toxic or irritating drug in management of IV extravasation; to diffuse anesthetics at site of injection (including dental surgical sites); and to increase absorption of SC-administered contrast media in excretion urography.

ROUTE & DOSAGE

Absorption and Dispersion of Injected Drugs

Adult/Child ≥3 y: **SC** 150 U added to each liter of drug solution or injected before clysis.
Child <3 y: **SC** Max volume of single clysis, 200 ml.

SC Urography

Adult: **SC** 75 U injected over each scapula followed by injection of contrast medium at same sites.

Management of Catecholamine Extravasation

Adult: **SC** 5–10 ml infiltrated around site of extravasation.
Child: **SC** 0.2 ml of 15 U/ml solution in 5 injections around site of extravasation.

CONTRAINDICATIONS & PRECAUTIONS **Contraindicated in:** injection into or around inflamed, infected, or cancerous areas; CHF; hypoproteinemia. Safe use during pregnancy (category C) and in nursing mothers not established.

ADVERSE/SIDE EFFECTS Infrequent: sensitivity, allergic reactions (urticaria), spread of infectious processes, overhydration. **Overdosage:** local edema, erythema, chills, nausea, vomiting, dizziness, hypotension, tachycardia.

DRUG INTERACTIONS When hyaluronidase is used to increase diffusion of a local anesthetic, bear in mind that absorption rate will be enhanced as much as 3- to 12-fold. Therefore, watch for adverse reactions and expect a shorter duration of drug action.

INCOMPATIBILITIES **Solution/additive: epinephrine, heparin.**

NURSING IMPLICATIONS

Administration

- Preliminary skin test for sensitivity is advised.
- Just before use, reconstitute 150- and 1500-U vials with 1 and 10 ml, respectively, of 0.9% NaCl to yield 150 U/ml.
- Store the lyophilized powder at controlled room temperature in a dry place. Lyophilized form is unstable in solution.

Assessment & Drug Effects

- Closely monitor for overhydration during hypodermoclysis.
- If S & S of hypersensitivity occur (see Appendix G) during IV infusion, discontinue drug and notify physician.

Patient & Family Education

- Advise to immediately report S & S of hypersensitivity (see Appendix G) or shortness of breath.

HYDRALAZINE HYDROCHLORIDE

(hye-dral′a-zeen)

Trade names: Alazine, Apresoline

Prototype for classifications: CARDIOVASCULAR AGENT; NONNITRATE VASODILATOR; ANTIHYPERTENSIVE

Pregnancy category: C

ACTIONS/PHARMACODYNAMICS Reduces BP mainly by direct effect on vascular smooth muscles of arterial-resistance vessels, resulting in vasodilation. Has little effect on venous-capacitance vessels. Diastolic reponse is often greater than systolic Vasodilation reduces peripheral resistance and substantially improves cardiac output, renal and cerebral blood flow. Hypotensive effect may be limited by sympathetic reflexes, which increase heart rate, stroke volume, and cardiac output. Postural hypotensive effect is reportedly less than that produced by ganglionic blocking agents.

USES Most commonly in stepped-care approach to treat moderate to severe hypertension. Also in early malignant hypertension and resistant hypertension that persists after sympathectomy. **Unlabeled uses:** conjunctively with cardiac glycosides and other vasodilators in short-term treatment of acute CHF; unexplained pulmonary hypertension.

ROUTE & DOSAGE

Hypertension
Adult: **PO** 10–50 mg q.i.d. **IM** 10–50 mg q4–6h. **IV** 10–20 mg q4–6h.
Geriatric: **PO** start with 10 mg 2–3 times/d.
Child: **PO** 3–7.5 mg/kg/d in 4 divided doses. **IM/IV** 1.7–3.5 mg/kg/d in 4 divided doses.

PHARMACOKINETICS **Absorption:** readily absorbed from GI tract. **Onset:** 20–30 min. **Peak:** 2 h. **Duration:** 2–6 h. **Distribution:** crosses placenta; distributed into breast milk. **Metabolism:** metabolized in intestinal wall and liver. **Elimination:** half-life: 2–8 h; 90% rapidly excreted in urine; 10% excreted in feces.

CONTRAINDICATIONS & PRECAUTIONS **Contraindicated in:** coronary artery disease, mitral valvular rheumatic heart disease, MI, tachycardia, SLE. Safe use during pregnancy (category C) or in nursing mothers not established. **Cautious use in:** cerebrovascular accident, advanced renal impairment, use with MAO INHIBITORS.

ADVERSE/SIDE EFFECTS **CNS:** *headache,* dizziness, tremors. **CV:** *palpitation,* angina, *tachycardia,* flushing, paradoxical pressor response. Overdose: arrhythmia, <u>shock</u>. **Eye:** lacrimation, conjunctivitis. **GI:** anorexia, nausea, vomiting, diarrhea, constipation, abdominal pain, paralytic ileus. **GU:** difficulty in urination, glomerulonephritis. **Hematologic:** decreased hematocrit and hemaglobin, anemia, <u>agranulocytosis</u> (rare). **Hypersensitivity:** rash, urticaria, pruritus, fever, chills, arthralgia, eosinophilia, cholangitis, hepatitis, obstructive jaundice. **Other:** nasal congestion, muscle cramps, SLE-like syndrome, fixed drug eruption, edema.

DRUG INTERACTIONS BETA BLOCKERS and other ANTIHYPERTENSIVE AGENTS compound hypotensive effects.

INCOMPATIBILITIES **Solution/additive: aminophylline, ampicillin, chlorothiazide, edetate calcium disodium, hydrocortisone, mephentermine, methohexital, nitroglycerin, phenobarbital, verapamil.**

DIAGNOSTIC TEST INTERFERENCE Positive ***direct Coombs' tests*** in patients with hydralazine-induced SLE. Hydralazine interferes with urinary ***17-OHCS*** determinations ***(modified Glenn-Nelson technique).***

NURSING IMPLICATIONS

Administration

- Bioavailability of PO hydralazine is increased by taking it with food. Give with food.
- IV administration: Administer undiluted solution by direct IV. Give each 10 mg or fraction thereof over 1 min. Do not add hydralazine to IV solutions.
- Discontinuation of hydralazine should be accomplished gradually to avoid sudden rise in BP and acute heart failure. Patients should be informed of the dangers of abrupt withdrawal.
- Store at 15–30C (59–86F) in tight, light-resistant containers unless otherwise directed. Avoid freezing.

Assessment & Drug Effects

- LE cell preparation and antinuclear antibody titer determinations are advised before initiation of therapy and periodically during prolonged therapy.
- Baseline and periodic determinations should also be made of BUN, creatinine clearance, uric acid, serum potassium, blood glucose, and ECG.
- Closely monitor BP and HR. Check every 5 min until it is stabilized at desired level, then every 15 min thereafter throughout hypertensive crisis.
- I&O should be monitored when drug is given parenterally and in those with renal dysfunction.

Patient & Family Education

- Instruct to monitor weight, check for edema, and report weight gain.
- Some patients experience headache and palpitations within 2–4 h after first PO dose. Symptoms usually subside spontaneously.
- Caution to make position changes slowly and to avoid standing still, hot baths/showers, strenuous exercise, and excessive alcohol intake.
- Advise caution with hazardous activities until reaction to drug is known.

HYDROCHLOROTHIAZIDE

(hye-droe-klor-oh-thye′a-zide)

Trade names: Apo-Hydro ♣, Diaqua, Esidrix, Hydro-Chlor, HydroDiuril, Hydromal, Hydro-T, Oretic, SK-Hydrochlorothiazide, HCTZ, Urozide ♣

Prototype for classifications: ELECTROLYTIC AND WATER BALANCE AGENT; THIAZIDE DIURETIC; ANTIHYPERTENSIVE

Pregnancy category: B

ACTIONS/PHARMACODYNAMICS

Similar to chlorothiazide. Diuretic action is associated with drug interference with transport of sodium ions across renal tubular epithelium. This enhances excretion of sodium, chloride, potassium, bicarbonates, and water. **Action site:** cortical dilution segment of nephron. **Other actions:** hypotensive action, elevated plasma renin activity, and precipitation of diabetes in the prediabetic patient.

USES Adjunct in treatment of edema associated with CHF, hepatic cirrhosis, renal failure, and in the stepped-care management of hypertension (step 1 and 2 agent). **Unlabeled uses:** nephrogenic diabetes insipidus, hypercalciuria, and treatment of electrolyte disturbances associated with renal tubular acidosis.

ROUTE & DOSAGE

Edema

Adult: **PO** 25–200 mg/d in 1–3 divided doses.

Hypertension

Adult: **PO** 12.5–100 mg/d in 1–2 divided doses.

Child: **PO** 2.2 mg/kg/d in 2 divided doses.
Neonate <6 mo: **PO** 2–4 mg/kg/d in 2 divided doses.

PHARMACOKINETICS Absorption: incompletely absorbed. **Onset:** 2 h. **Peak:** 4 h. **Duration:** 6–12 h. **Distribution:** distributed throughout extracellular tissue; concentrates in kidney; crosses placenta; distributed in breast milk. **Metabolism:** does not appear to be metabolized. **Elimination:** half-life: 45–120 min; excreted in urine.

CONTRAINDICATIONS & PRECAUTIONS Contraindicated in: hypersensitivity to thiazides or other sulfonamides; anuria, pregnancy (category B), lactation. **Cautious use in:** bronchial asthma, allergy; hepatic cirrhosis; renal dysfunction; history of gout, SLE; diabetes mellitus; the elderly.

ADVERSE/SIDE EFFECTS CNS: mood changes, unusual tiredness or weakness, dizziness, light-headedness, paresthesias. **CV:** irregular heartbeat, weak pulse, orthostatic hypotension. **GI:** dry mouth, increased thirst, nausea, vomiting, anorexia, diarrhea, pancreatitis, jaundice. **Hematologic:** agranulocytosis, thrombocytopenia, aplastic anemia, leukopenia. **Metabolic:** *hyperglycemia,* glycosuria, *hyperuricemia, hypokalemia.* **Other:** hypersensitivity reactions, photosensitivity, blurred vision, yellow vision (xanthopsia), muscle spasm.

DIAGNOSTIC TEST INTERFERENCE Falsely decreased value in ***total urinary estrogen*** by ***spectrophotometric assay.*** See chlorothiazide.

DRUG INTERACTIONS Amphotericin B, CORTICOSTEROIDS increase hypokalemic effects; SULFONYLUREAS, **insulin** may antagonize hypoglycemic effects; **cholestyramine, colistipol** decrease thiazide absorption; **diazoxide** intensifies hypoglycemic and hypotensive effects; increased potassium and magnesium loss may cause **digoxin** toxicity; decreases **lithium** excretion and increases toxicity; increases risk of NSAID-induced renal failure and may attenuate diuresis.

NURSING IMPLICATIONS

Administration

- May give with food or milk to reduce GI upset.
- Schedule doses to avoid nocturia and interrupted sleep. If given in 2 doses, schedule second dose no later than 3 PM.
- Store tablets in tightly closed container at 15–30C (59–86F) unless otherwise directed.

Assessment & Drug Effects

- Antihypertensive effects may be noted in 3–4 d; maximal effects may require 3–4 wk.
- Baseline and periodic determinations of serum electrolytes, blood counts, BUN, blood glucose, uric acid, CO_2, are recommended.
- Check BP before initiation of therapy and at regular intervals.
- Closely monitor for hypokalemia, which increases the risk of digoxin toxicity.
- Monitor I&O and check for edema.
- Be aware that drug may cause hyperglycemia and loss of glycemic control in diabetics.
- Drug may cause orthostatic hypotension, dizziness.

Patient & Family Education

- Advise to consult physician before using OTC drugs. Many contain large amounts of sodium as well as potassium.

- Instruct to monitor weight daily.
- Drug causes impaired glucose tolerance. Advise the diabetic patient to monitor blood glucose closely.
- Report signs of hypokalemia (see Appendix G) to physician.
- Instruct to change positions slowly, to avoid hot baths or showers, extended exposure to sunlight, and sitting or standing still for long periods.
- Warn about possibility of photosensitivity reaction—usually occurs 10–14 d after initial sun exposure.

HYDROCODONE BITARTRATE

(hye-droe-koe′done)

Trade names: Dihydrocodeinone Bitartrate, Hycodan, Robidone✤, Vicodin (with acetaminophen)

Classifications: CNS AGENT; NARCOTIC (OPIATE) AGONIST ANALGESIC; ANTITUSSIVE

Prototype: Morphine

Pregnancy category: C

Controlled substance: Schedule III

ACTIONS/PHARMACODYNAMICS Morphine derivative similar to codeine but more addicting and with slightly greater antitussive activity. Suppresses cough reflex by direct action on cough center in medulla. Available in the United States only in combination with other drugs.

USES Symptomatic relief of hyperactive or nonproductive cough and for relief of moderate to moderately severe pain. A common ingredient in a variety of proprietary mixtures.

ROUTE & DOSAGE

Mild to Moderate Pain, Cough

Adult: **PO** 5–10 mg q4–6h prn (max 15mg/dose).

Child 2–12 y: **PO** 1.25–5 mg q4–6h (max 10 mg/dose).

PHARMACOKINETICS **Onset:** 10–20 min. **Duration:** 3–6 h. **Distribution:** crosses placenta; distributed into breast milk. **Metabolism:** metabolized in liver. **Elimination:** half-life: 3.8 h; excreted in urine.

CONTRAINDICATIONS & PRECAUTIONS **Cautious use in:** respiratory depression, asthma, emphysema; history of drug abuse or dependence; postoperative patients; debilitated patients; children < 1 y; pregnancy (category C); patients with preexisting increased intracranial pressure.

ADVERSE/SIDE EFFECTS Dry mouth, *constipation, nausea,* respiratory depression, vomiting; light-headedness, sedation, dizziness, *drowsiness,* euphoria, dysphoria, rash, pruritus.

DRUG INTERACTIONS **Alcohol** and other CNS DEPRESSANTS compound sedation and CNS depression.

NURSING IMPLICATIONS

Administration

- Hydrocodone may be taken with food or milk to prevent GI irritation.
- Preserve in tight, light-resistant containers.

Assessment & Drug Effects

- Monitor for effectiveness of drug for pain relief.
- Monitor for nausea and vomiting, especially in ambulatory patients.
- Monitor respiratory status and bowel elimination.

Patient & Family Education

- Caution to avoid hazardous activities until response to drug is determined.
- Warn that alcohol and other CNS

depressants may cause additive depression.

- Advise adequate hydration.
- Caution patient not to take larger doses than prescribed.

HYDROCORTISONE

(hye-droe-kor′ti-sone)

Trade names: Aeroseb-HC, Alphaderm, Cetacort, Cortaid, Cort-Dome, Cortenema, Cortril, DermaCort, Dermolate, Hydrocortone, Hytone, Proctocort, Rectocort♣, Synacort

HYDROCORTISONE ACETATE

Trade names: Anusol HC, CaldeCort, Carmol HC, Colifoam, Cortaid, Cortamed, Cort-Dome, Cortef Acetate, Corticaine, Cortifoam, Cortiment♣ Epifoam, Hydrocortone Acetate

HYDROCORTISONE CYPIONATE

Trade name: Cortef Fluid

HYDROCORTISONE SODIUM PHOSPHATE

Trade name: Hydrocortone Phosphate

HYDROCORTISONE SODIUM SUCCINATE

Trade names: A-hydroCort, Solu-Cortef

HYDROCORTISONE VALERATE

Trade name: Westcort

Prototype for classifications: SKIN AND MUCOUS MEMBRANE AGENT; ANTIINFLAMMATORY; SYNTHETIC HORMONE; ADRENAL CORTICOSTEROIDS; GLUCOCORTICOID; MINERALOCORTICOID

Pregnancy category: C

ACTIONS/PHARMACODYNAMICS

Short-acting synthetic steroid with both glucocorticoid and mineralocorticoid properties that affect nearly all systems of the body. **Antiinflammatory (glucocorticoid) action:** stabilizes leukocyte lysosomal membranes; inhibits phagocytosis and release of allergic substances; suppresses fibroblast formation and collagen deposition; reduces capillary dilation and permeability; and increases responsiveness of cardiovascular system to circulating catecholamines. **Immunosuppressive action:** modifies immune response to various stimuli; reduces antibody titers; and suppresses cell-mediated hypersensitivity reactions. **Mineralocorticoid action:** promotes sodium retention, but under certain circumstances (e.g., sodium loading), enhances sodium excretion; promotes potassium excretion; and increases glomerular filtration rate (GFR). **Metabolic action:** promotes hepatic gluconeogenesis, protein catabolism, redistribution of body fat, and lipolysis.

USES Replacement therapy in adrenocortical insufficiency; to reduce serum calcium in hypercalcemia, to suppress undesirable inflammatory or immune responses, to produce temporary remission in nonadrenal disease, and to block ACTH production in diagnostic tests. Use as antiinflammatory or immunosuppressive agent largely replaced by synthetic glucocorticoids that have minimal mineralocorticoid activity.

ROUTE & DOSAGE

Adrenal Insufficiency, Antiinflammatory

Adult: **PO** 10–320 mg/d in 3–4 divided doses. **IM/IV** 15–800

mg/d in 3–4 divided doses up to 2 g/d.
Child: **PO** 2.5–10 mg/kg/d in 3–4 divided doses. **IM/IV** 1–5 mg/kg/d divided q12–24 h.

Intraarticular, Intralesional (Acetate Salt)

Adult: **IM** 5–50 mg q3–5d for bursae; once q1–4wk for joints.

Antiinflammatory Agent

Adult: **Topical** apply a small amount to the affected area 1–4 times/d. **PR** insert 1% cream, 10% foam, 10–25 mg suppository, or 100 mg enema nightly.

PHARMACOKINETICS **Absorption:** readily absorbed from GI tract and IM injection site. **Onset:** 1–2 h PO; immediately IV; 3–5 d PR. **Peak:** 1 h PO; 4–8 h IM. **Duration:** 1–1.5 d PO/IM; 0.5–4 wk intraarticular. **Distribution:** distributed primarily to muscles, liver, skin, intestines, kidneys; crosses placenta. **Metabolism:** hepatically metabolized. **Elimination:** half-life: 1.5–2 h; HPA suppression 8–12 h; metabolites excreted in urine; excreted in breast milk.

CONTRAINDICATIONS & PRECAUTIONS **Contraindicated in:** hypersensitivity to glucocorticoids, idiopathic thrombocytopenic purpura, psychoses, acute glomerulonephritis, viral or bacterial diseases of skin, infections not controlled by antibiotics, active or latent amebiasis, hypercorticism (Cushing's syndrome), smallpox vaccination or other immunologic procedures. (Topical steroids contraindicated in presence of varicella, vaccinia, on surfaces with compromised circulation, and in children <2 y). Safe use in nursing mothers, during pregnancy (category C) not established. **Cautious use in:** children; diabetes mellitus; chronic, active hepatitis positive for hepatitis B surface antigen; hyperlipidemia; cirrhosis; stromal herpes simplex; glaucoma, tuberculosis of eye; osteoporosis; convulsive disorders; hypothyroidism; diverticulitis; nonspecific ulcerative colitis; fresh intestinal anastomoses; active or latent peptic ulcer; gastritis; esophagitis; thromboembolic disorders; CHF; metastatic carcinoma; hypertension; renal insufficiency; history of allergies; active or arrested tuberculosis; systemic fungal infection; myasthenia gravis.

H

ADVERSE/SIDE EFFECTS Dose and treatment duration dependent. **CNS:** vertigo, headache, nystagmus, ataxia (rare), increased intracranial pressure with papilledema (usually after discontinuation of medication), mental disturbances, aggravation of preexisting psychiatric conditions, insomnia. **CV:** syncopal episodes, thrombophlebitis, thromboembolism or fat embolism, palpitation, tachycardia, necrotizing angiitis. **Endocrine:** suppressed linear growth in children, decreased glucose tolerance; hyperglycemia, manifestations of latent diabetes mellitus; hypocorticism; amenorrhea and other menstrual difficulties. **Eye:** posterior subcapsular cataracts (especially in children), glaucoma, exophthalmos, increased intraocular pressure with optic nerve damage, perforation of the globe, fungal infection of the cornea, decreased or blurred vision. **Fluid and electrolyte disturbances:** hypocalcemia; *sodium and fluid retention;* hypokalemia and hypokalemic alkalosis; CHF, hypertension. **GI:** *nausea,* increased appetite, ulcerative esophagitis, pancreatitis, abdominal distention, peptic ulcer with perforation and hemorrhage, melena. **Hematologic:**

thrombocytopenia. **Musculoskeletal (long-term use):** osteoporosis, compression fractures, muscle wasting and weakness, tendon rupture, aseptic necrosis of femoral and humeral heads. **Skin:** skin thinning and atrophy, *acne, impaired wound healing;* petechiae, ecchymosis, easy bruisings; suppression of skin test reaction; hypopigmentation or hyperpigmentation, hirsutism, acneiform eruptions, subcutaneous fat atrophy; allergic dermatitis, urticaria, angioneurotic edema, increased sweating. **Other:** negative nitrogen balance, hypersensitivity or anaphylactoid reactions; aggravation or masking of infections; malaise, weight gain, obesity; increased or decreased motility and number of sperm, decreased serum concentration of vitamins A and C; urinary frequency and urgency, enuresis. **Overdose:** anxiety, mental confusion, depression, hyperglycemia, hypokalemia, hypernatremia, polycythemia, hypertension, edema, GI cramping or bleeding, ecchymoses, "moon" facies. **With parenteral therapy:** ***IV site:*** pain, irritation, necrosis, atrophy, sterile abscess; Charcot-like arthropathy following intraarticular use; burning and tingling in perineal area (after IV injection).

DIAGNOSTIC TEST INTERFERENCE Hydrocortisone (corticosteroids) may increase serum ***cholesterol, blood glucose,*** serum ***sodium, uric acid*** (in acute leukemia) and ***calcium*** (in bone metastasis). It may decrease serum ***calcium, potassium, PBI, thyroxin (T_4), triiodothyronine (T_3) and reduce thyroid I 131*** uptake. It increases ***urine glucose*** level and ***calcium*** excretion; decreases ***urine 17-OHCS*** and ***17-KS*** levels. May produce false-negative results with nitroblue tetrazolium test for systemic bacterial infection and may suppress reactions to skin tests.

DRUG INTERACTIONS BARBITURATES, **phenytoin, rifampin** may increase hepatic metabolism, thus decreasing cortisone levels; ESTROGENS potentiate the effects of hydrocortisone; NSAIDS compound ulcerogenic effects; **cholestyramine, colestipol** decrease hydrocortisone absorption; DIURETICS, **amphotericin b** exacerbate hypokalemia; ANTICHOLINESTERASE AGENTS (e.g., **neostigmine**) may produce severe weakness; immune response to VACCINES and TOXOIDS may be decreased.

INCOMPATIBILITIES Solution/additive: amobarbital, ampicillin, bleomycin, colistimethate, dimenhydrinate, doxapram, doxorubicin, ephedrine, heparin, hydralazine, metaraminol, methicillin, nafcillin, pentobarbital, phenobarbital, prochlorperazine, promethazine, secobarbital, TETRACYCLINES. **Y-site: ergotamine, phenytoin.**

NURSING IMPLICATIONS

Administration

- Give oral drug with food.
- Administer retention enema preferably after a bowel movement. The enema should be retained at least 1 h or all night if possible.
- Inject IM preparation deep into gluteal muscle.
- IV administration: IV hydrocortisone may be given by direct IV undiluted or diluted in NS or D5W. Administer at a rate of 25 mg or a fraction thereof over 1 min.
- IV administration to infants, children: Verify correct IV concentration and rate of infusion/injection with physician.
- Solutions that have been diluted

for IV infusion should be administered within 24h of dilution.

Occlusive Dressing

- If an occlusive dressing is to be used, apply medication sparingly, rub until it disappears, and then reapply, leaving a thin coat over lesion. Completely cover area with transparent plastic or other occlusive device or vehicle.
- Avoid covering a weeping or exudative lesion.
- Usually, occlusive dressings are not applied to face, scalp, scrotum, axilla, and groin.
- Inspect skin carefully between applications for ecchymotic, petechial, and purpuric signs, maceration, secondary infection, skin atrophy, striae or miliaria; if present, stop medication and notify physician.
- Store medication at 15–30C (59–86F) unless otherwise directed by manufacturer. Protect drug from light and freezing.

Assessment & Drug Effects

- Establish baseline and continuing data regarding BP, weight, fluid and electrolyte balance, and blood glucose.
- The elderly and the patient with low serum albumin are especially susceptible to adverse or side effects.
- Be alert to signs of hypocalcemia (see Appendix G).
- Ophthalmoscopic examinations are recommended every 2–3 mo, especially if patient is receiving ophthalmic steroid therapy.
- Compression and spontaneous fractures of long bones and vertebrae present hazards. Monitor for persistent backache or chest pain.
- Monitor for and report changes in mood and behavior, emotional instability, or psychomotor activity, especially with long-term therapy.
- Be alert to possibility of masked infection and delayed healing (antiinflammatory and immunosuppressive actions).
- Dose adjustment may be required if patient is subjected to severe stress (serious infection, surgery, or injury).
- Single doses of corticosteroids or use for a short period (<1 wk) do not produce withdrawal symptoms when discontinued, even with moderately large doses.

Patient & Family Education

- Inform that a slight weight gain with improved appetite is expected, but after dosage is stabilized, a sudden slow but steady weight increase (2 kg [5 lb]/wk) should be reported.
- Encourage to avoid alcohol and caffeine, which may contribute to steroid-ulcer development in long-term therapy.
- Dyspepsia with hyperacidity should not be ignored. Encourage to report symptoms to physician and not to self-medicate to find relief.
- Warn not to use aspirin or other OTC drugs unless prescribed specifically by the physician.
- A high protein, calcium, and vitamin D diet may be advisable to reduce risk of corticosteroid-induced osteoporosis.
- Instruct to report slow healing, any vague feeling of being sick, or return to pretreatment symptoms.
- To prevent withdrawal symptoms, advise patient not to abruptly discontinue drug: doses are gradually reduced.
- Advise patient to report exacerbation of disease during drug withdrawal.
- Advise patient receiving corticosteroid to carry a medical identification card or jewelery with recorded diagnosis, drug therapy, and name of physician.

Topical Applications (Hydrocortisone and Its Esters)

- Warn patient not to self-dose with OTC topical preparations of a corticosteroid more than 7 d. They should not be used for children <2 y. If symptoms do not abate, consult physician.
- Usually, topical preparations are applied after a shower or bath when skin is damp or wet. Cleansing and application of prescribed preparation should be done with extreme gentleness because of fragility, easy bruisability, and poor healing skin.
- Hazard of systemic toxicity is higher in small children because of the greater ratio of skin surface area to body weight. Apply sparingly.
- Urge patient on long-term therapy with topical corticosterone to check shelf-life date.

H

HYDROFLUMETHIAZIDE

(hye-droe-floo-meth-eye'a-zide)

Trade names: Diucardin, Saluron

Classifications: ELECTROLYTIC AND WATER BALANCE AGENT; THIAZIDE DIURETIC; ANTIHYPERTENSIVE

Prototype: Hydrochlorothiazide

Pregnancy category: B

ACTIONS/PHARMACODYNAMICS Thiazide diuretic chemically related to sulfonamides. Similar to hydrochlorothiazide in actions, uses, contraindications, precautions, adverse reactions, and interactions.

USES Mild hypertension, management of edema associated with CHF.

ROUTE & DOSAGE

Edema

Adult: **PO** 25 mg–200 mg/d in 1–2 divided doses.

Hypertension

Adult: **PO** 50–100 mg/d in 1–2 divided doses.
Child: **PO** 1 mg/kg/d once/d.

PHARMACOKINETICS Absorption: incompletely absorbed. **Onset:** 1–2 h. **Peak:** 3–4 h. **Duration:** 18–24 h. **Distribution:** distributed throughout extracellular tissue; concentrates in kidney; crosses placenta; distributed in breast milk. **Metabolism:** does not appear to be metabolized. **Elimination:** half-life: 17 h; excreted in urine.

CONTRAINDICATIONS & PRECAUTIONS Contraindicated in: hypersensitivity to other thiazides or sulfonamide derivatives; anuria; pregnancy (category B), lactation; hypokalemia.

ADVERSE/SIDE EFFECTS Postural hypotension, photosensitivity, *hypokalemia, hyperglycemia,* hyponatremia, *asymptomatic hyperuricemia.* See also hydrochlorothiazide.

DRUG INTERACTIONS Amphotericin B, CORTICOSTEROIDS increase hypokalemic effects; may antagonize hypoglycemic effects of ORAL HYPOGLYCEMIC AGENTS, **insulin; cholestyramine, colestipol** decrease thiazide absorption; **diazoxide** intensifies hypoglycemic and hypotensive effects; increased potassium and magnesium loss may cause **digoxin** toxicity; decreases **lithium** excretion, thus increasing lithium toxicity; increases risk of NSAID-induced renal failure—NSAIDS may attenuate diuresis.

NURSING IMPLICATIONS

Administration

- Schedule diuretic dose early in the morning to prevent interrupted sleep. If two doses are taken each day, schedule dose 2 no later than 3 PM.

- Antihypertensive effects may be noted in 3–4 d, maximal effects may require 3–4 wk.

Assessment & Drug Effects

- Baseline and periodic determinations should be made for serum electrolytes, blood counts, BUN, blood glucose, uric acid, and CO_2.
- Monitor patient for hypokalemia and hyponatremia (see Appendix G).
- Elderly patients are especially susceptible to the hypotensive effects that may accompany excessive diuresis.
- Asymptomatic hyperuricemia can be produced because of interference with uric acid excretion. Report onset of joint pain and limitation of motion.
- Monitor for signs of diabetes. The diabetic patient should be watched for loss of control of diabetes.

Patient & Family Education

- Warn patient about the possibility of photosensitivity reaction. Thiazide-related photosensitivity is considered a photoallergy. It occurs $1\frac{1}{2}$–2 wk after initial sun exposure.
- Counsel patient to avoid use of OTC drugs unless approved by the physician.
- Store tablets in tightly closed container at 15–30C (59–86F) unless otherwise directed.

HYDROMORPHONE HYDROCHLORIDE

(hye-droe-mor′fone)

Trade names: Dilaudid, Dilaudid-HP

Classifications: CNS AGENT; ANALGESIC; NARCOTIC (OPIATE) AGONIST

Prototype: Morphine

Pregnancy category: C

Controlled substance: Schedule II

ACTIONS/PHARMACODYNAMICS Semisynthetic derivative structurally similar to morphine but with 8–10 times more potent analgesic effect. Has more rapid onset and shorter duration of action than morphine and is reported to have less hypnotic action and less tendency to produce nausea and vomiting. Has antitussive properties.

USES Relief of moderate to severe pain and control of persistent nonproductive cough.

ROUTE & DOSAGE

Moderate to Severe Pain

Adult: **PO/SC/IM/IV** 1–4 mg q4–6h prn. **Rectal** 3 mg q4–6h.
Child: **PO** 0.03–0.08 mg/kg q4–6h (max 5 mg/dose). **IV** 0.015 mg/kg q4–6h.

Antitussive

Adult: **PO** 1 mg q3–4h prn.
Child 6–12 y: **PO** 0.5 mg q3–4h prn.

PHARMACOKINETICS **Onset:** 15–30 min. **Peak:** 30–90 min. **Duration:** 4–5 h. **Distribution:** crosses placenta; distributed into breast milk. **Metabolism:** metabolized in liver. **Elimination:** excreted in urine.

CONTRAINDICATIONS & PRECAUTIONS **Contraindicated in:** intolerance to opiate agonists. Safe use in pregnancy (category C) or in children not established.

ADVERSE/SIDE EFFECTS **GI:** nausea, vomiting, constipation. **CNS:** euphoria, dizziness, sedation, *drowsiness.* **CV:** hypotension, bradycardia or tachycardia. **Respiratory:** respiratory depression. **Other:** blurred vision.

DRUG INTERACTIONS **Alcohol** and other CNS DEPRESSANTS compound sedation and CNS depression.

INCOMPATIBILITIES Solution/additive: prochlorperazine, sodium bicarbonate, thiopental. Y-site: minocycline, prochlorperazine, tetracycline.

NURSING IMPLICATIONS

Administration

- When narcotic therapy is initiated, a fixed schedule provides more effective management than a prn schedule.
- For direct IV injection, dilute in at least 5 ml of sterile water or 0.9% NaCl. Administer at a rate of 2 mg over 3–5 min.
- IV administration to infants, children: Verify correct IV concentration and rate of infusion with physician.
- A slight discoloration may develop in ampules or multidose vials with no loss of potency.
- Preserve in tight, light-resistant containers at 15–30C (59–86F).

Assessment & Drug Effects

- Before administration of drug, note respiratory rate, rhythm, and depth and size of pupils. Respirations of 12/min or less and mitosis are signs of toxicity. Withhold drug and promptly notify physician.
- Monitor vital signs at regular intervals. Drug-induced respiratory depression may occur even with small doses and increases progressively with higher doses.
- Assess effectiveness of pain relief 30 min after medication administration.
- Carefully monitor drug effects in elderly or debilitated patients and those with impaired renal and hepatic function.
- Drug depresses cough and sigh reflexes and may induce atelectasis, especially in postoperative patients and those with pulmonary disease. Assess effectiveness of cough.
- Nausea and orthostatic hypotension most often occur in ambulatory patients or when a supine patient assumes the head-up position.
- Monitor I&O ratio and pattern. Assess lower abdomen for bladder distension. Report oliguria or urinary retention.
- Monitor bowel pattern, as drug-induced constipation may require treatment.

Patient & Family Education

- Advise patient on prn schedule to request medication at the onset of pain and not to wait until pain is severe.
- Inform patient that drug may cause drowsiness, dizziness, and blurred vision. Advise caution with activities requiring alertness.
- Advise patient to avoid alcohol and other CNS depressants while receiving drug.

HYDROQUINONE

(hye′droe-kwin-one)

Trade names: Eldopaque, Eldoquin, Esoterica Regular, Melanex, Porcelana, Solaquin

Classifications: SKIN AND MUCOUS MEMBRANE AGENT; DEPIGMENTOR

Pregnancy category: C

ACTIONS/PHARMACODYNAMICS
Topical agent that causes reversible bleaching of hyperpigmented skin due to increased melanin. Interferes with formation of new melanin but does not destroy existing pigment. Depresses melanin synthesis and melanocytic growth, and possibly by increasing excretion of melanin from melanocytes.

USES Gradual bleaching of hyperpigmented skin conditions such as chloasma or melasma, severe freckling, senile lentigines (age spots or liver spots). Also as an antioxidant in topical preparations. Some formulations include a sunscreening agent (e.g., Porcelana with Sunscreen, Mercolized Cocrema, Pabaquinone, and Solaquin).

ROUTE & DOSAGE

Bleaching of Hyperpigmented Skin

Adult: **Topical** Apply thin layer and rub into hyperpigmented skin b.i.d., AM and PM.

CONTRAINDICATIONS & PRECAUTIONS **Contraindicated in:** prickly heat, sunburn, irritated skin, depilatory usage. Safe use during pregnancy (category C), in nursing women, and in children ≤ 12 y not established.

ADVERSE/SIDE EFFECTS Dryness and fissuring of paranasal and infraorbital areas, inflammatory reaction, erythema; stinging, tingling, burning sensations; irritation, sensitization, and contact dermatitis.

DRUG INTERACTIONS None established.

NURSING IMPLICATIONS

Administration

- Skin should be tested for sensitivity before treatment is initiated. Apply small amount of drug (about 25 mm in diameter) to an unbroken patch of skin and check in 24 h. If vesicle formation, itching, or excessive inflammation occurs, drug should not be used. Minor redness is not a contraindication.
- Applications should be limited to an area no larger than that of face and neck.

Assessment & Drug Effects

- In general, complete depigmentation occurs in 1–4 mo and lasts 2–6 mo after hydroquinone is discontinued. Once desired results are obtained, amount and frequency of applications should be reduced to the least that will maintain depigmentation.
- If bleaching or skin lightening does not occur after 2 or 3 mo of therapy, it should be discontinued.

Patient & Family Education

- Advise to use a sunscreen agent or a hydroquinone formulation containing a sunscreen for daytime applications.
- Instruct to wash drug off if rash or irritation develops and to consult physician.
- Advise to avoid contact of hydroquinone with the eyes and not to use on open lesions, sunburned, irritated, or otherwise damaged skin.
- Advise to continue use of protective clothing and sunscreening agent after treatment is terminated to reduce possibility of repigmentation.

HYDROXOCOBALAMIN (VITAMIN $B_{12\alpha}$)

(hye-drox-oh-koe-bal'a-min)

Trade names: Acti-B_{12} ✦, Alphamine, AlphaRedisol, Hydrobexan, Hydroxo-12, LA-12

Classification: VITAMIN B_{12}

Prototype: Cyanocobalamin

Pregnancy category: A (C if > RDA)

ACTIONS/PHARMACODYNAMICS Cobalamin derivative similar to cyanocobalamin (vitamin B_{12}) in actions, uses, contraindications, precautions, and adverse reactions. More slowly absorbed from injection site than cyanocobalamin and may be taken up by liver in larger quantities. **Unlabeled uses:** cyanide poisoning and tobacco amblyopia.

ROUTE & DOSAGE

Vitamin B_{12} Deficiency

Adult: **IM** 30 μg/d for 5–10 d and then 100–200 μg/mo *or* 1000 μg qod until remission and then 1000 μg/mo.
Child: **IM** 100 μg doses to a total of 1–5 mg over 2 wk and then 30–50 μg/mo.

H

PHARMACOKINETICS Distribution: widely distributed; principally stored in liver, kidneys, and adrenals; crosses placenta. **Metabolism:** converted in tissues to active coenzymes; enterohepatically cycled. **Elimination:** 50–95% of doses ≥ 100 μg are excreted in urine in 48 h; excreted in breast milk.

DRUG INTERACTION Chloramphenicol may interfere with therapeutic response to hydroxycobalamin.

NURSING IMPLICATIONS

See cyanocobalamin for additional nursing implications.

- Some patients experience mild pain at injection site after administration.

HYDROXYCHLOROQUINE SULFATE

(hye-drox-ee-klor'oh-kwin)
Trade name: Plaquenil Sulfate
Classifications: ANTIINFECTIVE; ANTIMALARIAL
Prototype: Chloroquine
Pregnancy category: C

ACTIONS/PHARMACODYNAMICS Derivative closely related to chloroquine and with similar actions, uses, contraindications, precautions, adverse reactions, and interactions.

USES Suppressive prophylaxis and treatment of acute malarial attacks due to all forms of susceptible malaria. Used adjunctively with primaquine for eradication of *Plasmodium vivax* and *Plasmodium malariae*. More commonly prescribed than chloroquine for treatment of rheumatoid arthritis and lupus erythematosus (usually in conjunction with salicylate or corticosteroid therapy). **Unlabeled use:** porphyria cutanea tarda.

ROUTE & DOSAGE

Doses are expressed in terms of hydroxychloroquine base: 400-mg tablet = 310-mg base; 800-mg tablet = 620-mg base

Acute Malaria

Adult: **PO** 620-mg base followed by 310 mg base at 6, 18, and 24 h.
Child: **PO** 10-mg base/kg and then 5-mg base/kg at 6, 18, and 24 h.

Malaria Suppression

Adult: **PO** 310-mg base the same day each week starting 2 wk before exposure and continuing for 4–6 wk after leaving the area of exposure.
Child: **PO** 5-mg base/kg the same day each week starting 2 wk before exposure and continuing for 4–6 wk after leaving the area of exposure.

Lupus Erythematosus

Adult: **PO** 310-mg base 1–2 times/d.

Child: **PO** 3–5 mg/kg/d in 1–2 divided doses (max 400 mg/d or 7 mg/kg/d).

Rheumatoid Arthritis

Adult: **PO** 400–600 mg/d until response and then decrease to lowest maintenance levels possible.
Child: **PO** 3–5 mg/kg/d in 1–2 divided doses (max 400 mg/d or 7 mg/kg/d).

PHARMACOKINETICS Absorption: rapidly and almost completely absorbed. **Peak:** 1–2 h. **Distribution:** widely distributed; concentrates in lungs, liver, erythrocytes, eyes, skin, and kidneys; crosses placenta. **Metabolism:** partially metabolized in liver to active metabolite. **Elimination:** half-life: 70–120 h; eliminated in urine; excreted in breast milk.

CONTRAINDICATIONS & PRECAUTIONS Contraindicated in: known hypersensitivity to, or retinal or visual field changes associated with, quinoline compounds; psoriasis, porphyria, long-term therapy in children; pregnancy (category C). Safe use in juvenile arthritis not established. **Cautious use in:** hepatic disease; alcoholism, with hepatotoxic drugs; impaired renal function; metabolic acidosis; patients with tendency to dermatitis.

ADVERSE/SIDE EFFECTS CNS: fatigue, vertigo, headache, mood or mental changes, anxiety, *retinopathy,* blurred vision, difficulty focusing. **GI:** anorexia, nausea, vomiting, diarrhea, abdominal cramps, weight loss. **Hematologic:** hemolysis in patients with G6PD deficiency, agranulocytosis (rare), aplastic anemia (rare), thrombocytopenia. **Skin:** bleaching or loss of hair, unusual pigmentation (blue-black) of skin or inside mouth, skin rash, itching.

DRUG INTERACTIONS Aluminum- and **magnesium**-containing ANTACIDS and LAXATIVES decrease hydroxychloroquine absorption—separate administrations by at least 4 h; hydroxychloroquine may interfere with response to **rabies vaccine.**

NURSING IMPLICATIONS

Administration

- Administration of drug with meals or milk may reduce incidence of GI distress.
- Administer antacids and laxatives at least 4 h before or after hydroxychloroquine.
- Store at 15–30C (59–86F) unless otherwise directed.

Assessment & Drug Effects

- All patients on long-term therapy should have baseline and periodic ophthalmoscopic examinations and blood cell counts.
- Therapeutic effect may not appear for several weeks, and maximal benefit may not occur for 6 mo.
- Patients receiving prolonged therapy should be informed about adverse symptoms. Drug should be discontinued if weakness, visual symptoms, hearing loss, unusual bleeding or bruising or skin eruptions occur.

Patient & Family Education

- Counsel patient to follow drug regimen as prescribed by the physician.
- Caution patients to keep drug out of reach of children.

HYDROXYPROGESTERONE CAPROATE

(hye-drox-ee-proe-jess′te-rone)

Trade names: Duralutin, Gesterol L.A., Hylutin, Hyprogest 250, Pro-Depo

Classifications: HORMONE; PROGESTIN
Prototype: Progesterone
Pregnancy category: X

ACTIONS/PHARMACODYNAMICS Long-acting synthetic progestational hormone. Has slower onset and longer action than progesterone. Has minimal estrogenic and androgenic activity. Induces and maintains endometrium, preventing uterine bleeding; inhibits production of pituitary gonadotropin, preventing ovulation; and produces thick cervical mucus resistant to passage of sperm.

USES Amenorrhea, abnormal uterine bleeding, advanced uterine cancer, and as "medical D & C" (conversion of proliferative endometrium to secretory endometrium and desquamation). Also as a test for endogenous estrogen production.

ROUTE & DOSAGE

Amenorrhea
Adult: **IM** 375 mg started anytime during cycle; after 4 d of desquamation or if no bleeding, 21 d after injection, start cyclic therapy; repeat cyclic therapy q4wk and stop after 4 cycles.

Advanced Uterine Adenocarcinoma
Adult: **IM** ≥ 1 g at once, and repeat 1 or more times/wk; stop at time of relapse or if no desirable results obtained after a total of 12 wk of therapy.

Test for Endogenous Estrogen Production
Adult: **IM** 250 mg at any time during cycle; repeat for confirmation 4 wk after first injection; stop after second injection.

PHARMACOKINETICS Duration: 9–17 d. **Distribution:** crosses placenta; distributed into breast milk. **Metabolism:** metabolized in liver. **Elimination:** eliminated in urine.

CONTRAINDICATIONS & PRECAUTIONS Contraindicated in: severe hepatic disease, carcinoma of breast or genital region; thromboembolic disorders, pregnancy (category X), missed abortion, abnormal vaginal bleeding. **Cautious use in:** diabetes mellitus; asthma; epilepsy; migraine; cardiac or renal dysfunction; mental depression.

ADVERSE/SIDE EFFECTS CNS: cerebral thrombosis or hemorrhage, migraine, depression. **CV:** hypertension, thromboembolic disorders, e.g., <u>pulmonary embolism.</u> **GI:** nausea, vomiting, cholestatic jaundice, abdominal cramps. **Reproduction:** breakthrough bleeding, changes in cervical erosion and secretions, changes in menstrual flow, dysmenorrhea, vaginal candidiasis. **Other:** edema, weight changes; breast tenderness, enlargement, or secretion; allergylike reactions (especially at high doses); female fetus masculinization; decreased glucose tolerance. **Respiratory:** coughing, dyspnea, chest constriction. **Skin:** photosensitivity, acne, melasma, hirsutism, some loss of scalp hair, rash.

DRUG INTERACTION Rifampin may decrease pharmacologic effects of progestins.

NURSING IMPLICATIONS

Administration
- Inject deep IM into a large muscle. Drug may cause local irritation at injection site.
- Protect drug preparation from light; store at 15–30C (59–86F).

Assessment & Drug Effects
- Record onset and duration of men-

strual flow when drug is used to treat amenorrhea.

Patient & Family Education

- Stress importance of reporting immediately suspected pregnancy, onset of vaginal bleeding, or thromboembolic implications (pain or numbness of legs, sudden onset of chest pain or shortness of breath, sudden severe headache or dizziness, visual problems).
- Teach breast self-examination.
- Advise diabetics to monitor blood glucose closely.
- Caution to use sunscreen and protective clothing to reduce risk of photosensitivity.
- Counsel that onset of normal menstrual cycles may not occur for 2 or 3 mo after cessation of drug.

HYDROXYUREA

(hye-drox′ee-yoo-ree-ah)

Trade name: Hydrea

Classifications: ANTINEOPLASTIC; ANTIMETABOLITE

Prototype: Fluorouracil

Pregnancy category: D

ACTIONS/PHARMACODYNAMICS Synthetic analogue of urea with antimetabolite activity. Blocks incorporation of thymidine into DNA and may damage already formed DNA molecules; does not affect synthesis of RNA or protein. Cytotoxic effect limited to tissues with high rates of cell proliferation. May reduce iron use by erythrocytes; has no effect on erythrocyte survival time. No cross resistance with other antineoplastics has been demonstrated.

USES Palliative treatment of metastatic melanoma, chronic myelocytic leukemia; recurrent metastatic, or inoperable ovarian cancer. Also used as adjunct to x-ray therapy for treatment of advanced primary squamous cell (epidermoid) carcinoma of head (excluding lip), neck, lungs. **Unlabeled uses:** psoriasis; combination therapy with radiation of lung carcinoma; sickle cell anemia.

ROUTE & DOSAGE

Palliative Therapy

Adult: **PO** 80 mg/kg q3d or 20–30 mg/kg/d.

Sickle Cell Anemia

Adult: **PO** 15 mg/kg/d; may increase by 5 mg/kg/d to a max of 35 mg/kg/d or until toxicity develops.

PHARMACOKINETICS Absorption: readily absorbed from GI tract. **Peak:** 2 h. **Distribution:** crosses blood–brain barrier. **Metabolism:** metabolized in liver. **Elimination:** eliminated as respiratory CO_2 and as urea in urine.

CONTRAINDICATIONS & PRECAUTIONS Contraindicated in: Pregnancy (category D), children, myelosuppression. **Cautious use in:** recent use of other cytotoxic drugs or irradiation; renal dysfunction; elderly patients; history of gout.

ADVERSE/SIDE EFFECTS CNS: Rare: headache, dizziness, hallucinations, convulsions. **GI:** stomatitis, anorexia, nausea, vomiting, diarrhea, constipation. **Hematologic:** <u>bone marrow suppression</u> (*leukopenia,* anemia, thrombocytopenia), megaloblastic erythropoiesis. **Skin:** maculopapular rash, facial erythema, postirradiation erythema. **Other:** renal tubular dysfunction, elevated BUN, serum, creatinine levels, hyperuricemia, fever, chills, malaise.

DRUG INTERACTIONS None established.

NURSING IMPLICATIONS

Administration

- If patient has difficulty swallowing capsule, open, mix with water, and give immediately.
- Store in tightly covered container at 15–30C (59–86F) unless otherwise directed.

Assessment & Drug Effects

- Status of kidney, liver, bone marrow functions should be determined before and periodically during therapy; hemoglobin, WBC, platelet counts are monitored at least once weekly.
- If WBC drops to 2500/mm^3 or platelets to 100,000/mm^3, therapy will be interrupted.
- Monitor I&O. Advise patients with high serum uric acid levels particularly to drink at least 10–12 240 ml (8 oz) glasses of fluid daily to prevent uric acid nephropathy.
- Patients with marked renal dysfunction may rapidly develop visual and auditory hallucinations and hematologic toxicity.

Patient & Family Education

- Toxicity incidence with use of hydroxyurea is as high as 66% with doses of 40 mg/kg body weight.
- Advise patient to report fever, chills, sore throat, nausea, vomiting, diarrhea, loss of appetite, and unusual bruising or bleeding.
- Advise patient to use barrier contraceptive during therapy. Drug is teratogenic.

HYDROXYZINE HYDROCHLORIDE

(hye-drox′i-zeen)

Trade names: Atarax, Hyzine-50, Quiess, Vistaril Intramuscular, Vistacon, Vistaject

HYDROXYZINE PAMOATE

Trade names: Hy-Pam, Vamate, Vistaril Oral

Prototype for classifications: ANTIHISTAMINE; ANTIPRURITIC

Pregnancy category: C

ACTIONS/PHARMACODYNAMICS

Piperazine derivative structurally and pharmacologically related to other cyclizines (e.g., buclizine, chlorcyclizine). In common with such agents, it causes CNS depression and has anticholinergic, antiemetic, bronchodilator, and antihistaminic activity. Its tranquilizing (ataractic) effect is produced primarily by depression of hypothalamus and brain-stem reticular formation, rather than cortical areas.

USES Emotional or psychoneurotic states characterized by anxiety, tension, or psychomotor agitation; to relieve anxiety, control nausea and emesis, and reduce narcotic requirements before or after surgery or delivery. Also used in management of pruritus due to allergic conditions, e.g., chronic urticaria, atopic and contact dermatoses, and in treatment of acute and chronic alcoholism with withdrawal symptoms or delirium tremens.

ROUTE & DOSAGE

Anxiety

Adult: **PO** 25–100 mg t.i.d. or q.i.d. **IM** 25–100 mg q4–6h.
Child: **PO** *<6 y,* 50 mg/d in divided doses; *>6 y,* 50 mg/d in divided doses. **IM** 1.1 mg/kg q4–6h.

Pruritus

Adult: **PO** 25 mg t.i.d. or q.i.d. **IM** 25 mg q4–6h.

Geriatric: **PO** 10 mg 3–4 times daily.
Child: **PO** >*6 y*, 50–100 mg/d in divided doses; <*6 y*, 50 mg/d in divided doses. **IM** 1.1 mg/kg q4–6h.

Nausea

Adult: **IM** 25–100 mg q4–6h.
Child: **IM** 1.1 mg/kg q4–6h.

PHARMACOKINETICS **Absorption:** readily absorbed from GI tract. **Onset:** 15–30 min PO. **Duration:** 4–6 h. **Distribution:** not known if it crosses placenta or is distributed into breast milk. **Metabolism:** metabolized in liver. **Elimination:** probably excreted in bile.

CONTRAINDICATIONS & PRECAUTIONS **Contraindicated in:** known hypersensitivity to hydroxyzine; use as sole treatment in psychoses or depression. Safe use during early pregnancy (category C) or in nursing mothers not established. **Cautious use in:** history of allergies; the elderly.

ADVERSE/SIDE EFFECTS *Drowsiness* (usually transitory), sedation, dizziness, injection site reactions, hypotension, *dry mouth,* headache, involuntary motor activity (rare). **Hypersensitivity:** urticaria, dyspnea, chest tightness, wheezing, erythematous macular eruptions, erythema multiforme. **Other:** Phlebitis, hemolysis, thrombosis, digital gangrene from inadvertent IV or intraarterial injection.

DIAGNOSTIC TEST INTERFERENCE Possibility of false-positive ***urinary 17-hydroxycorticosteroid*** determinations (modified Glenn-Nelson technique).

DRUG INTERACTIONS **Alcohol** and CNS DEPRESSANTS add to CNS depression; TRICYCLIC ANTIDEPRESSANTS and other ANTICHOLINERGICS have additive anticholinergic effects; may inhibit pressor effects of **epinephrine.**

INCOMPATIBILITIES **Solution/additive: aminophylline, amobarbital, chloramphenicol, dimenhydrinate, penicillin G, pentobarbital, phenobarbital.**

NURSING IMPLICATIONS

Administration

- Tablets may be crushed before administration and taken with fluid of patient's choice. Capsule may be emptied and contents swallowed with water or mixed with food. Liquid formulations are available.
- IM administration should be made deep into body of a relatively large muscle. The Z-track technique of injection is recommended to prevent SC infiltration.
- Recommended IM site: In adult, the gluteus maximus or vastus lateralis; in children, the vastus lateralis.
- Protect hydroxyzine from light. Store at 15–30C (59–86F) unless otherwise specified.

Assessment & Drug Effects

- Drowsiness may occur and usually disappears with continued therapy or following reduction of dosage.
- If patient is on high dosage of hydroxyzine, monitor condition of oral membranes daily.
- Usefulness of hydroxyzine should be reevaluated periodically.
- When CNS depressants are prescribed concomitantly, dosage of the depressant is reduced up to 50%.

Patient & Family Education

- Forewarn about the possibility of drowsiness and dizziness, and caution against hazardous activities until reaction to drug is known.
- Alcohol and hydroxyzine should not be taken at the same time.
- Women who become pregnant

should communicate with physician about the desirability of discontinuing the drug.

- Dry mouth may be relieved by frequent warm water rinses, increasing fluid intake, and by use of a salivary substitute (e.g., Moi-stir, Xero-Lube) if necessary.
- Urge patient to give scrupulous care to teeth. Avoid irritation or abrasion of gums and other oral tissues.
- Advise patient to consult physician before self-dosing with OTC medications.

H

HYOSCYAMINE SULFATE

(hye-oh-sye′a-meen)

Trade names: Anaspaz, Cystospaz, Levsin, Levsinex, Neoquess

Classifications: ANTICHOLINERGIC (PARASYMPATHOLYTIC); ANTIMUSCARINIC, ANTISPASMODIC

Prototype: Atropine

Pregnancy category: C

ACTIONS/PHARMACODYNAMICS Extremely potent belladonna alkaloid with anticholinergic and antispasmodic activity. Anticholinergic effect chiefly related to the levo isomer. Action is produced by competitive inhibition of acetylcholine at the parasympathetic neuroeffector junctions.

USES GI tract disorders caused by spasm and hypermotility, as conjunct therapy with diet and antacids for peptic ulcer management, and as an aid in the control of gastric hypersecretion and intestinal hypermotility. Also symptomatic relief of biliary and renal colic, as a "drying agent" to relieve symptoms of acute rhinitis, to control preanesthesia salivation and respiratory tract secretions, to treat symptoms of parkinsonism, and to reduce pain and hypersecretion in pancreatitis.

ROUTE & DOSAGE

GI Spasms

Adult: **IV/IM/SC** 0.25–0.5 mg q6h. **PO/SL** 0.125–0.25 mg t.i.d. or q.i.d. prn.
Child 2–12 y: **PO** 0.0625–0.125 mg q4h prn (max 0.75 mg/d).

PHARMACOKINETICS **Absorption:** well absorbed from all administration sites. **Onset:** 2–3 min IV; 20–30 min PO. **Peak effect:** 15–30 min IV; 30–60 min PO. **Duration:** 4–6 h (up to 12 h with sustained release form). **Distribution:** distributed in most body tissues; crosses blood–brain barrier and placenta; distributed in breast milk. **Metabolism:** metabolized in liver. **Elimination:** half-life: 3.5–13 h; excreted in urine.

CONTRAINDICATIONS & PRECAUTIONS **Contraindicated in:** hypersensitivity to belladonna alkaloids, narrow-angle glaucoma, prostatic hypertrophy, obstructive diseases of GI or GU tract, paralytic ileus or intestinal atony, myasthenia gravis. **Cautious use in:** diabetes mellitus, cardiac disease; pregnancy (category C).

ADVERSE/SIDE EFFECTS **CNS:** headache, unusual tiredness or weakness, confusion, *drowsiness,* excitement in elderly patients. **CV:** palpitations, tachycardia. **Eye:** *blurred vision,* increased intraocular tension, cycloplegia, mydriasis. **GI:** *dry mouth, constipation,* paralytic ileus. **Other:** *urinary retention,* anhidrosis, suppression of lactation.

DRUG INTERACTIONS **Amantadine,** ANTIHISTAMINES, TRICYCLIC ANTIDEPRESSANTS, **quinidine, disopyr-**

Common side effect in *italic,* life-threatening effects underlined: generic names in **bold;** drug class in SMALL CAPS

amide, procainamide add anticholinergic effects; decreases **levodopa** effects; **methotrimeprazine** may precipitate extrapyramidal effects; decreases antipsychotic effects of PHENOTHIAZINES (decreased absorption).

NURSING IMPLICATIONS

Administration

- Administer PO preparations about 1 h before meals and at bedtime (at least 2 h after last meal).
- A single IV dose may be given by direct IV undiluted over 60 s.
- Dose for the elderly patient should be less than the standard adult dose. Observe patient carefully for signs of paradoxic reactions.

Assessment & Drug Effects

- Monitor bowel elimination; may cause constipation.
- Monitor urinary output.
- Risk of urinary retention is lessened if patient voids prior to each dose.
- Assess for dry mouth and advise good oral hygiene.

Patient & Family Education

- Advise to avoid excessive exposure to high temperatures, since drug-induced heatstroke can develop.
- Advise patient to observe caution and to avoid driving and other potentially hazardous activities until response to drug is known.
- If patient complains about blurred vision, suggest use of dark glasses; but if this side effect persists, advise patient to report to physician for dose adjustment or possible change of drug.

IBUPROFEN

(eye-byoo′proe-fen)

Trade names: Advil, Amersol♣, Children's Motrin, Haltran, Ibuprin, Junior Strength Motrin Caplets, Medipren, Motrin, Nuprin, Pediaprofen, Pamprin-IB, Rufen, Trendar

Prototype for classifications: CNS AGENT; ANALGESIC; ANTIPYRETIC; NSAID

Pregnancy category: B

ACTIONS/PHARMACODYNAMICS

Prototype of the propionic acid NSAIDS with nonsteroidal antiinflammatory activity and significant antipyretic and analgesic properties. Blocks prostaglandin synthesis. Ibuprofen activity also includes modulation of T-cell function, inhibition of inflammatory cell chemotaxis, decreased release of superoxide radicals, or increased scavenging of these compounds at inflammatory sites. Inhibits platelet aggregation and prolongs bleeding time but does not affect prothrombin or whole blood clotting times. Cross-sensitivity with aspirin and other nonsteroidal antiinflammatory drugs has been reported.

USES Chronic, symptomatic rheumatoid arthritis and osteoarthritis; relief of mild to moderate pain; primary dysmenorrhea; reduction of fever. **Unlabeled use:** gout, juvenile rheumatoid arthritis, psoriatic arthritis, ankylosing spondylitis, vascular headache.

ROUTE & DOSAGE

Inflammatory Disease

Adult: **PO** 400–800 mg t.i.d. or q.i.d. (max 3200 mg/d).
Child: **PO** *< 20 kg,* up to 400 mg/d in divided doses; *20–30 kg,* up to 600 mg/d in divided doses; *30–40 kg,* up to 800 mg/d in divided doses.

Mild to Moderate Pain, Dysmenorrhea

Adult: **PO** 400 mg q4–6h up to 1200 mg/d.

Fever

Adult: **PO** 200–400 mg t.i.d. or q.i.d. (max 1200 mg/d).
Child 6 mo–12 y: **PO** 5–10 mg/kg q4–6h up to 40 mg/kg/d.

PHARMACOKINETICS Absorption: 80% absorbed from GI tract. **Onset:** 1 h antipyretic effect. **Peak:** 1–2 h. **Duration:** 6–8 h. **Metabolism:** metabolized in liver. **Elimination:** half-life: 2–4 h; excreted primarily in urine; some biliary excretion.

I

CONTRAINDICATIONS & PRECAUTIONS Contraindicated in: patient in whom urticaria, severe rhinitis, bronchospasm, angioedema, nasal polyps are precipitated by aspirin or other NSAIDS; active peptic ulcer, bleeding abnormalities. Safe use during pregnancy (category B), by nursing mothers, or by children < 6 mo not established. **Cautious use in:** hypertension, history of GI ulceration, impaired hepatic or renal function, chronic renal failure, cardiac decompensation, patients with SLE.

ADVERSE/SIDE EFFECTS CNS: headache, dizziness, light-headedness, anxiety, emotional lability, fatigue, malaise, drowsiness, anxiety, confusion, depression, aseptic meningitis. **CV:** hypertension, palpitation, congestive heart failure (patient with marginal cardiac function); peripheral edema. **Eye/ear:** amblyopia (blurred vision, decreased visual acuity, scotomas, changes in color vision); nystagmus, visual-field defects; tinnitus, impaired hearing. **GI:** dry mouth, gingival ulcerations, dyspepsia, *heartburn, nausea,* vomiting, anorexia, diarrhea, constipation, bloating, flatulence, epigastric or abdominal discomfort or pain, GI ulceration, *occult blood loss.* **Hematologic:** thrombocytopenia, neutropenia, hemolytic or <u>aplastic anemia</u>, leukopenia; decreased Hgb, Hct; transitory rise in AST, ALT, serum alkaline phosphatase; rise in (Ivy) bleeding time. **Renal:** acute renal failure, polyuria, azotemia, cystitis, hematuria, nephrotoxicity, decreased creatinine clearance. **Skin:** maculopapular and vesicobullous skin eruptions, erythema multiforme, pruritus, rectal itching, acne. **Other:** fluid retention with edema, Stevens-Johnson syndrome, <u>toxic hepatitis</u>, hypersensitivity reactions, <u>anaphylaxis</u>, bronchospasm, serum sickness, SLE, angioedema.

DRUG INTERACTIONS ORAL ANTICOAGULANTS, **heparin** may prolong bleeding time; may increase **lithium** and **methotrexate** toxicity.

NURSING IMPLICATIONS

Administration

- Give on an empty stomach, 1 h before or 2 h after meals.
- If GI intolerance occurs, ibuprofen may be taken with meals or milk.
- Tablet may be crushed if patient is unable to swallow it whole and mixed with food or liquid before swallowing.
- Store preferably at 15–30C (59–86F) in tightly closed, light-resistant container unless otherwise directed by manufacturer.

Assessment & Drug Effects

- Optimum therapeutic response generally occurs within 2 wk (e.g., relief of pain, stiffness, or swelling;

or improved joint flexion and strength).

- Patients with history of cardiac decompensation should be observed closely for evidence of fluid retention and edema.
- Baseline and periodic evaluations of Hgb, renal and hepatic function, and auditory and ophthalmologic examinations are recommended in patients receiving prolonged or high-dose therapy.
- Monitor for GI distress and S&S of GI bleeding.
- Symptoms of acute toxicity in children are apnea, cyanosis, response only to painful stimuli, dizziness, and nystagmus.

Patient & Family Education

- Instruct to report immediately passage of dark tarry stools, "coffee ground" emesis, frankly bloody emesis, or other GI distress.
- Advise to report immediately to physician the onset of skin rash, pruritus, jaundice.
- Instruct to report immediately blood or protein in urine.
- Inform about possible CNS effects (light-headedness, dizziness, drowsiness), and caution them to avoid dangerous activities until reaction to the drug has been determined.
- Avoid self-medication with ibuprofen if taking prescribed drugs or if being treated for a serious condition without consulting physician.
- Avoid taking aspirin or acetaminophen concurrently with ibuprofen.
- Inform patient that alcohol and NSAIDs may increase risk of GI ulceration and bleeding tendencies and, therefore, should be avoided, unless otherwise advised by physician.

IBUTILIDE FUMARATE

(i-bu′ti-lide)

Trade name: Corvert

Classifications: CARDIOVASCULAR AGENT; ANTIARRHYTHMIC AGENT

Prototype: Procainamide

Pregnancy category: C

ACTIONS/PHARMACODYNAMICS

Ibutilide is a class III antiarrhythmic agent. It prolongs the cardiac action potential and increases both atrial and ventricular refractoriness (i.e., class III antiarrhythmic electrophysiologic effects).

USES Rapid conversion of atrial fibrillation or atrial flutter of recent onset.

ROUTE & DOSAGE

Atrial Fibrillation or Flutter

Adult: **IV** *Weight ≥60 kg:* 1 mg (10 ml), may repeat in 10 min if inadequate response. *Weight <60 kg:* 0.01 mg/kg (0.1 ml/kg), may repeat in 10 min if inadequate response.

PHARMACOKINETICS **Onset:** 30 min. **Metabolism:** metabolized in liver. **Elimination:** half-life: 6 h (range 2–21 h); 82% excreted in urine, 19% in feces.

CONTRAINDICATIONS & PRECAUTIONS **Contraindicated in:** hypersensitivity to ibutilide, pregnancy (category C), hypokalemia, hypomagnesia. **Cautious use in:** history of CHF, low ejection fraction, recent MI, prolonged QT intervals, liver disease, cardiovascular disorder other than atrial arrhythmias, other drugs that prolong QT interval, lactation. Safety and effectiveness in children < 18 y not established.

ADVERSE/SIDE EFFECTS CNS: headache. **CV:** proarrhythmic effects (sustained and nonsustained polymorphic ventricular tachycardia), AV block, bundle branch block, ventricular extrasystoles, hypotension, postural hypotension, bradycardia, tachycardia, palpitations, prolonged QT segment. **GI:** nausea.

DRUG INTERACTIONS Increased potential for proarrhythmic effects when administered with **astemizole,** PHENOTHIAZINES, TRICYCLIC ANTIDEPRESSANTS, **terfenadine. Amiodarone, disopyramide, quinidine, procainamide, sotalol** may cause prolonged refractoriness if given within 4 h of ibutilide.

NURSING IMPLICATIONS

Administration

- IV preparation and administration: Contents of 1-mg vial may be given undiluted or diluted in 50 ml of 0.9% NaCl or 5% dextrose to a concentration of 0.017 mg/ml. Infuse over 10 min.
- Stop IV infusion as soon as presenting arrhythmia is terminated or with appearance of ventricular tachycardia or marked prolongation of QT or QT_c.
- Class Ia and other class III antiarrhythmic drugs should not be given concurrently or within 4 h of ibutilide.
- Diluted solution is stable for 24 h at 15–30C (59–86F) or 48 h refrigerated at 2–8C (36–46F).

Assessment & Drug Effects

- Hypokalemia and hypomagnesemia should be corrected prior to treatment with ibutilide.
- Observe with continuous ECG, BP, and HR monitoring during and for at least 4 h after infusion or until QT_c has returned to baseline. Monitor for longer periods with liver dysfunction or if proarrhythmic activity is observed.
- Conversion to normal sinus rhythm normally occurs within 30 min of initiation of infusion.

Patient & Family Education

- Patients should be well informed of the potential risks of ibutilide therapy.

IDARUBICIN

(i-da-a-roo′bi-cin)

Trade names: Idamycin, Idamycin PFS

Classifications: ANTINEOPLASTIC ANTIBIOTIC; IMMUNOSUPPRESSANT

Prototype: Doxorubicin

Pregnancy category: D

ACTIONS/PHARMACODYNAMICS Cytotoxic anthracycline antibiotic and derivative of daunorubicin. Idarubicin's potency is greater than that of daunorubicin or doxorubicin. It may be less cardiotoxic than other anthracyclines. Idarubicin exhibits inhibitory efforts on DNA and RNA polymerase and, therefore, on nucleic acid synthesis. Intensive maintenance with idarubicin is not recommended due to its considerable toxicity, including deaths while patient was in remission of acute myelogenous leukemia (AML).

USES In combination with other antineoplastic drugs for treatment of AML. **Unlabeled uses:** breast cancer, other solid tumors.

ROUTE & DOSAGE

Acute Myelogenous Leukemia (AML)

Adult: **IV** 8–12 mg/m^2 daily for 3 d injected slowly over 10–15 min.

Acute Nonlymphocytic Leukemia, Acute Lymphocytic Leukemia

Child: **IV** 10–12 mg/m²/d for 3 d.

PHARMACOKINETICS Onset: median time to remission 28 d. **Peak:** serum level 4 h. **Duration:** serum levels 120 h. **Distribution:** concentrates in nucleated blood and bone marrow cells. **Metabolism:** metabolized in liver to idarubicinol, which may be as active as idarubicin. **Elimination:** half-life: idarubicin 15–45 h, idarubicinol 45 h; 16% excreted in urine; 17% excreted in bile.

CONTRAINDICATIONS & PRECAUTIONS Contraindicated in: myelosuppression, hypersensitivity to idarubicin or doxorubicin, pregnancy (category D), lactation. **Cautious use in:** impaired renal or hepatic function; patients who have received irradiation or radiotherapy to areas surrounding heart. Safety and efficacy in children not established.

ADVERSE/SIDE EFFECTS CV: CHF, atrial fibrillation, chest pain, MI. **GI:** *nausea, vomiting, diarrhea, abdominal pain,* mucositis. **Hematologic:** *anemia, leukopenia,* thrombocytopenia. **Other:** nephrotoxicity, hepatotoxicity, *alopecia,* rash.

INCOMPATIBILITIES Solution/additive: acyclovir, ALKALINE SOLUTIONS (i.e., **sodium bicarbonate**), **ampicillin/sulbactam, cefazolin, ceftazidime, clindamycin, dexamethasone, etoposide, furosemide, gentamicin, heparin, hydrocortisone, imipenem/cilastatin, meperidine, methotrexate, mezlocillin, sargramostim, sodium bicarbonate, vancomycin, vincristine. Y-site:** same as above.

NURSING IMPLICATIONS

Administration

- Reconstitute 5- and 10-mg vials with 5 and 10 ml, respectively, of 0.9% sodium chloride to yield a concentration of 1 mg/ml. Bacteriostatic diluents are not recommended.
- Caution: Vials are under negative pressure; carefully insert needle into vial to reconstitute. Skin accidently exposed should be washed with soap and water.
- Diluted idarubicin should be given slowly over 10–15 min into tubing of IV 0.9% sodium chloride or 5% dextrose.
- IV administration to infants, children: Verify correct IV concentration and rate of infusion with physician.
- If extravasation is suspected, immediately stop infusion, elevate the arm, and apply ice pack for 1/2 h than q.i.d. for 1/2 h × 3 d.
- Reconstituted solutions are stable for 7 d refrigerated at 2–8C (36–46F) and 72 h at room temperature (15–30C/59–86F)

Assessment & Drug Effects

- Monitor infusion site closely, as extravasation can cause severe local tissue necrosis. Notify physician if pain, erythema, or edema develops at insertion site.
- Monitor hepatic and renal function.
- Monitor cardiac status closely, especially in elderly patients or those with preexisting cardiac disease.
- Carefully monitor hematologic status; during the period of myelosuppression, patients are at high risk for bleeding and infection.
- Monitor for development of hyperuricemia secondary to lysis of leukemic cells.

Patient & Family Education

- Inform patient about all potential adverse reactions to idarubicin.

- Advise patient to anticipate possible development of alopecia.
- Discuss interventions to minimize nausea, vomiting, diarrhea, and stomatitis.

IDOXURIDINE (IDU)

(eye-dox-yoor′i-deen)

Trade names: Herplex Liquifilm, IDU, Stoxil

Classifications: ANTIINFECTIVE; ANTIVIRAL

Prototype: Acyclovir

Pregnancy category: C

I

ACTIONS/PHARMACODYNAMICS Topical antiviral agent. Pyrimidine nucleoside structurally related to thymidine, a metabolite essential for synthesis of DNA. Antiviral activity is primarily due to inhibition of viral replication. Inhibits growth of herpes simplex types I and II, varicella-zoster, vaccinia, cytomegalovirus, and small animal viruses containing DNA. Not effective against RNA viruses. Epithelial viral infections characterized by a dendritic figure respond well to the antiviral activity especially during initial attacks. Chronic or recurrent viral infections that involve deep stromal structures (e.g., herpetic iritis) respond less well and do not heal. Some resistant strains of herpes simplex have been reported.

USE Herpes simplex keratitis as single agent or conjunctively with a corticosteroid. **Unlabeled use:** cutaneous herpes simplex.

ROUTE & DOSAGE

Herpes Simplex Keratitis

Adult/Child: **Topical** 1 drop instilled in conjunctival sac q1h during the day and q2h at night until improvement occurs; then decrease to q2h during the day and q4h at night; use ointment q4h during the day with the last dose at bedtime (5 applications/d).

PHARMACOKINETICS Absorption: poorly absorbed from eye tissues. **Distribution:** crosses placenta. **Metabolism:** metabolized in liver.

CONTRAINDICATIONS & PRECAUTIONS Contraindicated in: hypersensitivity to idoxuridine, iodine or iodine-containing preparations, or any components in the formulation. **Cautious use in:** pregnancy (category C), lactation; corticosteroid therapy.

ADVERSE/SIDE EFFECTS Eye: local irritation, pain, burning, lacrimation, pruritus, inflammation, or edema of eyes, lids, and surrounding face; follicular conjunctivitis, photophobia; corneal ulceration and swelling; delayed healing. **Systemic absorption:** stomatitis, anorexia, nausea, vomiting, alopecia, leukopenia, thrombocytopenia, iodism, hepatotoxicity. **Overdosage** (local): small defects in corneal epithelium. **Other:** sensitization.

NURSING IMPLICATIONS

Administration

- To prevent the possibility of systemic absorption, apply light finger pressure to head of lacrimal duct for 1 min when eyedrop is instilled.
- Follow manufacturer's directions regarding storage. Decomposed idoxuridine not only has reduced antiviral activity but also may be toxic.
- Ophthalmic solution should be refrigerated at 2–8C (36–46F) in a tight, light-resistant container unless otherwise directed. The oint-

ment should be stored at 2–15C (36–59F).

Assessment & Drug Effects

- Epithelial infections usually improve within 7–8 d. If patient continues to improve, therapy is generally continued ≤ 21 d.
- Patients should be closely supervised by ophthalmologist.

Patient & Family Education

- Instruct patient in proper technique for eye drop instillation.
- The recommended frequency and duration of therapy must not be exceeded.
- If photosensitivity is troublesome, advise patient to wear sunglasses.

IFOSFAMIDE

(i-fos′-fa-mide)

Trade name: Ifex

Classifications: ANTINEOPLASTIC; ALKYLATING AGENT

Prototype: Cyclophosphamide

Pregnancy category: D

ACTIONS/PHARMACODYNAMICS Ifosfamide is a chemotherapeutic agent chemically related to nitrogen mustards. The alkylated metabolites of ifosfamide interact with DNA. Cytotoxic action is primarily due to cross-linking of strands of DNA and RNA, as well as inhibition of protein synthesis.

USES In combination with other agents in various regimens for germ cell testicular cancer, soft tissue sarcomas, Ewing's sarcoma, and non-Hodgkin's lymphoma. Also for lung and pancreatic sarcoma.

ROUTE & DOSAGE

Antineoplastic

Adult: **IV** 1.2 g/m^2/d for 5 consecutive d; administer over at least 30 min; repeat q3wk or after recovery from hematologic toxicity (platelets ≥ 100,000/mm^3; WBC ≥ 4,000/mm^3).

PHARMACOKINETICS **Distribution:** distributed into breast milk. **Metabolism:** metabolized in liver to active form. **Elimination:** half-life: 7–15 h; 70–86% excreted in urine.

CONTRAINDICATIONS & PRECAUTIONS **Contraindicated in:** patients with severe bone marrow depression or who have demonstrated previous hypersensitivity to ifosfamide. **Cautious use in:** impaired renal function, prior radiation or prior therapy with other cytotoxic agents; pregnancy (category D) and nursing mothers.

ADVERSE/SIDE EFFECTS **CNS:** *somnolence, confusion, hallucinations,* coma, dizziness, seizures, cranial nerve dysfunction. **GI:** *nausea, vomiting,* anorexia, diarrhea, metabolic acidosis, hepatic dysfunction. **Hematologic:** neutropenia, thrombocytopenia. **GU:** hemorrhagic cystitis, nephrotoxicity. **Other:** *alopecia,* skin necrosis with extravasation.

DRUG INTERACTIONS HEPATIC ENZYME INDUCERS (BARBITURATES, **phenytoin, chloral hydrate**) may increase hepatic conversion of ifosfamide to active metabolite; CORTICOSTEROIDS may inhibit conversion to active metabolites.

NURSING IMPLICATIONS

Administration

- Prepare IV solution of drug by diluting 1 g in 20 ml of sterile water or bacteriostatic water with a final concentration of 50 mg/ml. Solution prepared with sterile water should be used within 6 h. Solution prepared with bacteriostatic

I

solution is stable for a week at 30C or 6 wk at 5C.

- Solutions for intermittent IV infusion may be prepared by further dilution of drug with 5% dextrose injection, 0.9% NaCl injection, or lactated Ringer's injection. Administer over 30 min.
- Reconstituted solutions are stable for 1 wk at 30C (86F) and 3 wk at 5C (41F).

Assessment & Drug Effects

- Monitor CBC with differential before each dose is given and at regular intervals.
- Hold ifosfamide if WBC count is below 2000/mm^3 or platelet count is below 50,000/mm^3.
- Monitor urinalysis prior to each dose for microscopic hematuria.
- To reduce the risk of hemorrhagic cystitis, hydration with 3000 ml of fluid daily is recommended prior to ifosfamide therapy and for at least 72 h following treatment to ensure ample urine output.
- Therapy should be discontinued if any of the following CNS symptoms occur: somnolence, confusion, depressive psychosis, and hallucinations.

Patient & Family Education

- Instruct patient to void frequently to lessen contact of irritating chemical with bladder mucosa.
- Advise patient that susceptibility to infection may increase and to avoid people with infection. Should report any infection, fever or chills, cough or hoarseness, lower back or side pain, painful or difficult urination.
- Advise patient to check with physician immediately if there is any unusual bleeding or bruising, black tarry stools, or blood in urine or if pinpoint red spots develop on skin.
- Advise patient of possible side effects (e.g., alopecia, nausea, and vomiting) and measures that can be taken to minimize them.

IMIPENEM-CILASTATIN SODIUM

(i-mi-pen'em sye-la-stat'in)

Trade name: Primaxin

Prototype for classifications: ANTIINFECTIVE; BETA-LACTAM ANTIBIOTIC

Pregnancy category: C

ACTIONS/PHARMACODYNAMICS

Fixed combination of imipenem, a beta-lactam antibiotic, and cilastatin, an inhibitor of dipeptidase inactivation of imipenem. Action of imipenem: inhibition of mucopeptide synthesis in bacterial cell walls leading to cell death. Has the greatest microbiologic spectrum of any beta-lactam antibiotic, surpassing that of all the third-generation cephalosporins. Acts synergistically with aminoglycoside antibiotics against some isolates of *Pseudomonas aeruginosa*. Infections resistant to cephalosporins, penicillins, and aminoglycosides have responded to treatment with this combination.

USES Treatment of serious infections caused by susceptible organisms in the urinary tract, lower respiratory tract, bones and joints, skin and skin structures; also intraabdominal, gynecologic, and mixed infections; bacterial septicemia and endocarditis.

ROUTE & DOSAGE

Serious Infections

Adult: **IV** 250–500 mg infused over 20–30 min q6–8h; up to 1 g

infused over 40–60 min q6h. **IM** 500 or 750 mg q12h.
Child: **IV** 10–15 mg/kg q6h. **IM** 15–25 mg/kg q12h.
Neonate: **IV** 20–40 mg/kg/d divided q12–24h.
Adjustment for Renal Impairment
Cl_{cr} 20–30 ml/min: dose q8–12h; <20 ml/min: dose q12h.

PHARMACOKINETICS Distribution: widely distributed; limited concentrations in CSF; crosses placenta; in breast milk. **Elimination:** half-life: 1 h; 70% of dose excreted in urine within 10 h.

CONTRAINDICATIONS & PRECAUTIONS Contraindicated in: hypersensitivity to any component of product, multiple allergens. Safe use in pregnancy (category C) or in children <12 y not established. **Cautious use in:** nursing mothers, patients with CNS disorders (e.g., seizures, brain lesions, history of recent head injury); renal impairment; patients with history of penicillin allergies.

ADVERSE/SIDE EFFECTS CNS: seizures, dizziness, confusion, somnolence, encephalopathy, myoclonus, tremors, paresthesia, headache. **GI:** *nausea, vomiting*, diarrhea, pseudomembranous colitis, hemorrhagic colitis, gastroenteritis, abdominal pain, glossitis, heartburn. **Hypersensitivity:** rash, fever, chills, dyspnea, pruritus. **Respiratory:** chest discomfort, hyperventilation, dyspnea. **Skin:** rash, pruritus, urticaria, candidiasis, flushing, increased sweating, skin texture change, facial edema. **Other:** hyponatremia, hyperkalemia, transient hearing loss, weakness, oliguria/anuria, polyuria, polyarthralgia; *phlebitis and pain at injection site.* Altered laboratory findings: increased WBC, AST, ALT, alkaline phosphatase, BUN, LDH, creatinine; decreased Hgb, Hct, eosinophilia, superinfections.

DRUG INTERACTIONS Aztreonam, cephalosporins, penicillins may antagonize the antibacterial effects.

INCOMPATIBILITIES Solution/additive: Ringer's lactate, stable in dextrose-containing solutions for only 4 h.

NURSING IMPLICATIONS

Administration

- IM administration: Administer IM suspension by deep injection into the gluteal muscle.
- Use reconstituted IM injection within 1 h after preparation.
- Caution: IM solution should not be given IV, and IV solution should not be given IM.
- IV preparation: Follow manufacturer's recommendation for preparation of infusion solution. Dilute each dose with 10 ml of D5W, NS, or other compatible infusion solution. After reconstitution the resulting solution contains 2.5 mg/ml, or 5 mg/ml. Agitate the solution until clear. Color should range from colorless to yellow. Further dilute with 100 ml of selected infusion solution.
- IV administration to neonates, infants, children: Verify correct IV concentration and rate of infusion with physician.
- Caution for IV administration: Imipenem-cilastatin is not intended for direct or bolus injection. Administer each 500 mg or fraction thereof over 20–30 min.
- Nausea appears to be related to infusion rate, and if it presents during infusion, slow the rate. Occurs most frequently with 1-g doses.
- Stability of IV solutions depends on diluent used for reconstitution.

Consult manufacturer's recommendations. Most IV solutions retain potency for 4 h at 15–30C (59–86F) or for 24 h if refrigerated at 4C (39F). Avoid freezing.

Assessment & Drug Effects

- Determine previous hypersensitivity reaction to beta-lactam antibiotics (penicillins and cephalosporins) or to other allergens.
- Monitor for S&S of hypersensitivity (see Appendix G). Discontinue drug and notify physician if S&S occur.
- Monitor closely patients vulnerable to CNS adverse effects.
- If focal tremors, myoclonus, or seizures occur, notify physician. Dosage modification may prevent seizure recurrence.
- Monitor for S&S of superinfection (see Appendix G).
- If severe diarrhea accompanied by abdominal pain and fever occurs, pseudomembranous enterocolitis (see Appendix G) should be ruled out. Notify physician promptly.
- The sodium content derived from cilastatin sodium and sodium bicarbonate buffer in the fixed combination is about 0.8 mEq (18.4 mg) in the 250 mg dose. This should be considered in patient on restricted sodium intake.
- Periodically monitor renal, hematologic, and liver function.

Patient & Family Education

- Instruct patient to immediately report pruritus or symptoms of respiratory distress.
- Instruct patient to report loose stools or diarrhea promptly.
- Instruct patient to report pain or discomfort at IV infusion site since phlebitis occurs in approximately 3% of patients.

IMIPRAMINE HYDROCHLORIDE

(im-ip′ra-meen)

Trade names: Impril ♣, Janimine, Novopramine ♣, Tofranil

IMIPRAMINE PAMOATE

Trade name: Tofranil-PM

Prototype for classifications: CNS AGENT; PSYCHOTHERAPEUTIC; TRICYCLIC ANTIDEPRESSANT

Pregnancy category: C

ACTIONS/PHARMACODYNAMICS

Tricyclic antidepressant (TCA) and tertiary amine, structurally related to the phenothiazines. In contrast with phenothiazines, which act on dopamine receptors, TCAs potentiate both norepinephrine and serotonin in the CNS by blocking their reuptake by presynaptic neurons. Decreases number of awakenings from sleep, markedly reduces time in REM sleep, and increases stage 4 sleep. Relief of nocturnal enuresis is perhaps due to anticholinergic activity and to nervous system stimulation, resulting in earlier arousal to sensation of full bladder.

USES Endogenous depression and occasionally for reactive depression. Imipramine is the only TCA used as temporary adjuvant treatment of enuresis in children > 6 y. **Unlabeled uses:** certain syndromes that mimic or overlap diagnostically with depression: alcoholism, cocaine withdrawal; attention deficit disorder with or without hyperactivity (children > 6 y and adolescents); with amphetamines or methylphenidate for narcolepsy; phobic anxiety syndromes such as panic disorders and agoraphobia; obsessive-compulsive neurosis; chronic intractable pain.

ROUTE & DOSAGE

Depression

Adult: **PO** 75–100 mg/d (up to 300 mg/d) in 1 or more divided doses. **IM** 50–100 mg/d in divided doses.
Child: **PO** 1.5 mg/kg/d; may increase by 1 mg/kg/d q3–4d to a max of 5 mg/kg/d.

Enuresis in Childhood

Child: **PO** 25 mg 1 h before bedtime; *< 12 y,* may increase to 50 mg nightly (max dose 2.5 mg/kg); *> 12 y,* may increase to 75 mg nightly (max dose 2.5 mg/kg).

PHARMACOKINETICS Absorption: Completely absorbed from GI tract. **Peak:** 1–2 h PO; 30 min IM. **Metabolism:** metabolized to the active metabolite desipramine in liver. **Elimination:** half-life: 8–16 h; primarily excreted in urine, small amount in feces; crosses placenta; may be secreted in breast milk.

CONTRAINDICATIONS & PRECAUTIONS Contraindicated in: hypersensitivity to tricyclic drugs; acute recovery period after MI, defects in bundle-branch conduction; severe renal or hepatic impairment; use of hydrochloride in children < 12 y except to treat enuresis; use of pamoate in children of any age. Safe use during pregnancy (category D) and in nursing mothers not established. **Cautious use in:** children, adolescents, the elderly; respiratory difficulties; cardiovascular, hepatic, or GI diseases; blood disorders; increased intraocular pressure, narrow-angle glaucoma; schizophrenia, hypomania or manic episodes, patient with suicidal tendency, seizure disorders; prostatic hypertrophy, urinary retention; alcoholism, hyperthyroidism; electroshock therapy.

ADVERSE/SIDE EFFECTS CNS: *sedation, drowsiness,* dizziness, headache, fatigue, numbness, tingling (paresthesias) of extremities; incoordination, ataxia, tremors, peripheral neuropathy, extrapyramidal symptoms (including parkinsonism effects and tardive dyskinesia); lowered seizure threshold, altered EEG patterns, delirium, disturbed concentration, confusion, hallucinations, anxiety, nervousness, insomnia, vivid dreams, restlessness, agitation, shift to hypomania, mania; exacerbation of psychoses; hyperpyrexia. **CV:** *orthostatic hypotension,* mild sinus tachycardia; *arrhythmias,* hypertension or hypotension, palpitation, MI, CHF, *heart block,* ECG changes, stroke, flushing, cold cyanotic hands and feet (peripheral vasospasm). **Endocrine:** testicular swelling, gynecomastia (men), galactorrhea and breast enlargement (women), increased or decreased libido, ejaculatory and erectile disturbances, delayed or absent orgasm (male and female); elevation or depression of blood glucose levels. **ENT:** nasal congestion, tinnitus. **Eye:** *blurred vision,* disturbances of accommodation, *slight mydriasis,* nystagmus. **GI:** *dry mouth,* constipation, heartburn, excessive appetite, weight gain, nausea, vomiting, diarrhea, slowed gastric emptying time, flatulence, abdominal cramps, esophageal reflux, anorexia, stomatitis, increased salivation, black tongue, peculiar taste, paralytic ileus. **GU:** *urinary retention,* delayed micturition, nocturia, paradoxic urinary frequency. **Hematologic:** bone marrow depression; agranulocytosis, eosinophilia, thrombocytopenia. **Hypersensitivity:** skin rash, erythema, petechiae, urticaria, pruritus, pho-

I

tosensitivity, angioedema (face, tongue, generalized); drug fever. **Other:** excessive perspiration, cholestatic jaundice, precipitation of acute intermittent porphyria; dyspnea, changes in heat and cold tolerance, hair loss, syndrome of inappropriate antidiuretic hormone secretion (SIADH).

DIAGNOSTIC TEST INTERFERENCE Imipramine elevates ***serum bilirubin, alkaline phosphatase*** and may increase or decrease ***blood glucose.*** It decreases ***urinary 5-HIAA*** and ***VMA*** excretion and may falsely increase excretion of ***urinary catecholamines.***

DRUG INTERACTIONS MAO INHIBITORS may precipitate hyperpyrexic crisis, tachycardia, or seizures; ANTIHYPERTENSIVE AGENTS potentiate orthostatic hypotension; CNS DEPRESSANTS, **alcohol** add to CNS depression; **norepinephrine** and other SYMPATHOMIMETICS may increase cardiac toxicity; **cimetidine** decreases hepatic metabolism, thus increasing imipramine levels; **methylphenidate** inhibits metabolism of imipramine and thus may increase its toxicity.

NURSING IMPLICATIONS

Administration

- Administer with or immediately after food.
- Single doses can be given h.s. or qAM, respectively, if drowsiness or insomnia results.
- Crystals may form in some ampuls of injectable imipramine. To dissolve them, immerse intact ampul in warm water for about 1 min.
- Dose adjustments are not made more frequently than q4d.
- Store at 15–30C (59–86F).

Assessment & Drug Effects

- Dose sensitivity and side effects are most likely to occur in adolescents and the elderly. A lower initial dose should be used for these patients.
- Signs of therapeutic effectiveness of TCAs may not occur for 2 wk or more after initiation of imipramine.
- Periodically monitor hepatic and renal function, CBC with differential, and fluid and electrolyte balance.
- Monitor HR and BP frequently. Orthostatic hypotension tends to be mild in normotensive individuals but may be marked in pretreatment hypertensive or cardiac patients.
- Accurate early reporting to physician about patient's response to drug therapy is essential to prevent serious adverse effects.
- During the first 2 wk of therapy, elderly patients sometimes develop confusional reaction: restlessness, disturbed sleep, forgetfulness. Symptoms last 3–20 d. Report to physician.
- Weigh patient under standard conditions at least biweekly: a gain of 0.5–1.0 kg ($1\frac{1}{2}$–2 lb) within 2–3 d and frank edema should be reported.
- Monitor urinary and bowel elimination, at least until maintenance dosage is stabilized, to detect urinary retention or frequency, constipation, or paralytic ileus.
- Report promptly early signs of agranulocytosis (see Appendix G).
- Report signs of cholestatic jaundice: flu-like symptoms, yellow skin or sclerae, dark urine, light-colored stools, pruritus.
- Extrapyramidal symptoms (tremors, twitching, ataxia, incoordination, hyperreflexia, drooling) may occur in patients receiving large doses and especially in the elderly. Notify physician if they are noted.
- Hyperglycemia or hypoglycemia (see Signs & Symptoms, Appendix

G) may occur in some patients. Diabetic patients should be monitored for loss of glycemic control, particularly during early therapy.

- Frequently inspect oral mucosa, especially gingival surfaces under dentures.
- Overdose onset may be sudden. Monitoring should focus on the following potential signs of toxicity: QRS prolongation (to 100 ms or greater), arrhythmias, hypotension, respiratory depression, altered level of consciousness, seizures.

Patient & Family Education

- Instruct patient to change position slowly and in stages, especially from recumbency to upright posture and to dangle legs over bed for a few minutes before ambulation.
- In some patients, effectiveness decreases with continued drug administration. Counsel parent to inform physician if this occurs.
- Advise not to use OTC drugs while on a TCA unless physician approves.
- Warn to avoid hazardous tasks until drug response is known.
- Exposure to strong sunlight should be avoided because of potential photosensitivity. Advise use of sunscreen lotion with sun protection factor (SPF) of 12–15 if allowed.

IMMUNE GLOBULIN INTRAMUSCULAR (IGIM, GAMMA GLOBULIN, IMMUNE SERUM GLOBULIN [ISG])

Trade names: Gamastan, Gammar

IMMUNE GLOBULIN INTRAVENOUS (IGIV)

Trade names: Gamimune N, Gammagard, Gammar-P IV, IGIV, Iveegam, Sandoglobulin, Venoglobulin-S

Classifications: SERUM; IMMUNIZING AGENT

Pregnancy category: C

ACTIONS/PHARMACODYNAMICS

Sterile concentrated solution containing globulin (primarily IgG) prepared from large pools of normal human plasma of either venous or placental origin and processed by a special fractionating technique. Like hepatitis B immune globulin (HBIG), contains antibody specific to hepatitis B surface antigen but in lower concentrations. Therefore, not considered treatment of first choice for postexposure prophylaxis against hepatitis B but usually an acceptable alternative when HBIG is not available. Also much less expensive than HBIG. Nonreactive when tested for hepatitis B.

USES IGIM: in susceptible persons to provide passive immunity or to modify severity of certain infectious diseases, e.g., rubeola (measles), rubella (German measles), varicella-zoster (chickenpox), type A (infectious) hepatitis, and as replacement therapy in congenital agammaglobulinemia or IgG deficiency diseases. May be used as an alternative to HBIG to provide passive immunity in hepatitis B infection. Also for post-exposure prophylaxis of hepatitis non-A, non-B, and nonspecific hepatitis. **IGIV:** principally as maintenance therapy in patients unable to manufacture sufficient quantities of IgG antibodies, in patients requiring an immediate increase in immunoglobulin levels, and when IM injections are contraindicated as in patients with bleeding disorders or who have small muscle mass. Also in chronic autoimmune thrombocytopenia and idiopathic thrombocytopenic purpura (ITP). **Unlabeled uses:** Kawasaki syndrome, chronic lymphocytic leukemia, AIDS, premature and low-birth-weight neonates, autoimmune neutropenia or hemolytic anemia.

ROUTE & DOSAGE

Hepatitis A Exposure

Adult: **IM** 0.02 ml/kg as soon as possible after exposure; if period of exposure will be ≥ 3 mo, give 0.05–0.06 ml/kg once q4–6mo.
Child: **IM** Same as for adult.

Hepatitis B Exposure

Adult: **IM** 0.02–0.06 ml/kg as soon as possible after exposure if HBIG is unavailable.
Child: **IM** Same as for adult.

Rubella Exposure

Adult: **IM** 20 ml as single dose in susceptible pregnant women.

Rubeola Exposure

Adult: **IM** 0.25 ml/kg within 6 d of exposure.
Child: **IM** Same as for adult.

Varicella-zoster Exposure

Adult: **IM** 0.6–1.2 ml/kg promptly.
Child: **IM** Same as for adult.

Immunoglobulin Deficiency

Adult: **IV** Gammagard, Gamimune: 100 mg/kg/mo; Sandoglobulin, Venoglobulin: 200 mg/kg/mo;
IM 1.2 ml/kg followed by 0.6 ml/kg q2–4wk.
Child: **IV** Gammagard, Gamimune; same as for adult; Sandoglobulin, Venoglobulin: same as for adult;
IM Same as for adult.

Idiopathic Thrombocytopenia Purpura

Adult: **IV** 400 mg/kg/d for 5 consecutive d *or* 1 g/kg qod for up to 3 doses.
Child: **IV** Same as for adult.

PHARMACOKINETICS **Peak:** 2 d. **Distribution:** rapidly and evenly distributed to intravascular and extravascular fluid compartments. **Elimination:** half-life: 21–23 d.

CONTRAINDICATIONS & PRECAUTIONS **Contraindicated in:** history of anaphylaxis or severe reaction to human immune serum globulin (IG) or to any ingredient in the formulation such as thimerosal (mercury derivative) preservative in IM formulations and maltose (stabilizing agent) in IV formulations; persons with clinical hepatitis A; IGIV for patients with class-specific anti-IgA deficiencies; IGIM in severe thrombocytopenia or other bleeding disorders. Safe use during pregnancy (category C) not established.

ADVERSE/SIDE EFFECTS **IGIM:** *pain, tenderness, muscle stiffness at IM site;* local inflammatory reaction, erythema, urticaria, angioedema, headache, malaise, fever, arthralgia, nephrotic syndrome, hypersensitivity (fever, chills, anaphylactic shock). **IGIV (mostly related to rate of administration):** *nausea, flushing, chills,* headache, chest tightness, wheezing, skeletal pain, back pain, abdominal cramps, anaphylaxis.

DRUG INTERACTIONS May interfere with antibody response to LIVE VIRUS VACCINES (measles/mumps/rubella); give vaccines 14 d before or 3 mo after immune globulins.

NURSING IMPLICATIONS

Administration

- Hepatitis A (infectious hepatitis): immune globulin is most effective when given before or as soon as possible after exposure but not more than 2 wk after (incubation period for hepatitis A is 15–50 d). Persons who are already presenting clinical manifestations of hepatitis A should not receive immune globulin.

- Hepatitis B (serum hepatitis): immune globulin is administered preferably within 24 h and not more than 7 d after exposure.
- Note that IGIM is intended only for IM use and that IGIV is meant only for IV use. They are not interchangeable.
- IM administration: For adults and older children, IM injections are made preferably into deltoid or anterolateral aspect of thigh; in neonates and small children, into anterolateral aspect of thigh.
- Gluteal injections are generally avoided; however, when large volumes of immune globulin are prescribed or when large doses must be divided into several injections, the upper outer quadrant of the gluteus has been used in adults.
- IV administration: Venoglobulin-1 and Gammagard are packaged with the diluent and transfer device. Gamimune N may be given undiluted or diluted to a 5% solution. Sandoglobulin is provided with enough diluent to make a 3% solution.
- Infusion flow rates vary with product being infused. Gamimune is generally started at 0.01–0.02 ml/kg/min for 30 min; if tolerated, rate is increased to 0.02–0.04 ml/kg/min. The initial flow rate for Sandoglobulin is 0.5–1 ml/min. If tolerated after 15–30 min, rate is increased to 1.5–2.5 ml/min.
- Refer to manufacturer's directions for information on reconstitution, dilution, and flow IV rates.
- Store Gamimune at 2–8C (36–46F); store Sandoglobulin below 20C (68F) unless otherwise directed. Avoid freezing. Do not use if turbidity has occurred or if product has been frozen. Do not mix with other drugs. Discard partially used vial.

Assessment & Drug Effects

- Emergency drugs and appropriate emergency facilities should be immediately available for treatment of anaphylaxis or sensitization.
- Hypersensitivity reactions (see Appendix G) are most likely to occur in patients receiving large IM doses, repeated injections, or rapid IV infusion of immune globulin.
- When patient is receiving IGIV, monitor vital signs continuously and closely monitor infusion rate.
- IGIV may have a mild diuretic effect in some patients because of the presence of maltose in the formulation.

Patient & Family Education

- Advise to immediately report S&S of hypersensitivity (see Appendix G).
- During IV infusion, instruct to report immediately such symptoms as nausea, chills, headache, and chest tightness during IV infusion. Such side effects may be an indication to slow rate of infusion.
- Measles (rubeola): After immune globulin administration, passive immunity lasts about 3–4 wk. In general, patients who are ≤ 15 mo should receive active immunization with measles virus vaccine (unless it is contraindicated) 3 mo after administration of IGIM.

INDAPAMIDE

(in-dap′a-mide)

Trade names: Lozide ♣, Lozol

Classifications: ELECTROLYTIC AND WATER BALANCE AGENT; THIAZIDE-LIKE DIURETIC

Prototype: Hydrochlorothiazide

Pregnancy category: B

ACTIONS/PHARMACODYNAMICS Sulfonamide derivative. Has both diuretic and direct vascular effects; action mechanism is similar to that of the thiazide diuretics. Principal site of action is on the proximal portion of the distal renal tubules. Enhances excretion of sodium, potassium, and water by interfering with sodium transfer across renal epithelium. Hypotensive activity in the hypertensive patient appears to result from a decrease in plasma and extracellular fluid volume, decreased peripheral vascular resistance, direct arteriolar dilation, and calcium channel blockade. Augments the action of other hypotensive agents.

USES Alone or with other antihypertensives as step 1 agent in the management of hypertension in patients who have failed to respond to diet, exercise, or weight reduction. **Unlabeled use:** edema associated with CHF.

ROUTE & DOSAGE

Hypertension, Edema

Adult: **PO** 2.5 mg once/d; may increase to 5 mg/d if needed.

PHARMACOKINETICS **Absorption:** readily absorbed from GI tract. **Peak:** 2–2.5 h. **Duration:** up to 36 h. **Metabolism:** metabolized in liver. **Elimination:** half-life: 14–18 h; 60% excreted in urine; 16–23% excreted in feces.

CONTRAINDICATIONS & PRECAUTIONS **Contraindicated in:** hypersensitivity to indapamide or other sulfonamide derivatives, anuria. Safe use during pregnancy (category B), lactation, and in children not established. **Cautious use in:** electrolyte imbalance, severe renal disease; impaired hepatic function or progressive liver disease; hypokalemia; prediabetic and type II diabetic patient, hyperparathyroidism, thyroid disorders; SLE; sympathectomized patient; history of gout.

ADVERSE/SIDE EFFECTS **CNS/Neuromuscular:** headache, dizziness, fatigue, weakness, muscle cramps or spasm, paresthesia, tension, anxiety, nervousness, agitation, vertigo, insomnia, mental depression, blurred vision, drowsiness. **CV:** orthostatic hypotension, PVCs, dysrhythmias, flushing, palpitation. **GI:** dry mouth, anorexia, nausea, vomiting, diarrhea, constipation, abdominal cramps or pain. **GU:** urinary frequency, nocturia, polyuria, glycosuria, impotence or reduced libido. **Skin:** rash, hives, pruritus, vasculitis, photosensitivity. **Other:** dilutional hyponatremia, *hyperuricemia,* exacerbation of gout; *hypokalemia,* hyperglycemia, hypochloremia, hypercalcemia, increased BUN or creatinine, weight loss, exacerbation of SLE; increased cholesterol.

DIAGNOSTIC TEST INTERFERENCE Since indapamide may cause hypercalcemia (and hypophosphatemia), it is generally withheld before tests for ***parathyroid function*** are performed.

DRUG INTERACTIONS Effects of **diazoxide** and indapamide intensified; increased risk of **digoxin** toxicity with hypokalemia; decreased renal **lithium** clearance may increase risk of lithium toxicity.

NURSING IMPLICATIONS

Administration

- Give with food or milk to reduce GI irritation.
- Administer in AM to prevent nocturia. Urge patient to take at least 240 ml (8 oz) of fluid (if allowed) with the medication.
- Store in tight, light-resistant con-

tainer at 15–30C (59–86F) unless otherwise directed.

Assessment & Drug Effects

- Periodically monitor BP throughout course of therapy.
- Obtain baseline data and periodically monitor BUN, serum creatinine, uric acid, blood glucose, serum electrolytes, and fluid balance.
- Monitor for digitalis toxicity in those on concurrent therapy.
- Electrolyte imbalances may become clinically serious in the following situations: protracted vomiting and diarrhea, excessive sweating, GI drainage, and paracentesis.
- Report promptly signs of hyponatremia or hypokalemia (see Appendix G).
- Monitor patients with diabetes for loss of glycemic control.

Patient & Family Education

- Advise how to take medication to avoid GI distress and sleep disturbance.
- Instruct to report decreased urine output, dizziness, weakness or muscle cramps, nausea, jaundice, or blurred vision.
- Inform of risk of photosensitivity; advise precaution with sun exposure.
- Record weight at least every other day and inspect ankles and legs for edema. Report unexplained, progressive weight gain (e.g., 1–1.5 kg [2–3 lb] in 2–3 d).

INDINAVIR SULFATE

(in-din'a-vir)

Trade name: Crixivan

Classifications: ANTIINFECTIVE; ANTIVIRAL; PROTEASE INHIBITOR

Prototype: Saquinavir

Pregnancy category: C

ACTIONS/PHARMACODYNAMICS

Indinavir is an HIV protease inhibitor. HIV protease is an enzyme required to produce the polyprotein precursors of the functional proteins in infectious HIV. Protease inhibitors prevent cleavage of the viral polyproteins, resulting in formation of immature noninfectious virus particles. Indinavir binds to the protease active site and thus inhibits activity of the enzyme.

USE Treatment of HIV infection, usually in combination with other antiretroviral agents or protease inhibitors.

I

ROUTE & DOSAGE

HIV

Adult: **PO** 800 mg (2 × 400 mg) q8h 1 h before or 2 h after meal.

PHARMACOKINETICS Absorption: rapidly absorbed from GI tract; a meal high in calories, fat, and protein significantly reduces absorption. **Distribution:** 60% protein bound. **Metabolism:** metabolized in liver by cytochrome P4503A4 (CYP3A4). **Elimination:** excreted primarily in feces (>80%), 20% excreted in urine.

CONTRAINDICATIONS & PRECAUTIONS Contraindicated in: hypersensitivity to indinavir, lactation. **Cautious use in:** hepatic dysfunction, renal impairment, history of nephrolithiasis, history of adverse responses to other protease inhibitors, pregnancy (category C). Safety and efficacy in children not established.

ADVERSE/SIDE EFFECTS CNS: fatigue, headache, insomnia, dizziness, somnolence, nervousness, agitation, anxiety, paresthesia, peripheral neuropathy, tremor, vertigo. **CV:** palpitations. **Hematologic:** anemia, splenomegaly, lymphadenopathy. **GI:** *nausea*, diarrhea, abdominal discomfort, dyspepsia, stomatitis, anorexia, dry mouth, cholecystitis, cholestasis, constipation, flatulence. **Skin:** body odor, rash, pruritus, seborrhea, skin ulceration, dry skin, sweating, urticaria. **Other:** myalgia, allergic reaction, bronchitis, cough, rhinitis, taste alterations, visual disturbances, hyperglycemia, diabetes, kidney stones.

DRUG INTERACTIONS **Rifabutin, rifampin** significantly decrease indinavir levels. **Ketoconazole** significantly increases indinavir levels. Indinavir could inhibit the metabolism and increase the toxicity of **astemizole, cisapride, midazolam, terfenadine, triazolam.** Indinavir and **didanosine** should be administered at least 1 h apart on empty stomach to permit full absorption of each.

NURSING IMPLICATIONS

Administration

- Preferably given with water on an empty stomach 1 h before or 2 h after meal; if needed, may be given with a very light meal or beverage.
- If didanosine and indinavir are ordered concurrently, give each on empty stomach at least 1 h apart.
- Do not administer concurrently with astemizole, cisapride, midazolam, terfenadine, or triazolam.
- Store tightly closed with desiccant in original bottle at 15–30C (59–86F).

Assessment & Drug Effects

- Periodically monitor CBC with differential and platelet count, liver function tests, CPK, urinalysis, and serum amylase.
- Assess for S&S of renal dysfunction, respiratory dysfunction, GI distress, and other common adverse effects.

Patient & Family Education

- Provide administration and storage directions. If a dose is missed, instruct to take next dose at regularly scheduled time and not to double the dose.
- Advise regarding drug interactions and potential adverse reactions. Encourage adequate hydration to minimize risk of renal stones.
- Advise to report flank pain, hematuria, S&S of jaundice, or other distressing adverse effects.

INDOMETHACIN

(in-doe-meth'a-sin)

Trade names: Indameth, Indocid♣, Indocin, Indocin SR

Classifications: CNS AGENT; ANALGESIC, ANTIPYRETIC; NSAID

Prototype: Ibuprofen

Pregnancy category: B (D in third trimester)

ACTIONS/PHARMACODYNAMICS

Potent nonsteroidal compound with antiinflammatory, analgesic, and antipyretic effects similar to those of aspirin. Antipyretic and antiinflammatory actions may be related to ability to inhibit prostaglandin biosynthesis. Appears to reduce motility of polymorphonuclear leukocytes, development of cellular exudates, and vascular permeability in injured tissue.

USES Palliative treatment in active stages of moderate to severe rheumatoid arthritis, ankylosing rheumatoid spondylitis, acute gouty arthritis, and osteoarthritis of hip in patients intolerant to or unresponsive to adequate trials with salicylates and other therapy. Also used IV to close patent ductus arteriosus in the premature infant. **Unlabeled uses:** to relieve biliary pain and dysmenorrhea, Paget's disease, athletic injuries, juvenile arthritis, idiopathic pericarditis.

ROUTE & DOSAGE

Rheumatoid Arthritis

Adult: **PO** 25–50 mg b.i.d or t.i.d. (max 200 mg/d) *or* 75 mg sustained release 1–2 times/d.

Pediatric Arthritis

Child: **PO** 1–2 mg/kg/d in 2–4 divided doses (max 4 mg/kg/d) or 150–200 mg/d.

Acute Gouty Arthritis

Adult: **PO/PR** 50 mg t.i.d. until pain is tolerable; then rapidly taper off.

Bursitis

Adult: **PO** 25–50 mg t.i.d. or q.i.d. (max 200 mg/d) *or* 75 mg sustained release 1–2 times/d.

Close Patent Ductus Arteriosus

Premature Infant: **IV** *<48 h,* 0.2 mg/kg followed by 2 doses of 0.1 mg/kg q12–24h; *2–7 d,* 0.2 mg/kg followed by 2 doses of 0.2 mg/kg q12–24h; *<7 d,* 0.2 mg/kg followed by 2 doses of 0.25 mg/kg q12–24h.

PHARMACOKINETICS **Absorption:** completely absorbed from GI tract. **Onset:** 1–2 h. **Peak:** 3 h. **Duration:** 4–6 h. **Metabolism:** metabolized in liver. **Elimination:** half-life: 2.5–124 h; excreted primarily in urine.

CONTRAINDICATIONS & PRECAUTIONS **Contraindicated in:** allergy to indomethacin, aspirin, or other NSAID; nasal polyps associated with angioedema, history of GI lesions; pregnancy (category B; D in third trimester), nursing mothers, children (≤14 y). **Cautious use in:** history of psychiatric illness, epilepsy, parkinsonism; impaired renal or hepatic function; uncontrolled infections; coagulation defects, CHF; elderly patients, persons in hazardous occupations.

ADVERSE/SIDE EFFECTS **CNS:** *headache, dizziness,* vertigo, light-headedness, syncope, fatigue, muscle weakness, ataxia, insomnia, nightmares, drowsiness, confusion, coma, convulsions, peripheral neuropathy, psychic disturbances (hallucinations, depersonalization, depression), aggravation of epilepsy, parkinsonism. **CV:** elevated BP, palpitation, chest pains, tachycardia, bradycardia, CHF. **Eye/ear:** blurred vision, lacrimation, eye pain, visual field changes, corneal deposits, retinal disturbances including macula, *tinnitus,* hearing disturbances. **GI:** *nausea, vomiting,* diarrhea, anorexia, bloating, abdominal distention, ulcerative stomatitis, proctitis, rectal bleeding, <u>GI ulceration</u>, <u>hemorrhage</u>, <u>perforation</u>. **Hematologic:** hemolytic anemia, <u>aplastic anemia</u> (sometimes fatal), <u>agranulocytosis</u>, leukopenia, thrombocytopenic purpura, inhibited platelet aggregation. **Hypersensitivity:** rash, purpura, pruritus, urticaria, angioedema, angiitis, rapid fall in blood pressure, dyspnea, asthma syndrome (in aspirin-sensitive patients). **Renal:** renal function impairment, hematuria, urinary frequency. **Other:** epistaxis, hair loss, exfoliative dermatitis, erythema nodosum, vaginal bleeding, breast changes, hyponatremia, hypokalemia, hyperkalemia, hypoglycemia or hyperglycemia, glycosuria (rare), <u>toxic hepatitis</u>, edema, weight gain, flushing, sweating; tissue irritation with extravasation.

DIAGNOSTIC TEST INTERFERENCE Increased ***AST, ALT, bilirubin, BUN;*** positive direct ***Coombs' test.***

DRUG INTERACTIONS ORAL ANTICOAGULANTS, **heparin, alcohol** may prolong bleeding time; may increase **lithium** toxicity; effects of ORAL ANTICOAGULANTS, **phenytoin,** SALICYLATES, SULFONAMIDES, SULFONYLUREAS increased because of protein-binding displacement; increased toxicity including GI bleeding with SALICYLATES, NSAIDS; may blunt effects of ANTIHYPERTENSIVES and DIURETICS.

NURSING IMPLICATIONS

I

Administration

- Administer immediately after meals, or with food, milk, or antacid (if prescribed) to minimize GI side effects.
- Indomethacin rectal suppository use is contraindicated with history of proctitis or recent bleeding.
- IV preparation: Dilute 1 mg with 1 ml of NS or sterile water for injection without preservatives. Resulting concentration (1 mg/ml) may be further diluted with an additional 1 ml for each 1 mg to yield 0.5 mg/ml.
- IV administration: Give diluted solution by direct IV with a single dose given over 5–10 s.
- Discard any unused IV indomethacin, since it contains no preservative.
- Store oral and rectal forms in tight, light-resistant containers at 15–30C (59–86F) unless otherwise directed. Do not freeze.

IV Administration for Patent Ductus Arteriosus

- Avoid extravasation or leakage. Indomethacin IV can be irritating to tissue. Monitor I&O closely and keep physician informed. Indomethacin can cause significant impairment of renal function. It is not unusual for urine output to decrease by 50% or more. Monitor BUN, serum creatinine, glomerular filtration rate, creatinine clearance, and serum electrolytes.

Assessment & Drug Effects

- Question patient carefully regarding aspirin sensitivity before initiation of therapy.
- Patient should be carefully observed and should be instructed to report adverse reactions to prevent serious and sometimes irreversible or fatal effects.
- Periodically monitor renal function, hepatic function, CBC with differential, BP and HR, visual and hearing acuity.
- In patients with underlying cardiovascular disease, the potential for sodium and water retention should be anticipated. Monitor weight and observe dependent areas for signs of edema.
- Green urine has been reported in patients who develop indomethacin-induced hepatitis.

Patient & Family Education

- Expected therapeutic effects in rheumatoid arthritis are reduced fever, increased strength, reduced stiffness, and relief of pain, swelling, and tenderness.
- Therapeutic effect in acute gouty attack (relief of joint tenderness and pain) is usually apparent in 24–36 h; swelling generally disappears in 3–5 d.
- Instruct to report S&S of GI bleeding, visual disturbance, tinnitus, weight gain, or edema.
- Advise not to take aspirin or other NSAIDS as they will potentiate ulcerogenic effects.
- Inform that frontal headache is the most frequent CNS side effect; if it persists, dosage reduction or cessation of drug may be indicated. A bedtime dose, with milk, may reduce the incidence of morning headache.

- Caution to avoid activities requiring mental alertness until reaction to drug is known.

INFLIXIMAB

(in-flix'i-mab)

Trade name: Remicade

Classifications: IMMUNOMODULATOR; TUMOR NECROSIS FACTOR-ALPHA ANTIBODY; IMMUNOGLOBULIN G1 ANTIBODY

Prototype: Basiliximab

Pregnancy category: C

ACTIONS/PHARMACODYNAMICS IgG1-K monoclonal antibody that binds specifically to TNF-alpha, a cytokine. Thus it prevents TNF-alpha from binding to its receptors. TNF-alpha induces proinflammatory cytokines such as interleukin 1 (IL-1) and IL-6. Treatment with infliximab reduces infiltration of inflammatory cells and TNF-alpha production in inflamed areas of the intestine. Elevated concentrations of TNF-alpha have been found in the stools of Crohn's disease patients and correlated with disease activity.

USES Moderately to severely active Crohn's disease, including fistulizing Crohn's disease.

ROUTE & DOSAGE

Crohn's Disease

Adult: **IV** 5 mg/kg infused over at least 2 h; may repeat at 2 and 6 wk for fistulizing disease.

PHARMACOKINETICS **Distribution:** distributed primarily to the vascular compartment. **Elimination:** half-life: 9.5 d.

CONTRAINDICATIONS & PRECAUTIONS **Contraindicated in:** hypersensitivity to infliximab; pregnancy (category C); lactation. **Cautious use in:** history of allergic phenomena or untoward responses to monoclonal antibody preparation; renal or hepatic impairment; muscular sclerosis (potential exacerbation); immunosuppressed patients; elderly. Safety and effectiveness of infliximab in pediatric patients not established.

ADVERSE/SIDE EFFECTS **CNS: Body as whole:** fatigue, fever, pain, myalgia, back pain, chills, hot flashes, arthralgia. **CNS:** *headache,* dizziness, involuntary muscle contractions, paresthesias, vertigo, anxiety, depression, insomnia. **CV:** chest pain, peripheral edema, hypotension, hypertension, tachycardia, anemia. **GI:** nausea, diarrhea, abdominal pain, vomiting, constipation, dyspepsia, flatulence, intestinal obstruction, ulcerative stomatitis, increased hepatic enzymes. **Respiratory:** URI, pharyngitis, bronchitis, rhinitis, coughing, sinusitis, dyspnea. **Skin:** rash, pruritus, acne, alopecia, fungal dermatitis, eczema, dry skin, increased sweating, urticaria. **Other:** infections, development of autoantibodies, lupus-like syndrome, conjunctivitis, dysuria, urinary frequency. **Infusion-related reactions:** fever, chills, pruritus, urticaria, chest pain, hypotension, hypertension, dyspnea.

INCOMPATIBILITIES **Solution/additive:** incompatible with PVC bags and tubing. **Y-site:** should not be infused with any other drugs.

NURSING IMPLICATIONS

Administration

- Do not administer to a patient who has known or suspected sepsis.
- Reconstitute each vial with 10 ml of sterile water for injection, USP, using a 21-gauge or smaller syringe. Inject sterile water against wall of vial, then gently swirl to

dissolve but do not shake. Let stand for 5 min. The solution should be colorless to light yellow with a few translucent particles. Discard if particles are opaque.

- IV preparation: Further dilute reconstituted solution by first removing from a 250-ml IV bag of 0.9% NaCl a volume of 0.9% NaCl equal to the volume of reconstituted infliximab to be added to the IV bag. Slowly add the total volume of reconstituted infliximab solution to the 250-ml infusion bag and gently mix. Infusion concentration should be 0.4 to 4 mg/ml. Begin infusion within 3 h of preparation.
- IV infusion: Administer over ≥2 h using a polyethylene-lined infusion set with an in-line, low-protein-binding filter (pore size 1.2 mm or less). Discard unused infusion solution.
- Store unopened vials at 2–8C (36–46F).

Assessment & Drug Effects

- Therapeutic effectiveness is indicated by improved symptomatology.
- Discontinue IV infusion and notify physician if any of the following develop: fever, chills, pruritus, urticaria, chest pain, dyspnea, hypo/hypertension.
- Monitor for and immediately report S&S of local IV site or more generalized infection.

Patient & Family Education

- Nursing mothers should not receive infliximab.
- Promptly report any infection to your physician.

INSULIN INJECTION (REGULAR)

(in'su-lin)

Trade names: Humulin R, Novolin R, Regular Insulin, Pork Regular Iletin II, Regular Purified Pork Insulin, Velosulin, Velosulin BR, Velosulin Human

Prototype for classifications: SYNTHETIC HORMONE; INSULIN ANTIDIABETIC

Pregnancy category: B

ACTIONS/PHARMACODYNAMICS

Short-acting, clear, colorless solution of exogenous unmodified insulin extracted from beta cells in pork pancreas or synthesized by recombinant DNA technology (human). Enhances transmembrane passage of glucose across cell membranes of most body cells and by unknown mechanism may itself enter the cell to activate selected intermediary metabolic processes. Promotes conversion of glucose to glycogen.

USES Emergency treatment of diabetic ketoacidosis or coma, to initiate therapy in patient with insulin-dependent diabetes mellitus, and in combination with intermediate-acting or long-acting insulin to provide better control of blood glucose concentrations in the diabetic patient. Used IV to stimulate growth hormone secretion (glucose counterregulatory hormone) to evaluate pituitary growth hormone reserve in patient with known or suspected growth hormone deficiency. Other uses include promotion of intracellular shift of potassium in treatment of hyperkalemia (IV) and induction of hypoglycemic shock as therapy in psychiatry.

ROUTE & DOSAGE

Diabetes Mellitus

Adult: **SC** 5–10 U 15–30 min a.c. and h.s.; dose adjustments based on blood glucose determinations.

Child: **SC** 2–4 U 15–30 min a.c. and h.s.; dose adjustments based on blood glucose determinations.

Ketoacidosis

Adult: **IV** 2.4–7.2 U loading dose; followed by 2.4–7.2 U/h continuous infusion.
Child: **IV** 0.1 U/kg load; followed by 0.1 U/h continuous infusion.

PHARMACOKINETICS **Absorption:** rapidly absorbed from IM and SC injections. **Onset:** 0.5–1 h. **Peak:** 2–3 h. **Duration:** 5–7 h. **Distribution:** throughout extracellular fluids. **Metabolism:** metabolized primarily in liver with some metabolism in kidneys. **Elimination:** half-life: biological, up to 13 h; < 2% excreted in urine.

CONTRAINDICATIONS & PRECAUTIONS **Contraindicated in:** Hypersensitivity to insulin animal protein. **Cautious use in:** pregnancy (category C).

ADVERSE/SIDE EFFECTS **Hypersensitivity (usually occurs when insulin is at peak action point):** localized allergic reactions at injection site; generalized urticaria or bullae, lymphadenopathy, <u>anaphylaxis</u> (rare). **Hypoglycemia (hyperinsulinism):** *profuse sweating,* hunger, headache, *nausea, tremulousness,* tremors, *palpitation,* tachycardia, weakness, fatigue, nystagmus, circumoral pallor; numb mouth, tongue, and other paresthesias; visual disturbances (diplopia, blurred vision, mydriasis), staring expression, confusion, personality changes, ataxia, incoherent speech, apprehension, irritability, inability to concentrate, personality changes, uncontrolled yawning, loss of consciousness, delirium, hypothermia, convulsions, Babinski reflex, <u>coma</u>. (Urine glucose tests will be negative.) **Other:** posthypoglycemia or rebound hyperglycemia (Somogyi effect), lipoatrophy and lipohypertrophy of injection sites; insulin resistance. **Overdosage:** psychic disturbances, i.e., aphasia, personality changes, maniacal behavior.

DIAGNOSTIC TEST INTERFERENCE Large doses of insulin may increase urinary excretion of ***VMA.*** Insulin can cause alterations in ***thyroid function tests*** and ***liver function test*** and may decrease ***serum potassium*** and ***serum calcium***.

DRUG INTERACTIONS **Alcohol,** ANABOLIC STEROIDS, MAO INHIBITORS, **guanethidine,** SALICYLATES may potentiate hypoglycemic effects; **dextrothyroxine,** CORTICOSTEROIDS, **epinephrine** may antagonize hypoglycemic effects; **furosemide,** THIAZIDE DIURETICS increase serum glucose levels; **propranolol** and other BETA BLOCKERS may mask symptoms of hypoglycemic reaction.

INCOMPATIBILITIES **Solution/additive: aminophylline, amobarbital, chlorothiazide, cytarabine, dobutamine, pentobarbital, phenobarbital, phenytoin, secobarbital, sodium bicarbonate, thiopental. Y-site: dobutamine.**

NURSING IMPLICATIONS

Administration

- Insulins should not be mixed unless prescribed by physician. In general, regular insulin is drawn up into syringe first.
- Any change in the strength (e.g., U–40, U–100), brand (manufacturer), purity, type (regular, etc.), species (pork, human), or sequence of mixing two kinds of insulin is made by the physician only, since a simultaneous change in dosage may be necessary.

SC Administration

- Always use an insulin syringe.

- Regular insulin is generally administered 30 min before a meal.
- Avoid injection of cold insulin; it can lead to lipodystrophy, reduced rate of absorption, and local reactions.
- Commonly used injection sites are upper arms, thighs, abdomen (avoid area over urinary bladder and 2 in. [5 cm] around navel), buttocks, and upper back (if fat is loose enough to pick up). Rotate sites.

IV Administration

- IV regular insulin may be given by direct IV undiluted. Administer 50 U or a fraction thereof over 1 min. When insulin is administered by continuous infusion, rate must be ordered by physician.
- Regular insulin may be adsorbed into the container or tubing when added to an IV infusion solution. Amount lost is variable and depends on concentration of insulin, infusion system, contact duration, and flow rate. Monitor patient response closely.
- Insulin is stable at room temperature up to 1 mo. Avoid exposure to direct sunlight or to temperature extremes (safe range is wide: 5–38C [40–100F]). Refrigerate but do not freeze stock supply. Insulin tolerates temperatures above 38C with less harm than freezing.

Assessment & Drug Effects

- Frequency of blood glucose monitoring is determined by the type of insulin regimen and health status of the patient.
- Usually, urine is tested for ketones in new, unstable, and juvenile diabetes, and if patient has lost weight, exercises vigorously, or has an illness and whenever blood glucose is substantially elevated.
- Presence of acetone without sugar in the urine usually signifies insufficient carbohydrate intake. Acetone with sugar may indicate onset of ketoacidosis. Notify physician promptly.
- Monitor for hypoglycemia (see Appendix G) at time of peak action of insulin. Onset of hypoglycemia (blood sugar: 50–40 mg/dl) may be rapid and sudden.
- During treatment for ketoacidosis with IV insulin, check BP, I&O ratio, and blood glucose and ketones every hour.
- Patients with severe hypoglycemia may receive glucagon, epinephrine, or IV glucose 10–50%. As soon as patient is fully conscious, oral carbohydrate (e.g., dilute corn syrup or orange juice with sugar, Gatorade, or Pedialyte) should be given to prevent secondary hypoglycemia.
- Morning hyperglycemia may be caused by (1) a simple waning of circulating insulin, (2) the Somogyi phenomenon, or (3) the "dawn" phenomenon. Dawn phenomenon: In normal individuals, an increase in circulating insulin during the 3–7 AM period is associated with surges in growth hormone. In the diabetic, there may be a greater-than-normal secretion of growth hormone, which predisposes to development of hyperglycemia. Somogyi phenomenon: Hypoglycemia caused by insulin excess stimulates release of glucose counterregulatory hormones, which cause hyperglycemia. Suspect Somogyi phenomenon if evening blood or urine glucose levels are low followed by morning hyperglycemia.
- With simple waning of insulin, blood glucose values increase progressively through the night; with the Somogyi phenomenon, blood glucose levels usually decrease to the hypoglycemic or near-hypoglycemic range around 3 AM, then rise by 7 or 8 AM. In the dawn phe-

nomenon, blood glucose values usually do not increase until after 3 AM.

- Dawn phenomenon and waning insulin are treated by increasing overnight insulin coverage. Somogyi phenomenon is treated by reducing dose of insulin that is active overnight or increasing prebedtime snack.

Patient & Family Education

- Teach correct injection technique.
- If patient is engaged in active sports, it has been suggested that injection of insulin be made into the abdomen rather than into a muscle that will be heavily taxed.

Special Points on Adverse Reactions:

- Local reactions at injection site sometimes develop 1–3 wk after therapy starts. Symptoms may last several hours to days but usually disappear with continued use. Advise to report symptoms.
- During early period of dosage regulation, some experience visual difficulties. Advise to delay changing prescription lenses until vision stabilizes (usually 3–6 wk).
- Hypoglycemia can result from excess insulin, insufficient food intake, vomiting, diarrhea, unaccustomed exercise, infection, illness, nervous or emotional tension, or overindulgence in alcohol.
- Severe hypoglycemia is an emergency situation. Instruct to respond promptly to beginning symptoms of hypoglycemia. Advise patient to take 4 oz (120 ml) of any fruit juice or regular carbonated beverage (1.5–3 oz [45–90 ml] for child) followed by a meal of longer-acting carbohydrate or protein food. Failure to show signs of recovery within 30 min indicates necessity for emergency treatment.
- Advise to carry some form of fast-acting carbohydrate (e.g., lump sugar, Life-Savers or other candy) at all times to treat hypoglycemia.
- Loss of diabetes control (hyperglycemia or hypoglycemia) occurs commonly at the beginning of a menstrual period. Advise to check blood glucose regularly during this time and to adjust insulin dosage accordingly, as prescribed by physician.
- Inform of signs and symptoms of diabetic ketoacidosis.
- In the event of an illness, advise to continue taking insulin, to go to bed, and to drink liberally (every hour if possible) of noncaloric liquids. Consult physician for insulin regulation if unable to eat prescribed diet.
- Caution patients to avoid OTC medications unless approved by physician.

INSULIN INJECTION CONCENTRATED

Trade names: Iletin II Regular (Concentrated), U-500

Classifications: SYNTHETIC HORMONE; INSULIN ANTIDIABETIC

Prototype: Insulin injection

Pregnancy category: B

ACTIONS/PHARMACODYNAMICS

Concentrated insulin from purified pork pancreas unmodified by any agent that might prolong its action. Because of its high concentration, duration of action is similar to that of an intermediate-acting insulin. See insulin injection for actions, contraindications, precautions, and adverse reactions.

USES Only for the occasional patient who develops insulin resistance and requires daily doses greater than 200 U (even as high as several thousand units).

ROUTE & DOSAGE

Diabetes Mellitus
Adult: **IM/SC** individualized doses; see insulin injection.

PHARMACOKINETICS **Onset:** 0.5–1 h regular. **Peak:** 2–3 h regular. **Duration:** 5–7 h regular. **Metabolism:** metabolized in liver and kidney. **Elimination:** half-life: up to 13 h; <2% excreted unchanged in urine.

ADVERSE/SIDE EFFECTS See insulin injection.

I

INCOMPATIBILITIES Regular insulin. Solution/additive: aminophylline, amobarbital, chlorothiazide, dobutamine, pentobarbital, phenobarbital, phenytoin, secobarbital, sodium bicarbonate, thiopental.

NURSING IMPLICATIONS

See also insulin injection for numerous nursing implications, diagnostic test interferences, and drug interactions.

Administration

- This preparation should not be administered IV because of the high risk of allergic or anaphylactoid reaction.
- Use a tuberculin syringe for accuracy in measurement. Even a slight variation can mean a large overdose or underdose.
- Store in a cold place, preferably a refrigerator, unless otherwise directed. Avoid freezing.

Assessment & Drug Effects

- Patients receiving concentrated insulin are kept under close surveillance until dosage is established. Close monitoring for symptoms of hypoglycemia, hyperglycemia, allergic or anaphylactoid reactions, and of water and electrolyte imbalance is essential.
- Severe secondary hypoglycemia reactions may develop 18–24 h after administration of drug. Have on hand glucagon, IV dextrose, epinephrine.
- Frequently, responsiveness to insulin effect is regained after a short period of therapy with concentrated insulin.

INSULIN, ISOPHANE (NPH)

Trade names: Humulin N, Iletin II (pork), Insulatard NPH, Mixtard, Novolin 70/30, Novolin N

Classifications: HORMONE; INSULIN ANTIDIABETIC

Prototype: Insulin injection

Pregnancy category: B

ACTIONS/PHARMACODYNAMICS Intermediate-acting, cloudy suspension of zinc insulin crystals modified by protamine in a neutral buffer. NPH Iletin II (pork), and Insulatard are "purified" or "single component" insulins that have been purified and are less likely to cause allergic reactions than nonpurified preparations. Therapeutic effect is prompt enough to control postprandial hyperglycemia, which formerly called for supplemental doses of insulin injection. See insulin injection for actions, contraindications, and adverse reactions.

USES Generally considered drug of choice to control hyperglycemia in the diabetic patient. Mixtard and Novolin 70/30 are fixed combinations of purified regular insulin 30% and NPH 70%.

ROUTE & DOSAGE

Diabetes Mellitus
Adult: **IM/SC** Individualized doses; see insulin injection.

PHARMACOKINETICS **Onset:** 1–2 h. **Peak:** 8–12 h NPH. **Duration:** 18–24 h NPH. **Metabolism:** metabolized in liver and kidney. **Elimination:** half-life: up to 13 h; < 2% excreted unchanged in urine.

ADVERSE/SIDE EFFECTS See insulin injection.

NURSING IMPLICATIONS

See also insulin injection for numerous nursing implications, diagnostic test interferences, and drug interactions.

Administration

- Isophane insulin is usually given 30 min before first meal of the day. If necessary, a second smaller dose may be prescribed 30 min before supper or at bedtime.
- To ensure complete dispersion, mix thoroughly by gently rotating vial between palms and inverting it end to end several times. Do not shake.
- Isophane insulin may be mixed with insulin injection without altering either solution.
- Isophane insulin should not be mixed with lente forms.
- Insulins should not be mixed unless prescribed by physician. In general, when insulin injection (regular insulin) is to be combined, it is drawn first.
- Store unopened vial at 2–8C (36–46F); store vial in use at 15–30C (59–86F). Avoid freezing and exposure to extremes in temperature or to direct sunlight.

Assessment & Drug Effects

- Suspect hypoglycemia if fatigue, weakness, sweating, tremor, or nervousness occur. See insulin injection for complete description.

Patient & Family Education

- If insulin was given before breakfast, a hypoglycemic episode is most likely to occur between midafternoon and dinnertime, when insulin effect is peaking. Advise to eat a snack in midafternoon and to carry sugar or candy to treat a reaction. A snack at bedtime will prevent insulin reaction during the night.
- Teach the signs and symptoms of hypoglycemia and hyperglycemia (see Appendix G).

INSULIN LISPRO

(in′su-lin lis′pro)

Trade name: Humalog

Classifications: SYNTHETIC HORMONE; INSULIN; ANTIDIABETIC

Prototype: Insulin injection (Regular)

Pregnancy category: B

ACTIONS/PHARMACODYNAMICS

Insulin lispro of recombinant DNA origin is a human insulin that is a rapid-acting, glucose-lowering agent. One unit of insulin lispro has the same glucose-lowering ability of human regular insulin, but the effect is more rapid and of shorter duration. Contraindications, precautions, adverse side effects, drug interactions, diagnostic test interference, and incompatibilities are similar to those for insulin injection (regular).

USE Treatment of IDDM.

ROUTE & DOSAGE

Diabetes Mellitus

Adult: **SC** 5–10 U 0–15 min a.c.; dose adjustments based on blood glucose determinations.

PHARMACOKINETICS **Absorption:** rapidly absorbed from IM and SC injection sites. **Onset:** < 15 min. **Peak:** 0.5–1 h. **Duration:** 3–4 h. **Distribution:**

throughout extracellular fluids. **Metabolism:** metabolized in liver with some metabolism in kidneys. **Elimination:** half-life: biological, up to 13 h; <2% excreted in urine.

NURSING IMPLICATIONS

See **insulin injection (regular)** for additional nursing implications.

Administration

- May administer 0–15 min before meals.
- May give in same syringe with longer-acting insulins but its absorption may be delayed.
- Store at 15–30C (59–86F).

Assessment & Drug Effects

- Assess for hypoglycemia from 1 to 3 h after injection.
- Assess highly insulin-dependent patients for need for increases in intermediate/long-acting insulins.

Patient & Family Education

- Advise that risk of hypoglycemia is greatest 1–3 h after injection.

INSULIN, PROTAMINE ZINC (PZI)

Trade name: Iletin II

Classifications: HORMONE; INSULIN ANTIDIABETIC

Prototype: Insulin injection

Pregnancy category: B

ACTIONS/PHARMACODYNAMICS

Long-acting, cloudy suspension of insulin modified by addition of zinc chloride and protamine sulfate, which has poor solubility and thus delays absorption. Derived from pork pancreas. May be used in combination with a shorter acting form. See insulin injection for actions, contraindications, precautions, and adverse/side effects.

USE Diabetes mellitus in patients who are not adequately controlled by unmodified insulin.

ROUTE & DOSAGE

Diabetes Mellitus

Adult: **IM/SC** Individualized doses; see insulin injection.

PHARMACOKINETICS Onset: 4–8 h. **Peak:** 14–24 h. **Duration:** 36 h. **Metabolism:** metabolized in liver and kidney. **Elimination:** half-life: up to 13 h; < 2% excreted unchanged in urine.

ADVERSE/SIDE EFFECTS Lymphedema around injection site, hypoglycemia, hypersensitivity reactions. Also see insulin injection.

NURSING IMPLICATIONS

See also insulin injection for numerous nursing implications, diagnostic test interferences, drug interactions.

Administration

- PZI is usually administered 30 min before breakfast.
- To ensure complete dispersion, mix thoroughly by gently rotating vial between palms and inverting it end to end several times. Do not shake.
- PZI is compatible with regular insulin. Insulins must not be mixed unless prescribed by physician.
- When mixing regular insulin with PZI, prepare solution immediately before administration. Withdraw insulin injection into syringe before PZI.
- Store unopened vial at 2–8C (36–46F); store vial in use at 15–30C (59–86F). Avoid freezing and exposure to extremes in temperature or to direct sunlight.

Patient & Family Education

- Teach that prolonged insulin effect requires careful distribution of carbohydrates in a balanced diet.

- The usual proportion of PZI to insulin injection prescribed is 1:2 or 1:3 to provide a preparation with both rapid onset and prolonged duration of action.
- Full therapeutic effect of PZI may be delayed several days following institution of treatment.
- Between-meal snacks may be necessary; bedtime snacks are essential.
- If injection is given in the morning, hypoglycemia is most likely to occur during the night or early morning.
- Blood glucose levels fall slowly after injection of PZI; thus, marked hypoglycemia may develop without producing an apparent cluster of symptoms. Teach to be alert to the significance of sweating or fatigue unwarranted by patient's activities, as well as other vague symptoms such as lassitude, drowsiness, tremulousness.
- Treatment of PZI-induced hypoglycemia requires both fast acting and complex carbohydrate (e.g., corn syrup or honey with bread) followed in 1–2 h by additional "slow" carbohydrates, such as milk and crackers.

INSULIN ZINC SUSPENSION (LENTE)

Trade names: Humulin L, Lente Iletin II (pork), Lente Purified Pork Insulin, Novolin

Classifications: HORMONE; INSULIN ANTIDIABETIC

Prototype: Insulin injection

Pregnancy category: B

ACTIONS/PHARMACODYNAMICS
Intermediate-acting, cloudy insulin suspension, equivalent to a mixture of 30% prompt insulin zinc (Semilente) and 70% extended zinc insulin (Ultralente) suspensions. Obtained from pork pancreas. Allergic reactions are rare. Time action is intermediate between those of prompt and extended insulins and is so close to that of isophane (NPH) insulin that the two forms may be used interchangeably. See insulin injection for contraindications, precautions, and adverse/side effects.

USES Hyperglycemia in diabetic patients allergic to other preparations of insulin. Also for patients with evidence of thrombotic phenomena in which protamine may be a factor.

ROUTE & DOSAGE

Diabetes Mellitus
Adult: **IM/SC** individualized doses; see insulin injection.

PHARMACOKINETICS **Onset:** 1–2 h. **Peak:** 8–12 h. **Duration:** 18–24 h. **Metabolism:** metabolized in liver and kidney. **Elimination:** half-life: up to 13 h; < 2 % excreted unchanged in urine.

ADVERSE/SIDE EFFECTS See insulin injection.

NURSING IMPLICATIONS

See also insulin injection for numerous nursing implications, diagnostic test interferences and drug interactions.

Administration
- Insulin zinc suspensions are usually administered 30 min before breakfast. Some patients require another injection 30 min before suppertime or at bedtime.
- Zinc insulin preparations (Ultralente, Lente, Semilente) can be mixed with one another if pre-

scribed by physician, but they must not be mixed with other modified insulins. Compatible with regular insulin.

- To ensure complete dispersion, mix thoroughly by gently rotating the vial between the palms and by inverting it end-to-end several times. Do not shake.
- Because time of action of insulin zinc suspension (Lente) approximates that of isophane insulin suspension (NPH), the patient can usually be transferred directly to the latter on a unit-for-unit basis.
- Store unopened vial at 2–8C (36–46F); store vial in use at 15–30C (59–86F). Avoid freezing and exposure to extremes in temperature or to direct sunlight.

Patient & Family Education

- Symptoms of hypoglycemia (see Appendix G) are most apt to occur between midafternoon and dinner time (an early symptom may be a sense of extreme fatigue). Immediately take soluble carbohydrate (e.g., orange juice, honey). If the time between the midday and evening meal is prolonged, an afternoon snack may be needed.
- The possibility of nocturnal hypoglycemia should not be overlooked, especially during dose adjustment. Teach to monitor for signs of restlessness or profuse sweating during sleep.

INSULIN ZINC SUSPENSION, EXTENDED (ULTRALENTE)

Trade names: Humulin U; Ultralente; Ultralente Insulin

Classifications: HORMONE; INSULIN ANTIDIABETIC

Prototype: Insulin injection

Pregnancy category: B

ACTIONS/PHARMACODYNAMICS

Long-acting cloudy suspension of insulin modified by addition of zinc chloride. Large particle size and high zinc content delay absorption and prolong action. Obtained from pork pancreas. Incidence of allergic reactions is low. Similar to protamine zinc insulin suspension (PZI) in actions and indications. Usually administered in combination with a shorter acting insulin preparation. See insulin injection for actions, uses, contraindications, and adverse/side effects.

ROUTE & DOSAGE

Diabetes Mellitus

Adult: **IM/SC** individualized doses; see insulin injection.

PHARMACOKINETICS **Onset:** 4–8 h. **Peak:** 16–18 h. **Duration:** 36 h. **Metabolism:** metabolized in liver and kidney. **Elimination:** half-life: up to 13 h; < 2% excreted unchanged in urine.

NURSING IMPLICATIONS

See also insulin injection for numerous nursing implications, diagnostic test interferences, and drug interactions.

Administration

- Administer 30 min before breakfast by deep SC injection.
- To ensure complete dispersion, mix thoroughly by gently rotating vial between palms and by inverting it end to end several times. Do not shake.
- Ultralente may be mixed with Semilente but not with other modified insulin preparations. Compatible with regular insulin. Insulins should not be mixed unless prescribed by physician.
- Store unopened vial at 2–8C

(36–46F); store vial in use at 15–30C (59–86F). Avoid freezing and exposure to extremes in temperature or to direct sunlight.

Patient & Family Education

- Hypoglycemia is most apt to occur during the night or early morning. Teach to watch sleeping patient carefully for signs of restlessness or profuse sweating and to notify physician if it occurs. Hypoglycemia is treated by administering soluble carbohydrate (orange juice, sugar, honey) plus a slowly digestible carbohydrate (bread, crackers). Supplemental feedings may be prescribed.

INSULIN ZINC SUSPENSION, PROMPT (SEMILENTE)

Trade names: Semilente Insulin, Semilente Purified Pork Insulin

Classifications: HORMONE; INSULIN ANTIDIABETIC

Prototype: Insulin injection

Pregnancy category: B

ACTIONS/PHARMACODYNAMICS Rapid-acting cloudy suspension of insulin modified by addition of zinc chloride so that solid phase of suspension is amorphous and therefore more quickly absorbed. Obtained from pork pancreas. Incidence of allergic reactions is low. See insulin injection for actions, contraindications, precautions, and adverse/side effects.

USES Most commonly to supplement intermediate and long-acting insulins. Also for routine management of diabetes, especially for patients allergic to other types of insulin, and for patients with evidence of thrombotic phenomena in which protamine may be a factor.

ROUTE & DOSAGE

Diabetes Mellitus

Adult: **IM/SC** individualized doses; see insulin injection.

PHARMACOKINETICS **Onset:** 0.5–1 h. **Peak:** 4–7 h. **Duration:** 12–16 h. **Metabolism:** metabolized in liver and kidney. **Elimination:** half-life: up to 13 h; < 2% excreted unchanged in urine.

ADVERSE/SIDE EFFECTS See insulin injection.

NURSING IMPLICATIONS

See also insulin injection for numerous nursing implications, diagnostic test interferences, and drug interactions.

Administration

- Semilente is usually administered once daily, 30 min before breakfast. Additional doses may be required for some patients 30 min before a meal or at bedtime.
- To ensure complete dispersion, mix thoroughly by gently rotating vial between palms and by inverting it end to end several times. Do not shake.
- The zinc insulin preparations (Ultralente, Lente, Semilente) can be mixed with one another, but they must not be mixed with other modified insulin. Insulins should not be mixed unless prescribed by physician.
- Store unopened vial at 2–8C (36–46F); store vial in use at 15–30C (59–86F). Avoid freezing and exposure to extremes in temperature or to direct sunlight.

Patient & Family Education

- Symptoms of hypoglycemia are most apt to appear before lunch; glycosuria is most apt to appear during the night.

INTERFERON ALFA-2a

(in-ter-feer'on)

Trade name: Roferon-A Injection

Prototype for classifications: IMMUNOMODULATOR; ANTIVIRAL

Pregnancy category: C

ACTIONS/PHARMACODYNAMICS Interferon (IFN) alfa-2a, one of 4 types of alpha interferon, is a highly purified protein and natural product of human leukocytes within 4–6 h after viral stimulation. Also produced by recombinant DNA technology (rIFN-A). Has a broad spectrum of antiviral, cytotoxic, and immunomodulating activity (i.e., favorably adjusts immune system to better combat foreign invasion of antigens and viruses). ***Antiviral action:*** reprograms virus-infected cells to inhibit various stages of virus replication. ***Antitumor action:*** suppresses cell proliferation. ***Immunomodulating action:*** enhances phagocytic activity of macrophages and augments specific cytotoxicity of lymphocytes for target cells. IFN is species specific but not virus specific; it partially inhibits viral replication and is immediately produced at site of viral entry by any cell; thus, the immune system and the interferon system of defense are complementary.

USES To induce hairy cell leukemia remission in splenectomized and nonsplenectomized patients; treatment of hepatitis C, adjunct to surgery for malignant melanoma. **Unlabeled uses:** chronic hepatitis B virus infection, solid tumors, human papillomavirus (HPV)-associated diseases, AIDS-associated Kaposi's sarcoma. **Orphan drug:** proposed use treatment of Kaposi's sarcoma in AIDS patients.

ROUTE & DOSAGE

Hairy Cell Leukemia

Adult: **SC/IM** 3 million U/d for 16–24 wk; may be reduced to 3 times/wk for maintenance therapy.

AIDS-related Kaposi's Sarcoma

Adult: **SC/IM** 36 million U/d for 10–12 wk; may then be reduced to 3 times/wk.

Genital and Anal Warts

Adult: **Intralesional** 1 million U injected in each lesion 3 times/wk on alternate days for 3 wk.

Chronic Viral Hepatitis

Adult: **SC/IM** 1–3 million U/d for 1 wk, then 3 times/wk for 48–52 wk.

PHARMACOKINETICS **Absorption:** well absorbed after IM or SC injection. **Peak:** 15–60 min IV; 1–8 h IM. **Distribution:** widely distributed, concentrating in spleen, kidney, liver, and lung. **Metabolism:** metabolized principally in kidney. **Elimination:** half-life: 5.1 h.

CONTRAINDICATIONS & PRECAUTIONS **Contraindicated in:** hypersensitivity to alpha interferons or any component of product and to mouse immunoglobulin. Safe use during pregnancy (category C), by nursing mothers, or by children < 18 y not established. **Cautious use in:** cardiac disease or history of cardiac illness, severe cardiac, renal, or hepatic disease; seizure disorders, compromised CNS function; myelosuppression; chickenpox (existing or recent, including recent exposure), herpes zoster.

ADVERSE/SIDE EFFECTS *Flu-like syndrome (fever, chills, myalgia,* *headache*). **CNS:** *fatigue, dizziness,* confusion, paresthesias, lethargy, psychosis, depression, nervousness, forgetfulness. **CV:** dyspnea, edema, hypertension, palpitations. **GI:** *nausea,* vomiting, *diarrhea, anorexia,* abdominal pain, change in taste. **Hematologic:** leukopenia, neutropenia, thrombocytopenia, myelosuppression. **Skin:** *rash,* dry skin, pruritus, partial alopecia (eyelash growth increases), urticaria, reactivation of herpes labialis. **Other:** dryness or inflammation of oropharynx, transient impotence, arthralgia, mild to moderate hepatotoxicity, *coughing.*

DIAGNOSTIC TEST INTERFERENCE

Decreased Hgb, Hct; elevated fasting blood sugar, serum phosphorus, serum creatinine, AST, ALT, alkaline phosphatase, LDH; hypocalcemia.

NURSING IMPLICATIONS

Administration

- IFN should be administered under the guidance of a qualified physician.
- After reconstitution, solutions must be used within 30 d. Inspect solution for particulate matter and discoloration before administration.
- SC administration is recommended especially for patient who is at risk for bleeding (platelet count less than 50,000).
- Store sterile powder and its accompanying diluent, reconstituted solution, and injectable solution in refrigerator at 2–8C (36–46F). Do not freeze or shake solution.

Assessment & Drug Effects

- Establish baseline data for CBC and platelet count, peripheral and bone marrow hairy cells, liver and renal function. Monitor monthly during treatment.
- Monitor I&O ratio and pattern. Patient should be well hydrated during early stages of treatment. Encourage increased intake to at least 2500 ml if tolerated.
- Be aware of potential side effects. If detected early, most are reversible.
- Flu-like syndrome (fever, chills) occurs in most patients 2–6 h after a dose of IFN. Anorexia may persist after such an episode. Symptoms tend to lessen with continued therapy.
- Monitor for ecchymoses, petechiae, unexplained bleeding.
- Monitor BP, vital signs, and cardiac function. The elderly are particularly susceptible to cardiotoxicity.
- Monitor for gait difficulty, dizziness, and hypotension. Advise against hazardous activity until reaction to drug is known.
- Monitor for oral superinfection with *Candida albicans.* If stomatitis (sore mouth with ulceration), gingivitis, or white patches on oropharyngeal membrane surfaces are evidenced, alert physician.

Patient & Family Education

- The patient should be informed of the risks of severe and even fatal adverse reactions as well as the benefits from IFN therapy.
- Drug may be self-administered after therapy is well established and effectiveness of patient teaching has been evaluated. Read patient information sheet about IFN with patient before his or her discharge from agency.
- Advise to avoid exposure to infection during nadir period
- Careful periodic neuropsychiatric monitoring of patient is recommended.
- Urge prompt reporting if symptoms of infection develop (sore throat, fever, vomiting, diarrhea).
- If IFN is being given to a fertile,

nonpregnant woman, she should be using effective contraception.
- Caution patient not to change brands of interferon alfa without first consulting the physician (because of risk of dosage change).

INTERFERON ALFA-2b

(in-ter-feer′on)

Trade name: Intron A

Classifications: IMMUNOMODULATOR; ANTINEOPLASTIC; ANTIVIRAL

Prototype: Interferon alfa-2a

Pregnancy category: C

I

ACTIONS/PHARMACODYNAMICS Alpha (leukocyte) interferon is a natural product induced virally in peripheral WBC or lymphoblastoid cells. The drug interferon alfa-2b is obtained by recombinant DNA technology from a strain of *Escherichia coli* bearing an interferon alfa-2b gene from human leukocytes. Has the same actions (antiviral, immunomodulating, antiproliferative) as interferon alfa-2a.

USES Hairy cell leukemia in splenectomized and nonsplenectomized patients ≥ 18 y, chronic hepatitis B or C. **Unlabeled use:** multiple sclerosis, condylomata acuminata, AIDS-related Kaposi's sarcoma.

ROUTE & DOSAGE

Hairy Cell Leukemia

Adult: **IM/SC** 2 million U/m^2 3 times/wk

Kaposi's Sarcoma

Adult: **IM/SC** 30 million U/m^2 3 times/wk

Condylomata Acuminata

Adult: **IM/SC** 1 million U/m^2 3 times/wk

Chronic Hepatitis B or C

Adult: **SC** 3 million U 3 times/wk × 18–24 mo.

PHARMACOKINETICS Peak: 6–8 h. **Metabolism:** metabolized in kidneys. **Elimination:** half-life: 6–7 h.

CONTRAINDICATIONS & PRECAUTIONS Contraindicated in: hypersensitivity to interferon alfa-2b or to any components of the product. Safe use during pregnancy (category C), by nursing mothers, or children <18 y not established. **Cautious use in:** severe, preexisting cardiac, renal, or hepatic disease; pulmonary disease (e.g., COPD); diabetes mellitus prone to ketoacidosis; coagulation disorders; severe myelosuppression; recent MI; previous dysrhythmias.

ADVERSE/SIDE EFFECTS CNS: depression, nervousness, anxiety, confusion, *dizziness, fatigue,* somnolence, insomnia, altered mental states, ataxia, tremor, paresthesias, *headache.* **CV:** hypertension, dyspnea, *hot flushes.* **ENT:** epistaxis, pharyngitis, sneezing. **Eye:** abnormal vision. **GI:** taste alteration, *anorexia,* weight loss, *nausea,* vomiting, stomatitis, *diarrhea,* flatulence. **Hematologic:** mild thrombocytopenia, transient granulocytopenia, <u>leukemia</u>. **Skin:** mild pruritus, mild alopecia, rash, dry skin, herpetic eruptions, nonherpetic cold sores, urticaria. **Other:** *flu-like symptoms (fever, chills) associated with myalgia and arthralgia,* leg cramps.

NURSING IMPLICATIONS

See interferon alfa-2a for additional nursing implications related to assessment and drug effects and patient and family education.

Administration

- Interferon alfa-2b should be administered under the guidance of a qualified physician.

- Reconstitution: The final concentration with the amount of required diluent is determined by the condition being treated (see manufacturer's directions). Inject diluent (bacteriostatic water for injection) into interferon alfa-2b vial; gently agitate solution before withdrawing dose with a sterile syringe. Reconstituted solution remains stable for 1 mo if refrigerated.
- Reconstituted solution should be clear and colorless to light yellow. Inspect visually for particulate material and discard solution if it is present or if solution is discolored.
- Store vials and reconstituted solutions at 2–8C (36–46F).

Assessment & Drug Effects

- Closely monitor CBC with differential and platelet counts. Monitor for ecchymoses, petechiae, and bruising.
- Assess hydration status; patient should be well hydrated especially during initial stage of treatment and if vomiting or diarrhea occurs.
- Assess for flu-like symptoms, which may be relieved by acetaminophen (if prescribed).
- Monitor level of GI distress and ability to consume fluids and food.
- Monitor mental status and alertness; implement safety precautions if needed.

Patient & Family Education

- Teach techniques for reconstitution and administration of drug.
- Caution not to change brands of interferon without first consulting the physician.
- If flu-like symptoms develop, advise acetaminophen (if not contraindicated) and instruct to take interferon h.s.
- If interferon is being given to a fertile woman, advise use of a reliable contraceptive.
- Advise caution with hazardous activities until reaction to drug is known.
- Instruct regarding adverse effects and advise to report those that cause significant discomfort.

INTERFERON BETA-1a

(in-ter-fer′on)

Trade name: Avonex

Classifications: IMMUNOMODULATOR; ANTIVIRAL

Prototype: Interferon alfa-2a

Pregnancy category: C

ACTIONS/PHARMACODYNAMICS

Interferon beta-1a is produced by recombinant DNA technology. Interferon beta exerts its biological effects by binding to specific receptors on the surface of human cells. The mechanisms by which Avonex exerts its effect on multiple sclerosis is not fully defined; however, time of onset of progression in disability was significantly longer in patients treated with Avonex. Contraindications, precautions, and adverse side effects are similar to those for interferon beta-1b.

USE Relapsing-remitting multiple sclerosis.

ROUTE & DOSAGE

Adult: **IM** 30 μg qwk.

PHARMACOKINETICS **Peak:** 7.8–9.8 h. **Metabolism:** rapidly inactivated in body fluids and tissue. **Elimination:** half-life: 8.6–10 h.

NURSING IMPLICATIONS

Administration

- Review extensive instructions for reconstitution and injection provided by manufacturer.
- Use within 6 h of reconstitution (store at 2–8C [36–46F]).
- Store unreconstituted vials at 2–8C (36–46F). May store for ≤30 d at room temperature up to 25C (77F). Do not use beyond expiration date.

Assessment & Drug Effects

- If depression or suicidal ideation develops withhold drug and notify physician.
- Carefully monitor those with cardiac disease for worsening cardiac function.
- Periodically monitor liver function tests, renal function tests, routine blood chemistry, and CBC.

Patient & Family Education

- Review manufacturer's instructions on reconstitution, administration, and storage.
- For missed dose, take as soon as possible but not within 2 d of next scheduled dose.
- Advise regarding common adverse effects, especially flu-like syndrome.
- Advise to withhold drug and notify physician of depression and/or suicidal ideation or exacerbation of a preexisting seizure disorder.
- Instruct women who wish to become pregnant to discontinue therapy.

INTERFERON BETA-1B (BETA INFERON)

(in-ter-fer′on)

Trade name: Betaseron

Classifications: IMMUNOMODULATOR; ANTINEOPLASTIC; ANTIVIRAL; ORPHAN DRUG

Prototype: Interferon alfa-2a

Pregnancy category: C

ACTIONS/PHARMACODYNAMICS

Interferon beta-1b is a glycoprotein produced by recombinant DNA techniques using a strain of *E. coli*. Naturally occurring interferon beta-1b is produced principally by fibroblasts. Both natural and recombinant DNA interferon-1b possess antiviral, antiproliferative, antitumor, and immunomodulatory activity as interferon alfa-2a. The use of interferon beta-1b for multiple sclerosis (MS) is based on the assumption that MS is an immunologically mediated illness.

USE Relapsing-remitting multiple sclerosis. **Unlabeled uses:** AIDS, AIDS-related Kaposi's sarcoma, metastatic renal cell carcinoma, malignant melanoma, cutaneous T-cell lymphoma, acute hepatitis C.

ROUTE & DOSAGE

Multiple Sclerosis

Adult: **SC** 0.25 mg (8 million IU) q.o.d.

PHARMACOKINETICS Absorption: about 50% absorbed from SC sites. **Distribution:** penetrates intact blood–brain barrier poorly; crosses placenta; distributed into breast milk. **Metabolism:** rapidly inactivated in body fluids and tissue.

CONTRAINDICATIONS & PRECAUTIONS Contraindicated in: previous hypersensitivity to interferon beta-1b or human albumin, pregnancy (category C) but may cause a spontaneous abortion, nursing mothers.

Cautious use in: suicidal/mental disorders. Safety and efficacy in children < 18 y of age not established. Safety and efficacy in chronic progressive MS not evaluated.

ADVERSE/SIDE EFFECTS CNS: *headache, fever,* fatigue, lethargy, depression, somnolence, weakness, agitation, malaise, confusion or reduced ability to concentrate, anxiety, dementia, emotional lability, depersonalization, suicide attempts. **CV:** tachycardia, CHF (rare). **GI:** nausea, vomiting, *diarrhea.* **Hematologic:** *leukopenia, thrombocytopenia,* anemia. **Other:** hypocalcemia, elevated serum creatinine, elevated liver transaminases; local skin necrosis at injection site, *pain at injection site,* alopecia, myalgias, *flu-like syndrome.*

DRUG INTERACTION Zidovudine (AZT) levels are increased, resulting in toxicity.

NURSING IMPLICATIONS

Administration

- To reconstitute, add 1.2 ml of the supplied diluent (0.54% NaCl) to vial and gently swirl. *Do not shake.* The resultant solution contains 0.25 mg (8 million units)/ml.
- Discard reconstituted solution if it contains particulate matter or is discolored. Unused solution should be discarded.
- Rotate injection sites; use 27-guage needle to administer drug.
- Store vials under refrigeration, 2–8C (36–46F).

Assessment & Drug Effects

- Monitor vital signs, neurologic status, and neuropsychiatric status frequently during therapy.
- Monitor liver function, renal function, complete blood counts, and serum electrolytes periodically during therapy.
- Assess for and promptly treat flu-like symptom complex (fever, chills, myalgia, etc.).
- Assess injection sites; pain and redness are common reactions. Report tissue ulceration promptly.

Patient & Family Education

- Fully inform patient of potential adverse drug reactions.
- Advise to self-medicate with acetaminophen (if not contraindicated) if flu-like symptom complex develops.
- Advise to avoid prolonged exposure to sunlight.
- Ensure that patient knows proper technique for solution preparation and injection.
- Caution against performing hazardous activities until response to drug is known.

IODOQUINOL

(eye-oh-do-kwin′ole)

Trade names: Diiodohydroxyquin, Dioquinol, Sebaquin, Yodoxin

Classifications: ANTIINFECTIVE; AMEBICIDE; ANTIPROTOZOAL

Prototype: Emetine

Pregnancy category: C

ACTIONS/PHARMACODYNAMICS Direct-acting (contact) amebicide effective against both trophozoites and cyst forms of *Entamoeba histolytica* in intestinal lumen. Not useful for extraintestinal amebiasis. Range of antiprotozoal action includes *Trichomonas vaginalis* and *Balantidium coli;* also has some antibacterial and antifungal properties.

USES Intestinal amebiasis and for asymptomatic passers of cysts. Commonly used either concurrently or in alternating courses with another intestinal amebicide. **Unlabeled uses:** balantidiasis and *Acrodermatitis enteropathica;* traveler's diarrhea; shampoo preparation (Sebaquin) used for control of seborrheic dermatitis of scalp.

ROUTE & DOSAGE

Intestinal Amebiasis

Adult: **PO** 630–650 mg t.i.d. for 20 d (max 2 g/d); may repeat after a 2–3 wk drug-free interval.
Child: **PO** 30–40 mg/kg/d in 2–3 divided doses for 20 d (max 1.95 g/d); may repeat after a 2–3 wk drug-free interval.

PHARMACOKINETICS Absorption: small amount absorbed from GI tract. **Elimination:** excreted in feces.

CONTRAINDICATIONS & PRECAUTIONS Contraindicated in: hypersensitivity to any 8-hydroxyquinoline or to iodine-containing preparations or foods; hepatic or renal damage; preexisting optic neuropathy. **Cautious use in:** severe thyroid disease; minor self-limiting problems; prolonged high-dosage therapy. Safe use during pregnancy (category C) and in nursing mothers not established.

ADVERSE/SIDE EFFECTS CNS: headache, agitation, retrograde amnesia, vertigo, ataxia, peripheral neuropathy (especially in children); muscle pain, weakness usually below T_{12} vertebrae, dysesthesias especially of lower limbs, paresthesias. **Eye:** blurred vision, <u>optic atrophy</u>, optic neuritis, <u>permanent loss of vision</u>. **GI:** nausea, vomiting, anorexia, abdominal cramps, diarrhea, constipation, rectal irritation and itching. **Hypersensitivity:** urticaria, pruritus. **Skin:** discoloration of hair and nails, acne, hair loss, urticaria, various forms of skin eruptions. **Other:** increased sense of warmth, thyroid hypertrophy, <u>agranulocytosis</u> (rare). **Iodism:** generalized furunculosis (iodine toxiderma), skin eruptions, fever, chills, weakness.

DIAGNOSTIC TEST INTERFERENCE
Iodoquinol can cause elevations of ***PBI*** and decrease of ***I-131 uptake*** (effects may last for several weeks to 6 mo even after discontinuation of therapy). ***Ferric chloride test for PKU*** (phenylketonuria) may yield false-positive results if iodoquinol is present in urine.

NURSING IMPLICATIONS

Administration

- Administer drug after meals. If patient has difficulty swallowing tablet, it may be crushed and mixed with applesauce.
- Shampoo preparation (Sebaquin) should not be used over large areas or for prolonged periods.
- Store at 15–30C (59–86F) unless otherwise directed.

Assessment & Drug Effects

- Monitor I&O ratio. Record characteristics of stools: color, consistency, frequency, presence of blood, mucus, or other material.
- Ophthalmologic examinations should be performed at regular intervals during prolonged therapy.
- Monitor and report immediately the onset of blurred or decreased vision or eye pain. Also report symptoms of peripheral neuropathy: pain, numbness, tingling, or weakness of extremities.

Patient & Family Education

- Instruct patient to report skin rash

and symptoms of agranulocytosis (see Appendix G).

- Advise to rinse sebaquin shampoo thoroughly from hair following shampoo and to avoid bringing it in contact with eyes.
- Advise patient to complete full course of treatment. Inform that stool should be examined again 1, 3, and 6 mo after termination of treatment.
- Intestinal amebiasis is spread mainly by contaminated water, raw fruits or vegetables, flies, roaches, and hand-to-mouth transfer of infected feces. Emphasize importance of handwashing after defecation and before eating.

IPECAC SYRUP

(ip′e-kak)

Classifications: GASTROINTESTINAL AGENT; EMETIC

Pregnancy category: C

ACTIONS/PHARMACODYNAMICS Derived from dried rhizomes and roots of *Cephaelis ipecacuanha*. Contains cephaeline (produces emesis) and emetine, a toxic alkaloid that is excreted slowly from the body. Emetine can cause potentially fatal cumulative toxicity with repeated use. It appears to inhibit protein synthesis and energy production in muscle tissue with resultant skeletal and cardiac muscle toxicity. Acts locally on gastric mucosa and centrally on chemoreceptor trigger zone (CTZ) in the medulla to induce vomiting.

USE Emergency emetic to remove unabsorbed ingested poisons.

ROUTE & DOSAGE

Emergency Emesis

Adult: PO 30 ml followed by 1–2 240 ml (8 oz) glasses of water; may repeat once in 20 min if necessary.

Child: **PO** > 1 y, 15 ml followed by 1–2 240 ml (8 oz) glasses of water; may repeat once in 20 min if necessary; < 1 y, 5–10 ml followed by 120–240 ml (4–8 oz) of water; may repeat once in 20 min if necessary.

PHARMACOKINETICS **Onset:** 15–30 min. **Duration:** 25 min. **Elimination:** metabolite can be detected in urine up to 60 d after excessive doses.

CONTRAINDICATIONS & PRECAUTIONS **Contraindicated in:** comatose, semicomatose, inebriated, deeply sedated patients; patients in shock; patients with depressed gag reflex; seizures, active or impending; impaired cardiac function; arteriosclerosis; treatment of ingested strong alkalis, acids, or other corrosives, strychnine, petroleum distillates, volatile oils, or rapid-acting CNS depressants. Safe use in pregnancy (category C), nursing mothers, infants under 6 mo not established.

ADVERSE/SIDE EFFECTS Diarrhea, mild GI upset. If drug is not vomited but absorbed or if ipecac overdosage: *persistent vomiting,* gastroenteritis, bloody diarrhea, sensory disturbances, stomach cramps, tremor; achy, stiff muscles, severe myopathy, including cardiomyopathy, cardiotoxicity, cardiac arrhythmias, atrial fibrillation, tachycardia, chest pain, dyspnea, hypotension, fatal myocarditis, convulsions, coma.

NURSING IMPLICATIONS

Administration

- Do not confuse with ipecac fluid extract, which is 14 times stronger and has caused deaths when mistakenly given at the same dosage as ipecac syrup.
- Vomiting should not be induced if victim is unconscious or semiconscious or is convulsing.
- Store in tight containers at temperature not exceeding 25C (77F).

Assessment & Drug Effects

- Emetic effect occurs in 15–30 min and continues for 20–25 min. If vomiting does not occur in 20–30 min, dose may be repeated once.
- If vomiting does not occur within 15–20 min after a second dose, contact physician immediately. Dosage should be recovered by gastric lavage and activated charcoal if necessary.
- Ipecac syrup can be cardiotoxic if not vomited and allowed to be absorbed.
- Most patients stop vomiting within 2–3 h after ipecac syrup is given; however, if vomiting persists, report immediately to physician.

Patient & Family Education

- Call an emergency room, poison control center, or physician before using ipecac syrup.

IPRATROPIUM BROMIDE

(i-pra-troe′pee-um)

Trade name: Atrovent

Classifications: AUTONOMIC NERVOUS SYSTEM AGENT; ANTICHOLINERGIC (PARASYMPATHOLYTIC); BRONCHODILATOR

Prototype: Atropine

Pregnancy category: B

ACTIONS/PHARMACODYNAMICS

Quaternary compound, chemically related to atropine, with low solubility; does not cross blood–brain barrier. Produces local, site-specific effects on the larger central airways. Bronchodilation inhibits acetylcholine at its receptor sites, thereby blocking cholinergic bronchomotor tone (bronchoconstriction); also abolishes vagally mediated reflex bronchospasm triggered by such nonspecific agents as cigarette smoke, inert dusts, cold air, and a range of inflammatory mediators (e.g., histamine).

USES Maintenance therapy in COPD including chronic bronchitis and emphysema; nasal spray for perennial rhinitis and symptomatic relief of rhinorrhea associated with the common cold. **Unlabeled use:** perennial nonallergic rhinitis.

ROUTE & DOSAGE

COPD

Adult: **Inhalation** 2 inhalations of MDI q.i.d. at no less than 4 h intervals (max 12 inhalations in 24 h); *or* 500 μg (1 unit dose vial q6–8h by oral nebulization.
Child 3–12 y: **Inhalation** 1–2 inhalations t.i.d. (max 6/d). **Nebulizer** 125–250 μg t.i.d.

Rhinitis

Adult: **Intranasal** 2 sprays of 0.03% each nostril b.i.d. or t.i.d.
Child ≥6 y: **Intranasal** Same as for adult.

Common Cold

Adult: **Intranasal** 2 sprays of 0.06% each nostril t.i.d. or q.i.d. up to 4 d.

PHARMACOKINETICS Absorption: 10% of inhaled dose reaches lower airway; approximately 0.5% of dose is systemically absorbed. **Peak effect:** 1.5–2 h. **Duration:** 4–6 h. **Elimination:** half-life: 1.5–2 h; 48% of dose excreted in feces; < 5% excreted in urine.

CONTRAINDICATIONS & PRECAUTIONS Contraindicated in: use as primary treatment for acute episodes; hypersensitivity to atropine or derivatives. Safe use in children <12 y not established. **Cautious use in:** pregnancy (category B), nursing mothers; narrow-angle glaucoma; prostatic hypertrophy, bladder neck obstruction.

ADVERSE/SIDE EFFECTS Eye: blurred vision (especially if sprayed into eye), difficulty in accommodation, acute eye pain, worsening of narrow-angle glaucoma. **GI:** bitter taste, dry oropharyngeal membranes. With higher doses: nausea, constipation. **Respiratory:** *cough*, hoarseness, exacerbation of symptoms, drying of bronchial secretions, mucosal ulcers, epistaxis, nasal dryness. **Other:** rash, hives, urinary retention, headache.

NURSING IMPLICATIONS

Administration

- Demonstrate aerosol use and check return demonstration.
- Store inhaler below 30C (86F). Avoid freezing and exposure to excess humidity or to sunlight.

Assessment & Drug Effects

- Monitor respiratory status; auscultate lungs before and after inhalation.
- Treatment failure (exacerbation of respiratory symptoms) should be reported to physician.

Patient & Family Education

- This medication is not an emergency agent because of its delayed onset and the time required to reach peak bronchodilation.
- Review patient information sheet on proper use of nasal spray.
- Instruct to allow 30–60 s between puffs for optimum results. Caution against medication–eye contact.
- Advise patient who is using other inhalations to wait 5 min between medications. Check with physician about sequence of administration.
- Advise to take medication only as directed, noting some leniency in number of puffs within 24 h. Parent should supervise child's administration until certain all of dose is being administered.
- Patient may find it helpful to rinse mouth after medication puffs to reduce bitter taste.
- The elderly patient may develop urinary problems and should be alerted to discuss changes in normal urinary pattern with the physician.
- Advise patients to call physician if they note changes in sputum color or amount, ankle edema, or significant weight gain.

I

IRBESARTAN

(ir-be-sar′tan)

Trade name: Avapro

Classifications: CARDIOVASCULAR AGENT; ANGIOTENSIN II RECEPTOR ANTAGONIST; ANTIHYPERTENSIVE

Prototype: Losartan

Pregnancy category: C (first trimester); D (second and third trimesters)

ACTIONS/PHARMACODYNAMICS Irbesartan is an angiotensin II receptor (type AT_1) antagonist. Angiotensin II is a hormone of the renin–angiotensin–aldosterone system. Irbesartan selectively blocks the binding of angiotensin II to the AT_1 receptors found in many tissues (e.g., vascular smooth muscle, adrenal glands). This results in blocking the vasoconstricting and aldosterone-secreting effects of angiotensin II, thus resulting in an antihypertensive effect.

USE Hypertension. **Unlabeled use:** CHF.

ROUTE & DOSAGE

Hypertension

Adult: **PO** Start with 150 mg once daily. May increase to 300 mg/d.

I

PHARMACOKINETICS Absorption: rapidly absorbed from GI tract, 60–80% bioavailability. **Distribution:** 90% protein bound. **Metabolism:** metabolized in the liver primarily by CYP2C9. **Elimination:** half-life: 11–15 h; primarily excreted in feces (80%).

CONTRAINDICATIONS & PRECAUTIONS Contraindicated in: hypersensitivity to irbesartan, losartan, or valsartan; pregnancy (category C [first trimester], category D [second and third trimesters]), lactation. **Cautious use in:** patients on diuretics, arterial stenosis of the renal artery, severe CHF.

ADVERSE/SIDE EFFECTS Body as a Whole: edema, fatigue, pain. **CNS:** dizziness, headache, anxiety, nervousness. **CV:** tachycardia, chest pain. **GI:** diarrhea, dyspepsia, nausea, vomiting, abdominal pain. **Respiratory:** upper respiratory infection, cough, sinus disorder, pharyngitis, rhinitis. **Skin:** rash. **Other:** UTI.

NURSING IMPLICATIONS

Administration

- To prevent hypotension, volume depletion should be corrected prior to initiation of therapy.
- The daily dose may be titrated up to 300 mg; larger doses, however, are not likely to provide additional benefit.
- Store at 15–30C (59–86F).

Assessment & Drug Effects

- Therapeutic effectiveness is indicated by decreases in systolic and diastolic BP.
- Monitor BP periodically; trough readings, just prior to the next scheduled dose, should be made when possible.
- Lab tests: periodically monitor BUN and creatinine, serum potassium, and CBC with differential.

Patient & Family Education

- Women who become pregnant should immediately inform their physicians.
- Maximum pressure lowering effect may not be evident for 6–12 wk.
- Report episodes of dizziness especially when making position changes.

IRINOTECAN HYDROCHLORIDE

(eye-ri-no′te-can)

Trade name: Camptosar

Classifications: ANTINEOPLASTIC; CAMPTOTHECIN; TOPOISOMERASE I INHIBITOR

Prototype: Topotecan

Pregnancy category: D

ACTIONS/PHARMACODYNAMICS

Irinotecan is a camptothecin analog that displays antitumor activity by inhibiting the intranuclear enzyme topoisomerase I. Thus, it is a strong inhibitor of DNA and RNA synthesis. Topoisomerase I is an essential intranuclear enzyme that relaxes the supercoiled DNA, thus enabling replication and transcription to take place. By inhibiting topoisomerase I, irinotecan and its active metabolite SN-38 cause double-stranded DNA damage during the synthesis phase of DNA.

USES Metastatic carcinoma of colon or rectum.

ROUTE & DOSAGE

Metastatic Carcinoma

Adult: **IV** 125 mg/m^2 once weekly for 4 wk, then a 2-wk rest period. Future courses may be adjusted to range from 50 to 150 mg/m^2 depending on tolerance (see complete prescribing information for specific dosage adjustment recommendations based on toxic effects).

PHARMACOKINETICS Peak levels 1 h. **Distribution:** irinotecan is 30% bound to plasma proteins; active metabolite SN-38 is 95% protein bound. **Metabolism:** metabolized in liver by carboxylesterase enzyme to active metabolite SN-38. **Elimination:** half-life: 6 h, 10 h for SN-38; approximately 20% excreted in urine.

CONTRAINDICATIONS & PRECAUTIONS Contraindicated in: previous hypersensitivity to irinotecan, topotecan, or other camptothecin analogs; acute infection, diarrhea, pregnancy (category D), lactation. **Cautious use in:** gastrointestinal disorders, myelosuppression, renal or hepatic function impairment, history of bleeding disorders, previous cytotoxic or radiation therapy. Safety and effectiveness in children not established.

ADVERSE/SIDE EFFECTS Body as whole: *asthenia, fever, pain,* chills, edema, abdominal enlargement, back pain. **CNS:** *headache, insomnia, dizziness.* **CV:** vasodilation/flushing. **GI:** *diarrhea (early and late onset), dehydration, nausea, vomiting, anorexia, weight loss, constipation, abdominal cramping and pain,* flatulence, stomatitis, dyspepsia, increased alkaline phosphatase and SGOT. **Hematologic:** <u>*leukopenia, neutropenia*</u>, *anemia*. **Respiratory:** *dyspnea*, cough, rhinitis. **Skin:** *alopecia*, sweating, rash.

NURSING IMPLICATIONS

Administration

- Administer only after premedication (at least 30 min prior) with an antiemetic.
- IV preparation and administration: dilute the ordered dose in 500 ml of 5% dextrose injection (preferred) or 0.9% NaCl injection to a final concentration of 0.12–1.1 mg/ml and infuse over 90 min.
- If skin contacts drug during preparation, wash immediately with soap and water.
- Closely monitor IV site; if extravasation occurs, immediately flush with sterile water and apply ice.
- Store undiluted at 15–30C (59–86F) and protect from light. Use reconstituted solutions within 24 h.

Assessment & Drug Effects

- Before each dose monitor WBC with differential, Hgb, and platelet count.
- Monitor for acute GI distress, especially early diarrhea (within 24 h of infusion), which may be preceded by diaphoresis and cramping, and late diarrhea (>24 h after infusion).
- During and after periods of diarrhea, closely monitor fluid and electrolyte balance.
- Periodically monitor liver and

renal function tests and blood glucose.

Patient & Family Education

- Advise regarding common adverse effects and provide information on measures to control or minimize when possible.
- Instruct to immediately report diarrhea, vomiting, and S&S of infection. Stress that diarrhea requires prompt treatment to prevent serious fluid and electrolyte imbalances.

I

IRON DEXTRAN

Trade names: Dexferrum, Imfed, Imferon

Classifications: BLOOD FORMER; IRON PREPARATION

Prototype: Ferrous sulfate

Pregnancy category: C

ACTIONS/PHARMACODYNAMICS

A dark brown, slightly viscous liquid complex of ferric hydroxide with dextran in 0.9% NaCl solution for injection. Reticuloendothelial cells of liver, spleen, and bone marrow dissociate iron from iron dextran complex; the released ferric ion combines with transferrin and is transported to bone marrow, where it is incorporated into hemoglobin.

USE

Only in patients with clearly established iron deficiency anemia when oral administration of iron is unsatisfactory or impossible. Each milliliter of iron dextran contains 50 mg elemental iron.

ROUTE & DOSAGE

Iron Deficiency

Adult: **IM/IV** dose is individualized and is determined from a table of correlations between patient's weight and hemoglobin (see package insert); no more than 100 mg (2 ml) of iron dextran should be administered within 24 h.
Child: **IM/IV** <5 kg, no more than 0.5 ml (25 mg)/d; 5–10 kg, no more than 1 ml (50 mg)/d; >10 kg, no more than 2 ml (100 mg)/d.

PHARMACOKINETICS **Absorption:** 60% absorbed from IM site by 3 d; 90% absorbed by 1–3 wk. **Distribution:** crosses placenta; distributed into breast milk. **Metabolism:** metabolized in reticuloendothelial system. **Elimination:** half-life: 6 h.

CONTRAINDICATIONS & PRECAUTIONS **Contraindicated in:** hypersensitivity to the product; all anemias except iron-deficiency anemia. Safe use during pregnancy (category C) not established. **Cautious use in:** rheumatoid arthritis, ankylosing spondylitis; impaired hepatic function; history of allergies or asthma.

ADVERSE/SIDE EFFECTS **CNS:** headache, shivering, transient paresthesias, syncope, dizziness, coma. **CV:** *peripheral vascular flushing (rapid IV), hypotension,* precordial pain or pressure sensation, tachycardia, fatal cardiac arrhythmias, circulatory collapse. **GI:** nausea, vomiting, transient loss of taste perception, metallic taste, diarrhea, melena, abdominal pain, hemorrhagic gastritis, intestinal necrosis. **Hypersensitivity:** urticaria, skin rash, allergic purpura, pruritus, fever, chills, dyspnea, arthralgia, myalgia; anaphylaxis. **Other:** sterile abscess and brown skin discoloration (IM site), local phlebitis (IV site), lymphadenopathy, hemosiderosis, metabolic acidosis, hyperglycemia, reactivation of quiescent rheumatoid arthritis, exogenous hemosiderosis, hepatic damage, seizures, bleeding disorder with severe toxicity, *pain at IM injection site*.

DIAGNOSTIC TEST INTERFERENCE

Falsely elevated ***serum bilirubin*** and falsely decreased ***serum calcium*** values may occur. Large doses of iron dextran may impart a brown color to serum drawn 4 h after iron administration. ***Bone scans*** involving Tc-99m diphosphonate have shown dense areas of activity along contour of iliac crest 1–6 d after IM injections of iron dextran.

NURSING IMPLICATIONS

Administration

Test Dose

- A test dose of 0.5 ml is given over a 5 min period before the first IM or IV therapeutic dose to observe patient's response to the drug. Epinephrine (0.5 ml of a 1:1000 solution) should be immediately available for hypersensitivity emergency.
- Although anaphylactic reactions (see Appendix G) usually occur within a few minutes after injection, it is recommended that 1 h or more elapse before remainder of initial dose is given following test dose.

IM Administration

- The multiple-dose vial is used *only* for IM injections. Since it contains a preservative (phenol), it is not suitable for IV use.
- IM injections should be given only into the muscle mass in upper outer quadrant of buttock (never in the upper arm or other exposed area). Use a 2- or 3-inch, 19- or 20-gauge needle. The Z-track technique is recommended. Use one needle to withdraw drug from container and another needle for injection.
- If patient is receiving IM in standing position, patient should be bearing weight on the leg opposite the injection site; if in bed, patient should be in the lateral position with injection site uppermost.

IV Administration

- If the IV injection does not exceed 100 mg, it is administered undiluted at a prescribed rate usually no more than 50 mg (1 ml) or less per minute.
- IV infusion: Calculated iron dextran dose is diluted in 250–1000 ml of 0.9% NaCl injection. Test dose of 25 mg (0.5 ml) is administered over 5 min. If no adverse reactions occur, remainder of dose is infused (e.g., over 1–6 h). After infusion is completed, flush vein with 10 ml of 0.9% NaCl injection. Increased frequency of adverse effects may be expected with large IV doses.
- After IV administration, patient should remain in bed at least 30 min to prevent orthostatic hypotension. Monitor BP and pulse.
- Store below 30C (86F) unless otherwise directed.

Assessment & Drug Effects

- Anticipated response to parenteral iron therapy is an average weekly hemoglobin rise of about 1 g/d. Peak levels are generally reached in about 4–8 wk.
- IV administration may exacerbate acute joint pain in patients with rheumatoid arthritis or ankylosing spondylitis. For this reason, the IM route is generally preferred in these patients.
- Systemic reactions may occur over

24 h after parenteral iron has been administered.

- Periodic determinations of Hgb and Hct, and reticulocyte count should be made.

Patient & Family Education

- Patients receiving iron injections should not take iron by mouth.
- Encourage to eat foods high in iron and vitamin C.
- Advise to notify physician of any of the following: backache or muscle ache, chills, dizziness, fever, headache, nausea or vomiting, paresthesias, pain or redness at injection site, skin rash or hives, or difficulty breathing.

I

ISOCARBOXAZID

(eye-soe-kar-box′a-zid)

Trade name: Marplan

Classifications: CNS AGENT; PSYCHOTHERAPEUTIC; ANTIDEPRESSANT; MAO INHIBITOR

Prototype: Phenelzine

Pregnancy category: C

ACTIONS/PHARMACODYNAMICS MAO INHIBITOR of the hydrazine group. Inhibits monoamine oxidase, the enzyme involved in the catabolism of catecholamine neurotransmitters and serotonin. Drug increases concentration of these amines in the body, the proposed basis for the antidepressent effect of MAOIs.

USE Symptomatic treatment of depressed patients refractory to or intolerant of TCAs or electroconvulsive therapy.

ROUTE & DOSAGE

Refractory Depression

Adult: **PO** 10–30 mg/d in 1–3 divided doses (max 30 mg/d).

PHARMACOKINETICS **Duration:** up to 2 wk. **Metabolism:** metabolized in liver.

CONTRAINDICATIONS & PRECAUTIONS **Contraindicated in:** hypersensitivity to MAO INHIBITORS; pheochromocytoma; CHF; children (<16 y); elderly (>60 y) or debilitated; severe renal or hepatic impairment. Safe use during pregnancy (category C) and in nursing mothers not established. **Cautious use in:** hypertension, hyperthyroidism, parkinsonism, cardiac arrhythmias, epilepsy, suicidal risks.

ADVERSE/SIDE EFFECTS **CNS:** dizziness, light-headedness, tiredness, weakness, *drowsiness,* vertigo, headache, *overactivity,* hyperreflexia, muscle twitching, tremors, mania hypomania, *insomnia,* confusion, memory impairment. **CV:** *orthostatic hypotension,* paradoxical hypertension, palpitation, tachycardia, other arrhythmias. **Eye:** *blurred vision,* nystagmus, glaucoma. **GI:** increased appetite, weight gain, *nausea,* diarrhea, *constipation, anorexia,* black tongue, *dry mouth,* abdominal pain. **GU:** dysuria, *urinary retention,* incontinence, sexual disturbances. **Other:** peripheral edema, excessive sweating, chills, skin rash, hepatitis, jaundice.

DRUG INTERACTIONS TRICYCLIC ANTIDEPRESSANTS, **fluoxetine,** AMPHETAMINES, **ephedrine, phenylpropanolamine, reserpine, guanethidine, buspirone, methyldopa, dopamine, levodopa, tryp-**

tophan may precipitate hypertensive crisis, headache, or hyperexcitability; **alcohol** and other CNS DEPRESSANTS compound CNS depressant effects; **meperidine** can cause fatal cardiovascular collapse; ANESTHETICS exaggerate hypotensive and CNS depressant effects; **metrizamide** increases risk of seizures; compounds hypotensive effects of DIURETICS and other ANTIHYPERTENSIVE AGENTS. **Food–drug:** all **tyramine**-containing foods (aged cheeses, processed cheeses, sour cream, wine, champagne, beer, pickled herring, anchovies, caviar, shrimp, liver, dry sausage, figs, raisins, overripe bananas or avacodos, chocolate, soy sauce, bean curd, yeast extracts, yogurt, papaya products, meat tenderizers, broad beans) may precipitate hypertensive crisis.

NURSING IMPLICATIONS

Administration

- Dosage is individually adjusted on basis of careful observations of patient.
- Physician will reduce dosage to maintenance level as soon as improvement is observed because drug has a cumulative effect.
- Store in a tight, light-resistant container at 15–30C (59–86F).

Assessment & Drug Effects

- Therapeutic effects may be apparent within 1 wk or less, but in some patients there may be a time lag of 3–4 wk before improvement occurs.
- Monitor BP. Monitor for orthostatic hypotension by evaluating BP with patient recumbent and standing.
- Check for peripheral edema daily and monitor weight several times weekly.
- Toxic symptoms from overdosage or from ingestion of contraindicated substances (e.g., foods high in tyramine) may occur within hours.
- Monitor I&O and bowel elimination patterns.

Patient & Family Education

- Caution to make position changes slowly and in stages and to lie down or sit down if faintness occurs.
- Because drowsiness or dizziness may occur, advise to use caution when performing potentially hazardous activities.
- Advise to consult physician before self-medicating with OTC agents (e.g., cough, cold, hay fever, or diet medications).
- Advise to avoid alcohol and excessive caffeine-containing beverages and tryptophan- and tyramine-containing foods.
- Tyramine-rich foods include cheeses, yeast, meat extracts, smoked or pickled meat, poultry, or fish, fermented sausages, and overripe fruit.

ISOETHARINE HYDROCHLORIDE

(eye-soe-eth'a-reen)

Trade names: Arm-a-Med Isoetharine, Beta-2, Bronkosol, Dey-Lute, Dispos-a-Med Isoethorine

ISOETHARINE MESYLATE

Trade name: Bronkometer

Classifications: AUTONOMIC NERVOUS SYSTEM AGENT; BETA-ADRENERGIC AGONIST (SYMPATHOMIMETIC); BRONCHODILATOR

Prototype: Isoproterenol

Pregnancy category: C

ACTIONS/PHARMACODYNAMICS

Synthetic sympathomimetic stimulant with relatively rapid onset and long duration of action. Has selective affinity for $beta_2$ adrenoceptors on bronchial and selected arteriolar musculature. Relieves reversible bronchospasm and by bronchodilation facilitates expectoration of pulmonary secretions. Increases vital capacity and decreases airway resistance.

USES Bronchial asthma and reversible bronchospasm occurring with bronchitis and emphysema.

ROUTE & DOSAGE

Bronchospasm

Adult: **Inhalation** 0.5–1 ml 0.5% or 0.5 ml 1% solution diluted 1:3 with normal saline, *or* 2–4 ml 0.125% solution undiluted, *or* 2–5 ml 0.2% solution undiluted, *or* 2 ml 0.25% solution undiluted per nebulizer q4h up to 5 times/d; 1–2 inhalations from an MDI q4h up to 5 times/d.
Child: **Inhalation** 0.01 ml/kg of 1% solution (max 0.5 ml) diluted in 2–3 ml normal saline.

PHARMACOKINETICS **Onset:** immediate. **Peak effect:** 5–15 min. **Duration:** 1–4 h. **Metabolism:** metabolized in lungs, liver, GI tract, and other tissues. **Elimination:** excreted by kidneys.

CONTRAINDICATIONS & PRECAUTIONS **Contraindicated in:** known hypersensitivity to sympathomimetic amines and to bisulfites; concomitant use with epinephrine or other sympathomimetic amines; patients with preexisting cardiac arrhythmias associated with tachycardia. Use during pregnancy (category C) and by nursing mothers requires judgment of risk/benefit ratio. **Cautious use in:** elderly patients; hypertension; acute coronary artery disease; CHF; cardiac asthma; hyperthyroidism, diabetes mellitus; tuberculosis; history of seizures.

ADVERSE/SIDE EFFECTS *Tachycardia, palpitations,* changes in BP, cardiac arrest; nausea, vomiting; headache, *anxiety,* tension, restlessness, insomnia, *tremor,* weakness, dizziness, excitement; cough, bronchial irritation and edema; tachyphylaxis.

DRUG INTERACTIONS **Epinephrine,** other SYMPATHOMIMETIC BRONCHODILATORS possibly have additive effects; MAO INHIBITORS, tricyclic antidepressants potentiate action on vascular system; effects of both BETA-ADRENERGIC BLOCKERS and isoetharine antagonized.

NURSING IMPLICATIONS

Administration

- Administer drug on arising in morning and before meals to reduce fatigue from activity by improving lung ventilation.
- Wait 1 full min after initial 1 or 2 inhalations (Bronkometer) to be sure of necessity for another dose. Action should begin immediately and peak within 5–15 min.
- Isoetharine inhalation may be alternated with epinephrine administration but may not be administered simultaneously because of danger of excessively rapid heartbeat.
- Do not use discolored or precipitated solutions.
- Protect solutions from light, freezing, and heat. Store at 15–30C (59–86F).

Assessment & Drug Effects

- The preservative sodium bisulfite is in the hydrochloride formulation. If patient has a history of allergy to sulfite agents, this product should not be used.

- Elderly patients may be especially sensitive to adrenergic drug effects. Monitor cardiac status and report tachycardia and palpitations.

Patient & Family Education
- Warn to close eyes when actuating the nebulizer.
- Caution to use inhalation therapy according to prescribed regimen. Overuse may decrease desired effect and cause symptoms including tachycardia, palpitations, headache, nausea, dizziness.
- Information and instructions are furnished with the aerosol form of isoetharine. Urge patient to read.
- Urge to increase daily fluid intake to aid in liquefaction of bronchial secretions.
- If a sudden increase in dyspnea occurs, instruct to discontinue and report to physician.
- Remind patient not to discard drug applicator. Refill units are available.

ISOFLUROPHATE

(eye-soe-flure′oh-fate)
Trade name: Floropryl
Classifications: EYE PREPARATION; MIOTIC; ANTIGLAUCOMA AGENT
Prototype: Pilocarpine
Pregnancy category: C
See Appendix A.

ISONIAZID (ISONICOTINIC ACID HYDRAZIDE)

(eye-soe-nye′a-zid)
Trade names: INH, Isotamine ♣, Laniazid, Nydrazid, PMS Isoniazid ♣, Teebaconin

Prototype for classifications: ANTIINFECTIVE; ANTITUBERCULOSIS AGENT
Pregnancy category: C

ACTIONS/PHARMACODYNAMICS Hydrazide of isonicotinic acid with highly specific action against *Mycobacterium tuberculosis.* Exerts bacteriostatic action against actively growing tubercle bacilli; may be bactericidal in higher concentrations. Postulated to act by interfering with biosynthesis of bacterial proteins, nucleic acid, and lipids.

USES Treatment of all forms of active tuberculosis caused by susceptible organisms and as preventive in high-risk persons (e.g., household members, persons with positive tuberculin skin test reactions). May be used alone or with other tuberculostatic agents. **Unlabeled use:** treatment of atypical mycobacterial infections; tuberculous meningitis; action tremor in multiple sclerosis.

ROUTE & DOSAGE

Treatment
Adult: **PO/IM** 5 mg/kg up to 300 mg/d.
Child: **PO/IM** 10–20 mg/kg up to 300–500 mg/d.

Preventive Therapy
Adult: **PO** 300 mg/d.
Child: **PO** 10 mg/kg up to 300 mg/d *or* 15 mg/kg 3 times/wk.

PHARMACOKINETICS Absorption: readily absorbed from GI tract; food may reduce rate and extent of absorption. **Peak:** 1–2 h. **Distribution:** distributed to all body tissues and fluids including the CNS; crosses placenta. **Metabolism:** inactivated by acetylation in liver. **Elimination:** half-life: 1–4 h; 75–96% excreted in urine in 24 h; excreted in breast milk.

CONTRAINDICATIONS & PRECAUTIONS **Contraindicated in:** history of isoniazid-associated hypersensitivity reactions, including hepatic injury; acute liver damage of any etiology; pregnancy (category C) unless risk is warranted. **Cautious use in:** chronic liver disease; renal dysfunction; history of convulsive disorders; chronic alcoholism; persons over 35 y.

I

ADVERSE/SIDE EFFECTS Usually dose related. **CNS:** *paresthesias, peripheral neuropathy,* headache, unusual tiredness or weakness, tinnitus, dizziness, hallucinations. **Eye:** blurred vision, visual disturbances, optic neuritis, atrophy. **GI:** nausea, vomiting, epigastric distress, dry mouth, constipation. **Hematologic:** agranulocytosis, hemolytic or aplastic anemia, thrombocytopenia, eosinophilia, methemoglobinemia. **Hepatotoxicity:** *elevated AST, ALT;* bilirubinemia, jaundice, hepatitis. **Hypersensitivity:** fever, chills, skin eruption, vasculitis. **Metabolic/endocrine:** decreased vitamin B_{12} absorption, pyridoxine (vitamin B_6) deficiency, pellagra, gynecomastia, hyperglycemia, glycosuria, hyperkalemia, hypophosphatemia, hypocalcemia, acetonuria, metabolic acidosis, proteinuria. **Other:** dyspnea, urinary retention (males), drug-related fever, rheumatic and lupus erythematosus-like syndromes, irritation at injection site.

DIAGNOSTIC TEST INTERFERENCE Isoniazid may produce false-positive results using ***copper sulfate tests*** (e.g., ***Benedict's solution, Clinitest***) but not with glucose oxidase methods (e.g., Clinistix, Dextrostix, TesTape).

DRUG INTERACTIONS **Cycloserine, ethionamide** enhance CNS toxicity; may increase **phenytoin** levels, resulting in toxicity; ALUMINUM-CONTAINING ANTACIDS decrease GI absorption; **disulfiram** may cause coordination difficulties or psychotic reactions; **alcohol** increases risk of hepatotoxicity. **Drug–food:** food decreases rate and extent of isoniazid absorption; should be taken 1 h before meals.

NURSING IMPLICATIONS

Administration

- PO isoniazid is best taken on an empty stomach at least 1 h before or 2 h after meals. If GI irritation occurs, drug may be taken with meals.
- Isoniazid in solution tends to crystallize at low temperatures; if this occurs, solution should be allowed to warm to room temperature to redissolve crystals before use.
- Local transient pain may follow IM injections. Rotate injection sites.
- Preserved in tightly closed, light-resistant containers at 15–30C (59–86F), unless otherwise directed by manufacturer.

Assessment & Drug Effects

- Appropriate susceptibility tests should be performed before initiation of therapy and periodically thereafter to detect possible bacterial resistance.
- Therapeutic effects usually become evident within the first 2–3 wk of therapy. Over 90% of patients receiving optimal therapy have negative sputum by the sixth month.
- Eye examinations are recommended initially and whenever visual symptoms appear.
- Inactivation of the drug is genetically determined. Slow inactiva-

tion leads to high plasma drug levels and increased risk of toxicity.

- Isoniazid-induced pyridoxine (vitamin B_6) depletion causes neurotoxic effects. B_6 supplementation (10–50 mg) usually accompanies isoniazid use.
- Peripheral neuritis, the most common toxic effect, is usually preceded by paresthesias of feet and hands (numbness, tingling, burning). Patients particularly susceptible include alcoholics and patients with liver disease, malnourished patients, diabetics, slow inactivators, pregnant women, and the elderly.
- Monitor BP during period of dosage adjustment. Some experience orthostatic hypotension; therefore, caution against rapid positional changes.
- Monitor diabetics for loss of glycemic control.
- Periodically monitor hepatic function. Isoniazid hepatitis (sometimes fatal) usually develops during the first 3–6 mo of treatment, but it may occur at any time during drug therapy. It is much more frequent in patients 35 y or older, especially in those who ingest alcohol daily.
- Check weight at least twice weekly under standard conditions.

Patient & Family Education

- Warn patient that concurrent ingestion of tyramine-containing foods (e.g., aged cheeses, smoked fish) may cause palpitation, flushing, and blood pressure elevation.
- Warn patient that histamine-containing foods (e.g., skipjack, tuna, sauerkraut juice, yeast extracts) may cause exaggerated drug response (headache, hypotension, palpitation, sweating, itching, flushing, diarrhea).
- Instruct patient to withhold medication and report promptly to physician if S&S of hepatotoxicity develop (e.g., dark urine, jaundice, clay-colored stools).
- Advise to avoid or at least to reduce alcohol intake while on isoniazid therapy because of increased risk of hepatotoxicity.
- Hypersensitivity reaction should be reported immediately and all drugs withheld. Generally, it occurs within 3–7 wk after initiation of therapy.

I

ISOPROTERENOL HYDROCHLORIDE

(eye-soe-proe-ter′e-nole)

Trade names: Dispos-a-Med Isoproterenol, Isuprel

ISOPROTERENOL SULFATE

Trade name: Medihaler-Iso

Prototype for classifications: AUTONOMIC NERVOUS SYSTEM AGENT; BETA-ADRENERGIC AGONIST (SYMPATHOMIMETIC); BRONCHODILATOR

Pregnancy category: C

ACTIONS/PHARMACODYNAMICS

Synthetic sympathomimetic amine. Acts directly on $beta_1$-adrenergic receptors with little or no effect on alpha-adrenoceptors. Drug induced stimulation of $beta_1$-adrenergic receptors results in increased cardiac output and work by increasing strength of cardiac contraction and, to a slight degree, rate of contraction. Produces slight increase in systolic BP and decrease in diastolic pressure. Reduces total peripheral resistance and increases venous return to the heart by mobilizing blood from vascular reservoirs. Stimulation of $beta_2$-adrenoceptors relaxes bronchospasm and, by increasing ciliary motion, facilitates expectoration of pulmonary secretions. May dilate trachea and main bronchi past the resting diameter.

USES Bronchodilator in treatment of bronchial asthma and reversible bronchospasm induced by anesthesia. Also used as cardiac stimulant in cardiac arrest, carotid sinus hypersensitivity, cardiogenic and bacteremic shock, Adams-Stokes syndrome, or ventricular arrhythmias. Used in treatment of shock that persists after replacement of blood volume. **Unlabeled use:** treatment of status asthmaticus in children.

I

ROUTE & DOSAGE

Bronchospasms

Adult: **MDI** 1–2 inhalations 4–6 times/d; no more than 6 inhalations in any hour during a 24 h period. **Compressed Air or IPPB** 0.5 ml of 0.5% solution diluted to 2–2.5 ml with water or saline over 10–20 min up to 5 times/d. **IV** 0.01-0.02 mg prn.
Child: **MDI** Same as for adult. **Compressed Air or IPPB** 0.5 ml of 0.5% solution diluted to 2–2.5 ml with water or saline over 10-20 min up to 5 times/d.

Cardiac Arrhythmias/Cardiac Resuscitation

Adult: **IV** 0.02–0.06 mg bolus, followed by 5µg/min infusion. **SC** 0.15–0.2 mg prn.
Child: **IV** 2.5 µg/min *or* 0.1µg/kg/min by continuous infusion.

PHARMACOKINETICS Absorption: rapidly absorbed from oral inhalation or parenteral administration. **Onset:** immediate. **Duration:** 1 h oral inhalation; 2 h SC. **Metabolism:** action terminated by tissue uptake and metabolized by COMT in liver, lungs, and other tissues. **Elimination:** 40–50% excreted in urine unchanged.

CONTRAINDICATIONS & PRECAUTIONS Contraindicated in: preexisting cardiac arrhythmias associated with tachycardia; tachycardia caused by digitalis intoxication, central hyperexcitability, cardiogenic shock secondary to coronary artery occlusion and MI; simultaneous administration with epinephrine. Safe use during pregnancy (category C), and by nursing mothers not established. **Cautious use in:** sensitivity to sympathomimetic amines, elderly and debilitated patients, hypertension, coronary insufficiency and other cardiovascular disorders, renal dysfunction, hyperthyroidism, diabetes, prostatic hypertrophy, glaucoma, tuberculosis, during anesthesia by cyclopropane.

ADVERSE/SIDE EFFECTS CNS: headache, mild tremors, nervousness, anxiety, insomnia, excitement, fatigue. **CV:** flushing, palpitations, tachycardia, unstable BP, anginal pain, <u>ventricular arrhythmias</u>. **GI:** swelling of parotids (prolonged use), bad taste, buccal ulcerations (sublingual administration), nausea. **Other:** severe prolonged asthma attack, sweating, bronchial irritation and edema. **Overdosage:** (especially after excessive use of aerosols): *tachycardia,* palpitations, nervousness, nausea, vomiting.

DRUG INTERACTIONS Epinephrine and other SYMPATHOMIMETIC AMINES increase effects and cause cardiac toxicity. HALOGENATED GENERAL ANESTHETICS exacerbate arrhythmias. BETA BLOCKERS antagonize effects.

INCOMPATIBILITIES Solution/additive: sodium bicarbonate, **aminophylline.**

NURSING IMPLICATIONS

Administration

Parenteral (IV)

- IV injection: Dilute 1 ml of 1:5000 solution to 10 ml with sodium chloride or 5% dextrose injection to produce a 1:50,000 solution.
- IV infusion: Dilute 10 ml 1:5000 solution in 500 ml 5% dextrose to produce a 1:250,000 solution.
- Microdrip or constant-infusion pump is recommended to prevent sudden influx of large amounts of drug.
- Infusion rate is generally decreased or infusion may be temporarily discontinued if heart rate exceeds 110 bpm, because of the danger of precipitating arrhythmias.
- IV adminstration is regulated by continuous ECG monitoring. Patient must be observed and response to therapy must be monitored continuously.
- Isoproterenol solutions lose potency with standing. Discard if precipitate or discoloration is present.

Sublingual Tablet

- Patient should be forewarned of potential transient facial flushing, palpitation, and precordial discomfort. (Systemic effects reported to occur more frequently by this route than by inhalation.) Instruct patient to allow tablet to dissolve under tongue, without sucking, and not to swallow saliva (may cause epigastric pain) until drug has been completely absorbed. Sublingual tablet may be administered rectally, if prescribed.

MDI: Instructions for Use

- Shake MDI thoroughly to activate.
- Breathe out through nose expelling as much air from lungs as possible.
- Close lips and teeth around open end of mouthpiece placed well into mouth aimed at back of throat.
- Inhale deeply while pressing down on canister to activate spray mechanism.
- Try to hold breath for 10 s; then slowly exhale through nose or pursed lips.
- Wait 2 full min before starting a second inhalation, if it is necessary.

IPPB (follow IPPB manufacturer's instructions)

- Patient will sit erect in chair or, if not able, lie in semi-Fowler's position.
- Instruct patient to *allow machine to do the work* (deliver medication into air passages and breath for the patient).
- Dentures should be left in place.
- Rinse mouth immediately after inhalation therapy to prevent dryness and throat irritation.

General

- Store in tight, light-resistant containers preferably between 15–30C (59–86F) unless otherwise directed.

Assessment & Drug Effects

- Incidence of arrhythmias is high, particularly when drug is administered IV to patients with cardiogenic shock or ischemic heart disease, digitalized patients, or to those with electrolyte imbalance. Check pulse before and during IV administration. Rate > 110 usually indicates need to slow infusion rate or discontinue infusion. Consult physician for guidelines.
- Tolerance to bronchodilating effect and cardiac stimulant effect may develop with prolonged use.
- Parotid swelling after prolonged

use has been reported. Drug should be discontinued if this occurs.
- Rebound bronchospasm may occur when effects of drug end. Once tolerance has developed, continued use can result in serious adverse effects.

Patient & Family Education
- Prolonged use of sublingual tablets may damage teeth, possibly because of drug acidity. Advise patient to rinse mouth with water after medication has been completely absorbed and between doses.
- Caution patients to take medication as prescribed; (i.e., they should not increase, decrease, or omit doses or change intervals between doses). Advise patients to report to physician if treatment fails to give satisfactory relief.
- Inform patient taking repeated doses of isoproterenol (as well as responsible family members) about adverse effects, and advise them to report onset of such reactions to physician.
- Inform patient that saliva and sputum may appear pink after inhalation treatment.

I

ISOSORBIDE
(eye-soe-sor′bide)
Trade name: Ismotic
Classifications: OSMOTIC DIURETIC; EYE PREPARATION; ANTIGLAUCOMA
Prototype: Mannitol
Pregnancy category: B

ACTIONS/PHARMACODYNAMICS Actions similar to those of other osmotic agents, e.g., mannitol, but produces greater diuresis and does not cause hyperglycemia. Reduces intraocular pressure (IOP) by increasing plasma osmotic pressure.

USES Short-term emergency treatment of acute angle-closure glaucoma and for reducing IOP before and after surgery for glaucoma and cataract.

ROUTE & DOSAGE

Acute Angle-closure Glaucoma
Adult: **PO** 1–3 g/kg b.i.d. to q.i.d.

PHARMACOKINETICS Absorption: readily absorbed from GI tract. **Onset:** 30 min. **Peak:** 1–1.5 h. **Duration:** up to 5–6 h. **Elimination:** eliminated unchanged in urine.

CONTRAINDICATIONS & PRECAUTIONS Contraindicated in: hypersensitivity to isosorbide; severe renal disease, anuria; severe dehydration; frank or impending pulmonary edema; hemorrhagic glaucoma. Safe use during pregnancy (category B) not established. **Cautious use in:** diseases associated with sodium retention.

ADVERSE/SIDE EFFECTS CNS: *headache,* lethargy, vertigo, dizziness, light-headedness, syncope, *confusion, disorientation,* irritability. **GI:** *nausea, vomiting,* diarrhea, anorexia, gastric discomfort. **Other:** thirst, hiccups, rash, hypernatremia, hyperosmolality.

NURSING IMPLICATIONS

Administration
- Isosorbide may be more palatable if poured over cracked ice and sipped.
- Apply gentle pressure to lacrimal sac during and immediately following drug instillation for about 1 min to lessen possibility of systemic absorption.

Assessment & Drug Effects
- Fluid and electrolyte balance should be carefully monitored.

Patient & Family Education
- Advise patient to keep follow-up appointments.

ISOSORBIDE DINITRATE

(eye-soe-sor'bide)

Trade names: Coronex♣, Dilatrate-SR, Iso-Bid, Isordil, Isotrate, Novosorbide♣, Sorbitrate, Sorbitrate SA

Classifications: CARDIOVASCULAR AGENT; NITRATE VASODILATOR

Prototype: Nitroglycerin

Pregnancy category: C

ACTIONS/PHARMACODYNAMICS Organic nitrate with pharmacologic actions similar to those of nitroglycerin. Relaxes vascular smooth muscle with resulting vasodilation. Dilation of peripheral blood vessels tends to cause peripheral pooling of blood, decreased venous return to heart, and decreased left ventricular end-diastolic pressure, with consequent reduction in myocardial oxygen consumption. Cross tolerance with other nitrates is possible.

USES Relief of acute anginal attacks and for management of long-term angina pectoris. **Unlabeled uses:** alone or in combination with a cardiac glycoside or with other vasodilators (e.g., hydralazine, prazosin, for refractory CHF; diffuse esophageal spasm without gastroesophageal reflux and heart failure).

ROUTE & DOSAGE

Angina Prophylaxis

Adult: **PO** regular tablets: 2.5–30 mg q.i.d. a.c. and h.s.; sublingual tablet: 2.5–10 mg q4–6h; chewable tablet: 5–30 mg chewed q2–3h; sustained-release tablets: 40 mg q6–12h.

Acute Anginal Attack

Adult: **PO** sublingual tablet: 2.5–10 mg q2–3h prn; chewable tablet: 5–30 mg chewed prn for relief.

PHARMACOKINETICS Absorption: significant first pass metabolism with PO absorption, with 10–90% reaching systemic circulation. **Onset:** 2–5 min SL; within 1 h regular tabs; within 3 min chewable tabs; 30 min sustained-release tabs. **Duration:** 1–2 h SL; 4–6 h regular tabs; 0.5–2 h chewable tabs; 6–8 h sustained-release tabs. **Metabolism:** metabolized in liver. **Elimination:** 80–100% excreted in urine within 24 h.

CONTRAINDICATIONS & PRECAUTIONS Contraindicated in: hypersensitivity to nitrates or nitrites; severe anemia; head trauma; increased intracranial pressure. Safe use during pregnancy (category C) and in nursing mothers not established. **Cautious use in:** glaucoma, hypotension, hyperthyroidism.

ADVERSE/SIDE EFFECTS CNS: *headache,* dizziness, weakness, *lightheadedness,* restlessness. **CV:** palpitation, postural hypotension, tachycardia. **GI:** nausea, vomiting. **Skin:** *flushing,* pallor, perspiration, rash, exfoliative dermatitis. **Other:** hypersensitivity reaction, paradoxical increase in anginal pain, methemoglobinemia (overdose).

DRUG INTERACTIONS Alcohol may enhance hypotensive effects and lead to cardiovascular collapse;

ANTIHYPERTENSIVE AGENTS, PHENOTHIAZINES add to hypotensive effects.

NURSING IMPLICATIONS

Administration

- Do not confuse with isosorbide, an oral osmotic diuretic.
- Regular oral forms are best taken on an empty stomach (1 h a.c. or 2 h p.c.). If patient complains of vascular headache, however, it may be taken with meals.
- Advise patient not to eat, drink, talk, or smoke while sublingual tablet is under tongue.
- Instruct patient to place sublingual tablet under tongue at first sign of an anginal attack. If pain is not relieved, repeat dose at 5–10 min intervals to a maximum of 3 doses. If pain continues, notify physician or go to nearest hospital emergency room.
- Chewable tablet must be thoroughly chewed before it is swallowed.
- Sustained-release forms should be swallowed whole and not crushed or chewed.
- Patient should be sitting when taking rapid-acting forms of isosorbide dinitrate (sublingual and chewable tablets) because of the possibility of faintness.
- Store in tightly closed container in a cool, dry place, preferably at 15–30C (59–86F) unless otherwise directed. Do not expose to extremes of temperature.

Assessment & Drug Effects

- Monitor effectiveness of drug in relieving angina.
- Headaches tend to decrease in intensity and frequency with continued therapy but may require administration of analgesic and reduction in dosage.
- Chronic administration of large doses may produce tolerance and thus decrease effectiveness of nitrate preparations.

Patient & Family Education

- Caution to make position changes slowly, particularly from recumbent to upright posture, and to dangle feet and ankles before ambulating.
- Instruct to lie down at the first indication of light-headedness or faintness.
- Therapeutic effectiveness of isosorbide dinitrate may be evaluated by having patient keep a record of anginal attacks and the number of sublingual tablets required to provide relief.
- Advise not to drink alcohol because it may increase possibility of light-headedness and faintness.

ISOSORBIDE MONONITRATE

(eye-soe-sor′bide)

Trade names: Ismo, Imdur, Monoket

Classifications: CARDIOVASCULAR AGENT; NITRATE VASODIALATOR

Prototype: Nitroglycerin

Pregnancy category: C (category B for sustained form)

ACTIONS/PHARMACODYNAMICS

Isosorbide mononitrate is a long-acting metabolite of the vasodilator isosorbide dinitrate. It is equally or more effective than isosorbide dinitrate in the treatment of chronic, stable angina. It is a potent venodialator with antianginal and antiischemic effects. It decreases preload as measured by pulmonary capillary wedge pressure (PCWP), and left ventricular end volume and diastolic pressure (LVEDV), with a consequent reduction in myocardial oxygen consumption.

USE Prevention of angina. Not indicated for acute attacks.

ROUTE & DOSAGE

Prevention of Angina

Adult: **PO** ***Regular release (ISMO, Monoket):*** 20 mg b.i.d. 7 h apart. ***Sustained release (Imdur):*** 30–60 mg every morning; may increase up to 120 mg once daily after several days if needed (max dose 240 mg).

PHARMACOKINETICS Absorption: completely and rapidly absorbed from GI tract; 93% reaches systemic circulation. **Onset:** 1h. **Peak:** regular release 30–60 min; sustained release 3–4 h. **Duration:** regular release 5–12h; sustained release 12h. **Metabolism:** metabolized in liver by denitration and conjugation to inactive metabolites. **Elimination:** half-life: 4–5 h; excreted primarily by kidneys.

CONTRAINDICATIONS & PRECAUTIONS Contraindicated in: hypersensitivity to nitrates; severe anemia; closed-angle glaucoma, postural hypotension, head trauma, cerebral hemorrhage (increases intracranial pressure). Safe use during pregnancy [(category C) and (category B for sustained form)] and in nursing mothers not established. **Cautious use in:** elderly, hypotension.

ADVERSE/SIDE EFFECTS CNS: *headache,* agitation, anxiety, confusion, loss of coordination, hypoesthesia, hypokinesia, insomnia or somnolence, nervousness, migraine headache, paresthesia, vertigo, ptosis, tremor. **CV:** aggravation of angina, abnormal heart sounds, mumurs, <u>MI</u>, transient hypotension, palpitations. **Hematologic:** hypochromic anemia, purpura, thrombocytopenia, methemoglobinemia (high doses). **GI:** nausea, vomiting, dry mouth, abdominal pain, constipation, diarrhea, dyspepsia, flatulence, tenesmus, gastric ulcer, hemorrhoids, gastritis, glossitis. **Metabolic:** hyperuricemia, hypokalemia. **GU:** renal calculus, UTI, atrophic vaginitis, dysuria, polyuria, urinary frequency, decreased libido, impotence. **Respiratory:** bronchitis, pneumonia, upper respiratory tract infection, nasal congestion, bronchospasm, coughing, dyspnea, rales, rhinitis. **Skin:** rash, pruritus, hot flashes, acne, abnormal texture. **Other:** diplopia, blurred vision, photophobia, conjunctivitis.

DRUG INTERACTIONS Alcohol may cause severe hypotension and cardiovascular collapse. **Aspirin** may increase nitrate serum levels. CALCIUM CHANNEL BLOCKERS may cause orthostatic hypotension.

NURSING IMPLICATIONS

Administration

- With twice daily dosing, recommended regimen is first dose in morning on arising and second dose 7 h later. With once daily dosing, give in morning on arising.
- Sustained-release tablets should be stored at room temperature, 15–30C (59–86F), in a tight container. Sustained-release tablets may be stored under refrigeration or at room temperature, 2–30C (36–86F).

Assessment & Drug Effects

- Monitor cardiac status, frequency and severity of angina, and BP.
- Assess for and report possible signs and symptoms of toxicity, including orthostatic hypotension, syncope, dizziness, palpitations, light-headedness, severe head-

ache, blurred vision, and difficulty breathing.
- Monitor serum electolytes periodically.

Patient & Family Education
- Advise not to crush or chew sustained-release tablets. The tablets may be broken in two and should be taken with adequate fluid (4–8 oz).
- Advise not to withdraw drug abruptly, as doing so may precipitate acute angina.
- Instruct regarding importance of maintaining correct dosing interval with twice daily dosing.
- Warn geriatric patients of the possibility of developing postural hypotension.
- Advise to avoid alcohol ingestion and aspirin unless specifically permitted by physician.

I

ISOTRETINOIN (13-*cis*-RETINOIC ACID)

(eye-soe-tret'i-noyn)

Trade name: Accutane

Prototype for classifications: SKIN AND MUCOUS MEMBRANE AGENT; ANTIACNE; RETINOID

Pregnancy category: X

ACTIONS/PHARMACODYNAMICS Highly toxic metabolite of retinol (vitamin A). Principal actions: regulation of cell (e.g., epithelial) differentiation and proliferation and of altered lipid composition on skin surface. Decreases sebum secretion by reducing sebaceous gland size; inhibits gland cell differentiation; blocks follicular keratinization.

USES Treatment of severe recalcitrant cystic or conglobate acne in patient unresponsive to conventional treatment, including systemic antibiotics. **Unlabeled uses:** lamellar ichthyosis, oral leukoplakia, hyperkeratosis, acne rosacea, scarring gram-negative folliculitis; adjuvant therapy of basal cell carcinoma of lung and cutaneous T-cell lymphoma (mycosis fungoides); psoriasis; chemoprevention for prostate cancer.

ROUTE & DOSAGE

Cystic Acne

Adult: **PO** 0.5-1 mg/kg/d in 2 divided doses; max recommended dose 2 mg/kg/d.

Disorders of Keratinization

Adult: **PO** up to 4 mg/kg/d in divided doses.

PHARMACOKINETICS Absorption: rapid absorption after slow dissolution in GI tract; 25% of administered drug reaches systemic circulation. **Peak:** 3.2 h. **Distribution:** not fully understood; appears in liver, ureters, adrenals, ovaries and lacrimal glands. **Metabolism:** metabolized in liver; enterohepatically cycled. **Elimination:** half-life: 10–20 h; excreted in urine and feces in equal amounts.

CONTRAINDICATIONS & PRECAUTIONS Contraindicated in: pregnancy (category X); sensitivity to parabens (preservatives in the formulation), nursing mothers. **Cautious use in:** coronary artery disease; diabetes mellitus; obesity; alcoholism; rheumatologic disorders; history of pancreatitis, hepatitis; retinal disease; elevated triglycerides.

ADVERSE/SIDE EFFECTS Most are dose-related, i.e., occurring at doses >1 mg/kg/d; reversible with termination of therapy. **CNS:** lethargy, headache, fatigue, visual disturbances, pseudotumor cerebri, paresthesias, dizziness, depression, psychosis, suicide (rare). **Eye:** reduced night vision, dry eyes, papilledema, eye irritation, *conjunctivitis*, corneal opacities. **GI:** *dry mouth*, anorexia, nausea, vomiting, abdominal pain, nonspecific GI symptoms, acute hepatotoxic reactions (rare), inflammation and bleeding of gums. **Hematologic:** decreased Hct, Hgb, elevated sedimentation rate. **Musculoskeletal:** arthralgia; bone, joint, and muscle pain and stiffness; chest pain, skeletal hyperostosis (especially in athletic people and with prolonged therapy). **Skin:** *cheilitis*, skin fragility, dry skin, pruritus, peeling of face, palms, and soles; photosensitivity (photoallergic and phototoxic), erythema, skin infections, petechiae, rash, urticaria, exaggerated healing response (painful exuberant granulation tissue with crusting), brittle nails, thinning hair. **Other:** epistaxis, *dry nose*, increased AST, ALT; hyperuricemia, mild bruising, acute pancreatitis, *increased serum concentrations of triglycerides by 50–70%*, serum cholesterol by 15–20%, VLDL cholesterol by 50–60%, LDL cholesterol by 15–20%.

DRUG INTERACTION VITAMIN A SUPPLEMENTS increase toxicity.

NURSING IMPLICATIONS

Administration

- Take isotretinoin with or shortly after meals.
- After 2 wk of treatment, regimen is reassessed and dose adjusted as warranted.
- A single course of therapy provides adequate control in many patients. If a second course is necessary, it is delayed at least 8 wk because improvement may continue without the drug.
- Isotretinoin is photosensitive. Store in tight, light-resistant container at 15–30C (59–86F). Capsules remain stable for 2 y.

Assessment & Drug Effects

- Baseline control values for blood lipids should be determined at outset of treatment with isotretinoin, then at 2 wk, 1 mo, and every month thereafter throughout course of therapy.
- Liver function tests are performed at 2- or 3-wk intervals for 6 mo and then once a month thereafter during treatment. Signs of liver dysfunction (jaundice, pruritus, dark urine) should be reported promptly.
- Blood glucose should be closely monitored in diabetic and diabetic-prone patients.
- Persistence of hypertriglyceridemia (levels above 500–800 mg/dl) despite a reduced dose indicates necessity to stop drug to prevent onset of acute pancreatitis.

Patient & Family Education

- During the first few weeks, transient exacerbations of acne may occur. Urge to maintain drug regimen, however, since recurring symptoms may signify response of deep unseen lesions to the drug.
- If visual disturbances occur along with nausea, vomiting, and headache, instruct to discontinue the medication at once and report to the physician to rule out benign intracranial hypertension. Patient should be screened for papilledema. If papilledema is present, isotretinoin should be discontinued.
- Visual disturbances may also sig-

nify development of corneal opacities, which should be ruled out by ophthalmic examination. If corneal opacities are present, drug will be discontinued. Urge to return for a follow-up examination.

- Pregnancy should be ruled out by pregnancy test within 2 wk of starting treatment. Patient should use a reliable contraceptive at least 1 mo before and throughout treatment and for 1 mo after therapy has been discontinued.
- Weight reduction and restriction of alcohol and dietary fat intake are prophylactic against development of hypertriglyceridemia.
- Advise not to self-medicate with multivitamins, which usually contain vitamin A. Toxicity of isotretinoin is enhanced by vitamin A supplements.
- Warn to avoid or minimize exposure of the treated skin to sun or sunlamps. Photosensitivity (photoallergic and phototoxic) potential is high. The risk of skin cancer may be increased by this drug.
- Report abdominal pain, rectal bleeding, or severe diarrhea, possible symptoms of drug-induced inflammatory bowel disease. Drug treatment will be discontinued.
- Dry mouth and cheilitis (inflamed, chapped lips), frequent side effects of isotretinoin, are distressing and are potential preconditions conducive to infections. Urge patient to keep lips moist and softened (use thin layer of lubricant such as petroleum jelly).
- Advise to report joint pain, such as pain in the great toe (symptom of gout and hyperuricemia).
- Caution not to share drug with friend because it is associated with side effects that necessitate medical supervision.

I

ISOXSUPRINE HYDROCHLORIDE

(eye-sox′syoo-preen)

Trade names: Vasodilan, Vasoprine

Classifications: AUTONOMIC NERVOUS SYSTEM AGENT; BETA-ADRENERGIC AGONIST; CARDIOVASCULAR AGENT; VASODILATOR

Prototype: Isoproterenol

Pregnancy category: C

ACTIONS/PHARMACODYNAMICS

Sympathomimetic with beta-adrenergic stimulant activity and with slight effect on alpha receptors. Vasodilating action on arteries within skeletal muscles is greater than on cutaneous vessels. Also causes cardiac stimulation and may produce bronchodilation, mild inhibition of GI motility, and uterine relaxation.

USES Adjunctive therapy in treatment of cerebral vascular insufficiency and peripheral vascular disease, such as arteriosclerosis obliterans, thromboangitis obliterans (Buerger's disease), and Raynaud's disease. **Unlabeled uses:** dysmenorrhea and threatened abortion and premature labor, but efficacy has not been established.

ROUTE & DOSAGE

Cerebral Vascular Insufficiency, Peripheral Vascular Disease

Adult: **PO** 10–20 mg t.i.d. or q.i.d.

PHARMACOKINETICS **Absorption:** readily absorbed from GI tract. **Peak:** 1 h. **Duration:** 3 h. **Distribution:** crosses placenta. **Metabolism:** metabolized in blood. **Elimination:** half-life: 1.25 h; excreted in urine.

CONTRAINDICATIONS & PRECAUTIONS **Contraindicated in:** immediately postpartum; presence of arterial bleeding; parenteral use in presence of hypotension, tachycardia. Safe use in pregnancy (category C) not established. **Cautious use in:** bleeding disorders; severe cerebrovascular disease, severe obliterative coronary artery disease, recent MI.

ADVERSE/SIDE EFFECTS CV: flushing, orthostatic hypotension with light-headedness, faintness; palpitation, tachycardia. **CNS:** dizziness, nervousness, trembling, weakness. **GI:** nausea, vomiting, abdominal distress, abdominal distention.

NURSING IMPLICATIONS

Administration

- Do not give isoxsuprine immediately after delivery, since it causes uterine relaxation, or in the presence of arterial bleeding.
- Store in tight containers at 15–30C (59–86F) unless otherwise directed.

Assessment & Drug Effects

- May cause hypotension and tachycardia. Monitor BP and pulse. Supervise ambulation.
- If isoxsuprine has been used to delay premature labor, hypotension and irregular and rapid heartbeat may be observed in both mother and baby. Hypocalcemia, hypoglycemia, and ileus have been observed in babies born of mothers taking isoxsuprine.
- Therapeutic response to isoxsuprine in treatment of peripheral vascular disorders may take several weeks. Evaluate clinical manifestations of arterial insufficiency.

Patient & Family Education

- Advise to report adverse reactions (skin rash, palpitation, flushing) promptly; symptoms are usually effectively controlled by dosage reduction or discontinuation of drug.
- To prevent orthostatic hypotension, instruct to make position changes slowly and in stages, particularly from recumbent to upright posture and to avoid standing still.
- For treatment of menstrual cramps, isoxsuprine is usually started 1–3 d before onset of menstruation and continued until pain is relieved or menstrual flow stops.

ISRADIPINE

(is-ra′di-peen)

Trade names: Dynacirc, DynaCirc CR

Classifications: CARDIOVASCULAR AGENT; CALCIUM CHANNEL BLOCKER

Prototype: Nifedipine

Pregnancy category: C

ACTIONS/PHARMACODYNAMICS Inhibits calcium ion influx into cardiac muscle and smooth muscle without changing calcium concentrations, thus affecting contractility. Isradipine relaxes coronary vascular smooth muscle with little or no negative inotropic effect. It significantly decreases systemic vascular resistance and reduces BP at rest and during isometric and dynamic exercise.

USES Mild to moderate hypertension. **Unlabeled uses:** angina, CHF.

ROUTE & DOSAGE

Hypertension

Adult: **PO** 1.25–10 mg b.i.d. (max 20 mg/d). DynaCirc CR dosed q.d.

Angina
Adult: **PO** 2.5–7.5 mg t.i.d. (max 15 mg/d).

PHARMACOKINETICS Absorption: rapidly and completely absorbed from GI tract, but only 15–24% reaches systemic circulation because of first-pass metabolism. **Onset:** 1 h. **Peak:** 2–3 h. **Duration:** 12 h. **Distribution:** not known if crosses placenta or is distributed into breast milk. **Metabolism:** extensive first-pass metabolism in liver. **Elimination:** half-life: 5–11 h; 70% excreted in urine as inactive metabolites; 30% excreted in feces.

I

CONTRAINDICATIONS & PRECAUTIONS Contraindicated in: hypersensitivity to isradipine. **Cautious use in:** patients with CHF, pregnancy (category C). It is not known if isradipine is excreted in human milk. Safety and effectiveness have not been established in children.

ADVERSE/SIDE EFFECTS CNS: *headache,* dizziness, fainting, fatigue, sleep disturbances, vertigo. **CV:** flushing, ankle edema, palpitations, tachycardia, hypotension, chest pain, CHF. **GI:** nausea, vomiting, abdominal discomfort, constipation. **Other:** increased liver enzymes, dyspnea, rash, decreased skin sensation.

DRUG INTERACTIONS Adenosine may prolong bradycardia. May increase **cyclosporine** levels and toxicity.

NURSING IMPLICATIONS

Administration
- After the first 2–4 wk of drug therapy, dose may be increased for improved BP control in increments of 5 mg/d at 2–4 wk intervals up to a maximum dose of 20 mg/d.
- Store at 15–30C (59–86F) in tight, light-resistant container.

Assessment & Drug Effects
- Monitor BP throughout course of therapy.
- Carefully monitor patients with a history of CHF, especially with concurrent beta blocker use. Promptly report signs and symptoms of worsening heart failure.
- Monitor ambulation, especially with elderly patients, until response to isradipine is known.

Patient & Family Education
- Advise to promptly report shortness of breath, palpitations, or other signs of adverse cardiovascular effects.
- Advise of the potential for dizziness and encourage appropriate precautions.

ITRACONAZOLE
(i-tra-con′-a-zole)
Trade name: Sporanox
Classifications: ANTIINFECTIVE; ANTIBIOTIC; ANTIFUNGAL
Prototype: Fluconazole
Pregnancy category: C

ACTIONS/PHARMACODYNAMICS Synthetic antifungal agent active against many fungi, including yeast and dermatophytes. Antifungal spectrum of activity is similar to fluconazole.

USES Treatment of systemic fungal infections caused by blastomycosis, histoplasmosis, aspergillosis, onychomycosis due to dermatophytes of the toenail with or without fingernail involvement; oropharyngeal and esophageal candidiasis; orally to treat superficial mycoses (*Candida,* pityriasis versicolor). **Unlabeled use:** systemic and vaginal candidiasis.

ROUTE & DOSAGE

Pulmonary and Extrapulmonary Blastomycosis, Nonmeningeal Histoplasmosis

Adult: **PO** 200 mg once daily, may increase to a max of 200 mg b.i.d. if no apparent improvement. Continue for at least 3 mo. For life-threatening infections, start with 200 mg t.i.d. for 3 d, then 200–400 mg/d.
Child: **PO** 3–5 mg/kg/d for 3–6 mo.

Oropharyngeal Candidiasis

Adult: **PO** 200 mg daily for 1–2 wk.

Esophageal Candidiasis

Adult: **PO** 100 mg daily for at least 3 wk (max 200 mg/d).

Vaginal Candidiasis

Adult: **PO** 200 mg q.d. for 3 d.

Onychomycosis

Adult: **PO** 200 mg q.d. for 3 mo.

PHARMACOKINETICS **Absorption:** well absorbed from GI tract when taken with food. **Onset:** 2 wk–3 mo. **Peak:** peak levels at 1.5–5 h. Steady-state concentrations reached in 10–14 d. **Distribution:** highly protein bound, minimal concentrations in CSF. Higher concentrations in tissues than in plasma. **Metabolism:** extensively metabolized in liver, may undergo enterohepatic recirculation. **Elimination:** half-life: 34–42 h; 35% in urine, 55% excreted in feces.

CONTRAINDICATIONS & PRECAUTIONS **Contraindicated in:** coadministration of terfenadine, hypersensitivity to itraconazole, nursing mothers. **Cautious use in:** hypersensitivity to other azole antifungal agents, hepatitis, HIV infection, pregnancy (category C). Safety and efficacy in children not established.

ADVERSE/SIDE EFFECTS: **CV:** hypertension with higher doses. **CNS:** headache, dizziness, fatigue, somnolence (euphoria, drowsiness <1%). **Endocrine:** gynecomastia, hypokalemia (especially with higher doses), hypertriglyceridemia. **GI:** *nausea, vomiting, dyspepsia, abdominal pain, diarrhea, anorexia, flatulence, gastritis.* **GU:** decreased libido, impotence. **Hepatic:** elevations of serum transaminases, alkaline phosphatase, and bilirubin. **Skin:** rash, pruritus. **Severe toxicity:** doses exceeding 400 mg daily have been associated with higher risk of severe toxicity (hypokalemia, hypertension, adrenal insufficiency).

DRUG INTERACTIONS May be more susceptible to hypoglycemia with ORAL HYPOGLYCEMIC AGENTS. **Carbamazepine, phenytoin, rifampin** significantly decrease itraconazole levels, resulting in antifungal failure. H_2-ANTAGONISTS, **isoniazid** may decrease itraconazole levels. May increase **cyclosporine** levels and toxicity. May increase **digoxin** levels. Coadministration with **terfenadine** or **cisapride** has resulted in elevated **terfenadine** or **cisapride** plasma concentrations, which have led to rare occurrences of life-threatening cardiac dysrhythmias. May enhance anticoagulant effects of **warfarin.**

NURSING IMPLICATIONS

Administration

- Capsules should be taken with a full meal.
- Oral solution should be taken without food. Liquid should be vigorously swished for several seconds and swallowed.

- Oral solution and capsules should not be interchanged.
- Dosages greater than 200 mg/d should be divided into two doses.
- Store capsules at room temperature (15–30C/59–86F) unless otherwise directed.
- Store liquid at or below 25C (77F).

Assessment & Drug Effects

- Culture and sensitivity tests should be done before initiation of therapy. Therapy may be initiated while results are pending.
- Monitor hepatic functions especially in those with preexisting hepatic abnormalities.
- When given concurrently with digoxin, monitor for digoxin toxicity.
- When given concurrently with warfarin, carefully monitor PT and INR.
- Monitor for signs and symptoms of hypersensitivity (see Appendix G); discontinue drug and notify physician if noted.

Patient & Family Education

- Instruct to take with food.
- Instruct to promptly report signs and symptoms of liver dysfunction, including anorexia, nausea, and vomiting; weakness and fatigue; dark urine and clay-colored stool.
- Advise diabetics on oral hypoglycemic agents that risk of hypoglycemia may increase.

IVERMECTIN

(i-ver-mec'tin)

Trade name: Stromectol

Classifications: ANTIINFECTIVE; ANTHELMINTIC

Prototype: Mebendazole

Pregnancy category: C

ACTIONS/PHARMACODYNAMICS A semisynthetic anthelmintic agent which is a broad-spectrum antiparasitic agent with a unique mode of action. It leads to an increase in the permeability to chloride ions of the cell membrane of the parasites, resulting in hyperpolarization of the nerve or muscle cell. This results in paralysis and death of the parasite.

USES Treatment of strongyloidiasis of the intestinal tract, onchocerciasis.

ROUTE & DOSAGE

Strongyloides

Adult & Child ≥ 15 kg: **PO** 200 μg/kg × 1 dose (supplied as 6-mg tablets)

Onchocerciasis

Adult & Child ≥ 15 kg: **PO** 150 μg/kg × 1 dose. May retreat q3–12 mo prn.

PHARMACOKINETICS **Peak:** 4 h. **Distribution:** distributed into breast milk. **Metabolism:** metabolized in the liver. **Elimination:** half-life: 16 h; excreted in feces over 12 d.

CONTRAINDICATIONS & PRECAUTIONS **Contraindicated in:** hypersensitivity to ivermectin. **Cautious use in:** pregnancy (category C), nursing mothers. Safety and efficacy in children ≤ 15 kg have not been established.

ADVERSE/SIDE EFFECTS **Body as whole:** *fever,* peripheral edema. **CNS:** dizziness. **CV:** tachycardia. **GI** diarrhea, nausea. **Skin:** *pruritus, rash.* **Other:** arthralgia/synovitis, lymphadenopathy.

NURSING IMPLICATIONS

Administration

- Tablets should be taken with water.
- Store below 30C (86F).

Assessment & Drug Effects

- Therapeutic effectiveness for strongyloidiasis is indicated by negative stool samples.
- Monitor for cardiovascular effects such as orthostatic hypotension and tachycardia.
- Monitor for and report inflammatory conditions of the eyes.

Patient & Family Education

- A follow-up stool examination is needed to determine effectiveness of treatment for strongyloidiasis.
- Onchocerciasis treatment does not kill adult parasites; repeated follow-up and retreatment are usually needed.
- Report to physician if eye discomfort develops.

KANAMYCIN

(kan-a-mye'sin)

Trade name: Kantrex

Classifications: ANTIINFECTIVE; ANTIBIOTIC, AMINOGLYCOSIDE

Prototype: Gentamicin

Pregnancy category: D

ACTIONS/PHARMACODYNAMICS Broad-spectrum, aminoglycoside antibiotic derived from *Streptomyces kanamyceticus*. Usually bacterial in action. Active against many gram-negative microorganisms, especially *Acinetobacter, Escherichia coli, Enterobacter aerogenes, Klebsiella pneumoniae, Proteus* sp, and *Serratia marcescens*. Also effective against many strains of *Staphylococcus aureus,* but it is not the drug of choice. Inhibits growth of *Mycobacterium tuberculosis* in vitro.

USES Orally to reduce ammonia-producing bacteria in intestinal tract, as adjunctive treatment of hepatic coma, and for preoperative bowel antisepsis; parenterally for short-term treatment of serious infections; intraperitoneally after fecal spill during surgery; as irrigation solution; and as aerosol treatment. Has been used with other drugs to treat tuberculosis in patients resistant to conventional therapy.

ROUTE & DOSAGE

Preoperative Intestinal Antisepsis

Adult: **PO** 1 g q1h for 4 doses, then q6h for 36–72 h.

Hepatic Coma

Adult: **PO** 8–12 g/d in divided doses.

Serious Infection

Adult: **IM/IV** 15 mg/kg/d in equally divided doses q8–12h.
Child: **IM/IV** Same as for adult.
Adult: **Intraperitoneal** 500 mg diluted in 20 ml sterile water instilled through wound catheter; **Inhalation** 250 mg diluted in 3 ml normal saline administered per nebulizer q6–12h; **Irrigation** 0.25% solution prn.

PHARMACOKINETICS Absorption: poorly absorbed from GI tract; readily absorbed from peritoneal cavity, bronchial tree, and wounds. **Peak:** 1–2 h. **Distribution:** crosses placenta; distributed into breast milk. **Elimination:** half-life: 2–4 h; 80–90% excreted in urine within 24 h.

CONTRAINDICATIONS & PRECAUTIONS Contraindicated in: history of hypersensitivity to kanamycin or other aminoglycosides; history of drug-induced ototoxicity, preexisting hearing loss, vertigo, or tinnitus; long-term therapy; PO use in intestinal obstruction or ulcerative bowel lesions; intraperitoneally to patients under effects of inhalation anesthetics or skeletal muscle relaxants. Safe use during pregnancy (category D) and in nursing women not established. **Cautious use in:** impaired renal function; elderly patients, neonates, and infants (immature renal systems); myasthenia gravis; parkinsonian syndrome.

ADVERSE/SIDE EFFECTS Dose related: **CNS:** dizziness, circumoral and other paresthesias, optic neuritis, peripheral neuritis, headache, restlessness, tremors, lethargy, convulsions; rarely: neuromuscular paralysis, respiratory depression. **ENT:** *ototoxicity:* deafness (can be irreversible), *tinnitus, vertigo* or *dizziness,* ataxia, nystagmus. **GI:** nausea, vomiting, diarrhea, appetite changes, abdominal discomfort, stomatitis, proctitis, malabsorption syndrome (with prolonged oral administration). **Hematologic:** anemia, increased or decreased reticulocytes, granulocytopenia, agranulocytosis, thrombocytopenia, purpura. **Hypersensitivity:** eosinophilia, maculopapular rash, pruritus, urticaria, drug fever, anaphylaxis. **Renal:** nephrotoxicity; hematuria, urine casts and cells, proteinuria; elevated serum creatinine and BUN. **Other:** superinfections; local pain; nodular formation at injection site. See gentamicin for other possible adverse/side effects.

DRUG INTERACTIONS Amphotericin B, cisplatin, methoxyflurane, vancomycin add to nephrotoxicity; GENERAL ANESTHETICS, SKELETAL MUSCLE RELAXANTS add to neuromuscular blocking effects; **capreomycin** compounds ototoxicity and nephrotoxicity; LOOP AND THIAZIDE DIURETICS may increase risk of ototoxicity.

INCOMPATIBILITIES Solution/additive: cephalothin, cephapirin, chlorpheniramine, colistimethate, heparin, hydrocortisone, methohexital, ampicillin, carbenicillin, methicillin, penicillin, mezlocillin, piperacillin. Y-site: heparin, methohexital.

NURSING IMPLICATIONS

Administration

- PO kanamycin can be taken on a full or empty stomach.
- Administer IM injection deep into upper outer quadrant of gluteal muscle (often painful). Observe sites daily for signs of irritation; rotate injection sites.
- IV preparation and administration: Each 500 mg must be diluted with at least 100 to 200 ml 0.9% NaCl or 5% dextrose injection and administered over 30–60 min.
- Kanamycin is stable for 24 h at room temperature in most IV solutions. Consult manufacturer's literature for storage and compatibility information.
- Store unopened vials and capsules at 15–30C (59–86F) unless otherwise directed. Some vials may darken with time, but this does not affect potency.

Assessment & Drug Effects

- Culture and susceptibility studies should be performed before initiation of therapy and periodically thereafter.
- Baseline weight, vital signs, urinalysis, and kidney function tests should be assessed before and at regular intervals during therapy.
- Monitor peak and trough serum kanamycin concentrations.
- Peak kanamycin concentrations are generally drawn 30–60 min after IM administration and 30 min after completion of a 30–60 min IV infusion. For trough levels, blood specimens are drawn just before the next IM or IV dose.
- Parenteral kanamycin is highly

concentrated in the urinary system; patient should be well hydrated to prevent chemical irritation of renal tubules.

- Monitor I&O. Report decrease in urine output or change in I&O ratio.
- Check urinalysis and kidney function and notify physician immediately of signs of renal irritation: albuminuria, casts, red and white cells in urine, increasing NPN, BUN, and serum creatinine, decreasing urine specific gravity, and creatinine clearance, oliguria, and edema.
- Risk of ototoxicity is high in patients with impaired renal function, the elderly, poorly hydrated patients, and when therapy is expected to last ≥5 d.
- Patient should be monitored for hearing and balance problems. Drug should be stopped if ototoxicity occurs.
- Tinnitus is not a reliable index of ototoxicity in the very old.
- In patients with impaired renal function, deafness has occurred 2–7 d or more after termination of therapy.
- Patients receiving kanamycin in the immediate postoperative period should be closely monitored for neuromuscular blockade (muscle weakness, apnea, and respiratory depression).
- Be alert to signs of superinfection (see Appendix G).

Patient & Family Education

- In treatment of UTI, physician may prescribe concomitant administration of an alkalinizing agent or patient may be advised to omit foods that enhance urine acidity (e.g., prunes and prune juice, cranberries and cranberry juice).
- Advise to report ototoxic symptoms.

KAOLIN AND PECTIN

(kay'oh-lin and pek'tin)

Trade names: Kao-tin, Kapectolin, Kaypectol, K-P, K-Pek, Pecto Kay

Classifications: GI AGENT; ANTIDIARRHEAL

Prototype: Diphenoxylate with atropine

Pregnancy category: C

ACTIONS/PHARMACODYNAMICS

Kaolin is native hydrated aluminum silicate, powdered and freed from impurities for pharmaceutical use. Kaolin is reported to have adsorbent, protectant, and demulcent properties. Pectin's mechanism of action is unknown; it is believed to act as an adsorbent and demulcent and may help consolidate stool. Efficacy of kaolin or pectin in diarrhea is not clearly established.

USES Adjunct in symptomatic treatment of mild to moderately severe acute diarrhea. Commonly used in antidiarrheal combination products.

ROUTE & DOSAGE

Diarrhea

Adult: **PO** 60–120 ml of regular suspension *or* 45–90 ml of concentrated suspension after each loose bowel movement.
Child: **PO** *3–5 y,* 15–30 ml regular suspension *or* 15 ml concentrated suspension after each loose bowel movement; *6–11 y,* 30–60 ml regular suspension *or* 30 ml concentrated suspension after each loose bowel movement; *≥ 12 y,* 60 ml regular suspension *or* 45 ml concentrated suspension after each loose bowel movement.

K

PHARMACOKINETICS Absorption: not absorbed from GI tract.

CONTRAINDICATIONS & PRECAUTIONS Contraindicated in: suspected obstructive bowel lesion, pseudomembranous colitis, diarrhea associated with bacterial toxins; presence of fever; use for more than 48 h without medical direction. Safe use during pregnancy (category C) and breast feeding not established. **Cautious use in:** infants or children ≤ 3 y, elderly patients.

ADVERSE/SIDE EFFECTS Constipation usually mild and transient.

K

DRUG INTERACTIONS Chloroquine, digoxin, penicillamine, tetracycline, ciprofloxacin, and most other drugs, since it may decrease absorption of any orally administered medication. Administer at least 2–4 h before other oral medications.

NURSING IMPLICATIONS

Administration

- Shake suspension well before pouring.
- Store in tightly closed container at 15–30C (59–86F) unless otherwise directed. Protect from freezing.

Assessment & Drug Effects

- Assess for abdominal distension and number of stools per day.
- Be aware that fecal impaction may result from taking kaolin and pectin, especially in the elderly.

Patient & Family Education

- Instruct patient not to exceed prescribed dosage.
- Advise patient to notify physician if diarrhea is not controlled within 48 h or if fever develops.
- Prolonged use of kaolin can interfere with normal absorption of nutrients.

KETOCONAZOLE

(ke-to-con′a-zol)

Trade names: Nizoral, Nizoral A-D

Classifications: ANTIINFECTIVE; ANTIBIOTIC; ANTIFUNGAL

Prototype: Fluconazole

Pregnancy category: C

ACTIONS/PHARMACODYNAMICS Synthetic imidazole derivative and broad-spectrum antifungal agent closely related to miconazole. Usually fungistatic but may be fungicidal in high concentrations. Studies suggest mode of action involves interference with synthesis of ergosterol with resultant increase in cell membrane permeability and ultimately inhibition of fungal growth.

USES Oral: severe systemic fungal infections including candidiasis (e.g., oral thrush, candiduria), chronic mucocutaneous candidiasis, pulmonary and disseminated coccidioidomycosis, histoplasmosis, paracoccidioidomycosis, blastomycosis, and chromomycosis. **Unlabeled oral uses:** onychomycosis, vaginal candidiasis, Cushing's syndrome associated with adrenal or pituitary adenoma; precocious puberty, dysfunctional hirsutism, and as swish and swallow preparation for prophylaxis against fungal infections in patients with neutropenia induced by cancer chemotherapy and in patients with AIDS. **Topically:** tinea corporis and tinea cruris (caused by *Epidermophyton floccosum, Trichophyton mentagrophytes,* and *Trichophyton rubrum*) and in treatment of tinea versicolor (pityriasis) caused by *Malassezia furfur (Pityrosporum obiculare),* seborrheic dermatitis. **Unlabeled topical uses:** tinea pedis, tinea manum, cutaneous candidiasis, psoriasis.

ROUTE & DOSAGE

Fungal Infections

Adult: **PO** 200–400 mg once/d; **Topical** Apply 1–2 times/d to affected area and surrounding skin.
Child> 2 y: **PO** 3.3–6.6 mg/kg/d as single dose.

Dandruff

Adult/Child: **Topical** shampoo twice a week for 4 wk with at least 3 d between shampoos; apply sufficient shampoo to produce enough lather to wash scalp and hair and gently massage it over the entire scalp area for 1 min; rinse hair thoroughly; Repeat, leaving shampoo on scalp for 3 min. Rinse thoroughly.

PHARMACOKINETICS Absorption: erratically absorbed from GI tract (needs an acid pH); minimal absorption topically. **Peak:** 1–2 h. **Distribution:** distributed to saliva, urine, sebum, and cerumen; CSF levels unpredictable; distributed into breast milk. **Metabolism:** metabolized in liver. **Elimination:** half-life: 8 h; primarily excreted in feces, 13% in urine.

CONTRAINDICATIONS & PRECAUTIONS Contraindicated in: hypersensitivity to ketoconazole or to any component in the formulation; chronic alcoholism, fungal meningitis. Safe use during pregnancy (category C), in nursing mothers, and in children < 2 y not determined. **Cautious use in:** achlorhydria, history of hepatic disease.

ADVERSE/SIDE EFFECTS Systemic (PO): GI: *nausea, vomiting,* anorexia, epigastric or abdominal pain, constipation, diarrhea. **Hematologic:** with high doses: lowering of serum testosterone and ACTH-induced corticosteroid serum levels; transient decreases in serum cholesterol and triglycerides; hyponatremia (rare). **Hepatic:** transient elevation in serum liver enzymes, fatal hepatic necrosis (rare). **Hypersensitivity:** skin rash, erythema, urticaria, pruritus, angioedema, anaphylaxis. **Reproductive:** gynecomastia (males), breast pain; uterine bleeding, loss of libido, impotence, oligospermia, hair loss. **Other:** acute hypoadrenalism (reduction of adrenal stress syndrome), renal hypofunction. **Topical:** mild transient erythema, severe irritation, pruritus, stinging.

DRUG INTERACTIONS Alcohol may cause sunburnlike reaction; ANTACIDS, ANTICHOLINERGICS, H_2-RECEPTOR ANTAGONISTS decrease ketoconazole absorption; **isoniazid, rifampin** increase ketoconazole metabolism, thus decreasing its activity; levels of **phenytoin** and ketoconazole decreased; may increase **cyclosporine** levels and toxicity; **warfarin** may potentiate hypoprothrombinemia; may increase levels of **carbamazepine, cisapride, terfenadine,** and possibly **astemizole,** resulting in arrhythmias.

NURSING IMPLICATIONS

Administration

- Nausea and vomiting occur frequently during early therapy. Measures that may help to reduce GI effects include taking ketoconazole with food and dividing daily dosage into 2 doses. Do not give with antacids.
- Give drug with water, fruit juice, coffee, or tea. Ketoconazole requires an acid medium for dissolution and absorption.
- Store in tightly covered container at 15–30C (59–86F) unless otherwise directed.

K

Assessment & Drug Effects

- Advise to refrain from potentially hazardous activities until response to the drug is known. Drowsiness and dizziness are early and time-limited side effects.
- Liver function tests—AST, ALT, alkaline phosphatase, and bilirubin—should be performed before treatment is initiated and at least monthly throughout therapy.

Patient & Family Education

- Report promptly to physician seizures or symptoms suggestive of hepatotoxicity (see Appendix G). Immediate discontinuation of ketoconazole is essential to prevent irreversible liver damage.
- Treatment is continued until all clinical and laboratory tests indicate that fungal infection has subsided.
- Instruct to avoid OTC drugs for gastric distress, such as Rolaids, Tums, Alka-Seltzer and to check with physician before taking any nonprescribed medicines.
- Caution not to alter the dose or dose interval and not to stop taking ketoconazole before consulting the physician.
- Instruct to notify physician if skin condition fails to respond to topical medication therapy or worsens or if signs of irritation or sensitivity occur.

K

KETOPROFEN

(kee-toe-proe′fen)

Trade names: Actron, Orudis, Orudis KT, Oruvail, Rhodis ♣

Classifications: CNS AGENT; ANALGESIC; ANTIPYRETIC; NSAID

Prototype: Ibuprofen

Pregnancy category: B

ACTIONS/PHARMACODYNAMICS

Nonsteroidal antiinflammatory drug structurally related to ibuprofen. Analgesic potency matches that of indomethacin and is stronger than that of aspirin. Inhibits platelet aggregation and prolongs bleeding time. Has fewer adverse GI effects than aspirin.

USES Acute or long-term treatment of rheumatoid arthritis and osteoarthritis; primary dysmenorrhea; headache; symptomatic relief of postoperative, dental, and postpartum pain; visceral pain associated with cancer. **Unlabeled uses:** Reiter's syndrome, juvenile arthritis, acute gouty arthritis, biliary pain, renal colic.

ROUTE & DOSAGE

Inflammatory Disease

Adult: **PO** 75 mg t.i.d. or 50 mg q.i.d. (max 300 mg/d) or 200 mg sustained-release q.d.
Geriatric: **PO** Start with 25 mg q.i.d. or 50 mg t.i.d.

Mild to Moderate Pain, Dysmenorrhea

Adult: **PO** 12.5–50 mg q6–8h.

PHARMACOKINETICS **Absorption:** readily absorbed from GI tract. **Onset:** 1–2 h. **Peak:** 1–2 h. **Duration:** 4–6 h. **Metabolism:** metabolized in liver. **Elimination:** half-life: 1.1–4 h; excreted primarily in urine, with some biliary excretion.

CONTRAINDICATIONS & PRECAUTIONS **Contraindicated in:** patient in whom aspirin or other NSAID induces asthma, urticaria, bronchospasm, severe rhinitis, shock. Safe use during pregnancy (category B), in nursing mothers, or in children < 12 y not established. **Cautious use in:** history of GI disease, GI bleeding, active ulcer; renal or hepatic impairment, patient who may be adversely affected by prolongation of bleeding time; heart failure, hypertension; patient receiving diuretics; geriatric patient; myasthenia gravis.

ADVERSE/SIDE EFFECTS CNS: trouble in sleeping, nervousness, *headache,* dizziness; depression, drowsiness, confusion, migraine, vertigo. **CV:** peripheral edema, palpitations, hypertension, tachycardia. **Eye/ENT:** visual disturbances, conjunctivitis, eye pain, retinal hemorrhage, pigmentation changes; dry nose or throat, tinnitus, hearing impairment. **GI:** *dyspepsia,* drug-induced peptic ulcer, GI bleeding, nausea, vomiting, diarrhea, constipation, flatulence, stomach pain, anorexia, dry mouth, gingivitis, rectal burning and hemorrhage, melena. **Hematologic:** prolonged bleeding time, anemia, purpura, agranulocytosis, thrombocytosis. **Hepatic:** jaundice, elevated ALT, AST. **Skin:** rash, pruritus, urticaria, erythema, photosensitivity. **Other:** gynecomastia, changes in libido, aggravation of diabetes mellitus, laryngospasm, bronchospasm, laryngeal edema, pharyngitis, urinary tract irritation (dysuria, frequency/urgency), renal impairment.

DRUG INTERACTIONS ORAL ANTICOAGULANTS, **heparin** may prolong bleeding time; may increase **lithium** toxicity; may increase **methotrexate** toxicity.

NURSING IMPLICATIONS

Administration

- Do not crush. To reduce GI irritation, give with food, milk, or prescribed antacid.
- Store drug at 15–30C (59–86F) in tightly closed, light-resistant container unless otherwise directed.

Assessment & Drug Effects

- Both baseline and periodic evaluations of hemoglobin, renal and hepatic function, and auditory and ophthalmologic status are recommended during prolonged or high-dose therapy.
- Monitor for signs and symptoms of GI ulceration (e.g., stool for occult blood, persistent indigestion).

Patient & Family Education

- Advise to report promptly signs of jaundice (see Appendix G) and the following symptoms: blurred vision, tinnitus, urinary urgency or frequency, unexplained bleeding, weight gain with edema.
- Inform about possible CNS effects (light-headedness, dizziness, drowsiness) and caution against dangerous activities until reaction to the drug has been determined.
- Inform that alcohol, aspirin, or other NSAIDS may increase risk of GI ulceration and bleeding tendencies and therefore should be avoided.
- Advise to tell dentist or surgeon that they are taking ketoprofen.

KETOROLAC TROMETHAMINE

(ke-tor′o-lac)

Trade names: Toradol, Acular
Classifications: CNS AGENT; ANALGESIC; ANTIPYRETIC; NSAID
Prototype: Ibuprofen
Pregnancy category: B

ACTIONS/PHARMACODYNAMICS Ketorolac exhibits analgesic, antiinflammatory, and antipyretic activity. It inhibits synthesis of prostaglandins and is a peripherally acting analgesic. Ketorolac does not have any known effects on opiate receptors.

USES *Short-term* management of pain; ocular itching due to seasonal allergic conjunctivitis.

ROUTE & DOSAGE

Pain

Adult: **IV loading dose** 30 mg (15 mg if ≥ 65 y or < 50 kg). **IM** 30–60 mg loading dose, then 15–30 mg q6h; maximum recommended daily dose is 150 mg first day and 120 mg subsequent days (30 mg load, then 15 mg q6h if ≥ 65 y or < 50 kg). **PO** 10 mg q6h prn (max 40 mg/d). **Total therapy (PO, IV, IM) not to exceed 5 d.**

Allergic Conjunctivitis

Adult: **Ophthalmic** 1 drop 0.5% solution q.i.d.

K

PHARMACOKINETICS **Peak:** 45–60 min. **Distribution:** distributed into breast milk. **Metabolism:** metabolized in liver. **Elimination:** half-life: 4–6 h; excreted in urine.

CONTRAINDICATIONS & PRECAUTIONS **Contraindicated in:** hypersensitivity to ketorolac; individuals with complete or partial syndrome of nasal polyps, angioedema, and bronchiospastic reaction to aspirin or other NSAIDS; during labor and delivery; patients with severe renal impairment or at risk for renal failure due to volume depletion; patients with risk of bleeding; active PUD; pre- or intraoperatively; intrathecal or epidural administration; in combination with other NSAIDS; nursing mothers. **Cautious use in:** history of peptic ulcers; impaired renal or hepatic function; elderly; debilitated patients; pregnancy (category B). Safety and effectiveness in children have not been established.

ADVERSE/SIDE EFFECTS **CNS:** *drowsiness,* dizziness, headache. **GI:** *nausea,* dyspepsia, GI pain, <u>hemorrhage</u>. **Other:** edema, sweating, pain at injection site.

DRUG INTERACTIONS May increase **methotrexate** levels and toxicity; may increase **lithium** levels and toxicity.

NURSING IMPLICATIONS

Administration

- When applying ophthalmic drops, care should be taken to avoid contaminating the solution container. Do not touch container to the eye.
- Do not administer IV, IM, or PO ketorolac longer than 5 d.
- When used for pain relief, reduced oral dosages may be necessary with the elderly because of renal effects of NSAIDS.
- Inject IM ketorolac slowly and deeply into a large muscle.
- Injection site pain has been reported in some patients receiving multiple doses. Rotate injection sites.
- Administer IV bolus dose over at least 15 s.
- Store at 15–30C (59–86F).

Assessment & Drug Effects

- Hypovolemia should be corrected prior to administration of ketorolac.
- Monitor urinalysis results. Hematuria and proteinuria have been observed with long-term use.
- Monitor urine output, which may be decreased by ketorolac in the elderly, patients with a history of renal impairment, heart failure, or liver dysfunction or who are taking diuretics. Discontinuation of drug will return urine output to pretreatment level.
- Monitor for changes in liver function studies.
- Monitor for signs and symptoms of bleeding. Ketorolac decreases platelet aggregation and thus may prolong bleeding time.
- Monitor for signs and symptoms of GI distress or bleeding including

nausea, GI pain, diarrhea, melena, or hematemesis. GI ulceration with perforation can occur anytime during treatment.
- Patients with a history of cardiac decompensation should be observed closely for evidence of fluid retention and edema.

Patient & Family Education
- Inform patients on long-term therapy to watch for the signs and symptoms of GI ulceration and bleeding (e.g., bloody emesis, black tarry stools).
- Inform about possible CNS effects (dizziness, drowsiness) and caution them to avoid dangerous activities until reaction to the drug is known.
- Advise not to use other NSAIDS while taking ketorolac.

LABETALOL HYDROCHLORIDE

(la-bet'a-lole)

Trade names: Normodyne, Trandate

Classifications: AUTONOMIC NERVOUS SYSTEM AGENT; ALPHA- AND BETA-ADRENERGIC ANTAGONIST (SYMPATHOLYTIC); ANTIHYPERTENSIVE

Prototype: Propranolol

Pregnancy category: C

ACTIONS/PHARMACODYNAMICS Adrenergic receptor blocking agent that combines selective alpha activity and nonselective beta-adrenergic blocking actions. Both activities contribute to blood pressure reduction. Alpha blockade results in vasodilation, decreased peripheral resistance, and orthostatic hypotension and only slightly affects cardiac output and coronary artery blood flow. Beta-blocking effects on sinus node, AV node, and ventricular muscle lead to bradycardia, delay in AV conduction, and depression of cardiac contractility.

USES Mild, moderate, and severe hypertension, primarily as a step-2 drug. May be used alone or in combination with other antihypertensive agents, especially thiazide diuretics.

ROUTE & DOSAGE

Hypertension

Adult: **PO** 100 mg b.i.d.; may gradually increase to 200–400 mg b.i.d. (max 1200–2400 mg/d); **IV** 20 mg slowly over 2 min, with 40–80 mg q10min if needed up to 300 mg total, *or* 2 mg/min continuous infusion up to 300 mg total dose.
Geriatric: **PO** Start with 100 mg daily. **IV** As for adult.

PHARMACOKINETICS Absorption: readily absorbed from GI tract, but only 25% reaches systemic circulation because of first pass metabolism. **Onset:** 20 min–2 h PO; 2–5 min IV. **Peak:** 1–4 h PO; 5–15 min IV. **Duration:** 8–24 h PO; 2–4 h IV. **Distribution:** crosses placenta; distributed into breast milk. **Metabolism:** metabolized in liver. **Elimination:** half-life: 3–8 h; 60% excreted in urine, 40% in bile.

CONTRAINDICATIONS & PRECAUTIONS Contraindicated in: bronchial asthma; uncontrolled cardiac failure, heart block (greater than first degree), cardiogenic shock, severe bradycardia. Safe use during pregnancy (category C), in nursing women, and in children not established. **Cautious use in:** nonallergic bronchospastic disease (COPD), well-compensated patients with history of heart failure; pheochromocytoma; impaired hepatic function, jaundice; diabetes mellitus; peripheral vascular disease.

ADVERSE/SIDE EFFECTS CNS: dizziness, fatigue/malaise, headache, tremors, transient paresthesias (especially scalp tingling), hypoesthesia (numbness) following IV, mental depression, drowsiness, sleep disturbances, nightmares. **CV:** *postural hypotension,* angina pectoris, palpitation, bradycardia, syncope, pedal or peripheral edema, pulmonary edema, CHF, flushing, cold extremities, arrhythmias (following IV), paradoxical hypertension (patients with pheochromocytoma). **Eye:** dry eyes, vision disturbances. **GI:** nausea, vomiting, dyspepsia, constipation, diarrhea, taste disturbances, cholestasis with or without jaundice, increases in serum transaminases, dry mouth. **GU:** acute urinary retention, difficult micturition, impotence, ejaculation failure, loss of libido, Peyronie's disease. **Respiratory:** dyspnea, bronchospasm. **Skin:** rashes of various types, increased sweating, pruritus. **Other:** nasal stuffiness, rhinorrhea, myalgia, muscle cramps, toxic myopathy, antimitochondrial antibodies, positive antinuclear antibodies (ANA), SLE syndrome, pain at IV injection site.

DIAGNOSTIC TEST INTERFERENCE False increases in ***urinary catecholamines*** when measured by ***nonspecific trihydroxyindole (THI) reaction*** (due to labetalol metabolites) but not with specific radioenzymatic or high-performance liquid chromatography assay techniques.

DRUG INTERACTIONS Cimetidine may increase effects of labetalol; **glutethimide** decreases effects of labetalol; **halothane** adds to hypotensive effects; may mask symptoms of hypoglycemia caused by ORAL SULFONYLUREAS, **insulin;** BETA AGONISTS antagonize effects of labetalol.

INCOMPATIBILITY Y-site: furosemide.

NURSING IMPLICATIONS

Administration

- Administer PO preparation preferably with or immediately after food. Food increases drug bioavailability. Advise consistency.
- Patient should be supine when receiving labetalol IV. Take BP immediately before administration.
- Drug may be given undiluted by direct IV or further diluted in most IV solutions and administered as a continuous infusion.
- Direct IV administration: Give a 20-mg dose slowly over 2 min. Maximum hypotensive effect occurs 5–15 min after each administration.
- Continuous IV infusion: Rate is adjusted according to BP response. Normal rate is 2 mg/min. Once the desired BP is attained, labetalol is discontinued.
- Controlled infusion pump device is recommended for maintaining accurate flow rate during IV infusion. Usually administered at rate of 2 mg/min.
- Store at 2–30C (36–86F) unless otherwise advised. Do not freeze. Protect tablets from moisture.

Assessment & Drug Effects

- Monitor BP and pulse during dosage adjustment period. Standing BP is used often as indicator for making dosage adjustments and for assessing patient's tolerance of dosage increases. Generally taken after patient stands for 10 min. Clarify with physician.
- After IV administration, (1) monitor BP at 5 min intervals for 30 min; (2) then at 30 min intervals for 2 h; (3) then hourly for about 6 h, and as indicated thereafter.

- PO therapy is usually started when supine diastolic pressure rises about 10 mm Hg.
- Supine position should be maintained for at least 3 h after IV administration. At the end of this time, determine patient's ability to tolerate elevated and upright positions before allowing ambulation. Manage this slowly.

Patient & Family Education

- Caution that postural hypotension is most likely to occur during peak plasma levels (i.e., 2–4 h after drug administration).
- Instruct to make all position changes slowly and in stages, particularly from recumbent to upright position. Elderly patients are especially sensitive to hypotensive effects.
- Since labetalol can cause dizziness and light-headedness, advise to avoid potentially hazardous activities until reaction to drug is known.
- Diabetic patients should be closely monitored. Labetalol may mask usual cardiovascular response to acute hypoglycemia, e.g., tachycardia.
- Reassure that most adverse effects (e.g., scalp tingling) are mild, transient, and dose related and occur early in therapy.
- Stress importance of keeping follow-up appointments. Tests of liver and renal function should be performed periodically during therapy.
- Discontinuation of labetalol after chronic administration should be done by gradual reduction of dosage over a 1–2 wk period. Patient should be closely monitored during this time.

LACTULOSE

(lak'tyoo-lose)

Trade names: Cephulac, Chronulac

Classifications: GI AGENT; HYPEROSMOTIC LAXATIVE

Pregnancy category: C

ACTIONS/PHARMACODYNAMICS

Action in reducing blood ammonia appears to involve metabolism of lactose to organic acids by resident intestinal bacteria. The result is acidification of colon contents, which retards diffusion of nonionic ammonia (NH_3) from colon to blood while promoting its migration from blood to colon. In the acidic colon, NH_3 is converted to nonabsorbable ammonia ions (NH_4) and is then expelled in feces by laxative action. Osmotic effect of organic acids causes laxative action, which moves water from plasma to intestines, softens stools, and stimulates peristalsis by pressure from stool water content.

L

USES Prevention and treatment of portal-systemic encephalopathy (PSE), including stages of hepatic precoma and coma, and by prescription for relief of chronic constipation. **Unlabeled uses:** to restore regular bowel habit posthemorrhoidectomy; to evacuate bowel in elderly patients with severe constipation after barium studies; and for treatment of chronic constipation in children.

ROUTE & DOSAGE

Prevention and Treatment of Portal-Systemic Encephalopathy

Adult: **PO** 30–45 ml t.i.d. or q.i.d. adjusted to produce 2 or 3 soft stools/d. *Infant:* **PO** 2.5–10 ml/d in divided doses adjusted to produce 2–3 soft stools/d.
Child/Adolescent: **PO** 40–90 ml/d in divided doses adjusted to produce 2–3 soft stools/d.
Infant: **PO** 2.5–10 ml/d in 3–4 divided doses.

Management of Acute Portal-Systemic Encephalopathy

Adult: **PO** 30–45 ml q1–2h until laxation is achieved, then adjusted to produce 2–3 soft stools/d; **Rectal** 300 ml diluted with 700 ml water given via rectal balloon catheter, and retained for 30–60 min; may repeat in 4–6 h if necessary or until patient can take PO.

Chronic Constipation

Adult: **PO** 30–60 ml/d prn.
Child: **PO** 7.5 ml/d after breakfast.

PHARMACOKINETICS **Absorption:** poorly absorbed from GI tract. **Metabolism:** metabolized in gut by intestinal bacteria.

L

CONTRAINDICATIONS & PRECAUTIONS **Contraindicated in:** low galactose diet; pregnancy (category C). Safe use in nursing mothers and in children not established. **Cautious use in:** diabetes mellitus; concomitant use with electrocautery procedures (proctoscopy, colonoscopy); elderly and debilitated patients; pediatric use.

ADVERSE/SIDE EFFECTS Initial dose: flatulence, borborygmi, belching, abdominal cramps, pain, and distention; *diarrhea* (excessive dose), nausea, vomiting, colon accumulation of hydrogen gas; hypernatremia.

DRUG INTERACTION LAXATIVES may incorrectly suggest therapeutic action of lactulose.

NURSING IMPLICATIONS

Administration

- Administer with fruit juice, water, or milk (if not contraindicated) to increase palatability. Laxative effect is enhanced by taking lactulose with ample liquids. Avoid meal times.
- Lactulose may be administered as a retention enema via a rectal balloon catheter. If solution is evacuated too soon, instillation may be promptly repeated.
- Store at room temperature; do not freeze. Avoid prolonged exposure to temperatures above 30C (86F) or to direct light. Normal darkening does not affect action, but discard solution that is very dark or cloudy.

Assessment & Drug Effects

- If the initial dose for children causes diarrhea, the dose is reduced immediately. If diarrhea persists, lactulose is discontinued.
- Therapeutic response (decreased blood ammonia) in patient with hepatic encephalopathy is marked by improved EEG patterns and mental state: clearing of confusion, apathy, and irritation. (Normal blood ammonia: 12–55 μmol/L.)
- Lactulose-induced osmotic changes in the bowel support intestinal water loss and potential hypernatremia. Fluid intake (often self-limited by the elderly) should be actively promoted (≤ 1500–2000 ml/d) during drug therapy for constipation. Discuss with physician.

Patient & Family Education

- Laxative action is not instituted until drug reaches the colon; therefore, transit time before reaching the colon and during passage through colon affects response time. About 24–48 h is needed.
- Warn patient who may be discouraged by slow onset of drug action not to self-medicate with another laxative.
- Advise patient on prolonged therapy to report to the physician if diarrhea (i.e., more than 2 or 3 soft

stools/d) persists more than 24–48 h. Diarrhea is a sign of overdosage. Dose adjustment is indicated.

LAMIVUDINE (3TC)

(lam-i-vu'deen)

Trade name: Epivir

Classifications: ANTIINFECTIVE; ANTIRETROVIRAL AGENT

Prototype: Zidovudine (AZT)

Pregnancy category: C

ACTIONS/PHARMACODYNAMICS Lamivudine (formerly 3TC) is a synthetic nucleoside analog. Its phosphorylated metabolite (L-TP) inhibits the transcription of the HIV viral DNA chain.

USE HIV infection in combination with zidovudine.

ROUTE & DOSAGE

HIV Infection

Adult: **PO** 150 mg b.i.d.; 2 mg/kg b.i.d. if weight < 50 kg.
Child 12–16 y: **PO** 150 mg b.i.d.; 2 mg/kg b.i.d. if weight < 50 kg.
3 mo–12 y: **PO** 4 mg/kg b.i.d. up to max of 150 mg b.i.d.

PHARMACOKINETICS Absorption: rapidly absorbed from GI tract (86% reaches systemic circulation). **Distribution:** low binding to plasma proteins. **Metabolism:** minimal metabolism. **Elimination:** half-life: 2–4 h; excreted primarily unchanged in urine.

CONTRAINDICATIONS & PRECAUTIONS Contraindicated in: hypersensitivity to lamuvidine, nursing mothers. **Cautious use in:** renal impairment, pregnancy (category C), children.

ADVERSE/SIDE EFFECTS CNS: neuropathy, insomnia, sleep disorders, dizziness, depression, *headache,* fatigue, fever. **GI:** *nausea, diarrhea,* vomiting, anorexia, abdominal pain, cramps, dyspepsia, increased liver function tests (ALT, amylase). **Hematologic:** neutropenia, anemia, thrombocytopenia. **Musculoskeletal:** myalgia, arthralgia, malaise. **Other:** rash, nasal symptoms, cough.

DRUG INTERACTIONS Increases the C_{max} of **zidovudine. Trimethoprim-sulfamethoxazole** increases serum levels of lamivudine.

NURSING IMPLICATIONS

Administration

- Lamivudine should be given concurrently with zidovudine (AZT) therapy.
- Dosage reduction is required with significant renal impairment (Cl_{cr} ≤ 50 ml/min) in patients > 16 y. Follow manufacturer's recommended adjustment.
- Store solution at 2–25C (36–77F) tightly closed.

Assessment & Drug Effects

- Monitor children closely for signs and symptoms of pancreatitis; if they occur, immediately stop lamivudine and notify physician.
- Throughout therapy, monitor CBC with differential, renal, and hepatic function, and serum amylase.
- Monitor for and report all significant adverse reactions.

Patient & Family Education

- Stress the importance of taking lamivudine exactly as prescribed.
- Advise caregivers to monitor pediatric patients for symptoms of pancreatitis.
- Ensure that patients realize that long-term effects of lamivudine are unknown.

LAMOTRIGINE

(la-mo'tri-geen)

Trade name: Lamictal

Classifications: CENTRAL NERVOUS SYSTEM AGENT; ANTICONVULSANT

Prototype: Phenytoin

Pregnancy category: C

ACTIONS/PHARMACODYNAMICS Lamotrigine is an antiepileptic drug. Its exact mechanism of action is not known. Lamotrigine is thought to act by inhibiting the release of glutamate, an excitatory neurotransmitter. This may be due to lamotrigine's acting at voltage-sensitive sodium channels to stabilize neuronal membranes and inhibit neurotransmitter release, i.e., glutamate in brain tissue.

L

USES Adjunctive therapy for partial seizures in adults (>16 y). Generalized tonic–clonic, absence, or myoclonic seizures in adults.

ROUTE & DOSAGE

Partial Seizures, Patients Receiving Anticonvulsants Other Than Valproic Acid

Adult: **PO** Start with 50 mg q.d. for 2 wk, then 50 mg b.i.d. for 2 wk; may titrate up to 300–500 mg/d in 2 divided doses (max 700 mg/d).
Child 2–16 y: **PO** 1 mg/kg b.i.d. × 2 wk, then 2.5 mg/kg b.i.d. × 2 wk, then 5 mg/kg b.i.d. (15 mg/kg/d or 400 mg/d).

Partial Seizures, Patients Receiving Valproic Acid

Adult: **PO** Start with 25 mg q.o.d. for 2 wk, then 25 mg q.d. for 2 wk; may titrate up to 150 mg/d in 2 divided doses (max 200 mg/d).
Child 2–16 y: **PO** 0.2 mg/kg/d × 2 wk, then 0.5 mg/kg/d × 2 wk, then 1 mg/kg/d (max 5 mg/kg/d or 250 mg/d).

PHARMACOKINETICS **Absorption:** readily absorbed from GI tract; 98% reaches systemic circulation. **Onset:** 12 wk. **Peak:** 1–4 h. **Distribution:** 55% protein bound; crosses placenta; distributed into breast milk. **Metabolism:** metabolized in liver to inactive metabolite. **Elimination:** half-life: 25–30 h; can induce own metabolism; excreted in urine.

CONTRAINDICATIONS & PRECAUTIONS **Contraindicated in:** hypersensitivity to lamotrigine, nursing mothers. **Cautious use in:** renal insufficiency, concomitant administration of other anticonvulsants, pregnancy (category C), cardiac or hepatic function impairment. Safety and efficacy in children < 16 y have not been established. Fatal rash has been reported in children < 16 y.

ADVERSE/SIDE EFFECTS **CNS:** *dizziness, ataxia, somnolence, headache,* aphasia, vertigo, confusion, slurred speech, irritability, depression, incoordination, hostility. **GI:** *nausea,* vomiting, anorexia, abdominal pain, diarrhea, dyspepsia, constipation. **GU:** hematuria, dysmenorrhea, vaginitis. **Ocular:** *diplopia, blurred vision.* **Musculoskeletal:** peripheral neuropathy, chills, tremor, arthralgia. **Skin:** RASH (including Stevens-Johnson syndrome, toxic epidermal necrolysis), urticaria, pruritus, alopecia, acne. **Other:** *rhinitis,* pharyngitis, cough.

DRUG INTERACTIONS **Carbamazepine, phenobarbital, primidone, phenytoin** may decrease lamotrigine levels. **Valproic acid** may increase lamotrigine levels. Lamotrigine may decrease serum levels of **valproic acid.**

NURSING IMPLICATIONS

Administration

- Reduced dose may be warranted with renal or hepatic impairment.
- Unless patient safety is at risk, drug withdrawal should occur gradually over a 2-wk period.
- Store at 15–30C (59–86F).

Assessment & Drug Effects

- If rash develops, withhold drug and immediately report to physician.
- When other anticonvulsants are also given, monitor the plasma levels of lamotrigine and other drugs.
- Monitor for adverse reactions especially when lamotrigine is used with other anticonvulsants, especially valproic acid.
- With long-term use, periodic ophthalmologic exams are suggested.

Patient & Family Education

- Instruct to report immediately any of the following to the physician: worsening seizure control, skin rash, ataxia, blurred vision or diplopia, fever or flu-like symptoms.
- Advise caution with hazardous activities until reaction to the drug is known.
- Caution about photosensitivity and instruct on need for protection from sunlight or ultraviolet light until tolerance is known.
- Warn not to discontinue lamotrigine abruptly.

LANSOPRAZOLE

(lan'so-pra-zole)

Trade name: Prevacid

Classifications: GASTROINTESTINAL AGENT; ANTISECRETORY; PROTON PUMP INHIBITOR

Prototype: Omeprazole

Pregnancy category: B

ACTIONS/PHARMACODYNAMICS Lansoprazole belongs to a class of antisecretory compounds that are gastric acid pump inhibitors. Specifically, it suppresses gastric acid secretion by inhibiting the H^+, K^+-ATPase enzyme (the acid [proton H^+] pump) in the parietal cells. Lansoprazole does not exhibit anticholinergic or H_2-histamine antagonist properties.

USES Short-term treatment of duodenal ulcer (up to 4 wk) and erosive esophagitis (up to 8 wk), pathologic hypersecretory disorders, gastric ulcers; in combination with clarithromycin and amoxicillin for *Helicobacter pylori*. Gastroesophageal reflux disease.

ROUTE & DOSAGE

Duodenal Ulcer

Adult: **PO** 15 mg q.d. × 4 wk.

Erosive Esophagitis

Adult: **PO** 30 mg q.d. × 8 wk, then decrease to 15 mg q.d.

Hypersecretory Disorder

Adult: **PO** 60 mg q.d. (up to 120 mg/d in divided doses); dose may need to be adjusted for hepatic impairment.

H. pylori

Adult: **PO** 30 mg b.i.d. × 2 wk, in combination with 2 antibiotics.

PHARMACOKINETICS **Absorption:** rapidly absorbed from GI tract after leaving stomach; unstable in acidic media. **Onset:** acid reduction within 2 h; ulcer relief within 1 wk. **Peak:** 1.5–3 h. **Duration:** 24 h. **Distribution:** 97% bound to plasma proteins. **Metabolism:** metabolized in liver by cytochrome P450 system. **Elimination:** half-life: 1.5 h; 14–25% excreted in urine as metabolites; part of dose eliminated in bile and feces.

CONTRAINDICATIONS & PRECAUTIONS **Contraindicated in:** hypersensitivity to lansoprazole, nursing mothers. **Cautious use in:** severe hepatic impairment, pregnancy (category B). Safety and efficacy in children < 18 y have not been established.

ADVERSE/SIDE EFFECTS **CNS:** fatigue, dizziness, headache. **GI:** nausea, *diarrhea,* constipation, anorexia, increased appetite, elevated serum transaminases (AST, ALT). **Other:** rash, thirst.

DRUG INTERACTIONS May decrease **theophylline** levels. **Sucralfate** decreases lansoprazole bioavailability. May interfere with absorption of **ketoconazole, digoxin, ampicillin,** or IRON SALTS. **Drug–food:** food reduces peak lansoprazole levels by 50%.

NURSING IMPLICATIONS

Administration

- Lansoprazole should be given before a meal.
- Capsules should not be crushed or chewed. Capsules can be opened and sprinkled on food or mixed with 40 ml of apple juice and administered through an NG tube.
- Store at 15–30C (59–86F).

Assessment & Drug Effects

- Periodically monitor CBC, renal and liver function tests, and serum gastric levels.
- Monitor for therapeutic effectiveness of concurrently used drugs that require an acid medium for absorption (e.g., digoxin, ampicillin, ketoconazole).

Patient & Family Education

- Instruct to swallow capsules whole on an empty stomach.
- Advise patients on concurrent sucralfate therapy to take lansoprazole at least 30 min prior to that drug.

LATANOPROST

(la-tan′-o-prost)

Trade name: Xalatan

Classifications: PROSTAGLANDIN; EYE PREPARATION; MIOTIC (ANTIGLAUCOMA AGENT); ANTIHYPERTENSIVE

Prototype: Dinoprostone

Pregnancy category: C

See Appendix A.

LEFLUNOMIDE

(le-flu′no-mide)

Trade name: Arava

Classification: IMMUNOMODULATOR

Pregnancy category: X

ACTIONS/PHARMACODYNAMICS Immunomodulator that demonstrates antiinflammatory effects. Reduces the S&S of rheumatoid arthritis (RA).

USE Active RA.

ROUTE & DOSAGE

Rheumatoid Arthritis

Adult: **PO** Initiate with a loading dose of 100 mg/d × 3 d; then maintenance dose of 20 mg q.d; may decrease to 10 mg/d if higher dose is not tolerated.

PHARMACOKINETICS **Absorption:** approximately 80% reaches systemic circulation. **Peak:** 6–12 h for active metabolite. **Distribution:** >99% protein bound. **Metabolism:** metabolized primarily to M1 (active metabolite). **Elimination:** half-life: 19 d for active metabolite; 43% excreted in urine, 48% in feces.

CONTRAINDICATIONS & PRECAUTIONS **Contraindicated in:** hepatic insufficiency; hypersensitivity to leflunomide; pregnancy (category X); lactation; patients with positive hepatitis B or C serology; malignancy, particularly lymphoproliferative disorders; immunosuppression. Use in patients <18 y not recommended. **Cautious use in:** renal insufficiency.

ADVERSE/SIDE EFFECTS **Body as whole:** allergic reaction, asthenia, flu-like syndrome, infection, pain, back pain, arthralgia, leg cramps, synovitis, tenosynovitis. **CNS:** dizziness, headache, paresthesias. **CV:** hypertension, chest pain. **GI:** *diarrhea,* increased liver function tests (ALT and AST), abdominal pain, anorexia, dyspepsia, gastroenteritis, nausea, mouth ulcer, vomiting, hypokalemia, weight loss. **Respiratory:** bronchitis, cough, respiratory infection, pharyngitis, pneumonia, rhinitis, sinusitis. **Skin:** rash, alopecia, eczema, pruritus, dry skin. **Other:** UTI.

DRUG INTERACTIONS **Rifampin** may significantly increase leflunomide levels; **cholestyramine, charcoal** decrease absorption; caution should be used with other hepatotoxic drugs.

NURSING IMPLICATIONS

Administration

- Therapy is initiated with a 3-d loading dose followed by a lower maintenance dose.
- Store at 15–30C (59–86F).

Assessment & Drug Effects

- Therapeutic effectiveness is indicated by improved RA symptomatology.
- Lab tests: Baseline screening for hepatitis B or C; baseline and monthly liver enzymes × 12 mo, then every 6 mo thereafter.
- Carefully monitor for and immediately report S&S of infection; withhold leflunomide if infection is suspected.
- Periodically monitor BP and weight. Doses greater than 25 mg/d are associated with a greater incidence of side effects such as alopecia, weight loss, and elevated liver enzymes.

Patient & Family Education

- Sexually active men and women should use reliable contraception and mothers should not nurse their infants while on leflunomide.
- Women who wish to conceive and men wishing to father a child should discontinue leflunomide and undergo a drug elimination procedure prescribed by the physician.
- If you develop an infection, withhold leflunomide and notify the physician before resuming the drug.
- Promptly report any of the following: hair loss, weight loss, GI distress, rash, or itching.

L

LEPIRUDIN

(le-pir'u-din)

Trade name: Refludan

Classifications: BLOOD FORMERS AND COAGULATORS; ANTICOAGULANT

Prototype: Heparin

Pregnancy category: B

ACTIONS/PHARMACODYNAMICS Highly specific direct inhibitor of thrombin. One molecule of lepirudin binds to one molecule of thrombin and thereby blocks the thrombogenic activity of thrombin.

aPTT values increase in relation to the dose given.

USE Anticoagulation in patients with heparin-induced thrombocytopenia (HIT).

ROUTE & DOSAGE

Anticoagulation

Adult: **IV** 0.4 mg/kg initial bolus (max 44 mg) followed by 0.15 mg/kg/h (max 16.5 mg/h) for 2–10 d; adjust rate to maintain aPTT of 1.5–2.5.

PHARMACOKINETICS Distribution: distributed primarily to extracellular compartment. **Metabolism:** metabolized by catabolic hydrolysis in serum. **Elimination:** half-life: 1.3 h; 48% excreted in urine.

L

CONTRAINDICATIONS & PRECAUTIONS Contraindicated in: hypersensitivity to lepirudin; lactation; pregnancy (category B); intracranial bleeding; patients with increased risk of bleeding (e.g., recent surgery, CVA, advanced renal impairment). Safety and efficacy in children not established. **Cautious use in:** serious liver injury (e.g., cirrhosis); concomitant administration with streptokinase; renal impairment.

ADVERSE/SIDE EFFECTS CNS: <u>intracranial bleeding</u>. **CV:** heart failure, ventricular fibrillation, pericardial effusion, <u>MI</u>. **GI:** abnormal liver function tests. **Hematologic:** bleeding from injection site, anemia, hematoma, bleeding, hematuria, GI and rectal bleeding, epistaxis, hemothorax, vaginal bleeding. **Respiratory:** pneumonia, cough, bronchospasm, stridor, dyspnea. **Skin:** allergic skin reactions. **Other:** sepsis, abnormal kidney function, multiorgan failure.

DRUG INTERACTIONS Warfarin increases risk of bleeding.

NURSING IMPLICATIONS

Administration

- IV preparation: Reconstitute by adding 1 ml of sterile water for injection or 0.9% NaCl to the 50-mg vial. To prepare bolus dose, withdraw reconstituted solution into a 10-cc syringe and dilute to 10 ml with sterile water for injection, 0.9% NaCl, or D5W to yield 5 mg/ml. To prepare a continuous infusion, transfer the contents of two reconstituted vials into 250 or 500 ml of 0.9% NaCl or D5W to yield concentrations of 0.4 or 0.2 mg/ml, respectively. Diluted solution is stable for 24 h during infusion.
- IV bolus injection: A properly diluted bolus dose may be injected over 15–20 s.
- IV infusion: A properly diluted solution may be infused continuously at a rate determined by body weight.
- Store unopened vials at 2–25C (36–77F).

Assessment & Drug Effects

- Therapeutic effectiveness is indicated by aPTT ratio in target range of 1.5 to 2.5.
- Lab tests: Baseline aPTT prior to initiation of therapy (withhold therapy and notify physician if baseline aPTT ratio ≥2.5.); aPTT 4 h after start of therapy and at least once daily (more often with renal or hepatic impairment) thereafter.
- If aPTT is above target range of 2.5, stop infusion immediately and notify physician.
- Give with extreme caution to those at increased risk for bleeding.
- Carefully monitor for and immediately report bleeding events (e.g.,

from puncture wounds, hematoma, hematuria).

- Oral anticoagulants should not be administered until the lepirudin dose has been reduced and aPTT ratio lowered to just above 1.5.

LETROZOLE

(le′tro-zole)

Trade name: Femara

Classifications: ANTINEOPLASTICS; HORMONES AND SYNTHETIC SUBSTITUTES; AROMATASE INHIBITOR

Prototype: Anastrozole

Pregnancy category: D

ACTIONS/PHARMACODYNAMICS Nonsteroid competitive inhibitor of the enzyme system that converts androgens to estrogens, thus causing regression of estrogen-dependent tumors. Causes a reduction in estrogen synthesis in all tissues.

USE Advanced breast cancer in postmenopausal women following antiestrogen therapy.

ROUTE & DOSAGE

Breast Cancer

Adult: **PO** 2.5 mg q.d.

PHARMACOKINETICS Absorption: rapidly absorbed from GI tract. **Metabolism:** metabolized in liver by cytochromes P450 3A4 and 2A6. **Elimination:** half-life: 2 d; 90% excreted in urine.

CONTRAINDICATIONS & PRECAUTIONS Contraindicated in: hypersensitivity to letrozole; pregnancy (category D). **Cautious use in:** moderate to severe hepatic impairment; lactation. Safety and efficacy in children not established.

ADVERSE/SIDE EFFECTS Body as whole: fatigue, peripheral edema, asthenia, weight increase, *musculoskeletal pain,* arthralgia. **CNS:** headache, somnolence, dizziness. **CV:** chest pain, hypertension, hypercholesterolemia. **GI:** nausea, vomiting, constipation, diarrhea, abdominal pain, anorexia, dyspepsia. **Respiratory:** dyspnea, cough. **Skin:** hot flushes, rash, pruritus.

NURSING IMPLICATIONS

Administration

- Letrozole may be given without regard to food.
- Store at 15–30C (59–86F).

Assessment & Drug Effects

- Lab tests: Periodically monitor serum calcium and CBC with differential.
- Carefully monitor for and immediately report S&S of thrombophlebitis or thromboembolism.

Patient & Family Education

- Immediately contact physician if S&S of thrombophlebitis (see Appendix G) develop.

LEUCOVORIN CALCIUM

(loo-koe-vor′in)

Trade names: Calcium Folinate, Citrovorum Factor, Folinic Acid, Wellcovorin

Classifications: BLOOD FORMER; ANTIANEMIC AGENT; ANTIDOTE

Pregnancy category: C

ACTIONS/PHARMACODYNAMICS Reduced form of folic acid. Unlike folic acid, it does not require enzymatic reduction and therefore is readily available to participate in reactions. Functions as an essential cell growth factor. When given during antineoplastic therapy, leucovorin prevents serious toxicity by protecting cells from the action of folic acid antagonists such as methotrexate.

USES Folate-deficient megaloblastic anemias due to sprue, pregnancy, and nutritional deficiency when oral therapy is not feasible. Also to prevent or diminish toxicity of antineoplastic folic acid antagonists, particularly methotrexate; and as adjunct with antifols (e.g., pyrimethamine) in pneumocystosis or toxoplasmosis to prevent significant bone marrow toxicity.

ROUTE & DOSAGE

Megaloblastic Anemia

Adult: **IM/IV** No more than 1 mg/d.
Child **IM/IV** Same as for adult.

Leucovorin Rescue for Methotrexate Toxicity

Adult: **PO/IM/IV** 10 mg/m^2 followed by 10 mg/m^2 q6h for 72 h; further doses based on serum methotrexate concentrations.
Child: **PO/IM/IV** Same as for adult.

Leucovorin Rescue for Other Folate Antagonist Toxicity

Adult: **PO/IM/IV** 5–15 mg/d.
Child: **PO/IM/IV** Same as for adult.

Adjunct for Treatment of Pneumocystosis or Toxoplasmosis

Adult: **PO/IM/IV** 3–6 mg t.i.d.
Child: **PO/IM/IV** Same as for adult.

PHARMACOKINETICS **Onset:** within 30 min. **Duration:** 3–6 h. **Distribution:** crosses placenta; distributed into breast milk. **Metabolism:** metabolized in liver and intestinal mucosa to tetrahydrofolic acid derivatives. **Elimination:** 80–90% excreted in urine, 5–8% in feces.

CONTRAINDICATIONS & PRECAUTIONS **Contraindicated in:** undiagnosed anemia, pernicious anemia, or other megaloblastic anemias secondary to vitamin B_{12} deficiency. Safe use during pregnancy (category C) and in nursing mothers not established. **Cautious use in:** renal dysfunction.

ADVERSE/SIDE EFFECTS Allergic sensitization (urticaria, pruritus, rash, wheezing); thrombocytosis.

INCOMPATIBILITIES **Solution/additive: droperidol. Y-site: droperidol.**

NURSING IMPLICATIONS

Administration

- For reconstitution, manufacturer recommends using 5 ml bacteriostatic water for injection, which contains benzyl alcohol, for each 50 mg vial. (Leucovorin calcium contains no preservatives.) When reconstituted as directed, solution must be used within 7 d. If reconstituted with sterile water for injection, use immediately.
- Reconstituted leucovorin is further diluted in 100–500 ml of most IV solutions.
- IV leucovorin solution is infused over 15–60 min, depending on the volume of solution.
- Store at 15–30C (59–86F) unless otherwise directed. Protect from light.

Assessment & Drug Effects

- Use of leucovorin alone in treatment of pernicious anemia or other megaloblastic anemias associated with vitamin B_{12} deficiency can result in an apparent hematological remission while allowing already present neurologic damage to progress.

- Plasma methotrexate levels may be used to determine dosage and duration of leucovorin rescue therapy. Creatinine clearance determinations prior to initiation of leucovorin rescue, urine pH prior to and about every 6 h throughout leucovorin rescue, and daily serum creatinine levels are recommended to detect onset of renal function impairment.

Patient & Family Education

- Instruct to report signs and symptoms of a hypersensitivity reaction immediately (see Appendix G).

LEUPROLIDE ACETATE

(loo-proe′lide)

Trade names: Lupron, Lupron Depot

Prototype for classification: GONADOTROPIN-RELEASING HORMONE ANALOG

Pregnancy category: X

ACTIONS/PHARMACODYNAMICS Synthetic analog of naturally occurring porcine or bovine gonadotropin-releasing hormone (GnRH); a new approach to manipulation of androgen-sensitive carcinoma. Leuprolide occupies and desensitizes pituitary GnRH receptors, resulting initially in release of gonadotropins LH and FSH and stimulation of ovarian and testicular steroidogenesis. During long-term administration, both gonadotropin secretion and steroidogenesis are suppressed, leading to prostatic and testicular atrophy. **Contraceptive effect:** by inhibiting gonadotropin release, ovulation or spermatogenesis is suppressed. **Antitumor effect:** may inhibit growth of hormone-dependent tumors.

USES Palliative treatment of advanced prostatic carcinoma as alternative to orchiectomy or estrogen administration; endometriosis; anemia caused by leiomyomata. **Unlabeled uses:** breast cancer; male contraceptive; delayed puberty.

ROUTE & DOSAGE

Palliative Treatment for Prostate Cancer

Adult: **SC** 1 mg/d; **IM** 7.5 mg/mo or 22.5 mg q3mo or 30 mg q4mo (depot preparation).

Endometriosis, Anemia

Adult: **IM** 3.75 mg qmo or 11.25 mg q3mo.

Precocious Puberty

Child: **IM** Depot 0.15–0.3 mg/kg q28d (min dose 7.5 mg); titrate by 3.75-mg increments q4wk.

PHARMACOKINETICS **Absorption:** readily absorbed from SC or IM sites. **Metabolism:** metabolized by enzymes in hypothalamus and anterior pituitary. **Elimination:** half-life: 3 h.

CONTRAINDICATIONS & PRECAUTIONS **Contraindicated in:** following orchiectomy or estrogen therapy; metastatic cerebral lesions; pregnancy (category X). **Cautious use in:** life-threatening carcinoma in which rapid symptomatic relief is necessary; known hypersensitivity to benzyl alcohol.

ADVERSE/SIDE EFFECTS *Disease flare (worsening of signs and symptoms of carcinoma).* **CNS:** dizziness, pain, headache, paresthesia. **CV:** *peripheral edema,* cardiac arrhythmias,

MI. **Endocrine:** *hot flushes, impotence, decreased libido,* gynecomastia, breast tenderness, amenorrhea, vaginal bleeding, thyroid enlargement, hypoglycemia. **GI:** nausea, vomiting, constipation, anorexia, sour taste, GI bleeding, diarrhea. **Musculoskeletal:** increased bone pain, myalgia. **Renal:** increased hematuria, dysuria, flank pain. **Other:** injection site irritation, pleural rub, pulmonary fibrosis flare; decreased Hct, Hgb; asthenia, fatigue, fever, facial swelling, pruritus, rash, hair loss.

NURSING IMPLICATIONS

Administration

- Preparation of solution for injection: Using a 22-gauge needle, withdraw 1.5 ml of diluent from the supplied ampul and inject it into the vial. Shake well to form a uniform suspension. Withdraw entire contents and administer immediately.
- Do not administer parenteral drug formulation if particulate matter or discoloration is present.
- Refrigerate unopened vials at 2–8C (36–46F). Store vial in use at 15–30C (59–86F) for several months with minimal loss of potency. Protect from light and freezing.

Assessment & Drug Effects

- Laboratory evidence of therapeutic response is reduction in concentrations of PSA and serum testosterone to levels equal to or less than pretreatment levels. A gradual rise in values after their decrease may signify treatment failure.
- Inspect injection site daily. If local hypersensitivity reactions occur (erythema, induration), suspect sensitivity to benzyl alcohol. Report to physician.
- Monitor I&O ratio and pattern. Report hematuria and decreased output. Carefully monitor voiding problems.

Patient & Family Education

- Patient may be instructed to self-medicate with leuprolide. Review package information and teach correct injection technique.
- Inform that bone pain and voiding problems (i.e., symptoms of tumor obstruction) usually increase during first several weeks of continuous treatment but are transient. Hot flushes may be experienced also.
- Caution to report worsening of neurologic signs and symptoms (paresthesia and weakness in lower limbs). Evaluate safety and capability to ambulate unassisted.
- Inform women that continuous treatment may cause amenorrhea and other menstrual irregularities.

LEVOBUNOLOL

(lee-voe-byoo′noe-lole)

Trade name: Betagan

Classifications: EYE PREPARATION; AUTONOMIC NERVOUS SYSTEM AGENT; BETA-ADRENERGIC ANTAGONIST (SYMPATHOLYTIC)

Prototype: Pilocarpine

Pregnancy category: C

See Appendix A.

LEVOCABASTINE HYDROCHLORIDE

(lev-o-ca-bas′teen)

Trade name: Livostin

Classifications: ANTIHISTAMINE; H_1-RECEPTOR ANTAGONIST

Prototype: Diphenhydramine

Pregnancy category: C

ACTIONS/PHARMACODYNAMICS Levocabastine is a potent antihistamine that competes for H_1-receptor sites on effector cells, thus blocking histamine release.

USE Temporary relief of seasonal allergic conjunctivitis.

ROUTE & DOSAGE

Allergic Conjunctivitis
Adult: **Ophthalmic** 1 drop in affected eye q.i.d.; shake well before using

PHARMACOKINETICS Absorption: significant systemic absorption; 30–60 % reaches systemic circulation. **Onset:** 15 min. **Duration:** 4 h. **Distribution:** slight distribution into breast milk. **Metabolism:** minimal metabolism in liver. **Elimination:** half-life: 33–40 h; 65–73% excreted in urine unchanged; up to 20% excreted in bile.

CONTRAINDICATIONS & PRECAUTIONS Contraindicated in: hypersensitivity to levocabastine, soft contact lenses. **Cautious use in:** hypersensitivity to other antihistamines, renal disease, pregnancy (category C), and nursing women. Safety and efficacy in children <12 y not established.

ADVERSE/SIDE EFFECTS CNS: drowsiness, fatigue, headache. **GI:** dry mouth. **Ocular:** *occular irritation, mild transient stinging and burning,* conjunctival congestion, eyelid edema, eye pain, photophobia, abnormal lacrimation.

NURSING IMPLICATIONS

Administration

- Shake well before using. Apply drops in the center of the lower conjunctional sac. Do not touch eyelids with dropper.
- Store at room temperature, 15–30C (59–86F), in a tightly closed bottle. Do not use if discolored.

Assessment & Drug Effects

- Monitor for signs and symptoms of hypersensitivity to the drug (see Appendix G).
- Evaluate safety, as drowsiness is a potential adverse effect.

Patient & Family Education

- Instruct patient on appropriate administration technique.
- Inform patient of potential adverse responses to drug.
- Eye drops contain benzalkonium chloride, which may damage soft contact lenses.

LEVODOPA (L-DOPA)

(lee-voe-doe′pa)

Trade names: Dopar, Larodopa

Prototype for classifications: AUTONOMIC NERVOUS SYSTEM AGENT; ANTICHOLINERGIC (PARASYMPATHOLYTIC); ANTIPARKINSONISM AGENT

Pregnancy category: C

ACTIONS/PHARMACODYNAMICS Metabolic precursor of dopamine, a catecholamine neurotransmitter. Unlike dopamine, levodopa readily crosses the blood–brain barrier. Precise mechanism of action unknown. Levodopa restores dopamine levels in extrapyramidal centers (believed to be depleted in parkinsonism).

USES Idiopathic Parkinson's disease, postencephalitic and arteriosclerotic parkinsonism, and parkinsonism symptoms associated with manganese and carbon monoxide poisoning. **Unlabeled uses:** to relieve pain of herpes zoster (shingles), hepatic coma (caused by cirrhosis or fulminating hepatitis), bone pain in metastatic breast carcinoma, adjunctive therapy in CHF.

ROUTE & DOSAGE

Parkinson's Disease

Adult: **PO** 500 mg to 1 g daily in 2 or more equally divided doses; may be increased by 100–750 mg q3–7d to maximal response or 8 g/d; if used in combination with carbidopa, decrease levodopa dose by 75–80%.

PHARMACOKINETICS Absorption: rapidly and well absorbed from GI tract; lower absorption if taken with food. **Peak:** 1–3 h. **Distribution:** widely distributed in body. **Metabolism:** most of drug is decarboxylated to dopamine in lumen of GI tract, liver, and serum. **Elimination:** half-life: 1 h; 80–85% of dose excreted in urine in 24 h.

CONTRAINDICATIONS & PRECAUTIONS Contraindicated in: known hypersensitivity to levodopa; narrow-angle glaucoma patients with suspicious pigmented lesion or history of melanoma; acute psychoses, severe psychoneurosis, within 2 wk of use of MAO INHIBITORS. Safe use during pregnancy (category C), in nursing mothers, and in children < 12 y not established. **Cautious use in:** cardiovascular, renal, hepatic, or endocrine disease, history of MI with residual arrhythmias; peptic ulcer; convulsions: psychiatric disorders; chronic wide-angle glaucoma; diabetes; pulmonary diseases, bronchial asthma; patients receiving antihypertensive drugs.

ADVERSE/SIDE EFFECTS Altered laboratory values: elevated BUN, AST, ALT, alkaline phosphatase, LDH, bilirubin, protein-bound iodine, serum level of growth hormone; decreased glucose tolerance; hypokalemia, decreased WBC, Hgb, Hct. **CNS:** *choreiform and involuntary movements,* increased hand tremor, bradykinetic episodes (on–off phenomena), trismus, grinding of teeth (bruxism), ataxia, muscle twitching, numbness, weakness, fatigue, headache, opisthotonos, confusion, agitation, anxiety, euphoria, insomnia, nightmares; psychotic episodes with paranoid delusions or hallucinations, severe depression, including suicidal tendencies, hypomania. **CV:** *orthostatic hypotension;* palpitations, tachycardia, hypertension. **Eye:** *blepharospasm,* diplopia, blurred vision, dilated pupils. **GI:** *anorexia, nausea, vomiting,* abdominal distress, flatulence, dry mouth, dysphagia, sialorrhea; burning sensation of tongue, bitter taste, diarrhea or constipation; GI bleeding. **Other:** rhinorrhea, flushing, skin rashes, dark sweat or urine, increased sweating, bizarre breathing patterns; urinary retention or incontinence, increased sexual drive, priapism, postmenopausal bleeding, weight gain or loss, edema; loss of hair; hepatotoxicity.

DIAGNOSTIC TEST INTERFERENCE ***Urine glucose:*** false-negative tests may result with use of glucose oxidase methods (e.g., Clinistix, Tes-Tape) and false-positive results with the copper reduction method (e.g., Clinitest), especially in patients receiving large doses. It is reported that Clinistix and TesTape may be used if reading is taken at margin of wet and dry tape. ***Urinary ketones:*** there is possibility of false-positive tests by dipsticks, e.g., Acetest (equivocal), Ketostix, Labstix; ***Serum and urinary uric acid:*** false elevations by colorimetric methods, but not with uricase; ***Uri-***

nary protein: false increases by Lowry method; ***Urinary VMA:*** false decreases by Pisano method; ***Urinary catecholamine:*** false increases by Hingerty method. ***PKU urine test:*** interference.

DRUG INTERACTIONS MAO INHIBITORS may precipitate hypertensive crisis; TRICYCLIC ANTIDEPRESSANTS augment postural hypotension; PHENOTHIAZINES, **haloperidol** may antagonize the therapeutic effects of levodopa; **pyridoxine** can reverse effects of levodopa; ANTICHOLINERGICS may exacerbate abnormal involuntary movements; **methyldopa** may increase toxic CNS effects; HALOGENATED GENERAL ANESTHETICS increase risk of arrhythmias. **Drug–food:** food decreases the rate and extent of levodopa absorption.

NURSING IMPLICATIONS

Administration

- Give with food to reduce nausea. Absorption is decreased with high-protein meals.
- Store in tight, light-resistant containers preferably between 15–30C (59–86F) unless otherwise directed by manufacturer.

Assessment & Drug Effects

- Therapeutic effects: Significant improvement usually occurs during second or third week of therapy, but it may not occur for 6 mo or more in some patients.
- Monitor vital signs, particularly during period of dosage adjustment. Report alterations in BP, pulse, and respiratory rate and rhythm.
- Orthostatic hypotension is usually asymptomatic, but some patients experience dizziness and syncope. Supervision of ambulation is indicated. Tolerance to this effect usually develops within a few months of therapy.
- Rate of dosage increase is determined primarily by patient's tolerance and response to levodopa. Make accurate observations and report promptly adverse reactions (generally dose related and reversible) and therapeutic effects.
- All patients should be closely monitored for behavior changes.
- Patients with chronic wide-angle glaucoma should be monitored during therapy for changes in intraocular pressure.
- Patients with diabetes should be observed carefully for loss of glycemic control.
- Periodically monitor blood glucose, CBC, Hgb and Hct, serum potassium, and hepatic and renal function tests.
- Patients on full therapeutic doses for ≥1 y may develop abnormal involuntary movements such as facial grimacing, rhythmic opening and closing of mouth, and jerky arm and leg movements. Symptoms tend to increase if dosage is not reduced.
- Muscle twitching and spasmodic winking (blepharospasm) are early signs of overdosage; report them promptly.
- Chronic management may be accompanied by the on–off phenomenon: rapid unpredictable swings in intensity of motor symptoms of parkinsonism evidenced by increase in bradykinesia (attacks of "leg freezing" or slow body movement). Report to physician.
- Monitor mental status for S&S of drug-induced neuropsychiatric adverse reactions.

Patient & Family Education

- Advise not to take with high-protein foods.
- Caution to make positional changes slowly, particularly from

recumbent to upright position, and to dangle legs a few minutes before standing.

- Advise to avoid high consumption of food sources of pyridoxine, including wheat germ, green vegetables, banana, whole-grain cereals, muscular and glandular meats (especially liver), legumes. Discuss dietary practices.
- Caution not to take OTC preparations or fortified cereals unless approved by physician. Multivitamins, antinauseants, and fortified cereals usually contain vitamin B_6.
- Elevation of mood and sense of well-being may precede objective improvement. Stress importance of resuming activities gradually and observing safety precautions to avoid injury.
- Urge to maintain prescribed drug regimen. Sudden withdrawal of medication can lead to parkinsonism crisis (with return of marked rigidity, akinesia, tremor, hyperpyrexia) or to NMS.
- Inform that a metabolite of levodopa may cause urine to darken on standing and may also cause sweat to be dark-colored.

L

LEVOFLOXACIN

(lev-o-flox'a-sin)

Trade name: Levaquin

Classifications: ANTIINFECTIVE; ANTIBIOTIC; FLUROQUINOLONE

Prototype: Ciprofloxacin

Pregnancy category: C

ACTIONS/PHARMACODYNAMICS Broad-spectrum antibiotic that inhibits DNA bacterial topoisomerase II, an enzyme required for DNA replication, transcription, repair, and recombination. Active against bacteria resistant to beta-lactam antibiotics.

USES Treatment of maxillary sinusitis, acute exacerbations of bacterial bronchitis, community-acquired pneumonia, uncomplicated skin/skin structure infections, UTI, acute pyelonephritis caused by susceptible bacteria.

ROUTE & DOSAGE

Infections

Adult: **PO** 500 mg q24h × 10 d. **IV** 500 mg infused over 60 min q24h × 7–14 d. Reduce dose in patients with renal insufficiency: give an initial dose of 500 mg; adjust maintenance doses as follows: Cl_{cr} 20–50 mg/min, 250 mg q24h; Cl_{cr} < 20 ml/min, 250 mg q48h.

UTI, Pyelonephritis

Adult: **PO** 250 mg q24h × 10 d. **IV** 250 mg infused over 60 min q24h × 10 d. Reduce dose in patients with renal insufficiency: give an initial dose of 250 mg; adjust maintenance doses as follows: Cl_{cr} < 20 ml/min, 250 mg q48h.

PHARMACOKINETICS **Absorption:** rapidly absorbed from GI tract. **Peak:** **PO** 1–2 h. **Distribution:** penetrates lung tissue, 24–38% protein bound. **Metabolism:** minimally metabolized in the liver. **Elimination:** half-life: 6–8 h; primarily excreted unchanged in urine.

CONTRAINDICATIONS & PRECAUTIONS **Contraindicated in:** hypersensitivity to levofloxacin and quinolone antibiotics; lactation. **Cautious use in:** known or suspected CNS disorders predisposed to seizure activity (e.g., severe cerebral atherosclerosis), risk factors associated with potential seizures (e.g., some drug therapy, renal insufficiency), diabetes; pregnancy (category C);

patients receiving theophylline or caffeine. Safety and efficacy in children < 18 y have not been established.

ADVERSE/SIDE EFFECTS CNS: headache, insomnia, dizziness. **GI:** nausea, diarrhea, constipation, vomiting, abdominal pain, dyspepsia. **Skin:** rash, pruritus. **Other:** vaginitis, injection site pain or inflammation, chest or back pain.

DRUG INTERACTIONS Magnesium- or aluminum-containing antacids, sucralfate, iron, zinc may decrease levofloxacin absorption; NSAIDS may increase risk of CNS reactions, including seizures; may cause hyper- or hypoglycemia in patients on ORAL HYPOGLYCEMIC AGENTS.

INCOMPATIBILITIES The manufacturer does not recommend that any drugs be added to the levofloxacin solution or be infused simultaneously through the same line (Y-site).

NURSING IMPLICATIONS

Administration

- Do not give oral drug within 2 h of drugs containing aluminum, magnesium, iron, zinc, or sucralfate.
- IV preparation: single-use vials must be diluted in 100 ml D5W or other compatible solutions to a concentration of 5 mg/ml. Discard any unused drug remaining in the vial.
- IV administration: give as IVPB over a period of not less than 60 min. Use caution not to give a bolus dose nor infuse too rapidly.
- Store tablets at 15–30C (59–86F) in a tightly closed container. IV solution is stable for 72 h at 25C (77F).

Assessment & Drug Effects

- Therapeutic effectiveness is indicated by negative cultures and resolution of S&S of infection.
- C&S test should be done prior to beginning therapy and periodically during therapy.
- Therapy should be discontinued and physician immediately notified if any of the following occur: skin rash or other signs of a hypersensitivity reaction (see Appendix G); CNS symptoms such as seizures, restlessness, confusion, hallucinations, depression; skin eruption following sun exposure; symptoms of colitis such as persistent diarrhea; joint pain, inflammation, or rupture of a tendon; hypoglycemic reaction in diabetic on an oral hypoglycemic agent.

Patient & Family Education

- Note important indications for discontinuing drug and immediately notifying physician.
- Fluids should be consumed liberally while taking levofloxacin.
- Allow a minimum of 2 h between any of the following: aluminum and/or magnesium antacids, iron supplements, multivitamins with zinc, or sucralfate.
- Avoid exposure to excess sunlight or artificial UV light.
- If possible, nonsteroidal antiinflammatory drugs should be avoided while taking levofloxacin.

LEVOMETHADYL ACETATE HYDROCHLORIDE

(lev-o-meth'a-dil)

Trade name: Orlaam

Classifications: CNS AGENT; NARCOTIC AGONIST ANALGESIC; OPIOID DETOXIFICATION AGENT

Prototype: Morphine

Pregnancy category: C

ACTIONS/PHARMACODYNAMICS Levomethadyl is a synthetic opioid analgesic (methadone derivative) with a long duration of action. Its pharmacologic effects are similar to those of morphine and other opioid analgesics. Tolerance to the analgesic and sedative effects of levomethadyl occurs with prolonged usage. It is used as a cross-substitute for morphine-like agents, including heroin.

USE Management of opiate dependence.

ROUTE & DOSAGE

Opiate Detoxification
Adult: **PO** 20–40 mg diluted in liquid q48–72h, may be adjusted by 5–10 mg in 1- to 2-wk intervals. Doses have ranged from 10 to 140 mg 3 times/wk.

PHARMACOKINETICS Absorption: rapidly absorbed from GI tract. **Onset:** 15–30 min. **Peak:** 1.5–2 h. **Duration:** 48–72 h. **Distribution:** approx 80% protein bound, crosses placenta. **Metabolism:** Extensive first-pass metabolism to active metabolite, norlaam. **Elimination:** half-life: 2.6 d; 72% eliminated in urine.

CONTRAINDICATIONS & PRECAUTIONS Contraindicated in: hypersensitivity to levomethadyl, lactation. **Cautious use in:** pregnancy (category C), concurrent use of other CNS depressants, hepatic or renal insufficiency, elderly, cardiac disease or hypertension, head injury or increased intracranial pressure, respiratory disorders (asthma, cor pulmonale, COPD), hypothyroidism, Addison's disease, prostatic hypertrophy, acute abdomen, anesthesia, previous hypersensitivity to methadone or other opioids. Safety and effectiveness in children < 18 y not established.

ADVERSE/SIDE EFFECTS Withdrawal reactions: nasal congestion, abdominal symptoms, diarrhea, muscle aches, anxiety. **Body as whole:** asthenia, arthralgia, back pain, chills, edema, hot flashes (especially males), flu syndrome, *malaise*. **CNS:** abnormal dreams, anxiety, decreased libido, depression, euphoria, headache, *insomnia, nervousness,* somnolence. **GI:** *abdominal pain, constipation,* diarrhea, dry mouth, nausea, vomiting. **Other:** cough, rhinitis, yawning, rash, *sweating,* blurred vision, *difficult ejaculation, impotence.*

DRUG INTERACTIONS NARCOTIC ANTAGONISTS **(naloxone, naltrexone)** or PARTIAL ANTAGONISTS (buprenorphine, butorphanol, nalbuphine, **pentazocine)** can induce withdrawal symptoms. **Carbamazepine, phenobarbital, phenytoin, rifabutin, rifampin** may increase peak activity or shorten the duration of action of levomethadyl. **Cimetidine, erythromycin, ketoconazole** may slow onset, lower activity, or increase duration of action of levomethadyl.

NURSING IMPLICATIONS

Administration

- Do not give daily doses; recommended doses are intended for q.o.d./q3d dosing only.
- Treatment of overdose: Cautiously give naloxone beginning with small doses of 0.1–0.2 mg; increase if needed at 2- to 3-min intervals to max of 10 mg. As levomethadyl has longer duration of action than naloxone, keep under prolonged observation following initial reversal.
- See manufacturer's guidelines for reinduction following a lapse of one or more doses.

- Store at 15–30C (59–86F). Protect from direct light.

Assessment & Drug Effects

- Carefully monitor throughout induction period for overdose and respiratory depression.
- Dosage adjustment is complex due to delayed onset of action; therefore, monitor for excessive opioid effect (i.e., sedation, incoordination, orthostatic hypotension).
- During interdose periods, monitor for and report S&S of withdrawal, as changes in dosing may be needed.

Patient & Family Education

- Provide administration directions and inform that daily use will lead to serious and potentially fatal overdose.
- Stress need to avoid abuse of psychoactive drugs and alcohol, especially during initial induction period, as full effect of drug requires 7–10 d.
- Advise regarding common adverse effects and possible drug interactions.
- Advise not to engage in hazardous activities until reaction to drug is known.

LEVONORGESTREL

(lev-o-nor-ges′trel)

Trade name: Norplant

Classifications: HORMONE; PROGESTIN

Prototype: Progesterone

Pregnancy category: X

ACTIONS/PHARMACODYNAMICS Levonorgestrel reduces the secretion of follicle-stimulating hormone (FSH) and lutenizing hormone (LH). This blocks follicular maturation and ovulation. Low-dose levonorgestrel also produces scanty, viscous cervical mucus, which retards sperm penetration of the uterus.

USE Contraceptive.

ROUTE & DOSAGE

Adult: **SC** Insert 6 Silastic capsules subdermally into the fleshy part of upper arm.

PHARMACOKINETICS **Absorption:** each capsule contains 36 mg of levonorgestrel; 80 μg is released per day during first 6–18 mo; rate of release decreases to 25–30 μg/d for the remainder of 5 y. **Onset:** 24 h to 1 mo, depending on time of insertion in relation to next menses. **Peak:** serum level, 24 h. **Duration:** up to 5 y. **Distribution:** distributed in small amounts in breast milk. **Metabolism:** metabolized in liver. **Elimination:** half-life: approx 37 h; 40–50% excreted in urine; 32% excreted in feces.

CONTRAINDICATIONS & PRECAUTIONS **Contraindicated in:** abnormal uterine bleeding, hemorrhagic disorders, known or suspected pregnancy (category X), hepatic disease, thrombophlebitis, thromboembolic disorders, known or suspected breast carcinoma. **Cautious use in:** anticonvulsant medications, diabetes mellitus, history of psychotic depression, conditions that may be aggravated by fluid retention (asthma, seizure disorders, cardiac or renal dysfunction, migraines).

ADVERSE/SIDE EFFECTS **CNS:** headaches (including migraine), depression, dizziness, vertigo, *mood changes,* nervousness, stroke. **CV:** hypertension, palpitations. **GI:** *nausea, appetite changes, weight gain.* **GU:** *irregular menstrual bleeding, amenorrhea, spotting, prolonged* and *heavy menstrual bleeding,* <u>ectopic pregnancy,</u> ovarian cyst, uter-

L

ine fibroids, vaginal candidiasis. **Hematologic:** blood clots, thrombocytopenia. **Skin:** acne, urticaria, dermatitis, pain at implant site.

DRUG INTERACTIONS ANTICONVULSANTS, **rifabutin, rifampin,** may decrease contraceptive efficacy.

NURSING IMPLICATIONS

Administration

- Sterile technique should be strictly adhered to when implanting or removing levonorgestrel.
- Manufacturer's directions for insertion and removal should be followed exactly.
- Store at room temperature, 15–30C (59–86F).

Assessment & Drug Effects

- Periodically assess mental status and report signs and symptoms of depression or other mood disturbances.
- Periodically monitor for weight gain and fluid retention; report significant changes.
- Monitor BP, serum lipids, and hepatic function periodically.

Patient & Family Education

- Inform of the potential adverse effects of levonorgestrel.
- Advise patients on concurrent anticonvulsant or rifampin therapy not to rely on levonorgestrel as the sole method of contraception.
- Inform patients prone to migraine headaches that levonorgestrel may increase the frequency and/or severity of headaches.
- Inform that contraceptive failure is possible and advise to report menstrual changes suggestive of pregnancy.

LEVORPHANOL TARTRATE

(lee-vor'fa-nole)

Trade name: Levo-Dromoran

Classifications: CNS AGENT; ANALGESIC; NARCOTIC (OPIATE) AGONIST

Prototype: Morphine sulfate

Pregnancy category: B

Controlled substance: Schedule II

ACTIONS/PHARMACODYNAMICS

Synthetic morphinan derivative with agonist activity only. Actions, uses, contraindications, precautions, and adverse reactions similar to those of morphine. More potent as an analgesic and has somewhat longer duration of action than morphine. Reported to cause less nausea, vomiting, and constipation than equivalent doses of morphine but may produce more sedation, smooth-muscle stimulation, and respiratory depression.

USES To relieve moderate to severe pain. Also preoperatively to allay apprehension.

ROUTE & DOSAGE

Moderate to Severe Pain

Adult: **PO/SC** 2–3 mg q6–8h prn.

PHARMACOKINETICS **Peak:** 60–90 min. **Duration:** 6–8 h. **Distribution:** crosses placenta; distributed into breast milk. **Metabolism:** metabolized in liver. **Elimination:** half-life: 1.2 h; excreted in urine.

ADVERSE/SIDE EFFECTS **CNS:** euphoria, *sedation, drowsiness,* nervousness, confusion. **CV:** hypotension, fast, slow, or pounding heartbeat. **GI:** *nausea,* vomiting, dry mouth, cramps, *constipation.* **GU:** urinary frequency, urinary retention, sedation. **Other:** blurred vision; respiratory depression, physical dependence.

DRUG INTERACTIONS **Alcohol** and other CNS DEPRESSANTS compound sedation and CNS depression.

INCOMPATIBILITIES **Solution/additive: aminophylline, ammonium chloride,** BARBITURATES, **chlorothiazide, heparin, methacillin, phenytoin, sodium bicarbonate.**

NURSING IMPLICATIONS

Administration

- Levorphanol should be given in the smallest effective dose to minimize the possibility of tolerance and physical dependence.
- Store tablets and injection at 15–30C (59–86F) unless otherwise directed. Tablets should be stored in tightly covered, light-resistant containers.

Assessment & Drug Effects

- Assess degree of pain relief. Drug is most effective when peaks and valleys of pain relief are avoided.
- Monitor bowel function.
- Monitor ambulation, especially in elderly patients.

Patient & Family Education

- Advise to avoid alcohol and other CNS depressants unless approved by physician.
- Caution to avoid driving and other potentially hazardous activities.
- Advise that ambulation may increase frequency of nausea and vomiting.
- Instruct to increase fluid and fiber intake to offset constipating effects of the drug.

LEVOTHYROXINE SODIUM (T_4)

(lee-voe-thye-rox′een)

Trade names: Eltroxin ♣, Levothroid, Levoxyl, Synthroid

Prototype for classifications: SYNTHETIC HORMONE; THYROID

Pregnancy category: A

ACTIONS/PHARMACODYNAMICS Synthetically prepared monosodium salt and levo isomer of thyroxine, with similar actions and uses. Thyroxine, principal component of thyroid gland secretions, determines normal thyroid function. Drug action not clearly understood, but principal effect is increase in the metabolic rate of all body tissues.

USES Specific replacement therapy for diminished or absent thyroid function resulting from primary or secondary atrophy of gland, surgery, excessive radiation or antithyroid drugs, congenital defect. Administered orally for hypothyroid state; administered IV for myxedematous coma or other thyroid dysfunctions demanding rapid replacement, as well as in failure to respond to oral therapy.

ROUTE & DOSAGE

Thyroid Replacement

Adult: **PO** 25–50 μg/d, gradually increased by 50–100 μg q1–4wk to usual dose of 100–400 μg/d. **IV** 1/2 of usual PO dose.
Child: **PO** *0–6 mo,* 8–10 μg/kg/d or 25–50 μg/d; *6–12 mo,* 6–8 μg/kg/d or 50–75 μg/d; *1–5 y,* 5–6 μg/kg/d or 75–100 μg/d; *6–12 y,* 4–5 μg/kd/d or 100–150 μg/d. *>12 y,* 2–3 μg/kg/d or >150 μg/d. **IV** 1/2 of usual PO dose.

Myxedema Coma

Adult: **IV** 250–500 μg IV stat; then 100–300 μg after 24 h if needed; then 50–200 μg/d until patient is stable and can take drug PO.

PHARMACOKINETICS **Absorption:** variable and incompletely absorbed from GI tract (50–80%). **Peak:** 3–4

wk. **Duration:** 1–3 wk. **Distribution:** gradually released into tissue cells. **Elimination:** half-life: 6–7 d.

CONTRAINDICATIONS & PRECAUTIONS **Contraindicated in:** hypersensitivity to levothyroxine; thyrotoxicosis, severe cardiovascular conditions, adrenal insufficiency. **Cautious use in:** angina pectoris, hypertension, impaired renal function, pregnancy (category A).

ADVERSE/SIDE EFFECTS **CNS:** irritability, nervousness, *insomnia,* headache (pseudotumor cerebri in children), tremors, craniosynostosis (excessive doses in children). **CV:** palpitations, tachycardia, arrhythmias, angina pectoris, hypertension. **GI:** nausea, diarrhea, change in appetite. **Other:** menstrual irregularities, weight loss, heat intolerance, sweating, fever, leg cramps, temporary hair loss (children).

DRUG INTERACTIONS **Cholestyramine, colestipol** decrease absorption of levothyroxine; **epinephrine, norepinephrine** increase risk of cardiac insufficiency; ORAL ANTICOAGULANTS may potentiate hypoprothrombinemia.

NURSING IMPLICATIONS

Administration

- Administer as single dose, preferably before breakfast, to prevent insomnia. Give consistently with respect to meals.
- Maintenance dosage for the elderly may be 25% lower than for heavier and younger adults.
- Parenteral preparation should be reconstituted with NaCl injection immediately before administration. Shake vial until solution is clear. Discard unused portion.
- IV solution is prepared by adding supplied diluent (5 ml NS without preservatives) to 0.5 mg of powder. Resulting concentration is 0.1 mg/ml.
- IV solution is administered by direct IV at a rate of 0.1 mg or a fraction thereof over 1 min.
- Store in tight, light-resistant container at 15–30C (59–86F).

Assessment & Drug Effects

- Assess for therapeutic effectiveness, which includes diuresis, loss of weight and puffiness, increased sense of well-being and activity tolerance, and rise of T_3 and T_4 serum levels toward normal.
- Pulse rate is an important index of drug effectiveness. During dose adjustment, count the pulse before each dose. If rate is > 100, consult physician.
- Monitor for adverse effects during early adjustment. If metabolism increases too rapidly, especially in elderly and heart disease patients, symptoms of angina or cardiac failure may appear.
- Levothyroxine may aggravate severity of previously obscured symptoms of diabetes mellitus, Addison's disease, or diabetes insipidus. Therapy for these disorders may require adjustment.
- Baseline and periodic tests of thyroid function and of bone age, growth, and psychomotor function in children are recommended.
- Some children have partial hair loss after a few months; it returns even with continued therapy.
- Closely monitor PT and INP and assess for evidence of bleeding if patient is receiving concurrent anticoagulant therapy.
- A decrease in anticoagulant dosage may be needed 1–4 wk after concurrent levothyroxine is started.
- Note that Synthroid 0.1 and 0.3 mg tablets contain tartrazine, which may cause an allergic-type reac-

tion in certain patients. It is frequently seen in persons who also have aspirin hypersensitivity.

Patient & Family Education

- Advise that optimal time to take drug is 1 h before or 2 h after breakfast.
- Inform that thyroid replacement therapy is usually lifelong.
- Teach how to self-monitor pulse rate. Instruct to notify physician if rate begins to increase above 100 or if rhythm changes are noted.
- Instruct to immediately report signs of toxicity (e.g., chest pain, palpitations, nervousness).
- Instruct not to accept brand change, as differences in bioequivalence exist among brands.
- Caution to avoid OTC medications unless approved by physician.

LIDOCAINE HYDROCHLORIDE

(lye′doe-kane)

Trade names: Anestacon, Dilocaine, L-Caine, Lida-Mantle, Lidoject-1, LidoPen Auto Injector, Nervocaine, Octocaine, Xylocaine, Xylocard♣

Classifications: CARDIOVASCULAR AGENT; ANTIARRHYTHMIC; CNS AGENT; LOCAL ANESTHETIC

Prototype: Procainamide hydrochloride

Pregnancy category: B

ACTIONS/PHARMACODYNAMICS Cardiac actions similar to those of procainamide and quinidine but has little effect on myocardial contractility, AV and intraventricular conduction, cardiac output, and systolic arterial pressure in equivalent doses. Exerts antiarrhythmic action (class Ib) by suppressing automaticity in His-Purkinje system and by elevating electrical stimulation threshold of ventricle during diastole. Progressive depression of CNS occurs with increasing blood concentrations; produces anticonvulsant, sedative, and analgesic effects. Action as local anesthetic is more prompt, more intense, and longer lasting than that of procaine. Suppresses cough and gag reflexes.

USES Rapid control of ventricular arrhythmias occurring during acute MI, cardiac surgery, and cardiac catheterization and those caused by digitalis intoxication. Also as surface and infiltration anesthesia and for nerve block, including caudal and spinal block anesthesia and to relieve local discomfort of skin and mucous membranes. **Unlabeled use:** refractory status epilepticus.

ROUTE & DOSAGE

Ventricular Arrhythmias

Adult: **IV** 50–100 mg bolus at a rate of 20–50 mg/min; may repeat in 5 min, then start infusion of 20–50 μg/kg/min (1–4 mg/min) immediately after first bolus. **IM/SC** 200–300 mg IM; may repeat once after 60–90 min. *Child:* **IV** 0.5–1 mg/kg bolus dose, then 10–50 μg/kg/min infusion.

Anesthetic Uses

Adult: **Infiltration** 0.5–1% solution. **Nerve block** 1–2% solution. **Epidural** 1–2% solution; **Caudal** 1–1.5% solution. **Spinal** 5% with glucose, **Saddle block** 1.5% with dextrose. **Topical** 2.5–5% jelly, ointment, cream, or solution.

PHARMACOKINETICS **Onset:** 45–90 s IV; 5–15 min IM; 2–5 min topical. **Duration:** 10–20 min IV; 60–90 min IM; 30–60 min topical; > 100 min injected for anesthesia. **Distribution:** crosses blood–brain barrier and placenta; distributed into breast milk. **Metabolism:** metabolized in liver. **Elimination:** half-life: 1.5–2 h; excreted in urine.

CONTRAINDICATIONS & PRECAUTIONS **Contraindicated in:** history of hypersensitivity to amide-type local anesthetics; application or injection of lidocaine anesthetic in presence of severe trauma or sepsis, blood dyscrasias, supraventricular arrhythmias, Stokes-Adams syndrome, untreated sinus bradycardia, severe degrees of sinoatrial, atrioventricular, and intraventricular heart block. Safe use during pregnancy (category B), in nursing mothers, and in children not established. **Cautious use in:** liver or renal disease, CHF, marked hypoxia, respiratory depression, hypovolemia, shock; myasthenia gravis; debilitated patients, the elderly; family history of malignant hyperthermia (fulminant hypermetabolism). Topical use in eyes, over large body areas, over prolonged periods, in severe or extensive trauma or skin disorders.

ADVERSE/SIDE EFFECTS **CNS:** drowsiness, dizziness, light-headedness, restlessness, confusion, disorientation, irritability, apprehension, euphoria, wild excitement, numbness of lips or tongue and other paresthesias including sensations of heat and cold, chest heaviness, difficulty in speaking, difficulty in breathing or swallowing, muscular twitching, tremors, psychosis. With high doses: convulsions, respiratory depression and arrest. **CV:** (with high doses): hypotension, bradycardia, conduction disorders including heart block, cardiovascular collapse, cardiac arrest. **Ears:** tinnitus, decreased hearing. **Eye:** blurred or double vision, impaired color perception. **Other:** anorexia, nausea, vomiting, excessive perspiration, soreness at IM site, local thrombophlebitis (with prolonged IV infusion), hypersensitivity reactions (urticaria, rash, edema, anaphylactoid reactions).

DIAGNOSTIC TEST INTERFERENCE Increases in ***creatine phosphokinase*** (CPK) level may occur for 48 h after IM dose and may interfere with test for presence of MI.

DRUG INTERACTIONS BARBITURATES decrease lidocaine activity; **cimetidine,** BETA BLOCKERS, **quinidine** increase pharmacologic effects of lidocaine; **phenytoin** increases cardiac depressant effects; **procainamide** compounds neurologic and cardiac effects.

INCOMPATIBILITIES **Solution/additive: phenytoin, cefazolin. Y-site: phenytoin.**

NURSING IMPLICATIONS

Administration

- Only lidocaine hydrochloride injection without preservatives or epinephrine that is specifically labeled for IV use should be used for IV injection or infusion.
- Bolus dose of lidocaine may be given undiluted by direct IV at a rate of 50 mg or fraction thereof over 1 min.
- Lidocaine may be added to D5W for infusion. For adults, add 1 g to 250–500 ml; for children, add 120 mg to 100 ml.
- For IV infusion, use microdropper and infusion pump. Rate of flow is usually no more than 4 mg/min.
- IV infusion should be terminated as soon as patient's basic cardiac rhythm stabilizes or at earliest signs and symptoms of toxicity (infusions are rarely continued beyond 24 h).

- Deltoid muscle is recommended as the preferred IM site.
- Topical lidocaine should not be applied to large areas of skin or to broken or abraded surfaces. Consult physician about whether area can be covered with a dressing.
- Avoid contacting eyes with topical preparation.
- Anesthetic use: Lidocaine solutions containing preservatives should not be used for spinal or epidural (including caudal) block.
- Partially used solutions of lidocaine without preservatives should be discarded after initial use.
- Inspect solutions for particulate matter and discoloration prior to administration and discard if either is present.
- Store all preparations at 15–30C (59–86F) unless otherwise directed.

Assessment & Drug Effects

- If ECG signs of excessive cardiac depression occur, such as prolongation of PR interval or QRS complex and the appearance or aggravation of arrhythmias, infusion should be stopped immediately.
- Constant ECG monitoring and frequent determinations of BP, respirations, and CNS status are essential to avoid potential overdosage and toxicity.
- Auscultate lungs for basilar rales, especially in patients who tend to metabolize the drug slowly (e.g., CHF, cardiogenic shock, hepatic dysfunction).
- In patients receiving IV infusions of lidocaine or those with high lidocaine blood levels, watch for neurotoxic effects: drowsiness, dizziness, confusion, paresthesias, visual disturbances, excitement, behavioral changes.
- Lidocaine blood levels of approximately 1.5 to 6 μg/ml are reported to provide "usually effective" antiarrhythmic activity. Blood levels greater than 7 μg/ml are potentially toxic.

Patient & Family Education

- Instruct patient using lidocaine solution for relief of mouth discomfort to swish and spit it out. For use in pharnyx, lidocaine solution should be gargled and may be swallowed (as prescribed).
- Patient should know that oral topical anesthetics, e.g., Xylocaine Viscous, may interfere with swallowing reflex. Food should not be ingested within 60 min after drug application, especially in pediatric, geriatric, or debilitated patients. Also, warn patient against chewing gum while buccal and throat membranes are anesthetized to prevent biting trauma.

L

LINCOMYCIN HYDROCHLORIDE

(lin-koe-mye′sin)

Trade name: Lincocin

Classifications: ANTIINFECTIVE; ANTIBIOTIC

Prototype: Clindamycin

Pregnancy category: B

ACTIONS/PHARMACODYNAMICS

Derived from *Streptomyces lincolnensis*. Bacteriostatic or bactericidal depending on concentration used and sensitivity of organism. Similar to clindamycin in antibacterial activity and demonstrates some cross-resistance with it. Effective against most of the common gram-positive pathogens, particularly streptococci, pneumococci, and staphylococci. Also effective against *Bacteroides* and other anaerobes; however, little activity against most gram-negative organisms and ineffective against viruses, yeasts, or fungi. Resistance by *Staphylococcus* is acquired in stepwise manner. Lincomycin is reported to have neuromuscular blocking properties.

USES Reserved for treatment of serious infections caused by susceptible bacteria in penicillin-allergic patients or patients for whom penicillin is inappropriate.

ROUTE & DOSAGE

Infections

Adult: **PO** 500 mg q6–8h (max 8 g/d). **IM** 600 mg q12–24h; **IV** 600 mg–1 g q8–12h.
Child: **PO** > *1 mo,* 30–60 mg/kg in 3–4 divided doses. **IM** 10 mg/kg q12–24h; **IV** 10–20 mg/kg/d in 2–3 divided doses.

L

PHARMACOKINETICS Absorption: partially absorbed from GI tract (20–30%). **Peak:** 2–4 h PO; 30 min IM. **Duration:** 6–8 h PO; 12–14 h IM; 14 h IV. **Distribution:** high concentrations in bone, aqueous humor, bile, and peritoneal, pleural, and synovial fluids; crosses placenta; distributed into breast milk. **Metabolism:** partially metabolized in liver. **Elimination:** half-life: 5 h; excreted in urine and feces.

CONTRAINDICATIONS & PRECAUTIONS Contraindicated in: previous hypersensitivity to lincomycin and clindamycin; impaired hepatic function, known monilial infections (unless treated concurrently); use in newborns. Safe use in pregnancy (category B) and nursing mothers not established. **Cautious use in:** impaired renal function; history of GI disease, particularly colitis; history of liver, endocrine, or metabolic diseases; history of asthma, hay fever, eczema, drug or other allergies; elderly patients.

ADVERSE/SIDE EFFECTS CV: hypotension, syncope, cardiopulmonary arrest (particularly after rapid IV). **GI:** glossitis, stomatitis, *nausea, vomiting,* anorexia, decreased taste acuity, unpleasant or altered taste, abdominal cramps, *diarrhea,* acute enterocolitis, pseudomembranous colitis (potentially fatal). **Hematologic:** neutropenia, leukopenia, agranulocytosis, thrombocytopenic purpura, aplastic anemia. **Hypersensitivity:** pruritus, urticaria, skin rashes, exfoliative and vesiculobullous dermatitis, erythema multiforme (rare), angioedema, photosensitivity, anaphylactoid reaction, serum sickness. **Other:** superinfections (proctitis, pruritus ani, vaginitis), tinnitus, vertigo, dizziness, headache, generalized myalgia, thrombophlebitis following IV use; pain at IM injection site.

DRUG INTERACTIONS Kaolin and pectin decreases lincomycin absorption; **tubocurarine, pancuronium** may enhance neuromuscular blockade.

INCOMPATIBILITIES Solution/additive: penicillin G, phenytoin, ampicillin, carbenicillin, methicillin.

NURSING IMPLICATIONS

Administration

- Absorption is reduced and delayed by presence of food in stomach. Administer oral drug with a full glass (240 ml [8 oz]) of water at least 1 h before or 2 h after meals.
- Administer IM injection deep into large muscle mass; inject slowly to minimize pain. Rotate injection sites.
- For IV administration, 1 g of lincomycin is diluted in at least 100 ml of D5W, NS, or other compati-

ble solution. Rate of infusion should not exceed 1 g/h.

- Follow manufacturer's directions for further information on reconstitution, storage time, compatible IV fluids, and IV administration rates.
- Store unopened vials and oral drug at 15–30C (59–86F) unless otherwise directed.

Assessment & Drug Effects

- Culture and susceptibility tests should be performed initially and during therapy to determine continued microbial susceptibility.
- A careful history should be taken of previous sensitivities to drugs or other allergens.
- Monitor BP and pulse. Have patient remain recumbent following drug administration until BP stabilizes.
- Monitor patients closely and report changes in bowel frequency. If significant diarrhea occurs, drug should be discontinued.
- Diarrhea, acute colitis, or pseudomembranous colitis (see Appendix G) may occur up to several weeks after cessation of therapy.
- Examine IM and IV injection sites daily for signs of inflammation.
- Serum drug levels should be monitored closely in patients with severe impairment of renal function (levels tend to be higher).
- Periodic hepatic and renal function studies and CBC are indicated during prolonged drug therapy.
- Superinfections by nonsusceptible organisms are most likely to occur when duration of therapy exceeds 10 d (see Appendix G).

Patient & Family Education

- Advise to report promptly the onset of perianal irritation, diarrhea, or blood and mucus in stools. Antiperistaltic agents may prolong and worsen diarrhea by delaying removal of toxins from colon.
- Advise to report immediately symptoms of hypersensitivity (see Appendix G). Drug should be discontinued.
- Instruct to take drug for full course of therapy as prescribed.

LINDANE

(lin′dane)

Trade names: Gamabenzene, Kwell, Scabene

Prototype for classifications: SKIN AGENT; SCABICIDE; PEDICULICIDE; ANTIINFECTIVE

Pregnancy category: C

L

ACTIONS/PHARMACODYNAMICS

Has ectoparasitic and ovicidal activity against the two variants of *Pediculus humanus—Pediculus capitis* (head louse) and *Pediculus pubis* (crab louse)—and the arthropod *Sarcoptes scabiei* (scabies). Action of drug follows its direct absorption by parasites and ova (nits). Drug absorption through the exoskeleton stimulates the nervous system, resulting in seizures and death. Lindane is not prophylactic for pediculosis.

USES To treat head and crab lice and scabies infestations and to eradicate their ova.

ROUTE & DOSAGE

Adult: **Topical** Apply to all body areas except the face; leave lotion on 8–12 h; then rinse off; leave shampoo on 5 min; then rinse thoroughly; do not repeat in < 1 wk.
Child: **Topical** Same as for adult.

PHARMACOKINETICS Absorption: slowly and incompletely absorbed through intact skin; maximum absorption from face, scalp, axillae. **Distribution:** stored in body fat. **Metabolism:** metabolized in liver. **Elimination:** excreted in urine and feces.

CONTRAINDICATIONS & PRECAUTIONS Contraindicated in: premature neonates, patient with known seizure disorders; application to eyes, face, mucous membranes, urethral meatus, open cuts or raw, weeping surfaces; prolonged or excessive applications or simultaneous application of creams, ointments, oils. Use during pregnancy (category B) or by nursing mothers not recommended by CDC. **Cautious use in:** children < 10 y.

L

ADVERSE/SIDE EFFECTS CNS: CNS stimulation (usually after accidental ingestion or misuse of product): restlessness, dizziness, tremors, convulsions. **Inhalation:** headache, nausea, vomiting, irritation of ENT. **Skin:** eczematous eruptions.

NURSING IMPLICATIONS

Administration

- To reduce percutaneous absorption, all skin lotions and creams and oil-based hair dressings should be completely removed, and skin should be allowed to dry and cool before application of lindane.
- Cream or lotion: Shake container well. *Scabies:* Apply thin film from neck down over entire body surface including soles of feet. Avoid face and urethral meatus. Pay particular attention to intertriginous areas (finger webs and other body creases and folds), wrists, elbows, and belt line. Rub drug in; allow skin to dry and cool after application. After 8–12 h, remove medication by bath or shower. *Crab lice:* Apply thin film of drug to hair and skin of pubic area and, if infected, to thighs, trunk, axillary areas. Leave in place 8–12 h and follow with bath or shower. Observation of living lice after 7 d indicates the need for reapplication.
- Shampoo (*head lice*): Apply quantity sufficient to wet hair and skin. Work drug thoroughly onto hair shafts and scalp and allow to remain in place 4 min. Add small amounts of water sufficient to make a thick lather; then rinse well with water. Pay particular attention to areas above and behind ears and occipital region. Use fine-tooth comb or tweezers to remove remaining nit shells. If necessary, treatment may be repeated after 7 d but not more than twice in 1 wk. *Crab lice:* see above. Repeat treatment after 7 d only if live lice can be demonstrated.
- The caregiver should wear plastic disposable or rubber gloves when applying lindane, especially if she is pregnant or if she is applying medication to more than one patient, to avoid prolonged skin contact.
- Store drug at 15–30C (59–86F) in tight container away from direct light and heat. Protect from freezing.

Assessment & Drug Effects

- Case-finding efforts should include not only the sex partner but also other family members and close-contact persons. Suspect scabies if a person complains of nocturnal itching (classic symptom).
- Both scabies and *P. pubis* infestation are sexually transmitted diseases. The sex partner should be identified and treated simultaneously.
- Burrows made by scabies mites (may or may not be visible) appear

as grayish black straight or S-shaped lines with a papule containing the mite at one end and surrounded by a mild erythematous area.

Patient & Family Education

- Instruct on proper application of medication.
- Lindane is highly toxic drug if topical applications are excessive or if swallowed or inhaled. Keep out of reach of children.
- Lindane shampoo is an effective disinfectant for personal items such as combs, brushes.
- Penetration of the skin with scabies mites causes an intolerable itching that may persist 2–3 wk after they have been killed.
- Instruct to discontinue medication and report to a physician if signs of irritation, sensitization, or itching occur.
- Caution against applying medication to face, mouth, open skin lesions, or to eyelashes; avoid contact with eyes. If accidental eye contact occurs, flush with water.
- Recurring limited infestations of scabies may indicate a domestic animal source (e.g., cat, dog, cattle, poultry).

LIOTHYRONINE SODIUM (T_3)

(lye-oh-thye′roe-neen)

Trade name: Cytomel

Classifications: SYNTHETIC HORMONE; THYROID

Prototype: Levothyroxine

Pregnancy category: A

ACTIONS/PHARMACODYNAMICS Synthetic form of natural thyroid hormone. Shares actions and uses of thyroid but has more rapid action and more rapid disappearance of effect, permitting quick dosage adjustment if necessary. May be used in T_3 suppression test to differentiate suspected hyperthyroidism from euthyroidism. See thyroid for contraindications and precautions.

USES Replacement or supplemental therapy for cretinism, myxedema, goiter, secondary (pituitary) or tertiary (hypothalamic) hypothyroidism, and T_3 suppression test.

ROUTE & DOSAGE

Thyroid Replacement

Adult: **PO** 25–75 µg/d.
Geriatric: **PO** 5 µg/d, increase by 5 µg/d every 1–2 wk.
Child: **PO** 5 µg/d gradually increased by 5 µg/d q3–4d until desired response.

Myxedema

Adult: **PO** 5–100 µg/d.
Geriatric: **PO** Start at 5 µg/d.

Goiter

Adult: **PO** 5–75 µg/d.
Geriatric: **PO** Start at 5 µg/d.
Child: **PO** 5 µg/d; increase by 5 µg q1–2wk (usual maintenance dose 15–20 µg/d).

T_3 Suppression Test

Adult: **PO** 75–100 µg/d × 7 d.

PHARMACOKINETICS **Absorption:** completely absorbed from GI tract. **Peak:** 24–72 h. **Duration:** up to 72 h. **Distribution:** gradually released into tissue cells. **Elimination:** half-life: 6–7 d.

ADVERSE/SIDE EFFECTS Result from overdosage; evidenced as signs and symptoms of hyperthyroidism (see Appendix G). ***Children:*** accelerated rate of bone maturation.

DRUG INTERACTIONS **Cholestyramine, colestipol** decrease absorption; **epinephrine, norepineph-**

rine increase risk of cardiac insufficiency; ORAL ANTICOAGULANTS may potentiate hypoprothrombinemia.

NURSING IMPLICATIONS

Administration

- Give daily before breakfast.
- When changing to liothyronine, discontinue other thyroid drug and initiate liothyronine at low dosage, with gradual increases according to patient's response.
- Store tablets in heat-, light-, and moistureproof container at 15–30C (59–86F).

Assessment & Drug Effects

- Note that metabolic effects persist a few days after drug withdrawal.
- Residual actions of other thyroid preparations may persist for weeks; therefore, during early period of liothyronine substitution for another preparation, watch for possible additive effects, particularly if the patient is elderly, has cardiovascular disease, or is a child.
- With onset of overdosage symptoms (hyperthyroidism; see Appendix G), drug is withheld for 1 or 2 d; usually therapy can be resumed with lower dosage.

Patient & Family Education

- Instruct to take medication exactly as ordered.
- Teach S&S of hyperthyroidism (see Appendix G) and advise to report their appearance to physician promptly.

LIOTRIX (T_3-T_4)

(lye′oh-trix)

Trade names: Euthroid, Thyrolar

Classifications: SYNTHETIC HORMONE; THYROID

Prototype: Levothyroxine

Pregnancy category: A

ACTIONS/PHARMACODYNAMICS

Synthetic levothyroxine (T_4) and liothyronine (T_3) combined in a constant 4:1 ratio by weight. Actions and pharmacokinetics as for thyroid. Products by different manufacturers differ in total amounts of each drug included in the formulation.

USES Replacement or supplemental therapy for cretinism, myxedema, goiter, and secondary (pituitary) or tertiary (hypothalamic) hypothyroidism. Also with antithyroid agents in thyrotoxicosis and to prevent goitrogenesis and hypothyroidism.

ROUTE & DOSAGE

Thyroid Replacement

Adult: **PO** 12.5–30 μg/d gradually increased to desired response.
Child: **PO** Same as for adult.

CONTRAINDICATIONS & PRECAUTIONS **Contraindicated in:** thyrotoxicosis, acute MI, morphologic hypogonadism, nephrosis, adrenal deficiency due to hypopituitarism. **Cautious use in:** concomitant anticoagulant therapy; myxedema; angina pectoris, hypertension, arteriosclerosis; renal dysfunction, pregnancy (category A).

ADVERSE/SIDE EFFECTS CNS: nervousness, headache, tremors, insomnia. **CV:** palpitation, tachycardia, angina pectoris, cardiac arrhythmias, hypertension, CHF. **GI:** nausea, abdominal cramps, diarrhea. **Other:** weight loss, heat intolerance, fever, sweating, menstrual irregularities. Infants, children: accelerated rate of bone maturation.

DRUG INTERACTIONS Cholestyramine, colestipol decrease absorption; **epinephrine, norepinephrine** increase risk of cardiac insufficiency; ORAL ANTICOAGULANTS may potentiate hypoprothrombinemia.

NURSING IMPLICATIONS

Administration

- Usually administered as a single daily dose, preferably before breakfast.
- Dose increases are made at 1- to 2-wk intervals.
- Store in heat-, light-, and moisture-proof container at 15–30C (59–86F). Shelf-life: 2 y.

Assessment & Drug Effects

- Note that metabolic effects persist a few days after drug withdrawal.
- Residual actions of other thyroid preparations may persist for weeks; therefore, during early period of liotrix substitution for another preparation, watch for possible additive effects, particularly if the patient is elderly, has cardiovascular disease, or is a child.
- With onset of overdosage symptoms (hyperthyroidism; see Appendix G), drug is withheld for 1 or 2 d; usually therapy can be resumed with lower dosage.

Patient & Family Education

- Diabetic patients may require an increase in insulin or oral hypoglycemic dosage while taking liotrix.
- Euthyroid patient should report headache, since this may indicate need for dosage adjustment or change to another thyroid preparation.
- Instruct to take medication exactly as ordered.
- Teach S&S of hyperthyroidism (see Appendix G) and advise to report their appearance to physician promptly.

LISINOPRIL

(ly-sin′-o-pril)

Trade names: Prinivil, Zestril

Classifications: CARDIOVASCULAR AGENT; ANGIOTENSIN-CONVERTING ENZYME INHIBITOR; ANTIHYPERTENSIVE

Prototype: Captopril

Pregnancy category: D

ACTIONS/PHARMACODYNAMICS Lowers BP by specific inhibition of the angiotensin-converting enzyme (ACE). This interrupts conversion sequences initiated by renin that form angiotensin II, a potent vasoconstrictor. ACE inhibition alters hemodynamics without compensatory reflex tachycardia or changes in cardiac output (except in patients with CHF). Inhibition of ACE also decreases circulating aldosterone, which is normally released in response to angiotensin II stimulation. Reduced aldosterone is associated with a potassium-sparing effect. Lisinopril decreases peripheral resistance (afterload) and pulmonary vascular resistance. There is improved cardiac output and exercise tolerance.

USES Hypertension, alone or concomitantly with other classes of antihypertensive agents; CHF; to improve MI survival.

ROUTE & DOSAGE

Hypertension

Adult: **PO** 10 mg once/d; may increase up to 20–40 mg 1–2 times/d (max 80 mg/d).
Geriatric: **PO** Inital 2.5–5 mg/d, may increase by 2.5–5 mg/d every 1–2 wk (max 40 mg/d).

PHARMACOKINETICS Absorption: 25% absorbed from GI tract. **Onset:** 1 h. **Peak:** 6–8 h. **Duration:** 24 h. **Distribution:** limited amount crosses blood-brain barrier; crosses placenta; small amount distributed in breast milk. **Metabolism:** is not metabolized. **Elimination:** half-life: 12 h; excreted primarily in urine.

CONTRAINDICATIONS & PRECAUTIONS Contraindicated in: patients with a history of angioedema related to treatment with an angiotensin converting enzyme inhibitor, pregnancy (category D), nursing mothers. **Cautious use in:** impaired renal function, hyperkalemia, patients on diuretic therapy; autoimmune diseases especially systemic lupus erythematosus (SLE).

L

ADVERSE/SIDE EFFECTS CNS: headache, dizziness, fatigue. **CV:** hypotension, chest pain. **GI:** nausea, vomiting, diarrhea, anorexia, constipation. **Other:** dyspnea, cough, rash, azotemia, hyperkalemia, increased BUN and creatinine levels.

DRUG INTERACTIONS Indomethacin and other NSAIDS may decrease antihypertensive activity; POTASSIUM SUPPLEMENTS, POTASSIUM-SPARING DIURETICS may cause hyperkalemia; may increase **lithium** levels and toxicity.

NURSING IMPLICATIONS

Administration

- For diuretic-treated patients an initial dose of 5 mg is usually given. Monitor drug effect for 2 h or until the BP is stabilized for at least 1 additional hour. Concurrent administration with a diuretic may compound hypotensive effect.
- It is recommended that previous diuretic therapy be withdrawn 2 to 3 d before therapy is initiated.
- Lisinopril is removed from blood by hemodialysis; therefore, administer following dialysis.

Assessment & Drug Effects

- Sudden and severe hypotension may occur within the first 1–5 h after the initial dose, particularly in patients who are sodium- or volume-depleted because of diuretic therapy. If excessive hypotension occurs, place patient in supine position and notify physician.
- It is usually effective in once daily dosing. However, if the antihypertensive effect is diminished in less than 24 h, an increase in dosage may be necessary.
- Evaluate effect of drug by measuring BP just prior to dosing to determine whether satisfactory control is being maintained for 24 h.
- Closely monitor for angioedema of extremities, face, lips, tongue, glottis, and larynx. Promptly discontinue drug and notify physician. Carefully monitor for airway obstruction until swelling is relieved.
- Monitor serum sodium and serum potassium levels for hyponatremia and hyperkalemia.
- Renal function studies are recommended at periodic intervals, especially in patients with severe volume or sodium replacement or those with severe CHF.
- WBC count determination should be made prior to initiation of treatment, every month for the first 3–6 mo of therapy, and at periodic intervals for 1 y. Therapy should be discontinued if neutropenia (neutrophil count <1000/mm^3) develops.

Patient & Family Education

- Instruct that severe hypersensitivity reaction to any ACE inhibitor may include hoarseness, swelling of the face, mouth, hands, or feet or sudden trouble breathing. If these occur, discontinue drug and contact physician immediately.

- Discuss importance of proper diet, including sodium and potassium restrictions. Advise not to use salt substitute containing potassium.
- Discuss importance of continued compliance with high BP medication. If a dose is missed, instruct to take it as soon as possible but not if too close to next dose.
- Instruct to avoid driving or other potential hazardous activity until reaction to the drug is known.
- Advise patients on lithium that lisinopril increases the risk of lithium toxicity.
- Promptly notify physician of any indication of infection (e.g., sore throat, fever).
- Instruct to check with physician before use of any new medicine (prescription or nonprescription).
- Advise not to store drug in a moist area. Heat and moisture may cause the medicine to break down.

LITHIUM CARBONATE

(li'thee-um)

Trade names: Carbolith ♣, Duralith ♣, Eskalith, Eskalith CR, Lithane, Lithizine ♣, Lithobid, Lithonate, Lithotabs

LITHIUM CITRATE

Trade name: Cibalith-S

Prototype for classifications: CNS AGENT; PSYCHOTHERAPEUTIC; ANTIMANIC

Pregnancy category: D

ACTIONS/PHARMACODYNAMICS The lithium ion behaves in the body much like the sodium ion; but its exact mechanism of action is unclear. Competes with various physiologically important cations: Na, K, Ca, Mg; therefore, it affects cell membranes, body water, and neurotransmitters. At the synapse, it accelerates catecholamine destruction, inhibits the release of neurotransmitters and decreases sensitivity of postsynaptic receptors. Thus, neurotransmitter overactivity assumed to occur in mania is corrected. Has antidepressant and antimanic effects.

USES Control and prophylaxis of acute mania and the acute manic phase of mixed bipolar disorder. **Unlabeled uses:** acute and recurrent depression (unipolar affective disorder), schizophrenic disorders, disorders of impulse control, alcohol dependence, antineoplastic drug-induced neutropenia, aplastic anemia, SIADH, cyclic neutropenia.

ROUTE & DOSAGE

Mania

Adult: **PO** *Initial:* 600 mg t.i.d. *or* 900 mg sustained-release b.i.d. *or* 30 ml (48 mEq) of solution t.i.d. **Maintenance:** 300 mg t.i.d. or q.i.d. *or* 15–20 ml (24–32 mEq) solution in 2–4 divided doses (max 2.4 g/d).
Child: **PO** 15–60 mg/kg/d in divided doses.

PHARMACOKINETICS **Absorption:** readily absorbed from GI tract. **Peak:** 0.5–3 h carbonate; 15–60 min citrate. **Distribution:** crosses blood–brain barrier and placenta; distributed into breast milk. **Metabolism:** not metabolized. **Elimination:** half-life: 20–27 h; 95% excreted in urine, 1% in feces, 4–5% in sweat.

CONTRAINDICATIONS & PRECAUTIONS **Contraindicated in:** significant cardiovascular or renal disease, brain damage, severe debilitation, dehydration or sodium depletion; patients on low-salt diet or receiving diuretics; pregnancy, especially first trimester (category D), nursing mothers, children <12 y. **Cautious use in:** elderly patients; thyroid disease; epilepsy; concomitant use with haloperidol and other antipsychotics; parkinsonism; diabetes mellitus; severe infections; urinary retention.

ADVERSE/SIDE EFFECTS CNS: dizziness, *headache, lethargy,* drowsiness, *fatigue,* slurred speech, psychomotor retardation, giddiness, incontinence, restlessness, seizures, confusion, blackout spells, disorientation, *recent memory loss,* stupor, coma, EEG changes. **CV:** arrhythmias, hypotension, vasculitis, peripheral circulatory collapse, ECG changes. **EENT:** impaired vision, transient scotomas, tinnitus. **Endocrine:** diffuse thyroid enlargement, hypothyroidism, *nephrogenic diabetes insipidus,* transient hyperglycemia, glycosuria, hyponatremia. **GI:** *nausea, vomiting, anorexia, abdominal pain, diarrhea, dry mouth,* metallic taste. **Neuromuscular:** *fine hand tremors,* coarse tremors, choreoathetotic movements; fasciculations, clonic movements, incoordination including ataxia, *muscle weakness,* hyperreflexia, encephalopathic syndrome (weakness, lethargy, fever, tremors, confusion, extrapyramidal symptoms). **Skin:** (thought to be toxicity rather than allergy): pruritus, maculopapular rash, hyperkeratosis, chronic folliculitis, transient acneiform papules (face, neck, intertriginous areas), anesthesia of skin, cutaneous ulcers, drying and thinning of hair, allergic vasculitis. **Other:** *reversible leukocytosis* (14,000 to 18,000/mm^3), albuminuria, oliguria, urinary incontinence, polyuria, polydipsia, increased uric acid excretion, edema, weight gain (common) or loss, exacerbation of psoriasis; flu-like symptoms.

DRUG INTERACTIONS Carbamazepine, haloperidol, PHENOTHIAZINES increase risk of neurotoxicity, extrapyramidal effects, and tardive dyskinesias; DIURETICS, NSAIDS, **methyldopa, probenecid,** TETRACYCLINES decrease renal clearance of lithium, increasing pharmacologic and toxic effects; THEOPHYLLINES, **urea, sodium bicarbonate, sodium or potassium citrate** increase renal clearance of lithium, decreasing its pharmacologic effects.

NURSING IMPLICATIONS

Administration

- GI symptoms may be minimized by taking drug with meals.
- Store at 15–30C (59–86F) unless otherwise directed and protect from light and moisture.

Assessment & Drug Effects

- Onset of therapeutic effects usually is preceded by lag of 1–2 wk. Therapeutic response to lithium therapy is evidenced by changed facial affect, improved posture, assumption of self-care, improved ability to concentrate, improved sleep pattern. Keep physician informed of progress.
- Monitor lithium level: (1) Generally dosage regimen is designed to maintain serum lithium levels of 1.0–1.5 mEq/L in acute mania and 0.6–1.6 mEq/L during maintenance treatment. (2) Blood sample for determining serum lithium level is drawn prior to next dose (8–12 h after last dose) when lithium level is fairly stable.
- Signs of lithium intoxication occur when lithium levels are between 1.5 and 2.0 mEq/L: vomiting, diarrhea, lack of coordination, drowsiness, muscular weakness, slurred speech. Withhold one dose, call physician. Drug should not be stopped abruptly.
- When lithium levels are above 2.0 mEq/L, symptoms may include

L

ataxia, blurred vision, giddiness, tinnitus, muscle twitching or coarse tremors, and a large output of dilute urine.

- Weigh patient daily; check ankles, tibiae, and wrists for edema. Report changes in I&O ratio, sudden weight gain, or edema.
- Polydipsia and polyuria, apparently not dose-related, are common early side effects, particularly in the elderly. Symptoms may lessen but then reappear after several months or even years of maintenance.
- The encephalopathic syndrome may be induced when lithium is given concomitantly with haloperidol or with other antipsychotic medication, particularly in the elderly. Promptly report to the physician early signs of extrapyramidal reactions.
- The fine tremor of hand or jaw, polyuria, mild thirst, transient mild nausea, and general discomfort that may occur in early treatment of mania sometimes persist throughout therapy. Usually, however, symptoms subside with temporary reduction of dose. If symptoms persist, drug is withdrawn. Keep physician informed of all presenting signs and symptoms.
- Periodically monitor thyroid function. Be alert to and report symptoms of hypothyroidism (see Appendix G).
- Neonates born of mothers who took lithium during pregnancy may have high serum lithium level manifested by flaccidity, poor reflexes, cardiac dysrhythmia, and chronic twitching.
- Note that Lithane contains tartrazine, which may cause an allergic-type reaction in susceptible patients.
- The elderly require special monitoring to prevent toxicity, which may occur at serum levels ordinarily tolerated by other patients.

Patient & Family Education

- Instruct to be alert to increased output of dilute urine and persistent thirst. Dose reduction may be indicated.
- Teach patient to establish and adhere to a schedule for testing renal function.
- Because dehydration is a possibility, advise to contact physician if diarrhea or fever develops. Avoid practices that may encourage dehydration: hot environment, excessive caffeine beverages (diuresis).
- Urge to drink plenty of liquids (2–3 L/d) during stabilization period and at least $1–1\frac{1}{2}$ L/d during remainder of therapy.
- Normal dietary salt intake can be inadvertently compromised by lack of understanding. Caution patient to avoid self-prescribed low-salt regimen, self-dosing with Rolaids, Soda-mints, or other sodium antacids, high-sodium foods (e.g., prepared meats and diet soda). Also warn against "crash" diets or diet pills that reduce appetite and food, salt, and fluid intake.
- Reduced intake of fluid and sodium can accelerate lithium retention with subsequent toxicity. Conversely, marked increase in sodium intake can increase lithium excretion and reduce drug effect.
- Lithium may impair both physical and mental ability. Caution against any activity demanding alertness (e.g., driving a car) until clinical response to drug has been established.
- Contraceptive measures should be used during lithium therapy but if the patient becomes pregnant she should be informed of the poten-

tial risks to the fetus. If therapy is continued, serum lithium levels must be closely monitored to prevent toxicity. Renal clearance of lithium increases during pregnancy but reverts to lower rate immediately after delivery; dose, therefore, will be reduced to prevent toxicity.

- Warn not to switch brands of lithium carbonate. Because of varying fillers, a different brand may introduce a change in dose requirement.
- Urge to adhere to established dosage regimen, i.e., not to change or omit doses and not to change dose intervals.
- Clinical follow-up and regular checks on serum lithium levels are essential if treatment is to be safe and effective. Emphasize importance to family and patient of keeping all appointments for clinic visits.

L

LODOXAMIDE

(lo-dox'a-mide)

Trade name: Alomide

Classifications: ANTIALLERGIC; MAST CELL STABILIZER

Prototype: Cromolyn sodium

Pregnancy category: B

ACTIONS/PHARMACODYNAMICS Lodoxamide has exhibited mast cell stabilizing properties, which may prevent antigen-induced release of histamine, thereby suppressing an allergic response. It is believed to act by interfering with calcium transport across the mast cell membrane and, thus, preventing antigen-stimulated release of histamine. In addition, it prevents the release of other mast cell inflammatory mediators (i.e., slow-reacting substances of anaphylaxis [SRS-A]), thereby suppressing an allergic response.

USES Treatment of vernal keratoconjunctivitis, vernal conjunctivitis, vernal keratitis.

ROUTE & DOSAGE

Keratoconjunctivitis

Adult: **Ophthalmic** 1–2 drops in affected eye(s) q.i.d. for up to 3 mo.

Child > 2 mo: **Ophthalmic** same as adult.

PHARMACOKINETICS Absorption: no systemic absorption. **Onset:** 72 h. **Elimination:** half-life: 8.5 h.

CONTRAINDICATIONS & PRECAUTIONS Contraindicated in: hypersensitivity to lodoxamide. **Cautious use in:** pregnancy (category B), nursing women. Safety and efficacy in children <2 y of age not established.

ADVERSE/SIDE EFFECTS CNS: headache. **GI:** nausea, stomach upset. **Ocular:** *burning, stinging, local discomfort,* itching, blurred vision, xerophthalmia, hyperemia, tearing or discharge, crystalline deposits, foreign body sensation, eye pain, edema/swelling, corneal abrasion, corneal erosion, corneal ulcer, keratopathy, keratitis, blepharitis, blepharedema, mucus formation, epitheliopathy, hypersensitivity.

NURSING IMPLICATIONS

Administration

- Apply eyedrops to the center of the lower conjunctival sac. Do not touch eyelids with dropper.
- Store at room temperature, 15–27C (59–80F), in a tightly closed container.

Common side effect in *italic,* life-threatening effects underlined: generic names in **bold;** drug class in SMALL CAPS

Assessment & Drug Effects

- Monitor for signs and symptoms of hypersensitivity to the drug (see Appendix G).
- Assess safety, as dizziness and light-headedness are possible adverse effects.

Patient & Family Education

- Instruct patient on appropriate administration technique.
- Inform patient of potential adverse responses to the drug.
- Eyedrops contain benzalkonium chloride, which may damage soft contact lenses.
- Advise patient to contact physician if burning or stinging persists with eye drop instillation.

LOMEFLOXACIN

(lo-me-flox′a-cin)

Trade name: Maxaquin

Classifications: ANTIINFECTIVE; QUINOLONE ANTIBIOTIC

Prototype: Ciprofloxacin

Pregnancy category: C

ACTIONS/PHARMACODYNAMICS An oral fluoroquinolone broad-spectrum bactericidal agent that inhibits DNA-gyrase, an enzyme necessary for bacterial DNA replication and some aspects of its transcription, repair, recombination, and transposition. Lomefloxacin's antibiotic spectrum of activity is similar to that of other quinolones.

USES Urinary tract infections, transurethral surgery prophylaxis. **Unlabeled use:** lower respiratory tract infections.

ROUTE & DOSAGE

Urinary Tract & Lower Respiratory Tract Infections

Adult: **PO** 400 mg q.d. × 10 d.

Transurethral Surgery Prophylaxis

Adult: **PO** 400 mg 2–6 h before surgery.

PHARMACOKINETICS Absorption: readily absorbed from GI tract. **Peak:** 1–2 h. **Distribution:** crosses placenta; distributed into breast milk. **Elimination:** half-life: 6.35–7.77 h; 76% excreted in urine within 48 h.

CONTRAINDICATIONS & PRECAUTIONS Contraindicated in: known hypersensitivity to lomefloxacin or any other quinolone. **Cautious use in:** renal disease; patients with a history of epilepsy, psychosis, or increased intracranial pressure; pregnancy (category C); children and adolescents.

ADVERSE/SIDE EFFECTS CNS: *headache.* **GI:** nausea, abdominal discomfort. **Other:** photosensitivity.

DRUG INTERACTIONS ALUMINUM and MAGNESIUM-CONTAINING ANTACIDS decrease systemic bioavailability of lomefloxacin.

NURSING IMPLICATIONS

Administration

- Avoid administering mineral supplements or vitamins with iron or zinc within 2 h of lomefloxacin.
- Antacids with magnesium, aluminum, or sucralfate should not be given within 4 h before or 2 h after lomefloxacin.
- Hemodialysis patients are usually given an initial 400 mg loading dose followed by a 200 mg/d maintenance dose.

Assessment & Drug Effects

- Culture and sensitivity tests should be done prior to initial dose. Treatment may be implemented pending results.

- Before therapy is instituted, determine history of hypersensitivity reactions to quinolones or other drugs.
- Discontinue lomefloxacin and notify physician at the first sign of a skin rash or other allergic reaction.
- Monitor for seizures, especially in patients with known or suspected CNS disorders. Discontinue lomefloxacin and notify physician immediately if a seizure occurs.
- Assess for signs and symptoms of superinfection (see Appendix G).

Patient & Family Education

- Instruct patient to report loose stools or diarrhea promptly.
- Encourage liberal fluids if not contraindicated.
- Inform patient that dizziness or light-headedness may occur; advise appropriate caution.
- Inform patient of the possibility of phototoxicity and advise patient to avoid excessive sunlight or artificial ultraviolet light.

L

LOMUSTINE

(loe-mus′teen)

Trade names: CeeNU, CCNU

Classifications: ANTINEOPLASTIC; ALKYLATING AGENT

Prototype: Cyclophosphamide

Pregnancy category: D

ACTIONS/PHARMACODYNAMICS Lipid-soluble alkylating nitrosourea with actions like those of carmustine. Inhibits synthesis of both DNA and RNA; has myelosuppressive effect.

USES Palliative therapy in addition to other modalities or with other chemotherapeutic agents in primary and metastatic brain tumors and as secondary therapy in Hodgkin's disease. **Unlabeled uses:** GI, lung, and renal carcinomas, non-Hodgkin's lymphomas, malignant melanoma, and multiple myelomas.

ROUTE & DOSAGE

Palliative Therapy

Adult: **PO** 130 mg/m^2 as single dose, repeated in 6 wk; subsequent doses based on hematologic response (WBC > 4000/mm^3, platelets > 100,000/mm^3).
Child: **PO** 75–150 mg/m^2 q6wk.

PHARMACOKINETICS Absorption: readily absorbed from GI tract. **Peak:** 1–6 h. **Distribution:** readily crosses blood–brain barrier; crosses placenta; distributed into breast milk. **Metabolism:** metabolized in liver to several active metabolites. **Elimination:** half-life: 16–48 h; excreted in urine.

CONTRAINDICATIONS & PRECAUTIONS Contraindicated in: immunization with live virus vaccines, viral infections. Safe use during pregnancy (category D) and in nursing mothers not established. Reported to be carcinogenic in laboratory animals. **Cautious use in:** patients with decreased circulating platelets, leukocytes, or erythrocytes; renal or hepatic function impairment; infection; previous cytotoxic or radiation therapy.

ADVERSE/SIDE EFFECTS CNS: lethargy, ataxia, disorientation. **GI:** anorexia, *nausea, vomiting,* stomatitis. **Hematologic:** delayed (cumulative) myelosuppression: (thrombocytopenia, leukopenia); anemia. **Other:** transient elevations of liver function tests, alopecia; nephrotoxicity, skin rash, itching; pulmonary toxicity (rare).

NURSING IMPLICATIONS

Administration

- Take on an empty stomach to reduce possibility of nausea. An antiemetic given before lomustine may prevent nausea.
- Store capsules away from excessive heat (over 40C).

Assessment & Drug Effects

- A repeat course is not given until platelets have returned to above 100,000/mm^3 and leukocytes to above 4000/mm^3.
- Blood counts should be monitored weekly for at least 6 wk after last dose. Liver and kidney function tests should be performed periodically.
- Avoid invasive procedures during nadir of platelets.
- Thrombocytopenia occurs about 4 wk and leukopenia about 6 wk after a dose, persisting 1–2 wk.
- Inspect oral cavity daily for symptoms of superinfections (see Appendix G) and for signs of stomatitis or xerostomia.

Patient & Family Education

- Nausea and vomiting may occur 3–5 h after drug administration, usually lasting less than 24 h.
- Anorexia may persist for 2 or 3 d after a dose.
- Advise patient to report signs of sore throat, cough, fever. Report unexplained bleeding or easy bruising.
- Contraceptive measures are recommended during therapy.
- The possibility of hair loss should be discussed.
- Pharmacist will prepare prescribed dose by combining various capsule strengths. Explain to patient that a given dose may include capsules of different colors.

LOPERAMIDE

(loe-per′a-mide)

Trade names: Imodium, Imodium AD

Classifications: GI AGENT; ANTIDIARRHEAL

Prototype: Diphenoxylate hydrochloride with atropine sulfate

Pregnancy category: B

ACTIONS/PHARMACODYNAMICS

Synthetic piperidine derivative chemically related to diphenoxylate and to meperidine. Reportedly as effective an antidiarrheal as diphenoxylate with longer duration of action. Inhibits GI peristaltic activity by direct action on circular and longitudinal intestinal muscles. Prolongs transit time of intestinal contents, increases consistency of stools, and reduces fluid and electrolyte loss.

USES Acute nonspecific diarrhea, chronic diarrhea associated with inflammatory bowel disease, and to reduce fecal volume from ileostomies.

ROUTE & DOSAGE

Acute Diarrhea

Adult: **PO** 4 mg followed by 2 mg after each unformed stool (max 16 mg/d).
Child: **PO** *2–6 y,* 1 mg t.i.d.; *6–8 y,* 2 mg b.i.d.; *8–12 y,* 2 mg t.i.d.

Chronic Diarrhea

Adult: **PO** 4 mg followed by 2 mg after each unformed stool until diarrhea is controlled (max 16 mg/d).
Child: **PO** 0.1 mg/kg after each unformed stool (usually 1 mg).

PHARMACOKINETICS Absorption: poorly absorbed from GI tract. **Onset:** 30–60 min. **Peak:** 2.5 h solution; 4–5 h capsules. **Duration:** 4–5 h. **Metabolism:** metabolized in liver. **Elimination:** half-life: 11 h; primarily excreted in feces, <2% excreted in urine.

CONTRAINDICATIONS & PRECAUTIONS Contraindicated in: conditions in which constipation should be avoided, severe colitis, acute diarrhea caused by broad-spectrum antibiotics (pseudomembranous colitis) or associated with microorganisms that penetrate intestinal mucosa, e.g., toxigenic *Escherichia coli, Salmonella,* or *Shigella*. Safe use during pregnancy (category B), in nursing mothers, and in children <2 y not established. **Cautious use in:** dehydration; diarrhea caused by invasive bacteria; impaired hepatic function; prostatic hypertrophy; history of narcotic dependence.

L

ADVERSE/SIDE EFFECTS CNS: drowsiness, fatigue, dizziness, CNS depression (overdosage). **GI:** abdominal discomfort or pain, abdominal distention, bloating, constipation, nausea, vomiting, anorexia, dry mouth. **Hypersensitivity:** skin rash. **Other:** fever, toxic megacolon (patients with ulcerative colitis).

NURSING IMPLICATIONS

Administration

- Note that with acute diarrhea, dosing for a child is not scheduled prn.
- Store at 15–30C (59–86F) unless otherwise specified.

Assessment & Drug Effects

- In acute diarrhea, loperamide should be discontinued if there is no improvement after 48 h of therapy.
- Patients with chronic diarrhea usually respond to loperamide therapy within 10 d. If improvement does not occur within this time, it is unlikely that symptoms will be controlled by further administration.
- Monitor fluid and electrolyte balance.
- If the patient with ulcerative colitis develops abdominal distention or other GI symptoms, notify physician promptly (possible signs of potentially fatal toxic megacolon).

Patient & Family Education

- Advise to notify physician if diarrhea does not stop in a few days or if abdominal pain, distension, or fever develops.
- Instruct to record number and consistency of stools.
- Caution to avoid driving and other potentially hazardous activities until drug response is known.
- Inform that alcohol and other CNS depressants may enhance drowsiness and therefore should not be taken concomitantly unless otherwise advised by physician.
- Provide guidance on measures to relieve dry mouth.

LORACARBEF

(lor-a-car′bef)

Trade name: Lorabid

Classifications: ANTIINFECTIVE; OTHER BETA-LACTAM ANTIBIOTIC

Prototype: Imipenem

Pregnancy category: B

ACTIONS/PHARMACODYNAMICS Second-generation cephalosporin antibiotic with drug structure characterized by a beta-lactam ring (like the penicillin structure); generally resistant to hydrolysis by beta-lactamases. Effective against gram-positive and gram-negative bacteria including staphylococci, beta-hemolytic streptococci, *Streptococcus pneumoniae, Hemophilus influenzae, Moraxella catarrhalis.*

USES Upper and lower respiratory tract infections, skin and skin structure infections, urinary tract infections.

ROUTE & DOSAGE

Upper & Lower Respiratory Tract Infections

Adult: **PO** 200–400 mg q12h taken 1 h a.c. or 2 h p.c.
Child: **PO** 15–30 mg/kg/d divided q12h taken 1 h a.c. or 2 h p.c.

Skin & Skin Structure Infections

Adult: **PO** 200 mg q12h taken 1 h a.c. or 2 h p.c.
Child: **PO** 15 mg/kg/d divided q12h taken 1 h a.c. or 2 h p.c.

Urinary Tract Infections

Adult: **PO** 200 mg q24h or 400 mg q12h taken 1 h a.c. or 2 h p.c.

Otitis Media

Child: **PO** 30 mg/kg/d divided q12h taken 1 h a.c. or 2 h p.c.

PHARMACOKINETICS/DYNAMICS **Absorption:** readily absorbed from GI tract. **Peak:** 45–60 min. **Distribution:** distributes into middle ear fluid. **Elimination:** half-life: 0.78–0.85 h; excreted in urine.

CONTRAINDICATIONS & PRECAUTIONS **Contraindicated in:** hypersensitivity to cephalosporins and related antibiotics. **Cautious use in:** renal impairment, seizures, pregnancy (category B), and nursing mothers.

ADVERSE/SIDE EFFECTS **CNS:** headache. **GI:** nausea, vomiting, diarrhea, diaper rash, abdominal pain. **Other:** rash, candidiasis.

NURSING IMPLICATIONS

Administration

- Reconstitute suspension by adding 30 or 60 ml of water to the 50- or 100-ml bottles, respectively, of dry mixture. Add the water in 2 portions and shake bottle after each portion.
- Administer at least 1 h a.c. or 2 h p.c.
- Administer half of the normal dose if creatinine clearance lies between 10 and 49 ml/min.
- Store suspension in a tightly closed container at 15–30C (59–86F). Discard after 14 d.

Assessment & Drug Effects

- A careful history should be elicited to determine previous hypersensitivity reaction to beta-lactam antibiotics (penicillins and cephalosporins) or to other allergens.
- When allergic reaction occurs (e.g., hives, wheezing, rash, pruritus), discontinue the drug and notify the physician immediately.
- Inspect patient's mouth on a regular basis to detect superinfection. (See Appendix G.)
- If severe diarrhea accompanied by abdominal pain and fever occurs, pseudomembranous enterocolitis (see Appendix G) should be ruled out. Call physician immediately.
- Monitor renal function throughout the course of therapy.

Patient & Family Education

- Instruct patient to immediately report a rash or any other allergic reaction.
- Instruct patient to report loose stools or diarrhea promptly.

LORATADINE

(lor′-a-ti-deen)

Trade name: Claritin

Classifications: ANTIHISTAMINE; H_1-RECEPTOR ANTAGONIST

Prototype: Diphenhydramine
Pregnancy category: B

ACTIONS/PHARMACODYNAMICS
Loratadine is a long-acting antihistamine with selective peripheral H_1-receptor sites, thus blocking histamine release. (Histamine promotes capillary permeability and edema formation and constriction of respiratory, GI, and vascular smooth muscle.)

USES Relief of symptoms of seasonal allergic rhinitis; idiopathic chronic urticaria.

ROUTE & DOSAGE

Allergic Rhinitis
Adult: **PO** 10 mg once daily on an empty stomach. Patients with liver disease should start with 10 mg every other day.
Child ≥3 y: **PO** *<30 kg:* 5 mg q.d., *>30 kg:* 10 mg q.d.

PHARMACOKINETICS **Absorption:** readily absorbed from GI tract. **Onset:** 1–3 h. **Peak:** 8–12 h; reaches steady state levels in 3–5 d. **Duration:** 24 h. **Distribution:** distributed into breast milk. **Metabolism:** metabolized to active metabolite, descarboethoxyloratidine, in the liver. **Elimination:** half-life: 12–15 h; excreted in urine and feces.

CONTRAINDICATIONS & PRECAUTIONS **Contraindicated in:** hypersensitivity to loratadine. **Cautious use in:** liver impairment, pregnancy (category B), and nursing mothers. Safety and effectiveness in children below the age of 12 years have not been established.

ADVERSE/SIDE EFFECTS **CNS:** dizziness, dry mouth, fatigue, headache, somnolence, altered salivation and lacrimation, thirst, flushing, anxiety, depression, impaired concentration. **CV:** hypotension, hypertension, palpitations, syncope, tachycardia. **GI:** nausea, vomiting, flatulence, abdominal distress, constipation, diarrhea, weight gain, dyspepsia. **Other:** arthralgia, myalgia, blurred vision, earache, eye pain, tinnitus, rash, pruritus, photosensitivity.

DRUG INTERACTIONS None reported to date.

NURSING IMPLICATIONS

Administration
- Give loratidine on an empty stomach, 1 h before or 2 h after a meal.
- Store in a tightly closed container at 15–30C (59–86F).

Assessment & Drug Effects
- A variety of adverse effects, although not common, are possible. Some are an indication to discontinue the drug. Carefully assess for and report distressing or dangerous signs and symptoms that occur after initiation of the drug.
- Monitor cardiovascular status and report significant changes in blood pressure and palpitations or tachycardia.
- When given concurrently with drugs known to inhibit hepatic metabolism, monitor for possible increase in adverse reactions.

Patient & Family Education
- Advise patients to take drug on empty stomach and not to eat any food for at least 1 h after taking drug.
- Advise elderly patients and those with hepatic or renal impairment that drug may cause significant drowsiness.
- Inform patients that concurrent use of alcohol and other CNS depressants may have an additive effect.

LORAZEPAM

(lor-a'ze-pam)

Trade name: Ativan

Prototype for classifications: CNS AGENT; ANXIOLYTIC; SEDATIVE-HYPNOTIC; BENZODIAZEPINE

Pregnancy category: D

Controlled substance: Schedule IV

ACTIONS/PHARMACODYNAMICS Most potent of the available benzodiazepines. Effects (anxiolytic, sedative, hypnotic, and skeletal muscle relaxant) are mediated by the inhibitory neurotransmitter GABA. Action sites: thalamic, hypothalamic, and limbic levels of CNS. Limitations and interactions similar to those of chlordiazepoxide.

USES Management of anxiety disorders and for short-term relief of symptoms of anxiety. Also used for preanesthetic medication to produce sedation and to reduce anxiety and recall of events related to day of surgery; for management of status epilepticus. **Unlabeled uses:** chemotherapy-induced nausea and vomiting.

ROUTE & DOSAGE

Antianxiety

Adult: **PO** 2–6 mg/d in divided doses (max 10 mg/d).
Geriatric: **PO** 0.5–1 mg/d (max 2 mg/d).
Child: **PO/IV** 0.05 mg/kg q4–8h (max 2 mg/dose).

Insomnia

Adult: **PO** 2–4 mg at bedtime.
Geratric: **PO** 0.5–1 mg h.s.

Premedication

Adult: **IM** 2–4 mg (0.05 mg/kg) at least 2 h before surgery. **IV** 0.044 mg/kg up to 2 mg 15–20 min before surgery.
Child: **PO/IV/IM** 0.05 mg/kg (range 0.02–0.09 mg/kg).

Status Epilepticus

Adult: **IV** 4 mg injected slowly at 2 mg/min. If inadequate response after 10 min, may repeat dose once.
Child: **IV** 0.1 mg/kg slow IV over 2–5 min (max 4 mg/dose); may repeat with 0.05 mg in 10–15 min if needed.
Neonate: **IV** 0.05 mg/kg over 2–5 min; may repeat in 10–15 min.

PHARMACOKINETICS Absorption: readily absorbed from GI tract. **Onset:** 1–5 min IV; 15–30 min IM. **Peak:** 60–90 min IM; 2 h PO. **Duration:** 12–24 h. **Distribution:** crosses placenta; distributed into breast milk. **Metabolism:** not metabolized in liver. **Elimination:** half-life: 10–20 h; excreted in urine.

CONTRAINDICATIONS & PRECAUTIONS Contraindicated in: known sensitivity to benzodiazepines; acute narrow-angle glaucoma; primary depressive disorders or psychosis; children <12 y (PO preparation); coma, shock, acute alcohol intoxication; pregnancy (category D), and nursing mothers. **Cautious use in:** renal or hepatic impairment; organic brain syndrome; myasthenia gravis; narrow-angle glaucoma; suicidal tendency; GI disorders; elderly and debilitated patients; limited pulmonary reserve.

ADVERSE/SIDE EFFECTS Usually disappear with continued medication or with reduced dosage. **CNS:** anterograde amnesia, *drowsiness, sedation,* dizziness, weakness, unsteadiness, disorientation, depression, sleep disturbance, restlessness, confusion, hallucinations. **CV:** hypertension or hypotension. **Eye:** blurred vision, diplopia. **Ear:** depressed hearing. **GI:** nausea, vomiting, abdominal discomfort, anorexia.

DRUG INTERACTIONS Alcohol, CNS DEPRESSANTS, ANTICONVULSANTS potentiate CNS depression; **cimetidine** increases lorazepam plasma levels, increases toxicity; lorazepam may decrease antiparkinsonism effects of **levodopa;** may increase **phenytoin** levels; smoking decreases sedative and antianxiety effects.

L

INCOMPATIBILITY Y-site: ondansetron.

NURSING IMPLICATIONS

Administration

- When higher oral dosage is required, the evening dose should be increased before the daytime doses.
- IM lorazepam is injected undiluted, deep into a large muscle mass.
- IV preparation: Prepare lorazepam immediately before use. Dilute with an equal volume of sterile water, D5W, or NS. Do not use a discolored solution or one that has a precipitate.
- IV administration: Diluted drug is injected directly into vein or into IV infusion tubing at rate not to exceed 2 mg/min and with repeated aspiration to confirm IV entry.
- IV administration to neonates, infants, children: Verify correct IV concentration and rate of infusion with physician.
- Extreme precautions should be taken to prevent intraarterial injection and perivascular extravasation.
- Patients >50 y may have more profound and prolonged sedation with IV lorazepam. Usually, an initial dose of 2 mg should not be exceeded.
- Keep parenteral preparation in refrigerator; do not freeze. Store tablets at 15–30C (59–86F) unless manufacturer specifies otherwise.

Assessment & Drug Effects

- Equipment for maintaining patent airway should be immediately available before IV administration.
- IM or IV lorazepam injection of 2–4 mg is usually followed by a depth of drowsiness or sleepiness that permits patient to respond to simple instructions whether patient appears to be asleep or awake.
- Supervise ambulation of elderly patient for at least 8 h after lorazepam injection to prevent falling and injury.
- Periodic blood counts and liver function tests are recommended for the patient on long-term therapy.
- Closely supervise patient who exhibits depression with anxiety; the possibility of suicide exists, particularly when there is apparent improvement in mood.

Patient & Family Education

- Most patients will have difficulty recalling perioperative events. This *retrograde amnesia* is optimum within 2 h after IM administration and 15–20 min after IV injection. Full recall and recognition may not return for about 8 h. Inform patient of this possibility.
- If a narcotic analgesic, another tranquilizer, or sedative is given

with injectable lorazepam, lack of recall may extend for as long as 48 h.

- Advise to refrain from any hazardous activity, for a least 24–48 h after receiving IM injection of lorazepam.
- Advise to avoid large-volume intake of coffee. Anxiolytic effects of lorazepam can significantly be altered by caffeine.
- Alcoholic beverages should not be consumed for at least 24–48 h after an injection and should be avoided when patient is on an oral regimen.
- If daytime psychomotor function is impaired, see physician; change in regimen or drug may be needed.
- Regimen should be terminated gradually over a period of several days. Warn patient on long-term therapy not to stop the drug abruptly because withdrawal may be induced: feelings of panic, tonic–clonic seizures, tremors, abdominal and muscle cramps, sweating, vomiting.
- Advise not to self-medicate with OTC drugs unless the physician approves.
- Tell women who wish to become pregnant to discuss drug continuation with physician.

LOSARTAN POTASSIUM

(lo-sar′tan)

Trade name: Cozaar

Prototype for classifications: CARDIOVASCULAR AGENT; ANGIOTENSIN II RECEPTOR ANTAGONIST; ANTIHYPERTENSIVE

Pregnancy category: C (first trimester); D (second and third trimesters)

ACTIONS/PHARMACODYNAMICS Losartan is an angiotensin II receptor (type AT_1) antagonist. Angiotensin II is a potent vasoconstrictor and primary vasoactive hormone of the renin–angiotensin–aldosterone system. Losartan selectively blocks the binding of angiotensin II to the AT_1 receptors found in many tissues (e.g., vascular smooth muscle, adrenal glands). This results in blocking the vasoconstricting and aldosterone-secreting effects of angiotensin II, thus resulting in an antihypertensive effect.

USE Hypertension.

ROUTE & DOSAGE

Hypertension

Adult: **PO** 25–50 mg in 1–2 divided doses (max 100 mg/d); start with 25 mg/d if volume depleted (i.e., on diuretics)

PHARMACOKINETICS **Absorption:** rapidly absorbed from GI tract; approx 25–33% reaches systemic circulation. **Peak effect:** 6 h. **Duration:** 24 h. **Distribution:** highly bound to plasma proteins; does not appear to cross blood–brain barrier. **Metabolism:** extensively metabolized in liver by cytochrome P450 enzymes to an active metabolite. **Elimination:** half-life: losartan 1.5–2 h; metabolite 6–9 h; 35% excreted in urine, 60% in feces.

CONTRAINDICATIONS & PRECAUTIONS **Contraindicated in:** hypersensitivity to losartan, pregnancy [category C (first trimester), category D (second and third trimesters)], lactation. **Cautious use in:** patients on diuretics, renal impairment, hepatic impairment.

ADVERSE/SIDE EFFECTS **CNS:** dizziness, insomnia, headache. **GI:** diarrhea, dyspepsia. **Musculoskeletal:** muscle cramps, myalgia, back or leg pain.

Respiratory: nasal congestion, cough, upper respiratory infection, sinusitis.

DRUG INTERACTION **Phenobarbital** decreases serum levels of losartan and its metabolite.

NURSING IMPLICATIONS

Administration

- The starting dose is reduced 50% in patients with possible volume depletion or a history of hepatic impairment.
- Store at 15–30C (59–86F).

Assessment & Drug Effects

- Monitor blood pressure at drug trough (prior to a scheduled dose).
- Monitor drug effectiveness, especially in African-Americans when losartan is used as monotherapy.
- Inadequate response may be improved by splitting the daily dose into twice-daily dose.
- Periodically monitor CBC, electrolytes, and liver and renal function tests with long-term therapy.

Patient & Family Education

- Instruct to report symptoms of hypotension.
- Advise women to report pregnancies immediately to the physician.

LOTEPREDNOL ETABONATE

(lo-te′pred-nol e-ta-bo′nate)

Trade names: Alrex, Lotemax

Classifications: SKIN AND MUCOUS MEMBRANE AGENT; ANTIINFLAMMATORY; SYNTHETIC HORMONE ADRENAL CORTICOSTEROID

Prototype: Hydrocortisone

Pregnancy category: C

See Appendix A.

LOVASTATIN

(loe-vah-stat′in)

Trade names: Mevacor, Mevinolin

Prototype for classifications: CARDIOVASCULAR AGENT; ANTILIPEMIC; HMG-COA REDUCTASE INHIBITOR (STATIN)

Pregnancy category: X

ACTIONS/PHARMACODYNAMICS Reduces plasma cholesterol levels by interfering with body's ability to produce its own cholesterol. This cholesterol-lowering effect triggers induction of LDL receptors, which promote removal of LDL and VLDL remnants (precursors of LDL) from plasma. Lovastatin therapy also results in an increase in plasma HDL concentrations. (HDLs collect excess cholesterol from body cells and transport it to liver for excretion.)

USES Adjunct to diet for treatment of primary moderate hypercholesterolemia (types IIa and IIb) when diet and other nonpharmacologic measures have failed to reduce elevated total LDL cholesterol levels. Lovastatin is less effective in treatment of homozygous familial hypercholesterolemia than primary hypercholesterolemia, possibly because in these persons LDL receptors are not functional.

ROUTE & DOSAGE

Hypercholesterolemia

Adult: **PO** 20–40 mg 1–2 times/d.

PHARMACOKINETICS **Absorption:** approximately 30% absorbed from GI tract; extensive first pass metabolism. **Onset:** 2 wk. **Peak:** 4–6 wk. **Distribution:** crosses blood–brain barrier and placenta; distributed into breast milk. **Metabolism:** metabolized in liver to active metabolites. **Elimination:** 83% excreted in feces; 10% excreted in urine.

CONTRAINDICATIONS & PRECAUTIONS Contraindicated in: active liver disease, unexplained elevations of serum transaminases. Safe use in pregnancy (category X) or by nursing mothers and children not established. **Cautious use in:** patient who consumes substantial quantities of alcohol; history of liver disease; patient with risk factor predisposing to development of renal failure secondary to rhabdomyolysis.

ADVERSE/SIDE EFFECTS Drug is generally well tolerated. **CNS:** dizziness, mild transient headache, insomnia, fatigue. **Eye:** blurred vision. **GI:** dyspepsia, dysgeusia, heartburn, nausea, constipation, diarrhea, flatus, abdominal pain and cramps. **Hematologic:** increases in serum transaminases, elevated creatine phosphokinase (CPK). **Skin:** rash, pruritus.

DRUG INTERACTIONS Cyclosporine, erythromycin, gemfibrozil increase risk of myopathy and rhabdomyolysis.

NURSING IMPLICATIONS

Administration

- Administer lovastatin with meals.
- Store tablets at 5–30C (41–86F) in light-resistant, tightly closed container.

Assessment & Drug Effects

- Blood cholesterol levels and lipid profile are monitored periodically.
- Liver function tests are performed q4–6wk during first 15 mo of therapy.
- Drug-induced increases in serum transaminases, usually not associated with jaundice or other clinical signs or symptoms, return to normal when drug is discontinued. If these values rise and remain at 3 times upper level of normal, drug will be discontinued and liver biopsy considered.

Patient & Family Education

- Caution not to interrupt, increase, decrease, or omit dosage without advice of physician.
- Patient should promptly report muscle tenderness or pain, especially if accompanied by fever or malaise. If CPK is elevated or if myositis is diagnosed, drug will be discontinued.
- Alcohol should be avoided or at least reduced.
- Be certain that patients understand that lovastatin is not a substitute for, but an addition to, diet therapy.

L

LOXAPINE HYDROCHLORIDE

(lox'a-peen)

Trade names: Loxitane C, Loxitane IM

LOXAPINE SUCCINATE

Trade names: Loxapac♣, Loxitane

Classifications: CNS AGENT; PSYCHOTHERAPEUTIC; ANTIPSYCHOTIC

Prototype: Chlorpromazine

Pregnancy category: C

ACTIONS/PHARMACODYNAMICS Dibenzoxazepine antipsychotic, chemically distinct from other antipsychotics. Exact mode of action not established. Stabilizes emotional component of schizophrenia by acting on subcortical level of CNS. Sedative action is less than that produced by chlorpromazine, but anticholinergic effects are comparable and extrapyramidal effects may be more intense. Also has antiemetic activity; lowers seizure threshold in patients with history of convulsive disorders.

USE Manifestations of psychotic disorders. **Unlabeled use:** anxiety associated with mental depression.

ROUTE & DOSAGE

Psychosis

Adult: **PO** Start with 10 mg b.i.d. and rapidly increase to maintenance levels of 60–100 mg/d in 2–4 divided doses (max 250 mg/d); **IM** 12.5–50 mg q4–6h.

Dementia Behavior

Geriatric: **PO** 5–10 mg 1–2 times/d, may increase q4–7d to max of 125 mg/d.

L

PHARMACOKINETICS **Absorption:** readily absorbed from GI tract. **Onset:** 20–30 min. **Peak:** 1.5–3 h. **Duration:** 12 h. **Distribution:** widely distributed; crosses placenta; distributed into breast milk. **Metabolism:** metabolized in liver. **Elimination:** half-life: 19 h; 50% excreted in urine, 50% excreted in feces.

CONTRAINDICATIONS & PRECAUTIONS **Contraindicated in:** severe drug-induced CNS depression; comatose states, children <16 y. Safe use during pregnancy (category C) and in nursing mothers not established. **Cautious use in:** glaucoma, prostatic hypertrophy, urinary retention, history of convulsive disorders, cardiovascular disease.

ADVERSE SIDE EFFECTS **CNS:** *drowsiness,* sedation, dizziness, syncope, EEG changes, paresthesias, staggering gait, muscle weakness, *extrapyramidal effects,* akathisia, <u>tardive dyskinesia,</u> <u>neuroleptic malignant syndrome.</u> **CV:** *orthostatic hypotension,* hypertension, tachycardia. **ENT:** nasal congestion, tinnitus. **Eye:** blurred vision, ptosis. **GI:** constipation, dry mouth. **Skin:** dermatitis, facial edema, pruritus, photosensitivity. **Other:** urinary retention, polydipsia, weight gain or loss, hyperpyrexia, transient leukopenia, menstrual irregularities.

DRUG INTERACTIONS **Alcohol** and other CNS DEPRESSANTS potentiate CNS depression; will inhibit vasopressor effects of **epinephrine.**

NURSING IMPLICATIONS

Administration

- Loxapine should be taken with food, milk, or water to reduce possibility of stomach irritation.
- Dilute oral concentrate in about 2–3 oz (60–90 ml) water or orange or grapefruit juice shortly before administration (do not store diluted solution). Measured with calibrated dropper dispensed with drug.
- When therapy is to be terminated, dosage should be gradually reduced over period of several days.
- Store at 15–30C (59–86F); protect from light and freezing. Intensification of straw color to light amber is acceptable. If solution is noticeably discolored, however, discard.

Assessment & Drug Effects

- Determine BP pattern before and during therapy: both hypotension and hypertension have been reported as adverse reactions.
- Observe carefully for extrapyramidal effects such as acute dystonia (see Appendix G) during early therapy with loxapine. Most symptoms disappear with dose adjustment or with antiparkinsonism drug therapy.
- If a patient is on long-term treatment with this drug, be alert to first signs of impending tardive dyskinesia: fine vermicular movements of the tongue. Discontinue therapy and report promptly.
- Monitor I&O and bowel elimination patterns and check for blad-

der distention. The depressed patient often fails to report urinary retention or constipation.

- Risk of seizures is increased in those with history of convulsive disorders.

Patient & Family Education

- Caution not to change the dosage regimen in any way unless the physician approves.
- Warn to avoid self-dosing with OTC drugs unless prescribed by the physician.
- Drowsiness usually decreases with continued therapy. If it persists and interferes with ADL, consult physician. A change in time of administration or dose may help to prevent interference with normal physical activities.
- Instruct to avoid hazardous activity until drug response is known.
- Provide guidance on measures to prevent dry mouth. If dry mouth occurs, avoid overuse of commercial mouth rinses, since many contain alcohol, which enhances drying and irritation.
- Report to physician if blurred or colored vision occurs.
- Advise to withhold drug dose if the following appear: light-colored stools, bruising, unexplained bleeding, prolonged constipation, tremor, restlessness and excitement, sore throat and fever, rash.
- Caution to stay out of bright sun. Exposed skin area should be covered with sunscreen lotion.

LYMPHOCYTE IMMUNE GLOBULIN

Trade names: Antithymocyte Globulin, ATG, Atgam

Classifications: IMMUNOSUPPRESSANT; SERUM

Prototype: Cyclosporine

Pregnancy category: C

ACTIONS/PHARMACODYNAMICS

Lymphocyte immune globulin is an immunoglobulin (IgG) and lymphocyte-selective immunosuppressant derived from serum of healthy horses that have been immunized with human thymus lymphocytes. Action mechanism is not clear. Alters the formation of T-lymphocytes (killer cells) and reduces their number. Has little effect on B-cells and is not associated with severe lymphopenia. Increases susceptibility of patient to viral infections: it may reactivate or support infection with cytomegalovirus, herpes simplex virus (especially labial infections), or with Epstein-Barr virus (EBV). As with other immunosuppressant agents, carcinogenicity of this drug may be expressed.

USES Primarily to prevent or delay onset or to reverse acute renal allograft rejection. **Unlabeled uses:** moderate and severe aplastic anemia in patients unsuitable for bone marrow transplantation, T-cell malignancy, acute and chronic graft-vs-host disease, and to prevent rejection of skin allografts.

ROUTE & DOSAGE

Renal Allotransplantation

Adult: **IV** 10–30 mg/kg/d by slow IV infusion.
Child: **IV** 5–25 mg/kg/d by slow IV infusion.

Prevention of Allograft Rejection

Adult: **IV** 15 mg/kg/d for 14 d followed by 15 mg/kg q.o.d. for 14 d.

Treatment of Allograft Rejection

Adult: **IV** 10–15 mg/kg/d for 14 d followed by 15 mg/kg q.o.d. for 14 d if needed.

Aplastic Anemia
Adult: **IV** 15 mg/kg/d for 14 d followed by 15 mg/kg q.o.d. for 14 d *or* 15 mg/kg/d for 10 d.
Child: **IV** 10–20 mg/kg/d × 8–14 d, then 10–30 mg/kg q.o.d. × 7 more doses.

PHARMACOKINETICS Distribution: poorly distributed into lymphoid tissues (spleen, lymph nodes); probably crosses placenta and into breast milk. **Elimination:** half-life: approximately 6 d; about 1% of dose is excreted in urine.

CONTRAINDICATIONS & PRECAUTIONS Contraindicated in: hypersensitivity to thimerosal (preservative) or to other equine gamma globulin preparations; history of previous systemic reaction to ATG, hemorrhagic diatheses; use in renal transplant patient not receiving a concomitant immunosuppressant. Safe use during pregnancy (category C) or by nursing mothers not established. **Cautious use in:** children (experience limited).

ADVERSE/SIDE EFFECTS CNS: headache, paresthesia, seizures. **CV:** peripheral thrombophlebitis, hypotension. **GI:** nausea, vomiting, diarrhea, stomatitis, hiccups, epigastric pain, abdominal distension. **Hematologic:** *leukopenia, thrombocytopenia.* **Musculoskeletal:** arthralgia, myalgias, chest or back pain. **Respiratory:** dyspnea, <u>laryngospasm, pulmonary edema</u>. **Skin:** *rash, pruritus,* urticaria, wheal and flare. **Other:** *chills, fever,* night sweats, pain at infusion site, hyperglycemia, hypertension, systemic infection, wound dehiscence; <u>anaphylaxis</u>, *serum sickness,* herpes simplex virus reactivation.

DRUG INTERACTIONS Azathioprine, CORTICOSTEROIDS, other IMMUNOSUPPRESSANTS increase degree of immunosuppression.

NURSING IMPLICATIONS

Administration

- Lymphocyte immune globulin (ATG) should be administered only by persons experienced with immunosuppressant therapy and management of renal transplant patients.
- Before first dose, it is usual to do an intradermal skin test to rule out allergy to the drug. Inject 0.1 ml of a 1:1000 dilution (5 µg equine IgG in normal saline) and a saline control. If local reaction occurs (wheal or erythema more than 10 mm) or if there is pseudopod formation, itching, or local swelling, use caution during infusion. If systemic reaction develops (generalized rash, tachycardia, dyspnea, hypotension, anaphylaxis), discontinue infusion.
- IV preparation (ATG is available as concentrate, 50 mg/ml in 5 ml ampul): Dilute required dose of ATG concentrate with 0.45% or 0.9% NaCl injection; final concentration preferably not to exceed 1 mg equine IgG/ml. Dextrose injection or highly acidic solutions not recommended as diluents. Invert IV solution container into which ATG concentrate is added to prevent its contact with air inside container.
- IV administration to infants, children: Verify correct IV concentration and rate of infusion with physician.
- Administration of ATG into high-flow veins decreases potential for phlebitis and thrombosis.
- Visually inspect concentrate and diluted solution for particulate matter (may develop during storage) and discoloration; discard if present. Inline filters (0.2–5 µm) are generally used. Infusion

should be timed to take at least 4 h (usually 4–8 h).
- Total storage time (including storage time and actual infusion time) to keep diluted solutions: no more than 12 h. Refrigerate ampules and diluted solutions (if prepared before time of infusion) at 2–8C (35–46F). Do not freeze.

Assessment & Drug Effects
- Discontinue infusion and initiate appropriate therapy promptly with onset of anaphylactic response (respiratory distress; pain in chest, flank, back; hypotension, anxiety).
- Predictive value of skin test is not proven. Observe patient carefully; allergic reaction can occur even when test is negative.
- Closely monitor BP, vital signs, and patient's complaints during entire administration period. Prompt treatment is indicated for observed and reported symptoms of anaphylaxis (incidence: 1%), serum sickness, or allergic response. Always have available at bedside equipment for assisted respiration, epinephrine, antihistamines, corticosteroid, vasopressor.
- Watch closely for signs and symptoms of serum sickness: fever, malaise, arthralgia, nausea, vomiting, lymphadenopathy and morbilliform eruptions on trunk and extremities. Rash begins as asymptomatic pale pink macules in periumbilical region, axilla, and groin, then rapidly becomes generalized, erythematous, and confluent. Bands of progressive erythema along the sides of hands, fingers, feet, toes, and at margins of palm or plantar skin are characteristic.
- In ATG-induced serum sickness, when platelet count is low, petechiae and purpura rapidly replace rash as distributed over the body. Petechial areas are especially noticeable on legs but also on palms and soles.
- Serum sickness may occur during drug administration or when treatment is stopped but usually occurs 6–18 d after initiation of therapy.
- Because patient is usually receiving concomitant corticosteroids and antimetabolites, monitor carefully for signs of thrombocytopenia, concurrent infection, leukopenia.
- Monitor patient's temperature and attend to complaints of sore throat or rhinorrhea. Physician may stop ATG treatment if these symptoms occur.

Patient & Family Education
- Instruct to immediately report pain in chest, flank, or back; chills; pruritus; night sweats; sore throat.

LYPRESSIN
(lye-pres′sin)
Trade name: Diapid
Classifications: SYNTHETIC HORMONE; PITUITARY (ANTIDIURETIC)
Prototype: Vasopressin
Pregnancy category: B

ACTIONS/PHARMACODYNAMICS
Lysine vasopressin with pharmacologic actions similar to those of vasopressin. Possesses antidiuretic activity, with little oxytocic and minimal cardiovascular pressor (vasopressor) activity in therapeutic doses. Promotes reabsorption of water in kidneys (antidiuretic hormone effect) by increasing permeability to water in renal distal tubule. As a result, urine increases in osmo-

lality with concurrent reduction in water (urine) output.

USES To control or prevent complications of central diabetes insipidus due to deficiency of endogenous posterior pituitary antidiuretic hormone. Particularly useful in patients who are nonresponsive to other forms of therapy and who experience allergic or other undesirable effects from vasopressin of animal origin.

ROUTE & DOSAGE

Diabetes Insipidus

Adult: **Intranasal** 1–2 sprays in each nostril q.i.d.
Child: **Intranasal** Same as for adult.

PHARMACOKINETICS **Onset:** 0.5–2 h. **Duration:** 3–8 h. **Metabolism:** metabolized in kidneys and liver. **Elimination:** half-life: 15 min; excreted in urine.

CONTRAINDICATIONS & PRECAUTIONS **Contraindicated in:** pregnancy (category B). **Cautious use in:** patients for whom pressor effects would be undesirable, coronary artery disease, known sensitivity to antidiuretic hormone.

ADVERSE/SIDE EFFECTS Infrequent and mild: **Local:** rhinorrhea, nasal congestion and irritation, pruritus and ulceration of nasal passages. **Systemic:** headache, conjunctivitis, heartburn secondary to excessive nasal administration with postnasal drip, abdominal cramps, increased bowel movements. **Other:** with inadvertent oral inhalation: substernal tightness, coughing, and transient dyspnea; marked but transient fluid retention (overdosage); hypersensitivity.

DRUG INTERACTIONS **Demeclocycline, lithium,** other VASOPRESSORS may decrease antidiuretic response; **carbamazepine, chlorpropamide, clofibrate** may prolong antidiuretic response.

NURSING IMPLICATIONS

Administration

- Instruct patient to clear nasal passages well before administering the spray. Warn patient not to inhale the spray.
- A uniform, well-diffused spray will be delivered by holding bottle upright and inserting nozzle into nostril with patient's head in a vertical position.
- Have patient close eyes before actuating spray to prevent inadvertent contact of drug with conjunctiva.

Assessment & Drug Effects

- At beginning of therapy, establish baseline for BP and weight.
- Monitor I&O, urine, and serum osmolality.
- Monitor for and report symptoms of water intoxication (see Appendix G). This occurs with overdose and is usually transient.

Patient & Family Education

- See instructions for use of intranasal spray under Administration.
- If nocturia is a problem, physician may prescribe an additional dose at bedtime.
- If the patient develops a cold or allergy, absorption of lypressin will be diminished. Advise patient to report to physician; adjustment of therapy may be required.
- Lypressin dosage is individualized to control symptoms of diabetes insipidus: frequent urination and excessive thirst.
- Skin tests may be performed for patients with history of hypersen-

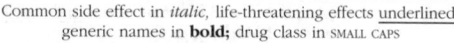

sitivity to antidiuretic hormones prior to initiation of therapy.

MAFENIDE ACETATE

(ma′fe-nide)

Trade name: Sulfamylon

Classifications: ANTIINFECTIVE; SULFONAMIDE DERIVATIVE

Prototype: Sulfisoxazole

Pregnancy category: C

ACTIONS/PHARMACODYNAMICS Topical sulfonamide derivative. Bacteriostatic against many gram-positive and gram-negative organisms, including *Pseudomonas aeruginosa,* and certain strains of anaerobes. Topical applications produce marked reduction of bacterial growth in avascular tissue. Active in presence of pus and serum and not affected by changes in pH of tissue environment. Cross-sensitivity with other sulfonamides not established.

USES Adjunctive therapy in second- and third-degree burns to prevent sepsis.

ROUTE & DOSAGE

Burns

Adult: **Topical** Apply aseptically to burn areas to a thickness of approximately 15 mm (1/16 in) once or twice daily.

PHARMACOKINETICS Absorption: rapidly absorbed from burn surface. **Peak:** 2–4 h. **Metabolism:** rapidly inactivated in blood to a weak carbonic anhydrase inhibitor. **Elimination:** eliminated through kidneys.

CONTRAINDICATIONS & PRECAUTIONS Contraindicated in: history of hypersensitivity to mafenide or to any ingredients in the formulation (e.g., metabisulfite); respiratory (inhalation) injury, pulmonary infection. Safe use during pregnancy (category C) not established. **Cautious use in:** impaired renal or pulmonary function.

ADVERSE/SIDE EFFECTS Hypersensitivity: pruritus, rash, urticaria, blisters, facial edema, eosinophilia. **Skin:** *intense pain, burning, or stinging at application sites,* bleeding of skin, excessive body water loss, delayed eschar separation, excoriation of new skin, superinfections. **Hematologic** (rare): hemolytic anemia, bone marrow suppression. **Other:** metabolic acidosis.

NURSING IMPLICATIONS

Administration

- Mafenide cream is applied aseptically to cleansed, debrided burn areas with sterile gloved hand.
- Burn areas must be covered with cream at all times. When necessary, reapplications should be made to areas from which cream has been removed.
- Store in tight, light-resistant containers. Avoid extremes of temperature.

Assessment & Drug Effects

- Monitor vital signs. Report immediately changes in BP, pulse, and respiratory rate and volume.
- Monitor I&O. Report oliguria or changes in I&O ratio and pattern.
- Acid–base balance should be monitored in patients with extensive burns and in those with pulmonary or renal dysfunction. Be alert to signs and symptoms of metabolic acidosis (see Appendix G).
- Be alert to evidence of superinfections (see Appendix G), particularly in and below burn eschar.
- It is frequently difficult to distinguish between adverse reactions to mafenide and the effects of se-

vere burns. Accurate observations are critical.

- Allergic reactions have reportedly occurred 10–14 d after initiation of mafenide therapy. Temporary discontinuation of drug may be necessary.
- Intensity of local pain caused by mafenide may require administration of analgesic. Report to physician.
- Mafenide therapy is usually continued until healing is progressing well (usually ≤ 60 d) or site is ready for grafting (after about 35–40 d). It is not withdrawn while there is a possibility of infection unless adverse reactions intervene.

M

MAGALDRATE

(mag′al-drate)

Trade names: Hydromagnesium Aluminate, Lowsium, Riopan

Classifications: GI AGENT; ANTACID

Prototype: Aluminum hydroxide

Pregnancy category: C

ACTIONS/PHARMACODYNAMICS Complex of aluminum and magnesium hydroxides. Nonsystemic antacid with true buffering action and high acid-neutralizing capacity. By reducing gastric acidity, stomach pH increases and proteolytic activity of pepsin is inhibited. Reportedly does not produce alkalosis or acid rebound and is not as likely to produce alterations of bowel function that occur with either aluminum or magnesium hydroxide alone.

USES Symptomatic relief of hyperacidity associated with peptic ulcer, gastritis, peptic esophagitis, and hiatal hernia, particularly in patients who need to restrict sodium.

ROUTE & DOSAGE

Antacid

Adult: **PO** 480–1080 mg (5–10 ml suspension or 1–2 tablets) q.i.d. (max 20 tablets or 100 ml/d).

PHARMACOKINETICS Absorption: minimally absorbed from GI tract. **Duration:** buffering action may persist for 60 min.

CONTRAINDICATIONS & PRECAUTIONS Contraindicated in: sensitivity to components, pregnancy (category C). **Cautious use in:** impaired renal function.

ADVERSE/SIDE EFFECTS Infrequent: constipation or diarrhea (with prolonged use), hypermagnesemia (in patients with impaired renal function).

NURSING IMPLICATIONS

Administration

- Shake suspension vigorously before pouring. Preferably administer between meals and at bedtime.
- Suspension should be taken with sufficient water to ensure passage of drug into stomach.
- Chewable tablet should be chewed thoroughly before it is swallowed. Tablet to be swallowed whole should be taken with enough water to ensure prompt swallowing without chewing.

Assessment & Drug Effects

- Question patient about effectiveness of medication in relieving GI distress.
- Patients on prolonged therapy should be periodically checked for electrolyte imbalance (i.e., hypermagnesemia).

Patient & Family Education

- In common with other antacids, magaldrate may cause premature dissolution and absorption of enteric-coated tablets and may interfere with the absorption of oral tetracyclines and other oral medications.

- In general, it is advisable not to take other oral drugs within 1–2 h of an antacid.

MAGNESIUM CITRATE

Trade names: Citrate of Magnesia, Citroma, Citro-Nesia

Classifications: GI AGENT; SALINE CATHARTIC

Prototype: Magnesium hydroxide

Pregnancy category: B

ACTIONS/PHARMACODYNAMICS Contains magnesium carbonate, citric acid, and potassium or sodium bicarbonate for added effervescence, in a lemon oil or cherry-flavored base. Promotes bowel evacuation by causing osmotic retention of fluid, which distends colon and stimulates peristaltic activity.

USES To evacuate bowel prior to certain surgical and diagnostic procedures and to help eliminate parasites and toxic materials after treatment with a vermifuge.

ROUTE & DOSAGE

Bowel Evacuation

Adult: **PO** 240 ml once.
Child: **PO** *2–6 y, 4–12 ml; 6–12 y,* 50–100 ml.

CONTRAINDICATIONS & PRECAUTIONS **Contraindicated in:** renal disease; nausea, vomiting, diarrhea, abdominal pain, acute surgical abdomen; intestinal impaction, obstruction or perforation; rectal bleeding; use of solutions containing sodium bicarbonate in patients on sodium-restricted diets. **Cautious use in:** pregnancy (category B).

ADVERSE/SIDE EFFECTS Abdominal cramps, nausea, fluid and electrolyte imbalance, hypermagnesemia (prolonged use).

NURSING IMPLICATIONS

Administration

- Magnesium citrate is most effective when taken on an empty stomach with a full (240 ml) glass of water. Time dosing so that it does not interfere with sleep. Drug produces a watery or semifluid evacuation in 2–6 h.
- To increase palatability manufacturer suggests chilling the solution by pouring it over ice or refrigerating it until ready to use.
- Once container is opened, magnesium citrate will lose some of its effervescence. This may affect palatability somewhat but not quality of preparation.
- Store in tightly covered containers at 2–30C (36–86F).

Assessment & Drug Effects

- Since drug may cause intense bowel evacuation, patient should be monitored for dehydration, hypokalemia, and hyponatremia (see Appendix G).
- Patients on prolonged therapy should be periodically checked for electrolyte imbalance (i.e., hypermagnesemia).

Patient & Family Education

- Advise all patients, especially the elderly, that this drug should not be used for routine treatment of constipation.
- Advise that some degree of abdominal cramping is to be expected.

MAGNESIUM HYDROXIDE

Trade names: Magnesia, Magnesia Magma, Milk of Magnesia, M.O.M.

Prototype for classifications: GI AGENT; SALINE CATHARTIC; ANTACID

Pregnancy category: B

ACTIONS/PHARMACODYNAMICS Milk of Magnesia is an aqueous suspension of magnesium hydroxide with rapid and long-acting neutralizing action. May cause slight acid rebound. Acts as antacid in low doses and as mild saline laxative at higher doses. Causes osmotic retention of fluid, which distends colon, resulting in mechanical stimulation of peristaltic activity.

M

USES Short-term treatment of occasional constipation, for relief of GI symptoms associated with hyperacidity, and as adjunct in treatment of peptic ulcer. Also has been used in treatment of poisoning by mineral acids and arsenic, and as mouthwash to neutralize acidity.

ROUTE & DOSAGE

Laxative

Adult: **PO** 2.4–4.8 g (30–60 ml)/d in 1 or more divided doses.
Child: **PO** *6–11 y,* 1.2–2.4 g (15–30 ml)/d in 1 or more divided doses; *2–5 y,* 0.4–1.2 g (5–15 ml)/d in 1 or more divided doses.

PHARMACOKINETICS Absorption: 15–30% of magnesium is absorbed. **Onset:** 3–6 h. **Distribution:** small amounts of magnesium distributed in saliva and breast milk. **Elimination:** excreted in feces; some renal excretion.

CONTRAINDICATIONS & PRECAUTIONS Contraindicated in: abdominal pain, nausea, vomiting, diarrhea, severe renal dysfunction, fecal impaction, intestinal obstruction or perforation, rectal bleeding, colostomy, ileostomy. Safe use during pregnancy (category B) and in children < 2 y not established.

ADVERSE/SIDE EFFECTS Excessive dosage: nausea, vomiting, abdominal cramps, *diarrhea,* alkalinization of urine, dehydration. **Hypermagnesemia:** weakness, nausea, vomiting, lethargy, mental depression, hyporeflexia, hypotension, bradycardia, complete heart block and other ECG abnormalities, respiratory depression, coma. **Prolonged use:** electrolyte imbalance.

DRUG INTERACTIONS Milk of Magnesia decreases absorption of **chlordiazepoxide, dicumarol, digoxin, isoniazid,** QUINOLONES, TETRACYCLINES.

NURSING IMPLICATIONS

Administration

- Shake bottle well before pouring to assure administration of suspension.
- For antacid action, Milk of Magnesia is usually given 20–60 min before meals and at bedtime. Mix suspension with water or follow with sufficient water to assure that it reaches the stomach.
- When intended for antacid use, laxative effect of Milk of Magnesia can be minimized by coadministering it or alternating it with an antacid with constipating effects (e.g., calcium carbonate or aluminum hydroxide). Consult physician.
- For laxative effect, follow the drug with at least a full glass of water to enhance drug action. Administer in the morning or at bedtime. Most

effective when taken on an empty stomach.

- Store at room temperature in tightly covered container. Slowly absorbs carbon dioxide on exposure to air. Avoid freezing.

Assessment & Drug Effects

- Evaluate the patient's continued need for drug. Prolonged and frequent use of laxative doses may lead to dependence. Additionally, even therapeutic doses can raise urinary pH and thereby predispose susceptible patients to urinary infection and urolithiasis.
- Monitor signs of elevated serum magnesium concentrations, which may cause bradycardia and other symptoms of hypermagnesemia (see Appendix G).

Patient & Family Education

- Inform that the cause of persistent or recurrent constipation or gastric distress should be investigated by a physician.
- Correct misconceptions about constipation. The omission of one day's evacuation is not constipation and will not cause poisons to accumulate in body.

MAGNESIUM OXIDE

Trade names: Mag-Ox, Maox, Par-Mag, Uro-Mag

Classifications: GI AGENT; ANTACID; SALINE CATHARTIC

Prototype: Magnesium hydroxide

Pregnancy category: B

ACTIONS/PHARMACODYNAMICS Nonsystemic antacid with high neutralizing capacity and relatively long duration of action. Its contraindications and precautions are essentially the same as those of magnesium hydroxide.

USES Essentially the same as those of magnesium hydroxide. May also be used as magnesium supplement.

ROUTE & DOSAGE

Antacid

Adult: **PO** 280–1500 mg with water or milk q.i.d., p.c. and h.s.

Laxative

Adult: **PO** 2–4 g with water or milk h.s.

Magnesium Supplement

Adult: **PO** 400–1200 mg/d in divided doses.

PHARMACOKINETICS Absorption: 30–50% absorbed from GI tract. **Elimination:** eliminated in urine.

ADVERSE/SIDE EFFECTS *Diarrhea,* abdominal cramps, nausea; hypermagnesemia, renal stones (chronic use).

DRUG INTERACTIONS See magnesium hydroxide.

NURSING IMPLICATIONS

Administration

- In common with other antacids, magnesium oxide can cause premature dissolution and absorption of enteric-coated and sustained release tablets and also may complex with and thus reduce absorption of PO tetracyclines and other oral drugs. In general, it is advisable not to take other oral medications within 1–2 h of an antacid.
- Store in airtight containers at 15–30C (59–86F) unless otherwise directed. On exposure to air, magnesium oxide rapidly absorbs moisture and carbon dioxide.

Assessment & Drug Effects

- Since drug may cause intense

M

bowel evacuation, patient should be monitored for dehydration, hypokalemia, and hyponatremia (see Appendix G).

- Patients on prolonged therapy should be periodically checked for electrolyte imbalance (i.e., hypermagnesemia).

Patient & Family Education

- As with other antacids, the liquid preparation is reportedly more effective than the tablet form.

MAGNESIUM SALICYLATE

Trade names: Doan's Pills, Magan, Mobidin

Classifications: CNS AGENT; ANALGESIC; ANTIPYRETIC; SALICYLATE; NSAID

Prototype: Aspirin

Pregnancy category: C

ACTIONS/PHARMACODYNAMICS Sodium-free salicylate derivative with low incidence of GI irritation. In equal doses, less potent than aspirin as an analgesic and antipyretic. Unlike aspirin, not associated with asthmatic reactions and does not inhibit platelet aggregation or increase bleeding time.

USES Relief of pain and inflammation in rheumatoid arthritis, osteoarthritis, bursitis, and other musculoskeletal disorders.

ROUTE & DOSAGE

Analgesic/Antipyretic

Adult: **PO** 650 mg t.i.d. or q.i.d.

Arthritic Conditions

Adult: **PO** Up to 9.6 g/d in divided doses.

CONTRAINDICATIONS & PRECAUTIONS **Contraindicated in:** hypersensitivity to salicylates, erosive gastritis, peptic ulcer; advanced renal insufficiency, liver damage, bleeding disorders, before surgery. Safe use during pregnancy (category C), in nursing mothers, and in children <12 y not established.

ADVERSE/SIDE EFFECTS **Salicylism:** dizziness, drowsiness, tinnitus, hearing loss, nausea, vomiting, hypermagnesemia (with high doses in patients with renal insufficiency).

DRUG INTERACTIONS **Aminosalicylic acid** increases risk of salicylate toxicity; **ammonium chloride** and other ACIDIFYING AGENTS decrease renal elimination and increase risk of salicylate toxicity; anticoagulants—added risk of bleeding with ANTICOAGULANTS; CARBONIC ANHYDRASE INHIBITORS enhance salicylate toxicity; CORTICOSTEROIDS compound ulcerogenic effects; increases **methotrexate** toxicity; low doses of salicylates may antagonize uricosuric effects of **probenecid, sulfinpyrazone.**

NURSING IMPLICATIONS

Administration

- Administer with a full glass of water or with food or milk to minimize gastric irritation.

Assessment & Drug Effects

- If used in high dosages or in patients with any degree of renal impairment, serum magnesium levels should be monitored because of risk of hypermagnesemia.
- Use of salicylates in children or teenagers with influenza or chickenpox may be associated with development of Reye's syndrome and is therefore not advised.

Patient & Family Education

- Advise to promptly report tinnitus, hearing loss, or dizziness.
- Advise not to take aspirin-containing drugs without consent of physician.
- Note: In Canada, Doan's pills contain acetaminophen plus salicylamide.

MAGNESIUM SULFATE

Trade name: Epsom Salt
Classifications: GI AGENT; SALINE CATHARTIC; REPLACEMENT AGENT; ANTICONVULSANT
Prototype: Magnesium hydroxide
Pregnancy category: A

ACTIONS/PHARMACODYNAMICS When taken PO, magnesium sulfate acts as laxative by osmotic retention of fluid, which distends colon, increases water content of feces, and causes mechanical stimulation of bowel activity. When given parenterally, it acts as CNS depressant and also depressant of smooth, skeletal, and cardiac muscle function. Anticonvulsant properties thought to be produced by CNS depression, principally by decreasing the amount of acetylcholine liberated from motor nerve terminals, thus producing peripheral neuromuscular blockade.

USES PO to relieve acute constipation and to evacuate bowel in preparation for x-ray of intestines. Parenterally to control seizures in toxemia of pregnancy, epilepsy, and acute nephritis and for prophylaxis and treatment of hypomagnesemia. Topically to reduce edema, inflammation, and itching. **Unlabeled uses:** to inhibit premature labor (tocolytic action) and as adjunct in hyperalimentation.

ROUTE & DOSAGE

Laxative
Adult: **PO** 10–15 g once/d.

Preeclampsia, Eclampsia
Adult: **IM/IV** 4 g in 250 ml D5W infused slowly, followed by 4–5 g IM in alternate buttocks q4h.

Hypomagnesemic Seizures
Adult: **IM/IV** ***Mild:*** 1 g q6h for 4 doses; ***Severe:*** 250 mg/kg infused over 4 h.
Child: **IV** 20–100 mg/kg q4–6h prn.

Total Parenteral Nutrition
Adult: **IV** 0.5–3 g/d.

PHARMACOKINETICS **Onset:** 1–2 h PO; 1 h IM. **Duration:** 30 min IV; 3–4 h PO. **Distribution:** crosses placenta; distributed into breast milk. **Elimination:** eliminated in kidneys.

CONTRAINDICATIONS & PRECAUTIONS **Contraindicated in:** myocardial damage; heart block; IV administration during the 2 h preceding delivery; PO use in patients with abdominal pain, nausea, vomiting, fecal impaction, or intestinal irritation, obstruction, or perforation; pregnancy (category A). **Cautious use in:** impaired renal function, digitalized patients, concomitant use of other CNS depressants or neuromuscular blocking agents.

ADVERSE/SIDE EFFECTS **Hypermagnesemia:** flushing, sweating, extreme thirst, hypotension, sedation, confusion, depressed reflexes or no reflexes, muscle weakness, flaccid paralysis, hypothermia, depressed cardiac function, complete heart block, circulatory collapse, respiratory paralysis; hypocalcemia. **Repeated laxative use:** dehydration, electrolyte imbalance including hypocalcemia.

DRUG INTERACTIONS NEUROMUSCULAR BLOCKING AGENTS add to respiratory depression and apnea.

INCOMPATIBILITIES Solution/additive: 10% fat emulsion; calcium gluceptate, clindamycin, dobutamine, polymyxin B sulfate, procaine, sodium bicarbonate.

NURSING IMPLICATIONS

Administration

- For laxative action, best administered in the morning or midafternoon in a glass of water. Bitter, salty taste may be disguised by chilling or flavoring with lemon or orange juice.
- A 10% solution may be given by direct IV at a rate of 1.5 ml/min or 150 mg/min.
- A solution of 4 g in 250 ml of D5W may be infused at a rate not to exceed 3 ml/min.
- IV administration to infants, children: Verify correct IV concentration and rate of infusion with physician.

Assessment & Drug Effects

- When magnesium sulfate is given IV, patient requires constant observation. Check BP and pulse q10–15min or more often if indicated.
- Monitoring of plasma magnesium levels is advised in patients receiving drug parenterally (normal: 1.8–3.0 mEq/L). Plasma levels in excess of 4 mEq/L are reflected in depressed deep tendon reflexes and other symptoms of magnesium intoxication. See adverse/side effects. Cardiac arrest occurs at levels in excess of 25 mEq/L.
- Early indicators of magnesium toxicity (hypermagnesemia) include cathartic effect, profound thirst, feeling of warmth, sedation, confusion, depressed deep tendon reflexes, and muscle weakness. Calcium and phosphorus levels should be monitored also.
- Monitor I&O (in patients receiving drug parenterally). Report oliguria and changes in I&O ratio.
- Before each repeated parenteral dose, patellar reflex should be tested. Depression or absence of reflexes is a useful index of early magnesium intoxication. Also check respiratory rate and character and urinary output, especially in patients with impaired renal function. Therapy is generally not continued if urinary output is less than 100 ml during the 4 h preceding each dose.
- Newborns of mothers who received parenteral magnesium sulfate within a few hours of delivery should be observed for signs of toxicity, including respiratory and neuromuscular depression.
- Patients receiving the drug for hypomagnesemia should be observed for improvement in these signs of deficiency: irritability, choreiform movements, tremors, tetany, twitching, muscle cramps, tachycardia, hypertension, psychotic behavior.

Patient & Family Education

- Sufficient water should be taken during the day when drug is administered orally to prevent net loss of body water.
- Recommended daily allowances of magnesium are obtained in a normal diet. Rich sources are whole-grain cereals, legumes, nuts, meats, seafood, milk, most green leafy vegetables, and bananas.

MANNITOL

(man'i-tole)

Trade name: Osmitrol

Prototype for classifications: ELECTROLYTIC AND WATER BALANCE AGENT; OSMOTIC DIURETIC

Pregnancy category: C

ACTIONS/PHARMACODYNAMICS

Induces diuresis by raising osmotic pressure of glomerular filtrate, thereby inhibiting tubular reabsorption of water and solutes. In large doses, may increase rate of electrolyte excretion, particularly sodium, chloride, and potassium. Reduces elevated intraocular and cerebrospinal pressures by increasing plasma osmolality, thus inducing diffusion of water from these fluids back into plasma and extravascular space.

USES To promote diuresis in prevention and treatment of oliguric phase of acute renal failure following cardiovascular surgery, severe traumatic injury, surgery in presence of severe jaundice, hemolytic transfusion reaction. Also used to reduce elevated intraocular (IOP) and intracranial pressure (ICP), to measure glomerular filtration rate (GFR), to promote excretion of toxic substances, to relieve symptoms of pulmonary edema, and as irrigating solution in transurethral prostatic reaction to minimize hemolytic effects of water. Commercially available in combination with sorbitol for urogenital irrigation.

ROUTE & DOSAGE

Acute Renal Failure

Adult: **IV** ***Test dose:*** 0.2 g/kg or 12.5 g as a 15–20% solution over 3–5 min. ***Positive response:*** 30–50 ml of urine over next 2–3 h, may repeat test dose 1 time; if still negative, do not use. ***Treatment:*** 50–100 g as 15–20% solution over 90 min to several hours.

Child: **IV** Test dose: 200 mg/kg (max 12.5 g) over 3–5 min. ***Positive response:*** urine flow of 1 ml/kg/h for 1–2 h. ***Maintenance:*** 0.25–0.5 g/kg q4–6 h.

Edema, Ascites

Adult: **IV** 100 g as a 10–20% solution over 2–6 h.

Elevated IOP or ICP

Adult: **IV** 1.5–2 mg/kg as a 15–25% solution over 30–60 min.

Acute Chemical Toxicity

Adult: **IV** 100–200 g depending on urine output.

Measurement of GFR

Adult: **IV** 100 ml of 20% solution diluted with 180 ml NaCl injection infused at a rate of 20 ml/min.

PHARMACOKINETICS **Onset:** 1–3 h diuresis; 30–60 min IOP; 15 min ICP. **Duration:** 4–6 h IOP; 3–8 h IC P. **Distribution:** confined to extracellular space; does not cross blood–brain barrier except with very high plasma levels in the presence of acidosis. **Metabolism:** small quantity metabolized to glycogen in liver. **Elimination:** half-life: 100 min; rapidly excreted by kidneys.

CONTRAINDICATIONS & PRECAUTIONS **Contraindicated in:** anuria; marked pulmonary edema or CHF; metabolic edema; organic CNS disease, intracranial bleeding; shock, severe dehydration, history of allergy; pregnancy (category C).

M

ADVERSE/SIDE EFFECTS CNS: headache, tremor, convulsions, dizziness, transient muscle rigidity. **CV:** edema, CHF, angina-like pain, hypotension, hypertension, thrombophlebitis. **Eye:** blurred vision. **GI:** dry mouth, nausea, vomiting. **GU:** marked diuresis, urinary retention, nephrosis, uricosuria. **Metabolic:** *fluid and electrolyte imbalance,* especially hyponatremia; dehydration, acidosis. **Other:** with extravasation: local edema, skin necrosis; chills, fever, allergic reactions.

NURSING IMPLICATIONS

Administration

- IV infusion flow rate is generally adjusted to maintain urine flow of at least 30–50 ml/h. See Route & Dosage for specific rates.
- A test dose is given to patients with marked oliguria to check adequacy of renal function. Response is considered satisfactory if urine flow of at least 30–50 ml/h is produced over 2–3 h after drug administration.
- IV administration to infants, children: Verify correct IV concentration and rate of infusion with physician.
- Concentrations higher than 15% have a greater tendency to crystallize. Administration set with an in-line IV filter should be used when infusing concentrations of 15% or above.
- Store preferably at 15–30C (59–86F) unless otherwise directed. Avoid freezing.

Assessment & Drug Effects

- Patients receiving urologic irrigations of mannitol should be observed closely for systemic reactions.
- Care should be taken to avoid extravasation. Observe injection site for signs of inflammation or edema.
- Serum and urine electrolytes and renal function should be closely monitored during therapy.
- I&O must be accurately measured and recorded to achieve proper fluid balance.
- Monitor allowable PO fluid intake volume.
- Monitor vital signs and carefully note possible indications of fluid and electrolyte imbalance (e.g., thirst, muscle cramps or weakness, paresthesias, and signs of CHF).
- Be alert to the possibility that a rebound increase in ICP sometimes occurs about 12 h after drug administration. Patient may complain of headache or confusion.
- Take accurate daily weight.

Patient & Family Education

- Advise to report any of the following: thirst, muscle cramps or weakness, paresthesia, dyspnea, or headache.
- Instruct family members to immediately report any evidence of confusion.

MAPROTILINE HYDROCHLORIDE

(ma-proe'ti-leen)

Trade name: Ludiomil

Classifications: CNS AGENT; PSYCHOTHERAPEUTIC; TETRACYCLIC ANTIDEPRESSANT

Prototype: Imipramine

Pregnancy category: B

ACTIONS/PHARMACODYNAMICS

Tetracyclic antidepressant pharmacologically and therapeutically similar to the tricyclic antidepressants. Has significant sedative effect and less prominent anticholinergic action; may lower seizure threshold. Useful in depression associated with anxiety and sleep disturbances.

USES Treatment of depressive neurosis (dysthymic disorder) and manic-depressive illness, depressed type (major depressive disorder).

ROUTE & DOSAGE

Mild to Moderate Depression

Adult: **PO** Start at 75 mg/d and gradually increase q2wk up to 150 mg/d in single or divided doses.
Geriatric: **PO** Start with 25 mg h.s. and gradually increase to 50–75 mg/d.

Severe Depression

Adult: **PO** Start at 100–150 mg/d and gradually increase up to 300 mg/d in single or divided doses if needed.

PHARMACOKINETICS Absorption: slowly absorbed from GI tract. **Peak:** 12 h. **Distribution:** distributed chiefly to brain, lungs, liver, and kidneys. **Metabolism:** metabolized in liver. **Elimination:** half-life: 51 h; 70% excreted in urine, 30% in feces.

CONTRAINDICATIONS & PRECAUTIONS Contraindicated in: patients < 18 y; history of seizure disorder; pregnancy (category B).

ADVERSE/SIDE EFFECTS CNS: seizures, exacerbation of psychosis, hallucinations, tremors, excitement, confusion, dizziness, *drowsiness.* **CV:** *orthostatic hypotension,* hypertension, tachycardia. **Eye:** accommodation disturbances, blurred vision, mydriasis. **GI:** nausea, vomiting, epigastric distress, *constipation, dry mouth.* **GU:** *urinary retention,* frequency. **Hypersensitivity:** skin rash, urticaria, photosensitivity.

DRUG INTERACTIONS May decrease some response to ANTIHYPERTENSIVES; CNS DEPRESSANTS, **alcohol,** HYPNOTICS, BARBITURATES, SEDATIVES potentiate CNS depression; may increase hypoprothombinemic effect of ORAL ANTICOAGULANTS; transient delirium with **ethchlorvynol;** with **levodopa,** SYMPATHOMIMETICS (e.g., **epinephrine, norepinephrine**) there is possibility of sympathetic hyperactivity with hypertension and hyperpyrexia; with MAO INHIBITORS there is possibility of severe reactions, toxic psychosis, cardiovascular instability; **methylphenidate** increases plasma TCA levels; THYROID DRUGS increase possibility of arrhythmias; **cimetidine** may increase plasma TCA levels.

NURSING IMPLICATIONS

Administration

- Drug may be given as single dose or in divided doses. Risk of seizures is reduced by initiating therapy with low dosages.
- Store drug at 15–30C (59–86F) unless otherwise specified.

Assessment & Drug Effects

- Therapeutic effects are sometimes seen in 3–7 d; 2–3 wk are usually necessary.
- Assess level of sedative effect. If recovering patient becomes too lethargic to care for personal hygiene or to maintain food intake and interactions with others, report to physician.
- Monitor bowel elimination pattern and I&O ratio. Severe constipation and urinary retention are potential problems, especially in the elderly. Advise increased fluid intake (at least 1500 ml/d).
- Risk of seizures appears to be high

in heavy drinkers. Observe seizure precautions.

- If patient uses excessive amounts of alcohol, it should be borne in mind that the potentiation of maprotiline effects may increase the danger of overdosage or suicide attempt.

Patient & Family Education

- Urge outpatient on high doses to report symptoms of stomatitis and dry mouth. Sore or dry mouth can be a major cause of lack of compliance.
- Caution that ability to perform tasks requiring alertness and skill may be impaired during early therapy.
- Urge not to change dose or dose schedule without consulting physician.
- Advise not to use OTC drugs unless physician approves.
- The actions of both alcohol and maprotiline are potentiated when they are used together during therapy and for ≤ 2 wk after maprotiline is discontinued. Consult physician about amount of alcohol, if any, that can be taken.

M

MASOPROCAL CREAM (10%)

(mas-o-pro′-cal)

Trade name: Actinex

Classifications: SKIN AND MUCOUS MEMBRANE AGENT

Pregnancy category: B

ACTIONS/PHARMACODYNAMICS Mechanism of action of masoprocal in the treatment of actinic keratoses is unknown. Dispensed as 10% cream.

USE Treatment of actinic keratosis. **Unlabeled use:** malignant melanoma.

ROUTE & DOSAGE

Actinic Keratosis

Adult: **Topical** Apply to lesions b.i.d. for 14–28 d.

PHARMACOKINETICS Absorption: <2% absorbed through intact skin. **Onset:** 2–4 wk.

CONTRAINDICATIONS & PRECAUTIONS Contraindicated in: hypersensitivity to masoprocal. **Cautious use in:** pregnancy (category B) and nursing mothers. Safety and efficacy in children have not been established.

ADVERSE/SIDE EFFECTS Skin: *inflammation, erythema, dryness, flaking,* itching, burning, tightness, bleeding, edema.

NURSING IMPLICATIONS

Administration

- Masoprocal is for external use only. Do not apply on mucous membranes. In case of eye contact, wash eye with water immediately.
- Before application, wash and dry affected areas. Gently massage masoprocol into area until it is evenly distributed.
- If cream is applied with an ungloved hand, wash immediately.
- Do not apply occlusive dressings over masoprocal cream.
- Store at room temperature, 15–30C (59–86F), unless otherwise directed.

Assessment & Drug Effects

- Assess for allergic contact dermatitis, which is an indication to discontinue.
- Severe skin reactions of any kind should be reported to the physician.

Patient & Family Education

- Instruct in proper technique for application of the cream.
- Inform that a transient local burning sensation may develop immediately following application.
- Inform that local skin reactions are common but usually disappear within 2 wk of discontinuing cream application.
- Advise patients with sulfite sensitivity that this product contains sulfites.
- Advise that masoprocal may stain clothing.

MAZINDOL

(may′zin-dole)

Trade names: Mazanor, Sanorex

Classifications: CNS AGENT; RESPIRATORY AND CEREBRAL STIMULANT

Prototype: Amphetamine sulfate

Pregnancy category: C

Controlled substance: Schedule IV

ACTIONS/PHARMACODYNAMICS Pharmacologic properties are similar to those of amphetamines. Produces CNS and cardiac stimulation in addition to amphetamine-like effects. Appears to exert primary effects on limbic system and to alter norepinephrine metabolism by inhibiting normal neuronal uptake mechanism.

USE Short-term management of exogenous obesity.

ROUTE & DOSAGE

Obesity

Adult: **PO** 1 mg t.i.d. a.c. or 2 mg q.d. 1 h before lunch.

PHARMACOKINETICS **Absorption:** readily absorbed from GI tract. **Onset:** 30–60 min. **Duration:** 8–15 h. **Metabolism:** metabolized in liver. **Elimination:** half-life: 2.5–9 h; 95% excreted in feces, 2–5% in urine.

CONTRAINDICATIONS & PRECAUTIONS **Contraindicated in:** glaucoma; severe hypertension; symptomatic cardiovascular disease, including arrhythmias; agitated states; history of drug abuse; during or within 14 d after administration of MAO inhibitors; children <12 y. Safe use during pregnancy (category C) not established. **Cautious use in:** hyperexcitability states.

ADVERSE/SIDE EFFECTS **CNS:** *restlessness,* dizziness, insomnia, dysphoria, depression, tremor, headache, drowsiness, weakness. **CV:** palpitation, tachycardia. **Endocrine:** impotence. **GI:** *dry mouth,* unpleasant taste, diarrhea, constipation, nausea, vomiting. **Skin:** rash, excessive sweating, clamminess.

DRUG INTERACTIONS **Acetazolamide, sodium bicarbonate** decrease mazindol elimination; **ammonium chloride, ascorbic acid** increase mazindol elimination; the effects of mazindol and BARBITURATES may be antagonized; **furazolidone** may increase BP effects of mazindol, and interaction may persist for several weeks after discontinuing furazolidone; antihypertensive effects of **guanethidine, guanadryl** antagonized; MAO INHIBITORS, **selegiline** can cause hypertensive crisis—do not administer mazindol during or within 14 d of administration of these drugs; PHENOTHIAZINES may inhibit mood elevating effects of mazindol; BETA-ADRENERGIC AGONISTS increase adverse cardiovascular effects of mazindol.

M

NURSING IMPLICATIONS

Administration

- Drug is given 1 h before meals if t.i.d. or 1 h before lunch if q.d. dose.
- Drug may be taken with meals if GI discomfort occurs.

Assessment & Drug Effects

- Monitor weight periodically.
- If patient experiences excessive restlessness or insomnia, drug may have to be taken early in the day.

Patient & Family Education

- Rate of weight loss is greatest during first few weeks of therapy and tends to decrease thereafter.
- Insulin requirements of patients with diabetes may be decreased in association with use of mazindol and concomitant caloric restriction and weight loss.
- Tolerance may develop within a few weeks. When it occurs, drug should be discontinued.
- Caution that mazindol may impair ability to perform hazardous activities such as driving a car or operating machinery.
- Instruct not to take more medication than prescribed.
- Instruct to report excessively dry mouth or constipation.

M

MEBENDAZOLE

(me-ben′da-zole)

Trade name: Vermox

Prototype for classifications: ANTIINFECTIVE; ANTHELMINTIC

Pregnancy category: C

ACTIONS/PHARMACODYNAMICS Carbamate with unusually broad spectrum of anthelmintic activity. Mechanism of action not known. Inhibits formation of worm's microtubules and inhibits glucose and other nutrient uptake by susceptible helminths.

USES Treatment of *Trichuris trichiura* (whipworm), *Enterobius vermicularis* (pinworm), *Ascaris lumbricoides* (roundworm), *Ancylostoma duodenale* (common hookworm), *Necator americanus* (American hookworm) in single or mixed infections. **Unlabeled uses:** beef, dwarf, and pork tapeworm and threadworm infections.

ROUTE & DOSAGE

Enterobiasis

Adult: **PO** 100 mg as single dose.
Child: **PO** 100 mg as single dose.

Other Infestations

Adult: **PO** 100 mg b.i.d. × 3 d.
Child: **PO** 100 mg b.i.d. × 3 d.

PHARMACOKINETICS **Absorption:** minimal absorption from GI tract (2–10% of oral dose). **Metabolism:** metabolized to inactive metabolite. **Elimination:** half-life: 3–9 h; primarily eliminated in feces.

CONTRAINDICATIONS & PRECAUTIONS **Contraindicated in:** safe use during pregnancy (category C), in nursing women, and in children <2 y not established.

ADVERSE/SIDE EFFECTS Transient abdominal pain, diarrhea, dizziness, fever (possibly due to tissue necrosis in cysts).

NURSING IMPLICATIONS

Administration

- Commercial chewable tablet may be chewed, crushed, mixed with food, or swallowed whole.

Assessment & Drug Effects

- If cure does not occur within 3 wk after initiation of therapy, second course of treatment is advised.
- Because pinworms are readily transmitted from person to person,

all family members should be examined and treated simultaneously.

Patient & Family Education

- Emphasize importance of washing hands thoroughly after toilet and before eating. Disinfect toilet facilities daily.
- Keep hands away from mouth; keep fingernails short.
- Handle bedding carefully without shaking it to avoid dispersing ova into the air.
- Advise to change underclothing, bedclothes, towels, and facecloths daily and to bathe frequently, preferably by showering. Infected person should sleep alone.

MECAMYLAMINE HYDROCHLORIDE

(mek-a-mill′a-meen)

Trade name: Inversine

Classifications: CARDIOVASCULAR AGENT; CENTRAL ACTING ANTIHYPERTENSIVE

Prototype: Methyldopa

Pregnancy category: C

ACTIONS/PHARMACODYNAMICS Potent, long-acting secondary amine nondepolarizing ganglionic blocking agent. Blocks neurotransmission at both sympathetic and parasympathetic ganglia by competing with ACh for cholinergic receptor sites on postsynaptic membranes. Reduces BP in both normotensive and hypertensive individuals, generally with greater decrease in standing or sitting BP than in supine BPs.

USES Moderately severe to severe hypertension and uncomplicated malignant hypertension.

ROUTE & DOSAGE

Moderately Severe to Severe Hypertension

Adult: **PO** 2.5 mg b.i.d. p.c. for 2 d, increased by increments of 2.5 mg at intervals of ≥ 2 d until desired BP response is attained (2.5–25 mg/d in 2–4 divided doses).

PHARMACOKINETICS **Absorption:** almost completely absorbed from GI tract. **Onset:** 30 min–2 h. **Peak:** 3–5 h. **Duration:** 6–12 h. **Distribution:** crosses blood-brain barrier and placenta; distributed into breast milk. **Metabolism:** metabolized in liver. **Elimination:** primarily excreted in urine.

CONTRAINDICATIONS & PRECAUTIONS **Contraindicated in:** coronary insufficiency, pyloric stenosis, glaucoma, uremia, chronic pyelonephritis, recent MI; mild labile hypertension; unreliable uncooperative patients; pregnancy (category C). **Cautious use in:** rising or elevated BUN; renal, cerebral, or coronary vascular pathology; recent CVA; prostatic hypertrophy, bladder neck obstruction, urethral stricture.

ADVERSE/SIDE EFFECTS Mostly dose-related. **CNS:** weakness, fatigue, sedation, headache, paresthesias. confusion, depression, choreiform movements, tremor. **CV:** *orthostatic hypotension,* changes in heart rate, dizziness, syncope, precipitation of angina. **EENT:** mydriasis, *blurred vision,* cyclopegia, nasal congestion, *dry mouth* with dysphagia, glossitis. **GI:** *anorexia, nausea, vomiting, constipation, diarrhea,* <u>adynamic ileus</u>. **Other:** decreased libido, impotence, *urinary retention*.

DRUG INTERACTIONS **Alcohol,** other ANTIHYPERTENSIVE AGENTS,

M

bethanechol, THIAZIDE DIURETICS potentiate hypotensive effects; **acetazolamide, sodium bicarbonate** increase mecamylamine toxicity because they decrease its elimination.

NURSING IMPLICATIONS

Administration

- Administration of drug after meals may result in more gradual absorption and smoother control of BP. Timing relative to meals should be consistent.
- Because of diurnal variations in BP, physician may prescribe a relatively small dose in the morning or omission of morning dose (morning BP usually lower) and larger doses for afternoon or evening.
- Sudden discontinuation of drug can result in severe hypertensive rebound with CVA and acute CHF. Usually, other antihypertensive therapy must be substituted gradually, and patient must be supervised daily during period of dosage adjustment.
- Store at 15–30C (59–86F) unless otherwise directed.

Assessment & Drug Effects

- Initial regulation of dosage should be dictated by BP readings in standing position at time of maximal drug effect, as well as symptoms of orthostatic hypotension (faintness, dizziness, light-headedness). Also note any changes in pulse rate.
- Partial tolerance may develop in some patients, necessitating dosage adjustment. Follow-up supervision is an essential part of therapy.
- Constipation, frequent loose stools with abdominal distension, or decreased bowel sounds may be the first signs of paralytic ileus (relatively frequent) and should be reported promptly. Paralytic ileus is sometimes preceded by small, frequent stools.

Patient & Family Education

- Instruct to make position changes slowly and in stages, particularly from recumbent to upright posture, and to sit on edge of bed and move ankles and feet before ambulating.
- Advise to lie down immediately if feeling light-headed or dizzy. Adverse reactions should be reported immediately, as drug effects may last hours to days after drug is discontinued.
- Inform of factors that may potentiate the action of mecamylamine: excessive heat, fever, infection, alcohol, vigorous exercise, salt depletion (vomiting, diarrhea, excessive sweating, diuresis). Hypotensive action may also be prominent during pregnancy, anesthesia, or surgery.
- Seasonal variations may alter the hypotensive effect, e.g., usually smaller doses are required in summer than in winter.
- Caution to avoid driving and other potentially hazardous activities until reaction to drug is known.
- Provide guidance on measures to prevent dry mouth.

MECHLORETHAMINE HYDROCHLORIDE

(me-klor-eth′a-meen)

Trade name: Mustargen

Prototype for classifications: ANTINEOPLASTIC; ALKYLATING AGENT; NITROGEN MUSTARD

Pregnancy category: D

ACTIONS/PHARMACODYNAMICS

Analog of mustard gas and standard of reference for nitrogen mustards. Forms highly reactive carbonium ion, which causes cross-linking and abnormal base-pairing in DNA, thereby interfering with DNA replication and RNA and protein synthesis. Cell-cycle nonspecific. Actions simulate those of x-ray therapy, but nitrogen mustards produce more acute tissue damage and more rapid recovery.

USES Generally confined to nonterminal stages of neoplastic disease. Employed as single agent or in combination with other agents in palliative treatment of Hodgkin's disease (stages III and IV), lymphosarcoma, mycosis fungoides, polycythemia vera, bronchogenic carcinoma, chronic myelocytic or chronic lymphocytic leukemia. Also for intrapleural, intrapericardial and intraperitoneal palliative treatment of metastatic carcinoma resulting in effusion.

ROUTE & DOSAGE

Advanced Hodgkin's Disease

Adult: **IV** 6 mg/m^2 on day 1 and 8 of a 28 d cycle.

Other Neoplasms

Adult: **IV** 0.4 mg/kg given as a single dose *or* in divided doses of 0.1–0.2 mg/kg/d; may repeat course in 3–6 wk.

PHARMACOKINETICS Metabolism: rapid transformation to metabolites. **Elimination:** not detectable in blood within a few minutes; <0.01% excreted in urine.

CONTRAINDICATIONS & PRECAUTIONS Contraindicated in: pregnancy (category D), lactation; myelosuppression; infectious granuloma; known infectious diseases, acute herpes zoster; intracavitary use with other systemic bone marrow suppressants. **Cautious use in:** bone marrow infiltration with malignant cells, chronic lymphocytic leukemia, men or women in childbearing age, use with x-ray treatment or other chemotherapy in alternating courses.

ADVERSE/SIDE EFFECTS CNS: neurotoxicity: vertigo, tinnitus, headache, drowsiness, peripheral neuropathy, light-headedness, paresthesias, cerebral deterioration, coma. **GI:** stomatitis, xerostomia, anorexia, *nausea, vomiting*, diarrhea. **Hematopoietic:** leukopenia, *thrombocytopenia,* lymphocytopenia, agranulocytosis, *anemia,* hyperheparinemia. **Skin:** pruritus, hyperpigmentation, herpes zoster, alopecia. **Other:** amenorrhea, azoospermia, chromosomal abnormalities, hyperuricemia, weakness, hypersensitivity reactions. *With extravasation: painful inflammatory reaction, tissue sloughing, thrombosis, thrombophlebitis.*

DRUG INTERACTIONS Mechlorethamine (nitrogen mustards) may reduce effectiveness of ANTIGOUT AGENTS by raising serum uric acid levels; dosage adjustments may be necessary.

NURSING IMPLICATIONS

Administration

- Surgical gloves should be worn to protect skin during preparation and administration of solution. Avoid inhalation of vapors and dust and contact of drug with eyes and skin.
- If drug contacts the skin, flush contaminated area immediately with copious amounts of water for at least 15 min, followed by 2% sodium thiosulfate solution. Irritation may appear after a latent period.
- If eye contact occurs, irrigate im-

mediately with copious amounts of 0.9% NaCl, followed by ophthalmologic examination as soon as possible.

- IV preparation: Prepare mechlorethamine solution immediately before administration by adding 10 ml sterile water for injection or 0.9% NaCl injection to drug vial. With needle still in rubber stopper, shake vial several times to hasten dissolving. Solution will contain 1 mg mechlorethamine per 1 ml of solution.
- Do not use discolored solution or contents of vial in which there are drops of moisture.
- IV administration: Reconstituted solution may be injected over 3–5 min directly into any suitable vein. However, to reduce risk of severe infections from extravasation or high concentration of the drug, injection is made preferably directly into tubing or sidearm of freely flowing IV infusion. Some clinicians flush vein with running IV solution for 2–5 min to clear tubing of any remaining drug.
- If drug extravasates, prompt subcutaneous or intradermal injection with isotonic sodium thiosulfate solution (1/6 molar) and application of ice compresses intermittently for a 6–12 h period may reduce local tissue damage and discomfort. Tissue induration and tenderness may persist 4–6 wk, and tissue may slough.

Assessment & Drug Effects

- Establish baseline data relative to body weight, I&O ratio and pattern, and blood picture as reference for design of drug and nursing care regimens.
- Mechlorethamine dosage is determined on basis of ideal dry body weight (i.e., unaugmented by edema or ascites). Record daily weight. Alert physician to sudden or slow, steady weight gain.
- Pain is rare with intrapleural injection, but transient cardiac irregularities may occur. Monitor cardiac function during and after treatment until cardiac status is stable.
- Pain is common with intraperitoneal injection and usually is associated with nausea, vomiting, and diarrhea lasting 2–3 d.
- Nausea and vomiting may occur 1–3 h after drug injection; vomiting usually subsides within 8 h, but nausea may persist. Attempt to schedule treatments, other drugs, and meals so as to avoid peak times of nausea.
- Prolonged vomiting and diarrhea can produce volume depletion. Carefully monitor and record patient's fluid losses.
- Monitor CBC with differential and platelet count.
- Petechiae, ecchymoses, or abnormal bleeding from intestinal and buccal membranes should be reported immediately. During period of thrombocytopenia, injections and other invasive procedures should be kept to a minimum.
- Report symptoms of unexplained fever, chills, sore throat, tachycardia, and mucosal ulceration, as they may signal onset of agranulocytosis (see Appendix G).
- Prevent exposure of patient to persons with infection, especially upper respiratory tract infections, and plan nursing interventions to keep patient's expenditure of energy at a minimum.
- Herpes zoster may be precipitated by mechlorethamine treatment and usually necessitates withdrawal of the drug. It occurs commonly in patients with lymphoma.
- Rapid neoplastic cell and leukocyte destruction leads to elevated

serum uric acid (hyperuricemia, see Appendix G) and potential renal urate calculi.

- Preventive measures against incidence of hyperuricemia include increased fluid intake, alkalinizing of urine, and administration of allopurinol.
- Establish baselines for oral care by inspecting oral cavity before chemotherapy begins. Note and record state of hydration of oral mucosa, condition of gingiva, teeth, tongue, mucosa, and lips. If prosthetic devices do not fit properly, record.

Patient & Family Education

- Laboratory studies of peripheral blood are essential guides for determining when to give another course of therapy. Urge patient to keep appointments for clinical evaluation.
- Explain the significance of thrombocytopenia with the development of bleeding tendencies and advise to report any signs of bleeding immediately.
- Warn to use caution to prevent falls or other traumatic injuries, especially during periods of thrombocytopenia.
- Encourage to increase fluid intake up to 3000 ml/d if allowed to minimize risk of renal stones. Urge prompt reporting of symptoms including flank or joint pain, swelling of lower legs and feet, changes in voiding pattern.
- High doses and regional infusion of mechlorethamine increase incidence of tinnitus and deafness. Alert patient to report symptoms promptly.
- Discuss the problem of alopecia (reversible) with the patient. If desired, facilitate cosmetic substitution.
- Encourage frequent oral hygiene. Brush teeth using soft-bristled toothbrush (softened with warm water); if gums are painful, consult physician.
- In presence of ulcerations or dysphagia, avoid hot or cold foods and drinks; avoid spicy, sour, dry, rough, or chunky foods as well as smoking and alcoholic beverages.
- Xerostomia may be relieved by use of a saliva substitute (available OTC) such as Xero-Lube, Moi-Stir, Orex, or Salivart.

MECLIZINE HYDROCHLORIDE

(mek′li-zeen)

Trade names: Antivert, Antrizine, Bonamine✦, Bonine, Dizmiss, Ru-Vert-M

Prototype for classifications: ANTIHISTAMINE; ANTIVERTIGO AGENT; H_1-RECEPTOR ANTAGONIST

Pregnancy category: B

ACTIONS/PHARMACODYNAMICS

Long-acting piperazine antihistamine, structurally and pharmacologically related to cyclizine compounds. Has marked effect in blocking histamine-induced vasopressive response but only slight anticholinergic action. Also exhibits CNS depression, antispasmodic, antiemetic, and local anesthetic activity. Has marked depressant action on labyrinthine excitability and on conduction in vestibular-cerebellar pathways.

USES Management of nausea, vomiting, and dizziness associated with motion sickness and in vertigo associated with diseases affecting vestibular system.

M

ROUTE & DOSAGE

Motion Sickness
Adult: **PO** 25–50 mg 1 h before travel, may repeat q24h if necessary for duration of journey.

Vertigo
Adult: **PO** 25–100 mg/d in divided doses.

PHARMACOKINETICS Absorption: readily absorbed from GI tract. **Onset:** 1 h. **Duration:** 8–24 h. **Distribution:** crosses placenta. **Elimination:** half-life: 6 h; excreted primarily in feces.

CONTRAINDICATIONS & PRECAUTIONS Contraindicated in: pregnancy (category B); and pediatric age group. **Cautious use in:** angle-closure glaucoma, prostatic hypertrophy.

M

ADVERSE/SIDE EFFECTS *Drowsiness,* dry mouth, blurred vision, fatigue.

NURSING IMPLICATIONS

Administration
- Drug may be given without regard to meals.

Assessment & Drug Effects
- Since drug may cause drowsiness, supervision of ambulation, particularly with the elderly, may be warranted.
- When meclizine is prescribed for vertigo, assess effectiveness of drug and inform physician, as dosage adjustment may be required.

Patient & Family Education
- Forewarn about side effects such as drowsiness, and advise not to drive a car or engage in other hazardous activities until reaction to the drug is known.
- Caution that the sedative action may be additive to that of alcohol, barbiturates, narcotic analgesics, or other CNS depressants.
- When meclizine is prescribed for motion sickness, instruct patient to take it 1 h before departure.

MECLOCYCLINE SULFOSALICYLATE

(me-kloe-sye'kleen)
Trade name: Meclan
Classifications: ANTIINFECTIVE; ANTIBIOTIC; TETRACYCLINE
Prototype: Tetracycline
Pregnancy category: B

ACTIONS/PHARMACODYNAMICS Synthetic derivative of oxytetracycline. Antibacterial action appears to be related to ability to suppress growth of susceptible organisms, principally *Propionibacterium acnes,* an anaerobic organism in sebaceous glands and follicles. Inactive against viruses and fungi.

USE Inflammatory acne vulgaris.

ROUTE & DOSAGE

Inflammatory Acne Vulgaris
Adult: **Topical** Apply to affected areas b.i.d., AM and PM.

PHARMACOKINETICS Absorption: not absorbed systemically in measurable amounts.

CONTRAINDICATIONS & PRECAUTIONS Contraindicated in: hypersensitivity to tetracyclines or to any ingredients in the formulation, e.g., formaldehyde. Safe use during pregnancy (category B), in nursing women, and in children < 11 y not established.

ADVERSE/SIDE EFFECTS Skin irritation; stinging, burning sensation; temporary yellow staining of skin around hair follicles (with excessive applications), superinfections.

NURSING IMPLICATIONS

Administration

- Apply cream generously morning and evening over affected skin areas.
- Less frequent applications may be used depending on patient's response.

Assessment & Drug Effects

- Since significant percutaneous absorption may result with prolonged use, carefully monitor patients with renal or hepatic dysfunction.
- Monitor for signs and symptoms of superinfection (see Appendix G).

Patient & Family Education

- Advise to apply medication as directed and to keep follow-up appointments. Overuse of tetracycline preparations can result in overgrowth of nonsusceptible organisms.
- Inform that excessive applications of meclocycline may cause temporary staining around hair roots and also can stain fabrics.
- Avoid use of meclocycline near or in eyes, ears, nose, mouth, or other mucous membranes.
- Advise to notify physician if noticeable improvement has not occurred by 6–8 wk. Maximum benefit may not be apparent for ≤ 12 wk.
- Inform that skin areas treated with meclocycline will fluoresce under ultraviolet light.
- Possibility of cumulative drying or irritant effects can occur with use of abrasive or medicated soaps and cleaners, other topical acne preparations, alcohol-containing preparations (e.g., after-shave astringents, lotions), "cover-up" medications, peeling agents (e.g., benzoyl peroxide, resorcinol, sulfur, salicylic acid, tretinoin). These preparations should be used with caution and only under medical guidance.

MECLOFENAMATE SODIUM

(me-kloe-fen-am′ate)

Trade names: Meclofen, Meclomen

Classifications: CNS AGENT; ANALGESIC; ANTIPYRETIC; NSAID

Prototype: Ibuprofen

Pregnancy category: B (D in third trimester)

ACTIONS/PHARMACODYNAMICS Has palliative antiinflammatory, analgesic, and antipyretic activity. Action mechanism unclear, but animal studies suggest that effects may result from inhibition of prostaglandin synthesis and competition for binding at prostaglandin receptor sites. Does not appear to alter course of arthritis.

USES Symptomatic treatment of acute or chronic rheumatoid arthritis and osteoarthritis. Also in combination with gold salts or corticosteroids in treatment of rheumatoid arthritis. **Unlabeled uses:** management of psoriatic arthritis, mild to moderate postoperative pain, dysmenorrhea.

ROUTE & DOSAGE

Inflammatory Disease

Adult: **PO** 200–400 mg/d in 3–4 divided doses (max 400 mg/d).

PHARMACOKINETICS **Absorption:** rapidly and completely absorbed from GI tract. **Peak:** 1–2 h. **Duration:** 2–4 h. **Distribution:** crosses placenta.

Metabolism: metabolized in liver. **Elimination:** half-life: 2–3.3 h; 60% excreted in urine, 30% in feces.

CONTRAINDICATIONS & PRECAUTIONS **Contraindicated in:** patient in whom bronchospasm, urticaria, and allergic rhinitis are induced by aspirin or other NSAIDS; pregnancy [first trimester (category B) and third trimester (category D)], nursing mothers, children < 14 y, patient designated as functional class IV rheumatoid arthritis (incapacitated, bedridden, or confined to wheelchair, little or no self-care); active peptic ulcer. **Cautious use in:** history of upper GI tract disease; compromised cardiac and renal function, or other conditions predisposing to fluid retention.

M

ADVERSE/SIDE EFFECTS **CNS:** *dizziness,* vertigo, lack of concentration, confusion, *headache,* tinnitus. **CV:** edema. **GI:** *severe diarrhea (dose-related),* peptic ulceration, GI bleeding, dyspepsia, abdominal pain, *nausea,* vomiting (may be severe), flatulence, eructation, pyrosis, anorexia, constipation. **Hepatic:** *abnormal liver function tests,* cholestatic jaundice. **Other:** blurred vision. **Renal:** elevated BUN and creatinine, renal failure. **Skin:** rash, pruritus, urticaria.

DRUG INTERACTIONS ORAL ANTICOAGULANTS, **heparin** may prolong bleeding time; may increase **lithium** toxicity; increases pharmacologic and toxic activity of **phenytoin,** SULFONYLUREAS, SULFONAMIDES, **warfarin** through protein-binding displacement.

NURSING IMPLICATIONS

Administration

- If patient complains of GI distress, suggest administration with food or milk, or an aluminum and magnesium hydroxide antacid (Maalox) may be prescribed. If symptoms persist, the physician should be consulted.
- Store in airtight, light-resistant container at 15–30C (59–86F) unless otherwise directed.

Assessment & Drug Effects

- Clinical improvement in the rheumatoid patient is evidenced within 2–3 wk with reduction in number of tender joints, severity of tenderness, and duration of morning stiffness.
- Improvement in the osteoarthritic patient is reflected by reduced night pain, pain on walking, starting pain, and pain with passive motion and improved joint function.
- With concurrent anticoagulant therapy, monitor PT, PTT, INP frequently.
- Diarrhea is the most frequent adverse effect and is usually dose related.
- Monitor renal function tests. Incidence of adverse reactions is potentially high because the drug is excreted primarily by the kidneys. Monitor I&O ratio. Encourage fluid intake of at least 8 glasses of liquid a day.
- The sodium content of meclofenamate tablets should be considered if the patient is on restricted sodium intake.

Patient & Family Education

- Instruct to stop taking this drug and promptly notify the physician if nausea, vomiting, severe diarrhea, and abdominal pain occur. Generally dose reduction or temporary withdrawal will control symptoms.
- Although incidence of side effects related to special senses is low, instruct to report without delay if blurred vision, tinnitus, or taste disturbances occur.
- Because visual disturbances have been reported with other NSAIDS,

ophthalmic examinations are recommended before and periodically during treatment and whenever patient experiences visual disturbances.

- Women who become pregnant while on meclofenamate therapy should notify physician.
- Patient should be weighed under standard conditions (similar clothing, same time of day) twice weekly. A weight gain of more than 2.5 to 3.5 kg (3–4 lb)/wk should be reported as well as signs of edema: swollen ankles, tibiae, hands, feet.
- Discourage use of OTC drugs without approval of physician.
- Dizziness, a troublesome early side effect, frequently disappears in time. Advise to avoid driving a car or using hazardous equipment until response to drug is known.
- Patient receiving a PO anticoagulant should immediately report any sign of bleeding (e.g., melena, epistaxis, ecchymosis).

MEDROXYPROGESTERONE ACETATE

(me-drox'ee-proe-jess'te-rone)

Trade names: Amen, Cycrin, Depo-Provera, Provera

Classifications: HORMONE; PROGESTIN

Prototype: Progesterone

Pregnancy category: X

ACTIONS/PHARMACODYNAMICS Synthetic derivative of progesterone with prolonged, variable duration of action and androgenic and antiestrogenic activity. Has no deleterious effects on lipid metabolism. Induces and maintains endometrium, preventing uterine bleeding; inhibits production of pituitary gonadotropin, preventing ovulation; and produces thick cervical mucus resistant to passage of sperm.

USES Dysfunctional uterine bleeding; secondary amenorrhea; parenteral form (Depo-Provera) used in adjunctive, palliative treatment of inoperable, recurrent, and metastatic endometrial or renal carcinoma; contraception. **Unlabeled use:** obstructive sleep apnea.

ROUTE & DOSAGE

Secondary Amenorrhea

Adult: **PO** 5–10 mg/d for 5–10 d beginning any time if endometrium is adequately estrogen primed (withdrawal bleeding occurs in 3–7 d after discontinuing therapy).

Abnormal Bleeding due to Hormonal Imbalance

Adult: **PO** 5–10 mg/d for 5–10 d beginning on the assumed or calculated 16th or 21st day of menstrual cycle; if bleeding is controlled, administer 2 subsequent cycles.

Carcinoma

Adult: **IM** 400–1000 mg/wk; continue at 400 mg/mo if improvement occurs and disease stabilizes.

Contraceptive

Adult: **IM** 100 mg q3mo.

CONTRAINDICATIONS & PRECAUTIONS **Contraindicated in:** pregnancy (category X); history of thromboembolic disorders. **Cautious use in:** asthma, seizure disorders, migraine, cardiac or renal dysfunction, liver disease.

ADVERSE/SIDE EFFECTS CNS: cerebral thrombosis or hemorrhage, depression. **CV:** hypertension, pulmonary embolism, edema. **GI:** vomiting, nausea, cholestatic jaundice, abdominal cramps. **Reproductive:** *breakthrough bleeding,* changes in menstrual flow, dysmenorrhea, vaginal candidiasis. **Skin:** angioneurotic edema. **Other:** weight changes; *breast tenderness,* enlargement or secretion.

NURSING IMPLICATIONS

See progesterone for numerous additional nursing implications.

Administration

- Oral drug may be given with food to minimize GI distress.
- Administer IM deep into a large muscle.
- Store at 15–30C (59–86F); protect from freezing.

Assessment & Drug Effects

- IM injection may be painful. Monitor sites for evidence of sterile abscess. A residual lump and discoloration of tissue may develop.
- Monitor for signs and symptoms of thrombophlebitis (see Appendix G).

Patient & Family Education

- After repeated IM injections, infertility and amenorrhea may persist as long as 18 mo.
- Planned menstrual cycling with medroxyprogesterone may benefit the patient with a history of recurrent episodes of abnormal uterine bleeding.
- Teach breast self-examination.
- Discuss package insert to ensure complete understanding of progestin therapy.

MEFENAMIC ACID

(me-fe-nam′ik)

Trade names: Ponstan, Ponstel

Classifications: CNS AGENT; ANALGESIC; ANTIPYRETIC; NSAID

Prototype: Ibuprofen

Pregnancy category: C

ACTIONS/PHARMACODYNAMICS

Anthranilic acid derivative with analgesic, antiinflammatory, and antipyretic actions similar to those of ibuprofen. Like ibuprofen, inhibits prostaglandin synthesis and affects platelet function. No evidence that it is superior to aspirin.

USE Short-term relief of mild to moderate pain including primary dysmenorrhea.

ROUTE & DOSAGE

Mild to Moderate Pain

Adult: **PO** 500 mg loading dose, then 250 mg q6h prn.

PHARMACOKINETICS Absorption: rapidly and completely absorbed from GI tract. **Peak:** 2–4 h. **Duration:** ≤ 6 h. **Distribution:** distributed in breast milk. **Metabolism:** partially metabolized in liver. **Elimination:** half-life: 2 h; 50% excreted in urine, 50% in feces.

CONTRAINDICATIONS & PRECAUTIONS Contraindicated in: hypersensitivity to drug, GI inflammation, or ulceration. Safe use in children < 14 y, during pregnancy (category C), and in nursing mothers not established. **Cautious use in:** history of renal or hepatic disease; blood dyscrasias; asthma; diabetes mellitus; hypersensitivity to aspirin. See also Drug Interactions.

ADVERSE/SIDE EFFECTS CNS: drowsiness, insomnia, dizziness, nervousness, confusion, headache. **GI:** *severe diarrhea,* ulceration, and bleeding; *nausea, vomiting,* abdominal cramps, flatus, constipation. **Hematologic:** prolonged prothrombin time, severe autoimmune hemolytic anemia (long-term use), leukopenia, eosinophilia, agranulocytosis, thrombocytopenic purpura, megaloblastic anemia, pancytopenia, bone marrow hypoplasia. **Renal:** nephrotoxicity, dysuria, albuminuria, hematuria, elevation of BUN. **Skin:** urticaria, rash, facial edema. **Other:** eye irritation, loss of color vision (reversible), blurred vision, ear pain, perspiration, hepatic toxicity, palpitation, dyspnea; acute exacerbation of asthma; bronchoconstriction (in patients sensitive to aspirin).

DIAGNOSTIC TEST INTERFERENCE False-positive reactions for ***urinary bilirubin*** (using diazo tablet test).

DRUG INTERACTIONS Mefenamic acid may prolong bleeding time with ORAL ANTICOAGULANTS, **heparin;** may increase **lithium** toxicity; increases pharmacologic and toxic activity of **phenytoin,** SULFONYLUREAS, SULFONAMIDES, **warfarin** because of protein binding displacement.

NURSING IMPLICATIONS

Administration

- Administer with meals, food, or milk to minimize GI adverse effects.
- Use of drug for a period exceeding 1 wk is not recommended (manufacturer's warning).

Assessment & Drug Effects

- Patients who develop severe diarrhea and vomiting should be assessed for dehydration and electrolyte imbalance.
- Patients on long-term therapy should have periodic blood counts, Hct and Hgb, and renal function tests.

Patient & Family Education

- Mefenamic acid should be discontinued promptly if diarrhea, dark stools, hematemesis, ecchymoses, epistaxis, or rash occur and should not be used thereafter. Advise to report these signs to the physician.
- Advise to notify physician if persistent GI discomfort, sore throat, fever, or malaise occurs.
- Since the drug may cause dizziness and drowsiness, caution to avoid driving a car and other potentially hazardous activities until response to drug is known.
- Diabetic patients may show increased need for insulin.

M

MEFLOQUINE HYDROCHLORIDE

(me-flo′quine)

Trade name: Lariam

Classification: ANTIMALARIAL

Prototype: Chloroquine

Pregnancy category: C

ACTIONS/PHARMACODYNAMICS Mefloquine is an antimalarial agent, structurally related to quinine. Mefloquine is effective against all types of malaria, including chloroquine resistant malaria.

USES Treatment of mild to moderate acute malarial infections, prevention of chloroquine-resistant malaria caused by *Plasmodium falciparum* and *P. vivax.*

ROUTE & DOSAGE

Treatment of Malaria

Adult: **PO** 1250 mg (5 tablets) as single oral dose taken with at least 8 oz of water.

Child: **PO** 20–30 mg/kg as single dose.

Prophylaxis for Malaria

Adult: **PO** 250 mg once a week × 4 wk (beginning 1 wk before travel), then 250 mg every other week for duration of exposure and for 2 doses after leaving endemic area.
Child: **PO** 1/4 tablet for 15–19 kg, 1/2 tablet for 20–30 kg, 3/4 tablet for 31–45 kg. The FDA has not approved the use of mefloquine in children, and the US Public Health Service does not recommend its use in children < 15 kg or in pregnant women.

PHARMACOKINETICS **Absorption:** 85% absorbed, concentrates in red blood cells. **Onset:** 59 and 28 h for parasite and fever clearance times in patients with *P. vivax* infections, respectively; 166 and 93 h in patients with *P. malariae* infections. **Distribution:** concentrated in red blood cells due to high-affinity binding to red blood cell membranes; 98% protein bound; distributed minimally into breast milk. **Metabolism:** metabolized in liver. **Elimination:** half-life: 10–21 d (shorter in patients with acute malaria); eliminated primarily in bile and feces.

CONTRAINDICATIONS & PRECAUTIONS **Contraindicated in:** hypersensitivity to mefloquine or a related compound; with a calcium channel blocking agent, severe heart arrhythmias, psychiatric depression, seizure disorders, pregnancy (category C), infancy. **Cautious use in:** lactation. Safety and efficacy in children not established.

ADVERSE/SIDE EFFECTS **CNS:** dizziness, nightmares, visual disturbances, headache, syncope, confusion, psychosis. **CV:** bradycardia. **GI:** nausea, vomiting. **Skin:** rash, itching.

DIAGNOSTIC TEST INTERFERENCE Transient increase in liver transaminases.

DRUG INTERACTIONS Mefloquine can prolong cardiac conduction in patients taking BETA BLOCKERS, CALCIUM CHANNEL BLOCKERS, and possibly **digoxin. Quinine** may decrease plasma mefloquine concentrations. Mefloquine may decrease **valproic acid** serum concentrations by increasing its hepatic metabolism. Administration with **chloroquine** may increase risk of seizures.

NURSING IMPLICATIONS

Administration

- Administer with food and at least 8 oz water.
- Do not administer concurrently with quinine or quinidine; wait at least 12 h beyond last dose of either drug before administering mefloquine.
- Store at room temperature, 15–30C (59–86F).

Assessment & Drug Effects

- During prophylactic use, carefully monitor for development of unexplained anxiety, depression, restlessness, or confusion; these manifestations may indicate a need to discontinue the drug.
- Cardiac and hepatic functions should be evaluated periodically with prolonged use.
- During prolonged use, periodically monitor CBC with differential.
- Patients on anticonvulsants should have blood levels of these drugs closely monitored while on mefloquine.

Patient & Family Education

- Instruct how to properly take this drug.
- Advise to take drug on the same day each week when used for malaria prophylaxis.
- Caution not to perform hazardous activities until reaction to the drug is known.
- Advise to report any of the following immediately: fever, sore throat, muscle aches, visual problems, anxiety, confusion, mental depression, hallucinations.

MEGESTROL ACETATE

(me-jess'trole)

Trade name: Megace

Classifications: ANTINEOPLASTIC; HORMONE; PROGESTIN

Prototype: Progesterone

Pregnancy category: X

ACTIONS/PHARMACODYNAMICS Progestational hormone with antineoplastic properties. Mechanism of action unclear; however, an antiluteinizing effect mediated via the pituitary has been postulated. Has local effect when instilled directly into the endometrial cavity.

USE Palliative agent for treatment of advanced carcinoma of breast or endometrium. **Unlabeled use:** appetite stimulant in patients with AIDS.

ROUTE & DOSAGE

Palliative Treatment for Advanced Breast Cancer

Adult: **PO** 40 mg q.i.d.

Palliative Treatment for Advanced Endometrial Cancer

Adult: **PO** 40–320 mg/d in divided doses.

Appetite Stimulation

Adult: **PO** 200 mg q6h.

PHARMACOKINETICS Absorption: appears to be well absorbed from GI tract. **Onset:** onset of objective response in breast cancer in 6–8 wk. **Peak:** 1–3 h. **Duration:** 3–12 mo. **Metabolism:** completely metabolized in liver. **Elimination:** 57–78% of dose excreted in urine within 10 d.

CONTRAINDICATIONS & PRECAUTIONS Contraindicated in: diagnostic test for pregnancy; use in neoplastic diseases other than cancer of endometrium and breast; first 4 mo of pregnancy (category X).

ADVERSE/SIDE EFFECTS Vaginal bleeding, breast tenderness, abdominal pain, nausea, vomiting, headache, increased appetite, weight gain, allergic-type reactions (including bronchial asthma), DVT.

NURSING IMPLICATIONS

Administration

- Drug may be given without regard to meals.
- Store in tightly closed container at 15–30C (59–86F) unless otherwise specified.

Assessment & Drug Effects

- Monitor weight periodically.
- Notify physician if abdominal pain, headache, nausea, vomiting, or breast tenderness become pronounced.
- Monitor for allergic reactions, including breathing distress characteristic of asthma, rash, urticaria, anaphylaxis, tachypnea, anxiety. Stop medication if they appear and notify physician.

Patient & Family Education

- Contraception measures are rec-

M

ommended during therapy for carcinoma with megestrol.

- Teach breast self-examination.
- Teach S&S of thrombophlebitis (see Appendix G).
- Discuss package insert to ensure understanding of megestrol therapy.

MELPHALAN

(mel'fa-lan)

Trade names: Alkeran, L-Pam, Phenylalanine Mustard, Alkeran IV

Classifications: ANTINEOPLASTIC; ALKYLATING AGENT

Prototype: Mechlorethamine

Pregnancy category: D

M

ACTIONS/PHARMACODYNAMICS Nitrogen mustard chemically and pharmacologically related to mechlorethamine. Has strong immunosuppressive and myelosuppressive effects but, unlike mechlorethamine, lacks vesicant propertes. Carcinogenic potential suspected.

USES Chiefly for palliative treatment of multiple myeloma. Also many other neoplasms, including Hodgkin's disease and carcinomas of breast and ovary. **Unlabeled use:** polycythemia vera.

ROUTE & DOSAGE

Multiple Myeloma

Adult: **PO** 6 mg/d for 2–3 wk; drug is then withdrawn for 4–5 wk; when WBC and platelet counts start to rise, restart at 2 mg/d. **IV** 16 mg/m^2 over 15 min q2wk for 4 doses.

Epithelial Ovarian Cancer

Adult: **PO** 0.2 mg/kg/d in divided doses for 5 d as single course; may repeat course q4–5 wk, depending on hematologic tolerance.

PHARMACOKINETICS Absorption: incompletely and variably absorbed from GI tract. **Peak:** 2 h. **Distribution:** widely distributed to all tissues. **Metabolism:** metabolized by spontaneous hydrolysis in plasma. **Elimination:** half-life: 1.5 h; 25–30% excreted in urine, 25–50% excreted in feces.

CONTRAINDICATIONS & PRECAUTIONS Contraindicated in: use during pregnancy (category D) or in men and women of childbearing age not established. **Cautious use in:** recent treatment with other chemotherapeutic agent; concurrent administration with radiation therapy; severe anemia, neutropenia, or thrombocytopenia, impaired renal function.

ADVERSE/SIDE EFFECTS Hematologic: leukopenia, agranulocytosis, thrombocytopenia, anemia, acute nonlymphatic leukemia. **Other:** uremia, angioneurotic peripheral edema, nausea, vomiting, stomatitis, temporary alopecia, pulmonary fibrosis.

DRUG INTERACTIONS Increases risk of nephrotoxicity with **cyclosporine.**

INCOMPATIBILITIES Y-site: amphotericin B, chlorpromazine.

NURSING IMPLICATIONS

Administration

- IV preparation: Reconstitute melphalan powder by *rapidly* injecting 10 ml of the diluent provided into the vial to produce a concentration of 5 mg/ml. Shake vigorously until clear. Immediately dilute further with 0.9% NaCl injection to a concentration of 0.45 mg/ml or less.

- IV administration: Infuse diluted solution over at least 15 min. Administration *must* be completed within 60 min of reconstitution of drug, because both reconstituted and diluted solutions are unstable.
- Do not refrigerate reconstituted solution.
- Administer PO drug with meals to reduce nausea and vomiting. An antiemetic may be ordered.
- Store in light-resistant, airtight containers at 15–30C (59–86F) unless otherwise directed.

Assessment & Drug Effects

- Monitor WBC and platelet counts are done 2–3 times/wk during dosage adjustment period; WBC is usually determined each week for 6–8 wk during maintenance therapy.
- Monitor laboratory reports to anticipate leukopenic and thrombocytopenic periods.
- A degree of myelosuppression is maintained during therapy so as to keep leukocyte count in range of 3000–3500/mm^3.
- Monitor serum uric acid levels and keep physician informed. Flank and joint pains may signal onset of hyperuricemia.

Patient & Family Education

- A favorable response to oral melphalan in patients with multiple myeloma may be gradual over many months.
- Instruct to be alert to onset of fever, profound weakness, chills, tachycardia, cough, sore throat, changes in kidney function, or prolonged infections and report them to physician.
- Inform that reversible alopecia is an expected side effect.

MENADIOL SODIUM DIPHOSPHATE (VITAMIN K_4)

(men-a-dye′ole)

Trade name: Synkayvite

Classification: VITAMIN K_4

Pregnancy category: C (X near term)

ACTIONS/PHARMACODYNAMICS

Synthetic, water-soluble analog of vitamin K analog derived from menadione. Has same actions, uses, contraindications, precautions, and adverse reactions as menadione but is about one-half as potent. Like menadione, it does not counteract action of heparin. In combination with radiotherapy, it may selectively increase radiosensitivity of tumor cells through an unknown action. Also reported to reduce adenosine triphosphate level in tumor cells.

USE Prevention and treatment of hypoprothrombinemia caused by vitamin K deficiency.

ROUTE & DOSAGE

Prevention and Treatment of Vitamin K Deficiency

Adult: **PO/SC/IM/IV** 5–15 mg/d.

PHARMACOKINETICS **Absorption:** readily absorbed from GI tract; converted to menadione in body. **Onset:** 1–2 h SC, IM.

ADVERSE/SIDE EFFECTS Nausea, vomiting, allergic reaction; pruritus, urticaria, rash.

NURSING IMPLICATIONS

Administration

- Menadiol may be given IV undiluted at a rate of a single dose over 60 seconds.
- It may be added to most IV infusion solutions.

- Store in tight, light-resistant containers at 15–30C (59–86F) unless otherwise directed.

Assessment & Drug Effects
- Dosage and duration of treatment are determined by prothrombin times and clinical response.
- Solutions of menadiol sodium diphosphate may be irritating to skin; monitor injection sites.

MENOTROPINS
(men-oh-troe′pins)
Trade names: Pergonal, Repronex
Classifications: HORMONE; GONADOTROPIN
Pregnancy category: X

M

ACTIONS/PHARMACODYNAMICS
Purified preparation of exogenous gonadotropins, extracted from human menopausal urinary gonadotropin and standardized biologically for follicle-stimulating hormone (FSH) and luteinizing hormone (LH) gonadotropic activities. Promotes growth of graafian follicles in women who do not have primary anovulation. With clinical proof of follicular maturation, ovulation is induced by menotropins followed by administration of human chorionic gonadotropin (HCG). Stimulates spermatogenesis in men with primary or secondary hypogonadotropic hypogonadism after pretreatment with HCG.

USES With HCG (in sequence) to induce ovulation and pregnancy in the infertile woman with functional anovulation (i.e., secondary to pituitary insufficiency). Also used in conjunction with HCG to treat male infertility.

ROUTE & DOSAGE

Induction of Ovulation
Adult: **IM** 1 ampul (75 IU of FSH and LH) daily for 9–12 d, followed by HCG 1 d after last dose of menotropins. If ovulation occurs without pregnancy, regimen may be repeated twice at same dosage before increasing dose to 2 ampuls daily continuing as before. If ovulation occurs without pregnancy, treatment may be repeated at monthly intervals for 2 more courses.

Stimulation of Spermatogenesis
Adult: **IM** Following pretreatment with HCG, 1 ampul 3 times/wk and 2000 U HCG 2 times/wk until detection of spermatozoa in the ejaculate (4–6 mo). If spermatogenesis does not increase, continue treatments or increase to 2 ampuls 3 times/wk.

PHARMACOKINETICS Distribution: testes in males, ovaries in females. **Elimination:** 8% excreted in urine within 24 h.

CONTRAINDICATIONS & PRECAUTIONS Contraindicated in: pregnancy (category X), primary anovulation; thyroid and adrenal dysfunction; organic intracranial lesion; infertility caused by factors other than anovulation; abnormal bleeding of unknown origin, ovarian cysts or enlargement not due to polycystic ovary syndrome; men with normal urinary gonadotropin concentrations, or primary testicular failure.

ADVERSE/SIDE EFFECTS Dose related: mild to *moderate ovarian enlargement,* abdominal distention and pain, ovarian hyperstimulation syndrome (sudden ovarian enlargement accompanied by ascites with or without pain or pleural effusion), hemoperitoneum, fever, nausea, vomiting, diarrhea, hypovolemia, multiple ovulations, follicular cysts, birth defects; gynecomastia (men).

NURSING IMPLICATIONS

Administration

- Drug is prepared immediately before administration by dissolving ampul contents in 1–2 ml of sterile NaCl injection. Unused portion should be discarded.
- When total estrogen excretion level is more than 100 μg/24 h, HCG is not administered because hyperstimulation syndrome is more likely to occur.

Assessment & Drug Effects

- Treatment for men is preceded by at least 4–6 mo of HCG or until normal serum testosterone concentration is achieved.
- Most reliable index of follicular maturation (estrogenic activity) is the rate of urinary estrogen excretion. Other indirect estimates include serial examination of vaginal smears and cervical mucus specimens.
- Patient should be examined frequently for 2 wk after HCG injection to detect excessive ovarian stimulation.
- Hyperstimulation syndrome, which generally occurs within 2 wk after initiation of treatment, develops rapidly over 3–4 d. This syndrome is an indication for discontinuation of treatment and hospitalization of patient.

Patient & Family Education

- Teach to recognize indirect indices of progesterone production: rise in basal body temperature (BBT), menstruation following shift in BBT, increased volume of thin and watery vaginal secretion.
- The couple should be encouraged to have intercourse daily beginning on day before administration of HCG until ovulation becomes apparent from indices of progestational activity.
- Warn to report immediately symptoms of hyperstimulation syndrome: abdominal distention and pain, dyspnea, vaginal bleeding.
- Advise to weigh herself every other day to detect sudden weight gain. Patient should understand the range of weight gain to be reported to physician.
- Mild ovarian enlargement (with or without abdominal distention and pain) usually regresses without treatment in 2–3 wk.
- Generally, pregnancy occurs within 4–6 courses of therapy.
- For the man receiving menotropin therapy, if there is no evidence of increased spermatogenesis after 4 mo, therapy can continue with increased dosage of menotropins.

MEPERIDINE HYDROCHLORIDE

(me-per′i-deen)

Trade names: Demerol, Pethadol♣, Pethidine Hydrochloride♣

Classifications: CNS AGENT; NARCOTIC (OPIATE) AGONIST ANALGESIC

Prototype: Morphine

Pregnancy category: B (D at term)

Controlled substance: Schedule II

ACTIONS/PHARMACODYNAMICS

Synthetic morphine-like compound. Chemically dissimilar to morphine, but in equianalgesic doses it is qualitatively comparable. Usual doses produce either no pupillary change or slight miosis, but overdosage results in marked miosis or mydriasis. Also, unlike morphine, has little or no antidiarrheic or antitussive action and produces CNS stimulation in toxic doses.

USES Relief of moderate to severe pain, for preoperative medication, for support of anesthesia, and for obstetric analgesia.

ROUTE & DOSAGE

Moderate to Severe Pain

Adult: **PO/SC/IM/IV** 50–150 mg q3–4h prn.
Child: **PO/SC/IM/IV** 1–1.5 mg/kg q3–4h (max ≤ 100 mg q4h) prn.

Preoperative

Adult: **IM/SC** 50–150 mg 30–90 min before surgery.
Child: **IM/SC** 1–2.2 mg/kg 30–90 min before surgery.

Obstetric Analgesia

Adult: **IM/SC** 50–100 mg when pains become regular; may be repeated q1–3h.

M

PHARMACOKINETICS Absorption: 50–60% absorbed from GI tract. **Onset:** 15 min PO; 10 min IM, SC; 5 min IV. **Peak:** 1 h PO, IM, SC. **Duration:** 2–4 h PO, IM, SC; 2 h IV. **Distribution:** crosses placenta; distributed into breast milk. **Metabolism:** metabolized in liver. **Elimination:** half-life: 3–5 h; excreted in urine.

CONTRAINDICATIONS & PRECAUTIONS Contraindicated in: hypersensitivity to meperidine, convulsive disorders, acute abdominal conditions prior to diagnosis, pregnancy prior to labor (category B), at term (category D), nursing mothers. **Cautious use in:** head injuries, increased intracranial pressure, asthma and other respiratory conditions, supraventricular tachycardias, prostatic hypertrophy, urethral stricture, glaucoma, elderly or debilitated patients, impaired renal or hepatic function, hypothyroidism, Addison's disease.

ADVERSE/SIDE EFFECTS Allergic: *pruritus,* urticaria, skin rashes, wheal and flare over IV site. **CNS:** *dizziness,* weakness, euphoria, dysphoria, *sedation,* headache, uncoordinated muscle movements, disorientation, decreased cough reflex, miosis, corneal anesthesia, respiratory depression. Toxic doses: muscle twitching, tremors, hyperactive reflexes, excitement, hypersensitivity to external stimuli, agitation, confusion, hallucinations, dilated pupils, convulsions. **CV:** facial flushing, light-headedness, hypotension, syncope, palpitation, bradycardia, tachycardia, cardiovascular collapse, cardiac arrest (toxic doses). **GI:** dry mouth, *nausea,* vomiting, *constipation,* biliary tract spasm. **Other:** oliguria, urinary retention, profuse perspiration, respiratory depression in newborn, bronchoconstriction (large doses), phlebitis (following IV use), pain, tissue irritation and induration, particularly following subcutaneous injection; increased levels of serum amylase, BSP retention, bilirubin, AST, ALT.

DIAGNOSTIC TEST INTERFERENCE High doses of meperidine may interfere with ***gastric emptying studies*** by causing delay in gastric emptying.

DRUG INTERACTIONS Alcohol and other CNS DEPRESSANTS, **cimetidine** cause additive sedation and CNS DEPRESSION; AMPHETAMINES may potentiate CNS STIMULATION; MAO INHIBITORS, **selegiline, furazolidone** may cause excessive and prolonged CNS depression, convulsions, cardiovascular collapse; **phenytoin** may increase toxic meperidine metabolites.

INCOMPATIBILITIES Solution/additive: aminophylline, BARBITURATES, **heparin, methicillin, morphine, phenytoin, sodium bicarbonate. Y-site: cefoperazone, heparin, mezlocillin, minocycline, tetracycline.**

NURSING IMPLICATIONS

Administration

- The syrup formulation should be taken in half a glass of water. Undiluted syrup may cause topical anesthesia of mucous membranes.
- SC route is painful and can cause local irritation. The IM route is generally preferred when repeated doses are required.
- Carefully aspirate before giving IM injection to avoid inadvertent IV administration. IV injection of undiluted drug can cause a marked increase in heart rate and syncope.
- IV injection: When meperidine is given by direct IV, dilute 50 mg in a minimum of 5 ml of NS or sterile water to yield 10 mg/ml. Inject it slowly at a rate not to exceed 25 mg/min. Slower injection preferred.
- IV infusion: When meperidine is given by continuous infusion, dilute it to a concentration of 1–10 mg/ml in NS, D5W, or other compatible solution. Infusion rate should not exceed 25 mg/min. Slower rate is preferred.
- IV administration to infants, children: Verify correct IV concentration and rate of infusion/injection with physician.
- Preserved in tightly closed, light-resistant containers preferably between 15–30C (59–86F), unless otherwise directed by manufacturer.

Assessment & Drug Effects

- Narcotic analgesics should be given in the smallest effective dose and for the least period of time compatible with patient's needs.
- Assess patient's need for prn medication. Record time of onset, duration, and quality of pain.
- In patients receiving repeated doses, note respiratory rate, depth, and rhythm and size of pupils. If respirations are 12/min or below and pupils are constricted or dilated (see actions and uses) or breathing is shallow, or if signs of CNS hyperactivity are present, consult physician before administering drug.
- Vital signs should be monitored closely. Heart rate may increase markedly, and hypotension may occur. Meperidine may cause severe hypotension in postoperative patients and those with depleted blood volume.
- Deep breathing, coughing (unless contraindicated), and changes in position at scheduled intervals may help to overcome the respiratory depressant effects of meperidine.
- Parenteral administration has caused corneal anesthesia and thus abolishment of corneal reflex in some patients. Be alert for this possibility.
- Chart the patient's response to meperidine and evaluate continued need for the drug. Suggest to physician a change to a milder analgesic when in your judgment it is indicated.
- Repeated use of meperidine can lead to tolerance and psychic and physical dependence of the morphine type.
- Abrupt discontinuation of meperidine following repeated use results in morphine-like withdrawal symptoms. Symptoms develop more rapidly (within 3 h, peaking in 8–12 h) and are of shorter duration than with morphine. Nausea, vomiting, diarrhea, and pupillary

M

dilatation are less prominent, but muscle twitching, restlessness, and nervousness are greater than produced by morphine.

Patient & Family Education

- Caution not to smoke and not to ambulate without assistance after receiving the drug. Side rails are advisable.
- Ambulatory patients are more likely than supine patients to manifest nausea, vomiting, dizziness, and faintness associated with fall in BP (these symptoms may also occur in patients without pain who are given meperidine). Symptoms are lessened by the recumbent position and aggravated by the head-up position.
- Caution ambulatory patients to avoid driving a car or engaging in other hazardous activities until any drowsiness and dizziness have passed.
- Caution not to take other CNS depressants or ingest alcohol because of their additive effects.

M

MEPHENTERMINE SULFATE

(me-fen′ter-meen)

Trade name: Wyamine

Classifications: AUTONOMIC NERVOUS SYSTEM AGENT; BETA-ADRENERGIC AGONIST (SYMPATHOMIMETIC)

Prototype: Isoproterenol

Pregnancy category: D

ACTIONS/PHARMACODYNAMICS Synthetic sympathomimetic with alpha- and predominant beta-adrenergic activity. Acts directly and chiefly indirectly by releasing norepinephrine from tissue storage sites. Elevation of blood pressure results primarily from positive inotropic action and increased cardiac output, and to lesser extent from increase in peripheral resistance caused by peripheral vasoconstriction. Heart rate may be reflexly slowed. Antiarrhythmic action results from decrease in AV conduction time, atrial refractory period, and conduction time in ventricular muscle.

USES Mainly as pressor agent in treatment of hypotension secondary to ganglionic blockade or spinal anesthesia. Also has been used as an emergency measure in therapy of shock secondary to hemorrhage until whole blood replacement is available; as adjunct in treatment of cardiogenic shock, and to abolish certain cardiac arrhythmias.

ROUTE & DOSAGE

Hypotension

Adult: **IM/IV** 10–80 mg.
Child: **IM/IV** 0.4 mg/kg.

Hypotensive Emergency

Adult: **IV** 20–60 mg as an IV infusion (1.2 mg/ml in D5W).

PHARMACOKINETICS **Onset:** 5–15 min IM; immediate IV. **Duration:** 1–4 h IM; 15–30 min IV. **Metabolism:** rapidly metabolized in liver. **Elimination:** excreted in urine.

CONTRAINDICATIONS & PRECAUTIONS **Contraindicated in:** shock secondary to hemorrhage (except in emergency). Safe use during pregnancy (category D) or lactation not established. **Cautious use in:** arteriosclerosis, cardiovascular disease, hypovolemia, hypertension, hyperthyroidism, patients with known hypersensitivities, chronically ill patients.

ADVERSE/SIDE EFFECTS **CNS:** euphoria, anorexia, weeping, nervousness, anxiety, tremor, seizures.

CV: tachycardia. With large doses: cardiac arrhythmias, marked elevation of blood pressure, incoherence, drowsiness.

DRUG INTERACTIONS Mephentermine may be ineffective in patients receiving **reserpine, guanethidine**, PHENOTHIAZINES; MAO INHIBITORS, SYMPATHOMIMETIC AMINES, **furazolidone, isoniazid** may potentiate pressor response; **methyldopa,** TRICYCLIC ANTIDEPRESSANTS may potentiate or inhibit pressor response; **cyclopropane, halothane** may cause serious arrhythmia; may increase risk of **digoxin**-induced arrhythmias.

INCOMPATIBILITIES Solution/additive: epinephrine, hydralazine.

NURSING IMPLICATIONS

Administration

- Mephentermine may be given by direct IV undiluted at a rate of 30 mg/min. It may be further diluted by adding 600 mg to 50 ml of D5W and infused at a rate of 1–5 mg/min. IV flow rate is usually prescribed by physician.
- Mephentermine is incompatible with epinephrine hydrochloride and hydralazine hydrochloride.
- Preserved in tightly closed, light-resistant containers preferably at 15–30C (59–86F), unless otherwise directed by manufacturer.

Assessment & Drug Effects

- Close observation and monitoring of BP, HR, ECG, and CVP are essential.
- During IV administration, check BP and pulse q2min until stabilized at prescribed level, then q5min thereafter during therapy. Continue monitoring vital signs for at least 45–60 min and longer if indicated after therapy.

MEPHENYTOIN

(me-fen′i-toyn)
Trade name: Mesantoin
Classifications: CNS AGENT; HYDANTOIN ANTICONVULSANT
Prototype: Phenytoin
Pregnancy category: D

ACTIONS/PHARMACODYNAMICS Reported to have lower incidence of ataxia, gingival hyperplasia, gastric distress, and hirsutism, but produces more sedative and hypnotic action than phenytoin; causes serious toxic reactions, including fatal blood dyscrasias, more frequently. Relatively ineffective for petit mal seizures.

USES Control of grand mal, focal, jacksonian, and psychomotor seizures in patients refractory to less toxic anticonvulsants. Usually used concomitantly with other antiepilepsy agents.

ROUTE & DOSAGE

Seizures

Adult: **PO** 50–100 mg/d during first week, increase weekly to 200–600 mg/d in 3 divided doses.
Child: **PO** 3–15 mg/kg/d in 3 divided doses, increase weekly to 100–400 mg/d in 3 divided doses.

PHARMACOKINETICS Absorption: readily absorbed from GI tract. **Onset:** 30 min. **Duration:** 24–48 h. **Metabolism:** metabolized in liver. **Elimination:** half-life: 144 h; excreted in urine.

CONTRAINDICATIONS & PRECAUTIONS Contraindicated in: use in conjunction with oxazolidinedione anticonvulsant agents, e.g., paramethadione, trimethadione (toxic synergism). Safe use during pregnancy (category D) not established.

Cautious use in: history of drug hypersensitivities.

ADVERSE/SIDE EFFECTS CNS: drowsiness, dizziness. **Dermatologic:** skin and mucous membrane manifestations (exfoliative dermatitis, erythema multiforme, toxic epidermal necrolysis, other skin rashes). **Hematologic:** blood dyscrasias: leukopenia, neutropenia, agranulocytosis, thrombocytopenia, aplastic anemia. **Other:** hepatic damage, periarteritis nodosa, systemic lupus erythematosus syndrome.

DRUG INTERACTIONS See phenytoin.

DIAGNOSTIC TEST INTERFERENCE See phenytoin.

NURSING IMPLICATIONS

Administration

- Mephenytoin may be given with food to reduce GI distress.
- Dose should not be increased until it is taken for at least 1 wk.
- Change from another anticonvulsant agent to mephenytoin is accomplished gradually by increasing dose at weekly intervals and reducing dose of drug to be discontinued over 3–6 wk.

Assessment & Drug Effects

- Patients should be kept under close supervision at all times, as drug is associated with severe adverse effects. Serious blood dyscrasias have occurred 2 wk–30 mo after initiation of therapy.
- Screening tests of liver function, total white cell count, and differential count should precede initiation of therapy.
- Blood studies should be performed q2wk and should be continued until patient is on maintenance dosage for 2 wk; then they should be repeated monthly for 1 y, and thereafter every 3 mo (unless neutrophil count drops to 2500/mm^3 or 1600/mm^3, then performed every 2 wk).
- Medication should be discontinued if neutrophil count falls to 1600/mm^3.

Patient & Family Education

- When mephenytoin replaces another antiepilepsy agent, the dosage of mephenytoin should be gradually increased while the drug being discontinued is gradually decreased over period of 3–6 wk.
- Caution to avoid hazardous activities until reactions to the drug have been determined. Supervision of ambulation and side rails may be indicated for some patients during early therapy.
- Advise to report immediately the onset of drowsiness, ataxia, skin rash, sore throat, fever, mucous membrane bleeding, or glandular swelling. All are indications of developing toxic reaction.
- Discontinuation of mephenytoin should be accomplished gradually to minimize the risk of precipitating seizures or status epilepticus.

MEPHOBARBITAL

(me-foe-bar'bi-tal)

Trade names: Mebaral, Methylphenobarbital

Classifications: CNS AGENT; BARBITURATE; ANTICONVULSANT; SEDATIVE-HYPNOTIC

Prototype: Phenobarbital

Pregnancy category: D

Controlled substance: Schedule IV

ACTIONS/PHARMACODYNAMICS Long-acting barbiturate with pharmacologic properties similar to those of phenobarbital; however, larger doses are required to produce comparable anticonvulsant effects.

Exerts strong sedative action, but relatively mild hypnotic effect.

USES To control grand mal and petit mal epilepsy, alone or in combination with other anticonvulsant agents, and for sedative effect in management of delirium tremens and other acute agitation and anxiety states.

ROUTE & DOSAGE

Anticonvulsant

Adult: **PO** 400–600 mg/d in divided doses.
Child: **PO** ≤ *5 y,* 16–32 mg t.i.d. or q.i.d.; ≥ *5 y,* 32–64 mg t.i.d. or q.i.d.

Sedative

Adult: **PO** 32–100 mg t.i.d. or q.i.d.
Child: **PO** ≤ *5 y,* 16–32 mg t.i.d. or q.i.d.; ≥ *5 y,* 32–64 mg t.i.d. or q.i.d.

Delirium Tremens

Adult: **PO** 200 mg t.i.d. or q.i.d.

PHARMACOKINETICS Absorption: 50% absorbed from GI tract. **Onset:** 60 min. **Duration:** 10–12 h. **Metabolism:** metabolized in liver to phenobarbital. **Elimination:** half-life: 34 h; excreted in urine. Alkalinization of urine or increase of urinary flow significantly increases the rate of phenobarbital excretion.

CONTRAINDICATIONS & PRECAUTIONS Contraindicated in: hypersensitivity to barbiturates. Safe use during pregnancy (category D) not established. **Cautious use in:** fever, hyperthyroidism, alcoholism; hepatic, renal, or cardiac dysfunction.

ADVERSE/SIDE EFFECTS CNS: *drowsiness,* dizziness, unsteadiness, hangover, paradoxical excitement. **GI:** nausea, vomiting, constipation. **Other:** hypersensitivity reactions, respiratory depression.

DRUG INTERACTIONS See phenobarbital.

NURSING IMPLICATIONS

Administration

- Change from other anticonvulsant to mephobarbital should be accomplished by gradually tapering off the former as mephobarbital doses are increased to maintain seizure control.
- When mephobarbital is prescribed concurrently with phenobarbital, the dose should be about one-half the amount of each used alone. When prescribed concurrently with phenytoin, the dose of phenytoin is usually reduced.
- When mephobarbital anticonvulsant therapy is to be discontinued, dosage should be reduced gradually over 4 or 5 days to avoid precipitating seizures of status epilepticus.

Assessment & Drug Effects

- Monitor respiratory status, especially with concurrent CNS therapy with other drug.
- The elderly or debilitated and children sometimes have a paradoxical response to barbiturate therapy, i.e., irritability, marked excitement (aggression in children), depression, and confusion.

Patient & Family Education

- Abrupt cessation after prolonged mephobarbital therapy may result in withdrawal symptoms (tremulousness, weakness, insomnia, delirium, convulsions).
- Caution to avoid hazardous activities such as driving a car until response to drug has stabilized.
- Alcohol in any amount should not be taken with a barbiturate.

MEPROBAMATE

(me-proe-ba'mate)

Trade names: Equanil, Meprospan, Miltown

Prototype for classifications: CNS AGENT; PSYCHOTHERAPEUTIC; CARBAMATE ANXIOLYTIC; SEDATIVE-HYPNOTIC

Pregnancy category: D

Controlled substance: Schedule IV

ACTIONS/PHARMACODYNAMICS Propanediol carbamate derivative structurally and pharmacologically related to carisoprodol. CNS depressant actions similar to those of barbiturates. Acts on multiple sites in CNS and appears to block corticothalamic impulses. Has no effect on medulla, reticular activating system, or autonomic nervous system. Hypnotic doses suppress REM sleep.

M

USES To relieve anxiety and tension of psychoneurotic states and as adjunct in disease states associated with anxiety and tension. Also used to promote sleep in anxious, tense patients.

ROUTE & DOSAGE

Sedative

Adult: **PO** 1.2–1.6 g/d in 3–4 divided doses (max 2.4 g/d).
Child: **PO** 100–200 mg b.i.d. or t.i.d.

Hypnotic

Adult: **PO** 400–800 mg.
Geriatric: **PO** 200 mg 2–3 times/d.
Child: **PO** 200 mg.

PHARMACOKINETICS **Absorption:** well absorbed from GI tract. **Peak:** 1–3 h. **Onset:** 1 h. **Distribution:** uniformly distributed throughout body; crosses placenta. **Metabolism:** rapidly metabolized in liver. **Elimination:** half-life: 10–11 h; renally excreted; excreted in breast milk.

CONTRAINDICATIONS & PRECAUTIONS **Contraindicated in:** history of hypersensitivity to meprobamate or related carbamates such as carisoprodol and tybamate; history of acute intermittent porphyria; pregnancy (category D), nursing women, children <6 y. **Cautious use in:** impaired renal or hepatic function; convulsive disorders; history of alcoholism or drug abuse; patients with suicidal tendencies.

ADVERSE/SIDE EFFECTS **Allergy or idiosyncrasy:** itchy, urticarial, or erythematous maculopapular rash; exfoliative dermatitis, petechiae, purpura, ecchymoses, eosinophilia, peripheral edema, angioneurotic edema, adenopathy, fever, chills, proctitis, bronchospasm, oliguria, anuria, Stevens-Johnson syndrome; anaphylaxis. **CNS:** *drowsiness and ataxia,* dizziness, vertigo, slurred speech, headache, weakness, paresthesias, impaired visual accommodation, paradoxic euphoria and rage reactions, seizures in epileptics, panic reaction, rapid EEG activity. **CV:** hypotensive crisis, syncope, palpitation, tachycardia, arrhythmias, transient ECG changes. **GI:** anorexia, nausea, vomiting, diarrhea. **Hematologic** (rare): aplastic anemia (rare): leukopenia, agranulocytosis, thrombocytopenia. **Other:** exacerbation of acute intermittent porphyria, grand mal attack, respiratory depression, and circulatory collapse (toxic doses).

DIAGNOSTIC TEST INTERFERENCE Meprobamate may cause falsely high ***urinary steroid*** determinations. ***Phentolamine*** tests may be falsely positive; meprobamate should be withdrawn at least 24 h and preferably 48–72 h before the test.

DRUG INTERACTIONS **Alcohol** and other CNS DEPRESSANTS potentiate CNS depression.

NURSING IMPLICATIONS

Administration

- Meprobamate may be administered with food to minimize gastric distress.
- Treatment of meprobamate physical dependence consists of gradual drug withdrawal over 1–2 wk to prevent onset of withdrawal symptoms.
- Store drug at 15–30C (59–86F), unless otherwise specified by manufacturer.

Assessment & Drug Effects

- The elderly and debilitated patients are prone to oversedation and to the hypotensive effects of meprobamate, especially during early therapy.
- Caution to make position changes slowly, especially from recumbent to upright, and to dangle legs for a few minutes before standing. Supervise ambulation, if necessary.
- Hypnotic doses may cause increased motor activity during sleep. Side rails are advisable for hospitalized patients.
- If daytime psychomotor function is impaired, consult physician. A change in regimen or drug may be indicated.
- Psychic or physical dependence may occur with long-term use of high doses.
- Sudden withdrawal in physically dependent patients may precipitate preexisting symptoms or withdrawal reactions within 12–48 h: vomiting, ataxia, muscle twitching, mental confusion, hallucinations, convulsions, trembling, sleep disturbances, increased dreaming, nightmares, insomnia. Symptoms usually subside within 12–48 h.

Patient & Family Education

- Warn that tolerance to alcohol will be lowered.
- Caution to avoid driving a car or engaging in other hazardous activities until drug response has been determined.
- Instruct to report immediately onset of skin rash, sore throat, fever, bruising, unexplained bleeding.
- Instruct to take drug as prescribed.

MERCAPTOPURINE (6-MP, 6-MERCAPTOPURINE)

(mer-kap-toe-pyoor′een)

Trade name: Purinethol

Classifications: ANTINEOPLASTIC; ANTIMETABOLITE; IMMUNOSUPPRESSANT

Prototype: Fluorouracil

Pregnancy category: D

ACTIONS/PHARMACODYNAMICS

Antimetabolite and purine antagonist. Inhibits purine metabolism by unclear mechanism. Blocks conversion of inosinic acid to adenine and xanthine ribotides within sensitive tumor cells. Also inhibits adenine-containing coenzymes, suggesting an influence over multiple cellular reactions. Has delayed immunosuppressive properties and carcinogenic potential.

USES Primarily for acute lymphocytic and myelogenous leukemia. Response in adults is less than in children, but mercaptopurine is initial drug of choice. In chronic granulocytic leukemia, produces temporary remission. **Unlabeled uses:** prevention of transplant graft rejection; SLE; rheumatoid arthritis; Crohn's disease.

ROUTE & DOSAGE

Leukemias

Adult: **PO** 2.5 mg/kg/d; may increase up to 5 mg/kg/d after 4 wk if needed. **Maintenance dose:** 1.25–2.5 mg/kg/d.
Child: **PO** Same as for adult.

PHARMACOKINETICS Absorption: approximately 50% absorbed from GI tract. **Peak:** 2 h. **Distribution:** distributes into total body water. **Metabolism:** rapidly metabolized by xanthine oxidase in liver. **Elimination:** half-life: 20–50 min; 11% excreted in urine within 6 h.

CONTRAINDICATIONS & PRECAUTIONS Contraindicated in: prior resistance to mercaptopurine; first trimester of pregnancy (category D), infections. **Cautious use in:** impaired renal or hepatic function; concomitant use with allopurinol.

M

ADVERSE/SIDE EFFECTS GI: stomatitis, esophagitis, anorexia, nausea, vomiting, diarrhea, intestinal ulcerations. **Hematologic:** leukopenia, anemia, eosinophilia, pancytopenia, thrombocytopenia, abnormal bleeding, bone marrow hypoplasia. **Other:** impaired liver function, hyperuricemia, skin rash, oliguria, renal impairment, drug fever, hepatic necrosis.

DRUG INTERACTIONS Allopurinol may inhibit metabolism and thus increase toxicity of mercaptopurine; may potentiate or antagonize anticoagulant effects of **warfarin.**

NURSING IMPLICATIONS

Administration

- The most effective dose with optimum therapeutic effect and least toxicity varies from patient to patient. Therefore careful titration of dosage is necessary.
- The total daily dose may be given at one time.
- The dose of mercaptopurine is usually reduced by 1/3–1/4 when allopurinol in given concurrently.
- Store tablets in light- and air-resistant container.

Assessment & Drug Effects

- Closely monitor CBC with differential, platelet count, Hgb, and Hct.
- Drug should be discontinued at the first sign of an abnormally large or rapid fall in platelet and leukocyte count. Notify physician.
- Record baseline data related to I&O ratio and pattern and body weight.
- Weigh patient under standard conditions once weekly and record weight.
- Check vital signs daily. Report febrile states promptly.
- During periods of leukopenia, protect patient from exposure to trauma, infections, or other stresses (restrict visitors and personnel who have colds).
- Nausea, vomiting, and diarrhea may signal excessive dosage, especially in adults.
- If thrombocytopenia develops, watch for signs of abnormal bleeding (ecchymoses, petechiae, melena, bleeding gums); report them immediately.
- Monitor liver function tests. Hepatic toxicity occurs most often when dose exceeds 2.5 mg/kg/d. Jaundice signals onset of hepatic toxicity and may necessitate terminating use.

Patient & Family Education

- Instruct to report any signs of bleeding (e.g., hematuria, bruising, bleeding gums).
- Instruct to report signs of hepatic toxicity (see Appendix G).
- Increase hydration (10–12 glasses of fluid daily) to reduce risk of hy-

peruricemia. Consult physician about desirable volume.
- Instruct to notify physician of onset of chills, nausea, vomiting, flank or joint pain, swelling of legs or feet, or symptoms of anemia.

MEROPENEM

(mer-o′pe-nem)
Trade name: Merrem
Classifications: ANTIINFECTIVE; CARBAPENEM ANTIBIOTIC
Prototype: Imipenem
Pregnancy category: B

ACTIONS/PHARMACODYNAMICS Meropenem is a broad-spectrum carbapenem antibiotic that inhibits the cell wall synthesis of gram-positive and gram-negative bacteria by its strong affinity for penicillin-binding proteins of bacterial cell wall. It has high resistance to most bacterial beta-lactamases. It should **not** be used to treat methicillin-resistant staphylococci.

USES Complicated appendicitis and peritonitis, bacterial meningitis caused by susceptible bacteria. **Unlabeled uses:** other intraabdominal infections, skin/soft tissue infections, febrile neutropenia.

ROUTE & DOSAGE

Intraabdominal Infections

Adult: **IV** 1 g q8h.
Child ≥3 mo: **IV** 20 mg/kg q8h (max 1 g q8h).

Bacterial Meningitis

Adult: **IV** 2 g q8h infused over 15–30 min.
Child ≥3 mo: **IV** 40 mg/kg q8h (max 2 g q8h).

Adjustment for Renal Impairment

Cl_{cr} 26–50 ml/min: 1 g q12h; 10–25 ml/min: 500 mg q12h; <10 ml/min: 500 mg q24h.

PHARMACOKINETICS Distribution: attains high concentrations in bile, bronchial secretions, cerebrospinal fluid. **Metabolism:** undergoes renal and extrarenal metabolism via dipeptidases or nonspecific degradation. **Elimination:** half-life: 0.8–1 h; excreted primarily in urine.

CONTRAINDICATIONS & PRECAUTIONS Contraindicated in: hypersensitivity to meropenem, other carbapenem antibiotics including imipenim, penicillins, cephalosporins, or other beta-lactams. **Cautious use in:** history of asthma or allergies, renal impairment, epileptics, history of neurologic disorders, elderly, pregnancy (category B). Safety and effectiveness in infants < 3 mo not established.

ADVERSE/SIDE EFFECTS GI: diarrhea, nausea, vomiting, constipation. **Local:** inflammation at injection site, phlebitis, thrombophlebitis. **Other:** headache, rash, pruritus, apnea, oral moniliasis, diaper rash.

DRUG INTERACTION Probenecid will delay meropenem excretion.

NURSING IMPLICATIONS

Administration

- IV bolus preparation and administration: To the 500-mg or 1-g vial, respectively, add 10 or 20 ml sterile water for injection to yield approximately 50 mg/ml. Shake to dissolve and let stand until clear. Give 5- to 20-ml bolus over 3–5 min.
- IV infusion preparation and administration: Dilute in 50–100 ml

of 5% dextrose or 0.9% NaCl and infuse over 15–30 min.

- Dosage reduction is recommended for elderly persons.
- Store undiluted at 15–30C (59–86F). Diluted IV solutions should generally be used within 1 h of preparation.

Assessment & Drug Effects

- Before therapy is initiated, perform C&S tests; determine history of hypersensitivity reactions to other beta-lactams, cephalosporins, penicillins, or other drugs.
- Discontinue drug and immediately report S&S of hypersensitivity (see Appendix G).
- Periodically monitor liver and renal function tests.
- Report S&S of superinfection or pseudomembranous colitis (see Appendix G).
- Monitor for seizures especially in the elderly and those with renal insufficiency.

Patient & Family Education

- Teach S&S of hypersensitivity, superinfection, and pseudomembranous colitis; instruct to promptly report any of these.

M

MESALAMINE

(me-sal'a-meen)

Trade names: Asacol, Rowasa, Salofalk♣, Pentasa

Classifications: MUCOUS MEMBRANE AGENT; ANTIINFLAMMATORY

Pregnancy category: C

ACTIONS/PHARMACODYNAMICS

Mesalamine provides topical antiinflammatory action in the colon of patients with ulcerative colitis. It is thought that the drug diminishes inflammation by blocking cyclooxygenase and inhibiting prostaglandin synthesis in the colon.

USES Indicated in active mild to moderate distal ulcerative colitis, proctosigmoiditis, or proctitis; maintenance of remission of ulcerative colitis. **Unlabeled use:** Crohn's disease.

ROUTE & DOSAGE

Ulcerative Colitis

Adult: **Rectal** 4 g once/d h.s.; enema should be retained for about 8 h if possible; *or* 1 suppository (500 mg) b.i.d. **PO** ***Asacol:*** 800 mg t.i.d. × 6 wk. ***Pentasa:*** 500 mg t.i.d. × 6 wk.

Child: **PO** 50 mg/kg/d divided q6–12h.

PHARMACOKINETICS **Absorption:** PR: 5–35% absorbed from colon depending on retention time of enema or suppository. PO (Asacol): approximately 28% absorbed; 80% of drug is released in colon 12 h after ingestion. PO (Pentasa): 50% of drug is released in colon at a pH < 6. **Peak:** 3–6 h. **Distribution:** rectal administration may reach as high as the ascending colon. Asacol is released in the ileum and colon; Pentasa is released in the jejunum, ileum, and colon. Low concentrations of mesalamine and higher concentrations of its metabolites are excreted in breast milk. **Metabolism:** mesalamine is rapidly acetylated in the liver and colon wall. **Elimination:** half-life: 2–15 h (depending on formulation); excreted primarily in feces; absorbed drug excreted in urine.

CONTRAINDICATIONS & PRECAUTIONS **Contraindicated in:** hypersensitivity to mesalamine. **Cautious use in:** renal impairment, pregnancy (category C). Sensitivity to sulfasalazine or salicylates. Not known if it is excreted in breast milk.

ADVERSE/SIDE EFFECTS CNS: *headache,* fatigue, asthenia, malaise, weakness, dizziness. **GI:** *abdominal pain, cramps, or discomfort,* flatulence, nausea, diarrhea, constipation, hemorrhoids, rectal pain. **Other:** sensitivity reactions, rash, pruritus, alopecia, fever, thrombocytopenia (rare), interstitial nephritis, hepatitis (rare), eosinophilia.

NURSING IMPLICATIONS

Administration

- Emptying bowel immediately prior to enema is important for best results.
- Shake the bottle well to make sure the suspension is homogenized.
- Mesalamine rectal suspension should be used at bedtime with the objective of retaining it all night.
- Store at 15–30C (59–86F).

Assessment & Drug Effects

- The kidney is the major target organ for mesalamine toxicity. Careful monitoring of urinalysis, BUN, and creatinine is essential, especially in patients with preexisting renal disease.
- Suspension contains a sulfite that may cause allergic-type reaction in asthmatics and some nonasthmatic persons; assess for signs and symptoms (e.g., hives, itching, wheezing, anaphylaxis).
- Response to therapy may occur within 3–21 d; however, the usual course of therapy is from 3–6 wk, depending on symptoms and sigmoidoscopic examinations.

Patient & Family Education

- Instruct to promptly report cramping, abdominal pain, or bloody diarrhea, which are indications for immediate drug withdrawal.
- Instruct to check with doctor if rectal irritation (e.g., bleeding, blistering, pain, burning, itching) occurs while they are using this drug.
- Advise to check with physician before they use any new medicine (prescription or OTC).
- Instruct to continue medication for full time of treatment even if they are feeling better.
- Store away from heat and light.

MESNA

(mes′na)

Trade name: Mesnex

Classifications: ANTIDOTE; DETOXIFYING AGENT

Pregnancy category: B

ACTIONS/PHARMACODYNAMICS

Mesna is a detoxifying agent used to inhibit the hemorrhagic cystitis induced by ifosfamide. It is analogous to the physiological cysteine-cystine system. In the kidney, the thiol compound mesna reacts chemically with urotoxic ifosfamide metabolites, resulting in their detoxification, and thus significantly decreases the incidence of hematuria.

USES Prophylaxis for ifosfamide-induced hemorrhagic cystitis. Not effective in preventing hematuria due to other pathologic conditions such as thrombocytopenia. **Unlabeled use:** reduces the incidence of cyclophosphamide-induced hemorrhagic cystitis.

ROUTE & DOSAGE

Use with Ifosfamide

Adult: **IV** Dose = 20% of ifosfamide dose and is given at time of ifosfamide administration and 4 and 8 h after ifosfamide administration.
Child: Not established.

PHARMACOKINETICS Metabolism: rapidly oxidized in liver to active metabolite dimesna; dimesna is further metabolized in kidney. **Elimination:** half-life: mesna 0.36 h, dimesna 1.17 h; 65% excreted in urine within 24 h.

CONTRAINDICATIONS & PRECAUTIONS Contraindicated in: hypersensitivity to mesna or other thiol compounds. **Cautious use in:** pregnant women (category B) and only if the benefits clearly outweigh any possible risk to fetus.

ADVERSE/SIDE EFFECTS GI: *bad taste in mouth, soft stools,* nausea, vomiting.

DIAGNOSTIC TEST INTERFERENCE May produce a false-positive result in test for ***urinary ketones.***

M

DRUG INTERACTIONS Not compatible with **cisplatin.** Can mix with ifosfamide.

INCOMPATIBILITY Solution/additive: cisplatin.

NURSING IMPLICATIONS

Administration
- To be effective, mesna must be administered with each dose of ifosfamide.
- IV preparation: Add 4 ml of 5% dextrose, 5% dextrose and NS, 0.9% NaCl, or lactated Ringer's solution for each 100 mg of mesna to produce a solution containing a final mesna concentration of 20 mg/ml.
- IV administration: Give a single dose by direct IV over 60 s.
- Parenteral drug products should be inspected visually for particulate matter and discoloration prior to administration.
- Any unused portion of the ampul of mesna should be discarded because drug oxidizes on contact with air.
- Diluted solutions of mesna are chemically and physically stable for 24 h at 25C (77F). However, it is recommended that diluted solutions be refrigerated or used within 6 h of mixing.
- Store below 40C (104F) at 15–30C (59–86F) unless otherwise specified.

Assessment & Drug Effects
- Examination of a morning specimen of urine for microscopic hematuria is recommended prior to each dose of ifosfamide or cyclophosphamide and mesna.
- A false-positive test for urinary ketones may arise in patients treated with mesna. In this test, a red-violet color develops that, with the addition of glacial acetic acid, will turn to violet.
- About 6% of patients treated with mesna along with ifosfamide still develop hematuria.

Patient & Family Education
- Inform that mesna prevents ifosfamide-induced hemorrhagic cystitis; it will not prevent or alleviate other adverse reactions or toxicities associated with ifosfamide therapy.
- Advise to report any unusual or allergic reactions to mesna.
- Advise to check with physician before they use any new prescription or OTC medicine.

MESORIDAZINE BESYLATE

(mez-oh-rid′a-zeen)

Trade name: Serentil

Classifications: CNS AGENT; PSYCHOTHERAPEUTIC; PHENOTHIAZINE ANTIPSYCHOTIC

Prototype: Chlorpromazine

Pregnancy category: C

ACTIONS/PHARMACODYNAMICS Piperidine derivative of phenothiazine. Major tranquilizer with stronger sedative action than produced by chlorpromazine but has more antiemetic action and lower incidence of extrapyramidal side effects. Produces psychomotor slowing and reduces emotional stress.

USES Schizophrenia, behavioral problems in mental deficiency and chronic brain syndrome, acute and chronic alcoholism. Also to reduce symptoms of anxiety and tension associated with many neurotic disorders.

ROUTE & DOSAGE

Psychotic Disorders

Adult: **PO** 10–50 mg b.i.d. or t.i.d.; may increase as needed up to 400 mg/d. **IM** 25 mg; may repeat in 30–60 min if necessary.

Dementia Behavior

Geriatric: **PO** 10 mg 1–2 times/d, may gradually increase q4–7d to max 250 mg/d.

Management of Hyperactivity

Adult: **PO** 25 mg t.i.d. up to 75–300 mg/d.

Alcohol Dependence

Adult: **PO** 25 mg b.i.d. up to 50–200 mg/d.

Anxiety & Tension

Adult: **PO** 10 mg b.i.d. up to 150 mg/d.

PHARMACOKINETICS **Absorption:** readily absorbed from GI tract. **Peak:** 2 h PO; 30 min IM. **Duration:** 4–6 h PO; 6–8 h IM. **Metabolism:** metabolized in liver. **Elimination:** half-life: 24–48 h; excreted in urine and bile.

CONTRAINDICATIONS & PRECAUTIONS **Contraindicated in:** known sensitivity to other phenothiazines; severely depressed (drug-induced) patient, comatose state, children < 12 y. Safe use during pregnancy (category C) and in nursing mothers not established. **Cautious use in:** previously detected cancer of breast; glaucoma; prostatic hypertrophy, urinary retention; history of cardiovascular disease.

ADVERSE/SIDE EFFECTS Dizziness, *sedation,* fainting, blurred vision, xerostomia, nasal congestion, urinary retention, constipation, decreased sweating, contact dermatitis, tachycardia, *orthostatic hypotension,* extrapyramidal effects.

NURSING IMPLICATIONS

Administration

- Just before administration, dilute PO concentrate in about 1/2 glass (120 ml) of fluid. Suggested diluents: fruit juices, water, soup, carbonated beverage. Measure drug with calibrated dispenser included in original package. Explain use of dispenser and dose to patient.
- Inject IM solution slowly and deeply into upper outer quadrant of buttock. Advise patient to lie still for 20–30 min after the injection to minimize possible dizziness.
- Slight yellowing of the solution will not change potency; however, darkened solution should be discarded.
- Protect solution from light and freezing. Store below 25C (77F); refrigeration is not necessary.

Assessment & Drug Effects

- Monitor I&O and bowel elimination patterns and check bladder

M

for distension. The depressed patient often fails to report urinary discomfort or constipation.

- If patient complains of blurred vision, report to physician. Periodic ophthalmic examinations are advisable with long-term therapy.
- Monitor BP with patient supine and standing.

Patient & Family Education

- Caution to avoid spilling drug on skin since it may cause contact dermatitis. Thoroughly rinse off with water if spilling occurs.
- Because of possible dizziness and drowsiness during early period of therapy, advise not to drive a car or engage in any dangerous activity until drug response is known.
- Drowsiness usually decreases with continued therapy. If it persists and interferes with ADL, consult physician. A change in time of administration or dose may help to prevent interference with normal physical activities.
- Warn of possibility of orthostatic hypotension. Advise patient to dangle legs over bedside upon arising from sleep.
- Alcohol should be avoided during mesoridazine therapy.
- Provide guidance on measures to prevent dry mouth.

METAPROTERENOL SULFATE

(met-a-proe-ter′e-nole)

Trade names: Alupent, Metaprel

Classifications: AUTONOMIC NERVOUS SYSTEM AGENT; BETA-ADRENERGIC AGONIST; BRONCHODILATOR

Prototype: Isoproterenol hydrochloride

Pregnancy category: C

ACTIONS/PHARMACODYNAMICS Potent synthetic sympathomimetic amine similar to isoproterenol in chemical structure and pharmacologic actions. Acts selectively on $beta_2$-adrenergic receptors to relax smooth muscle of bronchi, uterus, and blood vessels supplying skeletal muscles.

USES Bronchodilator in symptomatic relief of asthma and reversible bronchospasm associated with bronchitis and emphysema. **Unlabeled uses:** treatment and prophylaxis of heart block and to avert progress of premature labor (tocolytic action).

ROUTE & DOSAGE

Bronchospasm

Adult: **PO** 20 mg q6–8h; **Metered Dose Inhaler** 2–3 inhalations q3–4h (max 12 inhalations/d); **Nebulizer** 5–10 inhalations of undiluted 5% solution; **IPPB** 2.5 ml of 0.4–0.6% solution q4–6h.
Geriatric: **PO** 10 mg 3–4 times/d, may increase to 20 mg 3–4 times/d.
Child: **PO** *> 9 y,* 20 mg q6–8h; *6–9 y,* 10 mg q6–8h; *2–6 y,* 1.2–2.6 mg/kg/d in 3–4 divided doses; *<2 y,* 0.4 mg/kg t.i.d.–q.i.d.

PHARMACOKINETICS Absorption: 40% of PO doses reaches systemic circulation. **Onset:** inhaled: 1 min; PO 15 min. **Peak:** 1 h all routes. **Duration:** inhaled: 1–5 h; PO 4 h. **Metabolism:** metabolized in liver. **Elimination:** excreted in urine.

CONTRAINDICATIONS & PRECAUTIONS Contraindicated in: sensitivity to other sympathomimetic agents; cardiac arrhythmias associated with tachycardia; hyperthyroidism. Safe use during pregnancy (category C); by nursing mothers, and in children

< 12 y (for aerosol use) not established. **Cautious use in:** the elderly; hypertension, coronary artery disease; hyperthyroidism; diabetes.

ADVERSE/SIDE EFFECTS **CNS:** nervousness, weakness, drowsiness, *tremor (particularly after PO administration),* headache, fatigue. **CV:** *tachycardia,* hypertension, cardiac arrest, palpitation. **GI:** nausea, vomiting, bad taste. **Other:** occasional difficulty in micturition and muscle cramps, throat irritation, cough, exacerbation of asthma.

DRUG INTERACTIONS **Epinephrine,** other SYMPATHOMIMETIC BRONCHODILATORS may compound effects of metaproterenol; MAO INHIBITORS, TRICYCLIC ANTIDEPRESSANTS potentiate action of metaproterenol on vascular system; the effects of both metaproterenol and BETA-ADRENERGIC BLOCKERS are antagonized.

NURSING IMPLICATIONS

Administration

- Oral drug may be taken with food to reduce GI distress.
- Metered aerosol dose: Instruct patient to shake container, exhale through nose as completely as possible, administer aerosol while inhaling deeply through mouth, and to hold breath about 10 seconds before exhaling slowly. Administer second inhalation 10 min after first.
- Patient may use tablets and aerosol concomitantly.
- Protect from light and heat. Store at 15–30C (59–86F) unless otherwise directed.

Assessment & Drug Effects

- Monitor respiratory status. Auscultate lungs before and after inhalation to determine efficacy of drug in decreasing airway resistance.
- Monitor cardiac status. Report tachycardia and hypotension.

Patient & Family Education

- Drug may have shorter duration of action after long-term use. Instruct to report failure to respond to usual dose.
- Warn not to increase dose or frequency unless ordered by physician; there is the possibility of serious adverse effects.
- Advise that tremor is an anticipated side effect.

METARAMINOL BITARTRATE

(met-a-ram'i-nole)

Trade name: Aramine

Classifications: AUTONOMIC NERVOUS SYSTEM AGENT; ALPHA- AND BETA-ADRENERGIC AGONIST (SYMPATHOMIMETIC)

Prototype: Epinephrine

Pregnancy category: D

ACTIONS/PHARMACODYNAMICS Potent synthetic sympathomimetic amine. Overall effects similar to those of norepinephrine; but is not as potent, has more gradual onset and longer duration of action, and usually lacks CNS stimulant effects. Acts directly on alpha-adrenergic receptors (vasoconstriction) and also directly stimulates $beta_1$ receptors of heart (positive inotropic effect); indirectly causes release of norepinephrine from storage sites. Vasoconstrictor action increases pulmonary arterial pressure, produces sustained rise in systolic and diastolic pressures, and reduces blood flow to kidneys.

USES Prevention and treatment of acute hypotensive states occurring with spinal anesthesia and as adjunct in treatment of hypotension due to hemorrhage, reaction to medication, surgical complications, brain damage, cardiogenic shock, and septicemia. **Unlabeled uses:** provocative test for diagnosis of familial Mediterranean fever and to increase cardiac output in pericardial tamponade.

ROUTE & DOSAGE

Hypotension
Adult: **SC/IM** 2–10 mg; may repeat in 10 min if necessary. **IV** 0.5–5 mg followed by IV infusion of 15–100 mg in 500 ml of D5W or NS.
Child: **SC/IM** 0.1 mg/kg; may repeat in 10 min if necessary. **IV** 0.01 mg/kg followed by IV infusion of 0.04 mg/kg (each mg diluted in 25 ml of D5W or NS).

M

PHARMACOKINETICS **Onset:** 1–2 min IV; < 10 min IM; 5–20 min SC. **Duration:** 20–90 min. **Metabolism:** metabolized in tissues. **Elimination:** excreted in urine.

CONTRAINDICATIONS & PRECAUTIONS **Contraindicated in:** use with cyclopropane, halothane, within 14 d of MAO INHIBITOR therapy; peripheral or mesenteric thrombosis; pulmonary edema, cardiac arrest; untreated hypoxia, hypercapnia, and acidosis; as sole therapy in hypovolemia. Safe use during pregnancy (category D) not established. **Cautious use in:** digitalized patients; hypertension; thyroid disease; diabetes mellitus; cirrhosis of liver; history of malaria (may produce relapse).

ADVERSE/SIDE EFFECTS Apprehension, restlessness, headache, tremor, nausea, vomiting, weakness, flushing, pallor, sweating, precordial pain, palpitation, tachycardia, bradycardia, decreased urinary output, metabolic acidosis (hypovolemic patients), hyperglycemia. **Excessive dosage:** severe hypertension, headache, convulsions, acute pulmonary edema, arrhythmias, <u>cardiac arrest</u>. **Injection site reactions (especially following SC):** abscess formation, tissue necrosis, sloughing. **Prolonged use:** plasma volume depletion with recurrence of shock state, hypotension.

DRUG INTERACTIONS ERGOT ALKALOIDS, **furazolidone, guanethidine,** MAO INHIBITORS, TRICYCLIC ANTIDEPRESSANTS may cause an excessive pressor response; **phentolamine** may decrease pressor response; increases risk of arrhythmias with **halothane, cyclopropane.**

INCOMPATIBILITIES **Solution/additive: amphotericin B, dexamethasone, erythromycin, fibrinogen, hydrocortisone, methicillin, methylprednisolone, penicillin, thiopental, warfarin.**

NURSING IMPLICATIONS

Administration

- IV preparation: For adults, 15–100 mg may be dissolved in 500 ml of D5W, NS, or other compatible IV fluid and titrated to maintain BP at a desired level.
- For children, IV infusion is prepared to yield a concentration of 1 mg for each 25 ml of solution.
- IV administration: IV flow rate will be prescribed by physician (usually, systolic BP is maintained at 80–100 mm Hg for previously normotensive patients; for previously hypertensive patients it is maintained at 30–40 mm Hg below the usual pressure).
- Up to 5 mg may be given undiluted by direct IV over at least 1 min.
- When infusion is to be discontinued, flow rate should be reduced

gradually, and abrupt withdrawal avoided. Equipment for reinstituting therapy should be immediately available.

- Patients receiving drug IV must be constantly attended, with infusion flow rate being closely monitored. Changes in flow rate must be made cautiously, since the drug has cumulative effect and prolonged action.
- Care should be taken to avoid extravasation during IV infusion. Injury to local tissue and necrosis may result.
- Avoid exposure of drug to excessive heat, and protect it from light.

Assessment & Drug Effects

- Except in emergency situations, blood volume should be corrected as fully as possible before therapy is initiated.
- During IV infusion, check BP q5min until it is stabilized at prescribed level, then q15min thereafter throughout therapy. Also note pulse rate and quality. Continue monitoring at regular intervals for several hours after infusion is complete.
- Observe I&O ratio and pattern. Keep physician informed of renal response. Urinary output may decrease initially, then increase as BP approaches normal levels. With excessive dosage, output may again decrease.
- Carefully monitor injection sites for S&S of tissue damage.
- Metaraminol may cause diuresis in patients with cirrhosis of liver. Patients should be carefully monitored for excessive losses of water, sodium, and potassium.
- Patients with diabetes should be closely monitored for loss of diabetes control.

Patient & Family Education

- Instruct to immediately report pain at IV insertion site or site of SC injection.
- Instruct to immediately report respiratory distress, chest pain, or palpitations.

METFORMIN

(met-for′min)

Trade name: Glucophage

Classifications: ANTIDIABETIC; BIGUANIDE HYPOGLYCEMIC AGENT

Pregnancy category: B

ACTIONS/PHARMACODYNAMICS

Metformin is a biguanide oral hypoglycemic agent. Unlike sulfonylureas, biguanides do not stimulate the release of insulin from the beta cells of the pancreas. Mechanism of action is thought to be due to both increasing the binding of insulin to its receptor and potentiating insulin action. It is known that metformin has a direct effect on the glucose transport system, especially in skeletal muscle cells. Metformin increases glucose transport across the cell membrane, with enhanced glucose utilization in skeletal muscles.

USES Treatment of non-insulin-dependent diabetes mellitus (NIDDM) in patients not controlled with diet alone. May be used with an oral sulfonylurea.

ROUTE & DOSAGE

Adult: **PO** Start with 500 mg q.d. to t.i.d. May increase by 500 mg/d every 1–3 wk to a max of 3 g/d.

PHARMACOKINETICS **Absorption:** 50–60% of dose reaches systemic circulation. **Peak:** 1–3 h. **Distribution:** not bound to plasma proteins. **Me-**

tabolism: not metabolized. **Elimination:** half-life: 6.2–17.6 h; excreted in urine.

CONTRAINDICATIONS & PRECAUTIONS **Contraindicated in:** hypersensitivity to metformin; renal, hepatic, or cardiopulmonary insufficiency; alcoholism; concurrent infection. **Cautious use in:** previous hypersensitivity to phenformin or buformin, pregnancy (category B), lactation.

ADVERSE/SIDE EFFECTS **CNS:** headache, dizziness, agitation, fatigue. **Metabolic:** lactic acidosis. **GI:** *nausea, vomiting, abdominal pain, bitter or metallic taste, diarrhea, bloatedness, anorexia;* malabsorption of amino acids, vitamin B_{12}, and folic acid possible.

M

DRUG INTERACTIONS **Captopril, furosemide, nifedipine** may increase risk of hypoglycemia. **Cimetidine** reduces clearance of metformin. Concomitant therapy with AZOLE ANTIFUNGAL AGENTS (FLUCONAZOLE, KETOCONAZOLE, ITRACONAZOLE) and ORAL HYPOGLYCEMIC DRUGS has been reported in severe hypoglycemia. IODINATED RADIOCONTRAST DYES can cause lactic acidosis and acute renal failure. **Acarbose** may decrease metformin levels.

DIAGNOSTIC TEST INTEFERENCE Iodinated contrast dyes may cause lactic acidosis or acute renal failure.

NURSING IMPLICATIONS

Administration

- Hold metformin 48 h before and 48 h after receiving IV contrast dye.
- Metformin should be taken with or shortly after main meals.
- Dose increment, if needed, should be made at 2–3-wk intervals.
- Reduction of the metformin dose should be considered with concurrent cimetidine therapy.
- Temporarily withhold metformin 48 h prior to and 48 h after administration of iodinated radiocontrast dyes.
- Store at room temperature 15–30C (59–86F).

Assessment & Drug Effects

- Baseline and periodic renal and hepatic function tests should be done; the drug is contraindicated in the presence of renal or hepatic insufficiency.
- Carefully monitor known or suspected alcoholics for decreased hepatic function.
- Monitor cardiopulmonary status throughout the course of therapy; cardiopulmonary insufficiency may predispose to lactic acidosis.
- Periodically monitor blood glucose, total glycosylated hemoglobin, body weight, and lipid profile.

Patient & Family Education

- Inform that hypoglycemia is not a risk when metformin is taken in recommended therapeutic doses.
- Advise to report immediately S&S of infection, which increase the risk of lactic acidosis.

METHADONE HYDROCHLORIDE

(meth′a-done)

Trade name: Dolophine

Classifications: CNS AGENT; NARCOTIC (OPIATE) AGONIST ANALGESIC

Prototype: Morphine

Pregnancy category: B (D for use of high doses at term)

Controlled substance: Schedule II

ACTIONS/PHARMACODYNAMICS Synthetic derivative similar to those of morphine but is orally effective and has longer duration of action. A single oral dose produces less sedation and euphoria than does morphine, but repeated doses produce marked sedation. Causes less constipation than morphine, but respiratory depressant effect and antitussive actions are comparable. Highly addictive, with abuse potential that matches that of morphine; abstinence syndrome develops more slowly; withdrawal symptoms are less intense but more prolonged.

USES To relieve severe pain; for detoxification and temporary maintenance treatment in hospital and in federally controlled maintenance programs for ambulatory patients with narcotic abstinence syndrome.

ROUTE & DOSAGE

Moderate to Severe Acute Pain
Adult: **PO/SC/IM** 2.5–10 mg q3–4h prn.
Child: **PO/IV** 0.1 mg/kg q4h × 2–3 doses, then q6–12h prn (max 10 mg/dose).

Chronic Pain
Adult: **PO/SC/IM** 5–20 mg q6–8h.

Detoxification Treatment
Adult: **PO/SC/IM** 15–40 mg once/d; usually maintained at 20–120 mg/d.
Neonate: **PO/IV** 0.05–0.2 mg/kg q12–24h or 0.5 mg/kg/d divided q8h; taper dose by 10–20%/wk over 1–1½ mo.

PHARMACOKINETICS **Absorption:** well absorbed from GI tract. **Onset:** 30–60 min PO; 10–20 min IM/SC. **Peak:** 1–2 h. **Duration:** 6–8 h PO, IM, SC; may last 22–48 h with chronic dosing. **Distribution:** crosses placenta; distributed into breast milk. **Metabolism:** metabolized in liver. **Elimination:** half-life: 15–25 h; excreted in urine.

CONTRAINDICATIONS & PRECAUTIONS **Contraindicated in:** obstetric analgesia. Safe use during pregnancy (category B, category D for use of high doses at term), in nursing mothers, and for treatment of narcotic addiction in patients < 18 y not established. **Cautious use in:** hepatic, renal, or cardiac dysfunction.

ADVERSE/SIDE EFFECTS *Drowsiness,* nausea, vomiting, dry mouth, *constipation,* light-headedness, dizziness, transient fall in BP, bone and muscle pain, hallucinations, impotence, respiratory depression.

DRUG INTERACTIONS **Alcohol** and other CNS DEPRESSANTS, **cimetidine** add to sedation and CNS depression; AMPHETAMINES may potentiate CNS stimulation; with MAO INHIBITORS, **selegiline, furazolidone** causes excessive and prolonged CNS depression, convulsions, cardiovascular collapse.

INCOMPATIBILITIES **Solution/additive: aminophylline, ammonium chloride,** BARBITURATES, **chlorothiazide, heparin, methicillin, phenytoin, sodium bicarbonate.**

NURSING IMPLICATIONS

Administration

- For analgesic effect, methadone should be administered in the smallest effective dose to minimize the possibility of tolerance and physical and psychic dependence.
- IM route is preferred when repeated parenteral administration is required (SC injections may cause local irritation and induration). Rotate injection sites.
- IV administration to neonates, infants, children: Verify correct IV

concentration and rate of infusion with physician.

- Preserve in tight, light-resistant containers at 15–30C (59–86F) unless otherwise directed.

Assessment & Drug Effects

- Evaluate the patient's continued need for methadone for pain. Adjustment of dosage and lengthening of between-dose intervals may be possible.
- Monitor respiratory status. Principal danger of overdosage, as with morphine, is extreme respiratory depression.
- Because of the cumulative effects of methadone, abstinence symptoms may not appear for 36–72 h after last dose and may last 10–14 d. Symptoms are usually of mild intensity (anorexia, insomnia, anxiety, abdominal discomfort, weakness, headache, sweating, hot and cold flashes).
- Narcotic antagonists such as naloxone, naltrexone, and levallorphan terminate methadone intoxication. Since antagonist action is shorter (1–3 h) than that of methadone (36–48 h or more), repeated doses for 8–24 h may be required. Patient should be watched closely for recurrence of respiratory depression.

Patient & Family Education

- Orthostatic hypotension, sweating, constipation, drowsiness, GI symptoms, and other transient side effects of therapeutic doses appear to be more prominent in ambulatory patients. Most side effects disappear over a period of several weeks.
- Instruct to make position changes slowly, particularly from recumbent to upright position, and to sit or lie down if they feel dizzy or faint.
- Inform that methadone may impair mental and physical abilities required for performance of potentially hazardous activities, such as driving a car or operating machinery.

METHAMPHETAMINE HYDROCHLORIDE

(meth-am-fet′a-meen)

Trade names: Desoxyephedrine, Desoxyn

Classifications: CNS AGENT; RESPIRATORY AND CEREBRAL STIMULANT; ANOREXIANT; AMPHETAMINE

Prototype: Amphetamine sulfate

Pregnancy category: C

Controlled substance: Schedule II

ACTIONS/PHARMACODYNAMICS

Sympathomimetic amine chemically related to amphetamine. CNS stimulant actions approximately equal to those of amphetamine, but accompanied by less peripheral activity. However, larger doses produce increased cardiac output, possibly reflex slowing of heart rate, and sustained increase in BP, chiefly by cardiac stimulation.

USES Short-term adjunct in management of exogenous obesity, as adjunctive therapy in attention deficit disorder (ADD), narcolepsy, epilepsy, and postencephalitic parkinsonism, and in treatment of certain depressive reactions, especially when characterized by apathy and psychomotor retardation.

ROUTE & DOSAGE

Attention Deficit Disorder

Child ≥ 6 y: **PO** 2.5–5 mg 1–2 times/d; may increase by 5 mg at weekly intervals up to 20–25 mg/d.

Obesity

Adult: **PO** 2.5–5 mg 1–3 times/d 30 min before meals; *or* 5–15 mg of long-acting form once/d.

PHARMACOKINETICS Absorption: readily absorbed from the GI tract. **Duration:** 6–12 h. **Distribution:** all tissues especially the CNS; excreted in breast milk. **Metabolism:** metabolized in liver. **Elimination:** renal elimination.

CONTRAINDICATIONS & PRECAUTIONS Contraindicated in: during pregnancy, especially first trimester (category C), as anorexiant in children < 12 y; patients receiving MAO INHIBITORS; arteriosclerotic parkinsonism. **Cautious use in:** mild hypertension; psychopathic personalities; hyperexcitability states; history of suicide attempts; elderly or debilitated patients.

ADVERSE/SIDE EFFECTS CNS (stimulation): restlessness, tremor, hyperreflexia, insomnia, headache, nervousness, anxiety, dizziness, euphoria or dysphoria. **CV:** palpitation, arrhythmias, hypertension, hypotension, circulatory collapse. **GI:** dry mouth, unpleasant taste, nausea, vomiting, diarrhea, constipation, increased intraocular pressure.

DRUG INTERACTIONS Acetazolamide, sodium bicarbonate decrease amphetamine elimination; **ammonium chloride, ascorbic acid** increase amphetamine elimination; effects of both methamphetamine and BARBITURATES may be antagonized; **furazolidone** may increase BP effects of amphetamines—interaction may persist for several weeks after discontinuing furazolidone; antagonizes antihypertensive effects of **guanethidine, guanadryl;** MAO INHIBITORS, **selegiline** can cause hypertensive crisis (fatalities reported)—do not administer amphetamines during or within 14 d of administration of these drugs; PHENOTHIAZINES may inhibit mood elevating effects of amphetamines; TRICYCLIC ANTIDEPRESSANTS enhance amphetamine effects because they increase norepinephrine release; BETA-ADRENERGIC AGONISTS increase adverse cardiovascular effects of amphetamines.

NURSING IMPLICATIONS

Administration

- If possible, medication should be taken early in the day to avoid insomnia.
- When used for treatment of obesity, drug is administered 30 min before each meal. If insomnia results, advise patient to inform physician.
- Preserve in tight, light-resistant containers.

Assessment & Drug Effects

- Monitor weight throughout period of therapy.
- Paradoxic increase in depression or agitation sometimes occurs in depressed patients. Report immediately; drug should be withdrawn.
- Duration of methamphetamine use in treatment of obesity should not exceed a few weeks.

Patient & Family Education

- Tolerance develops readily, and prolonged use may lead to drug dependence. Abuse potential is high. Methamphetamine is commonly known as "speed" or "crystal" among drug abusers.
- Withdrawal after prolonged use is frequently followed by lethargy that may persist for several weeks.
- Instruct to weigh themselves every other day under standard conditions and maintain a record of weight loss.

M

METHAZOLAMIDE

(meth-a-zoe′la-mide)

Trade name: Neptazane

Classifications: EYE PREPARATION; CARBONIC ANHYDRASE INHIBITOR; SULFONAMIDE DERIVATIVE; ANTI-GLAUCOMA

Prototype: Acetazolamide

Pregnancy category: C

ACTIONS/PHARMACODYNAMICS Nonbactericidal sulfonamide derivative similar to acetazolamide but with slower onset and longer duration of action. Appears to cause more drowsiness and fatigue than acetazolamide does, and has less diuretic activity.

USES Adjunctive treatment in chronic simple (open-angle) glaucoma and secondary glaucoma and preoperatively in acute angle-closure glaucoma when delay of surgery is desired in order to lower intraocular pressure. May be used concomitantly with miotic and osmotic agents.

M

ROUTE & DOSAGE

Glaucoma

Adult: **PO** 50–100 mg b.i.d. or t.i.d.

PHARMACOKINETICS **Absorption:** slowly absorbed from GI tract. **Onset:** 2–4 h. **Peak:** 6–8 h. **Duration:** 10–18 h. **Distribution:** distributed throughout body, concentrating in RBCs, plasma, and kidneys; crosses placenta. **Metabolism:** partially metabolized in liver. **Elimination:** excreted primarily in urine.

CONTRAINDICATIONS & PRECAUTIONS **Contraindicated in:** glaucoma due to severe peripheral anterior synechiae, severe or absolute glaucoma, hemorrhagic glaucoma; hypokalemia, hyponatremia; pregnancy (category C).

ADVERSE/SIDE EFFECTS Malaise, drowsiness, fatigue, lethargy, mild GI disturbance, anorexia, headache, vertigo, paresthesias, mental confusion, depression.

DRUG INTERACTIONS Renal excretion of AMPHETAMINES, **ephedrine, flecainide, quinidine, procainamide,** TRICYCLIC ANTIDEPRESSANTS may be decreased, thereby enhancing or prolonging their effects; increases renal excretion of **lithium;** excretion of **phenobarbital** may be increased; **amphotericin B,** CORTICOSTEROIDS may add to potassium loss; hypokalemia caused by methazolamide may predispose patients on DIGITALIS GLYCOSIDES to digitalis toxicity; patients on high doses of SALICYLATES are at higher risk for salicylate toxicity.

NURSING IMPLICATIONS

Administration

- Drug may be given with meals to minimize GI distress.

Assessment & Drug Effects

- Supervise ambulation in elderly, since drug may cause vertigo.
- Since drug may cause fatigue and lethargy, assess patient's ability to perform ADL.

Patient & Family Education

- Instruct that drug may cause drowsiness. Advise caution with hazardous activities until reaction to drug is known.
- Brand interchange is not recommended without evidence of therapeutic equivalence.

METHENAMINE HIPPURATE

(meth-en′a-meen hip′yoo-rate)
Trade names: Hiprex, Urex

METHENAMINE MANDELATE

Trade names: Mandelamine, Mandameth
Classification: URINARY TRACT ANTIINFECTIVE
Prototype: Trimethoprim
Pregnancy category: C

ACTIONS/PHARMACODYNAMICS In an acid medium, this tertiary amine liberates formaldehyde, a nonspecific antibiotic agent with bactericidal activity. Most bacteria and fungi are susceptible to formaldehyde; however, bacteria that are urease-positive (e.g., *Proteus* sp) convert urea to ammonium hydroxide, which prevents the generation of formaldehyde from methenamine.

USES Prophylactic treatment of recurrent urinary tract infections (UTIs). Also long-term prophylaxis when residual urine is present (e.g., neurogenic bladder).

ROUTE & DOSAGE

UTI Prophylaxis

Adult: **PO *Hippurate:*** 1 g b.i.d.; ***mandelate:*** 1 g q.i.d.
Child: **PO** *6–12 y,* ***hippurate:*** 0.5–1 g b.i.d.; ***mandelate:*** 500 mg q.i.d. or 50 mg/kg/d in 3 divided doses; *≤ 6 y,* ***mandelate:*** 18.4 mg/kg q.i.d.

PHARMACOKINETICS Absorption: readily absorbed from GI tract, although 10–30% of dose is hydrolyzed to formaldehyde in stomach. **Peak:** 2 h. **Duration:** up to 6 h or until patient voids. **Distribution:** crosses placenta; distributed into breast milk. **Metabolism:** hydrolyzed in acid pH to formaldehyde. **Elimination:** half-life: 4 h; excreted in urine.

CONTRAINDICATIONS & PRECAUTIONS Contraindicated in: renal insufficiency; hepatic disease; gout; severe dehydration; combined therapy with sulfonamides. Safe use during pregnancy (category C), and in nursing mothers, not established. **Cautious use in:** PO suspension for patients susceptible to lipoid pneumonia (e.g., the elderly, debilitated patient).

ADVERSE/SIDE EFFECTS GI: nausea, vomiting, diarrhea, abdominal cramps, anorexia. **Renal:** bladder irritation, dysuria, frequency, albuminuria, hematuria, crystalluria.

DIAGNOSTIC TEST INTERFERENCE Methenamine (formaldehyde) may produce falsely elevated values for ***urinary catecholamines*** and ***urinary steroids*** (17-hydroxycorticosteroids) (by Reddy method). Possibility of false ***urine glucose determinations*** with Benedict's test. Methenamine interferes with ***urobilinogen*** and possibly ***urinary VMA*** determinations.

DRUG INTERACTIONS Sulfamethoxazole forms insoluble precipitate in acid urine; **acetazolamide, sodium bicarbonate** may prevent hydrolysis to formaldehyde.

NURSING IMPLICATIONS

Administration

- Administer after meals and at bedtime to minimize gastric distress.
- PO suspension contains a vegetable oil base; administer with caution to the elderly or the debilitated patient because of the pos-

M

sibility of lipid (aspiration) pneumonia.
- Reconstitute PO granules by dissolving 1 packet (500 mg or 1 g) in 60–120 ml water immediately before use. Solution may remain cloudy after reconstitution.
- Store at 15–30C (59–86F) in tightly closed container; protect from excessive heat.

Assessment & Drug Effects
- Monitor urine pH, since a value of 5.5 or less is required for optimum drug action.
- Monitor I&O ratio and pattern. Methenamine is most effective when fluid intake is maintained at 1500 or 2000 ml/d.
- Generally, fluids are not forced, as copious amounts with this drug may increase diuresis, elevate urine pH, and dilute formaldehyde concentration to subinhibitory levels.
- If patient complains of gastric distress, consult physician about changing formulation to enteric-coated tablet.
- Supplemental acidification to maintain pH of 5.5 or below required for drug action may be necessary. This can be accomplished by drugs (ascorbic acid, ammonium chloride) or by foods.

Patient & Family Education
- Caution not to self-medicate with OTC antacids containing sodium bicarbonate or sodium carbonate (to prevent raising urine pH).
- Supplementary acidification may be achieved by limited intake of foods that can increase urine pH: vegetables, fruits, and fruit juice (except cranberry, plum, prune) and liberal intake of foods that can decrease urine pH: proteins, cranberry juice, plums, prunes.

METHICILLIN SODIUM

(meth-i-sill′in)

Trade name: Staphcillin

Classifications: ANTIINFECTIVE; BETA-LACTAM ANTIBIOTIC; PENICILLIN; ANTISTAPHYLOCOCCAL PENICILLIN

Prototype: Penicillin G potassium

Pregnancy category: B

ACTIONS/PHARMACODYNAMICS Semisynthetic salt of penicillin with antimicrobial spectrum similar to that of penicillin G. Not as effective as penicillin G against non-penicillinase-producing staphylococci, streptococci, or pneumococci. A growing number of methicillin-resistant strains are reported to be developing.

USES Primarily in infections caused by penicillinase-producing staphylococci. May be used to initiate therapy in suspected staphylococcal infections pending results of culture and sensitivity tests.

ROUTE & DOSAGE

Staphylococcal Infections

Adult: **IM/IV** 1–2 g q4–6h up to 12 g/d.
Child: **IM/IV** 150–200 mg/kg/d divided q4–6h.
Neonate: **IM/IV** 50–100 mg/kg/d divided q6–12h.

PHARMACOKINETICS **Peak:** 30–60 min IM; 15 min IV. **Duration:** 4 h IM; 2 h IV. **Distribution:** distributes into CNS with inflamed meninges; crosses placenta; distributed into breast milk. **Metabolism:** small amount metabolized in liver. **Elimination:** half-life: 0.4–0.5 h; 80% excreted in urine, 20% in feces.

CONTRAINDICATIONS & PRECAUTIONS **Contraindicated in:** hypersensitivity to penicillins or cephalosporins. IV dosage in infants not established. Safe use during pregnancy (category B) not established. **Cautious use in:** history of allergy, asthma; nursing women, pediatric use; impaired renal function.

ADVERSE/SIDE EFFECTS Hypersensitivity reactions: *skin rash,* pruritus, urticaria, eosinophilia, serum sickness, anaphylactic reaction, *acute interstitial nephritis.* **Other:** irritation at IM site, thrombophlebitis (after IV administration); oral, rectal, vaginal candidal superinfections.

INCOMPATIBILITIES Solution/additive: amikacin, chlorpromazine, codeine, hydrocortisone, levorphanol, meperidine, metaraminol, methadone, methohexital, morphine, tetracyclines, promethazine, sodium bicarbonate, vancomycin, heparin, streptomycin.

NURSING IMPLICATIONS

Administration

- Give IM injection deep into a large muscle. Rotate injection sites.
- Methicillin is reconstituted with sterile water for injection or NaCl injection (1.5 ml/g; 5.7 ml/4g; 8.6 ml/6g). Resulting concentration is 500 mg/ml. Shake vial vigorously before withdrawing contents.
- IV administration: Each 1 ml (500 mg) is further diluted with 25 ml of sterile water or NS and given by direct IV at a rate of 10 ml/min.
- Solution may be further diluted by addition to a compatible IV infusion solution and given over 30 min–8 h.
- IV administration to neonates, infants, children: Verify correct IV concentration and rate of infusion with physician.
- Stability of diluted concentrations: 2 mg/ml, 4 h; 10–30 mg/ml, 8 h.
- Reconstituted methicillin solutions are stable for 24 h at room temperature (59–86F) and for 4 d under refrigeration (36–46F).

Assessment & Drug Effects

- Culture and susceptibility tests should be performed initially and periodically during therapy.
- Before starting therapy, obtain history of previous hypersensitivity reactions to penicillins, cephalosporins, or any other allergens.
- Observe all injection sites for evidence of irritation or inflammation.
- Periodic assessment of renal, hematopoietic, and hepatic function are advised during prolonged therapy.
- Frequent drug blood level measurements are advised in infants, as urinary excretion of drug is slower in this age group.
- Febrile reactions are reported to occur in some patients 1–2 h after IV administration.
- Monitor patients for signs and symptoms of interstitial nephritis, a hypersensitivity reaction that occurs 2–4 wk after initiation of therapy: spiking fever, anorexia, skin rash, oliguria, hematuria, cloudy urine (pyuria, albuminuria), eosinophilia. Usually reversible following prompt termination of drug.
- Monitor for signs and symptoms of superinfections (see Appendix G).

Patient & Family Education

- Instruct patient to immediately report symptoms of a hypersensitivity reaction (see Appendix G) or interstitial nephritis (see Assessment & Drug Effects).

METHIMAZOLE

(meth-im'a-zole)

Trade name: Tapazole

Classifications: SYNTHETIC HORMONE; ANTITHYROID AGENT
Prototype: Propylthiouracil
Pregnancy category: D

ACTIONS/PHARMACODYNAMICS Thioamide with actions and uses similar to those of propylthiouracil but 10 times as potent. Actions are less consistent, but effects appear more promptly than those of propylthiouracil. See propylthiouracil for adverse/side effects.

USES Hyperthyroidism and prior to surgery or radiotherapy of the thyroid; may be used cautiously to treat hyperthyroidism in pregnancy.

ROUTE & DOSAGE

Hyperthyroidism
Adult: **PO** 5–15 mg q8h.
Child: **PO** 0.2–0.4 mg/kg/d divided q8h.

PHARMACOKINETICS Absorption: readily absorbed from GI tract. **Onset:** 30–40 min. **Peak:** 1 h. **Duration:** 2–4 h. **Distribution:** crosses placenta; distributed into breast milk. **Elimination:** half-life: 5–13 h; 12% excreted in urine within 24 h.

CONTRAINDICATIONS & PRECAUTIONS Contraindicated in: pregnancy (category D), breastfeeding. **Cautious use in:** other drugs known to cause agranulocytosis.

NURSING IMPLICATIONS

Administration
- Take medication at same time each day relative to meals.
- Store drug in light-resistant container at 15–30C (59–86F).

Assessment & Drug Effects
- Periodic blood work is indicated, since agranulocytosis is a rare, but possible side effect.
- Monitor PT and INR in patients on oral anticoagulants. Anticoagulant activity may be potentiated.

Patient & Family Education
- Instruct to adhere to established dosage regimen (i.e., not to double, decrease, or omit doses and not to alter the interval between doses).
- Skin rash or swelling of cervical lymph nodes indicates need to discontinue drug and change to another antithyroid agent.
- Notify physician promptly if the following symptoms appear: bruising, unexplained bleeding, sore throat, fever, jaundice.
- Dosage may be suspended about 2 wk before anticipated delivery and restored in postpartum period if required.
- Advise patient who has had drug-induced jaundice that it may persist up to 10 wk after withdrawal of methimazole.
- Methimazole does not induce hypothyroiditis.

METHOCARBAMOL
(meth-oh-kar'ba-mole)
Trade names: Marbaxin, Robaxin
Classifications: AUTONOMIC NERVOUS SYSTEM AGENT; CENTRAL-ACTING SKELETAL MUSCLE RELAXANT
Prototype: Cyclobenzaprine
Pregnancy category: C

ACTIONS/PHARMACODYNAMICS Similar to those of cyclobenzaprine, but it produces higher plasma levels more rapidly and for longer periods. Exerts skeletal muscle relaxant action by depressing multisynaptic pathways in spinal cord and possibly by sedative effect. Has no direct action on skeletal muscles.

USES Adjunct to physical therapy and other measures in management of discomfort associated with acute musculoskeletal disorders. Also used intravenously as adjunct in management of neuromuscular manifestations of tetanus.

ROUTE & DOSAGE

Acute Musculoskeletal Disorders

Adult: **PO** 1.5 g q.i.d. for 2–3 d, then 4–4.5 g/d in 3–6 divided doses. **IM** 0.5–1 g q8h. **IV** 1–3 g/d in divided doses given at a max rate of 300 mg/min.

Tetanus

Adult: **PO** Up to 24 g/d in divided doses crushed and suspended in saline, flushed down a nasogastric tube. **IV** 1–2 g/d directly into IV tubing at a max rate of 300 mg/min; may be repeated q6h until nasogastric tube is possible. *Child:* **PO** 15 mg/kg repeated q6h as needed up to 1.8 $g/m^2/d$ for 3 consecutive d if necessary.

PHARMACOKINETICS Absorption: readily absorbed from GI tract. **Onset:** 30 min. **Peak:** 1–2 h. **Metabolism:** metabolized in liver. **Elimination:** half-life: 1–2 h; excreted in urine.

CONTRAINDICATIONS & PRECAUTIONS Contraindicated in: comatose states, CNS depression, acidosis, renal dysfunction (injectable methocarbamol contains polyethylene glycol 300 in vehicle, which may cause urea retention and acidotic problems). Safe use during pregnancy (category C), in nursing women, and in children < 12 y (except for tetanus) not established. **Cautious use in:** epilepsy.

ADVERSE/SIDE EFFECTS Allergic (parenteral or PO use): urticaria, pruritus, rash, conjunctivitis, nasal congestion, headache, blurred vision, fever, anaphylactic reaction. **PO use:** *drowsiness, dizziness, light-headedness,* headache, nausea. **Parenteral use:** thrombophlebitis, pain, sloughing (with extravasation), flushing, metallic taste, syncope, hypotension, bradycardia, convulsions. **Other:** slight reduction of white cell count with prolonged therapy.

DRUG INTERACTIONS Alcohol and other CNS DEPRESSANTS enhance CNS depression.

DIAGNOSTIC TEST INTERFERENCES Methocarbamol may cause false increases in ***urinary 5-HIAA*** (with nitrosonaphthol reagent) and ***VMA*** (Gitlow method).

NURSING IMPLICATIONS

Administration

- IM dose should not exceed 5 ml (0.5 g) into each gluteal region. Insert needle deep and carefully aspirate. Inject drug slowly. Rotate injection sites and observe daily for evidence of irritation.
- IV administration: IV methocarbamol may be given by direct IV undiluted or diluted in up to 250 ml of NS or D5W and infused at a rate of 300 mg/min for adults.
- Patient should be recumbent during and for at least 15 min after IV injection in order to reduce the possibility of orthostatic hypotension and other adverse reactions. Monitor vital signs and IV flow rate.
- Care should be taken to avoid extravasation of IV solution, which may result in thrombophlebitis and sloughing.

M

- Store at 15–30C (59–86F) unless otherwise directed.

Assessment & Drug Effects
- Periodic WBC counts are advised during prolonged therapy.
- Supervise ambulation following parenteral administration.

Patient & Family Education
- Advise to make position changes slowly, particularly from recumbent to upright position, and to dangle legs before standing.
- Adverse reactions after PO administration are usually mild and transient and subside with dosage reduction. Caution regarding drowsiness and dizziness. Advise against activities requiring mental alertness and physical coordination until response to drug action is known.
- Urine may darken to brown, black, or green on standing.

M

METHOHEXITAL SODIUM

(meth-oh-hex'i-tal)

Trade name: Brevital Sodium

Classifications: CNS AGENT; GENERAL ANESTHETIC; BARBITURATE

Prototype: Thiopental

Pregnancy category: B

Controlled substance: Schedule IV

ACTIONS/PHARMACODYNAMICS Rapid, ultra-short-acting barbiturate anesthetic agent. More potent than thiopental but has less cumulative effect and shorter duration of action, and recovery is more rapid. Abnormal muscle movements, coughing, sneezing, and laryngospasm reportedly occur more frequently than with thiopental. See thiopental for pharmacokinetics, contraindications and precautions, and adverse/side effects.

USES Induction of anesthesia, as supplement for other anesthetics, and as general anesthetic for brief operative procedures.

ROUTE & DOSAGE

Induction of Anesthesia

Adult: **IV** 5–12 ml of 1% solution (50–120 mg) at a rate of 1 ml (5 mg) q5min, then 2–4 ml (20–40 mg) q4–7min prn.
Child: **IV** 1–2 mg/kg. **PR** 20–35 mg/kg as 10% solution (max 500 mg/dose).

CONTRAINDICATIONS & PRECAUTIONS **Cautious use in:** pregnancy (category B).

DRUG INTERACTIONS **Alcohol** and other CNS DEPRESSANTS enhance CNS depression.

INCOMPATIBILITIES **Solution/additive: atropine, chlorpromazine, glycopyrrolate, hydralazine, kanamycin, lidocaine, methicillin, methyldopa, prochlorperazine, promazine, promethazine, streptomycin,** TETRACYCLINES.

NURSING IMPLICATIONS

Administration
- Patient should be recumbent during drug administration. Fall in BP may occur in susceptible patients receiving drug in upright position.
- Methohexital is stable in sterile water for injection at room temperature for at least 6 wk. Solutions prepared with isotonic NaCl injection or 5% dextrose injection are stable for about 24 h. Only clear, colorless solutions should be used.
- Methohexital solution is incompatible with acid solutions (e.g., atropine and with silicone). Do not allow contact with rubber stoppers or parts of syringes treated with silicone.

Assessment & Drug Effects

- Hiccups are common, particularly with rapid injection; they sometimes persist after anesthesia.
- Facilities for assisting respiration and administration of oxygen should be readily available in the event of respiratory distress.

METHOTREXATE

(meth-oh-trex'ate)

Trade names: Amethopterin, Mexate, MTX, Rheumatrex

METHOTREXATE SODIUM

Trade names: Folex, Mexate

Classifications: ANTINEOPLASTIC; ANTIMETABOLITE; IMMUNOSUPPRESSANT

Prototype: Fluorouracil

Pregnancy category: D

ACTIONS/PHARMACODYNAMICS Antimetabolite and folic acid antagonist. Blocks folic acid participation in nucleic acid synthesis, thereby interfering with mitotic process. Rapidly proliferating tissues (malignant cells, bone marrow) are sensitive to this effect. In psoriasis, reproductive rate of epithelial cells is higher than in normal cells. Induces remission slowly; use often preceded by other antineoplastic therapies.

USES Principally in combination regimens to maintain induced remissions in neoplastic diseases. Effective in treatment of gestational choriocarcinoma and hydatidiform mole and as immunosuppressant in kidney transplantation, for acute and subacute leukemias and leukemic meningitis, especially in children. Used in lymphosarcoma, in certain inoperable tumors of head, neck, and pelvis, and in mycosis fungoides. Also used to treat severe psoriasis nonresponsive to other forms of therapy, rheumatoid arthritis. **Unlabeled uses:** psoriatic arthritis, SLE, polymyositis.

ROUTE & DOSAGE

Trophoblastic Neoplasm

Adult: **PO** 15–30 mg/d for 5 d; repeat q12wk for 3–5 courses. **IM/IV** 15–30 mg/d for 5 d; repeat q12wk for 3–5 courses.

Leukemia

Adult: **IM/IV** Induction: 3.3 $mg/m^2/d$; **PO/IM/IV** Maintenance: 20–30 mg/m^2 2 times/wk.
Child: **PO/IM** 7.5–30 mg/m^2 q1–2 wk.

Lymphoma

Adult: **PO** 12–25 mg/d for 4–8 d with 7–10 d rest intervals.

Psoriasis

Adult: **PO** 2.5–5 mg q12h for 3 doses each wk up to 25–30 mg/wk. **IM/IV** 10–25 mg/wk.

Rheumatoid Arthritis

Adult: **PO** 2.5–5 mg q12h for 3 doses each wk or 7.5 mg once/wk.
Child: **PO/IM/SC** 5–15 mg/m^2/wk as single dose or in 3 divided doses 12 h apart.

PHARMACOKINETICS Absorption: readily absorbed from GI tract. **Peak:** 0.5–2 h IM/IV; 1–4 h PO. **Distribution:** widely distributed with highest concentrations in kidneys, gallbladder, spleen, liver, and skin; minimal passage across blood–brain barrier; crosses placenta; distributed into breast milk. **Metabolism:** metabolized in liver. **Elimination:** half-life: 2–4 h; excreted primarily in urine.

CONTRAINDICATIONS & PRECAUTIONS **Contraindicated in:** pregnancy (category D), men and women in childbearing age; hepatic and renal insufficiency; concomitant administration of hepatotoxic drugs and hematopoietic depressants; alcohol; ultraviolet exposure to psoriatic lesions; preexisting blood dyscrasias. **Cautious use in:** infections; peptic ulcer, ulcerative colitis; very young or old patients; cancer patients with preexisting bone marrow impairment, poor nutritional status.

ADVERSE/SIDE EFFECTS Dose-related and reversible. **CNS:** *headache,* drowsiness, blurred vision, dizziness, aphasia, hemiparesis; arachnoiditis, convulsions (after intrathecal administration); mental confusion, tremors, ataxia, coma. **GI:** hepatotoxicity, GI ulcerations and hemorrhage, *ulcerative stomatitis, glossitis, gingivitis,* pharyngitis, nausea, vomiting, diarrhea, hepatic cirrhosis. **GU:** defective oogenesis or spermatogenesis, nephropathy, hematuria, menstrual dysfunction, infertility, abortion, fetal defects. **Hematologic:** *leukopenia, thrombocytopenia,* anemia, marked myelosuppression, aplastic bone marrow, telangiectasis, thrombophlebitis at intraarterial catheter site, hypogammaglobulinemia, hyperuricemia. **Skin:** erythematous rashes, pruritus, urticaria, folliculitis, vasculitis, photosensitivity, depigmentation, hyperpigmentation, alopecia. **Other:** malaise, undue fatigue, systemic toxicity (after intrathecal and intraarterial administration), chills, fever, decreased resistance to infection, septicemia, osteoporosis, metabolic changes precipitating diabetes and sudden death, pneumonitis, pulmonary fibrosis.

DIAGNOSTIC TEST INTERFERENCE Severe reactions may occur when ***live vaccines*** are administered because of immunosuppressive activity of methotrexate.

DRUG INTERACTIONS **Alcohol** increases risk of hepatotoxicity; **chloramphenicol,** SALICYLATES, NSAIDS, SULFONAMIDES, SULFONYLUREAS, **phenylbutazone, phenytoin,** TETRACYCLINES, **PABA, penicillin, probenecid** may increase methotrexate levels with increased toxicity; **folic acid** may alter response to methotrexate.

INCOMPATIBILITIES **Solution/additive: bleomycin, prednisolone, droperidol, heparin, metoclopramide, ranitidine. Y-site: droperidol, ranitidine.**

NURSING IMPLICATIONS

Administration

- Oral preparations should be given 1 h before or 2 h after meals.
- A test dose (5–10 mg parenterally) 1 wk before therapy precedes treatment of psoriasis.
- Avoid skin exposure and inhalation of drug particles.
- IV preparation: Dilute by adding 5 mg to 2 ml of NS or D5W without preservatives to yield 2.5 mg/ml.
- IV administration: Give diluted drug by direct IV at rate of 10 mg or fraction thereof over 60 s.
- IV administration to children: Verify correct IV concentration and rate of infusion with physician.
- Preserve drug in tight, light-resistant container.

Assessment & Drug Effects

- Hepatic and renal function tests, blood tests, and chest x-rays should be part of the health data base. Tests are repeated at weekly intervals during methotrexate therapy.
- Prolonged treatment with small frequent doses may lead to hepa-

Common side effect in *italic,* life-threatening effects underlined: generic names in **bold;** drug class in SMALL CAPS

totoxicity, which is best diagnosed by liver biopsy.

- Ulcerative stomatitis with glossitis and gingivitis, often the first signs of toxicity, necessitate interruption of therapy or dosage adjustment. Inspect mouth daily; report patchy necrotic areas, bleeding and discomfort, or overgrowth (black, furry tongue).
- In presence of hyperuricemia, patient may be kept well hydrated (about 2000 ml/24 h) to dilute hyperuric fluids and given allopurinol to prevent urate deposition.
- Monitor I&O ratio and pattern. Severe nephrotoxicity (hematuria, dysuria, azotemia, oliguria) fosters drug accumulation and renal damage and requires dosage adjustment or discontinuation.
- During leukopenic periods, prevent exposure to personnel and visitors with infections or colds. Be alert to onset of agranulocytosis (cough, extreme fatigue, sore throat, chills, fever) and report symptoms promptly. Methotrexate therapy will be interrupted and appropriate antibiotic drugs prescribed.
- Be alert for and report symptoms of thrombocytopenia: ecchymoses, petechiae, epistaxis, melena, hematuria, vaginal bleeding, slow and protracted oozing following trauma.
- Bloody diarrhea necessitates interruption of therapy to prevent perforation or hemorrhagic enteritis. Report to physician.
- Diabetes may be precipitated; therefore, periodically monitor blood glucose.

Patient & Family Education

- Inform of dangers of this drug and warn to report promptly any abnormal symptoms.
- Alcohol ingestion increases the incidence and severity of methotrexate hepatotoxicity.
- Fastidious mouth care prevents infection, provides comfort, and is essential to maintenance of adequate nutritional status.
- Alopecia is reversible; hair regrowth begins after drug discontinuation, but it may require several months.
- Methotrexate may precipitate gouty arthritis. Instruct the patient to report joint pains to physician.
- Warn not to self-medicate with vitamins. Some OTC compounds may include folic acid (or its derivatives), which alters methotrexate response.
- Contraceptive measures should be used both during and for at least 8 wk following therapy.
- Exposure to ultraviolet light and to sunlight may aggravate psoriatic lesions in patients on methotrexate therapy.
- Burning and erythema may occur in psoriatic areas after each dose of methotrexate. Instruct to notify physician if psoriasis worsens.

METHOTRIMEPRAZINE

(meth-oh-trye-mep′ra-zeen)

Trade names: Levoprome, Nozinan ♣

Classifications: CNS AGENT; NONNARCOTIC ANALGESIC; PHENOTHIAZINE ANXIOLYTIC; SEDATIVE-HYPNOTIC

Prototype: Chlorpromazine

Pregnancy category: C

ACTIONS/PHARMACODYNAMICS

Methotrimeprazine, in addition to tranquilizing and sedative effects, also has prominent analgesic properties. Extrapyramidal symptoms and dry mouth reportedly uncommon, but orthostatic hypotension and sedation effects are more prominent. Raises pain threshold and may also produce amnesia.

USES To relieve moderate to severe pain in nonambulatory patients and for analgesia and sedation when respiratory depression is to be avoided, as in obstetrics and pre- and postoperatively.

ROUTE & DOSAGE

Analgesia, Sedation
Adult: **IM** 10–20 mg q4–6h.

Preoperative Medication
Adult: **IM** 2–20 mg 45 min–3 h before surgery.

Postoperative Analgesia
Adult: **IM** 2.5–7.5 mg q4–6h as needed.

M

PHARMACOKINETICS **Onset:** 20–40 min. **Peak:** 1–2 h. **Duration:** 4 h. **Distribution:** crosses CSF and placenta; distributed into breast milk. **Metabolism:** metabolized in liver. **Elimination:** slowly excreted in urine; elimination may continue for 1 wk after a single dose.

CONTRAINDICATIONS & PRECAUTIONS **Contraindicated in:** hypersensitivity to phenothiazines and to ingredients in the formulation, e.g., bisulfite; severe cardiac, renal, or hepatic disease; history of convulsive disorders; significant hypotension; comatose states; premature labor; children < 12 y; concomitant use with antihypertensive agents, including MAO inhibitors. **Cautious use in:** elderly and debilitated patients with heart disease; early pregnancy (category C).

ADVERSE/SIDE EFFECTS **CNS:** *excessive sedation, drowsiness, amnesia,* disorientation, euphoria, delirium, extrapyramidal symptoms. **CV:** *orthostatic hypotension with faintness,* weakness, dizziness; tachycardia, bradycardia, palpitation. **EENT:** blurred vision, nasal congestion. **GI:** nausea, vomiting, abdominal discomfort, dry mouth. **GU:** dysuria, hematuria. **Other:** headache, slurred speech, fever, chills, injection site reactions, <u>respiratory depression</u> (infrequent). **With prolonged high dosage:** increased weight, jaundice, severe blood dyscrasias including <u>agranulocytosis and pancytopenia</u>.

DRUG INTERACTIONS **Alcohol** and other CNS DEPRESSANTS enhance CNS depression; with ANTICHOLINERGIC AGENTS, aggravation of extrapyramidal symptoms, CNS stimulation, delirium, tachycardia, and hypotension; ANTIHYPERTENSIVE AGENTS, MAO INHIBITORS add to hypotensive effects; **epinephrine** may antagonize pressor effects; SKELETAL MUSCLE RELAXANTS may prolong duration of muscle relaxation.

INCOMPATIBILITIES **Solution/additive: ranitidine. Y-site: heparin.**

NURSING IMPLICATIONS

Administration

- Administer IM injection deep into large muscle mass.
- Pain at injection site and local inflammatory reaction commonly occur. Rotate injection sites and observe daily.
- The manufacturer states that methotrimeprazine may be mixed in the same syringe with either atropine or scopolamine, but not with any other drugs. (Dosage of atropine or scopolamine should be reduced.)
- Protect drug from light.

Assessment & Drug Effects

- Orthostatic hypotension with faintness, weakness, and dizziness may occur within 10–20 min after drug administration and may last 4–6 h and occasionally as long as 12 h. Ambulation should be avoided or carefully supervised for at least 6 h, but preferably 12 h. Tolerance to these effects usually develops with successive doses.
- Excessive sedation and amnesia also occur commonly during early drug therapy.
- BP and pulse should be checked frequently until dosage requirements and response are stabilized. Elderly and debilitated patients require close monitoring.
- When drug is used for prolonged periods, periodic blood studies and liver function tests are recommended.
- Injection formulation contains bisulfite, an allergen for some individuals.
- If severe hypotension occurs, treatment with epinephrine is specifically contraindicated.

METHOXAMINE HYDROCHLORIDE

(meth-ox'a meen)

Trade name: Vasoxyl

Prototype for classifications: AUTONOMIC NERVOUS SYSTEM AGENT; ALPHA-ADRENERGIC AGONIST (SYMPATHOMIMETIC)

Pregnancy category: C

ACTIONS/PHARMACODYNAMICS Direct-acting sympathomimetic amine pharmacologically related to phenylephrine. Acts almost exclusively on alpha-adrenergic receptors. Pressor action is due primarily to direct peripheral vasoconstriction, which in turn causes rise in arterial BP. Has no direct effect on heart but tends to slow ventricular rate by vagal stimulation in response to elevated BP. Large doses may produce bradycardia. Markedly reduces renal blood flow. CNS-stimulating action. True tachyphylaxis not reported.

USES To support, restore, or maintain BP during anesthesia and to terminate some episodes of paroxysmal supraventricular tachycardia.

ROUTE & DOSAGE

Hypotension During Anesthesia

Adult: **IM** 5–20 mg. **IV** 3–5 mg. *Child:* **IM** 0.25 mg/kg. **IV** 0.08 mg/kg.

Paroxysmal Supraventricular Tachycardia

Adult: **IM** 10–20 mg. **IV** 5–15 mg over 3–5min.

PHARMACOKINETICS **Onset:** immediately after IV. **Peak:** 0.5–2 min IV; 15–20 min IM. **Duration:** 5–15 min IV; 60–90 min IM. **Metabolism:** unknown. **Elimination:** unknown.

CONTRAINDICATIONS & PRECAUTIONS **Contraindicated in:** severe coronary or cardiovascular disease; hypovolemia, in combination with local anesthetics for tissue infiltration; within 2 wk of MAO inhibitors; pregnancy (category C). **Cautious use in:** history of hypertension or hyperthyroidism; following use of ergot alkaloids.

ADVERSE/SIDE EFFECTS Paresthesias, feeling of coldness (particularly with high dosage), restlessness, nervousness, high blood pressure, projectile vomiting, severe headache, pilomotor erection (gooseflesh), urinary urgency, bradycardia.

DRUG INTERACTIONS **Phentolamine** and PHENOTHIAZINES block vasopressor response. BETA BLOCKERS may increase amount of methoxamine available to receptor sites. **Atropine** blocks reflex bradycardia and enhances vasopressor effects. MAO INHIBITORS, **vasopressin**, and ERGOT ALKALOIDS may cause hypertensive crisis.

NURSING IMPLICATIONS

Administration

- Administer undiluted by direct IV at a rate of 5 mg/min if systolic BP is less than 60 mm Hg.
- Methoxamine may be diluted in 250 ml 5% dextrose and infused at rate needed to maintain blood pressure.
- Supplemental IM dose may be administered after emergency IV infusion.
- Antidote for extravasation: Area should be infiltrated as soon as possible with 10–15 ml normal saline solution containing 5–10 mg phentolamine.
- Protect drug from light.

Assessment & Drug Effects

- Patients should be under close supervision.
- Monitor vital signs. Report any increase in BP above level prescribed by physician; report slowing of heart rate.
- Be alert for sudden changes in blood pressure and pulse after drug has been discontinued.
- Monitor intake and output. Urinary frequency with retention is a possibility. Report oliguria or change in I&O ratio.
- Methoxamine injection contains a bisulfite, an allergen for some patients.

Patient & Family Education

- Instruct to report headache, which may be severe. This adverse effect may require analgesia for relief.
- Instruct to report nausea, since it may be accompanied by projectile vomiting.

METHOXSALEN

(meth-ox'a-len)

Trade names: 8-MOP, Oxsoralen, UltraMOP

Prototype for classifications: SKIN AGENT; PSORALEN

Pregnancy category: C

ACTIONS/PHARMACODYNAMICS

A psoralen derivative with strong photosensitizing effects: used with ultraviolet-A light (UVA) in therapeutic regimens called PUVA (P-psoralen). After photoactivation by long wavelength UVA, methoxsalen combines with epidermal cell DNA, causing photodamage (cytotoxic action) and inhibition of the rapid and uncontrolled epidermal cell turnover characteristic of psoriasis, and an inflammatory reaction with erythema. Methoxsalen is also strongly melanogenic.

USES With controlled exposure to UVA to repigment vitiliginous skin and for symptomatic treatment of severe disabling psoriasis that is refractory to other forms of therapy. **Unlabeled use:** (PUVA therapy) mycosis fungoides.

ROUTE & DOSAGE

Idiopathic Vitiligo

Adult: **Topical** Apply lotion 1–2 h before exposure to UV light once/wk.

Psoriasis

Adult: **PO** Administer 1.5–2 h before exposure to UV light 2–3 times/wk: <30 kg, 10 mg; 30–50 kg, 20 mg; 51–65 kg, 30 mg; 66–80 kg, 40 mg; 81–90 kg, 50 mg; 91–115 kg, 60 mg; >115 kg, 70 mg.

PHARMACOKINETICS Absorption: variably absorbed from GI tract. **Peak:** 2 h. **Duration:** 8–10 h. **Distribution:** preferentially taken up by epidermal cells; distributes into lens of eye. **Elimination:** half-life: 0.75–2.4 h; 80–90% excreted in urine within 8 h.

CONTRAINDICATIONS & PRECAUTIONS Contraindicated in: sunburn, sensitivity (or its history) to psoralens, diseases associated with photosensitivity (e.g., LE, albinism, melanoma or its history), invasive squamous cell cancer, cataract, aphakia, previous exposure to arsenic or ionizing radiation, pregnancy (category C); safe use (oral) in children not established. **Cautious use in:** hepatic insufficiency, GI disease, chronic infection, treatment with known photosensitizing agents; immunosuppressed patient, cardiovascular disease, nursing mothers; safe use (lotion) in children < 12 y not established.

ADVERSE/SIDE EFFECTS CNS: nervousness, dizziness, headache, mental depression or excitation, vertigo, insomnia. **Eye:** cataract formation, ocular damage. **GI:** cheilitis, *nausea* and other GI disturbances, toxic hepatitis. **Skin:** phototoxic effects: severe edema and erythema, *pruritus,* painful blisters; burning, peeling, thinning, freckling, and accelerated aging of skin; hyper- or hypopigmentation; severe skin pain (lasting 1–2 mo), photoallergic contact dermatitis (with topical use), exacerbation of latent photosensitive dermatoses, malignant melanoma (rare). **Other:** transient loss of muscular coordination, edema, leg cramps, systemic immune effects, drug fever.

DRUG INTERACTIONS Anthralin, coal tar, griseofulvin, PHENOTHIAZINES, **naladixic acid,** SULFONAMIDES, BACTERIOSTATIC SOAPS, TETRACYCLINES, THIAZIDES compound photosensitizing effects. **Drug–food:** food will increase peak and extent of absorption.

NURSING IMPLICATIONS

Administration

- Methoxsalen (PUVA therapy) should be under the complete control of a physician with special competence and experience in photochemotherapy.
- To prevent GI distress, oral doses are best administered with milk or food.
- Maintain a consistent time relationship between food–drug ingestion. Food digestion and absorption appear to affect drug serum levels.
- Only small (less than 10 cm^2), well-defined areas are treated with lotion. Systemic treatment is used for large areas.
- The lotion is applied with cotton swabs, allowed to dry 1–2 min, then reapplied. Borders of the lesion should be protected with petrolatum and sunscreen lotion to prevent hyperpigmentation.
- Finger cots or gloves should be used to apply lotion to prevent photosensitization and burned skin.
- During PUVA therapy, sunscreen lotion is applied to the skin for about one third of the initial exposure time until there is sufficient tanning. It should not be applied to psoriatric areas before the treatment.
- Store lotion and capsules in light-resistant containers at 15–30C

M

(59–86F) unless otherwise directed by manufacturer.

Assessment & Drug Effects

- A pretreatment ophthalmologic exam is performed to rule out cataracts; it should be repeated periodically during treatment and at yearly intervals thereafter.
- CBC, renal and hepatic function tests, and antinuclear antibody tests are monitored during PO psoralen therapy.
- Fair-skinned patients appear to be at greatest risk for photochemotherapeutic toxicity from PUVA therapy (see Adverse/Side Effects).
- Repigmentation is more rapid on fleshy areas, i.e., face, abdomen, buttocks, than on hands or feet.

Patient & Family Education

- Effective repigmentation may require 6–9 mo of treatment; periodic treatment usually is necessary to retain pigmentation. If, after 3 mo of treatment, there is no apparent response, methoxsalen is discontinued.
- After drug ingestion and UVA exposure, additional exposure to UV light (direct or indirect) should be avoided for at least 8 h.
- After topical application, the initial sunlight exposure is limited to 1 min, with subsequent gradual and incremental exposures by prescription. The patient should fully understand the intended schedule.
- After topical methoxsalen application and UVA exposure, the patient should not expose skin to additional UV light for 24–48 h.
- If sunlight cannot be avoided after the treatment, sunscreen lotion (with SPF 15 or higher) and protective clothing (hat, gloves) should cover all exposed areas including lips, to prevent burning or blistering.
- Sunbathing is contraindicated for at least 48 h after PUVA treatment. Sunburn and photochemotherapy are additive in the production of burning and erythema.
- Wraparound sunglasses with UVA-absorbing properties must be worn both indoors and outdoors during daylight hours for 24 h.
- Warn not to substitute prescription sunglasses or photosensitive darkening glasses; they may actually increase danger of cataract formation.
- Instruct to alert physician to appearance of new psoriatic areas, to flares, or to regressed cleared skin areas should they occur during treatment and maintenance periods.

METHSCOPOLAMINE BROMIDE

(meth-skoe-pol′a-meen)

Trade name: Pamine

Classifications: AUTONOMIC NERVOUS SYSTEM AGENT; ANTICHOLINERGIC (PARASYMPATHOLYTIC); ANTIMUSCARINIC; ANTISPASMODIC

Prototype: Atropine

Pregnancy category: C

ACTIONS/PHARMACODYNAMICS

Quaternary ammonium derivative of scopolamine but lacks scopolamine's CNS actions. Its spasmolytic and antisecretory actions are quantitatively similar to those of atropine, but they last longer. Has greater selectivity in blocking vagal impulses from GI tract than either scopolamine or atropine.

USES Adjunct in treatment of peptic ulcer, irritable bowel syndrome, and a variety of other GI conditions. Also may be used to control excessive sweating and salivation, migraine headaches, and premenstrual cramps.

Common side effect in *italic*, life-threatening effects underlined; generic names in **bold**; drug class in SMALL CAPS

ROUTE & DOSAGE

Adult: **PO** 2.5–5 mg 30 min a.c. and h.s.

PHARMACOKINETICS Absorption: erratic after PO administration. **Onset:** approximately 1 h. **Duration:** 4–6 h. **Elimination:** excreted primarily in urine and bile; some unchanged drug excreted in feces.

CONTRAINDICATIONS & PRECAUTIONS Contraindicated in: hypersensitivity to any of the drug's constituents, prostatic hypertrophy, pyloric obstruction, intestinal atony, tachycardia, cardiac disease. Safe use during pregnancy (category C) not established. **Cautious use in:** elderly and debilitated patients.

ADVERSE/SIDE EFFECTS Dry mouth, blurred vision, dizziness, drowsiness, constipation, flushing of skin, urinary hesitancy or retention.

NURSING IMPLICATIONS

Administration

- PO preparation is usually administered 30 min before meals and at bedtime.
- Preserve in tight, light-resistant containers.

Assessment & Drug Effects

- Incidence and severity of side effects are generally dose-related and therefore may be controlled by dosage reduction. Dosage is usually maintained at a level that produces slight dryness of mouth.
- Urinary retention may be an indication for discontinuation of the drug. Report promptly.

Patient & Family Education

- Warn not to engage in activities requiring mental alertness, such as driving a car, until response to drug is known.
- Caution to make position changes slowly and in stages.
- Dryness of mouth may be relieved by sugarless chewing gum or candy or by frequent rinsing of mouth with water.

METHSUXIMIDE

(meth-sux′i-mide)

Trade name: Celontin

Classifications: CNS AGENT; ANTICONVULSANT; SUCCINIMIDE

Prototype: Ethosuximide

Pregnancy category: C

ACTIONS/PHARMACODYNAMICS Succinimide derivative with actions, contraindications, precautions, and adverse reactions similar to those of ethosuximide. Associated with high incidence of adverse effects.

USES Control of absence (petit mal) seizures refractory to other anticonvulsants. May be used in combination with other anticonvulsants in mixed types of epilepsy.

ROUTE & DOSAGE

Absence Seizures

Adult: **PO** 300 mg/d; may increase q4–7d as needed (max 1.2 g/d in divided doses).
Child: **PO** 10–15 mg/kg/d in 3–4 divided doses; may increase to max of 30 mg/kg/d.

PHARMACOKINETICS Absorption: readily absorbed from GI tract. **Peak:** 1–3 h. **Metabolism:** metabolized in liver. **Elimination:** half-life: 3 h; excreted slowly in urine; small amounts excreted in bile and feces.

CONTRAINDICATIONS & PRECAUTIONS Contraindicated in: hypersensitivity to succinimides; drug allergies; hepatic or renal disease; blood dyscrasias; pregnancy (category C).

ADVERSE/SIDE EFFECTS **CNS:** *drowsiness, dizziness, ataxia;* headache, insomnia, diplopia, photophobia, severe mental depression, behavioral changes. **GI:** *nausea, vomiting, anorexia, diarrhea, constipation, epigastric* or *abdominal pain, weight loss.* **Hypersensitivity:** skin eruptions, fever, hiccups, periorbital edema and hyperemia, blood dyscrasias including aplastic anemia.

DRUG INTERACTIONS **Carbamazepine** decreases methsuximide levels; **isoniazid** significantly increases methsuximide levels; the levels of both **phenobarbital** and methsuximide may be altered, with increased seizure frequency.

M

NURSING IMPLICATIONS

Administration

- Drug should be taken exactly as prescribed.
- Store capsules away from heat at 15–30C (59–86F) unless otherwise directed.

Assessment & Drug Effects

- Drug tolerance varies among patients. Patient must be closely observed when dosage is increased or decreased or when other medication is being added or eliminated.
- Observe patient closely for behavioral changes. Drug should be withdrawn (slowly) at first appearance of depression, aggression, or other unusual behavioral manifestations to prevent progression to acute psychosis.
- Periodic blood cell counts, tests of liver function, and urinalysis should be performed during therapy.
- Caution patients to avoid potentially hazardous activities such as driving a car until drug response is known.

Patient & Family Education

- Advise to report immediately the onset of adverse effects (often controlled by dosage reduction). Development of a rash may herald more serious reactions.
- Advise to report immediately any signs of infection (e.g., sore throat, fever).
- Abrupt drug withdrawal may precipitate petit mal seizures.
- Advise to carry identification indicating that he or she has epilepsy and is taking medication.

METHYCLOTHIAZIDE

(meth-i-kloe-thye′a-zide)

Trade names: Aquatensen, Duretic ♣, Enduron, Ethon

Classifications: ELECTROLYTIC AND WATER BALANCE AGENT; THIAZIDE DIURETIC

Prototype: Hydrochlorothiazide

Pregnancy category: C

ACTIONS/PHARMACODYNAMICS Thiazide diuretic. Similar to hydrochlorothiazide in actions, uses, contraindications, adverse reactions, and interactions.

USES Primary (step 1) agent in stepped care approach to antihypertensive treatment and adjunctively in the management of edema associated with CHF, renal pathology, and hepatic cirrhosis.

ROUTE & DOSAGE

Edema

Adult: **PO** 2.5–10 mg once/d or 3–5 times/wk.

Hypertension

Adult: **PO** 2.5–10 mg/d.
Child: **PO** 0.05–0.2 mg/kg/d.

PHARMACOKINETICS **Absorption:** incompletely absorbed. **Onset:** 2 h. **Peak:** 6 h. **Duration:** > 24 h. **Distribution:** distributed throughout extracellular tissue; concentrates in kidney; crosses placenta; distributed in breast milk. **Metabolism:** does not appear to be metabolized. **Elimination:** excreted in urine.

CONTRAINDICATIONS & PRECAUTIONS **Contraindicated in:** hypersensitivity to thiazides, sulfonamide derivatives; anuria, hypokalemia, pregnancy (category C), nursing mothers. **Cautious use in:** impaired renal or hepatic function, gout, SLE, hypercalcemia, diabetes mellitus.

ADVERSE/SIDE EFFECTS Postural hypotension, sialadenitis, unusual fatigue, dizziness, paresthesias, photosensitivity, yellow vision, *hypokalemia,* agranulocytosis.

DRUG INTERACTIONS **Amphotericin B,** CORTICOSTEROIDS increase hypokalemic effects; may antagonize hypoglycemic effects of **insulin,** SULFONYLUREAS; **cholestyramine, colestipol** decrease thiazide absorption; intensifies hypoglycemic and hypotensive effects of **diazoxide;** increased potassium and magnesium loss may cause **digoxin** toxicity; decreases **lithium** excretion, increasing its toxicity; NSAIDS may attenuate diuresis, and risk of NSAID-induced renal failure increased.

NURSING IMPLICATIONS

Administration

- Administer drug early in AM after eating (to reduce gastric irritation) to prevent sleep interruption because of diuresis. If 2 doses are ordered, administer second dose no later than 3 PM.
- Store drug at 15–30C (59–86F) unless otherwise instructed.

Assessment & Drug Effects

- Antihypertensive effects may be noted in 3–4 d; maximal effects may require 3–4 wk.
- Monitor BP and I&O ratio during first phase of antihypertensive therapy. Report a sudden fall in BP, which may initiate severe postural hypotension and potentially dangerous perfusion problems, especially in the extremities.
- Monitor patient for signs of hypokalemia (see Appendix G). Report promptly. Physician may change dose and institute replacement therapy.

Patient & Family Education

- Hypokalemia is rarely severe in most patients even on long-term therapy with thiazides if they eat a balanced diet. To prevent onset, urge patient to eat potassium-rich foods (potatoes, whole grain cereals, beef, fruit juices, skim milk) and to include a banana (about 370 mg potassium) and at least 180 ml (6 oz) orange juice (about 330 mg potassium) every day.
- The diabetic patient should be watched carefully for loss of diabetes control or early signs of hyperglycemia (see Appendix G). The symptoms are slow to develop.
- Counsel to avoid use of OTC drugs unless they are approved by the physician. Many preparations contain both potassium and sodium, and electrolyte imbalance side effects may be induced.
- The elderly are more responsive to excessive diuresis; advise that orthostatic hypotension may be a problem.
- Instruct patient with orthostatic hypotension to change from recumbency to upright positions slowly and in stages; to avoid hot baths or showers, extended exposure to sunlight, and standing still. Provide

assistance as necessary to prevent falling.

- Advise to avoid driving a vehicle or working with dangerous equipment until adjustment to the hypotensive effects of this drug has been made.

METHYLDOPA

(meth-ill-doe'pa)

Trade names: Aldomet, Apo-Methyldopa♣, Dopamet♣, Novomedopa♣

METHYLDOPATE HYDROCHLORIDE

(meth-ill-doe'pate)

Trade name: Aldomet Ester HCl Injection

Prototype for classifications: CARDIOVASCULAR AGENT; CENTRAL-ACTING ANTIHYPERTENSIVE; AUTONOMIC NERVOUS SYSTEM AGENT; ALPHA-ADRENERGIC AGONIST (SYMPATHOMIMETIC)

Pregnancy category: C

ACTIONS/PHARMACODYNAMICS Structurally related to catecholamines and their precursors. Has weak neurotransmitter properties; inhibits decarboxylation of dopa, thereby reducing concentration of dopamine, a precursor of norepinephrine; also inhibits the precursor of serotonin. Lowers standing and supine BP, and unlike adrenergic blockers, it is not so prone to produce orthostatic hypotension, diurnal blood pressure variations, or exercise hypertension. Reduces renal vascular resistance; maintains cardiac output without acceleration, but may slow heart rate; tends to support sodium and water retention.

USES Step 2 agent in stepped-care approach in treatment of sustained moderate to severe hypertension, particularly in patients with renal dysfunction. Also used in selected patients with carcinoid disease. Parenteral form has been used for treatment of hypertensive crises but is not preferred because of its slow onset of action.

ROUTE & DOSAGE

Hypertension

Adult: **PO** 250 mg b.i.d. or t.i.d.; may be increased up to 3 g/d in divided doses. **IV** 250–500 mg q6h given over 30–60 min, up to 1 g q6h.
Geriatric: **PO** 125 mg b.i.d. or t.i.d., may increase gradually to max of 3 g/d.
Child: **PO** 10–65 mg/kg/d in 2–4 divided doses (max 3 g/d). **IV** 20–65 mg/kg/d in 4 divided doses.

PHARMACOKINETICS Absorption: about 50% absorbed from GI tract. **Peak:** 4–6 h. **Duration:** 24 h PO; 10–16 h IV. **Distribution:** crosses placenta, distributed into breast milk. **Metabolism:** metabolized in liver and GI tract. **Elimination:** half-life: 1.7 h; excreted primarily in urine.

CONTRAINDICATIONS & PRECAUTIONS Contraindicated in: active hepatic disease (hepatitis, cirrhosis), pheochromocytoma, blood dyscrasias. Safe use during pregnancy (category C) not established. **Cautious use in:** history of impaired liver or renal function or disease; angina pectoris, history of mental depression, young or elderly patients.

ADVERSE/SIDE EFFECTS Allergic: *fever,* skin eruptions, ulcerations of soles of feet, flu-like symptoms, lymphadenopathy, eosinophilia.

CNS: *sedation, drowsiness,* sluggishness, headache, weakness, fatigue, dizziness, vertigo, *decrease in mental acuity,* inability to concentrate, amnesia-like syndrome, parkinsonism, mild psychoses, depression, nightmares. **CV:** orthostatic hypotension, syncope, bradycardia, myocarditis, edema, weight gain *(sodium and water retention),* paradoxic hypertensive reaction (especially with IV administration). **GI:** diarrhea, constipation, abdominal distension, malabsorption syndrome, nausea, vomiting, dry mouth, sore or black tongue, sialadenitis. **Hematologic:** *positive direct Coombs' test* (common especially in blacks), granulocytopenia. **Hepatotoxicity** (believed to be allergic reaction): abnormal liver function tests, jaundice, hepatitis, hepatic necrosis (rare). **Other:** *nasal stuffiness,* gynecomastia, lactation, *decreased libido, impotence,* hypothermia (large doses), positive tests for lupus and rheumatoid factors, granulomatous skin lesions.

DRUG INTERACTIONS AMPHETAMINES, TRICYCLIC ANTIDEPRESSANTS, PHENOTHIAZINES may attenuate antihypertensive response; methyldopa may inhibit effectiveness of **ephedrine; haloperidol** may exacerbate psychiatric symptoms; with **levodopa,** additive hypotension, increased CNS toxicity, especially psychosis; increases risk of **lithium** toxicity; **methotrimeprazine** causes excessive hypotension; MAO INHIBITORS may cause hallucinations; **phenoxybenzamine** may cause urinary incontinence.

INCOMPATIBILITIES **Solution/additive: amphotericin B, methohexital, verapamil. Y-site:** fat emulsion.

DIAGNOSTIC TEST INTERFERENCE Methyldopa may interfere with ***serum creatinine*** measurements using alkaline picrate method, ***AST*** by colorimetric methods, and ***uric acid*** measurements by phosphotungstate method (with high methyldopa blood levels); it may produce false elevations of ***urinary catecholamines*** and increase in ***serum amylase*** in methyldopa-induced sialadenitis.

NURSING IMPLICATIONS

Administration

- IV methyldopa may be given diluted in 100–200 ml of D5W. Administer over 30–60 min.
- To minimize daytime sedation, physician may prescribe dosage increases to be made in the evening. Some patients maintain adequate BP control with a single evening dose.

Assessment & Drug Effects

- During IV infusion of methyldopate, check BP and pulse at least q30min until stabilized, and observe for adequacy of urinary output.
- During period of dosage adjustment, physician may request BP to be taken at regular intervals in lying, sitting, and standing positions.
- Transient sedation, drowsiness, mental depression, weakness, and headache commonly occur during first 24–72 h of therapy or whenever dosage is increased. Symptoms tend to disappear with continuation of therapy or dosage reduction.
- Elderly patients and patients with impaired renal function are particularly likely to manifest orthostatic hypotension with dizziness and light-headedness during period of dosage adjustment. Supervision of ambulation is advisable.

- Monitor fluid and electrolyte balance and I&O. Report oliguria and changes in I&O ratio. Weigh patient daily, and check for edema because methyldopa favors sodium and water retention.
- Baseline and regularly scheduled blood counts and liver function tests are advised during first 6–12 wk of therapy or if patient develops unexplained fever.
- Be alert to and report symptoms of mental depression (e.g., anorexia, insomnia, inattention to personal hygiene, withdrawal). Drug-induced depression may persist after drug is withdrawn.
- Rising BP indicating tolerance to drug effect may occur during week 2 or 3 of therapy.

Patient & Family Education

- Caution that hot baths and showers, prolonged standing in one position, and strenuous exercise may enhance orthostatic hypotension. Instruct patient to make position changes slowly, particularly from recumbent to upright posture and to dangle legs a few minutes before standing.
- Caution that methyldopa may affect ability to perform activities requiring concentrated mental effort, especially during first few days of therapy or whenever dosage is increased; patient should avoid potentially hazardous tasks such as driving a car until reaction to drug is known.
- Advise not to take OTC medications unless approved by physician.

METHYLERGONOVINE MALEATE

(meth-ill-er-goe-noe'veen)

Trade name: Methergine

Classifications: AUTONOMIC NERVOUS SYSTEM AGENT; ADRENERGIC ANTAGONIST (SYMPATHOLYTIC); ERGOT ALKALOID; OXYTOCIC

Prototype: Ergotamine

ACTIONS/PHARMACODYNAMICS Ergot alkaloid that induces rapid, sustained tetanic uterine contraction that shortens third stage of labor and reduces blood loss. Has minimal vasoconstrictive activity.

USES Routine management after delivery of placenta and for postpartum atony, subinvolution, and hemorrhage. With full obstetric supervision, may be used during second stage of labor.

ROUTE & DOSAGE

Postpartum Hemorrhage

Adult: **PO** 0.2–0.4 mg q6–12h until danger of atony passes (2–7 d). **IM/IV** 0.2 mg q2–4h up to a max of 5 doses.

PHARMACOKINETICS **Absorption:** readily absorbed from GI tract. **Onset:** 5–15 min PO; 2–5 min IM; immediate IV. **Duration:** 3 or more h PO; 3 h IM; 45 min IV. **Distribution:** distributed into breast milk. **Metabolism:** slowly metabolized in liver. **Elimination:** half-life: 0.5–2 h; excreted mainly in feces, small amount in urine.

CONTRAINDICATIONS & PRECAUTIONS **Contraindicated in:** hypersensitivity to ergot preparations, to induce labor, use prior to delivery of placenta, threatened spontaneous abortion, prolonged use, uterine sepsis, hypertension, toxemia.

ADVERSE/SIDE EFFECTS *Nausea, vomiting* (especially with IV doses), severe hypertensive episodes, bradycardia, allergic phenomena including shock, ergotism.

DRUG INTERACTIONS PARENTERAL SYMPATHOMIMETICS, other ERGOT ALKALOIDS add to pressor effects and carry risk of hypertension.

NURSING IMPLICATIONS

Administration

- IV methylergonovine may be given by direct IV undiluted at a rate of 0.2 mg over 60 seconds.
- Ampuls containing discolored solution or visible particles should not be used. Store at 15–30C (59–86F) unless otherwise directed. Protect from light.

Assessment & Drug Effects

- Monitor vital signs (particularly BP) and uterine response during and after parenteral administration of methylergonovine until partum period is stabilized (about 1–2 h).
- Notify physician if BP suddenly increases or if there are frequent periods of uterine relaxation.

METHYLPHENIDATE HYDROCHLORIDE

(meth-ill-fen′i-date)

Trade names: Ritalin, Ritalin-SR
Classifications: CNS AGENT; RESPIRATORY AND CEREBRAL STIMULANT
Prototype: Amphetamine
Pregnancy category: C
Controlled substance: Schedule II

ACTIONS/PHARMACODYNAMICS Piperidine derivative with actions and abuse potential qualitatively similar to those of amphetamine. Acts mainly on cerebral cortex. Exerts mild CNS and respiratory stimulation analeptic effect with potency intermediate between those of amphetamine and caffeine. Effects more prominent on mental than on motor activities. Also believed to have an anorexiant effect.

USES Adjunctive therapy in hyperkinetic syndromes characterized by attention deficit disorder, narcolepsy, mild depression, and apathetic or withdrawn senile behavior.

ROUTE & DOSAGE

Narcolepsy

Adult: **PO** 10 mg b.i.d. or t.i.d. 30–45 min p.c. (range 20–40 mg/d).

Attention Deficit Disorder

Child: **PO** 5–10 mg before breakfast and lunch, with a gradual increase of 5–10 mg/wk as needed (max 60 mg/d).

Depression

Geriatric: **PO** 2.5 mg in morning before 9 AM, may increase by 2.5–5 mg q2–3d to max 20 mg/d divided 7 AM and noon.

PHARMACOKINETICS Absorption: readily absorbed from GI tract. **Peak:** 1.9 h; 4–7 h extended release. **Duration:** 3–6 h; 8 h extended release. **Elimination:** excreted in urine.

CONTRAINDICATIONS & PRECAUTIONS Contraindicated in: hypersensitivity to drug; history of marked anxiety, agitation; motor tics, or Tourette's disease. Safe use in pregnancy (category C), by nursing mothers, or by children < 6 y of age not established. **Cautious use in:** the alcoholic; emotionally unstable patient; history of drug dependence; hypertension; history of seizures.

ADVERSE/SIDE EFFECTS CNS: dizziness, drowsiness, *nervousness, insomnia*. **CV:** palpitations, changes in BP and pulse rate, angina, cardiac arrhythmias. **Eye:** difficulty with accommodation, blurred vision. **GI:** dry throat, anorexia, nausea; hepatotoxicity; abdominal pain. **Other:** hypersensitivity reactions (rash, fever, arthralgia, urticaria, exfoliative dermatitis, erythema multiforme); growth suppression.

DRUG INTERACTIONS MAO INHIBITORS may cause hypertensive crisis; antagonizes hypotensive effects of **guanethidine, bretylium.**

NURSING IMPLICATIONS

Administration

- Administer 30–45 min before meals. To avoid insomnia, last dose should be taken before 6 PM.
- Sustained-release tablets: Swallow whole; do not crush.
- Store at 15–30C (59–86F).

Assessment & Drug Effects

- BP and pulse should be monitored at appropriate intervals.
- Periodic CBC and differential and platelet counts are advised during prolonged therapy.
- Chronic abusive use can lead to tolerance, psychic dependence, and psychoses.
- During prolonged therapy, periodic drug-free periods are recommended to assess the child's condition.
- Careful supervision is required for drug withdrawal following prolonged use. Abrupt withdrawal may result in severe depression and psychotic behavior.

Patient & Family Education

- Nervousness and insomnia may diminish with time or require reduction of dosage or omission of afternoon or evening dose. Advise to report these and other adverse effects.
- Advise to check weight at least 2 or 3 times weekly and to report weight loss. Height and weight should be checked in children, and failure to gain in either should be reported.

METHYLPREDNISOLONE

(meth-ill-pred-niss'oh-lone)

Trade name: Medrol

METHYLPREDNISOLONE ACETATE

Trade names: Depoject, Depo-Medrol, Depopred, Duralone, M-Prednisol, Rep-Pred

METHYLPREDNISOLONE SODIUM SUCCINATE

Trade names: A-MethaPred, Solu-Medrol

Classifications: SYNTHETIC HORMONE; ADRENAL CORTICOSTEROID; GLUCOCORTICOID; ANTIINFLAMMATORY

Prototype: Prednisone

Pregnancy category: C

ACTIONS/PHARMACODYNAMICS

Intermediate-acting synthetic adrenal corticosteroid with similar glucocorticoid activity but considerably fewer sodium and water retention effects than hydrocortisone. Acetate has longer duration of action and more rapid onset of activity than parent compound. Sodium succinate is characterized by rapid onset of action and is used for emergency therapy of short duration.

USES An antiinflammatory agent in the management of acute and chronic inflammatory diseases, for palliative management of neoplastic diseases, and for control of severe acute and chronic allergic processes. High-dose, short-term therapy: management of acute bronchial asthma, prevention of fat embolism in patient with long-bone fracture. **Unla-**

Common side effect in *italic*, life-threatening effects underlined; generic names in **bold**; drug class in SMALL CAPS

beled uses: acetate form used as a long-acting contraceptive and for spinal cord injury, lupus nephritis, multiple sclerosis.

ROUTE & DOSAGE

Inflammation

Adult: **PO** 2–60 mg/d in 1 or more divided doses. **IM** acetate: 4–80 mg/wk for 1–4 wk; succinate:–10–250 mg q6h. **IV** 10–250 mg q6h.
Child: **PO/IM/IV** 0.5–1.7 mg/kg/d divided q6–12h.

Acute Spinal Cord Injury

Adult: **IV** 30 mg/kg over 15 min, followed in 45 min by 5.4 mg/kg/h x 23 h.
Child: **IV** Same as for adult.

PHARMACOKINETICS Absorption: readily absorbed from GI tract. **Peak:** 1–2 h PO; 4–8 d IM. **Duration:** 1.25–1.5 d PO; 1–5 wk IM. **Metabolism:** metabolized in liver. **Elimination:** half-life: > 3.5 h; HPA suppression: 18–36 h.

CONTRAINDICATIONS & PRECAUTIONS Contraindicated in: systemic fungal infections. Safe use during pregnancy (category C) and lactation not established. **Cautious use in:** Cushing's syndrome; GI ulceration; hypertension; varicella, vaccinia; diabetes mellitus; emotional instability or psychotic tendencies.

ADVERSE/SIDE EFFECTS CNS: euphoria, headache, insomnia, confusion, psychosis. **CV:** CHF, edema. **GI:** nausea, vomiting, peptic ulcer. **Musculoskeletal:** muscle weakness, delayed wound healing, muscle wasting, osteoporosis, aseptic necrosis of bone, spontaneous fractures. **Endocrine:** cushingoid features, growth suppression in children, carbohydrate intolerance, hyperglycemia, **Other:** cataracts, leukocytosis, hypokalemia.

DRUG INTERACTIONS Amphotericin B, furosemide, THIAZIDE DIURETICS increase potassium loss; with ATTENUATED VIRUS VACCINES, may enhance virus replication or increase vaccine side effects; **isoniazid, phenytoin, phenobarbital, rifampin** decrease effectiveness of methylprednisolone because they increase metabolism of steroids.

INCOMPATIBILITIES Solution/additive: calcium gluconate, glycopyrrolate, metaraminol, nafcillin, penicillin G sodium, doxapram.

NURSING IMPLICATIONS

Administration

- Tablet may be crushed before administration and taken with fluid of patient's choice.
- The oral preparation will be less irritating if given with food.
- Alternate day therapy may be used when methylprednisolone is given over long period.
- Give IM injection deep into large muscle (not deltoid).
- Provided in Mix-O-Vial from which solution is withdrawn and given by direct IV at a rate of 500 mg or fraction thereof over 60 seconds or longer.
- IV administration to infants, children: Verify correct IV concentration and rate of infusion with physician.
- Methylprednisolone sodium succinate solution should be used within 48 h after preparation.
- Avoid contacting eyes with the ointment.
- Store at 15–30C (59–86F). Prevent freezing.

Assessment & Drug Effects

- Periodically monitor renal function, hepatic function, thyroid function, CBC, serum electrolytes, weight, and total cholesterol.

- Monitor urine for loss of glycemic control. The diabetic may require increased doses of insulin or sulfonylurea.
- Monitor serum potassium and report S&S of hypokalemia (see Appendix G).
- Monitor for and report S&S of Cushing's syndrome (see Appendix G).

Patient & Family Education

- Instruct not to alter established dosage regimen (i.e., not to increase, decrease, or omit doses or change dose intervals). Withdrawal symptoms (rebound inflammation, fever) can be induced with sudden discontinuation of therapy.
- Instruct to report immediately onset of signs of hypocorticism adrenal insufficiency: fatigue, nausea, anorexia, joint pain, muscular weakness, dizziness, fever.

M

METHYLTESTOSTERONE

(meth-ill-tess-toss′te-rone)

Trade names: Android, Metandren ♣, Oreton-Methyl, Testred, Virilon

Classifications: HORMONE; ANDROGEN/ANABOLIC STEROID

Prototype: Testosterone

Pregnancy category: X

Controlled substance: Schedule III

ACTIONS/PHARMACODYNAMICS Orally effective, short-acting steroid with androgen/anabolic activity ratio (1:1) similar to that of testosterone but less effective than its esters. Fails to produce full sexual maturation when administered to preadolescent male with complete testicular failure unless preceded by testosterone therapy.

USES Androgen replacement therapy, delayed puberty (male), palliation of female mammary cancer (1–5 y postmenopausal), postpartum breast engorgement.

ROUTE & DOSAGE

Replacement
Adult: **PO** 10–50 mg/d in divided doses.

Breast Cancer
Adult: **PO** 50–200 mg/d in divided doses for duration of therapeutic response or no longer than 3 mo if no remission.

Postpartum Breast Engorgement
Adult: **PO** 80 mg/d for 3–5 d.

PHARMACOKINETICS **Absorption:** readily absorbed from GI tract. **Metabolism:** metabolized in liver. **Elimination:** excreted in urine.

CONTRAINDICATIONS & PRECAUTIONS **Contraindicated in:** hepatic dysfunction; pregnancy (category X); prostate cancer. **Cautious use in:** hepatic, renal, or cardiac dysfunction.

ADVERSE/SIDE EFFECTS Cholestatic hepatitis with jaundice, renal calculi (especially in immobilized patient), irritation of oral mucosa with buccal administration, *acne, gynecomastia, edema,* oligospermia, priapism, menstrual irregularities.

DRUG INTERACTIONS Increases risk of bleeding associated with ORAL ANTICOAGULANTS; possibly increases risk of **cyclosporine** toxicity; may decrease glucose level, making adjustment of doses of **insulin,** SULFONYLUREAS necessary.

Common side effect in *italic,* life-threatening effects underlined; generic names in **bold;** drug class in SMALL CAPS

NURSING IMPLICATIONS

Administration

- Dosage is individualized according to age, sex, and diagnosis.
- Store drug at 15–30C (59–86F). Avoid freezing.

Assessment & Drug Effects

- Monitor hepatic function periodically; report signs of hepatic toxicity (see Appendix G).
- Monitor for flank pain, abdominal pain radiating to groin, or other symptoms of renal calculi.

Patient & Family Education

- Since dosage sufficient to produce remission in breast cancer is quantitatively similar to that used for androgen replacement in the male, women should be prepared for distressing and undesirable side effects of virilization.
- Advise to report promptly if signs of virilism appear. Voice change and hirsutism may be irreversible, even after drug is withdrawn.
- Instruct men to report priapism or other signs of excess sexual stimulation. The physician will terminate methyltestosterone therapy.
- Jaundice with or without pruritus appears to be dose related. Instruct to report symptoms to physician. If liver function tests are altered at the same time, this drug will be withdrawn.

METHYPRYLON

(meth-i-prye′lon)

Trade name: Noludar

Classifications: CNS AGENT; HYPNOTIC

Prototype: Secobarbital

Pregnancy category: B

Controlled substance: Schedule III

ACTIONS/PHARMACODYNAMICS Piperidine derivative structurally related to glutethimide. Produces CNS depressant effects similar to those of short-acting barbiturates. Hypnotic doses suppress REM sleep.

USES Hypnotic for relief of simple insomnia. Sometimes used as sedative, but value for this purpose not established.

ROUTE & DOSAGE

Hypnotic
Adult: **PO** 200–400 mg 15 min before retiring.
Adolescent: **PO** > 12 y, 50–200 mg h.s.

PHARMACOKINETICS **Absorption:** readily absorbed from GI tract. **Onset:** 45–60 min. **Peak:** 1 h. **Duration:** 5–8 h. **Metabolism:** metabolized in liver; some enterohepatic circulation. **Elimination:** half-life: 3–6 h; excreted in urine.

CONTRAINDICATIONS & PRECAUTIONS **Contraindicated in:** porphyria; known hypersensitivity to methyprylon; patient who is hallucinating or who is psychotic. Safe use during pregnancy (category B) and in nursing mothers and children < 12 y not established. **Cautious use in:** hepatic or renal impairment, addiction-prone individuals, mental depression, history of suicidal tendencies.

ADVERSE/SIDE EFFECTS *Morning drowsiness,* dizziness, nausea, vomiting, diarrhea, esophagitis, headache, paradoxic excitation, skin rash, exacerbation of intermittent porphyria. **Acute toxicity:** somnolence, confusion, constricted pupils, hyperpyrexia, hypothermia, <u>shock</u>, pulmonary edema, <u>respiratory depression</u>; occasionally during recovery: excitation, convulsions, delirium, hallucinations.

M

DIAGNOSTIC TEST INTERFERENCE Methyprylon may interfere with ***urinary steroid*** determinations.

DRUG INTERACTIONS **Alcohol** and other CNS DEPRESSANTS add to CNS depression.

NURSING IMPLICATIONS

Administration

- Hypnotic dose is administered 15 min before patient retires. Prepare patient for sleep before administering drug.
- Preserve in tightly closed, light-resistant containers.

Assessment & Drug Effects

- In some patients, suppression of REM sleep may cause irritability, tension, confusion, and tremors.
- Although tolerance develops to suppression of REM sleep, during chronic administration, REM rebound may occur when drug is withdrawn: increased dreaming, nightmares, insomnia, hallucinations.
- Tolerance may develop to hypnotic and sedative effects but not to toxic effects.
- Psychologic and physical dependence may occur, especially after prolonged use of large doses. Patient's continued need for methyprylon should be evaluated regularly.
- Periodic blood counts are advised if drug is used repeatedly or over prolonged periods.

Patient & Family Education

- Warn about possible additive effects with alcohol and other CNS depressants.
- Caution to avoid driving a car or engaging in other activities requiring mental alertness until response to drug is known.
- Gradual drug withdrawal is advised after prolonged use. Sudden discontinuation may result in withdrawal symptoms: confusion, marked nervousness, insomnia, sweating, polyuria, hyperreflexia, delirium, miosis, hallucinations, convulsion, death.

METHYSERGIDE

(meth-i-ser′jide)

Trade name: Sansert

Classifications: AUTONOMIC NERVOUS SYSTEM AGENT; ERGOT ALKALOID

Prototype: Ergotamine

Pregnancy category: C

ACTIONS/PHARMACODYNAMICS Ergot derivative and congener of LSD. Unlike ergotamine, has weak vasoconstrictor and oxytoxic actions. Action mechanism in migraine prevention unclear. Serotonin (a strong vasoconstrictor) levels are reduced during an attack. Methysergide replaces serotonin on cranial artery receptor sites during an attack, thereby preserving vasoconstriction afforded by serotonin.

USES Prophylactic management of severe recurrent migraine, cluster, and other vascular headaches unresponsive to other antimigraine drugs. **Unlabeled uses:** diarrhea and malabsorption associated with GI hypermotility in carcinoid disease; postgastrectomy dumping syndrome.

ROUTE & DOSAGE

Headache Prophylaxis

Adult: **PO** 4–8 mg/d in divided doses with meals; should not be administered continuously for > 6 mo; a drug-free interval of 3–4 wk must follow each 6 mo course.

Diarrhea Associated with Carcinoid Disease
Adult: **PO** 2–16 mg t.i.d.

PHARMACOKINETICS Absorption: readily absorbed from GI tract. **Distribution:** widely distributed, including into breast milk. **Metabolism:** metabolized in liver. **Elimination:** half-life: 10 h; excreted in urine.

CONTRAINDICATIONS & PRECAUTIONS Contraindicated in: fibrotic processes; pulmonary or collagen diseases; edema; serious infections; debilitated states. Pregnancy (category C), severe peripheral vascular disease, severe hypertension, severe arteriosclerosis, phlebitis or cellulitis of lower limbs, impaired liver or renal function.

ADVERSE/SIDE EFFECTS CNS: *insomnia,* drowsiness, vertigo, mild euphoria, confusion, excitement, feelings of unreality or depersonalization, distortions of body image, depression, anxiety, hallucinations, nightmares, ataxia, hyperesthesia, paresthesia. **CV:** peripheral edema, thrombophlebitis, claudication, impaired circulation, angina of effort, ECG changes, *postural hypotension,* tachycardia. **GI:** *nausea, vomiting, heartburn,* hyperchlorhydria, *abdominal pain, diarrhea,* constipation. **Skin:** facial flushing, telangiectasia, rash, excessive hair loss. **Other:** neutropenia, eosinophilia, weakness, arthralgia, myalgia, weight gain, scotomas, nasal stuffiness, positive direct Coombs' test. **Fibrotic complications:** retroperitoneal fibrosis, pleuropulmonary fibrosis, cardiac fibrosis.

NURSING IMPLICATIONS

Administration

- GI side effects can frequently be prevented by administering drug with meals.
- Preserve in tight, light-resistant containers at 15–30C (59–86F) unless otherwise directed.

Assessment & Drug Effects

- One or 2 d of drug therapy is required before protective drug action is realized; at end of therapy, protection continues 2 d beyond last dose.
- Therapeutic trial period of 3 wk is advised to determine patient's response to methysergide. If no response occurs in this time, it is unlikely that longer administration will be of benefit.
- Pretreatment and periodic assessments of cardiac status, renal function, blood count, and sedimentation rate are advised.
- Since incidence of side effects is relatively high (usually reversible with discontinuation of drug), patient should be examined regularly for fibrotic and vascular complications: auscultate heart and lungs; check peripheral pulses, and auscultate major vessels for bruits; observe for signs of phlebitis or venous obstruction. Also, question patient concerning presence of CNS symptoms and other adverse effects.

Patient & Family Education

- Instruct to report the following immediately: onset of abdominal, back, or chest pain; dyspnea; leg pains while walking; cold, numb, or painful extremities; fever; dysuria or other urinary problems; edema; weight gain.
- Counsel to weigh self daily and teach patient how to check extremities for edema.
- Caloric restriction and reduction of salt intake may be prescribed. Consult physician and instruct patient accordingly.
- Advise to make position changes

slowly, particularly from recumbent to upright posture, and to dangle legs a few minutes before standing. Also instruct patient to lie down if faintness occurs.

- To avoid "headache rebound," drug should be withdrawn gradually over 2- or 3-wk period.
- Patients with migraine should be helped to identify underlying emotional and physical stresses that may precipitate attacks.

METOCLOPRAMIDE HYDROCHLORIDE

(met-oh-kloe-pra'mide)

Trade names: Clopra, Emex ♣, Maxeran ♣, Maxolon, Reglan

Prototype for classifications: PROKINETIC AGENT, AUTONOMIC NERVOUS SYSTEM AGENT; DIRECT-ACTING CHOLINERGIC (PARASYMPATHOMIMETIC); GI AGENT; ANTIEMETIC

Pregnancy category: B

ACTIONS/PHARMACODYNAMICS Potent central dopamine receptor antagonist. Structurally related to procainamide but has little antiarrhythmic or anesthetic activity. Exact mechanism of action not clear but appears to sensitize GI smooth muscle to effects of acetylcholine by direct action. Increases resting tone of esophageal sphincter and tone and amplitude of upper GI contractions. As a result, gastric emptying and intestinal transit are accelerated with little effect if any on gastric, biliary, or pancreatic secretions. Antiemetic action results from drug-induced elevation of CTZ threshold and enhanced gastric emptying.

USES Management of diabetic gastric stasis (gastroparesis); to prevent nausea and vomiting associated with emetogenic cancer chemotherapy (e.g., cisplatin, dacarbazine); to facilitate intubation of small bowel; symptomatic treatment of gastroesophageal reflux.

ROUTE & DOSAGE

Gastroesophageal Reflux

Adult: **PO** 10–15 mg q.i.d. a.c. and h.s.
Child: **PO/IV/IM** 0.4–0.8 mg/kg/d in 4 divided doses.

Diabetic Gastroparesis

Adult: **PO** 10 mg q.i.d. a.c. and h.s. for 2–8 wk.
Geriatric **PO** 5 mg a.c and h.s.

Small-bowel Intubation, Radiologic Examination

Adult: **IM/IV** 10 mg administered over 1–2 min.
Child: **IM/IV** *6–14 y,* 2.5–5 mg over 1–2 min; *< 6 y,* 0.1 mg/kg over 1–2 min.

Chemotherapy-induced Emesis

Adult/Child: **PO** 2 mg/kg 1 h before antineoplastic administration; may repeat q2h for 3 more doses if needed. **IM/IV** 2 mg/kg 30 min before antineoplastic administration; may repeat q2h for 2 doses, then q3h for 3 doses if needed.

PHARMACOKINETICS **Absorption:** readily absorbed from GI tract. **Onset:** 30–60 min PO; 10–15 min IM; 1–3 min IV. **Peak:** 1–2 h. **Duration:** 1–3 h. **Distribution:** distributed to most body tissues including CNS; crosses placenta; distributed into breast milk. **Metabolism:** minimally metabolized in liver. **Elimination:** half-life: 2.5–6 h; 95% excreted in urine, 5% in feces.

CONTRAINDICATIONS & PRECAUTIONS **Contraindicated in:** sensitivity or intolerance to metoclopramide; allergy to sulfiting agents; history of seizure disorders; concurrent use of drugs that can cause extrapyramidal symptoms; pheochromocytoma; mechanical GI obstruction or perforation; history of breast cancer. Safe use during pregnancy (category B), and in nursing mothers not established. **Cautious use in:** CHF, hypokalemia; renal dysfunction; GI hemorrhage; history of intermittent porphyria.

ADVERSE/SIDE EFFECTS **CNS:** *mild sedation* (50% of patients), *fatigue, restlessness,* agitation, headache, insomnia, disorientation, *extrapyramidal symptoms* (acute dystonic type). **GI:** nausea, constipation, *diarrhea,* dry mouth. **Other:** urticarial or maculopapular rash, glossal or periorbital edema, methemoglobinemia, galactorrhea, gynecomastia, amenorrhea, impotence, altered drug absorption, hypertensive crisis (rare).

DIAGNOSTIC TEST INTERFERENCE Metoclopramide may interfere with gonadorelin test by increasing ***serum prolactin*** levels.

DRUG INTERACTIONS **Alcohol** and other CNS DEPRESSANTS add to sedation; ANTICHOLINERGICS, OPIATE ANALGESICS may antagonize effect on GI motility; PHENOTHIAZINES may potentiate extrapyramidal symptoms.

INCOMPATIBILITIES **Solution/additive: cisplatin, erythromycin,** TETRACYCLINES, **ampicillin, calcium gluconate, cephalothin, chloramphenicol, furosemide, methotrexate, penicillin G potassium, sodium bicarbonate. Y-site: furosemide.**

NURSING IMPLICATIONS

Administration

- Oral form is usually taken 30 min before meals and at bedtime.
- IV Administration: For cancer drug-induced emesis, doses > 10 mg IV should be diluted in 50 ml of compatible parenteral solution and administered over 15 min. Doses of 10 mg or less may be given undiluted by direct IV over 1–2 min.
- IV administration to infants, children: Verify correct IV concentration and rate of infusion with physician.
- Bags of metoclopramide should be protected from light during IV infusion (use of aluminum foil or a thick cotton cover).
- Discard open ampuls; do not store for future use.
- The injection form contains sodium metabisulfite as antioxidant. If patient has history of allergy to sulfiting agents, this product should be avoided.
- Store in light-resistant bottle at 15–30C (59–86F). Tablets are stable for 3 y; solutions and injections, for 5 y.

Assessment & Drug Effects

- Extrapyramidal symptoms are most likely to occur in children, young adults, and the elderly and with high-dose treatment of vomiting associated with cancer chemotherapy. Symptoms can take months to regress. Report immediately the onset of restlessness, involuntary movements, facial grimacing, rigidity, or tremors.
- Therapeutic effectiveness in patient with diabetic gastroparesis is indicated by relief of anorexia, nausea, vomiting, persistent fullness after meals.
- During early treatment period, serum aldosterone may be ele-

M

vated; however, after prolonged administration periods, it returns to pretreatment level.

- Monitor for possible hypernatremia and hypokalemia (see Appendix G), especially if patient has CHF or cirrhosis.
- Adverse reactions associated with increased serum prolactin concentration (galactorrhea, menstrual disorders, gynecomastia) usually disappear within a few weeks or months after drug treatment is stopped.

Patient & Family Education

- Caution to avoid driving and other potentially hazardous activities for a few hours after drug administration.
- Instruct to report signs of acute dystonia (see Appendix G) immediately.

M

METOCURINE IODIDE

(met-oh-kyoo′reen)

Trade name: Metubine Iodide

Classifications: AUTONOMIC NERVOUS SYSTEM AGENT; NONDEPOLARIZING SKELETAL MUSCLE RELAXANT

Prototype: Tubocurarine

Pregnancy category: C

ACTIONS/PHARMACODYNAMICS Semisynthetic nondepolarizing neuromuscular blocking agent. Pharmacologic effects almost identical to those of tubocurarine but is reportedly 2–3 times more potent. Has a slightly shorter duration of action, less histamine-releasing effect, and produces less ganglionic blockade.

USES Adjunct to anesthesia to induce skeletal muscle relaxation. Has been used to reduce intensity of skeletal muscle contractions in drug- or electrically induced convulsions and to facilitate endotracheal intubation.

ROUTE & DOSAGE

Adjunct to General Anesthesia
Adult: **IV** 0.1–0.3 mg/kg over 30–60 s with 0.5–1 mg q30–90 min prn.

Adjunct for Intubation
Adult: **IV** 0.2–0.4 mg/kg over 30–60 s.

Electroshock Therapy
Adult: **IV** 1.75–5.5 mg/kg.

PHARMACOKINETICS **Onset:** 1–4 min. **Peak:** 3–5 min. **Duration:** 35–90 min. **Distribution:** crosses placenta. **Elimination:** half-life: 3.6 h; primarily excreted in urine, small amount in feces.

CONTRAINDICATIONS & PRECAUTIONS **Contraindicated in:** hypersensitivity to metocurine or to iodides; allergy, asthma. **Cautious use in:** myasthenia gravis, renal, hepatic, or pulmonary impairment, respiratory depression, electrolyte disturbances; pregnancy (category C).

ADVERSE/SIDE EFFECTS Same toxic potential as for tubocurarine. *Hypotension,* dizziness, increased salivation, bronchospasm, respiratory depression, decreased GI motility and tone, hypersensitivity reactions.

INCOMPATIBILITIES **Solution/additive:** ALKALINE SOLUTIONS. **Y-site:** BARBITURATES, **meperidine, morphine.**

NURSING IMPLICATIONS

Administration

- Administer by direct IV injection over 30–60 s.
- Metocurine solution should be

protected from prolonged exposure to heat and direct sunlight.
- Store at 15–30C (59–86F).

Assessment & Drug Effects
- Complete recovery from IV dose may require several hours.
- A peripheral nerve stimulator may be used to monitor response.

METOLAZONE

(me-tole'a-zone)

Trade names: Diulo, Mykrox, Zaroxolyn

Classifications: ELECTROLYTIC AND WATER BALANCE AGENT; THIAZIDE-LIKE DIURETIC; ANTIHYPERTENSIVE

Prototype: Hydrochlorothiazide

Pregnancy category: D

ACTIONS/PHARMACODYNAMICS Diuretic structurally and pharmacologically similar to hydrochlorothiazide. Appears to be more effective as a diuretic than thiazides in patients with severe renal failure.

USES Management of hypertension as sole agent or to enhance effectiveness of other antihypertensives in severe form of hypertension; also edema associated with CHF and renal disease.

ROUTE & DOSAGE

Edema

Adult: **PO** 5–20 mg/d.
Child: **PO** 0.2–0.4 mg/kg/d divided q12–24h.

Hypertension

Adult: **PO** 2.5–5 mg/d; Mykrox: 0.5–1 mg/d.

PHARMACOKINETICS Absorption: incompletely absorbed; Mykrox has greater absorption. **Onset:** 1 h. **Peak:** 2–8 h. **Duration:** 12–24 h. **Distribution:** distributed throughout extracellular tissue; concentrates in kidney; crosses placenta; distributed in breast milk. **Metabolism:** does not appear to be metabolized. **Elimination:** half-life: 14 h; excreted in urine.

CONTRAINDICATIONS & PRECAUTIONS Contraindicated in: anuria, hypokalemia; hepatic coma or precoma; hypersensitivity to metolazone and sulfonamides; pregnancy (category D), nursing mothers. **Cautious use in:** history of gout; allergies; concomitant use of digitalis glycosides; renal and hepatic dysfunction.

ADVERSE/SIDE EFFECTS Cholestatic jaundice, vertigo, orthostatic hypotension, venous thrombosis, leukopenia, dehydration, *hypokalemia, hyperuricemia, hyperglycemia.*

DRUG INTERACTIONS Amphotericin B, CORTICOSTEROIDS increase hypokalemic effects; may antagonize hypoglycemic effects of SULFONYLUREAS, **insulin; cholestyramine, colestipol** decrease thiazide absorption; intensifies hypoglycemic and hypotensive effects of **diazoxide;** because of increased potassium and magnesium loss, may cause **digoxin** toxicity; decreases **lithium** excretion, increasing its toxicity; NSAIDS may attenuate diuresis—increased risk of NSAID-induced renal failure.

NURSING IMPLICATIONS

Administration
- Schedule doses to avoid nocturia and interrupted sleep. Administer PO early in AM after eating to prevent gastric irritation (if given in 2 doses, schedule second dose no later than 3 PM).
- Store tablets in tightly closed container at 15–30C (59–86F) unless otherwise specified.

M

Assessment & Drug Effects

- Geriatric patients may be more sensitive to effects of usual adult dose; thus overdosage and adverse reactions should be anticipated.
- When adverse reactions are moderate to severe, metolazone therapy should be terminated.
- Antihypertensive effects may be observed in 3 or 4 d, but 3–4 wk are required for maximum effect.
- Serum potassium should be determined at regular intervals. Prolonged treatment with metolazone and inadequate potassium intake increase potential for hypokalemia (see Signs & Symptoms, Appendix G).

Patient & Family Education

- Warn not to drink alcohol, since it potentiates orthostatic hypotension.
- Antihypertensive therapy may require as adjunct a high-potassium, low-sodium, and low-calorie diet.
- Encourage dietary inclusion of potassium-rich foods.
- If hypokalemia develops, dietary potassium supplement of 1000–2000 mg (25–50 mEq) is usually an adequate treatment.

M

METOPROLOL TARTRATE

(me-toe′proe-lole)

Trade names: Apo-Metoprolol ♣, Betaloc ♣, Lopressor, Norometoprol ♣, Toprol XL

Classifications: AUTONOMIC NERVOUS SYSTEM AGENT; BETA-ADRENERGIC ANTAGONIST (SYMPATHOLYTIC); ANTIHYPERTENSIVE

Prototype: Propranolol

Pregnancy category: C

ACTIONS/PHARMACODYNAMICS Beta-adrenergic blocking agent with preferential effect on $beta_1$ adrenoreceptors located primarily on cardiac muscle. At higher doses, metoprolol also inhibits $beta_2$ receptors located chiefly on bronchial and vascular musculature. Reduces heart rate and cardiac output at rest and during exercise; lowers both supine and standing BP, slows sinus rate and decreases myocardial automaticity. Antihypertensive action may be due to competitive antagonism of catecholamines at cardiac adrenergic neuron sites, drug-induced reduction of sympathetic outflow to the periphery, and to suppression of renin activity. Antianginal effect is like that of propranolol.

USES Management of mild to severe hypertension (monotherapy or in combination with a thiazide or vasodilator or both); long-term treatment of angina pectoris and prophylactic management of stable angina pectoris reduce the risk of mortality after an MI.

ROUTE & DOSAGE

Hypertension

Adult: **PO** 50–100 mg/d in 1–2 divided doses; may increase weekly up to 100–450 mg/d.
Geriatric: **PO** 25 mg/d; usual range 25–300 mg/d.

Angina Pectoris

Adult: **PO** 100 mg/d in 2 divided doses; may increase weekly up to 100–400 mg/d.

Myocardial Infarction

Adult: **IV** 5 mg q2min for 3 doses, followed by PO therapy. **PO** 50 mg q6h for 48 h, then 100 mg b.i.d.

PHARMACOKINETICS Absorption: readily absorbed from GI tract; 50% of dose reaches systemic circulation.

Onset: 15 min. **Peak:** 1.5 h. **Duration:** 13–19 h. **Distribution:** crosses blood–brain barrier and placenta; distributed into breast milk. **Metabolism:** extensively metabolized in liver. **Elimination:** half-life: 3–4 h; excreted in urine.

CONTRAINDICATIONS & PRECAUTIONS **Contraindicated in:** cardiogenic shock, sinus bradycardia, heart block greater than first degree, overt cardiac failure, right ventricular failure secondary to pulmonary hypertension. Safe use during pregnancy (category C), in nursing mothers, and in children not established. **Cautious use in:** impaired hepatic or renal function; cardiomegaly, CHF controlled by digitalis and diuretics; AV conduction defects; bronchial asthma and other bronchospastic diseases; history of allergy; thyrotoxicosis; diabetes mellitus; peripheral vascular disease.

ADVERSE/SIDE EFFECTS **Allergic:** erythematous rash, fever, headache, muscle aches, sore throat, laryngospasm, respiratory distress. **CNS:** *dizziness, fatigue, insomnia,* increased dreaming, mental depression. **CV:** *bradycardia,* palpitation, cold extremities, Raynaud's phenomenon, intermittent claudication, angina pectoris, CHF, intensification of AV block, AV dissociation, complete heart block, cardiac arrest. **GI:** nausea, *heartburn,* gastric pain, diarrhea or constipation, flatulence. **Hematologic:** eosinophilia, thrombocytopenic and nonthrombocytopenic purpura, agranulocytosis (rare). **Skin:** dry skin, pruritus, skin eruptions. **Other:** dry mouth and mucous membranes, hypoglycemia, bronchospasm (with high doses), *shortness of breath.*

DIAGNOSTIC TEST INTERFERENCE In common with other beta blockers, metoprolol may cause elevated ***BUN*** and ***serum creatinine levels*** (patients with severe heart disease), elevated ***serum transaminase, alkaline phosphatase, lactate dehydrogenase,*** and ***serum uric acid.***

DRUG INTERACTIONS BARBITURATES, **rifampin** may decrease effects of metoprolol; **cimetidine, methimazole, propylthiouracil,** ORAL CONTRACEPTIVES may increase effects of metoprolol; additive bradycardia with **digoxin;** effects of both metoprolol and **hydralazine** may be increased; **indomethacin** may attenuate hypotensive response; BETA AGONISTS and metoprolol mutually antagonistic; **verapamil** may increase risk of heart block and bradycardia.

NURSING IMPLICATIONS

Administration

- Ingestion with food slightly enhances absorption; however, administration with food is not essential. It is important that drug be given with or without food consistently to minimize possible variations in bioavailability.
- IV metoprolol may be given by direct IV undiluted at a rate of 5 mg over 60 seconds.
- Store at 15–30C (59–86F). Protect from heat, light, and moisture.

Assessment & Drug Effects

- Take apical pulse and BP before administering drug. Report to physician significant changes in rate, rhythm, or quality of pulse or variations in BP prior to administration.
- During IV administration, BP, heart rate, and ECG should be carefully monitored.
- Maximal effect on BP is achieved usually after 1 wk of therapy.

- For patients with hypertension, take several BP readings close to the end of a 12 h dosing interval to evaluate adequacy of dosage, particularly in patients on twice daily doses. Some patients require doses 3 times a day to maintain satisfactory control.
- Hypertensive patients with CHF controlled by digitalis and diuretics must be closely observed for impending heart failure: dyspnea on exertion, orthopnea, night cough, edema, distended neck veins. Monitor I&O, daily weight; auscultate daily for pulmonary rales.
- Drug should be withdrawn if patient presents symptoms of mental depression because it can progress to catatonia. Possible symptoms of depression: disinterest in people, surroundings, food, personal hygiene; withdrawal, apathy, sadness, difficulty in concentrating, insomnia.
- Since metoprolol masks signs of hyperthyroidism (see Appendix G), patients with thyrotoxicosis must be closely monitored. Abrupt withdrawal may precipitate thyroid storm.
- Baseline and regularly scheduled evaluations should be made of blood cell counts, blood glucose, cardiac function, hepatic and renal function.

Patient & Family Education

- Instruct patient receiving metoprolol should be instructed to take radial pulse before each dose. Advise to report to physician if it is slower than base rate (e.g., 60 bpm) or becomes irregular. Consult physician for parameters.
- Insomnia or increased dreaming may be reduced by avoiding late evening doses.
- Patients with diabetes mellitus should be monitored closely. Metoprolol may mask some symptoms of hypoglycemia (e.g., BP and heart rate changes) and may prolong hypoglycemia. Alert patient to other possible signs of hypoglycemia not affected by metoprolol that should be reported: sweating, fatigue, hunger, inability to concentrate.
- Instruct to protect extremities from cold and not to smoke. Advise to report cold, painful, or tender feet or hands or other symptoms of Raynaud's disease (intermittent pallor, cyanosis or redness, paresthesias). Physician may prescribe a vasodilator.
- Instruct to report immediately to physician the onset of ocular symptoms.
- If mouth dryness is bothersome, advise the following measures: rinse mouth frequently with clear warm water; increase noncalorie liquid intake if it has been inadequate; sugarless gum or lemon drops.
- Eye dryness may be relieved by use of sterile artificial tears available OTC.
- Advise to avoid driving and other potentially hazardous activities until drug effects are known.
- Emphasize importance of compliance and caution not to alter established dosage regimen.
- When metoprolol is to be discontinued, dosage should be reduced gradually over a period of 1–2 wk. Sudden withdrawal can result in increase in anginal attacks and MI in patients with angina pectoris and thyroid storm in patients with hyperthyroidism.

METRONIDAZOLE

(me-troe-ni′da-zole)

Trade names: Flagyl, Flagyl ER, Flagyl I.V. RTU, Flagyl 375, Meti-

zol, Metric 21, Metro I.V., MetroGel, MetroGel-vaginal, Protostat
Prototype for classifications: ANTIINFECTIVE; ANTITRICHOMONAL; AMEBICIDE
Pregnancy category: B

ACTIONS/PHARMACODYNAMICS

Synthetic compound with direct trichomonicidal and amebecidal activity against *Trichomonas vaginalis, Entamoeba histolytica,* and *Giardia lamblia*. Also exhibits antibacterial activity against obligate anaerobic bacteria, gram-negative anaerobic bacilli, and clostridia. Microaerophilic streptococci and most aerobic bacteria are resistant.

USES Asymptomatic and symptomatic trichomoniasis in females and males; acute intestinal amebiasis and amebic liver abscess; preoperative prophylaxis in colorectal surgery, elective hysterectomy or vaginal repair, and emergency appendectomy. IV metronidazole is used for the treatment of serious infections caused by susceptible anaerobic bacteria in intraabdominal infections, skin infections, gynecologic infections, septicemia, and for both pre- and postoperative prophylaxis, bacterial vaginosis. **Topical:** rosacea. **Unlabeled uses:** treatment of pseudomembranous colitis, Crohn's disease.

ROUTE & DOSAGE

Trichomoniasis, Giardiasis, *Gardnerella*

Adult: **PO** 2 g once; *or* 250 mg t.i.d., 375 mg b.i.d., *or* 500 mg b.i.d. for 7 d. **Vaginal** Apply once or twice daily × 5 d.
Child: **PO** 15 mg/kg/d in 3 divided doses for 7–10 d. *Infant:* **PO** 10–30 mg/kg/d for 5–8 d.

Amebiasis

Adult: **PO** 500–750 mg t.i.d.
Child: **PO** 35–50 mg/kg/d in 3 divided doses.

Anaerobic Infections

Adult: **PO** 7.5 mg/kg q6h (max 4 g/d). **IV** 15 mg/kg loading dose, then 7.5 mg/kg q6h (max 4 g/d).
Child: **PO/IV** 30 mg/kg/d divided q6h (max 4 g/d).
Neonate: **PO/IV** 7.5–15 mg/kg/d divided q12–48h.

Pseudomembranous Colitis

Adult: **PO** 250–500 mg t.i.d. **IV** 250–500 mg t.i.d. or q.i.d.
Child: **PO** 30 mg/kg/d divided q6h × 7 d.

Bacterial Vaginosis

Adult: **PO** (Flagyl ER) 750 mg q.d. × 7 d.

PHARMACOKINETICS Absorption: 80% of dose absorbed from GI tract. **Peak:** 1–3 h. **Distribution:** widely distributed to most body tissues, including CSF, bone, cerebral and hepatic abscesses; crosses placenta; distributed in breast milk. **Metabolism:** 30–60% metabolized in liver. **Elimination:** half-life: 6–8 h; 77% excreted in urine; 14% excreted in feces within 24 h.

CONTRAINDICATIONS & PRECAUTIONS Contraindicated in: blood dyscrasias, active CNS disease, first trimester of pregnancy (category B), nursing mothers. **Cautious use in:** coexistent candidiasis; second and third trimesters of pregnancy; alcoholism; hepatic disease.

ADVERSE/SIDE EFFECTS Allergic: rash, urticaria, pruritus, flushing. **CNS:** vertigo, headache, ataxia, con-

M

fusion, irritability, depression, restlessness, weakness, fatigue, drowsiness, insomnia, paresthesias, sensory neuropathy (rare). **GI:** *nausea,* vomiting, anorexia, epigastric distress, abdominal cramps, diarrhea, constipation, dry mouth, metallic or bitter taste. **GU:** polyuria, dysuria, pyuria, incontinence, cystitis, decreased libido, dyspareunia, dryness of vagina and vulva, sense of pelvic pressure. **Other:** nasal congestion, fever, fleeting joint pains, ECG changes (flattening of T wave); overgrowth of *Candida;* proctitis.

DIAGNOSTIC TEST INTERFERENCE **Metronidazole** may interfere with certain chemical analyses for AST, resulting in decreased values.

DRUG INTERACTIONS ORAL ANTICOAGULANTS potentiate hypoprothrombinemia; **alcohol** may elicit disulfiram reaction; **disulfiram** causes acute psychosis; **phenobarbital** increases metronidazole metabolism; may increase **lithium** levels; **fluorouracil, azathioprine** may cause transient neutropenia.

M

INCOMPATIBILITIES **Solution/additive:** TPN, **aztreonam, dopamine.**

NURSING IMPLICATIONS

Administration

- Tablets may be crushed before ingestion if patient cannot swallow them whole.
- Flagyl ER should not be crushed.
- Flagyl ER should be taken on an empty stomach, 1 h before or 2 h after meals.
- Administer oral preparation immediately before, with, or immediately after meals or with food or milk to reduce GI distress.
- Lower than normal doses should be given in the presence of hepatic disease.
- Therapy instituted during the second or third trimester of pregnancy should be over a 7 d period. The 2 g PO dose (1 d) produces a high serum level that may reach fetal circulation.

Parenteral (IV)

- Do not give direct IV bolus injection because of low pH of reconstituted product.
- IV preparation: Sequence for preparing solution (important) consists of (1) reconstitution with 4.4 ml sterile water or NS, (2) dilution in IV solution to yield 8 mg/ml in NS, D5W, or lactated Ringer's for infusion, (3) pH neutralization with approximately 5 mEq sodium bicarbonate injection for each 500 mg of Flagyl I.V. used.
- IV administration: Give IV solution slowly at a rate of one dose per hour.
- IV administration to neonates, infants, children: Verify correct IV concentration and rate of infusion with physician.
- Flagyl I.V. RTU does not require mixing, diluting, or neutralizing. Each container contains 14 mEq of sodium.
- Avoid use of aluminum-containing equipment when manipulating IV product (including syringes equipped with aluminum needles or hubs).
- Do not mix IV metronidazole with any other drug.
- CO_2 will be generated when neutralized with sodium bicarbonate; release of pressure within container may be necessary.
- Precipitation occurs if neutralized solution is refrigerated. Use diluted and neutralized solution within 24 h of preparation.
- Storage and stability: Reconstituted Flagyl I.V. is chemically stable for 96 h when stored below 30C (86F) in room light. Diluted and neutralized IV solutions con-

taining Flagyl I.V. should be used within 24 h of mixing. Flagyl I.V. RTU should be stored at 15–30C (59–86F); protect from light during storage.

Assessment & Drug Effects

- Total and differential WBC counts are recommended before, during, and after therapy, especially if a second course is necessary.
- Therapy should be discontinued immediately if symptoms of CNS toxicity (see Appendix G) develop. Monitor especially for seizures and peripheral neuropathy (e.g., numbness and paresthesia of extremities).
- Monitor for signs of sodium retention, especially in patients on corticosteroid therapy or with a history of CHF.
- Patients on lithium should be monitored for elevated lithium levels.
- Candidiasis may appear or become more prominent with metronidazole therapy. Report to physician promptly.
- Repeated feces examinations, usually up to 3 mo, are necessary to ensure that amebae have been eliminated.

Patient & Family Education

- Caution to adhere closely to the established regimen without schedule interruption or changing the dose.
- During therapy for trichomoniasis, it is recommended that the patient refrain from intercourse unless the male partner wears a condom to prevent reinfection.
- Sexual partners should receive concurrent treatment. Asymptomatic trichomoniasis in the male is a frequent source of reinfection of the female.
- Warn that ingestion of alcohol during metronidazole therapy may induce a disulfiram-type reaction (see Appendix G). Alcohol or alcohol-containing medications should be avoided for at least 48 h after treatment is completed.
- Inform that urine may appear dark or reddish brown (especially with higher than recommended doses). This appears to have no clinical significance.
- Advise to report symptoms of candidal overgrowth: furry tongue, color changes of tongue, glossitis, stomatitis; vaginitis, curdlike, milky vaginal discharge; proctitis. Treatment with a candicidal agent may be indicated.

METYROSINE

(me-tye'roe-seen)

Trade name: Demser

Classification: ENZYME INHIBITOR

Pregnancy category: C

ACTIONS/PHARMACODYNAMICS

By blocking the enzyme tyrosine hydroxylase, metyrosine inhibits the conversion of tyrosine to DOPA, which is the initial and rate-setting step in synthesis of catecholamines (dopamine, epinephrine, norepinephrine). In patients with pheochromocytoma, catecholamine synthesis may be reduced by as much as 80%, ameliorating hypertensive attacks and associated symptoms.

USES Short-term management of pheochromocytoma until surgery is performed, in long-term control when surgery is contraindicated, and in patients with malignant pheochromocytoma. **Unlabeled use:** has been used in selected patients with schizophrenia to potentiate antipsychotic effects of phenothiazines.

ROUTE & DOSAGE

Pheochromocytoma

Adult: **PO** 250 mg q.i.d.; may increase to 2–3 g/d in divided doses (max 4 g/d).

PHARMACOKINETICS Absorption: readily absorbed from GI tract. **Peak:** 2–3 d. **Duration:** 3–4 d. **Distribution:** crosses blood–brain barrier. **Elimination:** half-life: 3.4–7.2 h; excreted in urine.

CONTRAINDICATIONS & PRECAUTIONS Contraindicated in: control of essential hypertension. Safe use during pregnancy (category C), in nursing women, and in children <12 y not established. **Cautious use in:** impaired hepatic or renal function.

M

ADVERSE/SIDE EFFECTS CNS: *sedation,* fatigue; *extrapyramidal signs: drooling, difficulty in speaking (dysarthria), tremors,* jaw stiffness (trismus); frank parkinsonism, psychic disturbances (anxiety, depression, hallucinations, disorientation, confusion), headache, muscle spasms. **GI:** *diarrhea,* nausea, vomiting, abdominal pain, dry mouth. **Hypersensitivity:** rash, urticaria. **Renal:** transient dysuria, crystalluria, hematuria. **Reproductive:** impotence, failure of ejaculation, breast swelling, galactorrhea. **Other:** peripheral edema, nasal stuffiness, shortness of breath, eosinophilia.

DIAGNOSTIC TEST INTERFERENCE False increases in ***urinary catecholamines*** may occur because of catechol metabolites of metyrosine.

DRUG INTERACTIONS Alcohol and other CNS DEPRESSANTS add to sedation and CNS depression; **droperidol, haloperidol,** PHENOTHIAZINES potentiate extrapyramidal effects.

NURSING IMPLICATIONS

Administration

- Advise patient to take each dose with a full glass of water and to be consistent about time medication is to be taken.
- Store at 15–30C (59–86F) unless otherwise directed.

Assessment & Drug Effects

- Monitor I&O ratio and pattern. Fluid intake must be enough (e.g., 10–12 glasses or more) to maintain urinary output of 2000 ml or more to minimize risk of crystalluria.
- Routine urinalysis should be performed; if crystals occur, fluid intake should be increased further. If crystalluria persists, metyrosine dosage should be decreased or drug discontinued.
- Baseline and regularly scheduled measurements should be made of urinary catecholamines and their metabolites (metanephrines and VMA). Metabolite excretion should decrease in patients with pheochromocytoma. Other baseline and regular determinations should include vital signs, ECG, renal and hepatic function tests (in patients with dysfunction), BMR, and blood and urine sugar tests.
- Clinical effectiveness with pheochromocytoma is determined by decrease in frequency of hypertensive attacks and associated symptoms.
- Supervise ambulation. Sedative effects occur commonly within the first 24 h after drug is started. Maximal sedative effects in 2 or 3 d.

Patient & Family Education

- Advise to notify physician if the following metyrosine side effects occur: diarrhea, particularly if it is severe or persists, painful urination, jaw stiffness, drooling, difficult speech, tremors, disorientation.

Dosage reduction or discontinuation of drug may be indicated.

- Caution patient to avoid driving and other potentially hazardous activities until reaction to drug is determined.
- Abrupt discontinuation of metyrosine may result in psychic stimulation, feeling of increased energy, temporary changes in sleep pattern (usually insomnia). Symptoms may last for 2 or 3 d.
- Patient on prolonged therapy should be advised to carry medical identification and to notify all physicians and dentists involved in care about drug regimen.

MEXILETINE

(mex-il′e-teen)

Trade name: Mexitil

Classifications: CARDIOVASCULAR AGENT; ANTIARRHYTHMIC

Prototype: Procainamide

Pregnancy category: C

ACTIONS/PHARMACODYNAMICS

Analog of lidocaine with potent anesthetic action and class IB electrophysiologic properties similar to those of procainamide. Shortens action potential duration and refractory period and improves resting potential. Has little or no effect on atrial tissue and produces modest suppression of sinus node automatically and AV nodal conduction. Prolongs the His to ventricular interval (HQ) only if patient has preexisting conduction disturbance. It should be noted that lidocaine response is not a reliable predictor of mexiletine effectiveness.

USES Acute and chronic ventricular arrhythmias; prevention of recurrent cardiac arrests; suppression of PVCs due to ventricular tachyarrhythmias.

Unlabeled uses: Wolff-Parkinson-White syndrome and supraventricular arrhythmias.

ROUTE & DOSAGE

Ventricular Arrhythmias

Adult: **PO** 200–300 mg q8h (max 1200 mg/d).
Child: **PO** 1.4–5 mg/kg q8h.

PHARMACOKINETICS Absorption: readily absorbed from GI tract. **Peak:** 2–3 h. **Distribution:** distributed into breast milk. **Metabolism:** metabolized in liver. **Elimination:** half-life: 10–12 h; excreted in urine; renal elimination increases with urinary acidification.

CONTRAINDICATIONS & PRECAUTIONS Contraindicated in: severe left ventricular failure, cardiogenic shock, severe bradyarrhythmias. Pregnancy category C, preexisting second- or third-degree heart block.

ADVERSE/SIDE EFFECTS CNS: *dizziness, tremor, nervousness, incoordination,* headache, blurred vision, paresthesias, numbness. **CV:** exacerbated arrhythmias, palpitations, chest pain, syncope, hypotension. **GI:** *nausea, vomiting, heartburn,* diarrhea, constipation, dry mouth, abdominal pain. **Other:** rash, dyspnea, edema, arthralgia, fever, impotence, malaise, urinary retention, hiccups.

DRUG INTERACTIONS Phenytoin, phenobarbital, rifampin may decrease mexiletine levels; **cimetidine** may increase mexiletine levels.

NURSING IMPLICATIONS

Administration

- Administer with food or milk to reduce gastric distress.

Assessment & Drug Effects

- Check pulse and BP before administration of mexiletine, until both are stabilized. Patient should understand that changes in pulse rate and regularity may signal decreasing clinical effectiveness of drug.
- Effective serum concentration range is 0.5–2 μg/ml.
- CNS adverse reactions predominate (intention tremors, nystagmus, blurred vision, dizziness, ataxia, confusion, nausea). Supervise ambulation in the weak, debilitated patient or the elderly during drug stabilization period.
- Drug compliance with mexiletine is affected particularly by the distressing side effects of tremor, ataxia, and eye symptoms.
- Check frequently with patient about adherence to drug regimen. If side effects are increasing, consult physician. Dose adjustment or discontinuation may be needed.

Patient & Family Education

- Instruct about pulse parameters to be reported: changes in rhythm and rate (bradycardia = pulse below 60); symptomatic bradycardia (light-headedness, syncope, dizziness), and postural hypotension.

MEZLOCILLIN SODIUM

(mez-loe-sill'in)

Trade name: Mezlin

Prototype for classifications: ANTIINFECTIVE; ANTIBIOTIC; ANTIPSEUDOMONAL PENICILLIN

Pregnancy category: B

ACTIONS/PHARMACODYNAMICS Semisynthetic acylureidopenicillin with extended spectrum. Structurally resembles ampicillin and has similar but wider antibacterial spectrum than either ampicillin, carbenicillin, or ticarcillin. In common with other penicillins, mezlocillin is bactericidal and acts by interfering with bacterial cell wall synthesis. Active against a wide variety of gram-negative and gram-positive bacteria including aerobic and anaerobic strains. Broadened spectrum of activity includes strains of pathogenic aerobic gram-negative bacteria, e.g., *Bacteroides, Enterobacter, Escherichia, Hemophilus, Klebsiella, Pseudomonas, Proteus,* and *Serratia,* and gram-positive organisms such as *Streptococcus faecalis* (enterococcus). Inactive against penicillinase-producing strains of *Staphylococcus aureus.*

USES Primarily for serious infections caused by *Pseudomonas aeruginosa* alone or in combination with an aminoglycoside or a cephalosporin. Also used to treat other infections caused by susceptible strains.

ROUTE & DOSAGE

Uncomplicated UTI

Adult: **IM/IV** 1.5–2 g q6h (100–125 mg/kg/d).

Moderate to Severe Infections

Adult: **IM/IV** 4 g q6h (150–200 mg/kg/d).

Life-threatening Infection, *Pseudomonas* Infections

Adult: **IM/IV** 3 g q4h (max 24 g/d).
Child: **IM/IV** *1 mo–12 y,* 50–75 mg/kg q4h; *< 1 mo,* 75 mg/kg q8–12h.

PHARMACOKINETICS **Peak:** 45 min IM; 5 min IV. **Distribution:** widely distributed with highest concentrations in urine and bile; adequate CSF penetration with inflamed meninges; crosses placenta; distributed into breast milk. **Metabolism:** slightly metabolized in liver. **Elimination:** half-life: 50–55 min; 75% excreted in urine, up to 25% excreted in bile.

CONTRAINDICATIONS & PRECAUTIONS **Contraindicated in:** history of hypersensitivity to penicillins or cephalosporins. Safe use during pregnancy (category B) and in nursing mothers not established. **Cautious use in:** patients with known or suspected allergies to drugs or other substances; renal impairment, uremia; hypokalemia; bleeding tendencies.

ADVERSE/SIDE EFFECTS **CNS:** convulsive seizures, neuromuscular hyperirritability. **GI:** abnormal taste sensations, nausea, vomiting, *diarrhea*. **Hematologic:** neutropenia, leukopenia, eosinophilia, thrombocytopenia (infrequent); increases in AST, ALT, alkaline phosphatase, serum bilirubin, creatinine, BUN; decreased Hct and Hgb. **Hypersensitivity:** *rash,* pruritus, urticaria, drug fever, <u>anaphylactic reactions</u>. ***Local:*** pain (following IM), thrombophlebitis (IV injection); superinfections.

DRUG INTERACTIONS Mezlocillin increases risk of bleeding associated with ANTICOAGULANTS; **probenecid** decreases elimination of mezlocillin.

INCOMPATIBILITIES **Solution/additive: ciprofloxacin,** AMINOGLYCOSIDES. **Y-site: ciprofloxacin, meperidine, verapamil,** AMINOGLYCOSIDES.

NURSING IMPLICATIONS

Administration

- IM injections should be made into a relatively large muscle such as the gluteus maximus (upper outer quadrant). Discomfort associated with IM administration may be lessened by giving injection slowly (over 12–15 seconds) and by reconstituting solution with lidocaine 0.5–1% (lessens pain). Do not exceed 2 g per IM injection.
- IV preparation: Each 1 g of IV mezlocillin must be diluted with 10 ml of sterile water, D5W, or NS. Shake to dissolve.
- IV administration: Give by direct IV over 3–5 min or further diluted to a volume of 50–100 ml and infused over 30 min.
- Store unopened vials and infusion bottles at or below 30C (86F) unless otherwise directed. Powder and reconstituted solutions may darken slightly, but this does not indicate loss of potency. Solutions should be clear. If a precipitate should form under refrigeration, warm solution to 37C (98.6F) in a water bath and shake well.

Assessment & Drug Effects

- Culture and susceptibility tests should be performed before and periodically during therapy.
- Before initiation of therapy, a detailed history should be obtained to determine previous hypersensitivity, especially to penicillins and cephalosporins but also to other substances.
- Observe IV sites for evidence of thrombophlebitis (see Appendix G).
- Monitor carefully during first 30 min after initiation of IV therapy for signs of hypersensitivity and anaphylactoid reaction (see Appendix G).
- Bleeding abnormalities (thrombocytopenia), although rare, are particularly likely to occur in patients with impaired renal function. Observe and report ecchymoses, petechiae, bleeding gums, nosebleeds, or any other evidence of bleeding.

- Be alert to signs of superinfections (see Appendix G).
- Baseline and regularly scheduled studies of blood, renal, and hepatic function should be performed during long-term therapy.

Patient & Family Education

- Inform that therapy generally continues for at least 2 d after signs and symptoms of infection have subsided. Usual duration of therapy for serious infections is 7–10 d, but it may be longer in complicated infections.
- Advise women to report onset of symptoms of *Candida* vaginitis. *Candida* vaginitis symptoms are moderate amount of white, cheesy, nonodorous vaginal discharge, vaginal inflammation, and itching.
- Instruct to report a skin rash or pruritus. The patient should then be assessed for other signs of hypersensitivity (see Appendix G). Mezlocillin may need to be discontinued.

M

MICONAZOLE NITRATE

(mi-kon′a-zole)

Trade name: Monistat-Derm

Classifications: ANTIINFECTIVE; ANTIBIOTIC; ANTIFUNGAL

Prototype: Fluconazole

Pregnancy category: B

ACTIONS/PHARMACODYNAMICS Broad-spectrum agent with fungicidal activity against *Candida albicans* and other species of this genus. Inhibits growth of common dermatophytes *Trichophyton rubrum, Trichophyton mentagrophytes, Epidermophyton floccosum,* and organism responsible for tinea versicolor *(Malassezia furfur)*. Mode of action unclear but appears to inhibit uptake of components essential for cell reproduction and growth and to alter cell wall structure, thus promoting cell death.

USES Vulvovaginal candidiasis, tinea pedis (athlete's foot), tinea cruris, tinea corporis, and tinea versicolor caused by dermatophytes.

ROUTE & DOSAGE

Fungal Infection

Adult: Apply cream sparingly to affected areas twice a day, and once daily for tinea versicolor, for 2 wk. Improvement should be seen in 2–3 d. Tinea pedis should be treated for 1 mo to prevent recurrence.

PHARMACOKINETICS **Absorption:** small amount absorbed from vagina. **Metabolism:** rapidly metabolized in liver. **Elimination:** half-life: 2.1–24 h; excreted in urine and feces.

ADVERSE/SIDE EFFECTS Vulvovaginal burning, itching, or irritation; maceration, allergic contact dermatitis.

NURSING IMPLICATIONS

Administration

- Ask physician about how to cleanse affected area prior to application of cream.
- Massage affected area gently until cream disappears.
- Store at 15–30C (59–86F) unless otherwise directed.

Assessment & Drug Effects

- Clinical improvement from topical application should be expected in 1 or 2 wk. If no improvement in 4 wk, the diagnosis is reevaluated. Tinea pedis infection should be treated for 1 mo to assure permanent recovery.

Patient & Family Education

- The full course of treatment should be completed to ensure recovery.
- Avoid contact of drug with eyes.

MIDAZOLAM HYDROCHLORIDE

(mid′az-zoe-lam)
Trade name: Versed
Classifications: CNS AGENT; GENERAL ANESTHETIC; BENZODIAZEPINE ANXIOLYTIC; SEDATIVE-HYPNOTIC
Prototype: Lorazepam
Pregnancy category: D
Controlled substance: Schedule IV

ACTIONS/PHARMACODYNAMICS Short-acting parenteral benzodiazepine; CNS depressant with muscle relaxant, anticonvulsant, and anterograde amnestic effects. Mechanism of action unclear. Intensifies activity of gamma-aminobenzoic acid (GABA), a major inhibitory neurotransmitter of the brain, by interfering with its reuptake and promoting its accumulation at neuronal synapses. This calms the patient, relaxes skeletal muscles, and in high doses produces sleep.

USES Sedation before general anesthesia, induction of general anesthesia; to impair memory of perioperative events (anterograde amnesia); for conscious sedation prior to short diagnostic and endoscopic procedures; and as the hypnotic supplement to nitrous oxide and oxygen (balanced anesthesia) for short surgical procedures.

ROUTE & DOSAGE

Conscious Sedation

Adult: **IM** 0.07–0.08 mg/kg 30–60 min before procedure; **IV** 1–1.5 mg; may repeat in 2 min prn. ***For intubated patients*** 0.05–0.2 mg/kg/h by continuous infusion.
Child: **IM** 0.08 mg/kg × 1 dose. **PR** 0.3 mg/kg × 1 dose. ***For intubated patients*** 2 μg/kg/min by continuous infusion; may increase by 1 μg/kg/min q30min until light sleep is induced.
Neonate: **IV** 0.5–1 μg/kg/min.

IV Induction for General Anesthesia

Adult: **IV** ***Premedicated*** 0.15–0.25 mg/kg over 20–30 s; allow 2 min for effect.
IV Nonpremedicated 0.3–0.35 mg/kg over 20–30 s; allow 2 min for effect.
Child: **IV** 0.15 mg/kg followed by 0.05 mg/kg q2min × 1–3 doses.

Status Epilepticus

Child >2 mo: **IV** 0.15 mg/kg loading dose, then 1 μg/kg/min infusion; may titrate upward as needed q5min.

Preoperative Sedation

Child: **PO** *<5 y:* 0.5 mg/kg; *>5 y:* 0.4–0.5 mg/kg.

PHARMACOKINETICS **Onset:** 1–5 min IV; 5–15 min IM, 20–30 min PO. **Peak:** 20–60 min. **Duration:** < 2 h IV; 1–6 h IM. **Distribution:** crosses blood–brain barrier and placenta. **Metabolism:** metabolized in liver. **Elimination:** half-life: 1–4 h; excreted in urine.

CONTRAINDICATIONS & PRECAUTIONS **Contraindicated in:** intolerance to benzodiazepines; acute narrow-angle glaucoma; shock, coma; acute alcohol intoxication; intraarterial injection. Safe use in pregnancy (category D), labor and delivery or by nursing mothers not established. **Cautious use in:** patient with COPD; chronic renal failure; CHF; the elderly.

ADVERSE/SIDE EFFECTS **CNS:** *retrograde amnesia,* headache, euphoria, drowsiness, excessive sedation, confusion. **CV:** hypotension. **Eye:** blurred vision, diplopia, nystagmus, pinpoint pupils. **GI:** nausea, vomiting. **Respiratory:** coughing, laryngospasm (rare), respiratory arrest. **Skin:** hives, swelling, burning, pain, induration at injection site, tachypnea. **Other:** hiccups, chills, weakness.

DRUG INTERACTIONS **Alcohol,** CNS DEPRESSANTS, ANTICONVULSANTS potentiate CNS depression; **cimetidine** increases midazolam plasma levels, increasing its toxicity; may decrease antiparkinsonism effects of **levodopa;** may increase **phenytoin** levels; **smoking** decreases sedative and antianxiety effects.

INCOMPATIBILITIES **Solution/additive: dimenhydrinate, pentobarbital, perphenazine, prochlorperazine, ranitidine. Y-site: dimenhydrinate, pentobarbital, perphenazine, prochlorperazine, ranitidine.**

NURSING IMPLICATIONS

Administration

- Inject IM drug deep into a large muscle mass.
- IV midazolam is given diluted to a concentration of 0.25 mg/ml in NS or D5W. Avoid rapid injection, which may cause respiratory depression.
- IV administration to neonates, infants: Verify correct IV concentration and rate of infusion with physician.
- If stored at 15–30C (59–86F), therapeutic activity is retained for 2 y from date of manufacture.

Assessment & Drug Effects

- During IV infusion, inspect injection site for redness, pain, swelling, and other signs of extravasation.
- If the patient is premedicated with a narcotic agonist analgesic, the conscious sedation period may be marked by hypotension.
- Anterograde amnesia (dose related) correlates well with degree of drowsiness and is about the same as that for lorazepam. Most patients do not recall induction.
- In the obese patient, half-life is prolonged; therefore, duration of effects is prolonged (i.e., amnesia, postoperative recovery). Monitor vital signs for entire recovery period.
- Overdose symptoms include somnolence, confusion, sedation, diminished reflexes, coma, and untoward effects on vital signs.

Patient & Family Education

- Patient may feel drowsy, weak, or tired for 1–2 d after drug has been given. Warn not to drive a car or perform other tasks requiring alertness and coordination until effects of midazolam disappear.
- Prepare patient for the amnesia to prevent an upsetting postoperative period.
- Patient teaching during amnestic period may not be remembered. Even if dose is small and depth of amnesia is unclear, provide written instructions with verbal teaching to assure future understanding and compliance.

MIDODRINE HYDROCHLORIDE

(mid′o-dreen)

Trade name: ProAmatine

Classifications: AUTONOMIC NERVOUS SYSTEM AGENT; ALPHA$_1$ AGONIST

Prototype: Methoxamine

Pregnancy category: C

ACTIONS/PHARMACODYNAMICS

Midodrine is a vasopressor and an

$alpha_1$ agonist. It affects the alpha-adrenergic receptors of the arteries and veins, resulting in increased vascular tone and elevation in blood pressure. Midodrine affects standing, sitting, and supine systolic and diastolic blood pressures.

USE Treatment of symptomatic orthostatic hypotension.

ROUTE & DOSAGE

Orthostatic Hypotension

Adult: **PO** 10 mg t.i.d. during the daytime hours, dosed not less that 3 h apart; last dose should be taken at least 4 h before bedtime (max 20 mg/dose).

PHARMACOKINETICS **Absorption:** rapidly absorbed from GI tract. **Peak:** midodrine 0.5 h; desglymidodrine 1–2 h. **Metabolism:** rapidly metabolized to desglymidodrine, the active metabolite. **Elimination:** half-life: midodrine 25 min, desglymidodrine 3–4 h; excreted in urine.

CONTRAINDICATIONS & PRECAUTIONS **Contraindicated in:** severe organic heart disease, acute renal disease, urinary retention, pheochromocytoma, thyrotoxicosis, persistent and excessive supine hypertension. **Cautious use in:** renal impairment, history of visual problems, diabetes with hypotension or visual disorders, pregnancy (category C), nursing mothers. Safety and efficacy in children have not been established.

ADVERSE/SIDE EFFECTS **Body as whole:** *paresthesia,* chills, pain, facial flushing. **CNS:** confusion, nervousness, anxiety. **CV:** *hypertension.* **GI:** dry mouth. **Skin:** *pruritus, piloerection,* rash. **Other:** *dysuria, urinary retention, urinary frequency.*

NURSING IMPLICATIONS

Administration

- Drug should not be given 4 h before lying supine for any length of time (e.g., bedtime or napping).
- Give with caution in persons with pretreatment, supine systolic BP ≥ 170 mm Hg.
- Store at 15–30C (59–77F).

Assessment & Drug Effects

- Therapeutic effectiveness is indicated by an increase in 1-min standing systolic BP and subjective feelings of clinical improvement.
- Renal and hepatic function should be evaluated prior to initiating therapy.
- Regularly monitor supine and standing BP; drug should be stopped if supine BP increases excessively; determine acceptable parameters.
- Carefully monitor effect of the drug in diabetics with orthostatic hypotension and persons taking fludrocortisone acetate, which may increase intraocular pressure.

Patient & Family Education

- The last daily dose should be taken 4 h before bedtime.
- Immediately report to the physician sensations associated with supine hypertension (e.g., pounding in ears, headache, blurred vision, awareness of heart beating).
- Discontinue drug and report to physician if S&S of bradycardia develop (e.g., dizziness, pulse slowing, fainting).
- Do not take allergy drugs, cold preparations, or diet pills without consulting physician.

MILRINONE LACTATE

(mil′-ri-none)

Trade name: Primacor

Classifications: CARDIAC INOTROPIC

AGENT; ENZYME INHIBITOR; VASODILATOR
Pregnancy category: C

ACTIONS/PHARMACODYNAMICS Member of a new class of inotropic/vasodilator agents. Positive inotrope and vasodilator, with little chronotropic activity; mode of action and structure are different from digitalis and catecholamines as well as beta-adrenergic agonists.

Inhibitory action of milrinone is against cyclic-AMP phosphodiesterase in cardiac and smooth vascular muscle. In therapeutic dose, milrinone increases myocardial contractility. Therefore, milrinone increases cardiac output and decreases pulmonary wedge pressure and vascular resistance, without increasing myocardial oxygen demand or significantly increasing heart rate.

M

USE Short-term management of CHF. **Unlabeled uses:** short-term use to increase the cardiac index in patients with low cardiac output after surgery. To increase cardiac function prior to heart transplantation.

ROUTE & DOSAGE

Adult: **IV** ***Loading dose:*** 50 μg/kg IV over 10 min.
Maintenance infusion:
0.375–0.75 μg/kg/ min.

PHARMACOKINETICS Peak: 2 min. **Duration:** 2 h. **Distribution:** 70% protein bound. **Elimination:** half-life: 1.7–2.7 h; 80–85% excreted unchanged in urine within 24 h. Active renal tubular secretion is primary elimination pathway.

CONTRAINDICATIONS & PRECAUTIONS Contraindicated in: hypersensitivity to milrinone. **Cautious use in:** elderly, pregnancy (category C), nursing mothers. Safety and efficacy have not been established.

ADVERSE/SIDE EFFECTS CV: Increased ectopic activity, PVCs, ventricular tachycardia, ventricular fibrillation, supraventricular arrhythmias; possible increase in angina symptoms, hypotension.

DRUG INTERACTIONS Disopyramide may cause excessive hypotension.

INCOMPATIBILITIES Solution/additive: furosemide, procainamide. Y-site: furosemide.

NURSING IMPLICATIONS

Administration

- IV preparation: Dissolve 20 mg of milrinone in 0.45% NaCl or 0.9% NaCl injection, or 5% dextrose injection, to yield: 100 μg/ml with 180 ml diluent; 150 μg/ml with 113 ml diluent; 200 μg/ml with 80 ml diluent.
- IV administration: Give a loading dose of 50 μg/kg IV over 10 min followed by the ordered maintenance dose.
- Dosages may be titrated for maximum hemodynamic effect according to prescribed parameters.
- Do not administer the patients with preexisting hypokalemia until corrected.
- Dosage should be reduced in the presence of renal impairment according to creatinine clearance.
- Store according to manufacturer's directions.

Assessment & Drug Effects

- Closely monitor cardiac status during and for several hours following infusion. Supraventricular and ventricular arrhythmias have occurred.
- Monitor blood pressure and

promptly slow or stop infusion in presence of significant hypotension. Closely monitor those with recent aggressive diuretic therapy for decreasing blood pressure.
- Monitor fluid and electrolyte status. Hypokalemia should be corrected whenever it occurs during administration.

Patient & Family Education
- Advise to immediately report angina during drug infusion.
- Inform that drug may cause a headache, which can be treated with analgesics.

MINERAL OIL

Trade names: Agoral Plain, Heavy Mineral Oil, Kondremul Plain, Milkinol, Neo-Cultol, Zymenol

Classifications: GI AGENT; STOOL SOFTENER

Prototype: Docusate

Pregnancy category: C

ACTIONS/PHARMACODYNAMICS Mixture of hydrocarbons obtained from petroleum. Lubricates and softens feces, retards water absorption from fecal content, eases passage of stool.

USES Temporary relief of constipation, when straining at stool is contraindicated (e.g., hypertension, certain cardiac disorders, following anorectal surgery), and to relieve fecal impaction. Also used as pharmaceutical solvent and vehicle.

ROUTE & DOSAGE

Constipation
Adult: **PO** 15–30 ml prn. **Rectal** 90–120 ml.
Child ≥ 6 y: **PO** 5–15 ml once/d.

PHARMACOKINETICS **Absorption:** limited absorption from GI tract. **Distribution:** distributes to mesenteric lymph nodes, intestinal mucosa, liver, and spleen. **Elimination:** eliminated in stool in 6–10 h.

CONTRAINDICATIONS & PRECAUTIONS **Contraindicated in:** nausea, vomiting, abdominal pain, intestinal obstruction, oral administration to dysphagic patients; use with emollients. **Cautious use in:** oral use in elderly or debilitated patients; during pregnancy (category C).

ADVERSE/SIDE EFFECTS Occasionally, pruritus ani; interference with postoperative anorectal wound healing; with aspiration: pulmonary granuloma, lipid pneumonitis. Prolonged use: anorexia, nausea, vomiting, nutritional deficiencies, hypoprothrombinemia.

DRUG INTERACTIONS May potentiate effects of ORAL ANTICOAGULANTS by decreasing the absorption of Vitamin K; large doses may decrease the absorption of **warfarin;** STOOL SOFTENERS may form a concretion in the GI tract.

NURSING IMPLICATIONS

Administration
- Mineral oil is usually administered in the evening. Digestion and passage of food from stomach may be delayed if taken within 2 h of mealtime.
- Potential of lipid pneumonia from aspiration is especially high in the elderly and debilitated patient. Administer with patient in upright position and avoid giving just before patient retires.
- Administration of retention enema is generally followed by a cleansing enema in 30–60 min. Consult physician.

Patient & Family Education

- Prolonged use (> 2 wk) can reduce absorption of fat-soluble vitamins A, D, E, and K, carotene, calcium, and phosphates.
- Repeated oral use or rectal administration may result in oil seepage from rectum with soiling of clothing. Forewarn patient to be prepared for this possibility.
- Frequent or prolonged use of mineral oil may result in dependence.

MINOCYCLINE HYDROCHLORIDE

(mi-noe-sye′kleen)

Trade name: Minocin

Classifications: ANTIINFECTIVE; TETRACYCLINE ANTIBIOTIC; ANTIACNE

Prototype: Tetracycline

Pregnancy category: D

ACTIONS/PHARMACODYNAMICS Semisynthetic tetracycline derivative with actions, uses, contraindications, precautions, and adverse reactions as for tetracycline. Appears to be active against strains of staphylococci resistant to other tetracyclines, and photosensitivity occurs only rarely. Reported to be more completely absorbed than other tetracyclines because it is more lipid-soluble.

ROUTE & DOSAGE

Antiinfective

Adult: **PO/IV** 200 mg followed by 100 mg q12h.
Child > 8 y: **PO/IV** 4.4 mg/kg followed by 2 mg/kg q12h.

PHARMACOKINETICS Absorption: 90–100% absorbed from GI tract. **Peak:** 2–3 h. **Distribution:** tends to accumulate in adipose tissue; crosses placenta; distributed into breast milk. **Metabolism:** partially metabolized. **Elimination:** half-life: 11–26 h; 20–30% excreted in feces; about 12% excreted in urine.

CONTRAINDICATIONS & PRECAUTIONS Contraindicated in: hypersensitivity to tetracyclines; oral administration in meningococcal infections; children < 8 y. Safe use during pregnancy (category D) not established. **Cautious use in:** renal impairment.

ADVERSE/SIDE EFFECTS *CNS side effects (weakness, light-headedness, ataxia, dizziness, or vertigo),* nausea, cramps, diarrhea, flatulence.

DRUG INTERACTIONS ANTACIDS, **iron, calcium, magnesium, zinc, kaolin and pectin, sodium bicarbonate, bismuth subsalicylate** can significantly decrease minocycline absorption; effects of both **desmopressin** and minocycline antagonized; increases **digoxin** absorption, increasing risk of digoxin toxicity; **methoxyflurane** increases risk of renal failure. **Food–drug:** dairy products significantly decrease minocycline absorption; food may also decrease its absorption.

INCOMPATIBILITIES Solution/additive: doxapram. Y-site: hydromorphone, meperidine, morphine, TPN.

NURSING IMPLICATIONS

Administration

- IV preparation: Reconstitute 100 mg with 5 ml of sterile water for injection; may be further diluted with 500–1000 ml of compatible solutions (e.g., NaCl, dextrose, Ringer's).
- IV administration: Give diluted IV solution by intermittent infusion at

a rate determined by the total volume of solution.

- Check expiration date. Outdated tetracycline can cause severe adverse side effects.
- Reconstituted solution is stable at room temperature for 24 h; further diluted solution should be used immediately.

Assessment & Drug Effects

- Prior to administration, culture and sensitivity test should be done and repeated at regular intervals during drug therapy.
- Prior to administration, obtain history of hypersensitivity reactions; drug is contraindicated with known tetracycline hypersensitivity.
- Carefully monitor IV infusion site, since thrombophlebitis occurs relatively often (see Appendix G).
- Carefully monitor for signs of hypersensitivity response (see Appendix G), particularly in patients with history of allergies, especially to drugs.
- Monitor for signs of superinfection (see Appendix G).
- Risk of toxic effects increases with renal and hepatic impairment; carefully assess at-risk patients.
- Serum drug level determinations are advised in patients receiving prolonged therapy.
- Supervise ambulation, since lightheadedness, dizziness, and vertigo occur frequently.

Patient & Family Education

- Advise to avoid hazardous activities or those requiring alertness while on minocycline.
- Instruct to use a sunscreen when outdoors and to otherwise protect themselves from direct sunlight since photosensitivity reaction may occur.
- Advise to report vestibular side effects (e.g., dizziness), which usually occur during first week of therapy. Effects are reversible if drug is withdrawn.
- Instruct to promptly report loose stools or diarrhea or other signs of superinfection.
- Advise women to use nonhormonal methods of contraception while they are taking drug.

MINOXIDIL

(mi-nox′i-dill)

Trade names: Loniten, Rogaine

Classifications: CARDIOVASCULAR AGENT; NONNITRATE VASODILATOR; ANTIHYPERTENSIVE

Prototype: Hydralazine

Pregnancy category: C

M

ACTIONS/PHARMACODYNAMICS

Direct-acting vasodilator similar to other drugs of this class, but hypotensive effect is more pronounced. Appears to act by blocking calcium uptake through cell membrane. Reduces elevated systolic and diastolic blood pressures in supine and standing positions, by decreasing peripheral vascular resistance. Hypotensive action is accompanied by reflex activation of sympathetic, vagal inhibitory, and renal homeostatic mechanisms; increased sympathetic stimulation also activates the renin-angiotensin-aldosterone system. The net result is increased heart rate and cardiac output, sodium retention, and edema, which usually necessitates concomitant supportive drug therapy. Drug-induced hair growth with systemic minoxidil usually develops after 1 y of therapy: it is nonvirilizing, involving face and limbs of the female and generalized increase in body hair in men. Topical minoxidil reverses balding to some degree. Action mechanism is uncertain.

USES Step 4 agent in stepped care approach to treat severe hypertension that is symptomatic or associated with damage to target organs and is not manageable with maximum therapeutic doses of a diuretic plus two other antihypertensive drugs. Used with a diuretic to prevent fluid retention and a beta-adrenergic blocking agent (e.g., propranolol) or an alpha-adrenergic agonist (e.g., clonidine or methyldopa) to prevent tachycardia. (Topical) to treat alopecia areata and male pattern alopecia.

ROUTE & DOSAGE

Hypertension

Adult: **PO** 5 mg/d, increased q3–5d up to 40 mg/d in single or divided doses as needed (max 100 mg/d).
Child: **PO** 0.2 mg/kg/d (max 5 mg/d) initially, gradually increased to 0.25–1 mg/kg/d in divided doses (max 50 mg/d).

Male Pattern Alopecia

Adult: **Topical** Apply 1 ml of 2% solution to affected area b.i.d.

PHARMACOKINETICS **Absorption:** readily absorbed from GI tract. **Onset:** 30 min PO; at least 4 mo topical. **Peak:** 2–8 h PO. **Duration:** 2–5 d PO; new hair growth will remain 3–4 mo after withdrawal of topical. **Distribution:** widely distributed including into breast milk. **Metabolism:** metabolized in liver. **Elimination:** half-life: 4.2 h; 97% excreted in urine and feces.

CONTRAINDICATIONS & PRECAUTIONS **Contraindicated in:** pheochromocytoma; acute MI, dissecting aortic aneurysm. Safe use during pregnancy (category C) or in nursing mothers not established. **Cautious use in:** severe renal impairment; recent MI (within preceding month); coronary artery disease, chronic CHF.

ADVERSE/SIDE EFFECTS **CV:** *tachycardia,* angina pectoris, *ECG changes,* pericardial effusion and tamponade, rebound hypertension (following drug withdrawal); *edema,* including pulmonary edema; *CHF (salt and water retention).* **Skin:** *hypertrichosis,* transient pruritus, darkening of skin, hypersensitivity rash, Stevens-Johnson syndrome. With topical use: itching, flushing, scaling, dermatitis, folliculitis. **Other:** fatigue.

DIAGNOSTIC TEST INTERFERENCE ***Hematocrit, hemoglobin,*** and ***erythrocyte count*** usually decrease (about 7%) during early therapy; ***serum alkaline phosphatase, BUN,*** and ***creatinine*** may increase during early therapy.

DRUG INTERACTIONS **Epinephrine, norepinephrine** cause excessive cardiac stimulation; **guanethidine** causes profound orthostatic hypotension.

NURSING IMPLICATIONS

Administration

- Dose adjustment intervals are normally at least 3 d. If more rapid adjustment is necessary, adjustments can be made q6h with careful monitoring.
- Store in tightly covered container at 15–30C (59–86F) unless otherwise directed.

Assessment & Drug Effects

- Take BP and apical pulse before administering medication and report significant changes. Consult physician for parameters.

- Monitor BP and pulse at regular intervals during therapy. Abrupt reduction in BP can result in CVA and MI. Keep physician informed.
- Fluid and electrolyte balance should be closely followed throughout therapy. Sodium and water retention commonly occur. Consult physician regarding sodium restriction. If patient is on diuretic therapy, potassium intake and serum potassium levels will require monitoring.
- Monitor I&O and daily weight. Report unusual changes in I&O ratio or daily weight gain ≥ 1 kg (2 lb).
- Observe patient daily for edema and auscultate lungs for rales. Be alert to signs and symptoms of CHF (see Appendix G).
- Observe for symptoms of pericardial effusion or tamponade. Symptoms are similar to those of CHF, but additionally patient may have paradoxical pulse (normal inspiratory reduction in systolic BP may fall as much as 10–20 mm Hg).
- Rebound hypertension has followed minoxidil withdrawal. Conversion to conventional therapy must be accomplished gradually and with close observation of patient.

Patient & Family Education

- Tell patients usual pulse rate and instruct to count radial pulse for one full minute before taking drug. Advise patient to report an increase of 20 or more bpm.
- Instruct to notify physician promptly if the following signs or symptoms appear: increase of 20 or more bpm in resting pulse; breathing difficulty; dizziness; light-headedness; fainting; edema (tight shoes or rings, puffiness, pitting); weight gain, chest pain, arm or shoulder pain; easy bruising or bleeding.
- Thoroughly inform of possibility of hypertrichosis: elongation, thickening, and increased pigmentation of fine body hair, especially of face, arms, and back. It develops 3–9 wk after start of therapy and occurs in approximately 80% of patients. It is reversible within 1–6 mo following discontinuation of minoxidil.
- A history of hypertension is not a contraindication to use of topical minoxidil, but coronary heart disease, valvular dysfunction, and heart failure are.
- Report any dermatologic adverse effects or any other adverse effect promptly. Follow-up examinations are usually scheduled for q4–6mo.
- Stress strict compliance: regular use maximizes chance of at least some hair regrowth.

MIRTAZAPINE

(mir-taz′-a-peen)

Trade name: Remeron

Classifications: CNS AGENT; PSYCHOTHERAPEUTIC; TETRACYCLIC ANTIDEPRESSANT

Pregnancy category: C, D

ACTIONS/PHARMACODYNAMICS

Tetracyclic antidepressant pharmacologically and therapeutically similar to the tricyclic antidepressants. Mechanism of action is unknown. Tetracyclics enhance central nonadrenergic and serotonergic activity. Mirtazapine is a potent antagonist of 5-HT_2 and 5-HT_3 serotonin receptors.

USE Treatment of depression.

ROUTE & DOSAGE

Depression

Adult: **PO** 15 mg/d in single dose h.s. May increase q1–2wk to max 45 mg/d. Use lower doses in **geriatric** patients and patients with **renal** or **hepatic insufficiency.**

PHARMACOKINETICS **Absorption:** rapidly absorbed from GI tract, 50% reaches systemic circulation. **Peak:** 2 h. **Distribution:** 85% protein bound. **Metabolism:** metabolized in liver by cytochrome P450 system (CYP2D6, CYP1A2, CYP3A). **Elimination:** half-life: 20–40 h; 75% excreted in urine, 15% in feces.

CONTRAINDICATIONS & PRECAUTIONS **Contraindicated in:** hypersensitivity to mirtazapine or mianserin, hypersensitivity to other antidepressants (e.g., tricyclic antidepressants and MAOI depressants). **Cautious use in:** history of cardiovascular or GI disorders, BPH, narrow-angle glaucoma, hepatic or renal impairment, pregnancy (category C), lactation, elderly. Safety and effectiveness in children have not been established.

M

ADVERSE/SIDE EFFECTS **Body as whole:** asthenia, flu syndrome, back pain, general and peripheral edema, malaise. **CNS:** *somnolence,* dizziness, abnormal dreams, abnormal thinking, tremor, confusion, depression, agitation, vertigo, twitching. **CV:** hypertension, vasodilation. **GI:** nausea, vomiting, abdominal pain, *increased appetite/*weight gain, *dry mouth, constipation,* anorexia, cholecystitis, stomatitis, colitis, abnormal LFTs. **Respiratory:** dyspnea, cough, sinusitis. **Skin:** pruritus, rash. **Other:** urinary frequency.

DRUG INTERACTIONS Additive cognitive and motor impairment with alcohol or BENZODIAZEPINES.

NURSING IMPLICATIONS

Administration

- Preferably given prior to going to sleep to minimize injury potential.
- Begin drug no sooner than 14 d after discontinuation of an MAO inhibitor.
- Dosage reductions may be warranted with severe renal or hepatic impairment and in the elderly.
- Store at 20–25C (68–77F) in tight, light-resistant container.

Assessment & Drug Effects

- Therapeutic effectiveness is indicated by elevation of mood.
- Periodically monitor WBC count with differential, lipid profile, blood glucose, and ALT/SGPT.
- Assess for weight gain and excessive somnolence or dizziness.
- With a history of cardiovascular or cerebrovascular disease, monitor for orthostatic hypotension. Periodically monitor ECG especially in those with known cardiovascular disease.
- Carefully monitor those with a history of increased intraocular pressure or urinary retention for worsening or recurrence.
- Monitor persons with a history of seizures for lowering of the seizure threshold.

Patient & Family Education

- Warn of high potential for drowsiness and dizziness and advise caution with hazardous activities until reaction to drug is known. Advise against alcohol use while on mirtazapine.
- Advise to immediately report unexplained fever or S&S of infection, especially flu-like symptoms.
- Caution about taking any other drugs without informing physician.
- Alcohol in combination with mirtazapine can significantly impair cognitive and motor skills. Avoid alcohol while on this drug.
- Make position changes slowly especially when changing from lying or sitting to standing. Report dizziness, palpitations, and fainting.
- Women who become pregnant should immediately notify their physician. Mothers should not breast-feed while on mirtazapine.

- Monitor weight periodically and report significant weight gains.

MISOPROSTOL

(my-so-prost′ole)
Trade name: Cytotec
Classification: PROSTAGLANDIN
Prototype: Dinoprostone
Pregnancy category: X

ACTIONS/PHARMACODYNAMICS Misoprostol, a synthetic prostaglandin E_1 analog, has both antisecretory (inhibiting gastric acid secretion) and mucosal protective properties. It can increase bicarbonate and mucosal protective properties. It also increases bicarbonate and mucous production. Misoprostol inhibits basal and nocturnal gastric acid secretion and acid secretion in response to a variety of stimuli, including meals, histamine, pentagastrin, and coffee. Misoprostol produces uterine contractions that may endanger pregnancy and cause a miscarriage.

USES Prevention of NSAID (including aspirin)-induced gastric ulcers in patients at high risk of complications from a gastric ulcer, e.g., the elderly and patients with a concomitant debilitating disease or a history of ulcers. The drug is taken for the duration of NSAID therapy and does not interfere with the efficacy of the NSAID. **Unlabeled use:** short-term treatment of duodenal ulcers.

ROUTE & DOSAGE

Prevention of NSAID-induced Ulcers

Adult: **PO** 100–200 µg q.i.d. p.c. and h.s. *or* 200 µg b.i.d. or t.i.d.

PHARMACOKINETICS Absorption: readily absorbed from GI tract; extensive first pass metabolism. **Onset:** 30 min. **Peak:** 60–90 min. **Duration:** at least 3 h. **Metabolism:** metabolized in liver. **Elimination:** half-life: 20–40 min; primarily excreted in urine; small amount excreted in feces.

CONTRAINDICATIONS & PRECAUTIONS Contraindicated in: pregnant women (category X), history of allergies to prostaglandins, and nursing mothers. **Cautious use in:** renal impairment. Safety in children < 18 y has not been established.

ADVERSE/SIDE EFFECTS CNS: headache. **GI:** *diarrhea, abdominal pain,* nausea, flatulence, dyspepsia, vomiting, constipation. **GU:** spotting, cramps, dysmenorrhea, uterine contractions.

DRUG INTERACTION MAGNESIUM-CONTAINING ANTACIDS may increase diarrhea.

NURSING IMPLICATIONS

Administration

- Maximum plasma concentrations are diminished when misoprostol is taken with food. Because of GI side effects, however, manufacturer recommends that drug be taken with food.
- Store away from heat, light, and moisture.

Assessment & Drug Effects

- Diarrhea is a common side effect and is dose related. It is usually self-limiting (often resolving in 8 d). The incidence of diarrhea can be minimized by taking the drug after meals and at bedtime.

Patient & Family Education

- Avoid using magnesium-containing antacids because of increased incidence of diarrhea.
- Before using a new medicine (prescription or nonprescription) or if

a new medical problem develops, check with doctor.

- Postmenopausal bleeding may be drug related. Report to physician.
- Advise women of childbearing potential that they must not be pregnant when misoprostol therapy is initiated, and they must use an effective contraception method while taking the drug.
- Advise of the abortifacient property of the drug. If woman becomes pregnant, the drug should be discontinued and the doctor contacted immediately.

MITOMYCIN

(mye-toe-mye'sin)

Trade name: Mutamycin

Classifications: ANTINEOPLASTIC; ANTIBIOTIC

Prototype: Doxorubicin

Pregnancy category: D

ACTIONS/PHARMACODYNAMICS Potent antibiotic antineoplastic compound. Effective in certain tumors nonresponsive to surgery, radiation, or other chemotherapeutic agents. Action mechanism not clear but reportedly combines with DNA, thereby interfering with cellular and enzymatic RNA and protein synthesis.

USES In combination with other chemotherapeutic agents in palliative, adjunctive treatment of disseminated adenocarcinoma of breast, pancreas, or stomach, squamous cell carcinoma of head, neck, lung, and cervix. Not recommended to replace surgery or radiotherapy or as a single primary therapeutic agent.

ROUTE & DOSAGE

Cancer

Adult/Child: **IV** 20 $mg/m^2/d$ as a single dose q6–8wk; additional doses based on hematologic response.

PHARMACOKINETICS Metabolism: metabolized rapidly in liver. **Elimination:** half-life: 17 min; excreted in urine.

CONTRAINDICATIONS & PRECAUTIONS Contraindicated in: hypersensitivity or idiosyncracy reaction; thrombocytopenia; coagulation disorders or bleeding tendencies; pregnancy (category D). **Cautious use in:** renal impairment; myelosuppression.

ADVERSE/SIDE EFFECTS CNS: paresthesias. **GI:** stomatitis, *nausea, vomiting,* anorexia. **Hematologic:** bone marrow toxicity *(thrombocytopenia, leukopenia* occurring 4–8 wk after treatment onset). **Respiratory:** acute bronchospasm, hemoptysis, dyspnea, nonproductive cough, pneumonia, interstitial pneumonitis. **Skin:** desquamation; induration, pain, necrosis, cellulitis at injection site; reversible alopecia, purple discoloration of nail beds. **Other:** thrombophlebitis, anemia, pain, hemolytic uremic syndrome, renal toxicity, headache, fatigue, edema, hematemesis, diarrhea.

INCOMPATIBILITY Solution/additive: DEXTROSE-CONTAINING SOLUTIONS.

NURSING IMPLICATIONS

Administration

- Patient receiving mitomycin should be hospitalized so that emergency treatment will be available.
- IV preparation: Add sterile water for injection 10 ml to vial containing 5 mg mitomycin (and mannitol). Shake to dissolve. If product does not clear immediately, allow to stand at room temperature until

solution is obtained. Reconstituted solution is purple.

- IV administration: Give reconstituted solution by direct IV over 5–10 min or longer as determined by volume of solution.
- IV administration to children: Verify correct IV concentration and rate of infusion/injection with physician.
- Avoid extravasation to prevent extreme tissue reaction (cellulitis) to the toxic drug.
- Unreconstituted drug is stable for at least 4 y at room temperature. Drug reconstituted with sterile water for injection (0.5 mg/ml) is stable for 14 d refrigerated or 7 d at room temperature. Drug diluted in 5% dextrose injection (20–40 μg/ml) is stable at room temperature for 3 h.

Assessment & Drug Effects

- Usually, drug is not administered if serum creatinine is > 1.7 mg/dl.
- If platelet count falls below 150,000/mm^3 and WBC is down to 4000/mm^3 or if prothrombin or bleeding times are prolonged, treatment is suspended or modified.
- Laboratory studies of platelet counts, prothrombin and bleeding times, differential and hemoglobin studies, serum creatinine are performed frequently during treatment and for at least 7 wk after treatment is terminated.
- Monitor I&O ratio and pattern. Any sign of impaired kidney function should be reported: change in ratio, dysuria, hematuria, oliguria, frequency, urgency. Keep patient well hydrated (at least 2000–2500 ml orally daily if tolerated). Drug is nephrotoxic.
- Observe closely for signs of infection. Monitor body temperature frequently.
- Inspect oral cavity daily for signs of stomatitis or superinfection (see Appendix G).

Patient & Family Education

- Instruct to immediately report respiratory distress.
- Instruct to report immediately if signs of common cold present.
- Inform that alopecia is reversible with cessation of treatment.

MITOTANE

(mye′toe-tane)

Trade name: Lysodren

Classifications: ADRENOCORTICAL CYTOTOXIC; ANTINEOPLASTIC

Pregnancy category: C

ACTIONS/PHARMACODYNAMICS

Cytotoxic agent with suppressant action on the adrenal cortex. Modifies peripheral metabolism of steroids and reduces production of adrenal steroids. Extraadrenal metabolism of cortisol is altered, leading to reduction in 17-hydroxycorticosteroids (17-OHCS); however, plasma levels of corticosteroids do not fall.

USES Inoperable adrenal cortical carcinoma (functional and nonfunctional). **Unlabeled use:** Cushing's syndrome secondary to pituitary disorders.

ROUTE & DOSAGE

Adrenocortical Carcinoma

Adult: **PO** 9–10 g/d in divided doses t.i.d. or q.i.d.; tolerated doses range from 2–16 g/d.

PHARMACOKINETICS **Absorption:** approximately 40% absorbed from GI tract. **Onset:** 2–4 wk. **Peak:** 3–5 h. **Distribution:** deposits in most body tissues, especially adipose tissue. **Metabolism:** metabolized in liver.

M

Elimination: half-life: 18–159 d; small amount excreted in bile.

CONTRAINDICATIONS & PRECAUTIONS **Contraindicated in:** pregnancy (category C) and nursing women only after risk-benefit ratio to mother and fetus has been assessed. **Cautious use in:** hepatic disease.

ADVERSE/SIDE EFFECTS **CNS:** vertigo, dizziness, drowsiness, tiredness, depression, *lethargy, sedation,* headache, confusion, tremors. **CV:** hypertension, hypotension, flushing. **GI:** *anorexia, nausea, vomiting, diarrhea.* **GU:** hematuria, hemorrhagic cystitis, albuminuria. **Other:** adrenocortical insufficiency, blurred vision, diplopia, lens opacity, toxic retinopathy, generalized aching, fever, cutaneous eruptions and pigmentation, muscle twitching, hypersensitivity reactions, hyperpyrexia, *rash, hypouricemia, hypercholesterolemia.*

DIAGNOSTIC TEST INTERFERENCE Mitotane decreases ***protein-bound iodine (PBI)*** and ***urinary 17-OHCS levels.***

DRUG INTERACTIONS Potentiates sedative effects of **alcohol** and other CNS DEPRESSANTS; may increase the metabolism of **phenytoin, phenobarbital, warfarin,** decreasing their effectiveness.

NURSING IMPLICATIONS

Administration

- Nausea and vomiting may be reduced or alleviated by antiemetic therapy before and during drug therapy.
- If an emergency occurs, mitotane may be temporarily withdrawn, since adrenal suppression is its prime action. Exogenous steroids may be required until the already depressed adrenal starts secreting steroids.
- Store in tight, light-resistant containers at 15–30C (59–86F) unless otherwise directed.

Assessment & Drug Effects

- Monitor pulse and BP for early signs of shock (adrenal insufficiency).
- Observe for symptoms of hepatotoxicity (see Appendix G). Report them promptly, since reduced hepatic capacity can increase toxicity of mitotane and because dose may have to be decreased.
- Medication causes aching muscles, fever, flushing, and muscle twitching. If these symptoms persist and become more severe, the physician should be notified.
- Monitor the obese patient for symptoms of adrenal hypofunction. Because a large portion of the drug deposits in fatty tissue, this person is particularly susceptible to prolonged side effects.
- Neurologic and behavioral assessments should be made at regular intervals throughout therapy.

Patient & Family Education

- Mitotane does not cure but does reduce tumor mass, pain, weakness, anorexia, and steroid symptoms.
- Symptoms of adrenal insufficiency (weakness, fatigue, orthostatic hypotension, pigmentation, weight loss, dehydration, anorexia, nausea, vomiting, and diarrhea) should be reported to physician.
- Advise to use caution when driving or performing hazardous tasks requiring alertness because of drug-induced drowsiness, tiredness, dizziness. These symptoms tend to recede with continuation in therapy.
- Contraceptive measures are advised during therapy because of terato-

genic properties of the drug. If the woman suspects she is pregnant, she should notify the physician.

MITOXANTRONE HYDROCHLORIDE

(mi-tox'an-trone)

Trade name: Novantrone

Classifications: ANTINEOPLASTIC; ANTIBIOTIC; IMMUNOSUPPRESSANT

Prototype: Doxorubicin

Pregnancy category: D

ACTIONS/PHARMACODYNAMICS Mitoxantrone is a non-cell-cycle-specific antitumor agent with less cardiotoxicity than doxorubicin. It interferes with DNA synthesis by intercalating with the DNA double helix, blocking effective DNA and RNA transcription.

USES In combination with other drugs for the treatment of acute nonlymphocytic leukemia (ANLL) in adults, bone pain in advanced prostate cancer. **Unlabeled uses:** breast cancer, refractory lymphomas.

ROUTE & DOSAGE

Combination Therapy for ANLL

Adult: **IV** ***Induction therapy:*** 12 mg/m^2/d on days 1–3; may need to repeat induction course. ***Consolidation therapy:*** 12 mg/m^2 on days 1 and 2; total lifetime exposure should not exceed 80–120 mg/m^2.
Child: **IV** 8–33 mg/m^2 q3–4wk.

Solid Tumors

Child: **IV** 5–8 mg/m^2 once a week or 18–20 mg/m^2 q3–4wk.

PHARMACOKINETICS **Distribution:** rapidly taken up by tissues and slowly released into plasma, resulting in low renal, hepatic, and metabolic clearance rates; 95% protein bound. **Metabolism:** metabolized in liver. **Elimination:** half-life: 37 h; excreted primarily in bile.

CONTRAINDICATIONS & PRECAUTIONS **Contraindicated in:** hypersensitivity to mitoxantrone, myelosuppression, pregnancy (category D), lactation. **Cautious use in:** impaired cardiac function, impaired hepatic and renal function, systemic infections.

ADVERSE/SIDE EFFECTS **CV:** arrhythmias, decreased left ventricular function, CHF, tachycardia, ECG changes, MI (occurs with cumulative doses of >80–100 mg/m^2), edema. **GI:** *nausea, vomiting* diarrhea. **Hematologic:** *leukopenia, thrombocytopenia*. **Other:** discolors urine and sclera a blue-green color, hepatotoxicity, mild phlebitis, blue skin discoloration, alopecia.

DRUG INTERACTIONS May impair immune response to VACCINES such as influenza and pneumococcal. May have increased risk of infection with **yellow fever vaccine.**

INCOMPATIBILITIES **Solution/additive: heparin, hydrocortisone, paclitaxel. Y-site: TPN.**

NURSING IMPLICATIONS

Administration

- If mitoxantrone touches skin, wash immediately with copious amounts of warm water.
- IV preparation: Withdraw contents of vial and add to at least 50 ml of either 0.9% NaCl injection or 5% dextrose injection.
- IV administration: Diluted solution should be introduced into the tubing as a freely running IV of 0.9% NaCl or 5% dextrose and infused

over at least 3 min (usually 30–60 min).

- If extravasation occurs, stop infusion and immediately restart in another vein.
- Mitoxantrone should not be mixed in the same infusion with other drugs.
- The use of goggles, gloves, and protective gown is recommended during drug preparation and administration.
- Discard unused portions of diluted solution. Once opened, multiple-use vials may be stored refrigerated (2–8C/35–46F) for 14 d.

Assessment & Drug Effects

- Monitor IV insertion site. Transient blue skin discoloration may occur at site if extravasation has occurred.
- Carefully monitor CBC with differential prior to and during therapy.
- Monitor cardiac functioning throughout course of therapy; report signs and symptoms of CHF or cardiac arrhythmias.
- Hepatic function tests should be performed prior to and during course of treatment.
- Monitor serum uric acid levels and initiate hypouricemic therapy before antileukemic therapy.

Patient & Family Education

- Inform of potential adverse effects of mitoxantrone therapy.
- Advise patient to expect urine to turn blue-green for 24 h after drug administration; sclera may also take on a bluish color.
- Inform patient that stomatitis/mucositis may occur within 1 wk of therapy.
- Advise patient not to risk exposure to persons with known infections during the periods of myelosuppression.

M

MIVACURIUM CHLORIDE

(miv-a-cur′i-um)

Trade name: Mivacron

Classifications: AUTONOMIC NERVOUS SYSTEM AGENT; NONDEPOLARIZING SKELETAL MUSCLE RELAXANT

Prototype: Tubocurarine

Pregnancy category: C

ACTIONS/PHARMACODYNAMICS

Short-acting, skeletal muscle relaxant that combines competitively to cholinergic receptors on the motor neuron end-plate. This antagonizes the action of acetylcholine, and blocks neuromuscular transmission. Blocking action is readily reversible with an anticholinesterase agent.

USES Adjunct to general anesthesia, to facilitate tracheal intubation, and to provide skeletal muscle relaxation during surgery or mechanical ventilation.

ROUTE & DOSAGE

Tracheal Intubation and Mechanical Ventilation

Adult: **IV *Initial dose:*** 0.15 mg/kg given over 5–15 s (over 60 s in patients with cardiovascular disease). ***Maintenance dose:*** 0.1 mg/kg generally q15min. ***Continuous infusion:*** Initial infusion of 9–10 µg/kg/min, reduce infusion to 4 µg/kg/min if started with initial bolus. Infusion rates should be decreased by 50% in patients with impaired renal function.

Child 2–12 y: **IV *Initial dose:*** 0.2 mg/kg given over 5–15 s (range 0.09–0.2 mg/kg). ***Maintenance dose:*** Same as adult. ***Continuous infusion:*** 10–15 µg/kg/min.

PHARMACOKINETICS Peak: 2–6 min. **Duration:** 25–30 min in adults, 8–16 min in children. **Distribution:** limited tissue distribution. **Metabolism:** rapidly hydrolyzed by plasma cholinesterase.

CONTRAINDICATIONS & PRECAUTIONS Contraindicated in: allergic reactions to mivacurium or its ingredients. **Cautious use in:** renal function impairment, hepatic function impairment, elderly clients; pregnancy (category C), and nursing mothers.

ADVERSE/SIDE EFFECTS CV: transient decrease in arterial blood pressure, hypotension, increases and decreases in heart rate. **Skin:** *transient flushing about the face, neck, and/or chest* (especially with rapid administration).

DRUG INTERACTIONS GENERAL ANESTHETICS **(enflurane, halothane, isoflurane)** may enhance the degree of neuromuscular blockade produced by mivacurium. AMINOGLYCOSIDES, TETRACYCLINES, **bacitracin,** POLYMYXINS, **lincomycin, clindamycin, colistin, magnesium salts, lithium,** LOCAL ANESTHETICS, **procainamide,** and **quinidine** may enhance the neuromuscular blockade.

INCOMPATIBILITIES Solution/additive: ALKALINE SOLUTIONS pH ≥ 8.5 (BARBITURATES).

NURSING IMPLICATIONS

Administration

- IV preparaton: May dilute to a concentration of 0.5 mg/ml in any of the following: 5% dextrose injection, 0.9% NaCl injection, 5% dextrose and 0.9% NaCl injection, lactated Ringer's injection, or 5% dextrose in lactated injection.
- IV administration: See manufacturer's guidelines, as dosages and infusion rates differ depending on which other drugs are being concurrently administered.
- The use of a peripheral nerve stimulator permits optimal dosing and minimizes risks of overdose or underdose.
- Diluted solution may be stored from 5–25C (41–77F) for up to 24 h.

Assessment & Drug Effects

- Patients with neuromuscular disease may experience prolonged neuromuscular blocks. Carefully assess and adjust drug dosage using a peripheral nerve stimulator.
- Carefully monitor hemodynamic status in patients with significant cardiovascular disease or those with potentially greater sensitivity to release of histamine-type mediators (e.g., asthma).
- Because overdose may increase the risk of hemodynamic side effects, monitor such patients for significant decreases in blood pressure.

MOEXIPRIL HYDROCHLORIDE

(mo-ex′i-pril)

Trade name: Univasc

Classifications: CARDIOVASCULAR AGENT; ANGIOTENSIN-CONVERTING ENZYME INHIBITOR; ANTIHYPERTENSIVE

Prototype: Captopril

Pregnancy category: C (first trimester, D (second and third trimesters)

ACTIONS/PHARMACODYNAMICS Moexipril is an ACE inhibitor that results in decreased conversion of angiotensin I to angiotensin II. This results in decreased vasopressor activity and aldosterone secretion.

Both actions result in an antihypertensive effect.

USE Hypertension. **Unlabeled use:** CHF.

ROUTE & DOSAGE

Hypertension

Adult: **PO** 7.5 mg once/d; may increase up to 30 mg/d in divided doses; start with 3.75 mg q.d. if patient is volume depleted, on diuretics, or has renal insufficiency ($Cl_{cr} \leq 40$ ml/min).

PHARMACOKINETICS Absorption: readily absorbed from GI tract; approx 13% of active metabolite reaches systemic circulation; absorption greatly reduced by food. **Onset:** 1 h. **Duration:** 24 h. **Distribution:** approx 50% protein bound. **Metabolism:** metabolized in liver to moexiprilat (active metabolite). **Elimination:** half-life: 2–9 h; 13% excreted in urine, 53% excreted in feces.

CONTRAINDICATIONS & PRECAUTIONS Contraindicated in: hypersensitivity to moexipril, history of angioedema related to an ACE inhibitor, pregnancy [(category C) first trimester; (category D) second and third trimesters]. **Cautious use in:** hypersensitivity to any other ACE inhibitor, renal impairment, renal artery stenosis, volume-depleted patients; hypertensive patient with CHF, history of autoimmune disease, severe liver dysfunction, immunosuppressed patients, hyperkalemia, patients undergoing surgery/anesthesia, preexisting neutropenia, lactation, concurrent lithium therapy. Safety and efficacy in children have not been established.

ADVERSE/SIDE EFFECTS CNS: headache, *dizziness,* drowsiness, sleep disturbances, nervousness, anxiety, mood changes. **CV:** hypotension, chest pain, angina, peripheral edema, MI, palpitations, arrhythmias. **Endocrine:** hyperkalemia. **GI:** diarrhea, nausea, dyspepsia, abdominal pain, taste disturbances, constipation, vomiting, dry mouth, pancreatitis. **GU:** urinary frequency, increased BUN and serum creatinine. **Other:** neutropenia, hemolytic anemia, cough, pharyngitis, rhinitis, flu-like symptoms. **Skin:** angioedema (rare), rash, flushing.

DRUG INTERACTIONS Capsaicin may exacerbate cough. NSAIDS may reduce antihypertensive effects. May increase **lithium** levels and toxicity. POTASSIUM SUPPLEMENTS and POTASSIUM-SPARING DIURETICS may increase risk of hyperkalemia. **Food–drug:** food greatly reduces absorption of moexipril.

NURSING IMPLICATIONS

Administration

- Take 1 h before or 2 h after meals. Food greatly reduces absorption of moexipril.
- Starting dose reduced 50% in patients with possible volume depletion or a history of renal insufficiency.
- Store at 15–30C (59–86F).

Assessment & Drug Effects

- Systematic hypotension may occur within 1–3 h of first dose, especially in those with high blood pressure, on a diuretic or restricted salt intake, or otherwise volume depleted.
- Monitor blood pressure and heart rate frequently during initiation of therapy, whenever a diuretic is added, and periodically throughout therapy.
- Determine trough blood pressure (just before next dose) before dose adjustments are made.
- Periodically monitor serum electrolytes, WBC with differential, Hct

and Hgb, UA, and renal and liver function tests throughout therapy.
- Closely supervise therapeutic response in patients with CHF.

Patient & Family Education
- Instruct to report immediately swelling around face or neck or in extremities.
- Advise to report signs and symptoms of hypotension (e.g., dizziness, weakness, syncope); nonproductive cough; skin rash; flulike symptoms; jaundice; irregular heartbeat or chest pains; and dehydration from vomiting, diarrhea, or diaphoresis.
- Advise to consult physician before using potassium-containing salt substitutes.

MOLINDONE HYDROCHLORIDE

(moe-lin′done)

Trade name: Moban

Classifications: CNS AGENT; PSYCHOTHERAPEUTIC; PHENOTHIAZINE ANTIPSYCHOTIC

Prototype: Chlorpromazine

Pregnancy category: C

ACTIONS/PHARMACODYNAMICS Tranquilizer structurally unrelated but pharmacologically similar to the piperazine phenothiazines. Has less sedative but comparable anticholinergic activity and greater incidence of extrapyramidal side effects than chlorpromazine. EEG studies suggest that ascending reticular system is chief site of action. Reportedly lowers convulsive threshold and produces tranquilization without compromising alertness.

USE Management of manifestations of psychotic disorders.

ROUTE & DOSAGE

Psychotic Disorders

Adult: **PO** 50–75 mg/d in 3–4 divided doses; may be increased to 100 mg/d in 3–4 d; may be able to decrease to 15–60 mg/d in divided doses (max 225 mg/d).

PHARMACOKINETICS **Absorption:** readily absorbed from GI tract. **Peak:** 1 h. **Duration:** 24–36 h. **Distribution:** distributed into breast milk. **Metabolism:** metabolized in liver. **Elimination:** half-life: 1.5 h; excreted in urine and feces.

CONTRAINDICATIONS & PRECAUTIONS **Contraindicated in:** known hypersensitivity to molindone or to phenothiazines; severe CNS depression; comatose states; children < 12 y. Safe use during pregnancy (category C) and by nursing mothers has not been established. **Cautious use in:** persons who may be harmed by increase in physical activity; prostatic hypertrophy; cardiovascular disease; previously detected cancer of breast.

ADVERSE/SIDE EFFECTS *Transient drowsiness,* insomnia, *extrapyramidal symptoms* (dose related), dry mouth, tinnitus, blurred vision, nasal congestion, xerostomia, constipation, urinary retention, euphoria, mild photosensitivity, tachycardia, change in weight, SLE-like syndrome, heavy menses, amenorrhea, galactorrhea, gynecomastia, increased libido, premature ejaculation, <u>hepatotoxicity, neuroleptic malignant syndrome</u>.

NURSING IMPLICATIONS

Administration
- Be certain patient swallows the medication.
- Store medication in tightly capped,

light-resistant bottles. Protect from heat and moisture.

Assessment & Drug Effects

- Withhold dose and consult with physician if the following symptoms occur: tremor, involuntary twitching, exaggerated restlessness, changes in vision, light-colored stools, sore throat, fever, rash.
- Monitor bowel pattern and urinary output. The depressed patient may not report constipation or urinary retention, both side effects of this medicine.
- Since this drug increases motor activity, supervise ambulation and other ADL in the elderly or debilitated or patient with impaired vision to prevent injury or falling.
- In early treatment, be alert to onset of parkinsonism (extrapyramidal) symptoms: rigidity, immobility, reduction of voluntary movements, tremors, fine vermicular tongue movements. Withhold dose and report promptly to physician.

Patient & Family Education

- Counsel to take drug as prescribed: the patient should not alter the dose regimen or stop the medication without consulting his or her physician.
- Dizziness during early therapy usually disappears as treatment continues.
- Caution not to drive or engage in other activities requiring mental or physical coordination until response to the drug is known.
- Warn to avoid alcohol and self-medication with other depressants during therapy. Patient should receive the physician's approval before using any OTC drug.
- Xerostomia (dry mouth) may be relieved by frequent rinses with warm water and by increasing noncaloric fluid intake. Avoid use of commercial mouth rinses, which can change oral flora leading to *Candida* infection and tissue erosion.
- Caution patient with angina to avoid overexertion and to report increase in frequency of precordial pain.
- Recommend that the patient on long-term treatment have periodic ophthalmic examinations.
- Resumption of menses in previously amenorrheic patients has been reported.

MOMETASONE FUROATE

(mo-met'a-sone)

Trade name: Elocon

Classifications: SKIN AND MUCOUS MEMBRANE AGENT; ANTIINFLAMMATORY; SYNTHETIC HORMONE; STEROID

Prototype: Hydrocortisone

Pregnancy category: C

See Appendix A.

MONOOCTANOIN

(mon-oh-ock'ta-noyn)

Trade name: Moctanin

Classification: CHOLELITHOLYTIC

Pregnancy category: C

ACTIONS/PHARMACODYNAMICS

Cholesterol-solubilizing agent that shrinks, softens, and dissolves cholesterol gallstones, depending on size and number. An effective alternative to removal of gallstones in some patients, superior to other solvent-type medications (e.g., chenodiol). Clinical efficacy related mainly to amount of cholesterol in the stones. Complete dissolution is more likely when there is but one stone than when multiple stones are present.

USE To dissolve cholesterol (radiolucent) gallstones retained in the biliary tract after cholecystectomy when other means are not viable or are unsuccessful.

ROUTE & DOSAGE

Radiolucent Gallstones
Adult: **Biliary Instillation** 3–5 ml/h at pressure of 10 cm H_2O for 2–10 d (avg 5 d).

PHARMACOKINETICS Metabolism: metabolized by pancreatic lipase and other digestive enzymes to fatty acids and glycerol, which are readily absorbed by the portal vein.

CONTRAINDICATIONS & PRECAUTIONS Contraindicated in: noncholesterol gallstones; impaired hepatic function; obstructive jaundice; pancreatitis; history of intolerance of vegetable oils; recent duodenal ulcer, or jejunitis, infection. Safe use during pregnancy (category C) or by children not established. **Cautious use in:** nursing mothers, bile duct obstruction.

ADVERSE/SIDE EFFECTS CNS: drowsiness, depression. **GI:** *abdominal pain*, epigastric burning, anorexia, *nausea*, *vomiting*, *diarrhea*, reversible irritability of duodenal mucosa, pancreatitis (rare). **Hematologic:** bleeding from duodenal ulcer, hypokalemia, increase in serum amylase. **Other:** shortness of breath, pruritus, fatigue, diaphoresis, fever, facial flushing.

NURSING IMPLICATIONS

Administration

- Monooctanoin is administered by continuous perfusion through a percutaneous transhepatic catheter directly inserted into the common bile duct.
- Infusion is usually administered with a positive pressure or peristaltic perfusion pump equipped with an overflow manometer. Monitor pressure to prevent exceeding 15 cm H_2O.
- Monitor flow rate carefully and adjust if necessary. If rate is too fast, incidence of GI side effects are apt to increase. Be alert to persistent nausea and diarrhea.
- Perfusion temperature is brought to room temperature 21–27C (70–80F) before the perfusion is started.
- Perfusion of monooctanoin may be interrupted for 1–2 h at mealtimes to reduce GI side effects.
- Store at room temperature.

Assessment & Drug Effects

- Discomfort from side effects may be relieved by temporary interruption of the treatment. Abdominal pain does not appear to be dose- or perfusion-rate dependent. If side effects persist, drug may have to be discontinued.
- Monitor vital signs. An elevated temperature with chills combined with severe right upper quadrant abdominal pain and jaundice suggest onset of ascending cholangitis. Report to physician.
- Correlate lab studies of WBC with patient's complaint of sore throat accompanied by fever and chills; leukopenia should be ruled out.

MONTELUKAST

(mon-te-lu′cast)

Trade name: Singulair

Classifications: BRONCHODILATOR (RESPIRATORY SMOOTH MUSCLE RELAXANT); RESPIRATORY STIMULANT; LEUKOTRIENE RECEPTOR ANTAGONIST

Prototype: Zafirlukast

Pregnancy category: B

M

ACTIONS/PHARMACODYNAMICS Selective leukotriene receptor antagonist of leukotriene D_4, thus inhibiting bronchoconstriction. Leukotrienes are considered more important than prostaglandins as inflammatory agents; they induce bronchoconstriction and mucus production. Elevated sputum and blood levels of leukotrienes have been documented during acute asthma attacks.

USES Prophylaxis and chronic treatment of asthma.

ROUTE & DOSAGE

Asthma
Adult: **PO** 10 mg q.d. in evening.
Child 6–14 y: **PO** 5-mg chewable tablet q.d. in evening.

M

PHARMACOKINETICS Absorption: rapidly absorbed from GI tract, bioavailability 64%. **Peak:** 3–4 h for oral tablet, 2–2.5 h for chewable tablet. **Distribution:** >99% protein bound. **Metabolism:** extensively metabolized by cytochromes P450 3A4 and 2C9. **Elimination:** half-life: 2.7–5.5 h; excreted in feces.

CONTRAINDICATIONS & PRECAUTIONS Contraindicated in: hypersensitivity to montelukast; severe asthma attacks; bronchoconstriction due to asthma or NSAIDs; status asthmaticus. **Cautious use in:** hypersensitivity to other leukotriene receptor antagonists (e.g., zafirlukast, zileuton); severe liver disease; severe asthma; pregnancy (category B); children <6 y of age.

ADVERSE/SIDE EFFECTS Body as whole: asthenia, fever, trauma. **CNS:** dizziness, *headache*. **GI:** abdominal pain, dyspepsia, gastroenteritis, dental pain, abnormal liver function tests (ALT, AST), diarrhea, nausea. **Respiratory:** nasal congestion, cough, influenza, laryngitis, pharyngitis, sinusitis. **Skin:** rash **Other:** pyuria.

NURSING IMPLICATIONS

Administration
- Montelukast should be given in the evening for maximum effectiveness.
- Chewable tablets for children should not be swallowed whole.
- Store at 15–30C (59–86F) in a tightly closed container and protect from light.

Assessment & Drug Effects
- Therapeutic effectiveness is indicated by improved pulmonary functions and better-controlled asthma symptoms.
- Carefully monitor effectiveness of montelukast when used in combination with phenobarbital or other potent cytochrome P450 enzyme inducers.

Patient & Family Education
- Montelukast should not be used for reversal of an acute asthmatic attack.
- Inform physician if short-acting inhaled bronchodilators are needed more often than usual while on montelukast.
- Chewable tablets contain phenylalanine and should be used with caution by phenylketonurics.

MORICIZINE

(mor-i′ci-zeen)

Trade name: Ethmozine

Classifications: CARDIOVASCULAR AGENT; ANTIARRHYTHMIC AGENT

Prototype: Procainamide

Pregnancy category: B

ACTIONS/PHARMACODYNAMICS Class I antiarrhythmic agent with po-

tent local anesthetic effect and myocardial membrane stabilizing effects. Shortens phase II and phase III repolarization, resulting in a decreased action potential duration and effective refractory period. Decrease in the maximum rate of phase 0 depolarization (V_{max}) occurs. Sinus node and atrial tissue are not affected. Prolongs atrioventricular conduction in patients with ventricular tachycardia. In patients with impaired left ventricular functioning, has minimal effects on cardiac index, pulmonary wedge pressure, and ejection fraction, either at rest or during exercise.

USES Treatment of ventricular tachycardia and ventricular premature depolarizations. **Unlabeled use:** supraventricular arrthythmias.

ROUTE & DOSAGE

Ventricular and Supraventricular Arrhythmias

Adult: **PO** 200–300 mg q8h. Should start with 600 mg/d or less in patients with liver or renal disease.

PHARMACOKINETICS Absorption: readily absorbed from GI tract. 30–40% reaches systemic circulation due to extensive first-pass metabolism. **Onset:** 2 h. **Peak:** 10–14 h. **Duration:** 10 h. **Distribution:** 92–95% bound to plasma proteins. Distributed into breast milk. **Metabolism:** extensively metabolized in the liver. **Elimination:** half-life: elimination 10 h; 39% excreted in urine over 2 d, 56% excreted in feces over 4–5 d.

CONTRAINDICATIONS & PRECAUTIONS Contraindicated in: preexisting second- and third-degree AV block, right bundle branch block unless a pacemaker is used; cardiogenic shock, nursing mothers; hypersensitivity to moricizine. **Cautious use in:** non-life-threatening arrhythmia, hypokalemia, hyperkalemia, hypomagnesia, sick sinus syndrome, hepatic impairment, renal impairment, pregnancy (category B). Safety and efficacy in children < 18 y have not been established.

ADVERSE/SIDE EFFECTS CV: arrhythmias, including PVCs and ventricular tachycardia. **CNS:** *dizziness, light-headedness, anxiety, headache, euphoria, perioral numbness.* **GI:** nausea, diarrhea, dry mouth, abdominal discomfort. **Other:** hyperthermia (rare).

DRUG INTERACTIONS May decrease **theophylline** concentrations. May increase the hypoprothrombinemic effects of **warfarin.**

M

NURSING IMPLICATIONS

Administration

- When transferring to moricizine from another antiarrhythmic, it is recommended to withdraw previous drug for 1–2 half-lives before starting moricizine.
- Moricizine therapy is normally initiated.
- Dose increments are generally limited to 150 mg/d at 3-d intervals.
- Store at 15–30C/59–86F unless otherwise directed by manufacturer.

Assessment & Drug Effects

- Electrolyte imbalances, especially hypo/hyperkalemia and hypomagnesemia, should be corrected prior to beginning moricizine.
- Closely monitor cardiac status at beginning and throughout therapy, because moricizine may cause serious new arrhythmias or worsening of preexisting arrhythmias.
- Closely monitor patients with he-

patic or renal dysfunction for adverse effects.

- Carefully monitor patients with sick sinus syndrome or conduction abnormalities. Moricizine may interfere with sinus activity or cause AV block, both of which may necessitate prompt discontinuation of the moricizine.
- Because dizziness occurs in up to 15% of those taking moricizine, initiate precautions where appropriate.

Patient & Family Education

- Advise of seriousness of taking moricizine exactly as prescribed.
- Inform of importance of regular follow-up while on moricizine.
- Instruct to immediately report palpitations, irregular heartbeat, chest pains, or fever.
- Advise to take moricizine consistently with respect to meals.

M

MORPHINE SULFATE

(mor'feen)

Trade names: Astramorph PF, Duramorph, Epimorph ♣, Kadian, MSIR, MS Contin, Oramorph SR, Roxanol, RMS, Statex ♣,

Prototype for classifications: CNS AGENT; ANALGESIC; NARCOTIC (OPIATE) AGONIST

Pregnancy category: B; D in long-term use or high dose

Controlled substance: Schedule II

ACTIONS/PHARMACODYNAMICS A natural opium alkaloid with agonist activity through binding with the same receptors as endogenous opioid peptides. Narcotic agonist effects are identified with 3 types of receptors: analgesia at supraspinal level, euphoria, respiratory depression and physical dependence; analgesia at spinal level, sedation and miosis; and dysphoric, hallucinogenic and cardiac stimulant effects.

USES Symptomatic relief of severe acute and chronic pain after nonnarcotic analgesics have failed and as preanesthetic medication; also used to relieve dyspnea of acute left ventricular failure and pulmonary edema and pain of MI.

ROUTE & DOSAGE

Pain Relief

Adult: **PO** 10–30 mg q4h prn *or* 15–30 mg extended release q8–12h; (Kadian: dose q12–24h); increase dose prn for pain relief. **IV** 2.5–15 mg q4h *or* 0.8–10 mg/h by continuous infusion; dose may be increased prn to control pain *or* 5–10 mg given epidurally q24h. **IM/SC** 5–20 mg q4h. **PR** 10–20 mg q4h prn.

Child: **IV** 0.05–0.1 mg/kg q4h *or* 0.025–2.6 mg/kg/h by continuous infusion. **IM/SC** 0.1–0.2 mg/kg q4h (no more than 15 mg/dose). **PO** 0.2–0.5 mg/kg q4–6h. **Sustained release:** 0.3–0.6 mg/kg q12h.

Neonate: **IV/IM/SC** 0.05 mg/kg q4–8h (max 0.1 mg/kg) or 0.01–0.02 mg/kg/h.

PHARMACOKINETICS Absorption: variably absorbed from GI tract. **Peak:** 60 min PO; 20–60 min PR; 50–90 min SC; 30–60 min IM; 20 min IV. **Duration:** up to 7 h. **Distribution:** crosses blood–brain barrier and placenta; distributed in breast milk. **Metabolism:** metabolized primarily in liver. **Elimination:** 90% of drug and metabolites excreted in urine in 24 h; 7–10% excreted in bile.

CONTRAINDICATIONS & PRECAUTIONS **Contraindicated in:** hypersensitivity to opiates; increased intracranial pressure, convulsive disorders; acute alcoholism; acute bronchial asthma, chronic pulmonary diseases, severe respiratory depression; chemical-irritant-induced pulmonary edema; prostatic hypertrophy; diarrhea caused by poisoning until the toxic material has been eliminated; undiagnosed acute abdominal conditions; following biliary tract surgery and surgical anastomosis; pancreatitis; acute ulcerative colitis; severe liver or renal insufficiency; Addison's disease, hypothyroidism; during labor for delivery of a premature infant, in premature infants. Safe use during pregnancy (category B; D in long-term use or when high dose used) not established. **Cautious use in:** toxic psychosis; cardiac arrhythmias, cardiovascular disease; emphysema; kyphoscoliosis; cor pulmonale; severe obesity; reduced blood volume; very old, very young, or debilitated patients; labor.

ADVERSE/SIDE EFFECTS **Allergic:** *pruritus*, rash, urticaria, edema, hemorrhagic urticaria (rare), anaphylactoid reaction (rare). **CNS:** respiratory depression, euphoria, insomnia, disorientation, visual disturbances, dysphoria, paradoxic CNS stimulation (restlessness, tremor, delirium, insomnia), convulsions (infants and children); decreased cough reflex, drowsiness, dizziness, miosis. **CV:** bradycardia, palpitations, syncope; flushing of face, neck, and upper thorax; orthostatic hypotension. **GI:** *constipation*, anorexia, dry mouth, biliary colic, *nausea*, vomiting, elevated transaminase levels. **GU:** urinary retention or urgency, dysuria, oliguria, reduced libido or potency (prolonged use). **Other:** sweating, prolonged labor and respiratory depression of newborn, precipitation of porphyria. **Overdosage:** severe respiratory depression (as low as 2–4/min) or arrest; pulmonary edema, deep sleep, coma; skeletal muscle flaccidity; cold, clammy skin; hypotension, bradycardia, cardiac arrest, marked miosis, hypothermia.

DIAGNOSTIC TEST INTERFERENCE False-positive ***urine glucose*** determinations may occur using Benedict's solution. ***Plasma amylase*** and ***lipase*** determinations may be falsely positive for 24 h after use of morphine; transaminase levels may be elevated.

DRUG INTERACTIONS CNS DEPRESSANTS, SEDATIVES, BARBITURATES, **alcohol**, BENZODIAZEPINES, and TRICYCLIC ANTIDEPRESSANTS potentiate CNS depressant effects. Use MAO INHIBITORS cautiously; they may precipitate hypertensive crisis. PHENOTHIAZINES may antagonize analgesia.

INCOMPATIBILITIES **Solution/additive: aminophylline, amobarbital, chlorothiazide, heparin, meperidine, methicillin, phenobarbital, phenytoin, sodium bicarbonate, thiopental, pentobarbital. Y-site: minocycline, tetracycline.**

NURSING IMPLICATIONS

Administration

- When narcotic analgesic therapy is started, a fixed, individualized schedule provides effective management because blood levels can be maintained and peaks of pain can be prevented; usually a 4-h interval is adequate.
- Dosage for elderly or debilitated patients is lower than for adult.
- The extended release tablet should not be broken in half, crushed, or chewed. Patient scheduled for pain

M

relief surgical procedure should not receive extended-release tablet within 24 h of surgery.

- Oral solution: Dilute in approximately 30 ml or more of fluid or semisolid food. A calibrated dropper comes with the bottle. Read labels carefully when using liquid preparation; available solutions: 20 mg/ml; 100 mg/ml.
- IV administration: Morphine may be given by direct IV, diluted in 5 ml of sterile water for injection, over 4–5 min.
- IV administration to neonates, infants, children: Verify correct IV concentration and rate of infusion/injection with physician.
- Store at 15–30C (59–86F). Avoid freezing. Suppositories should be refrigerated. Protect all formulations from light.

Assessment & Drug Effects

- Before administering the drug, note respiratory rate, depth, and rhythm and size of pupils. Respirations of 12/min or below and miosis are signs of toxicity. Withhold drug and report to physician.
- Observe patient closely to be certain pain relief is achieved. Record relief of pain (preferably in patient's own words) and duration of analgesia for reference when dosage modification is being considered.
- Elevated pulse or respiratory rate, restlessness, anorexia, or drawn facial expression may indicate need for analgesia.
- Differentiate among restlessness as a sign of pain and the need for medication, restlessness associated with hypoxia, and restlessness caused by morphine-induced CNS stimulation (a paradoxic reaction that is particularly common in women and elderly patients).
- Respiratory depression can be severe for as long as 24 h after epidural or intrathecal administration.
- Patients in particular jeopardy for severe respiratory depression after epidural or intrathecal injection: the elderly or debilitated or those who have decreased respiratory reserve (e.g., emphysema, severe obesity, kyphoscoliosis).
- Patient monitoring for respiratory depression should be continued for at least 24 h after each epidural or intrathecal dose.
- Monitor vital signs at regular intervals. Morphine-induced respiratory depression may occur even with small doses, and it increases progressively with higher doses (generally reaching maximum within 90 min following SC, 30 min after IM, and 7 min after IV administration).
- Narcotic analgesics also depress cough and sigh reflexes and thus may induce atelectasis, especially in postoperative patients. Purposefully encourage changes in position, deep breathing, and coughing (unless contraindicated) at regularly scheduled intervals.
- Nausea and orthostatic hypotension (with light-headedness and dizziness) most often occur in ambulatory patients or when a supine patient assumes the head-up position or in patients not experiencing severe pain.
- Closely observe the patient with increased intracranial pressure or with head injury. Morphine effects may obscure neurologic signs of further increase in intracranial pressure.
- Monitor I&O ratio and pattern. Report oliguria or urinary retention. Morphine may dull perception of bladder stimuli; therefore, encourage the patient to void at least q4h. Palpate lower abdomen to detect bladder distention.

Patient & Family Education

- Advise to avoid alcohol and other CNS depressants while receiving morphine. Advise against use of any OTC drug unless it has been approved by the physician.
- Caution not to smoke or ambulate without assistance after receiving the drug. Bed side rails are advisable.
- Since morphine may cause drowsiness, dizziness, or blurred vision, caution to avoid tasks requiring alertness (e.g., driving a car) until drug response is known.

MOXALACTAM DISODIUM

(mox′a-lak-tam)

Trade name: Moxam

Classifications: ANTIINFECTIVE; BETA-LACTAM ANTIBIOTIC; THIRD-GENERATION CEPHALOSPORIN

Prototype: Cefotaxime sodium

Pregnancy category: C

ACTIONS/PHARMACODYNAMICS Synthetic, broad-spectrum beta-lactam antibiotic with prolonged action; usually classified as third-generation cephalosporin. In general, spectrum of activity resembles that of other third-generation members, particularly cefotaxime. Like cefotaxime, is less active than first and second generation cephalosporins against gram-positive cocci (e.g., *Staphylococcus aureus,* group A and B streptococci, *Streptococcus pneumoniae*). Active against most gram-negative aerobes especially *Escherichia coli, Klebsiella pneumoniae,* and *Serratia marcescens.* Activity against *Pseudomonas aeruginosa* is variable, and it is usually not active against *Acinetobacter.* More highly resistant to inactivation by beta-lactamases than cefotaxime and other cephalosporins.

USES Serious infections of lower respiratory and urinary tracts, skin and skin structure, bone and joint, and for intraabdominal infections, septicemia, and meningitis. Used alone or with an aminoglycoside.

ROUTE & DOSAGE

Moderate to Severe Infections

Adult: **IV/IM** 2–6 g/d divided q8–12h up to 4 g q8h.
Child: **IV/IM** 50 mg/kg q6–8h up to 200 mg/kg or 12 g/d.
Neonates: **IV/IM** 50 mg/kg q8–12h up to 200 mg/kg or 12 g/d.

PHARMACOKINETICS Peak: 0.5–2 h after IM; 15–20 min after IV. **Distribution:** crosses blood–brain barrier and placenta. **Elimination:** half-life: 2–3.5 h; 80% excreted unchanged in urine; small amount excreted in bile.

CONTRAINDICATIONS & PRECAUTIONS Contraindicated in: history of hypersensitivity to moxalactam or other cephalosporins. Safe use during pregnancy (category C) and in nursing women not established. **Cautious use in:** history of type I hypersensitivity to penicillins (urticaria, angioedema, anaphylaxis), history of other allergies, particularly to drugs; impaired renal or hepatic function; history of bleeding disorders or GI diseases, particularly colitis.

ADVERSE/SIDE EFFECTS GI: anorexia, diarrhea, nausea, vomiting, <u>pseudomembranous colitis</u>. **Hematologic:** *hypoprothrombinemia,* anemia, mild transient neutropenia, leukopenia, granulocytopenia, thrombocytopenia, thrombocytosis,

M

eosinophilia, elevation of hepatic enzymes. **Hypersensitivity:** skin rash, purpura, fever, urticaria, pruritus, serum sickness–like reactions, dyspnea, angioedema. **Other:** seizures, bleeding problems including pulmonary hemorrhage. Local (site) reactions: mild burning pain (IM site); phlebitis, thrombophlebitis (following IV administration).

DIAGNOSTIC TEST INTERFERENCE Positive ***direct Coombs' test*** may occur (can interfere with hematologic and crossmatching procedures). Unlike other cephalosporins, moxalactam does not interfere with ***urine glucose*** tests.

DRUG INTERACTIONS **Probenecid** decreases renal elimination of moxalactam; produces disulfiram reaction with **alcohol** and ALCOHOL-CONTAINING PREPARATIONS; increases risk of bleeding with **warfarin, heparin, aspirin.**

INCOMPATIBILITIES **Solution/additive:** AMINOGLYCOSIDES. **Y-site:** AMINOGLYCOSIDES, **labetalol, meperidine, perphenazine.**

NURSING IMPLICATIONS

Administration

- IM injections should be made deep into large muscle mass such as the upper outer quadrant of gluteus maximus. Rotate injection sites.
- For IM administration, moxalactam should be diluted with either sterile or bacteriostatic water, sterile or bacteriostatic 0.9% NaCl for injection, or 0.5% or 1.0% lidocaine hydrochloride injection (by prescription).
- For direct IV administration, dilute each 1 g in 10 ml D5W, NS, or other compatible solution; may be given by direct IV slowly over 3–5 min, or through tubing of a free-flowing compatible IV infusion solution.
- Initially diluted solution may be further diluted in 30–50 ml IV solution and given by intermittent infusion.
- Refer to manufacturer's directions for reconstitution, compatible solutions, storage, stability information, and for specific recommendations for IV administration.
- Frozen solutions of moxalactam should be allowed to thaw naturally at room temperature without warming. Do not refreeze.
- Store vials at < 26C (78F) unless otherwise directed. Protect from light.

Assessment & Drug Effects

- Culture and susceptibility tests should be performed prior to and periodically during therapy to monitor drug effectiveness and bacterial resistance. Therapy may be instituted pending test results.
- Before therapy is initiated, a careful inquiry should be made regarding previous hypersensitivity reactions to cephalosporins, penicillins, and history of previous allergies.
- Pseudomembranous colitis, a potentially life-threatening complication, should be considered a possible cause of diarrhea. Discontinuation of drug may be required.
- Monitor I&O ratio and pattern in patients with impaired renal function or who are receiving high dosages or an aminoglycoside antibiotic concomitantly. Renal status (serum creatinine, BUN, creatinine clearance) and bleeding time should be evaluated at regular intervals.
- Baseline and periodic hematologic, renal, and hepatic function tests should be performed for all

patients during prolonged therapy. Patients receiving concomitant therapy with an aminoglycoside antibiotic should also have periodic audiometric tests

- Monitor BT, PT, and PTT in patients receiving > 4 g/d for more than 3 d, in patients with significantly impaired renal function.
- Report signs of bleeding: petechiae, ecchymoses, nosebleeds, bleeding gums, hemoptysis, bleeding from IM or IV sites, cloudy urine (possibly hematuria).
- Platelet dysfunction and prolonged bleeding time are dose-dependent and usually can be avoided by limiting dosage to 4 g/d.
- Observe for and report onset of superinfections (see Appendix G).

Patient & Family Education

- Advise to promptly report any signs of prolonged bleeding time.
- Advise to promptly report onset of loose stools or diarrhea.
- Advise to abstain from alcohol or alcohol-containing beverages during drug therapy with moxalactam and for several days after last dose. Alcohol and moxalactam may cause a disulfiram-type reaction (see Appendix G).

MUPIROCIN

(mu-pi-ro′sin)

Trade names: Bactroban, Bactroban Nasal

Classifications: ANTIINFECTIVE; PSEUDOMONIC ACID ANTIBIOTIC

Pregnancy category: B

ACTIONS/PHARMACODYNAMICS Mupirocin, a topical antibacterial produced by fermentation of *Pseudomonas fluorescens*, inhibits bacterial protein synthesis by binding with the bacterial transfer-RNA. Susceptible bacteria are *Staphylococcus aureus* (including methicillin-resistant and beta-lactamase-producing strains), *Staphylococcus epidermidis, Staphylococcus saprophyticus,* and *Streptococcus pyogenes.*

USES Impetigo due to *Staphylococcus aureus,* beta-hemolytic streptococci, and *Streptococcus pyogenes;* nasal carriage of *S. aureus.* **Unlabeled use:** superficial skin infections.

ROUTE & DOSAGE

Impetigo

Adult: **Topical** Apply to affected area t.i.d.; if no response in 3–5 d, reevaluate; usually continue for 1–2 wk.
Child: **Topical** Same as for adult.

Elimination of Staphylococcal Nasal Carriage

Child: **Intranasal** Apply intranasally b.i.d. to q.i.d. for 5–14 d.

PHARMACOKINETICS **Absorption:** not systemically absorbed.

CONTRAINDICATIONS & PRECAUTIONS **Contraindicated in:** hypersensitivity to any of its components and for ophthalmic use. **Cautious use in:** pregnancy (category B) and nursing mothers, burn patients.

ADVERSE/SIDE EFFECTS Burning, stinging, pain, pruritus, rash, erythema, dry skin, tenderness, swelling. **Intranasal:** local stinging, soreness, dry skin, pruritus.

DRUG INTERACTIONS Incompatible with **salicyclic acid 2%;** do not mix in HYDROPHILIC VEHICLES (e.g., Aquaphor) or COAL TAR SOLUTIONS; **chloramphenicol** may interfere

M

with bactericidal action of mupirocin.

NURSING IMPLICATIONS

Administration

- A thin layer of medication should be applied to affected area.
- The area being treated may be covered with a gauze dressing if desired.

Assessment & Drug Effects

- Prolonged or repeated therapy may result in superinfection by nonsusceptible organisms. Watch for signs and symptoms of superinfection (see Appendix G).
- Patients should show a clinical response within 3–5 d; if they do not, drug use should be reevaluated.
- Discontinue the drug and notify physician if signs of contact dermatitis develop or if exudate production increases.

Patient & Family Education

- Advise mothers to temporarily discontinue nursing while using mupirocin.
- If a sensitivity reaction or chemical irritation should occur (e.g., increased redness, itching, burning), discontinue drug and contact physician.

M

MUROMONAB-CD3

(myoo-roe-moe′nab)

Trade name: Orthoclone OKT3

Classification: IMMUNOSUPPRESSANT

Prototype: Cyclosporine

Pregnancy category: C

ACTIONS/PHARMACODYNAMICS Murine monoclonal antibody (purified $IgG_{2\alpha}$). Specifically targets the T3 (CD3) molecule in the antigenic recognition site of the human T-cell membrane. Following this antigenic challenge, CD3-positive T-cells are rapidly removed from circulation, and T-lymphocyte action leading to renal inflammation and destruction is blocked, thus reversing graft rejection. Lymphomas may follow immunosuppression therapy with muromonab-CD3; incidence is related to intensity and duration of drug-induced immunosuppression.

USE Acute allograft rejection in renal transplant patients. **Unlabeled use:** acute allograft rejection in heart and liver transplant patients.

ROUTE & DOSAGE

Transplant Rejection

Adult: **IV** 5 mg/d administered in <1 min for 10–14 d.
Child: **IV** *<12 y:* 0.1 mg/kg q.d. × 10–14 d; or *≤30 kg:* 2.5 mg q.d.; *>30 kg:* 5 mg q.d.

PHARMACOKINETICS Onset: the number of circulating CD3-positive T-cells decreases within minutes. **Peak:** 2–7 d. **Duration:** 7 d.

CONTRAINDICATIONS & PRECAUTIONS Contraindicated in: intolerance to any product of murine origin, patient with fluid overload; weight gain of more than 3% within week prior to treatment; infection: chickenpox (existing, recent, including recent exposure), herpes zoster. Safe use during pregnancy (category C) and by nursing mothers not established. **Cautious use in:** repeated courses.

ADVERSE/SIDE EFFECTS (Especially during first 2 d of therapy) **GI:** *nausea, vomiting, diarrhea*. **Respiratory:** severe pulmonary edema, *dyspnea, chest pain, wheezing*. **Other:** *fever, chills,* malaise, *tremor,* tachycardia; *increased susceptibility to cytomegalovirus, herpes simplex, Pneumo-*

Common side effect in *italic*, life-threatening effects underlined; generic names in **bold**; drug class in SMALL CAPS

cystis carinii, Legionella, Cryptococcus, Serratia organisms, and gram-negative bacteria.

NURSING IMPLICATIONS

Administration

- Muromonab-CD3 should be administered only by persons experienced with immunosuppressive therapy and management of renal transplant patients and only in area equipped with staff and facilities to deal with cardiac resuscitation.
- IV preparation: Do not shake ampule. Draw sterile solution into syringe through a low protein-binding 0.2- or 0.22-μm filter. Discard filter; attach syringe to an appropriate needle for IV bolus injection.
- Drug is given by IV rapid (bolus) injection; should not be given by IV infusion or in conjunction with other drug solutions.
- IV administration to infants, children: Verify correct rate of IV injection with physician.
- Administration of IV methylprednisolone sodium succinate before and IV hydrocortisone sodium succinate 30 min after muromonab-CD3 is strongly suggested to decrease incidence of first dose reaction.
- Concomitant maintenance immunosuppressive therapy is reduced or discontinued during drug therapy with muromonab-CD3 and resumed about 3 d prior to end of therapy.
- Store at 2–8C (36–46F) unless otherwise stipulated. Avoid freezing.

Assessment & Drug Effects

- If patient has a fever exceeding 37.8C (100F) before treatment, consult physician. Immediate attempts are made to lower temperature to at least 37.8C (100F) with antipyretics before muromonab-CD3 is administered.
- The patient with pretreatment fluid overload is particularly susceptible to acute pulmonary edema (may be fatal). Should it occur, be prepared for prompt intubation, oxygenation, and corticosteroid drug administration.
- Closely monitor patient's response for 48 h for first dose reaction (occurs within 45–60 min after first dose and lasts several hours). It may occur (less severe) after second dose; then usually does not occur with subsequent doses. Symptoms: chills, dyspnea, malaise, high fever.
- Monitor vital signs. If temperature rises above 37.8C (100F), suspect infection (commonly observed in first 45 d of therapy). Take temperature before treatment and several hours after drug administration to detect first signs of infection.

MYCOPHENOLATE MOFETIL

(my-co-phen′o-late mo′fe-till)

Trade name: CellCept

Classification: IMMUNOSUPPRESSANT

Prototype: Cyclosporine

Pregnancy category: C

ACTIONS/PHARMACODYNAMICS Mycophenolate is a prodrug with immunosuppressant properties because it inhibits T- and B-lymphocyte proliferation responses, inhibits antibody formation, and blocks the generation of cytotoxic T cells. Antirejection effects have been attributed to a decreased number of activated lymphocytes in the graft site. Mycophenolate is synergistic with cyclosporine.

USE Prophylaxis of organ rejection in patients receiving allogeneic renal transplants or heart transplants. **Un-**

labeled uses: rejection prophylaxis for liver transplants, treatment of rheumatoid arthritis and psoriasis.

ROUTE & DOSAGE

Prophylaxis for Renal Transplant Rejection

Adult: **PO/IV** Start within 24 h of transplant; 1 g b.i.d. in combination with corticosteroids and cyclosporine.
Child: **PO** 600 mg m^2 b.i.d.

Prophylaxis for Heart Transplant Rejection

Adult: **PO/IV** 1.5 g b.i.d. started within 24 h of transplant.

PHARMACOKINETICS **Absorption:** rapidly absorbed from GI tract; 94% reaches systemic circulation; absorption decreased by food. **Onset:** 4 wk. **Metabolism:** metabolized in liver to active form, mycophenolic acid. **Elimination:** half-life: 11 h; 87% excreted in urine.

CONTRAINDICATIONS & PRECAUTIONS **Contraindicated in:** hypersensitivity to mycophenolate mofetil, lactation, pregnancy (category C). **Cautious use in:** viral or bacterial infections, presence or history of carcinoma, bone marrow suppression, active PUD, severe diarrhea, malabsorption syndromes, renal impairment. Safety and efficacy in children have not been established.

ADVERSE/SIDE EFFECTS **CNS:** *headache, tremor,* insomnia, dizziness, weakness. **CV:** *hypertension.* **Endocrine:** hyperglycemia, hypercholesterolemia, hypophosphatemia, hypokalemia, hyperkalemia, *peripheral edema.* **GI:** *diarrhea, constipation, nausea,* anorexia, vomiting, *abdominal pain, dyspepsia.* **GU:** *UTI, hematuria,* renal tubular necrosis, burning, frequency, vaginal burning or itching, vaginal bleeding, kidney stones. **Hematologic:** *leukopenia, anemia, thrombocytopenia,* hypochromic anemia, leukocytosis. **Respiratory:** *respiratory infection, dyspnea,* increased cough, pharyngitis. **Other:** rash, leg or hand cramps, bone pain, myalgias, *sepsis (bacterial, fungal, viral).*

DRUG INTERACTIONS **Acyclovir, ganciclovir** may increase mycophenolate serum levels. Antacids, **cholestyramine** decrease mycophenolate absorption. **Mycophenolate** may decrease protein binding of **phenytoin** or **theophylline,** causing increased serum levels.

INCOMPATIBILITIES Do not mix or infuse with other medications.

NURSING IMPLICATIONS

Administration

- Administer oral drug on an empty stomach.
- Dosage adjustments are needed with severe chronic renal failure.
- Do not open or crush capsules; avoid contact with powder in capsules, and wash thoroughly with soap and water if contact occurs.
- IV preparation: Reconstitute and dilute with D5W to 6 mg/ml.
- IV administration: Slowly infuse over ≥2 h.
- IV mycophenolate mofetil is begun ≤24 h after transplant and continued for up to 14 d. Patient should be switched to oral drug as soon as possible.
- Store at 15–30C (59–86F).

Assessment & Drug Effects

- Monitor CBC weekly for first month, biweekly for second and third months, then once per month for first year. If neutropenia develops (ANC < $1.3 \times 10^3/\mu l$), withhold dose and notify physician.

- Periodically monitor and report abnormalities for any of the following: renal and hepatic function tests; serum electrolytes, lipase, and amylase; blood glucose; and routine urinalysis.
- Monitor for and report signs and symptoms of GI intolerance (e.g., diarrhea, nausea, vomiting).
- Monitor for and report any signs and symptoms of sepsis or infection.

Patient & Family Education

- Stress importance of absolute compliance with dosing regimen and scheduled laboratory tests.
- Advise to report immediately signs and symptoms of infection, such as UTI or respiratory infection.
- Instruct to report all troubling adverse reactions, such as hematuria and peripheral edema, as soon as possible.
- Advise to avoid taking OTC antacids simultaneously with mycophenolate mofetil. Separate the two drugs by 2 h.

NABILONE

(na'bi-lone)

Trade name: Cesamet

Classifications: GI AGENT; ANTIEMETIC

Pregnancy category: B

Controlled substance: Schedule II

ACTIONS/PHARMACODYNAMICS Synthetic derivative of tetrahydrocannabinol (THC), the principal psychoactive constituent of marijuana. Action mechanism not clear; inhibits vomiting control mechanism in the medulla oblongata, producing potent antiemetic activity; nontherapeutic actions are exactly like those of marijuana *(Cannabis sativa)*. Has mild anxiolytic properties that may increase its efficacy. Produces dose-dependent hypotension and minimal bronchodilatation.

USES Chemotherapy-induced nausea and vomiting in patient who is refractory to conventional antiemetics. Is especially effective in treatment of cisplatin-induced nausea.

ROUTE & DOSAGE

Chemotherapy-induced Nausea

Adult: **PO** 2 mg b.i.d. beginning 1–3 h before initiation of chemotherapy and continuing up to 48 h after chemotherapy.

PHARMACOKINETICS Absorption: readily absorbed from GI tract. **Onset:** 30–60 min. **Peak:** 2 h. **Duration:** 8 h. **Metabolism:** extensively metabolized. **Elimination:** half-life: 2 h; 65% eliminated in bile, 20% in urine.

CONTRAINDICATIONS & PRECAUTIONS Contraindicated in: nausea and vomiting caused by other than chemotherapeutic agents; hypersensitivity to marijuana, sesame oil. Safe use during pregnancy (category B), by nursing mothers, or patients <18 y not established. **Cautious use in:** first exposure especially in elderly or cardiac patient; hypertension; psychiatric illness; hepatic dysfunction; patient receiving other psychoactive drugs.

ADVERSE/SIDE EFFECTS CNS: *dizziness, drowsiness, vertigo,* ataxia; *psychological high,* depression, asthenia, headache, *euphoria,* hallucinations, tremor, syncope, nightmares, confusion, seizures, toxic psychoses. **CV:** orthostatic hypotension, tachycardia. **GI:** *dry mouth* (30%), anorexia.

DRUG INTERACTIONS **Alcohol** and other CNS DEPRESSANTS add to CNS depression.

NURSING IMPLICATIONS

Administration

- Nabilone administration will be tailored and administered according to need.

Assessment & Drug Effects

- Symptoms of toxic psychosis, orthostatic hypotension, ataxia, and visual disturbances may necessitate withdrawal of drug.
- Nausea and vomiting can lead to fluid and electrolyte imbalance. Assess patient on antiemetic therapy for potential clinical problems (e.g., I&O ratio and pattern; vital signs including BP; skin turgor; urine-specific gravity; thirst; condition of oral membranes and tongue surface).

Patient & Family Education

- Encourage patient to sleep during expected periods of vomiting if possible. If patient awakes with nausea, give the prescribed antiemetic and urge patient to rest in bed for 30 min.
- Relaxation techniques, positive imagery, or hypnosis may help to decrease nausea and vomiting. If patient is willing, initiate learning program with a qualified practitioner.
- Advise on interventions to minimize dry mouth.
- Effects of nabilone may persist for 72 or more hours. Alert patient and family member of possible drug-induced mood swings, behavior changes, or other neurologic side effects, which may continue for at least 3 d after last dose of nabilone.
- Caution patient to avoid driving or other potentially hazardous activities that require judgment and skills until response to nabilone is known.

NABUMETONE

(na-bu-me'tone)

Trade name: Relafen

Classifications: CNS AGENT; ANALGESIC, ANTIPYRETIC; NSAID

Prototype: Ibuprofen

Pregnancy category: C

ACTIONS/PHARMACODYNAMICS Blocks prostaglandin synthesis by inhibiting cyclooxygenase, an enzyme that converts arachidonic acid to precursors of prostaglandins.

USES Rheumatoid arthritis and osteoarthritis.

ROUTE & DOSAGE

Rheumatoid & Osteoarthritis

Adult: **PO** 1000 mg/d as a single dose; may increase up to a max of 2000 mg/d in 1–2 divided doses.

PHARMACOKINETICS **Absorption:** readily absorbed from GI tract; approximately 35% is converted to its active metabolite on first pass through the liver. **Onset:** 1–3 wk for antirheumatic action. **Peak:** 3–6 h. **Distribution:** 99% protein bound; distributes into synovial fluid. **Metabolism:** metabolized in liver to its active metabolite, 6-methoxy-2-naphthylacetic acid (6MNA). **Elimination:** half-life: 24 h (6MNA); 80% of dose is excreted in urine as 6MNA; 10% excreted in feces.

CONTRAINDICATIONS & PRECAUTIONS **Contraindicated in:** patients in whom urticaria, severe rhinitis, bronchospasm, angioedema, or nasal polyps are precipitated by aspirin or other NSAIDs; active peptic ulcer; bleeding abnormalities. Safe use during pregnancy (category C), in nursing mothers, or in children <6 mo not established. **Cautious use in:** hypertension, history of GI ulceration, impaired hepatic or renal function, chronic renal failure, cardiac decompensation, patients with SLE.

ADVERSE/SIDE EFFECTS CNS: tinnitus, dizziness, headache, insomnia, vertigo, fatigue, diaphoresis, nervousness, somnolence. **GI:** diarrhea, abdominal pain, nausea, dyspepsia, flatulence, melena, ulcers, constipation, dry mouth, gastritis. **Other:** rash, pruritus.

DRUG INTERACTIONS May attenuate the antihypertensive response to DIURETICS. NSAIDS increase the risk of **methotrexate** toxicity. **Food–drug:** food may increase the peak but not the overall absorption of nabumetone.

NURSING IMPLICATIONS

Administration

- Nabumetone may be administered with food, milk, or antacid (if prescribed) to reduce the possibility of GI upset.
- Store at 15–30C (59–86F).

Assessment & Drug Effects

- Baseline and periodic evaluation of Hgb and Hct levels is advised with prolonged or high-dose therapy.
- Monitor for signs and symptoms of GI bleeding.

Patient & Family Education

- Advise patient to exercise caution with hazardous activities since nabumetone may cause dizziness, drowsiness, and blurred vision.
- Instruct patient to report abdominal pain, nausea, dyspepsia, or black tarry stools.
- Advise patient that alcohol and aspirin will increase the risk of GI ulceration and bleeding.
- Tell patient to notify physician if any of the following occur: persistent headache, skin rash or itching, visual disturbances, weight gain, or edema.

NADOLOL

(nay-doe′lole)

Trade name: Corgard

Classifications: AUTONOMIC NERVOUS SYSTEM AGENT; BETA-ADRENERGIC ANTAGONIST (SYMPATHOLYTIC, BLOCKING AGENT); ANTIHYPERTENSIVE

Prototype: Propranolol

Pregnancy category: C

ACTIONS/PHARMACODYNAMICS Nonselective beta-adrenergic blocking agent pharmacologically and chemically similar to propranolol. Inhibits response to adrenergic stimuli by competitively blocking beta-adrenergic receptors within heart. As a result, reduces heart rate and cardiac output at rest and during exercise, and also decreases conduction velocity through AV node and myocardial automaticity. Suppression of $beta_2$-adrenergic receptors in bronchial and vascular smooth muscle can cause bronchospasm and a Raynaud's-like phenomenon. Decreases standing and supine BPs by an unknown mechanism. Reduces plasma renin activity.

USES Hypertension either alone or in combination with a diuretic. Also long-term prophylactic management of angina pectoris.

ROUTE & DOSAGE

Hypertension, Angina

Adult: **PO** 40 mg once/d; may increase up to 240–320 mg/d in 1–2 divided doses.

N

PHARMACOKINETICS Absorption: 30–40% of PO dose absorbed. **Peak:** 2–4 h. **Duration:** 17–24 h. **Distribution:** widely distributed; crosses placenta; distributed in breast milk. **Metabolism:** no hepatic metabolism. **Elimination:** half-life: 10–24 h; 70% excreted in urine; also excreted in feces.

CONTRAINDICATIONS & PRECAUTIONS Contraindicated in: bronchial asthma, severe COPD, inadequate myocardial function, sinus bradycardia, greater than first-degree conduction block, overt cardiac failure, cardiogenic shock. Safe use during pregnancy (category C), in nursing mothers, and in children <18 y not established. **Cautious use in:** CHF; diabetes mellitus; hyperthyroidism; renal impairment.

N

ADVERSE/SIDE EFFECTS Allergic: rash, pruritus, laryngospasm, respiratory disturbances. **CNS:** *dizziness, fatigue,* sedation, headache, paresthesias, behavioral changes. **CV:** *bradycardia, peripheral vascular insufficiency (Raynaud's type),* palpitation, postural hypotension, conduction or rhythm disturbances, CHF. **Eyes:** blurred vision, dry eyes. **Other:** dry mouth, dry skin, impotence.

DRUG INTERACTIONS NSAIDS may decrease hypotensive effects; may mask symptoms of a hypoglycemic reaction to **insulin,** SULFONYLUREAS; **prazosin, terazosin** may increase severe hypotensive response to first dose.

NURSING IMPLICATIONS

Administration

- If nadolol is to be discontinued, dosage should be reduced over a 1–2-wk period. Abrupt withdrawal can precipitate MI or thyroid storm in susceptible patients.
- Protect drug from light. Store at room temperature.

Assessment & Drug Effects

- Assess heart rate and BP before administration of each dose. Withhold drug and notify physician if apical pulse drops below 60 bpm or systolic BP below 90 mm Hg.
- Monitor weight. Advise patient to report weight gain of 1–1.5 kg (2–3 lb) in a day and any other possible signs of CHF (e.g., cough, fatigue, dyspnea, rapid pulse, edema).
- Therapeutic effectiveness for patients with angina is evaluated by reduction in frequency of anginal attacks and improved exercise tolerance. Improvement should coincide with steady state serum concentration reached within 6–9 d. Keep physician informed of drug effect.
- Patients with diabetes mellitus should be closely monitored. Beta-adrenergic blockade produced by nadolol may prevent important clinical manifestations of hypoglycemia (e.g., tachycardia, BP changes).
- Monitor I&O ratio and creatinine clearance in patients with impaired renal function or with cardiac problems. Dosage intervals will be lengthened with decreases in creatinine clearance.

Patient & Family Education

- Tell usual pulse rate and teach to check it before taking each dose. Instruct to withhold medication and to consult physician if pulse rate drops below 60 or becomes irregular.
- Emphasize importance of compliance and caution patient not to stop medication or alter dosage without consulting physician.
- Caution to avoid driving and other potentially hazardous activities until reaction to drug is known.

NAFARELIN ACETATE

(na-fa′re-lin)
Trade name: Synarel
Classification: GONADOTROPIN-RELEASING HORMONE ANALOG
Prototype: Leuprolide
Pregnancy category: X

ACTIONS/PHARMACODYNAMICS Potent agonist analog of gonadotropin-releasing hormone (GnRH). Inhibits pituitary gonadotropin secretion of LH and FSH. Therefore, tissues and functions that depend on LH and FSH become quiescent.

USES Endometriosis and precocious puberty. **Unlabeled uses:** uterine leiomyomas, benign prostatic hypertrophy.

ROUTE & DOSAGE

Endometriosis

Adult: **Inhalation** 2 inhalations/d (200 μg/inhalation), one in each nostril; begin between days 2 and 4 of menstrual cycle. Patients with persistent regular menstruation after 2 mo of therapy can be increased to 800 μg/d as 2 inhalations (one in each nostril) twice a day. Continue therapy for 6 mo. Retreatment is not advised because of lack of safety data.

Precocious Puberty

Child: **Inhalation** 800–1200 μg/d divided q8h.

PHARMACOKINETICS Absorption: 21% absorbed from nasal mucosa. **Onset:** 4 wk. **Peak:** 12 wk. **Duration:** 30–50 d after discontinuing drug. **Distribution:** 78–84% bound to plasma proteins; crosses placenta. **Metabolism:** hydrolyzed in kidney. **Elimination:** half-life: 2.7 h; 44–55% excreted in urine over 7 d, 19–44% in feces.

CONTRAINDICATIONS & PRECAUTIONS Contraindicated in: pregnancy (category X), nursing mothers; hypersensitivity to GnRH or GnRH agonist analog; undiagnosed abnormal vaginal bleeding. **Cautious use in:** polycystic ovarian disease.

ADVERSE/SIDE EFFECTS CNS: transient headache, inertia, mild depression, moodiness, fatigue. **Endocrine:** *hot flashes, anovulation, amenorrhea, vaginal dryness,* galactorrhea. **GI:** *bloating, abdominal cramps,* weight gain, nausea. **GU:** *impotence, decreased libido,* dyspareunia. **Other:** nasal irritation, decreased bone mineral content (reversible).

DIAGNOSTIC TEST INTERFERENCE Increased ***alkaline phosphatase;*** marked increase in ***estradiol*** in first 2 wk, then decrease to below baseline; decreased ***FSH*** and ***LH*** levels; decreased ***testosterone*** levels.

NURSING IMPLICATIONS

Administration
- If a topical nasal decongestant is needed for rhinitis during nafarelin treatment, decongestant should be withheld until at least 30 min after nafarelin administration.
- Store at 15–30C (59–86F) in light-resistant container.

Assessment & Drug Effects
- Breakthrough bleeding may indicate that patient has missed successive drug doses. Make appropriate inquiries.

Patient & Family Education
- Give patient the information pamphlet provided with nafarelin.
- Inform physician if breakthrough

N

bleeding occurs or menstruation persists.

- Advise use of nonhormonal method of contraception during treatment.
- Caution not to use topical nasal decongestant within 30 min of nafarelin administration.

NAFCILLIN SODIUM

(naf-sill′in)

Trade names: Nafcil, Nallpen, Unipen

Classifications: ANTIINFECTIVE; BETA-LACTAM ANTIBIOTIC; PENICILLIN; ANTISTAPHYLOCOCCAL PENICILLIN

Prototype: Penicillin G potassium

Pregnancy category: B

ACTIONS/PHARMACODYNAMICS Semisynthetic, acid-stable, penicillinase-resistant penicillin. Mechanism of bactericidal action, contraindications, precautions, and adverse reactions as for penicillin G. Effective against both penicillin-sensitive and penicillin-resistant strains of *Staphylococcus aureus*. Also active against pneumococci and group A beta-hemolytic streptococci. Highly active against penicillinase-producing staphylococci but less potent than penicillin G against penicillin-sensitive microorganisms and generally ineffective against methicillin-resistant staphylococci.

USES Primarily, infections caused by penicillinase-producing staphylococci. May also be used to initiate treatment in suspected staphylococcal infections pending culture and sensitivity test results. As with other penicillins, serum concentrations are considerably enhanced by concurrent use of probenecid.

ROUTE & DOSAGE

Staphylococcal Infections

Adult: **IM/IV** 500 mg–2 g q4–6h up to 12 g/d. **PO** 250–1000 mg q4–6h.
Child: **IM/IV** 100–300 mg/kg/d divided q4–6h. **PO** 50–100 mg/kg/d in 4 divided doses.
Neonate: **IM/IV** 50–100 mg/kg/d divided q6–12h.

PHARMACOKINETICS **Absorption:** incompletely and erratically absorbed orally. **Peak:** 30–120 min IM; 15 min IV. **Duration:** 4 h PO; 4–6 h IM. **Distribution:** distributes into CNS with inflamed meninges; crosses placenta; distributed into breast milk. **Metabolism:** enters enterohepatic circulation. **Elimination:** half-life: 1 h; primarily excreted in bile; 10–30% excreted in urine.

CONTRAINDICATIONS & PRECAUTIONS **Contraindicated in:** hypersensitivity to penicillins, cephalosporins, and other allergens; use of oral drug in severe infections, gastric dilatation, cardiospasm, or intestinal hypermotility; IV use in neonates and infants. Safe use during pregnancy (category B) not established. **Cautious use in:** history of or suspected atopy or allergy (eczema, hives, hay fever, asthma).

ADVERSE/SIDE EFFECTS Nausea, vomiting, *diarrhea*. **Allergic:** urticaria, pruritus, rash, eosinophilia, drug fever, anaphylaxis (particularly following parenteral therapy), allergic interstitial nephritis. Pain and tissue irritation and increase in serum transaminase activity (following IM); hypokalemia (with high IV doses); thrombophlebitis following IV; neutropenia (long-term therapy).

DIAGNOSTIC TEST INTERFERENCE Nafcillin in large doses can cause false-positive ***urine protein*** tests using sulfosalicylic acid method.

DRUG INTERACTION May antagonize hypoprothrombinemic effects of **warfarin.**

INCOMPATIBILITIES Solution/additive: aminophylline, ascorbic acid, aztreonam, bleomycin, cytarabine, hydrocortisone, methylprednisolone, promazine. Y-site: droperidol, Innovar, labetalol, nalbuphine, pentazocine, verapamil.

NURSING IMPLICATIONS

Administration

- Oral dose is best taken on an empty stomach (at least 1 h before or 2 h after meals).
- Oral solution should be dated after reconstitution and refrigerated. Discard unused portions after 1 wk.
- For IM injection, reconstitute with sterile water for injection, 0.9% NaCl injection, or bacteriostatic water for injection (with benzyl alcohol or parabens). Follow manufacturer's directions for attaining desired concentration.
- Following reconstitution, IM solutions are stable for 7 d under refrigeration and for 3 d at room temperature. Vial should be labeled and dated.
- IM injection in adults: Inject deeply into gluteal muscle. Make certain solution is clear. Select site carefully. Rotate injection sites.
- IM injection in children: The preferred IM site in children <3 y is the midlateral or anterolateral thigh. Follow agency policy.
- IV injection: Required dose should be diluted with 15–30 ml sterile water for injection or isotonic NaCl for injection and administered over 5–10 min period, either directly or into tubing of running IV infusion.
- Continuous IV infusion: Concentration of drug should be within range of 2–40 mg/ml. Rate and volume of infusion should be adjusted so that desired dose is administered before solution loses its stability.
- IV administration to neonates, infants, children: Verify correct IV concentration and rate of infusion with physician.
- Compatible IV infusion solutions include isotonic NaCl; 5% dextrose in water or in 0.4% NaCl; Ringer's injection; and sodium lactate (30 mg/ml concentration). Discard unused portions 24 h after reconstitution.

Assessment & Drug Effects

- Culture and sensitivity tests should be performed prior to initiation of therapy and periodically thereafter.
- A careful history should be obtained before therapy to determine any prior allergic reactions to penicillins, cephalosporins, and other allergens.
- IV therapy is usually not given for more than 24–48 h because of the possibility of thrombophlebitis (see Appendix G), particularly in the elderly. Inspect IV site for inflammatory reaction. Also check IV site for leakage; in the elderly patient especially, loss of tissue elasticity with aging may promote extravasation around the needle.
- Allergic reactions, principally rash, occur most commonly. Nausea, vomiting, and diarrhea may occur with oral therapy.
- Twice weekly differential WBC counts are advised in patients receiving IV nafcillin therapy for longer than 2 wk. Nafcillin-induced neutropenia (agranulocytosis) oc-

N

curs commonly during third week of therapy. It may be associated with malaise, fever, sore mouth, or throat.

- Periodic assessments of hepatic and renal functions are advised during prolonged therapy.
- Be alert for signs of bacterial or fungal superinfections (see Appendix G) in patient on prolonged therapy.
- Nafcillin sodium contains approximately 3 mEq of sodium per gram. Determine IV sodium intake for patients with sodium restriction.

Patient & Family Education

- Instruct to promptly report signs and symptoms of neutropenia (see Assessment & Drug Effects), superinfection, or hypokalemia (see Appendix G).

NAFTIFINE

(naf′ti-feen)

Trade name: Naftin

Classifications: ANTIINFECTIVE; ANTIBIOTIC; ANTIFUNGAL

Prototype: Fluconazole

Pregnancy category: B

ACTIONS/PHARMACODYNAMICS Naftifine is a synthetic broad-spectrum antifungal agent. It may be fungicidal depending on the organism. Interferes in the synthesis of ergosterol; ergosterol, the principal sterol in the fungus cell membrane, becomes depleted and interferes with membrane function.

USES Treatment of tinea pedis, tinea cruris, and tinea corporis.

ROUTE & DOSAGE

Tinea Infections

Adult: **Topical** Apply cream once daily, or apply gel twice daily; may use up to 4 wk.

PHARMACOKINETICS Absorption: 2.5–6% absorbed through intact skin. **Onset:** 7 d. **Metabolism:** Metabolized in liver. **Elimination:** half-life: 2–3 d; excreted in urine and feces.

CONTRAINDICATIONS & PRECAUTIONS Contraindicated in: hypersensitivity to naftifine. **Cautious use in:** pregnancy (category B), lactation. Safety and efficacy in children not established.

ADVERSE/SIDE EFFECTS Skin: burning or stinging, dryness, erythema, itching, local irritation.

NURSING IMPLICATIONS

Administration

- Gently massage into affected area and surrounding skin. Wash hands before and after application.
- Do not apply occlusive dressing unless specifically directed to do so.
- Store at room temperature, 15–30C (59–86F)

Assessment & Drug Effects

- Assess for irritation or sensitivity to cream; these are indications to discontinue use.
- If no improvement is noted after 4 wk, use of the drug should be reevaluated.

Patient & Family Education

- Instruct in correct application technique.
- Warn to avoid contact with eyes or mucous membranes.

NALBUPHINE HYDROCHLORIDE

(nal′byoo-feen)

Trade name: Nubain

Classifications: CNS AGENT; ANALGESIC; NARCOTIC (OPIATE) AGONIST-ANTAGONIST

Prototype: Pentazocine

Pregnancy category: B

ACTIONS/PHARMACODYNAMICS Synthetic narcotic analgesic with agonist and weak antagonist properties. Analgesic potency is about 3 or 4 times greater than that of pentazocine and approximately equal to that produced by equivalent doses of morphine. On a weight basis, produces respiratory depression about equal to that of morphine; however, in contrast to morphine, doses > 30 mg produce no further respiratory depression. Antagonistic potency is approximately one fourth that of naloxone and about 10 times greater than that of pentazocine.

USES Symptomatic relief of moderate to severe pain. Also preoperative sedation analgesia and as a supplement to surgical anesthesia.

ROUTE & DOSAGE

Moderate to Severe Pain
Adult: **SC/IM/IV** 10–20 mg q3–6h prn (max 160 mg/d).
Child: **SC/IM/IV** 0.1–0.15 mg/kg q3–6h prn.

PHARMACOKINETICS **Onset:** 2–3 min IV; 15 min IM. **Peak:** 30 min IV. **Duration:** 3–6 h. **Distribution:** crosses placenta. **Metabolism:** metabolized in liver. **Elimination:** half-life: 5 h; eliminated in urine.

CONTRAINDICATIONS & PRECAUTIONS **Contraindicated in:** history of hypersensitivity to drug. Safe use during pregnancy (category B) not established. **Cautious use in:** history of emotional instability or drug abuse; head injury, increased intracranial pressure; impaired respirations; impaired renal or hepatic function; MI; biliary tract surgery.

ADVERSE/SIDE EFFECTS *Sedation; sweaty, clammy skin; nausea, vomiting, dizziness,* dry mouth, vertigo. **CNS:** nervousness, depression, restlessness, crying, euphoria, dysphoria, distortion of body image, unusual dreams, confusion, hallucinations; numbness and tingling sensations, headache, miosis. **CV:** hypertension, hypotension, bradycardia, tachycardia, flushing. **GI:** abdominal cramps, bitter taste. **Hypersensitivity:** pruritus, urticaria, burning sensation. **Respiratory:** dyspnea, asthma, <u>respiratory depression</u>. **Other:** speech difficulty, urinary urgency, blurred vision.

DRUG INTERACTIONS **Alcohol** and other CNS DEPRESSANTS add to CNS depression.

INCOMPATIBILITIES **Solution/additive: diazepam, pentobarbital, promethazine, thiethylperazine. Y-site: nafcillin.**

N

NURSING IMPLICATIONS

Administration

- Nalbuphine may be given by direct IV undiluted at a rate of 10 mg over 3–5 min.
- IV administration to infants, children: Verify correct rate of IV injection with physician.
- Protect nalbuphine from light and store at 15–30C (59–86F) unless otherwise directed.

Assessment & Drug Effects

- Assess respiratory rate before drug administration. Withhold drug and notify physician if respiratory rate falls below 12.
- Nalbuphine may produce allergic response in persons with sulfite sensitivity.
- Administer with caution to patients with hepatic or renal impairment.
- Nalbuphine may produce drowsiness. Monitor ambulatory patients.
- Use of drug during labor and de-

livery may cause respiratory depression of newborn.

- Abrupt termination of nalbuphine following prolonged use may result in symptoms similar to narcotic withdrawal: nausea, vomiting, abdominal cramps, lacrimation, nasal congestion, piloerection, fever, restlessness, anxiety.

Patient & Family Education

- Caution to avoid driving and other potentially hazardous activities until reaction to drug is determined.
- Inform that concurrent use of alcohol and other CNS depressants may result in additive effects.

NALIDIXIC ACID

(nal-i-dix′ik)

Trade name: NegGram

Classifications: URINARY TRACT ANTIINFECTIVE; ANTIBIOTIC; QUINOLONE

Prototype: Ciprofloxacin

Pregnancy category: B

N

ACTIONS/PHARMACODYNAMICS Synthetic quinolone with marked bactericidal activity against most gram-negative urinary tract pathogens with the exception of strains of *Pseudomonas*. Also effective against some strains of *Shigella* and *Salmonella*. Gram-positive bacteria are relatively resistant to drug action. Intracellular action (by unknown mechanism) inhibits microbial DNA replication and RNA synthesis.

USES Urinary tract infections caused by susceptible gram-negative organisms including most *Proteus* strains, *Klebsiella, Enterobacter,* and *Escherichia coli*. **Unlabeled uses:** GI tract infections caused by susceptible strains of *Shigella sonnei;* prophylaxis of bacteriuria and in bladder irrigation for low-grade cystitis.

ROUTE & DOSAGE

Urinary Tract Infections

Adult: **PO** ***Acute therapy:*** 1 g q.i.d. ***Chronic therapy:*** 500 mg q.i.d.
Child > 3 mo: **PO** acute therapy: 55 mg/kg/d in 4 divided doses; chronic therapy: 33 mg/kg/d in 4 divided doses.

PHARMACOKINETICS Absorption: readily absorbed from GI tract. **Peak:** urine: 3–4 h. **Distribution:** crosses placenta; distributed into breast milk. **Metabolism:** partially metabolized in liver; some metabolism in kidneys. **Elimination:** half-life: 1.1–2.5 h; excreted in urine.

CONTRAINDICATIONS & PRECAUTIONS Contraindicated in: history of convulsive disorders; first trimester of pregnancy; infants <3 mo of age. **Cautious use in:** prepubertal child; second and third trimesters of pregnancy (category B), renal or hepatic disease; epilepsy; cerebral arteriosclerosis; respiratory insufficiency, patients with G6PD deficiency.

ADVERSE/SIDE EFFECTS CNS: drowsiness, headache, malaise, dizziness, vertigo, syncope, weakness, myalgia, peripheral neuritis, confusion, excitement, mental depression, seizures, insomnia. **GI:** abdominal pain, *nausea, vomiting,* diarrhea. **Hematologic:** eosinophilia, hemolytic anemia (especially in G6PD deficiency). **Hypersensitivity:** photosensitivity, angioedema, pruritus, urticaria, rash, fever, chills, arthralgia, hypersensitivity pneumonitis, <u>anaphylaxis</u> (rare). **Other:** cholestasis, transient increase in AST.

DIAGNOSTIC TEST INTERFERENCE False-positive urine tests for ***glucose*** with cupric sulfate reagent (e.g., Benedict's or Clinitest) but not with glucose oxidase methods (e.g., Clinistix, TesTape). May cause elevation of ***urinary 17-ketosteroids*** (Zimmerman method) and urine ***vanillymandelic acid*** (VMA).

DRUG INTERACTIONS ANTACIDS may decrease absorption of nalidixic acid; may increase hypoprothrombinemic effects of **warfarin.**

NURSING IMPLICATIONS

Administration

- Reportedly, blood concentrations are increased when drug is administered at least 1 h before or 2 h after meals. If patient complains of GI distress, administer with food or milk.
- Store in tight container at 15–30C (59–86F). Avoid freezing.

Assessment & Drug Effects

- Culture and susceptibility tests are advised prior to initiation of treatment and periodically thereafter.
- CNS reactions tend to occur 30 min after initiation of treatment or after second or third dose. Infants, children, and the elderly are especially susceptible. Report immediately the onset of marked irritability, vomiting, bulging of anterior fontanelle, headache, excitement or drowsiness, papilledema, vertigo.
- Blood counts and renal and hepatic function tests are recommended if therapy is continued longer than 2 wk.

Patient & Family Education

- Caution to use drug exactly as prescribed and not to change dosage. Omitted doses, especially in early days of therapy, may promote development of bacterial resistance. Patient should take full amount of medication.
- Encourage to maintain adequate hydration (2000–3000 ml/d if tolerated) during treatment period. If I&O ratio or pattern changes, consult physician.
- Advise parent to observe how prepubertal child walks. If child limps or complains of joint pain, promptly report to physician.
- Caution to avoid exposure to direct sunlight or ultraviolet light while receiving drug. Therapy should be discontinued if photosensitivity occurs (erythema or bullae). Susceptible patients may be photosensitive up to 3 mo after termination of drug.
- Subjective visual disturbances may occur during first few days of therapy. Report to physician. Symptoms usually disappear promptly with reduction of dosage or discontinuation of therapy.

NALMEFENE HYDROCHLORIDE

(nal′me-feen)

Trade name: Revex

Classifications: CENTRAL NERVOUS SYSTEM AGENT; NARCOTIC (OPIATE) ANTAGONIST

Prototype: Naloxone

Pregnancy category: B

ACTIONS/PHARMACODYNAMICS Nalmefene, an opiate antagonist, prevents or reverses the effects of opiates, including respiratory depression, sedation, and hypotension; these effects are dose related. Nalmefene has no opioid agonist activity; it has no pharmacologic activity when given in the absence of an opioid agonist.

USES Complete or partial reversal of opioid drug effects, management of opioid overdose.

ROUTE & DOSAGE

Reversal of Postoperative Opioid Depression

Adult: **IV/IM/SC** Use 100 μg/ml concentration; 0.25 μg/kg followed by 0.25 μg/kg incremental doses q2–5min until desired degree of reversal or 1 μg/kg cumulative dose is reached.

Known/Suspected Opioid Overdose

Adult: **IV/IM/SC** Use 1 mg/ml concentration. For non-opioid-dependent patients: 0.5 mg/70 kg; may repeat with 1 mg/70 kg 2–5 min later. For opioid-dependent patients: 0.1 mg/70 kg; if no evidence of withdrawal in 2 min, continue with 0.5 mg/70 kg; may repeat with 1 mg/70 kg 2–5 min later. Doses > 1.5 mg/70 kg not likely to be more effective.

N

PHARMACOKINETICS Absorption: well absorbed from IM and SC sites. **Onset:** 2–5 min IV; 15 min IM/SC. **Peak:** 5 min IV; 2 h IM/SC. **Duration:** 4–8 h. **Distribution:** approx 45% protein bound; blocks > 80% of brain opioid receptors within 5 min; distributed into breast milk of rats. **Metabolism:** metabolized in liver by glucuronidation. **Elimination:** half-life: 8.5–10.8 h; metabolites excreted primarily in urine, 17% excreted in feces.

CONTRAINDICATIONS & PRECAUTIONS Contraindicated in: hypersensitivity to nalmefene. **Cautious use in:** patients at high cardiovascular risk or who have received potential cardiotoxic drugs; patients with known physical dependence on opioids, renal and/or hepatic impairment, pregnancy (category B), nursing mothers. Safety and efficacy in children have not been established.

ADVERSE/SIDE EFFECTS CNS: dizziness, headache, irritability, tremor, paresthesias, confusion, paranoia, drowsiness, fatigue, vertigo, agitation, nervousness. **CV:** tachycardia, hypotension, hypertension, pulmonary edema, ventricular arrhythmias (especially in patients with preexisting cardiovascular disease). **GI:** *nausea, vomiting,* diarrhea, dry mouth, dyspepsia, elevation of liver function tests. **Other:** blurred vision, fever, chills.

DRUG INTERACTION Potential risk of seizures when combined with **flumazenil.**

NURSING IMPLICATIONS

Administration

- To calculate a dose in milliliters equal to 0.25 μg/kg using the 100-μg/ml concentration, refer to the manufacturer's dosage table or multiply the weight in kilograms by 0.0025.
- To calculate a dose in milliliters equal to 0.5 mg/70 kg using the 1-mg/ml concentration, divide the patient's weight in kilograms by 70; multiply that result by the number of milligrams ordered per 70 kg.
- In patients with renal failure, administer doses by slow IV push over 60 s.
- If IV access is lost, a single 1-mg dose may be given IM or SC. Allow 5–15 min for effect to occur.

Assessment & Drug Effects

- Monitor carefully for reversal of opioid depression within 2–5 min of an IV dose or 5–15 min of an IM/SC dose.
- If following reversal recurrent respiratory depression occurs, the dose should again be titrated to avoid over-reversal.

Common side effect in *italic,* life-threatening effects underlined: generic names in **bold;** drug class in SMALL CAPS

- Monitor cardiovascular status closely, assessing for changes in blood pressure and heart rate and development of arrhythmias.

NALOXONE HYDROCHLORIDE

(nal-ox'one)

Trade name: Narcan

Prototype for classifications: CNS AGENT; NARCOTIC (OPIATE) ANTAGONIST

Pregnancy category: B

ACTIONS/PHARMACODYNAMICS Analog of oxymorphone. A "pure" narcotic antagonist, essentially free of agonistic (morphine-like) properties. Thus, unlike the narcotic antagonist levallorphan, produces no significant analgesia, respiratory depression, psychotomimetic effects, or miosis when administered in the absence of narcotics and possesses more potent narcotic antagonist action.

USES Narcotic overdosage and for complete or partial reversal of narcotic depression including respiratory depression induced by natural and synthetic narcotics and by pentazocine and propoxyphene. Drug of choice when nature of depressant drug is not known and for diagnosis of suspected acute opioid overdosage. **Unlabeled uses:** shock and to reverse alcohol-induced or clonide-induced coma or respiratory depression.

ROUTE & DOSAGE

Opiate Overdose

Adult: **IV** 0.4–2 mg; may be repeated q2–3min up to 10 mg if necessary.
Child: **IV** 0.01 mg/kg; may be repeated q2–3min up to 10 mg if necessary.

Postoperative Opiate Depression

Adult: **IV** 0.1–0.2 mg; may be repeated q2–3min for up to 3 doses if necessary.
Child: **IV** 0.005–0.01 mg/kg; may be repeated q2–3min up to 3 doses if necessary.

Asphyxia Neonatorum

Child: **IV** 0.01 mg/kg into umbilical vein; may be repeated q2–3min up to 3 doses if necessary.

PHARMACOKINETICS **Onset:** 2 min. **Duration:** 45 min. **Distribution:** crosses placenta. **Metabolism:** metabolized in liver. **Elimination:** half-life: 60–90 min; excreted in urine.

CONTRAINDICATIONS & PRECAUTIONS **Contraindicated in:** respiratory depression due to nonopioid drugs. Safe use during pregnancy (other than labor) (category B) and in nursing mothers not established. **Cautious use in:** neonates and children; known or suspected narcotic dependence; cardiac irritability.

ADVERSE/SIDE EFFECTS ***Excessive dosage in narcotic depression:*** reversal of analgesia, increased BP, tremors, hyperventilation, slight drowsiness, elevated partial thromboplastin time. ***Too rapid reversal:*** nausea, vomiting, sweating, tachycardia.

NURSING IMPLICATIONS

Administration

- Naloxone may be given rapidly by direct IV in 0.1–0.2 mg increments at 2–3-min intervals by direct IV in 0.1–0.2-mg increments at 2–3-min intervals until desired narcotic reversal is achieved.

- Compatible admixtures should be used within 24 h.
- Protect drug from excessive light. Store at 15–30C (59–86F).

Assessment & Drug Effects

- Duration of action of some narcotics may exceed that of naloxone; therefore, patient must be closely observed. Keep physician informed; repeat naloxone dose may be necessary.
- Narcotic abstinence symptoms induced by naloxone generally start to diminish 20–40 min after administration and usually disappear within 90 min.
- Monitor respirations and other vital signs.
- Surgical and obstetric patients should be closely monitored for bleeding. Naloxone has been associated with abnormal coagulation test results. Also observe for reversal of analgesia, which may be manifested by nausea, vomiting, sweating, tachycardia.

N

NALTREXONE HYDROCHLORIDE

(nal-trex'one)

Trade names: Trexan, ReVia

Classifications: CNS AGENT; NARCOTIC (OPIATE) ANTAGONIST

Prototype: Naloxone

Pregnancy category: C

ACTIONS/PHARMACODYNAMICS A pure opioid antagonist with prolonged pharmacologic effect; structurally and pharmacologically similar to naloxone. Weakens or completely and reversibly blocks the subjective effects (the "high") of IV opioids and analgesics possessing both agonist and antagonist activity. Mechanism of action not clearly delineated, but it appears that competitive binding at opioid receptor sites reduces euphoria and drug craving without supporting the addiction.

USES Adjunct to the maintenance of an opioid-free state in detoxified addicts who are and desire to remain narcotic free. Management of alcohol dependence as an adjunct to social and psychotherapeutic methods. **Unlabeled use:** obesity.

ROUTE & DOSAGE

Treatment of Opiate Cessation

Adult: **PO** 25 mg followed by another 25 mg in 1 h if no withdrawal response. Maintenance regimen is individualized (up to 800 mg/d).

Alcohol Dependence

Adult: **PO** 50 mg once/d.

PHARMACOKINETICS **Absorption:** rapidly absorbed from GI tract; 20% reaches systemic circulation (first pass effect). **Onset:** 15–30 min. **Peak:** 1 h. **Duration:** 24–72 h. **Metabolism:** metabolized in liver to active metabolite. **Elimination:** half-life: 10–13 h; excreted in urine.

CONTRAINDICATIONS & PRECAUTIONS **Contraindicated in:** patient who is receiving opioid analgesics or is in acute opioid withdrawal; the opioid-dependent patient; acute hepatitis, liver failure. Also contraindicated in any individual who (1) fails naloxone challenge, (2) has a positive urine screen for opioids, or (3) has a history of sensitivity to naltrexone. Safe use during pregnancy (category C), by children <18 y, or by nursing mothers not established.

ADVERSE/SIDE EFFECTS CNS: *difficulty sleeping, anxiety, headache, nervousness,* reduced or increased energy, irritability, dizziness, depression. **GI:** dry mouth, anorexia, *nausea, vomiting,* constipation, *abdominal cramps/pain,* hepatotoxicity. **Musculoskeletal:** *muscle and joint pains.* **Skin:** skin rash. **Other:** chills, increased thirst.

NURSING IMPLICATIONS

Administration

- Treatment is not started until naloxone challenge is negative, patient has been opioid free 7–10 d (as verified by urine analysis for opioids), and patient reports or manifests no withdrawal symptoms.
- Compliance may be improved by establishing a maintenance schedule of dosing q48–72h.

Assessment & Drug Effects

The naloxone challenge test (administered IV or SC) is given before starting the abstinence program with naltrexone:

- A portion of the IV dose is injected, and with the needle left in place the patient is observed for 30 seconds for withdrawal symptoms: stuffiness or runny nose, tearing, yawning, sweating, tremors, vomiting, gooseflesh, feeling of temperature change, bone, joint, and muscle pains, abdominal cramps. If none, remainder of dose is injected and patient is observed for the next 20 min.
- The SC dose is followed by an observation period of 45 min for symptoms of withdrawal.
- Question patient during observation periods to assist in recognition of withdrawal should it occur.
- Interpretation: Evidence of withdrawal symptoms indicates that the patient is a potential risk and should not enter a naltrexone program. If no signs or symptoms appear, drug therapy can begin. In case of doubt that the patient is opioid free, confirmatory rechallenge is done.
- Liver function tests are checked before the treatment is started, at monthly intervals for 6 mo, and then periodically as indicated.

Patient & Family Education

- Transfer from methadone to naltrexone may be desirable and can be done after gradual withdrawal and final discontinuation of methadone.
- Instruct to report promptly onset of signs of hepatic toxicity (see Appendix G). The drug will be discontinued.
- Advise not to self-dose with OTC drugs for treatment of cough, colds, diarrhea, or analgesia. Many available preparations contain small doses of an opioid. Consult physician for safe drugs if they are needed.
- A doctor or dentist who treats a naltrexone user should be informed of the drug use.
- Discuss with the patient the danger of overdosing with an opiate while on naltrexone therapy. Small doses even at frequent intervals will give no desired effects; however, a dose large enough to produce a high is dangerous and may be fatal.
- Advise to wear identification jewelry indicating naltrexone use.

NANDROLONE DECANOATE

(nan′droe-lone)

Trade names: Androlone-D, Deca-Durabolin, Hybolin Decaneate

NANDROLONE PHENPROPIONATE

Trade names: Durabolin, Hybolin Improved, Nandrobolic
Classifications: SYNTHETIC HORMONE; ANABOLIC/ANDROGEN STEROID
Prototype: Testosterone
Pregnancy category: X
Controlled substance: Schedule III

ACTIONS/PHARMACODYNAMICS Synthetic steroid with high ratio of anabolic activity to androgenic activity. Both esters have same actions and uses but differ in action duration: decanoate actions last 3–4 wk; phenpropionate ester continues to exert anabolic effect for 1–3 wk.

USES Control of metastatic breast cancer, management of anemia of renal insufficiency.

ROUTE & DOSAGE

Anemia (Decanoate)
Adult: **IM** 50–200 mg/wk.
Child 2–13 y: **IM** 25–50 mg q3–4wk.

Metastatic Breast Cancer (Phenpropionate)
Adult: **IM** 50–100 mg/wk.

CONTRAINDICATIONS & PRECAUTIONS Contraindicated in: pregnancy (category X); males with prostate or breast cancer, hepatic dysfunction, nephrotic syndrome, hypercalcemia. **Cautious use in:** benign prostatic hypertrophy, history of MI.

ADVERSE/SIDE EFFECTS GI: *nausea, vomiting,* diarrhea, anorexia, abdominal fullness, cholestatic jaundice, hepatic necrosis, hepatocellular neoplasms. **CNS:** excitation, insomnia, chills, toxic confusion. **Endocrine:** *acne, virilization*. **Metabolic:** sodium, chloride, water, potassium, phosphate, and calcium retention, ankle edema, glucose intolerance. **Other:** muscle cramps, increased cholesterol, leukopenia.

DRUG INTERACTIONS May increase hypoprothrombinemic effects of **warfarin;** may decrease **insulin** and SULFONYLUREA requirements; CORTICOSTEROIDS may increase edema.

NURSING IMPLICATIONS

Administration
- Inject drug deep IM, preferably into gluteal muscle in adult; follow agency policy regarding IM site in small child.
- Intermittent therapy is usually recommended (4-mo course of treatment followed by 6–8-wk rest period).

Assessment & Drug Effects
- Baseline and periodic liver function evaluations and electrolyte levels are recommended. Monitor for signs and symptoms of hepatic toxicity (see Appendix G) and electrolyte imbalance, especially hyperkalemia and hypercalcemia (see Appendix G).
- Drug may interfere with glycemic regulation in diabetics.

Patient & Family Education
- Inform women of the potential for virilization (e.g., increased facial and body hair, deepening of voice).

NAPHAZOLINE HYDROCHLORIDE

(naf-az′oh-leen)
Trade names: Ak-Con, Albalon, Allerest, Clear Eyes, Comfort,

Degest-2, Muro's Opcon, Nafazair, Naphcon, Privine, VasoClear, Vasocon
Prototype for classifications: EENT PREPARATION; VASOCONSTRICTOR; DECONGESTANT; AUTONOMIC NERVOUS SYSTEM AGENT; ALPHA-ADRENERGIC AGONIST (SYMPATHOMIMETIC)
Pregnancy category: C

ACTIONS/PHARMACODYNAMICS Direct-acting imidazoline derivative with marked alpha-adrenergic activity. Produces rapid and prolonged vasoconstriction of arterioles, thereby decreasing fluid exudation and mucosal engorgement. Differs from other sympathomimetic amines in that systemic absorption may cause CNS depression rather than stimulation.

USES Topically, as nasal decongestant and ocular vasoconstrictor.

ROUTE & DOSAGE

Congestion
Adult: **Nasal** 2 drops or sprays of 0.05% solution in each nostril q3–6h for no more than 3–5 d. **Ophthalmic** See Appendix A.
Child: **Nasal** 1–2 drops or sprays of 0.025% solution q3–6h for no more than 3–5 d.

PHARMACOKINETICS **Onset:** within 10 min. **Duration:** 2–6 h.

CONTRAINDICATIONS & PRECAUTIONS **Contraindicated in:** Narrow-angle glaucoma; concomitant use with MAO inhibitors or tricyclic antidepressants. Safe use during pregnancy (category C) and in infants not established. **Cautious use in:** hypertension, cardiac irregularities, advanced arteriosclerosis; diabetes; hyperthyroidism; elderly patients.

ADVERSE/SIDE EFFECTS **Nasal use:** transient stinging or burning, dryness of nasal mucosa, hypersensitivity reactions. **Ophthalmic use:** pupillary dilation, increased intraocular pressure, rebound redness of the eye, headache, hypertension, nausea, weakness, sweating. **Overdosage:** drowsiness, hypothermia, bradycardia, <u>shock-like hypotension, coma.</u>

NURSING IMPLICATIONS

Administration

- Instill nasal spray with patient in upright position. If administered in reclining position, a stream rather than a spray may be ejected, with possibility of systemic reaction.
- When nose drops are instilled, the amount of drug swallowed can be minimized by taking care not to direct the flow toward nasopharynx and by positioning patient properly. Position used depends on condition being treated. Consult physician. Parkinson position: patient supine, head over edge of bed and turned to affected side (used for treating nasal passages and frontal and maxillary sinuses). Proetz position: patient supine, with head hanging straight back over edge of bed (used to treat ethmoid and sphenoid sinuses). Both positions can also be accomplished by placing pillow under patient's shoulders.
- Following nasal instillation of spray, rinse dropper or spray top in hot water to prevent contamination of solution.
- Preserve in tight container preferably at 15–30C (59–86F) unless

N

otherwise specified by manufacturer. Protect from freezing.

Assessment & Drug Effects

- Rebound congestion and chemical rhinitis can occur with frequent and continued use.
- Periodically monitor BP for development or worsening of hypertension, especially with ophthalmic route.
- Overdose: Bradycardia and hypotension can result. Report promptly.

Patient & Family Education

- Advise not to exceed prescribed regimen. Explain that systemic effects can result from swallowing excessive medication.
- If nasal congestion is not relieved after 5 d, advise patient to discontinue medication and to contact physician.
- To prevent contamination of eye solution, care should be taken not to touch eyelid or surrounding area with dropper tip.

N

NAPROXEN

(na-prox′en)

Trade names: Apo-Naproxen ♣, EC-Naprosyn, Naprelan, Naprosyn, Naxen ♣, Novonaprox ♣

NAPROXEN SODIUM

Trade names: Aleve, Anaprox, Anaprox DS

Classifications: CNS AGENT; ANALGESIC; ANTIPYRETIC; NSAID

Prototype: Ibuprofen

Pregnancy category: B

ACTIONS/PHARMACODYNAMICS Propionic acid derivative. Nonsteroidal antiinflammatory drug (NSAID) with analgesic and antipyretic properties similar to those of other propionic acid derivatives, e.g., ibuprofen, fenoprofen, ketoprofen. Mechanism of action thought to be related to inhibition of prostaglandin synthesis. In common with other drugs of this group, inhibits platelet aggregation and prolongs bleeding time but does not alter whole blood clotting or prothrombin time or platelet count. Cross-sensitivity with other NSAIDs has been reported.

USES Antiinflammatory and analgesic effects in symptomatic treatment of acute and chronic rheumatoid arthritis, juvenile arthritis (naproxen only), and for treatment of primary dysmenorrhea. Also management of ankylosing spondylitis, osteoarthritis, and gout. **Unlabeled uses:** Paget's disease of bone, Bartter's syndrome.

ROUTE & DOSAGE

275 mg naproxen sodium = 250 mg naproxen

Inflammatory Disease

Adult: **PO** 250–500 mg b.i.d. (max 1000 mg/d naproxen, 1100 mg/d naproxen sodium). Naprelan is dosed q.d.
Child >2 y: **PO** 10–15 mg/kg/d in 2 divided doses (max 1000 mg/d).

Mild to Moderate Pain, Dysmenorrhea

Adult: **PO** 500 mg followed by 200–250 mg q6–8h prn up to 1250 mg/d.
Child >2 y: **PO** 5–7 mg/kg q8–12h.

PHARMACOKINETICS Absorption: almost completely absorbed from GI tract when taken on empty stomach. **Peak:** 2 h naproxen; 1 h naproxen sodium. **Duration:** 7 h. **Metabolism:** metabolized in liver. **Elimination:** half-life: 12–15 h; excreted primarily in urine; some biliary excretion (<1%).

CONTRAINDICATIONS & PRECAUTIONS **Contraindicated in:** active peptic ulcer; patients in whom asthma, rhinitis, urticaria, bronchospasm, or shock is precipitated by aspirin or other NSAIDs. Safe use during pregnancy (category B), in nursing mothers, or in children <2 y not established. **Cautious use in:** history of upper GI tract disorders; impaired renal, hepatic, or cardiac function; patients on sodium restriction (naproxen sodium); low pretreatment Hgb concentration; fluid retention, hypertension, heart failure; geriatric patients.

ADVERSE/SIDE EFFECTS **CNS:** *headache, drowsiness, dizziness,* lightheadedness, depression. **CV:** palpitation, dyspnea, peripheral edema, CHF, tachycardia. **Eye/ear:** blurred vision, tinnitus, hearing loss. **GI:** *anorexia, heartburn,* indigestion, *nausea,* vomiting, GI bleeding. **Hematologic:** thrombocytopenia, leukopenia, eosinophilia, inhibited platelet aggregation, agranulocytosis (rare). **Skin:** pruritus, rash, ecchymosis. **Other:** thirst, nephrotoxicity, pulmonary edema, elevated serum ALT, AST.

DIAGNOSTIC TEST INTERFERENCE Transient elevations in ***BUN*** and serum ***alkaline phosphatase*** may occur. Naproxen may interfere with some urinary assays of ***5-HIAA*** and may cause falsely high ***urinary 17-KGS*** levels (using *m*-dinitrobenzene reagent). Naproxen should be withdrawn 72 h before adrenal function tests.

DRUG INTERACTIONS Bleeding time effects of ORAL ANTICOAGULANTS, **heparin** may be prolonged; may increase **lithium** toxicity.

NURSING IMPLICATIONS

Administration

- Naproxen may be administered with food or an antacid (if prescribed) to reduce incidence of GI upset.
- Note that naproxen sodium should not be used concomitantly with the related drug naproxen since they both circulate in plasma as the naproxen anion.
- Store naproxen at 15–30C (59–86F) in tightly closed container. Avoid freezing.

Assessment & Drug Effects

- Take a detailed drug history prior to initiation of therapy. In those with aspirin or other NSAID sensitivity, observe for signs of allergic response.
- Baseline and periodic evaluations of hemoglobin and renal and hepatic function and auditory and ophthalmic examinations are recommended in patients receiving prolonged or high dose therapy.
- Patients with arthritis may experience symptomatic relief (reduction in joint pain, swelling, stiffness) within 24–48 h with naproxen sodium therapy and in 2–4 wk with naproxen.

Patient & Family Education

- Inform that full therapeutic effect of naproxen may not be experienced for 3–4 wk.
- Since naproxen may cause dizziness and drowsiness, advise to exercise caution when they are driving or performing other potentially hazardous activities.
- Inform that alcohol and aspirin may increase risk of GI ulceration

and bleeding and, therefore, should be avoided unless otherwise advised by physician.

- Since naproxen may prolong bleeding time, caution to inform dentist or surgeon that this drug is being taken.

NARATRIPTAN

(nar-a-trip′tan)

Trade name: Amerge

Classifications: AUTONOMIC NERVOUS SYSTEM AGENT; ALPHA-ADRENERGIC ANTAGONIST (SYMPATHETOLYTIC); SEROTONIN $5HT_1$ AGONIST; ERGOT ALKALOID

Prototype: Sumatriptan

Pregnancy category: C

ACTIONS/PHARMACODYNAMICS Binds to the serotonin receptors ($5HT_{1D}$ and $5HT_{1B}$), causing vasoconstriction of cranial carotid arteries, thus relieving the migraine headache.

USE Acute migraine headaches with or without aura.

ROUTE & DOSAGE

Acute Migraine

Adult: **PO** 1–2.5 mg; may repeat in 4 h if necessary (max 5 mg/24 h); patients with mild or moderate renal or hepatic impairment should not exceed 2.5 mg/24 h.

PHARMACOKINETICS Absorption: rapidly absorbed, 70% bioavailability. **Peak:** 2–4 h. **Distribution:** 28–31% protein bound. **Metabolism:** metabolized in liver. **Elimination:** half-life: 6 h; excreted primarily in urine.

CONTRAINDICATIONS & PRECAUTIONS Contraindicated in: severe renal impairment (creatinine clearance <15 ml/min); severe hepatic impairment; history of ischemic heart disease (i.e., angina pectoris, MI); cerebrovascular syndromes (i.,e., strokes or TIA); uncontrolled hypertension; patients with hemiplegic or basilar migraine; hypersensitivity to naratriptan; elderly. **Cautious use in:** cardiovascular disease; renal or hepatic insufficiency; pregnancy (category C); lactation. Safety and efficacy in children <18 y not established.

ADVERSE/SIDE EFFECTS Body as whole: asthenia, fatigue, malaise, pain, pressure sensation, paresthesias, throat pressure, warm/cold sensations. **CNS:** somnolence, dizziness, drowsiness, headache, hypesthesia, decreased mental acuity, euphoria, tremor. **CV:** coronary artery vasospasm, transient myocardial ischemia, <u>MI</u>, ventricular tachycardia, ventricular fibrillation, chest pain/tightness/heaviness, palpitations. **GI:** dry mouth, nausea, vomiting, diarrhea. **Respiratory:** dyspnea. **Skin:** flushing. **Other:** hot flushes.

DRUG INTERACTIONS Dihydroergotamine, methysergide, and other $5\text{-}HT_1$ AGONISTS may cause prolonged vasospastic reactions; SSRIS have rarely caused weakness, hyperreflexia, and incoordination; MAOIS should not be used with $5\text{-}HT_1$ agonists.

NURSING IMPLICATIONS

Administration

- Administer any time after symptoms of migraine appear. If the first tablet was effective but symptoms return, a second tablet may be given but no sooner than 4 h after the first. Do not exceed 5 mg in 24 h.
- If there is no response to the first tablet, contact physician before administering a second tablet.
- Do not give within 24 h of an

ergot-containing drug or other 5-HT_1 agonist.

- Store at 2–25C (36–77F) and protect from light.

Assessment & Drug Effects

- Therapeutic effectiveness is indicated by relief or reduction of migraine pain.
- Carefully monitor cardiovascular status following first dose in patients at risk for CAD (e.g., postmenopausal women, men over 40 y old, persons with known CAD risk factors) or coronary artery vasospasms.
- ECG is recommended following first administration of naratriptan to someone with known CAD risk factors and periodically with long-term use.
- Immediately report to the physician chest pain, nausea, or tightness in chest or throat that is severe or does not quickly resolve.
- Periodic cardiovascular evaluation is recommended with continued naratriptan use.

Patient & Family Education

- Carefully review patient information leaflet and guidelines for administration.
- Immediately contact physician if any of the following develop following naratriptan use: symptoms of angina (e.g., severe and/or persistent pain or tightness in chest or throat, severe nausea), hypersensitivity (e.g., wheezing, facial swelling, skin rash, or hives), or abdominal pain.
- Report any other adverse effects (e.g., tingling, flushing, dizziness) at next physician visit.

NATAMYCIN

(na-ta-mye'sin)

Trade name: Natacyn

Classifications: ANTIINFECTIVE; ANTIFUNGAL

Prototype: Fluconazole

Pregnancy category: C

ACTIONS/PHARMACODYNAMICS Derived from *Streptomyces natalensis*. Effective against many yeasts and filamentous fungi including *Candida, Aspergillus, Cephalosporium, Fusarium,* and *Penicillium*. Action mechanism simulates that of amphotericin B and nystatin by binding to sterols in the bacterial cell membrane. Has some activity in vivo against *Trichomonas vaginalis;* is not active against gram-positive or gram-negative bacteria or viruses.

USES Topically to treat blepharitis, conjunctivitis, and keratitis caused by susceptible fungi. Drug of choice for *Fusarium solani* keratitis. **Unlabeled uses:** oral, cutaneous, and vaginal candidiasis; intranasal treatment of pulmonary aspergillosis.

ROUTE & DOSAGE

Fungal Keratitis

Adult: **Ophthalmic** 1 drop in conjunctival sac of infected eye q1–2h for 3–4 d; then decrease to 1 drop q6–8h; then gradually decrease to 1 drop q4–7d.

PHARMACOKINETICS **Absorption:** drug adheres to ulcerated surface of the cornea and is retained in conjunctival fornices. Does not appear to be systemically absorbed.

CONTRAINDICATIONS & PRECAUTIONS **Contraindicated in:** concomitant administration of a corticosteroid. **Cautious use in:** pregnancy (category C) and nursing mothers.

Safety and efficacy in children have not been established.

ADVERSE/SIDE EFFECTS Reports scanty. Blurred vision, photophobia, eye pain. Uneven adherence of suspension to epithelial ulcerations or in fornices.

NURSING IMPLICATIONS

Administration

- Thorough handwashing before and after treatment is imperative. Infection is easily transferred from infected to noninfected eye and to other individuals.
- Store ophthalmic suspension at 2–24C (36–75F) unless otherwise directed. Shake well before using.

Assessment & Drug Effects

- Inspect eye for response and tolerance at least twice weekly.
- Lack of improvement in keratitis within 7–10 d suggests that causative organisms may not be susceptible to natamycin. Reevaluation is indicated and possibly a change in therapy.

Patient & Family Education

- Temporary photophobia should be anticipated. Tell patient to be prepared to wear sunglasses outdoors after drug administration and perhaps for a few hours indoors.
- Instruct to return to ophthalmologist for reevaluation of eye problem if he or she experiences symptoms of conjunctivitis: pain, discharge, itching, scratching "foreign body sensation," changes in vision.
- Teach appropriate technique for application of eye drops.
- Facecloths and hand towels should be used only by the patient to prevent transmission of the fungal infection.

N

NEDOCROMIL SODIUM

(ned'o-cro-mil)

Trade name: Tilade

Classifications: ANTIASTHMATIC; ANTIINFLAMMATORY; MAST CELL STABILIZER

Prototype: Cromolyn sodium

Pregnancy category: B

ACTIONS/PHARMACODYNAMICS Inhibits activation of and mediator released from inflammatory cell types associated with asthma (e.g., neutrophils, mast cells, monocytes). Inhibits release of mediators including histamine and prostaglandin D_2. Has no intrinsic bronchodilator, antihistamine, or glucocorticoid activity.

USE Maintenance therapy for patients with mild to moderate asthma.

ROUTE & DOSAGE

Asthma

Adult: **Inhaled** 2 inhalations q.i.d. at regular intervals. Not for acute asthma attacks.
Child ≥ *6 y:* **Inhaled** 2 inhalations q.i.d.

PHARMACOKINETICS **Absorption:** 90% of dose is deposited in throat and swallowed. Less than 7% is absorbed systemically in patients with asthma. **Onset:** 1 wk for therapeutic effect. **Peak:** 10–20 min. **Metabolism:** dose not appear to be metabolized. **Elimination:** half-life: 2.3 h; 6% excreted in urine in 72 h.

CONTRAINDICATIONS & PRECAUTIONS **Contraindicated in:** hypersensitivity to nedocromil, acute bronchospasm, particularly status asthmaticus. **Cautious use in:** pregnancy (category B), nursing mothers.

Safety and effectiveness in children <6 y have not been established.

ADVERSE/SIDE EFFECTS General: *abnormal bitter taste,* sore throat, irritation, cough, headache, nausea, vomiting, dizziness.

NURSING IMPLICATIONS

Administration

- Correct administration technique is essential for maximum drug efficacy. Review instruction leaflet supplied by manufacturer.
- Reductions in dosage should occur in stages, with each lower dose maintained for several weeks of good control prior to further decreasing dose.
- Store 2–30C (36–86F).

Assessment & Drug Effects

- Assess for coughing and bronchospasms induced by nedocromil. These are indications for discontinuation of drug and should be promptly reported.
- Monitor patients for whom systemic or inhaled steroid therapy has been reduced, as nedocromil may not fully substitute for the decrease in dose of steroid.

Patient & Family Education

- Because nedocromil is not a bronchodilator, instruct not to use drug to treat acute bronchospasms.
- Stress need to continue regular nedocromil therapy even during symptom-free periods.
- Instruct on proper method of drug administration. Review patient instruction leaflet with patient.

NEFAZODONE

(nef-a-zo′done)

Trade name: Serzone

Classifications: CNS AGENT; PSYCHOTHERAPEUTIC; SEROTONIN REUPTAKE INHIBITOR; ANTIDEPRESSANT

Prototype: Fluoxetine hydrochloride

Pregnancy category: C

ACTIONS/PHARMACODYNAMICS Nefazodone is an antidepressant with a dual mechanism of action. It inhibits neuronal serotonin (5-HT) reuptake and also possesses 5-HT_2 antagonist properties. It is unrelated to tricyclic, MAO, or other antidepressants. Nefazodone has minimal cardiovascular effects, fewer anticholergenic effects, less sedation, and less sexual dysfunction than other antidepressants.

USE Treatment of depression.

ROUTE & DOSAGE

Depression

Adult: **PO** 50–100 mg b.i.d.; may need to increase up to 300–600 mg/d in 2–3 divided doses; start elderly patients with 50 mg b.i.d.

PHARMACOKINETICS Onset: 1 wk **Peak:** 3–5 wk. **Metabolism:** metabolized in liver to at least two active metabolites. **Elimination:** half-life: nefazodone 3.5 h, metabolites 2–33 h.

CONTRAINDICATIONS & PRECAUTIONS Contraindicated in: hypersensitivity to nefazodone or alcohol. **Cautious use in:** elderly, women, history of seizure disorders, renal and hepatic impairment, pregnancy (category C), nursing mothers. Safety and efficacy in children < 18 y have not been established.

ADVERSE/SIDE EFFECTS CNS: *headache, dizziness, drowsiness,* asthenia, tremor, insomnia, agitation, anxiety. **GI:** dry mouth, constipation, nausea.

DRUG INTERACTIONS May increase plasma levels of some BENZODIAZEPINES, including **alprazolam** and **triazolam**. May decrease plasma levels and effects of **propranolol.** May increase levels and toxicity of **carbamazepine, digoxin.**

NURSING IMPLICATIONS

Administration

- Dosage adjustment may be warranted with elderly patients.
- Store at room temperature, 15–30C (59–86F).

Assessment & Drug Effects

- Monitor patients with a history of seizures for increased activity.
- Assess safety, as dizziness and drowsiness are common adverse effects.
- Periodically monitor HR, BP, hepatic function tests, and CBC during long-term therapy.

Patient & Family Education

- Advise that significant improvement in mood may not occur for several weeks following initiation of therapy.
- Caution about performing hazardous activities until response to the drug is known.
- Advise patient to report changes in visual acuity.

NELFINAVIR MESYLATE

(nel-fin'a-vir)

Trade names: Viracept

Classifications: ANTIINFECTIVE AGENT; ANTIRETROVIRAL AGENT; PROTEASE INHIBITOR

Prototype: Saquinavir

Pregnancy category: C

ACTIONS/PHARMACODYNAMICS Nelfinavir is an inhibitor of HIV-1 protease. Inhibition of the viral protease prevents the cleavage of the viral polypeptide, resulting in the production of an immature, noninfectious virus.

USE Treatment of HIV infection in combination with a nucleoside analog.

ROUTE & DOSAGE

HIV infection

Adult: **PO** 750 mg t.i.d. with food.
Child 2–13 y: **PO** 20–30 mg/kg t.i.d. with food (max 750 mg/dose).

PHARMACOKINETICS Absorption: Food increases the amount of drug absorbed. **Distribution:** > 98% protein bound. **Metabolism:** metabolized in the liver by CYP3A. **Elimination:** half-life: 3.5–5 h; primarily excreted in feces.

CONTRAINDICATIONS & PRECAUTIONS Contraindicated in: hypersensitivity to nelfinavir; concurrent administration with fenadine, astemizole, cisapride, rifampin, triazolam or midazolam, lactation. **Cautious use in:** hepatic function impairment, patients with hemophilia, pregnancy (category C). Safety and effectiveness have not been established in children < 2 y.

ADVERSE/SIDE EFFECTS Body as whole: allergic reactions, back pain, fever, malaise, pain, asthenia, myalgia, arthralgia. **CNS:** headache, anxiety, depression, dizziness, insomnia, seizures. **GI:** abdominal pain, *diarrhea,* nausea, flatulence, anorexia, dyspepsia, <u>GI bleeding</u>, hepatitis, vomiting, pancreatitis, increased LFTs. **Hematologic:** anemia, leukopenia, thrombocytopenia. **Respiratory:** dyspnea, pharyngitis, rhinitis. **Skin:** rash, pruritus, sweating, urticaria.

DRUG INTERACTIONS Other PROTEASE INHIBITORS, ketoconazole may increase nelfinavir levels; **rifabutin, rifampin** may decrease nelfinavir levels; nelfinavir will decrease ORAL CONTRACEPTIVE LEVELS.

NURSING IMPLICATIONS

Administration

- Drug should be taken with a meal or light snack.
- Oral powder may be mixed with a small amount of water, milk, soy milk, or dietary supplements; liquid should be consumed immediately. Do not mix oral powder in original container nor with acid food or juice (e.g., orange or apple juice, or apple sauce).
- Concurrent therapy with terfenadine or rifampin is contraindicated.
- Concurrent doses of rifabutin should be cut in half.
- Store tablets and powder at 15–30C (59–86F).

Assessment & Drug Effects

- Therapeutic effectiveness is indicated by decreased viral load.
- Hemophiliacs (type A or B) should be closely monitored for spontaneous bleeding.
- Carefully monitor patients with liver impairment for toxic drug effects.

Patient & Family Education

- Drug must be taken exactly as prescribed. Do not alter dose or discontinue drug without consulting physician.
- Women using oral contraceptives should use an alternative form of contraception while on nelfinavir.
- Diarrhea is a common adverse effect that can usually be controlled by over-the-counter medications.

NEOMYCIN SULFATE

(nee-oh-mye′sin)

Trade names: Mycifradin, Myciguent

Classifications: ANTIINFECTIVE; AMINOGLYCOSIDE ANTIBIOTIC

Prototype: Gentamicin

Pregnancy category: D

ACTIONS/PHARMACODYNAMICS Aminoglycoside antibiotic obtained from *Streptomyces fradiae;* reported to be the most potent in neuromuscular blocking action and the most toxic of this group. Broad spectrum of antibacterial activity, and actions similar to those of gentamicin.

USES Severe diarrhea caused by enteropathogenic *Escherichia coli;* preoperative intestinal antisepsis; to inhibit nitrogen-forming bacteria of GI tract in patients with cirrhosis or hepatic coma and for urinary tract infections caused by susceptible organisms. Also topically for short-term treatment of eye, ear, and skin infections. Available in a variety of creams, ointments, and sprays in combination with other antibiotics and corticosteroids.

ROUTE & DOSAGE

Intestinal Antisepsis

Adult: **PO** 1 g q1h x 4 doses, then 1 g q4h x 5 doses.
Child: **PO** 10.3 mg/kg q4–6h for 3 d.

Hepatic Coma

Adult: **PO** 4–12 g/d in 4 divided doses for 5–6 d.
Child: **PO** 437.5–1225 mg/m^2 q6h for 5–6 d.

Diarrhea

Adult: **PO** 50 mg/kg in 4 divided doses for 2–3 d; **IM** 1.3–2.6 mg/kg q6h.
Child: **PO** 8.75 mg/kg q6h for 2–3 d.

N

Cutaneous Infections
Adult: **Topical** Apply 1–3 times/d.

PHARMACOKINETICS Absorption: 3% absorbed from GI tract in adults; up to 10% absorbed in neonates. **Peak:** 1–4 h. **Elimination:** half-life: 3 h; 97% excreted unchanged in feces.

CONTRAINDICATIONS & PRECAUTIONS Contraindicated in: use of oral drug in patients with intestinal obstruction; ulcerative bowel lesions; topical applications over large skin areas; parenteral use in patients with renal disease or impaired hearing; parkinsonism; myasthenia gravis, pregnancy (category D), lactation. **Cautious use in:** topical otic applications in patients with perforated eardrum, children.

N

ADVERSE/SIDE EFFECTS Oral use: mild laxative effect, diarrhea, nausea, vomiting; prolonged therapy: malabsorption-like syndrome including cyanocobalamin (vitamin B_{12}) deficiency, low serum cholesterol. **Systemic absorption:** nephrotoxicity, ototoxicity, neuromuscular blockade with muscular and respiratory paralysis, hypersensitivity reactions. **Topical use:** *redness,* scaling, pruritus, dermatitis.

DRUG INTERACTION May decrease absorption of **cyanocobalamin.**

NURSING IMPLICATIONS

Administration

- Neomycin retention enema is sometimes prescribed for patients with hepatic coma. Recommended dilution for adults is 200 ml/L 1% solution or 100 ml 2% solution to be retained for 20 min to more than 1 h, as prescribed.
- Preoperative bowel preparation: Saline laxative is generally given immediately before neomycin therapy is initiated.
- For applications to skin, consult physician about what to use for cleansing the part to be treated before each neomycin application.
- Topical therapy of external ear is most effective if canal is clean and dry prior to instillation of neomycin. Consult physician. Duration of treatment should be limited to 7–10 d.
- Parenteral solutions should be refrigerated (2–15C/35–59F) to minimize possibility of contamination and discoloration and should be used as soon as possible, preferably within 1 wk after reconstitution.

Assessment & Drug Effects

- Patients with renal or hepatic dysfunction receiving IM or extended oral neomycin therapy should have audiometric studies twice weekly, daily urinalysis for albumin, casts, and cells, and BUN every other day. Baseline determinations should be done before initiation of therapy. Serum drug levels also are advised (toxic levels reportedly range from 8 to 30 μg/ml, although individual variations exist).
- Neomycin can cause irreversible damage to auditory branch of eighth cranial nerve. At first, loss of hearing most often involves high-frequency sounds, then may progress to normal hearing frequencies. Severity and persistence of ototoxic symptoms depend on dosage and duration of drug therapy. Early reporting is essential.
- Monitor I&O in patients receiving oral or parenteral therapy. Report oliguria or changes in I&O ratio. Inadequate neomycin excretion results in high serum drug levels and risk of nephrotoxicity and ototoxicity.

Patient & Family Education

- High incidence of allergic dermatitis is associated with topical neomycin. Sensitivity may be manifested as persistent dermatitis. Caution patient to stop treatment and report to physician if irritation occurs.

- Advise to report any unusual symptom related to ears or hearing, e.g., tinnitus, roaring sounds, loss of hearing acuity, dizziness.
- Patients who develop sensitivity should be informed that they will probably continue to be sensitive to neomycin and to other aminoglycoside antibiotics (gentamicin, kanamycin, neomycin, streptomycin).
- Caution not to exceed prescribed dosage or duration of therapy.

NEOSTIGMINE BROMIDE

(nee-oh-stig′meen)

Trade name: Prostigmin

NEOSTIGMINE METHYLSULFATE

Trade name: Prostigmin

Prototype for classifications: AUTONOMIC NERVOUS SYSTEM AGENT; CHOLINERGIC (PARASYMPATHOMIMETIC); CHOLINESTERASE INHIBITOR

Pregnancy category: C

ACTIONS/PHARMACODYNAMICS Produces reversible cholinesterase inhibition or inactivation and thus allows intensified and prolonged effect of acetylcholine at cholinergic synapses (basis for use in myasthenia gravis). Also produces generalized cholinergic response, including miosis, increased tonus of intestinal and skeletal muscles, constriction of bronchi and ureters, slower pulse rate, and stimulation of salivary and sweat glands. Has direct stimulant action on voluntary muscle fibers and possibly on autonomic ganglia and CNS neurons.

USES To prevent and treat postoperative abdominal distension and urinary retention; for symptomatic control of and sometimes for differential diagnosis of myasthenia gravis; and to reverse the effects of nondepolarizing muscle relaxants, e.g., tubocurarine.

ROUTE & DOSAGE

Diagnosis of Myasthenia Gravis

Adult: **IM** 0.022 mg/kg; may increase to 0.031 mg/kg if first test is inconclusive.
Child: **IM** 0.025–0.04 mg/kg.

Treatment of Myasthenia Gravis

Adult: **PO** 15–375 mg/d in 3–6 divided doses. **IM/IV** 0.5–2.5 mg.
Child: **PO** 7.5–15 mg t.i.d. or q.i.d. *or* 0.333 mg/kg or 10 mg/m^2 6 times/d. *Neonate:* **PO** 1–4 mg q2–3h. **IM** 0.03 mg/kg q2–4h.

Reversal of Nondepolarizing Neuromuscular Blockade

Adult: **IV** 0.5–2.5 mg slowly.
Child: **IV** 0.025–0.08 mg/kg.
Infant: **IV** 0.025–0.1 mg/kg.

Postoperative Distention and Urinary Retention

Adult: **IM** 0.25 mg q4–6h for 2–3 d.

PHARMACOKINETICS Absorption: poorly absorbed from GI tract (1–2%). **Onset:** 10–30 min IM or IV; 2–4 h PO. **Peak:** 20–30 min IM or IV; 1–2 h PO. **Distribution:** not reported to cross placenta or appear in breast milk. **Metabolism:** hydrolyzed by cholinesterases; also metabolized in liver. **Elimination:** half-life: 50–90 min;

80% of drug and metabolites excreted in urine within 24 h.

CONTRAINDICATIONS & PRECAUTIONS **Contraindicated in:** hypersensitivity to neostigmine, cholinergics, or bromides; bradycardia, hypotension; mechanical obstruction of intestinal or urinary tract; peritonitis; pregnancy (category C), lactation; administration with other cholingeric drugs. **Cautious use in:** recent ileorectal anastomoses; epilepsy; bronchial asthma; bradycardia, recent coronary occlusion; vagotonia; hyperthyroidism; cardiac arrhythmias; peptic ulcer.

ADVERSE/SIDE EFFECTS **Muscarinic effects:** *nausea,* vomiting, eructation, epigastric discomfort, abdominal cramps, diarrhea, involuntary or difficult defecation or micturition, *increased salivation* and bronchial secretions, tightness in chest, sneezing, cough, dyspnea, diaphoresis, lacrimation, miosis, blurred vision, bradycardia, hypotension. **Nicotinic effects:** muscle cramps, *fasciculations,* twitching, pallor, elevated BP, fatigability, generalized weakness, respiratory depression, paralysis. **Overdosage:** CNS stimulation, agitation, fear, death.

DRUG INTERACTIONS **Succinylcholine decamethonium** may prolong phase I block or reverse phase II block; neostigmine antagonizes effects of **tubocurarine, atracurium, vecuronium, pancuronium; procainamide, quinidine, atropine** antagonize effects of neostigmine.

NURSING IMPLICATIONS

Administration

- Note that size of oral dose is considerably larger than that of parenteral dose because drug is poorly absorbed when taken orally (15 mg of oral drug is approximately equivalent to 0.5 mg of parenteral form).
- IV Administration: IV neostigmine methylsulfate may be given by direct IV undiluted at a rate of 0.5 mg or a fraction thereof over 1 min.

Assessment & Drug Effects

- Check pulse before giving drug to bradycardic patients. If below 80/min, consult physician. Atropine will be ordered to restore heart rate.
- For treatment of myasthenia gravis, monitor pulse, respiration, and BP during period of dosage adjustment.
- Report promptly and record accurately the onset of myasthenic symptoms and drug side effects in relation to last dose in order to assist physician in determining lowest effective dosage schedule.
- GI (muscarinic) side effects occur especially during early therapy and may be reduced by taking drug with milk or food. Physician may prescribe atropine or other anticholinergic agent to suppress side effects (*note:* these drugs may mask toxic symptoms of neostigmine).
- In myasthenic patients, the time that muscular weakness appears may indicate whether patient is in cholinergic or myasthenic crisis. Weakness that appears approximately 1 h after drug administration suggests cholinergic crisis (overdose) and is treated by prompt withdrawal of neostigmine and immediate administration of atropine. Weakness that occurs 3 h or more after drug administration is more likely to be due to myasthenic crisis (underdose or drug resistance) and is treated by more intensive anticholinesterase therapy.

- Signs and symptoms of myasthenia gravis that may be relieved by neostigmine include lid ptosis; diplopia; drooping facies; difficulty in chewing, swallowing, breathing, or coughing; and weakness of neck, limbs, and trunk muscles. Record drug effect and duration of action.
- Manifestations of neostigmine overdosage often appear first in muscles of neck and those involved in chewing and swallowing, with muscles of shoulder girdle and upper extremities affected next.
- When neostigmine is used as antidote for tubocurarine or other nondepolarizing neuromuscular blocking agents (usually preceded by atropine), monitor respiration, maintain airway or assisted ventilation, and give oxygen as indicated. Respiratory assistance is continued until recovery of respiration and neuromuscular transmission is assured.
- When neostigmine is used to relieve urinary retention, report to physician if patient does not urinate within 1 h after first dose.

Patient & Family Education

- Inform that regulation of dosage interval is extremely difficult; dosage must be adjusted for each patient to deal with unpredictable exacerbations and remissions.
- Frequently, drug therapy is required both day and night, with larger portions of total dose being given at times of greater fatigue, as in the late afternoon and at mealtimes.
- Encourage to keep a diary of "peaks and valleys" of muscle strength.
- Patient and responsible family members should be taught to keep an accurate record for physician of patient's response to drug, as well as how to recognize side effects, how to modify dosage regimen according to patient's changing needs, or how to administer atropine if necessary.
- Patients should be aware that certain factors may require an increase in size or frequency of dose (e.g., physical or emotional stress, infection, menstruation, surgery), whereas remission requires a decrease in dosage.
- Some patients become refractory to neostigmine after prolonged use and require change in dosage or medication.

NETILMICIN SULFATE

(ne-til-mye′sin)

Trade name: Netromycin

Classifications: ANTIINFECTIVE; AMINOGLYCOSIDE ANTIBIOTIC

Prototype: Gentamicin

Pregnancy category: D

ACTIONS/PHARMACODYNAMICS

Rapid-acting, broad-spectrum, semisynthetic aminoglycoside derivative of sisomicin. Spectrum of activity comparable to that of gentamicin, but netilmicin is also effective against gentamicin-resistant bacteria. Not inactivated by most strains of bacteria resistant to other aminoglycosides. Bactericidal action primarily against gram-negative organisms including *Citrobacter, Enterobacter, Escherichia coli, Klebsiella, Proteus mirabilis, Pseudomonas aeruginosa, Salmonella, Serratia,* and certain gram-positive bacteria such as *Staphylococcus pyogenes* and *Streptococcus faecalis*. Like other aminoglycosides, not effective against most anaerobic bacteria

(*Bacteroides* and *Clostridium* species), viruses, or fungi.

USES Short-term treatment of serious or life-threatening infections including septicemia, peritonitis, intraabdominal abscess, lower respiratory tract infections, complicated urinary tract infection, and infections of bones, joints, and skin and its structures. May be administered in conjunction with a beta-lactam antibiotic (e.g., a penicillin or cephalosporin) for synergistic effect pending results of susceptibility testing.

ROUTE & DOSAGE

Moderate to Severe Infections (all doses based on ideal body weight)
Adult: **IV/IM** 1.3–2.2 mg/kg q8h or 2–3.25 mg/kg q12h.
Child: **IV/IM** *6 wk–12 y,* 1.8–2.7 mg/kg q8h or 2.7–4 mg/kg q12h; *<6 wk,* 2–3.5 mg/kg q12h.

Complicated UTI
Adult: **IV/IM** 1.5–2 mg/kg q12h.

PHARMACOKINETICS **Peak:** end of IV infusion; 30–60 min IM. **Distribution:** does not cross blood–brain barrier; accumulates in renal cortex; crosses placenta; distributed into breast milk. **Elimination:** half-life: 2–2.5 h; excreted in urine.

CONTRAINDICATIONS & PRECAUTIONS **Contraindicated in:** history of hypersensitivity or toxic reaction to netilmicin or other aminoglycosides or to bisulfites or any other ingredient in the formulation, pregnancy (category D), nursing infants, minor infections. **Cautious use in:** impaired renal function; premature infants; neonates, the elderly; patients with ascites, edema, dehydration; severe burns; cystic fibrosis; fever; anemia; myasthenia gravis, parkinsonism; history of ear disease; infant botulism.

ADVERSE/SIDE EFFECTS Low incidence in patients with normal renal function. **CNS:** headache, lethargy, drowsiness, paresthesias, tremors, muscle twitching, peripheral neuritis, disorientation, seizures, neuromuscular blockade; musculoskeletal weakness or paralysis, respiratory depression or paralysis. **CV:** palpitation, hypotension. **ENT:** ototoxicity (usually irreversible: eighth cranial nerve auditory branch: tinnitus, hearing loss, ringing, buzzing or fullness in ears; vestibular branch: vertigo, nystagmus, ataxia, nausea, and vomiting). **Eye:** blurred vision. **GI:** nausea, vomiting, diarrhea, stomatitis, proctitis, enterocolitis. **Hematologic:** increases in ALT, AST, alkaline phosphatase, bilirubin; anemia, eosinophilia, neutropenia, thrombocytopenia, thrombocytosis, agranulocytosis, leukopenia, leukemoid reaction. **Hypersensitivity:** rash, pruritus. **Renal:** nephrotoxicity, increase in serum creatinine and BUN; decrease in creatinine clearance; hematuria, proteinuria, urinary frequency, oliguria, polyuria. **Other:** fever, edema, arthralgia; pain, induration, and hematoma at injection site; hypokalemia.

DIAGNOSTIC TEST INTERFERENCE Concomitant netilmicin-cephalosporin therapy may cause false elevations of ***creatinine*** determinations. Concomitant use of beta-lactam antibiotics (cephalosporins, penicillins) may result in falsely low ***aminoglycoside levels*** (mutual inactivation may continue in body fluid specimen unless promptly assayed, or frozen, or treated with beta-lactamase).

DRUG INTERACTIONS ANESTHETICS, SKELETAL MUSCLE RELAXANTS add to neuromuscular blocking effects; **acyclovir, amphotericin B, bacitracin, capreomycin,** CEPHALOSPORINS, **colistin, cisplatin, carboplatin, methoxyflurane, polymyxin B, vancomycin, furosemide, ethacrynic acid** increase risk of ototoxicity or nephrotoxicity or both.

INCOMPATIBILITIES Solution/additive: furosemide, heparin. Y-site: furosemide.

NURSING IMPLICATIONS

Administration

- Netilmicin containing 100 mg/ml and preserved with benzyl alcohol should not be used for neonates, infants, or children (benzyl alcohol may be toxic to this age group). Netromycin pediatric injection 25 mg/ml and Netromycin neonatal injection 10 mg/ml do not contain benzyl alcohol. All preparations contain a metabisulfite or bisulfite to which some individuals may be allergic.
- For adults, prescribed dose for IV infusion is diluted with 50–200 ml of D5W, NS, or other compatible IV solution (see manufacturer's package insert); solution may be infused over 30–120 min, as prescribed.
- Diluted solutions retain potency for up to 72 h when stored in glass containers either at room temperature or refrigerated. Do not use solutions that are discolored or that contain particulate matter.
- Avoid mixing netilmicin with other drugs without first determining compatibility.
- Store at 2–30C (36–86F) unless otherwise directed by manufacturer. Avoid freezing.

Assessment & Drug Effects

- Culture and sensitivity tests should be done prior to initiation of therapy. Therapy may begin before test results are available.
- Renal function should be evaluated before and periodically during therapy. Close monitoring is particularly important for high-risk patients (i.e., renal function impairment, the elderly, dehydrated patients, burn patients, and patients receiving high doses or prolonged therapy).
- Monitor I&O ratio and pattern and report significant changes. Keep patient well hydrated throughout therapy to minimize possibility of chemical irritation of renal tubules and to reduce risk of toxicity.
- To determine peak serum drug levels, blood is drawn 1 h after IM injection or IV infusion begins. To determine trough serum drug levels, blood is drawn just before next scheduled dose. Desirable peak values: 6–10 μg/ml; desirable trough values: 0.5–2 μg/ml. Peak values > 16 μg/ml and trough values > 4 μg/ml are associated with a high potential for toxicity.
- Close monitoring of serum drug concentrations is especially important for patients with fever, edema, severe burns, and anemia. Peak serum drug levels tend to be significantly reduced in these patients.
- Patients should be evaluated before and during therapy for hearing acuity and vestibular status. Notify physician promptly if patient complains of any hearing loss, tinnitus, vertigo, or ataxia.
- If therapeutic effectiveness is not evident within 3–5 d, bacterial susceptibility tests should be repeated.
- Watch for signs of superinfection

(see Appendix G), especially of upper respiratory tract. Also suspect overgrowth of opportunistic organisms if patient develops sore rectum, diarrhea, vaginal discharge, sore mouth, fever.

NEVIRAPINE

(ne-vir'-a-peen)

Trade name: Viramune

Prototype for classifications: ANTIINFECTIVE; ANTIVIRAL; NONNUCLEOSIDE REVERSE TRANSCRIPTASE INHIBITOR

Pregnancy category: C

ACTIONS/PHARMACODYNAMICS Nonnucleoside reverse transcriptase inhibitor (NNRTI) of HIV-1. Binds directly to reverse transcriptase and blocks RNA- and DNA-dependent DNA polymerase activities. Thus, it prevents replication of the HIV-1 virus. HIV-2 reverse transcriptase and DNA polymerases such as polymerases α, β, γ, and δ are not inhibited by nevirapine. Resistant strains appear rapidly.

USE In combination with nucleoside analogs for treatment of HIV.

ROUTE & DOSAGE

HIV

Adult: **PO** 200 mg once daily for first 14 d, then increase to 200 mg b.i.d.
Child: **PO** 120 mg/m^2 q.d. × 14 d, then increase q12h, if tolerated, to 120–200 mg/m^2 q12h (max 200 mg/dose).

PHARMACOKINETICS Absorption: rapidly absorbed from GI tract. **Peak:** 4h. **Distribution:** 60% protein bound, crosses placenta, distributed into breast milk. **Metabolism:** metabolized in liver by cytochrome P45O3A (CYP3A). **Elimination:** half-life: 25–40 h; excreted primarily in urine.

CONTRAINDICATIONS & PRECAUTIONS Contraindicated in: hypersensitivity to nevirapine, lactation. **Cautious use in:** liver disease, CNS disorders, pregnancy (category C). Safety and efficacy in children not established.

ADVERSE/SIDE EFFECTS Body as whole: fever, paresthesia, myalgia. **CNS:** headache. **GI:** nausea, diarrhea, abdominal pain, hepatitis, increased liver function tests. **Hematologic:** anemia, neutropenia. **Skin:** *rash,* Stevens–Johnson syndrome.

DRUG INTERACTIONS May decrease plasma concentrations of PROTEASE INHIBITORS, ORAL CONTRACEPTIVES.

NURSING IMPLICATIONS

Administration

- When dosing is interrupted for > 7 d, reinitiate with 200 mg/d for 14 d, then increase to b.i.d. dosing.
- Store at 15–30C (59–86F) in tightly closed container.

Assessment & Drug Effects

- Prior to initiation of therapy and periodically thereafter, monitor liver function tests, renal function tests, routine blood chemistry, CBC.
- Monitor weight, temperature, respiratory status with chest x-ray throughout therapy.
- Carefully monitor, especially during first 6 wk of therapy, for severe rash (with or without fever, blistering, oral lesions, conjunctivitis, swelling, joint aches, or general malaise).
- Withhold drug and notify physician if rash develops or liver function tests are abnormal.

Patient & Family Education

- Advise regarding common adverse effects, and instruct to withhold drug and notify physician if severe rash appears.
- Warn of high potential for drowsiness and fatigue and advise caution with hazardous activities until reaction to drug is known.
- Advise women not to use hormonal methods of birth control while on nevirapine.

NIACIN (VITAMIN B_3, NICOTINIC ACID)

(nye'a-sin)

Trade names: Niac, Nicobid, Nico-400, Nicolar, Nicotinex, Novo-niacin♣, Tri-B3♣

NIACINAMIDE (NICOTINAMIDE)

Classifications: VITAMIN B_3; CARDIOVASCULAR AGENT; ANTILIPEMIC; LIPID-LOWERING AGENT

Pregnancy: Categories A and C

ACTIONS/PHARMACODYNAMICS Niacin is a water-soluble, heat-stable, B-complex vitamin (B_3). Functions with riboflavin as a control agent in coenzyme system that converts protein, carbohydrate, and fat to energy through oxidation-reduction. Produces vasodilation by direct action on vascular smooth muscles. Inhibits hepatic synthesis of VLDL, cholesterol and triglyceride, and, indirectly, LDL. Large doses effectively reduce elevated serum cholesterol and total lipid levels in hypercholesterolemia and hyperlipidemic states. Niacinamide, an amide of niacin, is used as an alternative in the prevention and treatment of pellagra.

USES In prophylaxis and treatment of pellagra, usually in combination with other B-complex vitamins, and in deficiency states accompanying carcinoid syndrome, isoniazid therapy, Hartnup's disease, and chronic alcoholism. Also in adjuvant treatment of hyperlipidemia (elevated cholesterol or triglycerides) in patient who does not respond adequately to diet or weight loss. Also as vasodilator in peripheral vascular disorders, Ménière's disease, and labyrinthine syndrome, as well as to counteract LSD toxicity and to distinguish between psychoses of dietary and nondietary origin.

ROUTE & DOSAGE

Niacin Deficiency

Adult: **PO** 10–20 mg/d. **SC/IM/Slow IV** 25–100 mg 2–5 times/d.

Pellagra

Adult: **PO** 300–500 mg/d in divided doses.
Child: **PO** 50–100 mg t.i.d.

Hyperlipidemia

Adult: **PO** 1.5–3 g/d in divided doses; may increase up to 6 g/d if necessary.
Child: **PO** 100–250 mg/d in 3 divided doses; may increase by 250 mg/d q2–3 wk as tolerated.

PHARMACOKINETICS Absorption: readily absorbed from GI tract. **Peak:** 20–70 min. **Distribution:** distributed into breast milk. **Metabolism:** metabolized in liver. **Elimination:** half-life: 45 min; excreted primarily in urine.

CONTRAINDICATIONS & PRECAUTIONS Contraindicated in: hypersensitivity to niacin; hepatic impairment; severe hypotension; hemorrhaging or arterial bleeding; active peptic ulcer. Used during pregnancy (category A); if dose is larger than RDA, category C; in nurs-

N

ing women not established. **Cautious use in:** history of gallbladder disease, liver disease, and peptic ulcer; glaucoma; angina; coronary artery disease; diabetes mellitus; predisposition to gout; allergy.

ADVERSE/SIDE EFFECTS CNS: *transient headache, tingling of extremities,* syncope. With chronic use: nervousness, panic, toxic amblyopia, proptosis, blurred vision, loss of central vision. **CV:** *generalized flushing with sensation of warmth,* postural hypotension, vasovagal attacks, arrhythmias (rare). **GI:** *abnormalities of hepatic function tests; jaundice, bloating, flatulence, nausea,* vomiting, GI disorders, activation of peptic ulcer, xerostomia. **Skin:** *increased sebaceous gland activity,* dry skin, skin rash, *pruritus,* keratitis nigricans. **Other:** hyperuricemia, hyperglycemia, glycosuria, hypoprothrombinemia, hypoalbuminemia.

N

DIAGNOSTIC TEST INTERFERENCE Niacin causes elevated serum ***bilirubin, uric acid, alkaline phosphatase, AST, ALT, LDH*** levels and may cause ***glucose intolerance.*** Decreases ***serum cholesterol*** 15–30% and may cause false elevations with certain fluorometric methods of determining ***urinary catecholamines.*** Niacin may cause false-positive ***urine glucose*** tests using copper sulfate reagents, e.g., Benedict's solution.

DRUG INTERACTION Potentiates hypotensive effects of ANTIHYPERTENSIVE AGENTS.

NURSING IMPLICATIONS

Administration

- Give oral drug with meals to decrease GI distress. Give with cold water (not hot beverage) if necessary to facilitate swallowing.
- For treatment of niacin deficiency, small doses given frequently during the day are more effective than a single large daily dose, since a considerable amount of the latter is excreted in urine.
- In treatment of hyperlipidemia, dosage is individualized according to effect on serum lipid levels.
- IV drug may be given by direct IV undiluted at a rate of 2 mg over 60 seconds; 50–100 mg of drug may be diluted in 500 ml of NS to yield concentrations of 0.1–0.2 mg/ml and infused over 12–24 h.
- Store drug at 15–30C (59–86F) in light- and moisture-proof container.

Assessment & Drug Effects

- Therapeutic response usually begins within 24 h. Note and record effect of therapy on clinical manifestations of deficiency (fiery red tongue, excessive saliva secretion and infection of oral membranes, nausea, vomiting, diarrhea, confusion).
- Baseline and periodic tests of blood glucose and liver function should be performed in patients receiving prolonged high dose therapy.
- Diabetics and patients on high doses will require close monitoring. Hyperglycemia, glycosuria, ketonuria, and increased insulin requirements have been reported.
- Observe patient closely for evidence of hepatic dysfunction (jaundice, dark urine, light-colored stools, pruritus) and hyperuricemia in patient predisposed to gout (flank, joint, or stomach pain; altered urine excretion pattern).

Patient & Family Education

- Inform that cutaneous warmth and flushing in face, neck, and ears may occur within first 2 h after oral ingestion and immediately after parenteral administration and may last several hours. Effects are usually transient and subside as therapy continues.

- Caution to sit or lie down and to avoid sudden posture changes if weakness or dizziness occurs. These symptoms and persistent flushing should be reported to the physician. Relief may be obtained by reduction of dosage, increasing subsequent doses in small increments, or by changing to sustained-action formulation.
- Alcohol and large doses of niacin cause increased flushing and sensation of warmth.
- Caution patient with skin manifestations to avoid exposure to direct sunlight until lesions have entirely cleared.

NICARDIPINE HYDROCHLORIDE

(ni-car′di-peen)

Trade names: Cardene, Cardene IV, Cardene SR

Classifications: CARDIOVASCULAR AGENT; CALCIUM CHANNEL BLOCKER; ANTIHYPERTENSIVE

Prototype: Nifedipine

Pregnancy category: C

ACTIONS/PHARMACODYNAMICS Nicardipine is a calcium entry blocker that inhibits the transmembrane influx of calcium ions into cardiac muscle and smooth muscle without changing calcium concentrations, thus affecting contractility, and it more selectively affects vascular smooth muscle than cardiac muscle. Thus, it relaxes coronary vascular smooth muscle with little or no negative inotropic effect. It significantly decreases systemic vascular resistance. It reduces BP at rest and during isometric and dynamic exercise.

USES Either alone or with beta blockers for chronic, stable (effort-associated) angina; either alone or with other antihypertensives for essential hypertension. **Unlabeled uses:** CHF, cerebral ischemia, migraine.

ROUTE & DOSAGE

Hypertension, Angina

Adult: **PO** 20–40 mg t.i.d., or 30–60 mg SR b.i.d. **IV** Initiation of therapy in a drug-free patient: 5 mg/h initially; increase dose by 2.5 mg/h q 15 min (or faster) to a maximum of 15 mg/h; for severe hypertension: 4–7.5 mg/h; for post-op hypertension: 10–15 mg/h initially; then 1–3 mg/h. *Child:* **IV** 1–3 µg/kg/min has been used in children 9 days old to 10 y.

As Substitute for Oral Nicardipine

Adult: **IV**	**PO Dose**	**IV Dose**
	20 mg q8h	0.5 mg/h
	30 mg q8h	1.2 mg/h
	40 mg q8h	2.2 mg/h

PHARMACOKINETICS Absorption: immediately 35% of oral dose reaches systemic circulation. **Onset:** 1 min IV; 20 min PO. **Peak:** 0.5–2 h. **Duration:** 3 h IV. **Distribution:** 95% protein bound; excreted in breast milk. **Metabolism:** rapidly and extensively metabolized in liver; there is an active metabolite that has <1% activity of parent compound. **Elimination:** half-life: 8.6 h; 35% in feces, 60% in urine; elimination not affected by hemodialysis.

CONTRAINDICATIONS & PRECAUTIONS Contraindicated in: hypersensitivity to nicardipine, advanced aortic stenosis, and nursing mothers. **Cautious use in:** CHF, pregnancy (category C), and renal or liver impairment.

ADVERSE/SIDE EFFECTS **CNS:** dizziness or headache, fatigue, anxiety, depression, parathesias, insomnia, somnolence, nervousness. **CV:** pedal edema, hypotension, flushing, palpatations, tachycardia, increased angina. **GI:** anorexia, nausea, vomiting, dry mouth, constipation, dyspepsia. **Skin:** rash and pruritus. **Other:** arthralgia or arthritis.

DRUG INTERACTIONS **Adenosine** prolongs bradycardia. **Amidarone** may cause sinus arrest and AV block. **Benazepril** blunts increase in heart rate and increase in plasma norepinephrine and aldosterone seen with nicardipine. BETA BLOCKERS cause hypotension and bradycardia. **Cimetidine** increases levels of nicardipine, resulting in hypotension. Concommitant nicardipine and **cyclosporine** result in significant increase in cyclosporine serum concentrations 1–30 d after initiation of nicardipine therapy; following withdrawal of nicardipine, cyclosporine levels decrease. **Magnesium,** when used to retard premature labor, may cause severe hypotension and neuromuscular blockade.

N

NURSING IMPLICATIONS

Administration

- Dosages are individualized and titrated for each patient until desired effect is achieved. Usual initial oral dose is 20 mg.
- Oral drug dose should be increased to desired level at 3 d intervals to ensure achievement of steady-state plasma levels.
- Oral nicardipine should be taken on empty stomach. High-fat meals may decrease blood nicardipine levels.
- Dose adjustment may be necessary for patients with impaired hepatic or renal function. Plasma drug levels will increase with decreased hepatic function.
- To prevent symptoms of withdrawal, do not abruptly discontinue drug.
- IV preparation: Dilute each 25 mg ampul with 240 ml of 5% dextrose or 0.9% sodium chloride to yield 25 mg/250 ml or a concentration of 0.1 mg/ml.
- Manufacturer recommends infusing diluted IV solution by slow continuous infusion. Therapy is usually initiated at 50 ml/h, with rate increases of 25 ml/h q5–15 min up to a maximum of 150 ml/h.
- IV infusion of nicardipine is usually slowed to 30 ml/h once the target BP is reached.
- When converting from IV to oral dose, give first dose of t.i.d. regimen 1 h before discontinuing infusion.

Assessment & Drug Effects

- Establish baseline data before treatment is started including BP, pulse, and lab evaluations of hepatic and renal function.
- Carefully monitor BP during initiation and titration of dosage. Hypotension with or without an increase in heart rate may occur, especially in patients who are hypertensive or who are already taking antihypertensive medication.
- Avoid too rapid reduction in either systolic or diastolic pressure during parenteral administration.
- Discontinue IV infusion if hypotension or tachycardia develop.
- Observe for large peak and trough differences in BP. Initially, BP should be measured at peak effect (1–2 h after dosing) and at trough effect (8 h after dosing).

Patient & Family Education

- Instruct to record and report any

increase in frequency, duration, and severity of angina when initiating or increasing dosage. Instruct to keep a record of nitroglycerin use and to report promptly any changes in previous anginal pattern. Increased incidence and severity of angina has occurred in some patients using nicardipine.

- Stress the importance of compliance. Warn not to change dosage regimen without consulting physician.
- Abrupt withdrawal may cause an increased frequency and duration of chest pain. Advise that drug must be gradually tapered under medical supervision.
- Caution to rise slowly from a recumbent position and to avoid driving or operating dangerous equipment until response to nicardipine is established.
- Instruct to notify physician if any of the following occur: irregular heart beat, shortness of breath, swelling of the feet, pronounced dizziness, nausea, or drop in BP.

NICOTINE NASAL SPRAY

(nik'o-teen)

Trade name: Nicotrol NS

NICOTINE POLACRILEX

Trade name: Nicorette Gum

NICOTINE TRANSDERMAL SYSTEM

Trade name: Habitrol, Nicoderm, Nicotrol, ProStep

Classifications: CNS AND AUTONOMIC NERVOUS SYSTEM AGENT; SMOKING DETERRENT; CHOLINERGIC (PARASYMPATHOMIMETIC)

Pregnancy category: X (polacrilex); D (nasal spray, transdermal system)

ACTIONS/PHARMACODYNAMICS

Nicotine, a ganglionic cholinergic receptor antagonist, has both adrenergic and cholinergic effects. Responses include stimulant and depressant effects on the peripheral nervous system and CNS; respiratory stimulation; peripheral vasoconstriction; increased heart rate, contractile force, output, and stroke volume; increased tone and motor activity of GI smooth muscles; increased bronchial secretions (initially); antidiuretic activity. Heavy smokers are tolerant of these effects. Rationale for use of nicotine is to reduce withdrawal symptoms accompanying cessation of smoking. Success rate appears to be greatest in smokers with high "physical" type of nicotine dependence.

USES In conjunction with a medically supervised behavior modification program, as a temporary and alternate source of nicotine by the nicotine-dependent smoker who is withdrawing from cigarette smoking.

ROUTE & DOSAGE

Smoking Cessation

Chewing Gum

Adult: **PO** Chew 1 piece of gum when patient has an urge to smoke; may be repeated as needed; max 30 pieces of gum/d.

Nasal Spray

Adult: **Intranasal** 1 dose = 2 sprays, one in each nostril. Start with 1–2 doses (2–4 sprays) each hour. Max 5 doses/h, 40 doses/d. May continue for 3 mo.

Transdermal System

Adult: **Topical** Apply 1 patch q24h by the following schedule: ***Habitrol, Nicoderm:*** 21 mg/d × 6

N

wk, 14 mg/d × 2 wk, 7 mg/d × 2 wk; if weigh <45 kg (100 lb), smoke < 1/2 pack/d, or have cardiovascular disease: 14 mg/d × 6 wk, 7 mg/d × 2–4 wk. ***ProStep:*** 22 mg/d × 4–8 wk, 11 mg/d × 2–4 wk; if weigh < 45 kg (100 lb), smoke < 1/2 pack/d, or have cardiovascular disease: 11 mg/d × 4–8 wk. ***Nicotrol:*** Apply 1 patch for 16 h/d by the following schedule: 15 mg/d × 4–12 wk, 10 mg/d × 2–4 wk, 5 mg/d × 2–4 wk.

PHARMACOKINETICS Absorption: approximately 90% of the nicotine in a piece of gum is released slowly over a 15- to 30-min period; rate of release is controlled by vigor and duration of chewing; readily absorbed from buccal mucosa; transdermal 75–90% absorbed through skin; 53–58% of nasal spray is absorbed. **Peak:** transdermal 8–9 h; nasal spray 4–15 min. **Distribution:** crosses placenta; distributed into breast milk. **Metabolism:** metabolized in liver, primarily to cotinine. **Elimination:** half-life: 30–120 min; excreted in urine.

N

CONTRAINDICATIONS & PRECAUTIONS Contraindicated in: nonsmokers, immediate post-MI period, life-threatening arrhythmias, active temporomandibular joint disease, severe angina pectoris, women with childbearing potential (unless effective contraception is used). *Nicotine Polacrilex:* pregnancy (category X); *Nicotine Nasal Spray and Nicotine Transdermal System:* pregnancy (category D). Safe use by children and adolescents not established. **Cautious use in:** vasospastic disease (e.g., Buerger's disease, Prinzmetal variant angina), cardiac arrhythmias, hyperthyroidism, Type I (IDDM) diabetes mellitus, pheochromocytoma, esophagitis, oral and pharyngeal inflammation; patient with dentures, denture caps, or partial bridges; hypertension and peptic ulcer disease (active or inactive) and by mother only if benefit of a smoking cessation program outweighs risks.

ADVERSE/SIDE EFFECTS CNS: *headache, dizziness, light-headedness,* insomnia, irritability, dependence on nicotine. **CV:** arrhythmias, tachycardia, palpitations hypertension. **GI:** air swallowing, *jaw ache, nausea,* belching, salivation, anorexia, dry mouth, laxative effects, constipation, *indigestion,* diarrhea, dyspepsia. **Other:** *sore mouth or throat,* coughing, *hiccups,* hoarseness; injury to mouth, teeth, temporomandibular joint, *irritation/tingling of tongue.* **Skin:** *erythema, pruritus, local edema, rash;* skin reactions may be delayed, occurring after 3 wk of patch use. **EENT:** *runny nose, nasal irritation, throat irritation, watering eyes, cough,* minor epistaxis, nasal ulceration. Acute overdose—***nicotine intoxication:*** nausea, vomiting, sialorrhea, abdominal pain, diarrhea, perspiration, severe headache, dizziness, disturbed hearing and vision, mental confusion, severe weakness, fainting, hypotension, dyspnea, weak, rapid irregular pulse, seizures, <u>death</u> (from <u>respiratory failure</u> secondary to drug-induced <u>respiratory muscle paralysis</u>).

DRUG INTERACTIONS May increase metabolism of **caffeine, theophylline, acetaminophen, insulin, pentazocine.**

NURSING IMPLICATIONS

Administration

Transdermal

- Immediately after removal of patch from protective container, apply it to a nonhairy, clean, dry skin site.

- Always remove the old patch before application of the next patch.
- Most adverse local effects (irritation of tongue, mouth, and throat, jaw-muscle aches, dislike of taste) are transient and subside in a few days. Modification of the chewing technique may help.
- Transdermal systems are heat sensitive. Store at or below 30C (86F).

Assessment & Drug Effects
Transdermal

- Be aware that transient erythema, pruritus, or burning is common and usually disappears 24 h after patch removal.
- Cutaneous hypersensitivity (contact sensitization), which does not resolve in 24 h, must be differentiated from a transient local reaction. The former is an indication to discontinue the patch.

Patient & Family Education
Chewing Gum

- Specific written instructions are packaged with the gum and patch. Review these carefully with the patient.
- The full dose of nicotine from a piece of gum is obtained through approximately 30 min of intermittent chewing.
- Chew only one piece of gum at a time. Chewing gum too rapidly can cause excessive buccal absorption and lead to adverse effects: nausea, hiccups, throat irritation.
- Gradually decrease number of pieces chewed in 24 h. Usually, a period of 3 mo is allowed before patient is advised to taper use of gum.

Transdermal

- Advise to promptly discontinue use of patch and notify physician if a severe or persistent local or generalized skin reaction occurs.
- Inform that smoking while using the nicotine patch increases the risk of adverse reactions.

NIFEDIPINE

(nye-fed'i-peen)

Trade names: Adalat, Adalat CC, Procardia, Procardia XL

Prototype for classifications: CARDIOVASCULAR AGENT; CALCIUM CHANNEL BLOCKER; ANTIARRHYTHMIC; NONNITRATE VASODILATOR

Pregnancy category: C

ACTIONS/PHARMACODYNAMICS

Calcium channel blocking agent that selectively blocks calcium ion influx across cell membranes of cardiac muscle and vascular smooth muscle without changing serum calcium concentrations. Reduces myocardial oxygen utilization and supply and relaxes and prevents coronary artery spasm; has little or no effect on SA and AV nodal conduction with therapeutic dosing. Decreases peripheral vascular resistance and increases cardiac output. Vasodilation of both coronary and peripheral vessels is greater than that produced by verapamil or diltiazem and frequently results in reflex tachycardia. Decreased peripheral vascular resistance also leads to a rise in peripheral blood flow, the basis for use of this drug in treatment of Raynaud's phenomenon. Has minimal effect on myocardial contractility. Class IV antiarrhythmic.

USES Vasospastic "variant" or Printzmetal's angina and chronic stable angina without vasospasm. Mild to moderate hypertension alone or in combination with a diuretic (steps 2, 3, 4 of stepped-care approach in antihypertensive therapy). **Unlabeled uses:** esophageal disorders; vascular headaches; Raynaud's phenomenon;

N

asthma; cardiomyopathy; primary pulmonary hypertension.

ROUTE & DOSAGE

Angina

Adult: **PO** 10–20 mg t.i.d. up to 180 mg/d.

Hypertension

Adult: **PO** 10–20 mg t.i.d. up to 180 mg/d or 30–90 mg sustained release once/d.

Hypertensive Emergency

Adult: **PO** 10–20 mg q20–30 min if necessary.
Child: **PO** 0.25–0.5 mg/kg (max 10 mg/dose) q4–6h prn (max 1–2 mg/kg/d).

PHARMACOKINETICS **Absorption:** readily absorbed from GI tract; 45–75% reaches systemic circulation (first pass metabolism). **Onset:** 10–30 min. **Peak:** 30 min. **Distribution:** distributed into breast milk. **Metabolism:** metabolized in liver. **Elimination:** half-life: 2–5 h; 75–80% excreted in urine, 15% in feces.

CONTRAINDICATIONS & PRECAUTIONS **Contraindicated in:** known hypersensitivity to nifedipine. Safe use during pregnancy (category C) and in children not established. **Cautious use in:** concomitant use with hypotensives; CHF; nursing mothers.

ADVERSE/SIDE EFFECTS **CNS:** *dizziness, light-headedness,* nervousness, mood changes, weakness, jitteriness, sleep disturbances, blurred vision, retinal ischemia, difficulty in balance, *headache.* **CV:** hypotension, *facial flushing, heat sensation,* palpitations, *peripheral edema,* MI (rare). **GI:** nausea, heartburn, *diarrhea,* constipation, cramps, flatulence. **Musculoskeletal:** inflammation, joint stiffness, muscle cramps. **Other:** sore throat, weakness, dermatitis, pruritus, urticaria, gingival hyperplasia, fever, sweating, chills, febrile reaction, nasal congestion, sexual difficulties, dyspnea, cough, wheezing. **Overdosage:** prolonged systemic hypotension.

DIAGNOSTIC TEST INTERFERENCE Nifedipine may cause mild to moderate increases of ***alkaline phosphatase, CPK, LDH, AST, ALT.***

DRUG INTERACTIONS BETA BLOCKERS may increase likelihood of CHF; may increase risk of **phenytoin** toxicity.

NURSING IMPLICATIONS

Administration

- Nifedipine should not be given within the first 1–2 wk following an MI.
- Nifedipine should not be used in a hypertensive emergency.
- Discontinuation of drug should be gradual, with close medical supervision to prevent severe hypertension and other side effects.
- Protect capsules from light and moisture; store at 15–25C (59–77F).

Assessment & Drug Effects

- Careful monitoring of BP during titration period is indicated. Severe hypotension may be produced, especially if patient is also taking other drugs known to lower BP. Withhold drug and notify physician if systolic BP <90.
- Monitor the blood sugar in patient who is diabetic. Nifedipine has diabetogenic properties.
- Monitor for gingival hyperplasia and report promptly. This is a rare but serious side effect (which is similar to phenytoin-induced hyperplasia).

Patient & Family Education

- Occasionally, a patient has developed increased frequency, duration, and severity of angina on starting treatment with this drug or when dosage is increased. Counsel patient to keep a record of nitroglycerin use and to report promptly if changes in previous pattern occur.

- Warn that withdrawal symptoms may occur with abrupt discontinuation of the drug (chest pain, increase in anginal episodes, MI, dysrhythmias).
- Patient should visually inspect gums every day. Changes in gingivae may be gradual, and bleeding may be exhibited only with probing.
- Symptoms of hyperplasia (easy bleeding of gingivae and gradual enlargening of gingival mass, especially on buccal side of lower anterior teeth) should be treated promptly.
- Drug will be discontinued if gingival hyperplasia occurs.
- It has been shown that smoking decreases the efficacy of nifedipine and that it has direct and adverse effects on the heart in the patient on nifedipine treatment.

NILUTAMIDE

(ni-lu′ta-mide)

Trade name: Nilandron

Classifications: ANTINEOPLASTIC; ANTIANDROGEN

Prototype: Flutamide

Pregnancy category: C

ACTIONS/PHARMACODYNAMICS

Nilutamide is nonsteroidal with antiandrogen activity. It blocks the effects of testosterone at teh androgen receptor sites, thus preventing the normal androgenic response.

USE Use with surgical castration for metastratic prostate cancer.

ROUTE & DOSAGE

Metastatic Prostate Cancer

Adult: **PO** 300 mg q.d. × 30 d, then reduce to 150 mg q.d.

PHARMACOKINETICS Absorption: rapidly absorbed from GI tract. **Metabolism:** metabolized in the liver. **Elimination:** half-life: 38–50 h; primarily excreted in urine.

CONTRAINDICATIONS & PRECAUTIONS Contraindicated in: severe hepatic impairment; severe respiratory insufficiency; hypersensitivity to nilutamide. **Cautious use in:** pregnancy (category C) and Asian patients relative to interstitial pneumonitis. Safety and effectiveness in children have not been established.

ADVERSE/SIDE EFFECTS Body as Whole: *hot flushes, impotence, decreased libido, malaise.* **CNS:** nervousness, paresthesias. **CV:** angina, heart failure, syncope. **GI:** diarrhea, GI hemorrhage, melena, dry mouth. **Respiratory:** cough, interstitial lung disease, rhinitis. **Skin:** pruritus. **Other:** alcohol intolerance, edema, weight loss, arthritis, cataracts, photophobia.

NURSING IMPLICATIONS

Administration

- First dose should be given on the day of or day after surgical castration.
- Store below 15–30C (59–86F) and protect from light.

Assessment & Drug Effects

- Baseline chest x-ray should be done before treatment and periodically thereafter.
- Closely monitor for S&S of pneumonitis; at the first sign of adverse pulmonary effects, withhold drug and notify physician. Abnormal

pulmonary function tests may indicate need to discontinue drug.

- Lab tests: hepatic function tests should be monitored before beginning treatment and at 3-mo intervals; if serum transaminases increase > 2–3 times upper limit of normal, treatment should be discontinued.
- Patients taking phenytoin, theophylline, or coumadin should be closely monitored for toxic levels of these drugs.

Patient & Family Education

- Immediately report S&S of adverse effects on lungs, such as development of chest pain, dyspnea, and cough with fever.
- Immediately report S&S of liver injury, such as jaundice, dark urine, fatigue, or signs of GI distress including nausea, vomiting, abdominal pain.
- Drug may slow visual adaptation to darkness; caution is advised when moving from lighted to dark areas. Tinted glasses may partially alleviate the problem.

N

NIMODIPINE

(ni-mo′di-peen)

Trade name: Nimotop

Classifications: CARDIOVASCULAR AGENT; CALCIUM CHANNEL BLOCKER

Prototype: Nifedipine

Pregnancy category: C

ACTIONS/PHARMACODYNAMICS Nimodipine, a calcium channel blocking agent, is relatively selective for cerebral arteries compared with arteries elsewhere in the body. This may be attributed to the drug's high lipid solubility and specific binding to cerebral tissue.

USES To improve neurologic deficits due to spasm following subarachnoid hemorrhage from ruptured congenital intracranial aneurysms in patients who are in good neurologic condition postictus (e.g., Hunt and Hess Grades I–III). **Unlabeled uses:** migraine headaches, ischemic seizures.

ROUTE & DOSAGE

Subarachnoid Hemorrhage

Adult: **PO** 60 mg q4h for 21 d; start therapy within 96 h of subarachnoid hemorrhage.

PHARMACOKINETICS Absorption: readily absorbed from GI tract; approximately 13% reaches systemic circulation (first pass metabolism). **Peak:** 1 h. **Distribution:** crosses blood–brain barrier; possibly crosses placenta; distributed into breast milk. **Metabolism:** 85% metabolized in liver; 15% metabolized in kidneys. **Elimination:** half-life: 8–9 h; > 50% excreted in urine, 32% in feces.

CONTRAINDICATIONS & PRECAUTIONS Contraindications: none known. **Cautious use in:** hepatic impairment, pregnancy (category C), and nursing mothers. Safety and effectiveness in children have not been established.

ADVERSE/SIDE EFFECTS CNS: headache. **CV:** *hypotension.* **GI:** hemorrhage, mild, transient increase in liver function tests.

DRUG INTERACTION Hypotensive effects may be increased when nimodipine combined with other calcium channel blockers.

NURSING IMPLICATIONS

Administration

- If patient is unable to swallow, make a hole in both ends of the capsule with an 18-gauge needle and extract the contents into a sy-

ringe. Empty the contents into an enteral (if in use) tube and wash down with 30 ml of NS.
- Store below 40C (104F), preferably at 15–30C (59–86F) in a tightly closed container. Protect from light.

Assessment & Drug Effects
- Take apical pulse prior to administering drug and hold it if pulse is below 60. Notify the physician.
- Establish baseline data before treatment is started: BP, pulse, and laboratory evaluations of hepatic and renal function.
- Monitor frequently for adverse drug effects, including hypotension, peripheral edema, tachycardia, or skin rash.
- In elderly patients, risk of hypotension is increased. Monitor frequently for dizziness or lightheadedness.

Patient & Family Education
- Advise to report gradual weight gain and evidence of edema (e.g., tight rings on fingers, ankle swelling).
- Instruct on importance of keeping follow-up appointments for monitoring of progress during therapy.
- Instruct women not to breast feed while taking this drug.

NISOLDIPINE

(ni-sol′di-peen)

Trade names: Nisocor, Sular

Classifications: CARDIOVASCULAR AGENT; CALCIUM CHANNEL BLOCKER; ANTIHYPERTENSIVE

Prototype: Nifedipine

Pregnancy category: C

ACTIONS/PHARMACODYNAMICS

Nisoldipine is structurally similiar to nifedipine. It inhibits calcium ion influx across cell membranes of cardiac muscle and vascular smooth muscle. This results in vasodilation, inotropism, and negative chronotropism. Nisoldipine is 10 times as potent as nifedipine as an inhibitor of vasoconstriction in the peripheral vasculature. It significantly reduces total peripheral resistance, decreases blood pressure, and increases cardiac output. It is also a potent coronary vasodilator.

USES Hypertension, angina. **Unlabeled use:** CHF.

ROUTE & DOSAGE

Hypertension, Angina
Adult: **PO** 10–20 mg/d in 2 divided doses (max 40 mg/d); may need to reduce dose in patients with liver disease (cirrhosis, chronic hepatitis).

PHARMACOKINETICS **Absorption:** rapidly absorbed from GI tract; 4–8% reaches systemic circulation; absorption not affected by food. **Peak effect:** 1–3 h. **Duration:** 8–12 h for hypertension, 7–8 h for angina. **Distribution:** 99% protein bound. **Metabolism:** extensively metabolized in liver. **Elimination:** half-life: 2–14 h; 70–75% excreted in urine as metabolites.

CONTRAINDICATIONS & PRECAUTIONS **Contraindicated in:** hypersensitivity to nisoldipine or other calcium blockers, pregnancy (category D), systolic BP < 90 mm, advanced aortic stenosis, advanced heart failure, cardiogenic shock, severe hypotension, sick sinus syndrome. **Cautious use in:** liver dysfunction; elderly; paroxysmal atrial fibrillation; digital ischemia, ulceration, or gangrene; nonobstructive hypertrophic cardiomyopathy; Duchenne muscular dystrophy.

ADVERSE/SIDE EFFECTS **CNS:** dizziness, anxiety, tremor, weakness, fatigue, *headache*. **CV:** hypotension, lower extremity edema, palpitations, orthostatic hypotension. **GI:** abdominal pain, cramps, constipation, dry mouth, diarrhea, nausea. **Skin:** *flushing,* rash, erythema, urticaria. **Other:** urinary frequency, pulmonary edema (patients with CHF), wheezing, dyspnea, myalgia.

DRUG INTERACTIONS May cause significant increase in **digoxin** level in patients with CHF. BETA BLOCKERS may cause hypotension and bradycardia. Phenytoin may significantly decrease nisoldipine levels.

NURSING IMPLICATIONS

Administration

- Drug may be given with food to decrease GI distress.
- Discontinuation of drug should be gradual to prevent adverse effects.
- Dosage reductions should be considered in the elderly; initiate therapy at lower doses and follow with gradual increases.
- Store at 15–30C (59–86F).

Assessment & Drug Effects

- Carefully monitor blood pressure during period of drug initiation and with dosage increments.
- Monitor cardiovascular status especially heart rate, frequency of angina attacks, or worsening heart failure.
- Assess for and report edematous weight gain.
- With concurrent digoxin use, closely monitor digoxin levels and watch for signs and symptoms of digoxin toxicity.

Patient & Family Education

- Instruct not to discontinue the drug abruptly.
- Advise to report symptoms of orthostatic hypotension or other bothersome adverse effects.
- Advise of potential for dizziness and urge caution until reaction to drug is known.

NITROFURANTOIN

(nye-troe-fyoor′an-toyn)

Trade names: Apo-Nitrofurantoin ♣, Furadantin, Furalan, Furanite, Nephronex♣, Nitrofan, Novofuran♣

NITROFURANTOIN MACROCRYSTALS

Trade names: Macrobid, Macrodantin

Classification: URINARY TRACT ANTIINFECTIVE

Prototype: Trimethoprim

Pregnancy category: B

ACTIONS/PHARMACODYNAMICS

Synthetic nitrofuran derivative active against wide variety of gram-negative and gram-positive microorganisms, including strains of *Escherichia coli, Staphylococcus aureus, Streptococcus faecalis,* enterococci, and *Klebsiella-Aerobacter. Pseudomonas aeruginosa* and many strains of *Proteus* are resistant. Presumed to act by interfering with several bacterial enzyme systems. Highly soluble in urine and reportedly most active in acid urine. Antimicrobial concentrations in urine exceed those in blood.

USES Pyelonephritis, pyelitis, and cystitis caused by susceptible organisms.

ROUTE & DOSAGE

Pyelonephritis, Cystitis

Adult: **PO** 50–100 mg q.i.d. *or* Macrobid 100 mg b.i.d.
Child 1 mo–12 y: **PO** 5–7 mg/kg/d in 4 divided doses.

Common side effect in *italic,* life-threatening effects underlined: generic names in **bold;** drug class in SMALL CAPS

Chronic Suppressive Therapy
Adult: **PO** 50–100 mg h.s.
Child 1 mo–12 y: **PO** 1 mg/kg/d in 1–2 divided doses.

PHARMACOKINETICS Absorption: readily absorbed from GI tract. **Peak:** urine: 30 min. **Distribution:** crosses placenta; distributed into breast milk. **Metabolism:** partially metabolized in liver. **Elimination:** half-life: 20 min; primarily excreted in urine.

CONTRAINDICATIONS & PRECAUTIONS Contraindicated in: anuria, oliguria, significant impairment of renal function (creatinine clearance <40 ml/min); G6PD deficiency; infants <3 mo. Safe use during pregnancy (category B), pregnancy at term, and in nursing mothers not established. **Cautious use in:** history of asthma, anemia, diabetes, vitamin B deficiency, electrolyte imbalance, debilitating disease.

ADVERSE/SIDE EFFECTS CNS: peripheral neuropathy, headache, nystagmus, drowsiness, vertigo. **GI:** *anorexia, nausea, vomiting,* abdominal pain, diarrhea. **Hematologic (rare):** hemolytic or megaloblastic anemia (especially in patients with G6PD deficiency), granulocytosis. **Hypersensitivity:** allergic pneumonitis, eosinophilia, skin eruptions, pruritus, urticaria, angioedema, anaphylaxis, asthmatic attack (patients with history of asthma), drug fever, arthralgia, cholestatic jaundice, exfoliative dermatitis. **Others:** transient alopecia, genitourinary superinfections (especially with *Pseudomonas*), tooth staining from direct contact with oral suspension and crushed tablets (infants), crystalluria (elderly patients); pulmonary sensitivity reactions (interstitial pneumonitis or fibrosis), hepatic necrosis, dark yellow or brown urine.

DIAGNOSTIC TEST INTERFERENCE Nitrofurantoin metabolite may produce false-positive ***urine glucose*** test results with Benedict's reagent.

DRUG INTERACTIONS ANTACIDS may decrease absorption of nitrofurantoin; **nalidixic acid,** other QUINOLONES may antagonize antimicrobial effects; **probenecid, sulfinpyrazone** increase risk of nitrofurantoin toxicity.

NURSING IMPLICATIONS

Administration

- Administer oral drug with food or milk to minimize gastric irritation.
- Because of the possibility of tooth staining, advise patient to avoid crushing tablets, to dilute oral suspension in milk, water, or fruit juice, and to rinse mouth thoroughly after taking drug.
- Dispensed in amber-colored containers; strong light darkens drug.

Assessment & Drug Effects

- Culture and sensitivity tests are performed prior to therapy and are recommended in patients with recurrent infections.
- Monitor I&O. Report oliguria and any change in I&O ratio. Drug should be discontinued if oliguria or anuria develops or creatinine clearance falls below 40 ml/min.
- Be alert to signs of urinary tract superinfections (e.g., milky urine, foul-smelling urine, perineal irritation, dysuria).
- Nausea occurs fairly frequently and may be relieved by using macrocrystalline preparation (Macrodantin) or by reduction in dosage.
- Acute pulmonary sensitivity reac-

N

tion usually occurs within first week of therapy and appears to be more common in the elderly. May be manifested by mild to severe flu-like syndrome. Eosinophilia generally develops in a few days. Recovery usually occurs rapidly after drug is discontinued.

- Subacute or chronic pulmonary sensitivity reaction is associated with prolonged therapy. Commonly manifested by insidious onset of malaise, cough, dyspnea on exertion, altered pulmonary function.
- Peripheral neuropathy can be severe and irreversible. Be alert for and advise the patient to report onset of muscle weakness, tingling, numbness, or other sensations. Drug should be discontinued immediately.

Patient & Family Education

- Forewarn that IM injection of nitrofurantoin may be painful (pain may be severe enough to warrant discontinuation of drug by this route).
- Inform that nitrofurantoin may impart a harmless brown color to urine.
- Advise to consult physician regarding fluid intake. Generally, fluids are not forced; however, intake should be adequate.

NITROFURAZONE

(nye-troe-fyoor'a-zone)

Trade name: Furacin

Classifications: ANTIINFECTIVE; SKIN AND MUCOUS MEMBRANE AGENT

Pregnancy category: C

ACTIONS/PHARMACODYNAMICS Synthetic nitrofuran related to nitrofurantoin. Bactericidal against most microorganisms causing surface infections, including many that have developed antibiotic resistance. Activity against *Pseudomonas aeruginosa* and certain strains of *Proteus* is limited; has no activity against fungi or viruses. Acts by inhibiting aerobic and anaerobic cycles in bacterial carbohydrate metabolism.

USES Topically as adjunctive therapy to combat bacterial infection in second- and third-degree burns; to prevent infection of skin grafts and donor sites. Has been used orally in other countries for treatment of late stage of African trypanosomiasis.

ROUTE & DOSAGE

Bacterial Infections Associated with Burns or Skin Grafts

Adult: **Topical** Apply directly to lesion or dressings; reapply dressings or solutions daily for second- or third-degree burns or q4–5d for second-degree burn with minimum exudation.

CONTRAINDICATIONS & PRECAUTIONS **Contraindicated in:** hypersensitivity to nitrofurazone, pregnancy (category C). **Cautious use in:** known or suspected renal impairment, G6PD deficiency.

ADVERSE/SIDE EFFECTS *Allergic contact dermatitis,* irritation, sensitization, superinfections.

NURSING IMPLICATIONS

Administration

- Confine applications of nitrofurazone to the part being treated. When wet dressings are used, normal skin surrounding the wound should be protected with an agent such as sterile petrolatum, petrolatum gauze, or zinc oxide. Consult physician.
- Dressing removal may be facili-

tated by flushing the gauze with sterile isotonic saline solution.

- Consult physician regarding procedure for cleaning wound following each dressing removal.
- Preserve in tight, light-resistant containers, away from heat. Drug darkens slowly on exposure to light, but reportedly this does not appreciably affect potency.

Assessment & Drug Effects

- Drug should be discontinued with onset of symptoms of sensitization or allergy (e.g., redness, itching, burning, swelling, rash, failure to heal), and superinfections (e.g., black furry tongue, thrush, malodorous vaginal discharge, anogenital itching, diarrhea).

Patient & Family Education

- Instruct patient or family in appropriate technique for application of medication to skin lesions.

NITROGLYCERIN

(nye-troe-gli'ser-in)

Trade names: Deponit, Minitran, Nitro-Bid, Nitro-Bid IV, Nitrocap, Nitrodisc, Nitro-Dur, Nitrogard, Nitrogard-SR, Nitroglyn, Nitrol, Nitrolingual, Nitrong, Nitrong SR, Nitrospan, Nitrostat, Nitrostat I.V., Nitro-T.D., Transderm-Nitro, Tridil

Prototype for classifications: CARDIOVASCULAR AGENT; NITRATE VASODILATOR

Pregnancy category: C

ACTIONS/PHARMACODYNAMICS Organic nitrate and potent vasodilator with antianginal, antiischemic, and antihypertensive effects. Relaxes vascular smooth muscle by unknown mechanism, resulting in dose-related dilation of both venous and arterial blood vessels. Promotes peripheral pooling of blood, reduction of peripheral resistance, and decreased venous return to the heart. Both left ventricular preload and afterload are reduced and myocardial oxygen consumption or demand is decreased. Therapeutic doses may reduce systolic, diastolic, and mean BP; heart rate is usually slightly increased.

USES Prophylaxis, treatment, and management of angina pectoris. IV nitroglycerin is used to control BP in perioperative hypertension, CHF associated with acute MI; to produce controlled hypotension during surgical procedures, and to treat angina pectoris in patient who has not responded to nitrate or beta-blocker therapy. **Unlabeled use:** sublingual and topical nitroglycerin: to reduce cardiac workload in patients with acute MI and in CHF; ointment: in adjunctive treatment of Raynaud's disease.

ROUTE & DOSAGE

Angina

Adult: **SL** 1–2 sprays (0.4–0.8 mg) *or* a 0.3–0.6-mg tablet q3–5min as needed to a max of 3 doses in 15 min. **PO** 1.3–9 mg q8–12h. **IV** Start with 5 μg/min and titrate q3–5min until desired response. **Transdermal unit** Apply once q24h *or* leave on for 10–12 h; then remove and have a 10–12 h nitrate free interval. **Ointment** Apply 1.5–5 cm (1/2–2 in) of ointment q4–6h.

Child: **IV** 0.25–0.5 μg/kg/min; titrate by 0.5–1 μg/kg/min q3–5 min.

PHARMACOKINETICS **Absorption:** significant loss to first pass metabolism after oral dosing. **Onset:** 2 min SL; 3 min PO; 30 min ointment. **Duration:** 30 min SL; 3–5 h PO; 3–6 h ointment. **Distribution:** widely distributed; not known if distributes to breast milk. **Metabolism:** extensively metabolized in liver. **Elimination:** half-life: 1–4 min; inactive metabolites excreted in urine.

CONTRAINDICATIONS & PRECAUTIONS **Contraindicated in:** hypersensitivity, idiosyncrasy, or tolerance to nitrates; severe anemia; head trauma, increased ICP; glaucoma (sustained release forms). Also (IV nitroglycerin): hypotension, uncorrected hypovolemia, constrictive pericarditis, pericardial tamponade. Safe use during pregnancy (category C) or in nursing mothers not established. **Cautious use in:** severe hepatic or renal disease, conditions that cause dry mouth, early MI.

ADVERSE/SIDE EFFECTS **CNS:** *headache (50%),* apprehension, blurred vision, weakness, vertigo, dizziness, faintness. **CV:** *postural hypotension,* palpitations, tachycardia (sometimes with paradoxical bradycardia), increase in angina, syncope, and circulatory collapse. **GI:** nausea, vomiting, involuntary passing of urine and feces, abdominal pain, dry mouth. **Hematologic:** methemoglobinemia (high doses). **Skin:** cutaneous vasodilation with flushing, rash, exfoliative dermatitis, contact dermatitis with transdermal patch; topical allergic reactions with ointment: pruritic eczematous eruptions, anaphylactoid reaction characterized by oral mucosal and conjunctival edema. **Other:** muscle twitching, pallor, perspiration, cold sweat; local sensation in oral cavity at point of dissolution of sublingual forms.

DIAGNOSTIC TEST INTERFERENCE Nitroglycerin may cause increases in determinations of ***urinary catecholamines*** and ***VMA;*** may interfere with the Zlatkis-Zak color reaction, causing a false report of decreased ***serum cholesterol.***

DRUG INTERACTIONS **Alcohol,** ANTIHYPERTENSIVE AGENTS compound hypotensive effects; IV nitroglycerin may antagonize **heparin** anticoagulation.

INCOMPATIBILITIES **Solution/additive: hydralazine, phenytoin.**

NURSING IMPLICATIONS

Administration

- Drug forms appropriate for angina prophylaxis include ointment, transdermal unit, translingual spray, transmucosal tablet, and oral sustained release forms. Drug forms appropriate for acute angina include sublingual tablet, translingual spray, or transmucosal tablet.

Sublingual Tablet

- Instruct patient to sit or lie down upon first indication of oncoming anginal pain and to place tablet under tongue or in buccal pouch (hypotensive effect of drug is intensified in the upright position).
- Instruct patient to allow tablet to dissolve naturally and not to swallow until drug is entirely dissolved. Advise patient with dry mouth to take a sip of water or place 1 ml saline under the tongue before taking the nitroglycerin tablet.
- If pain is not relieved after 1 tablet, additional tablets may be taken at 5-min intervals, but not more than 3 tablets should be taken in a 15-min period. Taking more tablets than necessary can further decrease coronary blood flow by producing systemic hypotension.
- For hospitalized patient, tablets should be kept at bedside. Allocate a specific number (usually 10 tablets) in an appropriate container, label, and make sure patient knows location and use. Re-

quest patient to report all attacks. Count tablets daily.

Extended-Release Buccal Tablet

- Tablet is placed between lip and gum above incisors or between cheek and gum allowing slow dissolution over 3–5 h.
- Inform patient that touching tongue to tablet or drinking hot fluids hastens tablet dissolution, which can lead to decreased duration of medication effect and onset of anginal pain.
- Tablet should not be chewed or swallowed or crushed.

Sustained-Release Tablet or Capsule

- Take on an empty stomach (1 h before or 2 h after meals), with a full glass of water, and swallowed whole.
- Sustained release form helps to prevent anginal attacks; it is not intended for immediate relief of angina.
- Do not crush or chew.

Translingual Spray

- Do not shake cannister. Spray preferably on or under tongue. Do not inhale spray.
- Spray may be repeated q5min for a maximum of 3 metered doses.
- Wait at least 10 seconds before swallowing.

Transdermal Ointment

- Using dose-determining applicator (patch) supplied with package, squeeze prescribed dose onto the applicator. Place patch with ointment-side down onto desired site. Using applicator spread ointment in a thin, uniform layer to premarked 5.5 by 9 cm (2 1/4 by 3 1/2 in.) square nonhairy skin surface (areas commonly used: chest, abdomen, anterior thigh, forearm). Cover with transparent wrap and secure with tape. Avoid getting ointment on fingers.
- Rotate application sites to prevent dermal inflammation and sensitization. Remove ointment from previously used sites before reapplication.
- Keep ointment container tightly closed and store in cool place.

Transdermal Unit

- Transdermal unit is applied at the same time each day, preferably to skin site free of hair and not subject to excessive movement. Avoid abraded, irritated, or scarred skin. Clip hair if necessary.
- Change application site each time to prevent skin irritation and sensitization.

Parenteral (IV)

- Parenteral form must be diluted in 5% dextrose injection or 0.9% NaCl injection prior to infusion.
- Use only glass bottles and manufacturer-supplied IV tubing. Regular IV tubing can absorb 40–80% of nitroglycerin.
- IV nitroglycerin, properly diluted, is administered by continuous infusion regulated exactly by an infusion pump.
- IV administration to infants, children: Verify correct IV concentration and rate of infusion with physician.
- IV dosage titration requires careful and continuous hemodynamic monitoring.
- IV nitroglycerin is available in differing concentrations. Be attentive to the dilution, dosage, and directions for administration on each vial or ampul.
- Check to see if patient has transdermal patch or ointment in place before starting IV infusion. The patch (or ointment) is usually removed to prevent overdosage. When there is to be a switch from IV to transdermal nitroglycerin, the IV infusion rate is reduced by 50% with simultaneous appli-

N

cation of 5 or 10 mg/24 h transdermal patch.

- Stable for at least 48 h when stored at controlled room temperature between 15–30C (59–86F) and mixed and stored in a glass container.
- Use only glass containers for storage of reconstituted IV solution. Polyvinyl chloride (PVC) plastic can absorb nitroglycerin and therefore should not be used. Non-polyvinyl-chloride (non-PVC) sets are recommended or provided by manufacturer.

Assessment & Drug Effects

- IV nitroglycerin should be administered with extreme caution to patients with hypotension or hypovolemia since the IV drug may precipitate a severe hypotensive state.
- IV nitroglycerin solution contains a substantial amount of ethanol as diluent. Ethanol intoxication can develop with high doses of IV nitroglycerin (vomiting, lethargy, coma, breath smells of alcohol). Monitor patient closely for change in levels of consciousness and for dysrhythmias. If intoxication occurs, infusion should be stopped promptly; patient recovers immediately with discontinuation of drug administration.
- Moisture on sublingual tissue is required for dissolution of sublingual tablet. However, because chest pain typically leads to dry mouth, a patient may be unresponsive to sublingual nitroglycerin.
- Approximately 50% of all patients experience mild to severe headaches following nitroglycerin. Assess patient and consult as needed with physician about analgesics and dosage adjustment.
- Transient headache usually lasts about 5 min after sublingual administration and seldom longer than 20 min. Assess degree of severity.
- Postural hypotension may occur even with small doses of nitroglycerin. Patient may complain of dizziness or weakness due to postural hypotension. Supervision of ambulation may be indicated especially with the elderly or debilitated patient.
- Before initiation of treatment with transdermal preparations, take baseline BP and heart rate, with patient in sitting position.
- One hour after transdermal (ointment or unit) medication has been applied, check BP and pulse again with patient in sitting position. Report measurements to physician.
- Assess for and report blurred vision or dry mouth.
- Assess for and report the following topical reactions to drug administration: contact dermatitis from the transdermal patch; pruritus and erythema from the ointment.
- Any local burning or tingling from the sublingual form has no clinical significance.
- Overdose symptoms include hypotension, tachycardia; warm, flushed skin becoming cold and cyanotic; headache, palpitations, confusion, nausea, vomiting, moderate fever, and paralysis. Tissue hypoxia leads to coma, convulsions, cardiovascular collapse. Death can occur from asphyxia.

Patient & Family Education

- Advise patient using sublingual tablet that as soon as pain is completely relieved, any remaining tablet may be expelled from mouth, especially if patient is experiencing unpleasant side effects such as headache. Advise patient to relax for 15–20 min after taking tablet to prevent dizziness or faintness.

- Advise that pain not relieved by 3 sublingual tablets over a 15-min period may indicate acute MI or severe coronary insufficiency. Advise patient to contact physician immediately or have someone take patient directly to emergency room.
- Sublingual tablets may be taken prophylactically 5–10 min prior to exercise or other stimulus known to trigger angina (drug effect lasts 30–60 min).
- Instruct to keep record for physician of number of angina attacks, amount of medication required for relief of each attack, and possible precipitating factors.
- Instruct patient using transdermal unit that contact with water (e.g., bathing, swimming) does not affect the unit.
- If faintness, dizziness, or flushing occurs following application of transdermal unit or ointment advise patient to remove unit immediately from skin and notify physician.
- Sublingual formulation can be administered while transdermal unit or ointment is in place.
- Advise patient to report blurred vision or dry mouth. Both warrant discontinuation of drug.
- Dizziness, light-headedness, and syncope (due to postural hypotension) occur most frequently in the elderly. Advise to make position changes slowly and to avoid prolonged standing.
- Inform that severe postural hypotension (sharp drop in BP), vertigo, flushing, or pallor may occur if alcohol is ingested too soon after taking nitroglycerin.
- Advise to report any increase in frequency, duration, or severity of anginal attack.
- Withdrawal following prolonged use must be gradual to prevent precipitating anginal attack.

NITROPRUSSIDE, SODIUM

(nye-troe-pruss′ide)

Trade names: Nipride, Nitropress

Classifications: CARDIOVASCULAR AGENT; ANTIHYPERTENSIVE; NONNITRATE VASODILATOR

Prototype: Hydralazine

Pregnancy category: C

ACTIONS/PHARMACODYNAMICS

Potent, rapid-acting hypotensive agent with effects similar to those of nitrates. Acts directly on vascular smooth muscle to produce peripheral vasodilation, with consequent marked lowering of arterial BP, associated with slight increase in heart rate, mild decrease in cardiac output, and moderate lowering of peripheral vascular resistance.

USES Short-term, rapid reduction of BP in hypertensive crises and for producing controlled hypotension during anesthesia to reduce bleeding. **Unlabeled uses:** refractory CHF or acute MI.

ROUTE & DOSAGE

Hypertensive Crisis

Adult/Child: **IV** 0.5–10 μg/kg/min (average 3 μg/kg/min).

PHARMACOKINETICS **Onset:** within 2 min. **Duration:** 1–10 min after infusion is terminated. **Metabolism:** rapidly converted to cyanogen in erythrocytes and tissue, which is metabolized to thiocyanate in liver. **Elimination:** half-life (thiocyanate): 2.7–7 d; excreted in urine primarily as thiocyanate.

CONTRAINDICATIONS & PRECAUTIONS **Contraindicated in:** compensatory hypertension, as in atriovenous shunt or coarctation of aorta, and for control of hypotension in patients with inadequate cerebral circulation. Safe use during pregnancy (category C) not established. **Cautious use in:** hepatic insufficiency, hypothyroidism, severe renal impairment, hyponatremia, elderly patients with low vitamin B_{12} plasma levels or with Leber's optic atrophy.

ADVERSE/SIDE EFFECTS Profound hypotension, nausea, retching, abdominal pain, nasal stuffiness, diaphoresis, headache, dizziness, apprehension, restlessness, muscle twitching, retrosternal discomfort, palpitation, increase or transient lowering of pulse rate. Irritation at infusion site, bradycardia, tachycardia, ECG changes, increase in serum creatinine, fall or rise in total plasma cobalamins. **Overdosage or prolonged use (> 48 h):** thiocyanate toxicity: profound hypotension, tinnitus, blurred vision, fatigue, metabolic acidosis, pink skin color, absence of reflexes, faint heart sounds, loss of consciousness.

N

NURSING IMPLICATIONS

Administration

- Solutions must be freshly prepared with D5W and used no later than 4 h after reconstitution.
- IV nitroprusside is diluted by dissolving 50 mg in 2–3 ml of D5W and then further diluted in 250 ml D5W (200 μg/ml) or 500 ml D5W (100 μg/ml).
- IV administration to infants, children: Verify correct IV concentration with physician.
- No other drug should be added to sodium nitroprusside infusion.
- Following reconstitution, solutions usually have faint brownish tint; if solution is highly colored, do not use it. Promptly wrap container with aluminum foil or other opaque material to protect drug from light.
- Administer by infusion pump or similar device that will allow precise measurement of flow rate required to lower BP.
- Protect drug from light, heat, and moisture; store at 15–30C (59–86F) unless otherwise directed.

Assessment & Drug Effects

- Constant monitoring is required to titrate IV infusion rate to BP response.
- Adverse effects are usually relieved by slowing IV rate or by stopping drug; they may be minimized by keeping patient supine.
- If BP begins to rise after drug infusion rate is decreased or infusion is discontinued, notify physician immediately.
- Monitor I&O.
- Monitoring blood thiocyanate level is recommended in patients receiving prolonged treatment or in patients with severe renal dysfunction (levels usually are not allowed to exceed 10 mg/dl). Determination of plasma cyanogen level following 1 or 2 d of therapy is advised in patients with impaired hepatic function.

NIZATIDINE

(ni-za′ti-deen)

Trade names: Axid, Axid AR

Classifications: GI AGENT; ANTISECRETORY (H_2-RECEPTOR ANTAGONIST)

Prototype: Cimetidine

Pregnancy category: C

ACTIONS/PHARMACODYNAMICS Nizatidine inhibits secretion of gastric acid by reversible, competitive blockage of histamine at the H_2 receptor, particularly those in the gastric parietal cells. Significantly reduces nocturnal gastric acid secretion for up to 12 h.

USES Active duodenal ulcers and maintenance therapy for duodenal ulcers.

ROUTE & DOSAGE

Active Duodenal Ulcer

Adult: **PO** 150 mg b.i.d. or 300 mg h.s.

Maintenance Therapy

Adult: **PO** 150 mg h.s.

PHARMACOKINETICS Absorption: > 90% absorbed from GI tract. **Peak:** 0.5–3 h. **Metabolism:** metabolized in liver. **Elimination:** half-life: 1–2 h; 60% excreted in urine unchanged.

CONTRAINDICATIONS & PRECAUTIONS Contraindicated in: hypersensitivity to nizatidine or other H_2-receptor antagonists. **Cautious use in:** renal impairment, pregnancy (category C). Distribution into breast milk is unknown.

ADVERSE/SIDE EFFECTS CNS: somnolence, fatigue. **Skin:** pruritus, sweating. **Other:** hyperuricemia.

NURSING IMPLICATIONS

Administration

- Drug is usually given once daily at bedtime. Dose may be divided and given twice daily.
- Antacids consisting of aluminum and magnesium hydroxides with simethicone decrease nizatidine absorption by about 10%. Administer the antacid 2 h after nizatidine.

Assessment & Drug Effects

- Monitor patient for alleviation of symptoms. Most ulcers should heal within 4 wk.
- Since asymptomatic ventricular tachycardia is a side effect of the drug, monitor cardiac patient's apical pulse.
- Monitor for persistence of ulcer symptoms in patients who continue to smoke during therapy.
- Monitor liver enzyme studies (AST, ALT) or alkaline phosphatase. Nizatidine may cause hepatocellular injury.

Patient & Family Education

- Instruct to take medications for the full course of therapy even though symptoms may be relieved.
- Instruct not to take other prescription or nonprescription medications without consulting with physician.
- Instruct in the importance of stopping smoking since smoking adversely affects healing of ulcers and effectiveness of the drug.

NONOXYNOL-9

(noe-nox′ee-nole)

Trade names: Conceptrol, Delfen, Gynol II, Koromex

Classification: SPERMICIDE CONTRACEPTIVE

ACTIONS/PHARMACODYNAMICS Nonionic surfactant spermicidal impregnated into a soft, pliable, and disposable polyurethane sponge or incorporated into foams, gels, jelly, or suppositories. Applied over the cervix, this agent blocks entrance to uterus by sperm, traps and absorbs seminal fluid, then releases the immediately available spermicide. Immobilizes sperm by cell membrane disruption.

USE As barrier contraceptive alone or in conjunction with a vaginal diaphragm or with a condom.

ROUTE & DOSAGE

Contraceptive
Adult: **Topical** Apply or insert 30–60 min before intercourse; sponge is effective for 24 h; other formulations should be repeated before each intercourse.

PHARMACOKINETICS **Onset:** spermicidal action is prompt upon contact with sperm; minimal systemic absorption.

CONTRAINDICATIONS & PRECAUTIONS **Contraindicated in:** cystocele, prolapsed uterus, sensitivity or allergy to polyurethane or to nonoxynol-9; vaginitis; history of TSS; pregnancy; immediately after delivery or abortion; during menstruation.

ADVERSE/SIDE EFFECTS *Candidiasis;* vaginal irritation and dryness; increase in vaginal infections; menstrual and nonmenstrual TSS.

N

NURSING IMPLICATIONS

Patient & Family Education

- Patient should stop using the contraceptive sponge or other forms of nonoxynol-9 if pregnancy is suspected.
- Since nonoxynol-9 antifungal properties are weaker than its antibacterial potency, vulvovaginal candidiasis frequently occurs. Symptoms should be reported: burning, inflammation, intense vaginal and vulvar itching, cheesy, curdlike discharge, dyspareunia, dysuria.

General Guidelines for Use of Vaginal Spermicide

- Use spermicide before the first and every subsequent act of intercourse.
- Foams, gels, jelly, cream: fully load intravaginal applicator and insert about 2/3 of its length (7.5–10 cm [3–4 in.]) into vagina.
- Avoid douching for 6–8 h after coitus to prevent dilution or removal of spermicide.
- Use with diaphragm: Place 1–3 tsp spermicide formulation in dome prior to insertion. After diaphragm is in place, additional spermicide is recommended. Spermicide and diaphragm should be left in place 6 h after intercourse.

Spermicide Sponge

- Use of the sponge has been associated with toxic shock syndrome (TSS). If the following symptoms develop, stop using the sponge: fever, myalgias, desquamating rash, chills, edema, nausea, vomiting, watery diarrhea. Most clinicians counsel against future use of the contraceptive sponge by the patient who has had TSS.
- Thoroughly moisten sponge with clear tap water; squeeze out excess fluid (will feel soapy and wet). Fold in half with convex side up and attached loop hanging down.
- Insertion: Slide sponge into vagina and place over external os of the cervix.
- Leave sponge in place at least 6 h after intercourse.
- Remove sponge within 24 h after its insertion.
- Vaginal irritation may be due to remnants of sponge left behind after difficult removal. Consult physician for vaginal examination and diagnosis.
- Store all forms of drug at 15–30C (59–86F) protected from moisture and light.

NOREPINEPHRINE BITARTRATE

(nor-ep-i-nef′rin)

Trade names: Levarterenol, Levophed, Noradrenaline

Classifications: AUTONOMIC NERVOUS SYSTEM AGENT; ALPHA- AND BETA-ADRENERGIC AGONIST (SYMPATHOMIMETIC)
Prototype: Epinephrine
Pregnancy category: D

ACTIONS/PHARMACODYNAMICS

Direct-acting sympathomimetic amine identical to body catecholamine norepinephrine. Acts directly and predominantly on alpha-adrenergic receptors; little action on beta receptors except in heart ($beta_1$ receptors). Main therapeutic effects are vasoconstriction and cardiac stimulation. Has powerful constrictor action on resistance and capacitance blood vessels. Peripheral vasoconstriction and moderate inotropic stimulation of heart result in increased systolic and diastolic blood pressure, myocardial oxygenation, coronary artery blood flow, and work of heart. Cardiac output varies reflexly with systemic BP.

USES To restore BP in certain acute hypotensive states such as shock, sympathectomy, pheochromocytomectomy, spinal anesthesia, poliomyelitis, MI, septicemia, blood transfusion, and drug reactions. Also used as adjunct in treatment of cardiac arrest.

ROUTE & DOSAGE

Hypotension

Adult: **IV** Initially: 8–12 μg/min; titrate to maintenance dose of 2–4 μg/min.
Child: **IV** Initially: 2 μg/min; titrate to maintenance dose of 0.1 μg/kg/min.

PHARMACOKINETICS **Onset:** very rapid. **Duration:** 1–2 min after termination of infusion. **Distribution:** localizes in sympathetic nerve endings; crosses placenta. **Metabolism:** metabolized in liver and other tissues by catechol-o-methyl transferase and monoamine oxidase. **Elimination:** excreted in urine.

CONTRAINDICATIONS & PRECAUTIONS **Contraindicated in:** use as sole therapy in hypovolemic states, except as temporary emergency measure; mesenteric or peripheral vascular thrombosis; profound hypoxia or hypercarbia; pregnancy (category D); use during cyclopropane or halothane anesthesia. **Cautious use in:** hypertension; hyperthyroidism; severe heart disease; elderly patients; within 14 d of MAOI therapy, patients receiving tricyclic antidepressants.

ADVERSE/SIDE EFFECTS Headache, palpitation, hypertension, reflex bradycardia, fatal arrhythmias (large doses), respiratory difficulty, restlessness, anxiety, *tremors,* dizziness, weakness, insomnia, pallor, tissue necrosis at injection site (with extravasation). **With prolonged administration:** plasma volume depletion, edema, hemorrhage, intestinal, hepatic, and renal necrosis. **Overdosage or individual sensitivity:** blurred vision, photophobia, hyperglycemia, retrosternal and pharyngeal pain, profuse sweating, vomiting, severe hypertension, violent headache, cerebral hemorrhage, convulsions.

DRUG INTERACTIONS ALPHA AND BETA BLOCKERS antagonize pressor effects; ERGOT ALKALOIDS, **furazolidone, guanethidine, methyldopa,** TRICYCLIC ANTIDEPRESSANTS may potentiate pressor effects; **halothane, cyclopropane** increase risk of arrhythmias.

N

INCOMPATIBILITIES Solution/additive: **aminophylline, amobarbital, whole blood, cephapirin, chlorothiazide, chlorpheniramine, pentobarbital, phenobarbital, phenytoin, secobarbital, sodium bicarbonate, sodium iodide, streptomycin, thiopental.**

NURSING IMPLICATIONS

Administration

- IV infusion of norepinephrine in saline alone is not recommended. Dextrose (in distilled water or saline solution) is used to prevent oxidation and thus loss of potency. Usual dilution is a 4 ml ampul in 1000 ml diluent to yield 4 μg/ml.
- Do not use solution if discoloration or precipitate is present. Protect from light.
- Initial rate of infusion is 2–3 ml/min (8–12 μg/min); then titrated to maintain BP, usually 0.5–1 ml/min (2–4 μg/min). An infusion pump is used. Consult physician for specific titration guidelines.
- Risk of extravasation is reportedly reduced if infusion is administered through a plastic catheter inserted deep into vein.
- Flow rate must be constantly monitored. Check infusion site frequently (tape should not obscure injection site). Report immediately any evidence of extravasation: blanching along course of infused vein (may occur without obvious extravasation), cold, hard swelling around injection site.
- Antidote for extravasation ischemia: Phentolamine, 5–10 mg in 10–15 ml NS injection, is infiltrated throughout affected area (using syringe with fine hypodermic needle) as soon as possible. Some physicians prefer to add phentolamine (5–10 mg) to each liter of infusion solution as a preventive against sloughing should extravasation occur.
- If therapy is to be prolonged, it is advisable to change infusion sites at intervals to allow effect of local vasoconstriction to subside.
- When therapy is to be discontinued, infusion rate is slowed gradually. Abrupt withdrawal should be avoided.

Assessment & Drug Effects

- Patient should be monitored constantly while receiving norepinephrine. Take baseline BP and pulse before start of therapy, then q2min from initiation of drug until stabilization occurs at desired level, then every 5 min during drug administration.
- In normotensive patients, it is recommended that flow rate be adjusted to maintain BP at low normal (usually 80–100 mm Hg systolic). In previously hypertensive patients, systolic is generally maintained no higher than 40 mm Hg below preexisting systolic level.
- In addition to vital signs, carefully observe and record mental status (index of cerebral circulation), skin temperature of extremities, and color (especially of earlobes, lips, nail beds).
- Monitor I&O. Urinary retention and renal shutdown are possibilities, especially in hypovolemic patients. Urinary output is a sensitive indicator of the degree of renal perfusion. Report decrease in urinary output or change in I&O ratio.
- Be alert to patient's complaints of headache, vomiting, palpitation, arrhythmias, chest pain, photophobia, and blurred vision as possible symptoms of overdosage. Reflex bradycardia may occur as a result of rise in BP.

- Continue to monitor vital signs and observe patient closely after cessation of therapy for clinical sign of circulatory inadequacy.

NORETHINDRONE

(nor-eth-in'drone)

Trade names: Micronor, Norlutin, Nor-Q.D.

NORETHINDRONE ACETATE

Trade names: Aygestin ♣, Norlutate ♣

Classifications: SYNTHETIC HORMONE; PROGESTIN

Prototype: Progesterone

Pregnancy category: X

ACTIONS/PHARMACODYNAMICS Synthetic progestational hormone with androgenic, anabolic, and estrogenic properties. (The acetate form is the most potent anabolic agent.) May produce excess estrogenic effect. Mechanism for prevention of contraception unclear. Progestin-only contraceptives alter cervical mucus, exert progestational effect on endometrium, interfere with implantation, and, in some cases, suppress ovulation.

USES To treat amenorrhea, abnormal uterine bleeding due to hormonal imbalance in absence of organic pathology; endometriosis. Also alone or in combination with an estrogen for birth control.

ROUTE & DOSAGE

Amenorrhea

Adult: **PO *Norethindrone:*** 5–20 mg on day 5 through day 25 of menstrual cycle; ***Acetate:*** 2.5–10 mg on day 5 through day 25 of menstrual cycle.

Endometriosis

Adult: **PO *Norethindrone:*** 10 mg/d for 2 wk; increase by 5 mg/d q2wk up to 30 mg/d; dose may remain at this level for 6–9 mo or until breakthrough bleeding. ***Acetate:*** 5 mg/d for 2 wk; increase by 2.5 mg/d q2wk up to 15 mg/d; dose may remain at this level for 6–9 mo or until breakthrough bleeding.

Progestin-only Contraception

Adult: **PO *Norethindrone:*** 0.35 mg/d starting on day 1 of menstrual flow, then continuing indefinitely.

PHARMACOKINETICS **Absorption:** readily absorbed from GI tract. **Metabolism:** metabolized in liver. **Elimination:** excreted in urine and feces as metabolites.

CONTRAINDICATIONS & PRECAUTIONS **Contraindicated in:** known or suspected pregnancy (category X), thromboembolic disorders, cerebral vascular or coronary vascular disease, carcinoma of breast, endometrium, or liver, and abnormal vaginal bleeding.

ADVERSE/SIDE EFFECTS **CNS:** <u>cerebral thrombosis or hemorrhage</u>, depression. **CV:** hypertension, <u>pulmonary embolism</u>, edema. **GI:** nausea, vomiting, cholestatic jaundice, abdominal cramps. **Reproductive:** *breakthrough bleeding,* cervical erosion, changes in menstrual flow, dysmenorrhea, vaginal candidiasis. **Other:** *weight changes; breast tenderness,* enlargement or secretion.

NURSING IMPLICATIONS

Administration

- Dosing schedule is based on a 28-day menstrual cycle.

- When starting the minipill regimen, the patient should use a second method of birth control for the first cycle or for 3 wk to ensure full protection.

Assessment & Drug Effects

- Monitor for signs and symptoms of thrombophlebitis (see Appendix G).
- Drug should be withheld and physician notified if any of the following occur: sudden, complete, or partial loss of vision, proptosis, diplopia, or migraine headache.

Patient & Family Education

Continuous regimen with progestin-only contraception (minipill), e.g., Micronor, Nor-Q.D.:

- Advise to wait at least 3 mo before becoming pregnant after stopping the minipill to prevent birth defects. A nonhormonal method of contraception should be employed until pregnancy is desired.
- In the event of a missed menstrual period: (1) If patient has not adhered to prescribed dosing regimen, the possibility of pregnancy should be considered after 45 d from the last menstrual period; progestin-only contraceptive should be withheld until pregnancy is ruled out. (2) If patient has adhered to prescribed regimen and misses 2 consecutive periods, pregnancy should be ruled out, and a nonhormonal method of birth control should be used before continuing the regimen.
- Review package insert with the patient to ensure understanding of use of norethindrone.
- Instruct to report promptly prolonged vaginal bleeding or amenorrhea.
- Teach breast self-examination.
- Urge to keep appointments for physical checkups (q6–12mo) during period of hormonal birth control.
- Store at 15–30C (59–86F); protect drug from light and from freezing.

N

NORFLOXACIN

(nor-flox'a-sin)

Trade names: Chibroxin, Noroxin

Classifications: ANTIINFECTIVE; QUINOLONE ANTIBIOTIC

Prototype: Ciprofloxacin

Pregnancy category: C

ACTIONS/PHARMACODYNAMICS

Potent broad-spectrum activity. Alters structure of bacterial DNA-gyrase, thus promoting double-stranded DNA breakage, interfering with synthesis of bacterial protein and blocking bacterial survival. Active against virtually all bacterial urinary tract pathogens including *Escherichia coli, Klebsiella pneumoniae, Enterobacter cloacae,* indole-positive *Proteus* sp, *Pseudomonas aeruginosa, Staphylococcus aureus,* group D streptococci, *Neisseria gonorrhoeae,* and against common GI pathogens (e.g., *Salmonella, Shigella*). Generally ineffective against obligate anaerobes. Development of resistance (especially to *P. aeruginosa, K. pneumoniae, Acinetobacter* sp, and enterococci) has been reported, but drug has strong activity against many strains of multiple-antibiotic-resistant bacteria.

USES Adults with complicated and uncomplicated urinary tract infection (UTI) caused by susceptible organisms. **Ophthalmic:** conjunctivitis. **Unlabeled uses:** gonorrhea, gastroenteritis, and prevention of travelers' diarrhea.

ROUTE & DOSAGE

Urinary Tract Infection
Adult: **PO** 400 mg b.i.d.

Conjunctivitis
Adult: **Ophthalmic** 1–2 drops q.i.d.

Gonorrhea or Gonococcal Urethritis
Adult: **PO** 800 mg once/d.

Bacterial Gastroenteritis
Adult: **PO** 400 mg q8–12h.

PHARMACOKINETICS Absorption: 30–40% absorbed from GI tract. **Peak:** 1–2 h. **Distribution:** renal parenchyma, gallbladder, liver, prostate; crosses placenta; distributed into breast milk. **Metabolism:** metabolized in liver. **Elimination:** half-life: 3–4 h; excreted in urine and feces.

CONTRAINDICATIONS & PRECAUTIONS Contraindicated in: use in individual with known factors that predispose to seizures; history of hypersensitivity to norfloxacin and other quinolone antiinfectives. Safe use during pregnancy (category C), by nursing mothers, and by children not established. **Cautious use in:** impaired renal function, adolescent children if skeletal growth is complete.

ADVERSE/SIDE EFFECTS (approximately 3–4% of patients). **Arthropathy:** joint swelling, cartilage erosion in weight-bearing joints, tendonitis. In immunosuppressed adult: acute ankle and hip pain followed by acute pain, tenderness, and swelling of tendon sheath of middle finger of both hands after 4 wk of therapy. **CNS:** *headache,* dizziness, lightheadedness, fatigue, drowsiness, somnolence, depression, insomnia, seizures. **GI:** *nausea,* abdominal pain, diarrhea, vomiting, anorexia, dyspepsia, dysphagia, dry mouth, bitter taste, heartburn, flatulence, pruritus ani. **Hematologic:** leukopenia, neutropenia. **Hepatic:** increased serum AST, ALT, alkaline phosphatase. **Renal:** with high doses: crystalluria (not associated with renal toxicity). **Other:** vulvar irritation.

DRUG INTERACTIONS ANTACIDS, **iron, sucralfate** decrease absorption; **nitrofurantoin** may antagonize antibacterial effects; may increase hypoprothrombinemic effects of **warfarin;** may cause slight increase in **theophylline** levels.

NURSING IMPLICATIONS

Administration

- Administer norfloxacin 1 h before or 2 h after meals with a full glass of water.
- If patient is also taking an antacid, administer it at least 2 h after norfloxacin to prevent interference with absorption. Aluminum or magnesium ions in the antacid may bind to and form insoluble complexes with the quinolone in GI tract.
- Store at 40C (104F) or less in tightly closed container. Do not freeze.

Assessment & Drug Effects

- Urine specimens are collected before starting and during therapy for culture and susceptibility testing.
- If patient is adequately hydrated, yet I&O ratio and pattern changes are noted, or if condition does not improve within a few days, report to the physician. Dosage may need to be modified.

Patient & Family Education

- Advise to take drug at same time each day (e.g., if drug is prescribed

N

for twice daily, take it 12 h apart: 8 AM and 8 PM). It should not be necessary to establish a schedule that interferes with sleep.

- Caution to take norfloxacin exactly as prescribed. Erratic dosing can encourage emergence of resistant bacteria; underdosing or premature discontinuation of treatment can cause return of UTI symptoms.
- Encourage high fluid intake (at least 2500–3000 ml/d if tolerated) to provide adequate urine output and hydration, important in the prevention of crystalluria (rare side effect).
- Patient should be made aware of what to do when a dose of norfloxacin is missed.
- Provide guidance on interventions to minimize dry mouth.

NORGESTREL

(nor-jess′trel)

Trade name: Ovrette

Classifications: HORMONE; PROGESTIN

Prototype: Progesterone

Pregnancy category: X

ACTIONS/PHARMACODYNAMICS Potent progestational hormone with androgenic, antiestrogenic, and anabolic properties. Induces and maintains endometrium, preventing uterine bleeding; inhibits production of pituitary gonadotropin, preventing ovulation; and produces thick cervical mucus resistant to passage of sperm.

USE A progestin-only contraceptive (minipill).

ROUTE & DOSAGE

Progestin-only Contraception

Adult: **PO** 0.075 mg/d starting on day 1 of menstrual flow, then continuing indefinitely.

PHARMACOKINETICS Absorption: readily absorbed from GI tract. **Metabolism:** metabolized in liver. **Elimination:** excreted in urine and feces as metabolites.

CONTRAINDICATIONS & PRECAUTIONS Contraindicated in: known or suspected pregnancy (category X), thromboembolic disorders, cerebral vascular or coronary vascular disease, carcinoma of breast, endometrium, or liver, and abnormal vaginal bleeding.

ADVERSE/SIDE EFFECTS CNS: <u>cerebral thrombosis or hemorrhage</u>, depression. **CV:** hypertension, <u>pulmonary embolism</u>, edema. **GI:** nausea, vomiting, cholestatic jaundice, abdominal cramps. **Reproductive:** *breakthrough bleeding,* cervical erosion, changes in menstrual flow, dysmenorrhea, vaginal candidiasis. **Other:** *weight changes; breast tenderness,* enlargement, or secretion.

NURSING IMPLICATIONS

Administration

- When starting the minipill regimen, the patient should use a second method of birth control for the first cycle or for 3 wk to insure full protection.
- The minipill can be started right after delivery in the nonnursing mother; however, she should be aware of an increased risk of thromboembolic disease during the postpartum period.
- Minipill is to be taken at same time each day, even if user is menstruating.
- Store at 15–30C (59–86F) in a tightly closed container.

Assessment & Drug Effects

- Monitor for signs and symptoms of thrombophlebitis (see Appendix G).
- Drug should be withheld and

physician notified if any of the following occur: sudden complete or partial loss of vision, proptosis, diplopia, or migraine headache.

Patient & Family Education

- Amount and duration of flow, cycle length, breakthrough bleeding, spotting, and amenorrhea vary greatly with use of the progestin-only contraceptive.
- Advise to wait at least 3 mo before becoming pregnant after stopping the minipill to prevent birth defects. A nonhormonal method of contraception should be employed until pregnancy is desired.
- In the event of a missed menstrual period: (1) If patient has not adhered to prescribed dosing regimen, the possibility of pregnancy should be considered after 45 d from the last menstrual period; progestin-only contraceptive should be withheld until pregnancy is ruled out. (2) If patient has adhered to prescribed regimen and misses 2 consecutive periods, pregnancy should be ruled out and a nonhormonal method of birth control should be used before continuation of the regimen.
- Review package insert with patient to assure understanding about use of norgestrel.
- Teach breast self-examination.

NORMAL SERUM ALBUMIN, HUMAN

(al-byoo'min)

Trade names: Albuminar, Albutein, Buminate, Plasbumin

Prototype for classifications: BLOOD DERIVATIVE; PLASMA VOLUME EXPANDER

Pregnancy category: C

ACTIONS/PHARMACODYNAMICS
Obtained by fractionating pooled venous and placental human plasma, which is then sterilized by filtration and heat to minimize possibility of transmitting hepatitis B virus or HIV. Risk of sensitization is reduced because it lacks cellular elements and contains no coagulation factors, Rh factor, or blood group antibodies. Expands volume of circulating blood by osmotically shifting tissue fluid into general circulation.

USES To restore plasma volume and maintain cardiac output in hypovolemic shock; for prevention and treatment of cerebral edema; as adjunct in exchange transfusion for hyperbilirubinemia and erythroblastosis fetalis; to increase plasma protein level in treatment of hypoproteinemia; and to promote diuresis in refractory edema. Also used for blood dilution prior to or during cardiopulmonary bypass procedures. Has been used as adjunct in treatment of adult respiratory distress syndrome (ARDS).

ROUTE & DOSAGE

Emergency Volume Replacement
Adult: **IV** 25 g; may repeat in 15–30 min if necessary (max 250 g).

Colloidal Volume Replacement (Nonemergency)
Child: **IV** 12.5 g; may repeat in 15–30 min if necessary.

Hyperbilirubinemia, Erythroblastosis Fetalis
Child: **IV** 1 g/kg of 25% solution 1–2 h before transfusion.

Hypoproteinemia Prophylaxis in Neonates
Child: **IV** 1.4–1.8 ml/kg of 25% solution.

N

CONTRAINDICATIONS & PRECAUTIONS **Contraindicated in:** severe anemia, cardiac failure, patients with normal or increased intravascular volume. Safe use during pregnancy (category C) not established. **Cautious use in:** low cardiac reserve, pulmonary disease, absence of albumin deficiency; hepatic or renal failure, dehydration, hypertension, restricted sodium intake.

ADVERSE/SIDE EFFECTS Possibly due to allergy or to protein overload: fever, chills, urticaria, rash, flushing, circulatory overload, pulmonary edema (with rapid infusion); hypotension, hypertension, dyspnea, tachycardia, nausea, vomiting, increased salivation, headache, back pain.

DIAGNOSTIC TEST INTERFERENCE False rise in ***alkaline phosphatase*** when albumin is obtained partially from pooled placental plasma (levels reportedly decline over period of weeks).

N

INCOMPATIBILITY **Solution/additive: verapamil.**

NURSING IMPLICATIONS

Administration

- Normal serum albumin, 5%, is infused without further dilution. Normal serum albumin, 25%, may be infused undiluted or diluted in NS or D5W (with sodium restriction). Specific flow rate should be ordered by physician.
- Administration rate for hypovolemic shock: Initially administer as rapidly as necessary to restore blood volume. As blood volume approaches normal, rate should be reduced to avoid circulatory overload and pulmonary edema; 5% concentration is administered undiluted at rate not exceeding 2–4 ml/min. Twenty-five percent concentration is given undiluted or diluted in 5% dextrose or 0.9% NaCl injection (as prescribed), no faster than 1 ml/min.
- Administration rate for patients with normal blood volume: 5% albumin human solution not to exceed 5–10 ml/min; 25% solution not to exceed 2 or 3 ml/min. Usual rate for children is 1/4–1/2 the adult rate.
- May be administered in combination or in conjunction with sterile water for injection, dextrose, sodium lactate, or NaCl injections, whole blood or plasma. Consult pharmacist for compatible IV infusion fluids.
- Once container is opened, solution should be used within 4 h, since it contains no preservatives or antimicrobials. Discard unused portion.
- Store at room temperature, but not exceeding 37C (98.6F).

Assessment & Drug Effects

- Monitor BP, pulse and respiration, and IV albumin flow rate. Flow rate adjustments may be required to avoid too rapid a rise in BP.
- Laboratory parameters used to monitor dosage of albumin include plasma albumin (normal): 3.5–5 g/dl; total serum protein (normal): 6–8.4 g/dl; Hgb; Hct; and serum electrolytes.
- Observe closely for signs of circulatory overload and pulmonary edema (see Signs & Symptoms, Appendix G). If signs and symptoms appear, slow infusion rate just sufficiently to keep vein open, and report immediately to physician.
- With injuries or surgery, as BP rises, observe for bleeding points that failed to bleed at lower BP.
- Monitor I&O ratio and pattern. Report changes in urinary output. In-

crease in colloidal osmotic pressure usually causes diuresis, which may persist 3–20 h.

- When albumin is given to patients with cerebral edema, fluids are generally withheld completely during succeeding 8 h.

Patient & Family Education

- Instruct to immediately report chills, nausea, headache, or back pain.

NORTRIPTYLINE HYDROCHLORIDE

(nor-trip′ti-leen)

Trade names: Aventyl, Pamelor

Classifications: CNS AGENT; PSYCHOTHERAPEUTIC; TRICYCLIC ANTIDEPRESSANT

Prototype: Imipramine

Pregnancy category: D

ACTIONS/PHARMACODYNAMICS Secondary amine derivative of amitriptyline. Tricyclic antidepressant (TCA) with less sedative and anticholinergic effects than imipramine. Action mechanism unclear; mood elevation may be due to its inhibition of reuptake of norepinephrine at the presynaptic membrane.

USES To treat endogenous depression. Similar in actions, uses, limitations, and interactions to imipramine.

ROUTE & DOSAGE

Antidepressant

Adult: **PO** 25 mg t.i.d. or q.i.d., gradually increased to 100–150 mg/d.
Geriatric: **PO** Start with 10–25 mg h.s., increase by 25 mg q3d to 75 mg h.s. (max 150 mg/d).
Adolescent: **PO** 30–50 mg/d in divided doses.
Child 6–12 y: **PO** 10–20 mg/d in 3–4 divided doses.

Nocturnal Enuresis

Child: **PO** *6–7 y,* 10 mg/d; *8–11 y,* 10–20 mg/d; *>11 y,* 25–35 mg/d given 30 min before h.s.

PHARMACOKINETICS Absorption: rapidly absorbed from GI tract. **Peak:** 7–8.5 h. **Distribution:** crosses placenta; distributed in breast milk. **Metabolism:** metabolized in liver. **Elimination:** half-life: 16–90 h; primarily excreted in urine.

CONTRAINDICATIONS & PRECAUTIONS Contraindicated in: children <12 y; pregnancy, lactation, during or within 14 d of MAO inhibitor therapy; acute recovery period after MI; pregnancy (category D). **Cautious use in:** narrow-angle glaucoma, hyperthyroidism, concurrent administration of thyroid medications, concurrent use with electroshock therapy.

ADVERSE/SIDE EFFECTS *Urinary retention,* paralytic ileus, *orthostatic hypotension,* drowsiness, confusional state (especially in the elderly and with high dosage), agranulocytosis (rare), tremors, hyperhydrosis, *dry mouth,* blurred vision, photosensitivity reaction.

DRUG INTERACTIONS May decrease some antihypertensive response to ANTIHYPERTENSIVES; CNS DEPRESSANTS, **alcohol,** HYPNOTICS, BARBITURATES, SEDATIVES potentiate CNS depression; may increase hypoprothrombinemic effect of ORAL ANTICOAGULANTS; **ethchlorvynol** may cause transient delirium; **levodopa,** SYMPATHOMIMETICS (e.g., epinephrine, norepinephrine) pose possibility of sympathetic hyperactivity with hypertension and hyper-

N

pyrexia; MAO INHIBITORS pose possibility of severe reactions—toxic psychosis, cardiovascular instability; **methylphenidate** increases plasma TCA levels; THYROID DRUGS may increase possibility of arrhythmias; **cimetidine** may increase plasma TCA levels.

NURSING IMPLICATIONS

Administration

- Administer drug with food to decrease gastric distress.
- In elderly, total daily dose may be given once a day h.s. (preferred).
- Aventyl is a 4% alcohol solution.
- Supervise drug ingestion to be sure patient swallows medication.
- Store drug in tightly closed container at 15–30C (59–86F) unless otherwise specified.

Assessment & Drug Effects

- Nortriptyline has a narrow therapeutic plasma level range, a characteristic called "therapeutic window." Drug levels above or below the therapeutic window are associated with decreased rate of response.
- Therapeutic response may not occur for 2 wk or more.
- Monitor BP and pulse rate during adjustment period of TCA therapy. If systolic BP falls more than 20 mm Hg or if there is a sudden increase in pulse rate, withhold medication and notify the physician.
- If psychotic signs increase, notify physician. Because of the therapeutic window effect of nortriptyline, a substitute TCA may be prescribed rather than an increase in dosage.
- Inspect oral membranes daily if patient is on high doses of TCA. Urge outpatient to report stomatitis or dry mouth. Sore mouth can be a major cause of poor nutrition and noncompliance. Consult physician about use of a saliva substitute (e.g., VA-Oralube, Moi-Stir).
- Monitor bowel elimination pattern and I&O ratio. Urinary retention and severe constipation are potential problems, especially in the elderly. Advise increased fluid intake; consult physician about stool softener.
- Observe patient with history of glaucoma. Symptoms that may signal acute attack (severe headache, eye pain, dilated pupils, halos of light, nausea, vomiting) should be reported promptly.
- Fine tremors may be reduced or alleviated by propranolol. Report symptom to physician.
- Alcohol potentiation may increase the danger of overdosage or suicide attempt.

Patient & Family Education

- Caution that ability to perform tasks requiring alertness and skill may be impaired.
- Urge not to use OTC drugs unless physician approves.
- The actions of both alcohol and nortriptyline are potentiated when used together and for up to 2 wk after the TCA is discontinued. Consult physician about safe amount of alcohol, if any, that can be taken.
- The effects of barbiturates and other CNS depressants are enhanced by nortriptyline.

NOVOBIOCIN SODIUM

(noe-voe-bye′o-sin)

Trade name: Albamycin

Classifications: ANTIINFECTIVE; ANTIBIOTIC

Pregnancy category: C

ACTIONS/PHARMACODYNAMICS

Antibiotic obtained from cultures of

Streptomyces niveus or *Streptomyces spheroides*. Bacteriostatic action appears to involve interference with synthesis of bacterial cell wall and inhibition of bacterial protein and nucleic acid synthesis. Active in vitro against many gram-positive bacteria including *Staphylococcus aureus, Streptococcus pneumoniae,* group A streptococci, and viridans streptococci, and against some gram-positive bacilli. Enterococci are usually resistant to novobiocin. Also active against gram-negative bacteria including *Hemophilus influenzae* and *Neisseria gonorrhoeae*. Resistant strains of *S. aureus* may develop rapidly during therapy.

USES Serious infections due to *S. aureus* in patients unresponsive to less toxic antiinfectives or not sensitive to other antiinfectives.

ROUTE & DOSAGE

***S. aureus* Infections**
Adult: **PO** 250 mg q6h or 500 mg q12h up to 2 g/d.
Child: **PO** 15–45 mg/kg/d in 2–4 divided doses.

PHARMACOKINETICS **Absorption:** readily absorbed from GI tract. **Peak:** 1–4 h. **Distribution:** highest concentrations in liver, small intestine, and bile; distributed into breast milk. **Elimination:** excreted primarily in bile and feces.

CONTRAINDICATIONS & PRECAUTIONS **Contraindicated in:** neonates, during pregnancy (category C). **Cautious use in:** hepatic dysfunction.

ADVERSE/SIDE EFFECTS **GI:** *nausea, vomiting, diarrhea, anorexia, abdominal distress.* **Hematologic:** pancytopenia, agranulocytosis, anemia, thrombocytopenia, hemolytic anemia. **Hepatic:** jaundice, elevated serum bilirubin. **Hypersensitivity:** *urticaria,* maculopapular dermatitis, swollen joints, Stevens-Johnson syndrome, erythema multiforme, pruritus, fever, eosinophilia. **Other:** dizziness, drowsiness, light-headedness.

DIAGNOSTIC TEST INTERFERENCE A yellow metabolite may appear if serum interferes with ***serum bilirubin*** determinations (Evelyn-Malloy method).

DRUG INTERACTION TETRACYCLINES may reduce novobiocin effectiveness.

NURSING IMPLICATIONS

Administration

- Drug must be taken at correct time intervals (i.e., q6h or q12h) to be effective.
- When novobiocin is given concurrently with tetracyclines, schedule the two drugs to be taken at least 3 h apart.

Assessment & Drug Effects

- Novobiocin is an extremely potent sensitizing agent. Side effects should be reported promptly.
- A yellow metabolite of novobiocin can cause jaundice-like skin coloration. Differentiation of drug-induced effect from frank jaundice will depend on other signs of hepatic dysfunction (i.e., dark urine, pruritus, elevated serum bilirubin). Advise patient to report symptoms promptly.
- Inspect skin for signs of thrombocyte dyscrasia: petechiae, ecchymoses, easy bruising; these signs or epistaxis or bleeding for unexplained reason should be reported promptly.

Patient & Family Education

- Drug resistance may develop rapidly. Advise to report if there is a reversal in prior evidence of therapeutic response to drug therapy.

- Duration of therapy depends on the infection but inform patient that it will continue about 48 h after febrile condition is past or when evidence of the infection is eradicated. Patient should not stop treatment just because he or she feels better.
- Patient should not alter regimen without consulting physician; sensitivity and adverse effects may occur as well as a loss of therapeutic effects.
- Warn not to use leftover novobiocin to self-medicate for another infection.
- Symptoms of superinfections (see Appendix G) should receive prompt attention and thus should be reported immediately.

N

NYSTATIN

(nye-stat'in)

Trade names: Mycostatin, Nadostine ♣, Nilstat, Nyaderm ♣, Nystex, O-V Statin

Classifications: ANTIINFECTIVE; ANTIBIOTIC; ANTIFUNGAL

Prototype: Fluconazole

Pregnancy category: C

ACTIONS/PHARMACODYNAMICS Nontoxic, nonsensitizing antifungal antibiotic produced by *Streptomyces noursei*. Has both fungistatic and fungicidal activity against a variety of yeasts and fungi; not appreciably active against bacteria, viruses, or protozoa. Binds to sterols in fungal cell membrane, thereby changing membrane potential and allowing leakage of intracellular components.

USES Local infections of skin and mucous membranes caused by *Candida* sp including *Candida albicans*: e.g., paronychia; cutaneous, oropharyngeal, vulvovaginal, and intestinal candidiasis.

ROUTE & DOSAGE

***Candida* Infections**

Adult: **PO** 500,000–1,000,000 U t.i.d.; 1–4 troches 4–5 times/d; Suspension: 400,000–600,000 U q.i.d. **Vaginal** 1–2 tablets daily for 2 wk.
Child: **PO** Suspension: 400,000–600,000 U q.i.d. *Infants:* **PO** 100,000–200,000 U q.i.d.

PHARMACOKINETICS **Absorption:** poorly absorbed from GI tract. **Elimination:** excreted in feces.

CONTRAINDICATIONS & PRECAUTIONS **Contraindicated in:** use of vaginal tablets during pregnancy (category C); vaginal infections caused by *Gardnerella vaginalis* or *Trichomonas* sp.

ADVERSE/SIDE EFFECTS Usually mild: nausea, vomiting, epigastric distress, diarrhea (especially with high oral doses).

NURSING IMPLICATIONS

Administration

- Note that nystatin vaginal tablets may be given PO for treatment of candidiasis.
- Preservatives in some formulations are associated with a high incidence of contact dermatitis.
- Store all formulations except vaginal tablets at 15–30C (59–86F), vaginal tablets in refrigerator below 15C (59F). Avoid freezing of any formulation. Protect from excess heat and light.

Patient & Family Education

- Advise that drug may cause contact dermatitis. Withhold drug and report to physician if redness, swelling, or irritation develops.

Oral Candidiasis (Thrush) Treatment

(after meals and at bedtime)

- Oral suspension: Rinse mouth with 1–2 tsp nystatin oral suspension. Keep in mouth (swish) as long as possible (at least 2 min), then expectorate. (Drug may be swallowed if patient cannot retain liquid in mouth or cannot expectorate or if ordered "swish and swallow.") Children, infants: Apply drug with swab to each side of mouth. Avoid food or drink for 30 min after treatment.
- Troche: Leave in mouth until dissolved (about 30 min). Do not chew or swallow. Avoid food and drink during period of dissolving and for 30 min after treatment.
- Care of dentures: Remove dentures before each rinse with oral suspension and before use of troche. Advise patient to remove dentures at night (infection occurs more frequently in person who wears dentures 24 h a day).

Candidiasis of Feet, Skin, and Nails

- Instruct to dust shoes and stockings, as well as feet, with nystatin dusting powder.
- Occlusive dressings (including tight-fitting underclothing) or applications of ointment preparation to moist, dark areas of body favor growth of yeast and therefore should be avoided.
- Cream is preferred to the ointment for intertriginous areas. For very moist lesions, powder is usually prescribed. Infected areas should be cleaned gently with tepid water before each application.
- Treatment of cutaneous candidal infections is continued for at least 2 wk and discontinued only after two negative tests for *Candida*.

Vulvovaginal Candidiasis

- Inform that medication should be continued during menstruation. In most cases, 2 wk of therapy are sufficient; however, some patients may require longer treatment.
- Vaginal tablets may be used up to 6 wk before term to prevent thrush in the newborn.

OCTREOTIDE ACETATE

(oc-tre′o-tide)

Trade name: Sandostatin

Classifications: SYNTHETIC HORMONE; ANTIDIARRHEAL

Pregnancy category: B

ACTIONS/PHARMACODYNAMICS

A long-acting octapeptide that mimics the natural hormone somatostatin. Octreotide suppresses secretion of serotonin, pancreatic peptides, gastrin, vasoactive intestinal peptide, insulin, glucagon, secretin, and motilin. It stimulates fluid and electrolyte absorption from the GI tract, prolongs intestinal transit time, and also inhibits the growth hormone.

USES Symptomatic treatment of severe diarrhea and flushing episodes associated with metastatic carcinoid tumors. Also watery diarrhea associated with vasoactive intestinal peptide (VIP) tumors. **Unlabeled uses:** acromegaly associated with pituitary tumors, fistula drainage, variceal bleeding.

ROUTE & DOSAGE

Carcinoid Syndrome

Adult: **SC** 100–600 µg/d in 2–4 divided doses; titrate to response.
Child: **SC** 1–10 µg/kg/d in 2–4 divided doses; titrate to response.

VIPoma

Adult: **SC** 200–300 μg/d in 2–4 divided doses; titrate to response.
Child: **SC** 1–10 μg/kg/d in 2–4 divided doses; titrate to response.

PHARMACOKINETICS Absorption: rapidly absorbed from SC injection site. **Peak:** 0.4 h. **Duration:** up to 12 h. **Metabolism:** 68% metabolized in liver. **Elimination:** half-life: 1.5 h; excreted in urine.

CONTRAINDICATIONS & PRECAUTIONS Contraindicated in: hypersensitivity to octreotide. **Cautious use in:** cholelithiasis, renal impairment, pregnancy (category B), diabetes, and hypothyroidism. It is not known whether it is excreted in breast milk.

ADVERSE/SIDE EFFECTS CNS: headache, fatigue, dizziness. **GI:** *nausea, diarrhea,* abdominal pain and discomfort. **Metabolic:** hypoglycemia, hyperglycemia, increased liver transaminases, hypothyroidism (after long-term use). **Other:** flushing, edema, injection site pain.

DRUG INTERACTIONS May decrease **cyclosporine** levels; may alter other drug and nutrient absorption because of alterations in GI motility.

NURSING IMPLICATIONS

Administration

- Do not use solution if particulates or discoloration is observed.
- Subcutaneous injection is the recommended route of administration. However, under emergency conditions, an IV bolus may be given by direct injection over 60 seconds.
- To reduce local irritation, allow solution to reach room temperature before injection and administer slowly.
- For prolonged storage, ampules should be refrigerated at 2–8C. Ampuls stored at room temperature should be used within 24 h.

Assessment & Drug Effects

- Monitor for hypoglycemia and hyperglycemia (see Appendix G), because octreotide may alter the balance between insulin, glucagon, and growth hormone.
- Monitor fluid and electrolyte balance, as octreotide stimulates fluid and electrolyte absorption from GI tract.
- Dietary fat absorption may be altered in some clients. Monitor fecal fat and serum carotene to aid in the assessment of possible drug-induced aggravation of fat malabsorption.

Patient & Family Education

- Provide instruction on proper technique for SC injection if self-medication is required.
- Inform that preferred sites for SC injections of octreotide are the hip, thigh, and abdomen.
- Inform that multiple injections at the same SC injection site within short periods of time are not recommended. This is to avoid irritating the area.
- To minimize GI side effects, instruct to give injections between meals and at bedtime.

OFLOXACIN

(o-flox'a-cin)

Trade names: Floxin, Ocuflox
Classifications: ANTIINFECTIVE; QUINOLONE ANTIBIOTIC
Prototype: Ciprofloxacin
Pregnancy category: C

ACTIONS/PHARMACODYNAMICS A fluoroquinolone antibiotic with a broad spectrum of activity against gram-positive and gram-negative aerobic and anaerobic bacteria. Is bactericidal by inhibiting DNA gyrase, an enzyme necessary for bacterial DNA replication and some aspects of its transcription, repair, recombination, and transposition.

USES *Chlamydia trachomatis* infection, uncomplicated gonorrhea, prostatitis, respiratory tract infections, skin and skin structure infections, urinary tract infections due to susceptible bacteria, superficial ocular infections, pelvic inflammatory disease. Otic: otitis externa, otitis media with perforated tympanic membranes. **Unlabeled uses:** ENT infections, *Helicobacter pylori* infections, *Salmonella* gastroenteritis.

ROUTE & DOSAGE

Uncomplicated Gonorrhea

Adult: **PO** 400 mg for 1 dose.

Urinary Tract, Respiratory Tract, and Skin and Skin Structure Infections

Adult: **PO** 200–400 mg q12h × 7–10 d. **IV** 400 mg q12h × 7 d.

Prostatitis

Adult: **PO** 300 mg b.i.d. × 6 wk. **IV** 300 mg q12h × 10 d, then switch to PO for 6 wk.

Superficial Ocular Infections

Adult: **Ophthalmic** Instill 1–2 drops q2–4h for first 2d, then q.i.d. for up to 5 additional d.

Otitis Media

Adult/Child ≥ 1 y: **Otic** 1 drop q12h.

PHARMACOKINETICS Absorption: 90–98% absorbed from GI tract. **Peak:** 1–2 h. **Distribution:** distributes to most tissues; 50% crosses into CSF with inflamed meninges; 20–32% protein bound; crosses placenta; distributed into breast milk. **Metabolism:** slightly metabolized in liver. **Elimination:** half-life: 5–7.5 h; 72–98% excreted in urine within 48 h.

CONTRAINDICATIONS & PRECAUTIONS Contraindicated in: hypersensitivity to ofloxacin or other quinolone antibacterial agents. Safety and effectiveness in children and adolescents < 18 y not established. **Cautious use in:** renal disease; patients with a history of epilepsy, psychosis, or increased intracranial pressure; pregnancy (category C).

ADVERSE/SIDE EFFECTS CNS: *headache, dizziness, insomnia,* hallucinations. **GI:** nausea, vomiting, diarrhea, GI discomfort. **GU:** pruritus, pain, irritation, burning, vaginitis, vaginal discharge, dysmenorrhea, menorrhagia, dysuria, urinary frequency. **Skin:** pruritus, rash.

DRUG INTERACTIONS Ofloxacin absorption decreased when it is administered with MAGNESIUM- or ALUMINUM-CONTAINING ANTACIDS. Other CATIONS, including **calcium, iron,** and **zinc,** also appear to interfere with ofloxacin absorption.

NURSING IMPLICATIONS

Administration

- Oral ofloxacin should not be given with meals.
- Avoid administering mineral supplements or vitamins with iron or zinc within 2 h of oral ofloxacin.
- Antacids with magnesium, aluminum, or sucralfate should not be given within 4 h before or 2 h after oral ofloxacin.
- Ocular preparation: Do not allow

tip of dropper to contact any surface.
- IV preparation: Ofloxacin must be diluted to a concentration of at least 4 mg/ml prior to administration. Add the contents of the 10- or 20-ml vial to 100 ml of diluent (5% dextrose, 0.9% NaCl, 5% dextrose/0.9% NaCl).
- IV administration: Infuse the diluted solution over at least 60 min. Do not infuse with other additives or medications.
- Diluted IV solutions are stable for 14 d under refrigeration.
- Store oral form at 15–30C (59–86F) in a tightly closed container.

Assessment & Drug Effects
- Culture and sensitivity tests should be done before initial dose is given. Treatment may be implemented pending results.
- Before therapy is instituted, determine if there is a history of hypersensitivity reactions to quinolones or other drugs.
- Discontinue ofloxacin and notify physician at first sign of a skin rash or other allergic reaction.
- Monitor for seizures, especially in patients with known or suspected CNS disorders. Discontinue ofloxacin and notify physician immediately if seizure occurs.
- Assess for signs and symptoms of superinfection (see Appendix G).

Patient & Family Education
- Advise to take ofloxacin on an empty stomach.
- Encourage liberal fluids if not contraindicated.
- Inform that dizziness or light-headedness may occur; advise appropriate caution.
- Inform of the possibility of phototoxicity and advise avoidance of excessive sunlight or artificial ultraviolet light.

O

OLANZAPINE
(o-lan′za-peen)
Trade name: Zyprexa
Classifications: CENTRAL NERVOUS SYSTEM (CNS) AGENT; PSYCHOTHERAPEUTIC; NEUROLEPTIC AGENT; SEROTONIN-REUPTAKE INHIBITOR; DOPAMINE-REUPTAKE INHIBITOR
Prototype: Clozapine
Pregnancy category: C

ACTIONS/PHARMACODYNAMICS
Has antipsychotic activity which is thought to be due to antagonism for both serotonin $5HT_{2A/2C}$ and dopamine D_{1-4} receptors. Is thought to inhibit the CNS presynaptic neuronal reuptake of serotonin and dopamine. Antagonism of alfa-adrenergic receptors results in the side effect of orthostatic hypotension. Also has anticholinergic properties.

USE Management of psychotic disorders.

ROUTE & DOSAGE
Psychotic Disorders
Adult: **PO** Start with 5–10 mg once daily, may increase by 2.5–5 mg qwk until desired response (usual range 10–15 mg/d, max 20 mg/d).
Geriatric: **PO** Start with 5 mg once daily.

PHARMACOKINETICS **Absorption:** Rapidly absorbed from GI tract, 60% reaches systemic circulation. **Peak:** 6 h **Distribution:** 93% protein bound, secreted into breast milk of animals (human secretion unknown). **Metabolism:** metabolized in liver, primarily by cytochrome P450 1A2 (CYP1A2). **Elimination:** half-life: 21–54 h; approximately 57% excreted in urine, 30% in feces.

CONTRAINDICATIONS & PRECAUTIONS **Contraindicated in:** hypersensitivity to olanzapine, lactation. **Cautious use in:** known cardiovascular disease, cerebrovascular disease, conditions that predispose to hypotension (i.e., dehydration, hypovolemia), history of breast cancer, hepatic impairment, renal impairment, predisposition to aspiration pneumonia, history of or high risk for suicide, pregnancy (category C). Safety and effectiveness in children < 18 y not established.

ADVERSE/SIDE EFFECTS **Body as whole:** *weight gain*, fever, back and chest pain, peripheral and lower extremity edema, joint pain, twitching, premenstrual syndrome. **CNS:** *somnolence, dizziness, headache, agitation, insomnia, nervousness, hostility,* anxiety, personality disorder, akathisia, hypertonia, tremor amnesia, euphoria, stuttering, extrapyramidal symptoms (dystonic events, *parkinsonism, akathisia*), tardive dyskinesia. **CV:** postural hypotension, hypotension, tachycardia. **Eye:** amblyopia, blepharitis. **GI:** abdominal pain, constipation, dry mouth, increased appetite, increased salivation, nausea, vomiting, elevated liver function tests. **GU:** premenstrual syndrome, hematuria, urinary incontinence, metrorrhagia. **Respiratory:** rhinitis, cough, pharyngitis, dyspnea. **Skin:** rash.

DRUG INTERACTIONS May enhance hypotensive effects of ANTIHYPERTENSIVES. May enhance effects of other CNS ACTIVE DRUGS, **alcohol. Carbamazepine, omeprazole, rifampin** may increase metabolism and clearance of olanzapine. **Fluvoxamine** may inhibit metabolism and clearance of olanzapine.

NURSING IMPLICATIONS

Administration

- Recommended starting dose is 5 mg in persons who are debilitated, predisposed to hypotension, or at risk for slow metabolism of olanzapine (e.g., female nonsmokers ≥ 65 y).
- Store at 20–25C (68–77F). Protect from light and moisture.

Assessment & Drug Effects

- Withhold drug and immediately report S&S of NMS (see Appendix G); assess for and report S&S of tardive dyskinesia (see Appendix G).
- Periodically monitor ALT/SGPT, especially in those with hepatic dysfunction or being treated with other potentially hepatotoxic drugs.
- Periodically monitor BP and HR. Monitor temperature, especially under conditions such as strenuous exercise, extreme heat, or treatment with other anticholinergic drugs.
- Monitor for seizures, especially in elderly and cognitively impaired persons.

Patient & Family Education

- Warn of risk of orthostatic hypotension and cognitive impairment; advise against engaging in hazardous activities until reaction to drug is known.
- Advise regarding common adverse effects and possible drug interactions.
- Instruct to avoid alcohol and take no additional medications without informing physician.
- Advise against overheating and conditions leading to dehydration.
- Advise mothers not to breastfeed while on olanzapine.

OLOPATADINE HYDROCHLORIDE

(o-lo-pa′ta-deen)

Trade name: Patanol

O

Classifications: ANTIHISTAMINE; H_1-RECEPTOR ANTAGONIST
Prototype: Diphenhydramine
Pregnancy category: C

ACTIONS/PHARMACODYNAMICS
Olopatadine is a selective H_1-receptor antagonist inhibiting the release of histamine from the mast cell. This action inhibits type 1 hypersensitivity reaction.

USE Allergic conjunctivitis.

ROUTE & DOSAGE

Allergic Conjunctivitis
Adult/Child ≥ *3 y:* **Topical** Instill 1–2 drops in affected eye(s) b.i.d. Dose at least 6–8 h apart.

PHARMACOKINETICS Absorption: low systemic exposure with ocular administration. **Elimination:** half-life: 3 h; primarily excreted in urine.

O

CONTRAINDICATIONS & PRECAUTIONS Contraindicated in: hypersensitivity to olopatadine and use with contact lens. **Cautious use in:** pregnancy (category C) and lactation. Safety and efficacy in children < 3 y have not been established.

ADVERSE/SIDE EFFECTS Body as whole: asthenia, cold syndrome. **CNS:** headache. **Ocular:** burning or stinging, dry eye, foreign body sensation, hyperemia, keratitis, lid edema, pruritus. **Respiratory:** pharyngitis, rhinitis, sinusitis. **Other:** taste perversion.

NURSING IMPLICATIONS

Administration
- Remove contact lenses prior to instillation of drops. Do not touch lids or eye tissue with dropper tip.
- Store at 4–30C (39–86F) in tightly closed bottle.

Assessment & Drug Effects
- Therapeutic effectiveness is indicated by decreased eye itching.

Patient & Family Education
- If eye irritation increases, withhold drug and notify physician.

OLSALAZINE SODIUM
(ol-sal'a-zeen)
Trade name: Dipentum
Classifications: MUCOUS MEMBRANE AGENT; ANTIINFLAMMATORY
Pregnancy category: C

ACTIONS/PHARMACODYNAMICS Is converted to 5-aminosalicylic acid (5-ASA) by colonic bacteria. The 5-ASA is absorbed slowly, resulting in very high local concentration in the colon. The 5-ASA has antiinflammatory activity in ulcerative colitis.

USE Maintenance therapy in patients with ulcerative colitis. **Unlabeled use:** acute flareup of ulcerative colitis.

ROUTE & DOSAGE

Ulcerative Colitis
Adult: **PO** 500 mg b.i.d.; may increase up to 1.5–3 g/d in 2–4 divided doses.

PHARMACOKINETICS Absorption: 1–3% absorbed from GI tract; high colonic concentrations are associated with efficacy. **Metabolism:** olsalazine, a prodrug, is composed of 2 molecules of 5-ASA, the proposed active antiinflammatory agent, connected by an azo bond; colonic bacterial azo-reductases break the azo bond, thus releasing 2 active molecules of 5-ASA. **Elimination:** half-life: at least 6 h; primarily eliminated in feces as 5-ASA.

CONTRAINDICATIONS & PRECAUTIONS **Contraindicated in:** hypersensitivity to salicylates. **Cautious use in:** patients with preexisting renal disease and pregnancy (category C). It is not known whether it is excreted in breast milk. Safety and effectiveness in children have not been established.

ADVERSE/SIDE EFFECTS **CNS:** headache. **GI:** *diarrhea,* nausea, abdominal pain, indigestion, vomiting, bloating. **Other:** rash, arthralgia.

NURSING IMPLICATIONS

Administration

- Olsalazine should be given with food.
- Store at 15–30C (59–86F).

Assessment & Drug Effects

- Renal function should be monitored in patients with preexisting renal disease.
- Monitor for signs and symptoms of a hypersensitivity reaction (see Appendix G). Discontinue olsalazine and notify physician at first sign of an allergic response.

Patient & Family Education

- Inform patient that diarrhea, a possible adverse effect, should be reported to the physician.
- Advise to always take olsalazine with food and to take in two evenly divided doses.

OMEPRAZOLE

(o-me′pra-zole)

Trade names: Losec ♣, Prilosec

Prototype for classifications: GASTROINTESTINAL AGENT; PROTON PUMP INHIBITOR

Pregnancy category: C

ACTIONS/PHARMACODYNAMICS Omeprazole belongs to a class of antisecretory compounds that are gastric acid pump inhibitors. Specifically, it suppresses gastric acid secretion by inhibiting the H^+, K^+-ATPase enzyme system [the acid (proton H^+) pump] in the parietal cells. Omeprazole does not exhibit anticholinergic or H_2-histamine antagonist properties.

USES Duodenal and gastric ulcer. Gastroesophageal reflux disease including severe erosive esophagitis (4 to 8 wk treatment). Long-term treatment of pathologic hypersecretory conditions such as Zollinger-Ellison syndrome, multiple endocrine adenomas, and systemic mastocytosis. In combination with clarithromycin to treat duodenal ulcers associated with *Helicobacter pylori*.

ROUTE & DOSAGE

Gastroesophageal Reflux, Erosive Esophagitis, Duodenal Ulcer

Adult: **PO** 20 mg once/d for 4–8 wk.

Gastric Ulcer

Adult: **PO** 20 mg b.i.d. × 4–8 wk.

Hypersecretory Disease

Adult: **PO** 60 mg once/d up to 120 mg t.i.d.

Duodenal Ulcer Associated with *H. pylori*

Adult: **PO** 40 mg once/d for 14 d, then 20 mg/d for 14 d, in combination with clarithromycin 500 mg t.i.d. for 14 d.

PHARMACOKINETICS **Absorption:** poorly absorbed from GI tract; 30–40% reaches systemic circulation. **Onset:** 0.5–3.5 h. **Peak:** peak inhibition of gastric acid secretion: 5

O

d. **Metabolism:** metabolized in liver. **Elimination:** half-life: 0.5–1.5 h; 80% excreted in urine, 20% in feces.

CONTRAINDICATIONS & PRECAUTIONS **Contraindicated in:** long-term use for gastroesophageal reflux disease, duodenal ulcers, lactation. **Cautious use in:** pregnancy (category C). Safety and effectiveness in children have not been established.

ADVERSE/SIDE EFFECTS **CNS:** headache, dizziness, fatigue. **GI:** diarrhea, abdominal pain, nausea, mild transient increases in liver function tests. **GU:** hematuria, proteinuria. **Other:** rash.

DRUG INTERACTIONS Concomitant administration of **diazepam** and omeprazole may increase diazepam concentrations. Concomitant administration of **phenytoin** and omeprazole may increase phenyoin levels. Concomitant administration of **warfarin** and omeprazole may increase warfarin levels.

O

DIAGNOSTIC TEST INTERFERENCE Omeprazole has been reported to significantly impair peak ***cortisol*** response to exogenous ACTH. This finding is undergoing further investigation.

NURSING IMPLICATIONS

Administration

- Capsules must be swallowed whole and should be taken before eating.
- Antacids may be administered with omeprazole.

Assessment & Drug Effects

- Symptomatic response to therapy with omeprazole does not preclude gastric malignancy.
- Monitor urinalysis for hematuria and proteinuria.

Patient & Family Education

- Instruct to swallow capsule whole—not to open, chew, or crush—and to take drug before eating, preferably before breakfast.
- Lactating women should discontinue nursing prior to taking the drug.
- Instruct to report any changes in urinary elimination such as pain or discomfort associated with urination.
- Instruct to report severe diarrhea. The drug may need to be discontinued.

ONDANSETRON HYDROCHLORIDE

(on-dan′si-tron)

Trade name: Zofran

Prototype for classifications: GI AGENT; ANTIEMETIC; 5-HT_3 ANTAGONIST

Pregnancy category: B

ACTIONS/PHARMACODYNAMICS Ondansetron is a selective serotonin (5-HT_3) receptor antagonist used for prevention of nausea and vomiting associated with cancer chemotherapy. Serotonin receptors are located centrally in the chemoreceptor trigger zone (CTZ) and peripherally on the vagal nerve terminals. Serotonin is released from the wall of the small intestine and stimulates the vagal efferents through the serotonin receptors and initiates the vomiting reflex.

USES Prevention of nausea and vomiting associated with initial and repeated courses of cancer chemotherapy, including high-dose cisplatin; postoperative nausea and vomiting.

ROUTE & DOSAGE

Nausea and Vomiting

Adult: **PO** 8 mg 30 min before chemotherapy, then q8h × 2 more

doses. **IV** 0.15 mg/kg infused over 15 min beginning 30 min before start of chemotherapy, followed by 0.15 mg/kg 4 and 8 h after first dose of ondansetron; may also give 8 mg bolus, then 1 mg/h by continuous infusion (max 32 mg/d), or 32 mg as single dose.
Child >4 y: **PO** 4 mg 30 min before chemotherapy, then q8h × 2 more doses. **IV** *4–18 y*, same as for adult.

Postoperative Nausea and Vomiting

Adult: **IV** 4 mg by slow IV push. May repeat q8h as needed. **PO** 8 mg 1 h preoperatively.
Child ≥2 y: **IV** 0.1 mg/kg.

PHARMACOKINETICS Peak: 1–1.5 h. **Metabolism:** metabolized in liver. **Elimination:** half-life: 3 h; 44–60% excreted in urine within 24 h; approximately 25% excreted in feces.

CONTRAINDICATIONS & PRECAUTIONS Contraindicated in: hypersensitivity to ondansetron. **Cautious use in:** pregnancy (category B), nursing mothers, and children ≤3 y.

ADVERSE/SIDE EFFECTS CNS: dizziness and light-headedness, *headache, sedation*. **GI:** *diarrhea*, constipation, dry mouth, transient increases in liver aminotransferases and bilirubin. **Other:** hypersensitivity reactions.

NURSING IMPLICATIONS

Administration

- Administer tablets 30 min prior to chemotherapy and 1–2 h prior to radiation therapy.
- IV solution for chemotherapy: Dilute IV injection in 50 ml of 5% dextrose or 0.9% NaCl solution before administering. When three separate doses are administered, infuse each over 15 min.
- IV push for postoperative nausea and vomiting: Give undiluted over ≥30 s but preferably over 2–5 min.
- IV administration to infants, children: Verify correct IV concentration and rate of infusion/injection with physician.
- The diluted IV solution is stable under normal lighting conditions at room temperature for 48 h. Store tablets at room temperature, 15–30C (59–86F).

Assessment & Drug Effects

- Monitor fluid and electrolyte status. Diarrhea, which may cause fluid and electrolyte imbalance, is a potential adverse effect of the drug.
- Monitor cardiovascular status, especially in patients with a history of coronary artery disease. Rare cases of tachycardia and angina have been reported.

Patient & Family Education

- Inform that headache requiring an analgesic for relief is a common adverse effect.

OPIUM ALKALOIDS HYDROCHLORIDES

(oh'pee-um)

Trade name: Pantopon

Classifications: CNS AGENT; NARCOTIC (OPIATE) AGONIST ANALGESIC

Prototype: Morphine

Pregnancy category: C

Controlled substance: Schedule II

ACTIONS/PHARMACODYNAMICS

A mixture of opium alkaloids that contains about 50% anhydrous morphine or about 5 times the amount found in opium powder. Analgesic activity results from the morphine component of the mixture; small doses have antidiarrheal effects.

USES To relieve severe pain. Pantopon, however, has been largely replaced by other narcotics.

ROUTE & DOSAGE

Severe Pain
Adult: **IM/SC** 5–20 mg q4–5h.

PHARMACOKINETICS **Peak:** 50–90 min SC; 30–60 min IM. **Duration:** up to 7 h. **Distribution:** crosses placenta; distributed into breast milk. **Metabolism:** metabolized in liver. **Elimination:** excreted in urine.

ADVERSE/SIDE EFFECTS See morphine.

DRUG INTERACTIONS **Alcohol** and other CNS DEPRESSANTS add to CNS effects.

INCOMPATIBILITIES **Solution/additive: dimenhydrinate, pentobarbital, perphenazine, ranitidine.**

O

NURSING IMPLICATIONS

See nursing implications for morphine.

Administration

- A dose of 20 mg opium alkaloids hydrochlorides is therapeutically equivalent to 15 mg morphine.

OPIUM, POWDERED

OPIUM TINCTURE (LAUDANUM)

(oh′pee-um)

Trade name: Deodorized Opium Tincture

Classifications: CNS AGENT; NARCOTIC (OPIATE) AGONIST ANALGESIC; ANTIDIARRHEAL

Pregnancy category: B

Controlled substance: Schedule II

ACTIONS/PHARMACODYNAMICS Opium obtained from the unripe capsules of *Papaver somniferum* or *Papaver album* contains several natural alkaloids including morphine, codeine, papaverine. Antidiarrheal effects are due to inhibition of GI motility and propulsion. These actions lead to prolonged transit of intestinal contents, desiccation of feces, and constipation.

USES Symptomatic treatment of acute diarrhea and to treat severe withdrawal symptoms in neonates born to women addicted to opiates.

ROUTE & DOSAGE

Acute Diarrhea
Adult: **PO** 0.6 ml q.i.d. up to 1 ml q.i.d. (max 6 ml/d).
Child: **PO** 0.005–0.01 ml/kg q3–4h (max 6 doses/24 h).

Neonatal Withdrawal
Child: **PO** make a 1:25 aqueous dilution; then give 3–6 drops q3–6h as needed or 0.2 ml q3h; dose may be increased by 0.05 ml q3h until withdrawal symptoms are controlled; gradually decrease dose after withdrawal symptoms have stabilized.

PHARMACOKINETICS **Absorption:** variable absorption from GI tract. **Distribution:** crosses placenta; distributed into breast milk. **Metabolism:** metabolized in liver. **Elimination:** excreted in urine.

CONTRAINDICATIONS & PRECAUTIONS **Contraindicated in:** diarrhea caused by poisoning (until poison is completely eliminated); pregnancy (category B). **Cautious use in:** history of opiate agonist dependence; asthma, severe prostatic hypertrophy, hepatic disease.

ADVERSE/SIDE EFFECTS Nausea and other GI disturbances. **Acute toxicity:** depression of CNS.

DRUG INTERACTIONS **Alcohol** and other CNS DEPRESSANTS add to CNS effects.

NURSING IMPLICATIONS

Administration

- Do not confuse this preparation with camphorated opium tincture (paregoric), which contains only 2 mg anhydrous morphine/5 ml, thus requiring a higher dose volume than that required for therapeutic dose of Deodorized Opium Tincture.
- Give drug diluted with about one third glass of water to ensure passage of entire dose into stomach.
- Preserve in tight, light-resistant containers.

Assessment & Drug Effects

- If respirations are 12/min or below or have changed in character and rate, withhold medication and report to physician.
- Note character and frequency of stools; drug should be discontinued as soon as diarrhea is controlled.
- Frequently offer small amounts of fluid but attempt to maintain 3000–4000 ml fluid total in 24 h.
- Monitor body weight, I&O ratio and pattern, and temperature. If patient develops fever of 38.8C (102F) or above, electrolyte and hydration levels may need to be evaluated. Consult physician.

Patient & Family Education

- Inform that constipation may be a consequence of antidiarrheal therapy but that normal habit pattern usually is reestablished with resumption of normal dietary intake.
- Addiction is possible with prolonged use or with drug abuse.

OPRELVEKIN

(o-prel′ve-kin)

Trade name: Neumega

Classifications: BLOOD FORMER; HEMATOPOIETIC GROWTH FACTOR

Prototype: Epoetin Alfa

Pregnancy category: C

ACTIONS/PHARMACODYNAMICS Oprelvekin (interleukin-11), produced by recombinant DNA, is a hematopoietic growth factor. Increases platelet count in a dose-dependent manner.

USE Prevention of severe thrombocytopenia following myelosuppressive chemotherapy.

ROUTE & DOSAGE

Thrombocytopenia

Adult: **SC** 50 μg/kg once daily starting 6–24 h after completing chemotherapy and continuing until platelet count is ≥50,000 cells/μl or up to 21 d.
Child 8 mo–17 y: **SC** 75–100 μg/kg once daily starting 6–24 h after completing chemotherapy and continuing until platelet count is ≥50,000 cells/μl or up to 21 d.

PHARMACOKINETICS **Absorption:** 80% absorbed from SC injection site. **Onset:** days 5–9. **Duration:** 7 d after last dose. **Distribution:** distributes to highly perfused organs. **Elimination:** half-life: 6.9 h; excreted in urine.

CONTRAINDICATIONS & PRECAUTIONS **Contraindicated in:** hypersensitivity to oprelvekin, pregnancy (category C), lactation, myeloablative chemotherapy. **Cautious use in:** patients with left ventricular dysfunction, CHF, history of atrial arrhythmias, or other arrhythmias; respiratory disease; thromboembolic disorders; elderly; hepatic or renal dysfunction.

ADVERSE/SIDE EFFECTS Body as whole: *edema, neutropenic fever, fever,* asthenia, pain, chills, myalgia, bone pain. **CNS:** *headache, dizziness, insomnia,* nervousness. **CV:** *tachycardia,* vasodilation, palpitations, syncope, atrial fibrillation/flutter. **GI:** *nausea, vomiting, mucositis, diarrhea,* oral moniliasis, anorexia, constipation, dyspepsia. **Hematologic:** ecchymosis. **Respiratory:** *dyspnea, rhinitis, cough, pharyngitis,* pleural effusion. **Skin:** alopecia, *rash,* skin discoloration, exfoliative dermatitis. **Other:** conjunctival injection, amblyopia, dehydration.

NURSING IMPLICATIONS

Administration

- Reconstitute solution by gently injecting 1 ml of sterile water for injection (without preservative) toward the sides of the vial. Keep needle in vial and gently swirl to dissolve but do not shake solution. Without removing needle, withdraw specified amount of oprelvekin for injection.
- SC injection: Give as single dose into the abdomen, thigh, hip, or upper arm.
- Reconstituted solution must be used within 3 h; store at 2–8C (36–46F) until used.
- Do not use if solution is discolored or if it contains particulate matter.
- Discard any unused portion of the vial. It contains no preservatives.
- Store unopened vials at 2–8C (36–46F). Do not freeze.

Assessment & Drug Effects

- Therapeutic effectiveness is indicated by return of postnadir platelet count toward normal (≥50,000).
- Lab tests: Monitor platelet counts until adequate recovery; periodically monitor CBC with differential and serum electrolytes.
- Carefully monitor for and immediately report S&S of fluid overload, hypokalemia, and cardiac arrhythmias.
- Carefully monitor persons with preexisting fluid retention (e.g., CHF, pleural effusion, ascites) for worsening of symptoms.

Patient & Family Education

- Carefully review patient information leaflet with special attention to administration directions.
- Report any of the following to the physician: shortness of breath, edema of arms and/or legs, chest pain, unusual fatigue or weakness, irregular heartbeat, blurred vision.

O

ORAL CONTRACEPTIVES (ESTROGEN–PROGESTIN COMBINATIONS)

Trade names: Alesse, Brevicon, Demulen, Enovid, Estrostep, Loestrin, Mircette, Modicon, Norinyl, Norlestrin, Ortho-Novum, Ovcon, Ovral, Tri-Norinyl, Triphasic, Desogen, Orthocept, Ortho-Cyclen, Ortho-Tri-Cyclen, Preven, and others

Classifications: HORMONES; ESTROGEN-PROGESTIN COMBINATIONS

Prototypes: Estradiol, progesterone

Pregnancy category: X

ACTIONS/PHARMACODYNAMICS

Fixed combination of estrogen and progestin produces contraception by preventing ovulation and rendering reproductive tract structures hostile to sperm penetration and zygote implantation. Three types of estrogen-progestin combinations are available: (1) monophasic, fixed dosage of estrogen-progestin throughout the cycle; (2) biphasic, amount of estrogen remains the same throughout cycle, less progestin in first half of cycle and increased progestin in second half; (3) triphasic, estrogen amount is the same or varies throughout cycle, progestin amount varies.

USES To prevent conception and to treat hypermenorrhea and endometriosis; postcoital contraceptive or "morning after pill"; moderate acne in females ≥ 15 y (Tri-Cylen).

ROUTE & DOSAGE

Contraception

Adult: **PO** 1 active tablet daily for 21 d; then placebo tablet or no tablets for 7 d; repeat cycle.

Postcoital Contraception (Preven, Ovral)

Adult: **PO** 2 tablets within 72 h of intercourse; then 2 tablets 12 h later.

PHARMACOKINETICS Absorption: readily absorbed from GI tract. **Distribution:** widely distributed; crosses placenta; small amount distributed into breast milk. **Metabolism:** metabolized in liver. **Elimination:** half-life: 6–45 h; excreted in urine and feces.

CONTRAINDICATIONS & PRECAUTIONS Contraindicated in: pregnancy (category X), nursing mothers, missed abortion. Familial or personal history of or existence of breast or other estrogen-dependent neoplasm, recurrent chronic cystic mastitis, history of or existence of thrombophlebitis or thromboembolic disorders, cerebral vascular or coronary artery disease, MI, serious hepatic dysfunction, hepatic neoplasm, family history of hepatic porphyria, undiagnosed abnormal vaginal bleeding, women age 40 and over, adolescents with incomplete epiphyseal closure. **Cautious use in:** history of depression, preexisting hypertension, or cardiac or renal disease; impaired liver function, history of migraine, convulsive disorders, or asthma; multiparous women with grossly irregular menses, diabetes, or familial history of diabetes; gallbladder disease, lupus erythematosus, rheumatic disease, varicosities, smokers.

ADVERSE/SIDE EFFECTS CV: malignant hypertension, thrombotic and thromboembolic disorders, *mild to moderate increase in BP,* increase in size of varicosities, edema. **Eye:** unexplained loss of vision, optic neuritis, proptosis, diplopia, change in corneal curvature (steepening), intolerance to contact lenses, retinal thrombosis, papilledema. **GI:** *nausea,* cholelithiasis, gallbladder disease, cholestatic jaundice, benign hepatic adenomas; diarrhea, constipation, abdominal cramps. **GU:** ureteral dilation, increased incidence of urinary tract infection, hemolytic uremia syndrome, renal failure. **Metabolic:** *decreased glucose tolerance,* pyridoxine deficiency (see also diagnostic test interferences). **Reproductive:** increased risk of congenital anomalies, decreased quality and quantity of breast milk, dysmenorrhea, increased size of preexisting uterine fibroids, *menstrual disorders.* **Estrogen excess:** *nausea;* bloating, menstrual tension, cervical mucorrhea, polyposis, *chloasma, hypertension,* migraine headache, breast fullness or tenderness, *edema.* **Estrogen deficiency:** hypomenorrhea, *early or midcycle breakthrough bleeding,* increased spotting. **Progestin excess:** hypomenorrhea, breast regression, *vaginal candidiasis,* depression, fa-

O

tigue, weight gain, increased appetite, acne, oily scalp, hair loss. **Progestin deficiency:** late-cycle breakthrough bleeding, amenorrhea. **Other:** rash (allergic), paresthesias, photosensitivity (photoallergy or phototoxicity), acute intermittent porphyria.

DIAGNOSTIC TEST INTERFERENCE Oral contraceptives increase ***BSP*** retention, ***prothrombin*** and ***coagulation factors II, VII, VIII, IX, X; platelet aggregability, thyroid-binding globulin, PBI, T_4; transcortin; corticosteroid, triglyceride*** and ***phospholipid*** levels; ***ceruloplasmin, aldosterone, amylase, transferrin; renin*** activity, ***vitamin A.*** OCs decrease ***antithrombin III, T_3*** resin uptake, ***serum folate, glucose tolerance, albumin, vitamin B_{12}*** and reduce the ***metyrapone*** test response.

O

DRUG INTERACTIONS Aminocaproic acid may increase clotting factors, leading to hypercoagulable state; BARBITURATES, ANTICONVULSANTS, ANTIBIOTICS, **rifampin,** ANTIFUNGALS reduce efficacy of OCs and increase incidence of breakthrough bleeding and risk of pregnancy.

NURSING IMPLICATIONS

Administration

- Medication may be given without regard to meals.
- Intervals between one dose and the next should not exceed 24 h.

Assessment & Drug Effects

- Complete medical and family history should be taken prior to initiation of OC therapy. Baseline and periodic physical examination should include BP, breasts, abdomen, pelvis, Pap smear, and other relevant tests.
- Pregnancy should be ruled out before oral contraceptive therapy is begun.
- Check BP periodically. In some women, changes in BP occur within each cycle; in others, slow increase of pressure, particularly diastolic, over several months is significant. Drug-induced BP elevation is usually reversible with cessation of OC.
- Nausea with or without vomiting occurs in approximately 10% of patients during the first cycle and is reportedly one of the major reasons for voluntary discontinuation of therapy. Most side effects tend to disappear in third or fourth cycle of use. Instruct patient to report symptoms that persist after fourth cycle. Dose adjustment or a different product may be indicated.
- Hirsutism and loss of hair are reversible with discontinuation of OC or by change of selected combination.
- Acne may improve, worsen, or develop for first time. In women on OC for at least 1 y, postcontraceptive acne sometimes occurs 3–4 mo after stopping drug and may continue for 6–12 mo.
- Anovulation or amenorrhea following termination of OC regimen may persist more than 6 mo. The user with pretreatment oligomenorrhea or secondary amenorrhea is most apt to have oversuppression syndrome.
- Oral contraception may mask onset of climacteric. To determine if it has started, physician may advise patient to discontinue pill and to use alternate method of contraception. If menstruation occurs, the pill is indicated.

Patient & Family Education

- Tablets should be taken regularly at 24-h intervals (e.g., with a meal or at bedtime).

- In the first week of the initial cycle, patient should also use an additional method of birth control.
- If user forgets to take a tablet, she should take it as soon as she remembers or should take 2 tablets the next day. If 2 consecutive tablets are omitted, she should take 2 tablets daily for the next 2 days, then resume the regular schedule. If 3 consecutive tablets are missed, she should begin a new compact of tablets, starting 7 d after last tablet was taken.
- Use an additional form of birth control for 7 d after 2 missed doses or 14 d after 3 missed doses.
- Ovulation is unlikely with omission of 1 daily dose; however, the possibility of escaped ovulation, spotting, or breakthrough bleeding increases with each missed dose.
- If intracycle bleeding resembling menstruation occurs, patient should discontinue medication, then begin taking tablets from a new compact on day 5. If bleeding persists, advise patient to see physician.
- If 2 consecutive periods should be missed, user should see physician to rule out pregnancy before continuing on OC.
- If possible, hormone contraception should not be used until infant is weaned; alternate method of birth control should be used during this period.
- Oral contraception can be started immediately after delivery in the nonnursing mother.
- Urge patient not to skip scheduled visits for physical checkups while on contraceptive therapy. Teach breast self-examination and emphasize importance of doing this every month.
- Users with clinical conditions worsened by fluid retention should report exacerbation of symptoms promptly. Frequent weight checks should be recorded to permit early recognition of fluid retention.
- Inform of the increased risk of thromboembolic and cardiovascular problems and increased incidence of gallbladder disease with OC use.
- Teach how to elicit Homans' sign and to be alert to other manifestations of thrombotic or thromboembolic disorders: severe headache (especially if persistent and recurrent), dizziness, blurred vision, leg or chest pain, respiratory distress, unexplained cough. Advise patient to withhold drug if any of these symptoms appear and to report them promptly to physician.
- Sudden abdominal pain should be reported immediately to rule out ectopic pregnancy.
- Ophthalmic sequelae can occur as soon as 24 h after initiation of oral contraception. Advise patient to stop the drug and contact physician if unexplained partial or complete, sudden or gradual loss of vision, protrusion of eyeballs (proptosis), or diplopia occurs.
- Leukorrhea is an expected physical reaction to the OC; however, if OC use is accompanied by vaginal itching and irritation, candidiasis should be ruled out. Caution patient to report discomfort promptly.
- Instruct the diabetic to report positive urine or blood glucose test to physician. Adjustment of antidiabetic medication may be necessary. The potential diabetic (family history) should also be closely observed for onset of diabetes.
- Smokers who are OC users have a fivefold greater risk of fatal MI than nonsmoker OC users and a tenfold greater risk than non-OC users who are nonsmokers. The risk increases with age (marked in

women >35 y) and with heavy smoking (15 or more cigarettes/d).

ORPHENADRINE CITRATE

(or-fen'a-dreen)

Trade names: Banflex, Flexon, Myolin, Norflex

Classifications: AUTONOMIC NERVOUS SYSTEM AGENT; ANTICHOLINERGIC (PARASYMPATHOLYTIC); CENTRAL-ACTING SKELETAL MUSCLE RELAXANT

Prototype: Cyclobenzaprine

Pregnancy category: C

ACTIONS/PHARMACODYNAMICS Tertiary amine anticholinergic agent and central-acting skeletal muscle relaxant. Relaxes tense skeletal muscles indirectly, possibly by analgesic action or by atropinelike central action. Has some local anesthetic and antihistaminic activity but less than that of diphenhydramine. Also produces slight euphoria.

O

USE To relieve muscle spasm discomfort associated with acute musculoskeletal conditions.

ROUTE & DOSAGE

Muscle Spasm

Adult: **PO** 100 mg b.i.d. **IM/IV** 60 mg; may repeat in 12 h if needed.

PHARMACOKINETICS Absorption: readily absorbed from GI tract. **Peak:** 2 h. **Duration:** 4–6 h. **Distribution:** rapidly distributed in tissues; crosses placenta. **Metabolism:** metabolized in liver. **Elimination:** half-life: 14 h; excreted in urine.

CONTRAINDICATIONS & PRECAUTIONS Contraindicated in: narrow-angle glaucoma; pyloric or duodenal obstruction, stenosing peptic ulcers; prostatic hypertrophy or bladder neck obstruction; myasthenia gravis; cardiospasm (megaloesophagus). Safe use during pregnancy (category C) and in the pediatric age group not established. **Cautious use in:** history of tachycardia, cardiac decompensation, arrhythmias, coronary insufficiency.

ADVERSE/SIDE EFFECTS CNS: *drowsiness,* weakness, headache, dizziness; mild CNS stimulation (high doses): restlessness, anxiety, tremors, confusion, hallucinations, agitation, tachycardia, palpitation, syncope. **Eye:** increased ocular tension, dilated pupils, blurred vision. **GI:** *dry mouth,* nausea, vomiting, abdominal cramps, constipation. **GU:** *urinary hesitancy or retention.* **Hypersensitivity:** pruritus, urticaria, rash, <u>anaphylactic reaction</u> (rare).

DRUG INTERACTIONS Propoxyphene may cause increased confusion, anxiety, and tremors.

NURSING IMPLICATIONS

Administration

- Sustained-release tablets must be swallowed whole.
- Orphenadrine citrate and orphenadrine hydrochloride are not interchangeable.
- IV orphenadrine may be given by direct IV undiluted at a rate of 60 mg (2 ml) over 5 min.
- Protect orphenadrine from light.

Assessment & Drug Effects

- Periodic studies of blood, urine, and liver function are recommended with prolonged therapy.
- Complaints of mouth dryness, urinary hesitancy or retention, headache, tremors, GI problems, palpitation, or rapid pulse should be communicated to physician. Dosage reduction or drug withdrawal is indicated.

- The elderly patient is particularly sensitive to anticholinergic effects (urinary hesitancy, constipation) and therefore should be closely observed. Have patient void before taking drug.
- Keep physician informed of therapeutic drug effect. In the patient with parkinsonism, orphenadrine reduces muscular rigidity but has little effect on tremors. Some reduction in excessive salivation and perspiration may occur, and patient may appear mildly euphoric.

Patient & Family Education

- Mouth dryness may be relieved by frequent rinsing with clear tepid water, increasing noncaloric fluid intake, sugarless gum, or lemondrops. If these measures fail, a saliva substitute may help.
- Caution to avoid potentially hazardous activities until reaction to drug is known.
- Warn that concomitant use of alcohol and other CNS depressants may potentiate depressant effects.

OXACILLIN SODIUM

(ox-a-sill'in)

Trade names: Bactocill, Prostaphlin
Classifications: ANTIINFECTIVE; BETA-LACTAM ANTIBIOTIC; PENICILLIN; ANTISTAPHYLOCOCCAL PENICILLIN
Prototype: Penicillin G
Pregnancy category: B

ACTIONS/PHARMACODYNAMICS Semisynthetic, acid-stable, penicillinase-resistant isoxazoyl penicillin. In common with other isoxazoyl penicillins (cloxacillin, dicloxacillin), it is highly active against most penicillinase-producing staphylococci, is less potent than penicillin G against penicillin-sensitive microorganisms, and is generally ineffective against gram-negative bacteria and methicillin-resistant staphylococci.

USES Primarily, infections caused by penicillinase-producing staphylococci and penicillin-resistant staphylococci. May be used to initiate therapy in suspected staphylococcal infections pending culture and sensitivity test results. As with other penicillins, serum concentrations are enhanced by concurrent use of probenecid.

ROUTE & DOSAGE

Staphylococcal Infections
Adult: **IM/IV** 500 mg–2 g q4–6h up to 12 g/d; **PO** 250–1000 mg q4–6h.
Child: **IM/IV** 50–150 mg/kg/d divided q4–6h; **PO** 50–100 mg/kg/d in 4 divided doses.
Neonate: **IV** 50–100 mg/kg/d divided q6–12h.

PHARMACOKINETICS Absorption: incompletely and erratically absorbed orally. **Peak:** 30–120 min IM; 15 min IV. **Duration:** 4 h PO; 4–6 h IM. **Distribution:** distributes into CNS with inflamed meninges; crosses placenta; distributed into breast milk. **Metabolism:** enters enterohepatic circulation. **Elimination:** half-life: 0.5–1 h; primarily excreted in urine, some in bile.

CONTRAINDICATIONS & PRECAUTIONS Contraindicated in: hypersensitivity to penicillins or cephalosporins. Safe use during pregnancy (category B) not established. **Cautious use in:** history of or suspected atopy or allergy (hives, eczema, hay fever, asthma); premature infants, neonates.

ADVERSE/SIDE EFFECTS Nausea, vomiting, flatulence, *diarrhea*. **High-dose therapy:** interstitial nephritis, transient hematuria, albuminuria, azotemia (newborns and infants on high doses); thrombophlebitis (IV therapy), superinfections. **Hypersensitivity:** pruritus, rash, urticaria, wheezing, sneezing, fever, anaphylaxis; hepatocellular dysfunction (elevated AST, ALT, hepatitis), eosinophilia, leukopenia, thrombocytopenia, granulocytopenia, agranulocytosis; neutropenia (reported in children).

DIAGNOSTIC TEST INTERFERENCE

Oxacillin in large doses can cause false-positive ***urine protein tests*** using sulfosalicylic acid methods.

INCOMPATIBILITIES

Solution/additive: cytarabine, TETRACYCLINES. **Y-site: verapamil.**

NURSING IMPLICATIONS

Administration

- Oral oxacillin is best taken with a full glass of water on an empty stomach (either 1 h before meals or 2 h after meals). Food reduces absorption.
- Following reconstitution of oral solution, it is stable for 3 d at room temperature and for 14 d if refrigerated. Container should be so labeled and dated.
- For IM administration, reconstitute each 250 mg with 1.4 ml sterile water for injection and indicate date and time of reconstitution on vial. Shake vial vigorously until drug is completely dissolved. Discard unused portions after 3 d at room temperature or 7 d under refrigeration. Do not use undated vials.
- IM administration: Administer IM to adults by deep intragluteal injection. Follow agency policy for IM site in young children and infants. Injection into or near a major peripheral nerve or blood vessel can cause neurovascular damage. Rotate injection sites.
- IV preparation: For direct IV administration, reconstitute with sterile water for injection or isotonic NaCl by adding 1.4 ml of diluent to each 250 mg. The resulting concentration (250 mg/1.5 ml) is further diluted by adding 5 ml to each 500 mg or fraction thereof.
- Reconstituted and properly diluted solution may be given by direct IV at a rate of 1 g or fraction thereof over 10 min.
- For IV infusion, the reconstituted solution is added to a compatible IV solution (e.g., isotonic NaCl, D5W, NS, lactated Ringer's injection, or others recommended by manufacturer) and infused over 6 h.
- IV administration to neonates, infants, children: Verify correct IV concentration and rate of infusion/injection with physician.
- The total sodium content (including that contributed by buffer) in each gram of oxacillin is approximately 3.1 mEq or 71 mg.

Assessment & Drug Effects

- Prior to first dose inquiry should be made concerning hypersensitivity reactions to penicillins, cephalosporins, and other allergens.
- Hepatic dysfunction (possibly a hypersensitivity reaction) has been associated with IV oxacillin; it is reversible with discontinuation of drug. Symptoms may resemble viral hepatitis or general signs of hypersensitivity and should be reported promptly: hives, rash, fever, nausea, vomiting, abdominal discomfort, anorexia, malaise, jaundice (with dark yellow to brown urine, light-colored or clay-colored stools, pruritus).
- Withhold next drug dose and report the onset of hypersensitivity

O

reactions and superinfections (see Appendix G).

Patient & Family Education

- Instruct to take the oral medication around the clock, not to miss a dose, and to continue taking it until it is all gone unless otherwise directed by physician.
- Instruct on prolonged therapy to report symptoms of agranulocytosis (see Appendix G).

OXAMNIQUINE

(ox-am′ni-kwin)

Trade name: Vansil

Classifications: ANTIINFECTIVE; ANTHELMINTIC

Prototype: Mebendazole

Pregnancy category: C

ACTIONS/PHARMACODYNAMICS Tetrahydroquinone derivative prepared in the presence of *Aspergillus sclerotiorum*. Mechanism of action not fully explained, but it appears that drug-induced strong contractions and paralysis of worm musculature leads to immobilization of their suckers and dislodgment from their usual residence in mesenteric veins to the liver. Dislodgment of schistosomes begins about 2 d after single oral dose of oxamniquine; movement is not complete until 6 d after treatment with the drug. After treatment, surviving unpaired females return to mesenteric vessels; however, oviposition (egg laying) seems to stop in 24–48 h after drug treatment, reducing egg load and removing principal cause of pathology associated with schistosomal infection.

USES All stages of *Schistosoma mansoni* infection, including acute and chronic phases with hepatosplenic involvement.

ROUTE & DOSAGE

Schistosomiasis

Adult: **PO** 12–15 mg/kg as single dose.
Child: **PO** <30 kg, 10 mg/kg x 2 doses at 2–8 h intervals.

PHARMACOKINETICS Absorption: readily absorbed from GI tract. **Peak:** 1–3 h. **Metabolism:** extensively metabolized in GI mucosa. **Elimination:** half-life: 1–2.5 h; excreted in urine.

CONTRAINDICATIONS & PRECAUTIONS Contraindicated in: safe use during pregnancy (category C) and lactation or in children not established. **Cautious use in:** history of convulsant disorders.

ADVERSE/SIDE EFFECTS CNS: *transitory dizziness, drowsiness, headache;* persistent fever (in patients being treated in Egypt); EEG abnormalities, convulsions (rare). **GI:** anorexia, nausea, vomiting, abdominal pain. **Hematologic:** increased erythrocyte sedimentation rate, reticulocyte count, and increased or decreased leukocyte count. **Other:** urticaria, elevated liver enzyme concentrations, red-orange urine.

FOOD–DRUG INTERACTION Rate and extent of absorption are decreased by food.

NURSING IMPLICATIONS

Administration

- Administer with food if necessary to reduce GI distress and improve tolerance.
- Store product in tightly closed container at controlled room temperature less than 30C (86F).

Assessment & Drug Effects

- Since > 30% of patients experience

O

dizziness or drowsiness, supervision of ambulation and other safety precautions may be warranted.

Patient & Family Education

- Because drug can cause dizziness or drowsiness, advise to use caution while driving or performing other tasks requiring alertness.
- Inform that drug may change the normal urine color to a harmless orange-red.
- If patient has a history of seizures, the possibility of seizures is increased because of drug action (occur within hours of drug administration).

OXANDROLONE

(ox-an′dro-lone)

Trade name: Oxadrin

Classifications: SYNTHETIC HORMONE; ANDROGEN/ANABOLIC STEROID

Prototype: Testosterone

Pregnancy category: X

Controlled substance: Schedule III

ACTIONS/PHARMACODYNAMICS Synthetic steroid with anabolic and androgenic activity. Pharmacodynamics, contraindications, and precautions are similar to those of testosterone.

USES Adjunctive therapy to promote weight gain, offset protein catabolism associated with prolonged administration of corticosteroids, relieve bone pain accompanying osteoporosis.

ROUTE & DOSAGE

Weight Gain

Adult: **PO** 2.5 mg b.i.d. to q.i.d. (max 20 mg/d) for 2–4 wk.
Child: **PO** ≤0.1 mg/kg/d.

ADVERSE/SIDE EFFECTS CNS: habituation, excitation, insomnia, depression, changes in libido. **GU:** *males:* phallic enlargement, increased frequency or persistence of erections, inhibition of testicular function, testicular atrophy, oligospermia, impotence, chronic priapism, epididymitis, bladder irritability; *females:* clitoral enlargement, menstrual irregularities. **Hepatic:** cholestatic jaundice with or without <u>hepatic necrosis and death, hepatocellular neoplasms, peliosis hepatitis (long-term use)</u>. **Skin:** hirsutism and male pattern baldness in females, acne. **Other:** gynecomastia, deepening of voice in females, premature closure of epiphyses in children , edema, decreased glucose tolerance.

DRUG INTERACTIONS May increase sensitivity to ORAL ANTICOAGULANTS. May inhibit metabolism of ORAL HYPOGLYCEMIC AGENTS. Concomitant STEROIDS may increase edema.

DIAGNOSTIC TEST INTERFERENCE May decrease levels of thyroxine-binding globulin (decreased total T_4 and increased T_3RU and free T_4).

NURSING IMPLICATIONS

Administration

- Doses may need to be individualized as great variations in response exist.
- Store at 15–30C (59–86F).

Assessment & Drug Effects

- Closely monitor weight throughout therapy.
- Assess for and report development of edema or S&S of jaundice (see Appendix G).
- Periodically monitor liver function tests, lipid profile, Hct and Hgb, PT and INR, fluid and electrolyte status, and CPK.
- If hypercalcemia develops in

breast cancer patient, withhold drug and notify physician.

- X-ray exams of bone age should be done every 6 months in children to monitor bone maturation.

Patient & Family Education

- Instruct women to report signs of virilization, including acne and changes in menstrual periods.
- Instruct men to report too frequent or prolonged erections or appearance/worsening of acne.
- Advise to report S&S of jaundice (see Appendix G) or edema.
- Advise diabetics using oral agents to closely monitor for S&S of hypoglycemia.

OXAPROZIN

(ox-a-pro′zin)

Trade name: Daypro

Classifications: CNS AGENT; ANALGESIC, ANTIPYRETIC, NSAID

Prototype: Ibuprofen

Pregnancy category: C

ACTIONS/PHARMACODYNAMICS Long-acting NSAID agent, effective prostaglandin synthetase inhibitor. Mode of action presumed due to inhibition of prostaglandin E_2 synthesis at site of inflammation. Has antipyretic and analgesic properties.

USES Treatment of osteoarthritis and rheumatoid arthritis. **Unlabeled uses:** ankylosing spondylitis, chronic pain, gout, oral surgery pain, temporal arteritis, tendinitis.

ROUTE & DOSAGE

Osteoarthritis, Rheumatoid Arthritis

Adult: **PO** 600–1200 mg q.d. (max 1800 mg/d).

PHARMACOKINETICS **Absorption:** readily absorbed from GI tract. **Onset:** 1–6 wk for therapeutic effect. **Distribution:** 99% protein bound. Distributes into synovial fluid, crosses placenta. Distributed into breast milk. **Metabolism:** metabolized in the liver. **Elimination:** half-life: 40 h; 60% excreted in urine, 30–35% excreted in feces.

CONTRAINDICATIONS & PRECAUTIONS **Contraindicated in:** hypersensitivity to oxaprozin or any other NSAID; complete or partial syndrome of nasal polyps; angioedema. **Cautious use in:** history of GI bleeding, alcoholism, smoking; history of severe hepatic dysfunction, renal insufficiency; photosensitivity; pregnancy (category C), nursing mothers, elderly patients. Safety and effectiveness in children have not been established.

ADVERSE/SIDE EFFECTS **CNS:** tinnitus, headache, insomnia, somnolence. **GI:** diarrhea, abdominal pain, nausea, dyspepsia, flatulence, melena, ulcers, constipation, dry mouth, gastritis. **Other:** rash, pruritus, dysuria, urinary frequency.

DIAGNOSTIC TEST INTERFERENCE May cause false positive reactions for BENZODIAZEPINES with urine drug-screening tests.

DRUG INTERACTIONS May attenuate the antihypertensive response to DIURETICS. NSAIDS increase the risk of **methotrexate or lithium** toxicity. May increase **aspirin** toxicity.

NURSING IMPLICATIONS

Administration

- Although specific starting doses are recommended, individual variations in response to oxaprozin warrant individualization of dosage.

- Divided doses may be tried in those unable to tolerate once-daily dosing.
- Lower starting doses are recommended for those with renal or hepatic dysfunction, advanced age, low body weight, or a predisposition to GI ulceration.
- Oxaprozin may be given with meals or milk to decrease GI distress.
- The maximum recommended daily dose is 1800 mg or 25 mg/kg, whichever is *lower*.
- Store below 30°C/86°F in a tight, light-resistant container.

Assessment & Drug Effects

- Monitor for signs and symptoms of GI bleeding, especially in patients with a history of inflammation or ulceration of upper GI tract, or those treated chronically with NSAIDs.
- Monitor patients with CHF for increased fluid retention and edema. Report rapid weight increases accompanied by edema.
- Baseline and periodic evaluation of Hgb, renal and hepatic function, and auditory and ophthalmologic examinations are recommended with prolonged or high-dose therapy.

Patient & Family Education

- Inform that alcoholism and smoking increase risk of GI ulceration.
- Instruct to report immediately dark tarry stools, "coffee ground" or bloody emesis, or other GI distress.
- Instruct to avoid aspirin or other NSAIDs without explicit permission of physician.
- Inform about possibility of photosensitivity, which results in a rash on sun-exposed skin.
- Instruct to immediately report tinnitus, decreased hearing, or blurred vision.
- Inform that goal of therapy is lowest effective dose.

OXAZEPAM

(ox-a′ze-pam)

Trade names: Ox-Pam♣, Serax, Zapex♣

Classifications: CNS AGENT; ANXIOLYTIC; SEDATIVE-HYPNOTIC; BENZODIAZEPINE

Prototype: Lorazepam

Pregnancy category: C

Controlled substance: Schedule IV

ACTIONS/PHARMACODYNAMICS Benzodiazepine derivative related to lorazepam with which it shares actions, uses, limitations, and interactions.

USES Management of anxiety and tension associated with a wide range of emotional disturbances. Also to control acute withdrawal symptoms in chronic alcoholism.

ROUTE & DOSAGE

Anxiety

Adult: **PO** 10–30 mg t.i.d. or q.i.d.

Acute Alcohol Withdrawal

Adult: **PO** 15–30 mg t.i.d. or q.i.d.

PHARMACOKINETICS **Absorption:** readily absorbed from GI tract. **Peak:** 2–3 h. **Distribution:** crosses placenta; distributed into breast milk. **Metabolism:** metabolized in liver. **Elimination:** half-life: 2–8 h; primarily excreted in urine, some in feces.

CONTRAINDICATIONS & PRECAUTIONS **Contraindicated in:** hypersensitivity to oxazepam and other benzodiazepines; psychoses, pregnancy (category C), nursing mothers, children < 12 y; acute-angle glaucoma, acute alcohol intoxication. **Cautious use in:** elderly and debilitated patients; impaired renal and hepatic function; addiction-prone patients; COPD; mental depression.

ADVERSE/SIDE EFFECTS Usually infrequent and mild. **CNS:** *drowsiness,* dizziness, mental confusion, vertigo, ataxia, headache, lethargy, syncope, tremor, slurred speech, paradoxic reaction (euphoria, excitement). **GI:** nausea, xerostomia, jaundice. **Other:** skin rash, edema, hypotension, leukopenia, altered libido, edema.

DRUG INTERACTIONS **Alcohol,** CNS DEPRESSANTS, ANTICONVULSANTS potentiate CNS depression; **cimetidine** increases oxazepam plasma levels, increasing its toxicity; may decrease antiparkinsonism effects of **levodopa;** may increase **phenytoin** levels; smoking decreases sedative and antianxiety effects.

NURSING IMPLICATIONS

Administration

- Oxazepam may be given with food if GI upset occurs.
- Store in tightly closed container at 15–30C (59–86F) unless otherwise specified.

Assessment & Drug Effects

- Elderly patients should be observed closely for signs of overdosage. Report to physician if daytime psychomotor function is depressed.
- Liver function tests and blood counts should be performed on a regular planned basis.
- Excessive and prolonged use may cause physical dependence.

Patient & Family Education

- Mild paradoxic stimulation of affect and excitement with sleep disturbances may occur within the first 2 wk of therapy. Report promptly. Dosage reduction is indicated.
- Instruct not to change dose or dose schedule and to refrain from using drug to treat a self-diagnosed condition.
- Advise to consult physician before self-medicating with OTC drugs.
- Caution against driving a car or operating dangerous machinery until response to drug has been evaluated.
- Warn not to drink alcoholic beverages while being treated with oxazepam. The CNS depressant effects of each agent may be intensified.
- Advise that if she becomes pregnant during therapy or intends to become pregnant, patient should communicate with her physician about the desirability of discontinuing the drug.
- Following prolonged therapy, drug should be withdrawn slowly to avoid precipitating withdrawal symptoms (seizures, mental confusion, nausea, vomiting, muscle and abdominal cramps, tremulousness, sleep disturbances, unusual irritability, hyperhidrosis).

OXICONAZOLE NITRATE

(ox-i-con′a-zole)

Trade name: Oxistat

Classifications: SKIN AGENT; ANTIFUNGAL

Prototype: Fluconazole

Pregnancy category: B

ACTIONS/PHARMACODYNAMICS Oxiconazole is a synthetic antifungal agent. It presumably works by altering cellular membranes, resulting in increased membrane permeability, secondary metabolic effects, and growth inhibition.

USES Topical treatment of tinea pedis, tinea cruris, and tinea corporis due to *Trichophyton rubrum* and *Trichophyton mentagrophytes;* also used for cutaneous candidiasis caused by *Candida albicans* and *Candida tropicalis.*

ROUTE & DOSAGE

Tinea and Other Dermal Infections
Adult: **Topical** Apply to affected area once daily in the evening.

PHARMACOKINETICS Absorption: < 0.3% is absorbed systemically.

CONTRAINDICATIONS & PRECAUTIONS Contraindicated in: hypersensitivity to oxiconazole. **Cautious use in:** pregnancy (category B) and nursing mothers.

ADVERSE/SIDE EFFECTS Transient burning and stinging, dryness, erythema, pruritus, and local irritation.

NURSING IMPLICATIONS

Administration

- Apply cream to cover the affected areas once daily (in the evening).
- Tinea corporis and tinea cruris should be treated for 2 wk and tinea pedis should be treated for 1 mo to reduce the possibility of recurrence.
- Store at 15–30C (59–86F).

Patient & Family Education

- Medication is for external use only. Do not use intravaginally.
- If irritation or sensitivity develops, discontinue drug and contact physician.
- Avoid contact with eyes.
- If no improvement is noted after the prescribed treatment period, the physician should be consulted.

OXTRIPHYLLINE

(ox-trye'fi-lin)
Trade names: Choledyl, Choledyl-SA, Choline Theophyllinate
Classifications: BRONCHODILATOR (RESPIRATORY SMOOTH MUSCLE RELAXANT); XANTHINE
Prototype: Theophylline
Pregnancy category: C

ACTIONS/PHARMACODYNAMICS Choline salt of theophylline. Contains 64% theophylline. Compared to aminophylline, reportedly more stable, more soluble, and more uniformly and predictably absorbed, and produces less gastric irritation. Development of tolerance reported infrequently; therefore useful in long-term therapy.

ROUTE & DOSAGE

Asthma, COPD
Adult: **PO** 4.7 mg/kg (usual dose 200 mg) q8h.
Child: **PO** *9–16 y and adult smoker,* 4.7 mg/kg (usual dose 200 mg) q6h; *1–9 y,* 6.2 mg/kg q6h.

PHARMACOKINETICS Absorption: well absorbed from GI tract. **Duration:** 4–8 h; varies with age, smoking, and liver function. **Distribution:** crosses placenta; distributed into breast milk. **Metabolism:** extensively metabolized in liver. **Elimination:** half-life: 4 h in adults; parent drug and metabolites excreted by kidneys.

CONTRAINDICATIONS & PRECAUTIONS Contraindicated in: hypersensitivity to xanthines; coronary artery disease; renal, liver impairment. Safe use during pregnancy (category C), in nursing women, and in children < 2 y not established. **Cautious use in:** peptic ulcer; prostatic hypertrophy; diabetes mellitus; glaucoma.

ADVERSE/SIDE EFFECTS CNS: restlessness, dizziness, insomnia, convulsions, *muscle twitching*. **CV:** palpitation, tachycardia, flushing, hypotension. **GI:** *nausea,* vomiting, anorexia, epigastric pain, diarrhea, activation of peptic ulcer. **GU:** transient urinary frequency, kidney irritation. **Other:** urticaria, fever, dehydration.

DRUG INTERACTIONS Increases **lithium** excretion, lowering lithium levels; **cimetidine,** high dose **allopurinol** (600 mg/d), **ciprofloxacin, erythromycin, troleandomycin** can significantly increase theophylline levels.

NURSING IMPLICATIONS

See theophylline for numerous additional nursing implications.

Administration

- Oxtriphylline is preferably taken on an empty stomach (30 min to 1 h before or 2 h after meals); however, it may be taken after meals and at bedtime to reduce GI distress. Sustained-release tablet permits dosing q12h.
- Preserve in tightly closed containers away from heat. Elixir should be protected from light.

Patient & Family Education

- Advise to report gastric distress, palpitation, and CNS stimulation (irritability, restlessness, nervousness, insomnia). Reduction in dosage may be indicated.

OXYBUTYNIN CHLORIDE

(ox-i-byoo′ti-nin)

Trade name: Ditropan

Classifications: AUTONOMIC NERVOUS SYSTEM AGENT; ANTICHOLINERGIC (PARASYMPATHOLYTIC); ANTIMUSCARINIC; ANTISPASMODIC

Prototype: Atropine

Pregnancy category: C

ACTIONS/PHARMACODYNAMICS Synthetic tertiary amine with prominent antispasmodic activity. Exerts direct antispasmodic action and inhibits muscarinic effects of acetylcholine on smooth muscle.

USES To relieve symptoms associated with voiding in patients with uninhibited neurogenic bladder and reflex neurogenic bladder. Also has been used to relieve pain of bladder spasm following transurethral surgical procedures.

ROUTE & DOSAGE

Neurogenic Bladder

Adult: **PO** 5 mg b.i.d. or t.i.d. (max 20 mg/d).
Geriatric: **PO** 2.5–5 mg b.i.d.
Child: **PO** > 5 y, 5 mg b.i.d. (max 15 mg/d). 1–5 y, 0.2 mg/kg b.i.d.–q.i.d.

PHARMACOKINETICS **Onset:** 0.5–1 h. **Peak:** 3–6 h. **Duration:** 6–10 h. **Metabolism:** metabolized in liver. **Elimination:** excreted primarily in urine.

CONTRAINDICATIONS & PRECAUTIONS **Contraindicated in:** glaucoma, myasthenia gravis, partial or complete GI obstruction, paralytic ileus, intestinal atony (especially elderly or debilitated patients), megacolon, severe colitis, GU obstruction, unstable cardiovascular status. Safe use during pregnancy (category C) and in children <5 y not established. **Cautious use in:** the elderly; autonomic neuropathy, hiatus hernia with reflex esophagitis; hepatic or renal dysfunction; urinary infection; hyperthyroidism; CHF, coronary artery disease, hypertension; prostatic hypertrophy.

ADVERSE/SIDE EFFECTS **CNS:** *drowsiness,* dizziness, weakness, insomnia, restlessness, psychotic behavior (overdosage). **CV:** palpitations, tachycardia, flushing. **Eye:** mydriasis, *blurred vision,* cyclopegia, increased ocular tension. **GI:** *dry mouth,* nausea, vomiting, *constipation,* bloated feeling. **GU:** urinary hesitancy or retention, impotence. **Hypersensitivity:** severe allergic reactions including urticaria, skin rashes. **Other:** suppression of lactation, decreased sweating, fever.

NURSING IMPLICATIONS

Administration

- Note that the maximum dose is 5 mg q.i.d.
- Store in tight containers at 15–30C (59–86F).

Assessment & Drug Effects

- The diagnosis of neurogenic bladder should be confirmed before initiation of therapy.
- Periodic interruptions of therapy are recommended to determine patient's need for continued treatment. Tolerance has occurred in some patients.
- Keep physician informed of expected responses to drug therapy (e.g., effect on urinary frequency, urgency, urge incontinence, nocturia, completeness of bladder emptying).
- Patients with colostomy or ileostomy should be closely monitored; abdominal distension and the onset of diarrhea in these patients may be early signs of intestinal obstruction or of toxic megacolon.

Patient & Family Education

- Since oxybutynin may cause dizziness, drowsiness, and blurred vision, caution to avoid driving and other potentially hazardous activities until reaction to drug is known.
- Advise to avoid hot environments. By suppressing sweating, oxybutynin can cause fever and heat stroke.

OXYCODONE HYDROCHLORIDE

(ox-i-koe′done)

Trade name: OxyContin

OXYCODONE TEREPHTHALATE

Trade names: Percocet-5, Percodan, Percodan-Demi, Roxicet, Roxicodone

Classifications: CNS AGENT; NARCOTIC (OPIATE) AGONIST ANALGESIC

Prototype: Morphine

Pregnancy category: B (D for prolonged use or use of high doses at term)

Controlled substance: Schedule II

ACTIONS/PHARMACODYNAMICS

Semisynthetic derivative of opium alkaloid thebaine with actions qualitatively similar to those of morphine. Most prominent actions involve CNS and organs composed of smooth muscle. Binds with stereo-specific receptors in various sites of CNS to alter both perception of pain and emotional response to pain, but precise mechanism of action not clear. Appears to be more effective in relief of acute than long-standing pain. As potent as morphine and 10–12 times more potent than codeine.

USES Relief of moderate to moderately severe pain such as may occur with bursitis, dislocations, simple fractures and other injuries, and neuralgia. Relieves postoperative, post-extractional, postpartum pain.

ROUTE & DOSAGE

Moderate to Severe Pain

Adult: **PO** 5–10 mg q6h prn. OxyContin can be dosed q8h.
Child: **PO** ≥ 12 y, 2.5 mg q6h prn; 6–12 y, 1.25 mg q6h prn.

PHARMACOKINETICS Absorption: readily absorbed from GI tract. **Onset:** 10–15 min. **Peak:** 30–60 min. **Duration:** 4–5 h. **Distribution:** crosses placenta; distributed into breast milk. **Metabolism:** metabolized in liver. **Elimination:** excreted primarily in urine.

CONTRAINDICATIONS & PRECAUTIONS Contraindicated in: hypersensitivity to oxycodone and principal drugs with which it is combined; during pregnancy (category B); for prolonged use or high doses at term (category D); nursing women, and children < 6 y. **Cautious use in:** alcoholism; renal or hepatic disease; viral infections; Addison's disease; cardiac arrhythmias; chronic ulcerative colitis; history of drug abuse or dependency; gallbladder disease, acute abdominal conditions; head injury, intracranial lesions; hypothyroidism; prostatic hypertrophy; respiratory disease; urethral stricture; elderly or debilitated patients; peptic ulcer or coagulation abnormalities (combination products containing aspirin).

ADVERSE/SIDE EFFECTS CNS: euphoria, dysphoria, light-headedness, dizziness, *sedation*. **GI:** anorexia, *nausea,* vomiting, *constipation*. **Other:** shortness of breath, pruritus, skin rash, bradycardia, unusual bleeding or bruising, jaundice, dysuria, frequency of urination, urinary retention, <u>respiratory depression, hepatotoxicity</u> (combinations containing acetaminophen).

DIAGNOSTIC TEST INTERFERENCE ***Serum amylase*** levels may be elevated because oxycodone causes spasm of sphincter of Oddi. ***Blood glucose determinations:*** false decrease (measured by glucose oxidase-peroxidase method). ***5-HIAA determination:*** false positive with use of nitrosonaphthol reagent (quantitative test is unaffected).

DRUG INTERACTIONS Alcohol and other CNS DEPRESSANTS add to CNS depressant activity.

NURSING IMPLICATIONS

Administration

- OxyContin tablets MUST be swallowed whole. They cannot be divided or crushed.
- Administer after meals or with milk to reduce gastric irritation.
- Percodan contains aspirin. Do not administer to person with aspirin hypersensitivity. Percocet contains acetaminophen.
- Store this dangerous medication in a place inaccessible to children at 15–30C (59–86F). Protect from light.

Assessment & Drug Effect

- Closely monitor patient's response, expecially to controlled-release preparations.
- Nausea may occur during first few days of therapy; if it continues, consult physician.
- Light-headedness, dizziness, sedation, or fainting appear to be more prominent in ambulatory than in nonambulatory patients and may be alleviated if patient lies down.
- Evaluate patient's continued need for oxycodone preparations. Psychic and physical dependence and tolerance may develop with repeated use. The potential for drug abuse is high.

O

- Laboratory studies of hepatic function and hematologic status should be checked periodically in patients on high dosage.
- The ingestion of large doses of Percodan and Percodan-Demi can result in acute salicylate intoxication. An overdose of Percocet-5 could lead to acetaminophen poisoning.
- Serious overdosage of any oxycodone preparation presents problems associated with a narcotic overdose (respiratory depression, circulatory collapse, extreme somnolence progressing to stupor or coma).

Patient & Family Education

- Oxycontin tablets MUST be swallowed whole. Do not break, chew, or crush.
- Warn not to alter dosage regimen by increasing, decreasing, or shortening intervals between doses. Habit formation and liver damage may be induced.
- Caution to avoid potentially hazardous activities such as driving a car or operating machinery while using oxycodone preparation.
- Caution that taking large amounts of alcoholic beverages while using oxycodone preparation increases risk of liver damage.
- Instruct to check with physician before taking OTC drugs for colds, stomach distress, allergies, insomnia, or pain while also taking oxycodone.
- Tell patient to inform surgeon or dentist that oxycodone preparation is being taken before any surgical procedure is undertaken.

0

OXYMETAZOLINE HYDROCHLORIDE

(ox-i-met-az′oh-leen)

Trade names: Afrin, Dristan Long Lasting, Duramist Plus, Duration, Nafrine♣, Neo-Synephrine 12 Hour, Nostrilla, Sinex Long Lasting

Classifications: NASAL DECONGESTANT; AUTONOMIC NERVOUS SYSTEM AGENT; ALPHA-ADRENERGIC AGONIST (SYMPATHOMIMETIC)

Prototype: Naphazoline

Pregnancy category: C

ACTIONS/PHARMACODYNAMICS

Sympathomimetic that acts directly on alpha receptors of sympathetic nervous system to constrict smaller arterioles in nasal passages and prolong decongestant effect. Has no effect on beta receptors.

USES Relief of nasal congestion in a variety of allergic and infectious disorders of the upper respiratory tract; used as nasal tampon to facilitate intranasal examination or before nasal surgery. Also used as adjunct in treatment and prevention of middle ear infection by decreasing congestion of eustachian ostia.

ROUTE & DOSAGE

Nasal Congestion

Adult: **Intranasal** 2–3 drops or 2–3 sprays of 0.05% solution into each nostril b.i.d. for up to 3–5 d.
Child: **Intranasal** *> 6 y,* same as for adult; *2–5 y,* 2–3 drops or 2–3 sprays of 0.025% solution into each nostril b.i.d. for up to 3–5 d.

PHARMACOKINETICS **Onset:** 5–10 min. **Duration:** 6–10 h.

CONTRAINDICATIONS & PRECAUTIONS **Contraindicated in:** use in children < 6 y. Safe use during pregnancy (category C) not established. **Cautious use in:** within 14 d of MAO inhibitors, coronary artery disease, hypertension, hyperthyroidism, diabetes mellitus.

ADVERSE/SIDE EFFECTS *Burning,* stinging, dryness of nasal mucosa, *sneezing*. With excessive use: headache, light-headedness, drowsiness, insomnia, palpitations, *rebound congestion.*

NURSING IMPLICATIONS

Patient & Family Education

- Oxymetazoline is usually administered in the morning and at bedtime. Effects appear within 30 min and last about 6–7 h.
- Nasal spray is delivered with patient in upright position. Instruct to place spray nozzle in nostril without occluding it and to bend head slightly forward and sniff briskly during administration.
- Lateral, head-low position is recommended for instillation of nose drops.
- Instruct to rinse dropper or spray tip in hot water after each use to prevent contamination of solution by nasal secretions.
- Instruct to wash hands carefully after handling oxymetazoline. Anisocoria (inequality of pupil size, blurred vision) can develop if eyes are rubbed with contaminated fingers.
- Caution not to exceed recommended dosage. Rebound congestion (chemical rhinitis) may occur with prolonged or excessive use.
- Systemic effects can result from swallowing excessive medication.

OXYMETHOLONE

(ox-i-meth'oh-lone)

Trade names: Anadrol, Anadrol-50, Anapolon ♣

Classifications: HORMONE; ANDROGEN/ANABOLIC STEROID

Prototype: Testosterone

Pregnancy category: X

Controlled substance: Schedule III

ACTIONS/PHARMACODYNAMICS Potent steroid with anabolic activity ratio approximately 1:3. Promotes body tissue building and inhibits tissue-depleting processes; supports nitrogen, potassium, chloride, and phosphorus conservation. Enhances weight gain and combats depression and weakness in debilitating conditions. Stimulates bone growth, aids in bone matrix reconstitution, and may support calcification of metastatic lesions of breast cancer. Mechanism of action in refractory anemias is unclear but may be due to direct stimulation of bone marrow or protein anabolic activity or to androgenic stimulation of erythropoiesis.

USE Aplastic anemia. **Unlabeled uses:** osteoporosis, catabolic conditions.

ROUTE & DOSAGE

Aplastic Anemia

Adult: **PO** 1–5 mg/kg/d.
Child: **PO** Same as for adult.

PHARMACOKINETICS **Absorption:** readily absorbed from GI tract. **Metabolism:** metabolized in liver. **Elimination:** half-life: 9 h; excreted in urine.

CONTRAINDICATIONS & PRECAUTIONS **Contraindicated in:** prostatic hypertrophy with obstruction; pregnancy (category X); use in nursing mothers not established; prostatic or male breast cancer; cardiac, renal, hepatic decompensation; nephrosis; premature infant. **Cautious use in:** prepubertal males; geriatric male patients; diabetes mellitus; coronary disease; patient taking ACTH, corticosteroids, anticoagulants.

ADVERSE/SIDE EFFECTS Androgenic in women: suppression of ovulation, lactation, or menstruation; *hoarseness or deepening of voice* (often irreversible); *hirsutism; oily skin; acne;* clitoral enlargement; regression of breasts; male-pattern baldness (in disseminated breast cancer). Men: prepubertal: premature epiphyseal closure, phallic enlargement, priapism. Postpubertal: testicular atrophy, decreased ejaculatory volume, azoospermia, oligospermia (after prolonged administration or excessive dosage), impotence, epididymitis, gynecomastia. **CV:** *edema,* skin flush. **GI:** *nausea, vomiting, anorexia,* diarrhea, jaundice, hepatotoxicity. **GU:** bladder irritability. **Hypoestrogenic:** female: flushing, sweating; vaginitis with pruritus, drying, bleeding; menstrual irregularities. **Other:** hypercalcemia.

NURSING IMPLICATIONS

Administration

- A course of therapy for treatment of osteoporosis is 7–21 d.
- For treatment of anemias, a minimum trial period of 3–6 mo is recommended, since response tends to be slow.
- Store at 15–30C (59–86F). Protect from heat and light.

Assessment & Drug Effects

- Closely monitor patient with a history of seizures, since an increase in their frequency may be noted.
- Monitor periodically for edema that may develop with or without CHF.
- Monitor for hypercalcemia (see Appendix G), especially in women with breast cancer.
- Periodic liver function tests are especially important for the elderly patient. Drug should be stopped with first sign of liver toxicity (jaundice).
- Optimal effects in treatment of osteoporosis are usually experienced in 4–6 wk.

Patient & Family Education

- Inform diabetic that glucose tolerance may be decreased; instruct patient to monitor blood and urine closely.
- Instruct women to notify physician of signs of virilization.

OXYMORPHONE HYDROCHLORIDE

(ox-i-mor′fone)

Trade name: Numorphan

Classifications: CNS AGENT; NARCOTIC (OPIATE) AGONIST ANALGESIC

Prototype: Morphine

Pregnancy category: B (D for prolonged use or high doses at term)

Controlled substance: Schedule II

ACTIONS/PHARMACODYNAMICS

Structurally and pharmacologically related to morphine. Analgesic action of 1 mg is reportedly equivalent to that of 10 mg of morphine. Produces mild sedation and, unlike morphine, has little antitussive action. In equianalgesic doses, may have less antitussive effect and may cause less constipation than does morphine but more nausea, vomiting, and euphoria.

USES Relief of moderate to severe pain, preoperative medication, obstetric analgesia, support of anesthesia, and relief of anxiety in patients with dyspnea associated with acute ventricular failure and pulmonary edema.

ROUTE & DOSAGE

Moderate to Severe Pain

Adult: **SC/IM** 1–1.5 mg q4–6h prn. **IV** 0.5 mg q4–6h. **PR** 5 mg q4–6h prn.

PHARMACOKINETICS **Onset:** 5–10 min IV; 10–15 min IM; 15–30 min PR. **Peak:** 1–1.5 h. **Duration:** 3–6 h. **Distribution:** crosses placenta. **Metabolism:** metabolized in liver. **Elimination:** eliminated in urine.

CONTRAINDICATIONS & PRECAUTIONS **Contraindicated in:** pulmonary edema resulting from chemical respiratory irritants. Safe use during pregnancy (category B [D for prolonged use and high doses]), in nursing mothers, and in children < 12 y not established.

ADVERSE/SIDE EFFECTS *Nausea, vomiting,* euphoria, *dizziness,* respiratory depression (see morphine).

DRUG INTERACTIONS **Alcohol** and other CNS DEPRESSANTS add to CNS depression.

NURSING IMPLICATIONS

Administration

- IV oxymorphone may be given by direct IV diluted in 5 ml of sterile water or NS and injected at a rate of 0.5 mg over 2–5 min.
- Protect drug from light. Store suppositories in refrigerator (2–15C, 36–59F).

Assessment & Drug Effects

- Monitor respiratory rate. Withhold drug and notify physician if rate falls below 12 breaths per minute.
- Supervise ambulation and advise patient of possible light-headedness.
- Evaluate patient's continued need for narcotic analgesic. Prolonged use can lead to dependence of morphine type.
- Medication contains sulfite and may precipitate a hypersensitivity reaction in susceptible patient.
- Elderly and debilitated patients are most susceptible to CNS depressant effects of drug.

Patient & Family Education

- Advise ambulatory patient to exercise caution because of potential for injury from dizziness.
- Advise not to consume alcohol while taking oxymorphone.

OXYTETRACYCLINE

(ox-i-tet-ra-sye′kleen)

Trade name: Terramycin

OXYTETRACYCLINE HYDROCHLORIDE

Trade names: Terramycin, Uri-Tet

Classifications: ANTIINFECTIVE; ANTIBIOTIC; TETRACYCLINE

Prototype: Tetracycline

Pregnancy category: D

ACTIONS/PHARMACODYNAMICS Broad-spectrum antibiotic with actions, uses, contraindications, precautions, and adverse reactions similar to those of tetracycline.

ROUTE & DOSAGE

Antiinfective

Adult: **PO** 250–500 mg q6–12h. **IM** 100 mg q8–12h. **IV** 250–500 mg q12h (max 500 mg q6h).
Child: **PO** > *8 y,* 25–50 mg/kg/d in 4 divided doses. **IM** > *8 y,* 15–25 mg/kg/d in 2–3 divided doses (max 250 mg/dose). **IV** > *8 y,* 10–20 mg/kg/d in 2 divided doses.

PHARMACOKINETICS **Absorption:** about 60% absorbed from GI tract and IM site. **Peak:** 2–4 h. **Distribution:** appears to concentrate in hepatic system; crosses placenta; distributed into breast milk. **Metabolism:** partially metabolized. **Elimination:** half-life: 6–10 h; excreted in feces and urine.

CONTRAINDICATIONS & PRECAUTIONS **Contraindicated in:** hypersensitivity to tetracyclines; during tooth development [last half of pregnancy (category D), infancy, childhood to age 8 y]. **Cautious use in:** impaired renal function.

ADVERSE/SIDE EFFECTS Nausea, vomiting, diarrhea, stomatitis, skin rash, superinfections, renal toxicity. (See also tetracycline.)

DRUG INTERACTIONS ANTACIDS, **iron, calcium, magnesium, zinc, kaolin and pectin, sodium bicarbonate, bismuth subsalicylate** can significantly decrease oxytetracycline absorption; effects of both **desmopressin** and oxytetracycline antagonized; increases **digoxin** absorption, increasing risk of digoxin toxicity; **methoxyflurane** increases risk of renal failure. **Food–drug:** dairy products significantly decrease oxytetracycline absorption; food may decrease drug absorption.

O

NURSING IMPLICATIONS

Administration

- Dosage is reduced in the presence of renal impairment. Normal doses may result in liver toxicity.
- Check expiration date. Degradation products of outdated tetracyclines can be highly nephrotoxic.
- Food may interfere with rate and extent of absorption of oral drug. Administer at least 1 h before or 2 h following meals. Do not give with antacids, milk, milk products, or other calcium-containing foods.
- The commercially available solution for IM use contains only 2% lidocaine. Administer by deep IM. Do not use IM solution for IV administration.
- Only oxytetracycline hydrochloride for injection can be given IV. IV solution is prepared by adding 10 ml of sterile water for injection or D5W to the 250 or 500 mg vial. Further dilute with a minimum of 100 ml D5W, NS, or Ringer's lactate. Infuse slowly over 15–30 min. A slower rate of infusion and a large amount of diluent will reduce vein irritation.
- Syrup formulation (oxytetracycline calcium) should be stored in a cool place protected from light.
- Dry powder for parenteral use is stable at room temperature. Reconstituted solutions are stable for 48 h refrigerated (2–8C, 36–46.4F).

Assessment & Drug Effects

- Monitor for signs and symptoms of superinfection (see Appendix G).
- Discontinue drug and notify physician at the first sign of a hypersensitivity response (see Appendix G).

Patient & Family Education

- Instruct patient to discard unused drug when course of therapy has ended.
- Caution patient to avoid excessive exposure to sunlight because of the possibility of photosensitivity.

OXYTOCIN INJECTION

(ox-i-toe′sin)

Trade names: Pitocin, Syntocinon, Syntocinon Nasal Spray

Prototype for classification: OXYTOCIC

ACTIONS/PHARMACODYNAMICS Synthetic, water-soluble polypeptide consisting of eight amino acids, identical pharmacologically to the oxytocic principle of posterior pituitary. By direct action on myofibrils, produces phasic contractions characteristic of normal delivery. Promotes milk ejection (letdown) reflex in nursing mother, thereby increasing flow (not volume) of milk; also facilitates flow of milk during period of breast engorgement. Uterine sensitivity to oxytocin increases during gestation period and peaks sharply before parturition. Not used for elective induction of labor.

USES To initiate or improve uterine contraction at term only in carefully selected patients and only after cervix is dilated and presentation of fetus has occurred; used to stimulate letdown reflex in nursing mother and to relieve pain from breast engorgement. Uses include management of inevitable, incomplete, or missed abortion; stimulation of uterine contractions during third stage of labor; stimulation to overcome uterine inertia; control of postpartum hemorrhage and promotion of postpartum uterine involution. Also used to induce labor in cases of maternal diabetes, preeclampsia, eclampsia, and erythroblastosis fetalis.

ROUTE & DOSAGE

Antepartum

Adult: **IV** Start at 1 mU/min; may increase by 1 mU/min q15 min up to a max of 20 mU/min.

Postpartum

Adult: **IV** Infuse a total of 10 U at a rate of 20–40 mU/min after delivery.

To Promote Milk Ejection

Adult: **Nasal** 1 spray or 1 drop in 1 or both nostrils 2–3 min before nursing or pumping.

PHARMACOKINETICS Absorption: destroyed in GI tract. **Onset:** immediately IV; few minutes nasal. **Duration:** 1 h IV; 20 min nasal. **Distribution:** distributed throughout extracellular fluid; small amount may cross placenta. **Metabolism:** rapidly destroyed in liver and kidneys. **Elimination:** half-life: 3–5 min; small amounts excreted unchanged in urine.

CONTRAINDICATIONS & PRECAUTIONS Contraindicated in: hypersensitivity to oxytocin, significant cephalopelvic disproportion, unfavorable fetal position or presentations that are undeliverable without conversion before delivery, obstetric emergencies in which benefit-to-risk ratio for mother or fetus favors surgical intervention, fetal distress in which delivery is not imminent, prematurity, placenta previa, prolonged use in severe toxemia or uterine inertia, hypertonic uterine patterns, previous surgery of uterus or cervix including cesarean section, conditions predisposing to thromboplastin or amniotic fluid embolism (dead fetus, abruptio placentae), grand multiparity, invasive cervical carcinoma, primipara > 35 y of age, past history of uterine sepsis or of traumatic delivery, intranasal route during labor, simultaneous administration of drug by two routes. **Cautious use in:** concomitant use with cyclopropane anesthesia or vasoconstrictive drugs.

ADVERSE/SIDE EFFECTS Fetus: bradycardia and other arrhythmias, hypoxia, <u>intracranial hemorrhage</u>, trauma from too rapid propulsion through pelvis, neonatal jaundice, <u>death</u>. **Mother:** hypersensitivity leading to uterine hypertonicity, tetanic contractions, <u>uterine rupture</u>, anaphylactic reactions, postpartum hemorrhage, cardiac arrhythmias, pelvic hematoma, nausea, vomiting, hypertensive episodes, <u>subarachnoid hemorrhage</u>, increased blood

O

flow, fatal afibrinogenemia, ADH effects leading to severe water intoxication and hyponatremia, hypotension, ECG changes, PVCs, anxiety, dyspnea, precordial pain, edema, cyanosis or redness of skin, cardiovascular spasm and collapse. ***Citrate:*** parabuccal irritation.

DRUG INTERACTIONS VASOCONSTRICTORS cause severe hypertension; **cyclopropane anesthesia** causes hypotension, maternal bradycardia, arrhythmias.

INCOMPATIBILITIES Solution/additive: fibrinolysin, warfarin.

NURSING IMPLICATIONS

Administration

- Oxytocin administration should be supervised by persons having thorough knowledge of the drug and the skill to identify complications. A qualified physician should be immediately available to manage complications.
- Time of administration of oxytocin in relation to delivery of baby or placenta varies with physician's preference. The nurse should have a clear understanding of when drug is to be administered with respect to progress of labor. Infusion flow rates are established by physician. Accurate control of infusion is critical.
- Oxytocin should never be administered by more than one route at a time.
- During delivery, IM oxytocin is most easily injected deep into deltoid muscle. Massage injection site to assist quick absorption.
- When diluting oxytocin for IV infusion, rotate bottle gently to distribute medicine throughout solution.
- IV preparation: For inducing labor, add 10 U (1 ml) of oxytocin to 1 L of D5W or NS to give 10 mU/ml. For postpartum bleeding, add 10–40 U of oxytocin to 1 L of D5W or NS to give 10–40 mU/ml.
- Administer properly diluted IV solution by continuous infusion only. See recommended rates (mU/min) in Route & Dosage table.
- Unless otherwise directed by manufacturer, store oxytocin solution in refrigerator but do not freeze.

Assessment & Drug Effects

- Before instituting treatment, start flow charts to record maternal BP and other vital signs, I&O ratio, weight, strength, duration, and frequency of contractions, as well as fetal heart tone and rate.
- During infusion period, monitor fetal heart rate and maternal BP and pulse at least q15min; evaluate tonus of myometrium during and between contractions and record on flow chart. Report change in rate and rhythm immediately.
- If contractions are prolonged (occurring at less than 2-min intervals) and if monitor records contractions about 50 mm Hg or if contractions last 90 seconds or longer, stop infusion to prevent fetal anoxia, turn patient on her side, and notify physician. Stimulation will wane rapidly within 2–3 min. Oxygen administration may be necessary.
- If local or regional (caudal, spinal) anesthesia is being given to the patient receiving oxytocin, be alert to the possibility of hypertensive crisis: sudden intense occipital headache, palpitation, marked hypertension, stiff neck, nausea, vomiting, sweating, fever, photophobia, dilated pupils, bradycardia or tachycardia, constricting chest pain.
- Monitor I&O during labor. If patient is receiving drug by prolonged IV infusion, watch for

symptoms of water intoxication (drowsiness, listlessness, headache, confusion, anuria, weight gain). Report changes in alertness and orientation and changes in I&O ratio (i.e., marked decrease in output with excessive intake).

- The fundus should be checked frequently during the first few postpartum hours and several times daily thereafter.
- Incidence of hypersensitivity or allergic reactions is higher when oxytocin is given by IM or IV injection rather than by IV infusion (diluted solution).

Patient & Family Education

- Inform of purpose and anticipated effect of oxytocin.
- Instruct to report sudden, severe headache immediately.

PACLITAXEL

(pac-li-tax′-el)

Trade name: Taxol

Classification: ANTINEOPLASTIC

Pregnancy category: X

ACTIONS/PHARMACODYNAMICS Antimicrotubule agent that interferes with microtubule network essential for interphase and mitosis. Induces abnormal spindle formation and multiple asters during mitosis. In addition, normal functioning microtubules are essential for cell shape and organelles present within cells.

USES Ovarian cancer, breast cancer, Kaposi's sarcoma, non-small cell lung cancer (NSCLC). **Unlabeled uses:** other solid tumors, leukemia, melanoma.

ROUTE & DOSAGE

Ovarian Cancer, NSCLC

Adult: **IV** 135 mg/m^2 24-h infusion repeated q22d.

Breast Cancer

Adult: **IV** 175 mg/m^2 over 3 h q3wk.

Solid Tumors, Malignant Melanoma

Adult: **IV** 250 mg/m^2 24-h infusion repeated q3wk.

Kaposi's Sarcoma

Adult: **IV** 135 mg/m^2 infused over 3 h q3wk or 100 mg/m^2 infused over 3 h q2wk.

Note: Premedication with dexamethasone, diphenhydramine, and H_2 antagonists (or ephedrine) is recommended to reduce hypersensitivity reactions, and consists of dexamethasone 20 mg PO or IV 14 and 7 h prior to taxol infusion; diphenhydramine 50 mg IV 30 min prior to taxol; and cimetidine 300 mg or ranitidine 50 mg IV 30 min before taxol infusion.

PHARMACOKINETICS Distribution: highly protein bound; does not cross CSF. **Metabolism:** metabolic pathways have yet to be identified. **Elimination:** half-life: 1–9 h; only 5–6% of dose is recovered in urine. Available data suggest that metabolism, biliary excretion, and/or extensive tissue binding account for majority of systemic clearance.

CONTRAINDICATIONS & PRECAUTIONS Contraindicated in: hypersensitivity to paclitaxel, and patient's with baseline neutropenia of < 1500 cells/mm^3; and nursing mothers. **Cautious use in:** cardiac arrhythmias; impaired hepatic function; pregnancy (category X). Safety and efficacy in children have not been established.

ADVERSE/SIDE EFFECTS CV: ventricular tachycardia, ventricular ectopy, *transient bradycardia,* chest pain. **CNS:** fatigue, headaches, *peripheral neuropathy,* weakness, seizures. **GI:** *nausea, vomiting,* diarrhea, taste changes, *mucositis.* **Hematologic:** *neutropenia, anemia, thrombocytopenia.* **Hypersensitivity:** *hypotension, dyspnea with bronchospasm, urticaria, abdominal and extremity pain, diaphoresis,* angioedema. **Skin:** *alopecia,* tissue necrosis with extravasation. **Other:** minor elevations in renal and hepatic function tests, elevations in serum triglycerides, *myalgias, arthralgias, alopecia.*

DRUG INTERACTION Increased myelosuppression if **cisplatin** is given before paclitaxel.

INCOMPATIBILITIES Solution/additive: PVC bags and **infusion sets** should be avoided due to leaching of DEHP (plasticizer). Do not mix with any other medications.

NURSING IMPLICATIONS

Administration

- Follow institutional or standard guidelines for preparation, handling, and disposal of cytotoxic agents.
- Do not use equipment or devices containing polyvinyl chloride (PVC) in preparation of solutions for infusion.
- Dilute paclitaxel to a final concentration of 0.3–1.2 mg/ml in any of the following: 0.9% NaCl injection; 5% dextrose injection; 5% dextrose and 0.9% NaCl injection; or 5% dextrose in Ringer's injection.
- Because tissue necrosis occurs with extravasation, frequently assess patency of peripheral IV site. Generally, however, paclitaxel is given through a central IV line.
- The prepared solution may be hazy. Administer through IV tubing containing inline (0.22 μm or less) filter.
- An ordered dose (e.g., 135 mg/m^2) is administered over 24 h every 3 wk. Do not administer subsequent doses unless neutrophil count is at least 1500/mm^3 and platelet count is at least 100,000/mm^3.
- Dose is usually reduced by 20% in those who develop severe neutropenia (less than 500/mm^3 for a week or longer) or severe peripheral neuropathy.
- Solutions diluted for infusion are stable at room temperature (approximately 25C/77F) for up to 27h.

Assessment & Drug Effects

- Monitor for hypersensitivity reactions, especially during first and second administrations of the paclitaxel. Signs and symptoms requiring treatment, but not necessarily discontinuation of the drug, include dyspnea, hypotension, and chest pain. Development of angioedema and generalized urticaria requires immediate discontinuation of paclitaxel and aggressive symptom management.
- Frequently monitor vital signs, especially during the first hour of infusion. Bradycardia occurs in approximately 12% of patients, usually during infusion. It does not normally require treatment. Cardiac monitoring is indicated for those with severe conduction abnormalities.
- Monitor hematologic status throughout course of treatment. Severe neutropenia is common but usually of short duration (less than 500/mm^3 for less than 7 d) with the nadir occurring about day 11. Thrombocytopenia occurs less often and is less severe with the nader around day 8 or 9. The incidence and severity of anemia increase with exposure to paclitaxel.

- Monitor for peripheral neuropathy, the severity of which is dose dependent. Severe symptoms occur primarily with higher than recommended doses.

Patient & Family Education

- Advise of the signs and symptoms of paclitaxel hypersensitivity. Instruct to immediately report dyspnea, chest pain, palpitations, angioedema (subcutaneous swelling usually around face and neck), and urticaria.
- Inform of range of adverse effects of the drug. Stress need for periodic blood work. Discuss measures that will be used to manage adverse GI effects.
- Inform of high probability of developing alopecia (> 80%).

PALIVIZUMAB

(pal-i-viz′u-mab)

Trade name: Synagis

Classifications: IMMUNOMODULATOR; IMMUNOGLOBULIN

Prototype: Basiliximab

Pregnancy category: C

ACTIONS/PHARMACODYNAMICS
Palivizumab is a monoclonal antibody ($IgG1_k$ produced by recombinant DNA technology) to the respiratory syncytial virus (RSV).

USE Prevention of serious lower respiratory tract infections in children susceptible to RSV.

ROUTE & DOSAGE

RSV
Child: **IM** 15 mg/kg q. mo. during RSV season.

PHARMACOKINETICS Elimination: half-life: 20 d.

CONTRAINDICATIONS & PRECAUTIONS Contraindicated in: hypersensitivity to palivizumab in pediatric patients. **Cautious use in:** hypersensitivity to other immunoglobulin preparations, blood products, or other medications; renal or hepatic dysfunction; acute RSV infection.

ADVERSE/SIDE EFFECTS Body as whole: *otitis media,* pain, hernia. **GI:** increased SGOT, diarrhea, nausea, vomiting, gastroenteritis. **Respiratory:** *URI, rhinitis,* pharyngitis, cough, wheeze, bronchiolitis, asthma, croup, dyspnea, sinusitis, apnea. **Skin:** *rash*.

NURSING IMPLICATIONS

Administration

- Reconstitute solution by gently injecting 1 ml of sterile water for injection (without preservative) toward the sides of the vial. Gently swirl for 30 s to dissolve (do not shake solution). Allow to stand at room temperature for at least 20 min until solution clears.
- Give IM only preferably into the anterolateral aspect of the thigh. Volumes >1 ml should be divided and given in different sites.
- Reconstituted solution must be used within 6 h. Discard any unused portion of the vial. It contains no preservatives.
- Store unopened vials at 2–8C (36–46F).

Assessment & Drug Effects

- Therapeutic effectiveness is indicated by prevention of lower respiratory tract infection.
- Lab tests: Periodic monitoring of liver functions may be warranted.
- Carefully monitor for and immediately report S&S of respiratory illness including fever, cough, wheezing, and retractions.

- Assess for and report erythema or induration at injection site.

Patient & Family Education

- Contact physician if S&S of respiratory illness, vomiting, diarrhea, or redness develop at injection site.

PAMIDRONATE DISODIUM

(pa-mi′dro-nate)

Trade name: Aredia

Classification: REGULATOR, BONE METABOLISM, BIPHOSPHONATE

Prototype: Etidronate

Pregnancy category: C

ACTIONS/PHARMACODYNAMICS A bone-resorption inhibitor that is thought to absorb calcium phosphate crystals in bone. It may also inhibit osteoclast activity, thus contributing to inhibition of bone resorption. It does not inhibit bone formation or mineralization.

USES Hypercalcemia of malignancy and Paget's disease, bone metastases in multiple myeloma. **Unlabeled use:** primary hyperparathyroidism.

ROUTE & DOSAGE

Moderate Hypercalcemia of Malignancy (corrected calcium 12–13.5 mg/dl)

Adult: **IV** 15–90 mg in 1000 ml NS or D5W infused over 4–24 h; may repeat in 7 d.

Severe Hypercalcemia of Malignancy (corrected calcium > 13.5 mg/dl)

Adult: **IV** 90 mg in 1000 ml NS or D5W infused over 4–24 h; may repeat in 7 d.

PHARMACOKINETICS Absorption: 50% of IV dose is retained in body. **Onset:** 24–48 h. **Peak:** 6 d. **Duration:** 2 wk–3 mo. **Distribution:** accumulates in bone; once deposited, remains bound until bone is remodeled. **Metabolism:** not metabolized. **Elimination:** half-life: unknown; 50% excreted in urine unchanged.

CONTRAINDICATIONS & PRECAUTIONS Contraindicated in: hypersensitivity to pamidronate. **Cautious use in:** chronic renal failure and pregnancy (category C). It is not known if pamidronate is excreted in breast milk. Safety and effectiveness in children have not been established.

ADVERSE/SIDE EFFECTS *Fever with or without rigors* (20–40%) generally occurs within 48 h and subsides within 48 h despite continued therapy; thrombophlebitis at injection site (18%); general malaise lasting for several weeks; *hypocalcemia* (20%). **GI:** nausea, abdominal pain, epigastric discomfort (15%). **Other:** hypertension, rash, transient increase in bone pain.

DRUG INTERACTION Concurrent use of **foscarnet** may further decrease serum levels of ionized calcium.

INCOMPATIBILITIES Solution/additive: CALCIUM-CONTAINING SOLUTIONS (including LACTATED RINGER'S).

NURSING IMPLICATIONS

Administration

- To reconstitute add 10 ml sterile water for injection to the 30 mg vial to produce a concentration of 30 mg/10 ml.
- Withdraw the recommended dose of reconstituted solution and dilute with 0.45% or 0.9% NaCl or D5W. Unless otherwise ordered, dissolve in 1000 ml of IV solution and infuse over 24 h.

- Do not add to calcium-containing solutions such as Ringer's injection.
- Reconstituted pamidronate solution should be refrigerated at 2–8C (36–46F); the IV solution may be stored at room temperature. Both are stable for 24 h.

Assessment & Drug Effects
- Assess IV injection site for thrombophlebitis.
- Serum calcium and phosphate levels, CBC, temperature and renal function should be monitored throughout course of therapy.
- Monitor for signs and symptoms of hypocalcemia, hypokalemia, hypomagnesemia, and hypophosphatemia.
- Monitor for seizures especially in those with a preexisting seizure disorder.
- Be aware that drug fever which may occur with pamidronate use is self-limiting, usually subsiding in 48 hours even with continued therapy.

Patient & Family Education
- Inform that transient, self-limiting fever with/without chills may develop.
- Inform that generalized malaise, which may last for several weeks following treatment, may develop.
- Advise to immediately report perioral tingling, numbness, and paresthesia.

PANCRELIPASE

(pan-kre-li'pase)

Trade names: Cotazym, Cotazym-S, Festal II, Ilozyme, Ku-Zyme-Hp, Pancrease, Ultrase, Viokase

Classifications: ENZYME; DIGESTANT

Pregnancy category: C

ACTIONS/PHARMACODYNAMICS Pancreatic enzyme concentrate of porcine origin standardized for lipase content. Similar to pancreatin but on a weight basis has 12 times the lipolytic activity and at least 4 times the trypsin and amylase content of pancreatin.

USE Replacement therapy in symptomatic treatment of malabsorption syndrome due to cystic fibrosis and other conditions associated with exocrine pancreatic insufficiency.

ROUTE & DOSAGE

Pancreatic Insufficiency
Adult: **PO** 1–3 capsules or tablets or 1–2 packets of powder 1–2 h before, during, or 1 h after meals, with an extra dose taken with any food eaten between meals.
Child: **PO** 1–2 capsules or tablets 1–2 h before, during, or 1 h after meals, with an extra dose taken with any food eaten between meals.

P

CONTRAINDICATIONS & PRECAUTIONS **Cautious use in:** history of allergy to hog protein or enzymes. Safe use during pregnancy (category C) not established.

ADVERSE/SIDE EFFECTS High doses: anorexia, nausea, vomiting, diarrhea, hyperuricosuria.

DRUG INTERACTION **Iron** absorption may be decreased.

NURSING IMPLICATIONS

Administration
- Enteric-coated preparations are not to be crushed or chewed.
- For children, powder form may be sprinkled on food.
- Cimetidine, ranitidine, or an antacid may be prescribed to be given before pancrelipase to pre-

vent its destruction by gastric pepsin and acid pH.
- Dosage is usually determined by fat content in diet (suggested ratio: 300 mg pancrelipase for each 17 g dietary fat).

Assessment & Drug Effects
- Monitor I&O and weight. Note appetite and quality of stools, weight loss, abdominal bloating, polyuria, thirst, hunger, itching. Pancreatic insufficiency is frequently associated with steatorrhea, bulky stools, and insulin-dependent diabetes.

Patient & Family Education
- Instruct in the proper timing of medication in relation to meals.

PANCURONIUM BROMIDE
(pan-kyoo-roe′nee-um)
Trade name: Pavulon
Classifications: AUTONOMIC NERVOUS SYSTEM AGENT; NONDEPOLARIZING SKELETAL MUSCLE RELAXANT
Prototype: Tubocurarine
Pregnancy category: C

P

ACTIONS/PHARMACODYNAMICS Synthetic curariform nondepolarizing neuromuscular blocking agent. Similar to tubocurarine chloride in actions, uses, and limitations. Reported to be approximately 5 times as potent as tubocurarine but produces little or no histamine release or ganglionic blockade and thus does not cause bronchospasm or hypotension. In high doses, has direct blocking effect on acetylcholine receptors of heart and may increase heart rate, cardiac output, and arterial pressure.

USES Adjunct to anesthesia to induce skeletal muscle relaxation. Also to facilitate management of patients undergoing mechanical ventilation.

ROUTE & DOSAGE

Skeletal Muscle Relaxation
Adult/Child: **IV** 0.04–0.1 mg/kg initial dose; additional doses of 0.01 mg/kg may be given at 30–60 min intervals.

PHARMACOKINETICS **Onset:** 30–45 s. **Peak:** 2–3 min. **Duration:** 60 min. **Distribution:** well distributed to tissues and extracellular fluids; crosses placenta in small amounts. **Metabolism:** small amount metabolized in liver. **Elimination:** half-life: 2 h; excreted primarily in urine.

CONTRAINDICATIONS & PRECAUTIONS **Contraindicated in:** hypersensitivity to the drug or bromides; tachycardia. Safe use during pregnancy (category C) not established. **Cautious use in:** debilitated patients; myasthenia gravis; pulmonary, hepatic or renal disease; fluid or electrolyte imbalance.

ADVERSE/SIDE EFFECTS *Increased pulse rate and BP,* ventricular extrasystoles, transient acneiform rash, burning sensation along course of vein, salivation, skeletal muscle weakness, <u>respiratory depression</u>.

DIAGNOSTIC TEST INTERFERENCE Pancuronium may decrease ***serum cholinesterase*** concentrations.

DRUG INTERACTIONS GENERAL ANESTHETICS increase neuromuscular blocking and duration of action; AMINOGLYCOSIDES, **bacitracin, polymyxin B, clindamycin, lidocaine,** parenteral **magnesium, quinidine, quinine, trimethaphan, verapamil** increase neuromuscular blockade; DIURETICS may increase or decrease neuromuscular blockade; **lithium** prolongs duration of neuromuscular blockade; NARCOTIC ANALGESICS possibly add to respiratory depression; **succinylcholine** increases onset and depth of neuromuscular blockade; **phenytoin** may cause resistance to or reversal of neuromuscular blockade.

NURSING IMPLICATIONS

Administration

- Plastic syringe may be used for administration, but drug may adsorb to plastic with prolonged storage.
- Pancuronium bromide may be given by direct IV undiluted over 30–90 seconds.
- IV administration to infants, children: Verify correct rate of IV injection with physician.
- Refrigerate at 2–8C (36–46F). Do not freeze.

Assessment & Drug Effects

- Observe patient closely for residual muscle weakness and signs of respiratory distress during recovery period. Monitor BP and vital signs.
- Peripheral nerve stimulator may be used to assess the effects of pancuronium and to monitor restoration of neuromuscular function.

PAPAVERINE HYDROCHLORIDE

(pa-pav′er-een)

Trade names: Cerespan, Genabid, Pavabid, Pavased, Pavatyme, Paverolan

Classifications: CARDIOVASCULAR AGENT; NONNITRATE VASODILATOR

Prototype: Hydralazine

Pregnancy category: C

ACTIONS/PHARMACODYNAMICS Exerts nonspecific direct spasmolytic effect on smooth muscles unrelated to innervation. Action is especially pronounced on coronary, cerebral, pulmonary, and peripheral arteries when spasm is present. Like quinidine, acts directly on myocardium, depresses conduction and irritability, and prolongs refractory period. Stimulates respiration by action on carotid and aortic body chemoreceptors.

USES Primarily for relief of cerebral and peripheral ischemia associated with arterial spasm and MI complicated by arrhythmias. Also visceral spasm as in ureteral, biliary, and GI colic. **Unlabeled uses:** impotence, cardiac bypass surgery.

ROUTE & DOSAGE

Cerebral and Peripheral Ischemia

Adult: **PO** 100–300 mg 3–5 times/d; 150 mg sustained release q8–12h. **IM/IV** 30–120 mg q3h as needed.
Child: **IM/IV** 6 mg/kg/24 h divided into 4 doses.

Impotence

Adult: **IM** 0.5–37.5 mg injected into the corpus cavernosum of the penis as needed for erection.

PHARMACOKINETICS **Absorption:** readily absorbed from GI tract. **Peak:** 1–2 h. **Duration:** 6 h regular tablets; 12 h sustained release. **Metabolism:** metabolized in liver. **Elimination:** half-life: 90 min; excreted in urine chiefly as metabolites.

CONTRAINDICATIONS & PRECAUTIONS **Contraindicated in:** parenteral use in complete AV block. Safe use during pregnancy (category C) and in nursing mothers not established. **Cautious use in:** glaucoma; myocardial depression; angina pectoris; recent stroke.

ADVERSE/SIDE EFFECTS PO: nausea, anorexia, constipation, diarrhea, abdominal distress, dizziness, drowsiness, headache. **Parenteral (low incidence):** general discomfort, facial flushing, sweating, dry mouth and throat, pruritus, skin rash, dizziness, headache, excessive drowsiness and sedation (large doses), slight rise in BP, increased depth of respiration, paroxysmal tachycardia, transient ventricular ectopic rhythms, hepatotoxicity (jaundice, eosinophilia, abnormal liver function tests); with rapid IV administration: respiratory depression, AV block, arrhythmias, fatal apnea; priapism. **Overdosage:** diplopia, nystagmus, weakness, drowsiness, coma, respiratory depression.

DRUG INTERACTIONS May decrease **levodopa** effectiveness; **morphine** may antagonize smooth muscle relaxation effect of papaverine.

NURSING IMPLICATIONS

Administration
- Oral formulations may be taken with or following meals; milk or prescribed antacid may be given to reduce possibility of nausea.
- Timed-release forms should be swallowed whole and must not be chewed or crushed.
- Aspirate carefully before injecting IM to avoid inadvertent entry into blood vessel, and administer slowly.
- When given IV, papaverine may be given undiluted or diluted in an equal volume of sterile water for injection; drug must be administered slowly over 1–2 min.
- Parenteral papaverine is incompatible with lactated Ringer's injection (forms precipitate).
- Preserve in tightly covered, light-resistant containers.

Assessment & Drug Effects
- Monitor pulse, respiration, and BP in patients receiving drug parenterally. If significant changes are noted, withhold medication and report promptly to physician.
- Hepatic function and blood tests should be performed periodically. Hepatotoxicity (thought to be a hypersensitivity reaction) is reversible with prompt drug withdrawal.

Patient & Family Education
- Instruct to notify physician if any side effect persists or if GI symptoms, jaundice, or skin rash appear. Hepatic function tests may be indicated. Because of the possibility of drowsiness and dizziness, advise patient to avoid driving and other potentially hazardous tasks until reaction to drug is known. Alcohol may increase drowsiness and dizziness.

PARALDEHYDE

(par-al′de-hyde)

Trade names: Paracetaldehyde, Paral

Classifications: CNS AGENT; ANTICONVULSANT; SEDATIVE-HYPNOTIC; BARBITURATE

Prototype: Phenobarbital

Pregnancy category: C

Controlled substance: Schedule IV

ACTIONS/PHARMACODYNAMICS Cyclic ether formed by polymerization of acetaldehyde. Potent CNS depressant with sedative and hypnotic actions similar to those of alcohol, barbiturates, and chloral hydrate.

USES Sedative and hypnotic in acute agitation due to alcohol withdrawal; used to control convulsions arising from tetanus, eclampsia, status epilepticus, and drug poisoning. Has been used rectally to induce basal anesthesia, particularly in children.

ROUTE & DOSAGE

Both oral and rectal doses must be diluted before they are administered.

Hypnotic

Adult: **PO** 10–30 ml prn.
Child: **PO** 0.3 ml/kg.

Sedative

Adult: **PO** 5–10 ml prn.
Child: **PO** 0.15 ml/kg.

Seizures Secondary to Tetanus

Adult: **PO** up to 12 ml diluted 1:10 q4h prn.

Seizures Secondary to Other Poisons

Adult: **PR** 5–15 ml diluted in 200 ml per rectal tube.

Status Epilipticus

Child: PR 1 ml/y of age up to 5 ml; may repeat in 1 h if necessary, then change to PO. PO 2–5 ml q2–4h.

Alcohol Withdrawal Seizures

Adult: **PO** 5–10 ml q4–6h for 24 h; then q6h prn.

PHARMACOKINETICS **Absorption:** readily absorbed from GI tract. **Onset:** 10–15 min. **Duration:** 6–8 h. **Distribution:** distributed into CNS; crosses placenta. **Metabolism:** 80–90% of doses metabolized in liver. **Elimination:** half-life: 7.5 h; excreted through lungs (11–28%) and urine.

CONTRAINDICATIONS & PRECAUTIONS **Contraindicated in:** severe hepatic insufficiency; respiratory disease; GI inflammation or ulceration; disulfiram therapy; pregnancy (category C).

ADVERSE/SIDE EFFECTS *Irritation of mucous membrane (oral and rectal routes),* nausea, vomiting, unpleasant taste and odor, hangover, dizziness, ataxia, *erythematous skin rash;* occasionally confusion and paradoxical excitement. **Prolonged use:** toxic hepatitis, nephrosis, metabolic acidosis. **Overdosage:** rapid labored breathing, respiratory depression, pulmonary hemorrhage and edema, hypotension, bleeding gastritis, renal and liver damage, acidosis, dilation and failure of right heart, cardiovascular collapse.

DIAGNOSTIC TEST INTERFERENCE Chronic use of alcohol (ethanol) and paraldehyde may cause false-positive ***serum ketones*** (nitroprusside tube dilution method) and ***urine ketones*** (Acetest) and may interfere with ***urinary steroid*** (17-OHCS) determinations by modification of Reddy, Jenkins, Thorn procedure.

P

DRUG INTERACTIONS **Disulfiram** may increase paraldehyde levels; **alcohol** and other CNS DEPRESSANTS add to CNS depressant effects—fatalities reported with alcohol.

NURSING IMPLICATIONS

Administration

- In some hospitals, physicians administer parenteral paraldehyde because of danger of circulatory collapse or pulmonary edema, sterile abscesses, nerve injury, and paralysis.
- Paraldehyde is a colorless clear liquid with a strong characteristic odor and a burning, disagreeable taste.
- On exposure to light, air, and heat, drug liberates acetaldehyde, which oxidizes to acetic acid. Do not use

solution if it is colored in any way or smells of acetic acid (vinegar odor).

- Decomposed paraldehyde is extremely corrosive to tissues and can cause fatal poisoning. Discard unused contents of any container that has been open for more than 24 h.
- Do not use plastics for measuring or administering paraldehyde. Contact with plastic materials can decompose paraldehyde to toxic compounds. Parenteral preparation should be drawn into a glass syringe; use rubber catheter for rectal administration.
- Give oral drug well diluted in iced fruit juice or milk to reduce irritation of GI tract and mask odor and taste. Oral capsules are available.
- When given rectally, drug should be diluted with at least 2 volumes of olive oil or cottonseed oil or dissolved in 200 ml of 0.9% NaCl solution to prevent rectal irritation.
- IM injection should be made deep into upper outer quadrant of buttock well away from nerve trunks. Paraldehyde can cause nerve injury and paralysis. Aspirate carefully before injecting drug, and massage injection site well. Rotate injection sites. Not to exceed 5 ml per injection site.
- Rapid withdrawal after prolonged use may produce delirium tremens and hallucinations.
- Preserve in tight, light-resistant containers in amounts not exceeding 30 ml and at temperatures not over 25C (77F). Keep away from heat, open flames, and sparks.

Assessment & Drug Effects

- When paraldehyde is given by IV route (infrequently used), CNS depression may be preceded by a brief period of excitement and coughing. The coughing that sometimes occurs when paraldehyde is given IV may be due to untoward effects on pulmonary capillaries. Monitor patient closely for hypotension and respiratory depression.
- Bronchial secretions may be increased. Keep the patient turned on side to prevent aspiration. Suctioning may be necessary.
- Patient's breath will have a characteristic odor for several hours.
- Tolerance and physical and psychologic dependence can occur with prolonged use. Paraldehyde addiction resembles alcoholism.

PARAMETHADIONE

(par-a-meth-a-dye′one)

Trade name: Paradione

Classifications: CNS AGENT; HYDANTOIN ANTICONVULSANT

Prototype: Phenytoin

Pregnancy category: D

ACTIONS/PHARMACODYNAMICS

Pharmacologic actions, uses, contraindications, precautions, and adverse reactions similar to those of trimethadione. Unlike trimethadione, chronic administration is not associated with myasthenia gravis–like syndrome, and although incidence of other toxic reactions is lower, it is reportedly less effective.

USE To control absence (petit mal) seizures refractory to other drugs.

ROUTE & DOSAGE

Absence Seizures

Adult: **PO** 300 mg t.i.d.; may increase by 300 mg/d at weekly intervals (max 2.4 g/d).
Child: **PO** > *6 y,* 300 mg t.i.d. or q.i.d.; *2–6 y,* 200 mg t.i.d.; < *2 y,* 100 mg t.i.d.

PHARMACOKINETICS Absorption: readily absorbed from GI tract. **Metabolism:** metabolized in liver to active metabolites. **Elimination:** excreted slowly in urine.

CONTRAINDICATIONS & PRECAUTIONS Contraindicated in: hypersensitivity to oxazolidinedione anticonvulsants; severe blood dyscrasias, renal and hepatic dysfunction. Safe use during pregnancy (category D) and in nursing mothers not established. **Cautious use in:** retinal or optic nerve disease.

ADVERSE/SIDE EFFECTS *Sedation, drowsiness.* Infrequent: ataxia, headache, dizziness, paresthesias, vaginal bleeding, changes in BP, visual symptoms, GI distress, rash, alopecia, lymphadenopathy, abnormal liver function tests, albuminuria, mild neutropenia, <u>aplastic anemia, exfoliative dermatitis</u>, erythema multiforme, nephrotic syndrome, hepatitis, lupus.

NURSING IMPLICATIONS

Administration

- Capsule form contains an oily liquid and must be swallowed whole and not chewed or crushed.
- Oral solution contains alcohol 65% and should be diluted with water before administration.
- Drug should be withdrawn gradually to avoid precipitating seizure activity.
- Store in tightly covered containers at 15–30C (59–86F) unless otherwise directed. Solution should be stored in light-resistant container.

Assessment & Drug Effects

- Liver function tests, urinalysis, and CBC should be done prior to and at monthly intervals during therapy. If blood counts remain normal for 12 mo, intervals may be increased. Blood counts are done more frequently if neutrophil count drops to < 3000/mm^3, and drug is withdrawn if count drops to 2500/mm^3 or less.

Patient & Family Education

- Advise to measure oral solution with graduated dropper provided by manufacturer.
- Since drug may cause drowsiness and visual symptoms, caution to avoid driving and other potentially hazardous activities until reaction to drug is known.
- Instruct to report any unusual symptom to physician. Drug should be discontinued if patient develops jaundice, swollen glands, skin rash, hair loss, unexplained fever, fatigue, tendency to bleed or bruise, or sore mouth or throat.

PARAMETHASONE ACETATE

(par-a-meth'a-sone)

Trade name: Haldrone

Classifications: SYNTHETIC HORMONE; ADRENAL CORTICOSTEROID; GLUCOCORTICOID; ANTIINFLAMMATORY

Prototype: Prednisone

Pregnancy category: C

ACTIONS/PHARMACODYNAMICS Long-acting synthetic steroid with antiinflammatory action but little sodium-retaining potency. Has no particular advantages over other corticosteroids. Similar to prednisone in actions, uses, absorption, and fate.

ROUTE & DOSAGE

Allergies, Inflammation

Adult: **PO** 2–24 mg/d in 3–4 divided doses; then decrease to lowest dose necessary.
Child: **PO** 58–200 µg/kg/d in 1–4 divided doses.

P

PHARMACOKINETICS **Absorption:** readily absorbed from GI tract. **Peak:** 1–2 h. **Duration:** 2 d. **Distribution:** crosses placenta; distributed into breast milk. **Elimination:** half-life: 3–45 h; HPA suppression: 36–54 h.

CONTRAINDICATIONS & PRECAUTIONS **Contraindicated in:** systemic fungal infections; ocular herpes simplex; keratitis; safe use during pregnancy (category C), lactation, and by children < 6 y not established.

ADVERSE/SIDE EFFECTS Increase in appetite, growth retardation, hypocalcemia (prolonged treatment), psychic derangement. Same as those of prednisone.

DRUG INTERACTIONS Since BARBITURATES, **phenytoin, rifampin** increase steroid metabolism, may need to increase paramethasone doses; **amphotericin B,** DIURETICS add to potassium loss; **ambenonium, neostigmine, pyridostigmine** may cause severe muscle weakness in patients with myasthenia gravis; may inhibit antibody response to VACCINES, TOXOIDS.

NURSING IMPLICATIONS

See prednisone for numerous additional nursing implications.

Administration

- If drug is to be stopped after long-term therapy, it should be withdrawn gradually to prevent onset of hypocortisolism.
- Store in light-resistant container at 15–30C (59–86F).

Assessment & Drug Effects

- At high dosage (> 15 mg/d), urinary excretion of calcium and nitrogen increases significantly.
- Monitor electrolytes, creatinine, and BUN periodically.

PAREGORIC (CAMPHORATED OPIUM TINCTURE)

(par-e-gor′ik)

Classifications: GI AGENT; ANTIDIARRHEAL; CNS AGENT; NARCOTIC (OPIATE); AGONIST ANALGESIC

Prototype: Diphenoxylate HCl with atropine sulfate

Pregnancy category: B (D for prolonged use or high doses at term)

Controlled substance: Schedule III

ACTIONS/PHARMACODYNAMICS Contains 2 mg anhydrous morphine, alcohol, benzoic acid, camphor, and anise oil. Pharmacologic activity is due to morphine content. Increases smooth muscle tone of GI tract, decreases motility and effective propulsive peristalsis, and diminishes digestive secretions. Delayed transit of intestinal contents results in desiccation of feces and constipation.

USES Short-term treatment for symptomatic relief of acute diarrhea and abdominal cramps.

ROUTE & DOSAGE

Acute Diarrhea
Adult: **PO** 5–10 ml after loose bowel movement; may be administered q2h up to q.i.d. if needed.
Child: **PO** 0.25–0.5 ml/kg 1–4 times/d.

PHARMACOKINETICS **Absorption:** readily absorbed from GI tract. **Duration:** 4–5 h. **Distribution:** crosses placenta; distributed into breast milk. **Metabolism:** metabolized in liver. **Elimination:** half-life: 2–3 h; excreted in urine.

CONTRAINDICATIONS & PRECAUTIONS **Contraindicated in:** hypersensitivity to opium alkaloids; diarrhea caused by poisons (until eliminated); pregnancy [(category B), with prolonged use or high doses at term (category D)]. **Cautious use in:** asthma; hepatic disease; history of opiate agonist dependence; severe prostatic hypertrophy.

ADVERSE/SIDE EFFECTS GI: anorexia, nausea, vomiting, *constipation,* abdominal pain. **Other:** with high doses: dizziness, faintness, drowsiness, facial flushing, sweating, physical dependence.

DRUG INTERACTIONS Alcohol and other CNS DEPRESSANTS add to CNS effects.

NURSING IMPLICATIONS

Administration

- Camphorated opium tincture (paregoric) is not to be confused with Deodorized Opium Tincture, which contains 25 times more anhydrous morphine.
- Administer paregoric in sufficient water (2 or 3 swallows) to ensure its passage into the stomach (mixture will appear milky).
- Preserve in tight, light-resistant container at 15–30C (59–86F) unless otherwise directed.

Assessment & Drug Effects

- Paregoric may worsen the course of diarrhea by delaying the elimination of pathogens.
- Adverse effects are primarily due to morphine content. Paregoric abuse results because of the narcotic content of the drug.
- Assess for fluid and electrolyte imbalance until diarrhea has stopped.

Patient & Family Education

- Instruct to adhere strictly to prescribed dosage schedule.
- Bed rest is advisable if diarrhea is severe with a high level of fluid loss.
- Replacement of fluids and electrolytes is a vital adjunct to drug therapy for diarrhea. Instruct patient to drink warm clear liquids and to avoid dairy products, concentrated sweets, and cold drinks until diarrhea stops.
- Advise to observe character and frequency of stools. Drug should be discontinued as soon as diarrhea is controlled. Urge patient to report promptly to physician if diarrhea persists more than 3 d, if fever is > 38.8C (102F), abdominal pain develops, or if mucus or blood is passed.
- Inform that constipation is often a consequence of antidiarrheal treatment and that normal pattern is usually established as dietary intake increases.

PARICALCITOL

(par-i-cal′ci-tol)

Trade name: Zemplar

Classifications: HORMONE; VITAMIN D ANALOG

Prototype: Calcitriol

Pregnancy category: C

ACTIONS/PHARMACODYNAMICS Synthetic vitamin D analog that reduces parathyroid hormone (PTH) levels in chronic renal failure (CRF) patients. Serum levels of calcium and phosphate are lowered with paricalcitol, and the serum calcium times phosphate cross product value may increase.

USES Prevention and treatment of secondary hyperparathyroidism associated with CRF.

ROUTE & DOSAGE

CRF-associated Secondary Hyperparathyroidism

Adult: **IV** 0.04–0.1 μg/kg IV bolus no more frequently than q.o.d.;

P

may increase dose by 2–4 μg at 2- to 4-wk intervals if necessary (max 16.8 μg/dose).

PHARMACOKINETICS **Onset:** 2–4 h. **Elimination:** half-life: 15 h; 74% excreted in feces, 16% in urine.

CONTRAINDICATIONS & PRECAUTIONS **Contraindicated in:** hypersensitivity to paricalcitol, concurrent administration of phosphate or vitamin D-related compounds, evidence of vitamin D toxicity, hypercalcemia, pregnancy (category C). **Cautious use in:** lactation, liver disease, abnormally low levels of PTH.

ADVERSE/SIDE EFFECTS **Body as whole:** chills, fever, malaise, flu, sepsis. **CNS:** light-headedness. **CV:** palpitation, edema. **GI:** dry mouth, GI bleeding, nausea, vomiting. **Respiratory:** pneumonia.

NURSING IMPLICATIONS

Administration

- IV administration: Withdraw ordered dose undiluted and give IV push. Discard unused portion.
- Store unopened vials at 15–30C (59–86F) in a tightly closed container and protect from light.

Assessment & Drug Effects

- Therapeutic effectiveness is indicated by PTH levels between 1.5 and 3 times the upper limit of normal.
- Lab tests: During initial therapy, monitor serum calcium and phosphorus at least twice weekly and monthly thereafter; monitor serum or plasma PTH q3mo.
- Carefully monitor for and immediately report S&S of hypercalcemia including weakness, headache, somnolence, nausea and vomiting, constipation, dry mouth or metallic taste, and muscle or bone pain.
- Withhold drug and notify physician if hypercalcemia is suspected (see Appendix G).
- Carefully monitor patients on digitalis as toxicity is potentiated by hypercalcemia.

Patient & Family Education

- It is important to adhere to a diet with calcium supplementation and phosphorus restriction.
- Immediately notify physician if S&S of hypercalcemia develop such as weakness, headache, drowsiness, nausea, vomiting, constipation, dry mouth, metallic taste, and muscle or bone pain.

PAROMOMYCIN SULFATE

(par-oh-moe-mye′sin)

Trade name: Humatin

Classifications: ANTIINFECTIVE; AMEBICIDE; AMINOGLYCOSIDE ANTIBIOTIC

Prototype: Emetine

Pregnancy category: C

ACTIONS/PHARMACODYNAMICS Aminoglycoside antibiotic produced by certain strains of *Streptomyces rimosus* with broad spectrum of antibacterial activity closely paralleling that of kanamycin and neomycin. Exerts direct bactericidal and amebicidal action, primarily in lumen of GI tract. Ineffective against extraintestinal amebiasis. Reportedly significantly reduces serum cholesterol.

USES Acute and chronic intestinal amebiasis and to rid bowel of nitrogen-forming bacteria in patients with hepatic coma; used preoperatively to suppress intestinal flora. Also tapeworm infestation.

ROUTE & DOSAGE

Intestinal Amebiasis
Adult: **PO** 25–35 mg/kg divided in 3 doses for 5–10 d.
Child: **PO** Same as for adult.

Hepatic Coma
Adult: **PO** 4 g/d in 2–4 divided doses for 5–6 d.

PHARMACOKINETICS **Absorption:** poorly absorbed from intact GI tract. **Elimination:** in feces.

CONTRAINDICATIONS & PRECAUTIONS **Contraindicated in:** intestinal obstruction; impaired renal function; pregnancy (category C). **Cautious use in:** GI ulceration.

ADVERSE/SIDE EFFECTS **CNS:** headache, vertigo. **GI:** *diarrhea, abdominal cramps,* steatorrhea, *nausea, vomiting, heartburn,* secondary enterocolitis. **Skin:** exanthema, rash, pruritus. **Other:** ototoxicity, nephrotoxicity (in patients with GI inflammation or ulcerations), eosinophilia, overgrowth of nonsusceptible organisms.

DIAGNOSTIC TEST INTERFERENCE Prolonged use of paromomycin may cause reduction in ***serum cholesterol.***

NURSING IMPLICATIONS

Administration
- Paromycin sulfate is usually administered after meals to prevent gastric distress.

Assessment & Drug Effects
- Be alert for appearance of a superinfection during therapy (see Appendix G).
- Patients with history of GI ulceration must be closely monitored for nephrotoxicity and ototoxicity (see Appendix G). Drug absorption can take place through diseased mucosa.
- Criterion of cure is absence of amebae in stool specimens examined at weekly intervals for 6 wk after completion of treatment, and thereafter at monthly intervals for 2 y.

Patient & Family Education
- Patients receiving drug for intestinal amebiasis should be excluded from preparing, processing, and serving food until treatment is complete. Isolation is not required.
- Emphasize personal hygiene, particularly handwashing after defecation and before eating food, and sanitary disposal of feces.

PAROXETINE

(par-ox′-e-teen)
Trade name: Paxil
Classifications: CNS AGENT; PSYCHOTHERAPEUTIC; ANTIDEPRESSANT; SELECTIVE SEROTONIN REUPTAKE INHIBITOR
Prototype: Fluoxetine
Pregnancy category: B

ACTIONS/PHARMACODYNAMICS Antidepressant structurally unrelated to other serotonin uptake inhibitors. Potent and highly selective inhibitor of serotonin reuptake by neurons in CNS.

USES Depression, obsessive-compulsive disorders, panic attacks. **Unlabeled uses:** diabetic neuropathy, myoclonus.

ROUTE & DOSAGE

Depression
Adult: **PO** 10–50 mg/d (max 80 mg/d). Lower starting doses recommended for patients with renal or hepatic insufficiency and geriatric patients.

P

Obsessive-compulsive Disorder
Adult: 20–60 mg/d.

Panic Attacks
Adult: **PO** 40 mg/d.

PHARMACOKINETICS **Absorption:** 99% absorbed from GI tract. **Onset:** 2 wk. **Peak:** 5–8 h. **Distribution:** very lipophilic. 95% protein bound. Distributes into breast milk. **Metabolism:** extensively metabolized in the liver. Oxidized initially to an unstable catechol intermediate, with catechol being methylated in part at meta-position and conjugated to a glucuronide or sulfate. Appearance of metabolites of paroxetine in plasma simultaneously with paroxetine following oral administration is suggestive of first-pass metabolism. Major metabolites of paroxetine are conjugates that are not pharmacologically active. **Elimination:** half-life: 24 h; less than 2% is excreted unchanged in urine. Approximately 65% of dose appears in urine as metabolites. Metabolites of paroxetine are also excreted in feces, presumably via bile.

P

CONTRAINDICATIONS & PRECAUTIONS **Contraindicated in:** concomitant use of MAO inhibitors. **Cautious use in:** renal/hepatic impairment, elderly, history of metabolic disorders, pregnancy (category B), nursing mothers. Safety and efficacy have not been established in children.

ADVERSE/SIDE EFFECTS **CV:** postural hypotension. **CNS:** *headache,* tremor, agitation or nervousness, anxiety, parethesias, dizziness, insomnia, *sedation.* **GI:** *nausea,* constipation, vomiting, anorexia, diarrhea, dyspepsia, flatulence, increased appetite, taste aversion, *dry mouth.* **GU:** urinary hesitancy or frequency. **Hepatic:** isolated reports of elevated liver enzymes. **Ocular:** blurred vision. **Skin:** diaphoresis, rash, pruritus. **Other:** hyponatremia in elderly.

DRUG INTERACTIONS **Activated charcoal** reduces absorption of paroxetine. **Cimetidine** increases paroxetine levels. MAO INHIBITORS **selegiline** may cause an increased vasopressor response leading to hypertensive crisis or death. **Phenytoin** can cause hepatic enzyme induction resulting in lower paroxetine levels and shorter half-life. **Warfarin** may increase risk of bleeding.

NURSING IMPLICATIONS

Administration

- Recommended initial dose with elderly, debilitated, or those with severe renal or hepatic impairment is 10 mg/d. Dose may be gradually increased at weekly intervals to a maximum of 40 mg/d.
- Dose may be increased (usually at intervals of at least a week) by increments of 10 mg/d.
- At least 14 d should elapse when switching a patient from/to a MAO inhibitor to/from paroxetine.
- Store at room temperature, 15–30C (59–86F), unless otherwise directed.

Assessment & Drug Effects

- Monitor for adverse effects, most common of which include headache, weakness, sedation, dizziness, insomnia; nausea, constipation, or diarrhea; dry mouth; sweating; male ejaculatory disturbance. These occur in more than 10% of all patients and may result in poor compliance with drug regimen.
- Monitor elderly for fluid and sodium imbalances.
- Monitor for significant weight loss.

- Monitor patients with history of mania for reactivation of condition.
- Carefully monitor patients with preexisting cardiovascular disease, because the paroxetine may adversely affect hemodynamic status.

Patient & Family Education

- Caution about operating hazardous machinery or equipment until reaction to paroxetine is known.
- Advise that concurrent use of alcohol may increase risk of adverse CNS effects.
- Inform that adaptation to some adverse effects (especially dizziness and nausea) may occur over a period of 4–6 wk.
- Stress need to continue with drug therapy after improvement in emotional status occurs.
- Advise to notify physician of any distressing adverse effects.

PEMOLINE

(pem′oh-leen)

Trade name: Cylert

Classifications: CNS AGENT; RESPIRATORY AND CEREBRAL STIMULANT

Prototype: Amphetamine

Pregnancy category: B

Controlled substance: Schedule IV

ACTIONS/PHARMACODYNAMICS Actions qualitatively similar to those of amphetamine but with weak sympathomimetic activity. Capable of producing increased motor activity, mental alertness, diminished sense of fatigue, and mild euphoria. Also thought to have anorexigenic effect.

USES Adjunctive therapy to other remedial measures (psychologic, educational, social) in minimal brain dysfunction (attention deficit disorder [ADD]) in carefully selected children. **Unlabeled use:** mild stimulant for geriatric patients.

ROUTE & DOSAGE

Attention Deficit Disorder

Child >6 y: **PO** 37.5 mg/d; may be increased by 18.75 mg at weekly intervals (max 112.5 mg/d).

PHARMACOKINETICS Absorption: readily absorbed from GI tract. **Onset:** 2–3 wk. **Peak:** 2–4 h. **Duration:** 8 h. **Metabolism:** metabolized in liver. **Elimination:** half-life: 9–14 h; excreted in urine.

CONTRAINDICATIONS & PRECAUTIONS Contraindicated in: known hypersensitivity to pemoline; children <6 y. Safe use during pregnancy (category B) and in nursing women not established. **Cautious use in:** impaired hepatic and renal function; history of drug abuse; psychosis; emotional instability.

ADVERSE/SIDE EFFECTS *Insomnia, anorexia,* abdominal discomfort, hepatic failure, malaise, nausea, diarrhea, skin rash, irritability, fatigue, mild depression, dizziness, headache, drowsiness, dyskinetic movements of eyes or other parts of body; convulsions. **Overdosage:** nervousness, tachycardia, hallucinations, excitement, agitation, restlessness. Also reported: elevated AST, ALT, and alkaline phosphatase (after several months of therapy); jaundice.

NURSING IMPLICATIONS

Administration

- Administer drug in morning to provide maximal effectiveness and to avoid insomnia.
- Chewable tablet may be chewed or swallowed whole.

- Store at 15–30C (59–86F) unless otherwise directed.

Assessment & Drug Effects

- Insomnia and anorexia (most frequent side effects) appear to be dose-related.
- Monitor weight and height (growth rate) throughout therapy. Anorexia is often accompanied by weight loss.
- Careful clinical evaluation and supervision of patient are essential. Patients receiving long-term therapy should have baseline and periodic liver function studies. Pemoline should be discontinued if significantly abnormal liver functions are noted.
- Occasional interruption of drug therapy is advised to determine if behavioral symptoms recur.

Patient & Family Education

- Immediately report any sign of liver malfunction such as dark urine, jaundice, loss of appetite. Avoid potentially hazardous activities until the reaction to drug is known.
- Significant benefits of drug therapy may not be evident until third or fourth week of drug administration.
- Pemoline can produce tolerance and physical and psychologic dependence.

P

PENBUTOLOL

(pen-bu'tol-ol)

Trade name: Levatol

Classifications: AUTONOMIC NERVOUS SYSTEM AGENT; BETA-ADRENERGIC ANTAGONIST (BLOCKING AGENT, SYMPATHOLYTIC); ANTIHYPERTENSIVE

Prototype: Propranolol

Pregnancy category: C

ACTIONS/PHARMACODYNAMICS Penbutolol is a synthetic $beta_1$- and $beta_2$-adrenergic blocking agent. It lowers both supine and standing BP in hypertensive patients. Hypotensive effect is associated with decreased cardiac output, suppressed renin activity, as well as beta blockage.

USES Mild to moderate hypertension. May be used alone or with other antihypertensive agents.

ROUTE & DOSAGE

Hypertension

Adult: **PO** 10–20 mg once/d; may increase to 40–80 mg/d if needed.

PHARMACOKINETICS **Absorption:** readily absorbed from GI tract. **Peak:** 2–3 h. **Duration:** 20 h. **Metabolism:** metabolized in liver. **Elimination:** half-life: 5 h; excreted in urine.

CONTRAINDICATIONS & PRECAUTIONS **Contraindicated in:** clients with cardiogenic shock, sinus bradycardia, second and third degree AV block, bronchial asthma, and hypersensitivity to the drug. **Cautious use in:** cardiac failure, chronic bronchitis, emphysema, diabetes, pregnancy (category C), and nursing mothers. Safety and effectiveness in children has not been established.

ADVERSE/SIDE EFFECTS **CNS:** dizziness, fatigue, *headache,* insomnia. **CV:** AV block, bradycardia. **GI:** nausea, diarrhea, dyspepsia. **Respiratory:** cough, dyspnea. **Other:** impotence.

DRUG INTERACTIONS DIURETICS and other HYPOTENSIVE AGENTS increase hypotensive effect; effects of **albuterol, metaproterenol, terbutaline, pirbuterol,** and penbutolol are antagonized; NSAIDS blunt hypotensive effect; decreases hypoglycemic effect of **glyburide;**

amiodarone increases risk of bradycardia and sinus arrest.

NURSING IMPLICATIONS

Administration

- Penbutolol may be taken without regard to meals.
- Penbutolol should be discontinued by reducing the dose gradually over 1 to 2 wk.

Assessment & Drug Effects

- Take apical pulse before administering drug. If pulse is below 60, hold the drug and contact physician.
- If BP is not stabilized, take a BP reading before giving drug. If systolic pressure is ≤ 90 mm Hg, hold drug and contact physician.
- Check BP near end of dosage interval or before administration of next dose to evaluate effectiveness.
- Apical pulse, respirations, BP, and circulation to extremities should be closely monitored throughout periods of dosage adjustment. Consult physician regarding acceptable parameters.
- The full effectiveness of the drug is not seen for 4–6 wk.
- Watch for signs and symptoms of bronchial constriction. Report promptly and withhold drug.
- Diabetics should be closely monitored. Penbutolol suppresses clinical signs of hypoglycemia (e.g., BP changes, increased pulse rate) and may prolong hypoglycemic state.
- During drug withdrawal, carefully monitor for exacerbation of angina.

Patient & Family Education

- Instruct not to interrupt or discontinue the drug without physician's advice because of the possible exacerbation of ischemic heart disease.
- Instruct diabetics to report signs and symptoms of hypoglycemia (see Appendix G).
- Since penbutolol may cause dizziness and light-headedness due to mild hypotension, caution to avoid driving or other potentially hazardous activities until reaction is known.
- Advise to make position changes slowly and to avoid prolonged standing. Notify physician if dizziness and light-headedness persist.
- Stress the importance of compliance and warn not to alter established regimen (i.e., not to omit, increase, or decrease dosage or change dosage interval).
- Caution to avoid prolonged exposure of extremities to cold.
- Counsel to avoid excesses of alcohol. Heavy alcohol consumption (i.e., > 60 ml [2 oz]/d) may elevate arterial pressure; therefore, to maintain treatment effectiveness, either avoid alcohol or drink moderately (<60 ml/d). Consult physician.

P

PENCICLOVIR

(pen-cy′clo-vir)

Trade names: Denavir

Classifications: ANTIINFECTIVE; ANTIVIRAL

Prototype: Acyclovir

Pregnancy category: B

ACTIONS/PHARMACODYNAMICS

Penciclovir is an antiviral agent active against herpes simplex virus type 1 (HSV-1) and type 2 (HSV-2). HSV-1 and HSV-2 infected cells phosphorylate penciclovir utilizing viral thymidine kinases. The resulting form of penciclovir competes with viral DNA, thus inhibiting both viral DNA synthesis and replication.

USE Treatment of recurrent herpes labialis (cold sores).

ROUTE & DOSAGE

Cold Sores
Adult: **Topical** Apply q2h while awake × 4 d.

PHARMACOKINETICS Absorption: minimally absorbed from cold sore.

CONTRAINDICATIONS & PRECAUTIONS Contraindicated in: hypersensitivity to penciclovir, lactation. **Cautious use in:** pregnancy (category B). Safety and efficacy in children have not been established. Safety in immunocompromised patients has not been established.

ADVERSE/SIDE EFFECTS CNS: headache. **Skin:** erythema.

NURSING IMPLICATIONS

Administration

- Should be applied as soon as possible to developing lesion. Do not apply to mucous membranes or near the eyes.
- Store at or below 30C (86F) but do not freeze.

Assessment & Drug Effects

- Therapeutic effectiveness is indicated by diappearance of lip lesion.

Patient & Family Education

- Wash hands before and after application. Avoid contact of drug with eyes.

PENICILLAMINE

(pen-i-sill′a-meen)

Trade names: Cuprimine, Depen

Classification: CHELATING AGENT

ACTIONS/PHARMACODYNAMICS Thiol compound prepared by hydrolysis of penicillin but lacking antibacterial activity. Forms stable soluble chelate with copper, zinc, iron, lead, mercury, and possibly other heavy metals and promotes their excretion in urine. Also combines chemically with cystine to form a soluble disulfide complex that prevents stone formation and may even dissolve existing cystitic stones. Mechanism of action in rheumatoid arthritis not known but appears to be related to inhibition of collagen formation. Cross-sensitivity between penicillin and penicillamine can occur.

USES To promote renal excretion of excess copper in Wilson's disease (hepatolenticular degeneration). Active rheumatoid arthritis in patients who have failed to respond to conventional therapy. Cystinuria. **Unlabeled uses:** scleroderma, primary biliary cirrhosis, porphyria cutanea tarda, lead poisoning.

ROUTE & DOSAGE

Wilson's Disease
Adult: **PO** 250 mg q.i.d., with 3 doses 1 h a.c. and the last dose at least 2 h after the last meal.
Child: **PO** 20 mg/kg/d in 2–4 divided doses (max 1 g/d).

Cystinuria
Adult: **PO** 250–500 mg q.i.d., with doses adjusted to limit urinary excretion of cystine to 100–200 mg/d.
Child: **PO** 30 mg/kg/d in 4 divided doses with doses adjusted to limit urinary excretion of cystine to 100–200 mg/d.

Rheumatoid Arthritis
Adult: **PO** 125–250 mg/d; may increase at 1–3 mo intervals up to 1–1.5 g/d.

Child: **PO** 3 mg/kg/d (≤250 mg/d) × 3 mo, then 6 mg/kg/d (≤500 mg/d) in 2 divided doses × 3 mo; increase to max of 10 mg/kg/d (≤1.5 g/d) in 3–4 divided doses.

Lead Poisoning

Child: **PO** 30–40 mg/kg/d in 3–4 divided doses (max 1.5 g/d); initiate at 25% target dose; gradually increase to full dose over 2–3 wk.

PHARMACOKINETICS Absorption: readily absorbed from GI tract. **Peak:** 1 h. **Distribution:** crosses placenta. **Metabolism:** metabolized in liver. **Elimination:** excreted in urine and feces.

CONTRAINDICATIONS & PRECAUTIONS Contraindicated in: hypersensitivity to penicillamine or to any penicillin; history of penicillamine-related aplastic anemia or agranulocytosis; patients with rheumatoid arthritis who have renal insufficiency or who are pregnant, during pregnancy in patients with cystinuria; nursing mothers; concomitant administration with drugs that can cause severe hematologic or renal reactions, e.g., antimalarials, gold salts, immunosuppressants, oxyphenbutazone, phenylbutazone. **Cautious use in:** allergy-prone individuals.

ADVERSE/SIDE EFFECTS Allergic: *generalized pruritus, urticaria, early and late occurring rashes,* pemphiguslike rash, fever, arthralgia, lymphadenopathy, thyroiditis, SLE-like syndrome. **GI:** *anorexia, nausea, vomiting,* epigastric pain, diarrhea, oral lesions, *reduction or loss of taste perception (particularly salt and sweet), metallic taste,* activation of peptic ulcer. **Hematologic:** thrombocytopenia, leukopenia, agranulocytosis, thrombotic thrombocytopenic purpura, hemolytic anemia, aplastic anemia. **Renal:** membranous glomerulopathy, *proteinuria,* hematuria. **Other:** tinnitus, optic neuritis, thrombophlebitis, hyperpyrexia, alopecia, myasthenia gravis syndrome, mammary hyperplasia, alveolitis, skin friability, excessive skin wrinkling, pancreatitis, pyridoxine deficiency, tingling of feet, ptosis, weakness.

DRUG INTERACTIONS ANTIMALARIALS, CYTOTOXICS, **gold** therapy may potentiate hematologic and renal adverse effects; **iron** may decrease penicillamine absorption.

NURSING IMPLICATIONS

Administration

- Take on an empty stomach (60 min before or 2 h after meals) to avoid absorption of metals in foods by penicillamine.
- If patient cannot swallow capsules or tablets, contents may be administered in 15–30 ml of chilled fruit juice.

Assessment & Drug Effects

- Penicillamine can produce severe toxic reactions involving skin, blood, kidneys, and liver.
- Allergic reactions occur in about one third of patients receiving penicillamine. Temporary interruptions of therapy increase possibility of sensitivity reactions.
- White and differential blood cell counts, direct platelet counts, hemoglobin, and urinalyses should be done prior to initiation of therapy and every 3 d during the first month of therapy, then every 2 wk thereafter. Liver function tests and eye examinations should be performed before start of therapy and at least twice yearly thereafter.
- Clinical evidence of therapeutic ef-

P

fectiveness may not be apparent until 1–3 mo of drug therapy.

- Therapeutic effectiveness in Wilson's disease is indicated by improvement in psychiatric and neurologic symptoms, visual symptoms, and hepatic function. In some patients, neurologic symptoms become more prominent during initial therapy and then subside.
- Rheumatoid arthritis: Record evidence of drug effectiveness such as improvement in grip strength, decrease in stiffness following immobility, reduction of pain, decrease in sedimentation rate and rheumatoid factor.
- Dosage should be reduced or drug discontinued if the patient with rheumatoid arthritis develops proteinuria >1 g (some clinicians accept ≤2 g) or if platelet count drops to <100,000/mm^3, or platelet count falls 3500–4000/mm^3, or neutropenia occurs.
- Temperature should be taken nightly during first few months of therapy. Fever is a possible early sign of allergy.
- Instruct patient to observe skin over pressure sites: knees, elbows, shoulder blades, toes, buttocks. Penicillamine increases skin friability. Report unusual bruising or bleeding, sore mouth or throat, fever, skin rash, or any other unusual symptoms.

P

PENICILLIN G BENZATHINE

(pen-i-sill'in)

Trade names: Bicillin, Bicillin L-A, Permapen

Classifications: ANTIINFECTIVE; BETA-LACTAM ANTIBIOTIC; NATURAL PENICILLIN

Prototype: Penicillin G potassium

Pregnancy category: B

ACTIONS/PHARMACODYNAMICS
Acid-stable, penicillinase-sensitive, long-acting form of penicillin G. Because it has extremely low water solubility, it is absorbed slowly in body. Produces lower blood concentrations than other penicillin G compounds but has the longest duration of antimicrobial activity of all other available parenteral or repository penicillins.

USES Infections highly susceptible to penicillin G, such as streptococcal, pneumococcal, and staphylococcal infections, venereal disease such as syphilis (including early, late, and congenital forms), and nonvenereal diseases (e.g., yaws, bejel, and pinta). Also used in prophylaxis of rheumatic fever.

ROUTE & DOSAGE

Mild to Moderate Infections

Adult: **IM** 1,200,000 U once/d.
Child: **IM** >27 kg: 900,000 U once/d; <27 kg: 300,000–600,000 U once/d.

Syphilis

Adult: **IM** <1 y duration: 2,400,000 U as single dose; >1 y duration: 2,400,000 U/wk for 3 wk.
Child: **IM** Congenital: 50,000 U/kg as single dose.

Prophylaxis for Rheumatic Fever

Adult: **IM** 1,200,000 U q4wk.
Child: **IM** 1,200,000 U q3–4wk.

PHARMACOKINETICS Absorption: slowly absorbed from IM site. **Peak:** 12–24 h. **Duration:** 26 d. **Distribution:** crosses placenta; distributed into breast milk. **Metabolism:** hydrolyzed to penicillin in body. **Elimination:** excreted slowly by kidneys.

CONTRAINDICATIONS & PRECAUTIONS **Contraindicated in:** hypersensitivity to penicillins or cephalosporins; pregnancy (category B). **Cautious use in:** history of or suspected atopy or allergy (eczema, hives, hay fever, asthma).

ADVERSE/SIDE EFFECTS *Local pain,* tenderness, and fever associated with IM injection, Jarisch-Herxheimer reaction in patients with syphilis. **Hypersensitivity:** pruritus, urticaria and other skin eruptions, chills, fever, wheezing, anaphylaxis, eosinophilia, hemolytic anemia and other blood abnormalities, neuropathy, nephrotoxicity; superinfections. Also see penicillin G.

NURSING IMPLICATIONS

See penicillin G potassium for numerous additional nursing implications.

Administration

- Penicillin G benzathine is not to be confused with preparations containing procaine penicillin G (e.g., Bicillin C-R).
- IM injection should be made deep into upper outer quadrant of buttock. In infants and small children, the preferred site is the midlateral aspect of the thigh.
- Shake multiple-dose vial vigorously before withdrawing desired IM dose. Shake prepared cartridge unit vigorously before injecting drug. Injection form is for IM use only.
- Select IM site with care. Injection into or near a major peripheral nerve can result in nerve damage. Inadvertent IV administration has resulted in arterial occlusion and cardiac arrest.
- Injections should be made at a slow steady rate to prevent needle blockage.
- Store at 15–30C (59–86F).

Assessment & Drug Effects

- Prior to initiation of drug therapy, determine history of hypersensitivity reactions to penicillins, cephalosporins, or other allergens.
- As with other penicillins, culture and sensitivity tests should be done prior to initiation of therapy and periodically thereafter.

Patient & Family Education

- Instruct to take medication around the clock, not to miss a dose, and to continue taking medication until it is all gone.
- Instruct to report immediately to physician the onset of an allergic reaction. There is great risk of severe and prolonged reactions because drug is absorbed so slowly.

PENICILLIN G POTASSIUM

Trade names: Megacillin ♣, Pentids, Pfizarpen

PENICILLIN G SODIUM

Prototype for classifications: ANTIINFECTIVE; BETA-LACTAM ANTIBIOTIC; NATURAL PENICILLIN
Pregnancy category: B

ACTIONS/PHARMACODYNAMICS Acid-labile, penicillinase-sensitive, natural penicillin derived from cultures of *Penicillium notatum* or related molds. Antimicrobial spectrum is relatively narrow compared to that of the semisynthetic penicillins. Bactericidal at therapeutic serum levels; bacteriostatic at lower concentrations. Acts by interfering with synthesis of mucopeptides essential to formation and integrity of bacterial cell wall. Action is inhibited by penicillinase; therefore, penicillin G is ineffective against many strains of *Staphylococcus aureus*. Highly active against gram-positive cocci (e.g., non-penicillinase-producing

Staphylococcus, Streptococcus groups A, C, G, H, L, M, and *Streptococcus pneumoniae*); and gram-negative cocci *(Neisseria gonorrhoeae, N. meningitidis)*. Also effective against gram-positive bacilli (*Bacillus anthracis, Clostridium* species including gas gangrene and tetanus, and certain species of *Corynebacterium, Erysipelothrix,* and *Listeria*); gram-negative bacilli (*Fusobacterium, Pasteurella, Streptobacillus,* and *Bacteroides* species). Parenteral penicillin G is effective against some strains of *Salmonella* and *Shigella* and spirochetes *(Treponema pallidum, T. pertenue, Leptospira)*.

USES Moderate to severe systemic infections caused by penicillin-sensitive microorganisms: actinomycosis, anthrax, diphtheria (carrier state), empyema, erysipelas, gas gangrene, gonorrheal infections, leptospirosis, mastoiditis, meningitis, acute osteomyelitis, otitis media, pinta, pneumonia, rat-bite fever, sinus infections; certain staphylococcal infections; streptococcal infections, including scarlet fever; syphilis (all stages), tetanus, urinary tract infections, Vincent's gingivostomatitis, yaws. Also used as prophylaxis in patients with rheumatic or congenital heart disease. Since oral preparations are absorbed erratically and thus must be given in comparatively high doses, this route is generally used only for mild or stabilized infections or long-term prophylaxis.

ROUTE & DOSAGE

Moderate to Severe Infections

Adult: **PO** 1.6–3.2 million U divided q6h. **IV/IM** 1.2–24 million U divided q4h.
Child: **PO** 25,000–100,000 U/kg divided q6h. **IV/IM** 25,000–300,000 U/kg divided q4h.

PHARMACOKINETICS **Absorption:** 15–30% of PO dose absorbed; very acid labile. **Peak:** 30–60 min PO; 15–30 min IM. **Distribution:** widely distributed; good CSF concentrations with inflamed meninges; crosses placenta; distributed in breast milk. **Metabolism:** 16–30% metabolized. **Elimination:** half-life: 0.4–0.9 h; 60% excreted in urine within 6 h.

CONTRAINDICATIONS & PRECAUTIONS **Contraindicated in:** hypersensitivity to any of the penicillins or cephalosporins; administration of oral drug to patients with severe infections, nausea, vomiting, hypermotility, gastric dilatation, cardiospasm. Use of penicillin G sodium in patients on sodium restriction; safe use during pregnancy (category B) or in nursing mothers not established. **Cautious use in:** history of or suspected atopy or allergy (asthma, eczema, hay fever, hives); history of allergy to cephalosporins; renal or hepatic dysfunction, myasthenia gravis, epilepsy, neonates, young infants. Use in nursing mothers may lead to sensitization of infants.

ADVERSE/SIDE EFFECTS **Electrolyte imbalance:** hyperkalemia (penicillin G potassium); hypokalemia, alkalosis, hypernatremia, CHF (penicillin G sodium). **Hypersensitivity: (1) immediate** (usually occurs within 2–30 min after drug administration): localized anaphylaxis: itchy palms or axilla or generalized pruritus or urticaria, flushed skin, coughing, sneezing, feeling of uneasiness; systemic anaphylaxis: fever, vomiting, diarrhea, severe abdominal cramps, widespread increase in capillary permeability and vasodilation with resulting edema (mouth, tongue, pharynx, larynx), laryngospasm, bronchospasm, hypotension, circulatory collapse, cardiac arrhythmias, cardiac arrest. **(2) Accelerated** (occurs in 1–72 h): malaise, fever, *urticaria*, erythema or other skin reactions and (less commonly) angioneurotic and laryngeal edema, asthma. **(3) Delayed or late** (develops after 72 h): serum sickness (fever, malaise, pruritus, urticaria, lymphadenopathy, arthralgia, angioedema of face and extremities, neuritis prostration, eosinophilia). *Skin rashes* ranging from urticaria to exfoliative dermatitis, Stevens-Johnson syndrome, fixed-drug eruptions, contact dermatitis; hemolytic anemia, thrombocytopenia, SLE-like syndrome, interstitial nephritis, Loeffler's syndrome, vasculitis. **Injection site reactions:** pain, inflammation, abscess, phlebitis. **Superinfections:** especially with *Candida* and gram-negative bacteria (e.g., *Proteus, Pseudomonas*). **Toxicity:** neuromuscular irritability: twitching, lethargy, confusion, stupor, hyperreflexia, multifocal myoclonus, localized or generalized seizures, coma. **With oral therapy:** nausea, vomiting, epigastric distress, diarrhea, flatulence, dark discoloration of tongue, sore mouth or tongue. **Other:** *Jarisch-Herxheimer reaction (syphilis)*, drug fever.

DIAGNOSTIC TEST INTERFERENCE ***Blood grouping and compatibility tests:*** possible interference associated with penicillin doses greater than 20 million units daily. ***Urine glucose:*** massive doses of penicillin may cause false-positive test results with Benedict's solution and possibly Clinitest but not with glucose oxidase methods, e.g., Clinistix, Diastix, TesTape. ***Urine protein:*** massive doses of penicillin can produce false-positive results when turbidity measures are used (e.g., acetic acid and heat, sulfo-salicylic acid); Ames reagent reportedly not affected. ***Urinary PSP excretion tests:*** false decrease in urinary excretion of PSP. ***Urinary steroids:*** large IV doses of penicillin may interfere with accurate measurement of urinary 17-OHCS (Glenn-Nelson technique not affected).

DRUG INTERACTIONS **Probenecid** decreases renal elimination; penicillin G may decrease efficacy of ORAL CONTRACEPTIVES; **colestipol** decreases penicillin absorption; POTASSIUM-SPARING DIURETICS may cause hyperkalemia with penicillin G potassium. **Drug–food:** food increases breakdown in stomach.

INCOMPATIBILITIES **Solution/additive: dextran 40, fat emulsion, aminophylline, amphotericin B, cephalothin, chlorpromazine, dopamine, hydroxyzine, metaraminol,** TETRACYCLINES, **pentobarbital, prochlorperazine, promazine, sodium bicarbonate, thiopental, metoclopramide.**

P

NURSING IMPLICATIONS

Administration

General

- Note whether physician has prescribed penicillin G potassium or sodium.
- Store penicillin G tablets at room temperature in tightly closed containers. Avoid excessive heat. Store oral suspensions and syrups in refrigerator and discard unused portions after 14 d. The dry powder (for parenteral use) may be stored at room temperature. After reconstitution (initial dilution), solutions may be stored for 1 wk under refrigeration. Intravenous infusion solutions containing penicillin G are stable at room temperature for at least 24 h.

Oral Administration

- Oral penicillin G should be taken

on an empty stomach, at least 1 h before or 2 h after meals to reduce possibility of destruction by gastric acid and delay in absorption by food.

- Administer with a full glass of water. Instruct patient to avoid acidic beverages 1 h before and after taking oral penicillin G.

Parenteral Administration (IM & IV)

- See manufacturer's labeling for directions on preparation of initial dilution. Loosen powder by tapping vial against palm of hand. Holding vial horizontally, rotate it while directing stream of diluent against wall of vial. Shake vial vigorously until powder is completely dissolved. (For IV administration, the initial dilution should be further diluted with 0.9% NaCl or 5% dextrose for IV use.)
- Carefully select IM site. Accidental injection into or near a nerve can cause irritation with severe pain and dysfunction. IM injection is made deep into a large muscle mass. Inject slowly. Rotate injection sites.
- IV penicillin G is given by continuous infusion. In high doses, IV penicillin G should be administered slowly to avoid electrolyte imbalance from potassium or sodium content. Physician will prescribe specific flow rate.

Assessment & Drug Effects

- Culture and sensitivity tests should be done prior to initiation of therapy; however, treatment may be started before results are known.
- Hypersensitivity reactions are more likely to occur with parenteral penicillin but may also occur with the oral drug. Skin rash is the most common type allergic reaction and should be reported promptly to physician.
- Before treatment with penicillin is initiated, an exact history should be obtained of patient's previous exposure and sensitivity to penicillins and cephalosporins and other allergic reactions of any kind.
- Observe all patients closely for at least 30 min following administration of parenteral penicillin. The rapid appearance of a red flare or wheal at the IM or IV injection site is a possible sign of sensitivity. Report to physician. Also suspect an allergic reaction if patient becomes irritable, has nausea and vomiting, breathing difficulty, or sudden fever.
- Reactions to penicillin may be rapid in onset or may not appear for days or weeks. Symptoms usually disappear fairly quickly once drug is stopped, but in some patients may persist for 5 d or more and require hospitalization for treatment.
- Allergy to penicillin is unpredictable. It has occurred in patients with a negative history of penicillin allergy and also in patients with no known prior contact with penicillin (sensitization may have occurred from penicillin used commercially in foods and beverages).
- Neuromuscular irritability occurs most commonly in patients receiving parenteral penicillin in excess of 20 million U/d who have renal insufficiency, hyponatremia, or underlying CNS disease, notably myasthenia gravis or epilepsy. Seizure precautions are indicated. Symptoms usually begin with twitching, expecially of face and extremities.
- Monitor I&O, particularly in patients receiving high parenteral doses. Report oliguria, hematuria, and changes in I&O ratio. Consult physician regarding optimum fluid intake. Dehydration increases the

concentration of drug in kidneys and can cause renal irritation and damage.

- Neonates, young infants, the elderly, and patients with impaired renal function receiving high-dose penicillin therapy should be closely observed for signs of toxicity. Urinary excretion of penicillin is significantly delayed in these patients.
- Patients on high-dose therapy should be closely observed for evidence of bleeding, and bleeding time should be monitored. (In high doses, penicillin interferes with platelet aggregation.)
- Patients receiving prolonged treatment should have renal, hepatic, and hematologic systems evaluated at regular intervals. Additionally, electrolyte balance and cardiovascular status should be checked periodically in patients receiving high parenteral doses.
- Cultures should be taken following completion of treatment to determine need for further medication.

Patient & Family Education

- Inform that hypersensitivity reaction may be delayed. Advise them to immediately report urticaria, pruritus, fever, malaise, and other signs of a delayed reaction (see adverse/side effects).
- When used for infection, penicillin is to be taken around the clock (i.e., t.i.d. means q8h, q.i.d. means q6h, etc.) Instruct not to miss any doses and to continue taking the medication until it is all gone, unless otherwise directed by the physician.
- Measure liquid dosage form with specially marked measuring device. Household teaspoons vary in measure and therefore are not advised.
- Some patients receiving penicillin for treatment of syphilis develop Jarisch-Herxheimer reaction. This reaction resembles penicillin allergy but is thought to be due to the toxic products released from spirochetes killed by penicillin. It occurs 8–24 h following treatment with penicillin and is characterized by headache, chills, fever, myalgia, arthralgia, malaise, and worsening of syphilitic skin lesions. Advise to notify physician if these symptoms appear. The reaction is usually self-limiting.
- Advise to check with physician if symptoms do not improve within a few days or if they get worse.
- Instruct to report signs and symptoms of superinfection (see Appendix G).
- Patients with diabetes who are receiving massive doses of penicillin should be advised of the possibility of obtaining false-positive urine glucose test results.
- Emphasize importance of medical follow-up; present evidence suggests that glomerulonephritis, a possible complication of streptococcal infection, may not be prevented by penicillin.

PENICILLIN G PROCAINE

Trade names: Crysticillin A.S., Pfizerpen-AS, Procaine Benzylpenicillin, Wycillin

Classifications: ANTIINFECTIVE; BETALACTAM ANTIBIOTIC; NATURAL PENICILLIN

Prototype: Penicillin G potassium

Pregnancy category: B

ACTIONS/PHARMACODYNAMICS

Long-acting form of penicillin G. The procaine salt has low solubility and thus creates a tissue depot from which penicillin is slowly absorbed.

Same actions and antibacterial activity as for penicillin G and is similarly inactivated by penicillinase and gastric acids. Onset of action is slower and produces lower serum concentrations than equivalent doses of penicillin G, but has longer duration of action.

USES Moderately severe infections due to penicillin G-sensitive microorganisms that are susceptible to low but prolonged serum penicillin concentrations. Commonly, uncomplicated pneumococcal pneumonia, 1-d treatment of uncomplicated gonorrheal infections, and all stages of syphilis. May be used concomitantly with penicillin G or probenecid when more rapid action and higher blood levels are indicated.

ROUTE & DOSAGE

Moderate to Severe Infections

Adult: **IM** 600,000–1,200,000 U once/d.
Child: **IM** 300,000 U once/d.

Pneumococcal Pneumonia

Adult: **IM** 600,000 U q12h.

Uncomplicated Gonorrhea

Adult: **IM** 4,800,000 U divided between 2 different injection sites at one visit preceded by 1 g of probenecid 30 min before injections.

Syphilis

Adult: **IM** Primary, secondary, latent: 600,000 U/d for 8 d; late latent, tertiary, neurosyphilis: 600,000 U/d for 10–15 d.
Child: **IM** 500,000–1,000,000 U/m^2 once/d.

PHARMACOKINETICS Absorption: slowly absorbed from IM site. **Peak:** 1–3 h. **Duration:** 15–20 h. **Distribution:** crosses placenta; distributed into breast milk. **Metabolism:** hydrolyzed to penicillin in body. **Elimination:** excreted by kidneys within 24–36 h.

CONTRAINDICATIONS & PRECAUTIONS Contraindicated in: history of hypersensitivity to any of the penicillins, cephalosporins, or to procaine or any other "caine-type" local anesthetic; neonates, pregnancy (category B). **Cautious use in:** history of or suspected atopy or allergy.

ADVERSE/SIDE EFFECTS Hypersensitivity (procaine toxicity): mental disturbances (anxiety, confusion, depression, combativeness, hallucinations), expressed fear of impending death, weakness, dizziness, headache, tinnitus, unusual tastes, palpitation, changes in pulse rate and BP, seizures. Also see Penicillin G.

NURSING IMPLICATIONS

Administration

- Multiple-dose vial should be shaken thoroughly before withdrawing medication to ensure uniform suspension of drug.
- Administer IM deeply into upper outer quadrant of gluteus muscle; in infants and small children midlateral aspect of thigh is generally preferred. Select IM site carefully. Accidental injection into or near major peripheral nerves and blood vessels can cause neurovascular damage.
- Aspirate carefully before injecting drug to avoid entry into a blood vessel. Inadvertent IV administration reportedly has resulted in pulmonary infarcts and death. Inject drug at a slow, but steady rate to prevent needle blockage. Rotate injection sites.
- Note manufacturer's directions for storage. Generally, penicillin G procaine aqueous suspension

(A.S.) is stored in refrigerator. Avoid freezing.

Assessment & Drug Effects

- Before treatment is initiated, an exact history should be obtained of patient's previous exposure and sensitivity to penicillins, cephalosporins, and to procaine, and other allergic reactions of any kind.
- If sensitivity is suspected, physician may test patient by injecting 0.1 ml of 1–2% procaine hydrochloride intradermally. The appearance of a wheal, flare, or eruption indicates procaine sensitivity.
- Be alert to the possibility of a transient toxic reaction to procaine, particularly when large single doses are administered. The reaction manifested by mental disturbance and other symptoms (see adverse/side effects) occurs almost immediately and usually subsides after 15–30 min.
- Report onset of rash, pruritus, fever, chills or other symptoms of an allergic reaction to physician. Reactions may be difficult to treat because drug action is relatively prolonged.

PENICILLIN V

PENICILLIN V POTASSIUM

Trade names: Apo-Pen-VK ♣, Beepen VK, Betapen-VK, Ledercillin VK, Nadopen-V ♣, Novopen-VK ♣, Penicillin VK, Pen-V, Pen-Vee K, Robicillin VK, V-Cillin K, Veetids

Classifications: ANTIINFECTIVE; BETA-LACTAM ANTIBIOTIC; NATURAL PENICILLIN

Prototype: Penicillin G potassium

Pregnancy category: B

ACTIONS/PHARMACODYNAMICS Acid-stable analog of penicillin G with which it shares actions; is bactericidal, and is inactivated by penicillinase. Less active than penicillin G against gonococci and other gram-negative microorganisms.

USES Mild to moderate infections caused by susceptible streptococci, pneumococci, and staphylococci. Also Vincent's infection and as prophylaxis in rheumatic fever.

ROUTE & DOSAGE

Mild to Moderate Infections

Adult: **PO** 125–500 mg q6h.
Child <12 y: **PO** 15–50 mg/kg/d in 3–6 divided doses.

Endocarditis Prophylaxis

Adult: **PO** 2 g 30–60 min before procedure; then 500 mg q6h for 8 doses.
Child <30 kg: **PO** 1 g 30–60 min before procedure; then 250 mg q6h for 8 doses.

PHARMACOKINETICS Absorption: 60–73% absorbed from GI tract. **Peak:** 30–60 min. **Duration:** 6 h. **Distribution:** highest levels in kidneys; crosses placenta; distributed into breast milk. **Elimination:** half-life: 30 min; excreted in urine.

CONTRAINDICATIONS & PRECAUTIONS Contraindicated in: hypersensitivity to any penicillin or cephalosporin. History of or suspected atopy or allergy (hay fever, asthma, hives, eczema); pregnancy (category B).

ADVERSE/SIDE EFFECTS Nausea, vomiting, *diarrhea,* epigastric distress. ***Hypersensitivity reactions:*** flushing, pruritus, urticaria or other skin eruptions, eosinophilia, <u>anaphylaxis</u>; hemolytic anemia, leukopenia, thrombocytopenia, neuropathy, superinfections.

NURSING IMPLICATIONS

See penicillin G potassium for numerous additional nursing implications.

Administration

- Drug may be better absorbed and result in higher blood levels when taken after a meal than on an empty stomach.
- Following reconstitution, oral solution is stable for 14 d under refrigeration. Date and time of reconstitution and discard date should appear on container. Shake well before pouring.
- If oral liquid preparation is not dispensed with a specially marked measuring device, question pharmacist. The average household measure is not accurate enough for this formulation.

Assessment & Drug Effects

- Culture and sensitivity tests should be obtained before initiation of therapy and at regular intervals throughout therapy.
- Before therapy begins, careful inquiry should be made concerning hypersensitivity reactions to penicillins, cephalosporins, and other allergens.
- Patients receiving prolonged therapy should have evaluations of renal, hepatic, and hematologic systems at regular intervals.

Patient & Family Education

- Inform that to maintain a constant blood level, penicillin V should be given around the clock at specific intervals.
- Instruct not to miss any doses and to continue taking medication until it is all gone unless otherwise directed by the physician.
- As with other penicillin preparations, advise to withhold medication and to report promptly to physician the onset of hypersensitivity reactions and superinfections (see Appendix G).

P

PENTAERYTHRITOL TETRANITRATE

(pen-ta-er-ith′ri-tole)

Trade names: Duotrate, Pentylan, Peritrate, P.E.T.N.

Classifications: CARDIOVASCULAR AGENT; NITRATE VASODILATOR

Prototype: Nitroglycerin

Pregnancy category: C

ACTIONS/PHARMACODYNAMICS

Nitric acid ester of a tetrahydric alcohol. Actions, contraindications, precautions, and adverse/side effects as for nitroglycerin. Slower acting than nitroglycerin but duration of action is longer. Not effective for control of acute attacks. Tolerance can occur, and cross tolerance with other nitrites and nitrates is possible.

USE Prophylactically for long-term management of angina pectoris.

ROUTE & DOSAGE

Angina

Adult: **PO** 10–20 mg t.i.d. or q.i.d. up to 40 mg q.i.d.; *or* 80 mg sustained release q12h.

PHARMACOKINETICS **Absorption:** 50–60% absorbed from GI tract. **Onset:** 20–60 min. **Duration:** 4–5 h; up to 12 h with sustained release. **Metabolism:** metabolized in liver. **Elimination:** half-life: 10 min; excreted primarily in urine; small amounts in feces.

NURSING IMPLICATIONS

Administration

- Pentaerythritol tetranitrate is not to be used to relieve an acute episode of anginal pain.
- Administer at least 30 min before or 1 h after meals and at bedtime.

Sustained-release forms are also taken on an empty stomach (1 dose on arising and second dose 12 h later).

- Avoid sudden discontinuation of pentaerythritol therapy; coronary vasospasm may be induced.
- Protect drug from exposure to heat and moisture to prevent loss of potency. Store at 15–30C (59–86F).

Assessment & Drug Effects

- Orthostatic hypotension can be particularly dangerous for the elderly. Evaluate incidence; if troublesome, notify physician.

Patient & Family Education

- Advise to report onset of skin rash or persistent headaches to physician. Discontinuation of therapy may be required.
- Inform that alcohol may enhance drug hypotensive effect.
- Chronic administration may produce tolerance and may impair response to nitroglycerin or other concomitantly administered nitrites or nitrates. Advise patient to report signs of decreasing therapeutic effect.
- Caution not to engage in activities requiring mental alertness and skill until drug response has stabilized.
- In presence of high environmental temperature, heat prostration can occur with use of this drug, especially in the elderly.

PENTAMIDINE ISOETHIONATE

(pen-tam′i-deen)

Trade names: Nebupent, Pentacarinat♣, Pentam 300

Classifications: ANTIINFECTIVE; ANTIPROTOZOAL

Pregnancy category: C

ACTIONS/PHARMACODYNAMICS Aromatic diamide antiprotozoal drug effective against the sporozoan parasite *Pneumocystis carinii*. Action mechanism is unclear, but drug appears to block parasite reproduction by interfering with nucleotide (DNA, RNA), phospholipid, and protein synthesis. This parasite rarely causes infection in the general population, but if the patient is immunocompromised (e.g., AIDS) *P. carinii* pneumocystosis can be fatal. Pentamidine also has trypanosomicidal and leishmanicidal activity, but required doses for these conditions are quite toxic.

USE *P. carinii* pneumonia (PCP). **Unlabeled uses:** African trypanosomiasis and visceral leishmaniasis. (Drug supplied for the latter uses is through the Centers for Disease Control and Prevention, Atlanta, GA.)

ROUTE & DOSAGE

Treatment of *Pneumocystis carinii* Pneumonia

Adult: **IM/IV** 4 mg/kg once/d for 14–21 d; infuse IV over 60 min. *Child:* **IM/IV** Same as for adult.

Prophylaxis of *Pneumocystis carinii* Pneumonia

Adult: **Inhaled** 300 mg per nebulizer q4wk.

PHARMACOKINETICS Absorption: readily absorbed after IM injection. **Distribution:** leaves bloodstream rapidly to bind extensively to body tissues. **Elimination:** 50–66% excreted in urine within 6 h; small amounts found in urine for as long as 6–8 wk.

CONTRAINDICATIONS & PRECAUTIONS Contraindicated in: safe use in pregnancy (category C) not established. **Cautious use in:** hypertension, hypotension; hyperglycemia; hypoglycemia; hypocalcemia; blood dyscrasias; hepatic or renal dysfunction; diabetes mellitus.

ADVERSE/SIDE EFFECTS CNS: confusion, hallucinations, neuralgia, dizziness, sweating. **CV:** sudden, severe hypotension, cardiac arrhythmias, ventricular tachycardia, phlebitis. **GI:** anorexia, nausea, vomiting, pancreatitis, unpleasant taste. **Hematologic:** leukopenia, thrombocytopenia, anemia. **Metabolic:** hypoglycemia, hypocalcemia, *hyperkalemia*. **Respiratory:** *cough, bronchospasm,* laryngitis, shortness of breath, chest pain, pneumothorax. **Other:** Stevens-Johnson syndrome, acute renal failure, facial flush (with IV injection), *local reactions at injection site.*

DRUG INTERACTIONS AMINOGLYCOSIDES, **amphotericin B, cyclosporine, vancomycin,** other NEPHROTOXIC DRUGS increase risk of nephrotoxicity.

INCOMPATIBILITY Y-site: CEPHALOSPORINS.

P

NURSING IMPLICATIONS

Administration

- IM preparation: Dissolve contents of 1 vial (300 mg) in 3 ml sterile water for injection.
- The IM injection is painful and frequently causes local reactions (pain, induration, swelling). Select alternate sites for daily doses and institute local treatment if indicated.
- IV preparation: Dissolve contents of 1 vial in 3–5 ml sterile water for injection or 5% dextrose solution. Further dilute in 50–250 ml of D5W and infuse over 60 min.
- IV solutions of 1.0–2.5 mg/ml prepared in 5% dextrose injection are stable at room temperature for up to 24 h. Dry product should be stored at 2–8C (35–46F). Protect solution and drug product from light. Discard unused portions.
- Administer inhaled medication according to manufacturer's directions. Caution: Healthcare personnel should take appropriate respiratory precautions when adminstering pentamidine aerosol therapy because of the possibility of exposure to tuberculosis in settings where cough-inducing procedures are performed on patients at risk for undiagnosed *Mycobacterium* infections.

Assessment & Drug Effects

- Severe sudden hypotension may develop after a single dose. The patient should be in a supine position while receiving the drug. Monitor BP continuously during the infusion, every half hour for 2 h thereafter, and then every 4 h until BP stabilizes.
- Renal, cardiac, and hepatic function may be changed by pentamidine. Monitor HR, blood glucose, and electrolyte balance.
- Measure and record I&O ratio and pattern and check patient's pulse (to detect arrhythmia) at least twice daily.
- Dosage adjustment is indicated in renal failure; therefore, signs of impending dysfunction should be promptly reported (e.g., changed I&O ratio, oliguria, edema).
- Characteristics of pneumonia in the immunocompromised patient include constant fever, scanty (if any) sputum, dyspnea, tachypnea, and cyanosis.
- Fever is a constant symptom in *P. carinii* pneumonia, but it may be rapidly elevated (as high as 40C [104F]) shortly after drug infusion. Monitor temperature changes and institute measures to lower the temperature as indicated.

Patient & Family Education

- Advise to promptly report increasing respiratory difficulty.

PENTAZOCINE HYDROCHLORIDE

(pen-taz'oh-seen)

Trade names: Talwin, Talwin NX

Prototype for classifications: CNS AGENT; NARCOTIC (OPIATE) AGONIST-ANTAGONIST; ANALGESIC

Pregnancy category: C

Controlled substance: Schedule IV

ACTIONS/PHARMACODYNAMICS Synthetic analgesic structurally related to phenazocine. Analgesic potency approximately one third that of morphine and somewhat greater than that of codeine. In general, adverse reactions are qualitatively similar to those of morphine. Unlike morphine, large doses may increase BP and heart rate. Also, acts as weak narcotic antagonist and has sedative properties.

USES Relief of moderate to severe pain; also used for preoperative analgesia or sedation, and as supplement to surgical anesthesia.

ROUTE & DOSAGE

Moderate to Severe Pain (Excluding Patients in Labor)

Adult: **PO** 50–100 mg q3–4h (max 600 mg/d). **IM/IV/SC** 30 mg q3–4h (max 360 mg/d).
Geriatric: **PO** 50 mg q4h. **IM** 30 mg q4h.

Women in Labor

Adult: **IM** 20–30 mg; 20 mg may be repeated 1 or 2 times at 2–3 h intervals.

PHARMACOKINETICS Absorption: readily absorbed from GI tract; 20% reaches systemic circulation (first pass metabolism). **Onset:** 15–30 min PO, IM, SC; 2–3 min IV. **Peak:** 1–3 h PO, IM; 15 min IV. **Duration:** 3 h PO, IM; 1 h IV. **Distribution:** crosses placenta. **Metabolism:** extensively metabolized in liver. **Elimination:** half-life: 2–3 h; excreted primarily in urine; small amount in feces.

CONTRAINDICATIONS & PRECAUTIONS Contraindicated in: head injury, increased intracranial pressure; emotionally unstable patients, or history of drug abuse. Safe use during pregnancy (other than labor) (category C) and in children <12 y not established. **Cautious use in:** impaired renal or hepatic function; respiratory depression; biliary surgery; patients with MI who have nausea and vomiting.

ADVERSE/SIDE EFFECTS *Drowsiness,* sweating, flushing, *dizziness, light-headedness, euphoria, nausea, vomiting,* constipation, dry mouth, alterations of taste, urinary retention, visual disturbances, allergic reactions, injection-site reactions (induration, nodule formation, sloughing, sclerosis, cutaneous depression), rash, pruritus. **High doses:** <u>respiratory depression</u>, hypertension, palpitation, tachycardia, <u>shock</u>, psychotomimetic effects, confusion, anxiety, hallucinations, disturbed dreams, bizarre thoughts, euphoria and other mood alterations.

DRUG INTERACTIONS Alcohol and other CNS DEPRESSANTS add to CNS depression; NARCOTIC ANALGESICS may precipitate narcotic withdrawal syndrome.

INCOMPATIBILITIES Solution/additive: aminophylline, BARBITURATES, **sodium bicarbonate, glycopyrrolate, heparin, nafcillin. Y-site: glycopyrrolate, heparin, nafcillin.**

P

NURSING IMPLICATIONS

Administration

- IM administration is preferable to SC route when frequent injections over an extended period are required. Observe injection sites daily for signs of irritation or inflammation.
- IV administration: IV pentazocine may be given by direct IV undiluted or diluted with 1 ml sterile water for injection for each 5 mg. Give slowly at a rate of 5 mg over 60 seconds.
- Preserve in tight, light-resistant containers. Store at 15–30C (59–86F).

Assessment & Drug Effects

- Tolerance to analgesic effect sometimes occurs. Psychologic and physical dependence have been reported in patients with history of drug abuse, but rarely in patients without such history. Addiction liability matches that of codeine.
- Pentazocine may produce acute withdrawal symptoms in some patients who have been receiving opioids on a regular basis.

P

Patient & Family Education

- Caution ambulatory patients to avoid potentially hazardous activities such as driving a car or operating machinery until response to drug is known.
- Abrupt discontinuation of drug following extended use may result in chills, abdominal and muscle cramps, yawning, rhinorrhea, lacrimation, itching, restlessness, anxiety, drug-seeking behavior.

PENTOBARBITAL

(pen-toe-bar'bi-tal)

Trade name: Nembutal

PENTOBARBITAL SODIUM

Trade names: Nembutal Sodium, Novopentobarb ♣

Classifications: CNS AGENT; ANXIOLYTIC; SEDATIVE-HYPNOTIC; BARBITURATE

Prototype: Secobarbital

Pregnancy category: D

Controlled substance: Schedule II

ACTIONS/PHARMACODYNAMICS Short-acting barbiturate with actions, contraindications, precautions, and adverse reactions as for other barbiturates. Potent respiratory depressant.

USES Sedative or hypnotic for preanesthetic medication, induction of general anesthesia, adjunct in manipulative or diagnostic procedures, and emergency control of acute convulsions.

ROUTE & DOSAGE

Sedative

Adult: **PO** 20–30 mg b.i.d. to q.i.d.
Child: **PO** 2–6 mg/kg/d in 3 divided doses (max 100 mg/d).

Preoperative Sedation

Adult: **PO** 150–200 mg in 2 divided doses. **IM** 150–200 mg in 2 divided doses. **IV** 100 mg; may increase to 500 mg if necessary.

Hypnotic

Adult: **PO** 120–200 mg. **IM** 150–200 mg.
Child: **PO** 30–120 mg. **IM** 2–6 mg/kg (max 100 mg).

PHARMACOKINETICS **Onset:** 15–30 min PO; 10–15 min IM; 1 min IV. **Duration:** 1–4 h PO; 15 min IV. **Distribution:** crosses placenta. **Metabolism:** metabolized primarily in liver. **Elimination:** half-life: 4–50 h; excreted in urine.

CONTRAINDICATIONS & PRECAUTIONS **Contraindicated in:** pregnancy (category D). See secobarbital.

ADVERSE/SIDE EFFECTS With rapid IV: respiratory depression, laryngospasm, bronchospasm, apnea, hypotension. Also see secobarbital.

DRUG INTERACTIONS **Phenmetrazine** antagonizes effects of pentobarbital; CNS DEPRESSANTS, **alcohol,** SEDATIVES add to CNS depression; MAO INHIBITORS cause excessive CNS depression; **methoxyflurane** creates risk of nephrotoxicity.

INCOMPATIBILITIES **Solution/additive: chlorpheniramine, codeine, ephedrine, hydrocortisone, hydroxyzine, insulin, levorphanol, methadone, norepinephrine,** TETRACYCLINES, **penicillin G, pentazocine, phenytoin, promazine, promethazine, sodium bicarbonate, streptomycin, succinylcholine, triflubromazine, vancomycin, cimetidine, benzquinamide, butorphanol, chlorpromazine, dimenhydrinate, diphenhydramine, droperidol, fentanyl, glycopyrrolate, meperidine, midazolam, morphine, nalbuphine, perphenazine, prochlorperazine, ranitidine. Y-site: cimetidine, butorphanol, glycopyrrolate, midazolam, nalbuphine, perphenazine, ranitidine.**

NURSING IMPLICATIONS

Administration

- Do not use parenteral solutions that appear cloudy or in which a precipitate has formed.
- IM injections should be made deep into large muscle mass, preferably upper outer quadrant of buttock. Aspirate needle carefully before injecting it to prevent inadvertent entry into blood vessel. No more than 5 ml (250 mg) should be injected in any one site because of possible tissue irritation.
- IV route should be used only when other routes are not feasible. May be given by direct IV undiluted or diluted (preferred) with sterile water, D5W, NS, or other compatible IV solutions.
- IV administration should be slow; rate should not exceed 50 mg/min.
- Parenteral solution is highly alkaline. Extreme care should be taken to avoid extravasation. Necrosis may result.

Assessment & Drug Effects

- During IV administration monitor BP, pulse, and respiration q3–5min. Observe patient closely; maintain airway. Equipment for artificial respiration should be immediately available.
- After IM administration of hypnotic dose, observe patient closely for adverse effects for at least 30 min.

Patient & Family Education

- Caution ambulatory patients against operating a motor vehicle or machinery for the remainder of day after taking drug.

PENTOXIFYLLINE

(pen-tox-i′fi-leen)

Trade name: Trental

Classifications: HEMORRHEOLOGIC AGENT; ANTIPLATELET AGENT

Pregnancy category: C

ACTIONS/PHARMACODYNAMICS Useful in restoration of blood flow through nutritive capillary microcirculation that has been compromised by structural and flow dynamic changes in cerebral and peripheral vascular disorders. Action mechanism is not clear but pentoxifylline administration is followed by decreased blood viscosity and improved blood flow, with consequent reduction of tissue hypoxia. Drug action interrupts the vicious cycle of tissue hypoxia, sludging and stasis of capillary blood flow, microthrombotic activity, reduced oxygen delivery to ischemic cells. With increased blood flow to the extremities, the limiting pain and paresthesia of intermittent claudication is reduced; further, psychopathologic conditions associated with cerebral hypoxia are improved.

USES Intermittent claudication associated with occlusive peripheral vascular disease; diabetic angiopathies. **Unlabeled uses:** to improve psychopathologic symptoms in patient with cerebrovascular insufficiency and to reduce incidence of stroke in the patient with recurrent TIAs.

ROUTE & DOSAGE

Intermittent Claudication
Adult: **PO** 400 mg t.i.d. with meals.

PHARMACOKINETICS Absorption: readily absorbed from GI tract; 10–50% reaches systemic circulation (first pass metabolism). **Peak:** 2–4 h. **Distribution:** distributed into breast milk. **Metabolism:** metabolized in liver and erythrocytes. **Elimination:** half-life: 0.4–0.8 h; excreted primarily in urine.

CONTRAINDICATIONS & PRECAUTIONS Contraindicated in: intolerance to pentoxifylline or to methylxanthines (caffeine and theophylline). Safe use in pregnancy (category C), in nursing mothers, or in children <18 y not established. **Cautious use in:** angina, hypotension, arrhythmias, cerebrovascular disease.

ADVERSE/SIDE EFFECTS CNS: agitation, nervousness, *dizziness,* drowsiness, headache, insomnia, tremor, confusion. **CV:** angina, chest pain, dyspnea, arrhythmias, palpitations, hypotension, edema, flushing. **Eye:** blurred vision, conjunctivitis, scotomas. **GI:** abdominal discomfort, belching, flatus, bloating, diarrhea, *dyspepsia, nausea, vomiting.* **Skin:** brittle fingernails, pruritus, rash, urticaria. **Other:** earache, unpleasant taste, excessive salivation, leukopenia, malaise, sore throat, swollen neck glands, weight change. **Overdosage:** fever, flushing, hypotension, convulsions, somnolence, loss of consciousness.

NURSING IMPLICATIONS

Administration

- When pentoxifylline is given with food, absorption is delayed, but total amount absorbed is not affected; serum levels are lowered, however. May be taken on an empty stomach or with food; be consistent with time of day and relationship to food in establishing the daily regimen.
- Store tablets at 15–30C (59–86F).

Assessment & Drug Effects

- Therapeutic effects may be evident within 2–4 wk, but treatment is continued at least 8 wk before therapeutic failure is admitted.
- Successful treatment provides relief from pain and cramping in calf muscles, buttocks, thighs, and feet during exercise and improves walking performance (time and duration).
- If patient is also on antihypertensive treatment, monitor BP. Pentoxifylline may slightly decrease an already stabilized BP, necessitating a reduced dose of the hypotensive drug.

Patient & Family Education

- Before patient reestablishes walking as exercise, the patient should be checked by the physician to determine CV status and capacity.
- Advise to pay particular attention to care of the feet because of arte-

rial insufficiency (diminished perfusion to feet).

- Bleeding and prolonged prothrombin time in treated with pentoxifylline have been reported. Advise to report promptly unexplained bleeding, easy bruising, epistaxis, petechiae.
- Because of potential side effects (i.e., somnolence, blurred vision, dizziness) advise to avoid driving or working with dangerous machinery until drug response has stabilized.

PERGOLIDE

(per′go-lide)

Trade name: Permax

Classification: ANTIPARKINSON AGENT

Prototype: Levodopa

Pregnancy category: B

ACTIONS/PHARMACODYNAMICS Pergolide is a potent dopamine receptor agonist at both D_1- and D_2-receptor sites. The reduced tonic stimulation of dopaminergic D_2 receptors located on intrastriatal cholinergic neurons is most likely the cause of parkinsonian symptoms. It is thought that stimulation of the D_2 receptor alleviates the majority of parkinsonian symptoms.

USE Adjunct to levodopa/carbidopa for the treatment of Parkinson's disease. **Unlabeled uses:** acromegaly, hyperprolactinemia.

ROUTE & DOSAGE

Parkinson's Disease

Adult: **PO** Initiate with 0.05 mg daily for 2 d; then increase by 0.1 or 0.15 mg/d every 3 d for the next 12 d; then dose may be increased by 0.25 mg every third day until the desired therapeutic response is achieved. Give in divided doses t.i.d. Max dose 5 mg/d.

Acromegaly

Adult: **PO** 0.1–1.5 mg once daily.

Hyperprolactinemia

Adult: **PO** 0.025–0.6 mg once daily.

PHARMACOKINETICS Absorption: readily absorbed from GI tract; extensive first-pass metabolism. **Onset:** prolactin levels decrease within 15–30 min. **Peak:** prolactin nadir in 15 h. **Duration:** 22–24 h. **Distribution:** 90% protein bound; crosses placenta; distributed into breast milk. **Metabolism:** metabolized in liver. **Elimination:** half-life:27 h; 55% excreted in urine within 48 h; 40–50% excreted in feces.

CONTRAINDICATIONS & PRECAUTIONS Contraindicated in: hypersensitivity to pergolide or other ergot derivatives, lactation. **Cautious use in:** cardiac dysrhythmias, pregnancy (category B). Safety and efficacy in children not established.

ADVERSE/SIDE EFFECTS CNS: *confusion, anxiety, light-headedness, headache,* transient somnolence, hallucinations, nightmares. **CV:** ventricular arrhythmias, PVCs, edema, *orthostatic hypotension.* **GI:** *nausea, vomiting,* constipation. **Other:** rhinitis, rash, withdrawal symptoms (hallucinations, confusion, paranoid ideations, worsening of parkinsonian symptoms).

DIAGNOSTIC TEST INTERFERENCE Suppresses ***prolactin*** levels.

DRUG INTERACTIONS Addition of pergolide to **levodopa** therapy has produced an increased incidence of dyskinesias in patients with Parkinson's disease.

NURSING IMPLICATIONS

Administration

- Initiate with a daily dose of 0.05 mg for the first 2 d. Subsequent increases should follow the recommendations in the Route & Dosage table.
- Store at room temperature, 15–30C (59–86F).

Assessment & Drug Effects

- When initiating therapy, carefully monitor for orthostatic hypotension and syncope.
- Assess neurologic status; concurrent levodopa and pergolide may increase incidence of dyskinesias. If this occurs, levodopa may need to be reduced.
- Monitor patients with cardiac arrhythmias carefully, as drug may induce certain arrhythmias in persons at risk.

Patient & Family Education

- Inform of ways to reduce risk of orthostatic hypertension.
- Inform of all potential adverse effects including hallucinations.
- Advise to report worsening neurologic status.
- Instruct patient on levodopa not to abruptly discontinue pergolide.

P

PERINDOPRIL ERBUMINE

(per-in'do-pril)

Trade name: Aceon

Classifications: CARDIOVASCULAR AGENT; ANGIOTENSION-CONVERTING ENZYME INHIBITOR; ANTIHYPERTENSIVE

Prototype: Captopril

Pregnancy category: C (first trimester); D (second and third trimesters)

ACTIONS/PHARMACODYNAMICS Perindopril is an angiotension-converting enzyme (ACE) inhibitor. ACE catalyzes the conversion of angiotension I to angiotension II, a vasoconstrictor substance. Therefore, angiotension II levels are decreased, thus decreasing vasopressor activity and aldosterone secretion. Reduced aldosterone is associated with potassium-sparing effect. Thus, perindopril lowers BP by inhibition of ACE. In addition, perindopril decreases systemic vascular resistance (afterload) and pulmonary capillary wedge pressure (PCWP), a measure of preload, and improves cardiac output as well as activity tolerance.

USES Hypertension, CHF

ROUTE & DOSAGE

Hypertension, CHF

Adult: **PO** 4 mg once daily, may be increased to 8 mg daily in 1 or 2 divided doses (max 16 mg/d). May need to use lower doses in patients with mild to moderate renal impairment

PHARMACOKINETICS **Absorption:** readily absorbed from GI tract, absorption significantly decreased when taken with food. **Peak:** perindopril: 1 h; perindoprilat: 3–7 h. **Duration:** 24 h. **Metabolism:** hydrolyzed in the liver to its active form, perindoprilat. **Elimination:** half-life perindopril: 0.8–1 h, perindoprilat: 30–120 h; primarily excreted in urine.

CONTRAINDICATIONS & PRECAUTIONS **Contraindicated in:** hypersensitivity to perindopril or any other ACE inhibitor; history of angioedema induced by an ACE inhibitor, pregnancy [category C (first trimester), category D (second and third trimester)], patients with hypertrophic cardiomyopathy, renal artery stenosis. **Cautious use in:** renal insufficiency, volume-depleted patients, severe hepatic dysfunction; autoimmune diseases, immunosuppressant drug therapy, hyperkalemia or potassium-sparing diuretics, elderly, surgery, neutropenia, lactation, febrile illness.

ADVERSE/SIDE EFFECTS CNS: dizziness, light-headedness (in the absence of postural hypotension), headache, mood and sleep disorders, fatigue. **CV:** palpitations. **Endocrine:** hyperkalemia. **GI:** nausea, vomiting, epigastric pain, diarrhea, taste disturbances, dyspepsia. **Other:** proteinuria, impotence, sexual dysfunction, dry eyes, blurred vision, *cough*, angioedema, rash, pruritus, muscle cramps, sinusitis, hypertonia, fever.

DRUG INTERACTIONS POTASSIUM-SPARING DIURETICS (**amiloride, spironolactone, triamterene**) may increase the risk of hyperkalemia. POTASSIUM SUPPLEMENTS increase the risk of hyperkalemia. **Drug–food:** food can decrease drug absorption 35%.

NURSING IMPLICATIONS

Administration

- If a concurrently ordered diuretic cannot be discontinued 2–3 days before beginning perinodopril, the initial dose should be 2–4 mg in 1 or 2 divided doses.
- Best taken on an empty stomach 1 h before meals.
- Dosage adjustments should generally be made at intervals of at least 1 wk.
- Store at 20–25C (68–77F) and protect from moisture.

Assessment & Drug Effects

- Following the initial dose, carefully monitor BP for several hours until stable, especially in patients using concurrent diuretics, on salt restriction, or volume depleted.
- If excess hypotension develops, immediately place the patient in a supine position.
- Therapeutic effectiveness is indicated by normalization of BP and cardiac status.
- Lab tests: periodically monitor serum potassium, serum sodium, BUN and creatinine, ALT/SGTP, blood glucose, lipid profile, and WBC with differential.
- Closely monitor renal function in patients with CHF.
- If concurrently used, frequently monitor serum lithium levels and assess for S&S of lithium toxicity; increased caution is needed when diuretic therapy is also used.

Patient & Family Education

- Discontinue drug and immediately report S&S of angioedema (i.e., swelling) of face or extremities. Seek emergency help for swelling of the tongue or any other signs of potential airway obstruction.
- Light-headedness can occur, especially during early therapy; excess fluid loss of any kind (e.g., vomiting, diarrhea) will increase risk of hypotension and syncope.
- Avoid using potassium supplements unless specifically directed to do so by physician.
- Promptly report S&S of infection (e.g., sore throat, fever).

PERMETHRIN

(per-meth′rin)

Trade name: Nix

Prototype for classifications: SKIN AGENT; PEDICULICIDE

Pregnancy category: B

ACTIONS/PHARMACODYNAMICS Pediculicidal and ovidical activity against *Pediculus humanus* var. *capitis* (head louse). Permethrin inhibits sodium ion influx through nerve cell membrane channels, resulting in delayed repolarization of the action potential and paralysis of the pest. Since lice are completely dependent on blood for survival, they die within 24–48 h if unable to burrow into the skin. Drug is also active against ticks, mites, and fleas.

USE Pediculosis capitis.

ROUTE & DOSAGE

Head Lice

Adult: **Topical** Apply sufficient volume to clean wet hair to saturate the hair and scalp; leave on 10 min; then rinse hair thoroughly.
Child > 2 y: **Topical** same as for adult.

PHARMACOKINETICS Absorption: < 2% of amount applied is absorbed through intact skin. **Metabolism:** rapidly hydrolyzed to inactive metabolites. **Elimination:** excreted primarily in urine.

CONTRAINDICATIONS & PRECAUTIONS Contraindicated in: hypersensitivity to pyrethrins, chrysanthemums, sulfites, or other preservatives or dyes; acute inflammation of the scalp; pregnancy (category B). Safe use in nursing mothers and children < 2 y of age or in the elderly not documented.

ADVERSE/SIDE EFFECTS On scalp: *pruritus, transient tingling,* burning, stinging, numbness; erythema, edema, rash.

NURSING IMPLICATIONS

Administration

- Drug action results from topical application of the formulation. It is not a shampoo. Scalp as well as hair should be saturated by the lotion.
- Prior to treatment with permethrin, use regular shampoo, thoroughly rinse and towel-dry hair and scalp. Shake lotion well before application. One container holds enough for at least one treatment, but two containers may be necessary if patient has long hair. Do not retain left-over medicine.
- Following 10 min exposure to the medication, hair and scalp should be thoroughly rinsed and dried with a clean towel. Head lice are usually eliminated with one treatment.
- Store drug away from heat at 15–25C (59–77F) and direct light. Avoid freezing.

Assessment & Drug Effects

- If patient is known to be sensitive to any pyrethrin or pyrethroid, therapy should not be attempted, or if a reaction occurs, treatment should be stopped.

Patient & Family Education

- When hair is dry, patient may want to comb it with a fine-tooth comb (furnished with medication) to remove dead lice and remaining nits or nit shells. While not a therapeutic requirement, this combing has cosmetic value.
- Permethrin remains on hair shaft up to 14 d; therefore, recurrence of infestation rarely occurs (<1%).
- Instruct patient or parent to inspect hair shafts daily for at least 1 wk to determine drug effectiveness. If live lice are observed after 7 d, contact physician. A renewed prescription for a second treatment may be ordered. Signs of inadequate treatment: pruritis, erythema, excoriation, infected scalp areas.
- Regular shampooing may be resumed after treatment; residual deposit of drug on hair is not reduced.

P

- Permethrin is usually irritating to the eyes and mucosa. Flush well with water if medicine accidentally gets into eyes.

PERPHENAZINE

(per-fen'a-zeen)

Trade names: Phenazine, Trilafon

Classifications: CNS AGENT; PSYCHOTHERAPEUTIC; PHENOTHIAZINE ANTIPSYCHOTIC

Prototype: Chlorpromazine

ACTIONS/PHARMACODYNAMICS Piperazine phenothiazine similar to chlorpromazine. Affects all parts of CNS, particularly the hypothalamus. Antipsychotic effect: antagonizes the neurotransmitter dopamine by action on dopaminergic receptors in brain. Antiemetic action results from direct blockade of dopamine in the chemoreceptor trigger zone (CTZ) in the medulla. Produces less sedation and hypotension, greater antiemetic effects, higher incidence of extrapyramidal effects, and lower levels of anticholinergic side effects than chlorpromazine.

USES Psychotic disorders, symptomatic control of severe nausea and vomiting, acute conditions such as violent retching during surgery, and intractable hiccups.

ROUTE & DOSAGE

Psychotic Disorders

Adult: **PO** 4–16 mg b.i.d. to q.i.d.; 8–32 mg sustained release b.i.d. (max 64 mg/d).
IM 5 mg q6h (max 15–30 mg/d).
IV Dilute to 0.5 mg/ml in NS; administer at not more than 1 mg q1–2min or 5 mg by slow infusion.
Child: **PO** 4 mg b.i.d. to q.i.d.; 8 mg sustained release b.i.d. (max 16 mg/d). **IM** Same as for adult.
IV Same as for adult.

Dementia Behavior

Geriatric: **PO** 2–4 mg 1–2 times/d, may increase q4–7d to max 32 mg/d.

Nausea

Adult: **PO** 8–16 mg b.i.d. to q.i.d.
IM 5 mg q6h (max 15 mg/d).

PHARMACOKINETICS Absorption: poorly absorbed from GI tract; 20% reaches systemic circulation. **Onset:** 10 min IM. **Peak:** 1–2 h IM; 4–8 h PO. **Duration:** 6–12 h. **Distribution:** crosses placenta. **Metabolism:** metabolized in liver with some metabolism in GI tract. **Elimination:** half-life: 9.5 h; excreted in urine and feces.

CONTRAINDICATIONS & PRECAUTIONS Contraindicated in: hypersensitivity to perphenazine and other phenothiazines; preexisting liver damage, suspected or established subcortical brain damage, comatose states; bone marrow depression. Safe use during pregnancy, in nursing mothers, and in children <12 y not established. **Cautious use in:** previously diagnosed breast cancer; hepatic or renal dysfunction, cardiovascular disorders, alcohol withdrawal, epilepsy, psychic depression, patients with suicidal tendency, glaucoma, history of intestinal or GU obstruction, geriatric or debilitated patients, patients who will be exposed to extremes of heat or cold, or to phosphorous insecticides.

ADVERSE/SIDE EFFECTS CNS: *extrapyramidal effects (dystonic reactions, akathisia, parkinsonian syndrome, tardive dyskinesia), sedation,* convulsions. **CV:** *orthostatic*

P

hypotension, tachycardia, bradycardia. **Eye:** mydriasis, blurred vision, corneal and lenticular deposits. **GI:** constipation, *dry mouth,* increased appetite, adynamic ileus. **GU:** *urinary retention,* gynecomastia, menstrual irregularities, inhibited ejaculation. **Hematologic:** agranulocytosis, thrombocytopenic purpura, aplastic or hemolytic anemia. **Hepatic:** abnormal liver function tests, cholestatic jaundice. **Hypersensitivity:** photosensitivity, itching, erythema, urticaria, angioneurotic edema, drug fever, anaphylactoid reaction. **Local:** pain at injection site, sterile abscess. **Other:** nasal congestion, decreased sweating, hyperprolactinemia, galactorrhea, weight gain.

DIAGNOSTIC TEST INTERFERENCE Perphenazine may cause falsely abnormal ***thyroid function*** tests because of elevations of thyroid globulin.

DRUG INTERACTIONS **Alcohol** and other CNS DEPRESSANTS enhance CNS depression; ANTACIDS, ANTIDIARRHEALS may decrease absorption of phenothiazines; ANTICHOLINERGIC AGENTS add to anticholinergic effects including fecal impaction and paralytic ileus; BARBITURATES, ANESTHETICS increase hypotension and excitation.

INCOMPATIBILITIES **Solution/additive: midazolam, pentobarbital, thiethylperazine. Y-site: cefoperazone, midazolam, pentobarbital.**

P

NURSING IMPLICATIONS

Administration

- Extended-release tablet should be swallowed whole.
- Oral concentrate: Before administration, each 5 ml (16 mg) must be diluted with 60 ml water, milk, saline solution, 7-Up, or other compatible carbonated beverages. Do not use liquids that cause color changes or precipitate.
- Administer deep IM into a large muscle with patient in recumbent position. Advise patient to continue lying down for at least 1 h after injection. Injection may be painful. Observe daily for signs of inflammation.
- IV perphenazine is given by direct IV, with each 5 mg diluted in 9 ml NS, at a rate of 0.5 mg (1 ml) over 60 seconds.
- Protect solutions from light. Do not use precipitated or darkened parenteral solution; however, slight yellowing does not alter potency or therapeutic effects.
- Store at 15–30C (59–86F) in tightly covered, light-resistant container unless otherwise specified. Protect from freezing.

Assessment & Drug Effects

- Establish baseline BP before initiation of drug therapy and check it at regular intervals, especially during early therapy.
- BP and pulse should be monitored continuously during IV administration. Keep patient supine until assured that vital signs are stable. Elderly patients in particular should be observed carefully for hypotension and extrapyramidal reactions. Have immediately available norepinephrine (Levophed) (epinephrine is contraindicated) and drugs for controlling extrapyramidal reactions (benztropine mesylate [Cogentin], and diphenhydramine).
- A high incidence of extrapyramidal effects accompanies use of perphenazine, particularly with high doses and parenteral administration. Report restlessness, weakness of extremities, dystonic reactions (spasms of neck and shoulder muscles, rigidity of back, difficulty

swallowing or talking); motor restlessness (akathisia: inability to be still); and parkinsonian syndrome (tremors, shuffling gait, drooling [hypersalivation], slow speech).

- Patients on long-term therapy are at high risk of developing irreversible tardive dyskinesia: fine, wormlike (vermicular) movements or rapid protrusions of the tongue, chewing motions, lip smacking. Withhold medication and report immediately to physician. Patients (if competent) and responsible family members should be informed about tardive dyskinesia. Early reporting is essential.
- Differential blood cell counts and hepatic, and renal function studies, ECG, and ophthalmologic examination should be done before initiation of therapy and periodically during therapy.
- If jaundice appears between weeks 2 and 4, suspect hypersensitivity, withhold drug, and report to physician.
- Monitor I&O ratio and bowel elimination pattern.
- Be alert to the patient's altered tolerance to environmental temperature changes. Be cautious with external heat devices. Conditioned avoidance behavior may be depressed, and a severe burn could result.
- Antiemetic effect of this drug may obscure signs of toxicity due to overdosage of other drugs or make it more difficult to diagnose conditions with nausea as a primary symptom.

Patient & Family Education

- Caution to make all position changes slowly and in stages, particularly from recumbent to upright posture, and to lie down or sit down if light-headedness or dizziness occurs.
- Caution to avoid potentially hazardous activities such as driving a car or operating machinery until reaction to drug is known. Perphenazine may produce hypotension (dizziness, light-headedness), and sedation especially during early therapy.
- Photosensitivity results in skin color changes from brown to blue-gray. Caution patient to avoid long exposure to sunlight and to sunlamps.
- Review dosage regimen with patient. Advise strict adherence to it and to consult physician before changing it for any reason.
- Discontinuation of perphenazine following prolonged therapy should be accomplished gradually over a period of several weeks.
- Caution to avoid OTC drugs unless physician prescribes them.
- Perphenazine may discolor urine reddish brown.

PHENAZOPYRIDINE HYDROCHLORIDE

(fen-az-oh-peer′i-deen)

Trade names: Azo-Standard, Baridium, Geridium, Phenazo ♣, Phenazodine, Pyridiate, Pyridium, Pyronium ♣, Urodine, Urogesic

Classification: URINARY TRACT ANALGESIC

Pregnancy category: B

ACTIONS/PHARMACODYNAMICS
Azo dye with local anesthetic action on urinary tract mucosa. Precise mechanism of action not known. Imparts little or no antibacterial activity.

USES Symptomatic relief of pain, burning, frequency, and urgency arising from irritation of urinary tract mucosa, as from infection, trauma, surgery, or instrumentation.

ROUTE & DOSAGE

Cystitis
Adult: **PO** 200 mg t.i.d.
Child: **PO** 12 mg/kg/d in 3 divided doses.

PHARMACOKINETICS Absorption: readily absorbed from GI tract. **Distribution:** crosses placenta in trace amounts. **Metabolism:** metabolized in liver and other tissues. **Elimination:** primarily excreted in urine.

CONTRAINDICATIONS & PRECAUTIONS Contraindicated in: renal insufficiency, glomerulonephritis, pyelonephritis during pregnancy (category B), severe hepatitis. **Cautious use in:** GI disturbances; glucose-6-phosphate dehydrogenase deficiency.

ADVERSE/SIDE EFFECTS Infrequent: headache, vertigo, mild GI disturbances; in patients with impaired renal function or with high dosage or prolonged therapy: methemoglobinemia, hemolytic anemia, skin pigmentation, renal stones, transient acute renal failure.

P

DIAGNOSTIC TEST INTERFERENCE Phenazopyridine may interfere with any urinary test that is based on color reactions or spectrometry: ***bromsulphalein*** and ***phenolsulfonphthalein*** excretion tests; urinary ***glucose*** test using Clinistix or TesTape (copper-reduction methods such as Clinitest and Benedict's test reportedly not affected); ***bilirubin*** using "foam test" or Ictotest; ***ketones*** using nitroprusside (e.g., Acetest, Ketostix, or Gerhardt ferric chloride); urinary ***protein*** using Albustix, Albutest, or nitric acid ring test; urinary ***steroids; urobilinogen;*** assays for ***porphyrins.***

NURSING IMPLICATIONS

Administration

- Phenazopyridine should be taken after meals.

Assessment & Drug Effects

- Patients on prolonged therapy or with impaired renal function should have periodic blood work and renal function tests.

Patient & Family Education

- Inform that drug will impart an orange to red color to urine and may stain fabric.
- Appearance of yellowish tinge to skin or sclerae may indicate drug accumulation due to renal impairment. Advise to report immediately. Drug should be discontinued.
- Phenazopyridine should be discontinued when pain and discomfort are relieved (usually 3–15 d). Instruct to keep physician informed.

PHENELZINE SULFATE

(fen′el-zeen)
Trade name: Nardil
Prototype for classifications: CNS AGENT; PSYCHOTHERAPEUTIC; ANTIDEPRESSANT; MAO INHIBITOR
Pregnancy category: C

ACTIONS/PHARMACODYNAMICS Potent hydrazine MAO inhibitor. Precise mode of action not known. Antidepressant and diverse effects believed to be due to irreversible inhibition of MAO, thereby permitting increased concentrations of endogenous epinephrine, norepinephrine, serotonin, and dopamine within presynaptic neurons and at receptor sites. Also thought to inhibit hepatic microsomal drug-metabolizing enzymes; thus may intensify and prolong the effects of many drugs. Termination of drug action depends on regeneration of MAO, which occurs 2–3 wk after discontinuation of therapy.

USES Management of endogenous depression, depressive phase of manic-depressive psychosis, and severe exogenous (reactive) depression not responsive to more commonly used therapy.

ROUTE & DOSAGE

Depression

Adult: **PO** 15 mg t.i.d.; rapidly increased to at least 60 mg/d; may need up to 90 mg/d.

PHARMACOKINETICS **Absorption:** readily absorbed from GI tract. **Onset:** 2 wk. **Metabolism:** rapidly metabolized. **Elimination:** half-life: unknown; 79% of metabolites excreted in urine in 96 h.

CONTRAINDICATIONS & PRECAUTIONS **Contraindicated in:** hypersensitivity to MAO inhibitors; pheochromocytoma; hyperthyroidism; CHF, cardiovascular or cerebrovascular disease; impaired renal function, hypernatremia; atonic colitis; glaucoma; history of frequent or severe headaches; history of liver disease, abnormal liver function tests; elderly or debilitated patients; paranoid schizophrenia. Safe use during pregnancy (category C) and lactation and in children < 16 y of age not established. **Cautious use in:** epilepsy; pyloric stenosis; diabetes; depression accompanying alcoholism or drug addiction; manic-depressive states; agitated patients; suicidal tendencies; chronic brain syndromes; history of angina pectoris.

ADVERSE/SIDE EFFECTS *Constipation, dry mouth,* dizziness or vertigo, headache, *orthostatic hypotension,* drowsiness or *insomnia,* weakness, fatigue, *nausea,* vomiting, *anorexia,* weight gain, edema, tremors, twitching, hyperreflexia, mania, hypomania, confusion, memory impairment, blurred vision, hyperhidrosis, skin rash. **Hypertensive crisis:** intense occipital headache, palpitation, marked hypertension, stiff neck, nausea, vomiting, sweating, fever, photophobia, dilated pupils, bradycardia or tachycardia, constricting chest pain, intracranial bleeding. **Other:** delirium, hallucinations, euphoria, acute anxiety reaction, akathisia, ataxia, toxic precipitation of schizophrenia, convulsions, peripheral neuropathy, photosensitivity, normocytic and normochromic anemia, leukopenia. **Severe overdosage:** faintness, hypotension or hypertension, hyperactivity, marked agitation, anxiety, seizures, trismus, opisthotonos, respiratory depression, coma, circulatory collapse.

DIAGNOSTIC TEST INTERFERENCE Phenelzine may cause a slight false increase in ***serum bilirubin.***

DRUG INTERACTIONS TRICYCLIC ANTIDEPRESSANTS may cause hyperpyrexia, seizures; **fluoxetine, sertraline, paroxetine** may cause hyperthermia, diaphoresis, tremors, seizures, delirium; SYMPATHOMIMETIC AGENTS (e.g., **amphetamine, phenylephrine, phenylpropanolamine**), **guanethidine,** and **reserpine** may cause hypertensive crisis; CNS DEPRESSANTS have additive CNS depressive effects; OPIATE ANALGESICS (especially **meperidine**) may cause hypertensive crisis and circulatory collapse; **buspirone,** hypertension; GENERAL ANESTHETICS, prolonged hypotensive and CNS depressant effects; hypertension, headache, hyperexcitability reported with **dopamine, methyl-**

dopa, levodopa, tryptophan; metrizamide may increase risk of seizures; HYPOTENSIVE AGENTS and DIURETICS have additive hypotensive effects. **Drug–food:** aged meats or aged cheeses, protein extracts, sour cream, alcohol, anchovies, liver, sausages, overripe figs, bananas, avocados, chocolate, soy sauce, bean curd, natural yogurt, fava beans—tyramine-containing foods—may precipitate hypertensive crisis.

NURSING IMPLICATIONS

Administration

- MAO inhibitors should be discontinued at least 10 d before elective surgery to allow time for recovery of MAO before anesthetics are given.
- Rapid withdrawal of MAO inhibitors should be avoided, particularly after high dosage, since a rebound effect may occur (headache, excitability, hallucinations, and possibly depression).
- Preserve in tightly covered containers away from heat and light.

P

Assessment & Drug Effects

- Before initiation of phenelzine treatment, it is advisable to evaluate patient's BP in standing and recumbent positions. Baseline blood cell counts and liver function tests should also be performed.
- Many adverse reactions associated with MAO inhibitors are dose-related. Physician will rely on accurate observations and prompt reporting of patient's response to therapy to determine spacing and lowest effective dosage.
- In titrating initial dosages, BP and pulse should be monitored between doses, and patient should be closely observed for evidence of adverse drug effects. Thereafter, monitor at regular intervals throughout therapy.
- Monitor I&O ratio and pattern until dosage is stabilized to identify indirect indices of edema and urinary dysfunction. Report changes and abnormalities; impaired renal function increases the possibility of toxicity from cumulative effects.
- Hypomania (exaggeration of motility, feelings, and ideas) may occur as depression improves. This reaction may also appear at higher than recommended doses or with long-term therapy. Report immediately.
- Observe for and report therapeutic effectiveness of drug: improvement in sleep pattern, appetite, physical activity, interest in self and surroundings, as well as lessening of anxiety and bodily complaints.
- Patient with diabetes should be closely observed for signs of hypoglycemia (see Appendix G). Reduced dosage of insulin or oral antidiabetic drug may be necessary.
- Patients on prolonged therapy should be checked periodically for altered color perception, visual fields, and fundi. Changes in red-green vision may be the first indication of eye damage.
- Periodic hematologic studies and liver function tests are recommended during prolonged therapy and high dosage.

Patient & Family Education

- If no therapeutic response occurs after 3 or 4 wk, drug is usually discontinued. Maximum antidepressant effects generally appear in 2–6 wk and persist several weeks after drug withdrawal.
- Advise to avoid self-medication. OTC preparations containing dextromethorphan, sympathomimetic agents, or antihistamines (e.g., cough, cold, and hay fever remedies, appetite suppressants) can

precipitate severe hypertensive reactions if taken during therapy or within 2–3 wk after discontinuation of an MAO inhibitor.

- Headache and palpitation, prodromal symptoms of hypertensive crisis, indicate need to discontinue drug therapy. Instruct to report immediately the onset of these symptoms or any other unusual effects.
- Ingestion of foods and beverages containing tyramine or tryptophan or drugs containing pressor agents can result in severe hypertensive reactions.
- Foods that must be avoided include red wine, particularly Chianti; some beers; cheese (except cottage, ricotta, cream); smoked or pickled fish (herring); beef or chicken liver, summer (dry) sausage; fava or broad bean pods; yeast vitamin supplements. Questionable foods are ripe avocado, ripe fresh banana, sour cream, yogurt, soy sauce.
- Advise against excessive drinking of caffeine beverages: coffee, tea, cocoa, or cola.
- Provide patient and responsible family members with a list of foods and beverages that may cause hypertensive reactions. These substances should be avoided during drug therapy and for at least 2–3 wk after therapy has been discontinued.
- Elastic stockings and elevation of legs when sitting may minimize hypotensive effects of drug (discuss with physician).
- Instruct to make position changes slowly, especially from recumbent to upright posture, and to dangle legs over bed a few minutes before ambulating. Also caution against standing still for prolonged periods. Patient should avoid hot showers and baths (resulting vasodilatation may potentiate hypotension) and should lie down immediately if feeling light-headed or faint.
- Instruct to check weight 2 or 3 times per week and report unusual gain.
- Instruct to report jaundice. Hepatotoxicity is believed to be a hypersensitivity reaction unrelated to dosage or duration of therapy.
- MAO inhibitors may suppress anginal pain that would otherwise serve as a warning sign of myocardial ischemia. Caution patient to avoid overexertion while receiving drug therapy.

PHENMETRAZINE HYDROCHLORIDE

(fen-met′ra-zeen)

Trade name: Preludin

Classifications: CNS AGENT; RESPIRATORY AND CEREBRAL STIMULANT; AMPHETAMINE; ANOREXIANT

Prototype: Amphetamine

Pregnancy category: C

Controlled substance: Schedule II

P

ACTIONS/PHARMACODYNAMICS

Sympathomimetic agent chemically and pharmacologically related to amphetamine that reportedly produces less CNS stimulation.

USE Solely for short-term management of endogenous obesity.

ROUTE & DOSAGE

Obesity

Adult: **PO** 75 mg once/d midmorning.

PHARMACOKINETICS **Absorption:** readily absorbed from GI tract. **Peak:** 5–12 h. **Duration:** 12 h. **Elimination:** excreted in urine.

CONTRAINDICATIONS & PRECAUTIONS **Contraindicated in:** history of hypersensitivity to sympathomimetic amines, hypertension, advanced arteriosclerosis, symptomatic cardiovascular disease; hyperthyroidism; glaucoma (narrow angle), hyperexcitable or psychotic states; concomitant use of CNS stimulants during or within 2 wk of MAO inhibitors. Safe use during pregnancy (category C) and in children <12 y not established.

ADVERSE/SIDE EFFECTS CNS: *nervousness,* dizziness, *insomnia,* headache. **CV:** palpitation, tachycardia, elevated BP. **ENT:** blurred vision, dry mouth. **GI:** nausea, abdominal cramps, constipation. **Other:** sweating, frequent urination, urticaria, changes in libido, impotence. Large doses for prolonged periods: marked insomnia, irritability, severe dermatoses, hyperactivity, severe mental depression, personality changes, psychosis.

DRUG INTERACTIONS Acetazolamide, sodium bicarbonate decrease phenmetrazine elimination, **ammonium chloride, ascorbic acid** increase phenmetrazine elimination; may antagonize the effects of both BARBITURATES and phenmetrazine; **furazolidone** may increase BP effects of amphetamines—interaction may persist for several weeks after discontinuation of furazolidone; antagonizes antihypertensive effects of **guanethidine, guanadryl;** MAO INHIBITORS, **selegiline** can cause hypertensive crisis (fatalities reported)—do not administer amphetamines during or within 14 d of these drugs; PHENOTHIAZINES may inhibit mood elevating effects; TRICYCLIC ANTIDEPRESSANTS enhance amphetamine effects because of increased norepinephrine release; BETA AGONISTS increase adverse cardiovascular effects.

P

NURSING IMPLICATIONS

Administration

- Conventional tablet is administered at least 1 h before meals.
- Do not administer along with or within 14 d of MAO inhibitors. Hypertensive crisis may result.
- Sustained-release form may be taken in the morning; administration time should be determined by period of day anorexiant effect is needed (generally taken at least 12 h before bedtime). Advise patient to swallow tablet whole.

Assessment & Drug Effects

- BP checks before and periodically during treatment are advised.
- Sustained-release tablets contain tartrazine, which may cause allergic type reactions including bronchial asthma in susceptible individuals. This reaction is frequently seen in patients with aspirin hypersensitivity.

Patient & Family Education

- Advise against excessive use of CNS stimulants such as coffee, tea, and cola drinks.
- Since drug may cause blurred vision and dizziness, caution to avoid potentially hazardous activities such as driving a car or operating machinery until reaction to drug is known.
- Instruct to notify physician if nervousness, dizziness, or palpitation occur.
- Mouth dryness may be relieved by rinsing with warm water.
- As with other amphetamines, physical and psychic dependence and tolerance may develop with prolonged use.

PHENOBARBITAL

(fee-noe-bar'bi-tal)

Trade names: Barbita, Luminal, Solfoton

PHENOBARBITAL SODIUM

Trade name: Luminal Sodium
Prototype for classifications: CNS AGENT; ANTICONVULSANT; SEDATIVE-HYPNOTIC; BARBITURATE
Pregnancy category: D
Controlled substance: Schedule IV

ACTIONS/PHARMACODYNAMICS Long-acting barbiturate. Sedative and hypnotic effects of barbiturates appear to be due primarily to interference with impulse transmission of cerebral cortex by inhibition of reticular activating system. Initially, barbiturates suppress REM sleep, but with chronic therapy REM sleep returns to normal. Has no analgesic properties, and small doses may increase reaction to painful stimuli. CNS depression may range from mild sedation to coma, depending on dosage, route of administration, degree of nervous system excitability, and drug tolerance. Phenobarbital limits spread of seizure activity by increasing threshold for motor cortex stimuli. Barbiturates are habit forming.

USES Long-term management of tonic-clonic (grand mal) seizures and partial seizures; status epilepticus, eclampsia, febrile convulsions in young children. Also used as a sedative in anxiety or tension states; in pediatrics as preoperative and postoperative sedation and to treat pylorospasm in infants. **Unlabeled uses:** treatment and prevention of hyperbilirubinemia in neonates and in the management of chronic cholestasis; benzodiazepine withdrawal.

ROUTE & DOSAGE

Anticonvulsant

Adult: **PO** 100–300 mg/d. **IV/IM** 200–600 mg up to 20 mg/kg.
Child: **PO/IV** 3–8 mg/kg or 125 $mg/m^2/d$.
Neonate: **PO/IV** 3–4 mg/kg/d (max 5 mg/kg/d).

Status Epilepticus

Adult/Child: **IV** 15–18 mg/kg in single or divided doses (max 20 mg/kg).
Neonate: **IV** 15–20 mg/kg in single or divided doses.

Sedative

Adult: **PO** 30–120 mg/d. **IV/IM** 100–200 mg/d.
Child: **PO** 6 mg/kg/d *or* 180 mg/m^2 in 3 divided doses. **IV/IM** 16–100 mg/d (1–3 mg/kg).

PHARMACOKINETICS Absorption: 70–90% absorbed slowly from GI tract. **Peak:** 8–12 h PO; 30 min IV. **Duration:** 4–6 h IV. **Distribution:** 20–45% protein bound; crosses placenta; enters breast milk. **Metabolism:** oxidized in liver to inactivated metabolites. **Elimination:** half-life: 2–6 d; excreted in urine.

CONTRAINDICATIONS & PRECAUTIONS Contraindicated in: sensitivity to barbiturates, manifest hepatic or familial history of porphyria; severe respiratory or renal disease; history of previous addiction to sedative hypnotics; uncontrolled pain; pregnancy (particularly early pregnancy) (category D), nursing mothers, timed-release formulation for children <12 y of age. **Cautious use in:** impaired hepatic, renal, cardiac, or respiratory function; history of allergies; elderly or debilitated patients; patients with fever; hyperthyroidism; diabetes mellitus or severe anemia; during labor and delivery, lactation; patient with borderline hypoadrenal function.

ADVERSE/SIDE EFFECTS CNS: *somnolence,* nightmares, insomnia, "hangover," headache, anxiety, thinking abnormalities, dizziness, nystagmus, irritability, paradoxic excitement and exacerbation of hyperkinetic behavior (in children); confusion or depression or marked excitement (elderly or debilitated patients); ataxia. **CV:** bradycardia, syncope, hypotension. **GI:** nausea, vomiting, constipation, diarrhea, epigastric pain. **Hypersensitivity:** rash, angioneurotic edema, fever, serum sickness, urticaria; hypoventilation, apnea, laryngospasm, bronchospasm, circulatory collapse. **Injection site** (extravasation): thrombosis, gangrene transient pain, tenderness, redness. **IV:** coughing, hiccuping, laryngospasm. **Skin:** mild maculopapular, morbilliform rash; erythema multiforme, Stevens-Johnson syndrome, exfoliative dermatitis (rare). **Other:** liver damage, megaloblastic anemia, hypocalcemia, osteomalacia, rickets, myalgic, neuralgic, agranulocytosis, thrombocytopenia, folic acid deficiency, vitamin D deficiency. **Overdosage:** respiratory depression, CNS depression, coma, death.

P

DIAGNOSTIC TEST INTERFERENCE Barbiturates may affect ***bromsulphalein*** retention tests (by enhancing hepatic uptake and excretion of dye) and increase ***serum phosphatase.***

DRUG INTERACTIONS **Alcohol,** CNS DEPRESSANTS compound CNS depression; phenobarbital may decrease absorption and increase metabolism of ORAL ANTICOAGULANTS; increases metabolism of CORTICOSTEROIDS, ORAL CONTRACEPTIVES, ANTICONVULSANTS, **digitoxin,** possibly decreasing their effects; ANTIDEPRESSANTS potentiate adverse effects of phenobarbital; **griseofulvin** decreases absorption of phenobarbital.

INCOMPATIBILITIES **Solution/additive: benzquinamide, cephalothin, chlorpromazine, codeine phosphate, ephedrine, hydralazine, hydrocortisone sodium succinate, hydroxyzine, insulin, levorphanol, meperidine, methadone, morphine, norepinephrine,** TETRACYCLINES, **procaine, prochlorperazine, promazine, promethazine, ranitidine, streptomycin, vancomycin.**

NURSING IMPLICATIONS

Administration

- When administering oral barbiturates, observe that patient actually swallows the pill and does not "cheek" it.
- If patient cannot swallow pill, it may be crushed before administration, then mixed with a fluid or with food. (Do not permit patient to swallow dry crushed drug.)
- Administer IM deep into large muscle mass; volume should not exceed 5 ml at any one site.
- Commercially prepared solutions for injection (sodium phenobarbital) may be diluted with most IV infusion solutions. If not absolutely clear, discard.
- IV preparation: Slowly introduce sterile water for injection into ampule with sterile syringe. Use at least 10 ml of diluent. Rotate ampule to hasten dissolving drug (may take several minutes). If solution not clear in 5 min or if a precipitate remains, discard.
- IV administration: No greater than 60 mg/min. Administer reconstituted IV solution no later than 30 min after preparation.
- IV administration to neonates, infants, children: Verify correct IV concentration and rate of infusion with physician.
- Extravasation of IV phenobarbital

may cause necrotic tissue changes that may necessitate skin grafting. Frequently check the injection site.

- Store at 15–30C (59–86F) unless otherwise directed by manufacturer.

Assessment & Drug Effects

- Patients receiving large doses should be closely observed for at least 30 min to ensure that narcosis is not excessive.
- Keep patient under constant observation when drug is administered IV, and record vital signs at least every hour or more often if indicated.
- Therapeutic serum concentrations of 15–40 μg/ml produce anticonvulsant activity in most patients. These values are usually attained after 2 or 3 wk of therapy with a dose of 100–200 mg/d.
- Serum concentrations >50 μg/ml may cause coma; concentrations >80 μg/ml are potentially lethal.
- Phenobarbital and other long-acting barbiturates may be cumulative in action. Doses in excess of 400 mg/d for more than 90 d are likely to cause some degree of physical dependence.
- Barbiturates do not have analgesic action, and they may be expected to produce restlessness when given to patients in pain.
- The elderly or debilitated patient and children sometimes have paradoxical response to barbiturate therapy, i.e., irritability, marked excitement (inappropriate tearfulness and aggression in children), depression, and confusion. Be alert to unexpected responses and report promptly. Protect the elderly patient from falling, irrational behavior, and effects of depression (anorexia, social withdrawal).
- Hepatic function and hematology tests and determinations of serum folate and vitamin D levels are advised during prolonged therapy.
- Barbiturates increase the metabolism of many drugs, leading to decreased pharmacologic effects of those drugs. Whenever a barbiturate is added to an established regimen of another drug, close observation for changes in effectiveness of the first drug is essential, at least during early phase of barbiturate use.
- Barbiturates decrease or reduce pharmacologic effects of the following drugs (groups): anticoagulants (coumarins), carbamazepine, corticosteroids, digitoxin, doxycycline, estradiol, griseofulvin, oral contraceptives, quinidine, phenothiazines, tricyclic antidepressants. See Drug Interactions for more information.
- Monitor for and report chronic toxicity symptoms: ataxia, slurred speech, irritability, poor judgment, slight dysarthria, nystagmus on vertical gaze, confusion, insomnia, somatic complaints.
- Acute toxicity (serum concentration >80 μg/ml) symptoms include profound CNS depression, respiratory depression that may progress to Cheyne-Stokes respirations, hypoventilation, cyanosis, cold, clammy skin; hypothermia, constricted pupils (but may be dilated in severe intoxication), shock, oliguria, tachycardia, hypotension, respiration arrest, circulatory collapse, and death.

Patient & Family Education

- Patients receiving anticonvulsant therapy may experience drowsiness during first few weeks of treatment, but this usually diminishes with continued use of the barbiturate.
- Caution to avoid potentially hazardous activities requiring mental

P

alertness such as driving a car or operating machinery, until response to drug is known.

- Alcohol in any amount given with a barbiturate may severely impair judgment and abilities; it should not be consumed by a patient on barbiturate therapy.
- Phenobarbital increases vitamin D metabolism, leading to subtherapeutic levels and possibly onset of osteomalacia, or rickets (long-term therapy). Advise to increase vitamin D–fortified foods (e.g., milk products). A vitamin D supplement may be prescribed.
- Long-term therapy may result in nutritional folate (B_9) deficiency. Laboratory confirmation is the basis for urging patient to maintain adequate dietary folate intake: fresh vegetables (especially green leafy), fresh fruits, whole grains, liver. A supplement of folic acid may be prescribed.
- Large doses over extended time may cause vitamin B_{12} deficiency.
- Caution to adhere to drug regimen (i.e., intervals between doses should not be changed and doses should not be increased or decreased) without advice.
- Warn not to stop taking drug abruptly because of danger of withdrawal symptoms (8–12 h after last dose), which can be fatal. Early symptoms include apprehension, hand and finger tremors, weakness, dizziness, disturbed vision, nausea, vomiting, sweating, orthostatic hypotension, insomnia. More severe symptoms may develop 2–8 d after withdrawal: delirium, convulsion, status epilepticus (patient with epilepsy). Withdrawal symptoms may occur after a course of therapy with 600–800 mg/d for 35 d and may last up to 15 d after abrupt cessation of drug therapy.
- Instruct patients on prolonged therapy to report to physician the onset of fever, sore throat or mouth, malaise, easy bruising or bleeding, petechiae, jaundice, rash.
- Advise patients taking barbiturates at home not to keep drug on bedside table or in a readily accessible place. Patients have been known to forget having taken the drug and in half-wakened conditions have accidentally overdosed themselves.
- It is important that pregnancy be avoided in patients receiving barbiturates (reportedly teratogenic). Patients on prolonged therapy should consider alternative methods of contraception in addition to or instead of oral contraceptives to prevent unplanned pregnancy. Neonates born to mothers who received barbiturate therapy throughout the last trimester may show withdrawal symptoms for 1–14 d after birth. Symptoms resemble congenital opiate withdrawal symptoms: hyperactivity, restlessness, tremor, hyperreflexia, disturbed sleep.

P

PHENOLPHTHALEIN

(fee-nol-thay′leen)

Trade names: Alophen, Correctol, Espotabs, Evac-U-Gen, Evac-U-Lax, Ex-Lax, Feen-a-Mint, Lax-Pill, Modane, Phenolax, Prulet

Classifications: GI AGENT; STIMULANT LAXATIVE

Prototype: Bisacodyl

Pregnancy category: C

ACTIONS/PHARMACODYNAMICS

Diphenylmethane laxative similar to bisacodyl in pharmacologic properties. Common ingredient in several OTC fixed combination laxative drugs. Used for temporary relief of simple constipation.

ROUTE & DOSAGE

Laxative
Adult: **PO** 30–200 mg as directed.

PHARMACOKINETICS **Absorption:** up to 15% of dose absorbed from GI tract. **Onset:** 6–8 h. **Metabolism:** metabolized in liver with some enterohepatic cycling. **Elimination:** 85% excreted in feces, 15% in urine.

CONTRAINDICATIONS & PRECAUTIONS **Contraindicated in:** hypersensitivity to phenolphthalein; abdominal pain, nausea, vomiting; fecal impaction, intestinal obstruction, or perforation; pregnancy (category C).

ADVERSE/SIDE EFFECTS **Allergic reactions:** skin eruptions, urticaria, Stevens-Johnson syndrome, SLE-like syndrome. **Large doses or chronic use:** electrolyte imbalance, impaired glucose tolerance from potassium loss.

DIAGNOSTIC TEST INTERFERENCE Phenolphthalein may interfere with ***BSP excretion*** test.

NURSING IMPLICATIONS

Patient & Family Education

- Phenolphthalein is usually administered at bedtime to produce effect the next morning (approximately 6–8 h later).
- Since drug enters enterohepatic circulation, inform that laxative effect may persist for several days.
- Advise to avoid prolonged or frequent use. Dependence on drug action, as well as electrolyte imbalance, can occur.
- Inform that drug may impart reddish or purplish pink discoloration to alkaline urine or feces (made alkaline by soapsuds enema).
- Instruct to discontinue drug immediately if skin rash appears.
- Skin lesions resulting from allergic reaction may persist for months or years and may leave residual pigmentation.

PHENOXYBENZAMINE HYDROCHLORIDE

(fen-ox-ee-ben'za-meen)
Trade name: Dibenzyline
Classifications: AUTONOMIC NERVOUS SYSTEM AGENT; ALPHA-ADRENERGIC ANTAGONIST (BLOCKING AGENT, SYMPATHOLYTIC)
Prototype: Prazosin
Pregnancy category: C

ACTIONS/PHARMACODYNAMICS Long-acting alpha-adrenergic blocking agent. Apparently produces noncompetitive blockade of alpha-adrenergic receptor sites at postganglionic synapse. Alpha-receptor sites are thus unable to react to endogenous or exogenous sympathomimetic agents. Blocks excitatory effects of epinephrine, including vasoconstriction, but does not affect adrenergic cardiac inhibitory actions. Causes orthostatic hypotension in both normotensive and hypertensive patients.

USE Management of pheochromocytoma. **Unlabeled uses:** to improve circulation in peripheral vasospastic conditions such as Raynaud's acrocyanosis and frostbite sequelae, for adjunctive treatment of shock, hypertensive crisis.

ROUTE & DOSAGE

Management of Pheochromocytoma
Adult: **PO** 5–10 mg b.i.d.; may increase by 10 mg/d at 4-d intervals to desired response (usual range 20–60 mg/d in 2–3 divided doses).

P

Child: **PO** 0.2 mg/kg/d in 1–2 divided doses; may increase by 0.2 mg/kg/d at 4 d intervals to desired response (usual range 0.4–1.2 mg/kg/d).

PHARMACOKINETICS **Absorption:** variably absorbed (approximately 30%) from GI tract. **Onset:** 2 h. **Peak:** 4–6 h. **Duration:** 3–4 d. **Distribution:** accumulates in adipose tissue. **Elimination:** half-life: 24 h; 80% excreted in urine and bile within 24 h.

CONTRAINDICATIONS & PRECAUTIONS **Contraindicated in:** instances when fall in BP would be dangerous; compensated congestive failure. **Cautious use in:** marked cerebral or coronary arteriosclerosis, CHF; renal insufficiency; respiratory infections. Safe use during pregnancy (category C) not established.

ADVERSE/SIDE EFFECTS *Nasal congestion,* dry mouth, *miosis,* drooping of eyelids, *postural hypotension, tachycardia,* palpitation, *dizziness,* fainting, inhibition of ejaculation, drowsiness, sedation, tiredness, weakness, lethargy, confusion, headache, shock, CNS stimulation (large doses), allergic contact dermatitis.

NURSING IMPLICATIONS

Administration
- Giving the drug with milk or in divided doses may reduce gastric irritation.
- Preserve in airtight containers protected from light.

Assessment & Drug Effects
- During period of dosage adjustment, monitor BP and note pulse quality, rate, and rhythm in recumbent and standing positions. (Hypotension and tachycardia are most likely to occur in standing position.) Patient should be closely observed for at least 4 d from one dosage increment to the next.
- Since phenoxybenzamine has cumulative action, onset of therapeutic effects may not occur until after 2 wk of therapy, and full therapeutic effects may not be apparent for several more weeks.
- Therapeutic effectiveness with pheochromocytoma is indicated by decreases in BP, pulse, and sweating. With peripheral vasospastic problems, observe for improvement in skin color, temperature, and quality of peripheral pulses, as well as less sensitivity to cold.

Patient & Family Education
- Instruct to make position changes slowly, particularly from recumbent to upright posture, and to dangle legs and exercise ankles and feet for a few minutes before standing.
- Inform that postural hypotension and palpitations usually disappear with continued therapy but that they may reappear under conditions that promote vasodilation, such as strenuous exercise or ingestion of a large meal or alcohol.
- Inform that miosis, nasal stuffiness, and inhibition of ejaculation generally decrease with continued therapy.
- Advise not to take OTC medications for coughs, colds, or allergy without approval of physician. (Many contain sympathomimetic agents that cause BP elevation.)

PHENSUXIMIDE

(fen-sux'i-mide)

Trade name: Milontin

Classifications: CNS AGENT; ANTICONVULSANT SUCCINIMIDE
Prototype: Ethosuximide
Pregnancy category: D

ACTIONS/PHARMACODYNAMICS Succinimide derivative reportedly less potent and less effective than other drugs of this class. Apparently depresses the motor cortex and elevates the threshold of CNS to seizure activity.

USES Management of petit mal epilepsy (absence seizures) and with other anticonvulsants when other forms of epilepsy coexist with petit mal.

ROUTE & DOSAGE

Absence Seizures
Adult: **PO** 0.5–1 g b.i.d. or t.i.d.
Child: **PO** Same as for adult.

PHARMACOKINETICS Absorption: readily absorbed from GI tract. **Peak:** 1–4 h. **Metabolism:** metabolized in liver. **Elimination:** half-life: 5–12 h; excreted slowly in urine; small amounts excreted in bile and feces.

CONTRAINDICATIONS & PRECAUTIONS Contraindicated in: intermittent porphyria; pregnancy (category D); hepatic or renal disease.

ADVERSE/SIDE EFFECTS *Drowsiness, dizziness, ataxia,* alopecia, muscle weakness, *anorexia, nausea, vomiting,* flushing, periorbital edema, pruritus, skin rash, reversible nephropathy, granulocytopenia.

DRUG INTERACTIONS Carbamazepine decreases phensuximide levels; **isoniazid** significantly increases phensuximide levels; levels of both **phenobarbital** and phensuximide may be altered with increased seizure frequency.

NURSING IMPLICATIONS

Administration
- Shake oral suspension well before pouring to ensure uniform dosage.
- Protect from light and heat and store at 15–30C (59–86F) unless otherwise advised.

Assessment & Drug Effects
- Monitor weight, especially in children, since anorexic effects of drug might cause weight loss.
- Periodic renal function and blood tests should be performed, especially with long-term therapy.

Patient & Family Education
- Advise to report onset of skin rash or other unusual symptoms to physician.
- Inform that phensuximide may color urine pink, red, or red-brown.
- Concomitant use of OTC drugs must be discouraged unless the physician approves; loss of seizure control can be induced by ingredients in some popular OTC drugs.
- Caution against potentially hazardous tasks such as driving a car or operating machinery until response to drug is known.

P

PHENTOLAMINE MESYLATE
(fen-tole′a-meen)
Trade names: Regitine, Rogitine ♣
Classifications: AUTONOMIC NERVOUS SYSTEM AGENT; ALPHA-ADRENERGIC ANTAGONIST (BLOCKING AGENT, SYMPATHOLYTIC)
Prototype: Prazosin
Pregnancy category: C

ACTIONS/PHARMACODYNAMICS Alpha-adrenergic blocking agent structurally related to tolazoline but with more potent blocking effects. Competitively blocks alpha-adrenergic receptors, but action is transient and incomplete. Prevents hypertension resulting from elevated levels of circulating epinephrine or norepinephrine. Causes vasodilation and decreases general vascular resistance and pulmonary arterial pressure, primarily by direct action on vascular smooth muscle. Through stimulation of beta-adrenergic receptors, produces positive inotropic and chronotropic cardiac effects and increases cardiac output.

USES Diagnosis of pheochromocytoma and to prevent or control hypertensive episodes prior to or during pheochromocytomectomy. **Unlabeled use:** prevention of dermal necrosis and sloughing following IV administration or extravasation of norepinephrine.

ROUTE & DOSAGE

To Prevent Hypertensive Episode During Surgery

Adult: **IV/IM** 2–5 mg as needed.
Child: **IV/IM** 1 mg or 0.1 mg/kg (max 5 mg/dose).

To Test for Pheochromocytoma

Adult: **IV/IM** 5 mg.
Child: **IV/IM** 0.1 mg/kg.

To Prevent Necrosis from Norepinephrine Infusions

Adult: **IV** 10 mg added to each liter of IV fluid containing norepinephrine.

To Treat Catecholamine Extravasation

Adult/Child: **Intradermal** 5–10 mg diluted in 10 ml of normal saline injected into affected area within 12 h of extravasation.
Neonate: **Intradermal** 2.5–5 mg diluted in 10 ml of normal saline injected into affected area within 12 h of extravasation (max dose 0.1 mg/kg or 2.5 mg total).

PHARMACOKINETICS **Peak:** 2 min IV; 15–20 min IM. **Duration:** 10–15 min IV; 3–4 h IM. **Elimination:** half-life: 19 min; excreted in urine.

CONTRAINDICATIONS & PRECAUTIONS **Contraindicated in:** MI (previous or present), coronary artery disease. Safe use during pregnancy (category C) and in nursing mothers and lactation not established. **Cautious use in:** gastritis, peptic ulcer.

ADVERSE/SIDE EFFECTS Weakness, dizziness, flushing, *orthostatic hypotension,* nasal stuffiness, conjunctival infection. **GI:** *abdominal pain, nausea, vomiting, diarrhea, exacerbation of peptic ulcer.* With parenteral administration especially, *acute and prolonged hypotension, tachycardia, anginal pain,* cardiac arrhythmias, <u>MI</u>, cerebrovascular spasm, <u>shocklike state</u>.

NURSING IMPLICATIONS

Administration

- Reconstitute 5 mg vial with 1 ml of sterile water for injection. May be further diluted with up to 10 ml of sterile water and given by direct IV over 60 seconds. Manufacturer recommends that reconstituted solutions be used immediately.
- Patient should be in supine position when receiving drug parenterally. Monitor BP and pulse q2min until stabilized.
- Store in tight, light-resistant containers at 15–30C (59–86F).

Assessment & Drug Effects

- Test for pheochromocytoma: (1) Medications not deemed absolutely essential should be withheld at least 24 h, preferably 48–72 h; antihypertensive agents withheld until BP returns to pretreatment level (rauwolfia drugs withdrawn at least 4 wk prior to testing). (2) Keep patient at rest in supine position throughout test, preferably in quiet darkened room. (3) Take BP q10min for at least 30 min; when BP stabilizes, injection should be administered by physician. (4) IV administration: Record BP immediately after injection and at 30-second intervals for first 3 min; then at 1-min intervals for next 7 min. IM administration: BP determinations at 5-min intervals for 30–45 min.

Patient & Family Education

- Advise to avoid sudden changes in position, particularly from recumbent to upright posture and to dangle legs and exercise ankles and toes for a few minutes before ambulating.
- Instruct to lie down or sit down in head-low position immediately if he or she feels light-headed or dizzy.

PHENYLBUTAZONE

(fen-ill-byoo′ta-zone)

Classifications: CNS AGENT; ANALGESIC; ANTIPYRETIC; NSAID

Prototype: Ibuprofen

Pregnancy category: D

ACTIONS/PHARMACODYNAMICS Pyrazolone derivative with antiinflammatory, antipyretic, analgesic, and mild uricosuric properties. Specific antiinflammatory action mechanism unknown but appears to be associated with prostaglandin synthesis, leukocyte migration, and release or activity of lysosomal enzymes. Inhibits platelet aggregation. Does not cure inflammatory condition but produces effective short-term symptomatic relief of pain and disability. Should not be used as a general analgesic or antipyretic.

USES Short-term treatment of acute gouty arthritis, active rheumatoid arthritis and ankylosing spondylitis, and acute attacks of degenerative joint disease of hips and knees.

ROUTE & DOSAGE

Rheumatoid Arthritis, Ankylosing Spondylitis, Osteoarthritis

Adult: **PO** 300–600 mg/d in 3–4 divided doses.

Acute Gouty Arthritis

Adult: **PO** 400 mg initially; then 100 mg q4h until relief.

PHARMACOKINETICS **Absorption:** rapidly and completely absorbed. **Peak:** 2.5 h. **Distribution:** widely distributed; crosses placenta; distributed into breast milk. **Metabolism:** metabolized in liver to oxyphenbutazone, an active metabolite. **Elimination:** half-life: 50–100 h; 60% excreted in urine, 30% in feces.

P

CONTRAINDICATIONS & PRECAUTIONS **Contraindicated in:** phenylbutazone or oxyphenbutazone sensitivity and idiosyncracy, history of peptic ulcer, GI inflammatory disease, pancreatitis; stomatitis; aspirin hypersensitivity; drug allergy; blood dyscrasias; renal disease; hepatic dysfunction; left ventricular failure, borderline cardiac failure, severe hypertension; edema; polymyalgia rheumatica; temporal arteritis; concomitant use with other drugs such as chemotherapeutic agents, use with long-term anticoagulant (oral) therapy, children <14 y, senile patient. Safe use during pregnancy (category D), especially during third trimester, not established. **Cautious**

use in: glaucoma, patients >40 y, asthma.

ADVERSE/SIDE EFFECTS CV: hypertension, pericarditis, cardiac decompensation. **Endocrine/metabolic:** hyperglycemia, thyroid hyperplasia, toxic goiter, myxedema; sodium, chloride, and fluid retention; rapid plasma volume expansion with plasma dilution, metabolic acidosis, respiratory alkalosis. **Eye/ear:** Optic neuritis, retinal hemorrhage and detachment, oculomotor palsy, toxic amblyopia, blurred vision, conjunctivitis, scotomas; hearing loss, tinnitus. **GI:** *recurring dyspepsia* (including heartburn and indigestion), *nausea,* vomiting, constipation, diarrhea, xerostomia, ulcerative stomatitis and esophagitis, salivary gland enlargement, epigastric pain, constipation, abdominal distension with flatulence, ulceration of bowel, reactivation of peptic ulcer, hepatitis (fatal and nonfatal), pancreatitis. **Hematologic:** bone marrow depression, pancytopenia, thrombocytopenia, agranulocytosis, aplastic anemia, leukopenia, leukemia. **Hypersensitivity:** asthma, urticaria, anaphylaxis, drug fever, serum sickness, Stevens-Johnson syndrome, activation of SLE, Lyell's syndrome. **Renal:** hematuria, proteinuria, glomerulonephritis, acute renal failure, nephrotic syndrome, renal calculi, azotemia. **Skin:** fixed drug eruptions, erythema nodosum and multiforme, nonthrombocytopenic purpura. **Other:** trembling, nervousness, taste disturbances, headache, confusion.

DIAGNOSTIC TEST INTERFERENCE Phenylbutazone reduces ***iodine uptake*** by thyroid gland.

DRUG INTERACTIONS Increases activity and toxicity of **warfarin,** ORAL HYPOGLYCEMIC AGENTS, **phenytoin,** salicylates, SULFONAMIDES; increases **digitoxin** metabolism; increases **methotrexate** toxicity.

NURSING IMPLICATIONS

Administration

- Possible GI irritation can be minimized by administering drug with meals, with full glass of milk, or with an antacid (prescribed).
- Tablet may be crushed and capsule may be emptied if patient cannot swallow it whole. Mix crushed powder or capsule contents with fluid of patient's choice or with food. Should not be swallowed dry.
- Store drug at 15–30C (59–86F) in light- and moisture-resistant container.

Assessment & Drug Effects

- Steady-state therapeutic serum levels (95 μg/ml) are reached in 3–4 d.
- Frequent regular blood studies are advisable when drug is given beyond 1 wk, the usual treatment period.
- Any significant change in hematology, i.e., fall in total white count, relative decrease in granulocytes, appearance of blast forms, fall in Hct, signals the necessity to stop treatment pending complete hematology studies.
- Although phenylbutazone increases action of oral anticoagulants when they are given concomitantly, it does not affect prothrombin activity when administered alone; however, the combination of antiplatelet and ulcerogenic action of phenylbutazone contributes to the hazard of serious hemorrhage during drug therapy.
- Monitor patient with asthma, especially if patient is also sensitive to aspirin. This drug like others

with prostaglandin-synthesis inhibition activity may precipitate an acute asthma attack.

- Smoking–drug relationships: Smoking shortens half-life and increases clearance rate of phenylbutazone. It is possible that the heavy smoker may require an adjusted dosage regimen.
- Overdose symptoms are: prompt onset of respiratory or metabolic acidosis with hyperventilation that can progress to trismus, tonic-clonic seizures, shock, coma, hypotension, and oliguria. Other symptoms include: nausea, vomiting, epigastric pain, excessive perspiration, euphoria, psychoses, headache, vertigo, insomnia, tinnitus, edema, cyanosis, agitation, hallucinations, convulsions, and hematuria. Buccal or GI mucosal ulcerations are late manifestations of massive overdosage.

Patient & Family Education

- Urge to report for all scheduled blood studies. Hematologic toxicity may occur suddenly or many days or weeks after drug use has been terminated.
- Warn to discontinue drug therapy immediately and report to physician: fever, stomatitis, oral ulcerations, salivary gland enlargement, severe sore throat, epigastric pain, dyspepsia, unusual unexplained bleeding and bruising, tarry stools, skin rashes, edema, pruritus, jaundice.
- Any eye symptom should be investigated. Drug should be discontinued and a complete ophthalmic examination scheduled.
- Phenylbutazone may cause drowsiness; therefore, advise to observe caution while driving or performing tasks requiring alertness until response to drug is known.
- Instruct to keep a record of daily weight and to check for lower leg, ankle, or facial edema. Advise patient to report sudden weight gain (i.e., gain of 2–3 lb within 2–3 d). Edema may signify hepatic or renal dysfunction or electrolyte imbalance and may indicate necessity of stopping therapy. In the elderly, reduction of dose may suffice to reduce edema of ankles and face.
- Check with physician about alcohol ingestion. Alcohol impairs motor coordination in the patient receiving phenylbutazone (probably an additive effect).
- Urge not to self-dose with OTC drugs unless advised to do so by physician. Many pain relief OTC preparations contain aspirin.

PHENYLEPHRINE HYDROCHLORIDE

(fen-ill-ef′rin)

Trade names: AK-Dilate Ophthalmic, Alconefrin, Isopto Frin, Mydfrin, Neo-Synephrine, Nostril, Prefrin Liquifilm, Rhinall, Sinarest Nasal, Sinex, Vacon

Classifications: AUTONOMIC NERVOUS SYSTEM AGENT; ALPHA-ADRENERGIC AGONIST; EYE AND NOSE PREPARATION; MYDRIATIC; DECONGESTANT

Prototype: Methoxamine

Pregnancy category: C

ACTIONS/PHARMACODYNAMICS

Potent, synthetic, direct-acting sympathomimetic with strong alpha-adrenergic and weak beta-adrenergic cardiac stimulant actions. Produces little or no CNS stimulation. Elevates systolic and diastolic pressures through arteriolar constriction; also constricts capacitance vessels and increases venous return to heart. Rise in BP causes reflex bradycardia. Topical applications to eye produce vasoconstriction and prompt mydriasis of short duration, usually without causing cycloplegia. Reduces intraocular pressure by increasing outflow and decreasing rate of aqueous humor secretion. Nasal decongestant action qualitatively similar to that of epinephrine but more potent and has longer duration of action.

USES Parenterally to maintain BP during anesthesia, to treat vascular failure in shock, and to overcome paroxysmal supraventricular tachycardia. Used topically for rhinitis of common cold, allergic rhinitis, and sinusitis; in selected patients with wide-angle glaucoma; as mydriatic for ophthalmoscopic examination or surgery, and for relief of uveitis.

ROUTE & DOSAGE

Hypotension

Adult: **IM/SC** 1–10 mg (initial dose not to exceed 5 mg) q10–15min as needed. **IV** 0.1–0.18 mg/min until BP stabilizes; then 0.04–0.06 mg/min for maintenance.

Ophthalmoscopy

See Appendix A.

Vasoconstrictor

Adult: **Ophthalmic** See Appendix A. **Intranasal** Small amount of nasal jelly placed into each nostril q3–4h as needed *or* 2–3 drops or sprays of 0.25–0.5% solution q3–4h as needed.
Child: **Intranasal** *<6 y,* 2–3 drops or sprays of 0.125% solution q3–4h as needed; *6–12 y,* 2–3 drops or sprays of 0.25% solution q3–4h as needed.

PHARMACOKINETICS **Onset:** immediate IV; 10–15 min IM/SC. **Duration:** 15–20 min IV; 30–120 min IM/SC; 3–6 h topical. **Metabolism:** metabolized in liver and tissues by monoamine oxidase.

CONTRAINDICATIONS & PRECAUTIONS **Contraindicated in:** severe coronary disease, severe hypertension, ventricular tachycardia; narrow-angle glaucoma (ophthalmic preparations); pregnancy (category C). **Cautious use in:** hyperthyroidism; diabetes mellitus; myocardial disease, cerebral arteriosclerosis, bradycardia; elderly patients; 21 d before or following termination of MAO inhibitor therapy. ***10% ophthalmic solution:*** cardiovascular disease; diabetes mellitus; hypertension; aneurysms, infants.

ADVERSE/SIDE EFFECTS **Eye:** *transient stinging,* lacrimation, browache, headache, blurred vision, conjunctival allergy (pigmentary deposits on lids, conjunctiva, and cornea with prolonged use), increased sensitivity to light. **Intranasal:** *rebound congestion* (hyperemia and edema of mucosa), *burning,* stinging, dryness, *sneezing.* **Systemic effects:** palpitation, tachycardia, bradycardia (overdosage), extrasystoles, hypertension, trembling, sweating, pallor, sense of fullness in head, tingling of extremities, sleeplessness, dizziness, light-headedness, weakness, restlessness, anxiety, precordial pain, *tremor,* <u>severe visceral or peripheral vasoconstriction</u>, necrosis if IV infiltrates.

DRUG INTERACTIONS ERGOT ALKALOIDS, **guanethidine, reserpine,** TRICYCLIC ANTIDEPRESSANTS increase pressor effects of phenylephrine; **halothane, digoxin** increase risk of arrhythmias; MAO INHIBITORS cause hypertensive crisis; **oxytocin** causes persistent hypertension; ALPHA BLOCKERS, BETA BLOCKERS antagonize effects of phenylephrine.

NURSING IMPLICATIONS

Administration

- Nasal preparations: Instruct patient to blow nose gently (with both nostrils open) to clear nasal passages before administration of medication.
- Instillation (drops): Tilt head back while sitting or standing up, or lie on bed and hang head over side. Stay in position a few minutes to permit medication to spread through nose. (Spray): With head upright, squeeze bottle quickly and firmly to produce 1 or 2 sprays into each nostril; wait 3–5 min, blow nose, and repeat dose. (Jelly): Place in each nostril and sniff it well back into nose.
- Clean tips and droppers of nasal solution dispensers with hot water after use to prevent contamination of solution. Droppers of ophthalmic solution bottles should not touch any surface including the eye.
- Ophthalmic preparations: To avoid excessive systemic absorption, instruct patient to apply pressure to lacrimal sac during and for 1–2 min after instillation of drops.
- A local anesthetic may be instilled in eyes before the phenylephrine to reduce discomfort of stinging and burning.
- IV administration: IV phenylephrine may be given by IV infusion by diluting each 10 mg in 500 ml D5W or NS (concentration: 0.2 mg/ml); titrate to maintain BP.
- Wash hands carefully after handling the drug. Anisocoria (inequality in pupil size, blurred vision) can be caused by rubbing the eye with phenylpropranolamine-contaminated finger.
- Solutions and jelly change color to brown, form a precipitate, and lose potency with exposure to air, strong light, or heat. Do not transfer solutions from original container to another.
- Store in original container at 15–30C (59–86F) protected from freezing, strong light, and exposure to air.

Assessment & Drug Effects

- During IV administration, monitor pulse, BP, and central venous pressure (q2–5min). IV overdoses can induce ventricular dysrhythmias. Control flow rate and dosage to prevent excessive increases.
- Instillation of 2.5–10% strength ophthalmic solution can cause burning and stinging.
- Observe for congestion or rebound miosis after topical administration to eye.

Patient & Family Education

- Caution not to exceed recommended dosage regardless of formulation.
- If no relief is experienced from preparation in 5 d, patient should inform the physician.
- Systemic absorption from nasal and conjunctival membranes can occur, though infrequently (see Adverse/Side Effects). Stop the drug and report to the physician if adverse effects occur.
- Inform that after instillation of ophthalmic drops, pupils will be large and eyes may be more sensitive to light than usual. Advise to use sunglasses in bright light and to stop medication and notify physician if this sensitivity persists beyond 12 h after drug has been discontinued.
- Caution that some ophthalmic solutions may stain contact lenses.

- Caution to avoid swallowing solutions or jelly; systemic effects may be induced.

PHENYLPROPANOLAMINE HYDROCHLORIDE

(fen-ill-proe-pa-nole′a-meen)

Trade names: Acutrim, Allerest Timed Release, Contac, Dex-A-Diet, Dexatrim, Diadax

Classifications: AUTONOMIC NERVOUS SYSTEM AGENT; ALPHA- AND BETA-ADRENERGIC AGONIST (SYMPATHOMIMETIC); NASAL DECONGESTANT; CNS AGENT; ANOREXIANT

Prototype: Epinephrine

Pregnancy category: C

ACTIONS/PHARMACODYNAMICS Indirect-acting sympathomimetic amine with prominent peripheral adrenergic effects similar to those of epinephrine, but its action is more prolonged and it causes less CNS stimulation. Acts by stimulating alpha-adrenergic (excitatory) receptors of vascular smooth muscles, causing vasoconstriction and blanching of nasal mucosa. Also depresses appetite center in CNS.

USES Symptomatic relief of nasal congestion associated with allergies, hay fever, common cold, sinusitis, nasopharyngitis. Used parenterally as vasopressor during surgery, particularly during spinal anesthesia; exogenous obesity.

ROUTE & DOSAGE

Appetite Suppressant

Adult: **PO** 25 mg t.i.d. 30 min a.c. or 75 mg sustained release once/d before breakfast (max 75 mg/d).

Decongestant

Adult: **PO** 25 mg q4h prn *or* 75 mg sustained release q12h prn (max 150 mg/d).
Child: **PO** *2–6 y,* 6.25 mg q4h prn (max 37.5 mg/d); *6–12 y,* 12.5 mg q4h prn (max 75 mg/d).

PHARMACOKINETICS Absorption: readily absorbed from GI tract. **Onset:** 15–30 min. **Peak:** 1–2 h (3.5 h sustained release). **Duration:** 3 h (12 h sustained release). **Metabolism:** small amount metabolized in liver. **Elimination:** half-life: 3–4 h; excreted in urine.

CONTRAINDICATIONS & PRECAUTIONS Contraindicated in: concomitant use with MAO inhibitors. **Cautious use in:** hypertension, cardiovascular disease, hyperthyroidism, diabetes, prostatic enlargement, tricyclic antidepressants, pregnancy (category C).

ADVERSE/SIDE EFFECTS Larger doses: *hypertension,* tachycardia, *palpitation,* nervousness, restlessness, *insomnia.* **Overdosage:** tachycardia, rapid respirations, disorientation, kidney failure, dilated pupils, headache, CNS stimulation, nausea, vomiting, anorexia, seizures.

DRUG INTERACTIONS Antagonizes antihypertensive effects of **guanethidine, guanadryl, reserpine.** MAO INHIBITOR, **selegiline** can cause hypertensive crisis (fatalities reported)—do not administer phenylpropanolamine during or within 14 d of these drugs, may inhibit mood elevating effects of PHENOTHIAZINES; TRICYCLIC ANTIDEPRESSANTS enhance pressor effects of phenylpropanolamine.

NURSING IMPLICATIONS

See epinephrine for additional nursing implications.

Administration

- Preserve in tight, light-resistant containers.

Patient & Family Education

- Caution not to exceed recommended dosage.
- The use of OTC combination drugs without physician's approval while patient is receiving phenylpropanolamine should be discouraged.

PHENYTOIN

(fen'i-toy-in)

Trade names: Dilantin-125, Dilantin-30 Pediatric, Dilantin Infatab

PHENYTOIN SODIUM EXTENDED

Trade name: Dilantin Kapseals

PHENYTOIN SODIUM PROMPT

Trade names: Dilantin, Diphenylan Sodium

Prototype for classifications: CNS AGENT; ANTICONVULSANT HYDANTOIN

Pregnancy category: D

ACTIONS/PHARMACODYNAMICS Hydantoin derivative chemically related to phenobarbital. Precise mechanism of anticonvulsant action not known, but drug use is accompanied by reduced voltage, frequency, and spread of electrical discharges within the motor cortex, resulting in seizure activity inhibition. Has class IB antiarrhythmic properties similar to those of lidocaine and tocainamide (also class IB agents); in abnormal tissue causes slight increase in AV conduction velocity depressed by digitalis glycosides, prolongs effective refractory period, suppresses ventricular pacemaker automaticity, and may slow conduction or cause complete block in abnormal ventricular fibers.

USES To control tonic-clonic (grand mal) seizures, psychomotor and nonepileptic seizures (e.g., Reye's syndrome, after head trauma). Also used to prevent or treat seizures occurring during or after neurosurgery. Is not effective for absence seizures. **Unlabeled uses:** antiarrhythmic agent (phenytoin IV) especially in treatment of digitalis-induced arrhythmias; treatment of trigeminal neuralgia (tic douloureux).

ROUTE & DOSAGE

Anticonvulsant

Adult: **PO** 15–18 mg/kg or 1 g loading dose; then 300 mg/d in 1–3 divided doses; may be gradually increased by 100 mg/wk until seizures are controlled. **IV** 15–18 mg/kg or 1 g loading dose; then 100 mg t.i.d.
Child: **PO/IV** 15–20 mg/kg loading dose; then 5 mg/kg or 250 mg/m^2 in 2–3 divided doses.

P

PHARMACOKINETICS **Absorption:** completely absorbed from GI tract. **Peak:** 1.5–3 h prompt release; 4–12 h extended release. **Distribution:** 95% protein bound; crosses placenta; small amount in breast milk. **Metabolism:** oxidized in liver to inactive metabolites. **Elimination:** half-life: 22 h; metabolites excreted by kidneys.

CONTRAINDICATIONS & PRECAUTIONS **Contraindicated in:** hypersensitivity to hydantoin products, rash, seizures due to hypoglycemia, sinus bradycardia, complete or incomplete heart block, Adams-Stokes syndrome, pregnancy (category D), nursing mothers. **Cautious use in:** impaired hepatic or renal function; alcoholism; blood dyscrasias; hypotension, heart block, bradycardia, severe myocardial insufficiency, impending or frank heart failure; elderly, debilitated, gravely ill patients; pancreatic adenoma; diabetes mellitus, hyperglycemia; respiratory depression; acute intermittent porphyria.

ADVERSE/SIDE EFFECTS **CNS:** Usually dose-related: nystagmus, *drowsiness,* ataxia, dizziness, mental confusion, tremors, insomnia, headache, seizures. **CV:** bradycardia, hypotension, cardiovascular collapse, ventricular fibrillation, phlebitis. **Eye:** photophobia, conjunctivitis, diplopia, blurred vision. **GI:** *gingival hyperplasia,* nausea, vomiting, constipation, epigastric pain, dysphagia, loss of taste, weight loss, hepatitis, liver necrosis. **Hematologic:** thrombocytopenia, leukopenia, leukocytosis, agranulocytosis, pancytopenia, eosinophilia; megaloblastic, hemolytic, or aplastic anemias. **Metabolic:** fever, hyperglycemia, glycosuria, weight gain, edema, transient increase in serum thyrotropic (TSH) level. **Skin:** alopecia, hirsutism (especially in young female); rash: scarlatiniform, maculopapular, urticarial, morbilliform; bullous, exfoliative, or purpuric dermatitis; Stevens-Johnson syndrome, toxic epidermal necrolysis, keratosis, neonatal hemorrhage. **Other:** acute renal failure, osteomalacia or rickets associated with hypocalcemia and elevated alkaline phosphatase activity; acute pneumonitis, pulmonary fibrosis; periarteritis nodosum, acute systemic lupus erythematosus, craniofacial abnormalities (with enlargement of lips); Peyronie's disease, lymphadenopathy.

DIAGNOSTIC TEST INTERFERENCE Phenytoin (hydantoins) may produce lower than normal values for ***dexamethasone*** or ***metyrapone*** tests; may increase serum levels of ***glucose, BSP,*** and ***alkaline phosphatase*** and may decrease ***PBI*** and ***urinary steroid*** levels.

DRUG INTERACTIONS **Alcohol** decreases phenytoin effects; OTHER ANTICONVULSANTS may increase or decrease phenytoin levels; phenytoin may decrease absorption and increase metabolism of ORAL ANTICOAGULANTS; phenytoin increases metabolism of CORTICOSTEROIDS, ORAL CONTRACEPTIVES, and **nisoldipine,** thus decreasing their effectiveness; **amiodarone, chloramphenicol, omeprazole,** and **ticlopidine** increase phenytoin levels; ANTITUBERCULOSIS AGENTS decrease phenytoin levels. **Drug–food:** folic acid, calcium, and vitamin D absorption may be decreased by phenytoin; phenytoin absorption may be decreased by enteral nutrition supplements.

INCOMPATIBILITIES **Solution/additive: 5% dextrose, amikacin, aminophylline, bretylium, cephapirin, codeine phosphate, dobutamine, insulin, levorphanol, lidocaine, lincomycin, meperidine, metaraminol, methadone, morphine, nitroglycerin, norepinephrine, pentobarbital, procaine, secobarbital, streptomycin, sufentanil. Y-site: amikacin, bretylium, dobutamine, lidocaine, heparin, potassium chloride, vitamin B complex with C.**

NURSING IMPLICATIONS

Administration

- If patient cannot take a whole tablet, it may be crushed before administration. Drug should be mixed with food (e.g., applesauce) or fluid; have patient swallow a fluid first; then follow with the diluted or mixed drug along with a full glass of water, milk, or with food. This drug is strongly alkaline, and should not be swallowed without prior preparation to prevent esophageal and gastric direct contact.

- Shake suspension vigorously before pouring to ensure uniform distribution of drug. Suspension is available in two concentrations: 120 mg/5 ml and 30 mg/5 ml and is dispensed in bottles or individual unit dose foil pouches.
- Prompt-release capsules and chewable tablets are not intended for once-a-day dosage since drug is too quickly bioavailable and can therefore lead to toxic serum levels.
- Extended-release capsules only are used for once-a-day dosage regimens.
- IV administration: Give by direct IV 50 mg or fraction thereof over 1 min (25 mg/min in elderly or when used as antiarrhythmic). Usually, phenytoin is not given as a continuous infusion.
- IV administration to infants, children: Verify correct rate of IV injection with physician.
- During IV phenytoin administration, observe injection site frequently to prevent infiltration. Local soft tissue irritation may be serious, leading to erosion of tissues. The elderly woman, especially with peripheral vascular disease, seems to be at high risk.
- To minimize local venous irritation, each IV injection is followed with an injection of sterile saline through the same in-place catheter or needle.
- To reduce side effects with IV administration, lower doses than the usual adult range are given to geriatric, severely ill, debilitated patients or those with liver damage, and the flow rate is reduced to 50 mg over a 2–3-min period.
- A slightly yellowed injectable solution may be used safely. Precipitation may be caused by refrigeration, but slow warming to room temperature restores clarity. Do not administer unclear solution.
- Store phenytoin at 15–30C (59–86F) in tightly closed container. Protect from light.

Assessment & Drug Effects

- Therapeutic serum concentration: 10–20 μg/ml; toxic level: 30–50 μg/ml; lethal level: 100 μg/ml. Steady-state therapeutic levels are not achieved for at least 7–10 d.
- Margin between toxic and therapeutic IV doses is relatively small. Continuously monitor vital signs and symptoms during IV infusion and for an hour afterward. Watch for respiratory depression. If patient is elderly or has cardiac disease, constant observation and a cardiac monitor are necessary.
- Observe patient closely for neurologic side effects. Have on hand oxygen, atropine, vasopressor, assisted ventilation, seizure precaution equipment (mouth gag, nonmetal airway, suction apparatus).
- Gingival hyperplasia appears most commonly in children and adolescents and never occurs in edentulous patients. Adjustment of phenytoin dosage for patients on insulin or of sulfonylurea dosage may be necessary.
- Patients on prolonged therapy should have adequate intake of vitamin D-containing foods and sufficient exposure to sunlight.
- Periodic checks are indicated for decrease in serum calcium levels. Particularly susceptible: black children, patients receiving other an-

ticonvulsants concurrently, who are inactive, have limited exposure to sun, or whose dietary intake is inadequate.

- Observe patient for symptoms of folic acid deficiency: neuropathy, mental dysfunction.
- Serum concentration of magnesium may be decreased by phenytoin therapy. Be alert to symptoms of hypomagnesemia (see Appendix G); neuromuscular symptoms: tetany, positive Chvostek's and Trousseau's signs, seizures, tremors, ataxia, vertigo, nystagmus, muscular fasciculations.

Patient & Family Education

- Inform that drug may make urine pink or red to red-brown.
- Phenytoin can unmask a low thyroid reserve. Advise patient on long-term therapy to report symptoms of fatigue, dry skin, deepening voice.
- Caution to report promptly onset of liver dysfunction as evidenced by jaundice. Since phenytoin is largely metabolized in the liver, impairment of liver function leads to increased serum levels and toxicity. Early recognition of a toxic reaction may save the patient's life.
- Caution not to alter prescribed drug regimen. Abrupt drug discontinuation may precipitate seizures and status epilepticus.
- Advise not to request change in drug brand when refilling prescription. Differences can alter phenytoin serum levels.
- Warn about the effects of alcohol: alcohol intake may increase phenytoin serum levels, leading to phenytoin toxicity. Dosage for chronic alcoholics needs to be higher.
- Phenytoin should be discontinued immediately if a measles-like skin rash appears.
- If patient is receiving phenytoin to prevent major seizures, it probably will not be stopped during pregnancy because of the risk of precipitated status epilepticus with attendant hypoxia, a danger to both mother and fetus.
- Influenza vaccine during phenytoin treatment may increase seizure activity. Patient should be alerted in case a change in dose is necessary.

PHYSOSTIGMINE SALICYLATE

(fi-zoe-stig′meen)

Trade names: Antilirium, Isopto Eserine

PHYSOSTIGMINE SULFATE

Trade name: Eserine Sulfate

Classifications: AUTONOMIC NERVOUS SYSTEM AGENT; CHOLINERGIC (PARASYMPATHOMIMETIC); CHOLINESTERASE INHIBITOR; EYE PREPARATION; MIOTIC (ANTIGLAUCOMA AGENT)

Prototype: Neostigmine

Pregnancy category: C

ACTIONS/PHARMACODYNAMICS

Reversible anticholinesterase and tertiary amine. Chief effect: increases concentration of acetylcholine at cholinergic transmission sites; prolongs and exaggerates its action. Similar to neostigmine in actions and adverse effects, but produces greater secretion of glands, constriction of pupil, and effect on BP and less action on skeletal muscle. Also has direct blocking action on autonomic ganglia. Parenteral physostigmine can produce transient decrease in manic symptoms as well as precipitate mental depression. Topical application to conjunctiva produces constriction of ciliary muscle and iris sphincter, as result of which the iris is pulled away from anterior chamber angle, thus facilitating drainage of aqueous humor, with lowering of intraocular pressure.

USES To reverse CNS and cardiac effects of tricyclic antidepressant overdose, to reverse CNS toxic effects of atropine, scopolamine, and similar anticholinergic drugs, and to antagonize CNS depressant effects of diazepam. Applied topically to eye to reduce intraocular tension in glaucoma. **Orphan drug:** for hereditary ataxias.

ROUTE & DOSAGE

Reversal of Anticholinergic Effects

Adult: **IM/IV** 0.5–3 mg (IV not faster than 1 mg/min); repeat as needed.
Child: **IV** 0.01–0.03 mg/kg; may repeat q15–20min to max total dose of 2 mg.

Glaucoma

Adult: **Topical** See Appendix A.

PHARMACOKINETICS **Absorption:** readily absorbed from mucous membranes, muscle, subcutaneous tissue; 10–12% absorbed from GI tract. **Onset:** 3–8 min IM/IV; 2 min ophthalmic. **Duration:** 0.5–5 h IM/IV; 12–36 h ophthalmic. **Distribution:** crosses blood–brain barrier. **Metabolism:** metabolized in plasma by cholinesterases. **Elimination:** half-life: 15–40 min; excretion not fully understood; small amounts excreted in urine.

CONTRAINDICATIONS & PRECAUTIONS **Contraindicated in:** asthma; diabetes mellitus; gangrene, cardiovascular disease; mechanical obstruction of intestinal or urogenital tract; any vagotonic state; secondary glaucoma; inflammatory disease of iris or ciliary body; concomitant use with choline esters (e.g., methacholine, bethanechol) or depolarizing neuromuscular blocking agents (e.g., decamethonium, succinylcholine). Safe use during pregnancy (category C) not established. **Cautious use in:** epilepsy; parkinsonism; bradycardia; hyperthyroidism; peptic ulcer; hypotension.

ADVERSE/SIDE EFFECTS **Acute toxicity:** cholinergic crisis. **CNS:** restlessness, hallucinations, twitching, tremors, *sweating,* weakness, ataxia, convulsions, collapse, respiratory paralysis, pulmonary edema. With rapid IV: bradycardia, hyperactivity, respiratory distress, convulsions. **Eye:** headache, eye and brow pain, *marked miosis,* twitching of eyelids, *lacrimation,* dimness and blurring of vision; prolonged use: changes in pigmented epithelium of iris, chronic conjunctivitis, follicular cysts, contact allergic dermatitis. **Systemic absorption:** *nausea, vomiting, epigastric pain, diarrhea,* involuntary urination or defecation, miosis, *salivation, sweating, lacrimation,* rhinorrhea, dyspnea, bronchospasm, irregular pulse, palpitation, bradycardia, rise in BP.

DRUG INTERACTIONS Antagonizes effects of **echothiophate, isoflurophate.**

NURSING IMPLICATIONS

Administration

- The patient with brown or hazel eyes may require a stronger ophthalmic solution or more frequent instillation for desired effects than the patient with blue eyes.
- Physostigmine ophthalmic ointment may be prescribed at bedtime for patients with glaucoma to

P

prevent nocturnal rise in ocular tension.

- To reduce the possibility of systemic effects, apply gentle pressure over lacrimal sac during and for 1 or 2 min following instillation. Instruct patient to avoid squeezing lids together. Blot excess medication with clean tissue.
- IV administration: Physostigmine is given by direct IV undiluted at a slow rate, no more than 1 mg/min. Rapid administration and overdosage can cause a cholinergic crisis.
- IV administration to infants, children: Verify correct rate of IV injection with physician.
- Preserve in tight, light-resistant container. Use only clear, colorless solutions. Red-tinted solution indicates oxidation, and such solutions should be discarded.
- Store at 15–30C (59–86F).

Assessment & Drug Effects

- Closely monitor vital signs and state of consciousness in patients receiving drug for atropine poisoning. Since physostigmine is usually rapidly destroyed, patient can lapse into delirium and coma within 1 to 2 h; repeat doses may be required.
- Monitor closely for side effects related to CNS and for signs of sensitivity to physostigmine. Have atropine sulfate readily available for clinical emergency.
- When used parenterally or orally, the following symptoms indicate need to discontinue drug: excessive salivation, emesis, frequent urination, or diarrhea. Excessive sweating or nausea may be eliminated by dose reduction.
- When used as topical ophthalmic agent, be alert to symptoms of systemic absorption (see Adverse/Side Effects). Dosage should be reduced or drug discontinued.

Patient & Family Education

- Inform that physostigmine ophthalmic preparations may produce annoying lid twitching, temporary blurring of vision, and difficulty in seeing in dimmed light; therefore, necessary safety precautions should be taken.
- Emphasize the need for following prescribed drug regimen for glaucoma, and urge patient to remain under medical supervision.
- Teaching plan for glaucoma should include proper administration of eyedrops and adverse symptoms to be reported.
- Advise to wear identification tag indicating the presence of glaucoma and the medication being taken.

P

PHYTONADIONE (VITAMIN K_1)

(fye-toe-na-dye′one)

Trade names: AquaMEPHYTON, Konakion, Mephyton, Phylloquinone

Classifications: SYNTHETIC VITAMIN; ANTIDOTE

Pregnancy category: C

ACTIONS/PHARMACODYNAMICS Fat-soluble naphthoquinone derivative chemically identical to and with similar degree of activity as naturally occurring vitamin K. Vitamin K is essential for hepatic biosynthesis of blood clotting factors II, VII, IX, and X. Promotes liver synthesis of clotting factors by unknown mechanism. Does not reverse anticoagulant action of heparin. Reportedly demonstrates wide margin of safety when used in newborns.

USES Drug of choice as antidote for overdosage of coumarin and indandione oral anticoagulants. Also reverses hypoprothrombinemia secondary to administration of oral antibiotics, quinidine, quinine, salicylates, sulfonamides, excessive vitamin A, and secondary to inadequate absorption and synthesis of vitamin K (as in obstructive jaundice, biliary fistula, ulcerative colitis, intestinal resection, prolonged hyperalimentation). Also prophylaxis of and therapy for neonatal hemorrhagic disease.

ROUTE & DOSAGE

Anticoagulant Overdose

Adult: **PO/SC/IM** 2.5–10 mg; rarely up to 50 mg/d; may repeat parenteral dose after 6–8 h if needed; PO dose may be repeated after 12–24 h. **IV** Emergency only: 10–15 mg at a rate ≤1 mg/min; may be repeated in 4 h if bleeding continues.

Hemorrhagic Disease of Newborns

Infant: **IM/SC** 0.5–1 mg immediately after delivery; may repeat in 6–8 h if necessary.

Other Prothrombin Deficiencies

Adult: **IM/SC** 2–25 mg.
Child: **IM/SC** 5–10 mg.
Infant: **IM/SC** 1 mg.

PHARMACOKINETICS Absorption: readily absorbed from intestinal lymph only if bile is present. **Onset:** 6–12 h PO; 1–2 h IM/SC; 15 min IV. **Peak:** hemorrhage usually controlled within 3–8 h; normal prothrombin time may be obtained in 12–14 h after administration. **Distribution:** concentrates briefly in liver after absorption; crosses placenta; distributed into breast milk. **Metabolism:** rapidly metabolized in liver. **Elimination:** excreted in urine and bile.

CONTRAINDICATIONS & PRECAUTIONS Contraindicated in: severe liver disease. Pregnancy (category C). Effect on fertility and teratogenic potential not known.

ADVERSE/SIDE EFFECTS Gastric upset, headache (after oral dose). **Following IV:** hypersensitivity or anaphylaxis-like reaction: facial flushing, cramp-like pains, convulsive movements, chills, fever, diaphoresis, weakness, dizziness, peculiar taste sensation, *bronchospasm,* dyspnea, sensation of chest constriction, shock, cardiac arrest, respiratory arrest. **Injection site:** pain, hematoma, and nodule formation, erythematous skin eruptions (with repeated injections). Paradoxic hypoprothrombinemia (patients with severe liver disease). **Newborns (following large doses):** hyperbilirubinemia, severe hemolytic anemia, kernicterus, brain damage, death.

DIAGNOSTIC TEST INTERFERENCE Falsely elevated ***urine steroids*** (by modifications of Reddy, Jenkins, Thorn procedure).

DRUG INTERACTIONS Antagonizes effects of **warfarin; cholestyramine, colestipol, mineral oil** decrease absorption of oral phytonadione.

NURSING IMPLICATIONS

Administration

- Note that Konakion (which contains a phenol preservative) is intended for IM use only. Aquamephyton may be given SC, IM, or IV as prescribed.
- IM injection: In adults and older children, IM injection should be given in upper outer quadrant of buttocks. For infants and young

children, anterolateral aspect of thigh or deltoid region is preferred. Carefully aspirate to avoid intravascular injection. Apply gentle pressure to site following injection. Swelling (internal bleeding) and pain sometimes occur with SC or IM administration.

- IV infusion: Dilution may be made with 0.9% NaCl, 5% dextrose, or 5% dextrose in 0.9% NaCl injection. Other diluents should not be used. Administer solution immediately after dilution at a rate not to exceed 1 mg/min. Discard unused solution and contents in open ampul.
- Phytonadione is photosensitive. Protect infusion solution from light by wrapping container with aluminum foil or other opaque material.
- Store in tight, light-resistant containers in a dark place at 15–30C (59–86F). Protect from light at all times.

Assessment & Drug Effects

- Severe reactions, including fatalities, have occurred during and immediately after IV injection (see Adverse/Side Effects). Patient should be under constant surveillance. Monitor vital signs.
- Frequency, dose, and therapy duration are guided by prothrombin times and clinical response.
- Therapeutic responses to phytonadione include shortened prothrombin, bleeding, and clotting times, as well as decreased hemorrhagic tendencies.
- Some patients with liver disease, especially women, develop an itchy erythematous rash at injection sites following repeated IM doses. The rash is at first localized and later may spread and corresponds to inadequate control of prothrombin time. It appears within a few days to several weeks after initiation of therapy and subsides with scaling in 2–12 wk. A change to another form of vitamin K such as menadiol sodium diphosphate (Synkayvite) has resolved the problem.
- Patients on large doses may develop temporary resistance to coumarin- or indandione-type anticoagulants. If oral anticoagulant is reinstituted, larger than former doses of anticoagulant may be needed. Some patients may require change to heparin.
- Use of phytonadione to correct anticoagulant-induced prothrombin deficiency may promote the same clotting hazards that existed prior to anticoagulant therapy.

Patient & Family Education

- Advise patient stabilized on phytonadione to maintain consistency in diet and to avoid significant increases in daily intake of vitamin K-rich foods. Good sources of vitamin K are asparagus, broccoli, cabbage, lettuce, turnip greens, pork or beef liver, green tea, spinach, watercress, and tomatoes.

PILOCARPINE HYDROCHLORIDE

(pye-loe-kar′peen)

Trade names: Adsorbocarpine, Isopto Carpine, Minims Pilocarpine ♣, Miocarpine ♣, Ocusert, Pilo, Pilocar, Salagen

Prototype for classifications: EYE PREPARATION; MIOTIC (ANTIGLAUCOMA AGENT); AUTONOMIC NERVOUS SYSTEM AGENT; DIRECT-ACTING CHOLINERGIC (PARASYMPATHOMIMETIC)

Pregnancy category: C

ACTIONS/PHARMACODYNAMICS

Tertiary amine that acts directly on cholinergic receptor sites, thus mimicking acetylcholine. Induces miosis, spasm of accommodation, and fall in intraocular pressure (IOP) that may be preceded by a transitory rise. Decrease in IOP results from stimulation of ciliary and pupillary sphincter muscles, which pull iris away from filtration angle, thus facilitating outflow of aqueous humor. Also decreases production of aqueous humor.

USES Open-angle and angle-closure glaucomas; to reduce IOP and to protect the lens during surgery and laser iridotomy; to counteract effects of mydriatics and cycloplegics following surgery or ophthalmoscopic examination; to treat xerostomia.

ROUTE & DOSAGE

Acute Glaucoma

Adult: **Ophthalmic** 1 drop of 1–2% solution in affected eye q5–10min for 3–6 doses, then 1 drop q1–3h until IOP is reduced.
Child: **Ophthalmic** Same as for adult.

Chronic Glaucoma

Adult: **Ophthalmic** 1 drop of 0.5–4% solution in affected eye q4–12h or 1 ocular system (Ocusert) q7d.
Child: **Ophthalmic** Same as for adult.

Miotic

Adult: **Ophthalmic** 1 drop of 1% solution in affected eye.
Child: **Ophthalmic** Same as for adult.

Xerostomia

Adult: **PO** 5 mg t.i.d.; may increase up to 10 mg t.i.d.

PHARMACOKINETICS **Absorption:** topical penetrates cornea rapidly; readily absorbed from GI tract. **Onset:** miosis 10–30 min; IOP reduction 60 min; salivary stimulation 20 min. **Peak:** miosis 30 min; IOP reduction 75 min; salivary stimulation 60 min. **Duration:** miosis 4–8 h; IOP reduction 4–14 h (7 d with Ocusert); salivary stimulation 3–5 h. **Metabolism:** inactivated at neuronal synapses and in plasma. **Elimination:** half-life: 0.76–1.35 h; excreted in urine.

CONTRAINDICATIONS & PRECAUTIONS **Contraindicated in:** secondary glaucoma, acute iritis, acute inflammatory disease of anterior segment of eye. Safe use during pregnancy (category C), and in nursing mothers has not been established. **Cautious use in:** bronchial asthma; hypertension. **Ocular therapeutic system:** not used in acute infectious conjunctivitis, keratitis, retinal detachment, or when intense miosis is required.

ADVERSE/SIDE EFFECTS **CNS** (oral): asthenia, headaches, dizziness, chills. **Eye:** ciliary spasm with browache, twitching of eyelids, eye pain with change in eye focus, miosis, *diminished vision in poorly illuminated areas,* blurred vision, reduced visual acuity, sensitivity, contact allergy, lacrimation, follicular conjunctivitis, conjunctival irritation, caratact, <u>retinal detachment.</u> **GI:** *nausea,* vomiting, abdominal cramps, diarrhea, epigastric distress, *salivation*. **Other:** bronchospasm, rhinitis, tachycardia, tremors, *increased sweating,* urinary frequency.

DRUG INTERACTIONS The actions of pilocarpine and **carbachol** are additive when used concomitantly. **Oral:** May cause conduction disturbances with BETA BLOCKERS. Antagonizes the effects of concurrent ANTICHOLINERGIC DRUGS (e.g., **atropine, ipratropium**). **Drug–food:** high-fat meal decreases absorption of pilocarpine.

P

NURSING IMPLICATIONS

Administration

- During acute phase, physician may prescribe instillation of drug into unaffected eye also, to prevent bilateral attack of acute glaucoma.
- During instillation of eyedrops, care should be taken to prevent contamination of dropper tip and solution and to avoid touching eyelids or surrounding area with the dropper tip.
- Immediately after instillation of drops, apply gentle digital pressure to periphery of nasolacrimal drainage system for 1–2 min to prevent delivery of drug to nasal mucosa and general circulation. Excess solution around eye or on hands should be removed immediately with a tissue.

Assessment & Drug Effects

- Hourly tonometric tests may be done during early treatment with pilocarpine because drug may cause an initial transitory increase in IOP.
- Brow pain and myopia tend to be more prominent in younger patients and generally disappear with continued use of drug.

Patient & Family Education

- The patient should understand that therapy for glaucoma is prolonged and that adherence to established regimen is crucial to prevent blindness.
- Since drug causes blurred vision and difficulty in focusing, caution to avoid hazardous activities such as driving a car or operating machinery until vision clears.
- Advise to withhold medication if symptoms of irritation or sensitization persist and to report to physician.

Ocular Therapeutic System (Ocusert)

- Releases 20 μg/h for 7 d. The unit is placed in the eye cul-de-sac, where it remains for a week. Slow release of drug provides a nonfluctuating concentration of pilocarpine in the ciliary body and iris.
- The 20 μg/h system produces reduction in IOP about equal to that produced by topical application of 28 mg pilocarpine as a 2% solution q6h.
- Induced myopia, miosis, and spasm of accommodation is less than that produced by eyedrops. However, since transient blurring and dimness of vision may occur following Ocusert insertion, have patient do so at bedtime; myopia will be at a stable level in the AM.
- Several hours after Ocusert insertion, induced myopia decreases to a low base level that persists for the life of the therapeutic system.
- Conjunctival irritation with mild erythema and increase in mucus secretion may accompany early use of Ocusert. Usually, these symptoms subside, but if they do not, notify physician.
- If the system contacts an unclean surface, wash it with cool tap water before replacing it into cul-de-sac.
- If retention of the system is a problem, the superior conjunctival cul-de-sac may be a preferred site for insertion. This location is also preferred during sleep.
- Ocusert may be transferred from the lower conjunctival sac to the superior sac by closing eyelids, rolling the eye toward the nose and, with gentle digital pressure through the closed eyelid, directly moving the system. Avoid moving it over the colored part of the eye.
- If an unexpected increase in drug action occurs (sudden miosis, ciliary spasm, decreased visual acuity), the system should be re-

moved and replaced with a new one.

- If system ruptures, is deformed or grossly contaminated, discard and replace with another.
- Instruct to check for presence of Ocusert before retiring at night and upon rising. If the ocular system slips out during sleep, its effect continues for a short time.
- While IOP increases immediately with removal of Ocusert, it does not reach uncontrolled levels for 2–3 d.
- Information about inserting the ocular system is included in the drug package. Review these directions carefully with patient and ask for demonstration to test patient's ability to adjust, insert, and remove the system.
- Advise to keep follow-up appointments.
- Store ocular system form at 2–8C (35–46F); avoid freezing. Store solutions in tight, light-resistant containers.

PIMOZIDE

(pi′moe-zide)

Trade name: Orap

Classifications: CNS AGENT; PSYCHOTHERAPEUTIC; ANTIPSYCHOTIC BUTYROPHENONE

Prototype: Haloperidol

Pregnancy category: C

ACTIONS/PHARMACODYNAMICS A potent central dopamine antagonist that alters release and turnover of central dopamine stores; has no effect on turnover of norepinephrine. Blockade of CNS dopaminergic receptors results in suppression of the motor and phonic tics that characterize Tourette's disorder. Produces less sedation and fewer extrapyramidal reactions than haloperidol; lowers seizure threshold.

USES To suppress severe motor and phonic tics in patient with Tourette's disorder who has failed to respond satisfactorily to standard treatment (e.g., haloperidol).

ROUTE & DOSAGE

Tourette's Disorder

Adult: **PO** 1–2 mg/d in divided doses; gradually increase dose q.o.d. up to 0.2 mg/kg/d or 7–16 mg/d in divided doses, whichever is less (max 0.2 mg/kg/d or 10 mg/d).

PHARMACOKINETICS **Absorption:** slowly and variably absorbed from GI tract (40–50% absorbed). **Peak:** 6–8 h. **Metabolism:** metabolized in liver to 2 major metabolites. **Elimination:** half-life: 55 h; 80–85% excreted in urine, 15–20% in feces.

CONTRAINDICATIONS & PRECAUTIONS **Contraindicated in:** treatment of simple tics other than those associated with Tourette′s disorder; drug-induced tics; history of cardiac dysrhythmias and conditions marked by prolonged QT syndrome, patient taking drugs that may prolong QT interval (e.g., quinidine); severe toxic CNS depression. Safe use in children <12 y, during pregnancy (category C), and by nursing mothers not established. **Cautious use in:** renal and hepatic dysfunction; patients receiving anticonvulsant therapy.

ADVERSE/SIDE EFFECTS **CNS:** headache, *sedation, drowsiness,* insomnia, *akathisia,* speech disorder, *torticollis, tremor,* handwriting changes, *akinesia,* fainting, hyperpyrexia, seizures, tardive dyskinesia, *rigidity, oculogyric crisis,* hyper-

P

reflexia; seizures, neuroleptic malignant syndrome; *extrapyramidal dysfunction,* hyperthermia, autonomic dysfunction; diaphoresis, dyspnea, respiratory failure, stupor. **CV:** prolongation of QT interval, inverted or flattened T wave, appearance of U wave, labile blood pressure. **GU:** loss of libido, impotence, nocturia, urinary frequency, amenorrhea, dysmenorrhea, mild glactorrhea, urinary retention, acute renal failure. **Skin:** sweating, skin irritation. **Special senses:** visual disturbances, photosensitivity, decreased accommodation, blurred vision, cataracts. **Other:** weight changes, asthenia, chest pain, periorbital edema, increased salivation, nausea, vomiting, diarrhea, anorexia, abdominal cramps, constipation.

DRUG INTERACTIONS **Alcohol** and other CNS DEPRESSANTS increase CNS depression; ANTICHOLINERGIC AGENTS (e.g., TRICYCLIC ANTIDEPRESSANTS, **atropine**) increase anticholinergic effects; PHENOTHIAZINES, TRICYCLIC ANTIDEPRESSANTS, ANTIARRHYTHMICS increase risk of arrhythmias and heart block; pimozide antagonizes effects of ANTICONVULSANTS—there is loss of seizure control.

NURSING IMPLICATIONS

See haloperidol for additional nursing implications.

Administration

- Drug dose is increased gradually, usually over 1–3 wk, until maintenance dose is reached.
- When drug is to be discontinued, the regimen should be adjusted by prescription: slow, gradual changes over a period of days or weeks (drug has a long half-life). Sudden withdrawal may cause reemergence of original symptoms (motor and phonic tics) and of neuromuscular side effects of the drug.

Assessment & Drug Effects

- ECG baseline data should be obtained at beginning of therapy and checked periodicaly, especially during period of dosage adjustment.
- One of the adverse effects is widening of the QT interval (QRS complex and T wave), representing both ventricular depolarization and repolarization. Widening or prolongation of the interval suggests developing cardiotoxicity.
- Risk of tardive dyskinesia appears to be greatest in women, in the elderly, and those on high dosage.
- Extrapyramidal reactions often appear within the first few days of therapy, are dose-related, and usually occur when dose is high.
- Anticholinergic effects (dry mouth, constipation) may increase as dose is increased.

Patient & Family Education

- Advise to adhere to established drug regimen (i.e., dose or intervals should not be changed and dose should be discontinued only with physician's guidance).
- Discuss measures to relieve dry mouth (frequent rinsing with water, saliva substitute, increased fluid intake) and constipation (increased dietary fiber, drink 6–8 glasses of water daily).
- Warn that drug-caused hand tremors, drowsiness, and blurred vision may impair alertness and ability to safely drive a car or to engage in dangerous activities.
- Pseudoparkinsonism symptoms (see Appendix G) are usually mild and reversible with dose adjustment.
- Alert both patient and family to the earliest symptom of tardive dyskinesia ("flycatching,"—an involuntary movement of the tongue), which should be reported promptly to the physician.

- Urge to return for periodic assessments of therapy benefit and cardiac status.
- Advise moderation or abstinence from alcohol to prevent augmenting CNS depressant effects of pimozide.

PINDOLOL

(pin′doe-lole)

Trade name: Visken

Classifications: BETA-ADRENERGIC ANTAGONIST (BLOCKING AGENT, SYMPATHOLYTIC); ANTIHYPERTENSIVE

Prototype: Propranolol

Pregnancy category: B

ACTIONS/PHARMACODYNAMICS Nonselective beta-adrenergic blocking agent. Possesses slight intrinsic sympathomimetic activity (ISA) or partial beta agonist effect in therapeutic dose ranges. Thus, pindolol exerts vasodilator as well as hypotensive effects. Hypotensive mechanism is similar to that of propranolol: competitively blocks beta-adrenergic receptors primarily in myocardium, and beta receptors within bronchial and smooth muscle. Has negative chronotropic and inotropic properties and slows conduction in AV node. Does not consistently affect cardiac output, resting heart rate, or renin release; it does, however, decrease peripheral vascular resistance.

USES Management of hypertension (in stepped-care approach: step 1) concurrently with a thiazide diuretic or as single agent. Used in patient who has failed to respond to diet, exercise, and weight reduction. **Unlabeled use:** stress and exercise-induced chronic stable angina pectoris.

ROUTE & DOSAGE

Hypertension

Adult: **PO** 5 mg b.i.d.; may increase by 10 mg/d q2–3wk if needed up to max of 60 mg/d in 2–3 divided doses.
Geriatric: **PO** Start with 5 mg q.d.

Angina Pectoris

Adult: **PO** 15–40 mg/d in 3–4 divided doses.

PHARMACOKINETICS Absorption: rapidly absorbed from GI tract; 50–95% reaches systemic circulation (first pass metabolism). **Onset:** 3 h. **Peak:** 1–2 h. **Duration:** 24 h. **Distribution:** distributed into breast milk. **Metabolism:** 40–60% metabolized in liver. **Elimination:** half-life: 3–4 h; excreted in urine.

CONTRAINDICATIONS & PRECAUTIONS Contraindicated in: bronchospastic diseases, severe bradycardia, cardiogenic shock, cardiac failure. Safe use in pregnancy (category B), nursing mothers, and children not established. **Cautious use in:** nonallergic bronchospasm, CHF, diabetes mellitus, hyperthyroidism, impaired hepatic and renal function.

ADVERSE/SIDE EFFECTS CNS: *fatigue,* dizziness, insomnia, drowsiness, confusion, fainting, decreased libido. **CV:** *bradycardia,* hypotension, CHF. **GI:** nausea, *diarrhea, constipation,* flatulence. **Respiratory:** <u>bronchospasm,</u> pulmonary edema, dyspnea. **Sensitivity reactions:** antinuclear antibodies (ANA) (10–30% of patients). **Other:** back or joint pain, <u>agranulocytosis</u>, impotence, hypoglycemia (may mask symptoms of a hypoglycemic reaction).

DRUG INTERACTIONS DIURETICS and other HYPOTENSIVE AGENTS increase hypotensive effect; effects of **al-**

P

buterol, metaproterenol, terbutaline, pirbuterol and pindolol antagonized; NSAIDS blunt hypotensive effect; decreases hypoglycemic effect of **glyburide; amiodarone** increases risk of bradycardia and sinus arrest.

NURSING IMPLICATIONS

Administration

- Food does not decrease bioavailability but may increase rate of absorption. Give drug at same time of day each day with respect to time of food intake for most predictable results.
- Withdrawal or discontinuation of treatment is gradual over a period of 1–2 wk.

Assessment & Drug Effects

- Monitor HR and BP. Report bradycardia and hypotension. Dosage adjustment may be indicated.
- Hypotensive effect may begin within 7 d but is not therapeutically maximum until about 2 wk after beginning of treatment with pindolol.

P

Patient & Family Education

- Pindolol masks the dizziness and sweating premonitory symptoms of hypoglycemia.
- Abrupt withdrawal of drug might precipitate a thyroid crisis in a patient with hyperthyroidism, and angina in the patient with ischemic heart disease, leading to an MI. Warn to adhere to the prescribed drug regimen. If a change is desired, consult physician first.

PIPECURONIUM BROMIDE

(pi-pe-cu-ron′i-um)

Trade name: Arduan

Classifications: AUTONOMIC NERVOUS SYSTEM AGENT; NONDEPOLARIZING SKELETAL MUSCLE RELAXANT

Prototype: Tubocurarine

Pregnancy category: C

ACTIONS/PHARMACODYNAMICS

Nondepolarizing neuromuscular blocking agent. Appears to lack vagolytic or autonomic activity and results in minimal cardiovascular effects. Tachycardia and elevated blood pressure have been observed with other neuromuscular blocking agents, but not with pipecuronium. Therefore, it is the drug of choice in coronary artery bypass surgery and patients with coronary artery disease.

USES Adjunct to general anesthesia, and to provide skeletal muscle relaxation during surgery. Should only be used for procedures expected to last ≥ 90 minutes. **Unlabeled use:** skeletal muscle relaxation for endotracheal intubation.

ROUTE & DOSAGE

Adjunct for General Anesthesia

Adult: **IV** 85 to 100 μg/kg, ideal body weight, given as rapid bolus over 5–10 s. May give over 1 min if desired. Smaller supplemental doses (usually 5–25 μg/kg) have been given to maintain muscle relaxation during long surgical procedures.
Child: **IV** Same as adult.

Adjustment for Renal Impairment

Dose based on ideal body weight. Cl_{cr} < 80 ml/min: 70 μg/kg; <60 ml/min: 55 μg/kg; <40 ml/min: 50 μg/kg.

PHARMACOKINETICS **Onset:** 2–3 min. **Peak:** 3–6 min. **Duration:** dose dependent: 50–70 μg/kg lasts approx 1 h. Concomitant anesthetic agents will also affect duration of action. **Distribution:** approximately 32% protein bound (animal studies). **Me-**

tabolism: partially metabolized in the liver. It is unknown if metabolites have any pharmacologic activity. **Half-life:** 137–161 min. **Elimination:** excreted by the kidneys. About 56% of the dose is excreted in the urine within 24 h.

CONTRAINDICATIONS & PRECAUTIONS **Contraindicated in:** hypersensitivity to pipecuronium or bromide. **Cautious use in:** patients with myasthenia gravis, renal failure, hepatic insufficiency, amyotrophic lateral sclerosis, burn patients, children, infants, and pregnancy (category C).

ADVERSE/SIDE EFFECTS **CV:** bradycardia, hypotension. **Musculoskeletal:** prolonged duration of action resulting in muscle weakness to paralysis resulting in respiratory insufficiency or apnea.

DRUG INTERACTIONS **Capreomycin** may increase the action of neuromuscular blocking agents. **Enflurane, isoflurane** may prolong the pipecuronium-induced neuromuscular blockade. Dose reductions of pipecuronium may be needed.

NURSING IMPLICATIONS

Administration

- Pipecuronium may be reconstituted for IV administration using any of the following: 0.9% NaCl solution; 5% dextrose in 0.9% NaCl solution; 5% dextrose in water; lactated Ringer's; sterile water for injection; or bacteriostatic water for injection (not for use in newborns).
- Pipecuronium should not be diluted into or administered from large-volume IV solutions.
- When reconstituted with bacteriostatic water, store refrigerated or at room temperature, and use within 5 d.
- When reconstituted with solutions other than bacteriostatic water, refrigerate and use within 24 h.

Assessment & Drug Effects

- Monitor hemodynamic status; clinically significant bradycardia, hypotension, and hypertension have occurred in a small percentage (~ 3%) of patients.
- A peripheral nerve stimulator should be used to monitor drug response.

PIPERACILLIN SODIUM

(pi-per'a-sill-in)

Trade name: Pipracil

Classifications: ANTIINFECTIVE; BETA-LACTAM ANTIBIOTIC; ANTI-PSEUDOMONAL PENICILLIN

Prototype: Mezlocillin

Pregnancy category: B

ACTIONS/PHARMACODYNAMICS

Extended-spectrum parenteral penicillin with antibiotic activity against most gram-negative and many gram-positive anaerobic and aerobic organisms including members of *Clostridium, Bacteroides, Klebsiella, Enterobacter, Pseudomonas, Proteus,* and *Serratia* species and the anaerobic and aerobic cocci. Action is similar to that of other penicillins: by interference with bacterial cell wall synthesis, promotes loss of membrane integrity, leading to death of the organism. Less active than penicillin G against pneumococci and group A streptococci but comparable to ampicillin against enterococci. Penicillinase-producing staphylococci are resistant to piperacillin.

USES Susceptible organisms that cause gynecologic, skin and skin structure, gonococcal, and streptococcal infections; lower respiratory tract, intraabdominal, and bone and joint infections; septicemia, urinary tract infections. Also prophylactically prior to and during surgery and as empiric antiinfective therapy in granulocytopenic patients.

ROUTE & DOSAGE

Uncomplicated Urinary Tract Infection

Adult: **IV/IM** 8–16 g/d divided q6–8h.

Mild to Moderate Infections

Child: **IV** 200–300 mg/kg/d divided q4–6h (max 24 g/d).
Neonate: **IV** 150–200 mg/kg/d divided q6–8h.

Moderate to Severe Infections

Adult: **IV/IM** 4 g q6h (150–200 mg/kg/d).
Geriatric: **IV** 2–4 g q6–8h. **IM** 1–2 g q8–12h.

Life-threatening Infection, *Pseudomonas* Infections

Adult: **IV/IM** 3 g q4h (max 24 g/d).

Uncomplicated Gonococcal Infections

Adult: **IM** 2 g with 1 g probenecid given 30 min before piperacillin.

PHARMACOKINETICS Peak: 45 min IM; 5 min IV. **Distribution:** widely distributed with highest concentrations in urine and bile; adequate CSF penetration with inflamed meninges; crosses placenta; distributed into breast milk. **Metabolism:** slightly metabolized in liver. **Elimination:** half-life: 0.6–1.35 h; primarily excreted in urine, partly in bile.

CONTRAINDICATIONS & PRECAUTIONS Contraindicated in: hypersensitivity to penicillins, cephalosporins, or other drugs. Safe use in children <12 y, lactating mother, and during pregnancy (category B) not established. **Cautious use in:** hepatic and renal dysfunction, hypersensitivity to cephalosporins.

ADVERSE/SIDE EFFECTS See penicillin G potassium.

DRUG INTERACTIONS May increase risk of bleeding with ANTICOAGULANTS; **probenecid** decreases elimination of piperacillin.

INCOMPATIBILITIES Solution/additive: AMINOGLYCOSIDES. **Y-site:** AMINOGLYCOSIDES.

NURSING IMPLICATIONS

Administration

- IM injections should be limited to 2 g/site. Use the gluteal muscle, preferably. The deltoid muscle should be used only if well developed. Diluents for reconstitution of drug include sterile or bacteriostatic water for injection, bacteriostatic NaCl injection, and sterile lidocaine HCl injection 0.5–1.0% without epinephrine for IM. When reconstituted, solution contains 1 g/2.5 ml.
- Reconstitution: Piperacillin for direct IV injection is reconstituted by diluting 1 g with 5 ml sterile water or NS for injection and is given over 3–5 min. Reconstituted solution may be further diluted with 50–100 ml NS or D5W and is infused over 30 min.
- IV administration to neonates, infants, children: Verify correct IV concentration and rate of infusion with physician.
- Patients undergoing hemodialysis usually receive a maximum dosage of 2 g piperacillin q8h and an additional 1 g dose after each dialysis period.
- Doses and frequency are usually

modified if creatinine clearance is <40 ml/min.

- Duration of therapy depends on type and severity of infection but usually continues for at least 48–72 h after patient is asymptomatic and evidence that infection is eradicated has been obtained.
- Store reconstituted solution at room temperature for 24 h, up to 1 wk refrigerated, and up to 1 mo frozen.

Assessment & Drug Effects

- Prior to administration inquire about history of hypersensitivity to penicillins, cephalosporins, or other drugs.
- Monitor for hypersensitivity response; discontinue drug and notify physician if allergic response noted.
- Since high doses may induce coagulation abnormalities, monitor for hemorrhagic manifestations.

PIPERACILLIN/TAZOBACTAM

(pi-per'a-cil-lin/taz-o-bac'tam)

Trade name: Zosyn

Classifications: ANTIINFECTIVE; BETA-LACTAM ANTIBIOTIC; ANTIPSEUDOMONAL PENICILLIN

Prototype: Mezlocillin

Pregnancy category: B

ACTIONS/PHARMACODYNAMICS Piperacillin/tazobactam is an antibacterial combination product consisting of the semisynthetic piperacillin and the beta-lactamase inhibitor tazobactam. The tazobactam component does not decrease the activity of the piperacillin component against susceptible organisms. Tazobactam is an inhibitor of a wide variety of bacterial beta-lactamases. It has little antibacterial activity itself; however, in combination with piperacillin, it extends the spectrum of bacteria that are susceptible to piperacillin. This two-drug combination has antibiotic activity against an extremely broad spectrum of gram-negative and anaerobic bacteria.

USES Treatment of moderate to severe appendicitis, uncomplicated and complicated skin and skin structure infections, endometritis, pelvic inflammatory disease, or nosocomial or community-acquired pneumonia caused by piperacillin-resistant, piperacillin/tazobactam-susceptible, beta-lactamase-producing bacteria.

ROUTE & DOSAGE

Adult: **IV** 3.375 g q6h, infused over 30 min, for 7–10 d. Dose should be reduced for patients with renal insufficiency: Cl_{cr} 20–40 ml/min, 2.25 g q6h; Cl_{cr} <20 ml/min, 2.25 g q8h.
Child: **IV** *≥6 mo:* 240 mg piperacillin component/kg/d divided q8h. *<6 mo:* 150–300 mg piperacillin/kg/d divided q6–8h.

PHARMACOKINETICS **Distribution:** distributes into many tissues, including lung, blister fluid, and bile; crosses placenta; distributed into breast milk. **Metabolism:** metabolized in liver. **Elimination:** half-life: 0.7–1.2 h; piperacillin and tazobactam are excreted in urine.

CONTRAINDICATIONS & PRECAUTIONS **Contraindicated in:** hypersensitivity to piperacillin, tazobactam, penicillins, cephalosporins, or beta-lactamase inhibitors such as clavulanic acid and sulbactam. **Cautious use in:** renal failure, pregnancy (category B), nursing mothers. Safety and efficacy in children < 12 y not established.

ADVERSE/SIDE EFFECTS CNS: headache, insomnia, fever. **GI:** diarrhea, constipation, nausea, vomiting, dyspepsia, pseudomembranous colitis. **Other:** rash, pruritus, hypersensitivity reactions.

INCOMPATIBILITIES Solution/additive: aminoglycosides. **Y-site:** aminoglycosides.

NURSING IMPLICATIONS

Administration

- Reconstitute powder with 5 ml of diluent (e.g., 0.9% NaCl, 5% dextrose); shake well until dissolved. Further dilute to at least 50 ml and administer over at least 30 min.
- IV administration to infants, children: Verify correct IV concentration and rate of infusion with physician.
- For hemodialysis patients, the maximum dose is 2.25 g q8h; give one extra 0.75g dose after each dialysis period.
- Use single-dose vials immediately after reconstitution. Discard after 24 h at room temperature or 48 h under refrigeration (2–8C/36–46F).

Assessment & Drug Effects

- Prior to administration inquire about hypersensitivity to penicillins, cephalosporins, or other drugs.
- Monitor patient carefully during the first 30 min after initiation of the infusion for signs of hypersensitivity (see Appendix G).
- With prolonged therapy, monitor hematologic status: Hct and Hgb, CBC with differential, PT and PTT.

Patient & Family Education

- Advise to report rash, pruritis, or other signs of hypersensitivity immediately.
- Instruct to report loose stools or diarrhea as these may indicate pseudomembranous colitis.

P

PIPERAZINE CITRATE

(pi'per-a-zeen)

Trade name: Antepar

Classifications: ANTIINFECTIVE; ANTHELMINTIC

Prototype: Mebendazole

Pregnancy category: B

ACTIONS/PHARMACODYNAMICS Appears to act by producing muscle paralysis in parasite, thus promoting elimination through intestinal peristalsis.

USES Pinworm disease *(Enterobius vermicularis)* and roundworm or ascariasis *(Ascaris lumbricoides)* infestations.

ROUTE & DOSAGE

Roundworms

Adult: **PO** 3.5 g once/d for 2 d.
Child: **PO** 75 mg/kg (max 3.5 g) once/d for 2 d.

Pinworms

Adult: **PO** 65 mg/kg (max 2.5 g) once/d for 7–8 d.
Child: **PO** Same as for adult.

PHARMACOKINETICS Absorption: readily absorbed from GI tract. **Elimination:** excreted in urine.

CONTRAINDICATIONS & PRECAUTIONS Contraindicated in: impaired renal or hepatic function, convulsive disorders. Safe use during pregnancy (category B) not established. **Cautious use in:** malnutrition; anemia.

ADVERSE/SIDE EFFECTS Low toxicity. Usually with excessive dosage: **CNS:** headache, vertigo, ataxia, tremors, choreiform movements, muscular weakness, hyporeflexia, paresthesia, sense of detachment, memory defect, EEG abnormalities, convulsions. **ENT:** blurred vision, paralytic strabismus, nystagmus, cataracts, lacrimation, rhinorrhea, accommodative defects. **GI:** nausea, vomiting, abdominal cramps, diarrhea. **Hypersensitivity:** urticaria, erythema multiforme, photosensitivity, purpura, fever, productive cough, bronchospasm, arthralgia, hemolytic anemia.

DRUG INTERACTION PHENOTHIAZINES may exaggerate extrapyramidal effects or cause seizures.

NURSING IMPLICATIONS

Administration

- Drug may be given with food to reduce gastric distress.
- Store at controlled room temperature protected from heat and light.

Patient & Family Education

- Caution not to exceed recommended dosage schedule because of danger of neurotoxicity with high dosages.
- Instruct to withhold medication if CNS, GI, or hypersensitivity reactions occur and report them to physician.
- In severe infections, course of therapy may be repeated after 1 wk rest period.
- Pinworms and roundworms are transmitted by direct and indirect transfer of ova (e.g., by hands, food, and contaminated articles). Instruct patient and family in personal hygiene.

PIPOBROMAN

(pi-poe-broe′man)

Trade name: Vercyte

Classifications: ANTINEOPLASTIC; ALKYLATING AGENT

Prototype: Cyclophosphamide

Pregnancy category: D

ACTIONS/PHARMACODYNAMICS Dicarboxylic acid neutral amide of piperazine with toxic hematopoietic depressant properties. Exact mechanism of action unknown but is classified as a polyfunctional alkylating agent. Blocks DNA, RNA, and protein synthesis in rapidly proliferating cells.

USES Primarily polycythemia. Also to produce remissions in chronic myelocytic leukemia.

ROUTE & DOSAGE

Polycythemia

Adult: **PO** 1 mg/kg/d for at least 30 d; may be increased to 1.5–3 mg/kg/d if no response; then reduce to 0.1–0.2 mg/kg/d.

Chronic Myelocytic Leukemia

Adult: **PO** 1.5–2.5 mg/kg/d until optimal clinical response; maintenance dose: 7–175 mg/d.

PHARMACOKINETICS **Absorption:** readily absorbed from GI tract. **Metabolism:** unknown. **Elimination:** unknown.

CONTRAINDICATIONS & PRECAUTIONS **Contraindicated in:** children <15 y, myelosuppression from radiation or previous cytotoxic chemotherapy, pregnancy (category D).

ADVERSE/SIDE EFFECTS Nausea, vomiting, abdominal cramps, diarrhea, anorexia (transient), skin rash, thrombocytopenia, anemia, leukopenia.

NURSING IMPLICATIONS

Administration

- Since patient requires close observation, therapy is usually initiated in the hospital.

Assessment & Drug Effects

- Maintenance therapy is usually

P

started when Hct is reduced 50–55% in polycythemia vera, or when leukocyte count approaches 10,000/mm^3 in chronic myelocytic leukemia.

- Bone marrow studies should be performed prior to therapy and repeated at time of maximum hematologic response. Liver and kidney function tests should also be performed before and during therapy.
- Leukocyte and thrombocyte counts are advised every other day and CBCs weekly until desired response is obtained or toxic effects intervene.
- Therapy is interrupted when platelet count falls to 150,000/mm^3 or WBC to 3000/mm^3.
- Therapy is discontinued if there is a rapid drop in hemoglobin, increased bilirubin levels, or reticulocytosis.
- Myelosuppression may not appear for 4 wk or more after treatment begins.
- Observe carefully for ecchymoses, petechiae, purpura, melena, and hemoptysis and report to physician promptly.
- If nausea, vomiting, diarrhea, and skin rash persist, therapy will be interrupted.

P

PIRBUTEROL ACETATE

(pir-bu′ter-ol)

Trade name: Maxair

Classifications: AUTONOMIC NERVOUS SYSTEM AGENT; BETA-ADRENERGIC AGONIST (SYMPATHOMIMETIC); BRONCHODILATOR

Prototype: Isoproterenol

Pregnancy category: C

ACTIONS/PHARMACODYNAMICS Pirbuterol has a preferential effect on beta$_2$-adrenergic receptors compared with isoproterenol and, consequently, a lengthened duration of action. Stimulation of beta$_2$-adrenoreceptors relaxes bronchospasm and increases ciliary motion. Activates adenyl cyclase, the enzyme that catalyzes the conversion of ATP to cyclic adenosine monophosphate (cAMP). Increased cAMP is associated with relaxation of bronchial smooth muscle and inhibition of the release of histamine and other mediators of hypersensitivity from mast cells.

USE Prevention and reversal of bronchospasm associated with asthma.

ROUTE & DOSAGE

Asthma

Adult: **Inhaled** 2 inhalations (0.4 mg) q6h; max 12 inhalations/d.
Child > *12 y:* **Inhaled** same as adult.

PHARMACOKINETICS Onset: 5 min. **Peak:** 30 min.. **Duration:** 3–4 h. **Metabolism:** metabolized in liver. **Elimination:** half-life: 2–3 h; eliminated by kidneys.

CONTRAINDICATIONS & PRECAUTIONS Contraindicated in: hypersensitivity to pirbuterol or any other adrenergic agent such as epinephrine, albuterol, or isoproterenol; lactation, pregnancy (category C), children <12 y. **Cautious use in:** heart disease, irregular heartbeat, high blood pressure, history of stroke or seizure, diabetes, Parkinson's disease, thyroid disease, prostate disease, or glaucoma.

ADVERSE/SIDE EFFECTS CNS: nervousness, headache, dizziness, tremor. **CV:** palpitations, tachycardia. **GI:** dry mouth, nausea, glossitis, abdominal pain, cramps, anorexia, diarrhea, stomatitis. **Other:** cough, tolerance.

DRUG INTERACTIONS **Epinephrine** and other SYMPATHOMIMETIC BRONCHODILATORS may have additive effects. BETA BLOCKERS may antagonize the effects.

NURSING IMPLICATIONS

Administration

- Shake inhaler canister well immediately before using.
- Direct patient to exhale deeply and loosely close lips around mouthpiece, then inhale slowly and deeply through mouthpiece while pressing top of canister.
- Store at room temperature.

Assessment & Drug Effects

- Periodically monitor arterial blood gases and pulmonary functions.
- Monitor vital signs. Report tachycardia, palpitations, and hypertension or hypotension.

Patient & Family Education

- Instruct on proper technique for using the inhaler.
- Advise to report palpitations, chest pain, nervousness, tremors, or other bothersome side effects promptly.
- Advise to contact physician immediately if symptoms of asthma worsen or if he or she does not respond to the usual dose.
- Instruct to adhere rigidly to dosing directions and to contact physician if breathing difficulty persists.

PIROXICAM

(peer-ox'i-kam)

Trade name: Feldene

Classifications: CNS AGENT; ANTIPYRETIC; ANALGESIC; NSAID

Prototype: Ibuprofen

Pregnancy category: C

ACTIONS/PHARMACODYNAMICS Exact mechanism of action not clear. Strongly inhibits enzyme cyclooxygenase, biogenic catalyst of prostaglandin synthesis. Drug-induced reduction in prostaglandin levels is associated with decreased inflammatory processes in bone-joint disease and with possible interference with platelet aggregation.

USES Acute and long-term relief of mild to moderate pain and for symptomatic treatment of osteoarthritis and rheumatoid arthritis. **Unlabeled use:** acute and chronic relief of mild to moderate pain.

ROUTE & DOSAGE

Arthritis, Pain

Adult: **PO** 10–20 mg 1–2 times/d.

PHARMACOKINETICS **Absorption:** well absorbed from GI tract. **Onset:** 1 h analgesia; 7 d for rheumatoid arthritis. **Peak:** 3–5 h analgesia; 2–4 wk antirheumatic. **Duration:** 48–72 h analgesia. **Distribution:** small amount distributed into breast milk. **Metabolism:** extensively metabolized in liver. **Elimination:** half-life: 30–86 h; excreted primarily in urine, some in bile (<5%).

CONTRAINDICATIONS & PRECAUTIONS **Contraindicated in:** hemophilia; syndrome (bronchospasm, nasal polyps, angioedema) precipitated by aspirin or other NSAID; active peptic ulcer, GI bleeding. Safe use in children, during pregnancy (category C), and in nursing mothers not established. **Cautious use in:** history of upper GI disease including ulcerative colitis; renal dysfunction; compromised cardiac function; hypertension or other conditions predisposing to fluid retention; coagulation disorders.

P

ADVERSE/SIDE EFFECTS CNS: somnolence, dizziness, vertigo, depression, insomnia, nervousness. **CV/respiratory:** peripheral edema, hypertension, worsening of CHF, exacerbation of angina. **ENT:** tinnitus, hearing loss. **Eye:** blurred vision, reduced visual acuity, changes in color vision, scotomas, corneal deposits, retinal disturbances. **GI:** *nausea, vomiting, dyspepsia,* GI bleeding, diarrhea, constipation, flatulence, dry mouth, peptic ulceration, anorexia, jaundice, hepatitis. **Hematologic:** anemia, decreases in Hgb, Hct; leukopenia, eosinophilia, aplastic anemia; thrombocytopenia, *prolonged bleeding time.* **Skin:** urticaria, erythema multiforme, maculopapular, vesiculobullous rash; photosensitivity, sweating, Stevens-Johnson syndrome, bruising, dermatitis. **Other:** bronchospasm, allergic rhinitis, angioedema, fever, hypoglycemia, hyperglycemia, hyperkalemia, weight gain; dysuria, dyspnea, palpitations, syncope, muscle cramps, fever, hypersensitivity reactions, acute renal failure, papillary necrosis, hematuria, proteinuria, nephrotic syndrome.

P

DRUG INTERACTIONS ORAL ANTICOAGULANTS, **heparin** may prolong bleeding time; may increase **lithium** toxicity; **alcohol, aspirin** increase risk of GI hemorrhage.

NURSING IMPLICATIONS

Administration

- Patient should take drug at the same time every day.
- Administration of capsule with food or fluid may help to reduce GI irritation.
- Concomitant administration of an antacid to reduce gastric distress does not interfere with piroxicam absorption or action.
- Dose adjustments, usually made on basis of clinical response, are made at intervals of weeks rather than days in order to prevent overdosage.
- Store in tightly closed container at 15–30C (59–86F) unless otherwise directed.

Assessment & Drug Effects

- Evaluation of antirheumatic effect cannot be made for at least 7 d.
- Clinical evidence of benefits from drug therapy: pain relief in motion and in rest, reduction in night pain, stiffness, and swelling; increased ROM (range of motion) in all joints.
- Appearance of adverse/side effects may be delayed for 7–10 d after start of therapy (except for an allergic reaction).
- Periodic laboratory test levels (BUN, ALT, AST) as well as cell counts, Hgb, and Hct should be evaluated in patient (especially the elderly) receiving piroxicam for an extended period.

Patient & Family Education

- If patient misses a dose, advise taking the drug when omission is discovered if it is 6–8 h before the next scheduled dose. Otherwise, omit the dose and reestablish regimen at next scheduled hour.
- Advise against self-dosing with aspirin or other OTC drug without physician's advice.
- Warn not to increase dosage beyond prescribed regimen. Patient should understand that long half-life of drug may cause delayed therapeutic effect. Higher than recommended doses are associated with increased incidence of GI irritation and peptic ulcer.
- Incidence of GI bleeding with this drug is relatively high. Instruct to promptly report symptoms of melena, hematemesis, or severe gastric pain.
- Be alert to symptoms of drug-induced anemia: profound fatigue,

skin and mucous membrane pallor, lethargy.

- Since alcohol may increase the risk of GI bleeding, its use should be avoided or at least modified.
- If piroxicam is used concomitantly with an anticoagulant, advise to be alert to signs of hypoprothrombinemia during and for several days after therapy has been discontinued: ecchymoses, petechiae, unexplained bleeding, epistaxis, hematuria.
- Since side effects (i.e., blurred vision, vertigo, dizziness) may impair ability to perform activities requiring mental alertness, caution to avoid driving a car or engaging in hazardous activities until response to drug is known.
- Because most of drug is excreted by kidneys, impaired renal function increases danger of toxicity. Patient should drink at least 6–8 full glasses of water daily and report signs of renal insufficiency (see Appendix G).

PLASMA PROTEIN FRACTION

Trade names: Plasmanate, Plasma-Plex; Plasmatein, PPF, Protenate

Classifications: BLOOD DERIVATIVE; PLASMA VOLUME EXPANDER

Prototype: Normal serum albumin, human

Pregnancy category: C

ACTIONS/PHARMACODYNAMICS

Five percent solution of stabilized human plasma proteins in NaCl. Oncotic action approximately equivalent to that of human plasma; does not provide coagulation factors or gamma globulins. Heat-treated to minimize hazard of transmitting serum hepatitis; risk of sensitization is reduced since it lacks cellular elements. Does not require cross matching.

USES Emergency treatment of hypovolemic shock due to burns, trauma, surgery, infections; temporary measure in treatment of blood loss when whole blood is not available; to replenish plasma protein in patients with hypoproteinemia (if sodium restriction is not a problem).

ROUTE & DOSAGE

Plasma Volume Expansion

Adult: **IV** 250–500 ml at a max rate of 10 ml/min.
Child: **IV** 6.6–33 ml/kg at a rate of 5–10 ml/min.

Hypoproteinemia

Adult: **IV** 1–1.5 L/d infused at a rate not to exceed 5–8 ml/min.

CONTRAINDICATIONS & PRECAUTIONS **Contraindicated in:** severe anemia, cardiac failure; patients undergoing cardiopulmonary bypass surgery. Pregnancy (category C). **Cautious use in:** patients with low cardiac reserve; absence of albumin deficiency; hepatic or renal failure.

ADVERSE/SIDE EFFECTS Low incidence: nausea, vomiting, hypersalivation, headache. **Hypersensitivity:** tingling, chills, fever, cyanosis, chest tightness, backache, urticaria, erythema, shock (systemic anaphylaxis). **With rapid IV infusion:** circulatory overload, pulmonary edema.

NURSING IMPLICATIONS

Administration

- Check expiration date on label. Solutions that show a sediment or appear turbid should not be used. Do not use solutions that have been frozen.

- Once container is opened, solution should be used within 4 h because it contains no preservatives. Discard unused portions.
- Rate of infusion and volume of total dose will depend on patient's age, diagnosis, degree of venous and pulmonary congestion, Hct, and Hgb determinations. Specific flow rate should be prescribed by physician.
- As with any oncotically active solution, infusion rate should be relatively slow. Range may vary from 1–10 ml/min.
- Plasma protein fraction is reportedly incompatible with solutions containing alcohol or norepinephrine (levarterenol bitartrate).
- Storage temperature varies with manufacturer. See package insert.

Assessment & Drug Effects

- Monitor BP and pulse. Frequency of readings will depend on patient's condition. Flow rate adjustments are made according to clinical response and BP. Slow or stop infusion if patient suddenly becomes hypotensive.
- A widening pulse pressure (difference between systolic and diastolic) correlates with increase in cardiac output and should be reported.
- Report changes in I&O ratio and pattern.
- Observe patient closely during and after infusion for signs of hypervolemia or circulatory overload (see Appendix G). Report these symptoms immediately to physician.
- Make careful observations of patient who has had either injury or surgery in order to detect bleeding points that failed to bleed at lower BP.

P

PLICAMYCIN

(plik-a-mi′cin)

Trade names: Mithracin, Mithramycin

Classifications: ANTINEOPLASTIC; ANTIBIOTIC

Prototype: Doxorubicin

Pregnancy category: C

ACTIONS/PHARMACODYNAMICS

Cytotoxic antibiotic produced by *Streptomyces plicatus,* with minimal immunosuppressive activity. Complexes with DNA, thus inhibiting DNA-directed RNA synthesis. May lower serum calcium levels by unclear mechanism. Appears to block hypercalcemic action of vitamin D, and may inhibit parathyroid hormone effect on osteoclasts. Interferes with synthesis of various clotting factors. High toxicity with low therapeutic index limits clinical use.

USES To treat hospitalized patients with hypercalcemia or hypercalciuria associated with advanced neoplasms and to treat testicular malignancy.

ROUTE & DOSAGE

Neoplasia

Adult: **IV** 25–30 μg/kg once/d for 8–10 d or until toxicity necessitates discontinuing (max 30 μg/kg/d for 10 d).

Malignant Hypercalcemia

Adult: **IV** 25 μg/kg once/d for 3–4 d; may repeat after 1 wk.

PHARMACOKINETICS **Distribution:** crosses blood–brain barrier; appears to localize in areas of bone active resorption. **Elimination:** excreted in urine.

CONTRAINDICATIONS & PRECAUTIONS **Contraindicated in:** bleeding and coagulation disorders, myelosuppression; electrolyte imbalance (especially hypocalcemia, hypokalemia, hypophosphatemia); pregnancy (category C). **Cautious use in:** patients with prior abdominal or mediastinal radiology; liver or renal impairment.

ADVERSE/SIDE EFFECTS CNS: drowsiness, irritability, dizziness, weakness, headache, mental depression. **GI:** *stomatitis, anorexia, nausea, vomiting, diarrhea,* widespread intestinal hemorrhage. **Hematologic:** thrombocytopenia, bleeding and coagulation disorders (dose-related), leukopenia (mild). **Other:** fever, marked facial flushing, hemoptysis, nonspecific or acneiform skin rash, phlebitis, hypophosphatemia, hypokalemia, hypocalciuria, abnormal liver and renal function tests.

DRUG INTERACTIONS Concomitant administration of ***vitamin D*** may enhance hypercalcemia.

NURSING IMPLICATIONS

Administration

- When edema, ascites, or hydrothorax is present, drug dose is based on ideal body weight.
- Dilute each 25 mg with 4.9 ml of sterile water to yield 500 μg/ml. May be further diluted in either 1000 ml 5% dextrose or 0.9% NaCl injection and infused over a 4–6 h period.
- Carefully regulate IV flow rate (established by physician); GI side effects increase when rate is too fast.
- Terminate infusion immediately if extravasation occurs. Apply moderate heat to disperse the drug and to minimize tissue irritation.
- Unused portions of reconstituted solution should be discarded and new ones prepared daily.
- Refrigerate unreconstituted vials at 2–8C (36–46F).

Assessment & Drug Effects

- Therapy is usually interrupted if leukocyte count is <4000/mm^3, if platelet count is <150,000/mm^3, or if prothrombin time is > 4 seconds higher than control (normal: 12–14 seconds).
- Establish flow chart at beginning of therapy, permitting continuous record of weight and I&O ratio and pattern.
- Frequent assessments of liver and hematologic (platelet count, bleeding and prothrombin times) and renal function are performed throughout therapy and for several days after last dose.
- Thrombocytopenia, frequently evidenced by a single or persistent episode of epistaxis or hematemesis, may be rapid in onset during or after a course of treatment. Report marked facial flushing, which is often an early symptom.
- Inspect skin daily for signs of purpura. Hemoptysis may occur because of bleeding into metastasis; report this immediately.
- Rebound hypercalcemia (normal: 9–10.6 mg/dl) following plicamycin-induced hypocalcemia may persist 2–4 d. See Appendix G for signs and symptoms of hypercalcemia.
- The hypercalcemia patient may be dehydrated. Monitor I&O ratio to assure adequate fluid intake.
- Signs of antiblastic action on GI mucosal cells (hematemesis, melena) necessitate stopping drug use.
- Check patient's bowel function daily to prevent high fecal impaction due to diminished peristalsis.
- Consult physician about dietary calcium intake and coordinate di-

P

etary planning with dietitian, patient, and family.

PODOPHYLLUM RESIN

(pode-oh-fill′um)

Trade names: Condylox, Pod-Ben-25, Podo-ben, Podofin

Classifications: SKIN AGENT; KERATOLYTIC AGENT

ACTIONS/PHARMACODYNAMICS Potent cytotoxic and keratolytic agent with caustic action, derived from rhizomes and roots of *Podophyllum peltatum* (mandrake, May apple). Directly affects epithelial cell metabolism, causing degeneration and arrest of mitosis. Slow disruption of cells and tissue erosion that follows (caustic action) selectively affects embryonic and tumor cells more than adult cells.

USES Benign growths including external genital and perianal warts, papillomas, fibroids.

P

ROUTE & DOSAGE

Condylomata Acuminata

Adult: **Topical** Use 10% solution; repeat 1–2 times/wk for up to 4 applications.

Verruca Vulgaris (Common Wart)

Adult: **Topical** Use 5% solution, 1–5 applications/d.

Multiple Superficial Epitheliomatosis, Keratoses

Adult: **Topical** Apply daily for several days.

Note: Use 10–25% solution for areas <10 cm^2 or 5% solution for areas of 10–20 cm^2, anal or genital warts; apply drug to dry surface; allow area to dry between drops; wash off after 1–4 h.

CONTRAINDICATIONS & PRECAUTIONS **Contraindicated in:** birthmarks, moles, or warts with hair growth from them; cervical, urethral, oral warts; normal skin and mucous membranes peripheral to treated areas; pregnancy; diabetes mellitus; patient with poor circulation; irritated, friable, or bleeding skin; application of drug over large area.

ADVERSE/SIDE EFFECTS Severe systemic toxicity (sometimes fatal), sensorimotor neuropathy (reversible), and bone marrow suppression similar to that caused by antineoplastic drug toxicity. Specifically: **CNS:** lethargy, mental confusion, disorientation, delirium, agitation, seizures, progressive stupor, polyneuritis, pyrexia, coma, visual and auditory hallucinations, acute psychotic reaction, ataxia, hypotonia, areflexia, increased CSF protein. **CV:** sinus tachycardia. **Hematologic:** leukopenia, thrombocytopenia. **GI:** *nausea, vomiting, diarrhea, abdominal pain,* hepatotoxicity. **Peripheral neuropathy:** paralytic ileus, urinary retention, symptomatic orthostatic hypotension, paresthesias and weakness of extremities, stocking-glove sensory loss, absent ankle reflexes, decreased response to painful stimuli. **Renal:** renal failure. **Respiratory:** decreased respirations, apnea, hyperventilation. **Other:** increased serum concentrations of LDH, AST, and alkaline phosphatase.

NURSING IMPLICATIONS

Administration

- This potent drug is usually applied by an experienced clinician.
- Podophyllum resin contact with

eyes or similar mucosal surfaces should be avoided; should it occur, flush thoroughly with lukewarm water for 15 min and remove film precipitated by the water.

- Avoid application of drug to normal tissue. If it occurs, remove with alcohol. Protect surfaces surrounding area to be treated with a layer of petrolatum or flexible collodion.
- Thorough removal of drug with soap and water should follow each treatment of accessible tissue surface.
- A protective coat of talcum powder may be applied after treatment and drying of anogenital area.
- If application causes extreme pain, pruritus, or swelling, remove drug with alcohol.
- Store podophyllum resin in tight, light-resistant container; avoid exposure to excessive heat.

Assessment & Drug Effects

- Treatment for external perianal warts is usually preceded by a proctologic evaluation. Podophyllin is delayed until test results are known.
- Warts become blanched, then necrotic within 24–48 h. Sloughing begins after about 72 h with no scarring. Frequently, a mild topical antiinfective agent, with or without a dressing, is applied until the healing is complete.
- Sensorimotor polyneuropathy, if it occurs, appears about 2 wk after application of drug, worsens for 3 mo, and may persist for up to 9 mo. Cerebral effects may persist for 7–10 d; ataxia, hypotonia, and areflexia improve more slowly than effects on sensorium.

Patient & Family Education

- If self-administered as for treatment of verruca vulgaris (common wart), instruct in the proper technique of treatment. Patient should also be fully aware of the need to report treatment failure.
- As with any STD, the patient's sex partner should be examined.
- Systemic toxicity may be severe and serious and is associated with application of drug to large areas, to tissue that is friable, bleeding, or recently biopsied, or for prolonged time. It may occur within hours of application. When patient is self-medicating with podophyllum resin, stress dangers of overuse or misuse of the drug.
- Review symptoms of toxicity with patient and advise prompt reporting should they appear. (See Adverse/Side Effects.)

POLYCARBOPHIL

(pol-i-kar'boe-fil)

Trade names: FiberCon, Mitrolan

Classifications: GI AGENT; BULK LAXATIVE; ANTIDIARRHEAL

Prototype: Psyllium

Pregnancy category: C

ACTIONS/PHARMACODYNAMICS Calcium polycarbophil is hydrophilic. Absorbs free water in intestinal tract and opposes dehydrating forces of bowel by forming a gelatinous mass, thereby restoring more normal moisture level and motility in the lower GI tract. Produces well-formed stool and reduces diarrhea.

USES Constipation or diarrhea associated with acute bowel syndrome, diverticulosis, irritable bowel and in patients who should not strain during defecation. Also choleretic diarrhea, diarrhea caused by small-bowel surgery or vagotomy, and disease of terminal ileum.

ROUTE & DOSAGE

Constipation or Diarrhea
Adult: **PO** 1 g q.i.d. prn (max 6 g/d).
Child: **PO** *6–12 y,* 500 mg t.i.d. prn (max 3 g/d); *3–6 y,* 500 mg b.i.d. prn (max 1.5 g/d).

PHARMACOKINETICS Absorption: not absorbed from GI tract. **Onset:** 12–24 h. **Peak:** 1–3 d.

CONTRAINDICATIONS & PRECAUTIONS Contraindicated in: partial or complete GI obstruction; fecal impaction; dysphagia; acute abdominal pain; rectal bleeding; undiagnosed abdominal pain, or other symptoms pathognomonic of appendicitis; pregnancy (category C); poisonings; before radiologic bowel examination; bowel surgery. Safety of use in children <3 y not established.

ADVERSE/SIDE EFFECTS GI: esophageal blockage, intestinal impaction, *abdominal fullness.* **Other:** low serum potassium, elevated blood glucose levels (with extended use), asthma, skin rash.

P

DRUG INTERACTIONS May decrease absorption and clinical effects of ANTIBIOTICS, **warfarin, digoxin, nitrofurantoin,** SALICYLATES.

NURSING IMPLICATIONS

Administration
- Crush tablets before administration or have patient chew tablets well before swallowing.
- Each dose should be administered with a full glass (240 ml [8 oz]) of water or other liquid.
- In severe diarrhea, dose may be repeated every 30 min up to the maximum dose in 24 h.
- Abdominal fullness may be prevented by taking smaller doses more frequently during the day.
- Store in tightly closed container at 15–30C (59–86F) unless otherwise directed.

Assessment & Drug Effects
- If patient is being treated for diarrhea, determine duration and severity of diarrhea before medical treatment in order to anticipate signs of fluid-electrolyte losses.
- Monitor and record number and consistency of stools per day, presence and location of abdominal discomfort (i.e., tenderness, distension), and bowel sounds.
- Monitor and record I&O ratio and pattern. Dehydration is indicated if urine specific gravity is >1,030 and if output is <30 ml/h.
- Daily weights provide a rough estimate of fluid loss.
- Dehydration from an episode of diarrhea appears rapidly in young children and the elderly. Inspect oral cavity for dryness, and be alert to systemic signs (e.g., thirst and fever).

Patient & Family Education
- If sudden changes in bowel habit persist more than 1 wk, action is minimal or ineffective for 1 wk, or if there is no antidiarrheal action within 2 d, consult physician.
- Extended use may cause dependence on the drug for normal bowel function.
- Diet and exercise as well as medication are important in a plan designed to restore a more normal bowel habit.
- If patient is also taking an oral anticoagulant, digoxin, salicylates, or nitrofurantoin, warn against discontinuing polycarbophil unless physician advises patient to do so. Established serum concentrations (and drug effects) may be altered

by physical binding of any of these drugs to polycarbophil.

- Inform that this OTC medication is packaged with manufacturer's directions for use and review them if necessary.

POLYESTRADIOL PHOSPHATE

(pol-ee-ess-tra-dye'ole)

Trade name: Estradurin

Classifications: ANTINEOPLASTIC; ESTROGEN HORMONE

Prototype: Estradiol

Pregnancy category: X

ACTIONS/PHARMACODYNAMICS Estrogen derivative. Provides a continuous active level of exogenous estradiol that functions to alter the hormonal milieu of a tumor originating from hormone-responsive tissue. Suppresses pituitary secretion of luteinizing or interstitial cell stimulating hormone (LH), an action that in turn depresses ("turns off") androgen secretion by the testes (antitumor effect). Tumor growth is interrupted, but existing neoplastic cells are not killed.

USE Palliative treatment of an inoperable, progressing prostatic carcinoma.

ROUTE & DOSAGE

Prostatic Carcinoma
Adult: **IM** 40 mg q2–4wk or less frequently depending on response; may increase dose up to 80 mg.

PHARMACOKINETICS Absorption: readily absorbed from IM site; leaves bloodstream within 24 h. **Distribution:** stored in reticuloendothelial system. **Metabolism:** metabolized in liver. **Elimination:** excreted in bile and urine.

CONTRAINDICATIONS & PRECAUTIONS Contraindicated in: pregnancy (category X); men with known or suspected cancer of the breast except in appropriately selected patients being treated for metastatic disease; known or suspected estrogen-dependent neoplasm; active thromboembolic disorders. **Cautious use in:** hypertension; gallbladder disease; diabetes mellitus; heart failure; hepatic or renal dysfunction.

ADVERSE/SIDE EFFECTS CNS: headache, dizziness, depression, libido changes. **CV:** thromboembolic disorders, *hypertension*. **GI:** *nausea,* vomiting, diarrhea, anorexia, weight changes, bloating, cholestatic jaundice. **GU:** mastodynia gynecomastia, impotence, testicular atrophy. **Metabolic:** reduced carbohydrate tolerance, hypercalcemia, *fluid retention*. **Other:** leg cramps.

NURSING IMPLICATIONS

Administration

- Reconstitution of IM solution: Introduce sterile diluent into vial of drug powder using a 20-gauge needle and 5-ml syringe. Swirl gently to produce clear solution; do not shake vigorously. Discard cloudy solution.
- Administer drug deeply into large muscle mass (e.g., gluteus maximus). A transitory burning sensation may occur, but this usually does not continue with subsequent doses. If it continues, thereafter the dose may be given with a local anesthetic. Consult physician.
- Increasing the dosage prolongs action but does not increase blood level.
- Store lyophilized powder and reconstituted solution at 15–30C (59–86F) away from direct light.

Stability remains about 10 d, as long as solution is clear.

Patient & Family Education

- Clinical response should be apparent within 3 mo. Hormone is usually continued until disease is again progressive, then stopped.
- Teach how to elicit Homans' sign: pain in calf and popliteal region with forced dorsiflexion of foot (early sign of thrombosis).
- Instruct to report a positive Homans' sign and the following symptoms of thromboembolic disorders immediately: tenderness, swelling, and redness in extremity; sudden, severe headache or chest pain, slurring of speech; change in vision; tenderness, pain, sudden shortness of breath. If physician is not available, patient should go to the nearest hospital emergency room.

POLYMYXIN B SULFATE

(pol-i-mix'in)

Trade name: Aerosporin

Classifications: ANTIINFECTIVE; ANTIBIOTIC

Pregnancy category: B

ACTIONS/PHARMACODYNAMICS Polymyxin antibiotic derived from strains of *Bacillus polymyxa*. Binds to lipid phosphates in bacterial membranes and, through cationic detergent action, changes permeability to permit leakage of cytoplasm. Bactericidal against susceptible gram negative organisms, particularly most strains of *Escherichia coli, Hemophilus influenzae, Enterobacter aerogenes,* and *Klebsiella pneumoniae*. Most species of *Proteus* and *Neisseria* are resistant, as are all gram-positive organisms and fungi.

USES Topically and in combination with other antiinfectives or corticosteroids for various superficial infections of eye, ear, mucous membrane, and skin. Concurrent systemic antiinfective therapy may be required for treatment of intraocular infection and severe progressive corneal ulcer. Used parenterally only in hospitalized patients for treatment of severe acute infections of urinary tract, bloodstream, and meninges; and in combination with neosporin for continuous bladder irrigation to prevent bacteremia associated with use of indwelling catheter.

ROUTE & DOSAGE

Infections

Adult: **IV** 15,000–25,000 U/kg/d divided q12h. **IM** 25,000–30,000 U/kg/d divided q4–6h. **GU** 1 ml/L 0.9% NaCl q24h. **Topical** 1–2 drops in eye q1h.

Child: **IV** 15,000–25,000 U/kg/d divided q12h. **IM** 25,000–30,000 U/kg/d divided q4–6h.

PHARMACOKINETICS **Absorption:** not absorbed from GI tract. **Peak:** 2 h IM. **Distribution:** widely distributed except to CSF, synovial fluid, and eye; does not cross placenta. **Metabolism:** unknown. **Elimination:** half-life: 4.3–6 h; 60% excreted unchanged in urine.

CONTRAINDICATIONS & PRECAUTIONS **Contraindicated in:** hypersensitivity to polymyxin antibiotics; concurrent and sequential use of other nephrotoxic and neurotoxic drugs; concurrent use of skeletal muscle relaxants, ether, or sodium citrate. Safe use during pregnancy (category B) not established. **Cau-**

tious use in: impaired renal function; myasthenia gravis.

ADVERSE/SIDE EFFECTS CNS: irritability, facial flushing, drowsiness, dizziness, vertigo, ataxia, circumoral, lingual, and peripheral paresthesias (stocking-glove distribution); blurred vision, nystagmus, slurred speech, dysphagia, ototoxicity (vestibular and auditory) with high doses; convulsions, coma; neuromuscular blockade (generalized muscle weakness, respiratory depression or arrest); meningeal irritation, increased protein and cell count in cerebrospinal fluid, fever, headache, stiff neck (intrathecal use). **Nephrotoxicity:** rising blood drug levels without increase in dosage; albuminuria, cylinduria, azotemia, hematuria. **Other:** GI disturbances, severe pain (IM site), thrombophlebitis (IV site), superinfections, electrolyte disturbances (prolonged use; also reported in patients with acute leukemia); local irritation and burning (topical use), anaphylactoid reactions (rare).

DRUG INTERACTIONS ANESTHETICS and NEUROMUSCULAR BLOCKING AGENTS may prolong skeletal muscle relaxation. AMINOGLYCOSIDES and **amphotericin B** have additive nephrotoxic potential.

INCOMPATIBILITIES Solution/additive: amphotericin B, cephalothin, chloramphenicol, chlorothiazide, heparin, magnesium sulfate, prednisolone, sodium phosphate, tetracycline.

NURSING IMPLICATIONS

Administration

- Routine administration by IM route not recommended because it causes intense discomfort, along the peripheral nerve distribution, 40–60 min after IM injection.
- In adults, IM injection should be made deep into upper outer quadrant of buttock. Select IM site carefully to avoid injection into nerves or blood vessels. Rotate injection sites. Follow agency policy for IM site used in children.
- To reconstitute for IV administration, dissolve 500,000 U in 5 ml sterile water for injection or NS to yield 100,000 U/ml. Withdraw a single dose and then further dilute the dose in 300–500 ml of D5W. Infuse over period of 60–90 min. Inspect injection site for signs of phlebitis and irritation.
- Protect unreconstituted product and reconstituted solution from light and freezing. Store in refrigerator at 2–8C (36–46F). Parenteral solutions are stable for 1 wk when refrigerated. Discard unused portion after 72 h.

Assessment & Drug Effects

- Culture and susceptibility tests should be done prior to first dose and periodically thereafter to determine continuing sensitivity of causative organisms.
- Baseline serum electrolytes and renal function tests should be performed before parenteral therapy. Frequent monitoring of renal function and serum drug levels is advised during therapy.
- Electrolytes should be monitored at regular intervals during prolonged therapy. Patients with low serum calcium and low intracellular potassium are particularly prone to develop neuromuscular blockade.
- Dosage is reduced (as indicated by creatinine clearance) in the patient with renal impairment.
- Inspect tongue every day. Assess for signs and symptoms of superinfection (see Appendix G). Polymyxin therapy supports the

P

growth of opportunistic organisms. Report symptoms promptly.

- Some degree of renal toxicity usually occurs within first 3 or 4 d of therapy even with therapeutic doses. Monitor I&O. Fluid intake should be sufficient to maintain daily urinary output of at least 1500 ml. Consult physician.
- Decreases in urine output (change in I&O ratio), proteinuria, cellular casts, rising BUN, serum creatinine, or serum drug levels (not associated with dosage increase) can be interpreted as signs of nephrotoxicity. If any of these signs occur, withhold drug and report findings to physician.
- Nephrotoxicity is generally reversible, but it may progress even after drug is discontinued. Therefore, close monitoring of kidney function is essential, even following termination of therapy.
- Respiratory arrest has occurred with first dose and also as long as 45 d after initiation of therapy. It occurs most commonly in patients with renal failure and high plasma drug levels and is often preceded by dyspnea and restlessness.

P

Patient & Family Education

- Encourage to report immediately muscle weakness, shortness of breath, dyspnea, depressed respiration. These symptoms are rapidly reversible if drug is withdrawn immediately.
- Eyelid irritation, itching, and burning with ophthalmic drops should be reported promptly to the physician. Stop drug administration immediately.
- Transient neurologic disturbances (paresthesias, numbness, dizziness) occur commonly and usually respond to dosage reduction. Report promptly.
- Warn to report promptly onset of stiff neck and headache (possible symptoms of neurotoxic reactions, including neuromuscular blockade). This response is usually associated with high serum drug levels and/or nephrotoxicity.
- Instruct to promptly report signs and symptoms of superinfection (see Appendix G).

POLYTHIAZIDE

(pol-i-thye'a-zide)

Trade name: Renese

Classifications: ELECTROLYTIC AND WATER BALANCE AGENT; THIAZIDE DIURETIC

Prototype: Hydrochlorothiazide

Pregnancy category: D

ACTIONS/PHARMACODYNAMICS

Benzothiadiazine (thiazide) derivative. Similar to hydrochlorothiazide in actions, uses, contraindications, adverse reactions, and interactions.

USES Primary agent in stepped-care approach to antihypertensive treatment and adjunctively in the management of edema associated with CHF, renal pathology, and hepatic cirrhosis. Available in fixed combination with prazosin (Minizide) and with reserpine (Renese-R).

ROUTE & DOSAGE

Edema

Adult: **PO** 1–4 mg/d *or* q.o.d.

Hypertension

Adult: **PO** 2–4 mg/d.
Child: **PO** 0.02–0.08 mg/kg/d.

PHARMACOKINETICS **Onset:** 2 h. **Peak:** 6 h. **Duration:** 24–48 h. **Distribution:** distributed throughout extracellular tissue; concentrates in kidney; crosses placenta; distributed into breast milk. **Metabolism:** does not appear to be metabolized. **Elimination:** excreted in urine.

CONTRAINDICATIONS & PRECAUTIONS **Contraindicated in:** hypersensitivity to other thiazides or sulfonamides; anuria, pregnancy (category D), nursing mothers. **Cautious use in:** renal and hepatic dysfunction, SLE, gout, diabetes mellitus.

ADVERSE/SIDE EFFECTS Agranulocytosis, vascular thrombosis, *hyperuricemia, hypokalemia, hyperglycemia,* orthostatic hypotension, hepatic encephalopathy, photosensitivity.

DRUG INTERACTIONS **Amphotericin B,** CORTICOSTEROIDS increase hypokalemic effects; may antagonize hypoglycemic effects of **insulin,** SULFONYLUREAS; **cholestyramine, colistipol** decrease thiazide absorption; intensifies hypoglycemic and hypotensive effects of **diazoxide.** Increased potassium and magnesium loss may cause **digoxin** toxicity; decreases **lithium** excretion, increasing its toxicity; NSAIDS may attenuate diuresis and increase risk of NSAID-induced renal failure.

NURSING IMPLICATIONS

Administration

- Administer drug early in AM after eating (to reduce gastric irritation) and to prevent interrupted sleep because of diuresis.
- Store drug in tightly closed container at 15–30C (59–86F) unless otherwise instructed.

Assessment & Drug Effects

- Elderly patients may be more sensitive to the average adult therapeutic dose. Excessive diuresis may induce sudden hypotension and serious electrolyte imbalance.
- Antihypertensive effects may be noted in 3–4 d; maximal effects may require 3–4 wk. Effects persist for at least 1 wk after drug is discontinued.
- Monitor for signs and symptoms of hypokalemia and hyperglycemia (see Appendix G).
- Monitor serum electrolytes and blood glucose periodically.

Patient & Family Education

- If orthostatic hypotension is a clinical problem, instruct to change from recumbency to upright positions slowly and in stages; to avoid hot baths or showers, extended exposure to sunlight, and standing still.
- Urge to include specific sources of potassium in daily diet such as a banana (about 370 mg potassium) and at least 180 ml (6 oz) orange juice (about 330 mg potassium).
- Advise to maintain prescribed dosage regimen.
- Warn about the possibility of photosensitivity reaction and instruct him or her to notify physician if it occurs. Thiazide-related photosensitivity is considered a photoallergy (ultraviolet radiation changes drug structure and makes it allergenic for some individuals) and occurs 10–14 d after initial sun exposure. Advise use of a sunscreen lotion with a high SPF (12–15).
- Counsel to avoid OTC drugs unless approved by the physician. Many preparations contain both potassium and sodium and if misused or if patient overdoses, electrolyte side effects could be induced.

P

POTASSIUM CHLORIDE

(poe-tass′ee-um)

Trade names: Apo-K♣, K-10, Kalium Durules♣, Kaochlor, Kaochlor-20 Concentrate, Kaon-Cl, Kato, Kay Ciel, KCl 5% and 20%, K-Long ♣, Klor, Klor-10%, Klor-Con, Kloride, Klorvess, Klotrix, K-Dur, K-Lyte/Cl, K-tab, Micro-K Extentabs, Novolente K♣, Roychlor 10% and 20%♣, Rum-K, SK-Potassium Chloride, Slo-Pot♣, Slow-K

POTASSIUM GLUCONATE

Trade names: Kaon, Kaylixir, K-G Elixir, Potassium Rougier♣, Royonate♣

Classifications: ELECTROLYTIC AND WATER BALANCE AGENT; REPLACEMENT SOLUTION

Pregnancy category: A

ACTIONS/PHARMACODYNAMICS Potassium, the principal intracellular cation, is essential for maintenance of intracellular isotonicity, transmission of nerve impulses, contraction of cardiac, skeletal, and smooth muscles, maintenance of normal renal function, and for enzyme activity. Plays a prominent role in both genesis and correction of imbalances in acid–base metabolism; thus, potassium salts assume special importance as therapeutic agents but are also dangerous if improperly prescribed and administered.

USES To prevent and treat potassium deficit secondary to diuretic or corticosteroid therapy. Also indicated when potassium is depleted by severe vomiting, diarrhea; intestinal drainage, fistulas, or malabsorption; prolonged diuresis, diabetic acidosis. Effective in the treatment of hypokalemic alkalosis (chloride, not the gluconate).

ROUTE & DOSAGE

Hypokalemia

Adult: **PO** 10–100 mEq/d in divided doses. **IV** 10–40 mEq/h diluted to at least 10–20 mEq/100 ml of solution to a max of 200–400 mEq/d; monitor higher doses carefully.

Child: **PO** 1–3 mEq/kg/d in divided doses; extended release tablets not recommended in children. **IV** up to 3 mEq/kg/24 h at a rate ≤ 0.02 mEq/kg/min.

PHARMACOKINETICS **Absorption:** readily absorbed from upper GI tract. **Elimination:** 90% excreted in urine, 10% in feces.

CONTRAINDICATIONS & PRECAUTIONS **Contraindicated in:** severe renal impairment; severe hemolytic reactions; untreated Addison's disease; crush syndrome; early postoperative oliguria (except during GI drainage); adynamic ileus; acute dehydration; heat cramps, hyperkalemia, patients receiving potassium-sparing diuretics, digitalis intoxication with AV conduction disturbance. **Cautious use in:** cardiac or renal disease; systemic acidosis; slow-release potassium preparations in presence of delayed GI transit or Meckel's diverticulum; extensive tissue breakdown (such as severe burns); pregnancy (category A).

ADVERSE/SIDE EFFECTS *Nausea, vomiting,* diarrhea, abdominal distension and pain, oliguria. Hyperkalemia (serum potassium > 5.5 mEq/L): mental confusion, irritability, listlessness, paresthesias of extremities, muscle weakness and heaviness of limbs, difficulty in swallowing, flaccid paralysis, anuria, respiratory distress, hypotension, bradycardia; cardiac depression, arrhythmias, or arrest; altered sensitivity to digitalis glycosides. ***ECG changes in hyperkalemia:*** tenting (peaking) of T wave (especially in right precordial leads), lowering of

R with deepening of S waves and depression of RST; prolonged P-R interval, widened QRS complex, decreased amplitude and disappearance of P waves, prolonged Q-T interval, signs of right and left bundle block, deterioration of QRS contour and finally ventricular fibrillation and death.

DRUG INTERACTIONS POTASSIUM-SPARING DIURETICS, ANGIOTENSIN-CONVERTING ENZYME (ACE) INHIBITORS may cause hyperkalemia.

INCOMPATIBILITIES Solution/additive: amphotericin B, dobutamine (potassium phosphate only). **Y-site: diazepam, ergotamine, methylprednisolone, phenytoin, promethazine.**

NURSING IMPLICATIONS

Administration

- Some patients find it difficult to swallow the large sized KCl tablet. Administer while patient is sitting up or standing (never in recumbent position) to prevent drug-induced esophagitis.
- No potassium salt tablets should be crushed and then taken dry or chewed. Be certain patient does not suck tablet (oral ulcerations have been reported if tablet is allowed to dissolve in mouth). Whole tablet should be swallowed with large glass of water or fruit juice (if allowed) to wash drug down and to start esophageal peristalsis.
- Follow instructions regarding dilution. In general, each 20 mEq potassium (chloride, gluconate) should be diluted in at least 90 ml water or juice. Liquids, powders, and effervescent tablets must be completely dissolved in a large glass of water or fruit juice before administration. Allow "fizzing" to stop before giving to patient to sip slowly with meal or immediately after eating over 5–10 min. Dilution minimizes saline cathartic effect, gastric distress, and unpleasant taste.
- Dilute elixir as directed before giving it through nasogastric tube.
- An antacid may improve the tolerance of KCl by decreasing its irritating effect on GI mucosa; 10 ml KCl flavored syrup mixed with 15 ml antacid has given relief. Consult physician.
- If potassium supplement is given in conjunction with a diuretic, it may be preferable to give the potassium on days other than when diuretic is given.
- Color in some commercial oral solutions fades with exposure to light, but drug effectiveness is reportedly not altered.

IV Administration

- For IV infusion, add desired amount to 100–1000 ml IV solution (compatible with all standard solutions). Usual maximum is 40 mEq/1000 ml. When IV concentration is 40 mEq/L or more, there is danger of irritation to veins.
- KCl is never administered by IV "push" or in concentrated amounts by any route. Add the drug to infusion fluid with plastic bag in upright (noninfusion) position to prevent delivery of excessive amount of KCl in first few minutes of the treatment.
- Infuse IV KCl at rate not to exceed 20 mEq/h.
- Potassium infusion should be administered slowly to prevent fatal hyperkalemia. Flow rate will be prescribed according to serial ECG and serum electrolyte determinations.
- Extreme care should be taken to prevent extravasation and infiltration. At first sign, discontinue infusion and immediately remove needle or catheter.

P

- Unless manufacturer advises otherwise, store all preparations of KCl at 15–30C (59–86F). Protect from light, and do not freeze.

Assessment & Drug Effects

- Monitor I&O ratio and pattern in patients receiving the parenteral drug. If oliguria occurs, stop infusion promptly and notify physician.
- Use of extended-release tablets reduces the danger of bowel ulcerations and potential compliance problems. However, esophageal and gastric ulceration in cardiac patients with esophageal compression from left atrial enlargement have been reported with use of this formulation. Report signs (esophageal or epigastric pain or hematemesis). A liquid preparation in such a patient could be more tolerable.
- Irregular heartbeat is usually the earliest clinical indication of hyperkalemia. Care of patient receiving parenteral potassium demands close surveillance of the cardiac monitor.
- The risk of hyperkalemia with potassium supplement increases (1) in the elderly because of decremental changes in kidney function associated with aging, (2) when dietary intake of potassium suddenly increases, and (3) when renal function is significantly compromised.
- Potassium intoxication (hyperkalemia, see Signs & Symptoms, Appendix G) may result from any therapeutic dosage, and the patient may be asymptomatic. Monitoring of potassium is of extreme importance.

Patient & Family Education

- The extended-release tablet (e.g., Slow-K) utilizes a wax matrix as carrier for KCl crystals. After absorption of drug, the tablet carcass appears in the stool. Inform the patient that this is no cause for alarm.
- When potassium supplement is prescribed, compliance may be a problem because of unpalatability, gastric distress following ingestion of drug, or mental confusion (associated with hypokalemia). Teach patient and family importance of this drug and adherence to established dose regimen.
- Before discharge from medical supervision, help patient to design an acceptable, feasible dosing schedule for KCl and other drugs being taken concomitantly (e.g., digitalis, diuretics).
- Inform about sources of potassium with special reference to foods and OTC drugs.
- Avoid licorice; large amounts can cause both hypokalemia and sodium retention.
- Salt substitutes contain a substantial amount of potassium and electrolytes other than sodium. Instruct patient not to use any substitute unless it is specifically ordered by the physician.
- Caution not to self-prescribe laxatives. Chronic laxative use has been associated with diarrhea-induced potassium loss.
- Large losses of potassium can also occur because of persistent vomiting. If this occurs, notify physician.
- Urge patient on long-term replacement therapy to report continuing signs of potassium deficit: weakness, fatigue, polyuria, polydipsia.
- Counsel to assume responsibility for informing dentist or new physician that a potassium drug has been prescribed as maintenance therapy.
- Foil-wrapped powders and tab-

lets should not be opened before use.

POTASSIUM IODIDE

Trade names: Pima, SSKI, Thyro-Block ♣

Classifications: EXPECTORANT; ANTITHYROID AGENT

Prototype: Guaifenesin

Pregnancy category: D

ACTIONS/PHARMACODYNAMICS Pharmacologic use primarily related to iodide portion of molecule. Exact mechanism not clear but it is believed that by direct action on bronchial tissue, potassium iodide (KI) increases secretion of respiratory fluids, thereby decreasing mucus viscosity. If patient is euthyroid, excess iodide causes minimal change in thyroid gland mass. Conversely, when thyroid is hyperplastic, excess iodide temporarily inhibits secretion of thyroid hormone, fosters colloid accumulation in thyroid follicles, and decreases vascularity of gland. "Escape" from temporary effects (i.e., return of thyrotoxic symptoms) may occur after 10–14 d continuous treatment; consequently iodide administration for hyperthyroidism is limited to short-term therapy.

USES To facilitate bronchial drainage and cough in emphysema, asthma, chronic bronchitis, bronchiectasis, and respiratory tract allergies characterized by difficult-to-raise sputum. Also used alone for hyperthyroidism or in conjunction with antithyroid drugs and propranolol in treatment of thyrotoxic crisis; in immediate preoperative period for thyroidectomy to decrease vascularity, fragility, and size of thyroid gland and for treatment of persistent or recurring hyperthyroidism that occurs in Graves' disease patients. Used as a radiation protectant in patients receiving radioactive iodine and to shield the thyroid from radiation in the wake of a serious nuclear plant accident. (Use as an expectorant has been largely replaced by other agents.)

ROUTE & DOSAGE

To Reduce Thyroid Vascularity

Adult: **PO** 50–250 mg t.i.d. for 10–14 d before surgery.
Child: **PO** Same as for adult.

Expectorant

Adult: **PO** 300–650 mg p.c. b.i.d. or t.i.d.
Child: **PO** 60–250 mg p.c. b.i.d. or t.i.d.

Thyroid Blocking in Radiation Emergency

Adult: **PO** 130 mg/d for 10 d.
Child: **PO** *>1 y,* 130 mg/d for 10 d; *<1 y,* 65 mg/d for 10 d.

Adjunct to Management of Thyroid Crisis

Adult: **IV** 500 mg q4h.

PHARMACOKINETICS Absorption: adequately absorbed from GI tract. **Distribution:** crosses placenta. **Elimination:** cleared from plasma by renal excretion or thyroid uptake.

CONTRAINDICATIONS & PRECAUTIONS Contraindicated in: hypersensitivity or idiosyncrasy to iodine; hyperthyroidism; hyperkalemia; acute bronchitis. Safe use during pregnancy (category D) and in nursing mothers and children <1 y not established. **Cautious use in:** renal impairment; cardiac disease; pulmonary tuberculosis; Addison's disease.

P

ADVERSE/SIDE EFFECTS **GI:** diarrhea, nausea, vomiting, stomach pain, nonspecific small bowel lesions (associated with enteric coated tablets). **Hypersensitivity:** angioneurotic edema, cutaneous and mucosal hemorrhage, fever, arthralgias, lymph node enlargement, eosinophilia. **Iodine poisoning (iodism):** metallic taste, stomatitis, salivation, coryza, sneezing; swollen and tender salivary glands (sialadenitis), frontal headache, vomiting (blue vomitus if stomach contained starches, otherwise yellow vomitus), bloody diarrhea. **Metabolic:** hyperthyroid adenoma, goiter, hypothyroidism, collagen disease–like syndromes. **Other:** irregular heartbeat, mental confusion, acneifom skin lesions (prolonged use), weakness, paresthesias, productive cough, pulmonary edema, periorbital edema, flare-up of adolescent acne.

DIAGNOSTIC TEST INTERFERENCE Potassium iodide may alter ***thyroid function*** test results and may interfere with *urinary 17-OHCS* determinations.

DRUG INTERACTIONS ANTITHYROID DRUGS, **lithium** may potentiate hypothyroid and goitrogenic actions; POTASSIUM-SPARING DIURETICS, POTASSIUM SUPPLEMENTS, ACE INHIBITORS increase risk of hyperkalemia.

NURSING IMPLICATIONS

Administration

- To disguise salty taste and to minimize gastric distress, drug is taken with meals in a full glass (240 ml) of water or fruit juice and at bedtime with food or juice.
- Avoid giving KI with milk; absorption of the drug may be decreased by dairy products.
- When iodide is administered to prepare thyroid gland for surgery, strict adherence to schedule and accurate dose measurements are essential, particularly at end of treatment period when possibility of "escape" (from iodide) effect on thyroid gland increases.
- If crystals form in the solution, they may be dissolved by placing container in warm water and gently agitating it.
- Solutions may turn brownish yellow on standing, especially if exposed to light, because of liberated trace of free iodine. Discard such solutions.
- Store in airtight, light-resistant container at 15–30C (59–86F) unless otherwise directed.

Assessment & Drug Effects

- Serum potassium levels should be determined before and periodically during therapy. (Normal serum potassium: 3.6–5.5 mEq/L.)
- Keep physician informed about characteristics of sputum: quantity, consistency, color.

Patient & Family Education

- Advise to report promptly the occurrence of GI bleeding, abdominal pain, distension, nausea, or vomiting.
- Instruct to report clinical signs of iodism (see Adverse/Side Effects). Usually, symptoms will subside with dose reduction and lengthened intervals between doses.
- Foods rich in iodine to be avoided if patient develops iodism are vegetables growing near seacoast, seafoods, fish liver oils, and iodized salt.
- Sudden withdrawal following prolonged use may precipitate thyroid storm.
- Warn to avoid use of OTC drugs without consulting physician. Many preparations contain iodides and could augment prescribed dose, e.g., cough syrups, gargles,

asthma medication, salt substitutes, cod liver oil, multiple vitamins (often suspended in iodide solutions).

- Impress on the patient taking KI as an expectorant that optimum hydration is the best expectorant. Encourage increased daily fluid intake.

PRALIDOXIME CHLORIDE

(pra-li-dox′eem)

Trade names: PAM, Protopam Chloride

Classification: ANTIDOTE

Pregnancy category: C

ACTIONS/PHARMACODYNAMICS Reactivates cholinesterase inhibited by phosphate esters by displacing the enzyme from its receptor sites; the free enzyme then can resume its function of degrading accumulated acetylcholine, thereby restoring normal neuromuscular transmission. Less effective against carbamate anticholinesterases (ambenonium, neostigmine, pyridostigmine). More active against effects of anticholinesterases at skeletal neuromuscular junction than at autonomic effector sites or in CNS respiratory center; therefore, atropine must be given concomitantly to block effects of acetylcholine and accumulation in these sites.

USES As antidote in treatment of poisoning by organophosphate insecticides and pesticides with anticholinesterase activity (e.g., parathion, TEPP, sarin) and to control overdosage by anticholinesterase drugs used in treatment of myasthenia gravis (cholinergic crisis). **Unlabeled use:** to reverse toxicity of echothiophate ophthalmic solution.

ROUTE & DOSAGE

Organophosphate Poisoning

Adult: **IV** 1–2 g in 100 ml NS infused over 15–30 min; or 1–2 g as 5% solution in sterile water over not less than 5 min; may repeat after 1 h if muscle weakness not relieved.
IM/SC 1–2 g if IV route is not feasible.
Child: **IV** 20–40 mg/kg as for adult.

Anticholinesterase Overdose in Myasthenia Gravis

Adult: **IV** 1–2 g in 100 ml NS infused over 15–30 min, followed by increments of 250 mg q5min prn.

PHARMACOKINETICS **Peak:** 5–15 min IV; 10–20 min IM. **Distribution:** distributed throughout extracellular fluids; crosses blood–brain barrier slowly if at all. **Metabolism:** probably metabolized in liver. **Elimination:** half-life: 0.8–2.7 h; rapidly excreted in urine.

CONTRAINDICATIONS & PRECAUTIONS **Contraindicated in:** use in poisoning by carbamate insecticide Sevin, inorganic phosphates, or organophosphates having no anticholinesterase activity; asthma, peptic ulcer, severe cardiac disease, patients receiving aminophylline, theophylline, morphine, succinylcholine, reserpine, or phenothiazines. Safe use during pregnancy (category C) not established. **Cautious use in:** myasthenia gravis; renal insufficiency; concomitant use of barbiturates in organophosphorous poisoning.

ADVERSE/SIDE EFFECTS **Most commonly following IV use (usually mild and transient):** dizziness, nausea, blurred vision, diplopia, impaired accommodation, tachycardia, hypertension (dose-related), hyperventilation, headache, drowsiness, muscular weakness. **With rapid IV:** tachycardia, laryngospasm, muscle rigidity.

NURSING IMPLICATIONS

Administration

- Reconstitute 1-g vial by adding 20 ml NS to produce a concentration of 50 mg/ml (a 5% solution). If pulmonary edema is present, give without further dilution slowly by direct IV over at least 5 min.
- Reconstituted solution may be further diluted in 100 ml NS and infused over 15–30 min (preferred).
- Infusion should be stopped or IV rate reduced if hypertension occurs.

Assessment & Drug Effects

- Monitor BP, vital signs, and I&O. Report oliguria or changes in I&O ratio.
- It is difficult to differentiate toxic effects of organophosphates or atropine from toxic effects of pralidoxime. Be alert for these signs and report them immediately: reduction in muscle strength, onset of muscle twitching, changes in respiratory pattern, altered level of consciousness, increases or changes in heart rate and rhythm.
- Excitement and manic behavior reportedly may occur following recovery of consciousness. Observe necessary safety precautions.
- Patient should be kept under close observation for 48–72 h, particularly when poison was ingested, because of likelihood of continued absorption of organophosphate from lower bowel.
- Pralidoxime is relatively short-acting. In patients with myasthenia gravis, overdosage with pralidoxime may convert cholinergic crisis into myasthenic crisis.

P

PRAMIPEXOLE DIHYDROCHLORIDE

(pra-mi-pex′ole)

Trade names: Mirapex

Classifications: AUTONOMIC NERVOUS SYSTEM AGENT; ANTICHOLINERGIC (PARASYMPATHOMIMETIC); ANTIPARKINSON AGENT

Prototype: Dopamine

Pregnancy category: C

ACTIONS/PHARMACODYNAMICS

Pramipexole is a nonergot dopamine receptor agonist structurally similar to ropinirole for treatment of Parkinson's disease. It has high affinity for the D_2 subfamily of dopamine receptors in the brain and higher binding affinity to D_3 than to D_2 or D_4 receptor subtypes. The precise mechanism of action and treatment for Parkinson's disease is not known.

USE Treatment of idiopathic Parkinson's disease.

ROUTE & DOSAGE

Parkinson's Disease

Adult: **PO** Start with 0.125 mg t.i.d. × 1 wk, then 0.25 mg t.i.d. × 1 wk, continue to increase by 0.25 mg/dose t.i.d. qwk to a target dose of 1.5 mg t.i.d. *Patients with renal insufficiency:* Cl_{cr} 35–60 ml/min: same titration schedule dosed b.i.d. (max 1.5 mg b.i.d.). Cl_{cr} 15–35 ml/min: same titration schedule dosed q.d. (max 1.5 mg q.d.).

PHARMACOKINETICS **Absorption:** rapidly absorbed from GI tract >90% bioavailability. **Peak:** 2 h. **Distribution:** 15% protein bound. **Metabolism:**

minimally metabolized in the liver. **Elimination:** half-life: 8–12 h; primarily excreted in urine.

CONTRAINDICATIONS & PRECAUTIONS **Contraindicated in:** hypersensitivity to pramipexole or ropinirole; lactation. **Cautious use in:** renal and hepatic function impairment, concomitant use of CNS depressants, pregnancy (category C). Safety and efficacy in children have not been established.

ADVERSE/SIDE EFFECTS **Body as whole:** *asthenia,* general edema, malaise, fever. **CNS:** *dizziness, somnolence, insomnia, hallucinations, dyskinesia, extrapyramidal syndrome,* headache, confusion, amnesia, hypesthesia, dystonia, akathesia, myoclonus. **CV:** *postural hypotension,* chest pain. **GI:** *nausea, constipation,* anorexia, dysphagia, dry mouth. **Respiratory:** dyspnea, rhinitis. **Other:** peripheral edema, decreased weight, decreased libido, impotence, vision abnormalities, urinary frequency or incontinence.

DRUG INTERACTIONS **Cimetidine** decreases clearance; BUTYROPHENONES, **metoclopramide,** PHENOTHIAZINES may antagonize effects.

NURSING IMPLICATIONS

Administration

- Dose increments should be titrated gradually with at least 5–7 d between increases.
- Doses are reduced for creatinine clearance > 60 ml/min.
- If nausea develops, give with food.
- Store at 15–30C (59–86F) unless otherwise indicated by the manufacturer.

Assessment & Drug Effects

- Therapeutic effectiveness is indicated by improved control of neuromuscular functioning.
- Carefully monitor for S&S of orthostatic hypotension, especially when the dosage is increased.
- Monitor cardiac status, especially in those with significant orthostatic hypotension.
- Lab tests: periodically monitor BUN and creatinine; with complaints of muscle pain, monitor CPK.
- Monitor for and report signs of tardive dyskinesia (see Appendix G).

Patient & Family Education

- Hallucinations are a side effect of this drug and occur more often in the elderly.
- Make position changes slowly especially from a lying or sitting to standing position.
- Drowsiness is a common side effect. Use caution with potentially dangerous activities until reaction to the drug is known.
- Alcohol and other CNS depressants may exaggerate drowsiness, dizziness, and orthostatic hypotension. Avoid alcohol and use extra caution if taking other prescribed CNS depressants.
- Do no abruptly stop taking this drug. It should be discontinued over a period of 1 wk.
- Women who intend to breast-feed should notify the physician.

PRAMOXINE HYDROCHLORIDE

(pra-mox′een)

Trade names: Fleet Relief Anesthetic Hemorrhoidal, Prax, ProctoFoam, Tronolane, Tronothane ♣

Classifications: CNS AGENT; LOCAL ANESTHETIC (MUCOSAL); ANTIPRURITIC

Prototype: Procaine

Pregnancy category: C

ACTIONS/PHARMACODYNAMICS Differs chemically from the amide- or ester-type anesthetics; therefore, can be used in patient sensitive to these classes of drugs. Produces anesthesia by blocking conduction and propagation of sensory nerve impulses in skin and mucous membranes. Potency matches that of benzocaine as a topical anesthetic. Does not abolish gag reflex.

USES To relieve pain caused by minor burns and wounds; for temporary relief of pruritus secondary to dermatoses, hemorrhoids, and anal fissures; and to facilitate sigmoidoscopic examination.

ROUTE & DOSAGE

Relief of Minor Pain and Itching
Adult: **Topical** Apply t.i.d. or q.i.d.
Child ≥ 2 y: **Topical** same as for adult.

PHARMACOKINETICS **Onset:** 3–5 min. **Duration:** up to 5 h.

CONTRAINDICATIONS & PRECAUTIONS **Contraindicated in:** application to large areas of skin; prolonged use; preparation for laryngopharyngeal examination; bronchoscopy, or gastroscopy. Safe use in children <2 y or during pregnancy (category C) not established. **Cautious use in:** extensive skin disorders.

ADVERSE/SIDE EFFECTS **Local:** burning, stinging, sensitization.

NURSING IMPLICATIONS

Administration

- Before use for temporary relief of hemorrhoidal pain and itching, thoroughly clean and dry rectal area. Administer rectal preparations in the morning and evening and after bowel movement or as directed by physician.
- Apply lotion or cream to affected surfaces with a gloved hand. Wash hands thoroughly before and after treatment.
- Do not apply to eyes or nasal membranes.
- Store at 15–30C (59–86F); protect from light; avoid freezing.

Patient & Family Education

- Advise to discontinue use of drug if condition being treated does not improve within 2–3 wk or if it worsens, or if rash or condition not present before treatment appears, or if treated area becomes inflamed or infected.
- If rectal bleeding and pain occur during hemorrhoid treatment, drug should be discontinued and physician consulted.

PRAVASTATIN

(pra-vah-stat′in)
Trade name: Pravachol
Classifications: CARDIOVASCULAR AGENT; ANTILIPEMIC; HMG-COA REDUCTASE INHIBITOR (STATIN)
Prototype: Lovastatin
Pregnancy category: X

ACTIONS/PHARMACODYNAMICS Competitively inhibits 3-hydroxy-3-methylglutaryl-coenzyme A (HMG-CoA) reductase, the enzyme that catalyzes cholesterol biosynthesis. HMG-CoA reductase inhibitors increase serum HDL cholesterol levels and decrease serum LDL cholesterol, VLDL cholesterol, and plasma triglyceride levels. It is effective in reducing total and LDL cholesterol in various forms of hypercholesterolemia.

USES Hypercholesterolemia (alone or in combination with bile acid sequestrants) and familial hypercholesterolemia.

ROUTE & DOSAGE

Adult: **PO** 10–40 mg q.d.

PHARMACOKINETICS **Absorption:** poorly absorbed from GI tract; 17% reaches systemic circulation. **Onset:** 2 wk. **Peak:** 4 wk. **Distribution:** 43–55% protein bound; does not cross blood–brain barrier; crosses placenta; distributed into breast milk. **Metabolism:** extensive first-pass metabolism in liver; has no active metabolites. **Elimination:** half-life: 1.8–2.6 h; 20% of dose excreted in urine, 71% in feces.

CONTRAINDICATIONS & PRECAUTIONS **Contraindicated in:** hypersensitivity to pravastatin; active liver disease or unexplained elevated liver function study results; pregnancy (category X) and nursing mothers. **Cautious use in:** alcoholics, history of liver disease; renal impairment. Safety and efficacy in individuals < 18 y is not known.

ADVERSE/SIDE EFFECTS **GI:** nausea, diarrhea, abdominal pain, vomiting, constipation, flatulence, heartburn, transient elevations in serum liver transaminase levels. **Other:** fatigue, rhinitis, cough, transient elevations in CPK.

DRUG INTERACTIONS May increase PT when administered with **warfarin.**

NURSING IMPLICATIONS

Administration

- Pravastatin may be given without regard to meals.
- Pravastatin should be given in the evening.
- Store at 15–30C (59–86F).

Assessment & Drug Effects

- Monitor choesterol levels throughout therapy.
- Liver function tests should be performed at start of therapy and then at 12 wk. If normal at 12 wk, may change to semiannual monitoring.
- Monitor coagulation studies with patients receiving concurrent warfarin therapy. PT may be prolonged.

Patient & Family Education

- Advise to promptly report unexplained muscle pain, tenderness, or weakness, especially if accompanied by malaise or fever.
- Advise patients on warfarin therapy to promptly report signs of bleeding.

PRAZIQUANTEL

(pray-zi-kwon′tel)

Trade name: Biltricide

Classifications: ANTIINFECTIVE; ANTHELMINTIC

Prototype: Mebendazole

Pregnancy category: B

ACTIONS/PHARMACODYNAMICS Synthetic agent with broad-spectrum anthelmintic activity against all developmental stages of schistosomes and other trematodes (flukes) and against cestodes (tapeworm). Increases permeability of parasite cell membrane to calcium. Leads to immobilization of their suckers and dislodgment from their residence in blood vessel walls. Praziquantel is active against all developmental stages of schistosomes, including cercaria (free-swimming larvae). Activity against other trematodes (flukes) not fully understood; activity against cestodes (tapeworms) not clear but may be similar to that against schistosomes.

USES All stages of schistosomiasis (bilharziasis) caused by all schistosoma species pathogenic to humans. Other trematode infections caused by Chinese liver fluke: **Unlabeled uses:** lung, sheep liver, and intestinal flukes and tapeworm infections.

P

ROUTE & DOSAGE

Schistosomiasis

Adult: **PO** 60 mg/kg in 3 equally divided doses at 4–6 h intervals on the same day; may repeat in 2–3 mo after exposure.
Child > 4 y: **PO** same as for adult.

Other Trematodes

Adult: **PO** 75 mg/kg in 3 equally divided doses at 4–6 h intervals on the same day.
Child > 4 y: **PO** same as for adult.

Cestodiasis (Adult or Intestinal Stage)

Adult: **PO** 10–20 mg/kg as single dose.

Cestodiasis (Larval or Tissue Stage)

Adult: **PO** 50 mg/kg in 3 divided doses/d for 14 d.

PHARMACOKINETICS Absorption: approximately 80% absorbed from GI tract. **Peak:** 1–3 h. **Distribution:** crosses blood–brain barrier; distributed into breast milk. **Metabolism:** extensively metabolized in liver, including first pass metabolism. **Elimination:** half-life: 0.8–1.5 h, metabolites 4–5 h; excreted in urine.

CONTRAINDICATIONS & PRECAUTIONS Contraindicated in: hypersensitivity to drug; ocular cysticercosis. Safe use in children <4 y not established; use during pregnancy (category B) only when clearly needed. Women should not nurse on day of praziquantel therapy or for 72 h after last dose of drug.

ADVERSE/SIDE EFFECTS CNS: *dizziness, headache, malaise,* drowsiness, lassitude, CSF reaction syndrome (exacerbation of neurologic signs and symptoms such as seizures, increased CSF protein concentration, increased anticysticercal IgG levels, hyperthermia, intracranial hypertension) in patient treated for cerebral cysticercosis. **GI:** *abdominal pain or discomfort with or without nausea;* vomiting, anorexia, diarrhea. **Hepatic:** *increased AST, ALT (slight).* **Other:** pruritus, urticaria, fever, sweating, symptoms of host-mediated immunologic response to antigen release from worms (fever, eosinophilia).

DIAGNOSTIC TEST INTERFERENCE

Be mindful that selected drugs may interfere with stool studies for ova and parasites: ***iron, bismuth, oil*** (***mineral*** or ***castor***), ***Metamucil*** (if ingested within 1 wk of test), ***barium, antibiotics, antiamebic*** and ***antimalarial drugs,*** and ***gallbladder dye*** (if administered within 3 wk of test).

NURSING IMPLICATIONS

Administration

- Scored tablets are easily subdivided. If 1/4 tablet is required, break the segment from the outer end.
- Administer oral dose preferably with food and fluids. Tablets can be broken into quarters but should not be chewed. Advise patient to take sufficient fluid to wash down the medication. Tablets are soluble in water; gagging or vomiting because of bitter taste may result if tablets are retained in the mouth.
- Treatment for cestodiasis (tapeworm) may be followed by gentle purgation 2 h after drug administration to facilitate rapid removal of tapeworms and ova. The patient should be reexamined in 2 or 3 mo to ensure complete eradication of the infections.
- Store tablets in tight containers at <30C (86F).

Patient & Family Education

- Because of potential drug-induced dizziness and drowsiness, warn patient not to drive a car or operate hazardous machinery on day of praziquantel treatment or the following day.
- Schistosomiasis can be acquired by swimming in cercaria-infested freshwater in many parts of the world, especially Africa and the Middle East (larvae enter the body through the skin). Diarrhea, urinary disturbances, hematuria, hepatic cirrhosis, chronic dysentery are the most common symptoms. Ova in urine, stool, and rectal and liver biopsy confirm the diagnosis.
- Usually, all schistosomal worms are dead 7 d following treatment with praziquantel.
- Cure rates are generally lower in children and in patients with the heavy worm burden characteristic of massive infection.
- Instruct patient being treated for cestode infection to contact physician if patient develops a sustained headache or high fever. Conjunctive treatment with corticosteroids may be employed for treatment of cerebral cysticercosis (caused by pork tapeworm) to hasten recovery and reduce symptoms of CSF reaction syndrome (see Adverse/Side Effects).

PRAZOSIN HYDROCHLORIDE

(pra'zoe-sin)

Trade name: Minipress

Prototype for classifications: AUTONOMIC NERVOUS SYSTEM AGENT; ALPHA-ADRENERGIC ANTAGONIST (BLOCKING AGENT, SYMPATHOLYTIC); CARDIOVASCULAR AGENT; ANTIHYPERTENSIVE; VASODILATOR

Pregnancy category: C

ACTIONS/PHARMACODYNAMICS By selective competitive inhibition of alpha$_1$-adrenoceptors produces vasodilation in both resistance (arterioles) and capacitance (veins) vessels with the result that both peripheral vascular resistance and blood pressure are reduced. Lowers blood pressure in supine and standing positions with most pronounced effect on diastolic pressure. Has minor effect on heart rate and cardiac output in the supine position and does not increase plasma renin activity. Tolerance to antihypertensive effect rarely occurs. Effective when used concomitantly with a beta-adrenergic blocking agent and a thiazide diuretic. Infrequently used in monotherapy because of its tendency to support sodium and water retention resulting in increased plasma volume.

USE Treatment of hypertension. **Unlabeled uses:** severe refractory congestive heart failure, Raynaud's disease or phenomenon, ergotamine-induced peripheral ischemia, pheochromocytoma, benign prostatic hypertrophy.

ROUTE & DOSAGE

Hypertension

Adult: **PO** Start with 1 mg h.s.; then 1 mg b.i.d. or t.i.d.; may increase to 20 mg/d in divided doses.
Child: **PO** Start with 5 µg/kg q6h; gradually increase to 25 µg/kg q6h (max 15 mg or 0.4 mg/kg/d).

PHARMACOKINETICS **Absorption:** approximately 60% of oral dose reaches the systemic circulation. **Onset:** 2 h. **Peak:** 2–4 h. **Duration:** <24 h. **Distribution:** widely distributed, including into breast milk. **Metabolism:**

extensively metabolized in liver. **Elimination:** half-life: 2–4 h; 6–10% excreted in urine, the rest in bile and feces.

CONTRAINDICATIONS & PRECAUTIONS **Contraindicated in:** safe use during pregnancy (category C), and in nursing mothers not established. **Cautious use in:** chronic renal failure; hypertensive patient with cerebral thrombosis; men with sickle cell trait.

ADVERSE/SIDE EFFECTS **CNS:** *dizziness, headache, drowsiness*, nervousness, vertigo, depression, paresthesia, insomnia. **CV:** edema, dyspnea, syncope *first-dose phenomenon*, postural hypotension, *palpitations*, tachycardia, angina. **Eye/ear:** blurred vision, tinnitus, reddened sclerae. **GI:** dry mouth, *nausea*, vomiting, diarrhea, constipation, abdominal discomfort, pain. **GU:** urinary frequency, incontinence, priapism (especially in men with sickle cell anemia), impotence. **Skin:** rash, pruritus, alopecia, lichen planus. **Other:** diaphoresis, epistaxis, nasal congestion, arthralgia, transient leukopenia, increased serum uric acid, and BUN.

P

DRUG INTERACTIONS DIURETICS and other HYPOTENSIVE AGENTS increase hypotensive effects.

NURSING IMPLICATIONS

Administration

- The initial dose of prazosin should be taken at bedtime to reduce possibility of side effects such as postural hypotension and syncope. However, if first dose is taken during the day, patient should be advised not to drive a car for about 4 h after drug ingestion.
- Food may delay absorption but does not affect extent of absorption. Taking drug with food may reduce incidence of faintness and dizziness.
- Store prazosin capsules at 15–30C (59–86F) in tightly closed container away from strong light. Do not freeze.

Assessment & Drug Effects

- First-dose phenomenon (rare side effect: 0.15% of patients) is characterized by a precipitous decline in BP, bradycardia, and consciousness disturbances (syncope) within 90–120 min after the initial dose of prazosin. Recovery is usually within several hours. Preexisting low plasma volume (from diuretic therapy or salt restriction), beta-adrenergic therapy, and recent stroke appear to increase the risk of this phenomenon.
- Monitor blood pressure. If it falls precipitously with first dose, notify physician promptly.
- Full therapeutic effect of prazosin may not be achieved until 4–6 wk of therapy.

Patient & Family Education

- During early phase of prazosin treatment, advise to avoid situations that would result in injury should syncope occur. In most cases, effect does not recur after initial period of therapy; however, it may occur during acute febrile episodes, when prazosin dose is increased, or when another antihypertensive drug is added to the medication regimen.
- Postural hypotension can pose a problem with ambulation. Advise to make position and direction changes slowly and in stages. Dangle legs and move ankles a minute or so before standing when arising in the morning or after a nap.
- Caution patient who is experiencing light-headedness, dizziness, a sense of impending loss of consciousness,

or blurred vision to lie down immediately. Attempting to stand or ambulate may result in a fall.

- Until reaction to prazosin therapy is known (i.e., potential development of side effects), patient should not undertake any activity that might become a hazard in the presence of dizziness, syncope, or weakness.
- Advise to take drug at same time(s) each day. Encourage patient who has been taught to monitor own BP to keep a daily record noting BP and time taken, when medication was taken, which arm was used, position (i.e., standing, sitting), and time of day. Take this record to physician for reference at checkup appointment.
- Encourage men to promptly report priapism or impotence. A change in the drug regimen usually reverses these difficulties. Since acute episodes of priapism followed by impotence spontaneously occur in men with sickle cell anemia, another antihypertensive should be selected. In these patients, drug-induced priapism is frequently irreversible.
- Advise not to take OTC medications, especially those that may contain an adrenergic agent (e.g., remedies for coughs, colds, allergy), until a physician has been consulted.
- Side effects usually disappear with continuation of therapy, but dosage reduction may be necessary.

PREDNISOLONE

(pred-niss′oh-lone)

Trade names: Delta-Cortef, Inflamase Forte, Prelone

PREDNISOLONE ACETATE

Trade names: Econopred, Key-Pred, Pred Forte, Predcor

PREDNISOLONE SODIUM PHOSPHATE

Trade names: AK-Pred, Hydeltrasol, Inflamase, Inflamase Mild, Pred Mild

PREDNISOLONE TEBUTATE

Trade names: Hydeltra-T.B.A., Prednisol TBA

Classifications: SYNTHETIC HORMONE; ADRENAL CORTICOSTEROID; GLUCOCORTICOID

Prototype: Prednisone

Pregnancy category: C

ACTIONS/PHARMACODYNAMICS

Intermediate-acting synthetic dehydrogenated analog of hydrocortisone with 3–5 times greater potency. Mineralocorticoid properties are minimal, and potential for sodium and water retention and potassium loss is reduced.

USE Principally as an antiinflammatory and immunosuppressant agent.

P

ROUTE & DOSAGE

Antiinflammatory

Adult: **PO** 5–60 mg/d in single or divided doses. **IM** Acetate/Phosphate: 6–60 mg/d; Tebutate: 2–60 mg q wk. **IV** Phosphate: 4–60 mg/d; **Ophthalmic** See Appendix A.
Child: **PO** 0.14–2 mg/kg/d in single or divided doses. **IM** Acetate/Phosphate: 0.04–0.25 mg/kg 1–2 times/d. **IV** Phosphate: 0.04–0.25 mg/kg 1–2 times/d.

PHARMACOKINETICS **Absorption:** readily absorbed from GI tract. **Peak:** 1–2 h. **Duration:** 1–1.5 d. **Distribution:** crosses placenta; distributed into breast milk. **Metabolism:** metabolized in liver. **Elimination:** half-life: 3.5 h; HPA suppression: 24–36 h; excreted in urine.

ADVERSE/SIDE EFFECTS Hirsutism (occasional); perforation of cornea (with topical drug); sensitivity to heat; fat embolism, adverse effects on growth and development of the individual and on sperm; hypotension and shock-like reactions; insomnia; gastric irritation or ulceration; ecchymotic skin lesions; vasomotor symptoms. Also see prednisone.

CONTRAINDICATIONS & PRECAUTIONS Safe use during pregnancy (category C) and by lactating women not established.

DRUG INTERACTIONS BARBITURATES, **phenytoin, rifampin** increase steroid metabolism—may need increased doses of prednisolone; **amphotericin B,** DIURETICS add to potassium loss; **ambenonium, neostigmine, pyridostigmine** may cause severe muscle weakness in patients with myasthenia gravis; VACCINES, TOXOIDS may inhibit antibody response.

INCOMPATIBILITIES **Solution/additive: calcium gluceptate, metaraminol, methotrexate, polymyxin B.**

NURSING IMPLICATIONS

Administration

- Administer oral drug with meals to reduce gastric irritation. If distress continues, consult physician about possible adjunctive antacid therapy.
- IV prednisolone sodium phosphate may be given by direct IV undiluted at a rate of 10 mg or fraction thereof over 60 s.
- IV prednisolone may be added to IV infusions of NS or D5W (50–1000 ml) and infused at ordered rate.
- Store in airtight containers protected from light at 15–30C (59–86F); do not freeze.

Assessment & Drug Effects

- In diseases caused by microorganisms, infection may be masked, activated, or enhanced by corticosteroids. Be alert to subclinical signs of lack of improvement such as continued drainage, low-grade fever, and interrupted healing. Observe and report exacerbation of symptoms after short period of therapeutic response.
- Temporary local discomfort may follow injection of prednisolone into bursa or joint.

Patient & Family Education

- Advise to adhere to established dosage regimen, i.e., should not increase, decrease, or omit doses or change dose intervals.

Alternate-Day Therapy (ADT) for Patient on Long-term Therapy

- With ADT, the 48-h requirement for steroids is administered as a single dose every other morning.
- ADT minimizes adverse/side effects associated with long-term treatment while maintaining the desired therapeutic effect.
- If patient becomes symptomatic during period of switching to dose consolidation on the off or drugless day, a single small dose of glucocorticoid should be given on the off day and gradually reduced.
- If an acute flare is precipitated (high fever, reactivation of inflammatory condition being treated), ADT may have to be abandoned.

See **prednisone** for numerous additional nursing implications.

PREDNISONE

(pred'ni-sone)

Trade names: Apo-Prednisone ♣, Deltasone, Meticorten, Orasone, Panasol, Prednicen-M, Sterapred, Winpred ♣

Prototype for classifications: SYNTHETIC HORMONE; ADRENAL CORTICOSTEROID; GLUCOCORTICOID

Pregnancy category: C

ACTIONS/PHARMACODYNAMICS Immediate-acting synthetic analog of hydrocortisone. Effect depends on biotransformation to prednisolone, a conversion that may be impaired in patient with liver dysfunction. Has less mineralocorticoid activity than hydrocortisone, but sodium retention and potassium depletion can occur. Shares contraindications and precautions and adverse/side effects with fludrocortisone.

USES May be used as a single agent or conjunctively with antineoplastics in cancer therapy; also used in treatment of myasthenia gravis and inflammatory conditions and as an immunosuppressant.

ROUTE & DOSAGE

Antiinflammatory

Adult: **PO** 5–60 mg/d in single or divided doses.
Child: **PO** 0.1–0.15 mg/kg/d in single or divided doses.

Acute Asthma

Child: **PO** 1–2 mg/kg/d × 3–5 d or < 1 y: 10 mg q12h, 1–4 y: 20 mg q12h, 5–13 y: 30 mg q12h, >13 y: 40 mg q12h × 3–5 d.

PHARMACOKINETICS **Absorption:** readily absorbed from GI tract. **Peak:** 1–2 h. **Duration:** 1–1.5 d. **Distribution:** crosses placenta; distributed into breast milk. **Metabolism:** metabolized in liver. **Elimination:** half-life: 3.5 h; hypothalamus-pituitary axis suppression: 24–36 h; excreted in urine.

CONTRAINDICATIONS & PRECAUTIONS **Contraindicated in:** systemic fungal infections and known hypersensitivity. **Cautious use in:** patients with infections, nonspecific ulcerative colitis, diverticulitis, active or latent peptic ulcer, renal insufficiency, hypertension, osteoporosis, myasthenia gravis. Safe use by pregnant women (category C) and nursing mothers is not established.

ADVERSE/SIDE EFFECTS **CNS:** euphoria, headache, insomnia, confusion, psychosis. **CV:** CHF, edema. **GI:** nausea, vomiting, peptic ulcer. **Musculoskeletal:** muscle weakness, delayed wound healing, muscle wasting, osteoporosis, aseptic necrosis of bone, spontaneous fractures. **Endocrine:** cushingoid features, growth suppression in children, carbohydrate intolerance, hyperglycemia. **Other:** cataracts, leukocytosis, hypokalemia.

DRUG INTERACTIONS BARBITURATES, **phenytoin, rifampin** increase steroid metabolism—increased doses of prednisone may be needed; **amphotericin B,** DIURETICS increase potassium loss; **ambenonium, neostigmine, pyridostigmine** may cause severe muscle weakness in patients with myasthenia gravis; may inhibit antibody response to VACCINES, TOXOIDS.

NURSING IMPLICATIONS

Administration

- Before administration, tablet may

be crushed and then taken with fluid of patient's choice.

- Oral drug may be taken at mealtimes or with a snack to reduce gastric irritation.
- The initial suppressive dosing regimen should be brief, especially if alternate-day therapy is anticipated. Usually, 4–10 d is sufficient for satisfactory clinical response in many allergic and collagen diseases.
- Alternate-day therapy (ADT, i.e., single dose administered every other day) is used when long-term PO glucocorticoid treatment is anticipated. ADT may be advised to keep daily dose at minimal levels and to reduce degree of "steroid rebound" with withdrawal.
- Cortisol plasma levels are maximal between 2 and 8 AM and minimal between 4 PM and midnight (normal: 7–28 μg/dl in AM and below 10 μg/dl at 8 PM). Exogenous corticosteroids suppress adrenal cortex activity less when given in the morning. To minimize HPA axis suppression, replacement steroid should be given before 9 AM.
- Dose adjustment may be required if patient is subjected to severe stress (serious infection, surgery, or injury) or if a remission or disease exacerbation occurs.
- To prevent withdrawal symptoms and permit adrenals to recover from drug-induced partial atrophy, doses are gradually reduced by scheduled decrements (various regimens).
- Protect drug from light and air in tightly closed, dark container.
- Store at temperature between 15–30C (59–86F).

P

Assessment & Drug Effects

- Establish baseline and continuing data regarding BP, I&O ratio and pattern, weight, and sleep pattern. Start flow chart as reference for planning individualized pharmacotherapeutic patient care.
- Check and record BP during dose stabilization period at least 2 times daily. Report an ascending pattern.
- Urine specimens every 24 h for studies of 17-KS may be prescribed to rule out Cushing's syndrome. Normal 17-KS values: men, 10–25 mg/24 h; women < 50 y: 5–15 mg/24 h; women > 50 y; 4–8 mg/24 h.
- During long-term therapy, patient should be monitored for evidence of HPA axis suppression by determining plasma cortisol levels at weekly intervals.
- Two-hour postprandial blood glucose, serum potassium, chest x-ray, and routine laboratory studies are performed at regular intervals during long-term steroid therapy.
- The elderly patient and the patient with low serum albumin are especially susceptible to adverse/side effects because of excess circulating free glucocorticoids.
- If patient has a history of diabetes mellitus, urine should be tested for glycosuria daily. Report positive findings; dietary and antidiabetic medication dose adjustments may be indicated.
- Be alert to signs of hypocalcemia (see Appendix G). Patients with hypocalcemia have increased requirements for pyridoxine (vitamin B_6), vitamins C and D, and folates.
- Be alert to possibility of masked infection and delayed healing (antiinflammatory and immunosuppressive actions). Prednisone suppresses early classic signs of inflammation that are diagnostically important: capillary dilation (heat, redness), phagocytosis (pus formation), swelling

(pain), fibrin deposition (clot formation). When patient is on an extended therapy regimen, incidence of oral *Candida* infection is high. Inspect mouth daily for symptoms: white patches, black furry tongue, painful membranes and tongue.

- Exaggerated sense of well-being and analgesic effects may encourage patient to increase physical activity even if acute disease process still exists. Discuss with physician and work with patient and family to plan reasonable and safe range of activities and daily living.
- Compression and spontaneous fractures of long bones and vertebrae present hazards, particularly in long-term corticosteroid treatment of rheumatoid arthritis or diabetes, in immobilized patients, and the elderly. Supervise getting out of bed or chair. Report persistent backache or chest pain (possible symptoms of vertebral or rib fracture). Patient's mattress should be firm or supported by a bedboard.
- Be aware of previous history of psychotic tendencies. Watch for changes in mood and behavior, emotional stability, sleep pattern, or psychomotor activity, especially with long-term therapy, that may signal onset of recurrence. Report symptoms to physician.
- If a patient is receiving aspirin concomitantly with a corticosteroid, salicylism may be induced when the corticosteroid dosage is decreased or discontinued.
- Ordinarily long-term corticosteroid therapy is not interrupted when patient undergoes major surgery, but dosage may be increased.
- Abrupt discontinuation of corticosteroids after long-term therapy may result in withdrawal syndrome (myalgia, fever, arthralgia, malaise) and hypocorticism (anorexia, vomiting, nausea, fatigue, dizziness, hypotension, hypoglycemia, myalgia, arthralgia).
- If during withdrawal the disease flares up, a dosage increase followed by a more gradual withdrawal may be necessary.
- Patient is supervised about 1 y after withdrawal from systemic corticosteroids or until HPA axis function is restored. During period of HPA axis suppression, severe stress (trauma, surgery, infections) may induce symptoms of adrenal insufficiency necessitating reinstitution of corticosteroid treatment.

Patient & Family Education

- Counsel to take drug as prescribed and not to alter dosing regimen or stop medication without consulting physician. Additionally, patient should not give any of the drug to another person.
- Inform that a slight weight gain with improved appetite is expected, but after dosage is stabilized, a sudden slow but steady weight increase (2 kg [5 lb]) wk) should be reported.
- Encourage to avoid alcohol and caffeine (secretagogues); may contribute to steroid-ulcer development in long-term therapy.
- Dyspepsia with hyperacidity should not be ignored. Encourage to report symptoms to physician and not to self-medicate to find relief.
- Warn not to use aspirin or other OTC drugs unless they are prescribed specifically by the physician.
- Warn to report slow healing, any vague feeling of being sick with-

out clear etiologic definition, or return of pretreatment symptoms.

- The immunocompromised patient should be fastidious about personal hygiene, give special attention to foot care, and be particularly cautious about bruising or abrading the skin.
- Single doses of corticosteroids or use for a short period (> 1 wk) does not produce withdrawal symptoms when drug is discontinued, even with moderately large doses.
- Advise patient or family to tell a dentist or new physician about recent prolonged corticosteroid treatment.
- Advise patient receiving corticosteroid to carry a medical identification card or jewelry with recorded diagnosis, drug therapy, and name of physician.
- Urge to adhere to scheduled appointments for regimen reevaluation.

P

PRIMAQUINE PHOSPHATE

(prim'a-kween)

Classifications: ANTIINFECTIVE; ANTIMALARIAL

Prototype: Chloroquine

Pregnancy category: C

ACTIONS/PHARMACODYNAMICS Acts on primary exoerythrocytic forms of *Plasmodium vivax* and *Plasmodium falciparum* by an incompletely known mechanism. Destroys late tissue forms of *P. vivax* and thus effects radical cure (prevents relapse). Also has gametocidal activity against all species of plasmodia that infect man and thus can interrupt transmission of malaria.

USES To prevent relapse ("radical" or "clinical" cure) of *P. vivax* and *P. ovale* malarias and to prevent attacks after departure from areas where *P. vivax* and *P. ovale* malarias are endemic.

ROUTE & DOSAGE

Malaria Relapse Prevention

Adult: **PO** 15 mg once/d for 14 d concomitantly or consecutively with chloroquine or hydroxychloroquine on first 3 d of acute attack.

Child: **PO** 0.3 mg/kg once/d for 14 d concomitantly or consecutively with chloroquine or hydroxychloroquine on first 3 d of acute attack.

Malaria Prophylaxis

Adult: **PO** 15 mg once/d for 14 d beginning immediately after leaving malarious area.

Child: **PO** 0.3 mg/kg once/d for 14 d beginning immediately after leaving malarious area.

PHARMACOKINETICS Absorption: readily absorbed from GI tract. **Peak:** 6 h. **Metabolism:** rapidly metabolized in liver to active metabolites. **Elimination:** half-life: 3.7–9.6 h; excreted in urine.

CONTRAINDICATIONS & PRECAUTIONS Contraindicated in: rheumatoid arthritis; lupus erythematosus; hemolytic drugs, concomitant or recent use of agents capable of bone marrow depression, e.g., quinacrine; patients with G6PD deficiency. NADH methemoglobin reductase deficiency, pregnancy (category C).

ADVERSE/SIDE EFFECTS Hematologic reactions including granulocytopenia and acute hemolytic anemia in patients with G6PD deficiency. **Overdosage:** nausea, vomiting, epigastric distress, abdominal cramps, pruritus, methemoglobinemia (cyanosis): headache, confusion, mental depression, moderate leukocytosis or leukopenia, anemia, granulocytopenia, agranulocytosis, disturbances of visual accommodation, hypertension, arrhythmias (rare).

DRUG INTERACTIONS Toxicity of both **quinacrine** and primaquine increased.

NURSING IMPLICATIONS

Administration

- Administration of drug at mealtime or with an antacid (prescribed) may prevent or relieve gastric irritation. Notify physician if GI symptoms persist.
- Preserve in tight, light-resistant containers.

Assessment & Drug Effects

- Primaquine may precipitate acute hemolytic anemia in persons with G6PD deficiency, an inherited error of metabolism carried on the X chromosome, present in about 10% of American black males and certain white ethnic groups: Sardinians, Sephardic Jews, Greeks, and Iranians. Whites manifest more intense expression of hemolytic reaction than do blacks.
- Patients whose ethnic origin indicates the possibility of G6PD deficiency should be screened prior to initiation of therapy.
- Repeated hematologic studies (particularly blood cell counts and hemoglobin) and urinalyses should be performed during therapy.

Patient & Family Education

- Advise to examine urine after each voiding and to report darkening of urine, red-tinged urine, and decrease in urine volume. Also report chills, fever, precordial pain, cyanosis (all suggest a hemolytic reaction). Sudden reductions in hemoglobin or erythrocyte count suggest an impending hemolytic reaction.

PRIMIDONE

(pri′mi-done)

Trade names: Apo-Primidone ♣, Mysoline

Classifications: CNS AGENT; BARBITURATE ANTICONVULSANT

Prototype: Phenobarbital

Pregnancy category: D

ACTIONS/PHARMACODYNAMICS

Not a true barbiturate but closely related chemically and with similar mechanism of action. Converted in body to phenobarbital. Appears to increase metabolism of vitamin D so that more is needed to fulfill normal requirements. May also impair calcium, folic acid, and vitamin B_{12} metabolism and utilization.

USES Alone or concomitantly with other anticonvulsant agents in the prophylactic management of complex partial (psychomotor) and generalized tonic-clonic (grand mal) seizures. **Unlabeled use:** essential tremor.

ROUTE & DOSAGE

Seizures

Adult: **PO** 250 mg/d, increased by 250 mg/wk up to a max of 2 g in 2–4 divided doses.
Child: **PO** *8–12 y,* same as for adult; *<8 y,* 125 mg/d, increased by 125 mg/wk up to a max of 1 g in 2–4 divided doses.

PHARMACOKINETICS **Absorption:** approximately 60–80% absorbed from GI tract. **Peak:** 4 h. **Distribution:** distributed into breast milk. **Metab-**

olism: metabolized in liver to phenobarbital and PEMA. **Elimination:** half-life: primidone 3–24 h, PEMA 24–48 h; phenobarbital 72–144 h; excreted in urine.

CONTRAINDICATIONS & PRECAUTIONS **Contraindicated in:** safe use during pregnancy (category D) and in nursing mothers not established. Hypersensitivity to barbiturates, porphyria. **Cautious use in:** chronic lung disease; hepatic or renal disease; hyperactive children.

ADVERSE/SIDE EFFECTS **CNS:** *drowsiness, sedation, vertigo, ataxia, headache,* excitement (children), confusion, unusual fatigue, hyperirritability, emotional disturbances, acute psychoses (usually patients with psychomotor epilepsy). **Eye:** diplopia, nystagmus, swelling of eyelids. **GI:** *nausea, vomiting, anorexia*. **Hematologic:** leukopenia, thrombocytopenia, eosinophilia, decreased serum folate levels, megaloblastic anemia (rare). **Other:** alopecia, impotence, maculopapular or morbilliform rash, edema, lupus erythematosus-like syndrome, lymphadenopathy, osteomalacia.

P

DRUG INTERACTIONS See phenobarbital.

NURSING IMPLICATIONS

Administration

- Tablet may be crushed before administration and taken with fluid of patient's choice.
- If drug causes GI distress, it may be taken with food.
- Transition from another anticonvulsant to primidone should not be completed in <2 mo.

Assessment & Drug Effects

- Baseline and periodic studies should be made of CBC, SMA-12 (q6mo), and primidone and phenobarbital blood levels. (Therapeutic blood level for primidone: 5–10 μg/ml; for phenobarbital: 15–40 μg/ml.)
- Dosage may be adjusted with reference to primidone or phenobarbital metabolite plasma levels (concentrations of primidone > 10 μg/ml are usually associated with significant ataxia and lethargy).
- Therapeutic response may not be evident for several weeks.
- Observe for signs and symptoms of folic acid deficiency: mental dysfunction, psychiatric disorders, neuropathy, megaloblastic anemia. When indicated, serum folate levels should be determined.
- Neonatal hemorrhage has been reported in newborns whose mothers were taking primidone. Monitor closely for bleeding.
- Presence of unusual drowsiness in nursing newborns of primidone-treated mothers is an indication to discontinue nursing.

Patient & Family Education

- Because drowsiness, dizziness, and ataxia may be severe at beginning of treatment, advise to avoid driving and other potentially hazardous activities. Symptoms tend to disappear with continued therapy; if they persist, dosage reduction or drug withdrawal may be necessary.
- Advise to avoid alcohol and other CNS depressants unless otherwise directed by physician.
- Caution not to take OTC medications unless approved by physician.
- Pregnant women should receive prophylactic vitamin K therapy for 1 mo prior to and during delivery to prevent neonatal hemorrhage.
- Primidone withdrawal should be done gradually to avoid precipitating status epilepticus.

- Advise to carry medical information card or jewelry with name of drug, physician's name, and telephone number.

PROBENECID

(proe-ben′e-sid)

Trade names: Benemid, Benuryl ✦, Probalan, SK-Probenecid

Classifications: ANTIGOUT AGENT; SULFONAMIDE; URICOSURIC AGENT

Prototype: Colchicine

Pregnancy category: B

ACTIONS/PHARMACODYNAMICS Sulfonamide-derivative renal tubular blocking agent. In sufficiently high doses, competitively inhibits renal tubular reabsorption of uric acid, thereby promoting its excretion and reducing serum urate levels. Prevents formation of new tophaceous deposits, and causes gradual shrinking of old tophi.

USES Hyperuricemia in chronic gouty arthritis and tophaceous gout. **Unlabeled uses:** adjuvant to therapy with penicillin G and penicillin analogs to elevate and prolong plasma concentrations of these antibiotics; to promote uric acid excretion in hyperuricemia secondary to administration of thiazides and related diuretics, furosemide, ethacrynic acid, pyrazinamide.

ROUTE & DOSAGE

Gout

Adult: **PO** 250 mg b.i.d. for 1 wk; then 500 mg b.i.d. (max 3 g/d).

Adjunct for Penicillin or Cephalosporin Therapy

Adult: **PO** 500 mg q.i.d. or 1 g with single dose therapy (e.g., gonorrhea).

Child 2–14 y or <50 kg: **PO** 25–40 mg/kg/d in 4 divided doses.

PHARMACOKINETICS Absorption: readily absorbed from GI tract. **Onset:** 30 min. **Peak:** 2–4 h. **Duration:** 8 h. **Distribution:** crosses placenta. **Metabolism:** metabolized in liver. **Elimination:** half-life: 4–17 h; excreted in urine.

CONTRAINDICATIONS & PRECAUTIONS Contraindicated in: blood dyscrasias; uric acid kidney stones; during or within 2–3 wk of acute gouty attack; overexcretion of uric acid (> 1000 mg/d), patients with creatinine clearance <50 mg/min; use with penicillin in presence of known renal impairment, use for hyperuricemia secondary to cancer chemotherapy. Safe use during pregnancy (category B), in nursing mothers, and in children <2 y not established. **Cautious use in:** history of peptic ulcer.

ADVERSE/SIDE EFFECTS *Headache, nausea, vomiting, anorexia,* sore gums, urinary frequency, flushing, dizziness, anemia, <u>hemolytic anemia (possibly related to G6PD deficiency)</u>. Exacerbations of gout, uric acid kidney stones. Rare: <u>aplastic anemia</u>, <u>hepatic necrosis</u>. **Hypersensitivity:** dermatitis, pruritus, fever, <u>anaphylaxis.</u> **Overdose:** <u>respiratory depression.</u>

DIAGNOSTIC TEST INTERFERENCE False-positive results ***urine glucose*** tests are possible with Benedict's solution or Clinitest (glucose oxidase methods not affected, e.g., Clinistix, TesTape).

DRUG INTERACTIONS SALICYLATES may decrease uricosuric activity; may decrease **methotrexate** elimination, causing increased toxicity;

P

decreases **nitrofurantoin** efficacy and increases its toxicity.

NURSING IMPLICATIONS

Administration

- GI side effects are minimized by taking drug after meals, with food, milk, or antacid (prescribed). If symptoms persist, dosage reduction may be required.
- PO sodium bicarbonate (3–7.5 g/d) or potassium citrate (7.5 g/d) may be prescribed to alkalinize urine until serum uric acid levels return to normal range (3–7 mg/dl).
- Because frequency of acute gouty attacks may increase during first 6–12 mo of therapy, physician may prescribe concurrent prophylactic doses of colchicine for first 3–6 mo of probenecid therapy (probenecid alone aggravates acute gout). Probenecid is available in combination with colchicine, e.g., Col-Benemid.
- Tablets should be stored in tightly closed containers at 15–30C (59–86F). Expiration date is 3–5 y after date of manufacture.

Assessment & Drug Effects

- When gouty attacks have been absent for 6 mo or more and serum urate levels are controlled, daily dosage may be cautiously decreased by 0.5 g q6mo to lowest effective dosage that maintains stable serum urate levels.
- When urinary alkalinizers are used, periodic determinations of acid–base balance are advised. Some physicians prescribe acetazolamide at bedtime to keep urine alkaline and dilute throughout night.
- Patients taking sulfonylureas may require dosage adjustment. Probenecid enhances hypoglycemic actions of these drugs. See also diagnostic test interferences.
- Urate tophaceous deposits should decrease in size with probenecid therapy. Classic locations are in cartilage of ear pinna and big toe, but they can occur in bursae, tendons, skin, kidneys, and other tissues.

Patient & Family Education

- Increased uric acid excretion promoted by probenecid predisposes to renal calculi. Therefore, during early therapy, high fluid intake (approximately 3000 ml/d) is recommended to maintain daily urinary output of at least 2000 ml or more.
- Physician may advise restriction of high-purine foods during early therapy until uric acid level stabilizes. Foods high in purine include organ meats (sweetbreads, liver, kidney), meat extracts, meat soups, gravy, anchovies, and sardines. Moderate amounts are present in other meats, fish, seafood, asparagus, spinach, peas, dried legumes, wild game.
- Alcohol may increase serum urate levels and therefore should be avoided.
- Caution patient not to stop taking drug without consulting physician. Irregular dosage schedule may sharply elevate serum urate level and precipitate acute gout.
- Lifelong therapy is usually required in patients with symptomatic hyperuricemia. Advise patient to keep scheduled appointments with physician and appointments for studies of renal function and hematology.
- Instruct to report symptoms of hypersensitivity to physician. Discontinuation of drug is indicated.
- Advise not to take aspirin or other OTC medications without consult-

ing physician. If a mild analgesic is required, acetaminophen is usually allowed.

PROCAINAMIDE HYDROCHLORIDE

(proe-kane-a′mide)

Trade names: Procan, Procanbid, Pronestyl, Pronestyl SR

Prototype for classifications: CARDIOVASCULAR AGENT; ANTIARRHYTHMIC

Pregnancy category: C

ACTIONS/PHARMACODYNAMICS Amide analog of procaine hydrochloride with cardiac actions similar to those of quinine. Class Ia antiarrhythmic agent. Depresses excitability of myocardium to electrical stimulation, reduces conduction velocity in atria, ventricles, and His-Purkinje system. Increases duration of refractory period, especially in the atria. Produces slight change in contractility of cardiac muscle and cardiac output; suppresses automaticity of His-Purkinje ventricular muscle. Produces peripheral vasodilaton and hypotension, especially with IV use.

USES Prophylactically to maintain normal sinus rhythm following conversion of atrial flutter or fibrillation by other methods. Also to prevent recurrence of paroxysmal atrial fibrillation and tachycardia, paroxysmal AV junctional rhythm, ventricular tachycardia, ventricular and atrial premature contractions. Also cardiac arrhythmias associated with surgery and anesthesia. **Unlabeled use:** malignant hyperthermia.

ROUTE & DOSAGE

Arrhythmias

Adult: **PO** 1 g followed by 250–500 mg q3h *or* 500 mg–1 g q6h sustained release (b.i.d. for Procanbid). **IM** 0.5–1 g q4–6h until able to take PO. **IV** 100 mg q5min at a rate of 25–50 mg/min until arrhythmia is controlled or 1 g given, then 2–6 mg/min.
Child: **PO** 40–60 mg/kg/d divided q4–6h. **IV** 3–6 mg/kg q10–30min (max 100 mg/ dose), then 0.02–0.08 mg/kg/ min.

PHARMACOKINETICS Absorption: 75–95% absorbed from GI tract. **Peak:** 15–60 min IM; 30–60 min PO. **Duration:** 3 h; 8 h with sustained release. **Distribution:** distributed to CSF, liver, spleen, kidney, brain, and heart; crosses placenta; distributed into breast milk. **Metabolism:** metabolized in liver to *N*-acetylprocainamide (NAPA), an active metabolite (30–60% metabolized to NAPA). **Elimination:** half-life: 3 h procainamide, 6 h NAPA; excreted in urine.

CONTRAINDICATIONS & PRECAUTIONS Contraindicated in: myasthenia gravis; hypersensitivity to procainamide or procaine; blood dyscrasias; complete AV block, second and third degree AV block unassisted by pacemaker. **Cautious use in:** patient who has undergone electrical reversion to sinus rhythm; hypotension, cardiac enlargement, CHF, MI, coronary occlusion, ventricular dysrhythmia from digitalis intoxication, hepatic or renal insufficiency, electrolyte imbalance, bronchial asthma, history of SLE. Safe use in pregnancy (category C) or in nursing mothers not established.

P

ADVERSE/SIDE EFFECTS **CNS:** dizziness, psychosis. **CV:** severe hypotension, pericarditis, ventricular fibrillation, AV block, tachycardia, flushing. **GI** (mostly PO): bitter taste, nausea, vomiting, diarrhea, anorexia. **Hematologic:** agranulocytosis with repeated use; thrombocytopenia. **Hypersensitivity:** fever, muscle and joint pain, angioneurotic edema, maculopapular rash, pruritus. **Other:** *SLE-like syndrome (50% of patients on large doses for 1 y):* polyarthralgias, pleuritic pain, pleural effusion, erythema, skin rash, myalgia, fever.

DIAGNOSTIC TEST INTERFERENCE Procainamide increases the plasma levels of ***alkaline phosphatase, bilirubin, lactic dehydrogenase*** and ***AST.*** It may also alter results of the ***edrophonium test.***

DRUG INTERACTIONS Other ANTIARRHYTHMICS add to therapeutic and toxic effects; ANTICHOLINERGIC AGENTS compound anticholinergic effects; ANTIHYPERTENSIVES add to hypotensive effects; **cimetidine** may increase procainamide and NAPA levels with increase in toxicity.

INCOMPATIBILITIES **Solution/additive: bretylium, ethacrynate.**

NURSING IMPLICATIONS

Administration

- Oral preparation is best taken on empty stomach 1 h before or 2 h after meals with a full glass of water to enhance absorption. If drug causes gastric distress, administer with food.
- Immediate-release (but not sustained-release) tablet may be crushed if patient is unable to swallow it whole.
- Sustained-release tablet must be swallowed whole. It has a wax matrix that is not absorbed but appears in the stool.
- First PO dose should be given at least 4 h after last IV dose.
- IV preparation: When procainamide is given direct IV, dilute each 100 mg with 10 ml of D5W or sterile water for injection. When procainamide is given by IV infusion, add 1 g of procainamide to 250–500 ml of D5W solution. Yields 4 mg/ml in 250 ml or 2 mg/ml in 500 ml.
- IV administration: IV dosage over a period of several hours is controlled by assessment of procainamide plasma levels. Effective nontoxic therapeutic level: 3–10 μg/ml (8–16 μg/ml is potentially toxic, and toxicity is common at plasma levels > 16 μg/ml).
- Procainamide administration by IV infusion pump requires constant monitoring to maintain desired flow rate. Keep patient in supine position. Be alert to signs of too rapid administration of drug—speed shock: irregular pulse, tight feeling in chest, flushed face, headache, loss of consciousness, shock, cardiac arrest.
- Procainamide solution is stable for 24 h at room temperature and for 7 d under refrigeration at 2–8C (36–46F). Avoid freezing the solution. Refrigeration will retard color changes in solution. Slight yellowing does not alter drug potency, but discard solution if it is markedly discolored or precipitated.
- Store tablets in dark, airtight containers. Procainamide is hygroscopic; therefore, do not store in bathroom medicine cabinet or in refrigerator where moisture levels are high.

Assessment & Drug Effects

- Apical radial pulses should be checked before each dose of procainamide during period of adjustment to the oral route.

P

- Patients at particular risk for adverse effects are those with severe heart, hepatic, or renal disease and hypotension.
- Monitor the patient's ECG and BP continuously during IV drug administration.
- IV drug is temporarily discontinued when (1) arrhythmia is interrupted, (2) severe toxic effects are present, (3) QRS complex is excessively widened (greater than 50%), (4) PR interval is prolonged, or (5) BP drops 15 mm Hg or more. Obtain rhythm strip and notify physician.
- A complication of procainamide infusion given to treat atrial dysrhythmia is the onset of ventricular tachycardia (a lethal arrhythmia) evidenced by increased rate to as high as 200 bpm.
- Ventricular dysrhythmias are usually abolished within a few minutes after IV dose and within an hour after PO or IM administration.
- Digitalization may have preceded procainamide in patients with atrial arrhythmias. Cardiotonic glycosides may induce sufficient increase in atrial contraction to dislodge atrial mural emboli, with subsequent pulmonary embolism. Report promptly complaints of chest pain, dyspnea, and anxiety.
- Therapeutic procainamide blood levels are reached in approximately 24 h if kidney function is normal but are delayed in presence of renal impairment.

Patient & Family Education

- Advise to monitor and report immediately evidence of kidney dysfunction: changes in I&O ratio and body weight, local edema (tight shoes or rings). Encourage keeping a record of weekly weight for comparison purposes. If weight gain of 1 kg (2 lb) or more is accompanied by local edema, patient should notify the physician.
- Instruct on maintenance doses to record and report date, time, and duration of fibrillation episodes: light-headedness, giddiness, weakness, or syncope.
- Instruct to keep a record of pulse rates. Report changes in rate or quality.
- Instruct to report to the physician signs of reduced procainamide control: weakness, irregular pulse, unexplained fatigability, anxiety.
- Before discharge, work with patient to design a 24-h dosing schedule for all prescribed drugs that will best fit into ADL at home.
- At no time should a dose be doubled or an interval changed because a previous dose was missed. Procainamide should be taken at evenly spaced intervals around the clock unless otherwise prescribed.

P

PROCAINE HYDROCHLORIDE

(proe'kane)

Trade name: Novocain

Prototype for classifications: CNS AGENT; LOCAL ANESTHETIC (ESTER-TYPE)

Pregnancy category: C

ACTIONS/PHARMACODYNAMICS

Decreases sodium flux into nerve cell, thus depressing initial depolarization and preventing propagation and conduction of the nerve impulse. This local anesthetic action produces loss of sensation and motor activity in circumscribed areas of the body close to the injection or application site.

USES Spinal anesthesia and epidural and peripheral nerve block by injection and infiltration methods.

ROUTE & DOSAGE

Spinal Anesthesia

Adult: **SC** 10% solution diluted with 0.9% NaCl at 1 ml/5 s.

Infiltration Anesthesia/ Peripheral Nerve Block

Adult: **SC** 0.25–0.5% solution.

PHARMACOKINETICS Absorption: rapidly absorbed from injection site. **Onset:** 2–5 min. **Duration:** 1 h. **Metabolism:** hydrolyzed by plasma pseudocholinesterases. **Elimination:** 80% of metabolites excreted in urine; half-life: 7.7 min.

CONTRAINDICATIONS & PRECAUTIONS Contraindicated in: known hypersensitivity to procaine or to other drugs of similar chemical structure, to PABA, and to parabens; generalized septicemia, inflammation, or sepsis at proposed injection site; cerebrospinal diseases (e.g., meningitis, syphilis); heart block, hypotension, hypertension; bowel pathology, GI hemorrhage. Safe use in early pregnancy (category C) has not been established. **Cautious use in:** debilitated, elderly, or acutely ill patients; obstetric delivery; increased intraabdominal pressure; known drug allergies and sensitivities, dysrhythmias; shock.

P

ADVERSE/SIDE EFFECTS CNS (excitatory): anxiety, nervousness, dizziness, tinnitus, circumoral paresthesia, blurred vision, tremors, drowsiness, sedation, convulsions, respiratory arrest. **CV:** myocardial depression, arrhythmias including bradycardia (also fetal bradycardia); hypotension. **GI:** nausea, vomiting. **Skin:** cutaneous lesions of delayed onset, urticaria, pruritus, angioneurotic edema, sweating, syncope, anaphylactoid reaction. **Other:** with caudal or epidural anesthesia: urinary retention, fecal or urinary incontinence, loss of perineal sensation and sexual function, slowing of labor and increased incidence of forceps delivery, headache, backache, high or total spinal block. With spinal anesthesia: postspinal headache, arachnoiditis, palsies, spinal nerve paralysis, meningism.

INCOMPATIBILITIES Solution/additive: aminophylline, amobarbital, chlorothiazide, magnesium sulfate, phenobarbital, phenytoin, secobarbital, sodium bicarbonate.

NURSING IMPLICATIONS

Administration

- Reconstitution of solution: To prepare 60 ml of a 0.5% solution (5 mg/ml), dilute 30 ml of 1% solution with 30 ml sterile distilled water. Add 0.5–1 ml epinephrine 1:1000/100 ml anesthetic solution for vasoconstrictive effect (1:200,000–1:100,000).
- Do not use solutions that are cloudy, discolored, or that contain crystals. Discard unused portion of solutions not containing a preservative. Avoid use of solution with preservative for spinal, epidural, or caudal block.
- Injection should be slow with frequent aspirations to avoid inadvertent intravascular administration, which can lead to a systemic reaction.
- When used as spinal anesthetic, procaine is injected into the subarachnoid space, usually in interspace between L2 and L5.
- Store at 10–30C (59–86F). Avoid freezing.

Assessment & Drug Effects

- Reactions during dental procedure are usually mild, transient, and produced by epinephrine added to local anesthetic (headache, palpitation, tachycardia, hypertension, dizziness).
- Procaine with epinephrine should be used with caution in body areas with limited blood supply (fingers, toes, ears, nose). If used, inspect particular area for evidence of reduced perfusion (vasospasm): pale, cold, sensitive skin.
- Hypotension is the most important complication of spinal anesthesia. Risk period is during first 30 min after induction and is intensified by changes in position that promote decreased venous return, or by preexisting hypertension, pregnancy, old age, or hypovolemia.
- Hypersensitivities and anaphylactic reactions are not usually dose related.

Patient & Family Education

- Inform that there will be temporary loss of sensation in the area of the injection.
- Caution patient given drug for dental procedure that hot liquids or foods should not be consumed until sensation returns.

PROCARBAZINE HYDROCHLORIDE

(proe-kar'ba-zeen)

Trade names: Matulane, Natulan ♣

Classifications: ANTINEOPLASTIC; ANTIMETABOLITE

Prototype: Fluorouracil

Pregnancy category: D

ACTIONS/PHARMACODYNAMICS Hydrazine derivative with antimetabolite properties; cell cycle-specific for the S phase of cell division. Precise mechanism of action unknown. Suppresses mitosis at interphase, and causes chromatin derangement. Highly toxic to rapidly proliferating tissue. Has immunosuppressive properties and exhibits MAO inhibition activity. May delay myelosuppression. Reportedly does not affect survival time but may produce remissions of at least 1 mo duration.

USE Adjunct in palliative treatment of Hodgkin's disease. **Unlabeled use:** solid tumors.

ROUTE & DOSAGE

Adjunct for Hodgkin's Disease

Adult: **PO** 2–4 mg/kg/d in single or divided doses for 1 wk, then 4–6 mg/kg/d until WBC <4000/mm^3 or platelets are <100,000/mm^3 or maximum response obtained; drug is then discontinued until bone marrow recovery is satisfactory; treatment is started again at 1–2 mg/kg/d.

Child: **PO** 50 mg/m^2/d in single or divided doses for 1 wk, then 100 mg/m^2/d until WBC is <4000/mm^3 or platelets are <100,000/mm^3 or maximum response obtained; drug is then discontinued until bone marrow recovery is satisfactory; treatment is started again at 50 mg/m^2/d.

PHARMACOKINETICS Absorption: readily absorbed from GI tract. **Peak:** 1 h. **Distribution:** widely distributed with high concentrations in liver, kidneys, intestinal wall, and skin. **Metabolism** metabolized in liver. **Elimination:** half-life: 1 h; excreted in urine.

CONTRAINDICATIONS & PRECAUTIONS Contraindicated in: myelosuppression; alcohol ingestion; foods high in tyramine content; sym-

P

pathomimetic drugs. MAO inhibitors should be discontinued 14 d prior to therapy; tricyclic antidepressants, 7 d before therapy. Safe use during pregnancy (category D) and lactation not established. **Cautious use in:** concomitant administration with CNS depressants; hepatic or kidney impairment; following radiation or chemotherapy before at least 1 mo has elapsed; hepatic and renal impairment; infection; diabetes mellitus.

ADVERSE/SIDE EFFECTS CNS: myalgia, arthralgia, paresthesias, weakness, fatigue, lethargy, drowsiness, neuropathies, mental depression, acute psychosis, hallucinations, dizziness, headache, ataxia, nervousness, insomnia, <u>coma</u>, confusion, seizures. **GI:** *severe nausea and vomiting,* anorexia, stomatitis, dry mouth, dysphagia, diarrhea, constipation, jaundice. **Hematologic:** <u>bone marrow suppression (leukopenia, anemia, thrombocytopenia)</u>, hemolysis, bleeding tendencies. **Infrequent:** apprehension, nightmares, footdrop, decreased reflexes, tremors. **Skin:** dermatitis, pruritus, herpes, hyperpigmentation, flushing, alopecia. **Other:** ascites, *pleural effusion, cough,* hoarseness, hypotension, tachycardia, chills, fever, sweating, gynecomastia, depressed spermatogenesis, atrophy of testes; photosensitivity; <u>intercurrent infections.</u> Rare: edema, retinal hemorrhage, papilledema, altered hearing.

DIAGNOSTIC TEST INTERFERENCE Procarbazine may enhance the effects of ***CNS depressants.*** A disulfiram-like reaction may occur following ingestion of ***alcohol.***

DRUG INTERACTIONS Alcohol, PHENOTHIAZINES, and other **CNS depressants** add to CNS depression; TRICYCLIC ANTIDEPRESSANTS, MAO INHIBITORS, SYMPATHOMIMETICS, **ephedrine, phenylpropanolamine** may precipitate hypertensive crisis, hyperpyrexia; seizures, or death. **Food–drug:** tyramine-containing foods may precipitate hypertensive crisis (see phenelzine sulfate [MAO inhibitor]).

NURSING IMPLICATIONS

Administration

- Toxicity is a serious problem and demands that patient be hospitalized and under close medical and nursing supervision during treatment induction period.
- Store at 15–30C (59–86F). Protect from freezing, moisture, and light.

Assessment & Drug Effects

- Start flow sheet and record baseline BP, weight, temperature, pulse, and I&O ratio and pattern.
- Hematologic status (Hgb, Hct, WBC, differential, reticulocyte, and platelet counts) should be determined initially and at least q3–4d. Hepatic and renal studies (transaminase, alkaline phosphatase, BUN, urinalysis) are also indicated initially and at least weekly during therapy.
- Patient's hematologic status should be monitored carefully for indicators that suggest special nursing interventions and need for dosage adjustment or drug withdrawal.
- As patient approaches nadir of leukopenia (<4000/mm^3), protect patient from exposure to infection and trauma. Alert patient to report any sign of impending infection. Note and report changes in voiding pattern, hematuria, and dysuria (possible signs of urinary tract infection). I&O ratio and temper-

ature should be closely monitored.

- Prompt cessation of therapy is usual with appearance of CNS signs and symptoms (paresthesias, neuropathies, confusion), leukopenia (WBC count <4000/mm^3), thrombocytopenia (platelet count <100,000/mm^3), hypersensitivity reaction, the first small ulceration or persistent spot soreness of oral cavity, diarrhea, and bleeding. Patient should be warned to report promptly any signs and symptoms of toxicity.
- Symptoms of pleural effusion, an allergic reaction to procarbazine (chills, fever, weakness, shortness of breath, productive cough) should be reported promptly. Drug will be discontinued.
- Be alert to signs of hepatic dysfunction: jaundice (yellow skin, sclerae, and soft palate), frothy or dark urine, clay-colored stools.
- Tolerance to nausea and vomiting (most common side effects) usually develops by end of first week of treatment. Doses are kept at a minimum during this time. If vomiting persists, therapy will be interrupted.

Patient & Family Education

- Since procarbazine has MAO inhibitory activity, OTC nose drops, cough medicines, and antiobesity preparations containing sympathomimetic drugs (e.g., ephedrine, amphetamine, epinephrine) and tricyclic antidepressants should be avoided because they may cause hypertensive crises. Warn not to use OTC preparations without physician's approval.
- Intake of foods high in tyramine content should be avoided.
- Warn that ingestion of any form of alcohol may precipitate a disulfiram-type reaction (see Appendix G).
- Instruct to report immediately signs of hemorrhagic tendencies: bleeding into skin and mucosa, epistaxis, hemoptysis, hematemesis, hematuria, melena, ecchymoses, petechiae. Bone marrow depression often occurs 2–8 wk after start of therapy.
- Advise to avoid excessive exposure to the sun because of potential photosensitivity reaction: cover as much skin area as possible with clothing, and use sunscreen lotion (SPF > 12) on all exposed skin surfaces.
- Since drowsiness, dizziness, and blurred vision are possible side effects, warn patient to use caution while driving or performing hazardous tasks until response to drug is known.
- Advise use of contraceptive measures during procarbazine therapy.

P

PROCHLORPERAZINE

(proe-klor-per'a-zeen)

Trade name: Compazine

PROCHLORPERAZINE EDISYLATE

Trade name: Compazine

PROCHLORPERAZINE MALEATE

Trade names: Compazine, Stemetil ♣

Prototype for classifications: GI AGENT; ANTIEMETIC; PSYCHOTHERAPEUTIC; ANTIPSYCHOTIC PHENOTHIAZINE

Pregnancy category: C

ACTIONS/PHARMACODYNAMICS

Phenothiazine derivative with similar actions, contraindications, and interactions as chlorpromazine. Has greater extrapyramidal effects and antiemetic potency but fewer sedative, hypotensive, and anticholinergic effects than chlorpromazine.

USES Management of manifestations of psychotic disorders, of excessive anxiety, tension, and agitation, and to control severe nausea and vomiting.

PHARMACOKINETICS **Absorption:** readily absorbed from GI tract. **Onset:** 30–40 min PO; 60 min PR; 10–20 min IM. **Duration:** 3–4 h PO; 10–12 h sustained release PO; 3–4 h PR; up to 12 h IM. **Distribution:** crosses placenta; distributed into breast milk. **Metabolism:** metabolized in liver. **Elimination:** excreted in urine.

ROUTE & DOSAGE

Severe Nausea, Vomiting, Anxiety, Psychotic Disorders

Adult: **PO** 5–10 mg t.i.d. or q.i.d.; sustained release: 10–15 mg q12h. **IM** 5–10 mg q3–4h up to 40 mg/d. **IV** 2.5–10 mg q6–8h; max 40 mg/d. **PR** 25 mg b.i.d.
Child: **PO** 2.5 mg 1–3 times/d *or* 5 mg b.i.d.; max 15 mg/d. **IM** 0.13 mg/kg q3–4h. **PR** 2.5 mg b.i.d. or t.i.d. up to 20–25 mg/d.

CONTRAINDICATIONS & PRECAUTIONS **Contraindicated in:** hypersensitivity to phenothiazines; bone marrow depression; comatose or severely depressed states; children < 9 kg (20 lb) or 2 y of age; pediatric surgery; short-term vomiting in children or vomiting of unknown etiology; Reye's syndrome or other encephalopathies; history of dyskinetic reactions or epilepsy; (pregnancy category C). **Cautious use in:** patient with previously diagnosed breast cancer, children with acute illness or dehydration.

ADVERSE/SIDE EFFECTS *Drowsiness,* dizziness, hypotension, contact dermatitis, photosensitivity, galactorrhea, amenorrhea, blurred vision, cholestatic jaundice, leukopenia, agranulocytosis, *extrapyramidal reactions (akathisia, dystonia or parkinsonism),* persistent tardive dyskinesia, acute catatonia.

DRUG INTERACTIONS **Alcohol,** CNS DEPRESSANTS increase CNS depression; ANTACIDS, ANTIDIARRHEALS decrease absorption—administer 2 h apart; **phenobarbital** increases metabolism of prochlorperazine; GENERAL ANESTHETICS increase excitation and hypotension; antagonizes antihypertensive action of **guanethidine; phenylpropanolamine** poses possibility of sudden death; TRICYCLIC ANTIDEPRESSANTS intensify hypotensive and anticholinergic effects; decreases seizure threshold—ANTICONVULSANT dosage may need to be increased.

INCOMPATIBILITIES **Solution/additive: aminophylline, amphotericin B, ampicillin, calcium gluceptate, calcium gluconate, cephalothin, chloramphenicol, chlorothiazide, hydrocortisone, methohexital, penicillin G sodium, phenobarbital, sodium bicarbonate, dimenhydrinate, hydromorphone, midazolam, pentobarbital, thiopental.**

NURSING IMPLICATIONS

Administration

- Dosage for elderly, emaciated patients and for children should be advanced slowly.
- Oral concentrate is not to be administered to children.
- Avoid skin contact with oral concentrate or injection solution because of possibility of contact dermatitis.

Common side effect in *italic,* life-threatening effects underlined; generic names in **bold;** drug class in SMALL CAPS

- To ensure stability and palatability of oral concentrate add prescribed dose to 60 ml or more of diluent just prior to administration. Suggested diluents: tomato or fruit juice, carbonated drinks, water, semisolid foods (e.g., puddings, soups).
- IM injection in adults should be made deep into the upper outer quadrant of the buttock. Do not mix IM solution in the same syringe with other agents. Follow agency policy regarding IM injection site for children.
- IV administration: Give direct IV by diluting in D5W, NS, or other compatible diluent to a concentration of 1 mg/ml and give at a maximum rate of 5 mg/min.
- Slight yellowing does not appear to alter potency; however, markedly discolored solutions should be discarded. Protect drug from light; do not freeze. Store at temperature between 15 and 30C (59 and 86F) unless otherwise instructed by manufacturer.

Assessment & Drug Effects

- Postoperative patients who have received prochlorperazine may have depressed cough reflex and should be carefully positioned to prevent aspiration of vomitus.
- Monitor I&O ratio and elimination pattern. Depressed patients frequently cut back on fluid intake and do not seek help for constipation.
- Most elderly and emaciated patients and children, especially those with dehydration or acute illness, appear to be particularly susceptible to extrapyramidal effects. Be alert to onset of symptoms: in early therapy watch for pseudoparkinson's and acute dyskinesia. After 1–2 mo, be alert to akathisia.
- Keep in mind that the antiemetic effect may mask toxicity of other drugs or make it difficult to diagnose conditions with a primary symptom of nausea, such as intestinal obstruction and increased intracranial pressure.
- It has been reported that although patient is not responsive during acute catatonia (side effect), everything that happens during the episode can be recalled. Approach patient accordingly.
- Exposure to high environmental temperature, to sun's rays, or to a high fever associated with serious illness places this patient at risk for heat stroke. Be alert to signs: red, dry, hot skin; full bounding pulse; dilated pupils; dyspnea; confusion; temperature over 40.6C (105F); elevated BP. Inform physician and institute measures to reduce body temperature rapidly.

Patient & Family Education

- Counsel to take drug as prescribed and not to alter dose or schedule. Consult physician before stopping the medication.
- Since drug may impair mental and physical abilities, especially during first few days of therapy, caution patient to avoid hazardous activities such as driving a car until response to drug is known.
- This drug may color urine reddish brown. It also may cause the sun-exposed skin to turn gray-blue.
- Advise to protect skin from direct sun's rays and to use a sunscreen lotion (SPF > 12) to prevent photosensitivity reaction.
- Instruct to withhold dose and report to the physician if the following symptoms persist more than a few hours: tremor, involuntary twitching, exaggerated restlessness. Other reportable symptoms include light-colored stools, changes in vision, sore throat, fever, rash.

PROCYCLIDINE HYDROCHLORIDE

(proe-sye'kli-deen)

Trade names: Kemadrin, Procyclid♣

Classifications: AUTONOMIC NERVOUS SYSTEM AGENT; ANTICHOLINERGIC (PARASYMPATHOLYTIC); ANTIMUSCARINIC; ANTISPASMODIC ANTIPARKINSONISM AGENT

Prototype: Atropine

Pregnancy category: C

ACTIONS/PHARMACODYNAMICS

Centrally acting synthetic anticholinergic agent with actions similar to those of atropine; closely related to trihexyphenidyl.

USES To relieve symptoms of parkinsonism syndrome (postencephalitic, arteriosclerotic, and idiopathic), and drug-induced extrapyramidal symptoms.

ROUTE & DOSAGE

Parkinsonism Symptoms

Adult: **PO** 2.5 mg t.i.d. p.c.; may be gradually increased to 5 mg t.i.d. if tolerated with an additional 5 mg h.s. (max 45–60 mg/d).
Geriatric: **PO** Start with 2.5 mg 1–2 times/d.

PHARMACOKINETICS **Onset:** 35–40 min. **Duration:** 4–6 h.

CONTRAINDICATIONS & PRECAUTIONS **Contraindicated in:** angle-closure glaucoma. Safe use during pregnancy (category C), in nursing mothers, and in children not established. **Cautious use:** hypotension; mental disorders; tachycardia; prostatic hypertrophy.

ADVERSE/SIDE EFFECTS *Dry mouth,* blurred vision, mydriasis, photophobia, palpitation, tachycardia, flushing of skin, decreased sweating, headache, *hypotension,* light-headedness, nausea, vomiting, epigastric distress, dizziness, urinary retention, feeling of muscle weakness, constipation, paralytic ileus, acute suppurative parotitis, skin eruptions; (occasionally): mental confusion, psychotic-like symptoms.

NURSING IMPLICATIONS

Administration

- Side effects may be minimized by administration of drug during or after meals.
- Store in tightly closed containers at 15–30C (59–86F) unless otherwise directed.

Assessment & Drug Effects

- Monitor heart rate and rhythm and BP. Report palpitations, tachycardia, paradoxical bradycardia, or decreasing BP. Dosage adjustment or discontinuation of drug may be indicated.
- Procyclidine is usually more effective in controlling rigidity than tremors. Tremors may temporarily appear to be exaggerated as rigidity is relieved, especially in patients with severe spasticity.
- Drug occasionally causes mental confusion, disorientation, agitation, and psychotic-like symptoms, particularly in elderly patients who have low BP. Observe for and report these symptoms to physician.
- Check for constipation and abdominal distention and provide information for preventing constipation.
- Since dosage is guided by clinical response, observe and record improvement (or lack of it) that accompanies therapy.

Patient & Family Education

- If urinary hesitancy or retention is a problem, advise to void before taking drug.
- Since procyclidine may cause

blurred vision and dizziness, caution to avoid potentially hazardous activities until reaction to drug is known.

- Drug-induced dryness of mouth may be relieved by sugarless gum or hard candy and by frequent rinses with warm water or by increasing noncaloric fluid intake. If these measures fail, a saliva substitute, available OTC, may help (e.g., Orex, Xero-Lube).
- Advise to avoid alcohol and not to take other CNS depressants unless otherwise advised by physician.

PROGESTERONE

(proe-jess′ter-one)

Trade names: Crinone Gel, Gesterol 50, Progestaject, Progestasert, Prometrium

Prototype for classifications: HORMONE; PROGESTIN

Pregnancy category: X

ACTIONS/PHARMACODYNAMICS Steroid hormone synthesized and released by testes, ovary, adrenal cortex, and placenta. Has estrogenic, anabolic, and androgenic activity. Physiologic precursor to estrogens, androgens, and adrenocortical steroids. Transforms endometrium from proliferative to secretory state; suppresses pituitary gonadotropin secretion, thereby blocking follicular maturation and ovulation. Acting with estrogen, promotes mammary gland development without causing lactation and increases body temperature 1F at time of ovulation. Relaxes estrogen-primed myometrium and prohibits spontaneous contraction of uterus. Sudden drop in blood levels of progestin (and estradiol) causes "withdrawal bleeding" from endometrium. Intrauterine placement of progesterone (intrauterine progesterone contraceptive system) hypothetically inhibits sperm capacitation or survival, alters uterine milieu so as to prevent nidation, and suppresses endometrial proliferation (antiestrogenic effect).

USES Secondary amenorrhea, functional uterine bleeding, endometriosis, and premenstrual syndrome. As an intrauterine agent (Progestasert) and in combination with estrogens provides fertility control. Largely supplanted by new progestins, which have longer action and oral effectiveness. Treatment of infertile women with progesterone deficiency.

ROUTE & DOSAGE

Amenorrhea

Adult: **IM** 5–10 mg for 6–8 consecutive days. **PO** 400 mg h.s. × 10 d.

Uterine Bleeding

Adult: **IM** 5–10 mg/d for 6 d.

Premenstrual Syndrome

Adult: **PR** 200–400 mg/d.

Intrauterine Contraceptive

Adult: **Intrauterine** Insert in uterus for 1 y.

PHARMACOKINETICS **Absorption:** rapid absorption from IM site; PO peaks at 3 h. **Metabolism:** extensively metabolized in liver. **Elimination:** half-life: 5 min; excreted primarily in urine; excreted in breast milk.

CONTRAINDICATIONS & PRECAUTIONS **Contraindicated in:** hypersensitivity to progestins, known or suspected breast or genital malignancy; use as a pregnancy test; thrombophlebitis, thromboembolic

P

disorders; cerebral apoplexy (or its history), severely impaired liver function or disease, undiagnosed vaginal bleeding, missed abortion, use during first 4 mo of pregnancy (category X), nursing mother. Progestasert: pregnancy or suspicion of pregnancy. Prometrium (oral): patients with peanut allergy. **Cautious use in:** anemia, diagnostic test for pregnancy; diabetes mellitus, history of psychic depression; persons susceptible to acute intermittent porphyria or with conditions that may be aggravated by fluid retention (asthma, seizure disorders, cardiac or renal function, migraine); impaired liver function, previous ectopic pregnancy, presence or history of salpingitis, venereal disease, unresolved abnormal Pap smear, genital bleeding of unknown etiology, previous pelvic surgery.

ADVERSE/SIDE EFFECTS **CNS:** migraine headache, *dizziness,* lethargy, mental depression, somnolence, insomnia. **CV:** <u>thromboembolic disorders, pulmonary embolism</u>. **Eye:** change in vision, proptosis, diplopia, papilledema, retinal vascular lesions. **GI:** hepatic disease, cholestatic jaundice; *nausea,* vomiting, *abdominal cramps*. **GU:** gynecomastia, galactorrhea, vaginal candidiasis, chloasma, cervical erosion and changes in secretions, *breakthrough bleeding,* dysmenorrhea, amenorrhea, pruritus valvae. **Metabolic:** hyperglycemia, decreased libido, transient increase in sodium and chloride excretion, pyrexia. **Skin:** *acne,* pruritus, allergic rash, photosensitivity, urticaria, hirsutism, alopecia. **Other:** *edema, weight changes;* pain at injection site; fatigue.

DIAGNOSTIC TEST INTERFERENCE Progestins may decrease levels of ***urinary pregnanediol,*** and increase levels of serum alkaline phosphatase, plasma amino acids, urinary nitrogen, and ***coagulation factors VII, VIII, IX*** and ***X.*** They also decrease ***glucose tolerance*** (may cause false-positive ***urine glucose*** tests) and lower ***HDL*** (high-density lipoprotein) levels.

NURSING IMPLICATIONS

Administration

- Immerse vial in warm water momentarily to redissolve crystals and to facilitate aspiration of drug into syringe.
- Inject deeply IM. Injection site may be irritated. Inspect used sites carefully and rotate areas systematically.
- Oral capsules contain peanut oil. Do not give to patients allergic to peanuts.
- Store drug at 15–30C (59–86F) unless otherwise specified by manufacturer. Protect from freezing and light.

Assessment & Drug Effects

- A physical examination with special reference to pelvic organs, breasts, hepatic function, and a Pap test should precede therapy with a progestin and should be performed q6–12mo while patient is taking the drug.
- Baseline data for comparative value about patient's weight, I&O ratio, BP, and pulse should be recorded at onset of progestin therapy. Deviations should be reported promptly.
- Monitor weight. Report a steady gain to physician.
- Progestins can affect endocrine and hepatic function tests. An interval of up to 60 d following cessation of therapy may be necessary before laboratory results can be considered definitive.
- In susceptible patients, progestins reportedly may precipitate attack of acute intermittent porphyria: com-

mon manifestations include severe, colicky abdominal pain, vomiting, distention, diarrhea, constipation.

Patient & Family Education

- Caution to avoid exposure to UV light and prolonged periods of time in the sun. Photosensitivity severity is related to both time of exposure and dose. A phototoxic drug reaction usually looks like an exaggerated sunburn but may also produce acute eczematous or urticarial reactions. The reaction can occur within 5–18 h after exposure to sun and is maximal by 36–72 h.
- Advise use of a sunscreen lotion (SPF > 12) that contains para-aminobenzoic acid (PABA) on exposed skin surfaces whenever patient goes outdoors, even on dark days.
- Advise to inform physician promptly if any of the following occur: sudden severe headache or vomiting, dizziness or fainting, numbness in an arm or leg, pain in calves accompanied by swelling, warmth, and redness; acute chest pain or dyspnea.
- Caution to report promptly unexplained sudden or gradual, partial or complete loss of vision, ptosis, or diplopia. The progestin should be discontinued and appropriate diagnostic and therapeutic measures instituted.
- Instruct a diabetic user of progestin or progestin combination drug to monitor clinical signs of loss of diabetes control. If blood glucose tests become positive or if hypoglycemic symptoms occur, the physician should be consulted.
- Instruct to notify physician if she suspects pregnancy while receiving progestational therapy. She should be apprised of the potential risk to the fetus from exposure to progestin.

Intrauterine Progesterone Contraceptive System (Progestasert)

- During the first 2 mo of Progestasert use, another method of birth control (foam or condom) should be used.
- Advise patient to return to physician within 3 mo of insertion of the system for evaluation of its placement and efficacy; thereafter unless untoward symptoms present, an annual visit for evaluation and replacement should be expected.
- Spotting, cramping, and discomfort during first 3 mo can be relieved by nonnarcotic analgesics.
- Regular cyclic pattern of ovulation continues while Progestasert is in place.
- The menstrual period during Progestasert use is frequently heavier and longer than usual. If increased menstrual bleeding continues, however, patient should consult her physician.
- The Progestasert threads should be checked frequently during first few months and after menstruation (times when expulsion is most likely to occur). If patient cannot feel threads, she should go to physician for an examination and prescription for another method of birth control.
- Warn against pulling on threads for any reason. If the IUD is partially expelled, it should be removed; however, the user should not try to remove it herself nor allow her partner to attempt to do so.
- Instruct to consult with physician if a period is missed and pregnancy is suspected. The device should be removed during pregnancy.
- Fever, acute pelvic pain and tenderness, unusual bleeding, severe cramping are symptoms that indicate infection. Report to the physician for immediate treatment.

- To prevent pregnancy, the system must be replaced 1 y after insertion. Pelvic examination must be done. Pap smear, breast examination, Hct evaluation should be done.

PROMAZINE HYDROCHLORIDE

(proe′ma-zeen)

Trade names: Prozine, Sparine

Classifications: CNS AGENT; PSYCHOTHERAPEUTIC; ANTIPSYCHOTIC PHENOTHIAZINE

Prototype: Chlorpromazine

Pregnancy category: C

ACTIONS/PHARMACODYNAMICS Aliphatic derivative of phenothiazine. Compared with chlorpromazine has weak antipsychotic activity and extrapyramidal effects occur less frequently. Although drug-induced agranulocytosis is rare, it occurs more often than with other phenothiazines.

USES Manifestations of psychotic disorders and for reducing agitation and paranoia associated with alcohol withdrawal.

ROUTE & DOSAGE

Psychotic Disorders

Adult: **PO/IM** 10–200 mg q4–6h up to 1000 mg/d.
Adolescent >12 y: **PO/IM** 10–25 mg q4–6h.

Dementia Behavior

Geriatric: **PO/IM** Start with 25 mg 1–2 times/d, may increase q4–7 d to max of 500 mg/d in divided doses.

CONTRAINDICATIONS & PRECAUTIONS Contraindicated in: hypersensitivity to phenothiazines; myelosuppression; CNS depression; children <12 y of age, Reye's syndrome. Safe use during pregnancy (category C) and by nursing mothers not established. **Cautious use in:** prostatic hypertrophy; cardiovascular or hepatic disease; paralytic ileus; xerostomia; angle closure glaucoma; persons exposed to extremes in temperature or to organophosphorous insecticides; convulsive disorders.

ADVERSE/SIDE EFFECTS *Drowsiness, orthostatic hypotension.* Also, blurred vision, photosensitivity, constipation, epileptic seizures in susceptible individuals, leukopenia, agranulocytosis (rare).

NURSING IMPLICATIONS

Administration

- Oral route should be used whenever possible. Parenteral administration is reserved for acutely disturbed or uncooperative patients or those who cannot tolerate an oral preparation.
- Absorption is inhibited by antacids; therefore administer promazine 1 h before or 2 h after antacid.
- Syrup (10 mg/5ml) or oral concentrate (30 mg/ml) may be prescribed when tablet is unsuitable or refused. Dilute the concentrate immediately before administration with fruit juice, chocolate-flavored drinks, carbonated drinks, or soup (for best taste, 10 ml of diluent for each 25 mg of drug). Avoid coffee or tea ingestion near time of taking oral preparation. Explain dosage and dilution to patient if drug is to be self-administered.
- IM injection is made deep into upper outer quadrant of buttock. Tissue irritation can occur if given SC. Carefully aspirate before injecting drug slowly. Intraarterial injection can cause arterial or arteriolar spasm and consequent

impairment of local circulation. Rotate injection sites.

- Store in light-resistant container at 15–30C (59–86F) unless otherwise directed.

Assessment & Drug Effects

- Incidence of postural hypotension and drowsiness is particularly high after parenteral administration. Monitor BP and pulse before administration and between doses. Keep patient recumbent for about 1 h after dose is given.
- Monitor I&O ratio and bowel elimination pattern. Check for abdominal distension and pain. Encourage adequate fluid intake as prophylaxis for constipation and xerostomia. The depressed patient may not seek help for either symptom or for urinary retention.
- Symptoms suggesting agranulocytosis should be reported promptly (see Appendix G).

Patient & Family Education

- Warn that dizziness or faintness may occur on arising. Advise making all position changes slowly, particularly from recumbent to upright position.
- Warn to avoid alcohol during therapy.
- Promazine may cause contact dermatitis. Caution patient to avoid spilling oral solutions on hands or clothing. Wash exposed skin well with soap and water.
- Promazine may color urine pink to red to reddish brown.
- OTC drugs should be approved by physician during antipsychotic therapy.

PROMETHAZINE HYDROCHLORIDE

(proe-meth'a-zeen)

Trade names: Histantil♣, Pentazine, Phenazine, Phencen, Phenergan, Phenoject-50, Prometh, Prorex, Prothazine, V-Gan

Classifications: GI AGENT; ANTIEMETIC; ANTIVERTIGO AGENT; PHENOTHIAZINE

Prototype: Prochlorperazine

Pregnancy category: C

ACTIONS/PHARMACODYNAMICS

Long-acting derivative of phenothiazine with marked antihistaminic activity and prominent sedative, amnesic, antiemetic, and anti-motion-sickness actions. Unlike other phenothiazine derivatives, it is relatively free of extrapyramidal side effects; however, in high doses it carries same potential for toxicity. In common with other antihistamines, exerts antiserotonin, anticholinergic, and local anesthetic action. Antiemetic action thought to be due to depression of CTZ in medulla.

USES Symptomatic relief of various allergic conditions, to ameliorate and prevent reactions to blood and plasma, and in prophylaxis and treatment of motion sickness, nausea, and vomiting. Preoperative, postoperative, and obstetric sedation and as adjunct to analgesics for control of pain.

ROUTE & DOSAGE

Motion Sickness

Adult: **PO/PR/IM/IV** 25 mg b.i.d.
Child: **PO/PR/IM/IV** 12.5–25 mg b.i.d.

Nausea

Adult: **PO/PR/IM/IV** 12.5–25 mg q4–6h prn.
Child: **PO/PR/IM/IV** 0.25–0.5 mg/kg q4–6h prn.

Allergies

Adult: **PO/PR/IM/IV** 12.5 mg q.i.d. *or* 25 mg h.s.

P

Child: **PO/PR/IM/IV** 6.25–12.5 mg q.i.d. *or* 25 mg h.s.

Sedation

Adult: **PO/PR/IM/IV** 25–50 mg preoperatively or h.s.
Child: **PO/PR/IM/IV** 12.5–25 mg preoperatively or h.s.

PHARMACOKINETICS **Absorption:** readily absorbed from GI tract. **Onset:** 20 min PO/PR/IM; 5 min IV. **Duration:** 2–8 h. **Distribution:** crosses placenta. **Metabolism:** metabolized in liver. **Elimination:** slowly excreted in urine and feces.

CONTRAINDICATIONS & PRECAUTIONS **Contraindicated in:** hypersensitivity to phenothiazines; narrow-angle glaucoma; stenosing peptic ulcer, pyloroduodenal obstruction; prostatic hypertrophy; bladder neck obstruction; epilepsy; bone marrow depression; comatose or severely depressed states; pregnancy (category C), nursing mothers, newborn or premature infants, acutely ill or dehydrated children. **Cautious use in:** impaired hepatic function; cardiovascular disease; asthma; acute or chronic respiratory impairment (particularly in children), hypertension; elderly or debilitated patients.

P

ADVERSE/SIDE EFFECTS **Acute toxicity:** deep sleep, coma, convulsions, cardiorespiratory symptoms, extrapyramidal reactions, nightmares (in children), CNS stimulation, abnormal movements, respiratory depression. Toxic potential as for other phenothiazines. **CNS:** sedation *drowsiness,* confusion, dizziness, disturbed coordination, restlessness, tremors. **CV:** transient mild hypotension or hypertension. **GI:** anorexia, nausea, vomiting, constipation. **Hematologic:** leukopenia, agranulocytosis. **Other:** photosensitivity, irregular respiration, *blurred vision,* urinary retention; *dry mouth,* nose, or throat.

DIAGNOSTIC TEST INTERFERENCE Promethazine may interfere with ***blood grouping*** in ABO system and may produce false results with ***urinary pregnancy tests*** (Gravindex, false-positive; Prepurex and Dap tests, false-negative). Promethazine can cause significant alterations of flare response in ***intradermal allergen tests*** if performed within 4 d of patient's receiving promethazine.

DRUG INTERACTIONS **Alcohol** and other CNS DEPRESSANTS add to CNS depression and anticholinergic effects.

INCOMPATIBILITIES **Solution/additive:** **aminophylline, carbenicillin, cefotetan, chloramphenicol, chlorothiazide, heparin, hydrocortisone, methicillin, methohexital, penicillin G sodium, pentobarbital, phenobarbital, thiopental, diatrizoate, dimenhydrinate, iodipamide, iothalamate, nalbuphine.** **Y-site:** **carbenicillin, cefotetan, heparin, TPN.**

NURSING IMPLICATIONS

Administration

- Administration of oral medication with food, milk, or a full glass of water may minimize GI distress.
- Tablet may be crushed and mixed with water or food before swallowing.
- Oral doses for allergy are generally prescribed before meals and on retiring or as single dose at bedtime.
- Inspect parenteral drug before preparation. Discard if it is darkened or contains precipitate.
- IM injection is made deep into large muscle mass. Aspirate care-

fully before injecting drug. Intraarterial injection can cause arterial or arteriolar spasm, with resultant gangrene. Subcutaneous injection (also contraindicated) can cause chemical irritation and necrosis. Rotate injection sites and observe daily.

- IV administration: IV promethazine in concentrations of 25 mg/ml or less may be given by direct IV undiluted over 2 min. More concentrated preparations should be diluted in NS to yield no more than 25 mg/ml.
- When promethazine is administered by IV infusion, wrap IV bottle with aluminum foil to protect drug from light.
- Promethazine injection is incompatible with a number of drugs, especially those with alkaline pH (see Incompatibilities).
- Store in tight, light-resistant container at 15–30C (59–86F) unless otherwise directed.

Assessment & Drug Effects

- Promethazine sometimes produces marked sedation and dizziness. Side rails and supervision of ambulation may be advisable.
- Antiemetic action may mask symptoms of unrecognized disease and signs of drug overdosage as well as dizziness, vertigo, or tinnitus associated with toxic doses of aspirin or other ototoxic drugs.
- Patients in pain may develop involuntary (athetoid) movements of upper extremities following parenteral administration. These symptoms usually disappear after pain is controlled.
- Respiratory function should be monitored in patients with respiratory problems, particularly children. Promethazine may suppress cough reflex and cause thickening of bronchial secretions.
- Dry mouth may be relieved by frequent rinses with warm water or by increasing noncaloric fluid intake (if allowed) or by sugarless gum or lemon drops. If these measures fail, a saliva substitute may help (e.g., Moi-Stir, Orex, Xero-Lube).

Patient & Family Education

- When administered as prophylaxis against motion sickness, initial dose should be taken 30–60 min before anticipated travel and repeated at 8–12 h intervals if necessary. For duration of journey, repeat dose on arising and again at evening meal.
- Advise ambulatory patient to avoid driving a car or engaging in other activities requiring mental alertness and normal reaction time until response to drug is known.
- Promethazine may cause photosensitivity. Advise to avoid sunlamps or prolonged exposure to sunlight. A sunscreen lotion may be advisable during initial drug therapy.
- Advise not to take OTC medications without physician's approval, and caution against alcohol and other CNS depressants.

PROPAFANONE

(pro-pa′fan-one)

Trade name: Rythmol

Classifications: CARDIOVASCULAR AGENT; ANTIARRHYTHMIC

Prototype: Procainamide

Pregnancy category: C

ACTIONS/PHARMACODYNAMICS

Class IC antiarrhythmic drug with a direct stabilizing action on myocardial membranes. Reduces spontaneous automaticity. Rate of single and multiple PVCs is decreased by

P

appropriate dose and concentration of propafanone. In addition, it suppresses ventricular tachycardia. Propafanone, like other class IC arrhythmics, exerts a negative inotropic effect on the myocardium.

USE Ventricular arrhythmias. **Unlabeled uses:** atrial tachyarrhythmias, reentrant arrhythmias, Wolff–Parkinson–White syndrome.

ROUTE & DOSAGE

Ventricular Arrhythmias
Adult: **PO** 150–300 mg q8h.

PHARMACOKINETICS **Absorption:** readily absorbed from GI tract. **Peak:** 3.5 h. **Distribution:** 97% protein bound, highest concentrations in the lung. Crosses placenta, distributed into breast milk. **Metabolism:** extensively metabolized in the liver. **Elimination:** half-life: 5–8h; 18.5–38% of dose excreted in urine as metabolites.

P

CONTRAINDICATIONS & PRECAUTIONS **Contraindicated in:** uncontrolled CHF, cardiogenic shock, sinoatrial, AV or intraventricular disorders (e.g., sick sinus node syndrome, AV block) without a pacemaker; bradycardia, marked hypotension, bronchospastic disorders; electrolyte imbalances; hypersensitivity to propafanone; non-life-threatening arrhythmias, chronic bronchitis, emphysema, nursing mothers. **Cautious use in:** CHF, AV block; hepatic/renal impairment, elderly patients, pregnancy (category C). Safety and efficacy in children have not been established.

ADVERSE/SIDE EFFECTS **CNS:** *Blurred vision, dizziness,* paresthesias, fatigue, somnolence, vertigo, headache. **CV:** arrhythmias, ventricular tachycardia, hypotension, bundle branch block, AV block, complete heart block, sinus arrest, CHF. **Hematologic** (Rare): leukopenia, granulocytopenia. **GI:** nausea, abdominal discomfort, constipation, vomiting, dry mouth, *taste alterations,* cholestate hepatitis. **Other:** rash.

DRUG INTERACTIONS **Amiodarone, quinidine** increase the levels and toxicity of propafenone. May increase levels and toxicity of TRICYCLIC ANTIDEPRESSANTS, **cyclosporine, digoxin,** BETA BLOCKERS, **theophylline,** and **warfarin** may increase levels of both **propafenone** and **diltiazem. Phenobarbital** decreases levels of propafenone.

NURSING IMPLICATIONS

Administration

- Dosage is usually initiated with 150 mg q8h and may be increased at 3–4 d intervals to a maximum of 300 mg q8h.
- Dosage increments should be more gradual with the elderly or those with previous extensive myocardial damage.
- Dosage reduction should be considered with significant widening of the QRS complex or development of second- or third-degree AV block.
- With severe liver dysfunction, significant dose reduction is warranted.
- Store at room temperature, 15–30C (59–56F), as directed.

Assessment & Drug Effects

- Monitor cardiovascular status frequently (e.g., ECG, holter monitor) to determine effectiveness of drug and development of new or worsened arrhythmias.
- Patients with preexisting CHF should be closely monitored for worsening of this condition. Monitor for digoxin toxicity with con-

current use, because propafanone may increase serum digoxin levels.
- Development of second- or third-degree AV block after initiation of therapy requires dosage reduction or discontinuation of the drug.

Patient & Family Education
- Advise to report any of the following: chest pain, palpitations, blurred or abnormal vision, dyspnea, or signs and symptoms of infection.
- Advise patients on concurrent warfarin therapy of the possible increase in plasma warfarin levels with increased bleeding risk. Instruct patient to report unusual bleeding or bruising.
- Instruct to monitor radial pulse daily and report decreased heart rate or development of an abnormal heart beat.
- Alert elderly or debilitated patients to possibility of developing dizziness and need for caution with ambulation.

PROPANTHELINE BROMIDE
(proe-pan'the-leen)
Trade names: Pro-Banthine, Propanthel ♣
Classifications: ANTISPASMODIC; ANTICHOLINERGIC
Prototype: Atropine
Pregnancy category: C

ACTIONS/PHARMACODYNAMICS Similar to atropine in peripheral effects, contraindications, precautions, and adverse reactions. Potent in antimuscarinic activity and in nondepolarizing ganglionic blocking action. Very high doses block neurotransmission at myoneural junction.

USES Adjunct in treatment of peptic ulcer, irritable bowel syndrome, pancreatitis, ureteral and urinary bladder spasm. Also used prior to radiologic diagnostic procedures to reduce duodenal motility.

ROUTE & DOSAGE

Irritable Bowel Syndrome
Adult: **PO** 15 mg 30 min a.c. and 30 mg h.s. (max 120 mg/d).
Geriatric: **PO** 7.5 mg 2–3 times/d a.c. (max 90 mg/d).

PHARMACOKINETICS **Absorption:** incompletely absorbed from GI tract. **Onset:** 30–45 min. **Duration:** 4–6 h. **Metabolism:** 50% metabolized in GI tract before absorption; 50% metabolized in liver. **Elimination:** half-life: 9 h; excreted primarily in urine; some excreted in bile.

CONTRAINDICATIONS & PRECAUTIONS **Contraindicated in:** pregnancy (category C).

ADVERSE/SIDE EFFECTS *Constipation,* difficult urination, *dry mouth,* blurred vision, mydriasis, increased intraocular pressure, drowsiness, decreased sexual activity.

NURSING IMPLICATIONS

Administration
- Oral preparation is generally administered 30–60 min before meals and at bedtime. Advise the patient not to chew tablet; drug is bitter.
- Sustained-release tablets should not be crushed or chewed. Regular tablets may be crushed and mixed with fluid or food before swallowing.
- If patient is also receiving an antacid (or antidiarrheal agent), propantheline should be taken at least 1 h before or 1 h after the other drug.
- Store dry powder and tablets at 15–30C (59–86F), protected from freezing and moisture.

Assessment & Drug Effects

- Assess bowel sounds, especially in presence of ulcerative colitis, since paralytic ileus may develop, predisposing to toxic megacolon.
- The elderly or debilitated patient may respond to a usual dose with agitation, excitement, confusion, drowsiness. If these symptoms are observed, stop the drug and report to physician.
- Patients with cardiac disease should have periodic checks of BP and heart sounds and rhythm.

Patient & Family Education

- Advise to avoid alcoholic beverages.
- Urinary hesitancy or retention (especially likely to occur in elderly patients) may be avoided by advising patient to void just prior to each dose. Instruct to note daily urinary volume and to report voiding problems to physician.
- Dry mouth may be relieved by frequent rinsing with warm tap water, by sugar-free gum or hard candy. If symptoms persist, report to physician.
- Caution to maintain adequate fluid and high-fiber food intake to prevent constipation.
- Postural hypotension and tachycardia may occur during early therapy. Instruct to make all position changes slowly and to lie down immediately if faintness, weakness, or palpitations occur. Advise the patient to report these symptoms to the physician.
- Caution to avoid potentially hazardous activities such as driving a car or operating machinery until response to drug is known.

P

PROPOFOL

(pro′po-fol)

Trade name: Diprivan

Classifications: CNS AGENT, GENERAL ANESTHESIA; SEDATIVE-HYPNOTIC

Prototype: Thiopental

Pregnancy category: B

ACTIONS/PHARMACODYNAMICS Sedative-hypnotic used in the induction and maintenance of anesthesia or sedation. Rapid onset (40 s) and minimal excitation during induction.

USES Induction and/or maintenance of anesthesia as part of a balanced anethesia technique; conscious sedation in mechanically ventilated patients.

ROUTE & DOSAGE

Induction of Anesthesia

Adult: **IV** 2–2.5 mg/kg q10s until induction onset. Reduce to 1–1.5 mg/kg for elderly and debilitated patients.
Child ≥3 y: **IV** 2.5–3.5 mg/kg over 20–30 s.

Maintenance of Anesthesia

Adult: **IV** 100–200 µg/kg/min. Reduce to 50–100 µg/kg/min for elderly and debilitated patients.
Child *≥3 y:* **IV** 125–300 µg/kg/min.

Conscious Sedation

Adult: **IV** 5 µg/kg/min for at least 5 min. May increase by 5–10 µg/kg/min q5–10 min until desired level of sedation is achieved. May need maintenance rate of 5–50 µg/ kg/min.

PHARMACOKINETICS Onset: 9–36 s. **Duration:** 6–10 min. **Distribution:** highly lipophilic, crosses placenta, excreted in breast milk. **Metabolism:** extensively metabolized in the liver.

Elimination: half-life: 5–12 h; Approximately 88% of the dose is recovered in the urine as metabolites.

CONTRAINDICATIONS & PRECAUTIONS **Contraindicated in:** hypersensitivity to propofol or propofol emulsion, which contains soybean oil and egg phosphatide; obstetrical procedures, nursing mothers; patients with increased intracranial pressure and/or impaired cerebral circulation; pregnancy (category B). **Cautious use in:** patients with severe cardiac or respiratory disorders or history of epilepsy or seizures.

ADVERSE/SIDE EFFECTS **CNS:** headache, dizziness, *twitching, bucking, jerking, thrashing, clonic/myoclonic movements*. Decreased intraocular pressure. **CV:** hypotension, ventricular asystole (rare), vomiting, abdominal cramping. **Respiratory:** cough, hiccups, apnea. **Other:** pain at injection site.

DRUG INTERACTIONS Concurrent continuous infusions of propofol and **alfentanil** produce higher plasma levels of alfentanil than expected. CNS DEPRESSANTS cause additive CNS depression.

DIAGNOSTIC TEST INTERFERENCE Propofol produces a temporary reduction in serum **cortisol** levels. However, propofol does not seem to inhibit adrenal responsiveness to **ACTH.**

NURSING IMPLICATIONS

Administration

- Strict aseptic technique must be used in preparing propofol for injection, because the drug emulsion will support rapid growth of microorganisms.
- Inspect ampuls and vials of the drug for particulate matter and discoloration. Discard if either is noted.
- Shake well before use. Inspect for separation of the emulsion. Do not use if there is evidence of separation of phases of the emulsion.
- Propofol must not be administered through filters with a pore size less than 5 μm.
- When drawing or administering propofol from vials, a sterile vent spike should be used.
- Propofol must be drawn up into a sterile syringe immediately after ampuls or vials are opened. Drug administration should begin immediately and be completed within 6 h.
- When propofol is given IV directly from the vial, administration should begin immediately following spiking the vial and be completed within 6 h.
- Injection site pain may be decreased by dilution with a compatible solution, such as 5% dextrose injection or lactated Ringer's injection.
- Store unopened between 4C (40F) and 22C (72F). Refrigeration is not recommended. Protect from light.

Assessment & Drug Effects

- Monitor hemodynamic status and assess for dose-related hypotension.
- Tonic-clonic seizures have occurred following general anesthesia with propafol. Seizure precautions may be warranted.
- Be alert to the potential for drug induced excitation (e.g., twitching, tremor, hyperclonus) and take appropriate safety measures.
- Pain at the injection site is quite common especially when small veins are used. Comfort measures may be warranted.

PROPOXYPHENE HYDROCHLORIDE

(proe-pox'i-feen)

Trade names: 642♣, Darvon, Novopropoxyn♣

PROPOXYPHENE NAPSYLATE

Trade name: Darvon-N

Classifications: CNS AGENT; NARCOTIC (OPIATE) AGONIST ANALGESIC

Prototype: Morphine

Pregnancy category: C (D for prolonged use)

Controlled substance: Schedule IV

ACTIONS/PHARMACODYNAMICS Centrally acting opioid structurally related to methadone. Analgesic potency about 1/2–2/3 that of codeine. Unlike codeine, propoxyphene has little or no antitussive effect. The hydrochloride is freely soluble in water and is more rapidly and completely absorbed than the napsylate, which is only slightly water soluble. Lower incidence of GI side effects reported with the napsylate salt.

P

USE Relief of mild to moderate pain. **Unlabeled use:** to suppress narcotic withdrawal symptoms.

ROUTE & DOSAGE

100 mg napsylate = 65 mg HCl

Mild to Moderate Pain

Adult: **PO** 65 mg HCl or 100 mg napsylate q4h prn (max: 390 mg HCl/d, 600 mg napsylate/d).

PHARMACOKINETICS Absorption: readily absorbed from upper part of small intestine. **Onset:** 15–60 min. **Peak:** 2–3 h. **Duration:** 4–6 h. **Distribution:** crosses placenta; distributed into breast milk. **Metabolism:** metabolized in liver. **Elimination:** half-life: 6–12 h, 30–36 h for metabolite; excreted in urine.

CONTRAINDICATIONS & PRECAUTIONS Contraindicated in: hypersensitivity to drug; suicidal individuals; alcoholism; dependence on opiates. Safe use during pregnancy (category C [D for prolonged use]) and in children not established. **Cautious use in:** renal or hepatic disease.

ADVERSE/SIDE EFFECTS CNS: dizziness, light-headedness, *drowsiness,* sedation, unusual fatigue or weakness, restlessness, tremor, euphoria, dysphoria, headache, paradoxic excitement. **GI:** nausea, vomiting, abdominal pain, constipation. **Other:** minor visual disturbances, headache, skin eruptions (hypersensitivity), hypoglycemia (patients with impaired renal function); liver dysfunction. **Overdosage:** mental confusion, toxic psychosis, <u>coma</u>, convulsions, <u>respiratory depression</u>, pulmonary edema, acidosis, pinpoint pupils (dilate with advancing hypoxia), <u>circulatory collapse</u>, ECG abnormalities, nephrogenic diabetes insipidus.

DRUG INTERACTIONS Alcohol and other CNS DEPRESSANTS add to CNS depression—fatalities reported with alcohol; may increase hypoprothrombinemic effects of **warfarin;** may increase **carbamazepine** toxicity through decreased metabolism; **orphenadrine** increases CNS stimulation, anxiety, tremors, confusion.

NURSING IMPLICATIONS

Administration

- Capsules may be emptied and contents mixed with water or food before they are swallowed.
- Absorption may be somewhat de-

layed by presence of food in stomach.

- Store at 15–30C (59–86F) unless otherwise directed.

Assessment & Drug Effects

- Evaluate patient's need for continued use of this drug. Propoxyphene is commonly abused.
- Overdose: Fatalities occur commonly within first hour following overdosage; therefore, prompt action is required.
- Effectiveness of propoxyphene may be reduced in smokers. Smoking induces liver enzymes responsible for metabolizing propoxyphene.
- When propoxyphene is included in combination products, precautions relative to each drug ingredient must be considered.
- Tremulousness, restlessness ("speeding"), and mild euphoria occur frequently.
- Dizziness, light-headedness, drowsiness, nausea, and vomiting appear to be more prominent in the ambulatory patient. Symptoms may be relieved if patient lies down.

Patient & Family Education

- Caution ambulatory patients not to drive a car and to avoid other potentially hazardous activities.
- Caution not to exceed recommended dose and to avoid alcohol and other CNS depressants.
- Tolerance and physical and psychic dependence of the morphine type can occur with excessive use.

PROPRANOLOL HYDROCHLORIDE

(proe-pran'oh-lole)

Trade names: Apo-Propranolol ♣, Detensol ♣, Inderal, Inderal LA, Novopranol ♣

Prototype for classifications: AUTONOMIC NERVOUS SYSTEM AGENT; BETA-ADRENERGIC ANTAGONIST (BLOCKING AGENT, SYMPATHOLYTIC); ANTIHYPERTENSIVE

Pregnancy category: C

ACTIONS/PHARMACODYNAMICS

Nonselective beta blocker of both cardiac and bronchial adrenoreceptors which competes with epinephrine and norepinephrine for available beta-receptor sites. Blocks cardiac effects of beta-adrenergic stimulation; as a result, reduces heart rate, myocardial irritability (class II antiarrhythmic) and force of contraction, depresses automaticity of sinus node and ectopic pacemaker, and decreases AV and intraventricular conduction velocity. In higher doses, exerts direct quinidine-like effects which depress cardiac function. Lowers both supine and standing blood pressures in hypertensive patients. Hypotensive effect is associated with decreased cardiac output, suppressed renin activity, as well as beta-blockade. Also decreases platelet aggregability. Mechanism of antimigraine action unknown but thought to be related to inhibition of cerebral vasodilation and arteriolar spasms.

USES Management of cardiac arrhythmias, myocardial infarction, tachyarrhythmias associated with digitalis intoxication, anesthesia, and thyrotoxicosis, hypertrophic subaortic stenosis, angina pectoris due to coronary atherosclerosis, pheochromocytoma, hereditary essential tremor; also treatment of hypertension alone, but generally with a thiazide or other antihypertensive as step 1 agent. Available in fixed-dose combination with **hydrochlorothiazide** (Inderide). **Unlabeled uses:**

P

anxiety states, migraine prophylaxis, essential tremors, schizophrenia, tardive dyskinesia, acute panic symptoms (e.g., stage fright), recurrent GI bleeding in cirrhotic patients, treatment of aggression and rage.

ROUTE & DOSAGE

Hypertension

Adult: **PO** 40 mg b.i.d.; usually need 160–480 mg/d in divided doses.
Child: **PO** 1 mg/kg/d in 2 divided doses (1–5 mg/kg/d).
Neonate: **PO** 0.25 mg/kg q6–8h; may increase to max of 5 mg/kg/d. **IV** 0.01 mg/kg slow IV push over 10 min q6–8h prn (max 0.15 mg/kg q6–8h).

Angina

Adult: **PO** 10–20 mg b.i.d. or t.i.d.; may need 160–320 mg/d in divided doses.

Arrhythmias

Adult: **PO** 10–30 mg t.i.d. or q.i.d. **IV** 0.5–3 mg q4h prn.
Child: **PO** 1–4 mg/kg/d in 4 divided doses (max 16 mg/kg/ d). **IV** 10–20 μg/kg/min over 10 min.

Acute MI

Adult: **PO** 180–240 mg/d in divided doses.

Migraine Prophylaxis

Adult: **PO** 80 mg/d in divided doses; may need 160–240 mg/d.

PHARMACOKINETICS **Absorption:** completely absorbed from GI tract but undergoes extensive first-pass metabolism. **Peak:** 60–90 min immediate release; 6 h sustained release; 5 min IV. **Distribution:** widely distributed including CNS, placenta, and breast milk. **Metabolism:** almost completely metabolized in liver. **Elimination:** half-life: 2.3 h; 90–95% excreted in urine as metabolites; 1–4% excreted in feces.

CONTRAINDICATIONS & PRECAUTIONS **Contraindicated in:** greater than first-degree heart block; CHF, right ventricular failure secondary to pulmonary hypertension; sinus bradycardia, cardiogenic shock, significant aortic or mitral valvular disease; bronchial asthma or bronchospasm, severe COPD, allergic rhinitis during pollen season; concurrent use with adrenergic-augmenting psychotropic drugs or within 2 wk of MAO inhibition therapy. Safe use during pregnancy (category C) and in nursing mothers not established. **Cautious use in:** peripheral arterial insufficiency; history of systemic insect sting reaction; patients prone to nonallergenic bronchospasm (e.g., chronic bronchitis, emphysema); major surgery; renal or hepatic impairment; diabetes mellitus; patients prone to hypoglycemia; myasthenia gravis; Wolff-Parkinson-White syndrome.

ADVERSE/SIDE EFFECTS **Allergic:** erythematous, psoriasis-like eruptions; pruritus; fever; pharyngitis; respiratory distress. **CNS:** drug-induced psychosis, sleep disturbances, depression, *confusion,* agitation, giddiness, light-headedness, *fatigue,* vertigo, syncope, weakness, *drowsiness,* insomnia, vivid dreams, visual hallucinations, delusions, reversible organic brain syndrome. **CV:** palpitation, profound *bradycardia,* AV heart block, cardiac standstill, hypotension, angina pectoris, tachyarrhythmia, acute CHF, peripheral arterial insufficiency resembling Raynaud's disease, myotonia, paresthesia of hands. **Eye/ear:** dry eyes (gritty sensation), visual disturbances, conjunctivitis, tinnitus, hearing loss, nasal stuffiness. **GI:** dry mouth, cheilostomatitis, nausea, vomiting, heartburn, diarrhea, constipation, flatulence, abdominal cramps, mesenteric arterial thrombosis, ischemic colitis. **Hematologic:** transient eosinophilia, thrombocytopenic or nonthrombocytopenic purpura, agranulocytosis, hypoglycemia, hyperglycemia, hypocalcemia (patients with hyperthyroidism). **Respiratory:** dyspnea, laryngospasm, bronchospasm. **Skin:** reversible alopecia, hyperkeratoses of scalp, palms, feet; nail changes, dry skin. **Other:** pancreatitis, weight gain, impotence or decreased libido, LE-like reaction, cold extremities, leg fatigue, arthralgia.

DIAGNOSTIC TEST INTERFERENCE

BETA-ADRENERGIC BLOCKERS may produce false-negative test results in exercise tolerance ECG tests, and elevations in ***serum potassium, peripheral platelet count, serum uric acid, serum transaminase, alkaline phosphatase, lactate dehydrogenase, serum creatinine, BUN***, and an increase or decrease in ***blood glucose*** levels in diabetic patients.

DRUG INTERACTIONS

PHENOTHIAZINES have additive hypotensive effects. BETA-ADRENERGIC AGONISTS (e.g., **albuterol**) antagonize effects. **Atropine** and TRICYCLIC ANTIDEPRESSANTS block bradycardia. DIURETICS and other HYPOTENSIVE AGENTS increase hypotension. High doses of **tubocurarine** may potentiate neuromuscular blockade. **Cimetidine** decreases clearance, increases effects. ANTACIDS may decrease absorption.

NURSING IMPLICATIONS

Administration

- Manufacturer recommends giving oral propranolol before meals and at bedtime. Food enhances bioavailability of propranolol. Advise patient to be consistent with regard to taking propranolol with food or on an empty stomach to minimize variations in absorption.
- Tablet may be crushed before administration and taken with fluid of patient's choice.
- Retitration may be necessary when patient is switched from Inderal to Inderal LA (sustained-release capsule). It is not a simple mg-for-mg substitution. Blood pressure monitoring until drug effectiveness is demonstrated will be necessary.
- IV administration: For direct IV, give each 1 mg over 1 min either undiluted or diluted in 10 ml of 5% dextrose. For intermittent infusion, further dilute in 50 ml of normal saline solution and give over 15–20 min.
- IV administration to neonates: Verify correct IV concentration and rate of infusion with physician.
- When propranolol is to be discontinued, dosage is reduced gradually over a period of 1–2 wk and patient is closely monitored.
- Preserve in tightly closed, light-resistant containers at 15–30C (59–86F).

Assessment & Drug Effects

- Take apical pulse and BP before administering drug.
- Withhold drug if heart rate < 60 bpm or systolic BP ≤ 90 mm Hg.
- Careful medical history and physical examination are essential to rule out allergies, asthma, and other obstructive pulmonary disease. Propranolol can cause bronchiolar constriction even in normal subjects.
- Apical pulse, respiration, BP, and circulation to extremities should be closely monitored throughout

P

period of dosage adjustment. Consult physician regarding acceptable parameters.

- For patients being treated for hypertension, checking blood pressure near end of dosage interval or before administration of next dose is a way of evaluating if control is adequate or whether more frequent dosage intervals are indicated.
- Bradycardia is the most common adverse cardiac effect especially in patients with digitalis intoxication and Wolff-Parkinson-White syndrome.
- When propranolol is administered IV, ECG, BP, and pulmonary wedge pressure must be carefully monitored. Reduction in sympathetic stimulation caused by beta-blocking action can result in cardiac standstill.
- Adverse reactions generally occur most frequently following IV administration; however, incidence is also high following oral use in the elderly and in patients with impaired renal function. Reactions may or may not be dose related and commonly occur soon after therapy is initiated.
- I&O ratio and daily weight are significant indexes for detecting fluid retention and developing heart failure.
- Plasma volume may increase with consequent risk of CHF if dietary sodium is not restricted in patients receiving propranolol without concomitant diuretic therapy. Consult physician regarding allowable salt intake.
- In patients taking propranolol for angina pectoris, exercise performance studies and ECGs are recommended before therapy to establish baseline data, and during therapy to determine dosage requirements and need to continue treatment. Therapy is not continued unless there is reduced pain and increased work capacity.
- Fasting for more than 12 h may induce hypoglycemic effects fostered by propranolol.
- Caution to avoid prolonged exposure of extremities to cold. If patient complains of cold, painful, or tender feet or hands, examine them carefully for evidence of impaired circulation. Peripheral pulses may still be present even though circulation is impaired.
- When propranolol is given for prolonged periods, periodic determinations should be made of hematologic, renal, hepatic, and cardiac function.

Patient & Family Education

- Inform patient receiving propranolol at home about usual pulse rate and instruct to take radial pulse before each dose. Advise to report to physician if it is slower than base level or becomes irregular. (Consult physician for parameters.)
- Propranolol suppresses clinical signs of hypoglycemia (e.g., BP changes, increased pulse rate) and may prolong hypoglycemia. Alert to other signs of possible hypoglycemia not affected by propranolol such as excessive sweating, hunger, fatigue, inability to concentrate. Instruct to report these easily overlooked and tolerated symptoms.
- Stress importance of compliance and warn not to alter established regimen, i.e., not to omit, increase, or decrease dosage or change dosage interval.
- Abrupt discontinuation of propranolol can precipitate withdrawal syndrome: tremulousness, sweating, severe headache, malaise, palpitation, rebound hypertension, MI, and life-threatening arrhyth-

P

mias (in patients with angina pectoris).

- Caution normotensive patients on prolonged therapy that propranolol may cause mild hypotension (experienced as dizziness or lightheadedness). Advise to make position changes slowly and to avoid prolonged standing and to notify physician if these symptoms persist.
- Since propranolol may cause dizziness and light-headedness, caution to avoid driving and other potentially hazardous activities until reaction to drug is known.
- Smoking increases hepatic metabolism of propranolol, leading to unpredictable or diminished drug effects. Advise to stop smoking; but if it continues, more frequent monitoring for clinical effects of the drug is indicated.
- Advise to consult physician before self-medicating with OTC drugs.
- Instruct to inform dentist, surgeon, or ophthalmologist (propranolol lowers normal and elevated intraocular pressure) that he or she is taking propranolol.

PROPYLTHIOURACIL (PTU)

(proe-pill-thye-oh-yoor'a-sill)

Trade name: Propyl-Thyracil ♣

Prototype for classifications: SYNTHETIC HORMONE; ANTITHYROID AGENT

Pregnancy category: D

ACTIONS/PHARMACODYNAMICS Interferes with organification of iodine and blocks synthesis of thyroxine (T_4) and triiodothyronine (T_3). Does not interfere with release and utilization of stored thyroid; thus antithyroid action is delayed days and weeks until preformed T_3 and T_4 are degraded. Drug-induced hormone reduction results in compensatory release of thyrotropin (TSH), which causes marked hyperplasia and vascularization of thyroid gland. With good adherence to drug regimen, chemical euthyroidism can be achieved 6–12 wk after start of thioamide therapy.

USES Hyperthyroidism, iodine-induced thyrotoxicosis, and hyperthyroidism associated with thyroiditis; to establish euthyroidism prior to surgery or radioactive iodine treatment; palliative control of toxic nodular goiter.

ROUTE & DOSAGE

Hyperthyroidism

Adult: **PO** 300–450 mg/d divided q8h; *may* need 600–1200 mg/d initially.
Geriatric: **PO** 150–300 mg/d divided q8h.
Child: **PO** *>10 y,* 150–300 mg/ d or 150 mg/m2/d; *6–10 y,* 50–150 mg/d. *Neonates:* 5–10 mg/kg/d.

Thyrotoxic Crisis

Adult: **PO** 200 mg q4–6h until full control achieved.

PHARMACOKINETICS **Absorption:** rapidly absorbed from GI tract. **Peak:** 1–1.5 h. **Distribution:** appears to concentrate in thyroid gland; crosses placenta; some distribution into breast milk. **Metabolism:** rapidly metabolized to inactive metabolites. **Elimination:** half-life: 1–2 h; 35% excreted in urine within 24 h.

CONTRAINDICATIONS & PRECAUTIONS **Contraindicated in:** last trimester of pregnancy (category D), nursing mothers, concurrent administration of sulfonamides or coal tar derivatives such as aminopyrine or antipyrine. **Cautious use in:** infection;

P

concomitant administration of anticoagulants or other drugs known to cause agranulocytosis; bone marrow depression; impaired hepatic function.

ADVERSE/SIDE EFFECTS CNS: paresthesias, headache, vertigo, drowsiness, neuritis, ototoxicity (rare). **GI:** nausea, vomiting, diarrhea, dyspepsia, loss of taste, sialoadenitis, hepatitis. **Hematologic:** myelosuppression, lymphadenopathy, periarteritis, hypoprothrombinemia, thrombocytopenia, leukopenia, agranulocytosis. **Hypothyroidism** (goitrogenic): enlarged thyroid, reduced GI motility, periorbital edema, puffy hands and feet, bradycardia, cool and pale skin, worsening of ophthalmopathy, sleepiness, fatigue, mental depression, dizziness, vertigo, sensitivity to cold, paresthesias, nocturnal muscle cramps, changes in menstrual periods, unusual weight gain. **Skin:** skin rash, urticaria, pruritus, hyperpigmentation, lightening of hair color, abnormal hair loss. **Other:** drug fever, lupus-like syndrome, arthralgia, myalgia, hypersensitivity vasculitis.

P

DIAGNOSTIC TEST INTERFERENCE Propylthiouracil may elevate ***prothrombin time*** and serum ***alkaline phosphatase, AST, ALT*** levels.

NURSING IMPLICATIONS

Administration

- Administer PTU at the same time each day with relation to meals. Food may alter drug response by changing absorption rate.
- If drug is being used to improve thyroid state before radioactive iodine (RAI) treatment, PTU should be discontinued 3 or 4 d before treatment to prevent interference with RAI uptake. PTU therapy may be resumed if necessary 3–5 d after the RAI administration.
- Store drug in light-resistant container at 15–30C (59–86F).

Assessment & Drug Effects

- About 10% of patients with hyperthyroidism have leukopenia <4000 cells/mm^3 and relative granulopenia.
- Objective signs of clinical response to PTU (usually within 2 or 3 wk): significant weight gain, reduced pulse rate, reduced serum T_4.
- When thyroid gland is greatly enlarged, satisfactory euthyroid state may be delayed for several months.
- Long-term PTU therapy is usually monitored by follow-up examinations and hematologic studies q2–3mo. As soon as patient is euthyroid, thyroid hormone (especially T_3) may be added to regimen to prevent goitrogenic-induced hypothyroidism and to suppress TSH production.
- Be alert to signs of hypoprothrombinemia: ecchymoses, purpura, petechiae, unexplained bleeding. Warn ambulatory patients to report these signs promptly.
- Important diagnostic signs of excess dosage: contraction of a muscle bundle when pricked, mental depression, hard and nonpitting edema, and need for high thermostat setting and extra blankets in winter (cold intolerance).
- Urticaria may occur (3–7% of patients) during weeks 2 to 8 of treatment. Switching to another thioamide is usual if rash is severe.

Patient & Family Education

- Generally, duration of therapy covers a period of 6 mo to several years, followed by remission in 25% of patients. Medication is then stopped in the hope that natural remission will occur.
- If surgery fails to render patient euthyroid, PTU treatment may be reinstituted.

- To prevent hypothyroidism in mother, thyroid may be given concomitantly with PTU throughout pregnancy and after delivery with little effect on fetus.
- Postpartum patients receiving PTU should not nurse their babies. Exacerbation of hyperthyroidism 3–4 mo postpartum in the mother is common; PTU therapy can be reinstituted.
- Advise to report severe skin rash or swelling of cervical lymph nodes. Therapy may be discontinued.
- Warn to report sore throat, fever, and rash immediately (most apt to occur in first few months of treatment). Drug will be discontinued and hematologic studies initiated. If agranulocytosis is diagnosed, patient may be given broad-spectrum antibiotics and placed on reverse isolation.
- Advise to avoid use of OTC drugs for asthma, coryza, or cough treatment without checking with the physician. Iodides sometimes included in such preparations are contraindicated.
- Teach how to take pulse accurately. Advise daily check.
- Clinical response is monitored through changes in weight and pulse. Advise to chart weight 2 or 3 times weekly. Continued tachycardia, diarrhea, fever, irritability, listlessness, vomiting, weakness, should be reported as signs of inadequate therapy or thyrotoxicosis.
- Instruct patient in remission to continue monitoring and recording weight and pulse rate. Patient should report onset of tremor, anxiety state, gradual ascending pulse rate, and loss of weight to the physician (signs of hormone deficiency).
- Urge not to alter drug regimen: not to increase, decrease, or omit doses nor change administration intervals.
- Check with physician about use of iodized salt and inclusion of seafood in the diet.

PROTAMINE SULFATE

(proe′ta-meen)

Classification: ANTIDOTE

Pregnancy category: C

ACTIONS/PHARMACODYNAMICS Purified mixture of simple, low-molecular-weight proteins obtained from sperm or testes of suitable fish species. When used alone, has anticoagulant effect. Because it is strongly basic, protamine combines with strongly acidic heparin to produce a stable complex, and thus anticoagulant effect of both drugs is neutralized.

USES Antidote for heparin calcium or heparin sodium overdosage (after heparin has been discontinued). **Unlabeled use:** antidote for heparin administration during extracorporeal circulation.

P

ROUTE & DOSAGE

Antidote for Heparin Overdose

Adult/Child: **IV** Each milligram of protamine will neutralize 90 U of beef-lung heparin, 115 U of intestinal mucosa–derived heparin, and 100 U of calcium heparin; calculate approximate dose and give the first 25–50 mg by slow IV push and the rest by continuous infusion over 8–16 h.

PHARMACOKINETICS **Onset:** 5 min. **Duration:** 2 h.

CONTRAINDICATIONS & PRECAUTIONS **Contraindicated in:** hemorrhage not induced by heparin overdosage; pregnancy (category C). **Cautious use in:** cardiovascular disease, history of allergy to fish, vasectomized or infertile males, patients who have received protamine-containing insulin.

ADVERSE/SIDE EFFECTS *Abrupt drop in BP* (with rapid IV infusion), bradycardia, dyspnea, nausea, vomiting, lassitude; transient flushing and feeling of warmth. **Bleeding:** protamine overdose or "heparin rebound" (hyperheparinemia). **Hypersensitivity reactions:** urticaria, angioedema, pulmonary edema, anaphylaxis.

NURSING IMPLICATIONS

Administration

- Since protamine has a longer half-life than heparin and also has some anticoagulant effect of its own, dose must be carefully titrated to prevent excess anticoagulation.
- Reconstitute each 50 mg with 5 ml of sterile water for injection. Shake until dissolved. May be given by direct IV over 1–3 min without further dilution.
- Reconstituted solution may be further diluted in NS or D5W and infused at a rate not to exceed 50 mg over 10 min.
- IV administration to infants, children: Verify correct IV concentration and rate of infusion with physician.
- Protamine sulfate injection should be stored at 2–8C (36–46F); protamine powder for injection and reconstituted solution at 15–30C (59–86F). Avoid freezing. Solutions are stable for 72 h at this temperature.

Assessment & Drug Effects

- Protamine is not used if only minor bleeding occurs during heparin therapy because withdrawal of heparin will usually correct minor bleeding within a few hours.
- Monitor BP and pulse q15–30min, or more often if indicated. Continue for at least 2–3 h after each dose, or longer as dictated by patient's condition. Be prepared to treat patient for shock as well as hemorrhage.
- The effect of protamine in neutralizing heparin is monitored by APTT or ACT values. Coagulation tests are usually performed 5–15 min after administration of protamine, and again in 2–8 h if desirable.
- Patients undergoing extracorporeal dialysis or patients who have had cardiac surgery must be observed carefully for bleeding (heparin rebound). Even with apparent adequate neutralization of heparin by protamine, bleeding may occur 30 min to 18 h after surgery. Monitor vital signs closely. Additional protamine may be required in these patients.

PROTRIPTYLINE HYDROCHLORIDE

(proe-trip'te-leen)

Trade names: Triptil ♣, Vivactil

Classifications: CNS AGENT; PSYCHOTHERAPEUTIC; TRICYCLIC ANTIDEPRESSANT

Prototype: Imipramine

Pregnancy category: C

ACTIONS/PHARMACODYNAMICS Tricyclic antidepressant (TCA) with more rapid onset of action than imipramine. Has little if any sedative properties characteristic of most other TCAs but causes tachycardia, CNS stimulation, and strong anticholinergic activity; orthostatic hypotension occurs frequently. Actions, limitations, and interactions are similar to those of imipramine.

USES Symptomatic treatment of endogenous depression in patient under close medical supervision. Particularly effective for depression manifested by psychomotor retardation, apathy, and fatigue.

ROUTE & DOSAGE

Antidepressant

Adult: **PO** 15–40 mg/d in 3–4 divided doses (max 60 mg/d).
Adolescent: **PO** 15 mg/d in divided doses.

PHARMACOKINETICS **Absorption:** rapidly absorbed from GI tract. **Peak levels:** 24–30 h. **Distribution:** crosses placenta; distributed into breast milk. **Metabolism:** metabolized in liver. **Elimination:** half-life: 54–98 h; primarily excreted in urine.

CONTRAINDICATIONS & PRECAUTIONS **Contraindicated in:** use in children; concurrent use of MAO inhibitors; during acute recovery phase following MI; pregnancy (category C). **Cautious use in:** hepatic, cardiovascular, or renal dysfunction; diabetes mellitus; hyperthyroidism; patients with insomnia.

ADVERSE/SIDE EFFECTS **Allergic:** photosensitivity, edema (general or of face and tongue). **Anticholinergic:** *xerostomia,* blurred vision, *constipation,* paralytic ileus, *urinary retention,* confusional states. **CNS:** insomnia, headache, confusion. **CV:** change in heat or cold tolerance; *orthostatic hypotension, tachycardia.*

DRUG INTERACTIONS May decrease some response to ANTIHYPERTENSIVES; CNS DEPRESSANTS, **alcohol,** HYPNOTICS, BARBITURATES, SEDATIVES potentiate CNS depression; ORAL ANTICOAGULANTS may increase hypoprothrombinemic effects; **ethchlorvynol** causes transient delirium; **levodopa,** SYMPATHOMIMETICS (e.g., **epinephrine, norepinephrine**) increase possibility of sympathetic hyperactivity with hypertension and hyperpyrexia; MAO INHIBITORS present possibility of severe reactions—toxic psychosis, cardiovascular instability; **methylphenidiate** increases plasma TCA levels; THYROID DRUGS may increase possibility of arrhythmias; **cimetidine** may increase plasma TCA levels.

NURSING IMPLICATIONS

Administration

- Tablet may be crushed before administration and taken with fluid or mixed with food.
- Increase in dosage should be made in the morning dose to prevent sleep interference and because this TCA has psychic energizing action.
- Last dose of day should be taken no later than midafternoon; insomnia rather than drowsiness is a frequent side effect.
- To reduce possibility of relapse, maintenance therapy is generally continued at least 3 mo after satisfactory improvement is noted.
- Store drug in tightly closed container at 15–30C (59–86F) unless otherwise directed.

Assessment & Drug Effects

- Onset of initial effect characterized by increased activity and energy is fairly rapid, usually within 1 wk after therapy is initiated.
- If the elderly patient has a dose higher than 20 mg/d, monitor CV system responses closely.
- Maximum antidepressant effect may not occur for 2 wk or more after therapy begins.
- Monitor vital signs closely during early therapy, particularly in patients with cardiovascular disorders and in elderly patients receiv-

P

ing daily doses in excess of 20 mg. If BP falls more than 20 mm Hg and if there is a sudden increase in pulse rate, withhold drug and inform physician.

- During early therapy and when patient is on large doses, monitor I&O ratio and question patient about bowel regularity.
- Anticholinergic effects are prominent (xerostomia, blurred vision, constipation, paralytic ileus, urinary retention, delayed micturition). Assess and advise physician as indicated.
- Xerostomia can interfere with appetite, fluid intake, and integrity of tooth surfaces. Assess condition of oral membranes frequently; institute symptomatic treatment if necessary.
- Suicide is an inherent risk with any depressed patient and may remain until there is significant improvement. Supervise patient closely during early treatment period.
- If a patient uses excessive amounts of alcohol, it should be borne in mind that the potentiation of TCA effects may increase the danger of overdosage or suicide attempt.
- Patients receiving large doses for prolonged periods or in combination with other drugs should have periodic determinations of liver function and blood cell counts.

Patient & Family Education

- The actions of both alcohol and protriptyline are potentiated when used together during therapy and for up to 2 wk after the TCA is discontinued. Consult physician about safe amount of alcohol, if any, that can be taken.
- Smoking increases the metabolism of TCAs and therefore reduces its effectiveness. Urge to stop or to reduce smoking. Apparent treatment failure may be due to the nicotine effect.
- Advise to consult physician before taking any OTC medications.
- The effects of barbiturates and other CNS depressants are enhanced by TCAs.
- Caution to avoid hazardous activities requiring alertness and skill until response to drug is known.
- Photosensitivity reactions may occur. Until this possibility is ruled out, advise to avoid exposure to the sun without protecting skin with sunscreen lotion (SPF ≥ 12), if allowed, and to avoid sun between the hours of 10 and 3 when sun's rays are nearest.

PSEUDOEPHEDRINE HYDROCHLORIDE

(soo-doe-e-fed'rin)

Trade names: Cenafed, Decongestant Syrup, Dorcol children's Decongestant, Eltor ♣, Eltor 120 ♣, Halofed, Novafed, PediaCare, Pseudofrin ♣, Robidrine ♣, Sudafed, Sudrin

Classifications: AUTONOMIC NERVOUS SYSTEM AGENT; ALPHA- AND BETA-ADRENERGIC AGONIST (SYMPATHOMIMETIC); DECONGESTANT

Prototype: Epinephrine

Pregnancy category: C

ACTIONS/PHARMACODYNAMICS

Sympathomimetic amine that, like ephedrine, produces decongestion of respiratory tract mucosa by action on sympathetic nerve endings. Unlike ephedrine, also acts directly on smooth muscle and constricts renal and vertebral arteries. Has fewer side effects, less pressor action, and longer duration of effects than ephedrine. Produces little, if any, congestive rebound or irritation that occur with nasal sprays and solutions.

USES Symptomatic relief of nasal congestion associated with rhinitis, coryza, and sinusitis and for eustachian tube congestion.

ROUTE & DOSAGE

Nasal Congestion
Adult: **PO** 60 mg q4–6h or 120 mg sustained release q12h.
Geriatric: **PO** 30–60 mg q6h prn.
Child: **PO** *6–11 y,* 30 mg q4–6h (max 120 mg/d); *2–6 y,* 15 mg q4–6h (max 60 mg/d).

PHARMACOKINETICS **Absorption:** readily absorbed from GI tract. **Onset:** 15–30 min. **Duration:** 4–6 h (8–12 h sustained release). **Distribution:** crosses placenta; distributed into breast milk. **Metabolism:** partially metabolized in liver. **Elimination:** excreted in urine.

CONTRAINDICATIONS & PRECAUTIONS **Contraindicated in:** hypersensitivity to sympathomimetic amines; severe hypertension; coronary artery disease; use within 14 d of MAO inhibitors; glaucoma; hyperthyroidism; prostatic hypertrophy. Safe use during pregnancy (category C), in nursing mothers, and in children <6 y not established. **Cautious use in:** hypertension, heart disease.

ADVERSE/SIDE EFFECTS *Transient stimulation,* tremulousness, difficulty in voiding, arrhythmias, palpitation, *tachycardia, nervousness,* dizziness, headache, sleeplessness, numbness of extremities, anorexia, dry mouth, nausea, vomiting.

DRUG INTERACTIONS Other SYMPATHOMIMETICS increase pressor effects and toxicity; MAO INHIBITORS may precipitate hypertensive crisis; BETA BLOCKERS may increase pressor effects; may decrease antihypertensive effects of **guanethidine, methyldopa, reserpine.**

NURSING IMPLICATIONS

Administration

- Non-sustained-release tablet may be crushed before administration and taken with fluid of patient's choice.

Asssessment & Drug Effects

- Monitor HR and BP, especially in those with a history of cardiac disease. Report tachycardia or hypertension.

Patient & Family Education

- Since drug may act as a stimulant, advise to avoid taking it within 2 h of bedtime.
- Advise to withhold medication if extreme restlessness or signs of sensitivity occur and to consult physician.
- Warn against concomitant use of OTC medications; many contain ephedrine or other sympathomimetic amines and might intensify action of pseudoephedrine. Consult physician.

P

PSYLLIUM HYDROPHILIC MUCILLOID

(sill′i-um)
Trade names: Hydrocil, Instant, Karasil ♣, Konsyl, Metamucil, Modane Bulk, Perdiem Plain, Reguloid, Serutan, Siblin, Syllact, V-Lax
Prototype for classifications: GI AGENT; BULK LAXATIVE
Pregnancy category: C

ACTIONS/PHARMACODYNAMICS Highly refined colloid of blond psyllium seed (*Plantago ovata*) with equal amount of dextrose added as dispersing agent. On contact with water, produces bland, lubricating, gelatinous bulk, which promotes peristalsis and natural elimination.

USES Chronic atonic or spastic constipation and constipation associated with rectal disorders or anorectal surgery.

ROUTE & DOSAGE

Constipation or Diarrhea

Adult: **PO** 1–2 rounded tsp or 1 packet 1–3 times/d prn.
Child ≥ 6 y: **PO** 1 tsp in water h.s.

PHARMACOKINETICS Absorption: not absorbed from GI tract. **Onset:** 12–24 h. **Peak:** 1–3 d.

CONTRAINDICATIONS & PRECAUTIONS Contraindicated in: esophageal and intestinal obstruction, fecal impaction, undiagnosed abdominal pain. Pregnancy (category C).

P

ADVERSE/SIDE EFFECTS Eosinophilia, nausea and vomiting, diarrhea, with excessive use; GI tract strictures when drug used in dry form, abdominal cramps.

DRUG INTERACTIONS Psyllium may decrease absorption and clinical effects of ANTIBIOTICS, **warfarin, digoxin, nitrofurantoin,** SALICYLATES.

NURSING IMPLICATIONS

Administration

- Fill an 8-oz (240-ml) water glass with cool water, milk, fruit juice, or other liquid; sprinkle powder into liquid; stir briskly; and drink immediately (if effervescent form is used, add liquid to powder). Granules should not be chewed.
- Best results are obtained if each dose is followed by an additional glass of liquid.
- Be cautious with elderly patient who may aspirate the drug.

Assessment & Drug Effects

- If patient complains of retrosternal pain after taking the drug, report this promptly to physician. The drug may be lodged as a gelatinous mass (because of poor mixing) in the esophagus.
- When psyllium is used as either a bulk laxative or to treat diarrhea, the expected effect is formed stools.
- Laxative effect usually occurs within 12–24 h. Administration for 2 or 3 d may be needed to establish regularity.
- Assess for complaints of abdominal fullness. Smaller, more frequent doses spaced throughout the day may be indicated to relieve discomfort of abdominal fullness.

Patient & Family Education

- Inform that drug works to relieve both diarrhea and constipation by restoring a more normal moisture level to stool.
- Inform that drug may reduce appetite if it is taken before meals.
- Note sugar and sodium content of preparation if patient is on low-sodium or low-calorie diet. Some preparations contain natural sugars, whereas others contain artificial sweeteners.
- Instruct patients on restricted-calorie diets to read the number of calories per dose, which can vary from 1 to approximately 100 calories.
- Instruct about prevention of constipation (e.g., proper hydration, increased fiber in diet, regulation of bowel pattern).

PYRANTEL PAMOATE

(pi-ran'tel)

Trade names: Antiminth, Combantriln ♣

Classifications: ANTIINFECTIVE; ANTHELMINTIC
Prototype: Mebendazole
Pregnancy category: C

ACTIONS/PHARMACODYNAMICS Exerts selective depolarizing neuromuscular blocking action, which results in spastic paralysis of worm; also inhibits cholinesterases.

USES *Enterobius vermicularis* (pinworm) and *Ascaris lumbricoides* (roundworm) infestations. **Unlabeled uses:** hookworm infestations; trichostrongylosis.

ROUTE & DOSAGE

Pinworm or Roundworm
Adult: **PO** 11 mg/kg as a single dose (max 1 g).
Child: **PO** Same as for adult.

PHARMACOKINETICS Absorption: poorly absorbed from GI tract. **Peak:** 1–3 h. **Metabolism:** metabolized in liver. **Elimination:** > 50% excreted in feces, 7% in urine.

CONTRAINDICATIONS & PRECAUTIONS Contraindicated in: safe use during pregnancy (category C) and in children <2 y not established. **Cautious use in:** liver dysfunction; malnutrition; dehydration; anemia.

ADVERSE/SIDE EFFECTS CNS: dizziness, headache, drowsiness, insomnia. **GI:** anorexia, *nausea,* vomiting, abdominal distention, diarrhea, *tenesmus,* transient elevation of AST. **Other:** skin rashes.

DRUG INTERACTIONS Piperazine and pyrantel may be mutually antagonistic.

NURSING IMPLICATIONS

Administration

- Shake suspension well before pouring it to ensure accurate dosage.
- Pyrantel pamoate may be taken with milk or fruit juices and without regard to prior ingestion of food or time of day.
- Purging is not necessary before, during, or after therapy.
- Store below 30C (86F). Protect from light.

PYRAZINAMIDE

(peer-a-zin′a-mide)
Trade name: Tebrazid ♣
Classifications: ANTIINFECTIVE; ANTITUBERCULOSIS AGENT
Prototype: Isoniazid
Pregnancy category: C

ACTIONS/PHARMACODYNAMICS Pyrazinoic acid amide, analog of nicotinamide and bacteriostatic against *Mycobacterium tuberculosis.* When employed alone, resistance may develop in 6–7 wk; therefore, administration with other effective agents is recommended. Appears to interfere with renal capacity to concentrate and excrete uric acid; thus may cause hyperuricemia.

USES Short-term therapy of advanced tuberculosis before surgery and to treat patients unresponsive to primary agents (e.g., isoniazid, streptomycin).

ROUTE & DOSAGE

Tuberculosis
Adult: **PO** 15–35 mg/kg/d in 3–4 divided doses (max 2 g/d).
Child: **PO** 20–40 mg/kg/d divided q12–24h (max 2 g/d).

PHARMACOKINETICS Absorption: readily absorbed from GI tract. **Peak:** 2 h. **Distribution:** crosses blood–brain barrier. **Metabolism:** metabolized in liver. **Elimination:**

P

half-life: 9–10 h; excreted slowly in urine.

CONTRAINDICATIONS & PRECAUTIONS **Contraindicated in:** severe hepatic damage. Safe use during pregnancy (category C) not established. **Cautious use in:** presence or family history of gout or diabetes mellitus; impaired renal function; history of peptic ulcer; acute intermittent porphyria.

ADVERSE/SIDE EFFECTS *Active gout,* arthralgia, dificulty in urination, headache, urticaria, hemolytic anemia, splenomegaly, lymphadenopathy, fatal hemoptysis, aggravation of peptic ulcer, ***rise in serum uric acid, hepatotoxicity, abnormal liver function tests,*** decreased plasma prothrombin, skin rash (rare).

DIAGNOSTIC TEST INTERFERENCE Pyrazinamide may produce a temporary decrease in ***17-ketosteroids*** and an increase in ***protein-bound iodine.***

NURSING IMPLICATIONS

Administration

- Drug should be discontinued if hepatic reactions (jaundice, pruritis, icteric sclerae, yellow skin) or hyperuricemia with acute gout (severe pain in great toe and other joints) occur.
- Store tightly closed container at 15–30C (59–86F).

Assessment & Drug Effect

- The patient receiving pyrazinamide requires close observation and medical supervision. He or she should receive at least one other effective antituberculosis agent concurrently.
- Patients should be examined at regular intervals and questioned about possible signs of toxicity: liver enlargement or tenderness, jaundice, fever, anorexia, malaise, impaired vascular integrity (ecchymoses, petechiae, abnormal bleeding).
- Hepatic reactions appear to occur more frequently in patients receiving high doses.
- Liver function tests (especially AST, ALT, serum bilirubin) should be done prior to and at 2–4 wk intervals during therapy. Blood uric acid determinations are advised before, during, and following therapy.

Patient & Family Education

- Report to physician the onset of difficulty in voiding. Urge to keep fluid intake at 2000 ml/d if possible.
- Advise diabetics of possible loss of glycemic control.

PYRETHRINS

(peer′e-thrins)

Trade names: A-200 Pyrinate, Barc, Blue, Pyrinate, Pyrinyl, R & C, RID, TISIT, Triple X

Classifications: SKIN AGENT; PEDICULICIDE ANTIINFECTIVE

Prototype: Permethrin

Pregnancy category: C

ACTIONS/PHARMACODYNAMICS Pediculicide solution comprised of pyrethrins and piperonyl butoxide in deodorized kerosene. Acts as a contact poison affecting the parasite's nervous system, causing paralysis and death. Controls head lice, pubic (crab) lice, and body lice and their eggs (nits).

USE External treatment of *Pediculus humanus* infestations.

ROUTE & DOSAGE

***Pediculus humanus* Infestations**

Adult: **Topical** See nursing implications for appropriate application.

CONTRAINDICATIONS & PRECAUTIONS **Contraindicated in:** sensitivity to solution components; skin infections and abrasions; pregnancy (category C). **Cautious use in:** ragweed-sensitized patient, infants, children.

ADVERSE/SIDE EFFECTS Irritation with repeated use.

NURSING IMPLICATIONS

Administration

- Apply enough solution to completely wet infested area, including hair. Allow to remain on area for 10 min.
- Wash and rinse with large amounts of warm water.
- Use fine-toothed comb to remove lice and eggs from hair.
- Shampoo hair to restore body and luster.
- Treatment may be repeated if necessary once in 24 h.
- Repeat treatment in 7–10 d to kill newly hatched lice.
- Do not apply to eyebrows or eyelashes without consulting physician.
- In accidental contact of eyes, flush with copious amounts of warm water.

Patient & Family Education

- Pyrethrins should not be swallowed, inhaled, or allowed to contact mucosal surfaces or the eyes.
- If treated area becomes irritated, discontinue use and consult physician.
- Each family member should be examined carefully; if infested, he or she should also be treated immediately to prevent spread or reinfestation of previously treated patient.
- Dry clean, boil, or otherwise treat contaminated clothing. Sterilize (soak in pyrethrins) comb and brushes used by patient.
- Teach not to share comb, brush, or headgear with another person.

PYRIDOSTIGMINE BROMIDE

(peer-id-oh-stig′meen)

Trade names: Mestinon, Regonol

Classifications: AUTONOMIC NERVOUS SYSTEM AGENT; CHOLINERGIC (PARASYMPATHOMIMETIC); CHOLINESTERASE INHIBITOR

Prototype: Neostigmine

Pregnancy category: C

ACTIONS/PHARMACODYNAMICS Analog of neostigmine; indirect-acting cholinergic with anticholinesterase activity. By blocking the destruction of acetylcholine, the drug facilitates transmission of impulses across myoneural junctions. Has fewer side effects and longer duration of action than neostigmine.

USES Myasthenia gravis and as an antagonist to nondepolarizing skeletal muscle relaxants (e.g., curariform drugs).

ROUTE & DOSAGE

Myasthenia Gravis

Adult: **PO** 60 mg–1.5 g/d spaced according to requirements and response of individual patient; sustained release: 180–540 mg 1–2 times/d at intervals of at least 6 h. **IM/IV** approximately 1/30th of PO dose.
Child: **PO** 7 mg/kg/d divided into 5–6 doses.
Neonates: **PO** 5 mg q4–6h. **IM/IV** 0.05–0.15 mg/kg q4–6h.

Reversal of Muscle Relaxants

Adult: **IV** 10–20 mg immediately preceded by IV atropine.

P

PHARMACOKINETICS Absorption: poorly absorbed from GI tract. **Onset:** 30–45 min PO; 15 min IM; 2–5 min IV. **Duration:** 3–6 h. **Distribution:** crosses placenta. **Metabolism:** metabolized in liver and in serum and tissue by cholinesterases. **Elimination:** excreted in urine.

CONTRAINDICATIONS & PRECAUTIONS Contraindicated in: hypersensitivity to anticholinesterase agents or to bromides. Mechanical obstruction of urinary or intestinal tract; bradycardia, hypotension. Safe use during pregnancy (category C) or in nursing mothers not established. **Cautious use in:** bronchial asthma; epilepsy; vagotonia; hyperthyroidism; peptic ulcer; cardiac dysrhythmias.

ADVERSE/SIDE EFFECTS Acneiform (bromide) rash, thrombophlebitis (following IV administration). **With large doses:** Muscarinic effects: *nausea, vomiting, diarrhea, miosis, excessive salivation and sweating,* increased bronchial secretion, bronchoconstriction, bradycardia, weakness, fasciculation and hypotension.

P

DRUG INTERACTION Atropine NONDEPOLARIZING MUSCLE RELAXANTS antagonize effects of pyridostigmine.

NURSING IMPLICATIONS

Administration

- Administer oral drug with food or fluid.
- Swallow sustained-release tablet whole.
- A syrup is available. Some patients may not like it because it is sweet; try to make it more palatable by giving it over ice chips. The syrup formulation contains 5% alcohol.
- Sustained-release tablets are generally prescribed only at bedtime for patients who complain of weakness on awakening.
- IV pyridostigmine is given by direct IV undiluted at a rate of 0.5 mg over 1 min for myasthenia gravis; 5 mg over 1 min for reversal of muscle relaxants. Do not add to IV solutions.
- Store at 15–30C (59–86F). Protect from light and moisture.

Assessment & Drug Effects

- Failure of patient to show improvement may reflect either underdosage or overdosage. Report increasing muscular weakness, cramps, or fasciculations.
- Atropine may be used to abolish GI side effects or other muscarinic side effects. Observe patient closely because atropine may mask signs of overdosage (cholinergic crisis): increasing muscle weakness, which through involvement of respiratory muscles can lead to death.
- Monitor vital signs frequently, especially respiratory rate.
- Observe for signs of cholinergic reactions (see Appendix G), particularly when drug is administered IV.
- Neonates of myasthenic mothers who have received pyridostigmine should be closely observed for difficulty in breathing, swallowing, or sucking.
- When used as muscle relaxant antagonist, patient should be continuously observed. Airway and respiratory assistance must be maintained until full recovery of voluntary respiration and neuromuscular transmission is assured. Complete recovery usually occurs within 30 min.

Patient & Family Education

- Duration of drug action reportedly may vary with physical and emotional stress, as well as with severity of disease.

- Report onset of rash. Drug discontinuation may be indicated.
- Sustained-release tablets may become mottled in appearance; this does not affect their potency.

PYRIDOXINE HYDROCHLORIDE (VITAMIN B_6)

(peer-i-dox′een)

Trade names: Beesix, hexaBetalin, NesTrex

Classification: VITAMIN

Pregnancy category: A (C if > RDA)

ACTIONS/PHARMACODYNAMICS Water-soluble complex of three closely related compounds with B_6 activity. Considered essential to human nutrition, although a deficiency syndrome is not well defined. Converted in body to pyridoxal, a coenzyme that functions in protein, fat, and carbohydrate metabolism and in facilitating release of glycogen from liver and muscle. In protein metabolism, participates in many enzymatic transformations of amino acids and conversion of tryptophan to niacin and serotonin. Aids in energy transformation in brain and nerve cells, and is thought to stimulate heme production.

USES Prophylaxis and treatment of pyridoxine deficiency, as seen with inadequate dietary intake, drug-induced deficiency (e.g., isoniazid, oral contraceptives), and inborn errors of metabolism (vitamin B_6-dependent convulsions or anemia). Also to prevent chloramphenicol-induced optic neuritis, to treat acute toxicity caused by overdosage of cycloserine, hydralzine, isoniazid (INH); alcoholic polyneuritis; sideroblastic anemia associated with high serum iron concentration. Has been used for management of many other conditions ranging from nausea and vomiting in radiation sickness and pregnancy to suppression of postpartum lactation.

ROUTE & DOSAGE

Dietary Deficiency

Adult: **PO/IM/IV** 2.5–10 mg/d for 3 wk, then may reduce to 2.5–5 mg/d.
Child: **PO** 5–25 mg/d × 3 wk, then 1.5–2.5 mg/d.

Pyridoxine Deficiency Syndrome

Adult: **PO/IM/IV** Initial: up to 600 mg/d may be required; **maintenance:** up to 50 mg/d.

Isoniazid-induced Deficiency

Adult: **PO/IM/IV** 100–200 mg/d for 3 wk, then 25–100 mg/d.
Child: **PO** 10–50 mg/d × 3 wk, then 1–2 mg/kg/d.

Pyridoxine-dependent Seizures

Neonate/Infant: **PO/IM/IV** 50–100 mg/d.

PHARMACOKINETICS **Absorption:** readily absorbed from GI tract. **Distribution:** stored in liver; crosses placenta. **Metabolism:** metabolized in liver. **Elimination:** excreted in urine.

CONTRAINDICATIONS & PRECAUTIONS **Contraindicated in:** safe use of large doses in pregnancy (category A [C if more than RDA]), in nursing mothers not established.

ADVERSE/SIDE EFFECTS Rarely: paresthesias, somnolence seizures (particularly following large parenteral doses), slight flushing or feeling of warmth, low folic acid levels,

P

temporary burning or stinging pain in injection site.

DRUG INTERACTIONS **Isoniazid, cycloserine, penicillamine, hydralazine,** and ORAL CONTRACEPTIVES may increase pyridoxine requirements; may reverse or antagonize therapeutic effects of **levodopa.**

NURSING IMPLICATIONS

Administration

- Oral drug may be given without regard to food.
- IV pyridoxine may be given by direct IV undiluted at a rate of 50 mg or fraction thereof over 60 seconds. May also be added to most IV infusions.
- Preserve in tight, light-resistant containers at 15–30C (59–86F). Avoid freezing.

Assessment & Drug Effects

- Therapeutic effectiveness of vitamin B_6 therapy is evaluated by improvement of B_6 deficiency manifestations: nausea, vomiting, skin lesions resembling those of riboflavin and niacin deficiency (seborrhea-like lesions about eyes, nose, and mouth, glossitis, stomatitis), edema, CNS symptoms (depression, irritability, peripheral neuritis, convulsions), hypochromic microcytic anemia.
- A complete dietary history should be recorded so that poor eating habits can be identified and corrected (a single vitamin deficiency is rare; patient can be expected to have multiple vitamin deficiencies).

Patient & Family Education

- Recommended dietary allowances of pyridoxine are 2.2 mg for adults and 2.6 mg during pregnancy and lactation. Need for pyridoxine increases with amount of protein in diet.
- Rich dietary sources of vitamin B_6 include yeast, wheat germ, whole grain cereals, muscle and glandular meats (especially liver), legumes, green vegetables, bananas.
- Advise not to self-medicate with vitamin combinations (OTC) without first consulting physician.

PYRIMETHAMINE

(peer-i-meth′a-meen)

Trade name: Daraprim

Classifications: ANTIINFECTIVE; ANTIMALARIAL

Prototype: Chloroquine

Pregnancy category: C

ACTIONS/PHARMACODYNAMICS

Long-acting folic acid antagonist chemically related to metabolite of chloroguanide. Selectively inhibits action of dehydrofolic reductate in parasite with resulting blockade of folic acid metabolism. Has no gametocidal activity but prevents development of fertilized gametes in mosquito and thus helps to prevent transmission of malaria. Because action against blood-borne schizonts is slow in onset, has little value as single agent in treatment of acute primary malarial attack. Cross-resistance with chloroguanide may occur.

USES Prophylaxis of malaria due to susceptible strains of plasmodia. May be used conjointly with fast-acting antimalarial (e.g., chloroquine, quinacrine, quinine) to initiate transmission control and suppressive cure. Used with a sulfonamide to provide synergistic action in treatment of toxoplasmosis.

ROUTE & DOSAGE

Malaria Chemoprophylaxis

Adult: **PO** 25 mg once/wk.
Child: **PO** > *10 y,* 25 mg once/wk;

4–10 y, 12.5 mg once/wk; *<4 y,* 6.25 mg once/wk.

Toxoplasmosis

Adult: **PO** 50–75 mg/d with a sulfonamide for 1–3 wk; then decrease dose by half and continue for 1 mo.
Child: **PO** 1 mg/kg/d divided into 2 doses with a sulfonamide for 1–3 wk; then decrease to 0.5 mg/kg/d for 1 mo (max 25 mg/d).

PHARMACOKINETICS Absorption: readily absorbed from GI tract. **Peak:** 2 h. **Distribution:** concentrates in kidneys, lungs, liver, and spleen; distributed into breast milk. **Elimination:** half-life: 54–148 h; excreted slowly in urine; excretion may extend over 30 d or longer.

CONTRAINDICATIONS & PRECAUTIONS Contraindicated in: chloroguanide-resistant malaria, megaloblastic anemia caused by folate deficiency. Safe use during pregnancy (category C) not established. **Cautious use in:** patients with convulsive disorders receiving high doses of an anticonvulsant (e.g., phenytoin).

ADVERSE/SIDE EFFECTS *With large doses or prolonged therapy:* anorexia, vomiting, atrophic glossitis, abdominal cramps, skin rashes, *folic acid deficiency (megaloblastic anemia, leukopenia, thrombocytopenia, pancytopenia,* diarrhea). ***Acute toxicity:*** CNS stimulation including convulsions, respiratory failure.

DRUG INTERACTIONS Folic acid, *para*-aminobenzoic acid (PABA) may decrease effectiveness against toxoplasmosis.

NURSING IMPLICATIONS

Administration

- GI distress may be minimized by taking drug with meals. If symptoms persist, dosage reduction may be necessary.
- For malaria prophylaxis, drug should be taken on same day each week. Administration should begin when individual enters malarious area and should continue for 10 wk after leaving the area.
- Some physicians prescribe leucovorin concurrently for patients on high-dosage therapy to prevent the hematologic complications of folic acid deficiency.

Assessment & Drug Effects

- Dosages required for treatment of toxoplasmosis approach toxic levels. Blood counts, including platelets, should be performed twice weekly during therapy. If hematologic abnormalities appear, dosage should be reduced or drug discontinued; parenteral leucovorin (folinic acid) (leucovorin rescue) will be administered until blood counts return to normal.

Patient & Family Education

- Folic acid deficiency may occur with long-term use of pyrimethamine. Instruct patient to report symptoms: weakness, and pallor (from anemia), ulcerations of oral mucosa, superinfections, glossitis; GI disturbances such as diarrhea and poor fat absorption, fever. Folate (folinic acid) replacement may be prescribed. Encourage patient to increase food sources of folates (if allowed) in diet.

QUAZEPAM

(qua′ze-pam)

Trade name: Doral

Classifications: CNS AGENT; BENZODIAZEPINE ANXIOLYTIC, SEDATIVE-HYPNOTIC

Prototype: Lorazepam
Pregnancy category: X

ACTIONS/PHARMACODYNAMICS Quazepam is believed to potentiate gamma-aminobutyric acid (GABA) neuronal inhibition in the limbic, neocortical, and mesencephalic reticular systems. It significantly decreases sleep latency and total wake time and significantly increases sleep time. REM sleep is essentially unchanged. No transient sleep disturbance such as "rebound insomnia" was observed after withdrawal of the drug.

USE Insomnia characterized by difficulty in falling asleep, frequent nocturnal awakenings, or early morning awakenings.

ROUTE & DOSAGE

Insomnia
Adult: **PO** 7.5–15 mg h.s.

PHARMACOKINETICS Absorption: readily absorbed from GI tract. **Onset:** 30 min. **Peak:** 2 h. **Distribution:** crosses placenta; distributed into breast milk. **Metabolism:** metabolized in liver to active metabolites. **Elimination:** half-life: 39 h; excreted in urine and feces.

Q

CONTRAINDICATIONS & PRECAUTIONS Contraindicated in: hypersensitivity to quazepam or benzodiazepines; sleep apnea; pregnancy (category X). **Cautious use in:** impaired hepatic and renal function. Not recommended for nursing mothers. Safety and effectiveness in children < 18 y not established.

ADVERSE/SIDE EFFECTS CNS: *drowsiness, headache,* fatigue, dizziness, dry mouth. **GI:** dyspepsia.

DRUG INTERACTIONS Alcohol, CNS DEPRESSANTS, ANTICONVULSANTS potentiate CNS depression; **cimetidine** increases quazepam plasma levels, increasing its toxicity; may decrease antiparkinsonism effects of **levodopa;** may increase **phenytoin** levels; **smoking** decreases sedative effects of quazepam.

NURSING IMPLICATIONS

Administration

- Initial dose is usually 15 mg but can often be effectively reduced after several nights of therapy.
- In the elderly, dose should be reduced to lowest effective dose as soon as possible.

Assessment & Drug Effects

- Monitor for respiratory depression in patients with chronic respiratory insufficiency.
- Monitor for suicidal tendencies in previously depressed clients.
- Daytime drowsiness is more likely to occur with the elderly client.

Patient & Family Education

- Instruct to inform physician about any alcohol consumption and prescription or nonprescription medication being taken. Alcohol generally should not be used since it potentiates CNS depressant effects.
- Instruct to inform physician if she is to become pregnant or if pregnancy occurs while she is taking this medicine. The drug causes birth defects.
- Until reaction to the drug is known, advise not to drive a car or operate potentially dangerous machinery.
- Instruct not to increase the dose and to inform the doctor if the drug "no longer works."
- Advise that drug may cause daytime sedation, which may persist for several days even after drug is discontinued.

QUETIAPINE FUMARATE

(que-ti-a′peen)

Trade name: Seroquel

Classifications: CNS AGENT; PSYCHOTHERAPEUTIC; SEROTONIN AND DOPAMINE-REUPTAKE INHIBITOR

Prototype: Clozapine

Pregnancy category: C

ACTIONS/PHARMACODYNAMICS

Quetiapine fumarate antagonizes multiple neurotransmitter receptors in the brain including serotonin ($5\text{-}HT_{1A}$ and $5\text{-}HT_2$) as well as dopamine D_1 and D_2 receptors. Its mechanism of action is unknown. However, it is thought that quetiapine fumarate's antagonism of dopamine and sertonin receptors is responsible for its antipsychotic properties.

Additionally, quetiapine antagonizes histamine H_1 receptors resulting in possible somnolence, and adrenergic $alpha_1$ and $alpha_2$ receptors which may lead to orthostatic hypotension.

USE Management of psychotic disorders.

ROUTE & DOSAGE

Psychosis

Adult: **PO** Initiate with 25 mg b.i.d.; may increase by 25–50 mg b.i.d. to t.i.d. on the second or third day as tolerated to a target dose of 300–400 mg/d divided b.i.d. to t.i.d. May adjust dose by 25–50 mg b.i.d. q2d as needed (max 800 mg/d). A lower target dose should be considered in elderly patients or patients with hepatic impairment.

PHARMACOKINETICS Absorption: rapidly and completely absorbed from GI tract. **Peak:** 1.5 h. **Distribution:** 83% protein bound. **Metabolism:** extensively metabolized in the liver by CYP3A4. **Elimination:** half-life: 6 h; 73% excreted in urine, 20% in feces.

CONTRAINDICATIONS & PRECAUTIONS Contraindicated in: hypersensitivity to quetiapine; lactation; alcohol use. **Cautious use in:** hepatic function impairment, elderly, pregnancy (category C); cardiovascular disease (history of MI or ischemic heart disease, heart failure, arrhythmias, CVA, hypotension, dehydration, treatment with antihypertensives; history of seizures, Alzheimer's, concurrent use of centrally acting drugs; patient at risk for aspiration pneunomia, elderly, debilitated patients.

ADVERSE/SIDE EFFECTS Body as whole: asthenia, fever, hypertonia, dysarthria, flu syndrome. **CNS:** *dizziness, headache, somnolence.* **CV:** postural hypotension, tachycardia, palpitations. **GI:** dry mouth, dyspepsia, abdominal pain, constipation, anorexia. **Respiratory:** rhinitis, pharyngitis, cough, dyspnea. **Skin:** rash, sweating. **Other:** weight gain, peripheral edema, leukopenia.

DRUG INTERACTIONS BARBITURATES, **carbamazepine, phenytoin, rifampin, thioridazine** may increase clearance of quetiapine. Quetiapine may potentiate the cognitive and motor effects of **alcohol,** enhance the effects of ANTIHYPERTENSIVE AGENTS, antagonize the effects of **levodopa** and DOPAMINE AGONISTS. **Ketoconazole, itraconazole, fluconazole, erythromycin** may decrease clearance of quetiapine.

NURSING IMPLICATIONS

Administration

- Dose is titrated over 4 d usually to a target range of 300–400 mg/d.

Further dose adjustments of 25–50 mg 2 times/d are made at intervals of at least 2 d.

- Persons who have been off the drug for >1 wk must be titrated to the desired dose.
- Lower doses and slower titration are recommended for the elderly, debilitated, those with hepatic impairment or a predisposition to hypotension.
- Store at 15–30C (59–86F)

Assessment & Drug Effects

- Therapeutic effectiveness is indicated by a reduction in psychotic behavior. Periodically reassess need for continued treatment.
- Withhold the drug and immediately report S&S of tardive dyskinesia (see Appendix G) or neuroleptic malignant syndrome (see Appendix G).
- Lab tests: Periodically monitor liver functions, lipid profile, thyroid function, blood glucose, CBC with differential.
- Periodically monitor ECG, especially in those with known cardiovascular disease.
- Cataract exam should be done when therapy is started and at 6-mo intervals thereafter.
- Monitor persons with a history of seizures for lowering of the seizure threshold.

Patient & Family Education

- Exercise caution with potentially dangerous activities requiring alertness, especially during the first week of drug therapy or during dose increments.
- Make position changes slowly, especially when changing from lying or sitting to standing to avoid dizziness, palpitations, and fainting.
- Women who become pregnant should immediately notify their physician. Mothers should not breast-feed while on quetiapine.
- Avoid alcohol consumption and activities that may cause overheating and dehydration.

QUINACRINE HYDROCHLORIDE

(kwin′a-kreen)

Trade name: Atabrine

Classifications: ANTIINFECTIVE; ANTHELMINTIC

Prototype: Mebendazole

Pregnancy category: C

ACTIONS/PHARMACODYNAMICS

Eradicates beef, pork, dwarf, and fish tapeworm and *Giardia lamblia* by causing worm scolex to detach from intestinal tract. Acts as suppressive agent and controls clinical attacks of malaria but is not a true prophylactic agent and does not produce a radical cure.

USES Tapeworm infestations and giardiasis. Use as antimalarial has been largely superseded by more effective and less toxic drugs.

ROUTE & DOSAGE

Beef, Pork, or Fish Tapeworm

Adult: **PO** 200 mg with 600 mg sodium bicarbonate q10min for 4 doses.
Child: **PO** *11–14 y,* 200 mg with 300 mg sodium bicarbonate q10min for 3 doses; *5–10 y,* 200 mg with 300 mg sodium bicarbonate q10min for 2 doses.

Dwarf Tapeworm

Adult: **PO** 300 mg q20min for 3 doses, then 100 mg t.i.d. for 3 d.
Child: **PO** *11–14 y,* 400 mg initially, then 100 mg t.i.d. for 3 d; *8–10 y,* 300 mg initially, then 100 mg b.i.d. for 3 d; *4–8 y,* 200 mg initially, then 100 mg after breakfast for 3 d.

Giardiasis

Adult: **PO** 100 mg t.i.d. for 5 d.
Child: **PO** 2 mg/kg t.i.d. for 5 d (max 300 mg/d).

Malaria Supression

Adult: **PO** 100 mg once/d.
Child: **PO** 50 mg once/d.

PHARMACOKINETICS **Absorption:** readily absorbed from GI tract. **Peak:** 8 h. **Duration:** detected in plasma for 4–6 wk. **Distribution:** concentrates in liver, lungs, pancreas, and erythrocytes; crosses placenta; distributed into breast milk. **Elimination:** slowly excreted in urine.

CONTRAINDICATIONS & PRECAUTIONS **Contraindicated in:** psoriasis, porphyria; pregnancy (category C); concomitant use of primaquine; intracavitary use in pneumothorax. **Cautious use in:** adults > 60 y, children < 1 y, history of psychosis; hepatic disease; alcoholism; concomitant use with hepatotoxic drugs; G6PD deficiency.

ADVERSE/SIDE EFFECTS **CNS:** *headache,* dizziness, vertigo, restlessness, confusion, irritability, emotional changes, insomnia, nightmares, psychotic reactions, convulsions (large doses). **GI:** *nausea, vomiting,* anorexia, *diarrhea, abdominal cramps.* **Skin:** *yellow pigmentation,* urticaria, exfoliative dermatitis, contact dermatitis, lichen planus–like eruptions. **Other:** (usually with prolonged therapy): aplastic anemia, agranulocytosis, hepatitis, corneal edema or deposits (reversible), fever, retinopathy (rare).

DIAGNOSTIC TEST INTERFERENCE Possibility of false-positive ***adrenal function tests*** using Mattingly method (quinacrine is fluorescent in aqueous media).

DRUG INTERACTIONS **Alcohol** may cause disulfiram-like reaction; increased toxicity with **primaquine.**

NURSING IMPLICATIONS

Administration

Tapeworm Infestations

- Patient is given a bland liquid or no-residue semisolid, nonfat diet for 24–48 h before start of drug therapy, with fasting after evening meal before and on morning of treatment.
- Generally, a saline purge and cleansing enema are given before treatment to reduce amount of stool that must be examined for scolex. Saline purge is repeated 1–2 h after quinacrine is administered. Sodium bicarbonate is prescribed with each dose of quinacrine to reduce tendency to nausea and vomiting.
- For pork tapeworm *(Taenia solium),* drug is administered by duodenal tube to prevent vomiting. Vomiting may cause passage of worm segments (proglottids) into stomach, with subsequent release of ova and invasion of tissue (cysticercosis).

Giardiasis

- Administer quinacrine after meals; stools are examined 2 wk after last dose. Repeat course may be given, if indicated.

Malaria

- Quinacrine should be taken after meals with a full glass of water, tea, or fruit juice.
- For suppression of malaria, medication should be taken for 1–3 mo.

Assessment & Drug Effects

- CBCs and ophthalmoscopic examinations should be done periodically in patients on prolonged drug therapy.
- Be alert for symptoms of drug-

induced behavioral changes and psychosis. Psychotic reactions may last 2–4 wk after drug is stopped.

Patient & Family Education

- Inform that drug colors skin a reversible yellow (not jaundice) and sometimes may give a grayish-blue tinge resembling cyanosis to ears, nasal cartilage, and fingernail beds. Skin discoloration usually disappears about 2 wk after drug is discontinued.
- Advise to report immediately the onset of skin eruptions or visual disturbances (e.g., halos of light, focusing difficulties, blurred vision).
- With tapeworm, entire stool specimen is collected for 48 h to find the scolex (worm head). Worm is usually passed within 4–10 h. Cure is presumed if scolex is found; dwarf tapeworm infestations are usually multiple and require more persistent treatment.
- If scolex is not found, stools should be examined periodically for tapeworm; stools must be free of worm eggs or segments for 3–6 mo to be certain of cure.

Q

QUINAPRIL HYDROCHLORIDE

(quin′a-pril)

Trade name: Accupril

Classifications: CARDIOVASCULAR AGENT; ANGIOTENSIN-CONVERTING ENZYME (ACE) INHIBITOR

Prototype: Captopril

Pregnancy category: D

ACTIONS/PHARMACODYNAMICS

A potent, long-acting second-generation ACE inhibitor that lowers BP by interrupting the conversion sequences initiated by renin to form angiotensin II, a vasoconstrictor. Inhibition of ACE also decreases circulating aldosterone, a secretory response to angiotensin II stimulation. Quinapril reduces pulmonary capillary wedge pressure, systemic vascular resistance, and mean arterial pressure, with concurrent increases in cardiac output, cardiac index, and stroke volume. Consequently it is effective in the treatment of CHF.

USES Mild to moderate hypertension, CHF.

ROUTE & DOSAGE

Hypertension, CHF

Adult: **PO** 10–20 mg q.d.; may increase up to 80 mg/d in 1–2 divided doses.
Geriatric: **PO** Start with 2.5–5 mg q.d.

PHARMACOKINETICS **Absorption:** rapidly absorbed from GI tract. **Onset:** 1 h. **Peak:** 2–4 h. **Duration:** up to 24 h. **Distribution:** 97% bound to plasma proteins; crosses placenta; not known if distributed into breast milk. **Metabolism:** extensively metabolized in liver to its active metabolite, quinaprilat. **Elimination:** half-life: 2 h; 50–60% excreted in urine, primarily as quinaprilat; 30% excreted in feces.

CONTRAINDICATIONS & PRECAUTIONS **Contraindicated in:** hypersensitivity to quinapril or other ACE inhibitors, pregnancy (category D). Not known if excreted in breast milk. **Cautious use in:** renal insufficiency, autoimmune disease, volume-depleted patients, renal artery stenosis, neutropenia.

ADVERSE/SIDE EFFECTS **CV:** edema, hypotension. **CNS:** dizziness, fatigue, headache. **GI:** nausea, vomiting, diarrhea. **Hematologic:** eosinophilia, neutropenia. **Other:** hyperkalemia, proteinuria, cough, angioedema, myalgia.

DIAGNOSTIC TEST INTERFERENCE May increase ***BUN*** or ***serum creatinine.***

DRUG INTERACTIONS POTASSIUM-SPARING DIURETICS may increase risk of hyperkalemia. May elevate serum **lithium** levels, resulting in lithium toxicity.

NURSING IMPLICATIONS

Administration

- If possible, diuretics should be discontinued 2–3 d before initiation of quinapril. If diuretics cannot be discontinued, the initial dose should not exceed 5 mg.
- Store at 15–30C (59–86F) and protect from moisture.

Assessment & Drug Effects

- Monitor BP at time of peak effectiveness, 2–4 h after dosing, and at end of dosing interval just before next dose.
- Report diminished antihypertensive effect toward end of dosing interval. Inadequate trough response may be an indication for dividing the daily dose.
- Monitor for first-dose hypotension, especially in salt- or volume-depleted persons.
- BUN and serum creatinine should be periodically monitored. Increases may necessitate dose reduction or discontinuation of quinapril.
- Monitor serum potassium values and observe for signs and symptoms of hyperkalemia (see Appendix G).

Patient & Family Education

- Advise to discontinue quinapril and report to physician signs and symptoms of angioedema (e.g., swelling of face or extremities, difficulty breathing or swallowing).
- Instruct to maintain adequate fluid intake and avoid potassium supplements or salt substitutes unless specifically prescribed by physician.
- Advise that taking quinapril with a high-fat meal may lessen its absorption.

QUINIDINE SULFATE

(kwin′i-deen sul-fate)

Trade names: Apo-Quinidine ♣, Novoquinidin ♣, Quinidex Extentabs, Quinora

QUINIDINE GLUCONATE

(kwin′i-deen)

Trade names: Duraquin, Quinaglute Duratabs

QUINIDINE POLYGALACTURONATE

(kwin′i-deen)

Trade name: Cardioquin

Classifications: CARDIOVASCULAR AGENT; ANTIARRHYTHMIC

Prototype: Procainamide

Pregnancy category: C

ACTIONS/PHARMACODYNAMICS Dextro isomer of quinine and alkaloid of *Cinchona.* Class I-A antiarrhythmic. Cardiac actions similar to those of procainamide. Depresses myocardial excitability, contractility, automaticity, and conduction velocity, and prolongs effective refractory period. Anticholinergic action blocks vagal stimulation of AV node, thus tending to increase ventricular rate, particularly in larger doses.

USES Premature atrial, AV junctional, and ventricular contraction; paroxysmal atrial tachycardia, chronic ventricular tachycardia (when not associated with complete heart block); maintenance therapy after electrical conversion of atrial fibrillation or flutter. **Unlabeled use:** quinidine gluconate for severe malaria.

ROUTE & DOSAGE

Sulfate contains 83% anhydrous quinidine base; polygalacturonate, 80%; and gluconate, 62%.

Ectopic Beats

Sulfate

Adult: **PO** 200–300 mg t.i.d. or q.i.d.
Child: **PO** 6 mg/kg 5 times/d.

Ventricular Arrhythmias

Sulfate

Adult: **PO** 400–600 mg q2–3h until arrhythmia terminates, then 200–300 mg 3–4 times/d.

Atrial Fibrillation or Flutter

Sulfate

Adult: **PO** 200 mg q2–3h for 5–8 doses until sinus rhythm restored or toxicity occurs (max 3–4 g); then 200–300 mg t.i.d. or q.i.d.

Polygalacturonate

Adult: **PO** 275–825 mg q3–4h for 4 or more doses until arrhythmia terminates; then 137.5–275 mg b.i.d. or t.i.d.

Acute Tachycardia

Gluconate

Adult: **PO** 324–660 mg q8–12h; **IM** 600 mg, then 400 mg q2h prn; **IV** 200–750 mg at a rate of 16 mg/min.

PHARMACOKINETICS Absorption: almost completely absorbed from GI tract. **Onset:** 1–3 h. **Peak:** 0.5–1 h. **Duration:** 6–8 h. **Distribution:** widely distributed to most body tissues except the brain; crosses placenta; distributed into breast milk. **Metabolism:** metabolized in liver. **Elimination:** half-life: 6–8 h; > 95% excreted in urine, < 5% in feces.

CONTRAINDICATIONS & PRECAUTIONS Contraindicated in: hypersensitivity or idiosyncrasy to quinine or *Cinchona* derivatives; safe use during pregnancy (category C) and during lactation not established. Thrombocytopenic purpura resulting from prior use of quinidine, intraventricular conduction defects, complete AV block, ectopic impulses and rhythms due to escape mechanisms; thyrotoxicosis; acute rheumatic fever; subacute bacterial endocarditis, extensive myocardial damage, frank CHF, hypotensive states; myasthenia gravis; digitalis intoxication. **Cautious use in:** incomplete heart block; impaired renal or hepatic function; bronchial asthma or other respiratory disorders; myasthenia gravis; potassium imbalance.

ADVERSE/SIDE EFFECTS CNS: headache, fever, tremors, apprehension, delirium, syncope with sudden loss of consciousness, disturbed hearing (tinnitus, auditory acuity). **CV:** hypotension, CHF, widened QRS complex, bradycardia, heart block, atrial flutter, ventricular flutter, fibrillation or tachycardia; quinidine syncope, torsades de pointes. **Eye:** mydriasis, blurred vision, disturbed color perception, reduced visual field, photophobia, diplopia, night blindness, scotomas, optic neuritis. **GI:** *nausea, vomiting, diarrhea, abdominal pain,* hepatic dysfunction. **Hematologic:** acute hemolytic anemia (especially in patients with G6PD deficiency), hypoprothrombinemia, leukopenia. Rare: Thrombocytopenia, agranulocytosis. **Hypersensitivity:** may include symptoms of cinchonism plus angioedema, vasculitis (rare), acute asthma, respiratory depression, vascular collapse. **Skin:** rash, urticaria, cutaneous flushing with intense pruritus, photosensitivity. **Other:** SLE; Cinchonism: nausea, vomiting, headache, dizziness, fever, tremors, vertigo, tinnitus, visual disturbances. **Overdosage:** hypokalemia, cinchonism, tachyarrhythmias, seizures.

DRUG INTERACTIONS May increase **digoxin** levels by 50%; **amiodarone** may increase quinidine levels, thus increasing its risk of heart block; other ANTIARRHYTHMICS, PHENOTHIAZINES, **reserpine** add to cardiac depressant effects; ANTICHOLINERGIC AGENTS add to vagolytic effects; CHOLINERGIC AGENTS may antagonize cardiac effects; ANTICONVULSANTS, BARBITURATES, **rifampin** increase the metabolism of quinidine, thus decreasing its efficacy; CARBONIC ANHYDRASE INHIBITORS, **sodium bicarbonate,** CHRONIC ANTACIDS decrease renal elimination of quinidine, thus increasing its toxicity; **verapamil** causes significant hypotension; may increase hypoprothrombinemic effects of **warfarin. Diltiazem** may increase levels and decrease elimination of quinidine.

NURSING IMPLICATIONS

Administration

- Oral administration: Test dose is used by some physicians to determine idiosyncrasy before establishing full dosage schedule.
- For optimum absorption, quinidine is taken with a full glass of water on an empty stomach (i.e., 1 h before or 2 h after meals). If GI symptoms occur (nausea, vomiting, diarrhea are most common), administer drug with food.
- Sustained-release tablet is usually reserved for maintenance and prophylactic therapy.
- Dosage is adjusted to maintain plasma concentration between 2 and 5 μg/ml. Levels of 8 μg/L or more are associated with myocardial toxicity.
- Preserve in tight, light-resistant containers away from excessive heat.
- Parenteral administration: Examine parenteral solution before preparation; use only if clear and colorless.
- When administering drug IM, aspirate syringe carefully before injection to avoid inadvertent entry into blood vessel.
- IV quinidine is prepared by diluting 800 mg (10 ml) in at least 40 ml D5W to yield a maximum concentration of 16 mg/ml. Administer via infusion pump at a rate not to exceed 16 mg (1 ml)/min.
- Severe hypotension is most likely to occur in patients receiving drug IV. Supine position during drug administration is advisable.
- Protect IV solutions from light and heat to prevent brownish discoloration and possibly precipitation.

Assessment & Drug Effects

- Observe cardiac monitor and report immediately the following indications for stopping quinidine: (1) sinus rhythm, (2) widening QRS complex in excess of 25% (i.e., > 0.12 seconds), (3) changes in QT interval or refractory period, (4) disappearance of P waves, (5) sudden onset of or increase in ectopic ventricular beats (extrasystoles, PVCs), (6) decrease in heart rate to 120 bpm. Also report immediately any worsening of minor side effects.
- Continuous monitoring of ECG and BP is required. Close observa-

Q

tion of patient (check sensorium and be alert for any sign of toxicity) and frequent determinations of plasma quinidine concentrations are indicated when large doses (more than 2 g/d) are used or when quinidine is given parenterally, i.e., quinidine gluconate.

- Observe patient closely following each parenteral dose. Amount of subsequent dose is gauged by response to preceding dose.
- During acute treatment, monitor vital signs q1–2h or more often as needed. Count apical pulse for a full minute. Report any change in pulse rate, rhythm, or quality or any fall in BP.
- Severe hypotension is most likely to occur in patients receiving high oral doses or parenteral quinidine, i.e., quinidine gluconate.
- Reversion to sinus rhythm in longstanding fibrillation or when fibrillation is complicated by CHF involves some risk of embolization from dislodgment of atrial mural emboli.
- Quinidine can cause unpredictable rhythm abnormalities in the digitalized heart. Patients with atrial flutter or fibrillation may be pretreated with digitalis (until ventricular rate is 100 bpm) to increase AV nodal block and thus reduce possibility of paradoxic tachycardia.
- Monitor I&O. Diarrhea occurs commonly during early therapy; most patients become tolerant to this side effect. If symptoms become severe, serum electrolytes and acid-base and fluid balance should be evaluated. Dosage adjustment may be required.
- During long-term therapy, periodic blood counts, serum electrolyte determinations, and kidney and liver function tests are advised.

Patient & Family Education

- Instruct to report feeling of faintness ("quinidine syncope") caused by quinidine-induced changes in ventricular rhythm resulting in decreased cardiac output and syncope.
- Hypersensitivity reactions usually appear 3–20 d after drug is started. Fever occurs commonly and may or may not be accompanied by other symptoms. Advise to inform physician if they occur.
- A diet high in alkaline ash foods (vegetables, citrus fruit, milk) may prolong half-life of quinidine by decreasing its excretion and increasing danger of toxicity. Advise to eat a balanced diet: no excesses in fruit or fruit juices, milk, or a vegetarian diet.
- Advise not to self-medicate with OTC drugs without advice from physician.
- Discuss medication schedule with patient. Advise not to increase, decrease, skip, or discontinue doses without consulting physician.
- Advise to notify physician immediately of disturbances in vision, ringing in ears, sense of breathlessness, onset of palpitations, and unpleasant sensation in chest and to note time of occurrence and duration of chest symptoms.

QUININE SULFATE

(kwye′nine)

Trade names: Novoquinine ♣, Quinamm, Quiphile

Classifications: ANTIINFECTIVE; ANTIMALARIAL

Prototype: Chloroquine

Pregnancy category: X

Q

ACTIONS/PHARMACODYNAMICS Chief alkaloid from bark of cinchona tree. Exact mechanism of antimalarial action uncertain. Inhibits protein synthesis and depresses many enzyme systems in malaria parasite. Has schizonticidal action and is gametocidal with *Plasmodium vivax* and *Plasmodium malariae* but not *Plasmodium falciparum*. Resembles salicylates in analgesic and antipyretic properties and exerts curare-like skeletalmuscle relaxant effect. Also has oxytocic action and hypoprothrombinemic effect. Qualitatively similar to quinidine in cardiovascular effects. Generally replaced by less toxic and more effective agents in treatment of malaria.

USES Chloroquine-resistant falciparum malaria and in combination with other antimalarials for radical cure of relapsing vivax malaria; also relief of nocturnal recumbency leg cramps.

ROUTE & DOSAGE

Acute Malaria

Adult: **PO** 650 mg q8h for 3 d.
Child: **PO** 25 mg/kg/d in three divided doses q8h for 3 d.

Malaria Chemoprophylaxis

Adult: **PO** 325 mg b.i.d. for 6 wk.

Nocturnal Leg Cramps

Adult: **PO** 260–300 mg h.s.

PHARMACOKINETICS **Absorption:** well absorbed from GI tract. **Peak:** 1–3 h. **Duration:** 6–8 h. **Distribution:** widely distributed to most body tissues except the brain; crosses placenta; distributed into breast milk. **Metabolism:** metabolized in liver. **Elimination:** half-life: 8–21 h; > 95% excreted in urine, < 5% in feces.

CONTRAINDICATIONS & PRECAUTIONS **Contraindicated in:** tinnitus, optic neuritis; myasthenia gravis; G6PD deficiency; pregnancy (category X). **Cautious use in:** cardiac arrhythmias. Same precautions as for quinidine sulfate when used in patients with cardiovascular conditions.

ADVERSE/SIDE EFFECTS **Cinchonism:** tinnitus, decreased auditory acuity, dizziness, vertigo, headache, visual impairment, *nausea, vomiting, diarrhea,* fever. **CNS:** confusion, excitement, apprehension, syncope, delirium. **CV:** angina. **Hematologic:** leukopenia, thrombocytopenia, <u>agranulocytosis</u>, hypoprothrombinemia, hemolytic anemia. **Hypersensitivity:** cutaneous flushing, visual impairment, pruritus, skin rash, fever, gastric distress, dyspnea, tinnitus. **Toxicity:** decrease in BP and respiration, tachycardia, <u>hypothermia</u>, convulsions, <u>cardiovascular collapse</u>, <u>coma</u>, blackwater fever (extensive intravascular hemolysis with renal failure), <u>death</u>.

DIAGNOSTIC TEST INTERFERENCE Quinine may interfere with determinations of ***urinary catecholamines*** (Sobel and Henry modification procedure) and ***urinary steroids*** (17-hydroxycorticosteroids) (modification of Reddy, Jenkins, Thorn method).

DRUG INTERACTIONS May increase **digoxin** levels; ANTICHOLINERGIC AGENTS add to vagolytic effects; CHOLINERGIC AGENTS may antagonize cardiac effects; ANTICONVULSANTS, BARBITURATES, **rifampin** increase the metabolism of quinine, thus decreasing its efficacy; CARBONIC ANHYDRASE INHIBITORS, **sodium bicarbonate,** CHRONIC ANTACIDS decrease renal elimination of quinine, thus increasing its toxicity; **warfarin** may increase hypoprothrombinemic effects.

NURSING IMPLICATIONS

Administration

- Administer drug with or after meals or a snack to minimize gastric irritation. Quinine has potent local irritant effect on gastric mucosa. Advise patients not to crush capsule; drug is not only irritating but also extremely bitter.
- Preserve in tight, light-resistant containers.

Assessment & Drug Effects

- Be alert to signs of rising plasma concentration of quinine: tinnitus and hearing impairment, which usually do not occur until concentration is 10 μg/ml or more.
- In patients with atrial fibrillation, follow the same precautions with quinine as are used with quinidine, since quinine may produce cardiotoxicity in these patients.

Patient & Family Education

- Inform about possible adverse reactions and advise to report promptly the onset of any unusual symptom.

RALOXIFENE HYDROCHLORIDE

(ra-lox′i-feen)

Trade name: Evista

Classifications: HORMONE AND SYNTHETIC SUBSTITUTE; SELECTIVE ESTROGEN RECEPTOR ANTAGONIST/AGONIST

Prototype: Tamoxifen

Pregnancy category: X

ACTIONS/PHARMACODYNAMICS Tamoxifen analog that exhibits selective estrogen receptor antagonist activity on uterus and breast tissue. Prevents tissue proliferation in both sites. Decreases bone resorption and increases bone density. Decreases serum total cholesterol and LDL cholesterol without lowering HDL cholesterol or triglycerides.

USE Prevention of osteoporosis in postmenopausal women.

ROUTE & DOSAGE

Prevention of Osteoporosis

Adult: **PO** 60 mg q.d.

PHARMACOKINETICS Absorption: 60% absorbed, absolute bioavailability 2%. **Metabolism:** extensive first-pass metabolism in liver. **Elimination:** half-life: 27.7–32.5 h; excreted primarily in feces.

CONTRAINDICATIONS & PRECAUTIONS Contraindicated in: active thromboembolic event, pregnancy (category X), hypersensitivity to raloxifene, lactation, children. **Cautious use in:** concurrent use of raloxifene and estrogen hormone replacement therapy and lipid-lowering agents.

ADVERSE/SIDE EFFECTS Body as whole: infection, flu syndrome, leg cramps, fever, arthralgia, myalgia, arthritis. **CNS:** migraine headache, depression, insomnia. **CV:** *hot flashes,* chest pain, peripheral edema, decreased serum cholesterol. **GI:** nausea, dyspepsia, vomiting, flatulence, GI disorder, gastroenteritis, weight gain. **Respiratory:** sinusitis, pharyngitis, cough, pneumonia, laryngitis. **Skin:** rash, sweating. **Other:** vaginitis, UTI, cystitis, leukorrhea, endometrial disorder, breast pain, vaginal bleeding.

DRUG INTERACTIONS Concomitant use of estrogens not recommended; absorption reduced by **cholestyramine.**

NURSING IMPLICATIONS

Administration

- Raloxifene may be taken at any time of day without regard to food.

- Raloxifene should be discontinued 72 h before and during prolonged immobilization.
- Store at 15–30C (59–86F) in a tightly closed container and protect from light.

Assessment & Drug Effects
- Therapeutic effectiveness is indicated by increased bone mineral density.
- Lab tests: Periodically monitor bone density and plasma lipids; with concurrent oral anticoagulants, carefully monitor PT and INR.
- Carefully monitor for and immediately report S&S of thromboembolic events.
- Raloxifene should not be given concurrently with cholestyramine; however, if unavoidable, space the two drugs as widely as possible.

Patient & Family Education
- Contact physician immediately if unexplained calf pain or tenderness occurs.
- Avoid prolonged restriction of movement during travel.
- Raloxifene does not prevent and may induce hot flashes.
- Do not take raloxifene with other estrogen-containing drugs.
- Tell prescriber if you are taking drugs to lower your cholesterol.

RAMIPRIL
(ram′i-pril)
Trade name: Altace
Classifications: CARDIOVASCULAR AGENT; ANGIOTENSIN-CONVERTING ENZYME (ACE) INHIBITOR
Prototype: Captopril
Pregnancy category: D

ACTIONS/PHARMACODYNAMICS By inhibiting the formation of angiotensin II, a potent vasoconstrictor, ramipril reduces peripheral vascular resistance and lowers BP. Inhibition of ACE also decreases serum aldosterone levels. ACE inhibitors also reduce peripheral arterial resistance (afterload) and improve cardiac output as well as exercise tolerance.

USES Mild to moderate hypertension, CHF.

ROUTE & DOSAGE

Hypertension, CHF
Adult: **PO** 2.5–5 mg q.d.; may increase up to 20 mg/d in 1–2 divided doses.

PHARMACOKINETICS Absorption: 60% absorbed from GI tract. **Onset:** 2 h. **Peak:** 6–8 h. **Duration:** up to 24 h. **Distribution:** crosses placenta; not known if distributed into breast milk. **Metabolism:** rapidly metabolized in liver to its active metabolite, ramiprilat. **Elimination:** half-life: 2–3 h; 40–60% excreted in urine, 40% in feces.

CONTRAINDICATIONS & PRECAUTIONS Contraindicated in: hypersensitivity to ramipril or any other ACE inhibitor, patients with history of angioneurotic edema, pregnancy (category D), nursing mothers. **Cautious use in:** impaired renal function, impaired liver function, surgery or anesthesia. Safety and effectiveness in children not established.

ADVERSE/SIDE EFFECTS CNS: dizziness, fatigue, headache. **GI:** nausea, vomiting, diarrhea, eructation. **Other:** hyperkalemia, hyponatremia, cough, erythema, pruritus, angioedema.

DRUG INTERACTIONS POTASSIUM-SPARING DIURETICS may increase risk of hyperkalemia. May elevate serum **lithium** levels, resulting in lithium toxicity.

NURSING IMPLICATIONS

Administration

- If possible, diuretics should be discontinued 2–3 d before initiation of ramipril. If diuretics cannot be discontinued, initial dose should not exceed 1.25 mg.
- Store at 15–30C (59–86F) and protect from moisture.

Assessment & Drug Effects

- Monitor BP at time of peak effectiveness, 3–6 h after dosing and at end of dosing interval just before next dose.
- Report diminished antihypertensive effect.
- Monitor for first-dose hypotension, especially in salt- or volume-depleted persons.
- BUN and serum creatinine should be periodically monitored. Increases may necessitate dose reduction or discontinuation of drug.
- Monitor serum potassium values and observe for signs and symptoms of hyperkalemia (see Appendix G).

R

Patient & Family Education

- Advise to discontinue ramipril and report to physician signs and symptoms of angioedema (e.g., swelling of face or extremities, difficulty breathing or swallowing).
- Instruct to maintain adequate fluid intake and avoid potassium supplements or salt substitutes unless specifically prescribed by the physician.

RANITIDINE HYDROCHLORIDE

(ra-nye′te-deen)

Trade names: Zantac, Zantac EFFERdose, Zantac GELdose, Zantac-75

Classifications: GI AGENT; ANTISECRETORY (H_2-RECEPTOR ANTAGONIST)

Prototype: Cimetidine

Pregnancy category: B

ACTIONS/PHARMACODYNAMICS

A potent antiulcer drug that competitively and reversibly inhibits histamine action at H_2-receptor sites on parietal cells. Blocks daytime and nocturnal basal gastric acid secretion stimulated by histamine and reduces gastric acid release in response to food, pentogastrin, and insulin. Indirectly reduces pepsin secretion but appears to have minimal effect on fasting and postprandial serum gastrin concentrations or secretion of gastric intrinsic factor or mucus.

USES Short-term treatment of active duodenal ulcer; maintenance therapy for duodenal ulcer patient after healing of acute ulcer; treatment of gastroesophageal reflux disease; short-term treatment of active, benign gastric ulcer; treatment of pathologic GI hypersecretory conditions (e.g., Zollinger-Ellison syndrome, systemic mastocytosis, and postoperative hypersecretion); heartburn.

ROUTE & DOSAGE

Duodenal Ulcer, Gastric Ulcer, Gastroesophageal Reflux

Adult: **PO** 150 mg b.i.d. *or* 300 mg h.s. **IV** 50 mg q6–8h; 150–300 mg/24 h by continuous infusion.
Child: **PO** 4–5 mg/kg/d divided q8–12h (max 6 mg/kg/d or 300 mg/d). **IM/IV** 2–4 mg/kg/d divided q6–8h; 0.1–0.125 mg/kg/h by continuous infusion.

Infants <2 wk: **PO** 2 mg/kg/d divided q12h. **IV** 1.5 mg/kg/d divided q12h or 0.04 mg/kg/h by continuous infusion.

Duodenal Ulcer, Maintenance Therapy

Adult: **PO** 150 mg h.s.

Pathologic Hypersecretory Conditions

Adult: **PO** 150 mg b.i.d. up to 6.3 g/d. **IV** 50 mg q6–8h.

Heartburn

Adult: **PO** 75 mg b.i.d.

PHARMACOKINETICS Absorption: incompletely absorbed from GI tract (50% reaches systemic circulation). **Peak:** 2–3 h PO. **Duration:** 8–12 h. **Distribution:** distributed into breast milk. **Metabolism:** metabolized in liver. **Elimination:** half-life: 2–3 h; excreted in urine, with some excreted in feces.

CONTRAINDICATIONS & PRECAUTIONS Contraindicated in: safe use during pregnancy (category B) and in nursing mothers not established. **Cautious use in:** hepatic and renal dysfunction.

ADVERSE/SIDE EFFECTS CNS: headache, malaise, dizziness, somnolence, insomnia, vertigo, mental confusion, agitation, depression, hallucinations in elderly patients. **CV** (rare): tachycardia, bradycardia (with rapid IV push). **GI:** constipation, nausea, abdominal pain, diarrhea. **Other:** rash, reversible decrease in WBC count, thrombocytopenia, hypersensitivity reactions, anaphylaxis (rare).

DIAGNOSTIC TEST INTERFERENCE Ranitidine may produce slight elevations in ***serum creatinine*** (without concurrent increase in BUN); (rare) increases in ***AST, ALT, alkaline phosphatase, LDH,*** and total ***bilirubin.*** Produces false-positive tests for ***urine protein*** with Multistix (use sulphosalicylic acid instead).

INCOMPATIBILITIES Solution/additive: amphotericin B, clindamycin, chlorpromazine, diazepam, hydroxyzine, methotrimeprazine, midazolam, nalbuphine, OPIUM ALKALOIDS, **phenobarbital. Y-site: methotrimepra-zine, midazolam,** OPIUM ALKALOIDS, **phenobarbital.**

NURSING IMPLICATIONS

Administration

- Simultaneous administration of food does not appear to reduce oral ranitidine absorption or serum concentrations.
- Adjunctive antacid treatment of pain may be necessary. Administer the antacid 2 h before or after ranitidine.
- IM ranitidine does not need to be diluted.
- IV ranitidine must be diluted prior to use; 50 mg ranitidine injection is diluted in 0.9% NaCl injection or other compatible IV solution to a total volume of 20 ml. Give by direct IV at a rate of 4 ml/min or 20 ml over not less than 5 min.
- For intermittent IV infusion, dilute 50 mg in 50–100 ml of NS, D5W, or other compatible IV solution and infuse over 15–30 min.
- IV administration to infants, children: Verify correct IV concentration and rate of infusion with physician.
- If patient is having hemodialysis treatments, the scheduled ranitidine dose should coincide with the end of hemodialysis.
- Store tablets in light-resistant,

R

tightly capped container at 15–30C (59–86F) in a dry place.

Assessment & Drug Effects

- It has been shown that to inhibit 50% of the stimulated gastric acid secretion, serum concentrations of ranitidine need to be 36–94 ng/ml. Concentrations in this range are maintained after a 150 mg dose for up to 12 h.
- The potential for toxicity resulting from decreased clearance (elimination) and therefore prolonged action is greatest in the elderly patient or the patient with hepatic or renal dysfunction.
- Creatinine clearance is monitored if renal dysfunction is present or suspected. When clearance is < 50 ml/min, manufacturer recommends reduction of the dose to 150 mg once q24h with cautious and gradual reduction of the interval to q12h or less, if necessary.
- The incidence of hepatotoxicity is low (and is thought to be a hypersensitivity reaction), but be alert to early signs: jaundice (dark urine, pruritus, yellow sclera and skin), elevated transaminases (especially ALT) and LDH.
- Long-term ranitidine therapy may lead to vitamin B_{12} deficiency.

Patient & Family Education

- Long duration of action provides ulcer pain relief that is maintained through the night as well as the day.
- Endoscopic examination is usually performed at end of 2 wk of therapy because about 37% of patients have been completely healed in that time.
- Most patients have healed ulcers by 4 wk; however, if healing cannot be confirmed endoscopically, treatment may be continued for up to 8 wk.
- Even if symptomatic relief is provided by ranitidine, this should not be interpreted as absence of gastric malignancy. Follow-up examinations will be scheduled after therapy is discontinued.
- Since a family member ordinarily recognizes jaundice from hepatotoxicity sooner than the patient does, discuss these possible symptoms with patient and family. Urge adherence to scheduled periodic laboratory checkups during ranitidine treatment.
- Instruct not to supplement therapy with OTC remedies for gastric distress or pain without physician's advice (e.g., Mylanta II reduces ranitidine absorption).
- Smoking has been shown to decrease ranitidine efficacy and adversely affect ulcer healing. Urge patient to stop smoking, informing him or her that giving it up may be more important in preventing ulcer recurrence than the medication.

R

REMIFENTANIL HYDROCHLORIDE

(rem-i-fent′a-nil)

Trade name: Ultiva

Classifications: CNS AGENT; ANALGESIC; NARCOTIC (OPIATE) AGONIST; GENERAL ANESTHESIA

Prototype: Morphine

Pregnancy category: C

ACTIONS/PHARMACODYNAMICS Synthetic, potent narcotic agonist analgesic similar to fentanyl. Since remifentanil is rapidly metabolized, respiratory depression is of shorter duration than fentanyl analogs when discontinued.

USES Analgesic during induction and maintenance of general anesthesia, as the analgesic component of monitored anesthesia care.

ROUTE & DOSAGE

Adjunct to Anesthesia
Adult & Child > 2 y: **IV** 0.025–2 µg/kg/min or 1 µg/kg injected over 30–60 s. See prescribing information for rate charts.

PHARMACOKINETICS Duration: 12 min. **Distribution:** 70% protein bound. **Metabolism:** hydrolyzed by nonspecific esterases in the blood and tissues. **Elimination:** half-life: 3–10 min; excreted in urine.

CONTRAINDICATIONS & PRECAUTIONS Contraindicated in: hypersensitivity to fentanyl analogs, epidural or intrathecal administration. **Cautious use in:** pregnancy (category C), nursing mothers, head injuries, increased intracranial pressure; elderly, debilitated, poor-risk patients; COPD, other respiratory problems, bradyarrhythmias. Safety in labor and delivery has not been demonstrated. Safety and efficacy in children < 2 y have not been established.

ADVERSE/SIDE EFFECTS Body as whole: muscle rigidity, shivering. **CNS:** dizziness, headache. **CV:** hypotension, hypertension, bradycardia. **GI:** *nausea,* vomiting. **Respiratory:** respiratory depression, apnea. **Skin:** pruritus.

NURSING IMPLICATIONS

Administration
- See manufacturer's guidelines for reconstitution information and infusion rates.
- For persons > 65 y, starting doses should be reduced by 50%. For obese persons, doses should be based on ideal body weight.
- Upon discontinuing the remifentanil infusion, IV tubing must be completely cleared of the drug to ensure that inadvertent administration of the drug will not occur at a later time.
- Reconstituted solution is stable for 24 h at room temperature. Store vials of powder at 2–25C (36–77F).

Assessment & Drug Effects
- During postoperative period monitor vital signs, observe for and immediately report any signs of respiratory distress or respiratory depression, or signs of skeletal and thoracic muscle rigidity and weakness.
- Monitor for adequate postoperative analgesia.

REPAGLINIDE
(rep-a-gli'nide)
Trade name: Prandin
Classifications: HORMONES; ANTIDIABETIC AGENT; MEGLITINIDES
Prototype: None
Pregnancy category: C

ACTIONS/PHARMACODYNAMICS Oral hypoglycemic agent that lowers blood glucose levels by stimulating release of insulin from the pancreatic islets. Significantly reduces postprandial blood glucose in type 2 diabetes. Minimal effects on fasting blood glucose were observed.

USES Adjunct to diet and exercise in type 2 diabetes. May also be used in combination with metformin.

ROUTE & DOSAGE

Type 2 Diabetes
Adult: **PO** 0.5–4 mg 15–30 min before meals (2–4 doses/d depending on meal pattern) max 16 mg/d).

PHARMACOKINETICS Absorption: rapidly absorbed from GI tract, 56%

R

bioavailability. **Peak:** 1 h. **Distribution:** 98% protein bound. **Metabolism:** metabolized in liver by cytochrome P450 3A4. **Elimination:** half-life: 1 h; 90% excreted in feces.

CONTRAINDICATIONS & PRECAUTIONS **Contraindicated in:** hypersensitivity to repaglinide; insulin-dependent diabetes, ketoacidosis; lactation, pregnancy (category C). **Cautious use in:** hypoglycemia; loss of glycemic control due to secondary failure; hepatic impairment. No studies have been done in children.

ADVERSE/SIDE EFFECTS **Body as whole:** arthralgia, back pain, paresthesia. **CNS:** headache. **CV:** chest pain, angina. **GI:** nausea, diarrhea, constipation, vomiting, dyspepsia. **Respiratory:** URI, sinusitis, rhinitis, bronchitis. **Other:** *hypoglycemia,* UTI, tooth disorder, allergy.

NURSING IMPLICATIONS

Administration

- Repaglinide may be given within 30 min of beginning a meal.
- Store at 15–30C (59–86F) in a tightly closed container and protect from moisture.

Assessment & Drug Effects

- Therapeutic effectiveness is indicated by preprandial blood glucose between 80 and 120 mg/dl and HbA_{1C} (glycosylated hemoglobin) <7%.
- Lab tests: Frequent FBS monitoring and HbA_{1C} q3mo to determine effective dose.
- Carefully monitor for S&S of hypoglycemia especially during the 1-wk period following transfer from a longer-acting sulfonylurea such as chlorpropamide.

Patient & Family Education

- Repaglinide should be taken only with meals to lessen the chance of hypoglycemia. If a meal is skipped, skip a dose, or if a meal is added, add a dose.
- When patient is transferred to repaglinide from another oral hypoglycemia drug, repaglinide should be started the morning after the other agent is stopped.
- Be alert for S&S of hyperglycemia or hypoglycemia (see Appendix G); report poor blood glucose control to physician.

RESERPINE

(re-ser′peen)

Trade names: Serpalan, Sk-Reserpine, and others

Prototype for classifications: CARDIOVASCULAR AGENT; RAUWOLFIA ALKALOID; ANTIHYPERTENSIVE

Pregnancy category: D

ACTIONS/PHARMACODYNAMICS Principal alkaloid of *Rauwolfia serpentina.* Interferes with binding of serotonin at receptor sites, decreases synthesis of norepinephrine by depleting dopamine (its precursor), and competitively inhibits their reuptake in storage granules. Depletes norepinephrine and serotonin in CNS, peripheral nervous system, heart, and other organs and tissues. Sympathetic inhibitory action is reflected in small but persistent decrease in BP, frequently associated with bradycardia, and reduced cardiac output. Central effect results in tranquilization and sedation similar to that produced by chlorpromazine.

USES Mild essential hypertension and as adjunctive therapy with other antihypertensive agents in the more severe forms of hypertension. Also used in agitated psychotic states, primarily in patients intolerant to phenothiazines or patients who also require antihypertensive medication. **Unlabeled uses:** to reduce vasospastic attacks in Raynaud's phenomenon and other peripheral vascular disorders, and for short-term symptomatic treatment of thyrotoxicosis.

ROUTE & DOSAGE

Hypertension

Adult: **PO** 0.5 mg/d initially; reduced to 0.1–0.25 mg/d.
Geriatric: **PO** Start with 0.05 mg q.d., increase by 0.05 mg weekly.

PHARMACOKINETICS **Peak:** 2 h. **Distribution:** widely distributed, especially to adipose tissue; crosses blood–brain barrier and placenta; distributed in breast milk. **Metabolism:** extensively metabolized to inactive compounds. **Elimination:** half-life: 4.5 and 11.3 h; slowly excreted, 60% in feces within 96 h and 10% in urine.

CONTRAINDICATIONS & PRECAUTIONS **Contraindicated in:** hypersensitivity to rauwolfia alkaloids; history of mental depression; acute peptic ulcer, ulcerative colitis; patients receiving electroconvulsive therapy; within 7–14 days of MAO inhibitor therapy. Safe use during pregnancy (category D) and in nursing mothers not established. **Cautious use in:** renal insufficiency; cardiac arrhythmias; cardiac damage; cerebrovascular accident; epilepsy; bronchitis, asthma; elderly patients, debilitated patients; gallstones; obesity; chronic sinusitis; parkinsonism; pheochromocytoma.

ADVERSE/SIDE EFFECTS **CNS:** *drowsiness,* sedation, *lethargy,* mental depression, nervousness, anxiety, nightmares, increased dreaming, headache, dizziness, increased appetite, dull sensorium; prolonged use of large doses: CNS stimulation (parkinsonian syndrome): tremors, muscle rigidity; <u>respiratory depression</u>, convulsions, hypothermia. **CV:** bradycardia, *edema,* orthostatic hypotension, increased AV conduction time (prolonged therapy); angina-like symptoms, arrhythmias, CHF (rare). **ENT:** *nasal congestion,* epistaxis, lacrimation, blurred vision; miosis, ptosis, conjunctival congestion (acute toxicity). **GI:** dry mouth or excessive salivation, nausea, vomiting, abdominal cramps, diarrhea, reactivation of peptic ulcer (hypersecretion), heartburn, biliary colic. **Hematologic:** thrombocytopenic purpura, anemia, prolonged BT. **Hypersensitivity:** pruritus, rash, asthma. **Reproductive:** menstrual irregularities, breast engorgement, galactorrhea, gynecomastia, feminization (males), impaired sexual function, impotence. **Other:** muscle aches, dysuria, fixed-drug eruptions.

DIAGNOSTIC TEST INTERFERENCE Possibility of elevated ***blood glucose*** values; however, it is also reported that reserpine may decrease thiazide-induced hyperglycemia. Increase in ***serum prolactin*** with chronic administration of rauwolfia alkaloids; overdoses may cause initial increase in excretion of ***urinary catecholamines;*** decreases with chronic administration. Large doses may cause initial rise in ***urinary 5 HIAA*** excretion. Initial IM doses may increase ***urinary VMA*** excretion followed by decrease by end of third day of therapy (with oral or parenteral administration). Possible interference with ***urinary steroid*** colorimetric determinations: ***17-OHCS*** and ***17-KS.***

DRUG INTERACTIONS **Diuretics,** other HYPOTENSIVE AGENTS compound hypotensive effects; CARDIAC GLYCOSIDES **(digoxin)** may increase risk of arrhythmias; MAO INHIBITORS may cause excitation and hypertension; CNS DEPRESSANTS compound depression; may decrease response to **levodopa.**

NURSING IMPLICATIONS

Administration

- Reserpine is administered with meals or with milk or other food to minimize possibility of gastric irritation (drug increases gastric secretions).
- Preserve in tight, light-resistant containers, preferably at 15–30C (59–86F), unless otherwise directed by manufacturer.

Assessment & Drug Effects

- Take BP and pulse at intervals prescribed by physician. Both should be taken before each parenteral dose. Compare readings with baseline determinations and keep physician informed. (Note: drop in BP may be accompanied by bradycardia.)
- Postural hypotension occurs rarely with usual PO doses but is not uncommon in patients receiving large parenteral doses. Supervise ambulation as indicated.
- Monitor I&O especially in patients with impaired renal function. Report changes in I&O ratio and pattern.
- Full therapeutic effect of oral drug for hypertension may not occur until 2–3 wk of therapy, and effects may persist for as long as 4–6 wk after drug is discontinued.
- Special precautions should be observed when reserpine is prescribed for the elderly and the obese patient (half-life is reportedly prolonged in obese patients). Anticipate increased incidence of adverse/side effects.
- Mental depression is a serious side effect and may be severe. It occurs most commonly in high dosage regimens, e.g., 0.5–1 mg/d or more; may not appear until 2–8 mo of therapy and may last for several months after drug is withdrawn.
- Because rauwolfia alkaloids are cumulative and have a long duration of action, dosage adjustments when necessary are usually made at 7–14 d intervals.
- Rauwolfia alkaloids tend to lower the threshold for convulsions. Patients with epilepsy should be monitored for possible need of adjustment in anticonvulsant dosage.
- Rauwolfia alkaloids should be discontinued 1 wk before electroconvulsive therapy.

Patient & Family Education

- Advise to take drug at the same time each day, not to skip or double doses, and not to stop therapy without advice of physician.
- Since drowsiness, sedation, and dizziness are possible side effects, caution to avoid driving and other potentially hazardous activities until reaction to drug has been determined.
- Counsel regarding possible side effects and importance of prompt reporting. Untoward effects are usually minimal with proper dosage and adequate supervision.
- Instruct patient and responsible family members to report the following possible beginning symptoms of depression: early morning insomnia, anorexia, inability to concentrate, despondency, self-deprecation, attitude of detachment, mood swings, or impotence. Hospitalization may be necessary.
- Instruct to report symptoms of dizziness, light-headedness to physician. Advise patient to make position changes slowly, particularly from recumbent to upright posture, and to lie down or sit down (head-low position) if patient feels faint. Also advise patient not to take hot show-

ers or hot tub baths, and not to stand still for prolonged periods.

- Advise to check for edema and to record weight daily. Distinction must be made between weight gain from edema and that from increased appetite. Consult physician about gain of 1–2 kg (3–5 lb) in 1 wk.
- Advise not to take OTC medications without prior approval of physician or pharmacist. Many preparations for coughs and colds contain adrenergic agents that affect the actions of rauwolfia alkaloids.
- Since reserpine decreases carbohydrate tolerance, diabetics should monitor blood glucose carefully and notify physician of hyperglycemic symptoms (see Appendix G).

RESPIRATORY SYNCYTIAL VIRUS IMMUNE GLOBULIN (RSV-IVIG)

(res-pir'a-tory sin-cy'ti-al)

Trade name: RespiGam

Classification: IMMUNE GLOBULIN

Pregnancy category: C

ACTIONS/PHARMACODYNAMICS Contains IgG immune globulin antibodies from human plasma. The preparation contains large amounts of RSV-neutralizing antibodies. Recipients should be high-risk premature infants and children.

USES Prevention of serious lower respiratory tract infection caused by RSV in children <24 mo with bronchopulmonary dysplasia or history of premature birth.

ROUTE & DOSAGE

RSV

Child/Infant/Neonate: **IV** 750 mg/kg infused at 1.5 ml/kg/h for first 15 min, then 3 ml/kg/h for next 15 min, then 6 ml/kg/h for rest of infusion. May repeat monthly as needed.

CONTRAINDICATIONS & PRECAUTIONS **Contraindicated in:** previous severe reaction to RespiGam or other human immunoglobulin preparation, selective IgA deficiency. **Cautious use in:** immunodeficiency, CHF, renal failure, pregnancy (category C).

ADVERSE/SIDE EFFECTS **Body as whole:** fever, pyrexia, fluid overload. **CV:** tachycardia, hypertension. **GI:** vomiting, diarrhea, gastroenteritis. **Respiratory:** respiratory distress, wheezing, rales, hypoxia, hypoxemia, tachypnea. **Other:** injection site inflammation.

DRUG INTERACTIONS May interfere with immune response to LIVE VIRUS VACCINES (mumps, rubella, measles), may need to repeat vaccine if given within 10 mo of RespiGam.

INCOMPATIBILITY Do not mix with other drugs.

NURSING IMPLICATIONS

Administration

- IV administration: Do not shake vial; infuse vial contents undiluted through a separate IV line if possible; if "piggyback" must be used, see manufacturer's directions.
- DO NOT EXCEED IV INFUSION RATES given in Route & Dosage table! Use a constant infusion pump.
- Store vials at 2–8C (35–46F). Infusion should begin within 6 h after vial is entered and be completed within 12 h.

Assessment & Drug Effects

- Assess vital signs and respiratory status prior to infusion, during and after each rate change, and at 30-

R

min intervals until 30 min after infusion is completed, and periodically therafter for 24 h.
- If S&S of fluid overload appear, slow infusion and immediately report.
- Monitor routine blood chemistry, serum electrolytes, blood gases, osmolality, protein.
- Monitor for aseptic meningitis syndrome, which may begin up to 2 d after infusion.

Patient & Family Education
- Advise regarding possibility of aseptic meningitis syndrome; instruct on S&S to report (headache, drowsiness, fever, photophobia, painful eye movements, muscle rigidity, nausea, vomiting).

RETEPLASE RECOMBINANT

(re′te-plase)

Trade name: Retavase

Classifications: BLOOD FORMERS AND COAGULATORS; THROMBOLYTIC ENZYME

Prototype: Streptokinase

Pregnancy category: C

ACTIONS/PHARMACODYNAMICS
Reteplase is a DNA recombinant human tissue-type plasminogen activator (TPA), which acts as a catalyst in the cleavage of plasminogen to plasmin. Plasmin is responsible for degrading the fibrin matrix of the clot, and thus it has antithrombolytic properties.

USES Thrombolysis management of acute MI to reduce the incidence of CHF and mortality.

ROUTE & DOSAGE

Thrombolysis During Acute MI

Adult: **IV** 10 U injected over 2 min. Repeat dose in 30 min (20 U total).

PHARMACOKINETICS Elimination: half-life: 13–16 min; excreted in urine.

CONTRAINDICATIONS & PRECAUTIONS Contraindicated in: active internal bleeding, history of CVA, recent neurologic surgery or trauma, intercranial neoplasm, or aneurysm, bleeding disorders, severe uncontrolled hypertension. **Cautious use in:** pregnancy (category C), lactation, any condition in which bleeding constitutes a significant hazard, i.e., severe hepatic or renal disease, CVA, hypertension, acute pancreatitis, septic thrombophlebitis. Safety and efficacy in children have not been established.

ADVERSE/SIDE EFFECTS Hematologic: <u>hemorrhage</u> (including <u>intracranial,</u> GI, genitourinary), anemia.

DRUG INTERACTIONS **Aspirin, abciximab, dipyridamole, heparin** may increase risk of bleeding.

DIAGNOSTIC TEST INTERFERENCE Causes decreases in plasminogen and fibrinogen, making coagulation and fibrinolytic tests unreliable.

INCOMPATIBILITIES Solution/additive: heparin. Y-site: heparin.

NURSING IMPLICATIONS

Administration
- Reconstitution should be carried out using only the diluent, syringe, needle, and dispensing pin provided with reteplase. It must be reconstituted only with sterile water for injection without preservatives. Follow manufacturer's directions.
- Administer each bolus IV injection over 2 min; do not give any other drug simultaneously through the same IV line.
- Store drug kit unopened at 2–25C (36–77F).

Assessment & Drug Effects

- Should serious bleeding not controllable by local pressure occur, concomitant heparin should be immediately discontinued and, if not already given, the second reteplase bolus should be withheld.
- Carefully monitor all potential bleeding sites; monitor for S&S of internal hemorrhage (e.g., GI, GU, intracranial, retroperitoneal, pulmonary).
- Carefully monitior cardiac status for arrhythmias associated with reperfusion.
- Invasive procedures, arterial and venous punctures, IM injections, and nonessential handling of the patient should be avoided during reteplase therapy.

Rh_o(D) IMMUNE GLOBULIN

Trade names: Gamulin Rh, HypRho-D, Rhesonativ, RhoGAM

Rh_o (D) IMMUNE GLOBULIN MICRO-DOSE

ACTIONS/PHARMACODYNAMICS Sterile nonpyrogenic gamma globulin solution containing immunoglobulins (IgG). The solution is at least 90% IgG. The globulin provides passive immunity by suppressing active antibody response and formation of anti-Rh_o(D) (isoimmunization) in Rh-negative (Rh_o(D)-negative, D^u-negative) individuals previously exposed to Rh-positive (Rh_o(D)-positive, D^u-positive) blood. Such exposure occurs in Rh-negative women when Rh-positive fetal RBCs enter maternal circulation: during third stage of labor, fetal-maternal hemorrhage (as early as second trimester), amniocentesis, or other trauma during pregnancy, termination of pregnancy, and following transfusion with Rh-positive RBC, whole blood, or components (platelets, WBC) prepared from Rh-positive blood.

USES To prevent isoimmunization in Rh-negative individuals exposed to Rh-positive RBC (see above). Rh_o(D) immune globulin microdose is for use only after spontaneous or induced abortion or termination of ectopic pregnancy up to and including 12 wk of gestation.

ROUTE & DOSAGE

Antepartum Prophylaxis

Adult: **IM** 1 vial at approximately 28 wk; followed by 1 vial within 72 h of delivery if infant is Rh-positive.

Postpartum Prophylaxis

Adult: **IM** 1 vial within 72 h of delivery if infant is Rh-positive.

Following Amniocentesis, Miscarriage, Abortion, Ectopic Pregnancy

Adult: **IM** 1 vial of the microdose, preferably within 3 h but at least within 72 h.

Transfusion Accident

Adult: **IM** 1 vial for each volume of RBCs infused divided by 15, given within at least 72 h of accident.

CONTRAINDICATIONS & PRECAUTIONS **Contraindicated in:** Rh_o(D)-positive or D^u-positive patient; person previously immunized against Rh_o(D) factor, hypersensitivity for thimerosal (in commercial preparations), thrombocytopenia, or bleeding disorders.

ADVERSE/SIDE EFFECTS Infrequent: injection site irritation, slight fever, myalgia, lethargy.

DRUG INTERACTIONS May interfere with immune response to **live virus vaccine;** should delay use of live virus vaccines for 3 mo after administration of Rh_o(D) immune globulin.

NURSING IMPLICATIONS

Administration

- Lot numbers of drug used for the cross-match and the drug to be administered must be the same.
- Rh_o(D) immune globulin is administered IM only to the mothers and not to the infant.
- Use the deltoid muscle. The IM may be given in divided doses at different sites, all at once or at intervals, as long as the entire dose is given within 72 h after delivery or termination of pregnancy.
- Follow manufacturer's directions for reconstitution and use supplied sterile water diluent. Administer immediately. Commercially prepared solutions should be refrigerated, although they may be stable up to 30 d at room temperature according to manufacturers. Solutions that have been frozen should be discarded.
- Each vial of Rh_o(D) immune globulin contains enough anti-Rh_o(D) to suppress the immunizing potential of 15 ml Rh-positive packed RBC. Each vial of micro-dose contains enough anti-Rh_o(D) to suppress the immune response to 2.5 ml of Rh-positive packed RBC.
- Although systemic allergic reactions occur rarely, epinephrine should be immediately available.
- Store powder at 2–8C (36–46F) unless otherwise directed. Avoid freezing.

Assessment & Drug Effects

- Obtain history of systemic allergic reactions to human immune globulin preparations prior to drug administration.
- Before administration of Rh_o(D) immune globulin and immediately after delivery, send sample of newborn's cord blood to laboratory for cross-match and typing. Confirm that mother is Rh_o(D) and D^u-negative. Infant must be Rh-positive.

Patient & Family Education

- Approximately 13% of white Americans lack Rh_o(D) completely and therefore are Rh-negative. About 7–10% of black Americans are Rh-negative. About 1% of American Indians and Asian Americans are Rh-negative.
- Administration of Rh_o(D) immune globulin (antibody) prevents hemolytic disease of the newborn in a subsequent pregnancy.

RIBAVIRIN

(rye-ba-vye'rin)

Trade name: Virazole

Classifications: ANTIINFECTIVE; ANTIVIRAL

Prototype: Acyclovir

Pregnancy category: X

ACTIONS/PHARMACODYNAMICS

Synthetic nucleoside with broad-spectrum antiviral activity against DNA and RNA viruses. Exact mode of virostatic action not fully understood but is believed to involve multiple mechanisms. Appears to exert selective antiviral action by interfering with viral ribonucleic protein synthesis, ultimately leading to inhibition of viral replication. It does not influence interferon synthesis. Active against many RNA and DNA viruses, including respiratory syncytial virus (RSV), influenza A and B, parainfluenza, measles, mumps, Lassa fever, enterovirus 72 (formerly called hepatitis A), yellow fever,

R

HIV, herpes simplex virus (HSV-1 and HSV-2), and vaccinia. Immune responses appear to depend on cellular drug concentrations: low concentrations seem to stimulate and high concentrations appear to inhibit immune responses. Generally not active against poliovirus and coxsackieviruses. Unlike other antiviral agents, virus resistance to ribavirin does not appear to develop.

USES Only for aerosol treatment of carefully selected hospitalized infants and young children with severe lower respiratory tract infection caused by respiratory syncytial virus (RSV). **Unlabeled uses:** prophylaxis and treatment of influenza A and B, pneumonia caused by adenovirus; Lassa fever, measles, HSV-1, HSV-2, hepatitis A, herpes zoster, and for carefully selected patients with AIDS and AIDS-related complex (ARC).

ROUTE & DOSAGE

RSV

Child: **Inhalation** 20 mg via SPAG nebulizer administered over 12–18 h/d for a minimum of 3 d and a max of 7 d.

PHARMACOKINETICS **Absorption:** rapidly absorbed systemically from lungs. **Peak:** 60–90 min. **Distribution:** crosses placenta; distributed into breast milk. **Metabolism:** metabolized in cells to an active metabolite. **Elimination:** half-life: 24 h in plasma, 16–40 d in RBCs; 85% excreted in urine, 15% in feces.

CONTRAINDICATIONS & PRECAUTIONS **Contraindicated in:** mild RSV infections of lower respiratory tract; infants requiring simultaneous assisted ventilation; severe cardiopulmonary disease; prolonged or multiple courses of ribavirin inhalation therapy. Safe use during pregnancy (category X) and in nursing mothers not established. **Cautious use in:** COPD, asthma.

ADVERSE/SIDE EFFECTS **CV:** hypotension (faintness, light-headedness, unusual fatigue), cardiac arrest. **Eye:** conjunctivitis, erythema of eyelids. **Hematologic:** reticulocytosis. **Respiratory:** deterioration of respiratory function, dyspnea, apnea, chest soreness, bacterial pneumonia, ventilator dependence. **Other:** transient increases in AST, ALT, bilirubin; abdominal cramps.

DRUG INTERACTION Ribavirin may antagonize the antiviral effects of **zidovudine** (formerly AZT) against HIV.

NURSING IMPLICATIONS

Administration

- Note that aerosol solution is prepared with either sterile water for injection or sterile water for inhalation, without preservatives or any other added substance. See manufacturer's package insert for preparation directions.
- Inspect solution for discoloration or presence of particulate matter. Discard discolored or cloudy solutions.
- Ribavirin for inhalation is administered only by SPAG-2 aerosol generator. Administer according to manufacturer's directions. CAUTION: ribavirin has demonstrated teratogenicity in animals. It would be prudent to advise pregnant health-care personnel of the potential teratogenic risks associated with exposure during ribavirin administration to patients. No other aerosol medication is to be given concomitantly with ribavirin.
- The solution in the SPAG-2 reservoir should be discarded at least

q24h and whenever liquid level is low before fresh reconstituted solution is added.

- Following reconstitution, solution may be stored at 20–30C (68–86F) for 24 h.
- Store unopened vial in a dry place at 15–25C (59–78F) unless otherwise directed.

Assessment & Drug Effects

- Specimens should be obtained for rapid diagnosis of RSV infection before therapy is initiated or at least during the first 24 h of ribavirin therapy. Ribavirin should not be continued without laboratory confirmation of RSV infection.
- Efficacy of ribavirin in RSV infections appears to be greatest if treatment is initiated within the first 3 d.
- Respiratory function and fluid status must be closely monitored during therapy. Note rate and character of respirations and pulse before treatment begins and at frequent intervals during therapy. Observe for signs of labored breathing: dyspnea, apnea; rapid, shallow respirations, intercostal and substernal retraction, nasal flaring, limited excursion of lungs, cyanosis. Auscultate lungs for abnormal breath sounds.
- Patients requiring simultaneous assisted ventilation should be closely observed for signs of worsening pulmonary function. Every 2 h, check equipment carefully, including endotracheal tube, for malfunctioning. Precipitation of ribavirin and accumulation of fluid in tubing can obstruct the apparatus and cause inadequate ventilation and gas exchange.
- Consult physician about management of fluid and food intake and keep an accurate record of I&O.

RIBOFLAVIN (VITAMIN B_2)

(rye'bo-flay-vin)

Classification: VITAMIN

Pregnancy category: A (C if > RDA)

ACTIONS/PHARMACODYNAMICS Water-soluble vitamin and component of the flavoprotein enzymes that work together with a wide variety of proteins to catalyze many cellular respiratory reactions by which the body derives its energy.

USES To prevent riboflavin deficiency and to treat ariboflavinosis; also to treat microcytic anemia and as a supplement to other B vitamins in treatment of pellagra and beriberi.

ROUTE & DOSAGE

Nutritional Supplement

Adult: **PO** 5–10 mg/d.
Child: **PO** 1–4 mg/d.

Nutritional Deficiency

Adult: **PO** 5–30 mg/d in divided doses.
Child: **PO** 3–10 mg/d.

PHARMACOKINETICS **Absorption:** readily absorbed from GI tract. **Distribution:** little is stored; excess amounts are excreted in urine. **Elimination:** half-life: 66–84 min; excreted in urine.

CONTRAINDICATIONS & PRECAUTIONS **Cautious use in:** pregnancy [(category A), (category C if > RDA)].

ADVERSE/SIDE EFFECTS Apparently nontoxic.

DIAGNOSTIC TEST INTERFERENCE In large doses, riboflavin may produce yellow-green fluorescence in

urine and thus cause false elevations in certain fluorometric determinations of ***urinary catecholamines.***

NURSING IMPLICATIONS

Administration

- Administer oral preparation with food to enhance absorption.
- Preserve in airtight containers protected from light.

Assessment & Drug Effects

- Therapeutic effectiveness of vitamin B_2 therapy is evaluated by improvement of clinical manifestations of deficiency: digestive disturbances, headache, burning sensation of skin (especially "burning" feet), cracking at corners of mouth (cheilosis), glossitis, seborrheic dermatitis (often at angle of nose and anogenital region) and other skin lesions, mental depression, corneal vascularization (with photophobia, burning and itchy eyes, lacrimation, roughness of eyelids), anemia, neuropathy.
- Collaborate with physician, dietitian, patient, and responsible family member in planning for diet teaching. A complete dietary history is an essential part of vitamin replacement so that poor eating habits can be identified and corrected. Deficiency in one vitamin is usually associated with other vitamin deficiencies.

Patient & Family Education

- Inform patient receiving large doses that an intense yellow discoloration of urine may occur.
- Rich dietary sources of riboflavin: liver, kidney, beef, pork, heart, eggs, milk and milk products, yeast, whole-grain cereals, vitamin A-enriched breakfast cereals, green vegetables, and mushrooms.

RIFABUTIN

(rif-a-bu′tin)

Trade names: Ansamycin, Mycobutin

Classifications: ANTIINFECTIVE; ANTITUBERCULOSIS AGENT

Prototype: Isoniazid

Pregnancy category: B

ACTIONS/PHARMACODYNAMICS

Semisynthetic bacteriostatic antibiotic effective against *Myocobacterium avium* complex (MAC) (or *M. avium-intracellulare*). Rifabutin is also effective against many strains of *Mycobacterium* tuberculosis. Its mode of action may be to inhibit DNA-dependent RNA polymerase (an enzyme) in susceptible bacterial cells but not in human cells.

USES The prevention of disseminated *Mycobacterium avium* complex (MAC) disease in patients with advanced HIV infection.

ROUTE & DOSAGE

Prevention of MAC

Adult: **PO** 300 mg q.d. May give 150 mg b.i.d. if nausea is a problem.
Child: **PO** 75 mg q.d.

PHARMACOKINETICS **Absorption:** 12–20% of oral dose reaches the systemic circulation. **Peak:** 2–3 h. **Distribution:** 85% protein bound. Widely distributed, high concentrations in the lungs, liver, spleen, eyes, and kidney. Crosses placenta, distributed into breast milk. **Metabolism:** Metabolized in the liver. Causes induction of hepatic enzymes. **Elimination:** half-life: 16–96 h (average 45 h); approximately 53% of dose is excreted in urine as metabolites, 30% is excreted in feces.

R

CONTRAINDICATIONS & PRECAUTIONS **Contraindicated in:** hypersensitivity to rifabutin or any other rifamycins, nursing mothers. **Cautious use in:** pregnancy (category B).

ADVERSE/SIDE EFFECTS: **CNS:** *headache,* **GI:** *abdominal pain, dyspepsia, nausea, taste perversion, increased liver enzymes.* **Hematologic:** thrombocytopenia, eosinophilia, leukopenia, neutropenia. **Skin:** rash. **Other:** *turns urine, feces, saliva, sputum, perspiration, and tears orange. Soft contact lenses may be permanently discolored.*

DRUG INTERACTIONS May decrease levels of BENZODIAZEPINES, BETA BLOCKERS, **clofibrate, dapsone,** NARCOTICS, ANTICOAGULANTS, CORTICOSTEROIDS, **cyclosporine, quinidine,** ORAL CONTRACEPTIVES, PROGESTINS, SULFONYLUREAS, **ketoconazole, fluconazole,** BARBITURATES, **theophylline,** and ANTICONVULSANTS, resulting in therapeutic failure.

NURSING IMPLICATIONS

Administration

- Usual dose of 300 mg/d may be given in two divided doses of 150 mg with food if needed to reduce GI upset.
- Store at room temperature, 15–30C (59–86F), unless otherwise directed.

Assessment & Drug Effects

- Immediately evaluate patients who develop signs and symptoms of TB while on rifabutin. Single-agent rifabutin should not be administered to persons with active TB.
- Periodic blood work is required to monitor for neutropenia and thrombocytopenia.
- Patients on concurrent oral hypoglycemic therapy should be evaluated for loss of glycemic control.
- Patient's complete drug regimen should be reviewed, because dosage adjustment of a significant number of drugs may be needed when rifabutin is added to regimen.

Patient & Family Education

- Inform of signs and symptoms of TB and MAC (e.g., persistent fever, progressive weight loss, anorexia, night sweats, diarrhea), and instruct to notify physician if any of these develop.
- Instruct to notify physician if any of following develop: muscle or joint pain, eye pain or other discomfort, chest pain with dyspnea, rash, or a flu-like syndrome.
- Inform that urine, feces, saliva, sputum, perspiration, tears, and skin may be colored brown-orange. Soft contact lens may be permanently discolored.
- Inform that rifabutin may reduce the activity of a wide variety of drugs. Advise patient to provide a complete and accurate list of concurrent drugs to the physician for evaluation.

RIFAMPIN

(rif'am-pin)

Trade names: Rifadin, Rimactane, Rofact ♣

Classifications: ANTIINFECTIVE; ANTIBIOTIC; ANTITUBERCULOSIS AGENT; ANTILEPROSY (SULFONE) AGENT

Prototype: Isoniazid

ACTIONS/PHARMACODYNAMICS Semisynthetic derivative of rifamycin B, an antibiotic derived from *Streptococcus mediterranei,* with bacteriostatic and bactericidal actions. Inhibits DNA-dependent RNA polymerase activity in susceptible bacterial cells, thereby suppressing RNA synthesis. Active against *Mycobacterium tuberculosis, Mycobacterium leprae, Neisseria meningitidis,* and a wide range of gram-negative and gram-positive organisms. Since resistant strains emerge rapidly when it is employed alone, it is used in conjunction with other antitubercular agents in treatment of tuberculosis.

USES Primarily as adjuvant with other antituberculosis agents in initial treatment and retreatment of clinical tuberculosis; as short-term therapy to eliminate meningococci from nasopharynx of asymptomatic carriers of *N. meningitidis* when risk of meningococcal meningitis is high. **Unlabeled uses:** chemoprophylaxis in contacts of patients with *Hemophilus influenzae* type B infection; alone or in combination with dapsone and other antiinfectives in treatment of leprosy (especially dapsone-resistant leprosy). Also infections caused by susceptible gram-negative and gram-positive bacteria that fail to respond to other antiinfectives; in combination with erythromycin or tetracycline for treatment of Legionnaire's disease.

ROUTE & DOSAGE

Pulmonary Tuberculosis

Adult: **PO/IV** 600 mg once/d in conjunction with other antituberculosis agents.
Child: **PO** 10–20 mg/kg/d (max 600 mg/d).

Meningococcal Carriers

Adult: **PO** 600 mg b.i.d. for 2 consecutive d.
Child: **PO** 10–20 mg/kg b.i.d. for 2 consecutive d (max 600 mg/d).

Prophylaxis for *H. influenzae* Type B

Adult: **PO** 600 mg/d for 4 d.
Child: **PO** 10–20 mg/kg/d for 4 d (max 600 mg/d).

Dapsone-sensitive Multibacillary Leprosy

Adult: **PO** 600 mg once/mo with clofazimine and dapsone for a minimum of 2 y.

PHARMACOKINETICS Absorption: readily absorbed from GI tract. **Peak:** 2–4 h. **Distribution:** widely distributed, including CSF; crosses placenta; distributed into breast milk. **Metabolism:** metabolized in liver to active and inactive metabolites; is enterohepatically cycled. **Elimination:** half-life: 3 h; up to 30% excreted in urine, 60–65% in feces.

CONTRAINDICATIONS & PRECAUTIONS Contraindicated in: obstructive biliary disease; intermittent rifampin therapy. Safe use during pregnancy and in children < 5 y not established. **Cautious use in:** hepatic disease; history of alcoholism; concomitant use of other hepatotoxic agents.

ADVERSE/SIDE EFFECTS CNS: fatigue, drowsiness, headache, ataxia, confusion, dizziness, inability to concentrate, generalized numbness, pain in extremities, muscular weakness. **Eye/ear:** visual disturbances, transient low-frequency hearing loss, conjunctivitis. **GI:** *heartburn, epigastric distress, nausea, vomiting, anorexia, flatulence, cramps, diarrhea,* <u>pseudomembranous colitis</u>. **Hematologic:** thrombocytopenia, transient leukopenia, anemia, including hemolytic anemia. **Hypersensitivity:** fever, pruritus, urticaria, skin eruptions, soreness of mouth

R

and tongue, eosinophilia, hemolysis. **Renal:** hemoglobinuria, hematuria, acute renal failure. **Other:** hemoptysis, light-chain proteinuria, flu-like syndrome, menstrual disorders, hepatorenal syndrome (with intermittent therapy), *transient elevations in liver function tests* (bilirubin, BSP, alkaline phosphatase, ALT, AST), pancreatitis. **Overdosage:** GI symptoms, increasing lethargy, liver enlargement and tenderness, jaundice, brownish-red or orange discoloration of skin, sweat, saliva, tears, and feces; unconsciousness.

DIAGNOSTIC TEST INTERFERENCE Rifampin interferes with contrast media used for ***gallbladder study;*** therefore, test should precede daily dose of rifampin. May also cause retention of ***BSP.*** Inhibits standard assays for ***serum folate*** and ***vitamin*** B_{12}.

DRUG INTERACTIONS Alcohol, isoniazid increase risk of hepatotoxicity; ***p*-aminosalicylic acid (PAS)** decreases concentrations of rifampin; decreases concentrations of BARBITURATES, BENZODIAZEPINES, **clofibrate,** CORTICOSTEROIDS, **dapsone, digitoxin, methadone, metoprolol, warfarin,** SULFONYLUREAS, ORAL CONTRACEPTIVES, PROGESTINS, **propranolol, quinidine, ketoconazole, fluconazole,** leading to potential therapeutic failure.

R

NURSING IMPLICATIONS

Administration

- Capsule may be emptied and contents swallowed with fluid or mixed with food.
- An oral suspension can be prepared from capsules for use in pediatric patients. Consult pharmacist for specific preparation directions.
- Administer 1 h before or 2 h after a meal. Peak serum levels are delayed and may be slightly lower when given with food.
- A desiccant should be kept in bottle containing capsules; they become unstable with moisture.
- IV administration: IV rifampin is diluted by adding 10 ml of sterile water for injection to each 600-mg vial to yield 60 mg/ml. The ordered dose is withdrawn and further diluted in 100–500 ml of D5W. Infuse over 30 min to 3 h, depending on volume of solution. A less concentrated solution infused over a longer period is preferred.

Assessment & Drug Effects

- Serology and susceptibility testing should be performed prior to and in the event of positive cultures.
- Periodic hepatic function tests are advised. Patients with hepatic disease must be closely monitored.
- If patient is also receiving an anticoagulant, prothrombin times should be performed daily or as necessary to establish and maintain required anticoagulant activity.

Patient & Family Education

- Caution not to interrupt prescribed dosage regimen. Hepatorenal reaction with flu-like syndrome has occurred when therapy has been resumed following interruption.
- Inform that drug may impart a harmless red-orange color to urine, feces, sputum, sweat, and tears. Soft contact lens may be permanently stained.
- Instruct to report onset of jaundice, hypersensitivity reactions, and persistence of GI adverse effects.
- Patients taking oral contraceptives (OCs) should consider alternative methods of contraception. Concomitant use of rifampin and OC leads to decreased effectiveness of the contraceptive and to menstrual

disturbances (spotting, breakthrough bleeding).
- Caution patient to keep drug out of reach of children.

RIFAPENTINE

(rif′a-pen-teen)
Trade name: Priftin
Classifications: ANTIINFECTIVE; ANTIBIOTIC; ANTITUBERCULOSIS AGENT
Prototype: Isoniazid
Pregnancy category: C

ACTIONS/PHARMACODYNAMICS Rifamycin derivative similar to rifampin. Inhibits *Mycobacterium tuberculosis*. As resistant strains emerge rapidly when employed alone, it is used in conjunction with other antitubercular agents.

USE Pulmonary tuberculosis in conjunction with at least one other antitubercular agent.

ROUTE & DOSAGE

Tuberculosis: Short-course Therapy
Adult: **PO** 600 mg twice weekly (at least 72 h apart) × 2 mo, then 600 mg once weekly × 4 mo.

PHARMACOKINETICS Absorption: approx 70% absorbed. **Peak:** 5–6 h. **Distribution:** 97.7% protein bound. **Metabolism:** hydrolyzed by esterase enzyme to active metabolite in liver; inducer of cytochromes P450 3A4 and 2C8/9. **Elimination:** half-life: 13.3 h; 70% excreted in feces, 17% in urine.

CONTRAINDICATIONS & PRECAUTIONS Contraindicated in: hypersensitivity to any rifamycins (e.g., rifampin, rifabutin, rifapentine); pregnancy (category C); lactation. **Cautious use in:** patients with abnormal liver function tests or liver disease; HIV disease, and/or concurrent use of protease inhibitors. Safety and efficacy in children <12 y not known.

ADVERSE/SIDE EFFECTS CNS: headache, dizziness. **CV:** hypertension. **GI:** increased liver function tests (ALT, AST), anorexia, nausea, vomiting, dyspepsia, diarrhea. **GU:** *hyperuricemia,* pyuria, proteinuria, hematuria, urinary casts. **Hematologic:** neutropenia, lymphopenia, anemia, leukopenia, thrombocytosis. **Respiratory:** hemoptysis. **Skin:** rash, pruritus, acne. **Other:** arthralgia, pain.

DRUG INTERACTIONS Decreased levels of **indinavir** and possibly other PROTEASE INHIBITORS; increased metabolism and decreased activity of ORAL CONTRACEPTIVES, **phenytoin, disopyramide, mexiletine, quinidine, tocainide, warfarin, fluconazole, itraconazole, ketoconazole, diazepam,** BETA BLOCKERS, CALCIUM CHANNEL BLOCKERS, CORTICOSTEROIDS, **haloperidol,** SULFONYLUREAS, **cyclosporine, tacrolimus, levothyroxine,** NARCOTIC ANALGESICS, **quinine,** REVERSE TRANSCRIPTASE INHIBITORS, TRICYCLIC ANTIDEPRESSANTS, **slidenafil, theophylline.**

NURSING IMPLICATIONS

Administration
- Rifapentine must be given with an interval of no less than 72 h between doses.
- Rifapentine may be given with food to minimize GI upset.
- Store at 15–30C (59–86F) in a tightly closed container and protect from excess moisture.

Assessment & Drug Effects
- Therapeutic effectiveness is indicated by improvement in clinical

R

S&S (e.g., fever, cough, pleuritic pain, fatigue) and on chest x-ray.
- Lab tests: Sputum smear and culture, CBC, baseline liver functions (especially serum transaminases) to rule out preexisting hepatic disease and serum creatinine and BUN.
- Carefully monitor for S&S of toxicity with concurrent use of oral anticoagulants, digitalis preparations, or anticonvulsants.

Patient & Family Education
- Strict adherence to the prescribed dosing schedule for this and other tuberculosis drugs is essential to prevent emergence of resistant strains of tuberculosis.
- Food may be useful in preventing GI upset.
- Immediately report any of the following to the physician: fever, weakness, nausea or vomiting, loss of appetitie, dark urine or yellowing of eyes or skin, pain or swelling of the joint, severe or persistent diarrhea.
- Women using hormonal contraceptives should use an alternative form of contraception.

R

RILUZOLE
(ri-lu′zole)
Trade name: Rilutek
Classifications: CENTRAL NERVOUS SYSTEM AGENT; ANTI-AMYOTROPHIC LATERAL SCLEROSIS AGENT
Pregnancy category: C

ACTIONS/PHARMACODYNAMICS Glutamate antagonist used for treating amyotrophic lateral sclerosis (ALS). Inhibits the presynaptic release of glutamic acid in the CNS. One hypothesis for the pathogenesis of ALS is that motor neurons are injured by glutamate, hence the possible effectiveness of riluzole. Also protects neurons against the excitotoxicity of glutamic acid.

USES Treatment of ALS, may extend survival and/or time to tracheostomy.

ROUTE & DOSAGE

ALS
Adult: **PO** 50 mg q12h at least 1 h before or 2 h after meals.

PHARMACOKINETICS Absorption: well absorbed from GI tract, 60% reaches systemic circulation. **Steady state:** 5 d. **Distribution:** 96% protein bound. **Metabolism:** metabolized in liver by cytochrome P4501A2 (CYP1A2). **Elimination:** half-life: 12 h; 90% eliminated in urine.

CONTRAINDICATIONS & PRECAUTIONS Contraindicated in: hypersensitivity to riluzole, lactation. **Cautious use in:** liver dysfunction, renal impairment; hypertension, history of other CNS disorders, pregnancy (category C). Safety and efficacy in children not established.

ADVERSE/SIDE EFFECTS Body as whole: *asthenia,* headache, back pain, malaise, arthralgia, weight loss, peripheral edema, flulike syndrome. **CNS:** hypertonia, depression, dizziness, dry mouth, insomnia, somnolence, circumoral paresthesia. **CV:** hypertension, tachycardia, phlebitis, palpitation. **GI:** abdominal pain, *nausea,* vomiting, dyspepsia, anorexia, diarrhea, flatulence, stomatitis. **Respiratory:** *decreased lung function,* rhinitis, increased cough, apnea, bronchitis, dysphagia, dyspnea. **Skin:** pruritus, eczema, alopecia, exfoliative dermatitis (rare). **Other:** UTI.

NURSING IMPLICATIONS

Administration

- Give at same time daily and at least 1 h before or 2 h after a meal. Do not administer before/after a high-fat meal.
- Store at room temperature; protect from bright light.

Assessment & Drug Effects

- Monitor liver function tests before and during course of therapy; evaluate ALT/SGPT every month for first 3 mo, every 3 mo for remainder of first year, and periodically thereafter.
- Withhold drug and notify physician if liver enzymes are elevated.
- Periodically monitor Hct and Hgb, routine blood chemistries, and alkaline phosphatase. If febrile illness develops, monitor WBC count.

Patient & Family Education

- Provide administration directions and stress that there is no increased benefit from daily doses >50 mg q12h.
- Instruct to report any febrile illness and advise caution with potentially hazardous activities until reaction to drug is known.
- Advise regarding common adverse effects and possible adverse interaction with alcohol.

RIMANTADINE

(ri-man′ta-deen)

Trade name: Flumadine

Classifications: ANTIINFECTIVE; ANTIVIRAL

Prototype: Acyclovir

Pregnancy category: C

ACTIONS/PHARMACODYNAMICS Rimantadine is an antiviral agent for the treatment and prophylaxis of influenza A infections. It is thought to exert its inhibitory effect early in the viral replication cycle, probably by interfering with the viral uncoating procedure of the influenza A virus, thus interfering in the replication cycle. Rimantadine inhibits synthesis of both viral RNA and protein.

USES Prophylaxis and treatment of influenza A in adults and prophylaxis of influenza A in children.

ROUTE & DOSAGE

Prophylaxis of Influenza A

Adult: **PO** 100 mg b.i.d.; reduce to 100 mg daily in the elderly or patients with hepatic disease.
Child: **PO** <*10 y*, 5 mg/kg once daily (not to exceed 150 mg/d); >*10 y*, same as adult.

Treatment of Influenza A

Adult: **PO** 100 mg b.i.d.; reduce to 100 mg daily in the elderly or patients with hepatic disease; initiate as soon as possible, preferably within 48 h of onset of symptoms, and continue for about 7 d.

PHARMACOKINETICS **Absorption:** readily absorbed from GI tract. **Peak:** serum levels 3.2–4.3 h. **Distribution:** concentrates in respiratory secretions. **Metabolism:** extensively metabolized in liver. **Elimination:** half-life: 20–36 h; excreted by kidneys.

CONTRAINDICATIONS & PRECAUTIONS **Contraindicated in:** hypersensitivity to rimantadine and amantadine, pregnancy (category C), lactation, children <1 y. **Cautious use in:** history of seizures. Safety and efficacy in treatment of symptomatic influenza infection in children not established.

ADVERSE/SIDE EFFECTS **CNS:** nervousness, dizziness, headache, sleep

R

disturbances, fatigue or malaise, drowsiness, anticholinergic effects. **GI:** nausea, vomiting, diarrhea, dyspepsia, dry mouth, anorexia, abdominal pain.

NURSING IMPLICATIONS

Administration

- In the elderly or those with renal or hepatic disease, dose reduction to 100 mg/d is recommended.
- Store at room temperature, 15–30C (59–86F).

Assessment & Drug Effects

- In patients with a history of seizures, carefully monitor for seizure activity. Seizures are an indication to discontinue the drug.
- Monitor cardiac, respiratory, and neurologic status while on drug. Report palpitations, hypertension, dyspnea, or pedal edema.

Patient & Family Education

- Advise to report bothersome side effects, especially hallucinations, palpitations, difficulty breathing, and swelling of legs.
- Advise caution with hazardous activities until reaction to drug is known.

R

RIMEXOLONE

(rim-ex′o-lone)

Trade name: Vexol

Classifications: SYNTHETIC HORMONE; OPHTHALMIC CORTICOSTEROID; ANTIINFLAMMATORY AGENT

Prototype: Hydrocortisone

Pregnancy category: C

See Appendix A.

RISEDRONATE SODIUM

(ri-se-dron′ate)

Trade name: Actonel

Classifications: REGULATOR, BONE METABOLISM; BISPHOSPHONATE

Prototype: Etidronate Disodium

Pregnancy category: C

ACTIONS/PHARMACODYNAMICS Diphosphate preparation with primary action on bone. Mechanism of action not fully understood. Slows rate of bone resorption and new bone formation in pagetic bone lesions and in normal remodeling process. Lowers serum alkaline phosphatase, presumably by decreasing release of phosphate from bone and increasing excretion of parthyroid hormone. One thousand times more potent than etidronate.

USE Paget's disease. **Unlabeled use:** osteoporosis.

ROUTE & DOSAGE

Paget's Disease

Adult: **PO** 30 mg q.d. at least 30 min before the first food or drink of the day × 2 mo; may repeat after 2 mo rest if necessary.

PHARMACOKINETICS **Absorption:** minimally absorbed from GI tract, bioavailability 0.63%. **Peak:** 1 h. **Distribution:** approx 60% of dose is distributed to bone. **Metabolism:** not metabolized. **Elimination:** half-life: 220 h; excreted in urine; unabsorbed drug excreted in feces.

CONTRAINDICATIONS & PRECAUTIONS **Contraindicated in:** hypersensitivity to risedronate or other bisphosphonates; hypocalcemia, vitamin D deficiency; lactation; severe renal impairment (creatinine clearance <30 ml/min); pregnancy (category C). **Cautious use in:** renal impairment; CHF; hyperphosphatemia; liver disease; fever related to infection or other causes. Safety and efficacy in children not established.

ADVERSE/SIDE EFFECTS Body as whole: flu syndrome, asthenia, arthralgia, bone pain, leg cramps, myasthenia. **CNS:** headache, dizziness. **CV:** chest pain, peripheral edema. **GI:** *diarrhea,* abdominal pain, nausea, constipation, belching, colitis. **Respiratory:** bronchitis, sinusitis. **Skin:** rash. **Other:** amblyopia, tinnitus, dry eyes.

DIAGNOSTIC TEST INTERFERENCE May interfere with the use of bone-imaging agents.

DRUG INTERACTIONS Calcium, ANTACIDS significantly decrease absorption.

NURSING IMPLICATIONS

Administration

- Give on an empty stomach (before first food or drink of the day) with at least 6–8 oz plain water.
- Patient should be upright. Maintain upright position and empty stomach for at least 30 min after administration.
- Space calcium supplements and antacids as far as possible from risedronate.
- Store at 15–30C (59–86F) in a tightly closed container and protect from light.

Assessment & Drug Effects

- Therapeutic effectiveness is indicated by decreased bone and joint pain and improved bone density.
- Lab tests: Baseline and periodic serum calcium, phosphorus, and alkaline phosphatase.
- Carefully monitor for and immediately report S&S of GI bleeding and hypocalcemia.

Patient & Family Education

- Administration guidelines regarding upright position, empty stomach, and spacing relative to calcium supplements and antacids must be strictly followed.
- Report any of the following to the prescriber: eye irritation, significant GI upset, or flu-like symptoms.

RISPERIDONE

(ris-per′-i-done)

Trade name: Risperdal

Classifications: CNS AGENT; ANTIPSYCHOTIC; NEUROLEPTIC AGENT

Prototype: Clozapine

Pregnancy category: C

ACTIONS/PHARMACODYNAMICS Mechanism is not defined. Interferes with binding of dopamine to D_2-interlimbic region of the brain, serotonin (5-HT_2) receptors, and alpha-adrenergic receptors in the occipital cortex. It has low to moderate affinity to the other serotonin (5-HT) receptors and no affinity to non-dopaminergic sites (e.g., cholinergic, muscarinic, or beta-adrenergic receptors).

USES Reduction or elimination of psychotic symptoms in schizophrenia and related psychoses. Seems to improve negative symptoms such as apathy, blunted affect, and emotional withdrawal. **Unlabeled use:** adjunctive treatment of behavioral disturbances in patients with mental retardation.

ROUTE & DOSAGE

Psychosis

Adult: **PO** 1–6 mg b.i.d. Begin with 1 mg b.i.d., increase by 1 mg b.i.d. daily to an initial target dose of 3 mg b.i.d. Elderly, debilitated, and patients with renal insufficiency should start with 0.5

mg b.i.d. and increase by 0.5 mg b.i.d. daily to an initial target of 1.5 mg b.i.d. (max 6 mg/d).

PHARMACOKINETICS **Absorption:** rapidly absorbed; not affected by food. **Onset:** therapeutic effect 1–2 wk. **Peak:** 1–2 h. **Distribution:** 0.7 L/kg; in animal studies, risperidone has been found in breast milk. **Metabolism:** metabolized primarily in liver by cytochrome P450 with an active metabolite, 9-hydroxyrisperidone. **Elimination:** half-life: 20 h for slow metabolizers, 30 h for fast metabolizers; 70% excreted in urine; 14% in feces.

CONTRAINDICATIONS & PRECAUTIONS **Contraindicated in:** hypersensitivity to risperidone, lactation. **Cautious use in:** arrhythmias, hypotension, history of seizures, breast cancer, blood dyscrasia, cardiac disorders, renal or hepatic impairment, pregnancy (category C). Safety and efficacy in children not established.

ADVERSE/SIDE EFFECTS **CNS:** *sedation, drowsiness,* headache, transient blurred vision, fatigue, insomnia, disinhibition, agitation, dizziness, catatonia. **GI:** dry mouth, constipation. **Other:** urinary retention, tachycardia, elevated liver function tests (AST, ALT), sweating, weakness.

DIAGNOSTIC TEST INTERFERENCE Liver function tests (AST, ALT) are elevated.

DRUG INTERACTIONS Risperidone may enhance the effects of certain ANTIHYPERTENSIVE AGENTS. May antagonize the effects of **levodopa** and **dopamine** agonists. **Carbamazepine** may decrease risperidone levels. **Clozapine** may increase risperidone levels.

NURSING IMPLICATIONS

Administration

- When dosage adjustments are made, increases/decreases should not exceed 1 mg b.i.d. in normal populations and 0.5 mg b.i.d. in the elderly or debilitated.
- When the target doses of 3 mg b.i.d. in normal populations and 1.5 mg b.i.d. in the elderly or debilitated are reached, further increases should be made at 1-wk or longer intervals.
- Store at room temperature, 15–30C (59–86F).

Assessment & Drug Effects

- Patients should be reassessed periodically and maintained on the lowest effective drug dose.
- Closely monitor cardiovascular status; assess for orthostatic hypotension, especially during initial dosage titration.
- Carefully monitor those at risk for seizures.
- Assess degree of cognitive and motor impairment, and assess for environmental hazards.
- Periodically monitor serum electrolytes, liver function tests, and complete blood counts.

Patient & Family Education

- Advise to exercise caution with hazardous activities until the reaction to the drug is known.
- Advise of adverse drug effects and instruct to report those that are bothersome.
- Discuss the risk of othostatic hypotension with the patient.
- Advise to wear sunscreen and protective clothing to avoid photosensitivity.
- Advise female patients to notify physician if they intend to become or become pregnant.

RITODRINE HYDROCHLORIDE

(ri'toe-dreen)

Trade name: Yutopar

Classifications: AUTONOMIC NERVOUS SYSTEM AGENT; BETA-ADRENERGIC AGONIST

Prototype: Isoproterenol

Pregnancy category: C

ACTIONS/PHARMACODYNAMICS
$Beta_2$-adrenergic agonist clinically effective in preventing or delaying of preterm labor (tocolytic effect). Preferentially stimulates $beta_2$ receptors in uterine smooth muscle, reducing intensity and frequency of uterine contractions and lengthening gestation period. (Actions may be eliminated by beta-adrenergic antagonists.) Transitory cardiovascular effects including increased cardiac output, increased maternal and fetal heart rates, and widening of maternal pulse pressure ($beta_1$ stimulation) are common.

USE To manage premature labor in selected patients.

ROUTE & DOSAGE

Premature Labor

Adult: **PO** Start 30 min before terminating infusion; 10 mg q2h for first 24 h, then 10–20 mg q4–6h (max 120 mg/d); **IV** 50–100 µg/min; may increase by 50 µg/min q10min until uterine relaxation is achieved; may continue for up to 12 h after contractions have ceased.

PHARMACOKINETICS **Absorption:** 30% absorbed from GI tract. **Peak:** 30–60 min. **Distribution:** crosses placenta. **Metabolism:** metabolized in liver. **Elimination:** half-life: 1.7–2.6 h; excreted in urine.

CONTRAINDICATIONS & PRECAUTIONS **Contraindicated in:** mild to moderate preeclampsia or eclampsia, intrauterine infection, cervix dilated 4 cm or more (in a singleton pregnancy); pregnancy (category C); hypertension; diabetes mellitus; prior to 20th wk or after 36th wk of pregnancy or if continuation of pregnancy would be hazardous to mother and fetus (e.g., antepartum hemorrhage, eclampsia, intrauterine fetal death, maternal cardiac disease, pulmonary hypertension, maternal hyperthyroidism, severe diabetes mellitus). Also hypovolemia, cardiac arrhythmias associated with tachycardia or digitalis intoxication, uncontrolled hypertension; thyrotoxicosis; bronchial asthma being treated with betamimetics or steroids. **Cautious use in:** concomitant use of potassium-depleting diuretics, cardiac disease.

ADVERSE/SIDE EFFECTS More pronounced and frequent following IV infusion: *altered maternal and fetal heart rates and maternal BP* (dose related); *temporary hyperglycemia, palpitations,* arrhythmias, tremor, nausea, vomiting, headache, erythema; *nervousness,* restlessness, anxiety, malaise, chest pain, pulmonary edema. Infrequent: <u>anaphylactic shock</u>, rash, epigastric distress, ileus, bloating, constipation, diarrhea, dyspnea, hyperventilation, glycosuria, hemolytic icterus, sweating, chills, drowsiness, weakness, myotonic and muscular dystrophies.

DIAGNOSTIC TEST INTERFERENCE Ritodrine (IV route) may produce an increase in ***serum*** levels of ***glucose, insulin,*** and ***free fatty acids,*** and a decrease in ***serum potassium.*** It temporarily elevates results of ***glucose tolerance test.***

DRUG INTERACTIONS CORTICOSTEROIDS may precipitate pulmonary edema; BETA AGONISTS add to cardiovascular adverse effects; effects of both ritodrine and BETA BLOCKERS antagonized.

NURSING IMPLICATIONS

Administration

- Preparation of IV solution: Add 150 mg ritodrine to 500 ml 5% dextrose or NS solution, giving a final concentration of 0.3 mg/ml (300 μg/ml).
- IV solution should be clear and should not be administered if it is cloudy or if a precipitate is present.
- Monitor IV infusion flow rate to prevent circulation overload. Use a microdrip and infusion pump.
- Place patient in left lateral recumbent position throughout the infusion period to reduce risk of hypotension.
- Store drug below 30C (86F). Do not freeze.

Assessment & Drug Effects

- Uterine contractions will decrease in frequency and intensity during treatment.
- Pronounced dose-related side effects require continuous monitoring of maternal and fetal heart rates and maternal BP while infusion is running.
- Occult cardiac disease has been unmasked by use of ritodrine.
- If patient is also on steroid therapy, hospitalization for treatment with ritodrine is advised. Be alert to signs and symptoms of pulmonary edema (see Appendix G).

R

RITONAVIR

(ri-ton′-a-vir)

Trade name: Norvir

Classifications: ANTIINFECTIVE; ANTIVIRAL; PROTEASE INHIBITOR

Prototype: Saquinavir

Pregnancy category: B

ACTIONS/PHARMACODYNAMICS Protease inhibitor of both HIV-1 and HIV-2 proteases. HIV protease is an enzyme required to produce the polyprotein procurers of functional proteins in infectious HIV. Protease inhibitors prevent cleavage of the viral polyproteins, resulting in the formation of immature noninfectious virus particles.

USE Alone or in combination with other antiretroviral agents or protease inhibitors for treatment of HIV infection.

ROUTE & DOSAGE

HIV

Adult: **PO** 600 mg b.i.d. 1 h before or 2 h after meal (may take with a light snack).
Child 2–16 y: **PO** 400 mg/m^2 b.i.d. (max 600 mg b.i.d.). Start with 250 mg/m^2 b.i.d. and increase by 50 mg/m^2 q2–3d.

PHARMACOKINETICS **Absorption:** rapidly absorbed from GI tract. **Peak:** 2–4 h. **Distribution:** 98–99% protein bound. **Metabolism:** metabolized in liver by cytochrome P4503A4 (CYP3A4). **Elimination:** excreted primarily in feces (>80%).

CONTRAINDICATIONS & PRECAUTIONS **Contraindicated in:** hypersensitivity to ritonavir, lactation. **Cautious use in:** pregnancy (category B), hepatic impairment, renal insufficiency. Safety and efficacy in children <2 y not established.

ADVERSE/SIDE EFFECTS **CNS:** *asthenia,* fatigue, headache, fever, malaise, circumoral or peripheral paresthesia, insomnia, dizziness, somnolence, abnormal thinking, amnesia, agitation, anxiety, confusion, convulsions, aphasia, ataxia, diplopia, emotional lability, euphoria, hallucinations, decreased libido, nervousness, neuralgia, neuropathy, peripheral neuropathy, paralysis, tremor, vertigo. **CV:** palpitations, vasodilation, hypotension, postural hypotension, syncope, tachycardia. **Hematologic:** anemia, thrombocytopenia, lymphadenopathy. **GI:** *nausea, diarrhea, vomiting,* abdominal pain, dyspepsia, stomatitis, anorexia, dry mouth, constipation, flatulence, cholecystitis, cholestasis, abnormal liver function tests, hepatitis. **Skin:** rash, sweating, acne, contact dermatitis, pruritus, urticaria, skin ulceration, dry skin. **Other:** myalgia, allergic reaction, bronchitis, cough, rhinitis, taste alterations, visual disturbances, dysuria, hyperglycemia, diabetes.

DRUG INTERACTIONS **Carbamazepine, dexamethasone, phenobarbital, phenytoin, rifabutin, rifampin,** smoking can decrease ritonavir levels. **Ritonavir** may increase serum levels and toxicity of **clarithromycin,** especially in patients with renal insufficiency (reduce **clarithromycin** dose in patients with Cl_{cr} <60 ml/min); **desipramine; saquinavir, amiodarone, astemizole, bepridil, buproprion, cisapride, clozapine, dihydroergotamine, flecainide, meperidine, pimozide, piroxicam, propoxyphene, quinidine, rifabutin. Ritonavir** decreases levels of ORAL CONTRACEPTIVES, **theophylline**. Liquid formulation may cause disulfiram-like reaction with **alcohol** or **metronidazole**. See the complete prescribing information for a comprehensive table of potential, but not studied, drug interactions.

NURSING IMPLICATIONS

Administration

- Preferably given with food; oral solution may be mixed with chocolate milk within 1 h of dosing to improve taste.
- Do not administer concurrently with any of the following drugs: alprazolam, amiodarone, astemizole, bepridil, bupropion, cisapride, clozapine, clorazepate, diazepam, encainide, estazolam, flecainide, flurazepam, meperidine, midazolam, piroxicam, propafenone, propoxyphene, quinidine, rifabutin, terfenadine, triazolam, zolpidem.
- Store refrigerated at 2–8C (36–46F). Protect from light in tightly closed container.

Assessment & Drug Effects

- Periodically monitor CBC with differential and platelet count, liver function, kidney function, serum albumin, lipid profile, CPK, serum amylase, electrolytes, blood glucose, and alkaline phosphatase.
- In the presence of abnormal liver functions, withhold drug and notify physician.
- Assess for S&S of GI distress, peripheral neuropathy, and other potential adverse effects.

Patient & Family Education

- Provide administration directions. If a dose is missed, instruct to take next dose as soon as possible unless near time for next dose; advise not to double a dose.
- Advise regarding potential adverse reactions and drug interactions; instruct to report to physician use of any other drugs, including OTC drugs.

RITUXIMAB
(rit-ux′i-mab)
Trade name: Rituxan
Classifications: ANTINEOPLASTIC; IMMUNOMODULATOR
Prototype: Basiliximab
Pregnancy category: C

ACTIONS/PHARMACODYNAMICS Genetically engineered monoclonal antibody that binds with the CD20 antigen on the surface of normal and malignant B lymphocytes. Administration results in a rapid and sustained depletion of circulating and tissue-based (e.g., thymus, spleen) B lymphocytes in non-Hodgkin's lymphoma.

USE Relapsed or refractory CD20 positive, B-cell non-Hodgkin's lymphoma.

ROUTE & DOSAGE

Non-Hodgkin's Lymphoma
Adult: **IV** 375 mg/m^2 infused at 50 mg/h; can increase infusion rate q30min to max of 400 mg/h if tolerated; repeat dose on days 8, 15, and 22 (total of 4 doses).

R

PHARMACOKINETICS Duration: 6–12 mo. **Elimination:** half-life: 60–174 h (increases with multiple infusions).

CONTRAINDICATIONS & PRECAUTIONS Contraindicated in: hypersensitivity to murine proteins or rituximab; pregnancy (category C); lactation. **Cautious use in:** prior exposure to murine-based monoclonal antibodies; history of allergies; asthma and other pulmonary disease (increased risk of bronchospasm); CAD; thrombocytopenia; history of cardiac arrhythmias; renal impairment. Safety and efficacy in children not established.

ADVERSE/SIDE EFFECTS Body as whole: angioedema, *fatigue,* asthenia, night sweats, *fever, chills,* myalgia. **CNS:** headache, dizziness, depression. **CV:** hypotension, tachycardia, peripheral edema. **GI:** *nausea,* vomiting, throat irritation, anorexia, abdominal pain. **Hematologic:** <u>leukopenia, thrombocytopenia, anemia,</u> neutropenia. **Respiratory:** bronchospasm, dyspnea, rhinitis. **Skin:** pruritus, rash urticaria. **Infusion-related reactions:** *fever, chills, rigors, pruritus, urticaria, pain, flushing,* chest pain, hypotension, hypertension, dyspnea; <u>fatal infusion-related reactions have been reported</u>.

NURSING IMPLICATIONS

Administration

- IV preparation: Dilute ordered dose to 1–4 mg/ml by adding to an infusion bag of 0.9% NaCl or D5W; gently invert bag to mix. Discard unused portion left in vial.
- IV infusion: Infuse first dose of diluted drug at a rate of 50 mg/h; increase rate at 50 mg/h increments q30min to maximum rate of 400 mg/h; for subsequent doses, infuse at a rate of 100 mg/h and increase by 100 mg/h increments q30min up to maximum rate of 400 mg/h.
- Do not administer IV push or as a bolus dose.
- Slow or stop infusion if S&S of hypersensitivity appear (see Appendix G).
- Store unopened vials at 2–8C (36–46F) and protect from light.

Assessment & Drug Effects

- Therapeutic effectiveness is indicated by rapid and sustained depletion of B lymphocytes.
- Lab tests: CBC with differential, peripheral CD20+ B lymphocytes.
- During infusion carefully monitor

BP and ECG status; immediately report S&S of hypersensitivity (e.g., fever, chills, urticaria, pruritus, hypotension, bronchospasms; see Appendix G for others).

Patient & Family Education

- Persons with childbearing potential should use effective contraception during and for up to 12 mo following rituximab therapy.
- During infusion report any of the following: itching, difficulty breathing, tightness in throat, dizziness, headache, nausea.

RIZATRIPTAN BENZOATE

(ri-za-trip′tan ben′zo-ate)

Trade names: Maxalt, Maxalt-MLT

Classifications: AUTONOMIC NERVOUS SYSTEM AGENT; ALPHA-ADRENERGIC ANTAGONIST (SYMPATHETOLYTIC) SEROTONIN $5HT_{1B/1D}$ RECEPTOR AGONIST; ERGOT ALKALOID

Prototype: Sumatriptan

Pregnancy category: C

ACTIONS/PHARMACODYNAMICS Selective ($5HT_{1B/1D}$) receptor agonist. The agonist effects at $5HT_{1B/1D}$ reverse the vasodilation of cranial blood vessels associated with a migraine. Activation of these receptors also reduces the pain pathways associated with the migraine headache.

USE Acute migraine headaches with or without aura.

ROUTE & DOSAGE

Acute Migraine

Adult: **PO** 5–10 mg; may repeat in 2 h if necessary (max 30 mg/24 h); patients also on propranolol should use 5 mg with max 15 mg/24 h.

PHARMACOKINETICS Absorption: 45% of oral dose reaches systemic circulation. **Peak:** 1–1.5 h for oral tabs; 1.6–2.5 h for orally disintegrating tablets. **Metabolism:** metabolized via oxidative deamination by monoamine oxidase A. **Elimination:** half-life: 2–3 h; excreted primarily in urine (82%).

CONTRAINDICATIONS & PRECAUTIONS Contraindicated in: hypersensitivity to rizatriptan; CAD; Prinzmetal's angina (potential for vasospasm); risk factors for CAD such as hypertension, hypercholesterolemia, obesity, diabetes, smoking, and strong family history; concurrent administration with ergotamine drugs or sumatriptan; concurrent administration with MAOIs; basilar or hemiplegic migraine. **Cautious use in:** hypersensitivity to sumatriptan; renal or hepatic impairment; pregnancy (category C); lactation; hypertension; asthmatic patients. Safety and effectiveness unknown in patients <18 y.

ADVERSE/SIDE EFFECTS Body as whole: asthenia, fatigue, pain, pressure sensation, paresthesias, throat pressure, warm/cold sensations. **CNS:** somnolence, dizziness, headache, hypesthesia, decreased mental acuity, euphoria, tremor. **CV:** coronary artery vasospasm, transient myocardial ischemia, MI, ventricular tachycardia, ventricular fibrillation, chest pain/tightness/heaviness, palpitations. **GI:** dry mouth, nausea, vomiting, diarrhea. **Respiratory:** dyspnea. **Skin:** flushing. **Other:** hot flashes.

DRUG INTERACTIONS Propranolol may increase concentrations of rizatriptan, use smaller rizatriptan doses; **dihydroergotamine, methysergide,** other $5\text{-}HT_1$ AGONISTS may cause prolonged vasospastic re-

R

actions; SSRIS have rarely caused weakness, hyperreflexia, and incoordination; MAOIS should not be used with 5-HT_1 agonists.

NURSING IMPLICATIONS

Administration

- Administer any time after symptoms of migraine appear. If symptoms return, a second tablet may be given but no sooner than 2 h after the first.
- If there is no response to the first tablet, contact physician before administering a second.
- Do not give within 24 h of an ergot-containing drug or another 5-HT_1 agonist.
- Store at 15–30C (59–86F) and protect from light and moisture.

Assessment & Drug Effects

- Carefully monitor cardiovascular status following first dose in patients at risk for CAD (e.g., postmenopausal women, men over 40 years old, persons with known CAD risk factors) or coronary artery vasospasms.
- ECG is recommended following first administration of rizatriptan to someone with known CAD risk factors.
- Immediately report to the physician chest pain or tightness in chest or throat that is severe or does not quickly resolve.
- Periodic cardiovascular evaluation is recommended with continued rizatriptan use.

Patient & Family Education

- Carefully review patient information leaflet and guidelines for administration.
- Do not exceed 30 mg in 24 h.
- Allow orally disintegrating tablets to dissolve on tongue; no liquid is needed.
- Immediately contact physician if any of the following develop following rizatriptan use: symptoms of angina (e.g., severe and/or persistent pain or tightness in chest or throat), hypersensitivity (e.g., wheezing, facial swelling, skin rash, or hives), abdominal pain.
- Report any other adverse effects (e.g., tingling, flushing, dizziness) at next physician visit.

ROPINIROLE HYDROCHLORIDE

(ro-pi′ni-role)

Trade name: Requip

Classifications: AUTONOMIC NERVOUS SYSTEM AGENT; ANTICHOLINERGIC (PARASYMPATHOMIMETIC); ANTIPARKINSONISM AGENT

Prototype: Levodopa

Pregnancy category: C

ACTIONS/PHARMACODYNAMICS

Ropinirole is a nonergot dopamine receptor agonist structurally similar to pramipixole, for treatment of Parkinson's disease. It has high affinity for the D_2 subfamily of dopamine receptors and higher binding affinity to D_3 than to D_2 or D_4 receptor subtypes. The precise mechanism of action and treatment for Parkinson's disease is not known.

USE Idiopathic Parkinson's disease.

ROUTE & DOSAGE

Parkinson's Disease

Adult: **PO** Start with 0.25 mg t.i.d.; may titrate up by 0.25 mg/dose t.i.d. qwk to a target dose of 1 mg t.i.d. If response is still not satisfactory, may continue to increase by 1.5 mg/d qwk to a dose of 9 mg/d, and then by ≤ 3 mg/d weekly to a max dose of 24 mg/d.

PHARMACOKINETICS Absorption: rapidly absorbed from GI tract; 55% bioavailability. **Peak:** 1–2 h. **Distribution:** 30–40% protein bound. **Metabolism:** metabolized in the liver by CYP1A2. **Elimination:** half-life: 6 h; primarily excreted in urine.

CONTRAINDICATIONS & PRECAUTIONS Contraindicated in: hypersensitivity to ropinirole or pramipixole; lactation. **Cautious use in:** renal and hepatic function impairment, concomitant use of CNS depressants, pregnancy (category C). Safety and efficacy in children have not been established.

ADVERSE/SIDE EFFECTS Body as whole: increased sweating, dry mouth, flushing, asthenia, *fatigue,* pain, edema, malaise. **CNS:** *dizziness, somnolence,* hallucinations, confusion, amnesia, hypesthesia, yawning, hyperkinesia, impaired concentration, vertigo. **CV:** *syncope,* chest pain, orthostatic symptoms, hypertension, palpitations, atrial fibrillation, extrasystoles, hypotension, tachycardia. **GI:** *nausea, vomiting, dyspepsia,* abdominal pain, anorexia, flatulence. **Respiratory:** pharyngitis, rhinitis, sinusitis, bronchitis, dyspnea. **Other:** peripheral edema, abnormal vision, exerophthalmia, eye abnormality, *viral infection,* UTI, impotence, peripheral ischemia.

DRUG INTERACTIONS Ropinirole levels may be increased by ESTROGENS, QUINOLONE ANTIBIOTICS, **cimetidine, diltiazem, erythromycin, fluvoxamine, mexiletine, tacrine;** effects may be antagonized by PHENOTHIAZINES, BUTYROPHENONES, METOCLOPRAMIDE.

NURSING IMPLICATIONS

Administration

- Giving with food may reduce occurrence of nausea.
- Dose is titrated as needed at weekly intervals: begin with 0.25 mg t.i.d., increase by 0.25 mg per dose each week up to 1 mg t.i.d. in week 4. Thereafter, if needed, increase dose at weekly intervals by 1.5 mg/d up to 9 mg/d. Further weekly increases of ≤ 3 mg/d up to a total dose of 24 mg/d may be made.
- Drug must be discontinued gradually over 7 d by decreasing from t.i.d. to b.i.d. dosing for 4 d, and then to q.d. dosing for 3 d.
- With moderate-to-severe renal impairment, initial and maintenance doses should be lowered.
- Store at 15–30C (59–86F).

Assessment & Drug Effects

- Therapeutic effectiveness is indicated by improvement in Parkinson's disease.
- Lab test: periodically monitor BUN and creatinine; hepatic function tests.
- Periodic eye exams and chest x-ray are indicated in long-term use.
- Carefully monitor for orthostatic hypotension, especially during dose escalation.

Patient & Family Education

- Hallucinations are a possible side effect and occur more often in elderly persons.
- Postural hypotension is common, especially during early treatment with ropinirole. Make position changes slowly, especially after long periods of lying or sitting.
- Exercise caution with hazardous activities requiring alertness since drowsiness and sedation are common side effects. Effects are additive with alcohol or other CNS depressants.
- Women who become pregnant should immediately notify their physician. Mothers should not breast-feed without discussing potential problems with the physician.

ROPIVACAINE HYDROCHLORIDE
(ro-piv'i-cane)
Trade name: Naropin
Classifications: CNS AGENT; LOCAL ANESTHETIC (ESTER-TYPE)
Prototype: Procaine hydrochloride
Pregnancy category: B

ACTIONS/PHARMACODYNAMICS Ropivacaine blocks the generation and conduction of nerve impulses, probably by increasing the threshold for electrical excitability. This local anesthetic action produces loss of sensation and motor activity in areas of the body close to the injection site.

USES Local and regional anesthesia, postoperative pain management, anesthesia/pain management for obstetric procedures.

ROUTE & DOSAGE

Surgical Anesthesia
Adult: **Epidural** 25–200 mg (0.5–1% solution). **Nerve block** 5–250 mg (0.5% solution).

Labor Pain
Adult: **Epidural infusion** 20–40 mg (0.2% solution).

Postoperative Pain Management
Adult: **Epidural infusion** 12–20 mg/h (0.2% solution). **Infiltration** 2–200 mg (0.2–0.5% solution).

PHARMACOKINETICS Onset: 1–30 min (average 10–20 min) depending on dose/route of administration. **Duration:** 0.5–8 h depending on dose/route of administration. **Distribution:** 94% protein bound. **Metabolism:** metabolized in the liver by CYP1A. **Elimination:** half-life: 1.8–4.2 h; excreted in urine.

CONTRAINDICATIONS & PRECAUTIONS Contraindicated in: hypersensitivity to ropivacaine or any local anesthetic of the amide type; generalized septicemia, inflammation or sepsis at the proposed injection site; cerebral spinal diseases (e.g., meningitis); heart block, hypotension, hypertension, GI hemorrhage. **Cautious use in:** pregnancy (category B), debilitated, elderly, or acutely ill patients; arrhythmias, shock.

ADVERSE/SIDE EFFECTS Body as whole: pain, fever, rigors, hypoesthesia **CNS:** paresthesia, headache, dizziness, anxiety. **CV:** *hypotension,* bradycardia, hypertension, tachycardia, chest pain, fetal bradycardia. **GI:** nausea. **Skin:** pruritus. **Other:** urinary retention, oliguria, anemia.

DRUG INTERACTIONS Additive adverse effects with other LOCAL ANESTHETICS.

NURSING IMPLICATIONS

Administration
- Avoid rapid injection of large volumes of ropivacaine. Incremental doses should always be used to achieve the smallest effective dose and concentration.
- For postoperative analgesia, use an infusion concentration of 2 mg/ml (0.2%).
- Disinfecting agents containing heavy metal ions (e.g., mercury, copper, zinc, etc.) should not be used on the skin insertion site or to clean the ropivacaine container top.
- Solutions contain no preservatives. Continuous infusions must be discarded after 24 h.
- Store unopened at 20–25C (68–77F).

Assessment & Drug Effects
- Therapeutic effectiveness for postoperative pain management is indicated by adequate analgesia.

- Throughout treatment period, carefully monitor cardiovascular and respiratory status. Assess for hypotension and bradycardia.
- Immediately report S&S of CNS stimulation (e.g, restlessness, anxiety, tinnitus, blurred vision, tremors) or CNS depression.

SALMETEROL XINAFOATE

(sal-me′ter-ol xin′a-fo-ate)

Trade name: Serevent

Classifications: AUTONOMIC NERVOUS SYSTEM AGENT; BETA-ADRENERGIC AGONIST (SYMPATHOMIMETIC); BRONCHODILATOR; RESPIRATORY SMOOTH MUSCLE RELAXANT

Prototype: Isoproterenol

Pregnancy category: C

ACTIONS/PHARMACODYNAMICS Salmeterol is a long-acting $beta_2$-adrenoceptor agonist and an analog of albuterol. Stimulation of $beta_2$-adrenoreceptors relaxes bronchospasm and increases ciliary motility, thus facilitating expectoration of pulmonary secretions. Salmeterol also decreases airway reaction to allergens and inhibits the release of mediators (i.e., histamine) from mast cells, macrophages, and eosinophils.

USES Maintenance therapy for asthma or bronchospasm. Prevention of exercise-induced bronchospasm. Should *not* be used to treat acute bronchospasm.

ROUTE & DOSAGE

Asthma/Bronchospasm

Adult: **Inhaled** 2 inhalations (42 µg) b.i.d. approximately 12 h apart.
Child > 12 y: **Inhaled** same as adult.

Prevention of Exercise-induced Bronchospasm

Adult: **Inhaled** 2 inhalations (42 µg) 30–60 min before exercise.
Child > 12 y: **Inhaled** same as adult.

PHARMACOKINETICS **Onset:** 10–20 min. **Peak:** effect 2 h. **Duration:** up to 12 h. **Distribution:** 94–95% protein bound. **Metabolism:** dissociates in solution; salmeterol base and xinafoate salt are metabolized, absorbed, distributed, and excreted independently; salmeterol is extensively metabolized by hydroxylation. **Elimination:** half-life: 3–4 h; eliminated primarily in feces.

CONTRAINDICATIONS & PRECAUTIONS **Contraindicated in:** hypersensitivity to salmeterol, lactation. **Cautious use in:** cardiovascular disorders, cardiac arrhythmias, hypertension, history of seizures or thyrotoxicosis, liver impairment, elderly, diabetes mellitus, sensitivity to other beta-adrenergic agonists, pregnancy (category C), laboring women. Safety and efficacy in children <12 y not established.

ADVERSE/SIDE EFFECTS **CNS:** dizziness, headache, tremor. **CV:** palpitations, sinus tachycardia. **Other:** <u>respiratory arrest</u> (rare), rash, tolerance (tachyphylaxis).

DRUG INTERACTION Effects antagonized by BETA BLOCKERS.

NURSING IMPLICATIONS

Administration

- Salmeterol should *not* be used to relieve symptoms of acute asthma.
- Shake canister well before using; lips should be tightly closed around the mouthpiece, and patient should deeply inhale during each actuation.

- Store at room temperature, 15–30C (59–86F).

Assessment & Drug Effects
- If bronchospasms occur following use of salmeterol, the drug should be immediately discontinued.
- Monitor cardiovascular status; report tachycardia.
- With long-term therapy, hepatic enzymes should be monitored periodically.

Patient & Family Education
- Advise to report immediately worsening asthma or failure to respond to the usual dose of salmeterol.
- Patients on twice-daily doses of salmeterol should be told *not* to use an additional dose prior to exercise.
- Advise patients who use a preexercise dose to use it 30–60 min before exercise and to wait 12 h before an additional dose.

SALSALATE

(sal′sal-ate)

Trade names: Artha-G, Disalcid, Mono-Gesic, Salflex, Salsitab

Classifications: CNS AGENT; ANALGESIC; ANTIPYRETIC; SALICYLATE

Prototype: Aspirin

Pregnancy category: C

S

ACTIONS/PHARMACODYNAMICS Actions similar to those of other salicylates. Clinical studies suggest that salsalate does not produce significant gastric irritation, and it has not been associated with reactions causing asthmatic attacks in susceptible individuals. The incidence of side effects in general appears to be lower than that of other salicylates. Unlike aspirin, it does not appear to inhibit platelet aggregation.

USES Symptomatic treatment, rheumatoid arthritis, osteoarthritis, and related rheumatic disorders.

ROUTE & DOSAGE

Arthritis
Adult: **PO** 325–3000 mg/d in divided doses (max 4 g/d).

PHARMACOKINETICS **Absorption:** readily absorbed from small intestine. **Peak:** 1.5–4 h. **Metabolism:** hydrolyzed in liver, GI mucosa, plasma, whole blood, and other tissues. **Elimination:** half-life: 1 h; excreted in urine.

CONTRAINDICATIONS & PRECAUTIONS **Contraindicated in:** hypersensitivity to salicylates, chronic renal insufficiency, peptic ulcer, pregnancy (category C), children < 12 y.

ADVERSE/SIDE EFFECTS Occasionally, nausea, dyspepsia, heartburn. **Overdosage** (salicylism): tinnitus, hearing loss (reversible), vertigo, flushing, headache, confusion, drowsiness, hyperventilation, sweating, vomiting, diarrhea.

NURSING IMPLICATIONS

Administration
- Administer with a full glass of water or with food or milk to reduce GI side effects.

Assessment & Drug Effects
- Symptom relief is gradual (may require 3–4 d to establish steady-state salicylate level).
- Monitor for adverse GI effects, especially in patient with a history of peptic ulcer disease.

Patient & Family Education
- Warn not to take another salicylate (e.g., aspirin) while on salsalate therapy.
- Inform diabetic that drug may induce hypoglycemia when it is used with sulfonylureas.

- Instruct to report tinnitus, hearing loss, vertigo, rash, or nausea.

SAQUINAVIR MESYLATE
(sa-quin'a-vir mes'y-late)
Trade names: Fortovase, Invirase
Prototype for classification: PROTEASE INHIBITOR
Pregnancy category: B

ACTIONS/PHARMACODYNAMICS
Saquinavir is a synthetic peptide that inhibits the activity of HIV protease and prevents the cleavage of viral polyproteins essential for the maturation of HIV.

USE Advanced HIV infection, usually in combination with zidovudine or zalcitabine.

ROUTE & DOSAGE

HIV
Adult: **PO** *Invirase* 600 mg (3 × 200 mg) t.i.d. taken 2 h after a full meal. *Fortovase* 1200 mg t.i.d. with meals.

PHARMACOKINETICS **Absorption:** rapidly absorbed from GI tract; only 4% reaches systemic circulation; food significantly reduces absorption. **Distribution:** 98% protein bound. **Metabolism:** metabolized in liver by cytochrome P450. **Elimination:** excreted primarily in feces (> 70%).

CONTRAINDICATIONS & PRECAUTIONS **Contraindicated in:** significant hypersensitivity to saquinavir, nursing mothers. **Cautious use in:** pregnancy (category B), hepatic insufficiency. Safety and effectiveness in HIV-infected children < 16 y have not been established.

ADVERSE/SIDE EFFECTS **CNS:** headache, paresthesia, numbness, dizziness, peripheral neuropathy, ataxia, confusion, convulsions, hyperreflexia, hyporeflexia, tremor, agitation, amnesia, anxiety, depression, excessive dreaming, hallucinations, euphoria, irritability, lethargy, somnolence. **CV:** chest pain, hypertension, hypotension, syncope. **Endocrine:** dehydration, hyperglycemia, xerophthalmia, weight changes. **Hematologic:** anemia, splenomegaly, thrombocytopenia, pancytopenia. **GI:** *nausea, diarrhea, abdominal discomfort,* dyspepsia, mucosal damage, change in appetite, dry mouth. **Skin:** rash, pruritus, acne, erythema, seborrhea, hair changes, photosensitivity, skin ulceration, dry skin. **Other:** myalgia, allergic reaction, bronchitis, cough, dyspnea, epistaxis, hemoptysis, laryngitis, rhinitis, earache, taste alterations, tinnitus, visual disturbances, hyperglycemia, diabetes.

DRUG INTERACTIONS **Rifampin, rifabutin** significantly decrease **saquinavir** levels. **Phenobarbital, phenytoin, dexamethasone, carbamazepine** may also reduce **saquinavir** levels. May increase serum levels of **cisapride, triazolam, midazolam,** ERGOT DERIVATIVES, **terfenadine** or **astemizole.**

NURSING IMPLICATIONS

Administration
- Drug should be taken with a full meal to ensure adequate absorption and bioavailability.
- Saquinavir should not be administered to anyone taking rifampin or rifabutin.
- Store Invirase at 15–30C (59–86F) in tightly closed bottle.
- Store Fortovase in refrigerator. Capsules are stable for 3 mo at room temperature (≤ 25C/<77F).

Assessment & Drug Effects
- Prior to initiating therapy and periodically thereafter, monitor

S

serum electrolytes, CBC with differential, liver function tests, blood glucose, CPK, and serum amylase.
- Monitor for and report signs and symptoms of peripheral neuropathy.
- Assess for buccal mucosa ulceration or other distressing GI signs and symptoms.
- Monitor weight periodically.
- Monitor for toxicity if any of the following drugs is used concomitantly with saquinavir: calcium channel blockers, clindamycin, dapsone, quinidine, triazolam.

Patient & Family Education
- Inform that saquinavir is not a cure for HIV infection and that its long-term effects are unknown.
- Instruct to take drug within 2 h of a full meal.
- Advise to report any distressing adverse effects.

SARGRAMOSTIM (GM-CSF)
(sar-gra′mos-tim)
Trade names: Leukine, Leukine Liquid, Prokine
Classification: HEMATOPOIETIC GROWTH FACTOR
Prototype: Epoetin alfa
Pregnancy category: C

S

ACTIONS/PHARMACODYNAMICS
Sargramostim is a recombinant human granulocyte-macrophage colony stimulating factor (GM-CSF) produced by recombinant DNA technology in a yeast. GM-CSF is a hematopoietic growth factor that stimulates proliferation and differentiation of hematopoietic progenitor cells in the granulocyte-macrophage pathways. Sargramostim increases the cytotoxity of monocytes to certain neoplastic cell lines and activates polymorphonuclear neutrophils (PMNs) to inhibit the growth of tumor cells.

USES Myeloid reconstitution after autologous bone marrow transplantation for patients with non-Hodgkin's lymphoma (NHL), acute lymphoblastic leukemia (ALL), and Hodgkin's disease; mobilization of peripheral blood stem cells (PBSCs) for autologous transplantation. **Unlabeled uses:** to increase WBC counts in AIDS patients; to decrease leukopenia secondary to myelosuppressive chemotherapy; to correct neutropenia in aplastic anemia and in liver and kidney transplantations.

ROUTE & DOSAGE

Autologous Bone Marrow Transplant

Adult: **IV** 250 μg/m²/d infused over 2 h for 21 d; begin 2–4 h after bone marrow transfusion and not less than 24 h after last dose of chemotherapy or 12 h after last radiation therapy.
Child: **IV/SC** 250 μg/m²/d × 21 d; begin 2–4 h after bone marrow infusion or not less than 24 h after chemotherapy.

Neutropenia

Adult: **SC** 3–15 μg/kg/d.
Child: **SC** Same as for adult.

PHARMACOKINETICS **Absorption:** readily absorbed from SC site. **Onset:** 3–6 h. **Peak:** 1–2 h. **Duration:** 5–10 d SC. **Elimination:** half-life: 80–150 min; probably excreted in urine.

CONTRAINDICATIONS & PRECAUTIONS **Contraindicated in:** excessive leukemic myeloid blasts in bone marrow or blood; known hypersensitivity to GM-CSF or yeast products. **Cautious use in:** history of cardiac arrhythmias, preexisting cardiac disease, hypoxia, CHF, pulmonary infiltrates; renal and hepatic dysfunction; pregnancy (category C), and nursing mothers. Safety and efficacy in children not established; however, adverse side effects have been comparable to those in adults.

ADVERSE/SIDE EFFECTS CNS: lethargy, malaise, headache, fatigue. **CV:** abnormal ST segment depression, supraventricular arrhythmias, edema, *hypotension, tachycardia,* pericardial effusion, pericarditis. **Hematologic:** anemia, *thrombocytopenia.* **GI:** nausea, vomiting, diarrhea, anorexia. **Other:** *bone pain, myalgia, arthralgias,* weight gain, hyperuricemia, *fever,* pleural effusion, *rash, pruritus,* ***first-dose reaction*** (some or all of the following symptoms: hypotension, tachycardia, fever, rigors, flushing, nausea, vomiting, diaphoresis, back pain, leg spasms, and dyspnea).

DRUG INTERACTIONS CORTICOSTEROIDS should be used cautiously with sargramostim because the myeloproliferative effects may be potentiated. **Lithium** should be used with caution with sargramostim because it may potentiate the myeloproliferative effects.

INCOMPATIBILITIES Solution/additive: hydrocortisone, hydroxyzine, haloperidol. Y-site: acyclovir, amphotericin B, cefonicid, cefoperazone, chlorpromazine, idarubicin, lorazepam, mitomycin, morphine, nalbuphine, ondansetron, vancomycin.

NURSING IMPLICATIONS

Administration

- Sargramostim should not be administered within 24 h preceding or following chemotherapy or within 12 h preceding or following radiotherapy.
- Reconstitute each 250 or 500 μg vial with 1 ml of sterile water for injection (without preservative). Direct sterile water against side of vial and swirl gently. Avoid excessive or vigorous agitation. Do not shake.
- IV preparation: To dilute for IV infusion, use 0.9% NaCl. If the final concentration is < 10 μg/ml, add albumin (human) to NS before addition of sargramostim. Use 1 mg albumin per 1 ml of 0.9% NaCl to give a final concentration of 0.1% albumin.
- IV infusion: Infuse diluted solution over 2 h.
- IV administration to infants, children: Verify correct IV concentration and rate of infusion with physician.
- Administer as soon as possible and within 6 h of reconstitution or dilution for IV infusion. After 6 h, discard it.
- Sargramostim vials are single-dose vials. Discard unused portion.
- If the absolute neutrophil count exceeds 20,000/mm^3 or if platelet count exceeds 500,000/mm^3, interrupt administration and reduce the dose by 50%. Notify the physician.
- If the patient experiences dyspnea during administration, reduce the IV rate 50%. If respiratory symptoms worsen, discontinue infusion. Notify physician.
- Refrigerate the sterile powder, the reconstituted solution, and the diluted solution at 2–8C (36–46F). Do not freeze or shake.

Assessment & Drug Effects

- Obtain a CBC and platelet count prior to initiation of therapy.
- Treatment should be discontinued if WBC $\geq$ 50,000 /mm^3. Notify the physician.
- Notify physician of any severe adverse reaction immediately.
- Occasional transient supraventricu-

S

lar arrhythmias have occurred during administration, particularly in those with a history of cardiac arrhythmias. Arrhythmias are reversed with discontinuation of drug.

- Give special attention to respiratory symptoms (dyspnea) during and immediately following infusion, especially in patients with preexisting pulmonary disease.
- Peripheral edema, pleural or pericardial effusion has occurred after administration. It is reversible with dose reduction. Use drug with caution in patients with preexisting fluid retention, pulmonary infiltrates, or CHF.
- Biweekly monitoring of renal and hepatic function is necessary in patients with renal or hepatic dysfunction prior to the initiation of therapy.
- Monitor serum creatinine, bilirubin, and liver enzymes.
- Biweekly monitoring of CBC with differential should be continued during therapy.
- Potentially, sargramostim can act as a growth factor for myeloid malignancies. Should disease progression be detected, discontinue therapy and notify physician.

Patient & Family Education

- Instruct to notify nurse or physician immediately of any adverse effect (e.g., dyspnea, palpitations) experienced during or after drug administration.

S

SCOPOLAMINE

(skoe-pol′a-meen)

Trade names: Transderm-Scōp, Transderm-V ♣

SCOPOLAMINE HYDROBROMIDE

Trade names: Hyoscine, Isopto-Hyoscine, Murocoll, Triptone

Classifications: AUTONOMIC NERVOUS SYSTEM AGENT; ANTICHOLINERGIC (PARASYMPATHOLYTIC); ANTIMUSCARINIC; ANTISPASMODIC

Prototype: Atropine

Pregnancy category: C

ACTIONS/PHARMACODYNAMICS

Alkaloid of belladonna with peripheral actions resembling those of atropine. In contrast to atropine, produces CNS depression, with marked sedative and tranquilizing effects, and is less effective in preventing reflex bradycardia during anesthesia. More potent in mydriatic and cycloplegic actions and in inhibiting secretions of salivary, bronchial, and sweat glands, but has less prominent effect on heart, intestines, and bronchial muscles.

USES In obstetrics with morphine to produce amnesia and sedation ("twilight sleep") and as preanesthetic medication. To control spasticity (and drooling) in postencephalitic parkinsonism, paralysis agitans, and other spastic states, as prophylactic agent for motion sickness and as mydriatic and cycloplegic in ophthalmology. Therapeutic system (Transderm-Scōp) is used to prevent nausea and vomiting associated with motion sickness.

ROUTE & DOSAGE

Preanesthetic

Adult: **PO** 0.5–1 mg. **IM/SC/IV** 0.3–0.6 mg.
Child: **PO/IM/SC/IV** 0.006 mg/kg.

Motion Sickness

Adult: **PO** 0.25–0.6 mg 1 h before anticipated travel. **Topical** 1 patch q72h starting 12 h before anticipated travel.
Child: **PO** 0.006 mg/kg 1 h before anticipated travel.

Refraction

Adult: **Ophthalmic** 1–2 drops in eye 1 h before refraction.

Uveitis

Adult: **Ophthalmic** 1–2 drops in eye up to q.i.d.

PHARMACOKINETICS **Absorption:** readily absorbed from GI tract and percutaneously. **Peak:** 20–60 min. **Duration:** 5–7 d. **Distribution:** crosses placenta; distributed to CNS. **Metabolism:** metabolized in liver. **Elimination:** excreted in urine.

CONTRAINDICATIONS & PRECAUTIONS **Contraindicated in:** asthma; hepatitis; toxemia of pregnancy; pregnancy (category C). **Cautious use in:** cardiac disease; patients over 40 y, pyloric obstruction, urinary bladder neck obstruction, angle-closure glaucoma, thyrotoxicosis, paralytic ileus.

ADVERSE/SIDE EFFECTS Sense of fatigue, dizziness, *drowsiness, dry mouth and throat, constipation,* urinary retention, disorientation, decreased heart rate, dilated pupils, photophobia, depressed respiration, restlessness, hallucinations, toxic psychosis. **Eye:** blurred vision, *local irritation,* follicular conjunctivitis. **Skin:** local irritation from patch adhesive, rash.

DRUG INTERACTIONS **Amantadine,** ANTIHISTAMINES, TRICYCLIC ANTIDEPRESSANTS, **quinidine, disopyramide, procainamide** add to anticholinergic effects; decreases **levodopa** effects; **methotrimeprazine** may precipitate extrapyramidal effects; decreases antipsychotic effects (decreased absorption) of PHENOTHIAZINES.

NURSING IMPLICATIONS

Administration

- To minimize possibility of systemic absorption, apply pressure against lacrimal sac during and for 1 or 2 min following instillation of eye drops.
- May be given by direct IV diluted in sterile water for injection. Inject diluted solution slowly.

Therapeutic System (Transderm-Scōp, a Controlled-Release System):

- Transdermal disc system should be applied to dry surface behind the ear.
- If disc system becomes dislodged, it can be replaced by another on another site behind the ear.
- Preserve in tight, light-resistant containers.

Assessment & Drug Effects

- Some patients manifest excitement, delirium, disorientation, and garrulousness shortly after drug is administered until sedative effect takes hold. Observe patient closely for these effects.
- Side rails are advisable, particularly for the elderly, because of amnesic effect of scopolamine.
- In the presence of pain, scopolamine may cause delirium, restlessness, and excitement unless given with an analgesic.
- Tolerance may develop with prolonged use.
- Ophthalmic use should be terminated if local irritation, edema, or conjunctivitis occur.

Patient & Family Education

- When used as mydriatic or cycloplegic, caution that vision will be blurred; instruct patient to avoid potentially hazardous activities such as driving a car or operating machinery until vision clears.
- Disc system is effective if applied as soon as 2–3 h before anticipated

S

motion; however, therapeutic effect is best with 12 h of application.

- Advise to place disc on skin site the night before an expected trip.
- Advise to wash hands carefully after handling scopolamine. Anisocoria (unequal size of pupils, blurred vision can develop by rubbing eye with drug-contaminated finger).

SECOBARBITAL

(see-koe-bar'bi-tal)

Trade names: Novosecobarb ♣, Seconal

SECOBARBITAL SODIUM

Trade name: Seconal Sodium

Prototype for classifications: CNS AGENT; ANXIOLYTIC; SEDATIVE-HYPNOTIC; BARBITURATE

Pregnancy category: D

Controlled substance: Schedule II

ACTIONS/PHARMACODYNAMICS

Short-acting barbiturate with CNS depressant effects and anticonvulsant action similar to that of phenobarbital.

USES Hypnotic for simple insomnia and preoperatively to provide basal hypnosis for general, spinal, or regional anesthesia. Effective in the emergency control of acute convulsive conditions (e.g., tetanus, toxic reactions to poisons) and in the management of acute agitated behavior.

ROUTE & DOSAGE

Sedative

Adult: **PO** 100–300 mg/d in 3 divided doses.
Child: **PO/PR*** 4–6 mg/kg/d in 3 divided doses.

Preoperative Sedative

Adult: **PO** 100–300 mg 1–2 h before surgery.
Child: **PO** 50–100 mg 1–2 h before surgery. **PR*** *>3 y,* 60–120 mg 1–2 h before surgery; *6 mo–3 y,* 60 mg 1–2 h before surgery; *<6 mo,* 30–60 mg 1–2 h before surgery. **IM** 4–5 mg/kg 1–2 h before surgery.

Hypnotic

Adult: **PO/IM** 100–200 mg.
Child: **IM** 3–5 mg/kg.

Acute Convulsive Episode

Adult: **IM** 5.5 mg/kg repeated q3–4h if needed. **IV** 5.5 mg/kg repeated q3–4h if needed; infuse at ≤50 mg/15 s.
Child: **IM** 3–5 mg/kg.

Adjunct to Spinal Anesthesia

Adult: **IV** 50–100 mg (max 250 mg/dose), infused at ≤50 mg/15 s.
Child: **PR*** *>40 kg,* 5 mg/kg; *<40 kg,* 4 mg/kg.

*Make the rectal solution by diluting the IV with lukewarm tap water to a concentration of 10–15 mg/ml and administer rectally following a cleansing enema.

PHARMACOKINETICS **Absorption:** 90% absorbed from GI tract. **Onset:** 15–30 min PO; 7–10 min IM; 1–3 min IV. **Duration:** 1–4 h PO; 15 min IV. **Distribution:** crosses placenta; distributed into breast milk. **Metabolism:** metabolized in liver. **Elimination:** half-life: 30 h; excreted in urine.

CONTRAINDICATIONS & PRECAUTIONS **Contraindicated in:** history of sensitivity to barbiturates; pregnancy (category D); parturition, fetal immaturity, uncontrolled pain. Use of sterile injection containing polyethylene glycol vehicle in patients with renal insufficiency. **Cautious use in:** pregnant women with toxemia or history of bleeding.

ADVERSE/SIDE EFFECTS Drowsiness, lethargy, hangover, paradoxical excitement in the elderly patient; respiratory depression, laryngospasm, fall in BP (with rapid IV).

DRUG INTERACTIONS **Phenmetrazine** antagonizes effects of secobarbital; CNS DEPRESSANTS, **alcohol,** SEDATIVES compound CNS depression; MAO INHIBITORS cause excessive CNS depression; **methoxyflurane** increases risk of nephrotoxicity.

INCOMPATIBILITIES **Solution/additive: benzquinamide, codeine, cimetidine, ephedrine, erythromycin, glycopyrrolate, hydrocortisone, insulin, levorphanol, methadone, norepinephrine, pentazocine, phenytoin, procaine, sodium bicarbonate, streptomycin, tetracycline, vancomycin. Y-site: cimetidine, glycopyrrolate.**

NURSING IMPLICATIONS

Administration

- Discard parenteral solutions that are not clear or that contain a precipitate.
- Administer IM injection deep into large muscle mass. Carefully aspirate before injecting drug to avoid inadvertent entry into blood vessel.
- Reconstitute secobarbital sodium powder with sterile water for injection (incompatible with bacteriostatic water for injection) to a concentration of 250 mg/5 ml. Following addition of water, rotate ampul; do not shake it. Several minutes are required to dissolve drug completely. If solution is not completely clear within 5 min, do not use. Consult package literature for details.
- IV administration: Secobarbital may be administered by direct IV at a rate of 50 mg or a fraction thereof over 30–60 seconds.
- Aqueous solutions of secobarbital sodium for injection are not stable; they must be freshly prepared and used within 30 min after container is opened.

Assessment & Drug Effects

- Patients receiving drug IV must be kept under constant observation. Monitor BP, pulse, and respiration q3–5min.
- Following IM injection of large hypnotic dose, observe patient closely for 20–30 min to assure that hypnosis is not excessive.
- When secobarbital is administered to pregnant patient, fetal heartbeat should be closely monitored. Report slowing or irregularities.
- If patient cannot swallow pill, it may be crushed before administration, then mixed with a fluid or with food. (Do not permit patient to swallow dry crushed drug.)
- The elderly or debilitated patient and children sometimes have paradoxical response to barbiturate therapy, i.e., irritability, marked excitement (inappropriate tearfulness and aggression in children), depression, and confusion. Be alert to unexpected responses and report promptly. Protect the elderly patient from falling, irrational behavior, and effects of depression (anorexia, social withdrawal).
- Although it is uncommon, the patient may become irritable, uncooperative, and restive after a subhypnotic dose of a short-acting barbiturate.
- Barbiturates do not have analgesic action, and they may be expected to produce restlessness when given to patients in pain.

S

- Alcohol in any amount given with a barbiturate may severely impair judgment and abilities; it should not be consumed by a patient on barbiturate therapy.
- Long-term therapy may result in nutritional folate (B_9) and vitamin D deficiency.
- Hepatic function and hematology tests and determinations of serum folate and vitamin D levels are advised during prolonged therapy.
- Barbiturates increase the metabolism of many drugs, leading to decreased pharmacologic effects of those drugs. Whenever a barbiturate is added to an established regimen of another drug, close observation for changes in effectiveness of the first drug is essential, at least during early phase of barbiturate use.
- Chronic toxicity (dependence, drug abuse) is characterized by behavior simulating that of the chronic alcoholic: desire or need to continue taking the drug without physician's knowledge; self-limited abstinence periods; patient begins to see a number of physicians, never admitting to multiple prescriptions. Symptoms include ataxia, slurred speech, irritability, poor judgment, slight dysarthria, nystagmus on vertical gaze, confusion, insomnia, and somatic complaints.
- Acute toxicity (intoxication) is characterized by profound CNS depression, respiratory depression that may progress to Cheyne-Stokes respirations, hypoventilation, cyanosis, cold clammy skin, hypothermia, constricted pupils (but may be dilated in severe intoxication), shock, oliguria, tachycardia, hypotension, respiration arrest, circulatory collapse, and death.

Patient & Family Education

- Advise ambulatory patient following drug administration to avoid driving a car or other potentially hazardous activities for the remainder of day.
- Advise patients taking barbiturates at home not to keep drug on bedside table or in a readily accessible place. Patients have been known to forget having taken the drug, and in half-wakened conditions have accidentally overdosed themselves.
- It is important that pregnancy be avoided in patients receiving barbiturates (reportedly teratogenic). Patients on prolonged therapy should consider alternative methods of contraception in addition to or instead of oral contraceptives to prevent unplanned pregnancy. Neonates born of mothers who receive barbiturate therapy throughout the last trimester may show withdrawal symptoms for 1–14 d after birth. Symptoms resemble congenital opiate withdrawal symptoms: hyperactivity, restlessness, tremor, hyperreflexia, disturbed sleep.
- Instruct on prolonged therapy to report to physician the onset of fever, sore throat or mouth, malaise, easy bruising or bleeding, petechiae, jaundice, rash.

S

SELEGILINE HYDROCHLORIDE (L-DEPRENYL)

(se-leg′i-leen)

Trade names: Carbex, Eldepryl

Classifications: AUTONOMIC NERVOUS SYSTEM AGENT; ANTICHOLINERGIC (PARASYMPATHOLYTIC); ANTIPARKINSONISM AGENT

Prototype: Levodopa (L-dopa)

Pregnancy category: C

ACTIONS/PHARMACODYNAMICS

Mechanism of action is not fully understood. Increase in dopaminergic activity is thought to be primarily due to inhibition of MAO type B activity. Although MAOs are widely distributed throughout the body, most of the MAO in the brain is type B. Selegiline may also increase dopaminergic activity by interfering with dopamine reuptake at the synapse.

USES Adjunctive therapy of Parkinson's disease for patients being treated with levodopa and carbidopa who exhibit deterioration in the quality of their response to therapy.

ROUTE & DOSAGE

Parkinson's Disease

Adult: **PO** 5 mg b.i.d. with breakfast and lunch. Doses >10 mg/d are associated with increased risk of toxicity due to MAO inhibition.
Geriatric: **PO** Start with 5 mg qAM.

PHARMACOKINETICS Absorption: rapidly absorbed; 73% reaches systemic circulation. **Onset:** 1 h. **Duration:** 1–3 d. **Distribution:** crosses placenta; not known if distributed into breast milk. **Metabolism:** metabolized in liver to *N*-desmethyldeprenyl, amphetamine, and methamphetamine. **Elimination:** half-life: 15 min (metabolites 2–20 h); excreted in urine.

CONTRAINDICATIONS & PRECAUTIONS Contraindicated in: hypersensitivity to selegiline. **Cautious use in:** hypertension and pregnancy (category C). Not known whether excreted in breast milk. Safety and efficacy in children have not been studied.

ADVERSE/SIDE EFFECTS CNS: sleep disturbances, psychosis, agitation, confusion, dyskinesia. **CV:** hypotension. **GI:** anorexia.

DRUG INTERACTIONS Same as with other MAO inhibitors, including severe reactions with **meperidine. Fluoxetine,** and possibly **sertraline** and **paroxetine,** increase risk of CNS toxicity and muscle rigidity. TRICYCLIC ANTIDEPRESSANTS can cause severe CNS toxicity.

NURSING IMPLICATIONS

Administration

- Do not administer daily doses exceeding 10 mg/d.
- Concurrent levodopa and carbidopa doses are usually reduced 10–30% after 2–3 d of selegiline therapy.
- Note that concurrent meperidine therapy is contraindicated and that other opioids as well are generally avoided with selegiline.
- Store at 15–30C (59–86F).

Assessment & Drug Effects

- Monitor vital signs, particularly during period of dosage adjustment. Report alterations in BP or pulse. Indications for discontinuation of the drug include orthostatic hypotension, hypertension, and arrhythmias.
- All patients should be closely monitored for behavior changes (e.g., hallucinations, confusion, depression, delusions).

Patient & Family Education

- Stress importance of not exceeding the prescribed dose of selegiline.
- Instruct to immediately report symptoms of MAO inhibitor-induced hypertension (e.g., severe headache, palpitations, neck stiffness, nausea, vomiting).
- Caution to avoid driving or other hazardous activities until reaction to selegiline is known.
- Orthostatic hypotension is possible,

S

and some individuals have experienced dizziness, light-headedness, and fainting. Advise to make positional changes slowly and in stages.

SELENIUM SULFIDE

(se-lee′nee-um)

Trade names: Exsel, Selsun, Selsun Blue

Classifications: SKIN AGENT; ANTI-INFECTIVE; ANTIBIOTIC; ANTIFUNGAL

Pregnancy category: C

ACTIONS/PHARMACODYNAMICS Has antibacterial and mild antifungal activity. Mechanism of action and causal relationships have not been established, but drug is active against *Pityrosporum ovale,* a yeast-like fungus found in the normal flora of the scalp. Absorption of selenium sulfide into epithelial tissue cells is followed by degradation of compound to selenium and sulfide ions. Selenium ions block enzyme systems involved in epithelial cell growth. As a result, rate of turnover in cells with normal or higher than normal turnover rates is reduced.

USES Itching and flaking of the scalp associated with dandruff, seborrheic dermatitis of the scalp, and tinea versicolor.

ROUTE & DOSAGE

Dandruff Control, Seborrheic Dermatitis

Adult/Child: **Topical** Massage 5–10 ml of a 1–2.5% solution into wet scalp and leave on for 2–3 min; rinse thoroughly; then repeat application and rinse well again; initially, shampoo 2 times/wk for 2 wk; then decrease to once q1–4wk prn.

Tinea Versicolor

Adult/Child: **Topical** Apply a 2.5% solution to affected area with a small amount of water to form a lather; leave on for 10 min; then rinse thoroughly; repeat once/d for 7 d.

PHARMACOKINETICS Absorption: no percutaneous absorption if skin is intact.

CONTRAINDICATIONS & PRECAUTIONS Contraindicated in: application to damaged or inflamed skin surfaces; as treatment of tinea versicolor during pregnancy. Use during pregnancy (category C) as antiseborrheic only when clearly needed. **Cautious use in:** prolonged skin contact; use in genital area or skin folds.

ADVERSE/SIDE EFFECTS *Skin irritation (stinging),* rebound oiliness of scalp, hair discoloration, diffuse hair loss (reversible), systemic toxicity (if applied to abraded, infected skin).

NURSING IMPLICATIONS

Administration

- Wash hands thoroughly after application of selenium sulfide to affected areas. Advise removing jewelry before treatment; drug will damage it.
- Genital areas and skin folds should be rinsed well with water and dried after treatment for tinea versicolor to prevent irritation.
- Store in tight container, protected from heat, at 15–30C (59–86F). Avoid freezing.

Patient & Family Education

- If lotion contacts the eyes, thoroughly rinse with water to prevent chemical conjunctivitis.
- Caution not to use this drug more

frequently than required to maintain control of dandruff.

- Hair loss is reversible, usually within 2–3 wk after treatment is discontinued.
- Systemic toxicity may result from application of lotion to damaged skin (percutaneous absorption), from prolonged use (overdosage), and from accidental ingestion. Warn to discontinue use if skin is irritated or if treatment fails. Toxicity symptoms: tremors, anorexia, occasional vomiting, lethargy, weakness, severe perspiration, garlicky breath, lower abdominal pain. Symptoms disappear 10–12 d after treatment is stopped.

SENNA

Trade names: Black-Draught, Gentlax B, Senexon, Senokot, Senolax

Classifications: GI AGENT; STIMULANT LAXATIVE

Prototype: Bisacodyl

Pregnancy category: C

ACTIONS/PHARMACODYNAMICS

Prepared from dried leaflet of *Cassia acutifolia* or *Cassia angustifolia*. Similar to cascara sagrada but with more potent action. Senna glycosides are converted in colon to active aglycones, which stimulate peristalsis. Standardized concentrate is purified and standardized for uniform action and is claimed to produce less colic than crude form.

USES Acute constipation and preoperative and preradiographic bowel evacuation.

ROUTE & DOSAGE

Constipation

Adult: **PO *Standard senna concentrate:*** 1–2 tablets or 1/2–1 tsp h.s. (max 4 tablets or 2 tsp b.i.d.); ***syrup, liquid:*** 10–15 ml at h.s.

Child: **PO *Standard senna concentrate:*** *>27 kg,* 1 tablet or 1/2 tsp h.s.; ***syrup, liquid:*** *5–15 y,* 5–10 ml h.s.; *1–5 y,* 2.5–5 ml h.s.; *1 mo–1 y,* 1.25–2.5 ml h.s.

PHARMACOKINETICS **Onset:** 6–10 h; may take up to 24 h. **Metabolism:** metabolized in liver. **Elimination:** excreted in feces.

CONTRAINDICATIONS & PRECAUTIONS **Contraindicated in:** irritable colon, nausea, vomiting, abdominal pain, intestinal obstruction, pregnancy (category C), nursing mothers.

ADVERSE/SIDE EFFECTS Abdominal cramps, flatulence, nausea. Prolonged use: watery diarrhea, excessive loss of water and electrolytes, weight loss, melanotic segmentation of colonic mucosa (reversible).

NURSING IMPLICATIONS

Administration

- Senna is generally administered at bedtime for relief of constipation.
- When used for preoperative or prediagnostic bowel preparation, senna is usually given between 2 and 4 PM on day prior to procedure. Diet is then confined to clear liquids.
- Avoid exposure of drug to excessive heat; fluid extracts should be protected from light.

Assessment & Drug Effects

- Some patients may experience considerable abdominal cramping; if medication is to be repeated, dose reduction may be indicated.

Patient & Family Education

- Inform that drug may color urine yellowish brown (acid urine) or

S

reddish brown (alkaline urine). Feces may be similarly colored.

- Caution that continued use may lead to dependence. If constipation persists, consult physician.

See bisacodyl for additional nursing implications.

SERTRALINE HYDROCHLORIDE

(ser′tra-leen)

Trade name: Zoloft

Classifications: CNS AGENT; PSYCHOTHERAPEUTIC; ANTIDEPRESSANT; SELECTIVE SEROTONIN REUPTAKE INHIBITOR

Prototype: Fluoxetine

Pregnancy category: B

ACTIONS/PHARMACODYNAMICS A potent inhibitor of serotonin reuptake and thus an antidepressant. It does not produce any sympathomimetic response or anticholinergic activity. Sertraline does not inhibit MAO.

USES Major depression, obsessive–compulsive disorder, panic disorder.

ROUTE & DOSAGE

Depression

Adult: **PO** Begin with 50 mg/d; gradually increase every few weeks according to response. Range: 50–200 mg.
Geriatric: **PO** Start with 25 mg/d.

PHARMACOKINETICS **Absorption:** slowly absorbed from GI tract. **Onset:** 2–4 wk. **Distribution:** 99% protein bound; not known if distributed into breast milk. **Metabolism:** extensive first-pass metabolism in liver to inactive metabolites. **Elimination:** half-life: 24 h; 40–45% excreted in urine, 40–45% in feces.

CONTRAINDICATIONS & PRECAUTIONS **Contraindicated in:** patients taking MAO inhibitors or within 14 d of discontinuing an MAO inhibitor. **Cautious use in:** seizure disorders, major affective disorders, suicidal patients; hepatic dysfunction, renal impairment; pregnancy (category B). It is not known if sertraline is excreted in breast milk. Safety and effectiveness in children not established.

ADVERSE/SIDE EFFECTS **CV:** palpitations, chest pain, hypertension, hypotension, edema, syncope, tachycardia. **CNS:** *agitation, insomnia, headache, dizziness, somnolence, fatigue,* ataxia, incoordination, vertigo, abnormal dreams, aggressive behavior, delusions, hallucinations, emotional lability, paranoia, suicidal ideation, depersonalization. **Endocrine:** gynecomastia, male sexual dysfunction. **GI:** nausea, vomiting, diarrhea, constipation, indigestion, anorexia, flatulence, abdominal pain, dry mouth. **Eye:** exophthalmos, blurred vision, dry eyes, diplopia, photophobia, tearing, conjunctivitis, mydriasis. **Skin:** rash, urticaria, acne, alopecia. **Other:** rhinitis, pharyngitis, cough, dyspnea, bronchospasm, myalgia, arthralgia, muscle weakness, hyponatremia in elderly.

DIAGNOSTIC TEST INTERFERENCE May cause asymptomatic elevations in ***liver function tests.*** Slight decrease in ***uric acid.***

DRUG INTERACTIONS MONOAMINE OXIDASE INHIBITORS (e.g., **selegiline, parnate**) should be stopped 14 d before sertraline is started because of serious problems with other serotonin-reuptake inhibitors (shivering, nausea, diplopia, confusion, anxiety). **Tolbutamide** and **diazepam** clearance may be reduced. Use cautiously with other centrally acting CNS drugs.

NURSING IMPLICATIONS

Administration

- Sertraline may be given in the morning or evening.
- It should not be given concurrently with a MAO inhibitor or within 14 d of discontinuing a MAO inhibitor.

Assessment & Drug Effects

- Close supervision of patients at risk for suicide should accompany initial sertraline therapy.
- Monitor the elderly for fluid and sodium imbalances.
- Closely monitor patients with a history of a seizure disorder.
- Monitor PT and INR with patients receiving concurrent warfarin therapy.

Patient & Family Education

- Advise to report diarrhea, nausea, dyspepsia, insomnia, drowsiness, dizziness, or persistent headache.
- Advise patients on warfarin therapy to promptly report signs of bleeding.

SIBUTRAMINE HYDROCHLORIDE MONOHYDRATE

(si-bu′tra-meen)

Trade name: Meridia

Classifications: CNS AGENT; SEROTONIN/NOREPINEPHRINE REUPTAKE INHIBITOR

Prototype: Fluoxetine

Pregnancy category: C

Controlled substance: Schedule IV

ACTIONS/PHARMACODYNAMICS Inhibits the reuptake of serotonin (5HT), monoamine reuptake, as well as norepinephrine and dopamine reuptake, by blocking their receptors. Its mechanism results in appetite suppression.

USE Management of obesity, including weight loss and maintenance of weight loss, in patients with BMI of at least 30 kg/m^2 or BMI of at least 27 kg/m^2 and other risk factors (hypertension, diabetes, dyslipidemia).

ROUTE & DOSAGE

Weight Loss

Adult: **PO** 10 mg once daily, preferably in morning, may be increased to 15 mg if inadequate weight loss (<4 lb) in 4 wk.

PHARMACOKINETICS **Absorption:** rapidly absorbed from GI tract. **Peak:** 1.2 h. **Distribution:** 97% protein bound; concentrates in liver and kidneys. **Metabolism:** metabolized in liver by cytochrome P450 3A4 to 2 active metabolites. **Elimination:** half-life: 14–16 h (active metabolites); excreted primarily in kidneys.

CONTRAINDICATIONS & PRECAUTIONS **Contraindicated in:** anorexia nervosa; arrhythmias; concurrent administration with other serotonin reuptake inhibitors (e.g., fluoxetine), MAOIs, lithium, tryptophan; severe hepatic or renal impairment; CHF, stroke, CAD; uncontrolled or poorly controlled hypertension; pregnancy (category C). **Cautious use in:** history of hypertension; elderly; narrow-angle glaucoma; seizures; lactation. Safety and efficacy in patients <16 y unknown.

ADVERSE/SIDE EFFECTS **Body as whole:** back pain, flu syndrome, asthenia. **CNS:** *headache,* insomnia, migraine headache, dizziness, nervousness, anxiety, depression, paresthesias, seizures (rare). **CV:** increase in BP, tachycardia, vasodilation, palpitations. **GI:** *dry mouth,* anorexia, constipation, abdominal pain, increased appetite, nausea, dyspepsia, taste perversion. **Respiratory:** rhinitis, pharyngitis, sinusitis, cough. **Skin:** rash, sweating. **Other:** arthralgia, dysmenorrhea, UTI.

DRUG INTERACTIONS DECONGESTANTS, COUGH AND ALLERGY MEDICATIONS may cause additional increase in BP; MAOIS, ERGOT DERIVATIVES, **sumatriptan, naratriptan, rizatriptan, zolmitriptan, dextromethorphan, meperidine, pentazocine, fentanyl, lithium;** SSRIS may predispose to serotonin syndrome (see Appendix G); **ketoconazole, erythromycin** may inhibit metabolism of sibutramine.

NURSING IMPLICATIONS

Administration

- Doses above 15 mg/d are not recommended.
- At least 2 wks should elapse between discontinuing an MAOI and beginning sibutramine.
- Store at 15–30C (59–86F) in a tightly closed container and protect from light.

Assessment & Drug Effects

- Therapeutic effectiveness is indicated by a loss of at least 4 lb during the first 4 wk of therapy.
- Carefully monitor weight changes to determine therapeutic effect.
- Lab tests: Periodic liver functions, bilirubin, alkaline phosphatases, lipid profile.
- Regularly monitor BR and HR; immediately report sustained increases in BP or HR.
- Monitor for and immediately report S&S of serotonin syndrome (see Appendix G).
- Closely monitor persons with narrow-angle glaucoma for worsening intraocular pressure.

Patient & Family Education

- Notify physician if any of the following develop: rash, hives, or other S&S of an allergic reaction; signs of hyperstimulation such as restlessness, shivering, profuse sweating, irritability, and tremor.
- Drug may cause less interference with sleep if taken in the morning.
- Check with physician prior to taking any over-the-counter cough, cold, allergy, or weight-loss drugs.
- Strict adherence to prescribed antihypertensives must be maintained while on sibutramine.
- Serious adverse effects may be experienced if sibutramine is taken with some drugs used to treat depression. Inform physician of all drugs being taken.

SILDENAFIL CITRATE

(sil-den′a-fil ci′trate)
Trade name: Viagra
Classification: IMPOTENCE AGENT
Prototype: None
Pregnancy category: B

ACTIONS/PHARMACODYNAMICS Oral treatment for erectile dysfunction, whether organic or psychogenic in origin. Enhances the vasodilation effect of nitric oxide in the corpus cavernosus of the penis, thus sustaining an erection.

USE Erectile dysfunction.

ROUTE & DOSAGE

Erectile Dysfunction

Adult: **PO** 50 mg approx 1 h before sexual activity (range 0.5–4 h before); dose may range from 25 to 100 mg once per day; 25 mg should be used if age >65 y, there is hepatic or severe

S

renal impairment, or there is concomitant use of erythromycin, ketoconazole, or itraconazole.

PHARMACOKINETICS **Absorption:** rapidly absorbed from GI tract. **Peak:** 30–120 min. **Distribution:** 96% protein bound. **Metabolism:** metabolized in liver by cytochromes P450 3A4 (primary) and 2C9 (minor). **Elimination:** half-life: 4 h; 80% excreted in feces, 12% in urine.

CONTRAINDICATIONS & PRECAUTIONS **Contraindicated in:** hypersensitivity to sildenafil; concurrent administration of organic nitrates and nitroglycerin; pregnancy (category B). Not recommeded for women or children. **Cautious use in:** CAD; hypotension and hypertension; risk factors for CVA; anatomic deformity of the penis; sickle cell anemia; multiple myeloma; leukemia; active bleeding or a peptic ulcer; retinitis pigmentosa; hepatitis, cirrhosis; severe renal impairment (Cl_{cr} <30 ml/min); elderly; concurrent use with other medicines for penile dysfunction.

ADVERSE/SIDE EFFECTS **Body as whole:** face edema, photosensitivity, shock, asthenia, pain, chills, fall, allergic reaction, arthritis, myalgia. **CNS:** *headache,* dizziness, migraine, syncope, cerebral thrombosis, ataxia, neuralgia, paresthesias, tremor, vertigo, depression, insomnia, somnolence, abnormal dreams. **CV:** flushing, chest pain, <u>MI</u>, angina, AV block, tachycardia, palpitation, hypotension, postural hypotension, <u>cardiac arrest, sudden cardiac death,</u> heart failure, cardiomyopathy, abnormal ECG, edema. **GI:** dyspepsia, diarrhea, abdominal pain, vomiting, colitis, dysphagia, gastritis, gastroenteritis, esophagitis, stomatitis, dry mouth, abnormal liver function tests, thirst. **Respiratory:** nasal congestion, asthma, dyspnea, laryngitis, pharyngitis, sinusitis, bronchitis, cough. **Skin:** rash, urticaria, pruritus, sweating, <u>exfoliative dermatitis</u>. **Other:** UTI, abnormal vision (color changes, photosensitivity, blurred vision), anemia, leukopenia, gout, hyperglycemia, hyperuricemia, hypoglycemia, hypernatremia.

DRUG INTERACTIONS NITRATES increase risk of serious hypotension; **cimetidine, erythromycin, ketoconazole, itraconazole** increased sildenafil levels; **rifampin** can decrease sildenafil levels.

NURSING IMPLICATIONS

Administration

- Sildenafil is usually taken 1 h prior to sexual activity.
- Sildenafil should not be taken more than once a day.
- Store at 15–30C (59–86F) in a tightly closed container and protect from light.

Assessment & Drug Effects

- Carefully monitor for and immediately report S&S of cardiac distress.

Patient & Family Education

- Sildenafil should not be taken by anyone on concurrent therapy with drugs containing nitrates.
- Sildenafil may be taken anytime from 0.5 to 4 h prior to sexual activity.
- A high-fat meal eaten before taking sildenafil may cause the drug to take longer to work.
- Report the following to your physician: headaches, flushing, indigestion, blurred vision, sensitivity to light, changes in color vision.

S

SILVER SULFADIAZINE

(sul-fa-dye'a-zeen)

Trade name: Silvadene

Classifications: ANTIINFECTIVE; SULFONAMIDE
Prototype: Sulfisoxazole
Pregnancy category: C

ACTIONS/PHARMACODYNAMICS Produced by reaction of silver nitrate with sulfadiazine. Mechanism of action differs from that of either component. Silver salt is released slowly and exerts bactericidal effect only on bacterial cell membrane and wall, rather than by inhibiting folic acid synthesis; antibacterial activity is not inhibited by *p*-aminobenzoic acid (PABA). Contact with sodium chloride in body tissues and fluids results in slow release of sulfadiazine, which may be systemically absorbed from application site. Has broad antimicrobial activity including many gram-negative and gram-positive bacteria and yeast.

USE Prevention and treatment of sepsis in second- and third-degree burns.

ROUTE & DOSAGE

Burn Wound Treatment
Adult/Child: **Topical** Apply 1% cream 1–2 times/d to thickness of approximately 1.5 mm (1/16 in.).

S

CONTRAINDICATIONS & PRECAUTIONS **Contraindicated in:** hypersensitivity to other sulfonamides; G6PD deficiency; pregnancy (category C), pregnant women at term, premature and newborn infants < 2 mo. **Cautious use in:** impaired renal or hepatic function.

ADVERSE/SIDE EFFECTS Pain (occasionally), burning, itching, rash, reversible leukopenia. Potential for toxicity as for other sulfonamides if applied to extensive areas of the body surface.

DRUG INTERACTION PROTEOLYTIC ENZYMES are inactivated by silver in cream.

NURSING IMPLICATIONS

Administration

- Silver sulfadiazine cream is water soluble and white; if it darkens, do not use.
- Apply with sterile, gloved hands to cleansed, debrided burned areas. Cream should be reapplied to areas where it has been removed by patient activity; burn wounds should be covered with medication at all times.
- If possible, patient should be bathed daily (in whirlpool or shower or in bed) as aid to debridement. Drug should then be reapplied.
- Dressings are not required but may be used if necessary. Silver sulfadiazine does not stain clothing.
- Preserve at room temperature away from heat.

Assessment & Drug Effects

- Observe for and report hypersensitivity reaction manifested by rash, itching, or burning sensation in unburned areas.
- When drug is applied to extensive areas, serum sulfa concentrations, urinalysis, and kidney function tests should be monitored, since significant quantities of drug may be absorbed. Observe patient for reactions attributed to sulfonamides.
- Occasionally, pain is experienced on application; intensity and duration depend on depth of burn. Analgesic may be required.
- Unless adverse reactions occur, treatment should continue until satisfactory healing or until burn site is ready for grafting.

SIMETHICONE

(si-meth'i-kone)

Trade names: Gas-x, Mylicon, Phazyme

Classifications: GI agent; antiflatulent

ACTIONS/PHARMACODYNAMICS A surfactant (surface-active agent) claimed to defoam gastric juice by causing small gas bubbles to break up and coalesce so they can be more easily removed by belching or passing flatus.

USES To relieve flatulence and functional gastric bloating.

ROUTE & DOSAGE

Gas

Adult: **PO** 40–125 mg p.c. and h.s. prn (max 500 mg/d).

NURSING IMPLICATIONS

Administration

- Shake suspension well before pouring.
- Instruct patients to chew tablet form thoroughly before they swallow it.

SIMVASTATIN

(sim-vah-stat'in)

Trade name: Zocor

Classifications: CARDIOVASCULAR AGENT; ANTILIPEMIC; HMG-COA REDUCTASE INHIBITOR (STATIN)

Prototype: Lovastatin

Pregnancy category: X

ACTIONS/PHARMACODYNAMICS An inhibitor of 3-hydroxy-3-methylglutaryl coenzyme A (HMG-CoA) reductase; is similar in action to lovastatin but more potent. HMG-CoA reductase inhibitors increase HDL cholesterol and decrease LDL cholesterol and total cholesterol synthesis.

USES Hypercholesterolemia (alone or in combination with bile acid sequestrants), familial hypercholesterolemia. Reduces risk of coronary death and nonfatal MI.

ROUTE & DOSAGE

Hypercholesterolemia

Adult: **PO** 5–40 mg q.d.

PHARMACOKINETICS Absorption: rapidly absorbed from GI tract. **Onset:** 2 wk. **Peak:** 4–6 wk. **Distribution:** 95% protein bound; achieves high liver concentrations; crosses placenta. **Metabolism:** extensive first-pass metabolism in liver to its active metabolite. **Elimination:** 13% excreted in urine, 60% in bile and feces.

CONTRAINDICATIONS & PRECAUTIONS Contraindicated in: hypersensitivity to simvastatin, pregnancy (category X), nursing mothers, active liver disease. **Cautious use in:** homozygous familial hypercholesterolemia, history of liver disease, alcoholics. Safety and effectiveness in children and adolescents not established.

ADVERSE/SIDE EFFECTS CV: angina. **CNS:** dizziness, headache, vertigo, asthenia, fatigue, insomnia. **GI:** nausea, diarrhea, vomiting, abdominal pain, constipation, flatulence, heartburn, transient elevations in liver transaminases. **Other:** fatigue, rhinitis, cough, transient elevations in CPK.

DRUG INTERACTION May increase PT when administered with warfarin.

NURSING IMPLICATIONS

Administration

- Simvastatin may be given without regard to meals.
- It should be given in the evening.
- Store at 15–30C (59–86F).

Assessment & Drug Effects

- Monitor cholesterol levels throughout therapy.
- Liver function tests should be performed at the start of therapy and then periodically (q6mo) for first year.
- Monitor coagulation studies with patients receiving concurrent warfarin therapy. PT may be prolonged.

Patient & Family Education

- Advise patient to promptly report unexplained muscle pain, tenderness, or weakness, especially if accompanied by malaise or fever.
- Advise patients on warfarin therapy to promptly report signs of bleeding.

SODIUM BICARBONATE ($NaHCO_3$)

Classifications: GI AGENT; ANTACID; ELECTROLYTIC BALANCE AGENT

Pregnancy category: C

S

ACTIONS/PHARMACODYNAMICS Short-acting, potent systemic antacid. Rapidly neutralizes gastric acid to form sodium chloride, carbon dioxide, and water. After absorption of sodium bicarbonate, plasma alkali reserve is increased and excess sodium and bicarbonate ions are excreted in urine, thus rendering urine less acid. Not suitable for treatment of peptic ulcer because it is short-acting, high in sodium, and may cause gastric distention, systemic alkalosis, and possibly acid-rebound.

USES Systemic alkalinizer to correct metabolic acidosis (as occurs in diabetes mellitus, shock, cardiac arrest, or vascular collapse), to minimize uric acid crystallization associated with uricosuric agents, to increase the solubility of sulfonamides, and to enhance renal excretion of barbiturate and salicylate overdosage. Commonly used as home remedy for relief of occasional heartburn, indigestion, or sour stomach. Used topically as paste, bath, or soak to relieve itching and minor skin irritations such as sunburn, insect bites, prickly heat, poison ivy, sumac, or oak. Sterile solutions are used to buffer acidic parenteral solutions to prevent acidosis. Also as a buffering agent in many commercial products (e.g., mouthwashes, douches, enemas, ophthalmic solutions).

ROUTE & DOSAGE

Antacid

Adult: **PO** 0.3–2 g 1–4 times/d or 1/2 tsp of powder in glass of water.

Urinary Alkalinizer

Adult: **PO** 4 g initially; then 1–2 g q4h.
Child: **PO** 84–840 mg/kg/d in divided doses.

Cardiac Arrest

Adult: **IV** 1 mEq/kg of a 7.5% or 8.4% solution initially; then 0.5 mEq/kg q10min depending on arterial blood gas determinations (8.4% solutions contain 50 mEq/50 ml); give over 1–2 min.
Child: **IV** 0.5–1 mEq/kg of a 4.2% solution q10min depending on ar-

terial blood gas determinations; give over 1–2 min.

Metabolic Acidosis

Adult: **IV** 2–5 mEq/kg by IV infusion over 4–8 h. *Infant:* **IV** 2–3 mEq/kg/d of a 4.2% solution over 4–8 h.

PHARMACOKINETICS **Absorption:** readily absorbed from GI tract. **Onset:** 15 min. **Duration:** 1–2 h. **Elimination:** excreted in urine within 3–4 h.

CONTRAINDICATIONS & PRECAUTIONS **Contraindicated in:** prolonged therapy with sodium bicarbonate; patients losing chlorides (as from vomiting, GI suction, diuresis); heart disease, hypertension; renal insufficiency; peptic ulcer; pregnancy (category C). **Cautious use in:** edema, sodium-retaining disorders; elderly patients.

ADVERSE/SIDE EFFECTS **GI:** *belching, gastric distention,* flatulence. **Metabolic:** metabolic alkalosis; electrolyte imbalance: sodium overload (pulmonary edema), hypocalcemia (tetany), hypokalemia. **Rapid IV in neonates:** hypernatremia, reduction in CSF pressure, <u>intracranial hemorrhage</u>. **Other:** milk-alkali syndrome, severe tissue damage following extravasation of IV solution, dehydration, renal calculi or crystals, impaired renal function, renal calculi.

DIAGNOSTIC TEST INTERFERENCE Small increase in ***blood lactate*** levels (following IV infusion of sodium bicarbonate); false-positive ***urinary protein*** determinations (using Ames reagent, sulfoacetic acid, heat and acetic acid or nitric acid ring method); elevated ***urinary urobilinogen*** levels (urobilinogen excretion increases in alkaline urine).

INCOMPATIBILITIES **Solution/additive: alcohol, 5% lactated Ringer's, ascorbic acid, bupivicaine, carmustine, cisplatin, codeine, corticotropin, dobutamine, dopamine, epinephrine, glycopyrrolate, hydromorphone, imipenem-cilastatin, insulin, isoproterenol, labetalol, levorphanol, magnesium sulfate, meperidine, methadone, methicillin, metoclopramide, morphine, norepinephrine, oxytetracycline, pentazocine, phenobarbital, procaine, secobarbital, streptomycin, succinylcholine, tetracycline, thiopental, vancomycin, vitamin B complex with C. Y-site: amrinone, verapamil.**

NURSING IMPLICATIONS

Administration

- Infusion should be stopped immediately if extravasation occurs. Severe tissue damage has followed tissue infiltration.
- IV administration: The 4.2% and 5% $NaHCO_3$ solutions may be given undiluted. The 7.5% and 8.4% solutions should be diluted with compatible IV solutions.
- IV infusion should not exceed 50 mEq/h.
- Topical use (manufacturer's directions): Bath or soak: 1/2 cup or more into tub of warm water. Footsoak: 4 tbsp/L(qt) warm water; soak 5–10 min. Paste: 3 parts sodium bicarbonate to 1 part water. Solutions in water slowly decompose; decomposition is accelerated by agitating or warming the solution.
- Store in airtight containers. Note expiration date.

Assessment & Drug Effects

- Long-term use of oral preparation with milk or calcium can cause milk-

S

alkali syndrome: anorexia, nausea, vomiting, headache, mental confusion, hypercalcemia, hypophosphatemia, soft tissue calcification, renal and ureteral calculi, renal insufficiency, metabolic alkalosis.

- Urinary alkalinization: Urinary pH should be monitored as a guide to dosage (pH testing with nitrazine paper may be done at intervals throughout the day and dosage adjustments made accordingly).
- Metabolic acidosis: Patient should be closely monitored by observations of clinical condition; measurements of acid-base status (blood pH, Po_2, Pco_2, Hco_3^-, and other electrolytes, are usually made several times daily during acute period). Observe for signs of alkalosis (overtreatment) (see Appendix G).
- Observe for and report improvement or reversal in signs and symptoms, of metabolic acidosis (see Appendix G).

Patient & Family Education

- Discourage use of sodium bicarbonate as antacid. A nonabsorbable alternative (OTC) for repeated use is safer.
- Caution patient who self-medicates that routine doses of sodium bicarbonate or soda mints may be sufficient to cause sodium retention and alkalosis, especially when renal function is impaired. Antacids should not be taken longer than 2 wk except under advice and supervision of a physician.
- Commonly used OTC antacid products containing sodium bicarbonate: Alka-Seltzer, Bromo-Seltzer, Gaviscon.

S

SODIUM CHLORIDE 20%

Classification: ABORTIFACIENT
Pregnancy category: X

ACTIONS/PHARMACODYNAMICS Hypertonic saline instillation into the amniotic sac induces abortion and fetal death. Mechanism is unclear, but abortifacient activity may be a response to prostaglandins released by hypertonic NaCl-damaged decidual cells. Uterine contractions, induced by the saline solution are sufficient to cause evacuation of fetus and placenta; however, in 25–40% of the patients, abortion may be incomplete.

USES To induce abortion late in the second trimester of pregnancy. Oxytocin may be used as an adjunct (concurrent) uterine stimulant.

ROUTE & DOSAGE

Abortion Induction

Adult: **Intraamniotic** Instill 20% solution in volumes equal to amount of amniotic fluid removed or a max of 200–250 ml administered slowly over 20–30 min; repeated in 48 h if uterine contractility, cervical effacement, or cervical dilation is inadequate or if labor has not begun.

PHARMACOKINETICS Absorption: some drug diffuses into maternal blood. **Onset:** within 51 h. **Distribution:** sodium concentration in amniotic fluid must be at least 2.2 mEq/ml to induce abortion; most of drug concentrates in decidua and fetal part of placenta.

CONTRAINDICATIONS & PRECAUTIONS Contraindicated in: pregnancy (category X) of less than 15 wk or more than 24 wk, prior uterine surgery (including cervix), pelvic adhesions, sickle cell disease, diabetes mellitus, increased intraamniotic pressure (as in contracting or hypertonic uterus), poor health, blood disorders, coagulation factor deficiencies. **Cautious use in:** malignant hypertension, cardiovascular and renal disease, thrombocytopenia, fibrinolytic defects.

ADVERSE/SIDE EFFECTS **Within first 12–24 h after instillation:** coagulation changes; increased plasma volume, fibrin levels, thrombin, prothrombin, and partial thromboplastin times. **With overdistention of amniotic cavity by excess NaCl:** ascites, hypervolemia, circulation failure, uterine necrosis, severe electrolyte disturbances. **With delayed abortion:** retained placenta, hemorrhagic fever, infection, sepsis. **Other:** mild self-limiting form of disseminated intravascular coagulation, cervical lacerations and perforation, uterine rupture, pulmonary embolism, fever, flushing, cortical necrosis of kidneys.

DRUG INTERACTIONS **Indomethacin** may delay onset time of abortion; **terbutaline, ritodrine** inhibit uterine activity induced by hypertonic NaCl.

NURSING IMPLICATIONS

Administration

- Preparatory to procedure, skin is surgically prepared. By transabdominal tap, about 1 ml amniotic fluid is withdrawn to confirm location of needle (amniotic fluid has pH 7.4 and ability to fern). If blood is present or if no amniotic fluid is withdrawn, needle is repositioned. Some clinicians then remove all amniotic fluid (30–250 ml); others prefer not to before NaCl instillation.
- Instillation is through a 3-way stopcock with needle and polyethylene catheter inserted into amniotic cavity.
- Within 1–2 h after hypertonic solution instillation and after uterine response to the solution has ceased, IV infusion of dilute solution of oxytocin may be administered; rate, 20–100 mU/min. Oxytocin action as an adjunctive uterine stimulant shortens the abortifacient-abortion interval.
- Treatment of extraamniotic injection: procedure stopped promptly; IV infusion of D5W, additional support for hypernatremic shock.

Assessment & Drug Effects

- Observe patient for at least 30 min after instillation procedure. Be available for complaints and to check vital signs (temperature, pulse rate, BP).
- Intraamniotic instillation is a painless procedure. No anesthetic or sedative is needed or given so that patient is able to report early signs of extraamniotic injection: mental confusion, hypotension, severe headache, vague distress, extreme nervousness, pain, sensation of heat, thirst, fingertip numbness, dry mouth, salty taste, tinnitus.
- Suspect accidental intraperitoneal, intravascular, or myometrial injection if patient begins vomiting. Cardiovascular collapse, seizures, and maternal death may follow.

Patient & Family Education

- Instruct to drink at least 2 L water on day of procedure to promote NaCl excretion.
- With onset of labor, signs of rupture of fetal membrane, vaginal bleeding, fever, or any other untoward symptom, patient should return promptly to treatment center.
- If labor has not begun within 48 h of hypertonic saline instillation, patient should return to physician for evaluation and treatment.

S

SODIUM FLUORIDE

Trade names: Fluor-A-Day♣, Fluorinse, Fluoritabs, Flura-Drops, Karidium, Pediaflor, Point-Two, Thera-Flur-N

Classification: PROPHYLACTIC: DENTAL

Pregnancy category: C

ACTIONS/PHARMACODYNAMICS Source of the fluorine ion, a trace element. Its incorporation into developing tooth enamel hardens surfaces and increases resistance to cariogenic microbial processes. Topical application reduces acid production by bacteria in dental plaque and promotes remineralization of acid-damaged enamel. Application to exposed root surfaces supports formation of insoluble materials within dentinal tubules, thereby blocking transport of offending stimuli. Arrests rapid dental decay associated with drug-, radiation-, or age-related xerostomia. One of the few agents known that stimulates osteoblastic activity, leading to increased bone mass.

USES When fluoride ion concentration in drinking water is 0.7 ppm or less, to prevent periodontal disease and dental caries, to treat dental cervical hypersensitivity, and to control dental caries associated with xerostomia. **Unlabeled uses:** adjunctive treatment of osteoporosis; management of bone lesions in multiple myeloma; to reduce bone pain in patient with metastatic prostatic carcinoma; to stabilize progression of hearing loss in a limited number of patients with otosclerosis.

ROUTE & DOSAGE

Prevent Periodontal Disease (Drinking Water Concentration < 0.3 ppm)

Child: **PO** *Birth–2 y,* 0.25 mg/d; *2–3 y,* 0.5 mg/d; *3–13 y,* 1 mg/d.

Prevent Periodontal Disease (Drinking Water Concentration 0.3–0.7 ppm)

Child: **PO** *Birth–2 y,* 0.125 mg/d; *2–3 y,* 0.25 mg/d; *3–13 y,* 0.5 mg/d.

Prevent Dental Caries

Child: **Topical** *6–12 y,* 5 ml of 0.2% solution daily; *> 12 y,* 10 ml of 0.2% solution daily.

Desensitization of Exposed Root Surfaces

Child: **Topical** 0.2% rinsing solution once nightly after brushing and flossing.

PHARMACOKINETICS Absorption: readily absorbed from GI tract. **Distribution:** fluoride is stored in bones and teeth; crosses placenta; distributed into breast milk. **Elimination:** rapidly excreted, primarily in urine with small amounts in feces.

CONTRAINDICATIONS & PRECAUTIONS Contraindicated in: when daily intake of fluoride from drinking water exceeds 0.7 ppm, low-sodium or sodium-free diets, hypersensitivity to fluoride, gels or dental rinses by children < 6 y, 1 mg tablet or rinse in children < 3 y, or 1 mg rinse in children < 6 y, pregnancy (category C).

ADVERSE/SIDE EFFECTS Topical application: rash, atopic dermatitis, urticaria, stomatitis, GI and respiratory allergic reactions. Acute toxicity: salty or soapy taste, dehydration, thirst, excessive salivation, muscle weakness, rash, tremors, <u>shock, death from cardiac and respiratory failure</u>. **Chronic overdose:** dental fluorosis (brown or white mottling of tooth enamel), osseous fluorosis (patchy mineralization and possible

S

decrease in bone strength). **Fatal dose:** 500 mg in children; 5–10 g in untreated adults.

NURSING IMPLICATIONS

Administration

- All fluorine preparations should be applied or taken after thorough brushing and flossing and preferably at bedtime.
- Avoid giving sodium fluoride with milk or dairy products. Calcium from these products combines with fluorine, decreasing its absorption.
- Drops or tablets are taken preferably after meals. Drops may be taken undiluted or mixed with fluids or foods.
- Tablets should be dissolved in the mouth or chewed before they are swallowed. Administer at bedtime (after brushing the teeth).
- If patient's mouth is sore, the neutral preparation (Thera-Flur N) is better tolerated.
- Treatment for dental cervical hypersensitivity: thoroughly brush teeth; then swish PO solution around and between teeth for 1 min; expectorate. If gel is used, apply a few drops to toothbrush and brush gently onto affected surfaces.
- Gel-drops may also be applied with applicators supplied by the dentist. Spread gel on inner surfaces of applicators, which are then placed over lower and upper teeth at the same time. Instruct user to bite down lightly for 6 min and to then remove applicators and rinse mouth thoroughly. Applicators are cleaned with cold water.
- Store in tight plastic or paraffin-lined glass containers (sodium fluoride reacts with ordinary glass at a slow but appreciable rate) at 15–30C (59–86F). Avoid freezing.

Patient & Family Education

- Topically applied or rinse preparations are not to be swallowed.
- Do not eat, drink, or rinse mouth for at least 30 min after using the rinsing solution.
- Advise not to exceed recommended dosage. If mottling of teeth occurs, notify dentist.

Prophylactic Fluorine Regimen

- Sodium fluoride gel or solution used in orthodontic treatment regimen is applied immediately before attachment or reattachment of the tooth-encircling bands.
- To be effective, fluorine supplementation must be consistent and continuous from infancy until 12–14 y.
- A high fluorine content in drinking water and water used in food processing in addition to prescribed fluoride therapy may be a cause of dental fluorosis.
- If the family moves or if there is a change in water supply, consult dentist about continuation of fluoride therapy. (Mottling may occur if drinking water has fluorine content >1.5 ppm.)
- Dental fluorosis occurs only during tooth development but remains throughout life. If mild, it appears as opaque paper-white areas on tooth surfaces; if moderate, as brown stains with pitting.
- Pregnant or lactating women should consult physician about continuing fluorine therapy.

SODIUM IODIDE-131

Trade name: Iodotope

Classifications: ANTINEOPLASTIC; RADIOPHARMACEUTICAL

Pregnancy category: X

ACTIONS/PHARMACODYNAMICS

Radiopharmaceutical with relatively

S

long half-life (8.06 d). Processed in form of sodium iodide from products of uranium fission or neutron bombardment of tellurium. Chemically and physiologically identical to stable, naturally occurring iodide. Affords relatively simple, effective, economic means of treating hyperthyroidism (Graves' disease) by ablation without surgery. Therapeutic doses of radioactive iodine (RAI) deliver ionizing radiation to follicular cells, thereby damaging and destroying thyroid and neoplastic tissues.

USES Hyperthyroidism and thyrotoxicosis and to suppress neoplastic disease of thyroid. As a diagnostic aid, tracer doses are used in thyroid function studies and imaging to evaluate suspected hyperthyroidism and to visualize thyroid malignancy and metastasis.

ROUTE & DOSAGE

Hyperthyroidism

Adult: **PO** 4–10 mCi as a single dose; second dose, if necessary, after 6 wk.

Carcinoma of Thyroid

Adult: **PO** 50 mCi as a single dose; subsequent doses of 100–150 mCi if necessary.

PHARMACOKINETICS **Absorption:** readily absorbed from GI tract. **Onset:** evident in blood within 3–6 min. **Distribution:** concentrates in thyroid gland; iodide secretion from this gland permits radioactivity detection in nasal secretion, oral cavity, trachea, female breast, gallbladder, liver, and intestines; crosses placenta; distributed into breast milk. **Metabolism:** disintegrates by beta and gamma emission. **Elimination:** half-life: 8.06 d; excreted primarily by kidneys, with small amounts in sweat and feces; radiation of therapeutic dose is expended within 56 d.

CONTRAINDICATIONS & PRECAUTIONS **Contraindicated in:** acute hyperthyroidism; large nodular goiter; preexisting vomiting or diarrhea; use of antithyroid, thyroid hormone, or iodine-containing preparations within 15 d, recent MI, pregnancy (category X), nursing mothers, lactation; sensitivity to iodine; patients <30 y unless indications are exceptional. **Cautious use in:** impaired renal and cardiac function.

ADVERSE/SIDE EFFECTS Primary hypothyroidism, thyroid nodules, thyroid cancer (in children), angioedema, petechiae, transient thyroiditis (marked thyroid tenderness with swelling, feeling of fullness, fever, malaise, aching of teeth, headache, transient decrease in erythrocyte sedimentation rate, pain referred to ear, chest, or throat), alopecia (reversible), genetically transmissible chromosomal abnormalities, myelosuppression, blood dyscrasias.

NURSING IMPLICATIONS

Administration

- All antithyroid, thyroid, or iodine-containing medications are stopped 5–7 d before sodium-iodide I 131 dose. After treatment, antithyroid drugs are not resumed, but other drugs taken to treat hyperthyroidism symptoms (e.g., propranolol) can be resumed until onset of full therapeutic effect of I 131 (normally 5–6 wk).
- Presence of food may delay absorption; therefore, patient should fast overnight prior to RAI administration.
- When administering oral liquid I 131, rinse container 2 or 3 times to

S

ensure delivery of total dose. Glass or plastic cups are preferable to wax cups or paper cups.
- Solution is clear and colorless; however, on standing, bottle and solution may darken (without interfering with efficacy).

Assessment & Drug Effects
- Expected pattern of response to therapy: In the first 2 wk, there is minimal chemical or clinical change in thyrotoxicosis; next 4–8 wk, decrease in thyroid function, which reaches nadir (acute effects of radiation) between 8 and 12 wk after treatment.
- If patient is hyperthyroid following treatment, treatment is repeated in 16 wk and q3–4mo thereafter until euthyroid state is achieved.

Patient & Family Education
- Urge to empty bladder frequently after therapeutic dosages of I 131 to reduce gonadal radiation.
- Urge to force fluids for first 48 h after treatment to aid in flushing out the radiopharmaceutical.
- Emphasize need for rest following I 131 therapy. Consult physician for activity guides.
- Frequently, thyroxine replacement is instituted after patient achieves euthyroid state as prophylaxis against myxedema. Patient should understand that this will be lifelong medication and that patient will need to return to physician at least once a year for medical surveillance. Consult physician about when to discuss this with the patient and family.
- Teach the symptoms of hypothyroidism.
- Transient thyroiditis (see Adverse/Side Effects) may occur within 1 wk after I 131 treatment. Patient should report symptoms promptly to permit treatment.
- Temporary thinning of hair may begin 2 or 3 mo after treatment.
- Urine is slightly radioactive for 24 h but may be flushed down toilet. Saliva and vomit are highly radioactive for 6–8 h. Urge patient to refrain from expectorating for 24 h if possible. Urine, saliva, and perspiration remain radioactive for 3 d.
- Instruct visitors to remain several feet away from the patient who is on therapeutic I 131. Usually, visiting is restricted the first day after treatment with > 30 mCi.
- Avoid extended contact with small children (do not cuddle or hold on lap) until 7 d after treatment with I 131.
- Avoid sleeping in same room with another person 7 d after the treatment date.

SODIUM POLYSTYRENE SULFONATE

(pol-ee-stye′reen)

Trade names: Kayexalate, SPS Suspension

Classifications: RESIN EXCHANGE AGENT; CATION

Pregnancy category: C

ACTIONS/PHARMACODYNAMICS
Sulfonic cation-exchange resin. Removes potassium from body by exchanging sodium ion for potassium, particularly in large intestine; potassium-containing resin is then excreted. Small amounts of other cations such as calcium and magnesium may be lost during treatment.

USE Hyperkalemia.

ROUTE & DOSAGE
Hyperkalemia

Adult: **PO** 15 g suspended in 70% sorbitol or 20–100 ml of other

S

fluid 1–4 times/d; **PR** 30–50 g/100 ml 70% sorbitol q6h as warm emulsion high into sigmoid colon.
Child: **PO** Calculate appropriate amount on exchange rate of 1 mEq of potassium per gram of resin and suspend in 70% sorbitol or other appropriate solution. Usual dose: **PO** 1 g/kg q6h; **PR** 1 g/kg q2–6h.

CONTRAINDICATIONS & PRECAUTIONS **Cautious use in:** elderly; acute or chronic renal failure; patients receiving digitalis preparations; patients who cannot tolerate even a small increase in sodium load, e.g., CHF, severe hypertension, and marked edema; pregnancy (category C).

ADVERSE/SIDE EFFECTS **GI:** *constipation, fecal impaction (in the elderly);* anorexia, gastric irritation, nausea, vomiting, diarrhea (with sorbitol emulsions). **Other:** sodium retention, hypocalcemia, hypokalemia, hypomagnesemia.

DRUG INTERACTIONS ANTACIDS, LAXATIVES containing **calcium** or **magnesium** may decrease potassium exchange capability of the resin.

S

NURSING IMPLICATIONS

Administration

- Oral dose should be given as a suspension in a small quantity of water or in syrup. Usual amount of fluid ranges from 20–100 ml or approximately 3–4 ml/g of drug.

Administration of Drug in Enema Form

- Use warm fluid (as prescribed) to prepare the emulsion.
- Administer at body temperature and introduce by gravity, keeping suspension particles in solution by stirring. Flush suspension with 50–100 ml of fluid; then clamp tube and leave it in place.
- Urge patient to retain enema at least 30–60 min but as long as several hours if possible.
- Irrigate colon (after enema solution has been expelled) with 1 or 2 quarts flushing solution (should be nonsodium containing). Drain returns constantly through a Y-tube connection.
- Store remainder of prepared solution for 24 h; then discard.

Assessment & Drug Effects

- Serum potassium levels should be determined daily throughout therapy. Acid–base balance, electrolytes, and minerals should also be monitored in patients receiving repeated doses.
- Serum potassium levels do not always reflect intracellular potassium deficiency. Therefore, observe patient closely for early clinical signs of severe hypokalemia (see Appendix G). ECGs are also recommended.
- Usually, a mild laxative is prescribed to prevent constipation (common side effect) and fecal impaction. Check bowel function daily. Elderly patients are particularly prone to fecal impaction.
- Since drug contains approximately 100 mg (4.1 mEq) of sodium per gram (1 tsp, 15 mEq sodium), sodium content from dietary and other sources may be restricted. Consult physician.

SODIUM SALICYLATE

Trade name: Uracel
Classifications: CNS AGENT; SALICYLATE ANALGESIC; ANTIPYRETIC; NSAID
Prototype: Aspirin
Pregnancy category: C

ACTIONS/PHARMACODYNAMICS Properties similar to those of aspirin but less effective. Liberates free salicylic acid in the stomach and therefore tends to cause gastric irritation. Unlike aspirin, does not inhibit platelet aggregation. Increases prothrombin time, like aspirin, but reportedly is associated with less occult blood loss.

USES Primarily in treatment of acute pain, rheumatoid arthritis, osteoarthritis. May be used as an alternative in individuals with GI intolerance to aspirin.

ROUTE & DOSAGE

Analgesia, Antipyresis
Adult: **PO** 325–650 mg q4h prn. **IV** 500 mg diluted in 1 L NS or lactated Ringer's and infused over 4–8 h; may repeat x 1.
Child 2–11 y: **PO** 25–50 mg/kg/d in 4–6 divided doses.

Arthritis
Adult: **PO** 3.6–5.4 g/d divided q4–6h.
Child: **PO** 80–100 mg/kg/d divided q4–6h (max 130 mg/kg/d).

PHARMACOKINETICS **Absorption:** 80–100% absorbed. **Peak:** 0.25–2 h. **Distribution:** widely distributed in most body tissues; crosses placenta. **Metabolism:** metabolized in liver. **Elimination:** half-life: 2–18 h (dose dependent); 50% of dose is eliminated in urine in 2–4 h (low doses) or 15–30 h (high doses); excreted in breast milk.

CONTRAINDICATIONS & PRECAUTIONS **Contraindicated in:** hypersensitivity to other salicylates, severe renal disease, heart failure, patients on low-sodium diets; pregnancy (category C).

ADVERSE/SIDE EFFECTS *Tinnitus,* diminished hearing, nausea, vomiting, hypersensitivity reactions, *thrombophlebitis (with rapid infusion),* <u>sloughing of soft tissues (with extravasation)</u>, pulmonary edema in patients with rheumatic fever.

DRUG INTERACTIONS **Aminosalicylic acid** increases risk of salicylate toxicity; **ammonium chloride** and other ACIDIFYING AGENTS decrease renal elimination and thus increase risk of salicylate toxicity; ANTICOAGULANTS add to risk of bleeding; aspirin doses >2 g/d increase hypoglycemic activity of SULFONYLUREAS; carbonic anhydrase inhibitors enhance salicylate toxicity; CORTICOSTEROIDS add to ulcerogenic effects of salicylates; increases **methotrexate** toxicity; low doses of salicylates may antagonize uricosuric effects of **probenecid, sulfinpyrazone.**

NURSING IMPLICATIONS

Administration

- Administer with food, milk, or a full glass (240 ml) of water to minimize risk of gastric irritation. Caution patient not to chew or crush tablet.
- Some physicians prescribe concurrent administration of sodium bicarbonate or other antacid to prevent gastric irritation, although it may increase urinary excretion of salicylate and thus lower blood salicylate levels.
- In the symptomatic treatment of rheumatic fever, the dosage of sodium salicylate is the same as that employed with aspirin.
- See Route & Dosage table for IV administration.
- For patients receiving sodium salicylate IV, frequent checks of infusion site for extravasation and pre-

scribed infusion rate (should be slow) are advised.
- Store in light-resistant containers. Turns pink on exposure to light.

Assessment & Drug Effects
- Serum salicylate levels may be required as a guide for adequate dosing of patients on long-term therapy.
- There are 2 mEq (46 mg) of sodium in each 325 mg tablet of sodium salicylate.
- Monitor for adverse GI effects, especially in patients with a history of peptic ulcer disease.

Patient & Family Education
- Warn not to self-dose with aspirin or any other OTC drug during sodium salicylate therapy.
- Instruct to report tinnitus, hearing loss, vertigo, rash, or nausea.

SODIUM THIOSALICYLATE

Trade names: Asproject, Rexolate, Tusal
Classifications: CNS AGENT; SALICYLATE ANALGESIC; ANTIPYRETIC
Prototype: Aspirin
Pregnancy category: C

ACTIONS/PHARMACODYNAMICS Sodium salt of thiosalicylic acid with analgesic activity that may be due to interference with transmission of peripheral pain impulse reaching cerebral level.

USES To ameliorate moderate pain in arthritis; also used in rheumatic fever. Has been used for acute gout, but other agents are more effective.

ROUTE & DOSAGE

Acute Gout
Adult: **IM** 100 mg q3–4h; then 100 mg/d.

Analgesia
Adult: **IM** 50–100 mg/d or q.o.d.

Rheumatic Fever
Adult: **IM** 100–150 mg q4–6h for 3 d; then 100 mg b.i.d.

CONTRAINDICATIONS & PRECAUTIONS **Contraindicated in:** pregnancy (category C).

ADVERSE/SIDE EFFECTS See aspirin.

DRUG INTERACTIONS **Aminosalicylic acid** increases risk of salicylate toxicity; **ammonium chloride** and other ACIDIFYING AGENTS decrease renal elimination, thus increasing risk of salicylate toxicity; ANTICOAGULANTS add to risk of bleeding; aspirin doses >2 g/d increase hypoglycemic activity of SULFONYLUREAS; CARBONIC ANHYDRASE INHIBITORS enhance salicylate toxicity; CORTICOSTEROIDS add to ulcerogenic effects of salicylates; increases **methotrexate** toxicity; low doses of salicylates may antagonize uricosuric effects of **probenecid, sulfinpyrazone.**

NURSING IMPLICATIONS

See aspirin for numerous nursing implications.

SOMATREM

(soe′ma-trem)
Trade name: Protropin
Classification: HORMONE
Pregnancy category: C

ACTIONS/PHARMACODYNAMICS Biosynthetic product of recombinant DNA technology. Contains exact sequence of 191 amino acids in pituitary-derived human growth hormone (GH) plus an amino terminal methionyl group not found in natural

GH. Therapeutically equivalent to natural GH (somatropin) of pituitary origin, a product removed from the market by the FDA in 1987. Somatrem affects metabolism and growth of most body tissues including red cell mass, with possible exception of eye and brain. In presence of GH deficiency, promotes skeletal growth at epiphyseal plates of long bones by increasing levels of the mediator somatomedin-C and by increasing synthesis of protein, chondroitin sulfate, and collagen. Increases number and size of muscle cells. May induce GH antibody formation (IgG), but effect of antibodies on endogenous GH activity is unknown.

USE Long-term treatment of children with growth failure due to deficiency of endogenous GH.

ROUTE & DOSAGE

Growth Hormone Deficiency

Child: **IM/SC** Doses up to 0.1 mg/kg (0.2 U/kg) 3 times/wk with a minimum of 48 h between doses; may be increased in older children if epiphyses have not closed.

PHARMACOKINETICS **Metabolism:** metabolized in liver. **Elimination:** half-life: 20–30 min; excreted in urine.

CONTRAINDICATIONS & PRECAUTIONS **Contraindicated in:** patient with closed epiphyses; underlying progressive intracranial tumor; pregnancy (category C). **Cautious use in:** diabetes mellitus or family history of the disease; concomitant use of glucocorticoids; concomitant or prior use of thyroid or androgens in prepubertal male; hypothyroidism. Patient with known sensitivity to benzyl alcohol.

ADVERSE/SIDE EFFECTS **Allergic reaction** (systemic): peripheral edema, headache, myalgia, weakness. **Excess dosage:** diabetes mellitus, atherosclerosis, organ enlargement, hypertension, acromegalic features in children. **Metabolic:** glucose intolerance, ACTH deficiency, hypothyroidism. **Other:** recurrent intracranial tumor growth, persistent antibodies to GH; pain, swelling at injection site.

DIAGNOSTIC TEST INTERFERENCE Somatrem may reduce ***glucose tolerance, serum T_4 (thyroxin) concentration, RAI uptake,*** and ***thyroxine-binding capacity.***

DRUG INTERACTIONS ANABOLIC STEROIDS, **thyroid hormone,** ANDROGENS, ESTROGENS may accelerate epiphyseal closure; **ACTH,** CORTICOSTEROIDS may inhibit growth response to somatrem.

NURSING IMPLICATIONS

Administration

- Reconstitute each vial (containing 5 ml lyophilized powder) with 1–5 ml bacteriostatic water for injection, aiming stream of water against vial wall. Swirl vial gently to mix contents. Do not shake. If reconstituted solution is cloudy or has crystals, do not administer. Refrigeration may cause cloudiness. pH of reconstituted solution: about 7.8.
- Use disposable syringe small enough to administer prescribed doses with accuracy and needle long enough to ensure injection into muscle layer.
- Benzyl alcohol is the preservative in bacteriostatic water for injection and may be toxic to the newborn. Water for injection USP is the preferred diluent for this age group.
- Discard unused reconstituted solution within 7 d.
- Refrigerate lyophilized powder

and reconstituted solution at 2–8C (36–46F). Do not freeze. Expiration dates are on labels.

Assessment & Drug Effects

- Annual bone age assessments are advised in all patients and especially those also receiving thyroid, androgen, or estrogen replacement therapy, since concurrent use of these agents may precipitate early epiphyseal closure. Urge parent to take child for growth assessment on appointed annual dates.
- Thyroid status should also be evaluated at regular intervals. Untreated hypothyroidism may interfere with response to somatrem.
- Diabetic patients or those with family history of diabetes should be observed closely. Blood or urine glucose determinations should be evaluated regularly to recognize glucose intolerance.
- Patient with GH deficiency secondary to intracranial lesion should be examined frequently for progression or recurrence of underlying disease. Somatrem should not be used if tumor has been active during the previous 12 mo.

Patient & Family Education

- First year growth of 17.5 cm (7 in) with somatrem has been reported, but average expectations are 7.5–12.5 cm (3–5 in) in first year, slightly less in second year, and after that, normal growth rate. Additionally, subcutaneous fat diminishes but returns to pretreatment level later.
- Instruct parent to record accurate height measurements at regular intervals and to report to physician if rate is less than expected.
- Instruct parent to report child's complaints of hip or knee pain or a limp. Slipped capital femoral epiphysis may occur in patient with endocrine disorders.

SOMATROPIN

(soe-ma-troe′pin)

Trade names: Bio-Tropin, Genotropin, Humatrope, Norditropin, Nutropin

Classifications: HORMONE; GROWTH HORMONE

Pregnancy category: D.

ACTIONS/PHARMACODYNAMICS

New recombinant growth hormone with the natural sequence of 191 amino acids characteristic of endogenous growth hormone (GH). Differs from somatrem by absence of an extra methionyl group in its structure. Somatropin appears to be less likely to produce serum antibodies to endogenous GH than somatrem is, but it is not clear whether lack of antigenicity is of clinical importance. Induces growth responses similar to those produced in children treated with somatrem or with GH obtained from human pituitary glands (removed from market in 1987 by FDA). (See somatrem for other pharmacodynamics and for nursing implications.)

USES Growth failure due to GH deficiency; replacement therapy prior to epiphyseal closure in patients with idiopathic GH deficiency; GH deficiency secondary to intracranial tumors or panhypopituitarism; inadequate GH secretion; short stature in girls with Turner's syndrome.

ROUTE & DOSAGE

Growth Hormone Deficiency

Child: **IM/SC** Doses up to 0.06 mg/kg (0.16 IU/kg) 3 times/wk with a minimum of 48 h between doses.

Inadequate Growth Hormone Secretion
Child: **SC** Nutropin 0.3 mg/kg every week.

PHARMACOKINETICS Metabolism: metabolized in liver. **Elimination:** half-life: 15–50 min; excreted in urine.

CONTRAINDICATIONS & PRECAUTIONS Contraindicated in: patient with closed epiphyses; underlying progressive intracranial tumor. **Cautious use in:** diabetes mellitus or family history of the disease; concomitant or prior use of thyroid or androgens in prepubertal male; hypothyroidism.

ADVERSE/SIDE EFFECTS Pain, swelling at injection site; myalgia, *hypercalciuria;* oversaturation of bile with cholesterol, high circulating GH antibodies with resulting treatment failure, hyperglycemia, ketosis, accelerated growth of intracranial tumor.

DRUG INTERACTIONS ANABOLIC STEROIDS, **thyroid hormone**, ANDROGENS, ESTROGENS may accelerate epiphyseal closure; **ACTH,** CORTICOSTEROIDS may inhibit growth response to somatropin.

NURSING IMPLICATIONS

Administration

- Reconstitute each vial (containing 10 IU of drug) with 5 ml bacteriostatic water for injection only. Record date of reconstitution on vial.
- Rotate IM sites to prevent tissue damage. Use needle long enough to ensure injection into muscle layer.
- Refrigerate drug at 2–8C (36–46F). Discard after 1 mo.

Assessment & Drug Effects

- Before initiating treatment, careful documentation is made of growth rate for at least 6–12 mo. In addition, GH deficiency may be confirmed by demonstrating failure of plasma GH levels to exceed 5–7 ng/ml in response to standard stimuli. Thyroid, adrenal, and gonadal functions are also evaluated to rule out multiple pituitary hormone deficiency.
- Annual bone age assessments are advised in all patients and especially those also receiving concurrent thyroid or androgen treatment, since these drugs may precipitate early epiphyseal closure. Urge parent to take child for bone age assessment on appointed annual dates.
- Hypercalciuria, a frequent side effect in the first 2–3 mo of therapy, may be symptomless; however, it may be accompanied by renal calculi, with these reportable symptoms: flank pain and colic, GI symptoms, urinary frequency, chills, fever, hematuria.
- In patients who respond initially but who later fail to respond to somatropin therapy, test for circulating GH antibodies (antisomatropin antibodies) should be performed.
- Diabetic patients or those with family history of diabetes should be observed closely. Regular testing of urine for glycosuria or fasting blood glucose levels is recommended.
- Patient with GH deficiency secondary to intracranial lesion should be examined frequently for progression or recurrence of underlying disease process.

Patient & Family Education

- During first 6 mo of successful treatment, linear growth rates may be increased 8–16 cm or more per year (average about 7 cm/y). Additionally, SC fat diminishes but returns to pretreatment value later.

- Instruct parent of child under treatment to record accurate height measurements at regular intervals and to report to physician if rate is less than expected.
- In general, growth response to somatropin is inversely proportional to duration of treatment. Somatropin should be discontinued when patient has reached satisfactory adult height, when epiphyses have fused, or when patient fails to exhibit growth response.

SOTALOL

(so-ta'lol)

Trade name: Betapace

Classifications: AUTONOMIC NERVOUS SYSTEM AGENT; BETA-ADRENERGIC ANTAGONIST (BLOCKING AGENT, SYMPATHOLYTIC); CARDIOVASCULAR AGENT; ANTIARRHYTHMIC

Prototype: Propanolol

Pregnancy category: B

ACTIONS/PHARMACODYNAMICS Class II and class III antiarrhythmic properties. Slows heart rate, decreases AV nodal conduction, and increases AV nodal refractoriness. Produces significant reductions in both systolic and diastolic blood pressure.

USE Treatment of life-threatening ventricular arrhythmias (sustained ventricular tachycardia). **Unlabeled uses:** hypertension, angina.

ROUTE & DOSAGE

Ventricular Arrhythmias

Adult: **PO** Initial dose of 80 mg b.i.d. or 160 mg q.d. taken prior to meals. May increase every 3–4 d in 40–160 mg increments. Most patients respond to 240–320 mg/d in 2 or 3 divided doses. Doses > 640 mg/d have not been studied.

Dose adjustment for renal function:

Cl_{cr}	Dose
>60 ml/min	q12h
30–60 ml/min	q24h
10–30 ml/min	q36–48 h
<10 ml/min	Individualize carefully

PHARMACOKINETICS Absorption: slowly and completely absorbed from GI tract. Negligible first-pass metabolism. Absorption of sotalol may be reduced by food, especially milk and milk products. **Peak:** 2–3 h. **Duration:** 24 h. **Distribution:** Drug is hydrophilic and will enter the CSF slowly (about 10%). Crosses placental barrier. Distributed in breast milk. Not appreciably protein bound. **Metabolism:** does not undergo significant hepatic enzyme metabolism and no active metabolites have been identified. **Elimination:** half-life: 7–18 h; excreted by glomerular filtration in the urine with 75% of the drug excreted unchanged within 72 h.

CONTRAINDICATIONS & PRECAUTIONS Contraindicated in: bronchial asthma, sinus bradycardia, second and third degree heart block, long QT syndromes, cardiogenic shock, uncontrolled CHF, chronic bronchitis, emphysema, hypersensitivity to sotalol. **Cautious use in:** CHF, electrolyte disturbances, recent MI, diabetes, sick sinus rhythms, renal impairment.

ADVERSE/SIDE EFFECTS CV: AV block, hypotension, aggravation of CHF, although the incidence of heart failure may be lower than for other beta-blockers, life-threatening ventricular arrhythmias, including polymorphous ventricular tachycardia or torsade de pointes, *bradycardia, dyspnea, chest pain, palpitation,* bleeding (<2%). **CNS:** headache, *fatigue, dizziness,* weakness, lethargy, depression, lassitude. **GI:** nausea, vomiting, diarrhea, dyspepsia, dry mouth. **GU:** impotence, decreased libido. **Metabolic:** hyperglycemia. **Other:** visual disturbances, respiratory complaints, rash.

DRUG INTERACTIONS Antagonizes the effects of BETA AGONISTS. **Amiodarone** may lead to symptomatic bradycardia and sinus arrest. **Astemizole** may prolong QT interval leading to arrhythmias. The hypoglycemic effects of ORAL HYPOGLYCEMIC AGENTS may be potentiated. May cause resistance to **epinephrine** in anaphylactic reactions. Should be used with caution with other ANTIARRHYTHMIC AGENTS. **Drug–food:** absorption of **sotalol** may be reduced by food, especially **milk** and MILK PRODUCTS.

NURSING IMPLICATIONS

Administration

- Give on an empty stomach 1 h before or 2 h after meals. Do not give with milk or milk products.
- Sotalol should be initiated and doses increased only in a hospital with cardiac rhythm monitoring and frequent assessment.
- Smallest effective dose should be used for patients with nonallergic bronchospasms.
- Discontinuation of sotalol should not be abrupt. Dose should gradually be reduced over 1–2 wk.
- Store at room temperature, 15–30C (59–86F).

Assessment & Drug Effects

- Initial and periodic (especially when doses are increased) ECG monitoring are essential, because proarrhythmic events most often occur within 7 d of initiating therapy or increasing dose of sotalol.
- Electrolyte imbalances of hypokalemia or hypomagnesemia should be corrected prior to administering sotalol.
- Carefully monitor cardiac status, including ECG, through course of therapy. Special caution is warranted when sotalol is used concurrently with other antiarrhythmics, digoxin, or calcium channel blockers.
- Carefully monitor patients with bronchospastic disease (e.g., bronchitis, emphysema) for inhibition of bronchodilation.
- Monitor diabetics for loss of glycemic control. Beta blockage reduces the release of endogenous insulin in response to hyperglycemia and may blunt symptoms of acute hypoglycemia (e.g., tachycardia, BP changes).

Patient & Family Education

- Advise of risk for hypotension and syncope, especially with concurrent treatment with catecholamine-depleting drugs (e.g., reserpine, guanethidine).
- Teach to take radial pulse daily and report marked bradycardia (pulse below 60).
- Inform type II diabetics of increased risk for hyperglycemia. Inform all diabetics of possible masking of symptoms of hypoglycemia.
- Advise not to abruptly discontinue sotalol due to the risk of exacerbation of angina, arrhythmias, and possible myocardial infarction.

SPARFLOXACIN

(spar-flox′-a-sin)

Trade name: Zagam

S

Classifications: ANTIINFECTIVE; QUINOLONE
Prototype: Ciprofloxacin
Pregnancy category: C

ACTIONS/PHARMACODYNAMICS Synthetic quinolone that is a broad-spectrum bactericidal agent. Inhibits DNA-gyrase, an enzyme necessary for bacterial DNA replication and some aspects of transcription, repair, recombination, and transposition. Effective against many gram-positive and gram-negative organisms.

USES Treatment of community-acquired pneumonia, acute exacerbations of chronic bronchitis caused by susceptible bacteria.

ROUTE & DOSAGE

Community-acquired Pneumonia, Bronchitis

Adult: **PO** 400 mg day 1, then 200 mg q.d. day 2–10.
Adjustment for renal impairment: Cl_{cr} < 50 ml/min: 400 mg day 1, then 200 mg q48h day 2–10.

PHARMACOKINETICS Absorption: rapidly absorbed from GI tract. 92% bioavailability. **Peak:** 3–6 h. **Distribution:** 45% protein bound. Penetrates lower respiratory tract tissues. Crosses placenta, distributed into breast milk. **Metabolism:** metabolized in the liver. Does not utilize Cyt P450 enzymes. **Elimination:** half-life: 20 h (16–30 h); excreted in urine.

CONTRAINDICATIONS & PRECAUTIONS Contraindicated in: history of hypersensitivity or photosensitivity reactions; patients with known QT_c prolongation, antiarrhythmic agents that prolong the QT_c interval; exposure to sun while taking sparfloxacin; nursing mothers; hypokalemia, significant bradycardia, CHF, myocardial ischemia, and atrial fibrillation. **Cautious use in:** history of seizures, renal dysfunction, severe cerebral arteriosclerosis, pregnancy (category C). Safety and effectiveness in children < 18 y are not known.

ADVERSE/SIDE EFFECTS CNS: headache, dizziness, insomnia, somnolence. **CV:** prolonged QT_c interval on ECG. **GI:** pseudomembranous colitis, diarrhea, nausea, dyspepsia, abdominal pain, taste perversion, vomiting, flatulence, dry mouth. **Skin:** *phototoxicity* (burning, redness, swelling, blisters, rash, itching, dermatitis), pruritus, rash. **Other:** vaginal moniliasis.

DRUG INTERACTIONS MAGNESIUM- or ALUMINUM-CONTAINING ANTACIDS decrease absorption; torsade de pointes arrhythmias in patients on **disopyramide, amiodarone, quinidine, procainamide, sotalol, bepridil.**

NURSING IMPLICATIONS

Administration

- Do not give drug within 4 h of drugs containing aluminum, magnesium, iron, zinc, calcium, or sucralfate.
- Store at 20–25C (68–77F) in a tightly closed container.

Assessment & Drug Effects

- Therapeutic effectiveness is indicated by negative cultures and resolution of S&S of infection.
- C&S test should be done prior to beginning therapy and periodically during therapy.
- Sparfloxacin should not be given to persons with pro-arrhythmic conditions such as hypokalemia, CHF, atrial fibrillation, etc.
- Discontinue therapy and notify physician immediately if any of the following occur: skin rash or other

S

signs of a hypersensitivity reaction (see Appendix G); skin eruption following sun exposure; symptoms of colitis such as persistent diarrhea; joint pain, inflammation, or other signs of rupture of a tendon; CNS symptoms such as seizures, restlessness, anxiety, confusion, hallucinations, depression, suicidal ideation.

- Carefully monitor persons at risk for seizures.

Patient & Family Education

- Note important indications for discontinuing drug and immediately notifying physician.
- Fluids should be consumed liberally while taking sparfloxacin.
- Allow a minimum of 4 h between sparfloxacin and any of the following: aluminum and/or magnesium antacids, iron and calcium supplements, multivitamins with zinc, or sucralfate.
- Avoid all exposure to direct or indirect sunlight or artificial UV light during treatment and for 5 d after therapy. If brief sunlight exposure is necessary, cover as much skin surface as possible with clothing. Discontinue drug at first sign of phototoxicity (e.g., burning skin, redness, swelling, itching) and notify physician.

SPECTINOMYCIN HYDROCHLORIDE

(spek-ti-noe-mye′sin)

Trade name: Trobicin

Classifications: ANTIINFECTIVE; ANTIBIOTIC

Pregnancy category: B

ACTIONS/PHARMACODYNAMICS Antibiotic produced by *Streptomyces spectabilis*. Action is usually bacteriostatic. Variable activity against a wide variety of gram-negative and gram-positive organisms. Inhibits majority of *Neisseria gonorrhoeae* strains; effective for urethral and anorectal infections, but not pharyngeal. Not active against syphilis or chlamydial and mycoplasmal infections.

USES Only for treatment of uncomplicated gonorrhea in patients sensitized or resistant to penicillin or other effective drugs approved by US Centers for Disease Control. **Unlabeled uses:** disseminated gonococcal infections caused by penicillinase-producing strains of *N. gonorrhoeae* (PPNG) and sexually transmitted epididymoorchitis.

ROUTE & DOSAGE

Uncomplicated Gonorrhea

Adult: **IM** 2 g as single dose.
Child: **IM** 40 mg/kg as single dose.

Disseminated Gonorrhea

Adult: **IM** 2 g q12h.

PHARMACOKINETICS Absorption: readily absorbed from IM site. **Peak:** 1 hr. **Metabolism:** metabolized in liver. **Eliminations:** half-life: 1.2–2.8 h; excreted in urine.

CONTRAINDICATIONS & PRECAUTIONS Contraindicated in: safe use during pregnancy (category B), in nursing mothers, and in infants and children not definitely established. **Cautious use in:** history of allergies.

ADVERSE/SIDE EFFECTS *Pain and soreness at injection site,* urticaria, pruritus, transient rash, headache, dizziness, nausea, vomiting, chills, fever, insomnia, nervousness. **Following multiple doses:** decrease in Hgb, Hct, Cl_{cr}, elevated serum alkaline phosphatase, ALT, BUN.

S

NURSING IMPLICATIONS

Administration

- Administer IM injection deep into upper outer quadrant of gluteus. No more than 5 ml should be injected into single site (20-gauge needle is recommeded). Injection may be painful.
- Reconstitute with supplied diluent (bacteriostatic water for injection with 0.9% benzyl alcohol). Shake vial vigorously immediately after adding diluent and before withdrawing drug. Solution should be used within 24 h of reconstitution.
- Store at 15–30C (59–86F) unless otherwise directed.

Assessment & Drug Effects

- Observe patient for 45–60 min after injection. Systemic anaphylaxis has been reported (apprehension, pruritus, hypertension, abdominal pain, collapse).
- Patients with gonorrhea should have serologic tests for syphilis at time of diagnosis and again after 3 mo.
- Clinical effectiveness of drug should be monitored to detect antibiotic resistance.
- All gonococcal infection sites should be cultured 3–7 d after spectinomycin therapy is completed to verify eradication of infection.

S

SPIRAPRIL

(spir'a-pril)

Trade name: Renormax

Classifications: CARDIOVASCULAR AGENT; ANGIOTENSIN-CONVERTING ENZYME INHIBITOR; ANTIHYPERTENSIVE

Prototype: Captopril

Pregnancy category: C (first trimester), D (second and third trimesters)

ACTIONS/PHARMACODYNAMICS Lowers blood pressure by inhibiting ACE. Spirapril interrupts conversion sequences initiated by renin that lead to formation of angiotensin II. Inhibition of angiotensin II also decreases aldosterone secretion and vasodilates arteriolar smooth muscles, thus reducing blood pressure.

USE Hypertension. **Unlabeled use:** CHF.

ROUTE & DOSAGE

Hypertension

Adult: **PO** 6–12 mg in 1–2 divided doses; may be increased q2–4wk up to 24 mg/d.

PHARMACOKINETICS **Absorption:** rapidly absorbed from GI tract; 42% reaches systemic circulation as active metabolite, spiraprilat. **Onset:** 1 h. **Peak effect:** 3–6 h. **Distribution:** 86–91% protein bound. **Metabolism:** metabolized in liver to active form, spiraprilat. **Elimination:** half-life: 35 h (spiraprilat); 37–45% excreted in urine, 40–60% excreted in bile.

CONTRAINDICATIONS & PRECAUTIONS **Contraindicated in:** hypersensitivity to spirapril. **Cautious use in:** hypersensitivity or adverse reactions to other ACE inhibitors; pregnancy (category C [first trimester], category D [second and third trimesters]); elderly; renal impairment; liver disease; hyperkalemia; history of angioedema due to an ACE inhibitor; patients on dialysis; patients with autoimmune disease.

ADVERSE/SIDE EFFECTS **CNS:** *headache, dizziness, fatigue,* paresthesia, hypesthesia, migraine. **CV:** tachycardia, hypotension. **GI:** nausea, vomiting, diarrhea, constipation. **Skin:** angioedema (rare), rash.

Other: upper respiratory tract infections, cough, back pain.

NURSING IMPLICATIONS

Administration

- Dosage adjustments may be indicated with severe renal impairment (Cl_{cr} < 30 ml/min) or hepatic impairment.
- Recommended initial dose in the elderly is 6 mg/d.
- Store at 15–30C (59–86F).

Assessment & Drug Effects

- A sudden exaggerated hypotensive response may occur within 1–3 h of the first dose, especially in those with high blood pressure, on a diuretic, or on a salt-restricted diet.
- Monitor blood pressure frequently, especially during initiation of therapy. If significant hypotensive effects occur, dosage reduction may be warranted.
- Monitor renal function, serum electrolytes, and WBC with differential periodically throughout therapy. Urinary protein determination should be made prior to beginning therapy, monthly for 9 mo, and periodically thereafter.

Patient & Family Education

- Advise to report to physician immediately any of the following: swelling of face, hands, or feet; difficulty swallowing or breathing; sore throat, fever, or chills; confusion; palpitation; numbness or tingling; weakness of legs; persistent dizziness or light-headedness.
- Advise to avoid using salt substitutes unless approved by physician.
- Inform about the possibility of developing ACE inhibitor-induced dry cough. Advise to consult physician if cough interferes with sleep.

SPIRONOLACTONE

(speer-on-oh-lak′tone)

Trade names: Aldactone, Novospiroton ♣

Prototype for classifications: ELECTROLYTIC AND WATER BALANCE AGENT; POTASSIUM-SPARING DIURETIC

Pregnancy category: D

ACTIONS/PHARMACODYNAMICS

Steroidal compound and specific pharmacologic antagonist of aldosterone. Presumably acts by competing with aldosterone for cellular receptor sites in distal renal tubule. Promotes sodium and chloride excretion without concomitant loss of potassium. Diuretic effect reportedly not associated with hyperuricemia or hyperglycemia. Activity depends on presence of endogenous or exogenous aldosterone. Lowers systolic and diastolic pressures in hypertensive patients by unknown mechanism.

USES Clinical conditions associated with augmented aldosterone production, as in essential hypertension, refractory edema due to CHF, hepatic cirrhosis, nephrotic syndrome, and idiopathic edema. May be used to potentiate actions of other diuretics and antihypertensive agents or for its potassium-sparing effect. Also used for treatment of (and as presumptive test for) primary aldosteronism. **Unlabeled use:** hirsutism in women with polycystic ovary syndrome or idiopathic hirsutism; adjunct in treatment of myasthenia gravis and familial periodic paralysis.

ROUTE & DOSAGE

Edema

Adult: **PO** 25–200 mg/d in divided doses; continued for at

S

least 5 d; dose adjusted to optimal response; if no response, a thiazide or loop diuretic may be added.
Child: **PO** 3.3 mg/kg/d in single or divided doses; continued for at least 5 d; dose adjusted to optimal response.
Neonate: **PO** 1–3 mg/kg/d divided q12–24h.

Hypertension

Adult: **PO** 25–100 mg/d in single or divided doses; continued for at least 2 wk; dose adjusted to optimal response.

Primary Aldosteronism: Diagnosis

Adult: **PO** Short Test: 400 mg/d for 4 d; long test: 400 mg/d for 3–4 wk.

Primary Aldosteronism: Treatment

Adult: **PO** 100–400 mg/d in divided doses.

PHARMACOKINETICS Absorption: approximately 73% absorbed from GI tract. **Onset:** gradual. **Peak:** 2–3 d; max effect may take up to 2 wk. **Duration:** 2–3 d or more. **Distribution:** crosses placenta, distributed into breast milk. **Metabolism:** metabolized in liver and kidneys to active metabolites. **Elimination:** half-life: 1.3–2.4 h parent compound, 18–23 h metabolites, 40–57% excreted in urine, 35–40% in bile.

CONTRAINDICATIONS & PRECAUTIONS Contraindicated in: anuria, acute renal insufficiency, progressing impairment of renal function, hyperkalemia. Safe use during pregnancy (category D) and lactation not established. **Cautious use in:** BUN of 40 mg/dl or greater, hepatic disease.

ADVERSE/SIDE EFFECTS CNS: lethargy, mental confusion, fatigue (with rapid weight loss), headache, drowsiness, ataxia. **Endocrine:** gynecomastia (both sexes), inability to achieve or maintain erection, androgenic effects (hirsutism, irregular menses, deepening of voice); parathyroid changes, decreased glucose tolerance. **GI:** abdominal cramps, nausea, vomiting, anorexia, diarrhea. **Skin:** maculopapular or erythematous rash, urticaria. **Other:** fluid and electrolyte imbalance (particularly hyperkalemia and hyponatremia); elevated BUN, mild acidosis, drug fever, agranulocytosis, SLE, hypertension (postsympathectomy patient), hyperuricemia, gout.

DIAGNOSTIC TEST INTERFERENCE Spironolactone may produce marked increases in ***plasma cortisol*** determinations by ***Mattingly fluorometric*** method; these may persist for several days after termination of drug (spironolactone metabolite produces fluorescence). There is the possibility of false elevations in measurements of ***digoxin serum levels*** by ***RIA*** procedures.

DRUG INTERACTIONS Combinations of spironolactone and acidifying doses of **ammonium chloride** may produce systemic acidosis; use these combinations with caution. Diuretic effect of spironolactone may be antagonized by **aspirin** and other SALICYLATES (possibly by competing for same receptor sites). Patients receiving spironolactone and **digitoxin** or similar CARDIAC GLYCOSIDES concurrently should be monitored for decreased effect of cardiac glycoside (spironolactone shortens its half-life, possibly by acting as enzyme inducing agent). Hyperkalemia may result with POTASSIUM

S

SUPPLEMENTS (spironolactone conserves potassium).

NURSING IMPLICATIONS

Administration

- Administer with food to enhance absorption.
- Tablet may be crushed before administration and taken with fluid of patient's choice.
- Preserve in tight, light-resistant containers. Suspension is stable for 1 mo under refrigeration.

Assessment & Drug Effects

- Check blood pressure before initiation of therapy and at regular intervals throughout therapy.
- Serum electrolytes should be monitored, especially during early therapy. Be alert for signs of fluid and electrolyte imbalance.
- Monitor daily I&O and check for edema. Report lack of diuretic response or development of edema; both may indicate tolerance to drug.
- Weigh patient under standard conditions before therapy begins and daily throughout therapy. Weight is a useful index of need for dosage adjustment. For patients with ascites, physician may want measurements of abdominal girth.
- Observe for and report immediately the onset of mental changes, lethargy, or stupor in patients with hepatic disease.
- Adverse reactions are generally reversible with discontinuation of drug. Gynecomastia appears to be related to dosage level and duration of therapy; it may persist in some after drug is stopped.

Patient & Family Education

- Inform that maximal diuretic effect may not occur until third day of therapy and that diuresis may continue for 2 or 3 d after drug is withdrawn.
- Instruct to report signs of hyponatremia (see Appendix G), most likely to occur in patients with severe cirrhosis.
- Instruct to avoid replacing fluid losses with large amounts of free water (can result in dilutional hyponatremia).
- Generally, patient should avoid excessive intake of high-potassium foods and salt substitutes.

STANOZOLOL

(stan-oh'zoe-lole)

Trade name: Winstrol

Classifications: SYNTHETIC HORMONE; ANDROGEN/ANABOLIC STEROID

Prototype: Testosterone

Pregnancy category: X

Controlled substance: Schedule III

ACTIONS/PHARMACODYNAMICS

Synthetic steroid with relatively strong anabolic and weak androgenic activity. Pharmacokinetics, contraindications, adverse effects similar to those for testosterone.

USES Primarily to increase hemoglobin in selected cases of aplastic anemia, prophylaxis to decrease the frequency and severity of hereditary angioedema.

ROUTE & DOSAGE

Anemia

Adult: **PO** 2 mg t.i.d.; young women: 2 mg 1–2 times/d.
Child: **PO** <6 *y*, 1 mg b.i.d.; *6–12 y*, 2 mg t.i.d.

ADVERSE/SIDE EFFECTS See testosterone.

NURSING IMPLICATIONS

Administration

- Administer just before or with meals to reduce incidence of gastric distress.
- Smaller dose for young women is given to prevent virilizing effects of the drug. If such effects appear (early sign: change of voice), physician should be notified.

Assessment & Drug Effects

- Monitor Hct & Hgb periodically to determine efficacy of drug.
- Patient may need to be on a restricted salt intake. Check with the physician.
- Be alert to symptoms of hypercalcemia (see Appendix G).

Patient & Family Education

- Use with high-calorie, high-protein diet unless contraindicated.
- Stanozolol does not enhance athletic ability.

STAVUDINE (D4T)

(sta'vu-deen)

Trade name: Zerit

Classifications: ANTIINFECTIVE; ANTIVIRAL

Prototype: Zidovudine (AZT)

Pregnancy category: C

ACTIONS/PHARMACODYNAMICS Synthetic analog of thymidine (a major nucleoside in DNA) with antiviral action against HIV, the causative agent of AIDS. Stavudine inhibits the replication of HIV in human cells. It is phosphorylated to stavudine triphosphate by endogenous thymidine kinase. It appears to act by being incorporated into the growing DNA chains by viral transcriptase, thus terminating viral replication.

USES Treatment of adults with advanced HIV infection who are intolerant of other antiretroviral agents (zidovudine, didanosine, zalcitabine) or who have deteriorated on the other agents.

ROUTE & DOSAGE

Advanced HIV Infection

Adult: **PO** *≥60 kg,* 40 mg q12h; *<60 kg,* 30 mg q12h. Reduce dose by 50% in patients with peripheral neuropathy or creatinine clearance of 25–50 ml/min.
Child: **PO** *< 30 kg* give 2 mg/kg/d in 2 divided doses. *≥ 30 kg,* same dose as adult.

PHARMACOKINETICS Absorption: readily absorbed from GI tract; 82% reaches systemic circulation. **Peak:** effect 6 wk. **Distribution:** distributes into CSF; excreted in breast milk of animals. **Metabolism:** metabolized in liver; in addition to hepatic metabolism, some investigators suggest that degradation and salvage by other pyrimidine pathways may contribute to elimination; intracellularly, stavudine is phosphorylated by cellular enzymes to its active triphosphate form. **Elimination:** half-life: 1–1.6 h; excreted primarily in urine.

CONTRAINDICATIONS & PRECAUTIONS Contraindicated in: hypersensitivity to stavudine. Safe use during pregnancy (category C) and lactation not established. **Cautious use in:** previous hypersensitivity to zidovudine, didanosine, or zalcitabine; folic acid or B_{12} deficiency; liver and renal insufficiency; peripheral neuropathy; history of pancreatitis.

ADVERSE/SIDE EFFECTS CNS: *peripheral neuropathy,* paresthesias, cramping, headache, chills/fever. **Hematologic:** anemia. **Other:** rash, elevated liver function tests, abdominal pain.

NURSING IMPLICATIONS

Administration

- The 1-h intervals between doses should be closely adhered to.
- Store at room temperature, 15–30C (59–86F).

Assessment & Drug Effects

- Monitor for peripheral neuropathy and report numbness, tingling, or pain, which may indicate a need to interrupt stavudine.
- Periodically monitor hepatic enzymes, CBC with differential, PT, and renal function.
- Monitor for development of opportunistic infection.

Patient & Family Education

- Inform of adverse drug effects and advise to report those that are bothersome.
- Advise to report symptoms of peripheral neuropathy immediately.

STREPTOKINASE

(strep-toe-kye'nase)

Trade names: Kabikinase, Streptase

Prototype for classifications: BLOOD FORMER; THROMBOLYTIC ENZYME

Pregnancy category: A

ACTIONS/PHARMACODYNAMICS Derivative of the beta-hemolytic streptococci. Promotes thrombolysis by activating the conversion of plasminogen to plasmin, the enzyme that degrades fibrin, fibrinogen, and other procoagulant proteins into soluble fragments. This fibrinolytic activity is effective both outside and within the formed thrombus/embolus. Decreases blood and plasma viscosity and erythrocyte aggregation tendency, thus increasing perfusion of collateral blood vessels.

USES Acute extensive deep venous thrombosis, acute arterial thrombosis or embolism, acute pulmonary embolus, coronary artery thrombosis, MI, and arteriovenous cannula occlusion.

ROUTE & DOSAGE

Coronary Artery Thrombosis, MI

Adult: **IV** 1.5 million IU infused over 60 min. **Intracoronary** 15,000–20,000 IU bolus, followed by 2000–4000 IU/min for 60 min.

Deep Vein Thrombosis, Pulmonary Embolism, Arterial Embolism

Adult: **IV** 250,000 IU over 30 min loading dose, then 100,000 IU/h for 48–72 h.

Occluded Cannula

Adult: **IV** 250,000 IU in 2 ml over 25–35 min; clamp for 2 h, then aspirate cannula.

PHARMACOKINETICS **Metabolism:** rapidly cleared from circulation by antibodies. **Elimination:** half-life: 83 min; does not cross placenta, but antibodies do.

CONTRAINDICATIONS & PRECAUTIONS **Contraindicated in:** active internal bleeding; very recent cardiopulmonary resuscitation; recent (within 2 mo) intraspinal, intracranial, intraarterial procedures; intracranial neoplasm; CVA, severe uncontrolled hypertension; history of allergic response to SK, recent streptococcal infection; obstetrical delivery; diabetic hemorrhagic retinopathy; ulcerative colitis, diverticulitis; any condition in which bleeding presents a hazard or would be difficult to manage because of location; pregnancy (category A); safe use during lactation or in children not established. **Cautious use in:** patient with preexisting hemostatic deficits; conditions accompanied by risk of cerebral embolism; septic thrombophlebitis; uremia; hepatic failure.

ADVERSE/SIDE EFFECTS **Allergic:** *major* (12%) (bronchospasm, periorbital swelling, angioneurotic edema, anaphylaxis); *mild* (urticaria, itching, headache, musculoskeletal pain, flushing, nausea, pyrexia). **Hematologic:** phlebitis, *bleeding or oozing at sites of percutaneous trauma;* prolonged systemic hypocoagulability; spontaneous bleeding (GU, GI, retroperitoneal); unstable blood pressure; reperfusion atrial or ventricular dysrhythmias.

DIAGNOSTIC TEST INTERFERENCE Streptokinase promotes increases in ***TT, APTT,*** and ***PT.***

DRUG INTERACTIONS ANTICOAGULANTS increase risk of bleeding; **aminocaproic acid** reverses the action of streptokinase.

S

NURSING IMPLICATIONS

Administration

- IV preparation: SK is reconstituted with 5 ml 0.9% NaCl injection (preferred) or 5 ml 5% dextrose injection. Roll or tilt vial; avoid shaking to prevent foaming or increase in flocculation. Reconstituted solution may be carefully diluted again, avoiding shaking or agitation of the solution. Slight flocculation does not interfere with drug action; discard solution with large amount of flocculant.
- For rate of IV administration refer to Route & Dosage table.
- Observe infusion site frequently. If phlebitis occurs, it can usually be controlled by diluting the infusion solution.
- Reconstituted solution should be stored at 2–4C (36–39F). Discard after 24 h. Store unopened vials at 15–30C (59–86F).

Assessment & Drug Effects

- Thrombi more than 7 d old respond poorly to SK therapy; therefore, IV infusion is started as soon as possible after the thrombotic event.
- Before SK treatment is started, heparin is discontinued and baseline control levels are established for thrombin time (TT), activated partial thromboplastin time (APTT), prothrombin time (PT), Hct, and platelet count. Treatment is delayed until TT and APTT are less than 2 times the normal control level.
- Spontaneous bleeding occurs about twice as often with SK as with heparin. Protect patient from invasive procedures: IM injections are contraindicated. Also prevent undue manipulation during thrombolytic therapy to prevent bruising.
- During treatment with SK, TT is generally kept at about 2 times or more baseline value and checked q3–4h.
- Monitor for excessive bleeding q15min for the first hour of therapy, q30min for second to eighth hour, then q8h.
- Patient is at risk for postthrombolytic bleeding for 2–4 d after intracoronary SK treatment. Continue monitoring vital signs until laboratory tests confirm anticoagulant control.
- Report signs of potential serious bleeding; gum bleeding, epistaxis,

hematoma, spontaneous ecchymoses, oozing at catheter site, increased pulse, pain from internal bleeding. SK infusion should be interrupted, then resumed when bleeding stops.

- Report promptly symptoms of a major allergic reaction; therapy will be discontinued and emergency treatment instituted. Minor symptoms (e.g., itching, nausea) respond to concurrent antihistamine or corticosteroid treatment or both without interruption of SK administration.
- Check pulse frequently. Be alert to changes in cardiac rhythm, especially during intracoronary instillation. Dysrhythmias signal need to stop therapy at once.
- Monitor BP. Mild changes can be expected, but report substantial changes (greater than ± 25 mm Hg). Therapy may be discontinued.
- Check patient's temperature during treatment. A slight elevation, 0.8C (1.5F), perhaps with chills, occurs in about one third of the patients. An elevation to 40C (104F) or more requires symptomatic treatment.
- If an analgesic-antipyretic is indicated, avoid giving aspirin because of its antiplatelet action.

Patient & Family Education

- Instruct to immediately report symptoms of hypersensitivity, e.g., dyspnea, urticaria, pruritus.

STREPTOMYCIN SULFATE

(strep-toe-mye′sin)

Classifications: ANTIINFECTIVE; AMINOGLYCOSIDE ANTIBIOTIC; ANTITUBERCULOSIS AGENT

Prototype: Gentamicin

Pregnancy category: C

ACTIONS/PHARMACODYNAMICS

Aminoglycoside antibiotic derived from *Streptomyces griseus,* with bactericidal and bacteriostatic actions. Active against a variety of gram-positive, gram-negative, and acid-fast organisms. Because of rapid emergence of resistant strains when streptomycin sulfate is used alone, it most commonly is used concurrently with other antimicrobial agents. Reportedly, it is the least nephrotoxic of the aminoglycosides.

USES Only in combination with other antitubercular drugs in treatment of all forms of active tuberculosis caused by susceptible organisms. Used alone or in conjunction with tetracycline for tularemia, plague, and brucellosis. Also used with other antibiotics in treatment of subacute bacterial endocarditis due to enterococci and streptococci (viridans group) and *Hemophilus influenzae* and in treatment of peritonitis, respiratory tract infections, granuloma inguinale, and chancroid when other drugs have failed.

ROUTE & DOSAGE

Tuberculosis

Adult: **IM** 15 mg/kg up to 1 g/d as single dose.
Geriatric: **IM** 10 mg/kg (max 750 mg/d).
Child: **IM** 20–40 mg/kg/d up to 1 g/d as single dose.
Infant: **IM** 10–15 mg/kg q12h.
Neonate: **IM** 10–20 mg/kg q24h.

Tularemia

Adult: **IM** 1–2 g/d in 1–2 divided doses for 7–10 d.
Child: **IM** 20–40 mg/kg/d divided q6–12h.

Plague
Adult: **IM** 2 g/d in 2–4 divided doses.
Child: **IM** 30 mg/kg/d divided q8–12h.

PHARMACOKINETICS **Peak:** 1–2 h. **Distribution:** diffuses into most body tissues and extracellular fluids; crosses placenta; distributed into breast milk. **Elimination:** half-life: 2–3 h adults, 4–10 h newborns; excreted in urine.

CONTRAINDICATIONS & PRECAUTIONS **Contraindicated in:** history of toxic reaction or hypersensitivity to aminoglycosides; labyrinthine disease; during pregnancy or lactation; myasthenia gravis; concurrent or sequential use of other neurotoxic or nephrotoxic agents. **Cautious use in:** impaired renal function (given in reduced dosages); use in the elderly and in prematures, neonates, and children.

ADVERSE/SIDE EFFECTS **CNS:** paresthesias (peripheral, facial). **Hypersensitivity:** skin rashes, pruritus, angioedema, drug fever, eosinophilia, exfoliative dermatitis, stomatitis, enlarged lymph nodes, anaphylactic shock, blood dyscrasias: leukopenia, neutropenia, pancytopenia, hemolytic or aplastic anemia. **Ototoxicity:** *labyrinthine damage,* auditory damage. **Other:** nephrotoxicity, hepatotoxicity, headache, inability to concentrate, lassitude, muscular weakness, optic nerve toxicity (scotomas), *pain and irritation at IM site,* superinfections, neuromuscular blockade, arachnoiditis, encephalopathy, **CNS depression syndrome (infants):** stupor, flaccidity, coma, paralysis, cardiac arrest); respiratory depression.

S

DIAGNOSTIC TEST INTERFERENCE Streptomycin reportedly produces false-positive ***urinary glucose*** tests using copper sulfate methods (Benedict's solution, Clinitest) but not with glucose oxidase methods (e.g., Clinistix, TesTape). False increases in protein content in ***urine*** and ***CSF*** using Folin-Ciocalteau reaction and decreased ***BUN*** readings with Berthelot reaction may occur from test interferences. ***Culture and sensitivity*** tests may be affected if patient is taking salts such as sodium and potassium chloride, sodium sulfate and tartrate, ammonium acetate, calcium and magnesium ions.

DRUG INTERACTION May potentiate anticoagulant effects of **warfarin.**

NURSING IMPLICATIONS

Administration

- Administer IM deep into large muscle mass to minimize possibility of irritation. Injections are painful.
- Avoid direct contact with drug; sensitization can occur. Gloves are advised during preparation of drug.
- Commercially prepared IM solution is intended only for IM injection (contains a preservative, and therefore is not suitable for other routes). It is stable at room temperature; expiration date is 1–2 y depending on manufacturer.
- Solutions made from streptomycin sulfate powder are preferably used immediately after reconstitution. See specific manufacturer's recommendations.
- Exposure to light may slightly darken solution, with no apparent loss of potency.

Assessment & Drug Effects

- Culture and sensitivity tests are

done prior to and periodically during course of therapy.

- Caloric stimulation and audiometric tests should be performed before, during, and 6 mo after discontinuation of streptomycin. Periodic renal and hepatic function tests are also recommended.
- Be alert for and report immediately symptoms of ototoxicity (see Appendix G). Symptoms are most likely to occur in patients with impaired renal function, patients receiving high doses (1.8–2 g/d) or other ototoxic or neurotoxic drugs, and the elderly. If drug is not discontinued promptly, irreversible damage may occur.
- Damage to vestibular portion of eighth cranial nerve (higher incidence than auditory toxicity) appears to occur in three stages. Acute stage may be preceded for 1 or 2 d by moderately severe headache, then by nausea, vomiting, vertigo in upright position, difficulty in reading, unsteadiness, and positive Romberg sign; acute stage lasts 1–2 wk and ends abruptly. Chronic stage is characterized by difficulty in walking or in making sudden movements and ataxia and lasts approximately 2 mo. In the compensatory stage, symptoms are latent and appear only when eyes are closed. Full recovery may take 12–18 mo; residual damage is permanent in some patients.
- Auditory nerve damage is usually preceded by vestibular symptoms and high-pitched tinnitus, roaring noises, impaired hearing (especially to high-pitched sounds), sense of fullness in ears. Audiometric test should be done if these symptoms appear, and drug should be discontinued. Hearing loss can be permanent if damage is extensive. Tinnitus may persist several days to weeks after drug is stopped.
- In patients with impaired renal function, drug accumulation reportedly occurs if administered more frequently than q8–12h. Frequent determinations of serum drug concentrations and periodic renal and hepatic function tests are advised (serum concentrations should not exceed 25 μg/ml in these patients).
- Although drug fever is uncommon, it is life threatening. Monitor temperature and BP. If either is altered, report to physician.
- Monitor I&O. Report oliguria or changes in I&O ratio (possible signs of diminishing renal function). Sufficient fluids to maintain urinary output of 1500 ml/24 h are generally advised. Consult physician.

Patient & Family Education

- Instruct to report any unusual symptom. Adverse reactions should be reviewed periodically, especially in patients on prolonged therapy. Inform patient of possibility of ototoxicity.
- Instruct to report immediately any of the following; nausea, vomiting, vertigo, tinnitus, fullness in ears, impaired hearing.

STREPTOZOCIN

(strep-toe-zoe′sin)

Trade name: Zanosar

Classifications: ANTINEOPLASTIC; ALKYLATING AGENT; ANTIBIOTIC

Prototype: Cyclophosphamide

Pregnancy category: C

ACTIONS/PHARMACODYNAMICS

Therapeutic product is synthetic and is similar to other nitrosourea antineoplastics (e.g., carmustine) but with weaker alkylating effects. In general, this drug is highly toxic and has a low therapeutic index; thus a clinically effective response is likely to be accompanied by some evidence of toxicity. Inhibits DNA synthesis in both bacterial and mammalian cells and prevents progression of cells into mitosis, affecting all phases of the cell cycle (cell-cycle nonspecific). Appears to have minimal effects on RNA or protein synthesis. Delays repair of DNA damaged by nitrosurea-induced alkylation. Unlike other nitrosoureas, has markedly significant specificity for pancreas beta and exocrine cells.

USES Metastatic functional and nonfunctional islet cell carcinoma of pancreas, as single agent or in combination with fluorouracil. **Unlabeled uses:** a variety of other malignant neoplasms including metastatic carcinoid tumor or carcinoid syndrome, refractory advanced Hodgkin's disease, and metastatic colorectal cancer.

ROUTE & DOSAGE

Islet Cell Carcinoma of Pancreas
Adult: **IV** 500 mg/m²/d for 5 consecutive days q6wk or 1 g/m²/wk for 2 wk; then increase to 1.5 g/m²/wk; infuse dose over 15 min to 6 h.

PHARMACOKINETICS Absorption: undetectable in plasma within 3 h. **Distribution:** metabolite enters CSF. **Metabolism:** metabolized in liver and kidneys. **Elimination:** half-life: 35–40 min; 70–80% of dose excreted in urine, 1% in feces, and 5% in expired air.

CONTRAINDICATIONS & PRECAUTIONS Contraindicated in: safe use in pregnancy (category C), during lactation, and in children has not been established; hepatic and renal dysfunction.

ADVERSE/SIDE EFFECTS CNS: confusion, lethargy, depression. **GI:** *nausea, vomiting,* diarrhea, duodenal ulcer (rare). **Hematologic:** *mild* to moderate myelosuppression (*leukopenia, thrombocytopenia, anemia*). **Hepatic:** transient increase in AST, ALT, or alkaline phosphatase; hypoalbuminemia. **Metabolic:** glucose tolerance abnormalities (moderate and reversible); glycosuria without hyperglycemia, insulin shock (rare). **Renal:** nephrotoxicity: azotemia, anuria, proteinuria, hypophosphatemia, hyperchloremia; ***Fanconi-like syndrome*** (proximal renal tubular reabsorption defects, alkaline pH of urine, glucosuria, acetonuria, aminoaciduria): hypokalemia, hypocalcemia. **Other:** local necrosis following extravasation.

DRUG INTERACTIONS MYELOSUPPRESSIVE AGENTS add to hematologic toxicity; nephrotoxic agents (e.g., AMINOGLYCOSIDES, **vancomycin, amphotericin B, cisplatin**) increase risk of nephrotoxicity; **phenytoin** may reduce cytotoxic effect on pancreatic beta cells.

NURSING IMPLICATIONS

Administration

- Use only under constant supervision by physician experienced in therapy with cytotoxic agents and only when the benefit:risk ratio is fully and thoroughly understood by patient and family.
- Persons handling streptozocin should wear gloves to protect against topical exposure, which may pose a carcinogen hazard. If solution or powder comes in contact with skin or mucosa, promptly flush the area thoroughly with soap and water.
- IV administration: Reconstitute streptozocin powder for injection

Common side effect in *italic,* life-threatening effects underlined: generic names in **bold;** drug class in SMALL CAPS

with 9.5% ml dextrose injection or 0.9% NaCl injection; resulting solution will contain 100 mg/ml streptozocin and will be pale gold. Dilute solution further with 10–200 ml if desired with the same diluents and administer over 15 min.

- Inspect injection site frequently for signs of extravasation: patient complaints of stinging or burning at site, swelling around site, no blood return or questionable blood return.
- If extravasation occurs, area requires immediate attention to prevent necrosis. Remove needle, apply ice, and contact physician regarding further treatment to infiltrated tissue. Teach patient to inspect site at weekly intervals and to report changes in tissue appearance.
- An antiemetic given routinely every 4 or 6 h and prophylactically 30 min before a treatment may provide sufficient control to maintain the treatment regimen (even if it reduces but not completely eliminates nausea and vomiting).
- Protect reconstituted solution and vials of drug from light. Reconstituted solutions should be discarded after 12 h (contains no preservative and not intended for multidose use).

Assessment & Drug Effects

- When patient is receiving medication on a weekly dosing regimen, onset of therapeutic response usually occurs about 17 d after start of therapy, reaching maximum response in about 35 d.
- Functional islet cell tumors produce and secrete a variety of hormones including glucagon, insulin, calcitonin, serotonin, and others. Successful therapy with streptozocin (alone or in combination) produces a biochemical response evidenced by decreased secretion of hormones as well as measurable tumor regression. Thus, serial fasting insulin levels during treatment indicate response to the antineoplastic.
- Renal function must be adequate to prevent drug toxicity. Serial urinalyses and determinations of BUN, creatinine clearance, and serum electrolytes are obtained prior to and weekly during therapy, then for 4 wk after termination of therapy.
- Evidence of drug-induced declining renal function should be reported promptly; changes are dose related and cumulative.
- Early laboratory evidence of renal dysfunction consists of hypophosphatemia, mild proteinurea, and changes in I&O ratio and pattern.
- Mild adverse renal effects may be reversible following discontinuation of streptozocin, but nephrotoxicity may be irreversible, severe, or fatal.
- CBC should be performed at least weekly, and liver function tests at least prior to each course of therapy. Dosage adjustment or discontinuation may be required if there is evidence of decreased hepatic or bone marrow function.
- Myelosuppression is severe in 10–20% of patients and may be cumulative and more severe if patient has had prior exposure to radiation or to other antineoplastics. Be alert to symptoms of sepsis and superinfections (leukopenia) or increased tendency to bleed (thrombocytopenia).
- Platelet and leukocyte nadirs generally occur 1–2 wk after beginning therapy with streptozocin.
- Monitor for signs and symptoms of superinfection (see Appendix G).

S

- Monitor and record temperature pattern to promptly recognize impending sepsis.
- Of patients receiving this antineoplastic drug, 90% experience severe nausea and vomiting within 1–4 h after drug therapy begins. It may last up to 24 h and occasionally necessitates discontinuation of treatment.
- Repeat courses of streptozocin treatment are not given until patient's hepatic, renal, and hematologic functions are within acceptable limits.

Patient & Family Education

- Although this drug has minimal, if any, diabetogenic action, advise to report symptoms of hypoglycemia (see Appendix G).
- Encourage adeqate fluid intake (2000–3000 ml/d). Hydration may protect against drug toxicity effects.
- Instruct to report signs of nephrotoxicity (see Appendix G).
- Instruct not to use aspirin without consulting physician. Advise patient to promptly report signs of bleeding: hematuria, epistaxis, ecchymoses, petechial.
- Instruct to report symptoms that suggest anemia: shortness of breath, pale mucous membranes and nail beds, exhaustion, rapid pulse.

S

SUCCINYLCHOLINE CHLORIDE

(suk-sin-ill-koe'leen)

Trade names: Anectine, Quelicin, Sucostrin

Prototype for classifications: AUTONOMIC NERVOUS SYSTEM AGENT; DEPOLARIZING SKELETAL MUSCLE RELAXANT

Pregnancy category: C

ACTIONS/PHARMACODYNAMICS Synthetic, ultrashort-acting depolarizing neuromuscular blocking agent with high affinity for acetylcholine (ACh) receptor sites. Initial transient contractions and fasciculations are followed by sustained flaccid skeletal muscle paralysis produced by state of accommodation that develops in adjacent excitable muscle membranes. Rapidly hydrolyzed by plasma pseudocholinesterase. May increase vagal tone initially, particularly in children and with high doses, and subsequently produce mild sympathetic stimulation.

USES To produce skeletal muscle relaxation as adjunct to anesthesia; to facilitate intubation and endoscopy, to increase pulmonary compliance in assisted or controlled respiration, and to reduce intensity of muscle contractions in pharmacologically induced or electroshock convulsions.

ROUTE & DOSAGE

Surgical and Anesthetic Procedures

Adult: **IV** 0.3–1.1 mg/kg administered over 10–30 s; may give additional doses prn. **IM** 2.5–4 mg/kg up to 150 mg.
Child: **IV** 1–2 mg/kg administered over 10–30 s; may give additional doses prn. **IM** 2.5–4 mg/kg up to 150 mg.

Prolonged Muscle Relaxation

Adult: **IV** 0.5–10 mg/min by continuous infusion.

PHARMACOKINETICS **Onset:** 0.5–1 min IV; 2–3 min IM. **Duration:** 2–3 min IV; 10–30 min IM. **Distribution:** crosses placenta in small amounts. **Metabolism:** metabolized in plasma by pseudocholinesterases. **Elimination:** excreted in urine.

CONTRAINDICATIONS & PRECAUTIONS **Contraindicated in:** hypersensitivity to succinylcholine; family history of malignant hyperthermia. Safe use in pregnancy (category C) not established. **Cautious use in:** during delivery by cesarean section; renal, hepatic, pulmonary, metabolic, or cardiovascular disorders; dehydration, electrolyte imbalance, patients taking digitalis, severe burns or trauma, fractures, spinal cord injuries, degenerative or dystrophic neuromuscular diseases, low plasma pseudocholinesterase levels (recessive genetic trait, but often associated with severe liver disease, severe anemia, dehydration, marked changes in body temperature, exposure to neurotoxic insecticides, certain drugs); collagen diseases, porphyria, intraocular surgery, glaucoma.

ADVERSE/SIDE EFFECTS **CNS:** *muscle fasciculations,* profound and prolonged muscle relaxation, muscle pain. **CV:** *bradycardia,* tachycardia, hypotension, hypertension, arrhythmias, sinus arrest. **Respiratory:** respiratory depression, bronchospasm, hypoxia, apnea. **Other:** malignant hyperthermia, increased IOP, excessive salivation, enlarged salivary glands, myoglobinemia, hyperkalemia; decreased tone and motility of GI tract (large doses).

DRUG INTERACTIONS **Aminoglycosides, colistin, cyclophosphamide, cyclopropane, echothiophate iodide, halothane, lidocaine,** MAGNESIUM SALTS, **methotrimeprazine,** NARCOTIC ANALGESICS, ORGANOPHOSPHAMIDE INSECTICIDES, MAO INHIBITORS, PHENOTHIAZINES, **procaine, procainamide, quinidine, quinine, propranolol** may prolong neuromuscular blockade; DIGITALIS GLYCOSIDES may increase risk of cardiac arrhythmias.

INCOMPATIBILITIES **Solution/additive: sodium bicarbonate, thiopental.**

NURSING IMPLICATIONS

Administration

- Only freshly prepared solutions should be used; succinylcholine hydrolyzes rapidly with consequent loss of potency.
- IM injections are made deeply, preferably high into deltoid muscle.
- Initial small test dose may be given to determine individual drug sensitivity and recovery time.
- IV preparation: IV succinylcholine chloride may be diluted, 1 g in 1 L of D5W or NS, and given by intermittent or continuous infusion at a rate not to exceed 10 mg/min.
- IV administration: IV succinylcholine chloride may be given by direct IV undiluted over 10–30 s.
- Expiration date and storage before and after reconstitution vary with the manufacturer.

Assessment & Drug Effects

- Baseline serum electrolyte determinations are advised. Electrolyte imbalance (particularly potassium, calcium, magnesium) can potentiate effects of neuromuscular blocking agents.
- Transient apnea usually occurs at time of maximal drug effect (1–2 min); spontaneous respiration should return in a few seconds or, at most, 3 or 4 min.
- Facilities for emergency endotracheal intubation, artificial respiration, and assisted or controlled respiration with oxygen should be immediately available. A nerve stimulator may be used to assess

S

nature and degree of neuromuscular blockage.
- Selective muscle paralysis following drug administration develops in the following sequence: levator eyelid muscles, mastication, limbs, abdomen, glottis, intercostals, diaphragm. Recovery generally occurs in reverse order.
- Tachyphylaxis (reduced response) may occur after repeated doses.
- Adverse effects are primarily extensions of pharmacologic actions.
- Monitor vital signs and keep airway clear of secretions.

Patient & Family Education
- Patient may experience postprocedural muscle stiffness and pain (caused by initial fasciculations following injection) for as long as 24–30 h.
- Inform that hoarseness and sore throat are common even when pharyngeal airway has not been used.
- Instruct to report residual muscle weakness.

SUCRALFATE

(soo-kral′fate)

Trade names: Carafate, Sulcrate ♣

Classifications: GI AGENT; ANTIULCER

Pregnancy category: B

ACTIONS/PHARMACODYNAMICS A complex of aluminum hydroxide and sulfated sucrose structurally related to heparin but lacks its anticoagulant activity. Its action is chemically unlike any other drug used for antiulcer therapy. Following oral administration, sucralfate and gastric acid react to form a viscous, adhesive, pastelike substance that is resistant to further reaction with acid. This "paste" adheres to the GI mucosa with a major portion binding electrostatically to the positively charged protein molecules in the damaged mucosa of an ulcer crater or an acute gastric erosion caused by alcohol or other drugs. Sucralfate absorbs bile, inhibits the enzyme pepsin, and blocks back diffusion of H^+ ions. These actions plus adherence of the pastelike complex protect damaged mucosa against further destruction from ulcerogenic secretions and drugs.

USES Short-term (up to 8 wk) treatment of duodenal ulcer. **Unlabeled uses:** short-term treatment of gastric ulcer, aspirin-induced erosions, suspension for chemotherapy-induced mucositis.

ROUTE & DOSAGE

Duodenal Ulcer
Adult: **PO** 1 g q.i.d. 1 h a.c. and h.s. **Maintenance:** 1 g b.i.d.

PHARMACOKINETICS Absorption: minimally absorbed from GI tract (<5%). **Duration:** up to 6 h (depends on contact time with ulcer crater). **Elimination:** 90% excreted in feces.

CONTRAINDICATIONS & PRECAUTIONS Contraindicated in: safe use during pregnancy (category B), by nursing mothers, or by children has not been established.

ADVERSE/SIDE EFFECTS GI: nausea, gastric discomfort, *constipation,* diarrhea.

DRUG INTERACTIONS May decrease absorption of QUINOLONES (e.g., **ciprofloxacin, norfloxacin), digoxin, phenytoin, tetracycline.**

NURSING IMPLICATIONS

Administration

- If drug is to be administered through nasogastric tube, it should be solubilized in an appropriate diluent by a pharmacist.
- Antacids may be prescribed for pain relief if needed. Administer 30 min before or after sucralfate.
- Sucralfate apparently binds to certain compounds in the intestinal tract, thereby reducing their bioavailability. To prevent this action, separate administration of these agents from that of sucralfate by 2 h.
- Store in tight container at room temperature. Stable for 2 y after manufacture.

Assessment & Drug Effects

- Successful short-term course of sucralfate therapy does not seem to alter the tendency of the duodenal ulcer to heal and then to recur.

Patient & Family Education

- Although healing has occurred within the first 2 wk of therapy, treatment is usually continued 4–8 wk (in absence of healing as demonstrated by x-ray or endoscopic examination).
- If constipation is a drug-related problem, advise use of the following measures (unless contraindicated): increase water intake to 8–10 glasses per day; increase physical exercise, increase dietary bulk. Consult physician; a suppository or bulk laxative (e.g., Metamucil) may be prescribed.
- Emphasize need to adhere to sucralfate regimen: patient should not omit, increase, or decrease dosage or change administration times.
- Advise to stop smoking. Smoking is a major factor in recurrence of duodenal ulcer. Giving up smoking may be more important in prevention of recurrence of the ulcer than medication.

SUFENTANIL CITRATE

(soo-fen′ta-nil)

Trade name: Sufenta

Classifications: CNS AGENT; NARCOTIC (OPIATE) AGONIST ANALGESIC; GENERAL ANESTHETIC

Prototype: Morphine

Pregnancy category: C

Controlled substance: Schedule II

ACTIONS/PHARMACODYNAMICS

Potent synthetic opioid related to fentanyl and with similar pharmacologic actions, but about 7 times more potent. Onset of action and recovery from anesthesia occur more rapidly with sufentanil than with fentanyl. In common with other opiate agonists, sufentanil can cause respiratory depression and suppression of cough reflex.

USES Analgesic supplement in maintenance of balanced general anesthesia and also as a primary anesthetic.

ROUTE & DOSAGE

Adjunct to General Anesthesia

Adult: **IV** 1–8 μg/kg, depending on duration of surgery; may give additional doses of 10–25 μg if needed.

As Primary Anesthetic

Adult: **IV** 1–30 μg/kg administered with 100% oxygen and a muscle relaxant; may give additional doses of 10–25 μg if needed.
Child <12 y: **IV** 10–25 μg/kg administered with 100% oxygen and a muscle relaxant; may give additional doses of 25–50 μg up to 1–2 μg/kg/dose if needed.

S

PHARMACOKINETICS **Onset:** 1.5–3 min. **Duration:** 40 min. **Distribution:** crosses blood–brain barrier. **Metabolism:** metabolized in liver and small intestine. **Elimination:** half-life: 2–3 h; excreted in urine and feces.

CONTRAINDICATIONS & PRECAUTIONS **Contraindicated in:** safe use during pregnancy (category C) and in nursing women not established. **Cautious use in:** pulmonary disease, reduced respiratory reserve; impaired hepatic or renal function.

ADVERSE/SIDE EFFECTS **CV:** bradycardia, tachycardia, hypotension, hypertension, arrhythmias. **GI:** nausea, vomiting, constipation. **Respiratory:** bronchospasm, <u>*respiratory depression,*</u> <u>apnea</u>. **Other:** *skeletal muscle rigidity (especially of trunk),* chills, *itching,* spasms of sphincter of Oddi, urinary retention.

DRUG INTERACTIONS BETA-ADRENERGIC ANTAGONISTS increase incidence of bradycardia; **alcohol** and other CNS DEPRESSANTS such as BARBITURATES, TRANQUILIZERS, OPIATES and INHALATION GENERAL ANESTHETICS add to CNS depression; **cimetidine** increases risk of respiratory depression.

S

INCOMPATIBILITIES **Solution/additive: diazepam, lorazepam, phenobarbital, phenytoin, sodium bicarbonate. Y-site: lorazepam, phenytoin.**

NURSING IMPLICATIONS

Administration

- Sufentanil is administered only by qualified personnel, specifically prepared in the use of IV anesthesia and in the management of respiratory depression.
- Have available a narcotic antagonist (e.g., naloxone) to reverse respiratory depression.
- Because sufentanil is an opioid, the need for preoperative analgesia is generally reduced.
- Store at 15–30C (59–86F) unless otherwise directed. Protect from light during storage. Examine solution for particulate matter and discoloration (solution should be clear) before administration.

Assessment & Drug Effects

- Monitor vital signs. Observe for skeletal muscle rigidity, especially of chest wall, and respiratory depression, particularly in the elderly, and in patients who are obese, debilitated, or who have received high doses.
- If naloxone is given to reverse respiratory depression, bear in mind that the duration of sufentanil-induced respiratory depression may exceed the duration of naloxone.
- Sufentanil can produce morphine-like dependence and is frequently abused. Tolerance can occur with prolonged use.

SULFACETAMIDE SODIUM

(sul-fa-see'ta-mide)

Trade names: AK-Sulf, Bleph 10, Cetamide, Isopto Cetamide, Ophthacet, Sebizon, Sodium Sulamyd, Sulf-10

Classifications: ANTIINFECTIVE; SULFONAMIDE

Prototype: Sulfisoxazole

Pregnancy category: C

ACTIONS/PHARMACODYNAMICS Highly soluble sulfonamide effective against a wide range of gram-positive and gram-negative microorganisms. Exerts bacteriostatic effect by interfering with bacterial utilization of PABA, thereby inhibiting folic acid biosynthesis required for bacterial growth.

USES Ophthalmic preparations are used for conjunctivitis, corneal ulcers, and other superficial ocular infections and as adjunct to systemic sulfonamide therapy for trachoma. The topical lotion is used for scaly dermatoses, seborrheic dermatitis, seborrhea sicca, and other bacterial skin infections.

ROUTE & DOSAGE

Conjunctivitis
Adult: **Ophthalmic** 1–3 drops of 10%, 15%, or 30% solution into lower conjunctival sac q2–3h; may increase interval as patient responds; or use 1.5–2.5 cm ($\frac{1}{2}$–1 in) of 10% ointment q6h and at h.s.

CONTRAINDICATIONS & PRECAUTIONS **Contraindicated in:** hypersensitivity to sulfonamides or to any ingredients in the formulation. Pregnancy (category C). **Cautious use in:** application of lotion to denuded or debrided skin.

ADVERSE/SIDE EFFECTS *Temporary stinging or burning sensation,* retardation of corneal healing associated with long-term use of ophthalmic ointment; hypersensitivity reactions: Stevens-Johnson syndrome, lupus-like syndrome; superinfections with nonsusceptible organisms.

DRUG INTERACTIONS **Tetracaine** and other LOCAL ANESTHETICS DERIVED FROM PABA may antagonize the antibacterial effects of sulfonamides; SILVER PREPARATIONS may precipitate sulfacetamide from solution.

NURSING IMPLICATIONS

Administration

- Note strength of medication prescribed and also note that ophthalmic preparations and skin lotion are not interchangeable.
- See patient instructions for instilling eye drops.
- Store in tightly closed containers at 8–15C (46–59F) unless otherwise directed. Solutions left standing for a long time may darken. If this occurs, medication should be discarded.

Assessment & Drug Effects

- Drug should be discontinued if symptoms of hypersensitivity appear (erythema, skin rash, pruritus, urticaria).

Patient & Family Education

- Wash hands thoroughly with soap and running water (before and after instillation).
- Patient should be sitting or lying down if another person is to administer medication. If patient is to instill own medication, have patient stand in front of mirror.
- Examine eye medication; discard if cloudy or dark in color. Avoid contaminating any part of eye dropper that is inserted in bottle.
- With head tilted back, pull down lower lid. At the same time, have patient look up while drop is being instilled into conjunctival sac.
- Immediately apply gentle pressure to punctum (inner canthus next to nose) for 1 min.
- As soon as pressure is applied to punctum, patient should close eyes gently, so as not to squeeze out medication.
- Report purulent eye discharge. Sulfacetamide sodium is inactivated by purulent exudates.

S

SULFADIAZINE

(sul-fa-dye'a-zeen)
Trade name: Microsulfon
Classifications: ANTIINFECTIVE; SULFONAMIDE
Prototype: Sulfisoxazole
Pregnancy category: B

ACTIONS/PHARMACODYNAMICS Short-acting sulfonamide, slightly less soluble than sulfisoxazole. Shares actions, uses, contraindications, precautions, and adverse reactions of other sulfonamides.

USES Used in combination with pyrimethamine for treatment of cerebral toxoplasmosis and chloroquine-resistant malaria.

ROUTE & DOSAGE

Mild to Moderate Infections
Adult: **PO** 2–4 g loading dose; then 2–4 g/d in 4–6 divided doses.
Child >2 mo: **PO** 75 mg/kg loading dose; then 150 mg/kg/d in 4–6 divided doses (max 6 g/d).

Rheumatic Fever Prophylaxis
Adult: **PO** *>30 kg,* 1 g/d; *<30 kg,* 500 mg/d.

Toxoplasmosis
Adult: **PO** 2–8 g/d divided q6h.
Child >2 mo: **PO** 100–200 mg/kg/d divided q6h.
Neonate: **PO** 50 mg/kg q12h × 12 mo.

PHARMACOKINETICS Absorption: readily absorbed from GI tract. **Peak:** 3–6 h. **Distribution:** distributed to most tissues, including CSF; crosses placenta. **Metabolism:** metabolized in liver. **Elimination:** excreted in urine.

ADVERSE/SIDE EFFECTS See sulfisoxazole.

NURSING IMPLICATIONS

Administration
- Fluid intake must be sufficient to support urinary output of at least 1500 ml/d. If this cannot be accomplished, urinary alkalinizer such as sodium bicarbonate may be prescribed to reduce risk of crystalluria and stone formation.
- Preserve in tight, light-resistant containers.

Patient & Family Education
- Urge to take drug exactly as prescribed. Patient should not alter the schedule or dose and should take all that is prescribed unless physician changes the regimen.
- Early signs of blood dyscrasias (sore throat, pallor, fever) should be reported promptly to the physician.

SULFAMETHOXAZOLE

(sul-fa-meth-ox'a-zole)
Trade name: Gantanol
Classifications: ANTIINFECTIVE; SULFONAMIDE
Prototype: Sulfisoxazole
Pregnancy category: B

ACTIONS/PHARMACODYNAMICS Intermediate-acting sulfonamide closely related chemically to sulfisoxazole and similar to it in actions, uses, contraindications, precautions, and adverse reactions. Intestinal absorption and urinary excretion are somewhat slower than those of sulfisoxazole, and thus it is given less frequently to avoid excessive blood levels.

USES Acute, recurrent, or chronic urinary tract infections, lymphogran-

S

uloma venereum, and other infections caused by susceptible organisms.

ROUTE & DOSAGE

Mild to Moderate Infections

Adult: **PO** 2 g loading dose; then 1 g q8–12h.
Child >2 *mo:* **PO** 50–60 mg/kg loading dose; then 25–30 mg/kg q12h (max 75 mg/kg/d).

PHARMACOKINETICS Absorption: incompletely absorbed from GI tract. **Peak:** 3–4 h. **Distribution:** distributed to most tissues, including CSF; crosses placenta. **Metabolism:** metabolized in liver. **Elimination:** half-life: 7–12 h; excreted in urine.

ADVERSE/SIDE EFFECTS See sulfisoxazole.

NURSING IMPLICATIONS

Administration

- Tablet may be crushed before administration and taken with fluid of patient's choice.
- Fluid intake must be sufficient to produce urinary output of at least 1500 ml/24 h (between 3000 and 4000 ml/24 h for adults). Concomitant administration of urinary alkalinizer may be prescribed to reduce possibility of crystalluria and stone formation.
- Preserve in tight, light-resistant containers at 15–30C (59–86F). Do not freeze.

Patient & Family Education

- Urge to take drug exactly as prescribed. Patient should not alter the schedule or dose and should take all that is prescribed unless physician changes the regimen.
- Early signs of blood dyscrasias (sore throat, pallor, fever) should be reported promptly to the physician.

SULFASALAZINE

(sul-fa-sal'a-zeen)

Trade names: Azulfidine, PMS Sulfasalazine ♣, PMS Sulfasalazine E.C. ♣, Salazopyrin ♣, SAS-Enema ♣, SAS Enteric-500 ♣, S.A.S.-500 ♣

Classifications: ANTIINFECTIVE; SULFONAMIDE

Prototype: Sulfisoxazole

Pregnancy category: B (D if near term)

ACTIONS/PHARMACODYNAMICS Locally acting sulfonamide. Believed to be converted by intestinal microflora to sulfapyridine (which has antibacterial action) and 5-aminosalicylic acid or mesalamine which may exert antiinflammatory effect. Other proposed mechanisms of action include inhibition of prostaglandins known to cause diarrhea and affect mucosal transport, interference with absorption of fluids and electrolytes from colon, and reduction in *Clostridium* and *Escherichia coli* in the stools. Contraindications, precautions, and adverse/side effects are as for other sulfonamides.

USES Ulcerative colitis and relatively mild regional enteritis; rheumatoid arthritis. **Unlabeled uses:** granulomatous colitis, Crohn's disease, scleroderma.

ROUTE & DOSAGE

Ulcerative Colitis, Rheumatoid Arthritis

Adult: **PO** 1–2 g/d in 4 divided doses; may increase up to 8 g/d if needed.
Child: **PO** 40–50 mg/kg/d in 4 divided doses (max 75 mg/kg/d).

Juvenile Rheumatoid Arthritis

Child: **PO** 10 mg/kg/d; increase weekly by 10 mg/kg/d; usual

S

dose: 15–25 mg/kg q12h (max 2 g/d).

PHARMACOKINETICS **Absorption:** 10–15% absorbed from GI tract unchanged; remaining drug is hydrolyzed in colon to sulfapyridine (most of which is absorbed) and 5-aminosalicylic acid (30% of which is absorbed). **Peak:** 1.5–6 h sulfasalazine; 6–24 h sulfapyridine. **Distribution:** crosses placenta; distributed into breast milk. **Metabolism:** metabolized in intestines and liver. **Elimination:** half-life: 5–10 h; all metabolites are excreted in urine.

CONTRAINDICATIONS & PRECAUTIONS **Contraindicated in:** sensitivity to sulfasalazine and other sulfonamides; agranulocytosis; children <2 y; intestinal and urinary tract obstruction; pregnancy (category B, category D near term).

ADVERSE/SIDE EFFECTS *Nausea, vomiting, bloody diarrhea; anorexia,* arthralgia, rash, anemia, oligospermia (reversible), blood dyscrasias, hepatic injury, infectious mononucleosis–like reaction, *allergic reactions.*

DRUG INTERACTIONS **Iron,** ANTIBIOTICS may alter absorption of sulfasalazine.

S

NURSING IMPLICATIONS

Administration

- If possible, drug should be taken after eating to provide longer intestine transit time for the drug.
- Sulfasalazine should be given in evenly divided doses over each 24-h period. Intervals between nighttime doses should not exceed 8 h.
- If GI intolerance occurs after first few doses, symptoms are probably due to irritation of stomach mucosa. Symptoms may be relieved by spacing total daily dose more evenly over the day or by administration of enteric-coated tablets. Consult physician.
- Preserve in tight, light-resistant containers; store at 15–30C (59–86F).

Assessment & Drug Effects

- GI symptoms that develop after a few days of therapy may indicate need for dosage adjustment. If symptoms persist, physician may withhold drug for 5–7 d and restart it at a lower dosage level.
- Desensitization of patient who has an allergic reaction to sulfasalazine can be accomplished safely to permit continued use of the drug. Usually, the process is started with one-eighth tablet daily; dose is doubled q3–7d.
- Adverse reactions generally occur within a few days to 12 wk after start of therapy and are most likely to occur in patients receiving high doses (4 g or more).
- High doses (more than 2 g/d) reduce tissue folate stores as shown by measurement of RBC folate. A daily supplement may be prescribed.

Patient & Family Education

- Some patients pass enteric-coated tablets intact in feces, possibly because they lack enzymes capable of dissolving them. Advise patient to examine stools and report to physician if tablet is intact. Conventional tablet will be ordered.
- Forewarn patient that drug may color alkaline urine and skin orange-yellow.
- Advise patient to remain under close medical supervision. Relapses occur in about 40% of patients after initial satisfactory response. Response to therapy and duration of treatment are governed by endoscopic examinations.

SULFINPYRAZONE

(sul-fin-peer'a-zone)

Trade names: Antazone ♣, Anturan ♣, Anturane, Apo-Sulfinpyrazone ♣, Novopyrazone ♣

Classifications: ANTIGOUT AGENT; URICOSURIC

Prototype: Colchicine

Pregnancy category: C

ACTIONS/PHARMACODYNAMICS

Potent renal tubular blocking agent. At therapeutic doses, promotes urinary excretion of uric acid and reduces serum urate levels by competitively inhibiting tubular reabsorption of uric acid. Like all uricosurics, low doses may inhibit tubular secretion of uric acid and cause urate retention. Inhibits release of adenosine diphosphate and 5-hydroxytryptophan, and thus decreases platelet adhesiveness and increases platelet survival time; has no effect on prothrombin or blood clotting time.

USES Maintenance therapy in chronic gouty arthritis and tophaceous gout. **Unlabeled uses:** drug-induced hyperuricemia, to decrease platelet aggregation and increase their survival in prevention of TIAs and stroke.

ROUTE & DOSAGE

Gout

Adult: **PO** 100–200 mg b.i.d. for 1 wk; then increase to 200–400 mg b.i.d.; may reduce to 200 mg/d after serum urate levels are controlled (max 800 mg/d).

Inhibition of Platelet Aggregation

Adult: **PO** 200 mg t.i.d. or q.i.d.

PHARMACOKINETICS **Absorption:** readily absorbed from GI tract. **Peak:** 1–2 h. **Duration:** 4–6 h; may persist up to 10 h. **Metabolism:** metabolized in liver to active and inactive metabolites. **Elimination:** half-life: 3 h; slowly excreted in urine; 5% excreted in feces.

CONTRAINDICATIONS & PRECAUTIONS **Contraindicated in:** known hypersensitivity to pyrazoline derivatives; active peptic ulcer; concurrent administration of salicylates; patients with creatinine clearance less than 50 mg/min, treatment of hyperuricemia secondary to neoplastic disease or cancer chemotherapy. **Cautious use in:** impaired renal function; pregnancy (category C); history of healed peptic ulcer, use in conjunction with sulfonamides and sulfonylureas.

ADVERSE/SIDE EFFECTS **GI:** *nausea,* vomiting, diarrhea, *epigastric pain, blood loss, reactivation or aggravation of peptic ulcer,* ataxia, dizziness, vertigo, tinnitus; edema, labored respirations, convulsions, coma, hypersensitivity, reactions (skin rashes, fever), jaundice, precipitation of acute gout, urolithiasis, renal colic.

DRUG INTERACTIONS May decrease efficacy of **nitrofurantoin** for UTI and increase its systemic toxicity. May displace SULFONYLUREAS from protein binding and increase risk of hypoglycemia; may augment prothrombin time increased by **warfarin; cholestyramine** decreases absorption of sulfinpyrazone; **aspirin** may inhibit uricosuric effects of sulfinpyrazone.

DIAGNOSTIC TEST INTERFERENCE Sulfinpyrazone decreases urinary excretion of ***aminohippuric acid*** and ***phenolsulfonphthalein.***

NURSING IMPLICATIONS

Administration

- Administer with meals, milk, or antacid (prescribed) to prevent local drug irritant effect. Severity and frequency of symptoms increase with dosage. Persistence of GI symptoms may require discontinuation of drug.
- During early therapy, fluid intake should be sufficient to support urinary output of at least 2000–3000 ml/d (consult physician), and urine should be alkalinized (e.g., with large doses vitamin C) to increase solubility of uric acid and minimize risk of uric acid stones.

Assessment & Drug Effects

- Serum urate levels are used to monitor therapy. Aim of therapy is to lower serum urate levels to about 6 mg/dl and thus to reduce joint changes, tophi formation, and frequency of acute attacks and to improve renal function.
- Periodic blood cell counts are advised during prolonged therapy. Patients with impaired renal function should have periodic assessments of renal function.
- Sulfinpyrazone may increase the frequency of acute gouty attacks during first 6–12 mo of therapy, even when serum urate levels appear to be controlled. Physician may prescribe prophylactic doses of colchicine concurrently during first 3–6 mo of treatment to prevent or at least lessen severity of attacks.

Patient & Family Education

- Patient must remain under close medical supervision while taking sulfinpyrazone. Therapy is continued indefinitely.
- Caution to avoid experimentation with dosage, since subtherapeutic doses may enhance urate retention, and large doses may increase risk of toxicity.
- Sulfinpyrazone therapy should be continued without interruption even when patient has an acute gouty attack, which may be treated with full therapeutic doses of colchicine or other antiinflammatory agent.
- Caution to avoid aspirin-containing medications. If an analgesic is required (in patients with normal renal function), generally acetaminophen is recommended.

SULFISOXAZOLE

(sul-fi-sox′a-zole)

Trade name: Gantrisin

Prototype for classifications: ANTIINFECTIVE; SULFONAMIDE

Pregnancy category: B (D if near term)

ACTIONS/PHARMACODYNAMICS Short-acting derivative of sulfanilamide. In common with other sulfonamides, has broad antimicrobial spectrum against both gram-positive and gram-negative organisms. Bacteriostatic action believed to be by competitive inhibition of *p*-aminobenzoic acid (PABA), thereby interfering with folic acid biosynthesis required for bacterial growth.

USES Acute, recurrent, and chronic urinary tract infections and chancroid; adjunctive therapy in trachoma, chloroquine-resistant strains of malaria, acute otitis media due to *Hemophilus influenzae,* and meningococcal and *H. influenzae* meningitis. Ophthalmic preparations used in treatment of conjunctivitis, corneal ulcer, and other superficial eye infections and as adjunct to systemic sulfonamide therapy for trachoma. Topical vaginal preparation used for *H. vaginalis* vaginitis.

ROUTE & DOSAGE

Infection by Susceptible Organisms

Adult: **PO** 2–4 g initially, followed by 4–8 g/d in 4–6 divided doses. **Vaginal** 1 applicator full 1–2 times/d.
Child >2 mo: **PO** 75 mg/kg initially, followed by 150 mg/kg/d in 4–6 divided doses (max 6 g/d).

PHARMACOKINETICS Absorption: readily absorbed from GI tract. **Peak:** 2–4 h. **Distribution:** distributed in extracellular space; crosses blood–brain barrier and placenta; detected in breast milk. **Metabolism:** metabolized in liver. **Elimination:** half-life: 4.6–7.8 h; 95% excreted in urine in 24 h.

CONTRAINDICATIONS & PRECAUTIONS Contraindicated in: history of hypersensitivity to sulfonamides, salicylates, or chemically related drugs; use in treatment of group A beta-hemolytic streptococcal infections; infants <2 mo of age (except in treatment of congenital toxoplasmosis); pregnancy (category B, category D if near term); nursing mothers; porphyria; advanced renal or hepatic disease; intestinal and urinary obstruction. **Cautious use in:** impaired renal or liver function; severe allergy; bronchial asthma; blood dyscrasias; patients with G6PD deficiency.

ADVERSE/SIDE EFFECTS Low toxicity level but may include the following: **CNS:** headache, peripheral neuritis, peripheral neuropathy, tinnitus, hearing loss, vertigo, insomnia, drowsiness, mental depression, acute psychosis, ataxia, convulsions, kernicterus (newborns). **GI:** *nausea, vomiting, diarrhea,* abdominal pains, hepatitis, jaundice, pancreatitis, stomatitis. **Hematologic:** acute hemolytic anemia (especially in patients with G6PD deficiency), <u>aplastic anemia</u>, methemoglobinemia, <u>agranulocytosis</u>, thrombocytopenia, leukopenia, eosinophilia, hypoprothrombinemia. **Hypersensitivity:** headache, *fever,* chills, arthralgia, malaise, pruritus, urticaria, conjunctival or scleral infection, rash, erythema multiforme including *Stevens-Johnson syndrome, exfoliative dermatitis,* allergic myocarditis, serum sickness, <u>anaphylactoid reactions</u>, photosensitivity, vascular lesions. **Renal:** *crystalluria,* hematuria, proteinuria, anuria, toxic nephrosis. **Other:** conjunctivitis, goiter, hypoglycemia, diuresis, overgrowth of nonsusceptible organisms, LE phenomenon, retardation of corneal healing (ophthalmic ointment), alopecia, reduction in sperm count, lymphadenopathy, local reaction following IM injection, fixed drug eruptions.

DIAGNOSTIC TEST INTERFERENCE Sulfonamides may interfere with ***BSP*** retention and ***PSP*** excretion tests and may affect results of ***thyroid function*** tests (***I-131*** may be decreased for about 7 d). Large doses of sulfonamides reportedly may produce false-positive ***urine glucose*** determinations with copper reduction methods (e.g., Benedict's and Clinitest). Sulfonamides may produce false-positive results for ***urinary protein*** (with sulfosalicylic acid test) and may interfere with ***urine urobilinogen*** determinations using Ehrlich's reagent or Urobilistix. Follow-up cultures are unreliable unless PABA is added to culture medium.

DRUG INTERACTIONS PABA-CONTAINING LOCAL ANESTHETICS may antagonize sulfa's effects; ORAL ANTI-

COAGULANTS potentiate hypoprothrombinemia; may potentiate SULFONYLUREA-induced hypoglycemia.

NURSING IMPLICATIONS

Administration

- Tablet may be crushed before administration and taken with full glass of water or other fluid.
- Administration with food appears to delay but reportedly does not reduce amount of drug absorbed.
- Preserve in tight, light-resistant containers. Store at 15–30C (59–86F).

Assessment & Drug Effects

- Monitor I&O. Report oliguria and changes in I&O ratio. Fluid intake should be adequate to support urinary output of at least 1500 ml/d to prevent crystalluria and stone formation.
- Since a fall in urinary pH (more acidic) increases risk of crystalluria, daily check of urine pH with Nitrazine paper or Labstix is advisable.
- Report increasing urine acidity. If urine is highly acidic, physician may prescribe a urinary alkalinizer.
- Monitor temperature. Sudden appearance of fever may signify sensitization (serum sickness) or hemolytic anemia (frequent in patients with G6PD deficiency, which is most common among black males and Mediterranean ethnic groups). These reactions generally develop within 10 d after start of drug. Agranulocytosis may develop after 10 d–6 wk of therapy.
- Fever with sore throat, malaise, unusual fatigue, joint pains, pallor, bleeding tendencies, rash, and jaundice are early manifestations of blood dyscrasias or hypersensitivity reactions. Report them immediately.
- Skin lesions, papular or vesiculobullous lesions, especially on sun-exposed areas, Stevens-Johnson syndrome (severe erythema multiforme) may be preceded by high fever, severe headache, stomatitis, conjunctivitis, rhinitis, urticaria, balanitis (inflammation of penis or clitoris). Termination of drug therapy is indicated.
- Frequent kidney function tests and urinalyses are recommended; complete blood tests and hepatic function tests are advised, especially in patients receiving sulfonamides for longer than 2 wk.
- Diabetic patients receiving oral hypoglycemic agents should be closely observed for hypoglycemic reactions. Determinations of blood glucose levels are advised before and shortly after initiation of sulfonamide therapy.

Patient & Family Education

- Ensure patient understands that established dosage regimen must be followed: patient should not omit, increase, interrupt, or decrease dose. Full course of treatment should be completed.
- Caution not to take OTC medications without consulting physician. Many analgesic mixtures contain aspirin in combination with *p*-aminobenzoic acid. Inform patients that excessive doses of vitamin C acidify urine and therefore should be avoided (to prevent crystalluria).
- Advise patients using topical applications to stop treatment if local irritation or sensitivity reaction develops and to report to physician. Patient should be informed that sensitization to topical application precludes future systemic use of sulfonamides.
- Oral contraceptives may be unreliable while patient is receiving a

S

sulfonamide. Advise an alternate method of contraception. Breakthrough bleeding should be considered evidence of an interaction.

- Advise to avoid exposure to ultraviolet light and excessive sunlight to prevent photosensitivity reaction during therapy and for several months after treatment is discontinued.
- Advise to inform dentist or new physician of taking a sulfonamide.

SULINDAC

(sul-in′dak)

Trade name: Clinoril

Classifications: CNS AGENT; ANALGESIC; ANTIPYRETIC; NSAID

Prototype: Ibuprofen

Pregnancy category: B (D in third trimester)

ACTIONS/PHARMACODYNAMICS Acetic acid derivative structurally and pharmacologically related to indomethacin. Pharmacologic properties are similar to those of aspirin but is chemically unrelated. In common with these drugs, exhibits antiinflammatory, analgesic, and antipyretic properties. Exact mechanism of antiinflammatory action not known but is thought to result from inhibition of prostaglandin synthesis. Comparable to aspirin in antiinflammatory activity but has longer half-life, lower incidence of GI intolerance and tinnitus, and less effect on bleeding time and platelet function. May prolong bleeding time, but prothrombin time, whole blood clotting time, and platelet count are not affected. Serum uric acid lowering effect is less than that of aspirin.

USES Acute and long-term symptomatic treatment of osteoarthritis, rheumatoid arthritis, ankylosing spondylitis; acute painful shoulder (acute subacromial bursitis or supraspinatus tendinitis); acute gouty arthritis.

ROUTE & DOSAGE

Arthritis, Ankylosing Spondylitis, Acute Gouty Arthritis

Adult: **PO** 150–200 mg b.i.d. (max 400 mg/d).

PHARMACOKINETICS **Absorption:** 90% absorbed from GI tract. **Peak:** 2 h without food, 3–4 h with food. **Duration:** 10–12 h. **Distribution:** minimal passage across placenta; distributed into breast milk. **Metabolism:** metabolized in liver to active sulfide metabolite. **Elimination:** half-life: 7.8 h sulindac, 16.4 h sulfide metabolite; 75% excreated in urine, 25% in feces.

CONTRAINDICATIONS & PRECAUTIONS **Contraindicated in:** hypersensitivity to sulindac; hypersensitivity to aspirin (patients with "aspirin triad": acute asthma, rhinitis, nasal polyps) or to other NSAIDs; significant renal or hepatic dysfunction. Safe use during pregnancy (category B; category D in third trimester); in nursing mothers, and in children not established. **Cautious use in:** history of upper GI tract disorders, compromised cardiac function, hypertension, hemophilia or other bleeding tendencies.

ADVERSE/SIDE EFFECTS **CNS:** drowsiness, *dizziness, headache,* anxiety, nervousness. **CV:** palpitation, peripheral edema, CHF, (patients with marginal cardiac function). **ENT:** blurred vision, amblyopia, vertigo, tinnitus, decreased hearing. **GI:** *abdominal pain, dyspepsia, nausea, vomiting, constipation,* diarrhea, ulceration, flatulence, anorexia; sto-

S

matitis, sore or dry mucous membranes, dry mouth; GI bleeding, gastritis. **Hematologic:** prolonged bleeding time, aplastic anemia, thrombocytopenia. **Hypersensitivity:** angioneurotic edema, rash, pruritus, fever, chills, leukopenia, eosinophilia, anaphylaxis. **Other:** Stevens-Johnson syndrome, toxic epidermal necrolysis syndrome, rash, renal impairment.

DIAGNOSTIC TEST INTERFERENCE Abnormalities in ***liver function tests*** may occur.

DRUG INTERACTIONS **Heparin,** ORAL ANTICOAGULANTS may prolong bleeding time; may increase **lithium** toxicity; **aspirin**, other NSAIDS add to ulcerogenic effects; may increase **methotrexate** toxicity; **dimethylsulfoxide (DMSO)** may decrease effects of sulindac.

NURSING IMPLICATIONS

Administration

- If patient cannot swallow tablet, it may be crushed prior to administration.
- Sulindac may be administered with food, milk, or antacid (if prescribed) to reduce possibility of GI upset. However, food retards absorption and delays and lowers peak concentrations.

S

Assessment & Drug Effects

- A detailed drug history should be elicited before initiation of therapy. See Contraindications & Precautions.
- Baseline and periodic evaluations of hemoglobin, renal and hepatic function, and auditory and ophthalmic examinations are recommended in patients receiving prolonged or high-dose therapy.
- Recommend an ophthalmoscopic examination if patient has eye complaints.

Patient & Family Education

- Because sulindac may cause dizziness, drowsiness, and blurred vision, advise patient to exercise caution when he or she is driving or performing other potentially hazardous activities.
- Advise to report the onset of skin rash, itching, hives, jaundice, black stools, swelling of feet or hands, sore throat or mouth, unusual bleeding or bruising, shortness of breath, or night cough.
- Inform that adverse GI effects are relatively common. Instruct him or her to report abdominal pain, nausea, dyspepsia, diarrhea, or constipation.
- Therapeutic effectiveness of sulindac may not be evidenced for up to 7 d; peak effect is usually experienced in 2–3 wk (relief of joint pain and stiffness, reduction in joint swelling, increase in grip strength, and improved mobility).
- Inform that alcohol and aspirin may increase risk of GI ulceration and bleeding tendencies and, therefore, should be avoided while taking sulindac.
- Because sulindac may prolong bleeding time, advise to inform dentist or surgeon that patient is taking this drug.

SUMATRIPTAN

(sum-a-trip′-tan)

Trade name: Imitrex

Prototype for classifications: AUTONOMIC NERVOUS SYSTEM AGENT; SEROTONIN 5-HT_1-RECEPTOR AGONIST; ALPHA-ADRENERGIC ANTAGONIST (SYMPATHOLYTIC); ERGOT ALKALOID

Pregnancy category: C

ACTIONS/PHARMACODYNAMICS Selective agonist for a serotonin receptor (probably 5-HT_{1D}). Causes vasoconstriction of cranial carotid arteries, thus relieving the migraine headache. This does not result in decreased arterial blood pressure or total peripheral resistance. Also relieves photophobia, phonophobia, nausea and vomiting associated with migraine attacks.

USES Treatment of acute migraine attacks with or without aura, cluster headache.

ROUTE & DOSAGE

Migraine or Cluster Headache

Adult: **SC** 6 mg SC any time after onset of migraine. If no relief, may repeat with 6 mg SC at least 1 h after first injection (max 12 mg/24 h). **PO** 25 mg × 1 dose (max 100 mg). **Intranasal** 5, 10, or 20 mg in one nostril. If no relief, may repeat once after 2 h (max 40 mg/24 h).

PHARMACOKINETICS **Onset:** 10–30 min after SC administration. **Duration:** 1–2 h. **Distribution:** widely distributed, 10–20% protein bound. May be excreted in breast milk. **Metabolism:** hepatically metabolized to inactive metabolite. **Elimination:** half-life: 2 h; 57% excreted in urine, 38% excreted in feces.

CONTRAINDICATIONS & PRECAUTIONS **Contraindicated in:** hypersensitivity to sumatriptan; IV use; coronary artery disease (CAD); risk factors for CAD such as hypertension, hypercholesterolemia, obesity, diabetes, smoking, and strong family history; concurrent use with ergotamine drugs; concurrent use of sumatriptan PO with MAO inhibitors; basilar or hemiplegic migraine. **Cautious use in:** impaired hepatic or renal function; concurrent use of sumatriptan SC and MAO inhibitors; pregnancy (category C); nursing mothers. Safety and effectiveness in children have not been established.

ADVERSE/SIDE EFFECTS **CV:** mild increases in systolic and diastolic blood pressure may occur after IV doses of 8 μg/kg or more, chest pressure and tightness. **CNS:** *tingling, warming sensation, pressure, numbness,* headache, *dizziness, vertigo,* drowsiness, sedation, seizure. **Other:** *pain on injection,* weakness.

DRUG INTERACTIONS **Dihydroergotamine** may cause a slight elevation in blood pressure. MAO INHIBITORS increase sumatriptan levels and toxicity (especially the oral form); do not use concurrently or within 2 wk of stopping MAO inhibitors.

NURSING IMPLICATIONS

Administration

- Administer anytime after symptoms of migraine appear.
- A second tablet may be given if symptoms return but no sooner than 2 h after the first tablet.
- Do not exceed 100 mg in a single PO dose or 300 mg/d PO.
- A second injection may be given 1 h or longer following first injection if initial relief is not obtained or if migraine returns.
- If side effects are dose limiting, a lower dose may be effective.
- Autoinjection device is available for use with 6 mg prefilled syringes.
- Do not give within 24 h of an ergot-containing drug.
- Store at room temperature, 2–30C (36–86F). Protect from light.

Assessment & Drug Effects

- Carefully monitor cardiovascular status following first dose in pa-

S

tients at relatively high risk for coronary artery disease (e.g., postmenopausal women, men over 40 years old, persons with known CAD risk factors) or who have coronary artery vasospasms.

- Immediately report to the physician chest pain or tightness in chest or throat that is severe or does not quickly resolve following a dose of sumatriptan.
- Pain relief usually begins within 10 min of injection, with complete relief in approximately 65% of all patients with 2 h.

Patient & Family Education

- Carefully review patient information leaflet with patient.
- Instruct in correct use of autoinjector if patient is to self-administer sumatriptan.
- Advise to immediately notify physician of symptoms of severe angina (e.g., severe and/or persistent pain or tightness in chest or throat) or hypersensitivity (e.g., wheezing, facial swelling, skin rash, or hives) occur.
- Advise to report any other adverse effects (e.g., tingling, flushing, dizziness) at next physician visit.
- Inform that pain or redness at injection site is common but usually disappears in less than 1 h.

SUTILAINS

(soo′ti-lains)

Trade name: Travase

Classification: ENZYME DEBRIDING AGENT

Pregnancy category: C

ACTIONS/PHARMACODYNAMICS Concentrate of proteolytic enzymes produced by *Bacillus subtilis*. As a result of enzymatic activity, sutilains selectively digests necrotic soft tissue, hemoglogin, and purulent exudate. Moisture and a pH of 6–6.8 must be present to support proteolytic activity. Action is unaffected by presence in site of topical bacitracin, gentamicin, mafenide, neomycin, penicillin, silver sulfadiazine, or streptomycin, nor is it affected by appropriate systemic antiinfectives.

USES Biochemical debridement of decubitus ulcers, second and third degree burns, pyogenic incisional or traumatic wounds, ulcers secondary to peripheral vascular disease; also used adjunctively with other measures to debride necrotic tissue (e.g., mechanical debridement).

ROUTE & DOSAGE

Ulcer and Burn Debridement
Adult: **Topical** Apply t.i.d. or q.i.d.

PHARMACOKINETICS Onset: 1 h. **Peak:** 6 h. **Duration:** 8–12 h.

CONTRAINDICATIONS & PRECAUTIONS Contraindicated in: Wounds communicating with major body cavities; wound containing exposed major nerves or nervous tissue; fungating neoplastic ulcers; bleeding; dermatitis; compromised cardiac or pulmonary reserves. Safe use in wounds during pregnancy (category C) or in woman who may become pregnant not established.

ADVERSE/SIDE EFFECTS Pain, paresthesia, bleeding, transient dermatitis.

DRUG INTERACTIONS Benzalkonium chloride, hexachlorophene, nitrofurazone, hydrogen peroxide, IODINE COMPOUNDS, **silver nitrate, thimerosal** will inactivate sutilains.

NURSING IMPLICATIONS

Administration

Treatment Protocol

- Wear gloves. Thoroughly cleanse and irrigate wound area with sterile water or 0.9% saline solution. Gently wipe away dissolved material. Be sure all medication has been removed. Thoroughly moisten wound area.
- Change gloves and apply ointment in very thin layer (a small dab will cover an area as large as back of hand). Cover every crevice and crack in wound and extend ointment 0.5–1 cm (1/4–1/2 in.) beyond areas being debrided. Cover area with loose, wet dressings (not occlusive) to maintain constant moisture.
- Repeat entire protocol 3 or 4 times a day or as ordered.
- If hydrogen peroxide is used to cleanse the wound, it should be used before application of sutilains (not concomitantly).
- If used in treatment of burns, it is most effective before eschar becomes hard and dry.
- Drug-induced eschar digestion leads to increased fluid and blood loss in treated area; therefore, no more than 10–15% of a burned area is treated with sutilains at one time.
- Proteolytic action produces a warm, moist, and nutritious environment for bacteria. Topical anti-infectives may be used concomitantly to prevent sepsis.
- If ointment gets into the patient's eyes, irrigate promptly and copiously with normal saline or with sterile water.
- Store at 2–8C (35–46F).

Assessment & Drug Effects

- Maximum effect is usually achieved in 5–7 d for burns and wounds and in 8–12 d for ulcers.
- Inspect wound for bleeding. If it occurs or if pain persists during interval between treatments, sutilains therapy will be discontinued.

TACRINE

(tac′rine)

Trade name: Cognex

Classifications: AUTONOMIC NERVOUS SYSTEM AGENT; CHOLINERGIC (PARASYMPATHOMIMETIC); CHOLINESTERASE INHIBITOR

Prototype: Neostigmine

Pregnancy category: C

ACTIONS/PHARMACODYNAMICS

In early stages of Alzheimer's disease, pathologic changes in neurons result in deficiency of acetylcholine. Tacrine, a cholinesterase inhibitor, presumably elevates acetylcholine concentration in the cerebral cortex by slowing degradation of acetylcholine release by remaining intact neurons.

USE Improvement of memory in mild to moderate Alzheimer's dementia. **Unlabeled uses:** HIV infection (severe dementia), tardive dyskinesia, acute anticholinergic syndrome with possible advantage over physostigmine.

ROUTE & DOSAGE

Adult: **PO** 10 mg q.i.d. (taken between meals if tolerated). Increase in 40 mg/d increments not sooner than q6wk to a max of 160 mg/d. Dose-related hepatotoxic effects have been observed; use with caution or not at all in patients with history of past or current liver disease.

PHARMACOKINETICS **Absorption:** approximately 17% absorbed from

GI tract. Food decreases rate and extent of absorption by 30–40%. **Onset:** 30–90 min.**Peak:** 2 h. Steady state in 24–36 h. **Distribution:** penetrates blood–brain barrier. Protein binding is 55%. **Metabolism:** metabolized in the liver by cytochrome P-450 system. At least three hydroxylated metabolites have been identified that may be biologically active. Females have lower activity in cytochrome P-450 isoenzymes so plasma levels are approximately 50% higher than men with same dose. **Elimination:** half-life: 3.5 h; less than 3% of dose recovered in urine in 24 h.

CONTRAINDICATIONS & PRECAUTIONS **Contraindicated in:** hypersensitivity to tacrine or patients who develop jaundice while taking tacrine. **Cautious use in:** anesthesia, sick sinus rhythm, bradycardia; history of ulcers, GI bleeding, abnormal liver function; patients with astham, hypotension, hyperthyroidism, urinary tract obstruction, intestinal obstruction; pregnancy (category C), nursing mothers. Safety and efficacy in children have not been established.

ADVERSE/SIDE EFFECTS **CNS:** agitation, dizziness and confusion, ataxia, insomnia, somnolence, hallucinations. **GI:** Nausea, *vomiting,* belching, *diarrhea,* abdominal discomfort, anorexia. **Other:** *hepatotoxicity,* purpura, excessive micturition and incontinence with UTI infections, diaphoresis.

DRUG INTERACTIONS Prolongs action of **succinylcholine** and possibly other NEUROMUSCULAR BLOCKING AGENTS due to inhibition of plasma pseudocholinesterase. Increases **theophylline** concentrations twofold. **Cimetidine** increases concentration of tacrine by 64%.

NURSING IMPLICATIONS

Administration

- If possible, administer at least 1 h before meals, because bioavailability of tracine is reduced by 30–40% when taken with food.
- Rate of recommended dose escalation may be slowed if patient is intolerant of recommended titration schedule.
- Doses may be titrated upward as long as serum transaminase (ALT) levels remain less than or equal to 3 times upper limit of normal (ULN).
- Reduce daily dose by 40 mg/d when ALT exceeds 3 times but is less than or equal to 5 times ULN. Resume titration when ALT returns to normal.
- If ALT exceeds 5 times ULN, stop treatment with tracine.
- Rechallenge with tacrine may be possible when ALT returns to normal (see manufacturer's guidelines).
- Store at room temperature, 15–30C (59–86F), away from moisture.

Assessment & Drug Effects

- Monitor for clinical improvement (defined as a 4-point improvement in Alzheimer's Disease Assessment Scale/Cognitive Subscale). Improvement has been observed after 1–4 wk; however, it may take up to 6 mo to assess maximum benefit.
- Monitor serum transaminase (ALT) levels according to following schedule: every 2 wk for first 16 wk, then monthly for 2 mo, then every 3 mo thereafter; resume weekly monitoring for 6 wk with each dose increase; continue weekly monitoring if ALT remains more than 2 times normal; if therapy is interrupted more than 4 wk then restarted, resume full ALT monitoring schedule.
- Monitor I&O because tacrine may cause bladder outflow obstruction.

- Monitor for seizure activity and take appropriate precautions.
- Patients with history of angle-closure glaucoma should be monitored for a worsening of this condition.
- Monitor for GI distress and bleeding, especially in patients with a history of peptic ulcer disease or on concurrent NSAID therapy.
- Monitor ambulation because dizziness occurs in more than 10% of patients.
- Monitor cardiovascular status including periodic ECG monitoring. Assess for fluid retention and worsening of CHF.
- Monitor periodically for development of drug-induced diabetes.

Patient & Family Education

- Inform patient/caregiver that effectiveness of tacrine therapy depends on its administration at regular intervals; therefore, stress taking tacrine as directed.
- Instruct patient/caregiver about adverse effects related to initiation of therapy or dosage increases (e.g., nausea, vomiting, diarrhea) as well as delayed effects (e.g., rash, GI bleeding, jaundice). Advise to report adverse effects to the physician.
- Inform patient/caregiver that abrupt discontinuation or dosage reduction of 80 mg/d or more may precipitate acute deterioration of cognitive function.
- Stress the importance of regular follow-up and liver function tests.
- Advise patient/caregiver that tacrine may induce seizures, vertigo, and syncope. Therefore, appropriate precautions are warranted.
- Inform patient/caregiver that tacrine therapy is not a cure and will become ineffective at some point as the disease progresses.

TACROLIMUS (FK-506)

(tac-rol′i-mus)

Trade name: Prograf

Classification: IMMUNOSUPPRESSANT

Prototype: Cyclosporine

Pregnancy category: C

ACTIONS/PHARMACODYNAMICS

Tacrolimus is a macrolide antibiotic produced by a soil fungus. Its immunosuppressant activity is more marked than that of cyclosporine. Action in reducing transplant rejection appears to be due to selective inhibition of helper T-lymphocytes. Tacrolimus inhibits helper T-lymphocytes by selectively inhibiting secretion of interleukin-2, interleukin-3, and interleukin-gamma. This creates an imbalance in favor of suppressor T-lymphocytes (which inhibit antibody production); thus, immune response is subdued.

USES Liver rejection prophylaxis; rejection prophylaxis for other organ transplants (kidney, heart, bone marrow, pancreas, small bowel). **Unlabeled use:** psoriasis.

ROUTE & DOSAGE

Rejection Prophylaxis

Adult: **PO** 0.15–0.3 mg/kg/d in 2 divided doses q12h; start no sooner than 6 h after transplant; give first oral dose 8–12 h after discontinuing IV therapy. **IV** 0.05–0.1 mg/kg/d as continuous IV infusion; start no sooner than 6 h after transplant; continue until patient can take oral therapy.

Child: **PO** Same as adult, but start with upper end of dosage range. **IV** Same as adult, but start with upper end of dosage range.

PHARMACOKINETICS Absorption: erratic and incompletely absorbed from GI tract; absolute bioavailability approximately 14–25%; absorption reduced by food. **Peak:** PO 1–4 h. **Duration:** IV 12 h. **Distribution:** within plasma, tacrolimus is found primarily in lipoprotein-deficient fraction; 75–97% protein bound, mainly to albumin and alpha$_1$-acid glycoprotein; distributed into red blood cells; blood:plasma ratio reported >4; animal studies have demonstrated high concentrations of tacrolimus in lung, kidney, heart, and spleen, and simlar tissue profile is to be expected in humans; distributed into breast milk. **Metabolism:** extensively metabolized in liver. **Elimination:** half-life: 8.7–11.3 h; metabolites excreted primarily in bile.

CONTRAINDICATIONS & PRECAUTIONS Contraindicated in: hypersensitivity to tacrolimus or castor oil, pregnancy (category C), lactation. **Cautious use in:** renal or hepatic insufficiency, hyperkalemia, diabetes mellitus, gout, history of seizures, hypertension.

ADVERSE/SIDE EFFECTS CNS: *headache, tremors, insomnia, paresthesia, hyperesthesia* and/or sensations of warmth, circumoral numbness. **CV:** *mild to moderate hypertension.* **Endocrine:** hirsutism, *hyperglycemia, hyperkalemia, hypokalemia, hypomagnesemia,* hyperuricemia, decreased serum cholesterol. **GI:** *nausea, abdominal pain, gas,* appetite changes, *vomiting, anorexia, constipation,* diarrhea. **Hematologic:** *anemia, leukocytosis, thrombocytopenia purpura.* **Renal:** UTI, oliguria, nephrotoxicity. **Respiratory:** *pleural effusion, atelectasis, dyspnea.* **Other:** ascites, blurred vision, photophobia, *flushing, rash, pruritis,* alopecia, *pain, fever, peripheral edema.*

DRUG INTERACTIONS Use with **cyclosporine** increases risk of nephrotoxicity. **Erythromycin** may increase tacrolimus levels. NSAIDS may lead to oliguria or anuria.

INCOMPATIBILITY Y-site: phenytoin.

NURSING IMPLICATIONS

Administration

- IV preparation: Contents of 5 mg/ml ampuls must be diluted with 0.9% NaCl or 5% dextrose to a concentration of 0.004–0.02 mg/ml. The diluted infusion should be stored in glass or polyethylene containers and discarded after 24 h.
- IV tacrolimus is given as a continuous infusion.
- The patient should be converted from IV to oral therapy as soon as possible.
- Cyclosporine must be discontinued at least 24 h before the first dose of tacrolimus.
- Store ampuls between 5 and 25C (41 and 77F); store capsules at room temperature, 15–30C (59–86F).

Assessment & Drug Effects

- Closely monitor renal function; report elevated serum creatinine or decreased urinary output.
- Monitor serum electrolyte, uric acid, and blood glucose levels.
- Monitor for neurotoxicity, and report tremors, changes in mental status, or other signs of toxicity.
- Monitor cardiovascular staus and report hypertension.

Patient & Family Education

- Inform of potential adverse effects of tacrolimus.
- Provide patient with complete dosing instructions.

T

TAMOXIFEN CITRATE

(ta-mox'i-fen)

Trade names: Nolvadex, Nolvadex-D ♣, Tamofen ♣

Prototype for classifications: ANTINEOPLASTIC; HORMONE; ANTI-ESTROGEN

Pregnancy category: C

ACTIONS/PHARMACODYNAMICS Nonsteroidal gonad-stimulating principle with potent antiestrogenic activity. Competes with estradiol at estrogen receptor sites in target tissues such as breast, uterus, vagina, anterior pituitary, tumor with high concentration of estrogen receptors. Tamoxifen-receptor complexes move into nucleus, decreasing DNA synthesis and estrogen responses. Ovulation may be induced by stimulation of the release of hypothalamic gonadotropic-releasing factor.

USES Palliative treatment of advanced breast cancer in postmenopausal women, adjunctively with surgery in the treatment of breast carcinoma with positive lymph nodes. **Unlabeled use:** investigationally to stimulate ovulation in selected anovulatory women desiring pregnancy.

ROUTE & DOSAGE

Breast Carcinoma

Adult: **PO** 10–20 mg 1–2 times/d (morning and evening).

Stimulation of Ovulation

Adult: **PO** 5–40 mg b.i.d. for 4 d.

PHARMACOKINETICS Absorption: slowly absorbed from GI tract. **Peak:** 3–6 h. **Metabolism:** metabolized in liver, enterohepatically cycled. **Elimination:** half-life: 7 d; excreted primarily in feces.

CONTRAINDICATIONS & PRECAUTIONS Contraindicated in: pregnancy (category C), especially during first trimester. **Cautious use in:** lactation; vision disturbances; cataracts; leukopenia; thrombocytopenia.

ADVERSE/SIDE EFFECTS CNS: depression, light-headedness, dizziness, headache, mental confusion, sleepiness. **CV:** thrombosis. **Eye:** retinopathy, decreased visual acuity, blurred vision. **GI:** *nausea and vomiting (about 25% of patients),* distaste for food, anorexia. **Hematologic:** leukopenia, thrombocytopenia. **Reproductive:** changes in menstrual period, milk production and leaking from breasts, vaginal discharge and bleeding, pruritus vulvae. **Other:** skin rash or dryness, increased bone pain, and transient local disease flair; loss of hair, weight gain, shortness of breath, photosensitivity, *hot flashes,* hypercalcemia.

DIAGNOSTIC TEST INTERFERENCE Tamoxifen may produce transient increase in ***serum calcium.***

DRUG INTERACTION May enhance hypoprothombinemic effects of **warfarin.**

NURSING IMPLICATIONS

Administration

- If side effects are severe, sometimes a simple reduction in dosage gives sufficient relief without losing control of disease. Consult physician.
- Store at 15–30C (59–86F) in container that protects drug from light.

Assessment & Drug Effects

- An objective response may require 4–10 wk of therapy, longer if there is bone metastasis.
- Bone and tumor pain and local disease flair often necessitate ad-

ministration of analgesics for pain relief. Reassure patient that this discomfort frequently signals a good tumor response.

- Soft-tissue-disease response to tamoxifen may be local swelling and marked erythema over preexisting lesions or the development of new lesions. These symptoms rapidly subside after tamoxifen treatment is initiated.
- CBCs including platelet counts are periodically assessed. Transient leukopenia and thrombocytopenia (50,000–100,000/mm^3) without hemorrhagic tendency have been reported.

Patient & Family Education

- Report to physician if marked weakness, sleepiness, mental confusion, edema, dyspnea, and blurred vision occur.
- Discuss the possibility of drug-induced menstrual irregularities with patient before starting treatment.
- Avoid prolonged sun exposure, especially if skin is unprotected. Sunscreen lotions (SPF ≥12) should be applied to all exposed skin surfaces.
- Caution patient not to change established dose schedule.
- OTC drugs should be avoided unless specifically prescribed by the physician. Discuss with patient, particularly with respect to OTC analgesics.
- Report onset of tenderness or redness in an extremity.
- Urge patient to adhere to scheduled appointments for clinical evaluation. Medical supervision is necessary during tamoxifen therapy.

TAMSULOSIN HYDROCHLORIDE

(tam′-su-lo-sin)

Trade name: Flomax

Classifications: AUTONOMIC NERVOUS SYSTEM AGENT; ALPHA$_{1A}$-ADRENERGIC ANTAGONIST (BLOCKING AGENT, SYMPATHOLYTIC AGENT)

Prototype: Prazosin hydrochloride

Pregnancy category: B

ACTIONS/PHARMACODYNAMICS

Tamsulosin is an antagonist of the alpha$_{1A}$-adrenergic receptors located in the prostate. Symptoms related to benign prostatic hypertrophy (BPH) are related to bladder outlet obstruction. Blockage of alpha$_{1A}$-adrenergic receptors can cause smooth muscles in the bladder outlet and the prostate gland to relax, resulting in improvement in urinary blood flow and a reduction in symptoms of BPH.

USE Benign prostatic hypertrophy.

ROUTE & DOSAGE

Benign Prostatic Hypertrophy

Adult: **PO** 0.4 mg q.d. 30 min before a meal. May increase up to 0.8 mg q.d.

PHARMACOKINETICS Absorption: rapidly absorbed from GI tract. > 90% bioavailability. **Peak:** 4–5 h fasting, 6–7 h fed. **Distribution:** widely distributed in body tissues, including kidney and prostate. **Metabolism:** metabolized in the liver. **Elimination:** half-life: 14–15 h; 76% excreted in urine.

CONTRAINDICATIONS & PRECAUTIONS Contraindicated in: hypersensitivity to tansulosin, in conjunction with another alpha$_{1A}$-adrenergic blocking agent, nursing mothers, pediatric patients. **Cautious use in:** pregnancy (category B), history of syncope, hypotension.

ADVERSE/SIDE EFFECTS Body as whole: asthenia, back or chest pain. **CNS:** *headache, dizziness,* insomnia. **CV:** *orthostatic hypotension (especially with first dose).* **GI:** diarrhea, nausea. **Respiratory:** *rhinitis,* pharyngitis, increased cough, sinusitis. **Other:** decreased libido, *abnormal ejaculation,* amblyopia.

DRUG INTERACTION Cimetidine may decrease clearance of **tamsulosin.**

NURSING IMPLICATIONS

Administration

- Give 30 min after the same meal each day.
- Capsules should be swallowed whole; they should not be crushed, chewed, or opened.
- Store at 20–25C (68–77F).

Assessment & Drug Effects

- Therapeutic effectiveness is indicated by improved voiding.
- Monitor for signs of orthostatic hypotension; take BP lying down, then upon standing. Report a systolic pressure drop of ≥15 mm Hg or a HR increase of ≥15 beats upon standing.
- Closely monitor patients on warfarin therapy.

Patient & Family Education

- Make position changes slowly to minimize orthostatic hypotension.
- Report dizziness, vertigo, or fainting to physician. Exercise caution with hazardous activities until reaction to drug is known.
- Concurrent use of cimetidine may increase the orthostatic hypotension side effect of tamsulosin.

TAZAROTENE

(ta-zar′o-teen)

Trade name: Tazorac

Classifications: SKIN AND MUCOUS MEMBRANE AGENT; ANTIACNE; RETINOID

Prototype: Isotretinon

Pregnancy category: X

ACTIONS/PHARMACODYNAMICS A retinoid prodrug that blocks epidermal cell proliferation and hyperplasia. Tazarotene suppresses inflammation present in the epidermis of psoriasis patients. Its mechanism of action in acne is not known.

USES Topical treatment of plaque psoriasis on up to 20% of the body, mild to moderate acne.

ROUTE & DOSAGE

Plaque Psoriasis

Adult: **Topical** Apply thin film to affected area once daily in evening.

Acne

Adult: **Topical** After cleansing and drying face, apply thin film to acne lesions once daily in evening.

PHARMACOKINETICS Absorption: rapidly absorbed through skin. **Distribution:** active metabolite >99% protein bound; crosses placenta, distributed into breast milk. **Metabolism:** undergoes esterase hydrolysis to active metabolite AGN 190299. **Elimination:** half-life: 18 h; eliminated in both urine and feces.

CONTRAINDICATIONS & PRECAUTIONS Contraindicated in: hypersensitivity to tazarotene, pregnancy (category X), women who are or may become pregnant. **Cautious use in:** lactation, concurrent administration with drugs that are photosensitizers (e.g., thiazide, tetracyclines).

Safety and efficacy in children < 12 y have not been established.

ADVERSE/SIDE EFFECTS **Skin:** *pruritus, burning/stinging, erythema, worsening of psoriasis, irritation, skin pain,* rash, desquamation of skin, irritant contact dermatitis, inflammation, fissuring, bleeding, dry skin, sunburn.

NURSING IMPLICATIONS

Administration

- Skin should be completely dry before application of a thin film of medication.
- Medication should be applied to no more than 20% of body surface in those with psoriasis.
- Apply only to affected areas, avoiding contact with eyes and mucous membranes.

Assessment & Drug Effects

- Therapeutic effectiveness is indicated by improvement in acne or psoriasis.
- Monitor for photosensitivity in those concurrently using any of the following: thiazides, tetracyclines, fluoroquinolones, phenothiazines, sulfonamides.

Patient & Family Education

- Women must be fully informed regarding risk of serious fetal harm. Reliable forms of effective contraception must be used and treatment discontinued if pregnancy occurs.
- If contact with eyes occurs, immediately rinse thoroughly with water.
- Avoid all unnecessary exposure to sunlight or artificial UV light. If brief exposure is necessary, cover as much skin surface as possible and use sunscreens (minimum SPF 15).
- Tazarotene should not be applied to sunburned skin.
- Discontinue medication and notify physician if any of the following occur: pruritus, burning, skin redness, excessive peeling, or worsening of psoriasis.
- Limit application of topicals with strong skin-drying effects to skin areas being treated with tazarotene.

TEMAZEPAM

(te-maz′e-pam)

Trade name: Restoril

Classifications: CNS AGENT; ANXIOLYTIC; SEDATIVE-HYPNOTIC; BENZODIAZEPINE

Prototype: Lorazepam

Pregnancy category: X

Controlled substance: Schedule IV

ACTIONS/PHARMACODYNAMICS Benzodiazepine derivative with hypnotic, anxiolytic, sedative effects. Principal effect is significant improvement in sleep parameters as evidenced by reduced night awakenings and early morning awakenings, increased total sleep times, and absence of rebound effects. Sleep latency is not reduced, and there is minimal change in REM sleep.

USE To relieve insomnia associated with frequent nocturnal awakenings or early morning awakenings.

ROUTE & DOSAGE

Insomnia

Adult: **PO** 7.5–30 mg h.s.
Geriatric: **PO** 7.5 mg h.s.

PHARMACOKINETICS **Absorption:** readily absorbed from GI tract. **Onset:** 30–50 min. **Peak:** 2–3 h. **Duration:** 10–12 h. **Distribution:** crosses placenta; distributed into breast milk. **Metabolism:** metabolized in liver to oxazepam. **Elimination:** half-life: 8–24 h; excreted in urine.

CONTRAINDICATIONS & PRECAUTIONS Contraindicated in: pregnancy (category X); safe use in children < 18 y not established; narrow-angle glaucoma; psychoses. **Cautious use in:** nursing mother, severely depressed patient or one with suicidal ideation, history of drug abuse or dependence, acute intoxication, hepatic or renal dysfunction, elderly patients, sleep apnea.

ADVERSE/SIDE EFFECTS Usually mild and transient. **CNS:** *drowsiness,* dizziness, lethargy, confusion, headache, euphoria, relaxed feeling, weakness. **GI:** anorexia, diarrhea. **Other:** palpitations.

DRUG INTERACTIONS Alcohol, CNS DEPRESSANTS, ANTICONVULSANTS potentiate CNS depression; **cimetidine** increases temazepam plasma levels, thus increasing its toxicity; may decrease antiparkinsonism effects of **levodopa;** may increase **phenytoin** levels; smoking decreases sedative effects.

NURSING IMPLICATIONS

Administration

- Administer 20–30 min before patient retires.
- Store at 15–30C (59–86F) in tight container unless otherwise specified by manufacturer.

Assessment & Drug Effects

- Psychoactive drugs are the most frequent cause of acute confusion in the elderly. Be alert to signs of paradoxical reaction (excitement, hyperactivity, and disorientation) in this age group.
- CNS side effects are more apt to occur in the patient with hypoalbuminemia, liver disease, and the elderly patient. Report promptly incidence of bradycardia, drowsiness, dizziness, clumsiness, lack of coordination. Supervise ambulation, especially at night.
- With long-term use of this drug, hepatic and renal function tests are advised.
- Signs of overdose are weakness, bradycardia, somnolence, confusion, slurred speech, ataxia, coma with reduced or absent reflexes, hypertension, and respiratory depression.

Patient & Family Education

- Advise that improvement in sleep will not occur until after 2 or 3 doses of drug.
- If dreams or nightmares interfere with rest, notify physician. An alternate drug or reduced dose may be prescribed.
- Inform that difficulty getting to sleep may continue. Drug effect is evidenced by the increased amount of rest once asleep.
- Instruct to avoid use of alcohol as a sedative.
- Advise to take a warm beverage (e.g., milk) or light snack before bedtime.
- If patient is elderly, suggest avoiding daytime "catnaps."
- If insomnia continues in spite of medication, physician should be consulted.
- Smoking should be discontinued after medication is taken.
- Use by nursing mothers may cause sedation and possibly feeding problems and weight loss in the infant.
- Warn patient not to use OTC drugs (especially for insomnia) during temazepam therapy without advice of physician.
- Advise to consult physician before discontinuing drug especially after long-term use. Gradual reduction

T

of dose may be necessary to avoid withdrawal symptoms.

- Use of alcohol and other CNS depressants should be avoided.
- Patient should use extreme caution when operating machinery or driving a car because this drug may depress psychomotor skills and causes sedation.

TERAZOSIN

(ter-ay′zoe-sin)

Trade name: Hytrin

Classifications: AUTONOMIC NERVOUS SYSTEM AGENT; ALPHA-ADRENERGIC ANTAGONIST (SYMPATHOLYTIC, BLOCKING AGENT); ANTIHYPERTENSIVE

Prototype: Prazosin

Pregnancy category: C

ACTIONS/PHARMACODYNAMICS

Quinazoline antihypertensive and vasodilator chemically similar to prazosin. Selectively blocks $alpha_1$-adrenergic receptors in vascular smooth muscle producing relaxation that leads to reduction of peripheral vascular resistance and lowered BP. Vasodilation is accompanied by minimal reflex increase in heart rate. Antihypertensive drug therapy reserved for the patient who has failed to respond to diet, exercise, and weight reduction and other drug therapy. Effective when used with a beta-adrenergic blocking agent and a thiazide diuretic.

USES To treat hypertension alone or in combination with other antihypertensive agents (beta-adrenergic blocking agents, diuretics). To treat benign prostatic hypertrophy. **Unlabeled use:** urinary outflow obstruction.

ROUTE & DOSAGE

Hypertension, Benign Prostatic Hypertrophy, Urinary Obstruction

Adult: **PO** Start with 1 mg h.s.; then 1–5 mg/d (max 20 mg/d).

PHARMACOKINETICS Absorption: readily absorbed from GI tract. **Peak:** 1–2 h. **Metabolism:** metabolized in liver. **Elimination:** half-life: 9–12 h; 60% excreted in feces, 40% in urine.

CONTRAINDICATIONS & PRECAUTIONS Contraindicated in: safe use during pregnancy (category C), in nursing mothers, and children not established.

ADVERSE/SIDE EFFECTS CNS: *asthenia (weakness), dizziness, headache,* drowsiness, weakness. **CV:** postural hypotension, palpitation, *first-dose phenomenon (syncope).* **Eye/ear:** blurred vision. **GI:** nausea. **Other:** weight gain, pain in extremities, nasal congestion, sinusitis, impotence, dyspnea, peripheral edema.

DRUG INTERACTION Antihypertensive effects may be attenuated by NSAIDS.

NURSING IMPLICATIONS

Administration

- Food has little or no effect on bioavailability of terazosin; administer tablet with food or fluid of patient's choice.
- The initial dose of terazosin is given at bedtime to reduce the potential for severe hypotensive effect. This may occur with first few doses. After the initial dose, most patients take the drug in the morning.
- Store at 15–30C (59–86F) in tightly closed container away from heat and strong light. Do not freeze.

Assessment & Drug Effects

- First-dose phenomenon (precipitous decline in BP with consciousness disturbance) is rare; occurs within 90–120 min of initial dose.
- Advise patient to avoid situations that would result in injury should syncope occur after first dose. If it does develop, patient should lie down promptly and be treated symptomatically.
- Monitor BP at end of dosing interval (just before next dose) to determine level of antihypertensive control. Check BP also 2–3 h after the dose to determine if maximum and minimal responses are similar.
- Drug-induced decrease in BP appears to be more position dependent (i.e., greater in the erect position) during the first few hours after dosing than at end of 24 h.
- A greatly diminished hypotensive response at end of 24 h indicates need for change in dosage (increased dose or twice daily regimen).

Patient & Family Education

- Orthostatic hypotension can pose a problem with ambulation. Advise to make position changes slowly (i.e., change in direction or from recumbent to upright posture). Dangle legs and move ankles a minute or so before standing when arising. The orthostatic effect of terazosin is greatest shortly after dosing.
- Caution not to drive or engage in hazardous activity for at least 12 h after first dose, after dosage increase, or when treatment is resumed after interruption of therapy. Twelve hours should be sufficient time for serious side effects (orthostatic hypotension, syncope, light-headedness, dizziness) to appear if they are going to do so.
- Instruct to monitor weight: a sudden gain of more than 0.5–1 kg (1–2 lb) accompanied by edema in extremities should be reported to physician. Dose adjustment may be indicated.
- Emphasize importance of uninterrupted maintenance of established drug regimen. If drug is omitted for several days, consult physician. Drug will be started with the initial dosing regimen.
- Patient should keep scheduled appointments for assessment of BP control and other clinically significant tests.
- Encourage patient who has been taught to monitor own BP to keep a daily record noting BP and time taken, when medication was taken, which arm was used, position (i.e., standing, sitting) and time of day and to take this record to physician for reference at checkup appointment.
- Advise not to take OTC medications, particularly those that may contain an adrenergic agent (e.g., remedies for coughs, colds, allergy) without first consulting physician.

TERBINAFINE HYDROCHLORIDE

(ter-bin′a-feen)

Trade names: Lamisil, Lamisil DermaGel

Classifications: ANTIINFECTIVE; ANTIBIOTIC; ANTIFUNGAL

Prototype: Fluconazole

Pregnancy category: B

ACTIONS/PHARMACODYNAMICS

Terbinafine HCl is a synthetic antifungal agent that inhibits sterol biosynthesis in fungi, which ultimately causes fungal cell death. Dispensed in a 1% cream.

USES Topical treatment of superficial mycoses such as interdigital tinea pedis, tinea cruris, and tinea corporis due to *Epidermophyton floccosum, Trichophyton mentagrophytes,* or *T. rubrum;* oral treatment of onychomycosis due to tinea unguium.

ROUTE & DOSAGE

Tinea Pedis, Tinea Cruris, or Tinea Corporis

Adult: **Topical** Apply q.d. or b.i.d. to affected and immediately surrounding areas until clinical signs and symptoms are significantly improved (1–7 wk).

Onychomycosis

Adult: **PO** 250 mg q.d. × 6 wk for fingernails or × 12 wk for toenails.

PHARMACOKINETICS Absorption: 70% PO; approximately 3.5% of topical dose is absorbed systemically. **Elimination:** half-life: 36 h; excreted in urine.

CONTRAINDICATIONS & PRECAUTIONS Contraindicated in: hypersensitivity to terbinafine, nursing mothers. **Cautious use in:** pregnancy (category B). Safety and efficacy in children <12 y have not been established.

ADVERSE/SIDE EFFECTS Skin: pruritus, local burning, dryness, rash, vesiculation, redness, contact dermatitis at application site. **CNS:** *headache.* **GI:** diarrhea, dyspepsia, abdominal pain, liver test abnormalities. **Other:** taste disturbances, neutropenia (rare).

NURSING IMPLICATIONS

Administration

- Terbinafine should only be applied externally. Avoid application to mucous membranes and avoid contact with eyes.
- Do not use occlusive dressings unless specifically directed by physician to do so.
- Store at 5–30C (41–86F).

Patient & Family Education

- Instruct in the correct application of cream.
- Advise to notify physician if terbinafine causes increased skin irritation or sensitivity.
- Advise that medication must be used for full treatment time to be effective.

TERBUTALINE SULFATE

(ter-byoo'te-leen)

Trade names: Brethaire, Brethine, Bricanyl

Classifications: AUTONOMIC NERVOUS SYSTEM AGENT; BETA-ADRENERGIC AGONIST; BRONCHODILATOR

Prototype: Isoproterenol

Pregnancy category: B

ACTIONS/PHARMACODYNAMICS Synthetic adrenergic stimulant with selective $beta_2$- and negligible $beta_1$-agonist (cardiac) activity. Exerts preferential effect on $beta_2$ receptors in bronchial smooth muscles, inhibits histamine release from mast cells, and increases ciliary motility. These effects lead to relief of bronchospasm in chronic obstructive pulmonary disease (COPD) and significant increase in vital capacity. Other adrenergic effects include relaxation of vascular smooth muscle, contraction of GI and urinary sphincters, increase in renin, in pancreatic beta-cell secretion, and in serum HDL-cholesterol concentration. Increases uterine relaxation (thereby preventing or abolishing high intrauterine pressure).

USES Orally or subcutaneously as a bronchodilator in bronchial asthma and for reversible airway obstruction associated with bronchitis and emphysema. **Unlabeled use:** (PO and IV infusion) to delay delivery in preterm labor.

ROUTE & DOSAGE

Bronchodilator

Adult: **PO** 2.5–5 mg t.i.d. at 6 h intervals (max 15 mg/d). **SC** 0.25 mg q15–30min up to 0.5 mg in 4 h. **Inhaled** 2 inhalations separated by 60 s q4–6h. *Adolescent:* **PO** 12–15 y, 2.5 mg t.i.d. at 6 h intervals (max 7.5 mg/d). **SC** 0.25 mg q15–30min up to 0.5 mg in 4 h. **Inhaled** 2 inhalations separated by 60 s q4–6h.
Child <12 y: **PO** 0.05 mg/kg q8h; gradually increase up to 0.15 mg/kg q8h (max 5 mg/d). **SC** 0.005–0.01 mg/kg (max 0.4 mg) q15–20min × 2 doses.

Premature Labor

Adult: **IV** 10 µg/min titrated up to a max of 80 µg/min; continue at minimum effective dose for 4 h; then switch to PO. **PO** 2.5 mg q4–6h.

PHARMACOKINETICS Absorption: 33–50% absorbed from GI tract. **Onset:** 30 min PO; < 15 min SC; 5–30 min inhaled. **Peak:** 2–3 h PO; 30–60 min SC; 1–2 h inhaled. **Duration:** 4–8 h PO; 1.5–4 h SC; 3–4 h inhaled. **Distribution:** distributed into breast milk. **Metabolism:** metabolized in liver. **Elimination:** half-life: 3–4 h; excreted primarily in urine, 3% in feces.

CONTRAINDICATIONS & PRECAUTIONS Contraindicated in: known hypersensitivity to sympathomimetic amines, severe hypertension and coronary artery disease, tachycardia with digitalis intoxication, within 14 d of MAO inhibitor therapy, children < 12 y, angle-closure glaucoma. Used only after evaluation of risk-benefit ratio in pregnancy (category B) and lactation. **Cautious use in:** angina, stroke, hypetension; diabetes mellitus; thyrotoxicosis; history of seizure disorders; cardiac arrhythmias; the elderly patient; renal and hepatic dysfunction.

ADVERSE/SIDE EFFECTS Dose related. **CNS:** *nervousness, tremor,* headache, *light-headedness,* drowsiness, fatigue, seizures. **CV:** *tachycardia,* hypotension or hypertension, *palpitation,* maternal and fetal tachycardia. **GI:** nausea, vomiting. **Other:** sweating, muscle cramps.

DIAGNOSTIC TEST INTERFERENCE Terbutaline may increase ***blood glucose*** and free ***fatty acids.***

DRUG INTERACTIONS Epinephrine, other SYMPATHOMIMETIC BRONCHODILATORS may add to effects; MAO INHIBITORS, TRICYCLIC ANTIDEPRESSANTS potentiate action on vascular system; effects of both BETA-ADRENERGIC BLOCKERS and terbutaline antagonized.

NURSING IMPLICATIONS

Administration

- Tablet may be crushed before administration and taken with fluid of patient's choice.
- Be certain about recommended doses: PO preparation, 2.5 mg; SC, 0.25 mg. A decimal point error can be fatal.
- SC injection is usually administered into lateral deltoid area.
- If GI symptoms occur, advise patient to take the tablets with food.
- IV administration: IV terbutaline is diluted by adding each 5 mg to

T

1000 ml D5W or NS (for diabetics) to yield a concentration of 5 μg/ml. Infuse with microdrip and infusion pump.

- Store at 15–30C (59–86F). Protect from light and freezing.

Assessment & Drug Effects

- Cardiovascular side effects are more apt to occur when drug is given by SC route and when it is used by a patient with cardiac arrhythmia. Check pulse and BP before each dose. If perceptively altered from baseline level, consult physician.
- Most side effects are transient. However, rapid heart rate may persist for a relatively long time.
- Onset and degree of effect and incidence and severity of side effects of the SC formulation resemble those of epinephrine. Oral terbutaline appears to be equally as effective as ephedrine; however, onset of action is more rapid, and its effects last longer.
- Aerosolized terbutaline produces little cardiac stimulation or tremors.
- Muscle tremor is a fairly common side effect that appears to subside with continued use.
- The neonate born of a mother who used terbutaline during pregnancy may have hypoglycemia. Monitor for symptoms if there is reason to suspect this condition.
- Treatment for premature labor: Monitor patient for CV signs and symptoms for 12 h after drug is discontinued. Report tachycardia promptly. Monitor I&O ratio. Fluid restriction may be necessary. Consult physician.

Patient & Family Education

- Inhalator therapy: Review and discuss the instructions for use of inhalator (included in the package).
- Teach the ambulatory patient on oral terbutaline how to take his or her own pulse and the limits of change that indicate need to notify the physician.
- Instruct to consult the physician if breathing difficulty is not relieved or if it becomes worse within 30 min after an oral dose of terbutaline.
- Terbutaline appears to have a short clinical period for sustained effectiveness. Advise to keep appointments with physician for evaluation of continued drug effectiveness and clinical condition.
- Tolerance can develop with chronic use of terbutaline. Advise to consult physician if symptomatic relief wanes. Usually, a substitute agent will be prescribed.
- Instruct to adhere to established dosage regimen (i.e., not to change dose intervals or omit, increase, or decrease the dose).
- Be alert to the pattern of self-dosing established by the patient on long-term therapy. Caution that in the face of waning response, increasing the dose may cause overdosage and will not improve the clinical condition. The patient should understand that decreasing relief with continued treatment indicates need for another bronchodilator, not an increase in dose.
- Contents of the aerosol (inhalator) are under pressure. Warn not to puncture container, not to use or store it near heat or open flame, and not to expose it to temperatures above 49C (120F), which may cause bursting.
- No other aerosol bronchodilator should be used while the patient is being controlled by aerosol terbutaline. Warn not to self-medicate with an OTC aerosol.
- Warn not to use OTC drugs unless the physician approves. Many cold and allergy remedies, for example,

contain a sympathomimetic agent that when combined with terbutaline may be deleterious to the patient.

TERCONAZOLE

(ter-con'a-zole)

Trade names: Terazol$_7$, Terazol$_3$

Classifications: ANTIINFECTIVE; ANTIFUNGAL

Prototype: Fluconazole

Pregnancy category: C

ACTIONS/PHARMACODYNAMICS Terconazole exhibits fungicidal activity against *Candida albicans*. The exact mechanism of action is uncertain; however, it may exert its antifungal activity by disruption of normal fungal cell membrane permeability.

USE Local treatment of vulvovaginal candidiasis.

ROUTE & DOSAGE

Candidiasis

Adult: **Intravaginal** One suppository (2.5 g) q.h.s. × 3 d; one applicatorful of 0.4% cream q.h.s. × 7 d or one applicatorful of 0.8% cream q.h.s. × 3 d.

PHARMACOKINETICS Absorption: slow minimal absorption from vagina. **Onset:** within 3 d. **Metabolism:** metabolized in liver. **Elimination:** half-life: 4–11 h; half eliminated in urine, half in feces.

CONTRAINDICATIONS & PRECAUTIONS Contraindicated in: hypersensitivity to terconazole, lactation. **Cautious use in:** pregnancy (category C). Safety and efficacy in children not established.

ADVERSE/SIDE EFFECTS CNS: *headache*. **GU:** vaginal itching, burning, irritation. **Other:** rash, flulike syndrome (fever, chills, headache, hypotension).

NURSING IMPLICATIONS

Administration

- Insert applicator high into the vagina (except during pregnancy).
- Wash applicator before and after each use.
- Store away from direct heat and light.

Assessment & Drug Effects

- Terconazole should not be used if patient has a history of allergic reaction to other antifungal agents, such as miconazole.
- Monitor for sensitization and irritation; they may be an indication to discontinue drug.

Patient & Family Education

- Advise in correct application technique.
- Inform of potential adverse reactions, including sensitization and allergic response.
- Inform that terconazole may interact with diaphragms and latex condoms; concurrent use within 72 h should be avoided.
- Advise to refrain from sexual intercourse while using terconazole.
- Advise to wear only cotton underwear, which are changed daily.

TESTOLACTONE

(tess-toe-lak'tone)

Trade name: Teslac

Classifications: ANTINEOPLASTIC; HORMONE

Pregnancy category: C

ACTIONS/PHARMACODYNAMICS Chemotherapeutic agent with chemical configuration similar to that of certain androgens but devoid of androgenic activity in therapeutic doses. Exact mechanism of antineoplastic action unknown. Action simulates that of androgens without producing virilization in recommended dosage. In breast cancer, effect may result from depression of ovarian function by inhibition of synthesis of pituitary gonadotropin.

USES Adjunctive treatment in palliation of breast carcinoma in postmenopausal women when hormone therapy is indicated. Also effective in women diagnosed before menopause in whom ovarian function has been subsequently terminated.

ROUTE & DOSAGE

Adjunctive Therapy for Breast Cancer

Adult: **PO** 250 mg q.i.d.

PHARMACOKINETICS **Absorption:** readily absorbed from GI tract. **Metabolism:** metabolized in liver. **Elimination:** excreted in urine.

CONTRAINDICATIONS & PRECAUTIONS **Contraindicated in:** pregnancy (category C), premenopausal women, breast cancer in males. **Cautious use in:** hypercalcemia, cardiorenal disease.

ADVERSE/SIDE EFFECTS **CNS:** paresthesias. **Endocrine:** deepening of the voice, acne, facial hair growth, clitoral enlargement. **GI:** glossitis, anorexia; nausea, vomiting. **Other:** hypertension, edema in extremities.

DIAGNOSTIC TEST INTERFERENCE ***Urinary 17-OHCS*** determinations may be elevated.

DRUG INTERACTION May enhance hypoprothrombinemic effects of ORAL ANTICOAGULANTS.

NURSING IMPLICATIONS

Administration

- Drug may be administered without regard to food.
- Store at 15–30C (59–86F) unless otherwise directed. Protect from freezing.

Assessment & Drug Effects

- Clinical response usually occurs in 6–12 wk and is measured according to the following criteria: decrease in size of tumor; more than 50% of nonosseous lesions decrease in size even though all bone lesions remain static.
- Plasma calcium levels are checked routinely and periodically (normal serum calcium: 8.5–10.6 mg/dl).
- Report signs that may suggest impending hypercalcemia (see Appendix G).
- Note I&O ratio and pattern.
- Encourage patient mobility if feasible; if not, assist with passive exercises.

Patient & Family Education

- Testalactone treatment is usually continued for a minimum of 3 mo (unless there is active progression of the disease) to evaluate response.
- Hypercalcemia represents active remission of bone metastasis; if it occurs, appropriate therapy is instituted.

TESTOSTERONE

(tess-toss'ter-one)

Trade names: Andro 100, Histerone, Malogen♣, Testoderm

TESTOSTERONE CYPIONATE

Trade names: Andro-Cyp, Andronate, depAndro, Depo-Testosterone, Depotest, Duratest

TESTOSTERONE ENANTHATE

Trade names: Andro L.A., Delatest, Delatestryl, Everone, Malogex ♣, Testone L.A., Testrin PA, and others

TESTOSTERONE PROPIONATE

Trade names: Malogen in oil♣, Testex

Prototype for classifications: SYNTHETIC HORMONE; ANDROGEN/ANABOLIC STEROID; ANTINEOPLASTIC

Pregnancy category: X

Controlled substance: Schedule III

ACTIONS/PHARMACODYNAMICS Synthetic steroid compound with both androgenic and anabolic activity (1:1). Controls development and maintenance of secondary sexual characteristics. **Androgenic activity:** responsible for the growth spurt of the adolescent and for growth termination by epiphyseal closure. In males and some females, reduces excretion of phosphorus, nitrogen, potassium, sodium, and chloride. Increases erythropoiesis, possibly by stimulating production of renal or extrarenal erythropoietin, and promotes vascularization and darkening of skin. Antagonizes effects of estrogen excess on female breast and endometrium. **Anabolic activity:** increases protein metabolism and decreases its catabolism. Large doses suppress spermatogenesis, thereby causing testicular atrophy.

USES Androgen replacement therapy, delayed puberty (male), palliation of female mammary cancer (1–5 y postmenopausal), and to treat postpartum breast engorgement. Available in fixed combination with estrogens in many preparations.

ROUTE & DOSAGE

Male Hypogonadism

Adult: **IM** 10–25 mg 2–3 times/wk; propionate: 10–25 mg 3 times/wk; cypionate, enanthate: 50–400 mg q2–4wk **Topical** Start with 6 mg/d system applied daily; if scrotal area inadequate, use 4 mg/d system. Androderm can be applied to torso.

Delayed Puberty

Adult: **IM** Cypionate, enanthate: 50–200 mg q2–4wk.

Metastatic Breast Cancer

Adult: **IM** 50–100 mg short-acting testosterone 3 times/wk; propionate: 100 mg 3 times/wk; cypionate, enanthate: 200–400 mg q2–4wk.

Postpartum Breast Engorgement

Adult: **IM** 25–50 mg/d for 3–4 d; propionate: 25–50 mg/d for 3–4 d.

PHARMACOKINETICS **Absorption:** **cypionate** and **enanthate** are slowly absorbed from lipid tissue. **Duration:** 2–4 wk **cypionate** and **enanthate.** **Distribution:** 98% bound to sex hormone–binding globulin. **Metabolism:** primarily metabolized in liver. **Elimination:** half-life: 10–100 min; 90% excreted in urine, 6% in feces.

CONTRAINDICATIONS & PRECAUTIONS **Contraindicated in:** hypersensitivity or toxic reactions to androgens; serious cardiac, hepatic, or renal disease; pregnancy (category X, possibility of virilization of external genitalia of female fetus); nursing mothers; hypercalcemia; known or suspected prostatic or breast cancer in male; benign prostatic hypertrophy with obstruction; patients easily stimulated sexually; elderly, asthenic males who may react adversely to androgenic overstimulation; conditions aggravated by fluid retention; hypertension. **Cautious use in:** cardiac, hepatic, and renal disease; prepubertal males, geriatric patients, acute intermittent porphyria.

ADVERSE/SIDE EFFECTS **CNS:** excitation, insomnia. **CV:** skin flushing and vascularization. **GI:** nausea, vomiting, anorexia, diarrhea, gastric pain, jaundice. **Hematologic:** leukopenia. **Metabolic:** hypercalcemia, hypercholesterolemia, *sodium and water retention (especially in elderly) with edema*. **Renal:** renal calculi (especially in the immobilized patient), bladder irritability. **Reproductive:** *increased libido*. **Skin:** *acne*, injection site irritation and sloughing. **Other:** hypersensitivity to testosterone, anaphylactoid reactions (rare), precipitation of acute intermittent porphyria. Androgenic: (virilization) female: suppression of ovulation, lactation, or menstruation; hoarseness or deepening of voice (often irreversible); hirsutism; oily skin; clitoral enlargement; regression of breasts; male-pattern baldness (in disseminated breast cancer). Male: prepubertal: premature epiphyseal closure, phallic enlargement, priapism. Postpubertal: testicular atrophy, decreased ejaculatory volume, azoospermia, oligospermia (after prolonged administration or excessive dosage), impotence, epididymitis, priapism, *gynecomastia*. Hypoestrogenic: female: flushing, sweating; vaginitis with pruritus, drying, bleeding; menstrual irregularities.

DIAGNOSTIC TEST INTERFERENCE Testosterone alters ***glucose tolerance*** tests; decreases ***thyroxine-binding globulin concentration*** (resulting in decreased total T_4 serum levels and increased resin of T_3 and T_4). Increases ***creatinine*** and ***creatinine*** excretion (lasting up to 2 wk after therapy is discontinued) and alters response to ***metyrapone test***. It suppresses ***clotting factors II, V, VII, X*** and decreases excretion of ***17-ketosteroids***. May increase or decrease ***serum cholesterol***.

DRUG INTERACTIONS ORAL ANTICOAGULANTS may potentiate hypoprothrombinemia. May decrease **insulin** requirements.

NURSING IMPLICATIONS

Administration

- IM injections should be made deep into gluteal musculature. A wet syringe or needle may cloud the solution, but potency of material reportedly is unaffected.
- Store IM formulations prepared in oil at room temperature. Warming and shaking vial will redisperse precipitated crystals.
- Apply transdermal system on clean, dry scrotal skin. Dry-shave scrotal hair for optimal skin contact. Do not use chemical depilatories. The patch should be worn for 22–24 h.
- Androderm patches may be applied to abdomen, back, thigh, or upper arm. Alternate application site q24h with ≥7 d between same site.
- Store at 15–30C (59–86F).

Assessment & Drug Effects

- Check I&O and weigh patient daily during dose adjustment period. Weight gain (due to sodium and water retention) suggests need for decreased dosage. When dosage is stabilized, urge patient to check weight at least twice weekly and to report increases, particularly if accompanied by edema in dependent areas. Dose adjustment and diuretic therapy may be started.

- Periodic serum cholesterol and calcium determinations as well as cardiac and liver function tests should be performed throughout testosterone therapy.
- Improvement from testosterone therapy is slow. Therapeutic response in patients with breast cancer is usually apparent within 3 mo after regimen begins. If signs of disease progression appear, therapy should be terminated. In patients with metastatic breast cancer, hypercalcemia usually indicates progression of bone metastasis.
- If serum calcium rises above 14 mg/dl, androgenic therapy is terminated.
- Promptly report signs and symptoms of hypercalcemia (see Appendix G). The immobilized patient is particularly prone to develop hypercalcemia. Treatment includes withdrawing testosterone. Calcium, phosphate, and BUN levels should be checked daily.
- Testosterone-induced anabolic action enhances hypoglycemia (hyperinsulinism). Instruct diabetic to report sweating, tremor, anxiety, vertigo. Dosage adjustment of antidiabetic agent may be required.
- Observe the patient who is on concomitant anticoagulant treatment for signs of overdosage (e.g., ecchymoses, petechiae). Report promptly to physician; anticoagulant dose may need to be reduced.
- Prepubertal or adolescent males should be monitored throughout therapy to avoid precocious sexual development and premature epiphyseal closure. Skeletal stimulation may continue 6 mo beyond termination of therapy.

Patient & Family Education

- Review directions for application of transdermal patches.
- Advise to report soreness at injection site, because postinjection furunculosis may be an associated adverse reaction.
- Instruct male to report priapism (sustained and often painful erections occurring especially in early replacement therapy), reduced ejaculatory volume, and gynecomastia. The symptoms indicate necessity for temporary withdrawal or discontinuation of testosterone therapy.
- Instruct to notify physician promptly if pregnancy is suspected or planned. Masculinization of the fetus is most likely to occur if testosterone (androgen) therapy is provided during first trimester of pregnancy.
- At dosage required to treat carcinoma, androgens may cause virilism in women. Advise them to report increase in libido (early sign of toxicity), growth of facial hair, deepening of voice, male-pattern baldness. The onset of hoarseness can easily be overlooked unless its significance as an early and possibly irreversible sign of virilism is appreciated. Reevaluation of treatment plan is indicated.

TETRACAINE HYDROCHLORIDE

(tet′ra-kane)

Trade name: Pontocaine

Classifications: CNS AGENT; LOCAL ANESTHETIC (ESTER TYPE)

Prototype: Procaine hydrochloride

Pregnancy category: C

ACTIONS/PHARMACODYNAMICS Local anesthetic approximately 10 times more potent and toxic than procaine. Depresses the initial depolarization phase of the action potential, thus preventing propagation and conduction of the nerve impulse. This results in loss of sensation and motor activity in circumscribed body areas close to injection or application site.

USES Spinal anesthesia (high, low, saddle block) and topically to produce surface anesthesia. **Eye:** to anesthetize conjunctiva and cornea prior to superficial procedures (including tonometry, gonioscopy, removal of foreign bodies or sutures, corneal scraping). **Nose and throat:** to abolish laryngeal and esophageal reflexes prior to bronchoscopy, esophagoscopy. **Skin:** to relieve pruritus, pain, burning.

ROUTE & DOSAGE

Local Anesthesia

Adult: **Topical** 1–2 drops of 0.5% solution or 1.25–2.5 cm of ointment in lower conjunctival fornix before procedure; *or* 0.5% solution or ointment to nose or throat before procedure. **Spinal** 1% solution diluted with equal volume of 10% dextrose injected in subarachnoid space.

T

PHARMACOKINETICS **Onset:** 1 min eye; 3 min mucosal surface; 3 min spinal. **Duration:** up to 15 min eye; 30–60 min mucosal surface; 1.5–3 h spinal. **Metabolism:** metabolized in liver and plasma. **Elimination:** excreted in urine.

CONTRAINDICATIONS & PRECAUTIONS **Contraindicated in:** elderly and debilitated patient; prolonged use of ophthalmic preparations; known hypersensitivity to tetracaine or other local anesthetics of ester type (e.g., procaine, chloroprocaine, cocaine) or to PABA or its derivatives; infection at application or injection site. Safe use during pregnancy (category C) or in children not established. **Cautious use in:** shock, in nursing mothers, cachexia, cardiac decompensation.

ADVERSE/SIDE EFFECTS Anaphylactic reactions, convulsions, faintness, syncope, hypotention. **CNS:** postspinal headache, headache, spinal nerve paralysis, anxiety, nervousness, seizures. **CV:** bradycardia, arrhythmias, hypotension. **Eye:** stinging. ***Prolonged use:*** corneal erosion, retardation or prevention of healing of corneal abrasion, transient pitting and sloughing of corneal surface, dry corneal epithelium. **Nose/throat:** dry membranes, prolonged depression of cough reflex.

NURSING IMPLICATIONS

Administration

- Avoid use of solutions that are cloudy, discolored, or crystallized.
- When tetracaine is used on mucosa of larynx, trachea, or esophagus, the manufacturer recommends adding 0.06 ml of a 0.1% epinephrine solution to each ml tetracaine solution to slow absorption of the anesthetic.
- Storage temperatures: ophthalmic solution and ointment: 15–30C (59–86F); topical: refrigeration. Avoid freezing. Store in tight, light-resistant containers.

Assessment & Drug Effects

- Recovery from anesthesia to the pharyngeal area is complete when patient has feeling in the hard and soft palates and when muscles in the faucial (tonsillar) pillars contract with stimulation. To test: (1) Ask patient if he or she can feel hard palate with tongue. (2) Gently stroke soft palate with moistened cotton swab and ask patient if he or she can feel it. (3) Gently stroke soft palate with a cotton swab moistened with iced lemon water and observe whether or not pharyngeal muscles contract.

- Do not administer food or liquids until these normal pharyngeal responses are present (usually about 1 h after anesthetic administration). The first small amount of liquid (water) should be administered under supervision of the care provider.
- Increased blood concentration of the drug may result from excess application of tetracaine to the skin (to relieve pruritus or burning), application to debrided or infected skin surfaces, or too rapid injection rate.
- High blood concentrations of tetracaine can lead to adverse systemic effects involving CNS and CV systems: convulsions, respiratory arrest, dysrhythmias, cardiac arrest.

Patient & Family Education

- Caution not to use ophthalmic tetracaine longer than prescribed period. Prolonged use to eye surface may cause corneal epithelial erosions and retard healing of corneal surface.
- Natural barriers to eye infection and injury are removed by the anesthesia. Warn patient not to rub eye after tetracaine instillation until anesthetic effect has dissipated (evidenced by return of blink reflex). Patching for temporary protection of the corneal epithelium may be ordered.
- Instruct patient who self-medicates to wash or disinfect hands before and after administration of solutions or ointment. Review procedure for administration of eye medication.

TETRACYCLINE HYDROCHLORIDE

(tet-ra-sye′kleen)

Trade names: Achromycin, Achromycin V, Nor-Tet, Novotetra ♣, Panmycin, Robitet, SK-Tetracycline, Sumycin, Tetracap, Tetracyn, Tetralan, Tetram, Topicycline

Prototype for classifications: ANTIINFECTIVE; ANTIBIOTIC; TETRACYCLINE

Pregnancy category: D

ACTIONS/PHARMACODYNAMICS

Broad spectrum antibiotic derived from *Streptomyces aureofaciens* or produced semisynthetically from oxytetracycline. Effective against a variety of gram-positive and gram-negative bacteria and against most chlamydiae, mycoplasmas, rickettsiae, and certain protozoa (e.g., amebae). Tetracyclines usually are bacteriostatic but may be bactericidal in high concentrations. Exerts antiacne action by suppressing growth of *Proprionibacterium acnes* within sebaceous follicles, thereby reducing free fatty acid content in sebum. Free fatty acids are thought to be produced by breakdown of triglycerides by lipases liberated from *P. acne* and are believed to be largely responsible for inflammatory skin lesions (papules, pustules, cysts) and comedones of acne. Evidence suggests that topical tetracycline may be as effective as the oral preparation for treatment of mild to moderate acne; moderate to severe acne may require oral and topical tetracycline.

USES Chlamydial infections (e.g., lymphogranuloma venereum, psittacosis, trachoma, inclusion conjunctivitis, nongonococcal urethritis); mycoplasmal infections (e.g., *Mycoplasma pneumoniae*); rickettsial infections (e.g., Q fever, Rocky Mt spotted fever, typhus); spirochetal infections: relapsing fever (*Borrelia*), leptospirosis, syphilis (penicillin-hypersensitive patients); amebiases; uncommon gram-negative bacterial infections (e.g., brucellosis, shigellosis, cholera, gonorrhea [penicillin-hypersensitive patients], granuloma inguinale, tularemia); gram-positive infections (e.g., tetanus). Also used orally and topically (solution) for inflammatory acne vulgaris; topical ointment is used for superficial skin infections. (See tetracycline hydrochloride, ophthalmic, for ophthalmic uses.) **Unlabeled uses:** actinomycosis, acute exacerbations of chronic bronchitis; Lyme disease; pericardial effusion (metastatic); acute PID; sexually transmitted epididymoorchitis; with quinine for multidrug-resistant strains of *Plasmodium falciparum* malaria; antiinfective prophylaxis for rape victims; recurrent cystic thyroid nodules; melioidosis; and as fluorescence test for malignancy.

ROUTE & DOSAGE

Systemic Infection

Adult: **PO** 250–500 mg b.i.d.–q.i.d. (1–2 g/d). **IM** 250 mg once/d *or* 300 mg/d in 2–3 divided doses.
Child: **PO** *>8 y*, 25–50 mg/kg/d in 2–4 divided doses. **IM** *>8 y*, 15–25 mg/kg/d in 2–3 divided doses (max 250 mg/injection).

Acne

Adult: **PO** 500–1000 mg/d in 4 divided doses. **Topical** Apply to cleansed areas twice daily.
Child >8 y: **PO** same as for adult. **Topical** Same as for adult.

PHARMACOKINETICS Absorption: 75–80% of dose absorbed orally. **Peak:** 2–4 h. **Distribution:** widely distributed, preferentially binds to rapid growing tissues; crosses placenta; enters breast milk. **Metabolism:** not metabolized; enterohepatic cycling. **Elimination:** half-life: 6–12 h; 50–60% excreted in urine within 72 h.

CONTRAINDICATIONS & PRECAUTIONS Contraindicated in: hypersensitivity to tetracyclines or to any ingredient in the formulation; severe renal or hepatic impairment, common bile duct obstruction; use during tooth development (last half of pregnancy) (category D), during infancy and childhood to the 8th year, and in nursing women. Safe use of topical tetracycline preparations in children <11 y not established. **Cautious use in:** history of renal or hepatic dysfunction; myasthenia gravis; history of allergy, asthma, hay fever, urticaria; undernourished patients.

ADVERSE/SIDE EFFECTS CNS: headache, intracranial hypertension (rare). **Eye:** pigmentation of conjunctiva due to drug deposit. **GI:** reported mostly for oral administration, but also may occur with parenteral tetracycline: *nausea, vomiting,* epigastric distress, heartburn, *diarrhea,* bulky loose stools, steatorrhea, *abdominal discomfort, flatulence,* dry mouth; dysphagia, retrosternal pain, esophagitis, esophageal ulceration with oral administration. **Hepatic:** particularly patients with impaired renal or hepatic function: abnormally high liver function test values, decrease in serum cholesterol, <u>fatty degeneration of liver (jaundice, increasing nitrogen retention [azotemia], hyperphosphatemia, acidosis, irreversible shock)</u>. **Hypersensitivity:** urticaria, angioedema, rash, <u>exfoliative dermatitis,</u> drug fever, serum sickness, <u>anaphylaxis</u>. **Renal:** (particularly in

T

patients with renal disease): increase in BUN/serum creatinine, renal impairment even with therapeutic doses; Fanconi-like syndrome (outdated tetracyclines). Characterized by polyuria, polydipsia, nausea, vomiting, glycosuria, proteinuria acidosis, aminoaciduria. **Skin:** dermatitis, *phototoxicity*: discoloration of nails, onycholysis (loosening of nails); cheilosis; fixed drug eruptions particularly on genitalia; thrombocytopenic purpura. With topical applications: skin irritation, dry scaly skin, transient stinging or burning sensation, slight yellowing of skin at application site, acute contact dermatitis. **Superinfections:** vulvovaginitis, pruritus vulvae or ani (possibly hypersensitivity), foul-smelling stools or vaginal discharge, stomatitis, glossitis; black hairy tongue (lingua nigra), pharyngitis, laryngitis, dysphagia, diarrhea: staphylococcal enterocolitis, gram-negative folliculitis (long-term therapy). **Other:** pancreatitis, local reactions: pain and irritation (IM site), Jarisch-Herxheimer reaction (see Nursing Implications).

DIAGNOSTIC TEST INTERFERENCE Tetracyclines may cause false increases in ***urinary catecholamines*** (by fluorometric methods), and false decreases in ***urinary urobilinogen***. Parenteral tetracyclines containing ascorbic acid reportedly may produce false-positive ***urinary glucose*** determinations by copper reduction methods (e.g., Benedict's reagent, Clinitest); tetracyclines may cause false-negative results with glucose oxidase methods (e.g., Clinistix, TesTape).

DRUG INTERACTIONS ANTACIDS, **calcium,** and **magnesium** bind tetracycline in gut and decrease absorption. ORAL ANTICOAGULANTS potentiate hypoprothrombinemia. ANTIDIARRHEAL AGENTS with kaolin and pectin may decrease absorption. Effectiveness of ORAL CONTRACEPTIVES decreased. **Methoxyflurane** may produce fatal nephrotoxicity. **Drug–food interactions:** dairy products and iron supplements decrease tetracycline absorption.

NURSING IMPLICATIONS

Administration

- Check expiration date for all tetracyclines. Fanconi-like syndrome (renal tubular dysfunction) and also an LE-like syndrome have been attributed to outdated tetracycline preparations.
- Tetracyclines decompose with age, exposure to light, and when improperly stored under conditions of extreme humidity, heat, or cold. The resultant product may be toxic. Tetracycline preparations should be stored in tightly covered containers, in a dry place, protected from light preferably between 15–30C (59–86F), unless otherwise directed by manufacturer.

Oral

- Give oral tetracyclines with a full glass of water on an empty stomach at least 1 h before or 2 h after meals (food, milk, and milk products can reduce absorption by 50% or more).
- Shake oral suspension well before pouring to ensure uniform distribution of drug. Preparation should be dispensed with a calibrated liquid measure.
- If patient is having GI symptoms (e.g., nausea, vomiting, anorexia), physician may prescribe taking oral tetracycline with food, (exception: not foods high in calcium such as milk or milk products). If symptoms persist, drug should be discontinued.
- If patient is bedridden or has diffi-

culty swallowing pills, consult physician about ordering the oral suspension formulation.

Parenteral (IM)

- IM tetracycline preparations are not to be given IV. Commerically prepared IM solution contains procaine HCl and therefore is not appropriate for IV administration.
- Ask patient if he or she is allergic to any of the "caine" local anesthetics. (Tetracycline for IM use contains 40 mg procaine HCl per vial.)
- Powder for IM injection is reconstituted by adding 2 ml sterile water for injection or 0.9% NaCl injection to 100- or 250-mg vial. Resultant solution may be stored at room temperature but should be discarded after 24 h. (Directions may vary with manufacturer.)
- Administer IM injection deep into body of a relatively large muscle mass, e.g., gluteus maximus or midlateral thigh. Alternate injection sites and observe daily for irritation and swelling.
- IM administration causes local irritation and is extremely painful.

Assessment & Drug Effects

- Culture and sensitivity tests are recommended prior to first dose and periodically to confirm susceptibility of infecting organism to tetracycline.
- Initial and periodic studies of renal, hepatic, and hematopoietic function should be performed, particularly during high-dose, long-term therapy.
- GI symptoms (e.g., nausea, vomiting, diarrhea) are generally dose-dependent, occurring mostly in patients receiving 2 g/d or more and in patients on prolonged therapy. These symptoms are associated chiefly with oral tetracycline but may occur also with parenteral preparations. GI symptoms that appear during the first few days of therapy probably are caused by direct drug irritation. Report to physician. Frequently, symptoms can be controlled by reducing dosage or by administration of oral drug with compatible foods.
- Be alert to evidence of superinfections (see Appendix G). Regularly inspect tongue and mucous membrane of mouth for candidiasis (thrush). Suspect superinfection if patient complains of irritation or soreness of mouth, tongue, throat, vagina, or anus or persistent itching of any area, diarrhea, or foul-smelling excreta or discharge.
- Superinfections occur most frequently in patients who are receiving prolonged tetracycline therapy, who are debilitated, or who have diabetes, leukemia, systemic LE, or lymphoma. Women taking oral contraceptives reportedly are more susceptible to vaginal candidiasis. Tetracycline should be discontinued if superinfection develops.
- Follow-up cultures should be obtained from all gonococcal infection sites 3–7 d after completion of tetracycline therapy to verify eradication of infection.
- Monitor I&O in patients receiving parenteral tetracycline. Report oliguria or any changes in appearance of urine or in I&O.
- Hepatotoxicity (sometimes associated with pancreatitis) occurs most frequently in patients receiving other hepatotoxic drugs or who have a history of renal or hepatic impairment. Periodic hepatic and renal function tests and serum tetracycline levels are recommended in these high-risk patients. Serum tetracycline concentrations should not be allowed to exceed 15 μg/ml.
- Patients with renal or hepatic impairment usually require lower

T

and less frequent doses and careful monitoring of renal and hepatic function. Serum tetracycline levels should be closely monitored.

Patient & Family Education

- Instruct to report the onset of diarrhea to physician. It is important to determine whether diarrhea is due to irritating drug effect or to superinfections or pseudomembranous colitis (caused by overgrowth of toxin-producing bacteria: *Clostridium difficile)* (see Appendix G). The latter two conditions can be life threatening and require immediate discontinuation of tetracycline and prompt initiation of symptomatic and supportive therapy.
- The incidence of superinfection (see Appendix G) may be reduced by meticulous care of mouth, skin, and perineal area. Encourage patient to rinse mouth of food debris after eating; advise daily flossing and use of a soft-bristled toothbrush. Instruct patient to wash hands several times a day, particularly after each bowel movement and before eating.
- Warn to avoid direct exposure to sunlight while taking tetracycline and for a few days after therapy is terminated to reduce possibility of photosensitivity reaction. The reaction appears like an exaggerated sunburn. It starts within a few minutes to hours following sun exposure and may begin with paresthesias (tingling, burning sensation).
- Advise patients on long-term therapy to report immediately the onset of severe headache or visual disturbances. These are possible symptoms of increased intracranial pressure and necessitate prompt discontinuation of tetracycline to prevent irreversible loss of vision.
- Tetracycline therapy for brucellosis or spirochetal infections may cause a Jarisch-Herxheimer reaction. Symptoms are believed to be caused by release of endotoxins from phagocytized organisms. The reaction is usually mild and appears abruptly within 6–24 h after initiation of therapy. It is manifested by malaise, fever, chills, headache, adenopathy, leukocytosis, exacerbation of skin lesions, arthralgia, transient hypotension. Treatment is symptomatic; recovery generally occurs within 24 h.
- Esophagitis and esophageal ulceration have been associated with bedtime administration of tetracycline capsules or tablets with insufficient fluid, particularly to patients with hiatal hernia or esophageal problems. Sudden onset of painful or difficult swallowing (dysphagia) should be reported immediately to physician.
- Avoid contact of topical medication with eyes, nose, or mouth. Warn patient that tetracycline may stain clothing.
- Clean affected skin area with soap and water; rinse and dry well before application of topical tetracycline, unless otherwise directed.
- Some patients experience stinging and burning sensation with topical applications. Advise to report symptoms to physician if they become pronounced or persist or if infection worsens.
- Skin treated with topical drug will exhibit bright yellow to green fluorescence under ultraviolet light and "black light."
- Topicycline contains a sulfite that can cause an allergic reaction (itching, wheezing, anaphylaxis) in susceptible persons, e.g., asth-

T

matics or atopic (allergic) individuals.
- Most patients respond to acne therapy in 2–8 wk, but maximal results may not be apparent for up to 12 wk of therapy.

TETRAHYDROZOLINE HYDROCHLORIDE

(tet-ra-hye-drozz′a-leen)

Trade names: Collyrium, Malazine, Murine Plus, Optigene, Soothe, Tyzine, Visine

Classifications: EYE, EAR, NOSE, AND THROAT PREPARATION; VASOCONSTRICTOR; DECONGESTANT

Prototype: Naphazoline

Pregnancy category: C

ACTIONS/PHARMACODYNAMICS Related to naphazoline. In common with naphazoline, has more marked alpha-adrenergic than beta-adrenergic activity; large doses cause CNS depression rather than the stimulation produced by other sympathomimetic amines.

USES Symptomatic relief of minor eye irritation and allergies and for nasopharyngeal congestion of allergic or inflammatory origin.

ROUTE & DOSAGE

Decongestant

Adult: **Ophthalmic** See Appendix A. **Nasal** 2–4 drops of 0.1% solution or spray in each nostril q3h prn.
Child: **Nasal** ≥ *6 y*, same as for adult; *2–6 y*, 2–4 drops of 0.05% solution or spray in each nostril q3h prn.

CONTRAINDICATIONS & PRECAUTIONS **Contraindicated in:** hypersensitivity to any component; use of ophthalmic preparation in glaucoma or other serious eye diseases; use of drug in children < 2 y; use of 0.1% or higher strengths in children < 6 y; use within 14 d of MAO inhibitor therapy. Safe use during pregnancy (category C) not established. **Cautious use in:** hypertension; cardiovascular disease; hyperthyroidism; diabetes mellitus; young children.

ADVERSE/SIDE EFFECTS *Transient stinging,* irritation, *sneezing,* dryness, headache, tremors, drowsiness, lightheadedness, insomnia, palpitation. **Overdosage:** CNS depression (marked drowsiness, sweating, coma, hypotension, shock, bradycardia).

NURSING IMPLICATIONS

Administration
- Since drug action lasts 4–8 h, interval between doses is at least 4–6 h.
- When using squeeze bottle, patient should be in upright position. When patient is reclining, a stream rather than a spray may be ejected, with consequent overdosage.
- Nasal drops are usually administered in lateral, head-low position.

Patient & Family Education
- Instruct to discontinue medication and to consult physician if relief is not obtained within 48 h or if symptoms for which drug was given persist or increase.
- Caution not to exceed recommended dosage. Rebound congestion and rhinitis may occur with frequent or prolonged use of nasal preparation.

THALIDOMIDE

(tha-lid′o-mide)

Trade name: Thalomid

Classifications: IMMUNOSUPPRES-

SIVE AGENT; CNS AGENT; SEDATIVE-HYPNOTIC AGENT
Pregnancy category: X

ACTIONS/PHARMACODYNAMICS Mechanism of action in inducing immunosuppression is unknown. However, it has several antiinflammatory and immunologic actions. Inhibits neutrophil chemotaxis and decreases monocyte phagocytosis. Is involved in suppression of excessive tumor necrosis factor-alpha (TNF-alpha) production. In addition it reduces helper T cells and increases suppressor T cells.

USES Acute and maintenance treatment of cutaneous manifestations of moderate to severe erythema nodosum leprosum. **Unlabeled use:** stimulate appetite in patients with HIV-associated cachexia.

ROUTE & DOSAGE

Erythema Nodosum Leprosum
Adult: **PO** 100–300 mg q.d (max 400 mg/d) × at least 2 wk.
Child 11–17 y: **PO** 100 mg q.d.

PHARMACOKINETICS Absorption: slowly absorbed from GI tract. **Peak:** 2.9–5.7 h. **Distribution:** crosses placenta; unknown if present in ejaculate in males. **Metabolism:** does not appear to be hepatically metabolized. **Elimination:** half-life: 6–7.5 h.

CONTRAINDICATIONS & PRECAUTIONS Contraindicated in: hypersensitivity to thalidomide; peripheral neuropathy; pregnancy (category X); lactation. **Cautious use in:** liver and kidney disease; CHF or hypertension; constipation or other GI disorders; neurologic disorders or history of neuritis.

ADVERSE/SIDE EFFECTS Body as whole: asthenia, back pain, chills, facial edema, *fever,* malaise, pain. **CNS:** drowsiness, *somnolence,* peripheral neuropathy (possibly irreversible), *dizziness,* orthostatic hypotension, headache, agitation, insomnia, nervousness, paresthesia, tremor, vertigo. **CV:** bradycardia, peripheral edema, hyperlipidemia. **GI:** abdominal pain, anorexia, constipation, *diarrhea,* dry mouth, flatulence, abnormal liver function tests, nausea, oral moniliasis. **Hematologic:** neutropenia, anemia, *leukopenia,* lymphadenopathy. **Respiratory:** pharyngitis, rhinitis, sinusitis. **Skin:** *rash,* acne, nail disorder, fungal dermatitis, pruritus, sweating. **Other:** hypersensitivity reaction (rash, fever, tachycardia, hypotension), teratogenicity, HIV viral load increase, infection, albuminuria, hematuria, impotence.

DRUG INTERACTIONS Enhances sedation associated with BARBITURATES, **alcohol, chlorpromazine, reserpine.**

NURSING IMPLICATIONS

Administration

- Give at bedtime and at least 1 h after the evening meal.
- Give this drug only to persons who understand and have signed the required consent form.
- Prior to administration, verify that this drug was prescribed and dispensed only by persons registered by the STEPS (System for Thalidomide Education and Prescribing Safety) program.
- Store at 15–30C (59–86F) and protect from light.

Assessment & Drug Effects

- Therapeutic effectiveness is indicated by control of cutaneous

T

manifestations of erythema nodosum leprosum.
- Lab tests: Prior to therapy and periodically thereafter, monitor WBC with differential.
- Carefully monitor for and immediately report S&S of peripheral neuropathy. Discontinue drug and notify prescriber if peripheral neuropathy is suspected.

Patient & Family Education
- Under no circumstances should this medication be shared with anyone.
- Effective methods of birth control must be used by women and men 1 mo before, during, and 1 mo following discontinuation of thalidomide therapy. Men must use latex condoms when engaging in sexual activity.
- Exercise caution while engaging in hazardous activities as drug may cause dizziness.
- Immediately report pain, numbness, or tingling in the hands or feet.

THEOPHYLLINE
(thee-off'i-lin)

Trade names: Bronkodyl, Elixophyllin, Lanophyllin, PMS Theophylline ♣, Pulmopylline ♣, Quibron-T, Respbid, Slo-Bid, Slo-Phyllin, Somophyllin, Somophyllin-12 ♣, Theo-Dur, Theo-24, Theolair, Theospan-SR, Uni-Dur, Uniphyl, and others

THEOPHYLLINE SODIUM GLYCINATE

Trade name: Synophylate

Prototype for classifications: BRONCHODILATOR (RESPIRATORY SMOOTH MUSCLE RELAXANT); CNS AGENT; RESPIRATORY AND CEREBRAL STIMULANT; XANTHINE

Pregnancy category: C

ACTIONS/PHARMACODYNAMICS

Xanthine derivative that relaxes smooth muscle by direct action, particularly of bronchi and pulmonary vessels, and stimulates medullary respiratory center with resulting increase in vital capacity. Also relaxes smooth muscles of biliary and GI tracts. Stimulates myocardium, thereby increasing force of contractions and cardiac output, and stimulates all levels of CNS, but to a lesser degree than caffeine.

USES Prophylaxis and symptomatic relief of bronchial asthma, as well as bronchospasm associated with chronic bronchitis and emphysema. Also used for emergency treatment of paroxysmal cardiac dyspnea and edema of CHF. **Unlabeled uses:** treatment of apnea and bradycardia of prematures and to reduce severe bronchospasm associated with cystic fibrosis and acute descending respiratory infection. Theophylline sodium glycinate is a mixture of sodium theophylline and aminoacetic (glycine). Contains 45–47% theophylline. Similar actions, uses, adverse reactions, and precautions as other theophylline derivatives but claimed to produce less gastric irritation.

ROUTE & DOSAGE

Bronchospasm (all doses based on ideal body weight)

Loading Dose

Adult/Child: **PO/IV** 5 mg/kg loading dose.

Maintenance Dose*

Adult nonsmoker: **PO/IV** 0.4 mg/kg/h. *Adult smoker:* **PO/IV** 0.6 mg/kg/h. *Adult with CHF or cirrhosis:* **PO/IV** 0.2 mg/kg/h.

Child: **PO/IV** 10–12 y, 0.6 mg/kg/h; 1–9 y, 0.8 mg/kg/h.
Infant: **PO/IV** 6–11 mo, 0.7 mg/kg/h; 2–6 mo, 0.4 mg/kg/h.
Neonate: **PO/IV** 0.13 mg/kg/h.

*IV by continuous infusion; PO divided q6h (immediate release) or q8–12h (sustained release)

PHARMACOKINETICS Absorption: most products are 100% absorbed from GI tract. **Peak:** IV 30 min; uncoated tablet 1 h; sustained release 4–6 h. **Duration:** 4–8 h; varies with age, smoking, and liver function. **Distribution:** crosses placenta. **Metabolism:** extensively metabolized in liver. **Elimination:** parent drug and metabolites excreted by kidneys; excreted in breast milk.

CONTRAINDICATIONS & PRECAUTIONS Contraindicated in: hypersensitivity to xanthines; coronary artery disease or angina pectoris when myocardial stimulation might be harmful; severe renal or liver impairment. Safe use during pregnancy (category C) and lactation not established. **Cautious use in:** children; compromised cardiac or circulatory function, hypertension; hyperthyroidism; peptic ulcer; prostatic hypertrophy; glaucoma; diabetes mellitus; the elderly and neonates.

ADVERSE/SIDE EFFECTS CNS: (stimulation): irritability, restlessness, insomnia, dizziness, headache, tremor, hyperexcitability, muscle twitching, drug-induced seizures. **CV:** palpitation, *tachycardia,* extrasystoles, flushing, marked hypotension, circulatory failure. **GI:** *nausea*, vomiting, anorexia, epigastric or abdominal pain, diarrhea, activation of peptic ulcer. **Renal:** transient urinary frequency, albuminuria, kidney irritation. **Respiratory:** tachypnea, respiratory arrest. **Other:** fever, dehydration, possibility of increased urinary catecholamine excretion.

DIAGNOSTIC TEST INTERFERENCE False-positive elevations of ***serum uric acid*** (Bittner or colorimetric methods). ***Probenecid*** may cause false high serum theophylline readings, and spectrophotometric methods of determining ***serum theophylline*** are affected by a furosemide, sulfathiazole, phenylbutazone, probenecid, theobromine.

DRUG INTERACTIONS Increases **lithium** excretion, lowering lithium levels; **cimetidine,** high-dose **allopurinol** (600 mg/d), **tacrine,** QUINOLONES, MACROLIDE ANTIBIOTICS, and **zileuton** can significantly increase theophylline levels.

INCOMPATIBILITIES Solution/additive: amikacin, bleomycin, CEPHALOSPORINS, **chlorpromazine, clindamycin, codeine phosphate, dimenhydrinate, dobutamine, dopamine, doxapram, doxorubicin, epinephrine, hydralazine, hydroxyzine, insulin, isoproterenol, levorphanol, meperidine, methadone, methylprednisolone, morphine, nafcillin, norepinephrine, oxytetracycline, papaverine, penicillin G, pentazocine, procaine, prochlorperazine, promazine, promethazine, tetracycline, verapamil, vitamin B complex with C. Y-site: amiodarone, codeine phosphate, clindamycin,** PHENOTHIAZINES (**chlorpromazine, prochlorperazine,** etc), **epinephrine, dobutamine, dopamine, levorphanol, meperidine, methadone, morphine, norepinephrine, verapamil.**

NURSING IMPLICATIONS

Administration

- Oral preparations should be administered with a full glass of water and may be given after meals to minimize gastric irritation.
- Sustained-release forms and enteric-coated tablets must be swallowed whole. Chewable tablets must be chewed thoroughly before swallowing. Slow-release theophylline Sprinkle granules can be taken on an empty stomach or mixed with applesauce or water.
- Timing of dose is critical. Be certain patient understands the necessity to adhere to the proper intervals between doses.

Parenteral (IV)

- IV solution of 100% theophylline is available in D5W in concentrations of 4 mg/ml, 2 mg/ml, 1.6 mg/ml, 0.8 mg/ml, and 0.4 mg/ml. Administer at a rate not to exceed 20 mg/min.
- IV theophylline ethylenediamine solution with a concentration of 25 mg/ml may be given undiluted by direct IV at a rate of 20 mg/min or diluted in up to 200 ml of D5W and infused over 30 min.

Assessment & Drug Effects

- Therapeutic theophylline plasma level ranges from 10–20 μg/ml (a narrow therapeutic range). Levels exceeding 20 μg/ml are associated with toxicity.
- Cigarette smoking induces hepatic microsomal enzyme activity, decreasing serum half-life and increasing body clearance of theophylline. This effect requires close monitoring of drug level in the heavy smoker. An increase of dosage from 50–100% is usual in heavy smokers.
- During early therapy, dizziness is a relatively common side effect in the elderly. Take necessary safety precautions and forewarn patient of this possibility.
- Monitor vital signs and I&O. Improvement in quality of pulse and respiration and diuresis are expected clinical effects.
- Observe and report early signs of possible toxicity: anorexia, nausea, vomiting, dizziness, shakiness, restlessness, abdominal discomfort, irritability, palpitation, tachycardia, marked hypotension, cardiac arrhythmias, seizures.
- If theophylline is given to a patient with severe cardiac disease, monitor for tachycardia. Conversely, theophylline toxicity may be masked in patients with tachycardia.
- Plasma clearance of xanthines may be reduced in patients with heart failure, renal or hepatic dysfunction, alcoholism, high fever. Dosage regulation must be closely monitored particularly in these patients.
- Overdose with prolonged release preparation necessitates observing patient for a longer period of time than if conventional formulation had been ingested. Continued slow absorption leads to high plasma concentrations for a prolonged period.
- In the neonate of a mother using this drug, slight tachycardia, jitteriness, and apnea have been observed.
- Theophylline metabolism in the infant <6 mo and in prematures is prolonged as is the half-life; therefore, close monitoring for side effects is especially crucial in this age group.

Patient & Family Education

- Take medication at the same time every day.

T

- Charcoal-broiled foods (high in polycyclic carbon content) may increase theophylline elimination and reduce the half-life as much as 50%.
- Limit caffeine intake, which may increase incidence of adverse effects.
- Inform that cigarette smoking may significantly lower theophylline plasma concentration.
- A low-carbohydrate, high-protein diet increases theophylline elimination, and a high-carbohydrate, low-protein diet decreases it.
- Urge to drink adequate fluids (at least 2000 ml/d) to decrease viscosity of airway secretions.
- Warn to avoid self-dosing with OTC medications, especially cough suppressants, which may cause retention of secretions and CNS depression.
- Since theophylline is distributed into breast milk, it may be advisable for the infant to be nursed just before mother takes the drug.

THIABENDAZOLE

(thye-a-ben'da-zole)

Trade name: Mintezol

Classifications: ANTIINFECTIVE; ANTHELMINTIC

Prototype: Mebendazole

Pregnancy category: C

ACTIONS/PHARMACODYNAMICS Benzimidazole with vermicidal properties; structurally related to mebendazole. Precise action mechanism not clear but has wide spectrum of anthelmintic activity. Has been shown to inhibit helminth-specific enzyme fumarate reductase. Demonstrates antiinflammatory, antipyretic, and analgesic effects in animals. Suppresses production of eggs or larvae by some parasites and may inhibit subsequent development of eggs or larvae passed in feces.

USES Enterobiasis (pinworm infestation), ascariasis (roundworm), strongyloidiasis (threadworm), cutaneous larva migrans (creeping eruption), and hookworm infestations caused by *Ancyclostoma duodenale* or *Necator americanus*. Used during invasive stage of trichinosis to relieve symptoms and for mixed helminthic infestations.

ROUTE & DOSAGE

Enterobiasis, Ascariasis, Strongyloidiasis, Hookworm

Adult: **PO** *<70 kg,* 25 mg/kg b.i.d. x 2 d; *>70 kg,* 1.5 g b.i.d. (max 3 g/d) x 2 d.
Child 14–70 kg: **PO** 25 mg/kg b.i.d. x 2 d.

PHARMACOKINETICS Absorption: readily absorbed from GI tract. **Peak:** 1–2 h. **Metabolism:** metabolized in liver. **Elimination:** > 90% excreted in urine; 5% in feces.

CONTRAINDICATIONS & PRECAUTIONS Contraindicated in: safe use during pregnancy (category C) and in nursing mothers not established. **Cautious use in:** hepatic or renal dysfunction, when vomiting can be dangerous, severe dehydration or malnutrition, anemia, children weighing < 15 kg.

ADVERSE/SIDE EFFECTS CNS: weariness, *dizziness*, drowsiness, headache. **CV:** hypotension, bradycardia. **GI:** *anorexia, nausea, vomiting,* epigastric distress, jaundice, cholestasis, parenchymal liver damage, diarrhea, perianal rash. **Renal:** malodor of urine, crystalluria, hematuria,

T

nephrotoxicity, enuresis. **Other:** transient rise in AST, transient leukopenia, hypersensitivity, hyperglycemia, pruritus.

NURSING IMPLICATIONS

Administration

- Administer drug after meals. Tablets should be chewed before they are swallowed. Shake suspension well before pouring.

Assessment & Drug Effects

- If patient is anemic, dehydrated, or malnourished, supportive treatment is indicated prior to start of thiabendazole therapy.
- Adverse/side effects generally occur 3–4 h after administration, are mild, and last for 2–8 h. Incidence tends to be related to dose and duration of treatment.
- Drug should be discontinued immediately if there are symptoms of hypersensitivity: fever, facial flush, chills, conjunctival infection, skin rashes, erythema multiforme (including Stevens-Johnson syndrome), which can be fatal.

Patient & Family Education

- CNS side effects occur frequently and may prevent the patient from driving a car or engaging in activities requiring mental alertness. Warn patient of the possibility.

T

THIAMINE HYDROCHLORIDE (VITAMIN B_1)

(thye′a-min)

Trade names: Betalins, Bewon ♣, Biamine

Classification: VITAMIN B

Pregnancy category: A

ACTIONS/PHARMACODYNAMICS Water-soluble vitamin and member of B-complex group. Functions as an essential coenzyme in carbohydrate metabolism. Also has role in conversion of tryptophan to nicotinamide.

USES Treatment and prophylaxis of beriberi, to correct anorexia due to thiamine deficiency states, and in treatment of neuritis associated with pregnancy, pellagra, and alcoholism, including Wernicke-Korsakoff syndrome. Therapy generally includes other members of vitamin B complex, since thiamine deficiency rarely occurs alone.

ROUTE & DOSAGE

Thiamine Deficiency

Adult: **IV/IM** 50–100 mg t.i.d.
Child: **IV/IM** 10–25 mg t.i.d.

Beriberi

Adult: **IV/IM** 10–500 mg t.i.d. for 2 wk.
Child: **IV/IM** 10–50 mg t.i.d.

Dietary Supplement

Adult: **PO** 15–30 mg/d.
Child: **PO** 10–50 mg/d.

PHARMACOKINETICS Absorption: limited absorption from GI tract. **Distribution:** widely distributed, including into breast milk. **Elimination:** excreted in urine.

ADVERSE/SIDE EFFECTS Feeling of warmth, weakness, urticaria, pruritus, sweating, nausea, restlessness, tightness of throat, angioneurotic edema, cyanosis, pulmonary edema, GI hemorrhage, cardiovascular collapse, anaphylaxis. Following rapid IV administration: slight fall in BP.

INCOMPATIBILITIES Solution/additive: amobarbital, diazepam, erythromycin, furosemide, phenobarbital.

NURSING IMPLICATIONS

Administration

- IM injections may be painful. Rotate sites and apply cold compresses to area if necessary for relief of discomfort.
- IV thiamine may be given by direct IV undiluted at a rate of 100 mg over 5 min. May also be added to IV solutions and infused at ordered rate.
- Preserve in tight, light-resistant, nonmetallic containers. Thiamine is unstable in alkaline solutions (e.g., solutions of acetates, barbiturates, bicarbonates, carbonates, citrates) and neutral solutions.

Assessment & Drug Effects

- Intradermal test dose is recommended prior to administration in suspected thiamine sensitivity. Deaths have occurred following IV use.
- Careful recording of patient's dietary history is an essential part of vitamin replacement therapy. Collaborate with physician, dietitian, patient, and responsible family member in developing a diet teaching plan that can be sustained by patient.
- Therapeutic effectiveness is evaluated by improvement of clinical manifestations of thiamine deficiency: anorexia, gastric distress, depression, irritability, insomnia, palpitations, tachycardia, loss of memory, paresthesias, muscle weakness and pain, elevated blood pyruvic acid level (diagnostic test for thiamine deficiency), and elevated lactic acid level. Severe deficiency is characterized by ophthalmoplegia, polyneuropathy, muscle wasting ("dry" beriberi), edema, serous effusions, and CHF ("wet" beriberi).
- Body requirement of thiamine is directly proportional to carbohydrate intake and metabolic rate; thus, requirement increases when diet consists predominantly of carbohydrates. Total absence of dietary thiamine can produce a deficiency state in about 3 wk.

Patient & Family Education

- Recommended daily allowance (RDA): children 4–6 y of age, 0.9 mg; adult males, 1.4 mg; adult females, 1 mg; pregnancy and lactation, 1.4 mg.
- Food–drug relationships: Instruct patient on rich dietary sources of thiamine: yeast, pork, beef, liver, wheat and other whole grains, nutrient-added breakfast cereals, fresh vegetables, especially peas and dried beans.

THIETHYLPERAZINE MALEATE

(thye-eth-il-per'a-zeen)

Trade name: Torecan

Classifications: GI AGENT; ANTIEMETIC

Prototype: Prochlorperazine

Pregnancy category: X

ACTIONS/PHARMACODYNAMICS
Piperazine phenothiazine derivative with contraindications, precautions, and toxic effects similar to those of prochlorperazine. Reported to have higher ratio of antiemetic action to tranquilizing action than other phenothiazines. Acts directly on chemoreceptor trigger zone as well as the vomiting center.

USE To control nausea and vomiting. **Unlabeled use:** treatment of vertigo.

ROUTE & DOSAGE

Nausea and Vomiting
Adult: **PO/PR/IM** 10 mg 1–3 times/d.

T

PHARMACOKINETICS Onset: 1 h PO, PR; 30 min IM.

CONTRAINDICATIONS & PRECAUTIONS Contraindicated in: hypersensitivity to phenothiazines, CNS depression or comatose states, pregnancy (category X), IV administration. Safe use in children < 12 y, in nursing mothers, or following intracardiac or intracranial surgery not established. **Cautious use in:** renal or hepatic disease.

ADVERSE/SIDE EFFECTS *Drowsiness,* dizziness, headache, *dry mouth and nose,* blurred vision, tinnitus, restlessness, fever, orthostatic hypotension. Occasionally: extrapyramidal symptoms including convulsions; sialorrhea with altered taste sensations, cholestatic jaundice.

NURSING IMPLICATIONS

Administration

- Examine parenteral solution and administer only if it is clear and colorless.
- Patient should be recumbent when drug is being administered IM. Postural hypotension (manifested by weakness, light-headedness, faintness) and drowsiness may occur, particularly after initial injection. Advise patient to remain in bed for about 1 h or longer, if indicated, and supervise ambulation. If vasopressor agent is required, levarterenol or phenylephrine is used. Epinephrine is contraindicated.
- Administer IM deep into large muscle mass and aspirate hypodermic carefully before injecting drug to avoid inadvertent entry into a blood vessel. IV administration is specifically contraindicated because it can cause severe hypotension.
- Store at room temperature, away from heat, in light-resistant containers. Suppositories should be stored below 25C (77F).

Assessment & Drug Effects

- Patients who have received drug preoperatively may manifest restlessness or depression during anesthesia recovery.
- Report immediately the onset of extrapyramidal effects: gait disturbances, difficulty in speaking, muscle spasms, torticollis, deviations in eye movements. Reduction in dosage or discontinuation of medication is indicated.

Patient & Family Education

- Caution to avoid potentially hazardous activities such as driving a car or operating machinery because of possibility of drowsiness and dizziness.

THIMEROSAL

(thye-mer'oh-sal)

Trade names: Mersol, Merthiolate

Classifications: SKIN AND MUCOUS MEMBRANE AGENT; ANTIINFECTIVE

Pregnancy category: C

ACTIONS/PHARMACODYNAMICS Topical organic mercurial with sustained bacteriostatic and fungistatic activity. Ineffective against spore-forming organisms.

USES First-aid treatment of contaminated wounds, in antisepsis of intact skin, before surgery, and in pustular dermatosis; as antifungal agent in athlete's foot for wound irrigations. Ophthalmic preparation is used to treat conjunctivitis and corneal ulcer and for prevention of infection following removal of foreign bodies. Used as preservative in most solutions sold for cleaning, wetting, soaking, and storage of contact lenses; also used as preser-

T

vative for biologic and pharmaceutical products.

ROUTE & DOSAGE

Antiseptic
Adult: **Topical** 1:1000 solution—apply locally 1–3 times/d.

CONTRAINDICATIONS & PRECAUTIONS **Contraindicated in:** history of sensitivity to thio or mercurial compounds, prolonged use, pregnancy (category C).

ADVERSE/SIDE EFFECTS **Hypersensitivity:** itching erythema, papular or vesicular eruptions. **Prolonged use:** mercury poisoning (metallic taste, salivation, stomatitis, lethargy, peripheral neuropathy).

NURSING IMPLICATIONS

Administration

- For first-aid treatment, appropriate cleansing should precede application of antiseptic.
- To prevent skin irritation, do not apply bandage or other occlusive dressing until tincture application has completely dried.
- Thimerosal is antagonized by whole blood and is incompatible when used concurrently or following applications of boric acid, iodine, strong acids, aluminum, silver, or other salts of heavy metals. It is compatible with sulfonamides.
- Preserve in tightly covered, light-resistant containers. Avoid exposure to excessive heat.

Assessment & Drug Effects

- Aqueous Merthiolate contains thimerosal and borate (0.14%). Both are toxic if absorbed systemically.
- Long-term use, especially as treatment of otitis media, may lead to potentially fatal toxicity due to inadvertent swallowing of solution.

THIOGUANINE (TG, 6-THIOGUANINE)

(thye-oh-gwah'neen)
Trade name: Lanvis ♣
Classifications: ANTINEOPLASTIC; ANTIMETABOLITE
Prototype: Fluorouracil
Pregnancy category: X

ACTIONS/PHARMACODYNAMICS
Antimetabolite and purine antagonist with immunosuppressive activity. A highly toxic drug with a low therapeutic index; therapeutic response is normally accompanied by evidence of toxicity. Delays myelosuppression; has potential mutagenic and carcinogenic properties.

USES In combination with other antineoplastics for remission induction in acute myelogenous leukemia and as treatment of chronic myelogenous leukemia. Has little advantage over mercaptopurine.

ROUTE & DOSAGE

Leukemia
Adult: **PO** 2 mg/kg/d; may increase to 3 mg/kg/d if no response after 4 wk.

PHARMACOKINETICS **Absorption:** variable and incomplete absorption from GI tract. **Peak:** 8 h. **Distribution:** crosses placenta. **Metabolism:** metabolized in liver. **Elimination:** half-life: 11 h; excreted in urine.

ADVERSE/SIDE EFFECTS **Hematologic:** <u>leukopenia, thombocytopenia</u>, anemia. **Hepatic:** jaundice. **Other:** *hyperuricemia,* nausea, vomiting, anorexia, stomatitis, diarrhea.

T

NURSING IMPLICATIONS

Administration

- Because there is no known antagonist to thioguanine, prompt discontinuation of the drug is essential in avoiding irreversible myelosuppression when toxicity develops.
- Store in airtight container at 15–30C (59–86F).

Assessment & Drug Effects

- Blood counts are determined weekly; monitor reports as indicators for adaptations in drug regimens.
- Patient receiving this drug experiences an increased incidence of infections and possibly hemorrhage complications. Therapy should be discontinued at first sign of altered blood cell counts.
- Monitor I&O ratio and report oliguria.
- Observe patient's skin and sclera for jaundice. It is thought to be a reversible clinical sign, but it should be reported promptly as a symptom of toxicity; drug will be discontinued promptly.
- Expect that the leukocyte count descent may be slow over a period of 2–4 wk. Treatment is interrupted if there is a rapid fall within a few days.

Patient & Family Education

- Maintenance doses are continued throughout remissions.

T

THIOPENTAL SODIUM

(thye-oh-pen′tal)

Trade name: Pentothal

Prototype for classifications: CNS AGENT; GENERAL ANESTHETIC; SEDATIVE-HYPNOTIC; BARBITURATE

Pregnancy category: C

Controlled substance: Schedule III

ACTIONS/PHARMACODYNAMICS

Ultrashort-acting barbiturate that induces brief general anesthesia without analgesia by depression of CNS. Loss of consciousness is rapid. Reduction in cardiac output and peripheral vasodilation frequently accompany anesthesia. Rapid redistribution of agent out of brain reduces anesthesia level and increases reflex airway hyperactivity to mechanical stimulation. Muscle relaxation is slight, and reflexes are poorly controlled. Since analgesia is slight, thiopental is seldom used alone except for brief minor procedures.

USES To induce hypnosis and anesthesia prior to or as supplement to other anesthetic agents or as sole agent for brief (15-min) operative procedures. Also used as an anticonvulsant and sedative-hypnotic and for narcoanalysis and narcosynthesis in psychiatric disorders.

ROUTE & DOSAGE

Induction

Adult: **IV** test dose of 25–75 mg; then 50–75 mg at 20–40 s intervals; an additional 50 mg may be given if needed.
Child: **IV** 3–5 mg/kg initially, followed by 1 mg/kg if needed.
Infant: **IV** 5–8 mg/kg.
Neonate: **IV** 3–4 mg/kg.

Convulsions

Adult: **IV** 75–125 mg.
Child: **IV** 2–3 mg/kg.

Narcoanalysis

Adult: **IV** 100 mg/min until confusion occurs.

PHARMACOKINETICS **Onset:** 30–60 s. **Duration:** 10–30 min. **Distribution:** distributed into muscle and liver;

crosses placenta. **Metabolism:** metabolized in liver. **Elimination:** half-life: 12 min; excreted in urine.

CONTRAINDICATIONS & PRECAUTIONS **Absolute contraindications:** hypersensitivity to barbiturates, history of paradoxic excitation, absence of suitable veins for IV administration, status asthmaticus, acute intermittent or other hepatic porphyrias. Safe use during pregnancy (category C), in nursing women, and in children not established. **Cautious use in:** coronary artery disease, hypotension, shock; conditions that may potentiate or prolong hypnotic effect including excessive premedication, hepatic or renal dysfunction, myxedema, Addison's disease, severe anemia, increased BUN; increased intracranial pressure; myasthenia gravis; asthma and other respiratory diseases.

ADVERSE/SIDE EFFECTS **CNS:** headache, retrograde amnesia, emergence delirium, prolonged somnolence and recovery. **CV:** myocardial depression, arrhythmias, circulatory depression. **GI:** nausea, vomiting, regurgitation of gastric contents. **Rectal:** irritation, cramping, rectal bleeding, diarrhea. **Respiratory:** respiratory depression with apnea; hiccups, sneezing, coughing, bronchospasm, laryngospasm. **Other:** hypersensitivity reactions, anaphylaxis (rare), hypothermia, thrombosis and sloughing (with extravasation); salivation, shivering, skeletal muscle hyperactivity.

DIAGNOSTIC TEST INTERFERENCE ***Thiopental*** may cause decrease in ***^{123}I and ^{131}I thyroidal uptake*** test results.

DRUG INTERACTIONS CNS DEPRESSANTS potentiate CNS and respiratory depression. PHENOTHIAZINES increase risk of hypotension. **Probenecid** may prolong anesthesia.

INCOMPATIBILITIES **Solution/additive:** DEXTROSE RINGER'S COMBINATIONS, **10% dextrose, amikacin, cephapirin, codeine phosphate, dimenhydrinate, diphenhydramine, ephedrine, fibrinolysin, hydromorphone, insulin, levorphanol, meperidine, metaraminol, methadone, morphine, norepinephrine, penicillin G, prochlorperazine, promazine, promethazine, succinylcholine, tetracycline, benzquinamide, chlorpromazine, doxapram, glycopyrrolate, sodium bicarbonate.**

NURSING IMPLICATIONS

Administration

- Test dose may be given to assess unusual sensitivity to thiopental. Following administration, patient should be observed for at least 1 min for unexpected deep anesthesia or respiratory depression.
- Reconstitution: To each 500 mg thiopental powder add at least 20 ml of sterile water for injection to produce a 2.5% solution (25 mg/1 ml).
- IV preparation: Add 20 ml of reconstituted solution to at least 100 ml of 0.9% NaCl or D5W.
- IV infusion: Infuse each 25 mg over 1 min or more. Do not infuse solution with a concentration <2.5%. If concentration is <2%; such a solution causes hemolysis.
- Solution should be freshly prepared and used promptly. If a precipitate is present, discard solution. Unused portions should be discarded within 24 h.
- IV administration to neonates, infants, children: Verify correct IV concentration and rate of infusion with physician.
- If intraarterial injection or extrava-

T

sation occurs, the site will require particular attention to prevent arteritis, neuritis, and skin slough. An intraarterial injection usually causes extreme pain before patient loses consciousness. Consult physician.

- Store at room temperature 15–30C (59–86F). Avoid excessive heat; protect from freezing.

Assessment & Drug Effects

- Monitor vital signs q3–5min before, during, and after anesthetic administration until recovery and into postoperative period, if necessary.
- Hypovolemia, cranial trauma, or premedication with opioids increases potential for apnea and symptoms of myocardial depression (decreased cardiac output and arterial pressure). Report increases in pulse rate or drop in blood pressure.
- Shivering, excitement, muscle twitching may develop during recovery period from thiopental anesthesia if patient is in pain.

Patient & Family Education

- Inform that onset of drug effect is rapid, with loss of consciousness within 30–60 s.

THIORIDAZINE HYDROCHLORIDE

T

(thye-or-rid'a-zeen)

Trade names: Mellaril, Novoridazine ♣

Classifications: CNS AGENT; PSYCHOTHERAPEUTIC; PHENOTHIAZINE ANTIPSYCHOTIC

Prototype: Chlorpromazine

Pregnancy category: C

ACTIONS/PHARMACODYNAMICS Phenothiazine with actions, uses, limitations, and interactions similar to those of chlorpromazine. Rarely produces extrapyramidal effects. Has weak antiemetic but strong anticholinergic and alpha-adrenergic agonist activity and potent sedative action.

USES Management of nonpsychotic behavioral disturbances of senility, manifestations of psychotic disorders, alcohol withdrawal; symptomatic treatment of organic brain disease. Short-term treatment of moderate to marked depression and for management of hyperkinetic behavior syndrome (attention deficit disorder).

ROUTE & DOSAGE

Psychotic Disorders

Adult: **PO** 50–100 mg t.i.d.; may increase up to 800 mg/d as needed or tolerated. *Elderly:* **PO** 10 mg t.i.d.; may increase up to 200 mg/d.
Child > *2 y:* **PO** 0.5–3 mg/kg/d in divided doses; if hospitalized, may start at 25 mg t.i.d.

Moderate to Marked Depression

Adult: **PO** 25 mg t.i.d.; may increase up to 200 mg/d in divided doses.

Dementia Behavior

Geriatric: **PO** 10–25 mg 1–2 times/d, may increase q4–7 d to max of 400 mg/d in divided doses.

PHARMACOKINETICS Absorption: well absorbed from GI tract. **Onset:** days to weeks. **Distribution:** crosses placenta; distributed into breast milk. **Metabolism:** metabolized in liver. **Elimination:** half-life: 26–36 h; excreted in urine.

CONTRAINDICATIONS & PRECAUTIONS Contraindicated in: hypersensitivity to phenothiazines. Severe CNS depression, CV disease, children < 2 y. Safe use during pregnancy (category C) and in nursing mothers not established. **Cautious use in:** premature ventricular contractions; previously diagnosed breast cancer; patients exposed to extremes in heat or to organophosphorous insecticides; respiratory disorders.

ADVERSE/SIDE EFFECTS **CNS:** *Sedation,* dizziness, drowsiness, lethargy, nasal congestion, blurred vision, pigmentary retinopathy. **GI:** xerostomia, *constipation,* paralytic ileus. **Reproductive:** amenorrhea, breast engorgement, gynecomastia, galactorrhea. **CV:** ventricular dysrhythmias, hypotension. **Renal:** *urinary retention.* Infrequent: extrapyramidal syndrome, nocturnal confusion, hyperactivity.

DRUG INTERACTIONS **Alcohol** and other CNS DEPRESSANTS add to CNS depression.

NURSING IMPLICATIONS

Administration

- Tablet may be crushed before administration and taken with fluid of patient's choice.
- If the patient is also receiving antacid or antidiarrheal medication, schedule the phenothiazine to be taken at least 1 h before or 1 h after the other medication.
- Liquid concentrate should be diluted just prior to administration with 1/2 glass of fruit juice, milk, water, carbonated beverage, or soup.
- Increases in dose should be added to the first dose of the day to prevent sleep disturbance.
- Preserve in tightly covered, light-resistant containers at 15–30C (59–86F) unless otherwise indicated.

Assessment & Drug Effects

- Orthostatic hypotension may occur in early therapy. Female patients appear to be more susceptible than male patients.
- The patient may be unable to adjust to extremes of temperature because of drug effect on the heat regulatory center in the hypothalamus. Patient may complain of being cold even at average room temperature. The elderly patient is particularly susceptible to this modified regulatory function.
- If patient has been exposed to extremes in heat or has had an elevated temperature for several hours, be alert to the signs of heat stroke: red, dry, hot skin; full bounding pulse; dilated pupils; temperature above 40.6C (105F); dyspnea. Report them to physician and be prepared to institute measures to reduce temperature rapidly.
- Monitor I&O ratio and bowel elimination pattern. Check for abdominal distension and pain. Encourage adequate fluid intake as prophylaxis for constipation and xerostomia. The depressed patient may not seek help for either symptom or for urinary retention.
- Periodic blood and hepatic function tests are advised during therapy.
- Suicide is an inherent risk with any depressed patient and may remain a problem until there is significant clinical improvement. Supervise patient closely during early course of therapy. Do not permit access to more than one dose of medication and watch to see that the dose is not hoarded.

Patient & Family Education

- Explain dosage and dilution to pa-

T

tient if he or she is responsible for administration.

- Warn against spilling drug on skin or clothing because of danger of contact dermatitis. Wash skin well in soap and water if liquid drug is spilled.
- Counsel to take drug as prescribed and not to alter dosing regimen or stop medication without consulting physician.
- Alcohol should be avoided during phenothiazine therapy. Concomitant use enhances CNS depression effects.
- Marked drowsiness generally subsides with continued therapy or reduction in dosage.
- Caution to avoid potentially hazardous activities such as driving a car or operating machinery until reaction to drug is known.
- Advise to make position changes slowly, particularly from recumbent to upright posture, and to dangle legs a few minutes before standing. Also inform patient that vasodilation produced by hot showers or baths or by long exposure to environmental heat may accentuate hypotensive effect.
- Do not apply heating pad or hot water bottles to the body for external heat. Because of depressed conditioned avoidance behaviors, a severe burn may result.
- Instruct to report to physician the onset of any change in visual acuity, brownish coloring of vision, or impairment of night vision. These symptoms suggest pigmentary retinopathy (observed primarily in patients receiving extremely high doses). An ophthalmic consultation may be indicated.
- Thioridazine may color urine pink-red to reddish brown.
- Warn to avoid use of all OTC drugs unless they are approved by the physician.

T

THIOTEPA

(thye-oh-tep'a)

Trade names: Thioplex, TSPA

Classifications: ANTINEOPLASTIC; ALKYLATING AGENT

Prototype: Cyclophosphamide

Pregnancy category: D

ACTIONS/PHARMACODYNAMICS

Cell cycle nonspecific alkylating agent that selectively reacts with DNA phosphate groups to produce chromosome cross-linkage and consequent blocking of nucleoprotein synthesis. Nonvesicant, highly toxic hematopoietic agent with a low therapeutic index. Myelosuppression is cumulative and unpredictable and may be delayed. Has some immunosuppressive activity.

USES To produce remissions in malignant lymphomas, including Hodgkin's disease, and adenocarcinoma of breast and ovary. Also in chronic granulocytic and lymphocytic leukemia, superficial papillary carcinoma of urinary bladder, bronchogenic carcinoma, and in malignant effusions secondary to neoplastic disease of serosal cavities. **Unlabeled uses:** prevention of pterygium recurrences following postoperative beta-irradiation; leukemia, malignant meningeal neoplasms.

ROUTE & DOSAGE

Malignant Lymphomas

Adult: **IV** 0.3–0.4 mg/kg q1–4wk. **Intratumor** 0.6–0.8 mg/kg directly into tumor q1–4wk. **Intracavitary** 0.6–0.8 mg/kg instilled through same tubing used for paracentesis at intervals of at least 1 wk. **Intravesicular** 60 mg in 30–60 ml of distilled water instilled into bladder to be retained for 2 h once/wk for 4 wk; **Intrathecal** 1–10 mg/m_2 1–2 times/wk.

PHARMACOKINETICS Absorption: rapidly cleared from plasma. **Onset:** gradual response over several wk. **Metabolism:** metabolized in liver. **Elimination:** 60% of IV dose excreted in urine within 24–72 h.

CONTRAINDICATIONS & PRECAUTIONS Contraindicated in: hypersensitivity to drug; acute leukemia, pregnancy (category D). **Cautious use in** (if at all): chronic lymphocytic leukemia; myelosuppression produced by radiation; with other antineoplastics; bone marrow invasion by tumor cells; impaired renal or hepatic function.

ADVERSE/SIDE EFFECTS GI: anorexia, nausea, vomiting, stomatitis, ulceration of intestinal mucosa. **Hematologic:** leukopenia, thrombocytopenia, anemia, pancytopenia. **Hypersensitivity:** hives, rash, pruritus. **Reproductive:** amenorrhea, interference with spermatogenesis. **Other:** headache, febrile reactions, pain and weeping of injection site, hyperuricemia, slowed or lessened response in heavily irradiated area, sensation of throat tightness. ***Reported with intravesical administration:*** lower abdominal pain, hematuria, hemorrhagic chemical cystitis, vesical irritability.

NURSING IMPLICATIONS

Administration

- Use only under constant supervision by physicians experienced in therapy with cytotoxic agents.
- Avoid exposure of skin and respiratory tract to particles of thiotepa during solution preparation.
- Reconstitute with sterile water for injection. Usual dilution: 1.5 ml of diluent to vial containing 15 mg of drug (resultant solution: 10 mg/ml). Other diluents may result in hypertonic solutions which can cause irritation on injection.
- Following reconstitution, solution may be clear to slightly opaque. (If markedly opaque or contains a precipitate, do not use.) May be administered over 1–3 min without further dilution.
- Reconstituted solutions may be further diluted with 50–100 ml NaCl, dextrose, dextrose and sodium chloride, Ringer's or lactated Ringer's injection for IV infusion, or for intracavitary or perfusion therapy.
- Powder for injection and reconstituted solutions should be refrigerated at 2–8C (35–46F) and protected from light. Reconstituted solutions are stable for 5 d under refrigeration.

Assessment & Drug Effects

- Most patients will manifest some evidence of toxicity; therefore, close monitoring is essential.
- Because of cumulative effects, maximum myelosuppression may be delayed 3 or 4 wk after termination of therapy.
- Manufacturer recommends discontinuing therapy if leukocyte count falls to 3000/mm^3 or below or if platelet count falls below 150,000/mm^3.
- Hemoglobin level and leukocyte and thrombocyte counts should be determined at least weekly during therapy and for at least 3 wk after therapy is discontinued.
- Monitor leukocyte and thrombocyte counts as indicators for adaptations in nursing and drug regimens.

Patient & Family Education

- Discuss possibility of amenorrhea

T

with patient (usually reversible in 6–8 mo).

- Warn to report onset of fever, bleeding, a cold or illness, no matter how mild; medical supervision may be necessary.

THIOTHIXENE HYDROCHLORIDE

(thye-oh-thix′een)

Trade name: Navane

Classifications: CNS AGENT; PSYCHOTHERAPEUTIC; PHENOTHIAZINE ANTIPSYCHOTIC

Prototype: Chlorpromazine

Pregnancy category: C

ACTIONS/PHARMACODYNAMICS Thioxanthene derivative chemically and pharmacologically similar to chlorprothixene and the piperazine phenothiazines. Possesses sedative, adrenolytic, antiemetic, and weak anticholinergic activity.

USE Manifestations of psychotic disorders. **Unlabeled use:** antidepressant.

ROUTE & DOSAGE

Psychotic Disorders

Adult: **PO** 2 mg t.i.d.; may increase up to 15 mg/d as needed or tolerated (max 60 mg/d). **IM** 4 mg b.i.d. to q.i.d. (max 30 mg/d).

Dementia Behavior

Geriatric: **PO** 1–2 mg 1–2 times/d, may increase q4–7d to max of 30 mg/d in divided doses.

PHARMACOKINETICS **Absorption:** slowly absorbed from GI tract. **Onset:** days to weeks PO; 1–6 h IM. **Duration:** up to 12 h. **Distribution:** may remain in body for several weeks; crosses placenta. **Metabolism:** metabolized in liver. **Elimination:** half-life: 34 h; excreted in bile and feces.

CONTRAINDICATIONS & PRECAUTIONS **Contraindicated in:** hypersensitivity to thioxanthenes and phenothiazines, children < 12 y; comatose states; CNS depression; circulatory collapse; blood dyscrasias. Safe use during pregnancy (category C) not established. **Cautious use in:** history of convulsive disorders; alcohol withdrawal; glaucoma; prostatic hypertrophy; cardiovascular disease; patients who might be exposed to organophosphorous insecticides or to extreme heat; concomitant use of atropine or related drugs or ototoxic medications (especially ototoxic antibiotics); previously diagnosed breast cancer.

ADVERSE/SIDE EFFECTS *Drowsiness,* insomnia, dizziness, cerebral edema, convulsions, *extrapyramidal symptoms (dose related),* paradoxical exaggeration of psychotic symptoms; depressed cough reflex; xerostomia, constipation, tachycardia, *orthostatic hypotension* (especially with IM), impotence, gynecomastia, galactorrhea, amenorrhea, rash, contact dermatitis, photosensitivity, blurred vision, pigmentary retinopathy, decreased serum uric acid levels; sudden death, neuroleptic malignant syndrome, tardive dyskinesia.

DRUG INTERACTIONS **Alcohol** and other CNS DEPRESSANTS add to CNS depression.

NURSING IMPLICATIONS

Administration

- Avoid contact of oral concentrate with skin and clothing to prevent contact dermatitis. If concentrate spills, wash skin promptly with water.

- Oral concentrate contains 7% alcohol; it must be diluted just before administration in a cupful of water, fruit juice, carbonated beverage, milk, or soup.
- Capsule may be emptied and contents swallowed with water or mixed with food if patient prefers or if he or she is unable or unwilling to swallow the capsule.
- Administer IM injection deep into upper outer quadrant of buttock. Aspirate hypodermic carefully before injection. Rotate injection sites.
- If patient has suicidal tendency, do not permit access to more than one dose of medication; supervise its ingestion to prevent hoarding.
- Store medication in light-resistant containers at 15–30C (56–89F) unless otherwise indicated.

Assessment & Drug Effects

- Although therapeutic response can be observed 1–6 h following IM injection, it may be days or several weeks before there is a response with the oral preparation.
- Because of the possibility of orthostatic hypotension, patient receiving IM drug should be recumbent for at least 1 h following injection. Periodically check BP during this time.
- When thiothixene is added to the drug regimen of a patient on hypertensive treatment, monitor BP for excessive hypotensive response until drug therapy has been stabilized.
- Dosage adjustment may be necessary when patient is changed from IM to PO forms (capsules, concentrate).
- Hyperreflexia has been reported in infants delivered from mothers having received thiothixene.
- Periodic ophthalmic examinations and blood and hepatic function tests are advisable with prolonged therapy.
- Extrapyramidal effects (pseudoparkinsonism, akathisia, dystonia) may occur during early therapy. Report them to physician; dose adjustment or short-term therapy with an antiparkinsonism agent may provide relief.
- Be alert to first symptoms of tardive dyskinesia (see Appendix G). Discontinue drug immediately and inform physician.

Patient & Family Education

- Because of danger of light-headedness, advise to make position changes slowly, particularly from recumbent to upright, and to sit a few minutes before ambulation. Supervise ambulation if necessary.
- Mild drowsiness, common during first few days of drug therapy, usually subsides with continued treatment. Caution to avoid potentially hazardous activities until response to drug is known.
- Warn to avoid alcohol and other depressants during therapy.
- Counsel to take drug as prescribed and not to alter dosing regimen or stop medication without consulting physician. Abrupt discontinuation can cause delirium.
- Advise that use of all OTC drugs should be approved by the physician during therapy with this drug.
- Inform that although hyperhidrosis is an uncomfortable side effect, it does not indicate need to terminate therapy.
- Advise to avoid excessive exposure to sunlight to prevent a photosensitivity reaction. If sun exposure is expected, protect skin with sunscreen lotion (SPF 12 or above).

THROMBIN

Trade names: Thrombinar, Thrombostat

Classifications: BLOOD FORMER AND COAGULATOR; HEMOSTATIC

Pregnancy category: C

ACTIONS/PHARMACODYNAMICS Sterile plasma protein prepared from prothrombin of bovine origin. Induces clotting of whole blood or a fibrinogen solution without addition of other substances. Converts fibrinogen to thrombin.

USES When oozing of blood from capillaries and small venules is accessible, as in dental extraction, plastic surgery, grafting procedures, and epistaxis; also to shorten bleeding time at puncture sites in heparinized patient (i.e., following hemodialysis).

ROUTE & DOSAGE

Oozing Blood

Adult: **Topical** 100–2000 NIH U/ml, depending on extent of bleeding; may be used as solution, in dry form, by mixing thrombin with blood plasma to form a fibrin "glue," or in conjunction with absorbable gelatin sponge.

T

CONTRAINDICATIONS & PRECAUTIONS **Contraindicated in:** known hypersensitivity to any of drug components or to material of bovine origin, parenteral use, entry or infiltration into large blood vessels, pregnancy (category C).

ADVERSE/SIDE EFFECTS Sensitivity, allergic and febrile reactions, intravascular clotting and death when thrombin is allowed to enter large blood vessels.

NURSING IMPLICATIONS

Administration

- Sponge recipient area free of blood before applying thrombin.
- Solutions may be prepared in sterile distilled water or isotonic saline.
- Solutions should be used within a few hours of preparation. If several hours are to elapse between time of preparation and use, solution should be refrigerated, or preferably frozen, and used within 48 h.
- Store lyophilized preparation at 2–8C (36–46F).

THYROID

(thye′roid)

Trade names: Armour Thyroid, Thyrar

Classifications: HORMONE; THYROID AGENT

Prototype: Levothyroxine sodium

Pregnancy category: A

ACTIONS/PHARMACODYNAMICS Preparation of desiccated animal thyroid gland containing active thyroid hormones, *l*-thyroxine (T_4) and *l*-triiodothyronine (T_3). Action mechanism unknown; T_4 is largely converted to T_3, which exerts principal effects. Influences growth and maturation of various tissues (including skeletal and CNS) at critical periods. Promotes a generalized increase in metabolic rate of body tissues.

USES Replacement or substitution therapy in primary hypothyroidism (cretinism, myxedema, simple goiter, deficiency states in pregnancy and in the elderly) and secondary hypothyroidism caused by surgery, excess radiation, or antithyroid drug therapy. May be given as adjunct to antithyroid agents when it is desirable to limit release of thyrotropic hormones and to prevent goitrogenesis and hypothyroidism.

ROUTE & DOSAGE

Mild to Moderate Hypothyroidism

Adult: **PO** 60 mg/d; may increase q30d to 60–180 mg/d.

Severe Hypothyroidism

Adult: **PO** 15 mg/d; increased q2wk to 60 mg/d; then may increase q30d if needed.
Child: **PO** 15 mg/d; may increase by 15 mg q2wk if needed.

PHARMACOKINETICS **Absorption:** variably absorbed from GI tract. **Peak:** 1–3 wk. **Distribution:** does not readily cross placenta; minimal amounts in breast milk. **Metabolism:** deiodinated in thyroid gland. **Elimination:** half-life: T_3, 1–2 d; T_4, 6–7 d; excreted in urine and feces.

CONTRAINDICATIONS & PRECAUTIONS **Contraindicated in:** thyrotoxicosis; acute MI uncomplicated by hypothyroidism, cardiovascular disease; morphologic hypogonadism; nephrosis; uncorrected hypoadrenalism. **Cautious use in:** angina pectoris, hypertension, elderly patients who may have occult cardiac disease; renal insufficiency; pregnancy (category A); concomitant administration of catecholamines; diabetes mellitus; hyperthyroidism (history of); malabsorption states.

ADVERSE/SIDE EFFECTS **Chronic overdosage:** hyperthyroidism. **Massive overdosage:** thyroid storm: high temperature (as high as 41C [106F]), tachycardia, vomiting, <u>shock</u>, <u>coma</u>. **Overdosage (thyrotoxicosis):** staring expression in eyes, CHF, angina, cardiac arrhythmias, palpitation, tachycardia; weight loss, tremors, headache, nervousness, fever, diarrhea or abdominal cramps, insomnia, warm and moist skin, heat intolerance, leg cramps, menstrual irregularities, <u>shock</u>, changes in appetite, hyperglycemia (usually offset by increased tissue oxidation of sugar).

DIAGNOSTIC TEST INTERFERENCE Thyroid increases ***basal metabolic rate;*** may increase ***blood glucose levels, creatine phosphokinase, AST, LDH, PBI.*** It may decrease ***serum uric acid, cholesterol, thyroid-stimulating hormone (TSH), iodine 131*** uptake. Many medications may produce false results in thyroid function tests.

DRUG INTERACTIONS ORAL ANTICOAGULANTS potentiate hypoprothrombinemia; may increase requirements for **insulin,** SULFONYLUREAS; **epinephrine** may precipitate coronary insufficiency; **cholestyramine** may decrease thyroid absorption.

NURSING IMPLICATIONS

Administration

- Take as a single dose, preferably on an empty stomach.
- Transfer from thyroid treatment to liothyronine: Discontinue thyroid and initiate treatment with low daily dose of liothyronine; in reverse direction, therapy is initiated with replacement several days before complete withdrawal of liothyronine to avoid collapse.
- Generally, dosage is initiated at low level and systematically increased in small increments to desired maintenance dose.
- Store in dark bottle to minimize spontaneous deiodination. Keep desiccated thyroid dry. Potency in this form reportedly persists for as long as 17 y.

T

Assessment & Drug Effects

- During institution of treatment, observe patient carefully for untoward reactions such as angina, palpitations, cardiac pain.
- Be alert for symptoms of overdosage (see Adverse/Side Effects) that may occur 1–3 wk after therapy is started. If they develop, treatment should be interrupted for several days and restarted with reduced dosage.
- Hypothyroidism is common in the elderly. Women generally require less thyroxine replacement than men. Monitor response until regimen is stabilized to prevent iatrogenic hyperthyroidism. In drug-induced hyperthyroidism, there may also be increased bone loss. Such a patient is vulnerable to pathologic fractures.
- Earliest clinical response to thyroid (adult) is diuresis, accompanied by loss of weight and puffiness, followed by sense of well-being, increased pulse rate, increased pulse pressure, increased appetite, increased psychomotor activity, loss of constipation, normalization of skin texture and hair, and increased T_3 and T_4 serum levels.
- Pulse rate is an important clue to drug effectiveness. Count pulse before each dose during period of dosage adjustment. Consult physician if rate is 100 or more or if there has been a marked change in rate or rhythm.
- Free thyroxine index (FTI) and total serum thyroxine concentration (RT_3U) q3mo are usual during dose adjustment period.
- If patient has taken hormone during pregnancy, dose is frequently discontinued in the postpartum period, with evaluation of thyroid function 6 wk later.
- Toxic effects of thyroid develop slowly and disappear gradually. T_4 effects require up to 3–6 wk to dissipate; T_3 effects last 6–14 d after drug withdrawal.

Patient & Family Education

- Instruct to adhere to established dosage regimen; the dose intervals should not be changed without approval of the physician.
- Emphasize that replacement therapy for hypothyroidism is lifelong; therefore, continued follow-up surveillance is important.
- The patient should not change brands of thyroid unless physician approves. Hormone content varies among brands.
- Teach euthyroid patient to take own pulse and record it periodically. If rate begins to increase or if rhythm changes, patient should notify physician.
- Onset of chest pain or other signs of aggravated CV disease (dyspnea, tachycardia) should be reported promptly.
- If patient is receiving anticoagulant therapy, a decrease in the requirement usually develops within 1–4 wk after starting treatment with thyroid. Close monitoring of prothrombin time (normal: 9–11 seconds) is necessary. Warn patient to report evidence of excess anticoagulant, evidenced by ecchymoses, petechiae, purpura, unexplained bleeding.
- Serial height measurement of the juvenile being treated with thyroid is an important means of monitoring influence of thyroid on growth.
- Prepare parent and juvenile hypothyroid patient for a dramatic response to therapy, e.g., initial rapid weight loss and catch-up growth.

TIAGABINE HYDROCHLORIDE

(ti-a′ga-been)

Trade name: Gabitril Filmtabs

T

Classifications: CNS AGENT; ANTICONVULSANT; GABA INHIBITOR
Prototype: Valproic Acid Sodium (Sodium Valproate)
Pregnancy category: C

ACTIONS/PHARMACODYNAMICS GABA inhibitor for the treatment of partial epilepsy. Potent and selective inhibitor of GABA uptake into presynaptic neurons. Consequently, it allows more GABA to bind to the surfaces of postsynaptic neurons in the CNS.

USE Adjunctive therapy for partial seizures.

ROUTE & DOSAGE

Seizures
Adult: **PO** Start with 4 mg q.d.; may increase dose by 4–8 mg/d q.wk. up to 56 mg/d in 2–4 divided doses.
Adolescent 12–18 y: **PO** Start with 4 mg q.d.; after 2 wk may increase dose by 4–8 mg/d q.wk. up to 32 mg/d in 2–4 divided doses.

PHARMACOKINETICS Absorption: rapidly absorbed; 90% bioavailability. **Peak:** 45 min. **Distribution:** 96% protein bound. **Metabolism:** metabolized in liver, probably by cytochrome P450 3A isoform. **Elimination:** half-life: 7–9 h (4–7 h with other enzyme-inducing drugs); 25% excreted in urine, 63% excreted in feces.

CONTRAINDICATIONS & PRECAUTIONS Contraindicated in: hypersensitivity to tiagabine; pregnancy (category C). **Cautious use in:** hepatic function impairment; lactation; history of spike and wave discharge on EEG; status epilepticus.

ADVERSE/SIDE EFFECTS Body as whole: infection, flu syndrome, pain, myasthenia, allergic reactions, chills, malaise, arthralgia. **CNS:** *dizziness, asthenia, tremor, somnolence, nervousness,* difficulty concentrating, ataxia, depression, insomnia, abnormal gait, hostility, confusion, speech disorder, difficulty with memory, paresthesias, emotional lability, agitation, dysarthria, euphoria, hallucinations, hyperkinesia, hypertonia, hypotonia, myoclonus, twitching, vertigo. **CV:** vasodilation, hypertension, palpitations, tachycardia, syncope, edema, peripheral edema. **GI:** abdominal pain, diarrhea, nausea, vomiting, increased appetite, mouth ulcers. **Respiratory:** pharyngitis, cough, bronchitis, dyspnea, epistaxis, pneumonia. **Skin:** rash, pruritus, alopecia, dry skin, sweating. **Other:** ecchymoses, amblyopia, nystagmus, UTI, tinnitus, dysmenorrhea, dysuria, metrorrhagia, incontinence, vaginitis.

DRUG INTERACTIONS Carbamazepine, phenytoin, phenobarbital decrease levels of tiagabine.

NURSING IMPLICATIONS

Administration
- Tiagabine should be taken with food.
- Store at 15–30C (59–86F) in a tightly closed container and protect from light.

Assessment & Drug Effects
- Therapeutic effectiveness is indicated by reduction in seizure activity.
- Lab tests: Measure plasma levels of tiagabine before and after changes are made in the drug regimen.
- Concurrent use of other anticonvulsants may decrease effective-

T

ness of tiagabine or increase the potential for adverse effects.
- Carefully monitor for S&S of CNS depression.

Patient & Family Education
- Do not abruptly stop taking drug as this may cause sudden onset of seizures.
- Exercise caution while engaging in hazardous activities as drug may cause dizziness.
- Use caution when taking other prescription or over-the-counter drugs that can cause drowsiness.
- Report any of the following to the physician: rash or hives; red, peeling skin; dizziness; drowsiness; depression; GI distress; nervousness or tremors; difficulty concentrating or talking.

TICARCILLIN DISODIUM

(ti-car-sill'in)

Trade name: Ticar

Classifications: ANTIINFECTIVE; ANTIBIOTIC; ANTIPSEUDOMONAL PENICILLIN

Prototype: Mezlocillin

Pregnancy category: C

ACTIONS/PHARMACODYNAMICS Ticarcillin disodium is a semisynthetic injectable penicillin. It is bactericidal against gram-positive and gram-negative organisms. Susceptible organisms include *Pseudomonas aeruginosa, Escherichia coli, Proteus mirabilis, Proteus vulgaris, Enterobacter* species, *Hemophilus influenzae, Staphylococcus pneumoniae.*

USES Primarily for gram-negative bacterial infections, bacterial septicemia, skin and soft-tissue infections, acute and chronic respiratory infections, genitourinary tract infection by susceptible organisms, intraabdominal infections and infections of the female pelvis and reproductive system.

ROUTE & DOSAGE

Urinary Tract Infections

Adult: **IM/IV** 200 mg/kg/d in 4 divided doses or 1–2 g q6h.
Child: **IM/IV** 50–200 mg/kg/d in 4 divided doses.

Systemic Infections

Adult: **IM/IV** 15–40 g/d in 6 divided doses (max 40 g/d).
Child: **IM/IV** 250–500 mg/kg/d in 6 divided doses (max 40 g/d).
Neonate: **IV** 150–300 mg/kg/d divided q6–12h.

PHARMACOKINETICS Peak: 1–2 h IM. **Distribution:** low concentrations in CSF unless meninges are inflamed; crosses placenta; distributed into breast milk. **Elimination:** half-life: 67 min; 80–90% excreted unchanged in urine within 24 h.

CONTRAINDICATIONS & PRECAUTIONS Contraindicated in: history of allergic reaction to any penicillin. **Cautious use in:** allergy to cephalosporins, pregnancy (category C).

ADVERSE/SIDE EFFECTS Hypersensitivity reactions. **CNS:** headache, blurred vision, mental deterioration, convulsions, hallucinations, seizures, giddiness, neuromuscular hyperirritability. **GI:** *diarrhea, nausea,* vomiting, disturbances of taste or smell, stomatitis, flatulence. **Hematologic:** eosinophilia, thrombocytopenia, leukopenia, neutropenia, hemolytic anemia. **Other:** pain, burning, swelling at injection site; phlebitis, thrombophlebitis; superinfections, hypernatremia, transient increases in serum AST, ALT, BUN, and alkaline phosphatase; increases in serum LDH, bilirubin, and creatinine and decreased serum uric acid.

INCOMPATIBILITIES Solution/additive: AMINOGLYCOSIDES, **amphotericin b, bleomycin, chloramphenicol, cytarabine, doxapram, lincomycin,** TETRACYCLINES, **vitamin B complex with C. Y-site:** AMINOGLYCOSIDES, **promethazine.**

NURSING IMPLICATIONS

Administration

- Intramuscular injections should not exceed 2 g/per injection.
- In children weighing less than 40 kg, data are insufficient to recommend an optimum dose.
- IM injection: Reconstitute each 1 g of ticarcillin with 2 ml of sterile water for injection or NaCl injection and use promptly. Resulting concentration is 1 g/2.6 ml.
- IV preparation: Reconstitute each 1 g of ticarcillin with 4 ml of sterile water for injection. Dilute reconstituted solution further with at least 20 ml of D5W, NS, or other compatible IV solution.
- IV administration: Give direct IV as slowly as possible (≤1 g over 5 min) to avoid vein irritation. Administer intermittent IV solutions over 30–120 min in equally divided doses.
- IV administration to neonates, infants, children: Verify correct IV concentration and rate of infusion with physician.
- Solutions refrigerated longer than 72 h should not be used for multidose purposes.
- Store dry powder at room temperature or below.

Assessment & Drug Effects

- Culture and susceptibility tests should be done before initiating therapy; ticarcillin may be started pending results.
- Frequently assess IV access site for vein irritation and phlebitis.
- Some patients receiving high doses of ticarcillin may develop hemorrhagic manifestations associated with abnormalities of coagulation tests, such as bleeding time and platelet aggregation. If bleeding manifestations occur, ticarcillin should be discontinued.
- During prolonged treatment with ticarcillin, renal and hepatic functions studies should be monitored.
- Electrolyte and cardiac status should be monitored because of the high sodium content in ticarcillin.
- Monitor for hypokalemia (see Appendix G). Serum potassium levels should be determined periodically.
- Serious and sometimes fatal anaphylactoid reactions have been reported in patients with penicillin hypersensitivity or with history of sensitivity to multiple allergens.

Patient & Family Education

- Frequent bacteriologic tests and clinical evaluation are necessary during treatment for chronic urinary tract infections and may be required for several months after therapy has been discontinued. Urge patients to keep all appointments.
- Instruct to immediately report urticaria, rashes, or pruritus.
- Instruct to report frequent loose stools, diarrhea, or other possible signs of pseudomembranous colitis (see Appendix G).

TICARCILLIN DISODIUM/ CLAVULANATE POTASSIUM

(tye-kar-sill'in/clav-yoo'la-nate)

Trade name: Timentin

Classifications: ANTIINFECTIVE; AN-

TIBIOTIC; ANTIPSEUDOMONAL PENICILLIN
Prototype: Mezlocillin
Pregnancy category: B

ACTIONS/PHARMACODYNAMICS

Injectable extended-spectrum penicillin and fixed combination of ticarcillin disodium with the potassium salt of clavulanic acid, a beta-lactamase inhibitor produced by fermentation of *Streptomyces clavuligerus*. Used alone, clavulanic acid antibacterial activity is weak but in combination with ticarcillin prevents degradation by beta-lactamase and extends ticarcillin spectrum of activity against many strains of beta-lactamase-producing bacteria (synergistic effect). Synergism between the two drugs does not occur against organisms susceptible to ticarcillin alone. Susceptible strains of organisms include beta-lactamase strains of *Klebsiella* sp, *Escherichia coli, Staphylococcus aureus, Pseudomonas aeruginosa, Hemophilus influenzae, Citrobacter* sp, *Enterobacter cloacae, Serratia marcescens.*

USES Infections of lower respiratory tract and urinary tract and skin and skin structures, infections of bone and joint, and septicemia caused by susceptible organisms. Also mixed infections and as presumptive therapy before identification of causative organism.

T

ROUTE & DOSAGE

Moderate to Severe Infections

Adult: **IM/IV** >60 kg, 3.1 g q4–6h.
Child >3 mo: **IV** 200–300 mg/kg/d divided q4–6h (based on ticarcillin).
Infant <3 mo: **IV** 200–300 mg/kg/d divided q6–8h (based on ticarcillin).

PHARMACOKINETICS Distribution: widely distributed with highest concentrations in urine and bile; crosses placenta; distributed into breast milk. **Metabolism:** slightly metabolized in liver. **Elimination:** half-life: 1.1–1.2 h ticarcillin, 1.1–1.5 h clavulanate; excreted in urine.

CONTRAINDICATIONS & PRECAUTIONS Contraindicated in: hypersensitivity to penicillins or to cephalosporins. Safe use during pregnancy (category B) not established. **Cautious use in:** nursing women.

ADVERSE/SIDE EFFECTS See ticarcillin disodium.

DIAGNOSTIC TEST INTERFERENCE

May interfere with test methods used to determine ***urinary proteins*** except for tests for urinary protein that use bromphenol blue. Positive direct ***antiglobulin (Coombs')*** test results, apparently caused by clavulanic acid, have been reported. This test may interfere with transfusion cross-matching procedures.

DRUG INTERACTIONS May increase risk of bleeding with ANTICOAGULANTS; **probenecid** decreases elimination of ticarcillin.

INCOMPATIBILITIES Solution/additive: AMINOGLYCOSIDES, **doxapram. Y-site:** AMINOGLYCOSIDES.

NURSING IMPLICATIONS

Administration

- Reconstitute IV solution by adding to 3.1 g of powder 13 ml sterile water for injection or NaCl injection; shake until drug is dissolved. Resulting concentration is 200 mg/ml ticarcillin with 6.7 mg/ml clavulanic acid. Further dilute solution with NaCl injection, 5% dextrose injection, or lactated Ringer's injection. Inspect reconstituted and diluted solution: do not use if discoloration or particulate matter is present.

- Administer IV infusion over 30 min.
- IV administration to infants, children: Verify correct IV concentration and rate of infusion with physician.
- IV solutions of ticarcillin and clavulanate potassium are incompatible with sodium bicarbonate.
- Store vial with sterile powder: 21–24C (69–75F) or colder. If exposed to higher temperature, powder will darken, indicating degradation of clavulanate potassium and loss of potency. Discard vial. See package insert for information about storage and stability of reconstituted and diluted IV solutions of drug.

Assessment & Drug Effects

- Culture and susceptibility tests should be done before therapy is begun; however, ticarcillin/clavulanate potassium may be started pending laboratory results.
- Serious and sometimes fatal anaphylactoid reactions have been reported in patient with penicillin hypersensitivity or with history of sensitivity to multiple allergens. Reported incidence is low with this combination drug.
- Generally, treatment is continued for at least 2 d after signs and symptoms have disappeared (usually 10–14 d).
- Frequent bacteriologic tests and clinical evaluation are necessary during treatment for chronic urinary tract infections and may be required for several months after therapy has been discontinued. Urge patient to keep all appointments.
- Overdose symptoms: This drug may cause neuromuscular hyperirritability or seizures.

TICLOPIDINE

(ti-clo′pi-deen)

Trade name: Ticlid

Prototype for classifications: BLOOD FORMER; ANTIPLATELET AGENT

Pregnancy category: B

ACTIONS/PHARMACODYNAMICS This platelet aggregation inhibitor prevents the release of platelet constituents and prolongs bleeding time. It interferes with platelet membrane functioning and therefore platelet interactions.

USE Reduction of the risk of thrombotic stroke in patients intolerant to aspirin. **Unlabeled uses:** prevention of venous thromboembolic disorders; maintenance of bypass graft patency and of vascular access sites in hemodialysis patients; improvement of exercise performance in patients with ischemic heart disease and intermittent claudication; prevention of postoperative deep venous thrombosis (DVT).

ROUTE & DOSAGE

Stroke Prevention

Adult: **PO** 250 mg b.i.d. with food.

PHARMACOKINETICS Absorption: 90% absorbed from GI tract; increased absorption when taken with food. **Onset:** antiplatelet activity, 24–48 h; maximal effect at 3–5 d. **Peak:** peak serum levels at 2 h. **Duration:** bleeding times return to baseline within 4-10 d. **Distribution:** 90% bound to plasma proteins. **Metabolism:** rapidly and extensively metabolized in liver. **Elimination:** half-life: 12.6 h; terminal half-life is 4–5 d with repeated dosing; only 1% excreted unchanged; 60% of metabolites excreted in urine, 23% in feces.

CONTRAINDICATIONS & PRECAUTIONS **Contraindicated in:** hypersensitivity to ticlopidine; hematopoietic disease, pathologic bleeding; severe liver impairment. **Cautious use in:** hepatic function impairment, renal impairment; patients at risk for bleeding from trauma, surgery, or a bleeding disorder; GI bleeding; pregnancy (category B). It is not known if ticlopidine is excreted in breast milk. Safety and effectiveness in patients <18 y not established.

ADVERSE/SIDE EFFECTS **CNS:** dizziness. **GI:** nausea, vomiting, abdominal cramps; dyspepsia, flatulence, anorexia; abnormal liver function tests (few cases of hepatotoxicity reported). **Hematologic:** neutropenia (resolves in 1–3 wk), thrombocytopenia, leukopenia, <u>agranulocytosis</u> (usually within first 3 mo), and <u>pancytopenia;</u> hemorrhage (ecchymosis, epistaxis, menorrhagia, GI bleeding), <u>thrombotic thrombocytopenia purpura</u> (usually within first month). **Skin:** urticaria, maculopapular rash, erythema nodosum (generally occur within the first 3 mo of therapy, with most occurring within the first 3–6 wk).

T

DRUG INTERACTIONS ANTACIDS decrease bioavailability of ticlopidine. ANTICOAGULANTS increase risk of bleeding. **Cimetidine** decreases clearance of ticlopidine. CORTICOSTEROIDS counteract increased bleeding time associated with ticlopidine. May decrease **cyclosporine** levels (one case report). Increases **theophylline** half-life by 42%, possibly increasing theophylline serum levels. May increase **phenytoin** levels. **Drug–food:** food may increase bioavailability of ticlopidine.

DIAGNOSTIC TEST INTERFERENCE Increases total ***serum cholesterol*** by 8–10% within 4 wk of beginning therapy. Lipoprotein ratios remain unchanged. Elevates ***alkaline phosphatase*** and ***serum transaminases.***

NURSING IMPLICATIONS

Administration

- Ticlopidine should be given with food or just after eating to minimize GI irritation.
- Anticoagulants or fibrinolytic drugs should be discontinued before ticlopidine administration.
- Store at 15–30C (56–86F).

Assessment & Drug Effects

- Monitor CBC with differentials q2wk from second week to end of third month of therapy and thereafter if signs and symptoms of infection develop.
- Promptly report laboratory values indicative of neutropenia, thrombocytopenia, or agranulocytosis.
- Monitor for signs of bleeding (e.g., ecchymosis, epistaxis, hematuria, GI bleeding).

Patient & Family Education

- Advise to report promptly to physician if any of the following occur: nausea, diarrhea, rash, sore throat, or other signs of infection, signs of bleeding, or signs of cholestasis (e.g., yellow skin or sclera, dark urine or clay-colored stools).
- Explain the risk of GI bleeding and advise patient not to take aspirin along with ticlopidine.
- Advise not to take antacids within 2 h of ticlopidine.
- Stress the importance of scheduled blood tests.
- Advise to take ticlopidine with food.

TILUDRONATE DISODIUM

(til-u′dro-nate)

Trade name: Skelid

Classifications: REGULATOR, BONE METABOLISM

Prototype: Etidronate disodium

Pregnancy category: C

ACTIONS/PHARMACODYNAMICS Tiludronate, a diphosphate, acts primarily by inhibiting normal or abnormal bone resorption, thus reducing bone formation. Its mechanism of action inhibits osteoclastic activity, which leads to resorption of the bone matrix.

USE Treatment of Paget's disease.

ROUTE & DOSAGE

Paget's Disease

Adult: **PO** 400 mg/d taken with 6–8 oz of water 2 h before or after food × 3 mo.

PHARMACOKINETICS **Absorption:** poorly absorbed from GI tract. **Steady-state:** 30 d. **Metabolism:** not metabolized. **Elimination:** half-life: 150 h; primarily excreted in urine.

CONTRAINDICATIONS & PRECAUTIONS **Contraindicated in:** hypersensitivity to diphosphonates (e.g., alendronate, etidronate, pamidronate, tiludronate; severe renal failure Cl_{cr} < 30 ml/min). **Cautious use in:** pregnancy (category C), nursing mothers, hypocalcemia, active UGI problems (e.g., gastritis, dysphagia, ulcer, esophageal disease), CHF. Safety and efficacy in children have not been established.

ADVERSE/SIDE EFFECTS **Body as Whole:** *pain,* flulike syndrome, edema. **CNS:** headache, dizziness, paresthesias. **CV:** chest pain. **GI:** *nausea, diarrhea,* dyspepsia, vomiting, flatulence. **Ocular:** cataract, conjunctivitis, glaucoma. **Respiratory:** rhinitis, sinusitis, coughing, pharyngitis. **Skin:** rash. **Other:** hyperparathyroidism, vitamin D deficiency, arthralgia, arthrosis.

DRUG INTERACTIONS Absorption decreased by CALCIUM, ALUMINUM- or MAGNESIUM-CONTAINING ANTACIDS, **aspirin**. Absorption increased by **indomethacin.**

NURSING IMPLICATIONS

Administration

- Drug should be taken with 6–8 oz of plain water and not within 2 h of eating food.
- Do not give drug within 2 h of drugs containing calcium, aspirin, or indomethacin. Aluminum- or magnesium-containing antacids should be given no sooner than 2 h after tiludronate.
- Store in manufacturer's packaging at 15–30C (59–86F).

Assessment & Drug Effects

- Therapeutic effectiveness is indicated by decreasing levels of alkaline phosphatase.
- Monitor for S&S of upper GI dysfunction or ulceration.

Patient & Family Education

- Tablets should not be removed from foil strips until time to be taken.
- Wait at least 2 h after taking tiludronate to take aluminum- and magnesium-containing antacids.
- Tiludronate is most effective when taken with adequate daily intake of vitamin D and calcium.

TIMOLOL MALEATE

(tye′moe-lole)

Trade names: Betimol, Blocadren, Timoptic, Timoptic XE

Classifications: AUTONOMIC NERVOUS SYSTEM AGENT; BETA-ADRENERGIC ANTAGONIST (SYMPATHOLYTIC, BLOCKING AGENT); EYE PREPARATION; MIOTIC (ANTIGLAUCOMA AGENT)
Prototype: Propranolol
Pregnancy category: C

ACTIONS/PHARMACODYNAMICS

Nonselective beta-adrenergic blocking agent similar to propranolol. Demonstrates antihypertensive, antiarrhythmic, and antianginal properties, and suppresses plasma renin activity. When applied topically, lowers elevated and normal intraocular pressure (IOP) by unknown mechanism but appears to act by reducing formation of aqueous humor and possibly by increasing outflow. In contrast to pilocarpine and other miotics, timolol does not constrict pupil and therefore does not cause night blindness, and it does not affect accommodation or visual acuity.

USES Topically (ophthalmic solution) to reduce elevated IOP in chronic, open-angle glaucoma, aphakic glaucoma, secondary glaucoma, and ocular hypertension. May be used alone or in conjunction with epinephrine, pilocarpine, or a carbonic anhydrase inhibitor such as acetazolamide. Oral preparation is used as step 1 antihypertensive agent in monotherapy or in combination with a thiazide diuretic to prevent reinfarction after MI and to treat mild hypertension. **Unlabeled uses:** prophylactic management of stable, uncomplicated angina pectoris and migraine headaches.

ROUTE & DOSAGE

Glaucoma
See Appendix A.

Hypertension
Adult: **PO** 10 mg b.i.d.; may increase to 60 mg/d in 2 divided doses.

Angina
Adult: **PO** 15–45 mg in 3 divided doses.

PHARMACOKINETICS **Absorption:** 90% absorbed from GI tract; 50% reaches systemic circulation; some systemic absorption from topical application. **Peak:** 1–2 h PO; 1–5 h topical. **Distribution:** distributed into breast milk. **Metabolism:** 80% metabolized in liver to inactive metabolites. **Elimination:** excreted in urine.

CONTRAINDICATIONS & PRECAUTIONS **Contraindicated in:** bronchospasm, severe COPD, bronchial asthma, heart failure. Safe use during pregnancy (category C), in nursing mothers, and in children not established. **Cautious use in:** bronchitis, patients subject to bronchospasm; sinus bradycardia, greater than first-degree heart block, cardiogenic shock, right ventricular failure secondary to pulmonary hypertension; myasthenia gravis; concomitant use with adrenergic augmenting drugs, e.g., MAO inhibitors.

ADVERSE/SIDE EFFECTS **CNS:** fatigue, lethargy, weakness, somnolence, anxiety, headache, dizziness, confusion, psychic dissociation, depression. **CV:** palpitation, bradycardia, hypotension, syncope, AV conduction disturbances, CHF. **Eye:** *eye irritation* including conjunctivitis, blepharitis, keratitis, superficial punctate keratopathy. **GI:** anorexia, dyspepsia, nausea. **Hypersensitivity:** rash, urticaria. **Other:** difficulty in breathing, fever, bronchospasm, hypoglycemia, hypokalemia, aggravation of peripheral vascular insufficiency.

DRUG INTERACTIONS ANTIHYPERTENSIVE AGENTS, DIURETICS potentiate hypotensive effects; NSAIDS may antagonize hypotensive effects.

NURSING IMPLICATIONS

Administration

- Tablet may be crushed before administration and taken with fluid of patient's choice.

Assessment & Drug Effects

- Check pulse before administering timolol, topical or oral. If there are extremes (rate or rhythm), withhold medication and call the physician.
- Monitor pulse rate and BP at regular intervals in patients with severe heart disease.
- Some patients develop tolerance during long-term therapy.

Patient & Family Education

- Inform that drug may cause slight reduction in resting heart rate. Patient should be informed about usual pulse rate and should be instructed to report significant changes. Consult physician for parameters.
- Emphasize importance of adhering to regimen exactly as prescribed. Drug should not be withdrawn abruptly; angina may be exacerbated. Dosage is reduced over a period of 1 or 2 wk.
- Advise to report difficulty in breathing promptly. Drug withdrawal may be indicated.

TIOCONAZOLE

(ti-o-con′a-zole)

Trade name: Vagistat-1

Classifications: ANTIINFECTIVE; ANTIFUNGAL

Prototype: Fluconazole

Pregnancy category: C

ACTIONS/PHARMACODYNAMICS Tioconazole is a broad-spectrum antifungal agent that inhibits the growth of human pathogenic yeasts, including *Candida albicans,* other species of *Candida,* and *Torulopsis glabrata.*

USE Local treatment of vulvovaginal candidiasis.

ROUTE & DOSAGE

Candidiasis

Adult: **Intravaginal** One applicatorful h.s. × 1 d.

PHARMACOKINETICS Absorption: minimal absorption from vagina.

CONTRAINDICATIONS & PRECAUTIONS Contraindicated in: hypersensitivity to tioconazole or other imidazole antifungal agents, lactation. **Cautious use in:** pregnancy (category C), diabetes mellitus. Safety and efficacy in children not established.

ADVERSE/SIDE EFFECTS GU: mild erythema, burning, discomfort, rash, itching.

NURSING IMPLICATIONS

Administration

- Insert applicator high into the vagina (except during pregnancy).
- Wash applicator before and after each use.
- Store away from direct heat and light.

Assessment & Drug Effects

- Tioconazole should not be used by the patient with a history of allergic reaction to other antifungal agents, such as miconazole.
- Monitor for sensitization and irritation; they may be a indication to discontinue drug.

Patient & Family Education

- Advise in correct application technique.

- Inform of potential adverse reactions, including sensitization and allergic response.
- Inform that tioconazole may interact with diaphragms and latex condoms; concurrent use within 72 h should be avoided.
- Advise to refrain from sexual intercourse while using tioconazole.
- Advise to wear only cotton underwear, which are changed daily.

TIROFIBAN HYDROCHLORIDE

(tir-o-fib′an)

Trade name: Aggrastat

Classifications: BLOOD FORMERS AND COAGULATORS; ANTIPLATELET AGENT; GLYCOPROTEIN IIB/IIIA RECEPTOR INHIBITOR

Prototype: Abciximab

Pregnancy category: C

ACTIONS/PHARMACODYNAMICS Antiplatelet agent that binds to the glycoprotein IIb/IIIa receptor of platelets and thus inhibits platelet aggregation.

USE Acute coronary syndromes (unstable angina, MI).

ROUTE & DOSAGE

Acute Coronary Syndromes

Adult: **IV** 0.4 μg/kg/min × 30 min, then 0.1 μg/kg/min for 12–24 h after angioplasty or arteriectomy.

PHARMACOKINETICS **Duration:** 4–8 h after stopping infusion. **Distribution:** 65% protein bound. **Metabolism:** minimally metabolized. **Elimination:** half-life: 2 h; 65% excreted in urine, 25% in feces.

CONTRAINDICATIONS & PRECAUTIONS **Contraindicated in:** active internal bleeding within 30 d; acute pericarditis; aortic dissection; concurrent use with another glycoprotein IIb/IIIa receptor inhibitor (e.g., eptfibatide, abciximab); history of aneurysm or AV malformation; history of intracranial hemorrhage or neoplasm; hypersensitivity to tirofiban; major surgery or trauma within 3 d; stroke within 30 d; history of hemorrhagic stroke; thrombocytopenia following administration of tirofiban. **Cautious use in:** concomitant use with thrombolytic agents or drugs that cause hemolysis; hemorrhagic retinopathy; platelet count <150,000 mm^3; severe renal insufficiency.

ADVERSE/SIDE EFFECTS **Body as whole:** edema, swelling, pelvic pain, vasovagal reaction, leg pain. **CNS:** dizziness. **CV:** bradycardia, coronary artery dissection. **GI:** GI bleeding. **Hematologic:** *bleeding* (major bleeding 2.2%), anemia, thrombocytopenia. **Skin:** sweating.

NURSING IMPLICATIONS

Administration

- IV preparation: From a 500-ml bag of 0.9% NaCl or D5W withdraw 100 ml of solution and replace with 100 ml of tirofiban HCl injection; if a 250-ml IV bag is used, withdraw 50 ml of IV solution and replace with 50 ml of tirofiban injection. Either preparation yields a final concentration of 50 μg/ml. Mix well before infusing.
- Commercially premixed IV tirofiban solutions (50 μg/ml) are available.
- IV infusion: An initial loading dose of 0.4 μg/kg/min for 30 min is usually followed by a maintenance infusion of 0.1 μg/kg/min.
- When creatinine clearance is <30 ml/min, rate of infusion should be reduced by 50%.

- Discard unused IV solution 24 h following start of infusion.
- Store unopened containers at 15–30C (59–86F). Do not freeze and protect from light.

Assessment & Drug Effects

- Therapeutic effectiveness is indicated by minimizing thrombotic events during treatment of acute coronary syndrome.
- Lab tests: Monitor platelet count, Hgb, and Hct before treatment, within 6 h of infusing loading dose, and frequently throughout treatment; monitor aPTT and ACT, adjusting heparin dose to keep aPTT at approximately two times control.
- Discontinue tirofiban and heparin if thrombocytopenia (platelets <100,000) is confirmed.
- Carefully monitor for and immediately report S&S of internal or external bleeding.
- Wait at least 3–4 h after heparin is stopped and until ACT <180 s and aPPT <45 s before removing the femoral catheter sheath.
- Use of unnecessary invasive procedures and devices should be minimized to reduce the risk of bleeding.

TIZANIDINE HYDROCHLORIDE

(ti-zan′i-deen)

Trade name: Zanaflex

Classifications: AUTONOMIC NERVOUS SYSTEM AGENT; CENTRAL-ACTING SKELETAL MUSCLE RELAXANT

Prototype: Cyclobenzaprine

Pregnancy category: C

ACTIONS/PHARMACODYNAMICS A centrally acting alpha-adrenergic agonist. Tizanidine reduces spasticity by increasing presynaptic inhibition of motor neurons. It has no effect on skeltal muscle fibers, the neuromuscular junction, or monosynaptic spinal reflexes. Tizanidine has its greatest effect on polysynaptic afferent reflex activity at the spinal cord level, thereby reducing skeletal muscle spasm.

USE Acute and intermittent management of increased muscle tone associated with spasticity.

ROUTE & DOSAGE

Spasticity

Adult: **PO** Start with 4 mg and gradually increase to 8 mg q6–8h prn (max 3 doses or 36 mg/24 h). Use lower doses in patients with Cl_{cr} < 25 ml/min.

PHARMACOKINETICS Absorption: rapidly absorbed from GI tract; 40% bioavailability. **Peak:** 1–2 h. **Duration:** 3–6 h. **Distribution:** crosses placenta, distributed into breast milk. **Metabolism:** metabolized in the liver. **Elimination:** half-life: 2.5 h; 60% excreted in urine, 20% in feces.

CONTRAINDICATIONS & PRECAUTIONS Contraindicated in: hypersensitivity to tizanidine, lactation. Safety in labor and delivery is unknown. **Cautious use in:** patients with hepatic impairment, renal insufficiency (Cl_{cr} < 25 ml/min); concurrent use of antihypertensive therapy, women taking oral contraceptives; pregnancy (category C), elderly patients because of renal impairment. Safety and efficacy in children have not been established.

ADVERSE/SIDE EFFECTS Body as whole: *asthenia (tiredness),* flu-like syndrome, fever, myasthenia, back pain. **CNS:** *somnolence, dizziness,* dyskinesia, nervousness, depression, anxiety, paresthesia. **CV:** *hypotension, bradycardia.* **GI:** *dry*

T

mouth, constipation, abnormal LFTs, vomiting, abdominal pain, diarrhea, dyspepsia. **Respiratory:** pharyngitis, rhinitis. **Skin:** rash, sweating, skin ulcer. **Other:** *UTI,* infection, speech disorder, blurred vision, urinary frequency.

DRUG INTERACTIONS ORAL CONTRACEPTIVES decrease clearance of **tizanidine. Alcohol** will increase peak levels and decrease clearance of tizanidine.

NURSING IMPLICATIONS

Administration

- Dose increments should be made gradually in 2- to 4-mg steps.
- Store at 15–30C (59–86F).

Assessment & Drug Effects

- Therapeutic effectiveness is indicated by decreased muscle tone.
- Lab tests: monitor liver function tests (ALT/SGTP, AST/SGOT) during the first 6 mo of treatment (baseline, 1, 3, and 6 mo) and periodically thereafter.
- Monitor cardiovascular status and report orthostatic hypotension or bradycardia.
- Because drug clearance is reduced in the elderly, in those with renal impairment, and in women taking oral contraceptives, closely monitor these persons for adverse effects such as dry mouth, somnolence, dizziness, etc.

Patient & Family Education

- Caution should be exercised with hazardous activities requiring alertness since sedation is a common side effect. Effects are additive with alcohol or other CNS depressants.
- Because of the risk of orthostatic hypotension, position changes should be made slowly.
- Immediately report unusual sensory experiences; hallucinations and delusions have occurred with tizanidine use.

TOBRAMYCIN SULFATE

(toe-bra-mye'sin)

Trade names: Nebcin, Tobrex

Classifications: ANTIINFECTIVE; AMINOGLYCOSIDE ANTIBIOTIC

Prototype: Gentamicin sulfate

Pregnancy category: D

ACTIONS/PHARMACODYNAMICS

Broad-spectrum, aminoglycoside antibiotic derived from *Streptomyces tenebrarius.* Closely related to gentamicin in spectrum of antibacterial activity and pharmacologic properties. Reportedly causes less nephrotoxicity than gentamicin, but incidence of ototoxicity is similar. Cross-allergenicity and some cross-resistance among aminoglycosides have been demonstrated. Has greater antibiotic activity against *Pseudomonas aeruginosa* than other aminoglycosides.

USE Treatment of severe infections caused by susceptible organisms.

ROUTE & DOSAGE

All doses based on ideal body weight.

Moderate to Severe Infections

Adult: **IV** 3 mg/kg/d divided q8h up to 5 mg/kg/d infused over 20–60 min. **IM** 3 mg/kg/d divided q8h up to 5 mg/kg/d. **Topical** 1–2 drops in affected eye q1–4h.
Child ≥5 y: **IV** 3 mg/kg/d divided q8h up to 5 mg/kg/d infused over 20–60 min; **IM** 3 mg/kg/d divided q8h up to 5 mg/kg/d.

Child <5 y: **IM/IV** 2.5 mg/kg q8h.
Neonate: **IM/IV** 2.5 mg/kg q12–24h.

Cystic Fibrosis

Child: **IM/IV** 2.5–3.5 mg/kg q6–8h.

PHARMACOKINETICS **Peak:** 30–90 min IM. **Duration:** up to 8 h. **Distribution:** crosses placenta; accumulates in renal cortex. **Elimination:** half-life: 2–3 h in adults; excreted in urine.

CONTRAINDICATIONS & PRECAUTIONS **Contraindicated in:** history of hypersensitivity to tobramycin and other aminoglycoside antibiotics. Safe use during pregnancy (category D) and in nursing mothers not established. **Cautious use in:** impaired renal function; premature and neonatal infants; concurrent use with other neurotoxic or nephrotoxic agents or potent diuretics.

ADVERSE/SIDE EFFECTS Neurotoxicity (including ototoxicity), *nephrotoxicity,* increased AST, ALT, LDH, serum bilirubin; anemia, fever, rash, pruritus, urticaria, nausea, vomiting, headache, lethargy, superinfections; hypersensitivity. **Eye:** *burning, stinging of eye after drug instillation;* lid itching and edema.

DRUG INTERACTIONS ANESTHETICS, SKELETAL MUSCLE RELAXANTS add to neuromuscular blocking effects; **acyclovir, amphotericin B, bacitracin, capreomycin,** CEPHALOSPORINS, **colistin, cisplatin, carboplatin, methoxyflurane, polymyxin B, vancomycin, furosemide, ethacrynic acid** increased risk of ototoxicity, nephrotoxicity.

INCOMPATIBILITIES **Solution/additive: alcohol 5% in dextrose,** CEPHALOSPORINS, PENICILLINS, **clindamycin, heparin. Y-site:** CEPHALOSPORINS, **clindamycin, penicillins, heparin.**

NURSING IMPLICATIONS

Administration

- Each IV dose is diluted in 50–100 ml or more of D5W, 0.9% NaCl, or DSW + 0.9% NaCl. Concentration should not exceed 1 mg/ml. Infuse diluted solution over 20–60 min.
- IV administration to neonates, infants, children: Verify correct IV concentration and rate of infusion with physician.
- Wash hands before and after instillation of eye medication. Apply gentle finger pressure to lacrimal sac for 1 min after drug has been instilled in eye.
- Prior to reconstitution, store vial at 15–30C (59–86F). After reconstitution, solution may be refrigerated and used within 96 h. If kept at room temperature, use within 24 h.

Assessment & Drug Effects

- Weigh patient before treatment for calculation of dosage (by physician).
- Bacterial culture and susceptibility tests are advised prior to and during tobramycin therapy.
- As with other aminoglycosides, patient receiving tobramycin must remain under close clinical observation because of the high potential for toxicity, even in conventional doses.
- Monitoring of serum drug concentrations is advised to minimize rise of toxicity. Prolonged peak serum concentrations >10 μg/ml or trough concentrations >2 μg/ml are not recommended.
- Renal, auditory, and vestibular functions should also be closely monitored, particularly in patients with known or suspected renal im-

T

pairment and patients receiving high doses.

- Drug-induced auditory changes are irreversible (may be partial or total); usually bilateral. In cochlear damage, the patient may be asymptomatic, and partial or bilateral deafness may continue to develop even after therapy has been discontinued.
- Evidence of renal insufficiency or ototoxicity (see Appendix G) or vestibular damage indicates need for discontinuation of drug or dosage adjustment.
- Monitor I&O. Report oliguria, changes in I&O ratio, and cloudy or frothy urine (may indicate proteinuria). The elderly patient is especially susceptible to renal toxicity. Patient is usually kept well hydrated to prevent chemical irritation in renal tubules. Consult physician.
- Therapy is generally continued for 7–10 d. Complicated infection may require longer course of therapy, in which case close monitoring of renal, auditory, and vestibular function and serum drug concentrations is essential.
- Monitor patient with neuromuscular disorder (e.g., myasthenia gravis) for muscular weakness. Observe ambulation and assist if necessary.
- Ophthalmic: Prolonged use of ophthalmic solution may encourage superinfection with nonsusceptible organisms including fungi.
- Overdose symptoms for eye medication are increased lacrimation, keratitis, and edema and itching of eyelids. Report symptoms to physician.

Patient & Family Education

- Advise to report symptoms of superinfections (see Appendix G). Prompt treatment with an antibiotic or antifungal medication may be necessary.
- Instruct to report signs and symptoms of hearing loss, tinnitus, or vertigo.

TOCAINIDE HYDROCHLORIDE

(toe-kay′nide)

Trade name: Tonocard

Classifications: CARDIOVASCULAR AGENT; ANTIARRHYTHMIC

Prototype: Procainamide hydrochloride

Pregnancy category: C

ACTIONS/PHARMACODYNAMICS

Antiarrhythmic agent (class IB) and analog of lidocaine, with similar electrophysiologic characteristics and hemodynamic properties. Effective orally. Suppresses PVCs and may have particular use in arrhythmias associated with a prolonged QT interval that do not respond to quinidine-like antiarrhythmics (class IA). Decreases active potential duration in Purkinje fibers and slightly decreases resting membrane potential. Shortens effective refractory periods of atria, AV node, and ventricles without affecting AV conduction. QRS and QT intervals do not change.

USES Refractory ventricular arrhythmia. To increase effectiveness, it may be combined with a class IA antiarrhythmic (e.g., quinidine, disopyramide) or with propranolol. Also used to prevent ventricular tachyarrhythmia after acute MI.

ROUTE & DOSAGE

Ventricular Arrhythmias

Adult: **PO** 1.2–1.8 g/d in 3 divided doses; may increase up to 2.4 g/d.

PHARMACOKINETICS **Absorption:** rapidly and completely absorbed from GI tract. **Peak:** 0.5–2 h. **Distribution:** not fully known; does distribute into CNS. **Metabolism:** metabolized in liver. **Elimination:** half-life: 10–17 h; 70–80% excreted in urine within 72 h.

CONTRAINDICATIONS & PRECAUTIONS **Contraindicated in:** hypersensitivity to tocainide and to local anesthetics of the amide type; second- or third-degree AV block (in absence of artificial ventricular pacemaker), hypokalemia; myasthenia gravis; pregnancy (category C), nursing mothers. Safe use in children not established. **Cautious use in:** multiple drug therapy, known heart failure patient with minimum cardiac reserve; renal or hepatic disease.

ADVERSE/SIDE EFFECTS **CNS:** *tremors, dizziness, light-headedness, visual disturbances, vertigo, tinnitus,* hearing loss, ataxia, paresthesia, confusion. **CV:** exacerbation of arrhythmias, complete heart block, sinus node slowing (in patient with preexisting conduction system disease); hypotension, palpitations, bradycardia, chest pain, left ventricular failure, PVCs, hot flashes. **GI:** nausea, vomiting, anorexia, abdominal pain, diarrhea, hepatitis (rare). **Respiratory:** pulmonary fibrosis, edema, embolism and alveolitis; pneumonia, dyspnea. **Other:** alopecia, sweating, night sweats, tiredness/drowsiness, sleepiness, hot/cold feelings, hematologic disorders (leukopenia, agranulocytosis, thrombocytopenia, hypoplastic anemia), claudication, cold extremities, leg cramps, urinary retention, polyuria, metallic or menthol taste, hiccups.

DRUG INTERACTIONS **Lidocaine** may increase risk of CNS toxicity, including seizures. BETA BLOCKERS may lead to paranoia.

NURSING IMPLICATIONS

Administration

- Administer with food to decrease GI distress. This also protects against high peak concentration and toxicity because absorption rate is slowed. Bioavailability is not affected by food.

Assessment & Drug Effects

- Effective serum concentration is 3.5–10 μg/ml.
- When steady-state drug level is attained (usually in about 70 h), plasma level monitoring is recommended, especially if patient has renal or hepatic dysfunction.
- Onset of tremors is a good clinical indicator that maximum dose is being approached.
- In patient with kidney or hepatic dysfunction, drug elimination is significantly decreased. Monitor I&O ratio and pattern. Instruct patient to report to physician if symptoms of renal dysfunction occur.
- Anticipate and report evidence of blood dyscrasia (see Appendix G).
- Blood counts may be monitored during first 6 mo of treatment; abnormal counts usually stabilize within 1 mo after discontinuation of treatment.

Patient & Family Education

- The patient should fully understand what an irregular pulse signifies and how often it should be checked.
- Since drug may cause dizziness and drowsiness, warn to avoid driving and other potentially hazardous activities until drug response is known.
- Symptomatic bradycardia should be reported. Dose adjustment or discontinuation will follow.
- Advise to report promptly chest

T

pain, exertional dyspnea, wheezing, and cough even if no fever is present. Pulmonary fibrosis is a serious side effect and should be ruled out. Drug is discontinued if pulmonary symptoms persist or if pulmonary disorder is diagnosed.

TOLAZAMIDE

(tole-az'a-mide)
Trade name: Tolinase
Classifications: HORMONE; SULFONYLUREA ANTIDIABETIC
Prototype: Tolbutamide
Pregnancy category: C

ACTIONS/PHARMACODYNAMICS Orally effective sulfonylurea hypoglycemic structurally and pharmacologically related to tolbutamide but about 5 times more potent. Lowers blood glucose primarily by stimulating pancreatic beta cells to secrete insulin. As with other sulfonylureas, is ineffective in the absence of functioning beta cells. Contraindications, precautions, pharmacokinetics, and adverse effects as for tolbutamide.

USES Mild to moderately severe type II non-insulin-dependent diabetes mellitus that cannot be controlled by diet and weight reduction and that is uncomplicated by acidosis, ketosis, coma. Effective in primary or secondary failures to other sulfonylurea.

ROUTE & DOSAGE

Non-insulin-dependent Diabetes Mellitus

Adult: **PO** 100 mg–1 g q.d. to b.i.d. a.c.; may adjust dose by 100–250 mg/d at weekly intervals (max 1 g/d).

PHARMACOKINETICS **Absorption:** slowly absorbed from GI tract. **Onset:** 60 min. **Peak:** 4–6 h. **Duration:** 10–15 h (up to 20 h in some patients). **Distribution:** distributed in highest concentrations in liver, kidneys, and intestines; crosses placenta; distributed into breast milk. **Metabolism:** metabolized extensively in liver. **Elimination:** half-life: 7 h; 85% excreted in urine, 15% in feces.

CONTRAINDICATIONS & PRECAUTIONS **Contraindicated in:** known sensitivity to sulfonylureas and to sulfonamides, Type I (IDDM) insulin-dependent diabetes, diabetes complicated by ketoacidosis; infection; trauma; pregnancy (category C); safe use in nursing mothers and in children not established.

ADVERSE/SIDE EFFECTS Nausea, vomiting, hypoglycemia, vertigo, photosensitivity, agranulocytosis, cholestatic jaundice.

DRUG INTERACTIONS **Alcohol** elicits disulfiram-type reaction in some patients; ORAL ANTICOAGULANTS, **chloramphenicol, clofibrate, phenylbutazone,** MAO INHIBITORS, SALICYLATES, **probenecid,** SULFONAMIDES may potentiate hypoglycemic actions; THIAZIDES may antagonize hypoglycemic effects; **cimetidine** may increase tolazamide levels, causing hypoglycemia.

NURSING IMPLICATIONS

Administration

- Give in the morning with or before meals.
- When a dose of more than 500 mg is ordered, it should be divided and given b.i.d.
- Tablet may be crushed if patient is unable to swallow it whole. Be sure it is swallowed with an allowable fluid, not dry.
- When patient is newly diagnosed,

dosage is guided by fasting blood sugar values: if less than 200 mg/dl, therapy is started with 100 mg/d before breakfast; if greater than 200 mg/dl, with 250 mg/d.

- Store at 15–30C (59–86F) in a tightly closed container unless otherwise directed. Keep drug out of the reach of children.

Assessment & Drug Effects

- Reduction of dose frequently alleviates most of the mild to moderately severe hypoglycemic symptoms.
- Unlike tolbutamide, tolazamide is effective in some patients with a history of ketoacidosis or coma; close observation of these patients is especially important during the early adjustment period.

Patient & Family Education

- Patient must be under close medical supervision for first 6 wk of treatment; should check urine daily for sugar and acetone.
- Doses > 1000 mg/d rarely provide improvement in diabetic control: patient then usually is maintained on insulin therapy only.
- Caution not to self-dose with OTC preparations unless approved or prescribed by physician.
- Be certain that patient understands that alcohol can precipitate a disulfiram-type reaction.

TOLAZOLINE HYDROCHLORIDE

(toe-laz′a-leen)

Trade name: Priscoline

Classifications: AUTONOMIC NERVOUS SYSTEM AGENT; ALPHA-ADRENERGIC ANTAGONIST (SYMPATHOLYTIC, BLOCKING AGENT); VASODILATOR

Prototype: Prazosin

Pregnancy category: C

ACTIONS/PHARMACODYNAMICS Structurally related to phentolamine. In addition to weak alpha-adrenergic blocking activity, beta-adrenergic action increases cardiac output and rate, cholinergic effect increases GI motility, and histamine-like activity stimulates gastric secretions and peripheral vasodilation. Vasodilation is primarily due to direct relaxant effect on vascular smooth muscle. Inhibits aldehyde dehydrogenase, and may increase or decrease pulmonary artery pressure and total pulmonary resistance.

USE Persistent pulmonary hypertension of the newborn. **Unlabeled uses:** to improve blood flow in thromboangiitis obliterans (Buerger's disease), diabetic arteriosclerosis gangrene, Raynaud's disease, causalgia, scleroderma, postthrombotic conditions, frostbite sequelae, and other peripheral vasospastic disorders; to improve visualization of vasculature during arteriography, treatment of neonatal hypoxemia, as diagnostic agent to differentiate vasospastic and obstruction components in occlusive peripheral vascular disease, and as a provocative test for glaucoma.

ROUTE & DOSAGE

Vasospastic Disorders

Adult: **SC/IV/IM** 10–50 mg q.i.d. **Intraarterial** 25 mg test dose infused slowly; then 50–75 mg 1–2 times/d; **maintenance:** 50–75 mg 2–3 times/wk.

Improve Visualization of Vasculature

Adult: **Intraarterial** 12.5–50 mg prior to arteriography.

T

Persistent Pulmonary Hypertension

Neonate: **IV** 1–2 mg/kg via scalp needle over 10 min followed by infusion of 1–2 mg/kg/h for 36–48 h.

PHARMACOKINETICS Absorption: well absorbed from all routes. **Peak:** 30–60 min IM, SC. **Duration:** 3–4 h. **Elimination:** half-life: 1.5–41 h; excreted in urine.

CONTRAINDICATIONS & PRECAUTIONS Contraindicated in: following cerebrovascular accident; coronary artery disease; alcohol ingestion. Safe use during pregnancy (category C) and in nursing mothers not established. **Cautious use in:** gastritis, peptic ulcer (previous or current); mitral stenosis.

ADVERSE/SIDE EFFECTS CV: tachycardia, arrhythmias, anginal pain, postural hypotension, BP changes, marked hypertension (particularly following parenteral use). **GI:** nausea, vomiting, diarrhea, epigastric discomfort, *abdominal pain,* exacerbation of peptic ulcer. **Hematologic:** agranulocytosis, leukopenia, thrombocytopenia, pancytopenia. **Intraarterial administration:** *feeling of warmth or burning at injection site,* transient weakness, postural vertigo, palpitation, formication, apprehension, transient paradoxic impairment of blood supply, peripheral vasodilation. **Skin:** profuse, sweating, flushing, increased pilomotor activity with tingling and chilliness, rash. **Other:** mydriasis, edema, headache. **Severe overdosage:** hypotension progressing to shock.

DRUG INTERACTIONS Alcohol may elicit disulfiram-type reaction; **epinephrine, norepinephrine** may cause paradoxic fall in BP followed by rebound increase.

INCOMPATIBILITY Solution/additive: ethacrynic acid.

NURSING IMPLICATIONS

Administration

- With neonate, administer initial dose of 1–2 mg/kg over 10–15 min via scalp vein using an infusion pump.
- With neonate, administer maintenance infusion of 1–2 mg/kg/h by infusion over 36–48 h.
- Drug may be diluted in D5W, 0.45–0.9% NaCl, Ringer's, or any combination thereof.
- Infant may be pretreated with antacids to minimize risk of GI bleeding.

Assessment & Drug Effects

- Closely monitor cardiovascular status for hypotension or hypertension and arrhythmias. Ask physician for BP parameters.
- Assess for signs of bleeding: hematuria, bloody or tarry stools, hematemesis, bruising, or petechiae.
- Monitor electrolytes and arterial blood gases (ABGs) for signs of hypochloremic metabolic acidosis.
- Monitor pulmonary artery pressure (PAP) and pulmonary capillary wedge pressure (PCWP) during drug administration. A drop in PAP should be seen in 30 min of the initial dose.

TOLBUTAMIDE

(tole-byoo'ta-mide)

Trade names: Mobenol ♣, Novobutamide ♣, Orinase

TOLBUTAMIDE SODIUM

Trade name: Orinase Diagnostic
Prototype for classifications: SYNTHETIC HORMONE; SULFONYLUREA ANTIDIABETIC
Pregnancy category: C

ACTIONS/PHARMACODYNAMICS
Short-acting sulfonylurea compound chemically related to sulfonamides, but without antiinfective activity. Lowers blood glucose concentration by stimulating pancreatic beta cells to synthesize and release insulin. No action demonstrated if functional beta cells are absent. Responsiveness to blood glucose–lowering effects with long-term therapy may decline in some patients. Alternatively, patient who has become poorly responsive to other sulfonylureas may be responsive to tolbutamide.

USES Management of mild to moderately severe, stable non-insulin-dependent diabetes (type II) that is not controlled by diet and weight reduction alone. Also used in treatment of patients who are unresponsive to other sulfonylureas and adjunctively with insulin to stabilize certain cases of labile diabetes. Used as diagnostic agent to rule out pancreatic islet cell adenoma or diabetes.

ROUTE & DOSAGE

Diabetes

Adult: **PO** 250 mg to 3 g/d in 1–2 divided doses.

Diagnosis of Functioning Insulinoma

Adult: **IV** 1 g over 2–3 min.

PHARMACOKINETICS **Absorption:** readily absorbed from GI tract. **Peak:** 3–5 h. **Distribution:** distributed into extracellular fluids. **Metabolism:** principally metabolized in liver. **Elimination:** half-life: 7 h; 75–85% excreted in urine; some elimination in feces.

CONTRAINDICATIONS & PRECAUTIONS **Contraindicated in:** hypersensitivity to sulfonylureas or to sulfonamides, history of repeated episodes of diabetic ketoacidosis (with or without coma), type I (IDDM) diabetes; as sole therapy; diabetic coma; severe stress, infection, trauma, or major surgery; severe renal insufficiency, hepatic or endocrine disease. Safe use during pregnancy (category C) or use in children not established. **Cautious use in:** cardiac, thyroid, pituitary, or adrenal dysfunction; history of peptic ulcer; alcoholism; the elderly, debilitated, malnourished, or uncooperative patient.

ADVERSE/SIDE EFFECTS **GI (dose related):** nausea, epigastric fullness, heartburn, anorexia, constipation, diarrhea, cholestatic jaundice (rare). **Hematologic:** <u>agranulocytosis</u>, thrombocytopenia, leukopenia, hemolytic anemia, <u>aplastic anemia</u>, pancytopenia. **Metabolic:** hepatic porphyria, disulfiram-like reactions, SIADH. **Skin:** allergic skin reactions: pruritus, erythema, urticaria, morbilliform or maculopapular eruptions; porphyria cutanea tarda, photosensitivity. **Other:** taste alterations, headache. **Overdosage:** hypoglycemia without loss of consciousness or neurologic symptoms: unusual fatigue, tremulousness, hunger, drowsiness, GI distress, sweating, anxiety, headache; severe: visual disturbances, ataxia, paresthesias, confusion, tachycardia, seizures, <u>coma</u>.

DIAGNOSTIC TEST INTERFERENCE The sulfonylureas may produce abnormal ***thyroid function test*** results and reduced ***RAI uptake*** (after long-term administration). A tolbutamide metabolite may cause false-positive ***urinary protein*** values when turbidity procedures are used (such as heat and acetic acid or sulfosalicylic acid); Ames reagent strips reportedly not affected.

DRUG INTERACTIONS **Phenylbutazone** increases hypoglycemic effects; THIAZIDE DIURETICS may attenuate hypoglycemic effects; **alcohol** may produce disulfiram reaction; BETA BLOCKERS may mask symptoms of a hypoglycemic reaction.

NURSING IMPLICATIONS

Administration

- Total dose may be taken before breakfast but preferably in divided doses after meals.
- Tablet may be crushed and taken with full glass of water if patient desires.
- Because of danger of nocturnal hypoglycemia, tolbutamide should not be taken at bedtime unless specifically prescribed.
- Transfer from insulin to tolbutamide (sulfonylurea) is best controlled in the hospital. For patients receiving 20 U or less of insulin daily, insulin may be stopped abruptly; oral drug is usually started at maintenance dose.
- For patients receiving 20 U of insulin daily, tolbutamide is started at maintenance level, with gradual reductions in daily insulin.
- If tolbutamide is used during pregnancy, it is discontinued at least 2 wk before the expected delivery date to prevent prolonged severe hypoglycemia (4–10 d) in the neonate.
- Store below 40C (104F), preferably between 15–30C (59–86F), in well-closed container; avoid freezing.

Assessment & Drug Effects

- During initial period of therapy, patient should be under close medical supervision until dosage is established. One or 2 wk of therapy may be required before full therapeutic effect is achieved.
- Elderly patients may be hyperresponsive to oral antidiabetic therapy; thus, the initial dose should be low and given before breakfast. If blood and urine glucose tests are negative during first 24 h of therapy, initial dose may be continued on a daily basis.
- If a patient stabilized on tolbutamide is exposed to stress (e.g., infection, surgery), loss of blood glucose control may occur. Tolbutamide may be discontinued and replaced by insulin.
- Detection of a hypoglycemic reaction in a diabetic patient also receiving a beta blocker, especially if elderly, is difficult. Monitor closely during adjustment period, watching for symptoms of impending hypoglycemia (see Appendix G).
- Hypoglycemic symptoms may be especially vague in the elderly; therefore, check out nondefinitive vague complaints. Observe patient carefully, especially 2–3 h after eating, check urine for sugar and ketone bodies and capillary blood glucose.
- Repetitive complaints of headache and weakness a few hours after eating may signal incipient hypoglycemia. Report to physician.
- The potential for hypoglycemia in nursing infants presents the necessity to decide whether to discontinue nursing or to temporarily transfer to insulin (if diet alone is inadequate for blood sugar control).
- Pruritus and rash, frequently reported side effects, may clear

spontaneously; however, if they persist, drug will be discontinued.

- Effectiveness of any hypoglycemic agent declines over time. This phenomenon is called secondary (drug) failure.
- Patients most prone to secondary failure may be underweight, erratic in their meal schedules, careless about dosage, or they may have developed drug resistance.

Patient & Family Education

- Impress on the patient and family that oral antidiabetic drug therapy controls diabetes but will never cure it.
- The patient or family member should fully understand that the physician must be informed promptly of symptoms of hyperglycemia and ketoacidosis: flushed, dry skin, weight loss, fatigue, Kussmaul respiration, double or blurred vision, soft eyeballs, irritability, fruity-smelling breath, abdominal cramps, nausea, vomiting, diarrhea, dyspnea, polydipsia, polyphagia, polyuria, headache, hypotension, weak and rapid pulse, positive ketonuria and glycosuria. Report symptoms promptly so that emergency antidiabetic therapy can be instituted. Hypoglycemia is frequently caused by overdosage of hypoglycemic drug, inadequate or irregular food intake, nausea, vomiting, diarrhea, and added exercise without caloric supplement or dose adjustment. Its occurrence indicates need for immediate reevaluation of patient's diet, medication regimen, and compliance. It is most likely to appear in patients > 50 y of age. Report to physician.
- Report promptly any illness. The physician may want to evaluate need for insulin.
- Avoid self-medication with OTC drugs unless approved or prescribed by physician.
- Alcohol, even in moderate amounts, can precipitate a disulfiram-type reaction (see Appendix G). The patient should be aware of becoming hypoglycemic after ingesting alcohol; an observer may mistakenly think he or she is inebriated, and therefore patient may be deprived of necessary emergency treatment.
- Because of potential photosensitivity (especially in the alcoholic), protect exposed skin areas from the sun with a sunscreen lotion (SPF 12–15).
- Report promptly signs of hepatic toxicity, renal insufficiency, or blood dyscrasia (see Appendix G).
- Weigh self at least weekly and report a progressive gain, especially if edema is present. These signs indicate the necessity to discontinue tolbutamide.
- When a drug that affects the hypoglycemic action of sulfonylureas (see Drug Interactions) is withdrawn or added to the tolbutamide regimen, the patient should be alerted to the added danger of loss of control (hyperglycemia). Urine tests and blood glucose tests and test for ketone bodies should be carefully monitored and possibly increased in frequency for several days to determine if antidiabetic drug dose adjustment is indicated.
- Advise patients using oral contraceptives to use another form of birth control.
- Advise patient who wishes to become pregnant that a transfer to insulin for blood glucose control is recommended by many clinicians.
- Instruct to carry medical identification card or jewelry at all times (available from most drug stores). Card information should include

T

patient and physician's names and addresses, diagnosis, medication, and dose being taken.

TOLCAPONE

(tol′ca-pone)

Trade name: Tasmar

Classifications: CNS AGENT; ANTIPARKINSON AGENT; COMT INHIBITOR

Pregnancy category: C

ACTIONS/PHARMACODYNAMICS

Tolcapone is a selective inhibitor of catecho-o-methyltransferase (COMT). COMT is responsible for metabolizing levodopa. Consequently, concurrent administration of tolcapone and levodopa increases the amount of levodopa available to control Parkinson's disease by increasing dopanergic brain stimulation.

USE Idiopathic Parkinson's disease as adjunct to levodopa/carbidopa.

ROUTE & DOSAGE

Parkinson's Disease

Adult: **PO** 100 mg t.i.d. (max 200 mg t.i.d.).

PHARMACOKINETICS Absorption: rapidly absorbed from GI tract, bioavailability 65%; food decreases bioavailability. **Peak:** 2 h. **Distribution:** >99% protein bound. **Metabolism:** extensively metabolized by COMT and glucuronidation. **Elimination:** half-life: 2–3 h; 60% excreted in urine, 40% in feces; clearance is reduced by 50% in patients with moderate cirrhotic liver disease.

CONTRAINDICATIONS & PRECAUTIONS Contraindicated in: hypersensitivity to tolcapone; pregnancy (category C); liver disease. **Cautious use in:** history of hypersensitivity to other COMT inhibitors (e.g., entacapone, nitecapone); lactation.

ADVERSE/SIDE EFFECTS Body as whole: muscle cramps, orthostatic complaints, fatigue, falling, balance difficulties, hyperkinesia, stiffness, arthritis, hypokinesia. **CNS:** *dyskinesia, sleep disorder, dystonia, excessive dreaming,* somnolence, confusion, dizziness, headache, hallucination, syncope, paresthesias. **CV:** chest pain, hypotension. **GI:** *nausea,* anorexia, diarrhea, vomiting, constipation, <u>fulminant hepatic failure, severe hepatocellular injury,</u> dry mouth, abdominal pain, dyspepsia, flatulence. **Respiratory:** URI, dyspnea, sinus congestion. **Skin:** sweating. **Other:** UTI, urine discoloration, micturition disorder.

DRUG INTERACTIONS Will increase **levodopa** levels when taken simultaneously.

NURSING IMPLICATIONS

Administration

- Tolcapone may be given with food if GI upset occurs.
- Tolcapone should be given only in conjunction with levodopa/carbidopa therapy.
- Doses >100 mg t.i.d. are not recommended with moderate/severe liver impairment.
- Store at 20–25C (68–77F) in a tightly closed container.

Assessment & Drug Effects

- Lab tests: Monitor liver functions monthly for first 3 mo, every 6 wk for the next 3 mo, and periodically thereafter.
- When given concurrently with warfarin, carefully monitor PT and INR.
- Carefully monitor for and immedi-

T

ately report S&S of hepatic impairment (e.g., jaundice, dark urine).

Patient & Family Education

- Do not engage in hazardous activities until response to the drug is known. Avoid the use of alcohol or sedative drugs while on tolcapone.
- To avoid a rapid drop in BP with possible weakness or fainting, rise slowly from a sitting or lying position.
- Nausea is a possible side effect especially at the beginning of therapy.
- Do not suddenly stop taking this drug. Doses must be gradually reduced over time.
- Promptly notify the physician if any of the following are noted: increased loss of muscle control, fainting, yellowing of skin or eyes, darkening of urine, severe diarrhea, hallucinations.

TOLMETIN SODIUM

(tole′met-in)

Trade names: Tolectin, Tolectin DS

Classifications: CNS AGENT; ANALGESIC; ANTIPYRETIC; NSAID

Prototype: Ibuprofen

Pregnancy category: B (D in third trimester)

ACTIONS/PHARMACODYNAMICS Related to indomethacin. Possesses analgesic, antiinflammatory, and antipyretic activity. Exact mode of antiinflammatory action not known. Inhibition of platelet aggregation is less than that produced by equal therapeutic doses of aspirin. Comparable to aspirin and indomethacin in antirheumatic activity, but incidence of GI symptoms and tinnitus is less than in aspirin-treated patients, and CNS effects are less than in patients receiving indomethacin.

USES In acute flares and management of chronic rheumatoid arthritis. May be used alone or in combination with gold or corticosteroids.

ROUTE & DOSAGE

Arthritis

Adult: **PO** 400 mg t.i.d. (max 2 g/d).
Child ≥2y: **PO** 20 mg/kg/d in 3–4 divided doses (max 30 mg/kg/d).

PHARMACOKINETICS **Absorption:** rapidly absorbed from GI tract. **Peak:** 30–60 min. **Distribution:** crosses blood–brain barrier and placenta; distributed into breast milk. **Metabolism:** metabolized in liver. **Elimination:** half-life: 60–90 min; excreted in urine.

CONTRAINDICATIONS & PRECAUTIONS **Contraindicated in:** history of intolerance or hypersensitivity to tolmetin, aspirin, and other NSAIDs; active peptic ulcer, patients with asthma, nasal polyps, rhinitis ("aspirin triad"), in patients with functional class IV rheumatoid arthritis (severely incapacitated, bedridden, or confined to a wheelchair). Safe use not established during pregnancy (category B, category D in third trimester), in nursing mothers, and in children < 2 y. **Cautious use in:** history of upper GI tract disease; impaired renal function; compromised cardiac function.

ADVERSE/SIDE EFFECTS **CNS:** *headache, dizziness, vertigo, lightheadedness,* mood elevation or depression, tension, nervousness, weakness, drowsiness, insomnia,

T

tinnitus. **CV:** mild edema (about 7% patients), sodium and water retention, mild to moderate hypertension. **GI:** epigastric or abdominal pain, dyspepsia, *nausea,* vomiting, heartburn, constipation, peptic ulcer, GI bleeding. **Hematologic:** transient and small decreases in hemoglobin and hematocrit, purpura, petechiae, granulocytopenia, leukopenia. **Renal:** hematuria, proteinuria, increased BUN. **Skin:** toxic epidermal necrolysis, morbilliform eruptions, urticaria, pruritus. **Other:** anaphylaxis (especially after drug is discontinued and then reinstituted).

DIAGNOSTIC TEST INTERFERENCE

Tolmetin prolongs ***bleeding time,*** inhibits ***platelet aggregation,*** elevates ***BUN, alkaline phosphatase,*** and ***AST*** levels; may decrease ***hemoglobin*** and ***hematocrit*** values. Metabolites may produce false-positive results for ***proteinuria*** (with tests that rely on acid precipitation, e.g., sulfosalicylic acid).

DRUG INTERACTIONS ORAL ANTICOAGULANTS, **heparin** may prolong bleeding time; may increase **lithium** toxicity; **aspirin,** other NSAIDS add to ulcerogenic effects; may increase **methotrexate** toxicity.

NURSING IMPLICATIONS

Administration

- Treatment is preferably scheduled to include a morning dose (on arising) and a bedtime dose.
- Tablet may be crushed before administration and taken with fluid of patient's choice; capsule may be emptied and contents swallowed with water or mixed with food.
- Food delays absorption but does not affect total amount absorbed.
- Store drug in tightly capped light-resistant container at 15–30C (59–86F) unless otherwise instructed.

Assessment & Drug Effects

- The patient with renal damage should be closely monitored and perhaps given lower doses. I&O ratio should be evaluated and the patient encouraged to increase fluid intake to at least 8 full glasses of fluid per day.
- Periodic renal function tests (routine urinalysis, creatinine clearance, and serum creatinine) are recommended for patient on long-term therapy.
- Sodium bicarbonate alkalinizes the urine, which increases urinary excretion of tolmetin. Thus, degree and duration of effectiveness may be reduced. Check self-medicating habits of the patient.
- Therapeutic response in patient during treatment for rheumatoid arthritis or osteoarthritis generally occurs within 1 wk with progressive improvement in succeeding week: reduced joint pain and swelling, reduction in duration of morning stiffness, improved functional capacity (increase in grip strength, delayed onset of fatigue).

Patient & Family Education

- If GI disturbances occur, instruct to take drug with meals or milk. Advise patient to notify physician if symptoms persist; dosage reduction may be necessary, or an antacid may be prescribed.
- Instruct patient with impaired renal or cardiac function to monitor weight (an increase of more than 2 kg [4 lb]/wk should be reported) and to check for swelling in ankles, tibiae, hands, and feet.
- Because of possible enhanced bleeding, warn to inform surgeon or dentist before treatment that patient is taking tolmetin.
- Warn to report promptly signs of abnormal bleeding (ecchymosis, epistaxis, melena, petechiae), itch-

ing, skin rash, persistent headache, edema.
- Dizziness and drowsiness are common side effects; therefore, caution to avoid potentially hazardous activities until response to the drug is known.

TOLNAFTATE

(tole-naf′tate)

Trade names: Aftate, Pitrex♣, Tinactin

Classifications: SKIN AND MUCOUS MEMBRANE AGENT; ANTIINFECTIVE; ANTIFUNGAL ANTIBIOTIC

Prototype: Fluconazole

Pregnancy category: C

ACTIONS/PHARMACODYNAMICS

Synthetic topical antifungal agent. Action mechanism not clear, but it has been shown that tolnaftate distorts hyphae and stunts mycelial growth on susceptible fungi. Toxicity and susceptibility rates are low. Fungistatic or fungicidal to *Microsporum*, specifically *M. gypseum, M. canis, M. audouinii, M. japonicum, Trichophyton, T. rubrum, T. schoenleinii, T. tonsurans,* and *Epidermophyton floccosum,* but ineffective against *Candida albicans, Cryptococcus neoformans, Aspergillus fumigatus,* bacteria, protozoa, and viruses.

USES Tinea pedis (athlete's foot), tinea cruris (jock itch), tinea corporis (body ringworm); also tinea capitis and tinea unguium if infection is superficial, plantar or palmar lesions adjunctively with keratolytic agents, and tinea versicolor (caused by *Malassezia furfur*).

ROUTE & DOSAGE

Tinea Infestations

Adult/Child: **Topical** Apply 0.5–1 cm ($\frac{1}{4}$–$\frac{1}{2}$ in) of cream or 3 drops of solution b.i.d. in morning and evening; powder may be used prophylactically in normally moist areas.

CONTRAINDICATIONS & PRECAUTIONS **Contraindicated in:** skin irritations prior to therapy, nail and scalp infections; safe use during pregnancy (category C) and lactation or by children < 2 y not established. **Cautious use in:** excoriated skin.

ADVERSE/SIDE EFFECTS Local irritation, stinging of skin from aerosol formulation.

NURSING IMPLICATIONS

Administration

- Thoroughly cleanse site with water and dry completely before applying tolnaftate. Massage a thin layer of drug gently into skin. Area should not be wet from excess drug after application.
- Shake aerosol powder container well before use.
- The cream and powder are not recommended for nail or scalp infection.
- Liquids (solutions) are recommended for scalp infection or to treat hairy areas.
- Store cream, gel, powder, and topical solution in light-resistant containers at 15–30C (59–86F); store aerosol container at 2–30C (38–86F). Avoid freezing and exposure to light.

Patient & Family Education

- Tolnaftate does not stain skin or clothing.
- Emphasize importance of personal cleanliness. Daily bathing, thorough rinsing, and complete drying of skin destroys the kind of environment conducive to growth of fungi.

T

- If hair follicles or nail beds are involved, a systemic antifungal (e.g., griseofulvin) will be necessary concomitant treatment.
- Powder and powder aerosol are effective in treatment of athlete's foot and in daily hygiene to reduce natural moisture in groin and intertriginous areas.
- If patient has athlete's foot, patient should put socks on before putting on underclothes to avoid spread of infection to groin area (jock itch).
- Pruritus, soreness, burning should be relieved within 24–72 h after start of treatment.
- Explain that treatment should be continued for 2–3 wk after disappearance of all symptoms to prevent recurrence.
- In the absence of improvement within 4 wk, patient should return to physician for reevaluation of prescribed treatment.
- If skin has thickened as a result of the infection, desired clinical response may be delayed for 4–6 wk.
- Avoid contact of all drug forms with eyes.
- If solution solidifies, place container in warm water to liquefy contents. Potency is unaffected.
- Do not puncture or store aerosol near heat or an open flame or expose to temperature above 49C (120F). Do not place aerosol container in fire or incinerator for disposal.

T

TOLTERODINE TARTRATE

(tol-ter′o-deen tar′trate)

Trade name: Detrol

Classifications: AUTONOMIC NERVOUS SYSTEM AGENT; ANTICHOLINERGIC AGENT; ANTIMUSCARINIC AGENT; MUSCARINIC RECEPTOR ANTAGONIST

Prototype: Atropine

Pregnancy category: C

ACTIONS/PHARMACODYNAMICS Selective muscarinic urinary bladder receptor antagonist. Controls urinary bladder incontinence by controlling contractions.

USE Overactive bladder (urinary frequency, urgency, urge incontinence).

ROUTE & DOSAGE

Overactive Bladder

Adult: **PO** 2 mg b.i.d.; may decrease to 1 mg b.i.d. in those with significantly reduced hepatic function or taking drugs that inhibit cytochrome P450 3A4 (see Administration).

PHARMACOKINETICS **Absorption:** 77% absorbed, significantly decreased with food. **Peak:** 1–2 h. **Distribution:** 96% protein bound. **Metabolism:** metabolized in liver by cytochrome P450 2D6 enzymes to active metabolite. **Elimination:** half-life: 1.9–3.7 h; 77% excreted in urine, 17% in feces.

CONTRAINDICATIONS & PRECAUTIONS **Contraindicated in:** gastric retention; hypersensitivity to tolterodine; uncontrolled narrow-angle glaucoma; urinary retention; pregnancy (category C). **Cautious use in:** lactation; cardiovascular disease; liver disease; controlled narrow-angle glaucoma; obstructive GI disease; obstructive uropathy; paralytic ileus or intestinal atony; renal impairment; ulcerative colitis.

ADVERSE/SIDE EFFECTS **Body as whole:** back pain, fatigue, flu-like syndrome, falls, arthralgia. **CNS:** headache, paresthesias, vertigo, dizziness, nervousness, somnolence. **CV:** chest pain, hypertension. **GI:** *dry mouth,* dyspepsia, constipation, abdominal pain, diarrhea, flatulence, nausea, vomiting. **GU:** dysuria, micturition frequency, urinary retention, UTI. **Respiratory:** bronchitis, cough, pharyngitis, rhinitis, sinusitis, URI. **Skin:** pruritus, rash, erythema, dry skin. **Other:** dry eyes, vision abnormalities, weight gain.

NURSING IMPLICATIONS

Administration

- Doses >1 mg b.i.d. should not be given to those with significantly reduced hepatic function or concurrently receiving macrolide antibiotics, azole antifungal agents, or other cytochrome P450 3A4 inhibitors.
- Store at 20–25C (68–77F) in a tightly closed container.

Assessment & Drug Effects

- Therapeutic effectiveness is indicated by reduced urinary incontinence, urgency, and frequency.
- More frequent monitoring of intraocular pressure is required with glaucoma patients.
- Carefully monitor HR and BP, especially in those with cardiovascular disease.

Patient & Family Education

- Promptly notify the prescriber if you experience eye pain, rapid heartbeat, difficulty breathing, skin rash or hives, confusion, or incoordination.
- Blurred vision, sensitivity to light, and dry mouth are common side effects. Report these if they become bothersome.
- Avoid the use of alcohol or over-the-counter antihistamines.

TOPIRAMATE

(to-pir′a-mate)

Trade name: Topamax

Classifications: CENTRAL NERVOUS SYSTEM AGENT; ANTICONVULSANT

Pregnancy category: C

ACTIONS/PHARMACODYNAMICS Sulfamate-substituted monosaccharide with a broad spectrum of anticonvulsant activity. Its precise mechanism of action is unknown. Topiramate has sodium channel–blocking action, as well as enhancing the ability of GABA to induce a flux of chloride ions into the neurons, thus potentiating the activity of this inhibitory neurotransmitter (GABA).

USE Adjunctive therapy for partial-onset seizures in adults.

ROUTE & DOSAGE

Partial-onset Seizures

Adult: **PO** Initiate with 25 mg b.i.d.; increase by 50 mg/wk to efficacy. Average maintenance dose 200–400 mg/d divided b.i.d. (max 1600 mg/d).

In Renal Impairment

Cl_{cr} < 70 ml/min, decrease dose by 50%.

PHARMACOKINETICS **Absorption:** rapidly absorbed from GI tract; 80% bioavailability. **Peak:** 2 h. **Distribution:** 13–17% protein bound. **Metabolism:** minimally metabolized in the liver. **Elimination:** half-life: 21 h; excreted primarily in urine.

T

CONTRAINDICATIONS & PRECAUTIONS **Contraindicated in:** hypersensitivity to topiramate. Topiramate's effect on labor and delivery is unknown. **Cautious use in:** renal impairment, hepatic function impairment, lactation, pregnancy (category C). Topiramate has been studied in patients 4–17 y of age. Safety and effectiveness in children have not been established.

ADVERSE/SIDE EFFECTS **Body as whole:** *fatigue.* **CNS:** *somnolence, dizziness, ataxia, psychomotor slowing, confusion, nystagmus, paresthesia, memory difficulty, difficulty concentrating, nervousness,* depression, anxiety, tremor. **GI:** anorexia. **Other:** *speech problems,* weight loss.

DRUG INTERACTIONS Increased CNS depression with **alcohol** and other CNS DEPRESSANTS; may increase **phenytoin** concentrations; may decrease ORAL CONTRACEPTIVE, **valproate** concentrations; may increase risk of renal stone formation with other CARBONIC ANHYDRASE INHIBITORS. **Carbamazepine, phenytoin, valproate** may decrease topiramate concentrations.

NURSING IMPLICATIONS

Administration

- Dosage increments of 50 mg should be made at weekly intervals to the recommended dose, usually 400 mg/d.
- Because of bitter taste, tablets should not be broken unless absolutely necessary.
- In patients with moderate-to-severe renal impairment, the dose should be reduced by half.
- Store at 15–30C (59–86F) in a tightly closed container. Protect from light and moisture.

Assessment & Drug Effects

- Therapeutic effectiveness is indicated by a decrease in seizure activity.
- Monitor mental status and report significant cognitive impairment.
- Lab tests: periodically monitor CBC with Hgb and Hct.

Patient & Family Education

- Drug should not be abruptly stopped. It should be discontinued gradually to minimize seizures.
- To minimize risk of kidney stones, at least 6–8 full glasses of water should be consumed daily.
- Caution should be exercised with hazardous activities. Sedation is common, especially with concurrent use of alcohol or other CNS depressants.
- While on topiramate, oral contraceptives may not be reliable as a sole method of birth control.
- Psychomotor slowing and speech/language problems may develop while on topiramate therapy.
- Report adverse effects that interfere with activities of daily living.

TOPOTECAN HYDROCHLORIDE

(toe-po-tee′can)

Trade name: Hycamtin

Prototype for classifications: CAMPTOTHECIN ANTINEOPLASTIC AGENT; TOPOISOMERASE I INHIBITOR

Pregnancy category: D

ACTIONS/PHARMACODYNAMICS The antitumor mechanism of topotecan is related to inhibition of activity of topoisomerase I, an enzyme required for DNA replication. Topoisomerase I is essential for the relaxation of supercoiled double-stranded DNA which enables replication and transcription to proceed. Topotecan binds to the DNA–topoisomerase I complex. It permits uncoiling but prevents recoiling of the two strands of DNA, thus resulting in a permanent break in the DNA strands.

USE Metastatic ovarian cancer.

ROUTE & DOSAGE

Metastatic Ovarian Cancer

Adult: **IV** 1.5 mg/m^2 daily for 5 d starting on day 1 of a 21-d course.

Four courses of therapy recommended. Subsequent doses can be adjusted by 0.25 mg/m^2 depending on toxicity.

PHARMACOKINETICS Distribution: 35% bound to plasma proteins. **Metabolism:** undergoes pH-dependent hydrolysis. **Elimination:** half-life: 2–3 h; approx 30% excreted in urine.

CONTRAINDICATIONS & PRECAUTIONS Contraindicated in: previous hypersensitivity to topotecan, irinotecan, or other camptothecin analogs; acute infection; pregnancy (category D); lactation. **Cautious use in:** myelosuppression, history of bleeding disorders, previous cytotoxic or radiation therapy.

ADVERSE/SIDE EFFECTS Body as a whole: *asthenia, fever, fatigue.* **GI:** *nausea, vomiting, diarrhea, constipation, abdominal pain, stomatitis, anorexia,* transient elevations in liver function tests. **Hematologic:** *leukopenia, neutropenia, anemia, thrombocytopenia.* **Respiratory:** *dyspnea.* **Skin:** *alopecia.*

NURSING IMPLICATIONS

Administration

- Initiate therapy only if baseline neutrophil count ≥1500/mm^3 and platelet count ≥ 100,000/mm^3. Do not give subsequent doses until neutrophils >1000/mm^3, platelets >100,000/mm^3, and Hgb ≥ 9.0 mg/dl.
- Dosage adjustments to 0.75 mg/m^2 are recommended with moderate renal impairment.
- Preparation and administration of IV solution: Reconstitute each 4-mg vial with 4 ml sterile water for injection. Inject required amount of diluted solution into a 100-ml bag of 0.9% NaCl Injection or 5% Dextrose Injection, and infuse immediately over 30 min.
- If skin contacts drug during preparation, wash immediately with soap and water.
- Store vials at 20–25C (68–77F). Protect from light. Reconstituted vials are stable for 24 h.

Assessment & Drug Effects

- Frequently monitor complete blood cell counts with differential; periodically monitor ALT/SGPT.
- Throughout therapy, assess for GI distress, respiratory distress, neurosensory symptoms, and S&S of infection.

Patient & Family Education

- Advise regarding common adverse effects and provide information on measures to control or minimize when possible. Instruct to immediately report any distressing adverse effects.
- Advise women to avoid pregnancy during therapy; advise lactating women to discontinue nursing prior to taking the drug.

TOREMIFENE CITRATE

(tor-em′i-feen ci′trate)

Trade name: Fareston

Classifications: ANTINEOPLASTIC; HORMONE; ANTIESTROGEN

Prototype: Tamoxifen

Pregnancy category: D

ACTIONS/PHARMACODYNAMICS Nonsteroidal antiestrogen chemical derivative of tamoxifen. Antitumor activity thought to be due to its ability to compete with estrogen for binding sites in the cancer cells.

USE Metastatic breast cancer in postmenopausal women who are estrogen receptor positive.

T

ROUTE & DOSAGE

Breast Cancer
Adult: **PO** 60 mg q.d.

PHARMACOKINETICS Absorption: rapidly absorbed from GI tract. **Peak:** 3 h. **Distribution:** >99% protein bound; crosses placenta. **Metabolism:** metabolized in liver by cytochrome P450 3A4. **Elimination:** half-life: 5 d; excreted primarily in feces.

CONTRAINDICATIONS & PRECAUTIONS Contraindicated in: hypersensitivity to toremifene; pregnancy (category D). **Cautious use in:** preexisting endometrial hyperplasia; lactation; bone metatases (may result in hypercalcemia); geriatric patients; leukopenia and thrombocytopenia; liver disease; history of thrombolytic disease.

ADVERSE/SIDE EFFECTS Body as whole: *hot flashes, sweating,* edema. **CNS:** dizziness. **GI:** *nausea,* vomiting, abnormal LFTs. **Respiratory:** pulmonary embolism. **Other:** *vaginal discharge,* vaginal bleeding, cataracts, dry eyes, corneal keratopathy.

DRUG INTERACTIONS THIAZIDE DIURETICS increase risk of hypercalcemia; increased PT on **warfarin; carbamazepine, phenobarbital, phenytoin** may increase toremifene metabolism.

T

NURSING IMPLICATIONS

Administration
- Toremifene should not generally be given to anyone with a history of thromboembolic disease.
- Store at 15–30C (59–86F) in a tightly closed container and protect from light.

Assessment & Drug Effects
- Lab tests: Periodically monitor CBC with differential, serum calcium, liver functions, and renal functions.
- Carefully monitor patients with bone metastases or those on drugs that decrease calcium excretion (e.g., thiazide diuretics) for S&S of hypercalcemia (see Appendix G).
- When given concurrently with warfarin, carefully monitor PT and INR.

Patient & Family Education
- Promptly report any of the following: unexplained weakness or fatigue, musculoskeletal pain or calf pain and tenderness, sudden chest pain, vaginal bleeding.
- Periodic eye exams are recommended with long-term therapy.

TORSEMIDE
(tor′se-mide)
Trade name: Demadex
Classifications: ELECTROLYTE AND WATER BALANCE AGENT; LOOP DIURETIC
Prototype: Furosemide
Pregnancy category: B

ACTIONS/PHARMACODYNAMICS
Long-acting potent sulfonamide "loop" diuretic and antihypertensive agent. Similarly to other loop diuretics, it inhibits reabsorption of sodium and chloride primarily in the loop of Henle, but also in the proximal and distal renal tubules. It binds to the sodium/potassium/chloride carrier in the loop of Henle and in the renal tubules. It has lower potassium-wasting effects than furosemide and a longer half-life.

USES Management of edema associated with CHF, chronic renal failure, hepatic cirrhosis; hypertension.

ROUTE & DOSAGE

CHF, Chronic Renal Failure
Adult: **PO/IV** 10–20 mg once daily; may increase up to 200 mg/d as needed.

Hepatic Cirrhosis
Adult: **PO/IV** 5–10 mg once daily administered with an aldosterone antagonist or potassium-sparing diuretic; may increase up to 40 mg/d as needed.

Hypertension
Adult: **PO/IV** 5 mg once daily; may increase to 10 mg/d if no response after 4–6 wk.

PHARMACOKINETICS Absorption: readily absorbed from GI tract. **Onset:** IV 10 min; PO 60 min. **Peak:** IV within 60 min; PO 60–120 min. **Duration:** 6–8 h. **Metabolism:** metabolized in liver by cytochrome P450 system. **Elimination:** half-life: 210 min; 80% excreted in bile; 20% excreted in urine.

CONTRAINDICATIONS & PRECAUTIONS Contraindicated in: hypersensitivity to torsemide or sulfonamides, anuria, fluid and electrolyte depletion states, hepatic coma, pregnancy (category B). **Cautious use in:** renal impairment, concurrent use of other ototoxic drugs, gout or hyperuricemia, diabetes mellitus or history of pancreatitis, liver disease, hearing impairment.

ADVERSE/SIDE EFFECTS CNS: headache, dizziness, fatigue, insomnia. **CV:** orthostatic hypotension. **Endocrine:** *hypokalemia,* hyponatremia, hyperuricemia. **GI:** nausea, diarrhea. **Skin:** rash, pruritus. **Other:** muscle cramps, rhinitis.

DRUG INTERACTIONS NSAIDS may reduce diuretic effects. Also see furosemide for potential drug interactions such as increased risk of **digoxin** toxicity due to hypokalemia, prolonged neuromuscular blockade with NEUROMUSCULAR BLOCKING AGENTS, and decreased **lithium** elimination with increased toxicity.

NURSING IMPLICATIONS

Administration
- Torsemide may be given by direct IV, undiluted and administered slowly over 2 min.
- Oral and IV doses are therapeutically equivalent; patients may be switched between the two forms with no change in dosage.
- Store at room temperature 15–30C (59–86F).

Assessment & Drug Effects
- Monitor BP often and assess for orthostatic hypotension; periodically assess weight as an index of fluid retention.
- Monitor serum electrolytes, uric acid, blood glucose, BUN, and creatinine periodically throughout the course of therapy.
- Torsemide may increase blood levels of anticoagulants and lithium; monitor patients at risk with coagulation studies and lithium levels.

Patient & Family Education
- Instruct patient to check weight at least weekly and to report abrupt gains or losses.
- Advise patient of the risk of orthostatic hypotension.
- Instruct patient to report symptoms of hypokalemia (see Appendix G) or hearing loss immediately.
- Inform diabetics of the potential for loss of glycemic control.

TRAMADOL HYDROCHLORIDE

(tra′ma-dol)

Trade names: Ultram, Zydol ♣

Classifications: CENTRAL NERVOUS SYSTEM AGENT; OPIATE AGONIST; ANALGESIC

Prototype: Morphine sulfate

Pregnancy category: C

ACTIONS/PHARMACODYNAMICS

Tramadol is a centrally acting opiate receptor agonist. It inhibits the uptake of norepinephrine and serotonin, suggesting both opioid and nonopioid mechanisms of pain relief. It may produce opioid-like effects, but causes less respiratory depression than morphine.

USE Management of moderate to moderately severe pain.

ROUTE & DOSAGE

Pain

Adult: **PO** 50–100 mg q4–6h prn (max 400 mg/d or 300 mg/d in patients ≥75 y); should decrease to 50–100 mg q12h in patients with Cl_{cr} < 30 ml/min or cirrhosis.

PHARMACOKINETICS Absorption: rapidly absorbed from GI tract; 75% reaches systemic circulation. **Onset:** 30–60 min. **Peak:** 2 h. **Duration:** 3–7 h. **Distribution:** approx 20% bound to plasma proteins; probably crosses blood–brain barrier; crosses placenta; 0.1% excreted into breast milk. **Metabolism:** metabolized extensively in liver by cytochrome P450 system. **Elimination:** half-life: 6–7 h; excreted primarily in urine.

CONTRAINDICATIONS & PRECAUTIONS Contraindicated in: hypersensitivity to tramadol or other opioid analgesics; patients on MAO inhibitors; patients acutely intoxicated with alcohol, hypnotics, centrally acting analgesics, opioids, or psychotropic drugs; patients on obstetric preoperative medication; nursing mothers. **Cautious use in:** elderly debilitated patients; chronic respiratory disorders; liver disease; renal impairment; myxedema, hypothyroidism, or hypoadrenalism; acute abdominal conditions; increased ICP or head injury; history of seizures; pregnancy (category C); patients > 75 y. Safety and efficacy in children have not been established.

ADVERSE/SIDE EFFECTS CNS: drowsiness, *dizziness, vertigo, fatigue, headache, somnolence,* restlessness, euphoria, confusion, anxiety, coordination disturbance, sleep disturbances, seizures. **CV:** palpitations, vasodilation. **GI:** *nausea, constipation,* vomiting, xerostomia, dyspepsia, diarrhea, abdominal pain, anorexia, flatulence. **Other:** sweating, rash, visual disturbances, urinary retention/frequency, menopausal symptoms, <u>anaphylactic reaction</u> (even with first dose).

DRUG INTERACTIONS Carbamazepine significantly decreases tramadol levels (may need up to twice usual dose). Tramadol may increase adverse effects of MAO INHIBITORS. TRICYCLIC ANTIDEPRESSANTS, **cyclobenzaprine,** PHENOTHIAZINES, SELECTIVE SEROTONIN-REUPTAKE INHIBITORS (SSRIS), MAO INHIBITORS may enhance seizure risk with tramadol. May increase CNS adverse effects when used with other CNS DEPRESSANTS.

DIAGNOSTIC TEST INTERFERENCE Increased creatinine, liver enzymes; decreased hemoglobin; proteinuria.

T

NURSING IMPLICATIONS

Administration

- Note that dosage reduction is recommended for patients with renal insufficiency.
- Store at 15–30C (59–86F).

Assessment & Drug Effects

- Assess for level of pain relief and administer prn dose as needed but not to exceed the recommended total daily dose.
- Monitor vital signs and assess for orthostatic hypotension or signs of CNS depression.
- Discontinue drug and notify physician if signs and symptoms of hypersensitivity occur.
- Assess bowel and bladder function; report urinary frequency or retention.
- Use seizure precautions for patients who have a history of seizures or who are concurrently using drugs that lower the seizure threshold.
- Monitor ambulation and take appropriate safety precautions.

Patient & Family Education

- Advise caution with potentially hazardous activities until reaction to the drug is known.
- Inform of potential adverse effects and instruct to report problems with bowel and bladder function, CNS impairment, and any other bothersome adverse effects.

TRANDOLAPRIL

(tran-do′la-pril)

Trade name: Mavik

Classifications: CARDIOVASCULAR AGENT; ANGIOTENSIN-CONVERTING ENZYME INHIBITOR; ANTIHYPERTENSIVE

Prototype: Captopril

Pregnancy category: C (first trimester), D (second and third trimester)

ACTIONS/PHARMACODYNAMICS Lowers blood pressure by specific inhibition of ACE. This interrupts conversion sequences initiated by renin which leads to the formation of angiotensin II from angiotensin I. Angiotensin II is a potent endogenous vasoconstrictor. Peripheral vascular resistance is lowered by vasodilation. Inhibition of ACE also leads to decreased circulating aldosterone. Decreased aldosterone leads to diuresis and a slight increase in serum potassium. Unlike other ACE inhibitors, all racial groups respond to trandolapril, including low-renin hypertensives.

USE Treatment of hypertension, alone or in combination with other antihypertensive agents. **Unlabeled use:** CHF.

ROUTE & DOSAGE

Hypertension

Adult: **PO** 1 mg in nonblack patients, 2 mg in black patients once daily. May increase weekly to 2–4 mg once daily (max 8 mg/d). Diuretics should be discontinued 2–3 d before starting trandolapril.

Adjustment for Renal or Hepatic Impairment

Cl_{cr} <30 ml/min or hepatic cirrhosis: start with 0.5 mg once daily.

PHARMACOKINETICS **Absorption:** rapidly absorbed from GI tract and converted to active form, trandolaprilat, in liver; 70% of dose reaches systemic circulation as trandolaprilat. **Peak:** 4–10 h. **Distribution:** 80% protein bound; crosses placenta, secreted into breast milk of animals (human secretion unknown). **Metabolism:** metabolized in liver to active metabolite, trandolaprilat. **Elimination:** half-life: 6 h trandolapril, 10 h trandolaprilat; 33% excreted in urine, 66% in feces.

CONTRAINDICATIONS & PRECAUTIONS **Contraindicated in:** hypersensitivity to trandolapril, history of angioedema related to previous treatment with an ACE inhibitor, pregnancy (category C, first trimester; category D, second and third trimesters), lactation. **Cautious use in:** renal impairment, hepatic insufficiency, patients prone to hypotension (e.g, CHF, ischemic heart disease, aortic stenosis, CVA, dehydration), SLE, scleroderma. Safety and effectiveness in children < 18 y not established.

ADVERSE/SIDE EFFECTS **Body as whole:** fatigue, angioedema. **CNS:** dizziness, headache. **CV:** hypotension. **GI:** diarrhea. **Respiratory:** cough. **Skin:** rash, pruritus. **Other:** hyperkalemia.

DRUG INTERACTIONS DIURETICS may enhance hypotensive effects. POTASSIUM-SPARING DIURETICS (amiloride, spironolactone, triamterene), POTASSIUM SUPPLEMENTS, POTASSIUM-CONTAINING SALT SUBSTITUTES may increase risk of hyperkalemia. May increase serum levels and toxicity of **lithium**.

T

NURSING IMPLICATIONS

Administration

- If concurrently ordered diuretic cannot be discontinued 2–3 d before beginning trandolapril therapy, initial dose should be reduced to 0.5 mg.
- Dosage adjustments should generally be made at intervals of at least 1 wk.
- Store at 20–25C (68–77F).

Assessment & Drug Effects

- Following initial dose, carefully monitor BP for 1–3 h, especially in patients using concurrent diuretics, on salt restriction, or volume depleted.
- Periodically monitor BP and cardiac status; serum potassium, sodium, creatinine, and ALT/SGTP; and WBC with differential.
- If concurrently used, frequently monitor serum lithium levels and assess for S&S of lithium toxicity; increase caution when diuretic therapy is also used.

Patient & Family Education

- Instruct patients to discontinue drug and immediately report S&S of angioedema of face or extremities. Advise to seek emergency help for swelling of the tongue or any other sign of potential airway obstruction.
- Caution that light-headedness can occur, especially during early therapy. Inform that excess fluid loss of any kind will increase risk of hypotension and syncope.

TRANYLCYPROMINE SULFATE

(tran-ill-sip′roe-meen)

Trade name: Parnate

Classifications: CNS AGENT; PSYCHOTHERAPEUTIC; ANTIDEPRESSANT; MAO INHIBITOR

Prototype: Phenelzine

Pregnancy category: C

ACTIONS/PHARMACODYNAMICS Potent nonhydrazine MAO inhibitor structurally similar to amphetamine. Actions and toxicity similar to those of hydrazine MAO inhibitors but also has rapid and direct amphetamine-like CNS stimulatory action, is less likely to cause hepatotoxicity and does not produce prolonged MAO inhibition (reversible binding).

USE Owing to its toxic potential, use is reserved for treatment of severe mental depression in hospitalized patients who have not responded to other antidepressant therapy.

ROUTE & DOSAGE

Severe Depression

Adult: **PO** 30 mg/d in 2 divided doses (20 mg in AM, 10 mg in PM); may increase by 10 mg/d at 3 wk intervals up to max of 60 mg/d.

CONTRAINDICATIONS & PRECAUTIONS **Contraindicated in:** pregnancy (category C), patients > 60 y, confirmed or suspected cerebrovascular defect, cardiovascular disease, hypertension, pheochromocytoma, history of severe or recurrent headaches.

ADVERSE/SIDE EFFECTS **CNS:** vertigo, dizziness, tremors, muscle twitching, headache, blurred vision. **CV:** *orthostatic hypotension,* arrhythmias, hypertensive crisis. **GI:** dry mouth, anorexia, constipation, diarrhea, abdominal discomfort. **Other:** rash, impotence, peripheral edema, sweating.

DRUG INTERACTIONS TRICYCLIC ANTIDEPRESSANTS, **fluoxetine,** AMPHETAMINES, **ephedrine, phenylpropanolamine, reserpine, guanethidine, buspirone, methyldopa, dopamine, levodopa, tryptophan** may precipitate hypertensive crisis, headache, or hyperexcitability; **alcohol** and other CNS DEPRESSANTS add to CNS depressant effects; **meperidine** can cause fatal cardiovascular collapse; ANESTHETICS exaggerate hypotensive and CNS depressant effects; **metrizamide** increases risk of seizures; DIURETICS and other ANTIHYPERTENSIVE AGENTS add to hypotensive effects. **Food–drug:** tyramine-containing foods—aged cheeses, processed cheeses, sour cream, wine, champagne, beer, pickled herring, anchovies, caviar, shrimp, liver, dry sausage, figs, raisins, overripe bananas or avocados, chocolate, soy sauce, bean curd, yeast extracts, yogurt, papaya products, meat tenderizers, broad beans—may precipitate hypertensive crisis.

NURSING IMPLICATIONS

Administration

- Tablet may be crushed before administration and taken with fluid or mixed with food if patient has difficulty swallowing a pill.
- Because of possibility of insomnia, usually not given in the evening.

Assessment & Drug Effects

- Incidence of severe hypertensive reactions appears to be greater with tranylcypromine than with other MAO inhibitors.
- This drug usually produces therapeutic response within 3 d, but full antidepressant effects may not be obtained until 2 or 3 wk of drug therapy.

Patient & Family Education

- Emphasize importance of avoiding tyramine-containing foods (see Food–Drug Interactions).
- Inform that excessive use of caffeine-containing beverages (chocolate, coffee, tea, cola) can contribute to development of rapid heartbeat, arrhythmias, and hypertension.
- Instruct to make position changes slowly, particularly from recumbent to upright posture.
- Instruct to avoid hazardous activities until reaction to drug is known.
- Advise to avoid alcohol or other

T

CNS depressants because of their possible additive effects.

TRASTUZUMAB

(tra-stu'zu-mab)

Trade name: Herceptin

Classifications: IMMUNOMODULATOR; ANTI-HER MONOCLONAL ANTIBODY

Pregnancy category: B

ACTIONS/PHARMACODYNAMICS Recombinant DNA monoclonal antibody that selectively binds to the human epidermal growth factor receptor 2 protein (HER2). It is an IgG1 kappa antibody that binds to HER2. Trastuzumab inhibits the growth of human tumor cells that overexpress HER2 proteins.

USE Metastatic breast cancer in those whose tumors overexpress the HER2 protein.

ROUTE & DOSAGE

Metastatic Breast Cancer

Adult: **IV** 4 mg/kg as loading dose, then 2 mg/kg qwk as a maintenance dose.

PHARMACOKINETICS **Elimination:** half-life: 5.8 d.

T

CONTRAINDICATIONS & PRECAUTIONS **Contraindicated in:** concurrent administration of anthracycline or radiation; discontinue nursing during and for 6 mo following administration of trastuzumab. **Cautious use in:** preexisting cardiac dysfunction; previous administration of cardiotoxic therapy (e.g., anthracycline or radiation); pregnancy (category B); elderly; hypersensitivity to benzyl alcohol (preservative in bacteriostatic water).

ADVERSE/SIDE EFFECTS **Body as whole:** *pain, asthenia, fever, chills,* flu syndrome, allergic reaction, bone pain, arthralgia. **CNS:** *headache, insomnia, dizziness, paresthesias,* depression, peripheral neuritis, neuropathy. **CV:** CHF, cardiac dysfunction (dyspnea, cough, paroxysmal nocturnal dyspnea, peripheral edema, S3 gallop, reduced ejection fraction), tachycardia, edema. **GI:** *diarrhea, abdominal pain, nausea, vomiting,* anorexia. **Hematologic:** *anemia, leukopenia.* **Respiratory:** *cough, dyspnea,* rhinitis, pharyngitis, sinusitis. **Skin:** *rash,* herpes simplex, acne. **Other:** increased incidence of infections. **Infusion reaction:** *chills, fever,* nausea, vomiting, pain, rigors, headache, dizziness, dyspnea, hypotension, rash.

DRUG INTERACTIONS **Paclitaxel** may increase trastuzumab.

INCOMPATIBILITIES **Solution/additive:** dextrose solution; do not mix or coadminister with other drugs.

NURSING IMPLICATIONS

Administration

- IV preparation: Reconstitute each vial with 20 ml of supplied diluent (bacteriostatic water) to produce a multidose vial containing 21 mg/ml; immediately label vial with date and write "Do not use after . . ." with a future date 28 days from the date of reconstitution. Note: For patients with a hypersensitivity to benzyl alcohol, reconstitute with sterile water for injection; this solution must be used immediately with any unused portion discarded. Withdraw the number of milligrams needed for reconstituted vial and add to a 250-ml infusion bag of 0.9% NaCl and invert bag to mix. DO NOT give or mix with dextrose solutions.

- IV infusion: Infuse loading dose (4 mg/kg) over 90 min; infuse subsequent doses (2 mg/kg) over 30 min. DO NOT give IV push or as a bolus dose.
- Store unopened vials and reconstituted vials at 2–8C (36–46F). Discard reconstituted vials 28 days after reconstitution.

Assessment & Drug Effects

- Lab/diagnostic tests: Periodically monitor CBC with differential, platelet count, and Hgb.
- During the first IV infusion, monitor for chills and fever; these adverse events usually respond to prompt treatment without the need to discontinue the infusion. Notify physician immediately.
- Carefully monitor cardiovascular status at baseline and throughout course of therapy, assessing for S&S of heart failure (e.g, dyspnea, increased cough, PND, edema, S3 gallop). Persons with preexisting cardiac dysfunction are at high risk for cardiotoxicity.

Patient & Family Education

- Promptly report any unusual symptoms (e.g., chills, nausea, fever) during infusion.
- Promptly report any of the following: shortness of breath, swelling of feet or legs, persistent cough, difficulty sleeping, loss of appetite, abdominal bloating.

TRAZODONE HYDROCHLORIDE

(tray′zoe-done)

Trade names: Desyrel, Desyrel Dividose

Classifications: CNS AGENT; PSYCHOTHERAPEUTIC; ANTIDEPRESSANT

Prototype: Imipramine

Pregnancy category: C

ACTIONS/PHARMACODYNAMICS Centrally acting triazolepyridine derivative antidepressant chemically and structurally unrelated to tricyclic, tetracyclic, or other antidepressants. Potentiates serotonin effects by selectively blocking its reuptake at presynaptic membranes in CNS. Does not stimulate CNS and causes fewer anticholinergic genitourinary and neurologic effects as compared with other antidepressants. Produces varying degrees of sedation in normal and mentally depressed patient, increases total sleep time, decreases number and duration of awakenings in depressed patient, and decreases REM sleep. Has anxiolytic effect in severely depressed patient.

USES Both inpatient and outpatient with major depression with or without prominent anxiety. **Unlabeled uses:** adjunctive treatment of alcohol dependence, anxiety neuroses, drug-induced dyskinesias.

ROUTE & DOSAGE

Depression

Adult: **PO** 150 mg/d in divided doses; may increase by 50 mg/d q3–4d (max 400–600 mg/d).
Geriatric: **PO** 25–50 mg h.s., may increase q3–7d to usual range of 75–150 mg/d.
Child 6–18 y: **PO** 1.5–2 mg/kg/d in divided doses; increase q3–4d prn (max 6 mg/kg/d).

PHARMACOKINETICS **Absorption:** readily absorbed from GI tract. **Onset:** 1–2 wk. **Peak:** 1–2 h. **Distribution:** distributed into breast milk. **Metabolism:** metabolized in liver. **Elimination:** half-life: 5–9 h; 75% excreted in urine, 25% in feces.

CONTRAINDICATIONS & PRECAUTIONS **Contraindicated in:** initial re-

covery phase of MI, ventricular ectopy; electroshock therapy. Safe use in children < 18 y not established; pregnancy (category C). **Cautious use in:** patient with suicidal ideation, cardiac arrhythmias or disease; nursing mother.

ADVERSE/SIDE EFFECTS Appears to be dose related. **CNS:** *drowsiness,* light-headedness, tiredness, dizziness, insomnia, headache, agitation, impaired memory and speech, disorientation. **CV:** *hypotension (including orthostatic hypotension),* hypertension, syncope, shortness of breath, chest pain, tachycardia, palpitations, bradycardia, PVCs, ventricular tachycardia (short episodes of 3–4 beats). **ENT:** nasal and sinus congestion, blurred vision, eye irritation, sweating or clamminess, tinnitus. **GI:** *dry mouth,* anorexia, constipation, abdominal distress, nausea, vomiting, dysgeusia, flatulence, diarrhea. **GU:** hematuria, increased frequency, delayed urine flow, early or absent menses, male priapism, ejaculation inhibition. **Hematologic:** anemia. **Musculoskeletal:** skeletal aches and pains, muscle twitches. **Skin:** skin eruptions, rash, pruritus, acne, photosensitivity. **Other:** weight gain or loss.

DRUG INTERACTIONS ANTIHYPERTENSIVE AGENTS may potentiate hypotensive effects; **alcohol** and other CNS DEPRESSANTS add to depressant effects; may increase **digoxin** or **phenytoin** levels; MAO INHIBITORS may precipitate hypertensive crisis.

NURSING IMPLICATIONS

Administration

- Taking drug with food increases amount of absorption by 20% and appears to decrease incidence of dizziness or light-headedness. Urge patient to maintain the same schedule for food-drug intake throughout treatment period to prevent variations in serum concentration.
- Store in tightly closed, light-resistant container at 15–30C (59–86F).

Assessment & Drug Effects

- If patient has preexisting cardiac disease, monitor pulse rate and regularity before administration of drug.
- When trazodone is given at the same time as an MAO inhibitor, therapy is initiated cautiously, and dose is adjusted according to clinical response. No interaction has been documented, but the potential for hypertensive crisis is recognized until ruled out.
- Adverse/side effects generally are mild and tend to decrease and disappear after the first few weeks of treatment.
- Observe patient's level of activity. If it appears to be increasing toward sleeplessness and agitation with changes in reality orientation, report to physician. Manic episodes have been reported.
- Check patient for symptoms of hypotension. If orthostatic hypotension is troublesome, suggest measures to reduce danger of falling and to help patient to tolerate the effects. Discuss with physician; a reduction of dose or discontinuation of the drug may be prescribed.
- Ask male patient if he is having inappropriate or prolonged penile erections. If he is, the drug should be discontinued and physician consulted.
- Overdose is characterized by an extension of common adverse/side effects: vomiting, lethargy, drowsiness, and exaggerated anticholinergic effects. Seizures or arrhythmias are unusual. Death rarely

occurs except when other drugs are being taken concomitantly (such as alcohol, meprobamate).

Patient & Family Education

- Therapeutic effects usually begin in 1 wk but may require 2–4 wk to reach maximum levels. Teach patient importance of adhering to regimen and have family member reenforce this teaching with patient in the home.
- Urge not to alter dose or intervals between doses.
- If drowsiness becomes a distressing side effect, patient should consult physician. Dose regimen may be adjusted so that largest dose is at bedtime.
- Advise to limit or abstain from alcohol use. The depressant effects of CNS depressants and alcohol may be potentiated by this drug.
- Warn not to self-medicate with OTC drugs for colds, allergy, or insomnia treatment without advice of physician. Many of these drugs contain CNS depressants.
- Adherence to follow-up appointment is important to permit dose adjustment or discontinuation, as indicated.
- Alert dentist, surgeon, or emergency personnel that drug is being used. Trazodone is discontinued as long as possible prior to elective surgery.

TRETINOIN

(tret′i-noyn)

Trade names: Avita, Renova, Retin-A, Retin-A Micro, Retinoic Acid, Vesanoid, Vitamin A Acid

Classifications: SKIN AND MUCOUS MEMBRANE AGENT; ANTIACNE (RETINOID); ANTIPSORIATIC; ORPHAN DRUG

Prototype: Isotretinoin

Pregnancy category: B

ACTIONS/PHARMACODYNAMICS

A contact irritant containing retinoic acid and vitamin A acid. Reverses retention hyperkeratosis and comedo formation, primary events in acne pathology. Exact action mechanism unknown, but it is suggested that keratinocytes in the sebaceous follicle become less adherent, and turnover of follicular epithelial cells is increased. These two processes promote easy extrusion of the comedo and prevent it from reformation. Tretinoin also increases permeability of skin and support conversion of follicular epithelium into less sturdy and almost fragile condition.

USES Topical treatment of acne vulgaris grades I–III, especially during early stages when number of comedones is greatest; adjunctively in management of associated comedones and in treatment of flat warts; oral for remission induction treatment of acute promyelocytic leukemia; cream as adjunctive therapy for mitigation of fine wrinkles. **Unlabeled uses:** psoriasis, senile keratosis, ichthyosis vulgaris, keratosis palmaris and plantaris, basal cell carcinoma, photodamaged skin (photoaging), and other skin conditions. **Orphan drug:** for squamous metaplasia of conjunctiva or cornea with mucous deficiency and keratinization.

ROUTE & DOSAGE

Acne

Adult: **Topical** Apply once/d h.s.

Acute Promyelocytic Leukemia

Adult: **PO** 45 mg/m^2/d; PO is 60% absorbed.

Antiwrinkle Cream

Adult: **Topical** (0.05% cream) Apply to face once daily h.s.

T

PHARMACOKINETICS **Absorption:** minimally absorbed from intact skin; PO 60% absorbed. **Elimination:** half-life: 45 min; about 0.1% of topical dose is excreted in urine within 24 h. PO half-life: 2.5–2h; 63% excreted in urine, 31% in feces.

CONTRAINDICATIONS & PRECAUTIONS **Contraindicated in:** eczema, exposure to sunlight or ultraviolet rays (as with sunlamp), sunburn, pregnancy (category B). **Cautious use in:** patient in an occupation necessitating considerable sun exposure or weather extremes, nursing mothers.

ADVERSE/SIDE EFFECTS **Note:** Listed adverse effects occur primarily with oral administration; only skin effects with topical administration. **CNS:** *dizziness, paresthesias, anxiety, insomnia, depression, headache, fever, weakness, fatigue,* cerebral hemorrhage, intracranial hypertension, hallucinations. **CV:** *arrhythmias, flushing, hypotension, hypertension,* CHF. **Eye:** visual disturbances, ocular disturbances, change in visual acuity. **GI:** *nausea, vomiting, abdominal pain, diarrhea, constipation, dyspepsia,* *<u>GI hemorrhage.</u>* **Respiratory:** *dyspnea, respiratory insufficiency, pneumonia, rales, pleural effusion, wheezing.* **Skin:** local inflammatory reactions, transient stinging or warmth on site, *redness, scaling, severe erythema,* blistering, crusting and peeling, temporary hypopigmentation or hyperpigmentation, *increased sweating.* **Other:** *bone pain, malaise, shivering, hemorrhage, peripheral edema, pain, chest discomfort, weight gain or loss,* <u>DIC,</u> renal insufficiency, dysuria, acute renal failure, earache.

DRUG INTERACTIONS TOPICAL ACNE MEDICATIONS (including **sulfur, resorcinol, benzoyl peroxide,** and **salicylic acid**) may increase inflammation and peeling; topical products containing **alcohol** or **menthol** may cause stinging.

NURSING IMPLICATIONS

Administration

Topical

- If patient has been using a desquamative agent, a waiting period long enough for recovery from its action should intervene before starting treatment with tretinoin.
- Cleanse using a mild bland soap, and thoroughly dry areas being treated before applying drug. Avoid use of medicated, drying, or abrasive soaps and cleansers.
- Wash hands before and after treatment. Do not apply to nonaffected skin area.
- Avoid contact of drug with eyes, mouth, angles of nose, open wounds, mucous membranes.
- Store gel and liquid formulations below 30C (86F) and solution below 27C (80F).

Assessment & Drug Effects

- Tretinoin treatment to black individuals may cause unsightly postinflammatory hyperpigmentation; dark-complexioned whites may have a mild hypopigmentary effect. Both are reversible with termination of drug treatment.
- Clinical response to tretinoin should be evident in 2 or 3 wk, but a complete and satisfactory response (in 75% of the patients) may require a period of 3 or 4 mo. Once achieved, control is maintained by less frequent applications or a change in formulation or dosage.

Patient & Family Education

- Inform patient that erythema and desquamation during the first 1–3 wk of treatment do not represent exacerbation of the skin problem but a probable response to the drug from deep previously unseen lesions.

- Urge compliance with therapy.
- As treatment is continued, lesions gradually disappear, leaving an inflammatory background; scaling and redness decrease after 8–10 wk of therapy.
- Instruct the patient to wash face no more often than 2–3 times daily.
- Topical preparations with high concentrations of alcohol, astringents, spices or lime, perfumes and shaving lotions, should not be used during treatment period.
- Inform patient that the drug is not curative; relapses commonly occur within 3–6 wk after treatment has been discontinued.
- Nonmedicated cosmetics may be used during therapy, but they should be removed thoroughly before drug is applied.
- If exposure to sun cannot be avoided, it is advisable to use a sunscreen product with SPF 15 or higher.
- Warn patient against self-medication with additional acne treatment because of danger of drug interactions.
- Inform physician if even the mildest side effects occur rather than terminating the treatment prematurely. Keep appointments for assessment of progress to permit regimen adjustment when needed.

TRIAMCINOLONE

(trye-am-sin′oh-lone)

Trade names: Aristocort, Atolone, Kenacort, Kenalog-E

TRIAMCINOLONE ACETONIDE

Trade names: Azmacort, Cenocort A_2, Kenalog, Triam-A, Triamonide, Tri-kort, Trilog

TRIAMCINOLONE DIACETATE

Trade names: Amcort, Aristocort Forte, Articulose LA, Cenocort Forte, Kenacort, Triam-Forte, Trilone, Tristoject

TRIAMCINOLONE HEXACETONIDE

Trade name: Aristospan

Classifications: HORMONE; ADRENAL CORTICOSTEROID; ANTIINFLAMMATORY

Prototype: Hydrocortisone

Pregnancy category: C

ACTIONS/PHARMACODYNAMICS

Immediate acting synthetic fluorinated adrenal corticosteroid with glucocorticoid and antirheumatic activity 7–13 times more potent than that of hydrocortisone. Possesses minimal sodium and water retention properties in therapeutic doses.

USES An inflammatory or immunosuppressant agent. Orally inhaled: bronchial asthma in patient who has not responded to conventional inhalation treatment. Therapeutic doses do not appear to suppress HPA (hypothalamic-pituitary-adrenal) axis.

ROUTE & DOSAGE

Inflammation, Immunosuppression

Adult: **PO/IM/SC** 4–48 mg/d in divided doses. **Intraarticular/Intradermal** 4–48 mg/d. **Inhaled** 2–4 inhalations q.i.d. **Topical** See Appendix A.
Child: **PO/IM/SC** 3.3–50 mg/m_2/d in divided doses. **Intraarticular/Intradermal** 3.3–50 mg/m^2/d.

Acetonide

Adult: **IM** 60 mg; may repeat with 20–100 mg q6wk. **Intradermal** 1 mg per injection site (max 30 mg total). **Intraarticular** 2.5–4.0 mg; **Inhalation** See Appendix A.
Child 6–12 y: **IM** 0.03–0.2 mg q1–7d. **Inhalation** See Appendix A.

Diacetate

Adult: **PO** 4–48 mg/d in 1–4 divided doses. **IM** 40 mg once/wk. **Intradermal** 5–48 mg (max 75 mg/wk) may repeat q1–2wk if needed. **Intraarticular** 2–40 mg q1–8wk.
Child: **PO** 0.117–1.66 mg/kg/d.

Hexacetonide

Adult: **Intralesional** Up to 0.5 mg/in^2 of skin. **Intraarticular** 2–20 mg q3–4wk.

PHARMACOKINETICS **Absorption:** readily absorbed from all routes. **Onset:** 24–48 h PO, IM. **Peak:** 1–2 h PO; 8–10 h IM. **Duration:** 2.25 d PO; 1–6 wk IM. **Metabolism:** metabolized in liver. **Elimination:** half-life: 2–5 h; HPA suppression: 18–36 h; excreted in urine.

CONTRAINDICATIONS & PRECAUTIONS **Contraindicated in:** safe use during pregnancy (category C), by lactating women, and by children < 6 y not established. Renal dysfunction. Also see hydrocortisone.

ADVERSE/SIDE EFFECTS Muscle weakness and loss of tissue mass. **Local:** burning, itching, folliculitis, hypertrichosis, hypopigmentation. Also see prednisone.

DRUG INTERACTIONS BARBITURATES, **phenytoin, rifampin** increase steroid metabolism—may need increased doses of triamcinolone; **amphotericin B,** DIURETICS add to potassium loss; **ambenonium, neostigmine, pyridostigmine** may cause severe muscle weakness in patients with myasthenia gravis; may inhibit antibody response to VACCINES, TOXOIDS.

NURSING IMPLICATIONS

Administration

- Tablet may be crushed before administration and taken with fluid of patient's choice.
- Protect drug from light. Store at 15–30C (59–86F). See hydrocortisone for numerous additional nursing implications.

Assessment & Drug Effects

- This preparation may cause natriuresis, negative nitrogen balance, with weight loss in most patients (along with headache, fatigue, and dizziness) and sodium retention with weight gain and moon facies in others. Adequate diet to counter these effects should be designed. Plan with dietitian, patient, and physician. High-protein, high-potassium diet is often needed.
- If a local infection develops at site of application, occlusive dressing should be discontinued and appropriate antimicrobial treatment started.
- Systemic absorption may occur after topical application, especially in children and if used over extensive areas for prolonged periods or if occlusive dressings are used. Reportable symptoms include hypercortisolism or Cushing's syndrome (see Appendix G), hyperglycemia (see Appendix G), and glucosuria.

Patient & Family Education

- Warn that postural hypotension may accompany sodium loss and weight loss.
- Caution to adhere to drug regimen, i.e., not to increase or de-

crease established regimen and not to abruptly discontinue taking or using the drug.

TRIAMTERENE

(trye-am′ter-een)

Trade name: Dyrenium

Classifications: WATER BALANCE AGENT; POTASSIUM-SPARING DIURETIC

Prototype: Spironolactone

Pregnancy category: B

ACTIONS/PHARMACODYNAMICS Structurally related to folic acid. Like spironolactone, has weak diuretic action and a potassium-sparing effect. Promotes excretion of sodium, chloride (to lesser extent), and carbonate. Unlike spironolactone, blocks potassium excretion by direct action on distal renal tubule rather than by inhibiting aldosterone. Decreased glomerular filtration rate and elevated BUN are associated with daily administration.

USES Adjunct in the management of edema associated with CHF, hepatic cirrhosis, nephrotic syndrome, idiopathic edema, steroid-induced edema, and edema due to secondary hyperaldosteronism. Also alone or in conjunction with a thiazide or loop diuretic in patients with hypertension because of its potassium-sparing activity.

ROUTE & DOSAGE

Edema

Adult: **PO** 100 mg b.i.d. (max 300 mg/d); may be able to decrease to 100 mg/d or q.o.d.
Geriatric: **PO** 50 mg/d (max 100 mg/d in 1–2 divided doses).
Child: **PO** 2–4 mg/kg/d in divided doses or q.o.d. (max 300 mg/d).

PHARMACOKINETICS **Absorption:** rapidly but variably absorbed from GI tract. **Onset:** 2–4 h. **Duration:** 7–9 h. **Metabolism:** metabolized in liver to active and inactive metabolites. **Elimination:** half-life: 100–150 min; excreted in urine.

CONTRAINDICATIONS & PRECAUTIONS **Contraindicated in:** hypersensitivity to drug; anuria, severe or progressive kidney disease or dysfunction; severe hepatic disease; elevated serum potassium. Safe use during pregnancy (category B) and in nursing mothers not established. **Cautious use in:** impaired renal or hepatic function; history of gouty arthritis; diabetes mellitus, history of kidney stones.

ADVERSE/SIDE EFFECTS Diarrhea, nausea, vomiting, and other GI disturbances; dizziness, headache, dry mouth, pruritus, rash, anaphylaxis, photosensitivity, weakness and hypotension (large doses), muscle cramps, *hyperkalemia* and other electrolyte imbalances, elevated BUN, elevated uric acid (patients predisposed to gouty arthritis), hyperchloremic acidosis, blood dyscrasias: granulocytopenia, eosinophilia, megaloblastic anemia, patients with reduced folic acid stores (e.g., hepatic cirrhosis).

DIAGNOSTIC TEST INTERFERENCE Pale blue fluorescence in urine interferes with fluorometric assay of ***quinidine*** and ***lactic dehydrogenase activity.*** Triamterene may cause increases in ***blood glucose*** levels (diabetic patients), ***BUN, serum potassium, magnesium,*** and ***uric acid*** and ***urinary calcium excretion.***

DRUG INTERACTIONS May increase **lithium** levels, thus increasing its toxicity; **indomethacin** may de-

T

crease renal elimination of triamterene; ANGIOTENSIN-CONVERTING ENZYME (ACE) INHIBITORS, other POTASSIUM-SPARING DIURETICS may cause hyperkalemia.

NURSING IMPLICATIONS

Administration

- If patient cannot swallow capsule, it may be emptied and contents swallowed with fluid or mixed with food.
- Give drug with or after meals to prevent or minimize nausea.
- Schedule doses to prevent interruption of sleep from diuresis, e.g., with or after breakfast if a single dose is taken, or no later than 6 PM if more than one dose is prescribed. Consult physician.
- Drug should be withdrawn gradually in patients on prolonged therapy or in patients who have received high doses, in order to prevent rebound increased urinary excretion of potassium.
- Preserve in tight, light-resistant containers at 15–30C (59–86F) unless otherwise directed.

Assessment & Drug Effect

- Monitor BP during period of dosage adjustment. Hypotensive reactions, although rare, have been reported. Implications for ambulation should be noted, particularly for elderly patients.
- Weigh patient under standard conditions, prior to drug initiation and daily during therapy.
- Diuretic response usually occurs on first day of therapy, but maximum effect may not occur for several days.
- Monitor and report oliguria and unusual changes in I&O ratio. Consult physician regarding allowable fluid intake.
- Renal stone formation has been reported in patients taking high doses or who have low urine volume and increased urine acidity.
- Observe for signs and symptoms of hyperkalemia (see Appendix G), particularly in patients with renal insufficiency, in patients on high-dose or prolonged therapy, in the elderly, and in patients with diabetes. Baseline and periodic determinations of serum potassium and other electrolytes should be done.
- Periodic evaluations of renal function (BUN, serum creatinine) are advised in patients with known or suspected renal insufficiency.
- Patients with cirrhosis are usually hospitalized during triamterene therapy because rapid alterations in fluid and electrolyte balance can precipitate hepatic coma or precoma: irritability, restlessness, confusion, stupor, liver flap (asterixis), coma.
- Periodic blood studies are advised in patients on prolonged therapy and in patients with cirrhosis since they are prone to develop megaloblastic anemia.
- Triamterene may increase blood glucose; therefore, it should not be given to a diabetic patient unless blood glucose is controlled. Patients should be closely monitored.

Patient & Family Education

- Unlike most diuretics, triamterene promotes potassium retention. Therefore, potassium supplements, potassium-rich diet, and salt substitutes are usually not prescribed.
- Generally, salt restriction is not stressed because of the possibility of low-salt syndrome (hyponatremia). Consult physician.
- Instruct to report overpowering fatigue or weakness, malaise, fever, sore throat, or mouth (possible

T

 Common side effect in *italic,* life-threatening effects underlined; generic names in **bold;** drug class in SMALL CAPS

symptoms of granulocytopenia) and unusual bleeding or bruising (thrombocytopenia).

- Warn that triamterene may cause photosensitivity and therefore to avoid exposure to sun and sunlamps.
- Inform that triamterene may impart a harmless pale blue fluorescence to urine.

TRIAZOLAM

(trye-ay'zoe-lam)

Trade name: Halcion

Classifications: CNS AGENT; BENZODIAZEPINE ANXIOLYTIC; SEDATIVE-HYPNOTIC

Prototype: Lorazepam

Pregnancy category: X

Controlled substance: Schedule IV

ACTIONS/PHARMACODYNAMICS Benzodiazepine derivative with hypnotic effects with fewer residual daytime effects. Blockade of cortical and limbic arousal results in hypnotic activity. Drug-induced effects on sleep include decreased sleep latency and number of nocturnal awakenings, decreased total nocturnal wake time, and increased duration of sleep.

USES Short-term management of insomnia characterized by difficulty in falling asleep, frequent wakeful periods. Following long-term use, tolerance or adaptation may develop.

ROUTE & DOSAGE

Insomnia

Adult: **PO** 0.125–0.25 mg h.s. (max 0.5 mg/d).
Geriatric: **PO** 0.0625–0.125 mg h.s.

PHARMACOKINETICS **Absorption:** readily absorbed from GI tract. **Onset:** 15–30 min. **Peak:** 1–2 h. **Duration:** 6–8 h. **Distribution:** crosses placenta; distributed into breast milk. **Metabolism:** metabolized in liver to active metabolites. **Elimination:** half-life: 2–3 h; excreted in urine.

CONTRAINDICATIONS & PRECAUTIONS **Contraindicated in:** hypersensitivity to triazolam and benzodiazepines; pregnancy (category X). **Cautious use in:** depression; elderly and debilitated patients; patients with suicidal tendency; impaired renal or hepatic function; chronic pulmonary insufficiency.

ADVERSE/SIDE EFFECTS **CNS:** *drowsiness,* light-headedness, headache, dizziness, ataxia, visual disturbances, confusional states, *memory impairment, "rebound insomnia," anterograde amnesia.* **GI:** nausea, vomiting, constipation. **Other:** paradoxical reactions, minor changes in EEG patterns.

DRUG INTERACTIONS **Alcohol,** CNS DEPRESSANTS, ANTICONVULSANTS, **nefazodone,** BENZODIAZEPINES potentiate CNS depression; **cimetidine** increases triazolam plasma levels, thus increasing its toxicity; may decrease antiparkinsonism effects of **levodopa.**

NURSING IMPLICATIONS

Administration

- Patient should take triazolam immediately before retiring; onset of drug action is rapid.
- Recommended doses should not be exceeded.
- Store at 15–30C (59–86F).

Assessment & Drug Effects

- Because of short half-life, under normal circumstances dose is usually cleared before next bedtime dose; therefore, "morning after" grogginess rarely occurs.
- Signs of developing tolerance or adaptation (with long-term use)

T

include increased daytime anxiety, increased wakefulness during last one third of the night.
- Periodic blood counts, urinalysis, and blood chemistries are advised during long-term use of triazolam.
- Although the drug has minimum abuse potential, it should not be used by addiction-prone patients (drug addicts, alcoholics) unless careful surveillance by health personnel is available. Habituation and dependence can occur.
- As with other benzodiazepines, smoking may decrease hypnotic effects of triazolam.
- Overdosage (accidental or by intent) will develop with 4 times the maximum recommended therapeutic dose (0.5 mg), or 2 mg.
- Overdose symptoms are slurred speech, somnolence, confusion, impaired coordination, and coma.

Patient & Family Education
- Engaging in hazardous activities (driving a car, use of machinery) until drug response has been defined should be avoided.
- Advise that use of alcohol or other CNS depressants while on this drug increases sedative effects.
- Warn not to stop taking drug suddenly, especially if patient is subject to seizures. Withdrawal symptoms may occur. These range from mild dysphoria to more serious symptoms such as tremors, abdominal and muscle cramps, convulsions. Consult physician about schedule for discontinuing therapy.
- Caution not to increase dose without physician's advice because of toxic potential of drug.

TRICHLORMETHIAZIDE

(trye-klor-meth-eye′a-zide)

Trade names: Diurese, Metahydrin, Naqua, Niazide, Trichlorex

Classifications: WATER BALANCE AGENT; THIAZIDE DIURETIC; ANTIHYPERTENSIVE

Prototype: Hydrochlorothiazide

Pregnancy category: B

ACTIONS/PHARMACODYNAMICS Benzothiadiazine (thiazide) derivative. Similar to hydrochlorothiazide in pharmacologic actions, uses, contraindications, precautions, adverse effects, and interactions.

USES To treat hypertension as sole agent or to enhance the effects of another antihypertensive when given in combination. Also to treat edema associated with CHF, renal decompensation, and hepatic cirrhosis.

ROUTE & DOSAGE

Edema

Adult: **PO** 1–4 mg 1–2 times/d.

Hypertension

Adult: **PO** 2–4 mg/d in 1–2 divided doses.
Child: **PO** 0.07 mg/kg/d in 1–2 divided doses.

PHARMACOKINETICS **Onset:** 2 h. **Peak:** 6 h. **Duration:** 24 h. **Distribution:** crosses placenta; distributed into breast milk. **Elimination:** excreted in urine.

CONTRAINDICATIONS & PRECAUTIONS **Contraindicated in:** anuria; hypersensitivity to thiazides, sulfonamides; pregnancy (category B), lactation. **Cautious use in:** history of allergy; renal and hepatic disease; gout; diabetes mellitus.

ADVERSE/SIDE EFFECTS Anorexia, paresthesias, photosensitivity, vasculitis; exacerbation of gout, SLE. Also see hydrochlorothiazide.

Common side effect in *italic*, life-threatening effects underlined: generic names in **bold**; drug class in SMALL CAPS

T

DRUG INTERACTIONS Amphotericin B, CORTICOSTEROIDS increase hypokalemic effects; may antagonize hypoglycemic effects of SULFONYLUREAS, insulin; **cholestyramine, colestipol** decrease thiazide absorption; intensifies hypoglycemic and hypotensive effects of **diazoxide**; increased potassium and magnesium loss with **digoxin**—may cause digoxin toxicity; decreases **lithium** excretion, thus increasing its toxicity; NSAIDS may attenuate diuresis—risk of NSAID-induced renal failure increased.

NURSING IMPLICATIONS

Administration

- Drug should be taken early in AM after breakfast to reduce gastric irritation and to prevent interruption of sleep because of diuresis. If 2 doses are ordered, schedule second dose no later than 3 PM.
- Store in tightly closed container at 15–30C (59–86F) unless otherwise instructed.

Assessment & Drug Effects

- Monitor BP and I&O ratio during first phase of antihypertensive therapy. Report a sudden fall in BP, which may initiate severe postural hypotension and potentially dangerous perfusion problems, especially in the extremities.
- Antihypertensive effects may be noted in 3–4 d; maximal effects may require 3–4 wk.
- Older patients may be more sensitive to the average adult dose. Monitor them closely.
- Monitor patient for signs of hypokalemia (see Appendix G). Report them promptly. Hypokalemia is rarely severe in most patients even on long-term therapy, but the elderly are especially susceptible.
- The prediabetic or diabetic patient should be watched carefully for loss of control of diabetes or early signs of hyperglycemia: drowsiness, polyuria, anorexia, polydipsia. These symptoms are slow to develop and to recognize. Check urine for glycosuria.

Patient & Family Education

- To prevent onset of hypokalemia, urge patient to eat a balanced diet (usually includes potassium-rich foods such as fruits and fruit juices).
- Counsel to avoid use of OTC drugs unless they are approved by the physician. Many preparations contain both potassium and sodium and if misused, or if patient overdoses, electrolyte imbalance side effects may be induced.
- Advise to maintain prescribed dosage regimen, not to skip, reduce, or double doses or change dose intervals.

TRIFLUOPERAZINE HYDROCHLORIDE

(trye-floo-oh-per′a-zeen)

Trade names: Novoflurazine♣, Solazine♣, Stelazine, Terfluzine♣

Classifications: CNS AGENT; PSYCHOTHERAPEUTIC; ANTIPSYCHOTIC PHENOTHIAZINE

Prototype: Chlorpromazine

Pregnancy category: C

ACTIONS/PHARMACODYNAMICS

Phenothiazine similar to chlorpromazine in most actions, uses, limitations, and interactions. Produces less sedative, cardiovascular, and anticholinergic effects and more prominent antiemetic and extrapyramidal effects than other phenothiazines do. Total pharmacologic effects are more prolonged than those of chlorpromazine. Lowers convulsive threshold.

USES Management of manifestations of psychotic disorders; "possibly effective" control of excessive anxiety and tension associated with neuroses or somatic conditions.

ROUTE & DOSAGE

Psychotic Disorders

Adult: **PO** 1–2 mg b.i.d.; may increase up to 20 mg/d in hospitalized patients. **IM** 1–2 mg q4–6h (max 10 mg/d).
Child: **PO** 6–12 y, 1 mg 1–2 times/d; may increase up to 15 mg/d in hospitalized patients. **IM** 6–12 y, 1 mg 1–2 times/d; may increase up to 15 mg/d.

Dementia Behavior

Geriatric: **PO** 0.5–1 mg 1–2 times/d, may increase q4–7d to max of 40 mg in divided doses. **IM** 1 mg q4–6h (max 6 mg/d).

PHARMACOKINETICS **Absorption:** well absorbed from GI tract. **Onset:** rapid onset. **Peak** 2–3 h. **Duration:** up to 12 h. **Metabolism:** metabolized in liver. **Elimination:** excreted in bile and feces.

CONTRAINDICATIONS & PRECAUTIONS **Contraindicated in:** hypersensitivity to phenothiazines; comatose states, CNS depression; blood dyscrasias; children < 6 y; bone marrow depression; preexisting hepatic disease; pregnancy (category C). **Cautious use in:** previously detected breast cancer; compromised respiratory function; seizure disorders.

T

ADVERSE/SIDE EFFECTS Nasal congestion, *dry mouth,* sweating, blurred vision, *drowsiness,* insomnia, dizziness, agitation, *extrapyramidal effects,* agranulocytosis, photosensitivity, skin rash, constipation, tachycardia, *hypotension,* pigmentary retinopathy, depressed cough reflex, gynecomastia, galactorrhea, neuroleptic malignant syndrome.

DRUG INTERACTIONS **Alcohol** and other CNS DEPRESSANTS add to CNS depression.

NURSING IMPLICATIONS

Administration

- Separate antacid and phenothiazine doses by at least 2 h.
- Dilute oral concentrate just before administration with about 60–120 ml suitable diluent (e.g., water, fruit juices, carbonated beverage, milk, soups, puddings). Avoid coffee or tea near time of taking oral preparation. Explain dosage and dilution to patient if drug is to be self-administered.
- Tablet may be crushed before administration and taken with fluid or mixed with food if patient will not or cannot swallow a pill.
- Monitor ingestion of tablet to see that patient does not hoard medication.
- Administer IM injection deep into upper outer quadrant of buttock.
- Slight yellow discoloration of injectable drug reportedly does not alter potency. If color is markedly changed, discard solution.
- Wash hands if undiluted concentrate is spilled on skin to prevent contact dermatosis.
- Store in light-resistant container at 15–30C (59–86F) unless otherwise directed.

Assessment & Drug Effects

- Hypotension and extrapyramidal effects (especially akathisia and dystonia) are most likely to occur in patients receiving high doses or parenteral administration and in the elderly patient. Stop drug if patient has dysphagia, neck muscle spasm, or if tongue protrusion occurs.

- Reduction in dosage or temporary discontinuation of drug usually reverses extrapyramidal symptoms.
- Monitor I&O ratio and bowel elimination pattern. Check for abdominal distention and pain. Encourage adequate fluid intake as prophylaxis for constipation and xerostomia. The depressed patient may not seek help for either symptom or for urinary retention.
- Since trifluoperazine potentiates analgesics, its use may reduce amount of narcotic required in painful long-term illness such as cancer.
- Agitation, jitteriness, and sometimes insomnia may simulate original neurotic or psychotic symptoms. (They may disappear spontaneously.) Dosage should not be increased until side effects have subsided.
- Maximum therapeutic response generally occurs within 2 or 3 wk after initiation of therapy.

Patient & Family Education

- Counsel to take drug as prescribed and not to alter dosing regimen or stop medication without consulting physician.
- Advise to consult physician about use of any OTC drugs during therapy.
- Alcohol and other depressants should not be taken during phenothiazine therapy.
- Caution to avoid potentially hazardous activities such as driving a car or operating machinery, especially during first days of therapy. (Drowsiness and dizziness may be prominent during this time.)
- Increase in mental and physical activity is an expected result of therapy. Caution patients with angina to avoid overexertion and to report increase in frequency of original pain.
- Patient may be unable to adjust to temperature extremes because of drug effect on thermoregulatory center. Advise not to apply heating pad or hot water bottles; because of depressed conditioned avoidance behaviors, a severe burn may result.
- Advise to cover as much skin surface as possible with clothing when he or she must be in direct sunlight. A sunscreen lotion (SPF > 12) should be applied to exposed skin.
- Inform that urine may be discolored or reddish brown and that this is harmless.

TRIFLURIDINE

(trye-flure'i-deen)

Trade name: Viroptic

Classifications: ANTIINFECTIVE; ANTIVIRAL

Prototype: Acyclovir

Pregnancy category: C

ACTIONS/PHARMACODYNAMICS

Pyrimidine nucleoside active against herpes simplex virus (HSV) types 1 and 2, vaccinia virus, and certain strains of *Adenovirus*. Mechanism of antiviral action not completely known but appears to involve inhibition of viral DNA synthesis and viral replication. Not effective against bacteria, fungi, or *Chlamydia*.

USES Topically to eyes for treatment of primary keratoconjunctivitis and recurring epithelial keratitis caused by herpes simplex virus types 1 and 2. Also for other herpetic ophthalmic infections including stromal keratitis, uveitis, and for infections caused by vaccinia and *Adenovirus*, but clinical effectiveness has not been established.

T

ROUTE & DOSAGE

Viral Infections of Eye

Adult: **Ophthalmic** 1 drop 1% ophthalmic solution into affected eye q2h during waking hours until healing (reepithelialization) has occurred (max 9 drops/d); when healing appears to be complete, dosage reduced to 1 drop q4h during waking hours for an additional 7 d (max 5 drops/d); continuous administration beyond 21 d not recommended.

PHARMACOKINETICS Absorption: Following topical application to eye, trifluridine penetrates cornea and aqueous humor (inflammation enhances penetration). Systemic absorption does not appear to be significant.

CONTRAINDICATIONS & PRECAUTIONS Contraindicated in: safe use during pregnancy (category C) and in nursing women not established. **Cautious use in:** dry eye syndrome.

ADVERSE/SIDE EFFECTS Mild transient burning or stinging, mild irritation of conjunctiva or cornea, photophobia, edema of eyelids and cornea, punctal occlusion, superficial punctate keratopathy, epithelial keratopathy, stromal edema, keratitis sicca, hyperemia, increased intraocular pressure.

NURSING IMPLICATIONS

Administration

- Consult pharmacist regarding concurrent use with other topical ophthalmic preparations.
- Refrigerate at 2–8C (36–46F) unless otherwise directed.

Assessment & Drug Effects

- Epithelial eye infections usually respond to therapy within 2–7 d, with complete healing occurring in 1–2 wk.
- If improvement has not occurred after 7 d of treatment or if healing has not taken place after 14 d, other therapy should be considered.

Patient & Family Education

- Urge to keep physician informed of progress and to keep follow-up appointments. Herpetic eye infections have a tendency to recur and can lead to corneal damage if not adequately treated.

TRIHEXYPHENIDYL HYDROCHLORIDE

(trye-hex-ee-fen′i-dill)

Trade names: Aparkane ♣, Apo-Trihex ♣, Artane, Novohexidyl ♣, Trihexy

Classifications: AUTONOMIC NERVOUS SYSTEM AGENT; ANTICHOLINERGIC (PARASYMPATHOLYTIC); ANTIPARKINSONISM AGENT; ANTIMUSCARINIC; ANTISPASMODIC

Prototype: Atropine

Pregnancy category: C

ACTIONS/PHARMACODYNAMICS Synthetic tertiary amine anticholinergic agent with actions, contraindications, precautions, and adverse reactions similar to those of atropine. Thought to act by blocking excess of acetylcholine at certain cerebral synaptic sites. Relaxes smooth muscle by direct effect and by atropine-like blocking action on parasympathetic nervous system. Small doses cause CNS depression; larger doses produce CNS stimulation. Antispasmodic action appears to be one-half that of atropine, and side effects are usually less frequent and less severe.

USES Symptomatic treatment of all forms of parkinsonism (arteriosclerotic, idiopathic, postencephalitic). Also to prevent or control drug-induced extrapyramidal disorders. **Unlabeled uses:** Huntington's chorea, spasmodic torticollis.

ROUTE & DOSAGE

Parkinsonism

Adult: **PO** 1 mg day 1, 2 mg day 2, then increase by 2 mg q3–5d up to 6–10 mg/d in 3 or more divided doses (max 15 mg/d).

Extrapyramidal Effects

Adult: **PO** 5–15 mg/d in divided doses.

PHARMACOKINETICS Absorption: readily absorbed from GI tract. **Onset:** within 1 h. **Peak:** 2–3 h. **Duration:** 6–12 h. **Elimination:** excreted in urine.

CONTRAINDICATIONS & PRECAUTIONS Contraindicated in: narrow-angle glaucoma. Safe use during pregnancy (category C), in nursing mothers, and children not established. **Cautious use in:** history of drug hypersensitivities; arteriosclerosis; hypertension; cardiac disease, renal or hepatic disorders; obstructive diseases of GI or genitourinary tracts; elderly patients with prostatic hypertrophy.

ADVERSE/SIDE EFFECTS *Dry mouth, dizziness, blurred vision,* mydriasis, photophobia, *nausea, nervousness,* insomnia, constipation, drowsiness, urinary hesitancy or retention. **CNS:** stimulation (usually with high doses): confusion, agitation, delirium, psychotic manifestations, euphoria. **CV:** tachycardia, palpitations, hypotension, orthostatic hypotension. **Other:** hypersensitivity reactions, angle-closure glaucoma.

DRUG INTERACTIONS Reduces therapeutic effects of **chlorpromazine, haloperidol,** PHENOTHIAZINES; increases bioavailability of **digoxin;** MAO INHIBITORS potentiate actions of trihexyphenidyl.

NURSING IMPLICATIONS

Administration

- Trihexyphenidyl HCl may be taken before or after meals, depending on how patient reacts. Elderly patients and patients prone to excessive salivation (e.g., postencephalitic parkinsonism) may prefer to take drug after meals. If drug causes excessive mouth dryness, it may be better taken before meals, unless it causes nausea.
- Once stabilized on conventional dosage forms, patient may be switched to sustained-release capsules to permit once-a-day or twice-a-day dosing.
- Store at 15–30C (59–86F) in tight container unless otherwise directed.

Assessment & Drug Effects

- Incidence and severity of side effects are usually dose related and may be minimized by dosage reduction. Elderly patients appear to be more sensitive to usual adult doses.
- Monitor vital signs. Pulse is a particularly sensitive indicator of patient's response to drug. Report tachycardia, palpitations, paradoxical bradycardia, or fall in BP.
- CNS stimulation (see Adverse/Side Effects) may occur with high doses and in patients with arteriosclerosis or history of hypersensitivity to other drugs. If severe, drug may be discontinued for a few days and then resumed at lower dosage.
- In patients with severe rigidity, tremors may appear to be accen-

tuated during therapy as rigidity diminishes.

- Monitor daily I&O if patient develops urinary hesitancy or retention. Voiding before taking drug may relieve problem.
- If constipation is a problem, check for abdominal distention and bowel sounds.
- Close monitoring of intraocular pressure at regular intervals is advised.
- Close follow-up care is advisable. Tolerance may develop, necessitating dosage adjustment or use of combination therapy. Patients > 60 y frequently develop sensitivity to trihexyphenidyl action.

Patient & Family Education

- Drug-induced mouth dryness may be relieved by ice chips, sugarless gum, or hard candy, by frequent sips of water, and by maintaining adequate total daily fluid intake.
- Warn to avoid excessive heat because drug suppresses perspiration and, therefore, heat loss.
- Caution not to engage in activities requiring alertness and skill, as drug causes dizziness, drowsiness, and blurred vision. Supervision of ambulation may be indicated.

TRIMEPRAZINE TARTRATE

T

(trye-mep'ra-zeen)

Trade names: Panectyl ♣, Temaril

Classifications: ANTIHISTAMINE; ANTIPRURITIC

Prototype: Hydroxyzine

Pregnancy category: C

ACTIONS/PHARMACODYNAMICS Structural analog of the phenothiazines. Similar to hydroxyzine, with prominent antipruritic activity. Also shares sedative and antihistaminic effects of hydroxyzine. In common with antihistamines, exerts both anticholinergic and antiserotonin action. Suppresses the cough reflex; may exert ulcerogenic effect.

USE Primarily for symptomatic relief of pruritic symptoms in a variety of dermatologic and nondermatologic conditions. **Unlabeled use:** preoperative sedation in children.

ROUTE & DOSAGE

Pruritus

Adult: **PO** 2.5 mg q.i.d. or 5 mg sustained-release q12h.
Geriatric: **PO** 2.5 mg b.i.d.
Child: **PO** *>6 y,* 5 mg sustained-release once/d; *>3 y,* 2.5 mg h.s. or t.i.d.; *6 mo–3 y,* 1.25 mg h.s. or t.i.d.

CONTRAINDICATIONS & PRECAUTIONS **Contraindicated in:** hypersensitivity to phenothiazines; acute asthma attack; sleep apnea; pregnancy (category C), premature or full-term infants < 6 mo; use of extended-release form in children ≤ 6 y. **Cautious use in:** hepatic disease; history of GI ulceration; history of convulsive disorders in the elderly or debilitated patient; upper respiratory tract infection.

ADVERSE/SIDE EFFECTS *Drowsiness,* dizziness, *dry mucous membranes,* GI upset, allergic skin reactions, cholestatic jaundice, extrapyramidal reactions, leukopenia. In some children: paradoxic hyperactivity, irritability, insomnia, hallucinations. **Acute poisoning:** CNS depression with hypotension, hypothermia. Toxic potential as for other phenothiazines.

NURSING IMPLICATIONS

Administration

- Trimeprazine tartrate is usually ad-

ministered after each meal and at bedtime.
- Preserve in tight, light-resistant containers.

Assessment & Drug Effects
- Incidence and severity of adverse effects are generally dose-related; however, in some patients individual sensitivity is involved.
- Toxic manifestations of phenothiazine derivatives are most likely to occur between 4 and 10 wk of therapy.
- If child or elderly patient has a severe upper respiratory tract infection, this drug should be used only with caution because it suppresses the cough reflex.

Patient & Family Education
- Caution not to administer more than the prescribed dose to children.
- Drowsiness occurs frequently, but it generally disappears after a few days of medication. If it persists, dosage adjustment is indicated.
- Patient should know that sedative action of trimeprazine is additive to that of alcohol, barbiturates, narcotics, analgesics, and other CNS depressants.
- Warn to avoid activities requiring mental alertness and normal reaction time, such as operating a car or other hazardous activities, until drug response is known.

TRIMETHAPHAN CAMSYLATE

(trye-meth′a-fan)

Trade name: Arfonad

Classifications: CARDIOVASCULAR AGENT; NONNITRATE VASODILATOR; ANTIHYPERTENSIVE

Prototype: Hydralazine

Pregnancy category: X

ACTIONS/PHARMACODYNAMICS
Potent, short-acting ganglionic blocking agent. Blocks transmission in both adrenergic and cholinergic ganglia by competing with acetylcholine for receptor sites on postganglionic membranes. Adrenergic blockade results in vasodilation, improved peripheral blood flow, and thus decrease in BP. Also has direct peripheral vasodilation action and thus can produce marked hypotension. BP is significantly lower in head-up position because venous dilation and peripheral pooling reduce cardiac output.

USES To produce controlled hypotension for certain surgical procedures (e.g., neurologic, ophthalmic, and plastic surgery) and for short-term treatment of hypertensive crises associated with pulmonary edema. **Unlabeled uses:** acute dissecting aneurysm of aorta and ischemic heart disease.

ROUTE & DOSAGE

Controlled Hypotension, Short-term Treatment of Hypertensive Crisis

Adult: **IV** Dilute 500 mg in 500 ml of 5% dextrose; infuse at 0.5–1 mg/min with gradual increase until BP control is achieved.
Child: **IV** 50–150 μg/kg/min at a rate of 0.3–6 mg/min.

PHARMACOKINETICS Onset: immediate. **Duration:** 10 min. **Distribution:** crosses placenta. **Metabolism:** metabolized by pseudocholinesterases in plasma. **Elimination:** excreted in urine.

CONTRAINDICATIONS & PRECAUTIONS Contraindicated in: anemia, hypovolemia, shock; asphyxia, respiratory insufficiency; glaucoma;

during pregnancy. **Cautious use in:** history of allergy; elderly and debilitated patients, children; cardiac disease, arteriosclerosis; hepatic or renal disease; degenerative CNS disease; Addison's disease; diabetes mellitus; patients receiving steroids, antihypertensives, anesthetics (especially spinal), and diuretics.

ADVERSE/SIDE EFFECTS **CV:** tachycardia or decrease in heart rate, orthostatic hypotension, angina. **GI:** nausea, vomiting, anorexia. **Hypersensitivity:** urticaria, pruritus, histamine-like reaction along course of vein. **Symptoms due to cholinergic blockade:** atony of urinary bladder or GI tract, urinary retention, cycloplegia, mydriasis, dry mouth, suppression of perspiration. **Other:** restlessness, extreme weakness; respiratory depression, respiratory arrest (following large doses).

DIAGNOSTIC TEST INTERFERENCE Trimethaphan may decrease ***serum potassium*** and may prevent elevation of ***blood glucose*** that usually occurs during postoperative period.

DRUG INTERACTIONS DIURETICS, ANESTHETICS, **procainamide** add to hypotensive effects.

INCOMPATIBILITY **Solution/additive: tubocurarine.**

NURSING IMPLICATIONS

Administration

- Dilute one 10 ml ampule of Arfonad (50 mg/ml) to 500 ml with D5W, 0.9% NaCl, or Ringer's injection.
- IV infusion is started at 3–4 ml (3–4 mg)/min and then adjusted to maintain desired effect.
- IV flow rate is prescribed by physician to maintain desired BP level. Rate of infusion should be monitored constantly. Individuals vary considerably in response to drug.
- Use of an infusion pump, microdrip regulator, or similar device is recommended for precise measurement of flow rate.
- Infusion should be terminated gradually while BP is closely monitored. It is stopped before wound closure in surgery to allow BP to return to normal.
- Trimethaphan is stable under refrigeration, but freezing should be avoided. The diluted solution (500 mg/500 ml) is stable at room temperature for 24 h. Store at 15–30C (59–86F).

Assessment & Drug Effects

- Take vital signs prior to initiation of therapy as a baseline for comparison during drug administration.
- Patient must be observed continuously while receiving infusion. BP should be checked q2min until stabilized at desired level, then q5min for duration of treatment. Pulse and respiration should also be monitored closely.
- Intensity of hypotensive effect is largely dependent on positioning. Decrease in BP is most marked in sitting or standing position. Excessive hypotension can be reversed by having patient assume head-low position or elevate legs.
- Continue to monitor vital signs at regular intervals after completion of treatment. Since BP returns to pretreatment level within 10 min after the infusion is terminated, an oral antihypertensive is usually initiated in patients with hypertension as soon as desired BP level is achieved with trimethaphan.
- Monitor I&O. Ganglionic blockade may reduce renal blood flow initially as well as voiding contractions and urge to void. Check

T

lower abdomen for bladder distension.

- Some patients become refractory to trimethaphan (tachyphylaxis) within 48 h after initiation of therapy. Notify physician promptly if BP fails to respond.

TRIMETHOBENZAMIDE HYDROCHLORIDE

(trye-meth-oh-ben′za-mide)

Trade names: Arrestin, Ticon, Tigan, T-Gen

Classifications: GI AGENT; ANTIEMETIC

Prototype: Prochlorperazine

Pregnancy category: C

ACTIONS/PHARMACODYNAMICS Structurally related to ethanolamine antihistamines, but in therapeutic doses antihistamine activity is weak. Has sedative and antiemetic actions. Less effective than phenothiazine antiemetics but produces fewer side effects. Must be used with other agents when vomiting is severe. Primary locus of action is thought to be the chemoreceptor trigger zone (CTZ) in medulla.

USE Control of nausea and vomiting.

ROUTE & DOSAGE

Nausea and Vomiting

Adult: **PO** 250 mg t.i.d. or q.i.d. **Rectal/IM** 200 mg t.i.d. or q.i.d.
Child: **PO/Rectal** *15–45 kg,* 100–200 mg t.i.d. or q.i.d. **Rectal** *<15 kg,* 100 mg t.i.d. or q.i.d.

PHARMACOKINETICS **Onset:** 10–40 min PO; 15 min IM. **Duration:** 3–4 h PO; 2–3 h IM. **Elimination:** 30–50% of dose excreted unchanged in urine within 48–72 h.

CONTRAINDICATIONS & PRECAUTIONS **Contraindicated in:** uncomplicated vomiting in viral illness, parenteral use in children, rectal administration in prematures and newborns; known sensitivity to benzocaine (in suppository) or to similar local anesthetics. Safe use during pregnancy (category C) and in nursing mothers not established. **Cautious use in:** patients who have recently received other centrally acting drugs; in presence of high fever, dehydration, electrolyte imbalance.

ADVERSE/SIDE EFFECTS Hypersensitivity reactions (including allergic skin eruptions), hypotension, diarrhea, exaggeration of nausea, acute hepatitis, jaundice, muscle cramps. **Other:** pain, stinging, burning, redness, irritation at IM site; local irritation following rectal administration.

DRUG INTERACTIONS **Alcohol** and other CNS DEPRESSANTS add to depressant activity; BELLADONNA ALKALOIDS may intensify anticholinergic effects; PHENOTHIAZINES may precipitate extrapyramidal syndrome.

NURSING IMPLICATIONS

Administration

- Capsule may be emptied and contents swallowed with water or mixed with food (if patient has difficulty swallowing capsule).
- Administer IM deep into upper outer quadrant of buttock. To minimize possibility of irritation and pain, avoid escape of solution along needle track. This can be accomplished by Z-track injection or by drawing a small bubble of air into syringe after drug is measured; when medication is in-

T

jected, air bubble will clear needle of drug.

Assessment & Drug Effects

- Hypotension is reported, particularly in surgical patients receiving drug parenterally. Monitor BP.
- If an acute febrile illness accompanies or begins during therapy with trimethobenzamide, report promptly and stop drug therapy.
- The antiemetic effect of drug may obscure diagnoses of GI or other pathologic conditions or signs of toxicity from other drugs.

Patient & Family Education

- Advise to report promptly to physician the onset of rash or other signs of hypersensitivity (see Appendix G). Drug should be discontinued immediately.
- Since drug may cause drowsiness and dizziness, caution to avoid driving a car or other potentially hazardous activities.
- Advise not to drink alcohol or alcoholic beverages during therapy with this drug.

TRIMETHOPRIM

(trye-meth'oh-prim)

Trade names: Proloprim, Trimpex

Prototype for classification: URINARY TRACT ANTIINFECTIVE

Pregnancy category: C

T

ACTIONS/PHARMACODYNAMICS Antiinfective and folic acid antagonist with slow bactericidal action. Binding and interference with cell growth is 1000 times stronger in bacterial than in mammalian cells. Most pathogens causing urinary tract infection (UTI) are in normal vaginal and fecal flora. Thus, drug is effective against most common UTI pathogens, including *Escherichia coli, Enterobacter* species, *Klebsiella pneumoniae, Proteus mirabilis,* most strains of *Hemophilus influenzae, Streptococcus pneumoniae, Streptococcus pyogenes, Staphylococcus* organisms (including *S. saprophyticus*). Not effective against *Bacteroides, Lactobacillus* species, *Chlamydia* or *Pneumocystis carinii, Pseudomonas aeruginosa*. Resistant strains of Enterobacteriaceae (*E. coli* and *Klebsiella* and *Proteus* species) may develop during therapy.

USE Initial episodes of acute uncomplicated UTIs. **Unlabeled uses:** treatment and prophylaxis of chronic and recurrent UTI in both men and women; treatment in conjunction with dapsone of initial episodes of *Pneumocystis carinii* pneumonia; treatment of travelers' diarrhea.

ROUTE & DOSAGE

Urinary Tract Infection

Adult: **PO** 100 mg b.i.d. or 200 mg once/d.
Child: **PO** 2–3 mg/kg q12h × 10 d.

Travelers' Diarrhea

Adult: **PO** 200 mg b.i.d.

PHARMACOKINETICS Absorption: almost completely absorbed from GI tract. **Peak:** 1–4 h. **Distribution:** widely distributed, including lung, saliva, middle ear fluid, bile, bone, CSF; crosses placenta; appears in breast milk. **Metabolism:** metabolized in liver. **Elimination:** half-life: 8–11 h; 80% excreted in urine unchanged.

CONTRAINDICATIONS & PRECAUTIONS Contraindicated in: megaloblastic anemia secondary to folate deficiency; creatinine clearance <15 ml/min, impaired renal or hepatic function, possible folate deficiency; pregnancy (category C), nursing mothers, children with fragile X chromosome associated with mental retardation. Safe use in infants < 2 mo old and efficacy in children < 12 y old have not been established.

ADVERSE/SIDE EFFECTS GI: epigastric discomfort, nausea, vomiting, glossitis, abnormal taste sensation. **Hematologic:** neutropenia, *megaloblastic anemia,* methemoglobinemia, leukopenia, thrombocytopenia (rare). **Skin:** *rash, pruritus,* exfoliative dermatitis, photosensitivity. **Other:** fever, increased serum transaminases (ALT, AST), bilirubin, creatinine, BUN.

DIAGNOSTIC TEST INTERFERENCE Interferes with serum ***methotrexate assays*** that use a competitive binding protein technique with a bacterial dehydrofolate reductase as the binding protein. May cause falsely elevated creatinine values when Jaffe reaction is used.

DRUG INTERACTION May inhibit **phenytoin** metabolism causing increased levels.

NURSING IMPLICATIONS

Administration

- Administer with 240 ml (8 oz) of fluid if not contraindicated.
- Store at 15–30C (59–86F) in dry, light-protected place.

Assessment & Drug Effects

- Culture and susceptibility tests are conducted before trimethoprim therapy is initiated; however, therapy may be started before test results have been received.
- Recurrent infection after terminating prophylactic treatment of UTI may occur even after 6 mo of therapy. A possible reason may be noncompliance. Reinforce necessity to adhere to established drug regimen.
- Periodic urine cultures are recommended. Follow-up cultures may be ordered at end of treatment to verify elimination of causative organism.
- Monitor creatinine clearance tests.
- Assess urinary pattern during treatment. Altered pattern (frequency, urgency, nocturia, retention, polyuria) may reflect emerging drug resistance, necessitating change of drug regimen. Periodically check for bladder distention.
- Trimethoprim may worsen the psychomotor regression associated with mental retardation because of potential drug-induced folate deficiency.
- Elderly, malnourished, alcoholic, pregnant, or debilitated patients are especially susceptible to the hematologic toxic effects. Changes in temperature pattern and I&O ratio pattern should be recognized and reported.
- Drug-induced rash, a common side effect, is usually maculopapular, pruritic, or morbilliform and appears 7–14 d after start of therapy with daily doses of 200 mg or less.
- Overdose symptoms are nausea, vomiting, diarrhea, mental depression, confusion, facial swelling, and elevated serum transaminases.

Patient & Family Education

- Uncomplicated UTIs usually respond to treatment if patient takes all of prescribed medication.
- Discuss fluid intake pattern with the patient. Frequently, the elderly self-limit fluids; therefore, teaching should focus on fluid intake as an important adjunct to drug therapy.
- Usually, the adult patient should attempt to maintain fluid intake of 2000–3000 ml/d (if not contraindicated) to help flush out urinary bacteria.

T

- Before full drug effects are experienced, patient may have pain and discomfort with voiding, which can be relieved by a urinary analgesic. Pain and hematuria should be reported immediately.
- Tell not to postpone voiding even though increases in fluid intake may cause more frequent urination.
- Caution against use of douches or sprays during treatment periods, and stress careful perineal hygiene to prevent reinfection.
- Symptoms of a hematologic disorder (fever, sore throat, pallor, purpura, ecchymosis) should be reported promptly.
- If severe traveler's diarrhea does not respond to 3–5 d therapy with trimethoprim (i.e., persistence of symptoms of severe nausea, abdominal pain, diarrhea with mucus or blood, and dehydration), patient should consult a physician.

TRIMETHOPRIM-SULFAMETHOXAZOLE (TMP-SMZ)

Trade names: Bactrim, Co-Trimoxazole, Septra

Classifications: URINARY TRACT ANTIINFECTIVE; SULFONAMIDE

Prototype: Trimethoprim

Pregnancy category: C

T

ACTIONS/PHARMACODYNAMICS

Fixed combination of sulfamethoxazole (SMZ), an intermediate acting antiinfective sulfonamide, and trimethoprim (TMP), a synthetic antiinfective. Both components of the combination are synthetic folate antagonist antiinfectives. Mechanism of action is principally enzyme inhibition, which prevents bacterial synthesis of essential nucleic acid and proteins. Bacterial resistance to the combined drugs develops more slowly than to either of the drugs alone.

USES *Pneumocystis carinii* pneumonitis, shigellosis enteritis, and severe complicated UTIs due to most strains of the Enterobacteriaceae. Also children with acute otitis media due to susceptible strains of *Hemophilus influenzae,* and acute episodes of chronic bronchitis in adults. **Unlabeled uses:** isosporiasis; prevention of traveler's diarrhea; cholera; treatment of infections caused by *Nocardia, Legionella micdadei,* and *Legionella pneumophila* and genital ulcers caused by *Hemophilus ducreyi;* prophylaxis for *P. carinii* pneumonia in neutropenic patients.

ROUTE & DOSAGE

Systemic Infections

Adult: **PO** 160 mg TMP/800 mg SMZ (1 double strength [DS] tablet) q12h; **IV** 8–10 mg/kg/d TMP divided q6–12h infused over 60–90 min.
Child: **PO** *>2 mo, <40 kg,* 4 mg/kg/d TMP q12h; *>40 kg,* 160 mg TMP/800 mg SMZ (1 DS tablet) q12h; **IV** *>2 mo,* 8–10 mg/kg/d TMP divided q6–12h infused over 60–90 min.

***Pneumocystis carinii* Pneumonia**

Adult: **IV** 20 mg/kg/d TMP divided q6h infused over 60–90 min.

Prophylaxis for *Pneumocystis carinii* Pneumonia

Adult: **PO** 160 mg TMP/800 mg SMZ q24h.

Child: **PO** 150 mg/m² TMP/750 mg/m² SMZ b.i.d. 3 consecutive d/wk. Max 320 mg TMP/d.

PHARMACOKINETICS Absorption: readily absorbed from GI tract. **Peak:** 1–4 h PO. **Distribution:** widely distributed, including CNS; crosses placenta; distributed into breast milk. **Metabolism:** metabolized in liver. **Elimination:** half-life: 8–10 h TMP, 10–13 h SMZ; excreted in urine.

CONTRAINDICATIONS & PRECAUTIONS Contraindicated in: hypersensitivity to TMP, SMZ, sulfonamides, or bisulfites; group A betahemolytic streptococcal pharyngitis; megaloblastic anemia due to folate deficiency; creatinine clearance <15 ml/min; pregnancy (category C), lactation. **Cautious use in:** impaired renal or hepatic function; possible folate deficiency; severe allergy or bronchial asthma; G6PD deficiency, hypersensitivity to sulfonamide derivative drugs (e.g., acetazolamide, thiazides, tolbutamide). Not recommended for infants <2 mo.

ADVERSE/SIDE EFFECTS *Mild to moderate rashes (including fixed drug eruptions).* **GI:** *nausea, vomiting,* diarrhea, *anorexia,* hepatitis, pseudomembranous enterocolitis, stomatitis, glossitis, abdominal pain. **GU:** renal failure, oliguria, anuria, crystalluria. **Hematologic:** agranulocytosis (rare), aplastic anemia (rare), megaloblastic anemia, hypoprothrombinemia, thrombocytopenia (rare). **Other:** weakness, arthralgia, myalgia, photosensitivity, toxic epidermal necrolysis, allergic myocarditis.

DIAGNOSTIC TEST INTERFERENCE May elevate levels of serum creatinine, transaminase, bilirubin, alkaline phosphatase.

DRUG INTERACTIONS May enhance hypoprothombinemic effects of ORAL ANTICOAGULANTS; may increase **methotrexate** toxicity.

INCOMPATIBILITIES Solution/additive: stability in dextrose and normal saline is concentration dependent; **verapamil. Y-site:** fluconazole.

NURSING IMPLICATIONS

Administration

- Advise patient to take PO medication with a full glass of desired fluid and to maintain adequate fluid intake (at least 1500 ml/d) during therapy.
- Dosage may be adjusted in patient with renal dysfunction on basis of creatinine clearance tests. (Some clinicians reduce adult daily dose by 50% if creatinine clearance is between 15 and 30 ml/min).
- IV infusion must be diluted by adding contents of 5-ml ampul to 125 ml D5W. Use within 6 h. If a dilution of 5 ml/100 ml D5W is desired, use solution within 4 h. Do not refrigerate. Administer solution over 60–90 min, avoiding bolus or rapid injection.
- Do not mix other drugs or solutions with IV infusion. Discard solution if cloudy or if crystallization appears after mixing.
- Prophylaxis for travelers' diarrhea is usually reserved for the medically compromised patient: 160 mg/800 mg as a single dose. Nondrug prevention is preferable.
- Store at 15–30C (59–86F) in dry place protected from light. Avoid freezing.

Assessment & Drug Effects

- IV Septra contains sodium metabisulfite, which produces allergic-type reactions in susceptible pa-

T

tients: hives, itching, wheezing, anaphylaxis. Susceptibility (low in general population) is seen most frequently in asthmatics or atopic nonasthmatic persons.

- Monitor coagulation tests and prothrombin times in patient also receiving warfarin. Change in warfarin dosage may be indicated.
- Monitor I&O volume and pattern. Significant changes should be reported to forestall renal calculi formation. Also, failure of treatment (i.e., continued UTI symptoms) should be reported.
- Frequent urinalysis with macroscopic examination during therapy is advised.
- The elderly patient is at risk for severe adverse reactions, especially if liver or renal function is compromised or if certain other drugs are given. Most frequently observed: thrombocytopenia (with concurrent thiazide diuretics); severe decrease in platelets (with or without purpura); bone marrow suppression; severe skin reactions.
- Overdose symptoms (no extensive experience has been reported) are nausea, vomiting, anorexia, headache, dizziness, mental depression, confusion, and bone marrow depression.

T

Patient & Family Education

- Urge to report stat if rash appears. Other reportable symptoms are sore throat, fever, purpura, jaundice (early signs of serious reactions).
- This drug can cause fixed eruptions at the same sites each time the drug is administered. Every contact with drug may not result in eruptions; therefore, patient may overlook the relationship. Instruct patient to monitor for and report fixed eruptions.

TRIMETREXATE

(tri-me-trex′ate)

Trade name: Neotrexin

Classifications: ANTINEOPLASTIC; ANTIMETABOLITE

Prototype: Methotrexate

Pregnancy category: D

ACTIONS/PHARMACODYNAMICS

Antimetabolite and folic acid antagonist. Blocks folinic acid (active form of folic acid) participation in nucleic acid synthesis, thereby interfering with miotic process. Trimetrexate acts as a dihydrofolate reductase (DHFR) inhibitor in a similar manner to methotrexate; it disrupts DNA, RNA, and protein synthesis, with consequent cell death.

USES Used with concurrent leucovorin administration, as an alternate therapy for moderate-to-severe *Pneumocystis carinii* pneumonia (PCP) in immunocompromised patients, including AIDS patients. **Unlabeled uses:** advanced non-small cell lung cancer, metastatic cancer of the head and neck, metastatic colorectal adenocarcinoma, pancreatic carcinoma.

ROUTE & DOSAGE

***Pneumocystis carinii* Pneumonia**

Adult: **PO** 60 mg/m²/d prepared as the IV solution has been given orally to AIDS patients with PCP. **IV** 45 mg/m² once daily by IV infusion over 60–90 min with concurrent leucovorin 20 mg/m² q6h (IV or PO). Trimetrexate should be administered for 21 d and leucovorin for 24 d.

PHARMACOKINETICS Absorption: approximately 44% absorbed from GI tract. **Onset:** 3 d. **Distribution:** very

Common side effect in *italic*, life-threatening effects underlined: generic names in **bold**; drug class in SMALL CAPS

low CSF concentrations; distributes into lung tissue; 98% protein bound. **Metabolism:** extensively metabolized in liver. **Elimination:** half-life: 15–17 h; excreted in urine and feces.

CONTRAINDICATIONS & PRECAUTIONS **Contraindicated in:** hypersensitivity to trimetrexate, leucovorin, or methotrexate; profound myelosuppression; pregnancy (category D); lactation. **Cautious use in:** seizures; mild myelosuppression; severe renal or hepatic dysfunction; hypoalbuminemia or hypoproteinemia; concomitant use of myelosuppressive, hepatoxic, or renal toxic drugs; previous radiation of bone marrow or extensive chemotherapy with myelotoxic agents. Safety and efficacy in children <18 y not established.

ADVERSE/SIDE EFFECTS **Hematologic:** *myelosuppression, granulocytopenia, thrombocytopenia*. **GI:** *nausea, vomiting, stomatitis*. **Skin:** erythematous rash with posteruption hyperpigmentation. **Other:** mild transient elevations in serum creatinine and liver function tests.

DIAGNOSTIC TEST INTERFERENCE Mild increases in serum creatinine and liver function tests.

DRUG INTERACTIONS **Cimetidine, erythromycin, fluconazole** (and other AZOLE ANTIFUNGAL AGENTS) may increase trimetrexate levels and toxicity. Rifabutin, rifampin may decrease trimetrexate levels. Zidovudine may cause additive hematologic toxicity.

INCOMPATIBILITIES **Solution/additive, Y-site:** CHLORIDE-CONTAINING SOLUTIONS (including **sodium chloride**), **foscarnet.**

NURSING IMPLICATIONS

Administration

- Reconstitute trimetrexate with 2 ml of 5% dextrose injection or sterile water for injection; the resulting concentration is 12.5 mg/ml; allow 30 s for complete dissolution.
- Manufacturer recommends filtering (0.22 μm) reconstituted solution prior to dilution.
- Further dilute reconstituted solution with 10–100 ml of 5% dextrose injection to a final concentration of 0.25–2 mg of trimetrexate/ml and infuse over 60–90 min.
- The IV line should be flushed with at least 10 ml of 5% dextrose injection before and after administering trimetrexate.
- If drug contacts skin, immediately wash with soap and water.
- The reconstituted solution may be kept at room temperature or refrigerated for 24 h.

Assessment & Drug Effects

- Monitor complete blood count at least twice a week during therapy. Myelosuppression nadir occurs around day 8.
- Monitor renal and hepatic functions; impaired functioning may indicate need for dosage reduction.

Patient & Family Education

- Inform of potential adverse effects and instruct to report those that are bothersome.
- Inform that myelosuppression is the primary dose-limiting side effect.

TRIMIPRAMINE MALEATE

(tri-mip′ra-meen)

Trade name: Surmontil

Classifications: CNS AGENT; PSYCHOTHERAPEUTIC; TRICYCLIC ANTIDEPRESSANT

Prototype: Imipramine

Pregnancy category: C

T

ACTIONS/PHARMACODYNAMICS Tricyclic antidepressant (TCA) pharmacologically similar to imipramine in actions, uses, pharmacokinetics, limitations, and interactions. Has moderate anticholinergic and strong sedative effects; therefore is useful in depression associated with anxiety and sleep disturbances. More effective in alleviation of endogenous depression than other depressive states. Recent studies suggest strong, active H_2-receptor antagonism is a characteristic of TCAs.

USES Similar to those for imipramine. **Unlabeled use:** peptic ulcer disease.

ROUTE & DOSAGE

Depression
Adult: **PO** 75–100 mg/d in divided doses; may increase gradually up to 300 mg/d if needed; maintenance dose usually 50–150 mg/d.
Geriatric: **PO** 25 mg h.s., may increase q3d to max of 100 mg/d.

PHARMACOKINETICS **Absorption:** rapidly absorbed from GI tract. **Peak:** 2 h. **Metabolism:** metabolized in liver. **Elimination:** half-life: 9.1 h; excreted in urine and feces.

T

CONTRAINDICATIONS & PRECAUTIONS **Contraindicated in:** prostatic hypertrophy; during recovery period after MI. Safe use during pregnancy (category C) and by nursing mothers not established. **Cautious use in:** schizophrenia, with electroshock therapy, suicidal tendency; cardiovascular, hepatic, thyroid, renal disease.

ADVERSE/SIDE EFFECTS **CNS:** seizures, tremor, confusion, *sedation*, blurred vision. **CV:** tachycardia, *orthostatic hypotension*, hypertension. **GI:** *xerostomia, constipation*, paralytic ileus. **Other:** *urinary retention*, photosensitivity, sweating.

DRUG INTERACTIONS May decrease some antihypertensive response to ANTIHYPERTENSIVES; CNS DEPRESSANTS, **alcohol,** HYPNOTICS, BARBITURATES, SEDATIVES potentiate CNS depression; may increase hypoprothombinemic effect of ORAL ANTICOAGULANTS; **ethchlorvynol** may cause transient delirium; with **levodopa,** SYMPATHOMIMETICS (e.g., **epinephrine, norepinephrine**), possibility of sympathetic hyperactivity with hypertension and hyperpyrexia; with MAO INHIBITORS, possibility of severe reactions, toxic psychosis, cardiovascular instability; **methylphenidate increases plasma TCA levels;** THYROID AGENTS may increase possibility of arrhythmias; **cimetidine** may increase plasma TCA levels.

NURSING IMPLICATIONS

Administration

- Administer drug with food to decrease gastric distress.
- Supervise drug ingestion to be sure patient does not "hoard" the drug.
- Store in tightly closed container at 15–30C (59–86F) unless otherwise specified.

Assessment & Drug Effects

- Monitor BP and pulse rate during adjustment period of tricyclic antidepressant (TCA) therapy. If BP falls more than 20 mm Hg or if there is a sudden increase in pulse rate, withhold medication and notify physician.
- Orthostatic hypotension may be sufficiently severe to require protective assistance when patient is ambulating. Instruct patient to change position from recumbency to standing slowly and in stages.

- Report signs of hepatic dysfunction: yellow skin and sclerae, light-colored stools, pruritus, abdominal discomfort.
- Fine tremors, a distressing extrapyramidal side effect, should be reported to the physician.
- Monitor bowel elimination pattern and I&O ratio. Severe constipation and urinary retention are potential problems, especially in the elderly. Advise increased fluid intake to at least 1500 ml/d (if allowed).
- Inspect oral membranes daily if patient is on high doses. Urge outpatient to report symptoms of stomatitis or xerostomia.
- If xerostomia is a problem, institute symptomatic therapy. Sore or dry mouth can be a major cause of poor food intake and noncompliance. Consult physician about use of a saliva substitute (e.g., Moi-stir).
- Drug may cause intolerance to heat or cold. Regulate environmental temperature and patient's clothing accordingly.
- The severely depressed patient may need assistance with personal hygiene, particularly because of excessive sweating caused by the drug.
- If a patient uses excessive amounts of alcohol, it should be borne in mind that the potentiation of TCA effects may increase the danger of overdosage or suicide attempt.

Patient & Family Education

- Caution that ability to perform tasks requiring alertness and skill may be impaired.
- Urge not to use OTC drugs unless physician approves.
- The actions of both alcohol and trimipramine are potentiated when used together during therapy and for up to 2 wk after the TCA is discontinued. Consult physician about safe amount of alcohol, if any, that can be taken.
- Advise that the effects of barbiturates and other CNS depressants may also be enhanced by trimipramine.
- Alert to the fact that because TCAs have a "lag period" of 2–4 wk, therapeutic response will be delayed. (Increased dosage does not shorten period but rather increases incidence of adverse reactions.) This period is one that fosters noncompliance. Monitor drug intake to see that therapy is not interrupted.

TRIOXSALEN

(trye-ox'sa-len)

Trade name: Trisoralen

Classifications: SKIN AGENT; PSORALEN

Prototype: Methoxsalen

ACTIONS/PHARMACODYNAMICS

Systemic psoralen derivative structurally and pharmacologically related to methoxsalen but that produces less intense melanogenic and erythemic responses. Produces resistance to solar damage in persons particularly susceptible to painful reactions with exposure to sunlight. Accelerates pigmentation only when followed by exposure of skin to sunlight or ultraviolet irradiation, and may reach equivalence of a full summer of sun exposure.

USES In conjunction with controlled exposure to ultraviolet light or sunlight to repigment vitiliginous skin, to improve tolerance to sunlight in patients with albinism, and to enhance pigmentation.

ROUTE & DOSAGE

Repigment Vitiliginous Skin

Adult: **PO** 10 mg/d as single dose 2–4 h before controlled exposure to ultraviolet-A (UVA) or sunlight.

CONTRAINDICATIONS & PRECAUTIONS **Contraindicated in:** see methoxsalen.

ADVERSE/SIDE EFFECTS **Skin:** severe edema and erythema, painful blisters, burning and peeling of skin. **GI:** GI distress, nausea, vomiting. **CNS:** nervousness, vertigo, mental depression or excitation.

DRUG INTERACTIONS **Coal tar, griseofulvin,** SULFONAMIDES, PHENOTHIAZINES, THIAZIDES may increase photosensitivity reactions.

NURSING IMPLICATIONS

Administration

- Administer with milk or after a meal to reduce gastric distress.
- If trioxsalen is used to increase tolerance of skin to sunlight, treatment is continued no longer than 14 d, with dosage not exceeding 140 mg.
- Store in tightly closed, light-resistant container at 15–30C (59–86F).

Assessment & Drug Effects

- Repigmentation of idiopathic vitiligo may begin a few weeks after start of treatment, but significant effects require 6–9 mo of therapy.
- If repigmentation is not apparent after 3 mo of treatment, drug is discontinued.

Patient & Family Education

- Following successful repigmentation with PUVA (P = psoralen) therapy, pigmentation can be maintained by periodic exposure to sunlight and trioxsalen.
- Concomitant ingestion of furocoumarin-containing foods may intensify adverse reactions. Warn patient to avoid the following foods: figs, limes, parsley, parsnips, mustard, carrots, celery.
- Urge to adhere to dosage and exposure time prescribed by physician. Severe burning may occur with overdosage.

TRIPELENNAMINE HYDROCHLORIDE

(tri-pel-enn'a-meen)

Trade names: PBZ-SR, Pelamine, Pyribenzamine ♣

Classification: ANTIHISTAMINE (H_1-RECEPTOR ANTAGONIST)

Prototype: Diphenhydramine

Pregnancy category: B

ACTIONS/PHARMACODYNAMICS Antihistamine with mild CNS depressant effects and relatively high incidence of GI side effects. Antagonizes histamine action (i.e., increased capillary permeability, edema formation, itching, and constriction of respiratory, GI, and vascular smooth muscle). Does not inhibit gastric secretion. Has antiemetic, antitussive, anticholinergic, and local anesthetic action.

USES To relieve symptoms of various allergic conditions, to ameliorate reactions to blood or plasma, and in anaphylaxis as adjunct to epinephrine and other standard measures after acute symptoms have been controlled. Also to provide oral mucous membrane analgesia in young children with herpetic gingivostomatitis.

ROUTE & DOSAGE

Allergic Conditions

Adult: **PO** 25–50 mg q4–6h; or 100 mg sustained-release q8–12h (max 600 mg/d).

T

Child: **PO** 5 mg/kg/d in 4–6 divided doses (max 300 mg/d) (each 5 ml of tripelennamine citrate elixir is equal to 25 mg HCl).

PHARMACOKINETICS Absorption: readily absorbed from GI tract. **Onset:** 15–30 min. **Peak:** 2–3 h. **Duration:** 4–6 h (up to 8 h with sustained-release). **Distribution:** crosses placenta; distributed into breast milk. **Metabolism:** metabolized in liver. **Elimination:** excreted in urine.

CONTRAINDICATIONS & PRECAUTIONS Contraindicated in: narrow-angle glaucoma; symptomatic prostatic hypertrophy; bladder neck obstruction; GI obstruction or stenosis; lower respiratory tract symptoms, including asthma; within 14 d of MAO inhibitor therapy. Safe use during pregnancy (category B), in nursing mothers, and in neonates and prematures not established. **Cautious use in:** history of asthma; convulsive disorders; increased intraocular pressure; hyperthyroidism; cardiovascular disease; hypertension; diabetes mellitus.

ADVERSE/SIDE EFFECTS Atropine-like effects: *dry mouth, nose, and throat;* thickened bronchial secretions, wheezing, sensation of chest tightness, blurred vision, diplopia, headache; urinary hesitancy or retention; dysuria; palpitation, tachycardia, mild hypotension or hypertension. **CNS:** *drowsiness,* dizziness, tinnitus, vertigo, fatigue, disturbed coordination, tingling, tremors, euphoria, nervousness, restlessness, insomnia. **GI:** *epigastric distress, anorexia, nausea, vomiting, constipation* or diarrhea. **Hematologic:** leukopenia, hemolytic anemia. **Other:** skin rash, urticaria, photosensitivity, anaphylactic shock. **Overdosage (especially in children):** hallucinations, excitement, fever, ataxia, athetosis, convulsions, coma, cardiovascular collapse.

DRUG INTERACTIONS Alcohol and other CNS DEPRESSANTS add to CNS depression; MAO INHIBITORS may intensify anticholinergic effects.

NURSING IMPLICATIONS

Administration

- GI side effects may be lessened by administration of drug with or immediately after meals or food or with a glass of milk or water.
- Note that the sustained-release formulation (100 mg) is not intended for use in children of any age.
- Patients taking the sustained-release tablet should be instructed to swallow tablet whole and not to crush, break, or chew it.
- Preserve in tight, light-resistant containers.

Assessment & Drug Effects

- Dizziness, sedation, and hypotension are more likely to occur in the elderly. Assistance during ambulation may be necessary.
- Patients receiving long-term therapy with antihistamines should have periodic blood cell counts.

Patient & Family Education

- Urinary hesitancy can be reduced if patient voids just before taking drug.
- Mild to moderate drowsiness, blurred vision, and dizziness occur in some patients. Caution against operating motor vehicle or engaging in hazardous activities until drug response has been determined.
- Patient should know that the effects of antihistamines may be augmented by alcohol ingestion and by use of other CNS depressants.

- Caution not to take OTC preparations without consulting physician.
- Antihistamines should be discontinued within 4 d before skin testing procedure for allergy because they may obscure otherwise positive reactions.

TRIPROLIDINE HYDROCHLORIDE

(trye-proe′li-deen)

Trade name: Actidil

Classification: ANTIHISTAMINE (H_1-RECEPTOR ANTAGONIST)

Prototype: Diphenhydramine

Pregnancy category: B

ACTIONS/PHARMACODYNAMICS

Long-acting, potent antihistamine, similar to diphenhydramine in actions, uses, contraindications, precautions, and adverse effects. Has rapid onset of action, with maximum effect in about 3.5 h and duration up to 12 h. Low incidence of drowsiness and other side effects. See diphenhydramine for contraindications and precautions and adverse/side effects.

ROUTE & DOSAGE

Allergies, Colds

Adult: **PO** 2.5 mg b.i.d. or t.i.d. (max 10 mg/d).
Child: **PO** *6–12 y,* 1.25 mg b.i.d. or t.i.d. (max 5 mg/d); *2–5 y,* 0.6 mg t.i.d. or q.i.d. (max 2.5 mg/d); *4 mo–2 y,* 0.3 mg t.i.d. or q.i.d. (max 1.25 mg/d).

NURSING IMPLICATIONS

- The product Actifed combines the antihistaminic action of triprolidine and the decongestant effect of pseudoephedrine.
- Preserve in tight, light-resistant containers.

See diphenhydramine for numerous additional nursing implications.

TROGLITAZONE

(tro-glit′a-zone)

Trade name: Rezulin

Classifications: ANTIDIABETIC AGENT; THIAZOLIDINEDIONE

Pregnancy category: B

ACTIONS/PHARMACODYNAMICS

Troglitazone lowers blood sugar by improving target cell response to insulin. It decreases insulin resistance. Troglitazone decreases hepatic glucose output and increases glucose disposal in skeletal muscle and possibly in liver and adipose tissue.

USE Management of type II diabetes in patients not adequately controlled despite at least 30 U of insulin per day.

ROUTE & DOSAGE

Diabetes

Adult: **PO** Start with 200 mg q.d. with a meal in patients on insulin; may increase by 200 mg q2–4wk if needed (max 600 mg/d. Discontinue if no response at 600 mg/d × 1 mo).

PHARMACOKINETICS **Absorption:** rapidly absorbed from GI tract; food increases bioavailability. **Peak:** 2–3 h. **Distribution:** >99% protein bound. **Metabolism:** metabolized in the liver. **Elimination:** half-life: 16–34 h; primarily excreted in feces.

CONTRAINDICATIONS & PRECAUTIONS **Contraindicated in:** hypersensitivity to troglitazone, type I diabetics, or treatment of DKA; lactation. **Cautious use in:** New York

Heart Association (NYHA) Class III and Class IV cardiac status (e.g., congestive heart failure); hepatic disease, pregnancy (category B). Safety and efficacy in children have not been established.

ADVERSE/SIDE EFFECTS **Body as whole:** *infection, pain,* asthenia, back pain. **CNS:** *headache,* dizziness. **CV:** peripheral edema. **GI:** hepatotoxicity, nausea, diarrhea. **Respiratory:** rhinitis, pharyngitis. **Other:** UTI.

DRUG INTERACTIONS Decreased concentration of ORAL CONTRACEPTIVES; absorption decreased by **cholestyramine;** increased risk of hypoglycemia with concurrent SULFONYLUREAS.

NURSING IMPLICATIONS

Administration

- Drug should be taken with a meal.
- Co-administration of troglitazone with cholestyramine is not recommended.
- Store at 20–25C (68–77F) in tightly closed container. Protect from moisture and humidity.

Assessment & Drug Effects

- Therapeutic effectiveness is indicated by lower FBS and glycosylated Hgb levels.
- Closely monitor blood glucose level; concurrent insulin dose should be reduced by 10–25% when FBS < 120 mg/dl.
- Lab tests: check serum transaminase levels at the start of therapy, monthly for the first 6 mo, every 2 mo for the next 6 mo. Thereafter, periodically monitor liver function throughout therapy.
- Withhold troglitazone and notify physician at the first sign of liver dysfunction.

Patient & Family Education

- If the daily dose is missed with the usual meal, it may be taken with the next meal.
- Co-administration of troglitazone with insulin or other hypoglycemia agents may increase the risk of hypoglycemia. Promptly report hypoglycemic episodes or FBS levels < 120 mg/dl.
- Promptly report S&S of liver impairment (e.g., jaundice, dark urine, clay-colored stool).
- Women using oral contraceptives may need higher contraceptive doses or alternative means of birth control.

TROLEANDOMYCIN

(troe-lee-an-doe-mye′sin)

Trade name: Tao

Classifications: ANTIINFECTIVE; MACROLIDE ANTIBIOTIC

Prototype: Erythromycin

ACTIONS/PHARMACODYNAMICS Derivative of oleandomycin, a macrolide antibiotic prepared from cultures of *Streptomyces antibioticus.* Chemically related to erythromycin and has similar range of antibacterial activity, but reportedly less effective; has high potential for toxicity. Cross-sensitivity with erythromycin reported.

USES Acute, severe infections of upper respiratory tract caused by susceptible strains of pneumococci and group A beta-hemolytic streptococci.

ROUTE & DOSAGE

Upper Respiratory Tract Infections

Adult: **PO** 250–500 mg q6h.
Child: **PO** 6.6–11 mg/kg (125–250 mg) q6h.

PHARMACOKINETICS **Absorption:** incompletely absorbed from GI tract. **Peak:** 2 h. **Distribution:** distributed throughout body fluids; diffusion into CSF is poor unless meninges are inflamed. **Metabolism:** metabolized in liver. **Elimination:** excreted in bile and urine.

CONTRAINDICATIONS & PRECAUTIONS **Contraindicated in:** use for prophylaxis or for minor infections. Safe use during pregnancy not established. **Cautious use in:** impaired hepatic function.

ADVERSE/SIDE EFFECTS *Abdominal cramps and discomfort, nausea,* vomiting, diarrhea; allergic reactions (urticaria, skin rash, anaphylaxis); cholestatic jaundice, superinfections.

DIAGNOSTIC TEST INTERFERENCE Troleandomycin may cause false elevations of ***urinary 17-ketosteroids*** (Drekter), and ***17-hydroxycorticosteroids*** (Porter-Silver method).

DRUG INTERACTIONS May increase levels of **carbamazepine,** CYCLOSPORINES, and **theophylline** and their toxicity; ORAL CONTRACEPTIVES may cause cholestatic jaundice; **warfarin** may increase prothrombin time (PT); **ergotamine** may induce ischemia and peripheral vasospasm.

T

NURSING IMPLICATIONS

Administration

- Advise patient to take drug on an empty stomach (1 h before or 2 h after meals).
- To maintain effective blood levels, drug should be taken at evenly spaced intervals throughout the day, preferably around the clock.
- Generally, drug therapy does not exceed 10 d. For streptococcal infections, therapy should continue for 10 d to prevent development of rheumatic fever or glomerulonephritis.

Assessment & Drug Effects

- Periodic liver function tests are advised in patients receiving drug longer than 10 d or in repeated courses.
- Some patients develop an allergic type of hepatitis with right upper quadrant pain, fever, nausea, vomiting, jaundice, eosinophilia, and leukocytosis. Liver changes are reversible if drug is discontinued immediately.
- Superinfections are most likely to occur in patients on prolonged or repeated therapy. Drug should be discontinued if symptoms present (see Appendix G), and appropriate therapy should be started.

Patient & Family Education

- Instruct to report signs of jaundice: acholic stools, pruritus, icteric sclerae.
- Instruct not to stop drug before full course of therapy is completed. Patient should not interrupt then restart therapy or increase or decrease dose or interval.

TROMETHAMINE

(troe-meth′a-meen)

Trade names: Tham, Tham-E

Classifications: ELECTROLYTIC BALANCE AGENT; SYSTEMIC ALKALINIZER

Pregnancy category: C

ACTIONS/PHARMACODYNAMICS Sodium-free organic amine that acts as a proton acceptor in the body buffering system, thereby preventing or correcting acidosis. As a weak base, it combines with hydrogen ions from carbonic, lactic, pyruvic, and other metabolic acids and penetrates the cell membrane to combine with intracellular acid. Also acts as a weak osmotic diuretic increasing urine pH and excretion of fixed acids, CO_2, and electrolytes. May be preferable to sodium bicarbonate in treatment of severe metabolic acidosis when sodium or CO_2 elimination is restricted.

USES To prevent or correct metabolic acidosis associated with cardiac bypass surgery and cardiac arrest and to correct excess acidity of stored blood (preserved with acid citrate dextrose [CD]) and used in cardiac bypass surgery. (Stored blood has a pH range of 6.8–6.22.) **Unlabeled uses:** metabolic acidosis of status asthmaticus and neonatal respiratory distress syndrome.

ROUTE & DOSAGE

Dosage may be estimated from buffer base deficit of extracellular fluid using the following formula as a guide: ml of 0.3-M tromethamine solution = body weight (kg) × base deficit (mEq/L)

Metabolic Acidosis Associated with Cardiac Arrest

Adult: **IV** 3.5–6 ml/kg (126–216 mg/kg) of a 0.3-M solution into large peripheral vein; if chest is open, 55–165 ml (2–6 g) 0.3-M solution into ventricular cavity.

Systemic Acidosis During Cardiac Bypass Surgery

Adult: **IV** 9 ml/kg or approximately 500 ml (18 g) 0.3-M solution; a single dose of up to 1000 ml (36 g) may be necessary in severe acidosis.

Excess Acidity of ACD Priming Blood

Adult: **IV** 14–70 ml (0.5–2.5 g) 0.3-M solution added to each 500 ml blood.

PHARMACOKINETICS Metabolism: no appreciable metabolism. **Elimination:** rapidly and preferentially excreted by kidneys; 75% excreted within 8 h.

CONTRAINDICATIONS & PRECAUTIONS Contraindicated in: anuria, uremia; chronic respiratory acidosis; pregnancy (category C), children, neonates. **Cautious use in:** > 1 d of therapy.

ADVERSE/SIDE EFFECTS Injection site: *local irritation,* tissue inflammation, *chemical phlebitis,* extravasation. **Respiratory:** respiratory depression. **Other:** transient decrease in blood glucose, hypervolemia, hyperkalemia (with depressed renal function).

NURSING IMPLICATIONS

Administration

- Maximum allowable concentration for IV infusion is 0.3 M. Available as a 0.3-M solution or may be prepared by adding 36 g to 1 L of sterile water.
- A large antecubital vein should be selected for drug administration by slow IV infusion or via pump-oxygenator. Usually, an IV catheter is used. The limb should be elevated.
- Drug administration is usually over a period of no less than 1 h. Except in life-threatening situations, drug administration is limited to 1 d.
- Observe entry site carefully. Perivascular infiltration of the highly alkaline solution may lead to vasospasm, necrosis, and tissue sloughing. Stop infusion if extravasation occurs.
- Extravasation may be treated with a procaine and hyaluronidase infiltration to reduce vasospasm and to dilute tromethamine remaining in tissues. If necessary, local infiltration of an alpha-adrenergic block-

T

ing agent (e.g., phentolamine) into the area may be ordered.

- Tromethamine solution is highly alkaline and can erode glass; discard solution 24 h after reconstitution.
- Protect drug (available as solution or powder) from freezing or extreme heat.

Assessment & Drug Effects

- Hypoxia and hypoventilation may result from drug-induced reduction of CO_2 tension (a potent stimulus to breathing), particularly if respiratory acidosis is also present. Watch for signs of hypoxia (see Appendix G).
- Drug-induced hypoxia is a particular risk for the patient who is on other respiratory depressants or who has COPD or impaired renal function.
- Blood pH, Pco_2, Po_2, bicarbonate, glucose, and electrolytes should be monitored before, during, and after treatment. Dosage is controlled to raise blood pH to normal limits (arterial: 7.35–7.45) and to correct acid–base imbalance.
- Monitor ECG and serum potassium if drug is given to patient with imparied renal function (reduced drug elimination). Since hyperkalemia is often associated with metabolic acidosis, be alert to early signs (see Appendix G).
- Overdose symptoms (total drug or too rapid administration): alkalosis, overhydration, prolonged hypoglycemia, solute overload.

T

TROPICAMIDE

(troe-pik′a-mide)

Trade names: Mydriacyl, Tropicacyl

Classifications: EYE PREPARATION; MYDRIATIC; CYCLOPLEGIC

Prototype: Homatropine

Pregnancy category: C

See Appendix A.

TROVAFLOXACIN/ ALATROVAFLOXACIN

(tro-va-flox′a-sin/a-la-tro-va-flox′a-sin)

Trade names: Trovan, Trovan IV

Classifications: ANTIINFECTIVE; QUINOLONE

Prototype: Ciprofloxacin

Pregnancy category: C

ACTIONS/PHARMACODYNAMICS

Fluoroquinolone bactericidal agent. Interferes with the DNA enzyme gyrase needed for bacterial DNA replication. Has high potency against gram-negative bacteria including *Pseudomonas* and a very broad spectrum to include most gram-positive organisms.

USES Treatment of the following infections caused by susceptible bacteria: nosocomial pneumonia, community-acquired pneumonia, chronic bronchitis, acute sinusitis, complicated intraabdominal infections, endomyometritis, septic abortion, postpartum infections, surgical prophylaxis, complicated and uncomplicated skin and skin structure infections, PID, uncomplicated UTI, chronic bacterial prostatitis, uncomplicated gonorrhea, cervicitis.

ROUTE & DOSAGE

Nosocomial Pneumonia; Gynecologic, Pelvic, or Complicated Intraabdominal Infections

Adult: **IV** 300 mg infused over 60 min q.d. followed by **PO** 200 mg q.d. for total of 10–14 d.

Community-acquired Pneumonia; Complicated Skin and Skin Structure Infections (including Diabetic Foot Ulcers)

Adult: **IV** 200 mg infused over 60 min q.d. followed by **PO** 200 mg q.d. for total of 7–14 d (may initiate therapy with 200 mg PO q.d.)

Chronic Bronchitis; Uncomplicated Skin Infections

Adult: **PO** 100 mg q.d. × 7–10 d.

Acute Sinusitis

Adult: **PO** 200 mg q.d. × 10 d.

Surgical Prophylaxis

Adult: **IV/PO** 200 mg 30 min to 4 h prior to surgery.

Uncomplicated UTI

Adult: **PO** 100 mg q.d. × 3 d.

Chronic Bacterial Prostatitis

Adult: **PO** 200 mg q.d. × 28 d.

Gonorrhea

Adult: **PO** 100 mg × 1 dose.

Cervicitis

Adult: **PO** 200 mg q.d. × 5 d.

PID

Adult: **PO** 200 mg q.d. × 14 d. (*Note:* In patients with chronic hepatic disease, decrease 300-mg dose to 200 mg and 200-mg dose to 100 mg; no change for 100-mg doses.)

PHARMACOKINETICS Absorption: well absorbed from GI tract (88% bioavailability). **Peak:** 1 h. **Distribution:** 76% protein bound, widely distributed throughout target body tissues. **Metabolism:** metabolized in liver. **Elimination:** half-life: 9–12 h; 52% excreted in feces, 19% in urine.

CONTRAINDICATIONS & PRECAUTIONS Contraindicated in: hypersensitivity to trovafloxacin, alatrovafloxacin, other quinolone antibiotics; pregnancy (category C). **Cautious use in:** lactation; children < 18 y; hepatic insufficiency.

ADVERSE/SIDE EFFECTS CNS: dizziness, lightheadedness, headache. **GI:** nausea, vomiting, diarrhea, abdominal pain. **Skin:** rash, pruritus. **Other:** pain at injection site, vaginitis.

DRUG INTERACTIONS Absorption reduced by concomitant aluminum- or magnesium-containing ANTACIDS, **sucralfate,** IRON SALTS, and IV **morphine.**

INCOMPATIBILITIES Solution/additive: 0.9% NaCl, Ringer's lactate. **Y-site:** solutions containing multivalent cations (e.g., magnesium, calcium).

NURSING IMPLICATIONS

Administration

- Give oral dose at least 2 h before or 2 h after magnesium/aluminum-containing antacid, sucralfate, or iron preparations.
- If patient is receiving IV morphine, wait at least 2 or 4 h, respectively, after oral trovafloxacin is given on an empty stomach or with food to give IV morphine.
- IV preparation: Concentrate in vials is 5 mg/ml; dilute to a final concentration of 1–2 mg/ml by adding to 0.45% NaCl, D5W, D5W + 0.45% NaCl, or D5W + lactated Ringer's. To prepare a 50-ml solution with a concentration of 2 mg/ml, add 20 ml (100 mg) of concentrate to 30 ml of diluent to yield 100 mg in 50 ml total volume. To prepare a 200-ml solution with a concentration of 1 mg/ml, add 40 ml (200 mg) of concentrate to 160 ml of diluent to yield 200 mg in

T

200 ml total volume. See manufacturer's directions for other options.
- IV infusion: Diluted solution must be infused over 60 min. Avoid rapid or bolus infusion.
- Store tablets and IV solution at 15–30C (59–86F) in a tightly closed container and protect from light. Discard any unused portion left in single-dose IV vials.

Assessment & Drug Effects
- Therapeutic effectiveness is indicated by resolution of infection.
- Before drug is initiated, determine previous hypersensitivity to quinolones and other drugs.
- Lab tests: Baseline C&S prior to and periodically during therapy; CBC with differential; liver functions for therapy ≥21 d.
- Discontinue drug and notify prescriber immediately if S&S of hypersensitivity, including skin rash (see Appendix G), or CNS overstimulation occur.

Patient & Family Education
- Avoid hazardous activities until reaction to the drug is known.
- Taking drug at bedtime with food will reduce the risk of dizziness. Note instructions about antacids and iron preparations or multivitamins with iron.
- Discontinue drug and promptly notify prescriber if any of the following occur: S&S of a ruptured tendon (e.g., pain or inflammation in hand, shoulder, or foot), S&S of an allergic reaction (e.g., as rash, hives, difficulty swallowing or breathing, swelling of face, lips, tongue), S&S of phototoxicity (e.g., painful sunburn or skin eruptions after exposure to sun or UV light).
- Avoid sunlight or UV light while taking this drug.

TUBOCURARINE CHLORIDE
(too-boe-kyoo-ar′een)

Prototype for classifications: AUTONOMIC NERVOUS SYSTEM AGENT; NONDEPOLARIZING SKELETAL MUSCLE RELAXANT

Pregnancy category: C

ACTIONS/PHARMACODYNAMICS
Curare alkaloid, nondepolarizing neuromuscular blocking agent extracted from the plant *Chondodendron tomentosum*. Produces skeletal muscle relaxation or paralysis by competing with acetylcholine at cholinergic receptor sites on skeletal muscle endplate and thus blocks nerve impulse transmission. Also has histamine-releasing and ganglionic blocking properties. Has no known effect on intellectual functions, consciousness, or pain threshold.

USES To induce skeletal muscle relaxation as adjunct to general anesthesia, to facilitate management of mechanical ventilation, to reduce intensity of muscle contractions in tetanus and in pharmacologically or electrically induced convulsions, to treat spastic states in children, and for diagnosis of myasthenia gravis when conventional tests have been inconclusive.

ROUTE & DOSAGE

Adjunct to General Anesthesia

Adult: **IV** 6–9 mg followed by 3–4.5 mg in 3–5 min if necessary.
Child: **IV** 0.2–0.5 mg/kg followed by 0.04–0.1 mg/kg prn to maintain paralysis.
Neonate <1 mo: 0.3 mg/kg followed by 0.1 mg/kg prn to maintain paralysis.

T

Electroshock
Adult: **IV** 0.165 mg/kg administered slowly IV.

Diagnosis of Myasthenia Gravis
Adult: **IV** 0.004–0.033 mg/kg.

PHARMACOKINETICS **Peak:** 2–5 min. **Duration:** 20–30 min if used alone. **Metabolism:** demethylated in liver. **Elimination:** half-life: 1–3 h; 33–75% excreted in urine within 24 h; 11% excreted in bile; crosses placenta.

CONTRAINDICATIONS & PRECAUTIONS **Contraindicated in:** hypersensitivity to curare preparations; when histamine release is a hazard; hyperthermia; electrolyte imbalance; acidosis; neuromuscular disease; renal disease. Safe use during pregnancy (category C) not established. **Cautious use in:** impaired cardiovascular, renal, hepatic, pulmonary, or endocrine function; hypotension; carcinomatosis; thyroid disorders; collagen diseases; porphyria; familial periodic paralysis; history of allergies; myasthenia gravis; elderly or debilitated patients.

ADVERSE/SIDE EFFECTS Slight dizziness, feeling of warmth, profound and prolonged muscle weakness and flaccidity, respiratory depression, hypoxia, apnea, increased bronchial and salivary secretions, bronchospasm, decreased GI motility, *hypotension,* circulatory collapse, malignant hyperthermia, hypersensitivity reactions.

DRUG INTERACTIONS SKELETAL MUSCLE RELAXANTS, INHALED ANESTHETICS, AMINOGLYCOSIDES, **polymyxin B, clindamycin, quinidine, quinine, procainamide**, DIURETICS, **amphotericin B** may potentiate neuromuscular blockade.

INCOMPATIBILITIES **Solution/additive:** BARBITURATES, **sodium bicarbonate; trimethaphan.**

NURSING IMPLICATIONS

Administration

- Tubocurarine may be given undiluted (3 mg/ml) by direct IV over 60–90 s.
- IV administration to neonates, infants, children: Verify correct IV dilution and rate of IV injection with physician.
- Solutions of drug should not be used if more than faintly discolored.
- Tubocurarine is incompatible with solutions that have a high pH such as barbiturates and sodium bicarbonate; therefore, do not mix in same syringe.

Assessment & Drug Effects

- Baseline tests of renal function and determinations of serum electrolytes are generally done before drug administration. Electrolyte imbalance (particularly potassium and magnesium) can potentiate the effects of nondepolarizing neuromuscular blocking agents.
- Monitor BP, vital signs, and airway until assured of patient's recovery from drug effects. Ganglionic blockade (hypotension) and histamine liberation (increased salivation, bronchospasm) and neuromuscular blockade (respiratory depression) are known effects of tubocurarine.
- Selective muscle paralysis following drug administration occurs in the following sequence: jaw muscles, levator eyelid muscles and other muscles of head and neck, limbs, intercostals and diaphragm, abdomen, trunk. Facial and diaphragm muscles are first to recover, followed in order by legs, arms, shoulder girdle, trunk, lar-

T

ynx, hands, feet, pharynx. Muscle function is usually restored within 90 min.

- Measure and record I&O ratio during day of drug administration. Renal dysfunction will prolong drug action. Peristaltic action may be suppressed. Check for bowel sounds.

Patient & Family Education

- Tubocurarine is retained in the body long after effects of neuromuscular blockade appear to have dissipated. Instruct to report residual muscle weakness.

URACIL MUSTARD

(yoor'a-sill)

Classifications: ANTINEOPLASTIC; ALKYLATING AGENT

Prototype: Cyclophosphamide

Pregnancy category: X

ACTIONS/PHARMACODYNAMICS Nitrogen mustard agent thought to react selectively with phosphate groups of DNA, causing chromosomal cross-linkage and interference with normal mitosis. Lacks vesicant properties; ineffective in treatment of acute leukemia or acute blastic crisis. Has cumulative hematopoietic depressive properties at therapeutic dosage levels. Maximum bone marrow depression may not occur until 2–4 wk after uracil has been discontinued. Like other alkylating agents, uracil may be carcinogenic.

USES Chronic lymphocytic and myelocytic leukemia, non-Hodgkin's lymphomas, reticulum cell cancer. **Unlabeled uses:** carcinoma of lung, cervix, or ovary. Beneficial in early stages of polycythemia vera and in therapy of mycosis fungoides.

ROUTE & DOSAGE

Antineoplastic

Adult: **PO** 0.15 mg/kg qwk for 4 wk.
Child: **PO** 0.30 mg/kg qwk for 4 wk.

Thrombocytosis

Adult: **PO** 1–2 mg/d for 14 d.

PHARMACOKINETICS **Absorption:** incompletely absorbed from GI tract. **Elimination:** plasma concentrations decrease rapidly with no evidence after 2 h; <1% recovered unchanged in urine.

CONTRAINDICATIONS & PRECAUTIONS **Contraindicated in:** severe leukopenia, thrombocytopenia, aplastic anemia, pregnancy (category X). **Cautious use in:** history of gout or urate renal stones; leukopenia, thrombocytopenia.

ADVERSE/SIDE EFFECTS **CNS:** irritability, nervousness, mental confusion. **GI:** *anorexia, epigastric distress, nausea, vomiting, diarrhea, oral ulcerations.* **Hematologic:** leukopenia, thrombocytopenia, <u>bone marrow depression</u> (sometimes irreversible). **Skin:** pruritus, dermatitis, pigmentation. **Other:** <u>hepatotoxicity</u>, hyperuricemia, amenorrhea, azoospermia.

NURSING IMPLICATIONS

Administration

- Uracil mustard is administered at least 2 or 3 wk after maximum effect of previous antineoplastic or radiation has been achieved.
- It is usually administered at bedtime to alleviate GI side effects. Severe nausea and vomiting may necessitate discontinuation of drug.

Assessment & Drug Effects

- As total cumulative dose of uracil approaches 1 mg/kg body weight, irreversible bone marrow damage may occur.

- Depression of platelets is apt to be more serious than that of leukocytes; watch carefully for beginning signs of bleeding into skin and mucosa and gingival bleeding with tooth brushing. Report immediately.
- CBCs, including platelets, are advised 1 or 2 times weekly during and at least 1 mo after end of therapy. (Maximum bone marrow depression may not occur until 2–4 wk after discontinuation of therapy.)
- If possible, avoid invasive procedures that could lead to bleeding during thrombocytopenic period (IM, SC, rectal temperatures).
- In some patients, drug appears to act slowly, and response may not be apparent for 2–3 mo after drug therapy is initiated.

Patient & Family Education

- Urge to increase fluid intake so that renal flushing occurs. Changes in I&O ratio and pattern and flank, stomach, or joint pain should be reported promptly.
- Notify physician of the following symptoms: fever, chills, oral ulcerations, sore throat, bleeding and bruising, swelling of lower legs and feet.
- Frank alopecia is not a usual side effect as with other nitrogen mustards.

UREA

(yoor-ee′a)

Trade names: Aquacare, Carbamide, Carmol, Nutraplus, Ureacin, Ureaphil

Classifications: WATER BALANCE AGENT; OSMOTIC DIURETIC; OXYTOCIC

Prototype: Mannitol

Pregnancy: Category C

ACTIONS/PHARMACODYNAMICS

When present in high concentrations in blood, induces diuresis by elevating osmotic pressure of glomerular filtrate, with subsequent decrease in sodium and water reabsorption and promotion of chloride and potassium excretion. Volume and rate of urine flow is increased. Increased blood toxicity results in transudation of fluid from tissue, including brain, cerebrospinal, and intraocular fluid, into the blood. When used as an abortifacient, urea (in dextrose) is injected into amniotic sac, followed by IV oxytocin about 400 mU/min or by prostaglandin F_2.

USES To reduce or prevent intracranial pressure (cerebral edema) and intraocular pressure and to prevent acute renal failure during prolonged surgery or trauma. Also transabdominally for aborting second trimester of pregnancy. Topical preparation promotes hydration and removal of excess keratin in dry skin and hyperkeratotic conditions. **Unlabeled uses:** severe migraine attacks; acute sickle cell crisis.

ROUTE & DOSAGE

Reduction of Intracranial or Intraocular Pressure, Diuresis

Adult: **IV** 1–1.5 g/kg of 30% solution infused slowly over 1–2.5 h at a rate not to exceed 4 ml/min (max 120 g/24 h).
Child: **IV** >*2 y,* 0.5–1.5 g/kg of 30% solution infused slowly over 1–2.5 h at a rate not to exceed 4 ml/min; <*2 y,* 0.1–0.5 g/kg of 30% solution infused slowly over 1–2.5 h at a rate not to exceed 4 ml/min.

Hydration of Dry Skin

Adult: **Topical** Apply 2–40%

U

cream or lotion to affected area 1–3 times/d.

Second-Trimester Abortion

Adult: **Intraamniotic** Instill 40–50% urea solution in 5% dextrose in volumes equal to amount of amniotic fluid removed to a max of 200–250 ml.

PHARMACOKINETICS **Peak:** 1–2 h. **Duration:** 3–10 h for diuresis and intracranial pressure reduction; 5–6 h for intraocular pressure. **Distribution:** 10% of intraamniotic instillation diffuses into maternal blood; distributed widely; good ocular penetration; crosses placenta; distributed into breast milk. **Elimination:** half-life: 1 h; excreted in urine; 50% may be reabsorbed.

CONTRAINDICATIONS & PRECAUTIONS **Contraindicated in:** severely impaired renal or hepatic function; CHF; active intracranial bleeding; marked dehydration; IV injection into lower extremities, especially in elderly patients; topical use for viral skin diseases or impaired circulation. Safe use in pregnancy (category C), lactation, or in children not established. (Contraindications for intraamniotic urea: impaired renal function, frank liver failure, active intracranial bleeding; marked dehydration, diabetes mellitus, sickle cell anemia.) **Cautious use in:** use on face or broken skin.

ADVERSE/SIDE EFFECTS **CNS:** somnolence (prolonged use in patients with renal dysfunction), *headache,* acute psychosis, confusion, disorientation, nervousness. **CV:** tachycardia, hypotension, syncope. **GI:** *nausea, vomiting,* increased thirst. **Metabolic:** fluid and electrolyte imbalance, dehydration. **Other:** intraocular hemorrhage (rapid IV), pain, irritation, sloughing, venous thrombosis, chemical phlebitis at injection site; hyperthermia, skin rash, hemolysis (rapid IV).

DRUG INTERACTION May increase rate of **lithium** excretion, decreasing its effectiveness.

NURSING IMPLICATIONS

Administration

- Solution should be freshly prepared for each patient; discard unused portion. Urea may be reconstituted with 5% or 10% dextrose injection or 10% invert sugar in water.
- Reconstituted solution should be used within a few hours if stored at room temperature. If refrigerated at 2–8C (36–46F), solution should be used within 48 h; prolonged storage leads to ammonia formation. Discard unused portions.
- Infusion flow rate will be prescribed by physician. Rapid administration may be associated with increased capillary bleeding and hemolysis.
- Urea should not be administered by same IV set through which blood is being infused.
- Urea has the potential for causing tissue damage because of its osmotic properties. Extreme care must be taken to avoid extravasation; thrombosis and tissue necrosis can occur. Inspect injection site frequently. If extravasation is suspected, discontinue the IV line stat. Consult physician about removal of needle or cannula. Institute local treatment (according to institution protocol or physician's instructions); elevate part even if extravasation is minor.
- Action of topical preparation is enhanced by applying it to skin that

is still moist following washing or bathing.

Assessment & Drug Effects

- Monitor I&O. If diuresis does not occur within 6–12 h following administration or if BUN exceeds 75 mg/dl, drug should be withheld until renal function is evaluated.
- Monitor vital signs and mental status; promptly report any changes.
- Observe postoperative patients closely for signs of hemorrhage. Urea reportedly may increase prothrombin time and promote internal oozing at suture sites.
- Patient should be encouraged to drink fluids so as to hasten excretion of urea. However, if patient complains of a headache, do not allow him or her to drink as this will counteract the osmotic effects of the drug. Consult physician about fluid volume parameters.
- Determinations of serum and urinary sodium should be performed q12h. Frequent BUN and kidney function studies are advised, particularly in patients suspected of having renal dysfunction.
- Be alert for signs of hyponatremia, hypokalemia, dehydration, or transient overhydration (due to hyperosmotic activity) (see Appendix G).
- There is minimal systemic absorption of intraamniotic-instilled drug when given in the intraamniotic sac and minimal systemic effects. If patient complains of lower abdominal pain, it may be that drug is going into abdomen rather than into the amniotic sac.

See mannitol for additional nursing implications.

UROKINASE

(yoor-oh-kin'ase)

Trade names: Abbokinase, Open-Cath

Classifications: BLOOD FORMER; THROMBOLYTIC ENZYME

Prototype: Streptokinase

Pregnancy: Category B

ACTIONS/PHARMACODYNAMICS

Enzyme produced by kidneys and isolated from human kidney tissue cultures. Promotes thrombolysis by acting directly on the endogenous fibrinolytic system to convert plasminogen to the enzyme plasmin, an action that occurs within as well as on the surface of a thrombus or embolus. Urokinase also has an anticoagulant effect because its action leads to high plasma levels of fibrin and fibrinogen degradation products. Most effective action is on fresh, recently formed thrombi.

USES Lysis of acute massive pulmonary emboli and peripheral emboli and restoration of patency in occluded IV catheters (including central venous catheter); acute MI, retinal vessel occlusion, lysis of clot-occluded arteriovenous cannulas, and various other conditions associated with thromboembolization phenomenon.

ROUTE & DOSAGE

Pulmonary Embolus

Adult: **IV** 4400 IU/kg diluted in 0.9% NaCl or 5% dextrose infused over 10 min, followed by continuous infusion of 4400 IU/kg/h for 12 h; administer through in-line 0.22- or 0.45-μm filter using a constant infusion pump.

Occluded Coronary Artery

Adult: **IV** Precede urokinase with bolus of heparin (2500–10,000 U IV); then instill urokinase 6000 IU/min for periods up to 2 h; continue until artery is maximally

U

opened (usually 15–30 min using about 500,000 IU); administer through in-line 0.22- or 0.45-μm filter using a constant infusion pump.

Central Venous Catheter Clearance

Adult: **IV** Instill 5000 IU/ml solution into catheter port; after 5 min attempt to aspirate urokinase and clot; if no success after 30 min, cap port and wait 30–60 min and try again; instruct patient to exhale and hold breath any time catheter is disconnected from syringe or IV tubing; avoid excessive pressure of instillation to prevent rupture of catheter or forcing clot into circulation.

PHARMACOKINETICS Absorption: rapidly cleared from circulation. **Peak:** 3–4 h. **Elimination:** half-life: 10–20 min; small amount excreted in urine and bile.

CONTRAINDICATIONS & PRECAUTIONS Contraindicated in: pregnancy (category B), during lactation, and in children. See streptokinase for additional contraindications, adverse/side effects, diagnostic test interferences, and drug interactions.

ADVERSE/SIDE EFFECTS See streptokinase.

NURSING IMPLICATIONS

See streptokinase for additional nursing implications.

Administration

- Reconstitute by adding 5.2 ml sterile water for injection to vial containing 250,000 IU (resulting solution contains 50,000 IU/ml). Roll or tilt vial to mix; avoid agitating or shaking to prevent foaming and filament formation. Prepare further dilutions by adding 190 ml of 0.9% NaCl or D5W.
- Urokinase should be reconstituted immediately before use. Since the product contains no preservatives, discard unused portion. Total volume of administered fluid should not exceed 200 ml.
- Avoid adding other medication to urokinase solution.
- Store vials at 2–8C (36–46F).

Assessment & Drug Effects

- Measurable signs of clinical response may not occur for 6–8 h after therapy is started.
- Anticoagulant therapy with heparin is reinstituted at end of urokinase therapy and when TT has decreased to less than twice normal control value (usually within 3–4 h).
- Severe spontaneous bleeding, including fatality from cerebral hemorrhage, has occurred during urokinase treatment. Risk is estimated to be twice that associated with heparin therapy.

VALACYCLOVIR HCL

(val-a-cy'clo-vir)

Trade name: Valtrex

Classifications: ANTIINFECTIVE; ANTIVIRAL

Prototype: Acyclovir

Pregnancy category: B

ACTIONS/PHARMACODYNAMICS

Valacyclovir is an antiviral agent hydrolyzed in the intestinal wall and/or liver to acyclovir. Because of increased GI absorption, the plasma level of this drug is substantially higher than that of acyclovir when both are taken orally. It is active against herpes simplex virus types I (HSV-1) and 2 (HSV-2), varicella-zoster virus (VZV), and cytomegalovirus (CMV). Acyclovir interferes with DNA synthesis and thus inhibits viral replication.

USE Herpes zoster (shingles) in immunocompetent adults. Treatment and suppression of recurrent genital herpes.

ROUTE & DOSAGE

Herpes Zoster

Adult: **PO** 1 g (2 × 500 mg) t.i.d. for 7 d; should be started within 48 h of onset of zoster rash; dose should be reduced for patients with Cl_{cr} < 50 ml/min.

Treatment of Recurrent Genital Herpes

Adult: **PO** 500 mg b.i.d. × 5 d.

Suppression of Recurrent Genital Herpes

Adult: **PO** 1 g q.d.

PHARMACOKINETICS Absorption: rapidly absorbed from GI tract; 54% reaches systemic circulation as acyclovir. **Peak:** 1.5 h. **Distribution:** 13.5–17.9% bound to plasma proteins; distributes into plasma, cerebrospinal fluid, saliva, and major body organs; crosses placenta; excreted in breast milk. **Metabolism:** rapidly converted to acyclovir during first pass through intestine and liver. **Elimination:** half-life: 2.5–3.3 h; 40–50% excreted in urine.

CONTRAINDICATIONS & PRECAUTIONS Contraindicated in: hypersensitivity to or intolerance of valacyclovir or acyclovir; pregnancy (category B), nursing mothers, immunocompromised patients. **Cautious use in:** renal impairment, patients receiving nephrotoxic drugs, nursing mothers. Safety and efficacy in children have not been established.

ADVERSE/SIDE EFFECTS CNS: *headache,* weakness, somnolence, dizziness, fatigue, lethargy, confusion. **GI:** *nausea, vomiting, diarrhea,* abdominal pain, dyspepsia, flatulence. **GU:** glomerulonephritis, renal tubular damage, acute renal failure. **Skin:** rash, urticaria, pruritus.

DRUG INTERACTIONS Probenecid, cimetidine decrease acyclovir elimination. **Zidovudine** may cause increased drowsiness and lethargy.

NURSING IMPLICATIONS

Administration

- Drug should be initiated as soon as possible after diagnosis of herpes zoster, preferably within 48 h of onset of rash.
- Note that dosage reduction is recommended for patients with renal impairment.
- Give valacyclovir after hemodialysis.
- Store at 15–30C (59–86F).

Assessment & Drug Effects

- Monitor renal function in patients with renal impairment or those receiving potentially nephrotoxic drugs.
- If signs and symptoms of hypersensitivity occur, withhold drug and report to physician.

Patient & Family Education

- Inform patient of potential adverse effects and advise not to discontinue drug until full course is completed.
- Advise that postherpetic pain is likely to be present for several months after completion of therapy.

VALPROIC ACID (DIVALPROEX SODIUM, SODIUM VALPROATE)

(val-proe′ic)

Trade names: Depacon, Depa-

V

kene, Depakote, Depakote Sprinkle, Epival ♣
Prototype for classifications: ANTICONVULSANT; GABA INHIBITOR
Pregnancy category: D

ACTIONS/PHARMACODYNAMICS Anticonvulsant unrelated chemically to other drugs used to treat seizure disorders. Mechanism of action unknown; may be related to increased bioavailability of the inhibitory neurotransmitter GABA to brain neurons. Inhibits secondary phase of platelet aggregation.

USES Alone or with other anticonvulsants in management of absence (petit mal) and mixed seizures; mania; migraine headache prophylaxis. **Unlabeled uses:** status epilepticus refractory to IV diazepam, petit mal variant seizures, febrile seizures in children, other types of seizures including psychomotor (temporal lobe), myoclonic, akinetic and tonic-clonic seizures, photosensitivity seizures, and those refractory to other anticonvulsants.

ROUTE & DOSAGE

Management of Seizures, Mania

Adult: **PO/IV** 15 mg/kg/d in divided doses when total daily dose > 250 mg; increase at 1 wk intervals by 5–10 mg/kg/d until seizures are controlled or side effects develop (max 60 mg/kg/d).
Child: **PO/IV** Same as for adult.

Migraine Headache Prophylaxis

Adult: **PO** 250 mg b.i.d., may increase to max of 1000 mg/d.

Mania

Adult: **PO** 250 mg t.i.d., may increase to max of 60 mg/kg/d.

PHARMACOKINETICS Absorption: readily absorbed from GI tract. **Peak:** 1–4 h valproic acid; 3–5 h divalproex. **Therapeutic range:** 50–100 g/ml. **Distribution:** crosses placenta; distributed into breast milk. **Metabolism:** metabolized in liver. **Elimination:** half-life: 5–20 h; excreted primarily in urine; small amount excreted in feces and expired air.

CONTRAINDICATIONS & PRECAUTIONS Contraindicated in: patient with bleeding disorders or hepatic dysfunction or disease, pregnancy (category D), nursing mothers. **Cautious use in:** history of renal disease; adjunctive treatment with other anticonvulsants.

ADVERSE/SIDE EFFECTS CNS: breakthrough seizures, *sedation, drowsiness,* dizziness, increased alertness, hallucinations, emotional upset, aggression. **GI:** *nausea, vomiting, indigestion (transient),* hypersalivation, anorexia with weight loss, increased appetite with weight gain, abdominal cramps, diarrhea, constipation, <u>hepatic failure</u>. **Hematologic:** *prolonged bleeding time,* leukopenia, lymphocytosis, thrombocytopenia, hypofibrinogenemia, <u>bone marrow depression</u>, anemia. **Other:** skin rash, transient hair loss, curliness or waviness of hair, irregular menses, secondary amenorrhea, photosensitivity; hyperammonemia (usually asymptomatic). **Overdosage:** <u>deep coma</u>, pulmonary edema, <u>death</u>.

DIAGNOSTIC TEST INTERFERENCE Valproic acid produces false-positive results for ***urine ketones,*** elevated ***AST, ALT, LDH,*** and ***serum alkaline phosphatase,*** prolonged ***bleeding time,*** altered ***thyroid function*** tests.

DRUG INTERACTIONS Alcohol and other CNS DEPRESSANTS potentiate depressant effects; other ANTICONVULSANTS, BARBITURATES increase anticonvulsant and barbiturate levels and toxicity; **aspirin, dipyridamole, warfarin** increase risk of spontaneous bleed and decrease clotting; **clonazepam** may precipitate absence seizures; SALICYLATES **cimetidine** may increase valproic acid levels and toxicity. **Cholestyramine** may decrease absorption.

NURSING IMPLICATIONS

Administration

- Tablets and capsules should not be chewed. Medication should be swallowed whole. Patient should avoid using a carbonated drink as diluent for the syrup because it will release drug from delivery vehicle. Free drug painfully irritates oral and pharyngeal membranes.
- Serious GI side effects can lead to discontinuation of therapy with valproic acid. To reduce gastric irritation, administer drug with food. Enteric-coated tablet or syrup formulation is usually well tolerated.
- Abrupt discontinuation of therapy can lead to loss of seizure control. Warn patient not to stop or alter dosage regimen without consulting physician.

Assessment & Drug Effects

- Effective therapeutic serum levels of valproic acid are 50–100 μg/ml.
- Monitor alertness in patient on multiple drug therapy for seizure control. Plasma levels of the adjunctive anticonvulsants should be evaluated periodically as indicators for possible neurologic toxicity.
- Increased dosage increases frequency of adverse effects. Monitor patient carefully when dose adjustments are being made and report promptly if side effects persist.
- Platelet counts and bleeding time determinations are recommended prior to initiating treatment and at periodic intervals. Liver function tests, including serum ammonia, should be performed initially and at least q2mo, especially during the first 6 mo of therapy.

Patient & Family Education

- Inform the diabetic patient that this drug may cause a false-positive test for urine ketones. Should that occur, notify the physician; a differential diagnostic blood test may be indicated.
- If spontaneous bleeding or bruising (petechiae, ecchymotic areas, otorrhagia, epistaxis, melena) occurs, notify physician promptly.
- Instruct to withhold dose and report to the physician if the following symptoms appear: visual disturbances, rash, jaundice, light-colored stools, protracted vomiting, diarrhea. Fatal hepatic failure has occurred in patients receiving this drug.
- Warn to avoid alcohol and self-medication with other depressants during therapy. The use of all OTC drugs should be approved by the physician during anticonvulsant therapy. Particularly unsafe are combination drugs containing aspirin, sedatives, and medications for hay fever or other allergies.
- Advise not to drive a car or engage in other activities requiring mental alertness and physical coordination until reaction to drug is known.
- Patients on multiple drug therapy are at risk from hyperammonemia (lethargy, anorexia, asterixis, increased seizure frequency, vomiting). These symptoms should be reported promptly. If they persist with decreased dosage, the drug will be discontinued.
- Before any kind of surgery (in-

V

cluding dental surgery), the patient should inform the doctor or dentist of taking valproic acid.
- Advise to carry medical identification card or jewelry bearing information about medication in use and the epilepsy diagnosis.

VALSARTAN

(val-sar'tan)

Trade name: Diovan

Classifications: CARDIOVASCULAR AGENT; ANGIOTENSIN II-RECEPTOR ANTAGONIST; ANTIHYPERTENSIVE

Prototype: Losartan

Pregnancy category: C (first trimester); D (second and third trimester)

ACTIONS/PHARMACODYNAMICS Valsartan is an angiotensin II receptor (type AT_1) antagonist. Angiotensin II is a potent vasoconstrictor and primary vasoactive hormone of the renin–angiotensin–aldosterone system. Valsartan selectively blocks the binding of angiotensin II to the AT_1 receptors found in many tissues (e.g., vascular smooth muscle, adrenal glands). This results in blocking the vasoconstricting and aldosterone-secreting effects of angiotensin II, thus resulting in an antihypertensive effect.

USE Treatment of hypertension.

ROUTE & DOSAGE

Hypertension

Adult: **PO** 80 mg q.d., may increase up to 320 mg q.d.

PHARMACOKINETICS Absorption: rapidly absorbed from GI tract, 25% bioavailability. **Onset:** blood pressure decreased in 2 wk. **Peak:** plasma levels, 2–4 h; blood pressure effect 4 wk. **Distribution:** 99% protein bound. **Metabolism:** metabolized in the liver. **Elimination:** half-life: 6h, excreted primarily in feces.

CONTRAINDICATIONS & PRECAUTIONS Contraindicated in: hypersensitivity to valsartan or losartin; pregnancy [(category C) first trimester and (category D) second and third trimester], lactation. **Cautious use in:** severe renal or hepatic impairment. Safety and efficacy in children < 18 y have not been established.

ADVERSE/SIDE EFFECTS Body as whole: arthralgia. **CNS:** headache, dizziness. **GI:** diarrhea, nausea. **Respiratory:** cough, sinusitis. **Other:** hyperkalemia.

NURSING IMPLICATIONS

Administration
- Best taken on an empty stomach.
- To prevent hypotension, volume depletion should be corrected prior to initiation of therapy.
- Dosage reductions are needed in severe hepatic or renal impairment.
- The daily dose may be titrated up to 320 mg.
- Store at 15–30C (59–86F).

Assessment & Drug Effects
- Therapeutic effectiveness is indicated by decreases in systolic and diastolic BP.
- Monitor BP periodically; trough readings, just prior to the next scheduled dose, should be made when possible.
- Lab tests: Periodically monitor liver functions, BUN and creatinine, serum potassium, and CBC with differential.

Patient & Family Education
- Women who become pregnant should immediately inform their physicians.

- Maximum pressure lowering effect is usually evident between 2 and 4 wk.
- Report episodes of dizziness, especially those that occur when making position changes.

VANCOMYCIN HYDROCHLORIDE

(van-koe-mye′sin)

Trade names: Vancocin, Vancoled

Classifications: ANTIINFECTIVE; ANTIBIOTIC

Pregnancy category: C

ACTIONS/PHARMACODYNAMICS Glucopeptide antibiotic prepared from *Streptomyces orientalis,* with bactericidal and bacteriostatic actions. Action interferes with cell membrane synthesis in multiplying organisms. Active against many gram-positive organisms, including group A beta-hemolytic streptococci, staphylococci, pneumococci, enterococci, clostridia, and corynebacteria. Gram-negative organisms, mycobacteria, and fungi are highly resistant. Cross-resistance with other antibiotics or resistance to vancomycin has not been reported.

USES Parenterally for potentially life-threatening infections in patients allergic, nonsensitive, or resistant to other less toxic antimicrobial drugs. Used orally only in *Clostridium difficile* colitis (not effective by oral route for treatment of systemic infections).

ROUTE & DOSAGE

Systemic Infections

Adult: **IV** 500 mg q6h or 1 g q12h; infuse over 60–90 min.
Child: **IV** 40 mg/kg/d divided q6h; infuse over 60–90 min.
Neonate: **IV** 10 mg/kg/d divided q8–12h; infuse over 60–90 min.

***Clostridium difficile* Colitis**

Adult: **PO** 125–500 mg q6h.
Child: **PO** 40 mg/kg/d divided q6h (max 2 g/d).

PHARMACOKINETICS **Absorption:** not absorbed from GI tract. **Peak:** 30 min after end of infusion. **Distribution:** diffuses into pleural, ascitic, pericardial, and synovial fluids; small amount penetrates CSF if meninges are inflamed; crosses placenta. **Elimination:** half-life: 4–8 h; 80–90% of IV dose excreted in urine within 24 h; PO dose excreted in feces.

CONTRAINDICATIONS & PRECAUTIONS **Contraindicated in:** known hypersensitivity to vancomycin, previous hearing loss, concurrent or sequential use of other ototoxic or nephrotoxic agents, IM administration. Safe use during pregnancy (category C) not established. **Cautious use in:** neonates; impaired renal function.

ADVERSE/SIDE EFFECTS Ototoxicity (auditory portion of eighth cranial nerve), nephrotoxicity leading to uremia, hypersensitivity reactions (chills, fever, skin rash, urticaria, shock-like state); transient leukopenia, eosinophilia, anaphylactoid reaction with vascular collapse; superinfections, severe pain, thrombophlebitis at injection site; nausea, warmth, and generalized tingling following rapid IV infusion, *hypotension accompanied by flushing and erythematous rash on face and upper body* ("red-neck syndrome") following rapid IV infusion.

DRUG INTERACTIONS Adds to toxicity of OTOTOXIC and NEPHROTOXIC

DRUGS (AMINOGLYCOSIDES, **amphotericin B, colistin, polymyxin B**).

INCOMPATIBILITIES Solution/additive: aminophylline, BARBITURATES, **cefotaxime, chloramphenicol, chlorothiazide, dexamethasone, heparin, methicillin, sodium bicarbonate, warfarin. Y-site: heparin.**

NURSING IMPLICATIONS

Administration

- For oral administration, contents of vial (500 mg) may be diluted in 30 ml of water. It may also be administered at this dilution via nasogastric tube.
- IV preparation: Reconstitute 500 mg vial with 10 ml sterile water for injection (add 20 ml to 1-g vial). Further dilute 500 mg with 100 ml and 1 g with 200 ml of D5W, 0.9% NaCl, or Ringer's lactate.
- Administer a single dose of 500 mg over 60–90 min.
- Vancomycin may be given as a continuous infusion over 24 h (1–2 g/24h).
- Rapid infusion may cause sudden hypotension.
- Extravasation of IV infusion must be avoided; severe irritation and necrosis can result.
- Oral and parenteral solutions are stable for 14 d in refrigerator; after further dilution, parenteral solution is stable 24 h at room temperature.

Assessment & Drug Effects

- Monitor BP and heart rate continuously through period of drug administration.
- Periodic urinalyses, renal and hepatic function tests, and hematologic studies are advised in all patients.
- Serial tests of vancomycin blood levels are recommended in patients with borderline renal function and in patients > 60 y (target range is peak of 20–30 μg/ml and trough of <15 μg/ml).
- Assess hearing, as vancomycin may cause damage to auditory branch (not vestibular branch) of eighth cranial nerve, with consequent deafness, which may be permanent.
- Serum levels of 60–80 μg/ml are associated with ototoxicity. Tinnitus and high-tone hearing loss may precede deafness, which may progress even after drug is withdrawn. The elderly and those on high doses are especially susceptible
- Monitor I&O; report changes in I&O ratio and pattern. Oliguria or cloudy or pink urine may be a sign of nephrotoxicity (also manifested by transient elevations in BUN, albumin, and hyaline and granular casts in urine).

Patient & Family Education

- Warn to report ringing in ears promptly.
- Instruct to adhere to drug regimen, i.e., not to increase, decrease, or interrupt dosage. The full course of prescribed drug therapy should be completed.

VARICELLA VACCINE

(var-i-cel′la)

Trade name: Varivax

Classifications: VACCINE; VIRAL

Prototype: Hepatitis B

Pregnancy category: C

ACTIONS/PHARMACODYNAMICS

Both chickenpox and shingles (zoster) are caused by varicella-zoster infection. Varicella vaccine is a live attenuated vaccine and is effective in protecting healthy children from varicella.

Common side effect in *italic,* life-threatening effects underlined: generic names in **bold;** drug class in SMALL CAPS

USE Vaccination against varicella in individuals ≥ 12 mo.

ROUTE & DOSAGE

Varicella Protection
Adult: **SC** Primary immunization: 0.5 ml followed by 0.5 ml 4–8 wk after first dose; may need to revaccinate 3 mo after initial series if patient fails to seroconvert.
Child 12 mo–12 y: **SC** Single dose of 0.5 ml.

PHARMACOKINETICS **Onset:** seroconversion approx 42 d after vaccination. **Duration:** 5–10 y in healthy children. **Distribution:** crosses placenta; distributed into breast milk.

CONTRAINDICATIONS & PRECAUTIONS **Contraindicated in:** hypersensitivity to any component of the vaccine; history of anaphylactoid reaction to neomycin; individuals with blood dyscrasia, leukemia, lymphomas, bone marrow or lymphatic system malignancies, concomitant immunosuppression therapy; individuals with primary or acquired immunodeficient states; active untreated tuberculosis; any febrile respiratory illness or other febrile infection; pregnancy (category C); children < 1 y. **Cautious use in:** nursing mothers, acute lymphoblastic leukemia in remission.

ADVERSE/SIDE EFFECTS **CNS:** headache, fever. **Hematologic:** mild thrombocytopenia. **Skin:** *redness, swelling, or rash at injection site.* **Other:** herpes zoster infection (rare).

DRUG INTERACTIONS **Acyclovir** decreases vaccine's effectiveness. It is recommended that **yellow fever vaccine** be given at least 1 mo apart from varicella or any other live virus vaccine. Avoid **salicylates** for 6 wk after vaccination to decrease risk of developing Reye's syndrome.

NURSING IMPLICATIONS

Administration
- Reconstitute vaccine with 0.7 ml of supplied diluent; gently agitate the vial to mix. Withdraw entire contents of vial (0.5 ml) into syringe for injection. Change needle on syringe and administer immediately or within 30 min of reconstitution.
- Give SC into the outer aspect of the deltoid. Exercise caution not to inject IV.
- Store powder vaccine in frost-free freezer at −15C (+5F) or colder. Store diluent separately at room temperature or in the refrigerator.

Assessment & Drug Effects
- Withhold vaccine and notify physician if patient has a history of hypersensitivity to neomycin or a current febrile infection.
- Monitor for signs and symptoms of hypersensitivity (see Appendix G) and administer epinephrine if an anaphylactoid reaction occurs.

Patient & Family Education
- Advise to avoid use of salicylates (e.g., acetylsalicylic acid) for 6 wk after vaccination, especially with children and adolescents.
- Instruct to report all adverse reactions (i.e., fever, rash, respiratory illness).

VASOPRESSIN INJECTION
(vay-soe-press'in)
Trade name: Pitressin

VASOPRESSIN TANNATE
Trade name: Pitressin Tannate
Prototype for classifications: HORMONE; PITUITARY; ANTIDIURETIC
Pregnancy category: X

ACTIONS/PHARMACODYNAMICS Polypeptide hormone extracted from animal posterior pituitaries. Possesses pressor and antidiuretic (ADH) principles, but is relatively free of oxytocic properties. Produces concentrated urine by increasing tubular reabsorption of water (ADH activity), thus preserving up to 90% water. May increase sodium and decrease potassium reabsorption but plays no causative role in edema formation. Small doses may produce anginal pain; large doses may precipitate MI, decrease heart rate and cardiac output, and increase pulmonary arterial pressure and BP. The tannate (in peanut oil) is preferred for chronic therapy; intranasal aqueous vasopressin is effective for daily maintenance of mild diabetes insipidus.

USES Antidiuretic to treat diabetes insipidus, to dispel gas shadows in abdominal roentgenography, and as prevention and treatment of postoperative abdominal distension. Also given to treat transient polyuria due to ADH deficiency (related to head injuries or to neurosurgery). **Unlabeled uses:** test for differential diagnosis of nephrogenic, psychogenic, and neurohypophyseal diabetes insipidus; test to elevate ability of kidney to concentrate urine, and provocative test for pituitary release of corticotropin and growth hormone; emergency and adjunct pressor agent in the control of massive GI hemorrhage (e.g., esophageal varices).

ROUTE & DOSAGE

Diabetes Insipidus

Adult: **IM/SC** 5–10 U aqueous solution 2–4 times/d (5–60 U/d) *or* 1.25–2.5 U in oil q2–3d.
Intranasal Apply to cotton pledget or intranasal spray.
Child: **IM/SC** 2.5–10 U aqueous solution 2–4 times/d.

Abdominal Distention, Abdominal Radiographic Procedures

Adult: **IM/SC** 5 U with 5–10 U q3–4h prn *or* 5–15 U 2 h and 30 min prior to procedure.

GI Hemorrhage

Adult: **IV** 0.1–1 U/ml in D5W or NS at 0.2–0.4 U/min up to 0.9 U/min.

PHARMACOKINETICS **Duration:** 2–8 h in aqueous solution, 48–72 h in oil, 30–60 min IV infusion. **Distribution:** extracelluar fluid. **Metabolism:** metabolized in liver and kidneys. **Elimination:** half-life: 10–20 min; excreted in urine.

CONTRAINDICATIONS & PRECAUTIONS **Contraindicated in:** chronic nephritis accompanied by nitrogen retention; ischemic heart disease, PVCs, advanced arteriosclerosis; pregnancy (category X); during first stage of labor. **Cautious use in:** epilepsy; migraine; asthma; heart failure, angina pectoris; any state in which rapid addition to extracellular fluid may be hazardous; vascular disease; preoperative and postoperative polyuric patients, renal disease; goiter with cardiac complications; elderly patients, children.

ADVERSE/SIDE EFFECTS Infrequent with low doses. **Hypersensitivity:** rash, urticaria, <u>anaphylaxis</u>; *tremor,* sweating, bronchoconstriction, *circumoral and facial pallor,* angioneurotic edema, *eructations, passage of gas, nausea, vomiting, pounding in head,* anginal (in patient with coronary vascular disease), <u>cardiac arrest</u>, uterine cramps, *water intoxication* (especially with tannate). **Intraarterial infusion:** cardiac arrhythmia, pulmonary edema, bradycardia, gangrene at injection site. **Intranasal:** congestion, rhinorrhea, irritation, mucosal ulceration and pruritus, headache, conjunctivitis, heartburn, postnasal drip, abdominal cramps, increased bowel movements secondary to excessive use. **Large doses:** blanching of skin, abdominal cramps, nausea (almost spontaneously reversible), hypertension, bradycardia, minor arrhythmias, premature atrial contraction, heart block, peripheral vascular collapse, coronary insufficiency, MI.

DIAGNOSTIC TEST INTERFERENCE Vasopressin increases ***plasma cortisol*** levels.

DRUG INTERACTIONS **Alcohol, demeclocycline, epinephrine, heparin, lithium, phenytoin** may decrease antidiuretic effects of vasopressin; **guanethidine, neostigmine** increase vasopressor actions; **chlorpropamide, clofibrate, carbamazepine,** THIAZIDE DIURETICS may increase antidiuretic activity.

NURSING IMPLICATIONS

Administration

- Administration of 1 or 2 glasses of water with vasopressin tannate may reduce side effects and improve therapeutic response.
- Vasopressin tannate should never be administered IV. Before withdrawing drug for IM administration, warm ampul to body temperature and shake vigorously to disperse active principle.
- The tannate injection is often painful, and allergic reactions may develop. It is preferred for use in chronic therapy because of its longer duration of action.
- IV administration: Vasopressin aqueous injection may be given by continuous IV diluted with NS or D5W (0.1–1 U/ml) at a rate titrated to patient's response.

Assessment & Drug Effects

- Infants and children are more susceptible to volume disturbances (such as sudden reversal of polyuria) than adults are. Monitor closely.
- At beginning of therapy, establish baseline data of BP, weight, I&O pattern and ratio. Monitor both BP and weight throughout therapy. Report sudden changes in pattern to physician.
- Be alert to the fact that even small doses of vasopressin may precipitate MI or coronary insufficiency, especially in elderly patients. Emergency equipment and drugs (antiarrhythmics) should be readily available.
- Dose used to stimulate diuresis has little effect on BP.
- Check patient's alertness and orientation frequently during therapy. Lethargy and confusion associated with headache may signal onset of water intoxication, which, although insidious in rate of development, can lead to convulsions and terminal coma.
- If water intoxication (see Appendix G) occurs, vasopressin is withdrawn and fluid intake is restricted until specific gravity is at least 1.015 and polyuria occurs. With severe overhydration, osmotic diuresis is effected by drug therapy (e.g., mannitol, alone or in conjunction with furosemide).
- Urine output, specific gravity, and serum osmolality are monitored while patient is hospitalized.

Patient & Family Education

- Polyuria and thirst of diabetes insipidus are usually controlled for

36–48 h with a single dose of the tannate.

- Patient with vascular disease and diabetes insipidus may receive small doses of vasopressin. Patient should be prepared for possibility of anginal attack and should have available a coronary vasodilator (e.g., nitroglycerin). Such pain should be reported to the physician.
- At home, patient must measure and record data related to polydipsia and polyuria. Teach patient to determine specific gravity and how to keep an accurate record of output. Patient should understand that intense thirst should diminish with treatment and that undisturbed normal sleep should be restored.
- Patient should avoid hypertonic fluids (e.g., undiluted syrups), since these increase urine volume.

VECURONIUM

(vek-yoo-roe′nee-um)

Trade name: Norcuron

Classifications: AUTONOMIC NERVOUS SYSTEM AGENT; NONDEPOLARIZING SKELETAL MUSCLE RELAXANT

Prototype: Tubocurarine

Pregnancy category: C

ACTIONS/PHARMACODYNAMICS

Intermediate-acting nondepolarizing skeletal muscle relaxant structurally similar to pancuronium. Unlike older neuromuscular blocking agents, demonstrates negligible histamine release and therefore has minimal direct effect on cardiovascular system. Similar to atracurium in having unique metabolic and excretion pathways. In common with other drugs of this class, inhibits neuromuscular transmission by competitive binding with acetylcholine to motor endplate receptors. Given only after induction of general anesthesia.

USES Adjunct for general anesthesia to produce skeletal muscle relaxation during surgery. Especially useful for patients with severe renal disease, limited cardiac reserve, and history of asthma or allergy. Also to facilitate endotracheal intubation. **Unlabeled use:** continuous infusion for facilitation of mechanical ventilation.

ROUTE & DOSAGE

Skeletal Muscle Relaxation

Adult: **IV** 0.04–0.1 mg/kg initially; then after 25–40 min, 0.01–0.15 mg/kg q12–15min or 0.001 mg/kg/min by continuous infusion.
Child ≥1 y: **IV** Same as for adult.
Neonate: **IV** 0.1 mg/kg, followed by 0.03–0.15 mg/kg q1–2h prn.

PHARMACOKINETICS **Onset:** <1 min. **Peak:** 3–5 min. **Duration:** 25–40 min. **Distribution:** well distributed to tissues and extracellular fluids; crosses placenta; distribution into breast milk unknown. **Metabolism:** rapid nonenzymatic degradation in bloodstream. **Elimination:** half-life: 30–80 min; 30–35% excreted in urine, 30–35% in bile.

CONTRAINDICATIONS & PRECAUTIONS **Contraindicated in:** safe use during pregnancy (category C), in nursing mother, and in neonate not established. **Cautious use in:** severe hepatic disease; impaired acid–base, fluid, and electrolyte balance; severe obesity; adrenal or neuromuscular disease (myasthenia gravis, Eaton-Lambert syndrome); patients with slow circulation time (cardiovascular disease, old age, edematous states); malignant hyperthermia.

ADVERSE/SIDE EFFECTS Generally well tolerated. Skeletal muscle weakness, respiratory depression, malignant hyperthermia.

DRUG INTERACTIONS GENERAL ANESTHETICS increase neuromuscular blockade and duration of action; AMINOGLYCOSIDES, **bacitracin, polymyxin B, clindamycin, lidocaine, parenteral magnesium, quinidine, quinine, trimethaphan, verapamil** increase neuromuscular blockade; DIURETICS may increase or decrease neuromuscular blockade; **lithium** prolongs duration of neuromuscular blockade; NARCOTIC ANALGESICS increase possibility of additive respiratory depression; **succinylcholine** increases onset and depth of neuromuscular blockade; **phenytoin** may cause resistance to or reversal of neuromuscular blockade.

NURSING IMPLICATIONS

Administration

- Vecuronium is administered only by qualified clinicians.
- Following reconstitution, refrigerate or store solution below 30C (86F) unless otherwise directed. Discard solution after 24 h.

Assessment & Drug Effects

- Baseline determinations of serum electrolytes, acid–base balance, renal and hepatic function are generally done as part of preanesthetic assessment.
- Peripheral nerve stimulator may be used during and following drug administration to avoid risk of overdosage and to identify residual paralysis during recovery period. It is especially indicated when cautious use of vecuronium is specified.
- Monitor vital signs at least q15min until stable, then every 30 min for the next 2 h. Also monitor airway patency until assured that patient has fully recovered from drug effects. Note rate, depth, and pattern of respirations. Obese patients and patients with myasthenia gravis or other neuromuscular disease may pose ventilation problems.
- Evaluate patients for recovery from neuromuscular blocking (curare-like) effects as evidenced by ability to breathe naturally or take deep breaths and cough, to keep eyes open, and to lift head keeping mouth closed and by adequacy of hand grip strength. Notify physician if recovery is delayed.
- Note that recovery time may be delayed in patients with cardiovascular disease, edematous states, and in the elderly.

VENLAFAXINE

(ven-la-fax′een)

Trade name: Effexor

Classifications: CNS AGENTS; PSYCHOTHERAPEUTIC ANTIDEPRESSANT; SELECTIVE SEROTONIN REUPTAKE INHIBITOR

Prototype: Fluoxetine

Pregnancy category: C

ACTIONS/PHARMACODYNAMICS Venlafaxine is a bicyclic "second-generation" antidepressant. It is chemically unrelated to tricyclic, tetracyclic, or other antidepressants. It selectively inhibits neuronal uptake of serotonin, norepinephrine, and dopamine in decreasing order of potency. Antidepressant effect is presumed to be linked to its inhibition of CNS presynaptic neuronal uptake of serotonin. It does not cause anticholinergic, sedative, or cardiovascular effects.

USE Depression. **Unlabeled use:** obsessive-compulsive disorder.

ROUTE & DOSAGE

Depression

Adult: **PO** 25–125 mg t.i.d.; start with lower doses in the elderly.

PHARMACOKINETICS Absorption: well absorbed from GI tract. **Onset:** 2 wk. **Peak:** venlafaxine 1–2 h; metabolite 3–4 h. **Duration:** approximately 30% protein bound, but extensively tissue bound. **Metabolism:** undergoes substantial first-pass metabolism to its major active metabolite, *O*-desmethylvenlafaxine, with similar actvity to venlafaxine. **Elimination:** half-life: venlafaxine 3–4 h, *O*-desmethylvenlafaxine 10 h; approximately 60% excreted in urine as parent compound and metabolites.

CONTRAINDICATIONS & PRECAUTIONS Contraindicated in: hypersensitivity to venlafaxine, concurrent administration with MAO inhibitors. **Cautious use in:** renal and hepatic impairment, anorexia, history of mania, suicidal ideations, cardiac disorders, recent MI. Safety in pregnancy (category C), in lactation, and in children <18 y not established.

ADVERSE/SIDE EFFECTS CV: *increased blood pressure and heart rate,* palpitations. **CNS:** *dizziness,* fatigue, headache, anxiety, insomnia, *somnolence.* **Endocrine:** small but statistically significant increase in serum cholesterol, weight loss (approx 3 lb). **GI:** *nausea, vomiting, dry mouth,* constipation. **GU:** sexual dysfunction, erectile failure, delayed orgasm, anorgasmia, impotence, abnormal ejaculation **Other:** blurred vision, *sweating,* asthenia.

DRUG INTERACTIONS Cimetidine decreases clearance of venlafaxine. Should not use in combination with MAO INHIBITORS: do not start until 14 d after stopping MAO inhibitor; do not start MAO inhibitor until 7 d after stopping venlafaxine.

NURSING IMPLICATIONS

Administration

- It is recommended that venlafaxine be taken with food.
- With hepatic or renal impairment, the usual daily dose is reduced by 25–50% or greater.
- Dosage increments of up to 75 mg/d should be done at 4-d or longer intervals.
- Allow 14 d after discontinuing an MAO inhibitor before starting venlafaxine.
- After 1 wk or more of therapy with venlafoxine, drug should not be abruptly withdrawn.
- Store at room temperature, 15–30C (59–86F).

Assessment & Drug Effects

- Periodically monitor cardiovascular status with measurements of HR, BP, and serum lipids.
- Monitor neurologic status and report excessive anxiety, nervousness, and insomnia.
- Periodically monitor weight and report excess weight loss.
- Assess safety, as dizziness and sedation are common.

Patient & Family Education

- Inform of potential adverse effects and advise to report those that are bothersome.
- Advise caution with hazardous activity until reaction to the drug is known.
- Advise to avoid using alcohol while on venlafaxine.

VERAPAMIL HYDROCHLORIDE

(ver-ap′a-mill)

Trade names: Calan, Calan SR, Co-

Common side effect in *italic,* life-threatening effects underlined; generic names in **bold;** drug class in SMALL CAPS

vera-HS, Isoptin, Isoptin SR, Verelan, Veralen PM
Classifications: CARDIOVASCULAR AGENT; CALCIUM CHANNEL BLOCKER
Prototype: Nifedipine
Pregnancy category: C

ACTIONS/PHARMACODYNAMICS Inhibits calcium ion influx through slow channels into cell of myocardial and arterial smooth muscle. Verapamil dilates coronary arteries and arterioles and inhibits coronary artery spasm; thus, myocardial oxygen delivery is increased (antianginal effect). Decreases and slows SA and AV node conduction (antiarrhythmic effect) without effect on normal arterial action potential or intraventricular conduction. By vasodilation of peripheral arterioles, drug decreases total peripheral vascular resistance and reduces arterial BP at rest. May slightly decrease heart rate.

USES Supraventricular tachyarrhythmias; Prinzmetal's (variant) angina, chronic stable angina; unstable, crescendo or preinfarctive angina and essential hypertension. **Unlabeled use:** paroxysmal supraventricular tachycardia, atrial fibrillation; prophylaxis of migraine headache; and as alternate therapy in manic depression.

ROUTE & DOSAGE

Angina
Adult: **PO** 80 mg q6–8h; may increase up to 320–480 mg/d in divided doses. Covera-HS must be given once daily h.s.

Hypertension
Adult: **PO** 40–80 mg t.i.d. *or* 90–240 mg sustained release 1–2 times/d up to 480 mg/d.Covera-HS must be given once daily h.s.

Supraventricular Tachycardia, Atrial Fibrillation
Adult: **PO** 240–480 mg/d in divided doses; **IV** 5–10 mg IV push; may repeat in 15–30 min if needed.
Child <1 y: **IV** 0.1–0.2 mg/kg; 1–15 y, 0.1–0.3 mg/kg (2–5 mg).

PHARMACOKINETICS **Absorption:** 90% absorbed, but only 25–30% reaches systemic circulation (first pass metabolism). **Peak:** 1–2 h PO; 4–8 h extended release; 5 min IV. **Distribution:** widely distributed, including CNS; crosses placenta; present in breast milk. **Metabolism:** metabolized in liver. **Elimination:** half-life: 2–8 h; 70% excreted in urine; 16% in feces.

CONTRAINDICATIONS & PRECAUTIONS **Contraindicated in:** severe hypotension (diastolic <90 mm Hg), cardiogenic shock, cardiomegaly, digitalis toxicity, second- or third-degree AV block; Wolff-Parkinson-White syndrome including atrial flutter and fibrillation; accessory AV pathway, left ventricular dysfunction, severe CHF, sinus node disease, sick sinus syndrome (except in patient with functioning ventricular pacemaker). Safe use during pregnancy (category C), in nursing mothers, or in children (oral) not established. **Cautious use in:** Duchenne's muscular dystrophy; hepatic and renal impairment; MI followed by coronary occlusion, aortic stenosis.

ADVERSE/SIDE EFFECTS **CNS:** dizziness, vertigo, *headache,* fatigue, sleep disturbances, depression, syncope. **CV:** *hypotension,* congestive heart failure, bradycardia, severe tachycardia, peripheral edema, <u>AV block</u>. **GI:** nausea, abdominal discomfort, *constipation*. **Other:** pruri-

V

tus, flushing, pulmonary edema, muscle fatigue, diaphoresis, elevated liver enzymes.

DIAGNOSTIC TEST INTERFERENCE Verapamil may cause elevations of serum ***AST, ALT, alkaline phosphatase.***

DRUG INTERACTIONS BETA BLOCKERS increase risk of CHF, bradycardia, or heart block; significantly increased levels of **digoxin** and **carbamazepine** and toxicity; potentiates hypotensive effects of HYPOTENSIVE AGENTS; levels of **lithium** and **cyclosporine** may be increased, increasing their toxicity; **calcium salts** (IV) may antagonize verapamil effects.

INCOMPATIBILITIES Solution/additive: albumin, aminophylline, amphotericin B, hydralazine, cotrimoxazole. Y-site: ampicillin, mezlocillin, nafcillin, oxacillin, sodium bicarbonate.

NURSING IMPLICATIONS

Administration

- Administer oral dose with food to reduce gastric irritation.
- Verelan capsules can be opened and contents sprinkled on food. Do not dissolve or chew capsule contents.
- Covera-HS must be given in the evening.
- Abrupt withdrawal of verapamil may increase and extend duration of pain in the angina patient.
- IV injection: IV verapamil may be given by direct IV diluted in 5 ml of sterile water for injection at a rate of 10 mg/min.
- Inspect parenteral drug preparation before administration. Solution should be clear and colorless.
- Store at 15–30C (59–86F) and protect from light.

Assessment & Drug Effects

- Establish baseline data and periodically monitor: BP, pulse, and hepatic and renal function.
- Transient asymptomatic hypotension may accompany IV bolus. Instruct patient to remain in recumbent position for at least 1 h after dose is given to diminish subjective effects of hypotension.
- If IV verapamil is given concurrently with digitalis, monitor for AV block or excessive bradycardia.
- Monitor I&O ratio during IV and early oral maintenance therapy. Renal function impairment prolongs duration of action, increasing potential for toxicity and incidence of side effects. Advise patient to report gradual weight gain and evidence of edema.
- The incidence of adverse reactions is highest with IV administration, in the elderly, in patients with impaired renal function and patients of small stature. Drug action may be prolonged in these patients. Continuous ECG monitoring during IV administration is essential.
- During early treatment for hypertension, check BP shortly before administration of next dose to evaluate degree of control.
- Verapamil should decrease angina frequency, nitroglycerin consumption, and episodes of ST segment deviation.

Patient & Family Education

- Inform patient receiving verapamil at home about usual pulse rate and instruct to take radial pulse before each dose. An irregular pulse or one slower than base level should be reported.
- Caution to take drug exactly as prescribed.

- Warn to adhere to established guidelines for exercise program.
- Caution against driving or operating dangerous equipment until patient's response to verapamil is established. Dizziness (experienced as light-headedness) during early treatment period is common.
- Advise to decrease caffeine-containing beverage intake (i.e., coffee, tea, chocolate).
- Until tolerance to reduced BP is established, advise patient to change positions slowly from recumbent to standing to prevent falls because of vertigo.
- Instruct to report easy bruising, petechiae, unexplained bleeding.
- Advise not to use OTC drugs, especially aspirin, unless they are specifically prescribed.

VIDARABINE

(vye-dare'a-been)

Trade names: Adenine Arabinoside, ARA-A, Vira-A

Classifications: ANTIINFECTIVE; ANTIVIRAL

Prototype: Zidovudine

Pregnancy category: C

ACTIONS/PHARMACODYNAMICS Pyrimidine nucleoside obtained from *Streptomyces antibioticus*. Mechanism of action not known but appears to block early stages of DNA synthesis by inhibiting DNA polymerase. Has antiviral activity against herpes simplex virus types 1 and 2, varicella zoster, vaccinia, cytomegalovirus, hepatitis B virus, and Epstein-Barr virus. Not active against smallpox, adenovirus, DNA or RNA viruses, bacteria, and fungi.

USES Systemically for treatment of herpes simplex encephalitis and herpes zoster infections in patients with suppressed immunologic responses. Used topically (ophthalmic) for treatment of acute keratoconjunctivitis and recurrent epithelial keratitis caused by herpes simplex virus types 1 and 2. Topical antibiotics and topical corticosteroids may be used concurrently.

ROUTE & DOSAGE

Herpes Simplex Encephalitis, Herpes Zoster

Adult/Child: **IV** 15 mg/kg/d infused over 12–24 h.
Neonate: **IV** 15–30 mg/kg/d as 18- to 24-h infusion.

Herpes Keratitis

Adult: **Ophthalmic** Instill 1 cm (1/2 in) ribbon of ointment into lower conjunctival sac q3h 5 times/d.

PHARMACOKINETICS Distribution: widely distributed in body tissues and fluid; crosses blood–brain barrier; trace amounts of ophthalmic application found in aqueous humor; crosses placenta. **Metabolism:** rapidly deaminated to ara-hypoxanthine (Ara-Hx), a less active metabolite. **Elimination:** half-life: 1.5 h vidarabine, 3.3 h Ara-Hx; excreted primarily in urine.

CONTRAINDICATIONS & PRECAUTIONS Contraindicated in: safe use during pregnancy (category C) and breast feeding not established. **Cautious use in:** impaired renal or hepatic function, patients susceptible to fluid overload or cerebral edema.

ADVERSE/SIDE EFFECTS *IV:* **CNS:** (with high doses): hallucinations, confusion, psychosis, dizziness, ataxia, weakness, tremor, fatal metabolic encephalopathy. **GI (usually**

V

transient): *nausea, vomiting, anorexia, diarrhea, weight loss.* **Hematologic:** anemia, thrombocytopenia, neutropenia, decrease in WBC, Hgb, Hct. **Hepatic:** *elevated bilirubin and AST.* **Other:** malaise, pruritus, painful injection site. ***Ophthalmic:*** burning, itching, mild irritation, lacrimation, foreign body sensation, pain, photophobia, punctal occlusion, superficial punctate keratitis.

DRUG INTERACTION **Allopurinol** may increase potential for CNS side effects.

NURSING IMPLICATIONS

Administration

Intravenous Administration

- Dilute the vidarabine just before administration and use within 48 h.
- Shake vial well before withdrawing dose and transfer it to appropriate IV fluid. Most IV infusion fluids are suitable. Blood products, protein, or other colloidal fluids should not be used. Follow manufacturer's directions.
- A large volume of fluid is required to dissolve vidarabine as it is only slightly soluble (1 L of IV infusion fluid will solubilize a maximum of 450 mg of vidarabine, or 1 mg of drug to 2.22 ml of IV fluid). Agitate thoroughly until drug is completely dissolved. Prewarming the IV infusion fluid to 35–40C (95–100F) will facilitate dissolution. Once dissolved, subsequent shaking is unnecessary. Do not refrigerate the dilution.
- IV administration to neonates, infants, children: Verify correct IV concentration and rate of infusion with physician.
- Final dilution is administered through an in-line membrane filter (pore size of 0.45 μm or smaller).
- Infusion should be administered at a constant rate over 12–24h.

Assessment & Drug Effects

- Diagnosis of meningitis should be established before initiation of IV vidarabine therapy by studies of CSF, brain scan, EEG, or CAT. Vidarabine therapy is reportedly most effective when started before patient becomes semicomatose or comatose.
- Periodic hematologic tests are recommended during IV vidarabine therapy: Hgb, Hct, WBC, platelets.

Patient & Family Education

Ophthalmic Use

- Instruct to wash hands before and after treatment.
- Caution that vision may be temporarily hazy following instillation and to avoid potentially hazardous activities until vision clears.
- Advise that drug may cause sensitivity to bright light and to use sunglasses if necessary.
- Caution not to exceed recommended dose, frequency, and duration of treatment.

VINBLASTINE SULFATE

(vin-blast′een)

Trade names: Velban, Velbe ♣, VLB

Classifications: ANTINEOPLASTIC; MITOTIC INHIBITOR

Prototype: Vincristine

Pregnancy category: D

ACTIONS/PHARMACODYNAMICS

Cell cycle-specific alkaloid, extracted from periwinkle plant *Vinca rosea.* Arrests mitosis in metaphase by combination with microtubule proteins; may also interfere with other microtubular functions such as phagocytosis and cell mobility. In contrast to vincristine, has potent myelosuppressive and immunosuppressive properties but produces less neurotoxicity. Spectrum of activity not completely established.

USES Palliative treatment of Hodgkin's disease and non-Hodgkin's lymphomas, choriocarcinoma, lymphosarcoma, neuroblastoma, mycosis fungoides, advanced testicular germinal cell cancer, histiocytosis, and other malignancies resistant to other chemotherapy. Used singly or in combination with other chemotherapeutic drugs.

ROUTE & DOSAGE

Antineoplastic

Adult: **IV** 3.7 mg/m^2 infused over 1 min q wk; dose may be increased up to 18.5 mg/m^2 if tolerated.
Child: **IV** 2.5 mg/m^2 infused over 1 min q wk; dose may be increased up to 12.5 mg/m^2 if tolerated.

PHARMACOKINETICS **Distribution:** concentrates in liver, platelets, and leukocytes; poor penetration of blood–brain barrier. **Metabolism:** partially metabolized in liver. **Elimination:** half-life: 24 h; excreted in feces and urine.

CONTRAINDICATIONS & PRECAUTIONS **Contraindicated in:** leukopenia, bacterial infection, pregnancy (category D), men and women of childbearing potential, elderly patients with cachexia or skin ulcers. **Cautious use in:** malignant cell infiltration of bone marrow; obstructive jaundice, hepatic impairment; history of gout; use of small amount of drug for long periods; use in eyes.

ADVERSE/SIDE EFFECTS Generally dose related and short lived. **CNS (uncommon):** mental depression, peripheral neuritis, numbness and paresthesias of tongue and extremities, loss of deep tendon reflexes, headache, convulsions. **GI:** vesiculation of mouth, stomatitis, pharyngitis, anorexia, *nausea, vomiting,* diarrhea, ileus, abdominal pain, constipation, rectal bleeding, hemorrhagic enterocolitis, bleeding of old peptic ulcer. **Hematologic:** leukopenia, thrombocytopenia and anemia. **Skin:** *alopecia (reversible),* vesiculation. **Other:** phlebitis, cellulitis, and sloughing following extravasation (at injection site); fever, weight loss, muscular pains, weakness, urinary retention, *hyperuricemia,* parotid gland pain and tenderness, tumor site pain, aspermia, Raynaud's phenomenon, photosensitivity, bronchospasm.

INCOMPATIBILITIES **Solution/additive: furosemide, heparin. Y-site: furosemide.**

NURSING IMPLICATIONS

Administration

- To prepare solution, add 10 ml NaCl injection to 10 mg of drug (yields 1 mg/ml). Other diluents not advised.
- Drug is usually injected into tubing of running IV infusion of NS or D5W over period of 1 min. If vinblastine is given directly into vein, fresh, dry needle is used. To ensure no spillage into extravascular tissue, needle and syringe should be rinsed with venous blood before withdrawal from vein.
- If extravasation occurs, stop infusion promptly; applications of moderate heat and local injection of hyaluronidase are advised to help disperse extravasated drug. Infusion should be restarted in another vein. Observe injection site; sloughing may occur.

V

- Avoid contact with eyes. Severe irritation and persisting corneal changes may occur. Copious amounts of water should be applied immediately and thoroughly. Wash both eyes; do not assume one eye escaped contamination.
- Reconstituted solution may be refrigerated in tight, light-resistant containers up to 30 d without loss of potency.

Assessment & Drug Effects

- Recovery from leukopenic nadir follows rapidly, usually within 7–14 d. With high doses, total leukocyte count may not return to normal for 3 wk.
- Even if 7 d have passed, drug is not administered unless WBC count has not returned to at least $4000/mm^3$.
- Thrombocyte reduction seldom occurs unless patient has had prior treatment with other antineoplastics. However, be alert for unexplained bruising or bleeding, which should be promptly reported.
- With exception of epilation, leukopenia, and neurologic side effects, adverse reactions seldom persist beyond 24 h.
- Monitor bowel elimination pattern and bowel sounds to recognize severe constipation or paralytic ileus. A stool softener may be necessary.
- Skin surfaces over pressure areas should be inspected daily if patient is not ambulating. Note condition of skin of the elderly especially.
- Drug should be stopped if oral tissues break down.

Patient & Family Education

- Course of therapy may be continued 12 wk or more for adequate clinical trial. Encourage community-based patient to keep all appointments so that course of treatment is not interrupted.
- Temporary mental depression sometimes occurs on second or third day after treatment begins.
- Instruct to avoid exposure to infection, injury to skin or mucous membranes, and excessive physical stress, especially during leukocyte nadir period.
- Alopecia is frequently not total; in some patients, regrowth begins during maintenance therapy period.
- Instruct to report promptly onset of symptoms of agranulocytosis (see Appendix G). Appropriate treatment should not be delayed.
- Avoid exposure to sunlight unless protected with sunscreen lotion (SPF > 12) and clothing.

VINCRISTINE SULFATE

(vin-kris'teen)

Trade names: Oncovin, VCR

Prototype for classifications: ANTINEOPLASTIC; MITOTIC INHIBITOR

Pregnancy category: D

ACTIONS/PHARMACODYNAMICS Cell cycle–specific vinca alkaloid (obtained from periwinkle plant *Vinca rosea*); analog of vinblastine. Antineoplastic mechanism unclear; arrests mitosis at metaphase, thereby inhibiting cell division. In contrast to vinblastine, has relatively low toxic effect on normal cells and thus produces minimal myelosuppression; however, neurologic and neuromuscular effects are more severe.

USES Acute lymphoblastic and other leukemias, Hodgkin's disease, lymphosarcoma, neuroblastoma, Wilms' tumor, lung and breast cancer, reticular cell carcinoma, and osteogenic and other sarcomas. **Un-**

V

labeled use: for idiopathic thrombocytopenic purpura, alone or adjunctively with other antineoplastics.

ROUTE & DOSAGE

Antineoplastic

Adult: **IV** 1.4 mg/m^2 (max 2 mg/m^2) at weekly intervals.
Child: **IV** 2 mg/m^2 at weekly intervals.

PHARMACOKINETICS Distribution: concentrates in liver, platelets, and leukocytes; poor penetration of blood–brain barrier. **Metabolism:** partially metabolized in liver. **Elimination:** half-life: 10–155 h; excreted primarily in feces.

CONTRAINDICATIONS & PRECAUTIONS Contraindicated in: obstructive jaundice; pregnancy (category D), men and women of childbearing age; patient with demyelinating form of Charcot-Marie-Tooth syndrome. **Cautious use in:** leukopenia; preexisting neuromuscular disease; hypertension; infection; patients receiving drugs with neurotoxic potential.

ADVERSE/SIDE EFFECTS Usually dose-related and reversible. **CNS:** *peripheral neuropathy,* neuritic pain, *paresthesias, especially of hands and feet;* foot and hand drop, sensory loss, athetosis, ataxia, loss of deep tendon reflexes, muscle atrophy, dysphagia, weakness in larynx and extrinsic eye muscles, ptosis, diplopia, mental depression. **Eye:** optic atrophy with blindness; transient cortical blindness, ptosis, diplopia, photophobia. **GI:** stomatitis, pharyngitis, anorexia, nausea, vomiting, diarrhea, abdominal cramps, *severe constipation (upper-colon impaction), paralytic ileus, (especially in children),* rectal bleeding; hepatotoxicity. **GU:** urinary retention, polyuria, dysuria, SIADH (high urinary sodium excretion, hyponatremia, dehydration, hypotension); uric acid nephropathy. **Skin:** urticaria, rash, *alopecia,* cellulitis and phlebitis following extravasation (at injection site). **Other:** convulsions with hypertension, malaise, fever, headache, pain in parotid gland area, hyperuricemia, hyperkalemia, weight loss, hypertension, hypotension, bronchospasm.

INCOMPATIBILITIES Solution/additive: furosemide. Y-site: furosemide.

NURSING IMPLICATIONS

Administration

- IV preparation: Reconstitute with provided solution (bacteriostatic NaCl) or with sterile water or physiologic saline to concentrations of 0.01 to 1.0 mg/ml.
- Vincristine is available in solution form, which does not require reconstitution. Vincristine solution must be stored in the refrigerator.
- IV administration: Administration directly into vein or into running infusion should be over a 1 min period. Syringe and needle should be rinsed with venous blood before needle is withdrawn.
- If extravasation occurs, drug administration is discontinued immediately and restarted in another vein. Hyaluronidase should be injected locally into surrounding tissue. Apply moderate heat to the area to disperse drug and to minimize danger of sloughing. Be cautious because of possible sensory loss. Check agency policy or consult physician.

Assessment & Drug Effects

- Monitor I&O ratio and pattern, BP, and temperature daily. Record on flow chart as indicators for adap-

V

tations in nursing and drug regimen.

- Weigh patient under standard conditions weekly or more often if ordered. In the presence of edema or ascites, patient's ideal weight is used to determine dosage. Report a steady gain or sudden weight change to physician.
- Complete bone marrow remission in leukemia varies widely and may not occur for as long as 100 d after therapy is started.
- Neuromuscular side effects, most apt to appear in the patient with preexisting neuromuscular disease, usually disappear after 6 wk of treatment. Children are especially susceptible to neuromuscular side effects.
- Grasp hands of patient each day to detect onset of hand muscular weakness, and check deep tendon reflexes (depression of Achilles reflex is the earliest sign of neuropathy). Also observe for and report promptly: mental depression, ptosis, double vision, hoarseness, paresthesias, neuritic pain, and motor difficulties.
- Leukopenia occurs in a significant number of patients; leukocyte count in children usually reaches nadir on fourth day and begins to rise on fifth day after drug administration. Provide special protection against infection or injury during leukopenic days.
- To prevent injury to rectal mucosa, use of rectal thermometer or intrusive tubing should be avoided if possible.
- Walking may be impaired; check patient's ability to ambulate, and supply support if necessary.
- Care should be taken to distinguish between the depression associated with realization of neoplastic disease and that which is drug-induced.
- Dental caries or periodontal disease should be treated, since patient is highly susceptible to superinfections.

Patient & Family Education

- Advise to report promptly stomach, bone, or joint pain, and swelling of lower legs and ankles.
- A prophylactic regimen against constipation and paralytic ileus (adequate fluids, high-fiber diet, laxatives) is usually started at beginning of treatment with vincristine. Encourage to report changes in bowel habit as soon as manifested. Paralytic ileus is most likely to occur in young children.
- Alopecia (reversible) (up to 70% of patients) is reportedly the most common adverse reaction and may persist for the duration of therapy. However, regrowth of hair may start before end of treatment. Before therapy begins, discuss this side effect with patient. Inform that scalp hair will drop out in large clumps on pillow at night. This is a distressing side effect.

VINORELBINE TARTRATE

(vin-o-rel'been)

Trade name: Navelbine

Classifications: ANTINEOPLASTIC AGENT; MITOTIC INHIBITOR

Prototype: Vincristine

Pregnancy category: D

ACTIONS/PHARMACODYNAMICS

Vinorelbine is a semisynthetic vinca alkaloid with antineoplastic activity. It inhibits polymerization of tubules into microtubules, which disrupts mitotic spindle formation. Neurotoxicity is less than with other vinca alkaloids (e.g., vincristine).

USE Non-small cell lung cancer. **Unlabeled uses:** breast cancer, ovarian cancer, Hodgkin's disease.

ROUTE & DOSAGE

Non-Small Cell Lung Cancer, Breast Cancer
Adult: **IV** 30 mg/m^2 weekly.

PHARMACOKINETICS **Distribution:** 60–80% bound to plasma proteins (including platelets and lymphocytes); sequestered in tissues, especially lung, spleen, liver, and kidney, and released slowly. **Metabolism:** metabolized in liver. **Elimination:** half-life: 42–45 h; excreted primarily in bile and feces (50%), 10% excreted in urine.

CONTRAINDICATIONS & PRECAUTIONS **Contraindicated in:** hypersensitivity to vinorelbine, pregnancy (category D), nursing mothers. **Cautious use in:** hypersensitivity to vincristine or vinblastine; infection, leukopenia, or other indicator(s) of bone marrow suppression; chickenpox or herpes zoster infection; hepatic insufficiency; preexisting neurologic or neuromuscular disorders. Safety and efficacy in children have not been established.

ADVERSE/SIDE EFFECTS **CNS:** *decreased deep tendon reflexes, paresthesia, fatigue, asthenia, peripheral neuropathy,* myalgia, jaw pain. **Hematologic:** *anemia, neutropenia, granulocytopenia,* thrombocytopenia. **GI:** paralytic ileus, *constipation, nausea, vomiting, diarrhea,* stomatitis, mucositis. **Other:** hepatotoxicity *(elevated liver function tests), pain on injection,* venous pain, thrombophlebitis, *alopecia,* myalgia, muscle weakness.

DRUG INTERACTIONS Increased severity of granulocytopenia in combination with **cisplatin;** increased risk of acute pulmonary reactions in combination with **mitomycin.**

INCOMPATIBILITIES **Solution/additive: acyclovir, aminophylline/theophylline, amphotericin B, ampicillin, cefoperazone, ceforanide, cefotetan, ceftriaxone, fluorouracil, furosemide, ganciclovir, methylprednisolone, mitomycin, piperacillin, sodium bicarbonate, thiotepa, trimethoprim–sulfamethoxazole. Y-site: acyclovir, aminophylline/theophylline, amphotericin B, cefoperazone, ceforanide, cefotetan, ceftriaxone, fluorouracil, furosemide, ganciclovir, methylprednisolone, mitomycin, piperacillin, sodium bicarbonate, thiotepa, trimethoprim–sulfamethoxazole.**

NURSING IMPLICATIONS

Administration

- Use caution to prevent contact with skin, mucous membranes, or eyes during preparation.
- IV preparation: Dilute in a syringe with D5W or 0.9% NaCl to a final concentration of 1.5–3 mg/ml; or dilute in an IV bag with D5W, 0.9% NaCl, or Ringer's lactate to a final concentration of 0.5–2 mg/ml.
- IV administration: Administer the diluted solution over 6–10 min into the side port closest to an IV bag with free-flowing IV solution; follow by flushing with at least 75–125 ml of IV solution over 10 min.
- Take every precaution to avoid extravasation. If suspected, discontinue IV immediately and begin in a different site.
- Store at 2–8C (36–46F).

Assessment & Drug Effects

- Monitor CBC with differential throughout therapy and on the day of treatment prior to each dose of vinorelbine. Do not administer if the granulocyte count is below 1000 cells/mm^3.

- Monitor for signs and symptoms of infection, especially during period of granulocyte nadir 7–10 d after dosing.
- Periodically monitor renal and hepatic function tests and serum electrolytes.

Patient & Family Education

- Inform of potential and inevitable adverse effects.
- Advise to report distressing side effects, especially symptoms of leukopenia (e.g., chills, fever, cough) and peripheral neuropathy.

VITAMIN A

(vye'ta-min)

Trade names: Aquasol A, Del-Vi-A

Classification: VITAMIN A

Pregnancy category: A (X if >RDA)

ACTIONS/PHARMACODYNAMICS Synthetic fat-soluble vitamin available for clinical use as retinol or retinol esters. Formulation includes vitamin A as well as its precursors. Vitamin A is essential for normal growth and development of bones and teeth, for integrity of epithelial and mucosal surfaces, and for synthesis of rhodopsin (visual purple) necessary for visual dark adaptation. Stimulates healing of cortisone-retarded wounds when applied topically.

USES Vitamin A deficiency and as dietary supplement during periods of increased requirements, such as pregnancy, lactation, infancy, and infections. Used as replacement therapy in conditions that affect absorption, mobilization, or storage of vitamin A, e.g., steatorrhea, severe biliary obstruction, hepatic cirrhosis, total gastrectomy. Used in skin disorders (e.g., folliculosis keratosis [Darier's disease], psoriasis); however, other retinoids are being preferentially selected. Also used as a screening test for fat malabsorption.

ROUTE & DOSAGE

Severe Deficiency

Adult: **PO** 500,000 IU/d for 3 d followed by 50,000 IU/d for 2 wk, then 10,000–20,000 IU/d for 2 mo; **IM** 100,000 IU/d for 3 d followed by 50,000 IU/d for 2 wk.
Child: **PO/IM** *>8 y,* same as for adult; *1–8 y,* 10,000 IU/kg/d for 3 d followed by 17,000–35,000 IU/d for 2 wk; *<1 y,* 10,000 IU/kg/d for 3 d followed by 7500–15,000 IU/d for 10 d.

Dietary Supplement

Child: **PO** *4–8 y,* 15,000 IU/d; *<4 y,* 10,000 IU/d.

PHARMACOKINETICS Absorption: readily absorbed from GI tract in presence of bile salts, pancreatic lipase, and dietary fat. **Distribution:** stored mainly in liver; small amounts also found in kidney and body fat; distributed into breast milk. **Metabolism:** metabolized in liver. **Elimination:** excreted in feces and urine.

CONTRAINDICATIONS & PRECAUTIONS Contraindicated in: history of sensitivity to vitamin A or to any ingredient in formulation, hypervitaminosis A, oral administration to patients with malabsorption syndrome. Safe use in amounts exceeding 6000 IU during pregnancy (category A [category X if >RDA]) not established. **Cautious use in:** women on oral contraceptives, high doses in nursing mothers.

ADVERSE/SIDE EFFECTS **CNS:** irritability, headache, intracranial hypertension (pseudotumor cerebri), increased intracranial pressure, bulging fontanelles, papilledema, exophthalmos, miosis, nystagmus. **Hypervitaminosis A syndrome (general manifestations):** malaise, lethargy, abdominal discomfort, anorexia, vomiting. **Skeletal:** slow growth; deep, tender, hard lumps (subperiosteal thickening) over radius, tibia, occiput; migratory arthralgia; retarded growth; premature closure of epiphyses. **Skin:** gingivitis, lip fissures, excessive sweating, drying or cracking of skin, pruritus, increase in skin pigmentation, massive desquamation, brittle nails, alopecia. **Other:** hypomenorrhea, hepatosplenomegaly, hypercalcemia, polydipsia, polyurea, jaundice, leukopenia, hypoplastic anemias, vitamin A plasma levels > 1200 IU/dl, elevations of sedimentation rate and prothrombin time; <u>anaphylaxis</u>, <u>death</u> after IV use.

DIAGNOSTIC TEST INTERFERENCE Vitamin A may falsely increase ***serum cholesterol*** determinations (Zlatkis-Zak reaction); may falsely elevate ***bilirubin*** determination (with Ehrlich's reagent).

DRUG INTERACTIONS **Mineral oil, cholestyramine** may decrease absorption of vitamin A.

NURSING IMPLICATIONS

Administration

- Vitamin A should be taken on empty stomach or following food or milk if GI upset occurs.
- Preserve in tight, light-resistant containers.

Assessment & Drug Effects

- Evaluation of dosage is made with consideration of patient's average daily intake of vitamin A. Dietary and drug history is advisable, e.g., intake of fortified foods, dietary supplements, self-administration or prescription drug sources. Women taking oral contraceptives tend to have significantly high plasma vitamin A levels.
- Vitamin A deficiency is often associated with protein malnutrition as well as other vitamin deficiencies. It may manifest as night blindness, retardation of growth and development, epithelial alterations, susceptibility to infection, abnormal dryness of skin, mouth, and eyes (xerophthalmia) progressing to keratomalacia (ulceration and necrosis of cornea and conjunctiva), and urinary tract calculi.

Patient & Family Education

- Recommended daily allowances are for adult females, 4000 IU; adult males, 5000 IU; lactating women, 6000 IU; children 4–6 y, 2500 IU; and infants, 2100 IU.
- Avoid use of mineral oil while on vitamin A therapy.
- Instruct to report to physician symptoms of overdosage: nausea, vomiting, anorexia, drying and cracking of skin or lips, headache, loss of hair.
- Patients receiving therapeutic doses should be closely supervised. Inform patient and family that self-medication with vitamin A is potentially harmful.

V

VITAMIN B_1

See thiamine hydrochloride.

VITAMIN B_2

See riboflavin.

VITAMIN B_3

See niacin.

VITAMIN B_6

See pyridoxine.

VITAMIN B_9

See folic acid.

VITAMIN B_{12}

See cyanocobalamin.

VITAMIN B_{12A}

See hydroxycobalamin.

VITAMIN C

See ascorbic acid.

VITAMIN D

See calcitriol.

VITAMIN E (TOCOPHEROL)

Trade names: Aquasol E, Vita-Plus E, Vitec

Classification: VITAMIN

Pregnancy category: A

ACTIONS/PHARMACODYNAMICS Vitamin E refers to a group of naturally occurring fat-soluble substances known as tocopherols. Alpha tocopherol, comprising 90% of the tocopherols, is the most biologically potent and has been synthesized. It prevents peroxidation, a process that gives rise to free radicals, highly reactive chemical structures that damage cell membranes and alter nuclear proteins. Vitamin E is essential to the digestion and metabolism of polyunsaturated fats; it maintains the integrity of cell membranes, protects against blood clot formation by decreasing platelet aggregation, enhances vitamin A utilization, and promotes normal growth, development, and tone of muscles. Vitamin E deficiency causes no specific disease in humans but has been associated with increased susceptibility of RBC to hemolysis.

USES To treat and prevent hemolytic anemia due to vitamin E deficiency in premature neonates; to prevent retrolental fibroplasia secondary to oxygen treatment in neonates, and in treatment of diseases with secondary erythrocyte membrane abnormalities, e.g., sickle cell anemia, and G6PD deficiency and as supplement in malabsorption syndromes. Used in patients on diets containing large amounts of polyunsaturated fats for long periods and in the patient who abruptly discontinues such a diet. Also used topically for dry or chapped skin and minor skin disorders. **Unlabeled uses:** muscular dystrophy and a number of other conditions with no conclusive evidence of value. A component of many multivitamin formulations and of topical deodorant preparations as an antioxidant.

ROUTE & DOSAGE

Vitamin E Deficiency

Adult: **PO/IM** 60–75 IU/d.
Child: **PO** 1 IU/kg/d.

Prophylaxis for Vitamin E Deficiency

Adult: **PO** 12–15 IU/d.
Child: **PO** 7–10 IU/d.
Neonate: **PO** 5 IU/d.

PHARMACOKINETICS **Absorption:** 20–60% absorbed from GI tract if fat absorption is normal; enters blood via lymph. **Distribution:** stored mainly in adipose tissue; crosses placenta. **Metabolism:** metabolized in liver. **Elimination:** excreted primarily in bile.

ADVERSE/SIDE EFFECTS Appears to be nontoxic at therapeutic dosage range. With excessive doses for prolonged periods: skeletal muscle weakness, headache, blurred vision, fatigue, nausea, diarrhea, intestinal cramps, gonadal dysfunction; increased serum creatine kinase, cholesterol, triglycerides; decreased serum thyroxine and triiodothyronine; increased urinary estrogens, androgens; creatinuria; sterile abscess, thrombophlebitis, contact dermatitis.

DRUG INTERACTIONS **Mineral oil, cholestyramine** may decrease absorption of vitamin E; may enhance anticoagulant activity of **warfarin.**

NURSING IMPLICATIONS

Administration

- Vitamin E should be taken on empty stomach or following food or milk if GI upset occurs.
- Preserve in tight containers protected from light.

Patient & Family Education

- The estimated daily requirement is usually provided by the normal adult diet, but requirements are higher with increased intake of unsaturated fats.
- RDA of vitamin E may be increased if patient is also taking a large dose of iron.
- In sufficient doses, vitamin E may induce vitamin K deficiency.
- Wheat germ is the richest source of vitamin E; it is also found in vegetable oils (sunflower, corn, soybean, cottonseed); green leafy vegetables, nuts, dairy products, eggs, cereals, meat, and liver.

VITAMIN K_1

See phytonadione.

VITAMIN K_4

See menadiol sodium diphosphate.

WARFARIN SODIUM

(war'far-in)

Trade names: Coumadin Sodium, Panwarfin, Warfilone ♣

Classifications: BLOOD FORMER; ORAL ANTICOAGULANT

Pregnancy category: D

ACTIONS/PHARMACODYNAMICS Indirectly interferes with blood clotting by depressing hepatic synthesis of vitamin K–dependent coagulation factors: II, VII, IX, and X. Deters further extension of existing thrombi and prevents new clots from forming. Has no effect on already synthesized circulating coagulation factors or on circulating thrombi. Does not reverse ischemic tissue damage and has no effect on platelets. Unlike heparin, action is cumulative and more prolonged. Warfarin is not cross allergenic with other coumarin derivatives.

USES Prophylaxis and treatment of deep venous thrombosis and its extension, pulmonary embolism; treatment of atrial fibrillation with embolization. Also used as adjunct in treatment of coronary occlusion, cerebral transient ischemic attacks (TIAs), and as a prophylactic in patients with prosthetic cardiac valves. Used extensively as rodenticide.

W

ROUTE & DOSAGE

Adult: **PO/IV** 10–15 mg/d for 2–5 d, then 2–10 mg once/d with dose adjusted to maintain a PT 1.2–2 times control or INR of 2–3.
Child: **PO** 0.1–0.3 mg/kg/d; adjust to maintain INR of 2–3.

PHARMACOKINETICS **Absorption:** well absorbed from GI tract. **Onset:** 2–7 d. **Peak:** 0.5–3 d. **Distribution:** 97% protein bound; crosses placenta. **Metabolism:** metabolized in liver. **Elimination:** half-life: 0.5–3 d; excreted in urine and bile.

CONTRAINDICATIONS & PRECAUTIONS **Contraindicated in:** hemorrhagic tendencies: vitamin C or K deficiency, hemophilia, coagulation factor deficiencies, dyscrasias; active bleeding; open wounds, active peptic ulcer, visceral carcinoma, esophageal varices, malabsorption syndromes; hypertension (diastolic BP >110 mm Hg), cerebral vascular disease; pregnancy (category D); pericarditis with acute MI; severe hepatic or renal disease; continuous tube drainage of any orifice; subacute bacterial endocarditis; recent surgery of brain, spinal cord, or eye; regional or lumbar block anesthesia; threatened abortion; unreliable patients. **Cautious use in:** alcoholism, allergic disorders, during menstruation, nursing mother, elderly, debilitated patients; ***endogenous factors that may increase prothrombin time response (enhance anticoagulant effect):*** carcinoma, CHF, collagen diseases, hepatic and renal insufficiency, diarrhea, fever, pancreatic disorders, malnutrition, vitamin K deficiency, alcoholism; ***endogenous factors that may decrease prothrombin time response (decrease anticoagulant response):*** edema, hypothyroidism, hyperlipidemia, hypercholesterolemia, chronic alcoholism, hereditary resistance to coumarin therapy.

ADVERSE/SIDE EFFECTS <u>Major or minor hemorrhage from any tissue or organ.</u> **GI:** anorexia, nausea, vomiting, abdominal cramps, diarrhea, steatorrhea, stomatitis. **Hypersensitivity:** dermatitis, urticaria, pruritus, fever. **Other:** increased serum transaminase levels, hepatitis, jaundice, burning sensation of feet, transient hair loss. **Overdosage:** internal or external bleeding, paralytic ileus; skin necrosis of toes (purple toes syndrome), tip of nose, buttocks, thighs, calves, female breast, abdomen, and other fat-rich areas.

DIAGNOSTIC TEST INTERFERENCE Warfarin (coumarins) may cause alkaline urine to be red-orange; may enhance ***uric acid*** excretion, cause elevation of ***serum transaminases,*** and may increase ***lactic dehydrogenase*** activity.

DRUG INTERACTIONS In addition to the drugs listed in the table, many other drugs have been reported to alter the expected response to warfarin; however, clinical importance of these reports has not been substantiated. The addition or withdrawal of any drug to an established drug regimen should be made cautiously, with more frequent PT determinations than usual and with careful observation of the patient and dose adjustment as indicated.

INCOMPATIBILITIES **Solution/additive: ammonium chloride, 5% dextrose, Ringer's lactate,** AMINOGLYCOSIDES, **ascorbic acid, epinephrine, metaraminol, oxytocin, promazine, tetracycline, vancomycin, vitamin B complex with C.**

W

DRUGS THAT MAY ENHANCE ANTICOAGULANT EFFECT

Acetohexamide
Acetaminophen
Alcohol (acute intoxication)*
ALKYLATING AGENTS
Allopurinol
AMINOGLYCOSIDES
AMINOSALICYLIC ACID
Amiodarone
ANABOLIC STEROIDS
ANTIBIOTICS (ORAL)
ANTIMETABOLITES
ANTIPLATELET DRUGS
Aspirin
Asparaginase
BROMELAINS
Chloral hydrate*†
Chloramphenicol
Chlorpropamide
Chymotrypsin
Cimetidine
Cincophen
Clofibrate
Co-trimoxazole
Danazol
Dextran
Dextrothyroxine†
Diazoxide
Dietary deficiencies
Disulfiram†
DIURETICS*
DRUGS AFFECTING BLOOD ELEMENTS
Erythromycin
Ethacrynic acid
Fluconazole
Glucagon
Guanethidine
HEPATOTOXIC DRUGS
Influenza vaccine
Isoniazid
Itraconazole
Ketoconazole
MAO INHIBITORS
Meclofenamate
Mefenamic acid
Methyldopa
Methylphenidate
Metronidazole†
Miconazole
Mineral oil
Nalidixic acid
Neomycin (oral)
NONSTEROIDAL ANTIINFLAMMATORY DRUGS
Plicamycin
Potassium products
PROLONGED NARCOTICS
Propoxyphene
Propylthiouracil
PYRAZOLONES
Quinidine
Quinine
SALICYLATES
Streptokinase†
Sulindac
SULFONAMIDES
SULFONYLUREAS
TETRACYCLINES
THIAZIDES
THYROID DRUGS
Tolbutamide
TRICYCLIC ANTIDEPRESSANTS
Urokinase
Vitamin E
Zileuton

*Increased or decreased response.
†Avoid concurrent use if possible.

DRUGS THAT MAY REDUCE ANTICOAGULANT EFFECT

Alcohol (chronic alcoholism)*†
BARBITURATES
Carbamazepine
Chloral hydrate*†
Cholestyramine†
CORTICOSTEROIDS
Corticotropin
DIURETICS
Ethchlorvynol
Glutethimide†
Griseofulvin
LAXATIVES
Mercaptopurine
ORAL CONTRACEPTIVES (containing ESTROGENS)†
Rifampin
Spironolactone
Vitamin C
Vitamin K (dietary)

*Increased or decreased response.
†Avoid concurrent use if possible.

NURSING IMPLICATIONS

Administration

- Tablet may be crushed before administration and taken with fluid of patient's choice.
- IV administration: For IV administration add 2 ml of supplied diluent to 50 mg of warfarin powder. Administer immediately by direct IV at a rate of 25 mg (1 ml)/min.
- Antidote: In the event of bleeding, anticoagulant effect usually is reversed by omitting 1 or more doses of warfarin and by administration of specific antidote phytonadione (vitamin K_1) 2.5–10 mg orally. Physician may advise patient to carry vitamin K_1 at all times but not to take it until after consultation. If bleeding persists or progresses to a severe level, vitamin K_1 5–25 mg IV is given, or a fresh whole blood transfusion may be necessary.
- Protect all preparations from light and moisture (tablets). Discard discolored or precipitated solutions.

Assessment & Drug Effects

- PT should be determined before initiation of therapy and then daily until maintenance dosage is established.
- Start flow chart indicating prothrombin activity data, control values, and administered anticoagulant doses.
- Usual aim of therapy is to adjust dose so as to maintain PT at 1 1/2–2 1/2 times the control (12–15 s), or 15–35% of normal prothrombin activity, or an INR of 2–4 depending on diagnosis.
- When patient is receiving maintenance dosage, PT determinations may be prescribed at 1–4-wk intervals depending on patient's response. Periodic urinalyses, stool guaiac, and liver function tests are also usually performed. Optimum time to draw blood sample is 12–18 h after last dose.
- Since so many drugs interfere with the activity of anticoagulant drugs, a careful medication history should be obtained before start of therapy and whenever altered responses to therapy require interpretation.
- Elderly, psychotic, or alcoholic patients require close monitoring because they present serious noncompliance problems.

- Continued anticoagulant therapy is not advised in the absence of laboratory facilities or patient compliance.
- Patients with greatest risk of hemorrhage include those whose PT is difficult to regulate, who have an aortic valve prosthesis, or who are receiving long-term anticoagulant therapy and the elderly and debilitated.
- Suspect skin necrosis (local gangrene) and report to physician immediately if area is painful and skin appears purple-black surrounded by redness. Lesions usually occur within 3 d after initiation of therapy. Incidence is high in elderly, obese patients.

Patient & Family Education

- Inform that bleeding can occur even though PT is within therapeutic range. Advise patient to withhold dose and to notify physician immediately if bleeding or signs of bleeding appear: hematuria, bright red or black tarry stools, hematemesis, gingival bleeding with tooth brushing, ecchymoses, petechiae (often occur in ankle areas), epistaxis, bloody sputum, chest pain (hemopericardium), abdominal or lumbar pain or swelling (retroperitoneal bleeding), menorrhagia, pelvic pain, severe or continuous headache, faintness or dizziness (intracranial bleeding); prolonged oozing from any minor injury (e.g., nicks from shaving).
- Instruct patient and family to withhold dose and to report immediately any symptoms of hepatitis (dark urine, itchy skin, jaundice, abdominal pain, light stools) or hypersensitivity reaction.
- Instruct to avoid brand interchange, to take drug at same time each day, and not to alter dose.
- Menstrual flow is generally normal but may be slightly increased or prolonged. Advise to notify physician if there is an unusual increase in bleeding. PT should be checked at least monthly in menstruating women.
- Smoking increases metabolism and therefore may increase dose requirement. Patient should stop smoking or at least greatly modify amount of smoking during anticoagulant therapy.
- Influenza vaccine decreases hepatic metabolism of warfarin, leading to augmented anticoagulant effect as evidenced by hemorrhage. Patient is at risk of bleeding for up to 1 mo after receiving the vaccine.
- PT may be lengthened (enhanced anticoagulant effect) by fever, prolonged hot weather, malnutrition, diarrhea.
- PT may be shortened by a high-fat diet, sudden increase in vitamin K-rich foods (cabbage, cauliflower, broccoli, asparagus, lettuce, turnip greens, onions, spinach, kale, fish, liver), coffee or green tea (caffeine), or by tube feedings with high vitamin K content.
- Urge to maintain a well-balanced diet and to avoid excess intake of alcohol.
- Advise to inform dentist or any new physician about anticoagulant therapy and duration of treatment.
- Instruct to use a soft toothbrush and to floss teeth gently with waxed floss. Also advise use of electric razor for shaving.
- Inform patient who becomes pregnant while on anticoagulant therapy of the potential risk of congenital malformations.
- Warn against taking any other drug unless specifically approved by physician or pharmacist. Anticoagulant action is affected by many

prescription drugs as well as commonly used OTC preparations, e.g., antacids, antihistamines, aspirin, mineral oil, oral contraceptives, or vitamin C (in large doses).

- Patient should carry on his or her person medical identification card or jewelry, such as Medic Alert, that notes medications and physician's name, address, and telephone number (may be purchased in a pharmacy).

XYLOMETAZOLINE HYDROCHLORIDE

(zye-loe-met-az′oh-leen)

Trade names: Neosynephrine II, Otrivin

Classifications: NASAL DECONGESTANT; VASOCONSTRICTOR

Prototype: Naphazoline

Pregnancy category: C

ACTIONS/PHARMACODYNAMICS Markedly constricts dilated arterioles of nasal membrane. Has little or no beta-adrenergic activity. Structurally related to naphazoline. Decreases fluid exudate and mucosal engorgement associated with rhinitis and may open up obstructed eustachian ostia in patient with ear inflammation.

USES Temporary relief of nasal congestion associated with common cold, sinusitis, acute and chronic rhinitis, and hay fever and other allergies.

ROUTE & DOSAGE

Nasal Congestion

Adult: **Nasal** 1–2 sprays or 1–2 drops of 0.1% solution in each nostril q8–10h (max 3 doses/d).

Child: **Nasal** *6 mo–12 y,* 1 spray or 2–3 drops of 0.05% solution in each nostril q8–10h (max 3 doses/d); *<6 mo,* 1 drop of 0.05% solution in each nostril q6h (max 3 doses/d).

PHARMACOKINETICS Onset: 5–10 min. **Duration:** 5–6 h.

CONTRAINDICATIONS & PRECAUTIONS Contraindicated in: sensitivity to adrenergic substances; angle-closure glaucoma; concurrent therapy with MAO inhibitors or tricyclic antidepressants. Safe use during pregnancy (category C) not established. **Cautious use in:** hypertension; hyperthyroidism; heart disease, including angina; advanced arteriosclerosis, the elderly, and children.

ADVERSE/SIDE EFFECTS Usually mild and infrequent: local stinging, burning, dryness and ulceration, sneezing, headache, insomnia, drowsiness. **With excessive use:** *rebound nasal congestion* and vasodilation, tremulousness, hypertension, palpitations, tachycardia, arrhythmia, somnolence, sedation, <u>coma</u>.

NURSING IMPLICATIONS

Administration

- Instruct to clear each nostril gently before administering spray or drops.
- Spray: Do not shake container. Hold tube vertically (spray end up) so that solution is delivered in a fine spray. Head should be erect; spray into each nostril; 3–5 min later, clear (blow) nose thoroughly.
- Drops: Patient should be in a lateral, head-low position to permit application of drops to lower nostril surface. Have patient remain in this position for 5 min, then apply drops to opposite nostril surface in same manner; or drops may be

instilled with patient in reclining position with head tilted back as far as possible.

- Preserve in tight, light-resistant containers at 15–30C (59–86F).

Patient & Family Education

- To prevent contamination of nasal solution and to prevent spread of infection, rinse dropper and tip of nasal spray in hot water after each use and restrict use to the individual patient.
- Prolonged use may cause rebound congestion and chemical rhinitis. Caution patient not to exceed prescribed dosage and to report to physician if drug fails to provide relief within 3 or 4 d.
- Warn not to self-medicate with OTC drugs, sprays, or drops without physician's approval.
- Excessive use by child may lead to CNS depression.

ZAFIRLUKAST

(za-fir-lu′kast)

Trade name: Accolate

Prototype for classifications: BRONCHODILATOR (RESPIRATORY SMOOTH MUSCLE RELAXANT); RESPIRATORY STIMULANT; 5-LIPOXYGENASE INHIBITOR; LEUKOTRIENE RECEPTOR ANTAGONIST

Pregnancy category: B

ACTIONS/PHARMACODYNAMICS Selective peptide leukotriene receptor antagonist (LTRA) of leukotriene D_4 and E_4, thus inhibiting bronchoconstriction. Leukotriene production and receptor affinity have been correlated with the pathogenesis of asthma. These signs and symptoms include airway edema, smooth muscle constriction, and altered cellular activity due to inflammation.

USES Prophylaxis and chronic treatment of asthma in adults and children > 12 y (**not** for acute bronchospasm).

ROUTE & DOSAGE

Asthma

Adult: **PO** 20 mg b.i.d. 1 h before or 2 h after meals.
Child >12 y: **PO** Same as adult.

PHARMACOKINETICS **Absorption:** rapidly absorbed from GI tract, bioavailability significantly reduced by food. **Onset:** 1 wk. **Peak:** 3 h. **Distribution:** >99% protein bound; secreted into breast milk. **Metabolism:** metabolized in liver via cytochrome P450 2C9 (CYP2C9) and possibly CYP3A4. **Elimination:** half-life: 10 h; 90% excreted in feces, 10% in urine.

CONTRAINDICATIONS & PRECAUTIONS **Contraindicated in:** hypersensitivity to zafirlukast, lactation, acute asthma attacks. **Cautious use in:** hepatic impairment, patients ≥ 65 y, pregnancy (category B). Safety and effectiveness in children < 12 y not established.

ADVERSE/SIDE EFFECTS **Body as whole:** generalized pain, asthenia, myalgia, fever, back pain. **CNS:** *headache,* dizziness. **GI:** nausea, diarrhea, abdominal pain, vomiting, dyspepsia; liver dysfunction, increased liver function tests. **Other:** <u>Churg-Strauss syndrome</u> (fever, muscle aches and pains, weight loss).

DRUG INTERACTIONS May increase prothrombin time (PT) in patients on **warfarin. Erythromycin** decreases bioavailability of zafirlukast.

NURSING IMPLICATIONS

Administration

- Give 1 h before or 2 h after meals.

Z

- Store at 20–25C (68–77F); protect from light and moisture.

Assessment & Drug Effects
- Regularly assess respiratory status and airway function.
- Periodically monitor liver function tests.
- With concurrent warfarin therapy, closely monitor PT and INR.
- With concurrent phenytoin therapy, closely monitor phenytoin level.

Patient & Family Education
- Stress importance of taking medication regularly, even during symptom-free periods.
- Inform that drug is not intended to treat acute episodes of asthma.
- Advise to promptly report S&S of hepatic toxicity (see Appendix G) or flulike symptoms. Stress importance of follow-up lab work.
- Instruct to immediately notify physician if condition worsens while using prescribed doses of all antiasthmatic medications.
- Advise nursing mothers not to take this drug.

ZALCITABINE (ddC, DIDEOXYCYTIDINE)

(zal-cit′a-been)

Trade name: Hivid

Classifications: ANTIINFECTIVE; ANTIVIRAL

Prototype: Zidovudine

Pregnancy category: C

ACTIONS/PHARMACODYNAMICS A synthetic pyrimidine nucleotide that inhibits the replication of HIV by inhibition of viral DNA synthesis.

USES Combination therapy with zidovudine for AIDS. Second-line monotherapy for AIDS. **Unlabeled use:** can be used in children.

ROUTE & DOSAGE

Combination Therapy for HIV

Adult: **PO** 0.75 mg q8h given with zidovudine 200 mg q8h.
Child: **PO** 0.015 to 0.04 mg/kg q6h for 8 wk; after 8 wk of monotherapy an alternating regimen of zalcitabine and zidovudine is begun (a 4-wk cycle of zidovudine for 3 wk and zalcitabine for 1 wk).

Monotherapy for HIV

Adult: **PO** 0.01 mg/kg q8h.

PHARMACOKINETICS **Absorption:** readily absorbed from GI tract. **Onset:** 2 wk. **Distribution:** distributes somewhat into CSF. **Metabolism:** does not appear to be metabolized. **Elimination:** half-life: 1.2–1.8 h; 62% excreted unchanged in urine.

CONTRAINDICATIONS & PRECAUTIONS **Contraindicated in:** hypersensitivity to zalcitabine. **Cautious use in:** moderate to severe neuropathy; history of pancreatitis; CHF, cardiomyopathy; renal impairment, hepatic impairment, alcohol abuse; pregnancy (category C). It is not known if zalcitabine is excreted in breast milk. Safety and effectiveness in HIV-infected children <13 y not established.

ADVERSE/SIDE EFFECTS **CV:** may exacerbate existing CHF and cardiomyopathy. **CNS:** *peripheral neuropathy,* numbness. **GI:** diarrhea, mouth and esophageal ulcers, <u>pancreatitis</u>, may exacerbate existing hepatic dysfunction. **Hematologic:** neutropenia, thrombocytopenia. **Skin:** *transient symptom complex of cutaneous eruptions (maculovesicular in nature), fever, malaise, and aphthous mouth ulcers,* arthralgia, urticaria, <u>anaphylaxis</u>.

DRUG INTERACTION May cause additive peripheral neuropathy with **didanosine.**

NURSING IMPLICATIONS

Administration

- Should be taken on an empty stomach.
- Store at 15–30C (56–86F).

Assessment & Drug Effects

- Promptly discontinue drug and notify physician if patient experiences numbness, tingling, burning, or pain in extremities.
- Patients with history of pancreatitis or elevated serum amylase should be closely monitored with baseline and periodic tests for serum amylase, serum glucose, triglycerides, and serum calcium levels.

Patient & Family Education

- Advise of early symptoms of pancreatitis and peripheral neuropathy and instruct patient to promptly report if these occur.
- Instruct women of childbearing age to use contraception while on zalcitabine.

ZIDOVUDINE (AZIDOTHYMIDINE, AZT)

(zye-doe′vyoo-deen)

Trade name: Retrovir

Prototype for classifications: ANTIINFECTIVE; ANTIVIRAL

Pregnancy category: C

ACTIONS/PHARMACODYNAMICS Analog of thymidine (a major nucleoside in DNA). On entering host cell, zidovudine is converted to a triphosphate (the active form) by endogenous thymidine kinase and other cellular enzymes. Appears to act by being incorporated into growing DNA chains by viral reverse transcriptase, thereby terminating viral replication. Zidovudine has antiviral action against HIV (human immunodeficiency virus), the causative agent of AIDS (acquired immune deficiency syndrome), formerly referred to as HTLV III (human T-cell lymphotropic virus, type III), LAV (lymphadenopathy-associated virus), and ARV (AIDS-associated retrovirus).

USES Patients who are HIV positive and have a CD4 count ≤ 500/mm^3, asymptomatic HIV infection, early and late symptomatic HIV disease, prevention of perinatal transfer of HIV during pregnancy. **Unlabeled uses:** pediatric patients, postexposure chemoprophylaxis.

ROUTE & DOSAGE

Symptomatic HIV Infection

Adult: **PO** 200 mg q4h (1200 mg/d); after 1 mo may reduce to 100 mg q4h (600 mg/d); **IV** 1–2 mg/kg q4h (1200 mg/d).
Child: **PO/IV** 3 mo–13 y, 100–180 mg/m^2 q6h.

Asymptomatic HIV Infection, Postexposure Prophylaxis

Adult: **PO** 100 mg q4h while awake, 5 times/d.

PHARMACOKINETICS **Absorption:** readily absorbed from GI tract; 60–70% reaches systemic circulation (first-pass metabolism). **Peak:** 0.5–1.5 h. **Distribution:** crosses blood–brain barrier and placenta. **Metabolism:** metabolized in liver. **Elimination:** half-life: 1 h; 63–95% excreted in urine.

CONTRAINDICATIONS & PRECAUTIONS **Contraindicated in:** life-threatening allergic reactions to any of the

Z

drug components. Safe use during pregnancy (category C), in nursing mothers, and in children ≤ 13 y not established. **Cautious use in:** impaired renal or hepatic function, bone marrow depression.

ADVERSE/SIDE EFFECTS CNS: headache, insomnia, dizziness, paresthesias, mild confusion, anxiety, restlessness, agitation. **GI:** *nausea,* diarrhea, vomiting, *anorexia,* GI pain. **Hematologic:** *bone marrow depression (25% of patients):* granulocytopenia, anemia. **Skin:** rash, itching, diaphoresis. **Other:** fever, dyspnea, *malaise,* weakness, *myalgia.*

DRUG INTERACTIONS Acetaminophen may enhance bone marrow suppression; **amphotericin B** increases risk of AZT toxicity; **aspirin, dapsone, doxorubicin, flucytosine, indomethacin, interferon alfa, pentamidine, vincristine** may increase risk of AZT toxicity; **probenecid** will decrease AZT elimination, resulting in increased serum levels and thus toxicity. **Atovaquone** may increase bone marrow toxicity.

NURSING IMPLICATIONS

Administration

- For IV administration, withdraw required dose from vial and dilute with D5W to a concentration not to exceed 4 mg/ml. Administer over 60 min; avoid rapid infusion.
- Store at 15–25C (59–77F) protected from light unless otherwise directed.

Assessment & Drug Effects

- During the first month of therapy, patient should be evaluated at least weekly.
- Baseline and frequent (at least q2wk) blood counts should be performed. CD_4 (T_4) lymphocyte number, Hgb, and granulocyte count are strongly recommended to detect hematologic toxicity.
- Myelosuppression results in anemia, which commonly occurs after 4–6 wk of therapy, and granulocytopenia in 6–8 wk. Frequently, both respond to dosage adjustment. Significant anemia (Hgb <7.5 g/dl or reduction > 25% of baseline value), or granulocyte count < 750/mm^3 (or reduction > 50% of baseline) may require temporary interruption of therapy and transfusions.
- Monitor for common adverse effects, especially severe headache, nausea, insomnia, and myalgia.

Patient & Family Education

- Advise to contact physician promptly if health status changes for the worse or any unusual symptoms develop.
- Tell patients that the drug is not a cure for HIV infection and that they continue to be at risk for opportunistic infections.
- Advise not to share drug and to take it exactly as prescribed.
- Inform that the drug does not reduce the risk of transmission of HIV infection through body fluids.
- It is not known if the drug is secreted in human milk. Instruct nursing mothers to discontinue nursing.

ZILEUTON

(zi-leu′ton)

Trade names: Leutrol, Zyflo

Classifications: BRONCHODILATOR (RESPIRATORY SMOOTH MUSCLE RELAXANT); RESPIRATORY STIMULANT; 5-LIPOXYGENASE INHIBITOR; LEUKOTRIENE RECEPTOR ANTAGONIST

Prototype: Zafirlukast

Pregnancy category: C

ACTIONS/PHARMACODYNAMICS Inhibits 5-lipoxygenase, the enzyme needed to start the conversion of arachidonic acid to leukotrienes. Leukotrienes are considered more important than prostaglandins as inflammatory agents; they induce bronchoconstriction and mucus production. Elevated sputum and blood levels of leukotrienes have been documented during acute asthma attacks.

USES Prophylaxis and chronic treatment of asthma in adults and children >12 y.

ROUTE & DOSAGE

Asthma

Adult: **PO** 600 mg q.i.d.
Child (> 12 y): **PO** 600 mg q.i.d.

PHARMACOKINETICS **Absorption:** rapidly absorbed from GI tract. **Peak:** 1.7 h. **Duration:** 5–8 h. **Distribution:** 93% protein bound; secreted in the breast milk of rats. **Metabolism:** metabolized in liver primarily via glucuronide conjugation. **Elimination:** half-life: 2.5 h; excreted primarily in urine (94%).

CONTRAINDICATIONS & PRECAUTIONS **Contraindicated in:** hypersensitivity to zileuton or zafirlukast, active liver disease, lactation. **Cautious use in:** hepatic insufficiency, pregnancy (category C). Safety and effectiveness in children >12 y not established.

ADVERSE/SIDE EFFECTS **Body as whole:** pain, asthenia, myalgia, arthralgia, fever, malaise, neck pain/rigidity. **CNS:** *headache,* dizziness, insomnia, nervousness, somnolence. **CV:** chest pain. **GI:** abdominal pain, *dyspepsia,* nausea, constipation, flatulence, vomiting, elevated liver function tests, asymptomatic hepatitis. **Skin:** pruritus. **Other:** conjunctivitis, hypertonia, lymphadenopathy, vaginitis, UTI, leukopenia.

DRUG INTERACTIONS: May double **theophylline** levels and increase toxicity. Increases hypoprothrombinemic effects of **warfarin**. May increase levels of BETA BLOCKERS (especially **propranolol**), leading to hypotension and bradycardia. May increase **terfenadine** levels, leading to prolongation of QT_c interval.

NURSING IMPLICATIONS

Administration

- Drug is generally taken at meals and bedtime.
- Store at room temperature, 20–25C (68–77F); protect from light.

Assessment & Drug Effects

- Regularly assess respiratory status and airway function.
- Periodically monitor CBC and routine blood chemistry. Liver function tests should be monitored monthly for 3 mo, then every 2–3 mo for rest of first year, then periodically thereafter.
- With concurrent therapy, theophylline dose should be reduced and theophylline levels closely monitored.
- With concurrent warfarin therapy, closely monitor PT and INR.
- With concurrent phenytoin therapy, closely monitor phenytoin level.
- With concurrent propranolol therapy, closely monitor HR and BP for excessive beta blockade.

Patient & Family Education

- Stress importance of taking medication regularly even during symptom-free periods.
- Inform that drug is not intended to treat acute episodes of asthma.
- Advise to promptly report S&S of

hepatic toxicity (see Appendix G) or flulike symptoms. Stress importance of follow-up lab work.

- Instruct to immediately notify physician if condition worsens while using prescribed doses of all antiasthmatic medications.

ZOLMITRIPTAN

(zol-mi-trip′tan)

Trade name: Zomig

Classifications: AUTONOMIC NERVOUS SYSTEM AGENT; ALPHA-ADRENERGIC ANTAGONIST (SYMPATHOLYTIC) SEROTONIN $5\text{-}HT_{1B/1D}$ RECEPTOR AGONIST; ERGOT ALKALOID

Prototype: Sumatriptan

Pregnancy category: C

ACTIONS/PHARMACODYNAMICS

Seletive serotonin ($5\text{-}HT_{1B/1D}$) receptor agonist. The agonist effects at $5\text{-}HT_{1B/1D}$ reverse the vasodilation of cranial blood vessels associated with a migraine. Activation of these receptors also reduces the pain pathways associated with migraine headache.

USE Acute migraine headaches with or without aura.

ROUTE & DOSAGE

Acute Migraine

Adult: **PO** 2.5–5 mg; may repeat in 2 h if necessary (max 10 mg/24 h).

PHARMACOKINETICS **Absorption:** rapidly absorbed, 40% bioavailability. **Peak:** 2–3 h. **Distribution:** 25% protein bound. **Metabolism:** metabolized in liver to active metabolite. **Elimination:** half-life: 3 h; excreted primarily in urine (65%), 30% excreted in feces.

CONTRAINDICATIONS & PRECAUTIONS **Contraindicated in:** hypersensitivity to zolmitriptan; ischemic heart disease (angina pectoris, ECG changes, history of MI or Prinzmetal's angina); uncontrolled hypertension; hemiplegia or basilar migraine; pregnancy (category C); concurrent administration of ergotamine or sumatriptan. **Cautious use in:** men >40 y; postmenopausal women; patients with other cardiac risk factors, such as diabetes, obesity, cigarette smoking, high cholesterol levels, strong family history of CAD; lactation.

ADVERSE/SIDE EFFECTS **Body as whole:** asthenia, fatigue, malaise, pain, pressure sensation, paresthesias, throat pressure, warm/cold sensations, hypesthesia. **CNS:** somnolence, dizziness, drowsiness, headache, hypesthesia, decreased mental acuity, euphoria, tremor. **CV:** coronary artery vasospasm, transient myocardial ischemia, <u>MI</u>, ventricular tachycardia, ventricular fibrillation, chest pain/tightness/heaviness, palpitations. **GI:** dry mouth, nausea, vomiting. **Respiratory:** dyspnea. **Skin:** flushing. **Other:** hot flushes.

DRUG INTERACTIONS: **Dihydroergotamine, methysergide,** other $5\text{-}HT_1$ AGONISTS may cause prolonged vasospastic reactions; SSRIS have rarely caused weakness, hyperreflexia, and incoordination; MAOIS should not be used with $5\text{-}HT_1$ agonists; **cimetidine** increases half-life of zolmitriptan.

NURSING IMPLICATIONS

Administration

- Administer anytime after symptoms of migraine appear. Give ≤2.5 mg by breaking a 2.5-mg tablet in half. If headache returns, may repeat q2h up to 10 mg in 24 h.

Z

- If no relief with the first dose, do not give a second dose without first consulting the physician.
- Do not give zolmitriptan within 24 h of an ergot-containing drug or other 5-HT_1 agonist.
- Unused tablets that have been removed from the blister packaging should be discarded.
- Store at 2–25C (36–77F) and protect from light.

Assessment & Drug Effects

- Therapeutic effectiveness is indicated by relief or reduction of migraine pain within 1–4 h.
- Carefully monitor cardiovascular status following first dose in patients at risk for CAD (e.g., postmenopausal women, men over 40 y old, persons with known CAD risk factors) or coronary artery vasopasms.
- ECG is recommended periodically with long-term use.
- Immediately report chest pain, nausea, or tightness in chest or throat that is severe or does not quickly resolve.
- Periodic cardiovascular evaluation is recommended with continued zolmitriptan use.

Patient & Family Education

- Carefully review patient information leaflet and guidelines for administration.
- Do not take zolmitriptan during the aura phase but as early as possible after onset of migraine.
- Concurrent oral contraceptive use may increase incidence of adverse effects.
- Immediately contact physician if any of the following occur after zolmitriptan use: symptoms of angina (e.g., severe and/or persistent pain or tightness in chest or throat, sudden nausea), hypersensitivity (e.g., wheezng, facial swelling, skin rash, hives), fainting, or abdominal pain.
- Report any other adverse effects (e.g., tingling, flushing, dizziness) at next physician visit.

ZOLPIDEM

(zol′-pi-dem)

Trade name: Ambien

Classifications: CNS AGENT; ANXIOLYTIC; SEDATIVE-HYPNOTIC

Prototype: Lorazepam

Pregnancy category: B

ACTIONS/PHARMACODYNAMICS Nonbenzodiazepine hypnotic. Does not have muscle relaxant or anticonvulsant effects. Preserves deep sleep (stages 3 through 4) at hypnotic doses.

USE Short-term treatment of insomnia.

ROUTE & DOSAGE

Short-term Treatment of Insomnia

Adult: **PO** 5–10 mg h.s. Limit use to 7–10 d; start with 5 mg in the elderly.

PHARMACOKINETICS Absorption: readily absorbed from GI tract. 70% reaches systemic circulation. Food decreases rate and extent of absorption. **Onset:** 7–27 min. **Peak:** 0.5–2.3 h. **Duration:** 6–8 h. **Distribution:** highly protein bound. Lowest concentrations in CNS, highest concentrations in glandular tissue and fat. Crosses placenta, very small amounts (<0.02%) distributed into breast milk. **Metabolism:** metabolized in the liver to 3 inactive metabolites. **Elimination:** half-life: 1.7–2.5 h; 79–96% of dose appears as metabolites in the bile, urine, and feces.

CONTRAINDICATIONS & PRECAUTIONS **Contraindicated in:** nursing mothers. **Cautious use in:** depressed patients, hepatic/renal impairment, elderly patients, pregnancy (category B), patients with compromised respiratory status. Safety and efficacy in children <18 y have not been established.

ADVERSE/SIDE EFFECTS **CNS:** headache on awakening, drowsiness or fatigue, lethargy, drugged feeling, depression, anxiety, irritability, dizziness, double vision. Confusion and falls reported in elderly. Doses > 10 mg may be associated with anterograde amnesia or memory impairment. **GI:** dyspepsia, nausea, vomiting. **Other:** myalgia.

DRUG INTERACTIONS: CNS DEPRESSANTS, **alcohol,** PHENOTHIAZINES by augmenting CNS depression. **Food–drug:** Extent and rate of absorption of zolpidem is significantly decreased.

NURSING IMPLICATIONS

Administration

- Zolpidem should be administered immediately before bedtime.
- A dosage reduction to 5 mg is recommended for elderly or debilitated patients.
- For more rapid sleep onset, do not administer with or immediately after a meal.
- Store at room temperature, 15–30C (59–86F).

Assessment & Drug Effects

- Assess respiratory function in patients with compromised respiratory status. Report immediately significantly depressed respiratory rate (less than 12/min).
- Monitor patients who exhibit signs and symptoms of depression, because zolpidem may increase level of depression.
- Closely monitor elderly or debilitated patients for impaired cognitive or motor function and unusual sensitivity to the effects of zolpidem.

Patient & Family Education

- Advise to avoid taking alcohol or other CNS depressants while on zolpidem.
- Inform that zolpidem may cause daytime drowsiness or dizziness; therefore, caution is needed when performing hazardous tasks.
- Inform to report vision changes to physician.
- Inform that onset of drug is more rapid when taken on an empty stomach.

APPENDICES

GENERIC NAME	BRAND NAMES	INDICATIONS/ADULT DOSE	CLINICAL IMPLICATIONS*
Beta-Adrenergic Blockers **Prototype: Propranolol HCl**		Intraocular hypertension and chronic open-angle glaucoma	May cause *mild ocular stinging* and discomfort; tearing; may also have the adverse effects of systemic beta blockers.
Betaxolol HCl	Betoptic, Betoptic-S	1 drop of 0.5% solution or 0.25% suspension in affected eye twice daily.	May mask symptoms of acute hypoglycemia in diabetic patients (tachycardia, tremor, but not sweating). May precipitate thyroid storm in patients with hyperthyroidism.
Levobunolol	Betagan	1–2 drops 1–2 times/d.	Patients with impaired cardiac function and the elderly should report to physician signs and symptoms of CHF (see Appendix G).
Timolol maleate	Timoptic, Timoptic XE	1 drop of 0.25–0.5% solution b.i.d.; may decrease to q.d. Apply gel q.d.	Monitor BP for hypotension and heart rate for bradycardia.
Mitotics **Prototype for classification:** Pilocarpine HCl		**USES** Open-angle and angle-closure glaucomas; to reduce IOP and to protect the lens during surgery and laser iridotomy; to counteract effects of mydriatics and cycloplegics following surgery or ophthalmoscopic examination.	**Ocular:** ciliary spasm with browache, twitching of eyelids, eye pain with change in eye focus, miosis, *diminished vision in poorly illuminated areas,* blurred vision, reduced visual acuity, sensitivity, contact allergy, lacrimation, follicular conjunctivitis, conjunctival irritation, cataract, retinal detachment.

Apraclonidine	Iopidine	**Intraoperative and Postsurgical Increase in IOP:** 1 drop of 1% solution in affected eye 1 h before surgery and 1 drop in same eye immediately after surgery. **Open-angle Glaucoma:** 1 drop of 0.5% solution in affected eye q12h.	**CNS:** *headache, drowsiness,* depression, syncope. **GI:** abnormal taste, dry mouth. Wait 15 min after instillation before inserting soft contact lenses to avoid staining the lenses. MAOIs may have increased risk of hypertensive emergency. May increase the effects of beta blockers and other antihypertensives on blood pressure and heart rate. TCAs may reduce the effects of **brimonidine.**
Brimonidine tartrate	Alphagan	**Glaucoma:** 1 drop in affected eye(s) t.i.d. approximately 8h apart.	
Brinzolamide	Azopt	**Ocular Hypertension or Open-angle Glaucoma:** 1 drop in affected eye(s) t.i.d.	**Brinzolamide** is a carbonic anhydrase inhibitor (prototype: acetazolamide) and is a sulfonamide. It should not be used by patients with sulfa allergies.
Carbachol	Isopto Carbachol, Miostat	**Topical** 1–2 drops of 0.75–3% solution in lower conjunctival sac q4–8h. **Intraocular** 0.5 ml of 0.01% solution injected into anterior chamber of eye.	
Demecarium bromide	Humorsol	**Glaucoma:** 1–2 drops of 0.125–0.25% solution 2 times/wk up to b.i.d. **Convergent Strabismus:** *Child:* 1 drop of 0.125% solution in each eye daily for 2–3 wk; then decrease to 1 drop q.o.d. for 2–3 wk; then 1 drop 2 times/wk.	**Demecarium bromide** is capable of producing cumulative systemic effects. It is essential to adhere precisely to prescribed drug concentration, dosage schedule, and technique of administration.

*Clinical implications apply to all drugs in the group unless otherwise noted.

GENERIC NAME	BRAND NAMES	INDICATIONS/ADULT DOSE	CLINICAL IMPLICATIONS*
Echothiophate iodide	Phospholine Iodide	**Glaucoma:** 1 drop of 0.03–0.25% solution in conjunctival sac 1–2 times/d. **Accommodative Esotropia:** ***Diagnosis:*** 1 drop of 0.125% solution in both eyes once/d at bedtime for 2–3 wk. ***Treatment:*** 1 drop of 0.125% solution q.o.d. or 1 drop of 0.06% solution daily (max 1 drop 0.125% solution daily).	Reconstituted solutions of **echothiophate** remain stable for 1 mo at room temperature. Expiration date should appear on label. The time solutions remain stable under refrigeration varies with manufacturer. **Echothiophate** therapy is generally discontinued 2–6 wk before surgery. If necessary, alternate miotic therapy is substituted.
Isoflurophate	Fluoropryl	**Glaucoma:** 0.5 cm (1/4 in.) strip of ointment in conjunctival sac q8–72h. **Strabismus:** 0.5 cm (1/4 in.) strip of ointment in conjunctival sac of each eye at bedtime for 2 wk; when accommodative factor is evident, decrease frequency to q2–7d for 2 wk.	
Latanoprost	Xalatan	1 drop (1.5 mg) in affected eye(s) once daily in the evening.	**Latanoprost** is a prostaglandin analogue; may cause increased pigmentation of iris (increased brown pigment). Medication should be given in the evening. Give at least 5 min apart from other topical ophthalmic drugs.

Piolcarpine HCl	Adsorbocarpine, Isopto Carpine, Minims PilocarpineA, MiocarpineA, Ocusert, Pilo, Pilocar	**Acute Gluacoma:** 1 drop of 1–2% solution in affected eye q5–10min for 3–6 doses, then 1 drop q1–3h until IOP is reduced. **Chronic Glaucoma:** 1 drop of 0.5–4% solution in affected eye q4–12h or 1 ocular system (Ocusert) q7d. **Miotic:** 1 drop of 1% solution in affected eye.	
Physostigmine	Isopto Eserine	**Glaucoma:** Instill ointment in conjunctival sac at bedtime or instill 1–2 drops of 0.25–0.5% solution 3–4 times/d.	The patient with brown or hazel eyes may require a stronger ophthalmic solution or more frequent instillation of **physostigmine** for desired effects than the patient with blue eyes.
Mydriatic **Prototype for classification:** Homatropine HBr		**USES** Mydriatic for ocular examination and as cycloplegic to measure errors of refraction. Also inflammatory conditions of uveal tract, ciliary spasm, as a cycloplegic and mydriatic in preoperative and postoperative conditions, and as an optical aid in select patients with axial lens opacities.	**Contraindicated in:** primary (narrow-angle) glaucoma or predisposition to glaucoma; children <6 y. **Cautious use in:** increased IOP, infants, children, pregnancy (category C), the elderly or debilitated; hypertension; hyperthyroidism; diabetes; cardiac disease.

*Clinical implications apply to all drugs in the group unless otherwise noted.

GENERIC NAME	BRAND NAMES	INDICATIONS/ADULT DOSE	CLINICAL IMPLICATIONS*
Cyclopentolate HCl	Ak-Pentolate, Cyclogyl, Pentalair	**Cycloplegic Refraction:** *Adult:* 1 drop of 1% solution in eye 40–50 min before procedure followed by 1 drop in 5 min; may need 2% solution in patients with darkly pigmented eyes. *Child:* 1 drop of 0.5–1% solution in eye 40–50 min before procedure, followed by 1 drop in 5 min; may need 2% solution in patients with darkly pigmented eyes.	**ADVERSE/SIDE EFFECTS** Increased IOP, *blurred vision, photophobia.* **Prolonged use:** local irritation, congestion, edema, eczema, follicular conjunctivitis. **Excessive dosage/systemic absorption:** symptoms of atropine poisoning (flushing; dry skin, mouth, nose; decreased sweating; fever; rash; rapid, irregular pulse; abdominal and bladder distention; hallucinations; confusion). **CNS:** psychotic reaction, behavior disturbances, ataxia, incoherent speech, restlessness, hallucinations, somnolence, disorientation, failure to recognize people, grand mal seizures. Carefully monitor **cyclopentolate** patients with seizure disorders, since systemic absorption may precipitate a seizure.
Dipivefrin HCl	Propine	**Glaucoma:** 1 drop in eye q12h.	
Epinephrine borate	Epinal, Eppy/N	1–2 drops as needed	
Homatropine HBr	AK-Homatropine, Homatrine, Isopto Homatropine	**Cycloplegic Refraction:** 1–2 drops of 2% or 5% solution in eye repeated in 5–10 min if necessary. **Ocular Inflammation:** 1–2 drops of 2% or 5% solution in eye up to q3–4h.	Photophobia associated with mydriasis may require patient to wear dark glasses. Since drug causes blurred vision, supervision of activity may be indicated.

Phenylephrine HCl	Ak-Dilate Ophthalmic, Alconefrin, Isopto Frin, Mydfrin, Neo-Synephrine, Prefrin Liquifilm, Vacon	**Ophthalmoscopy:** *Adult:* 1 drop of 2.5% or 10% solution before examination. *Child:* 1 drop of 2.5% solution before examination. **Vasoconstrictor:** 2 drops of 0.12–0.15% solution q3–4h as necessary.	
Tropicamide	Mydriacyl, Tropicacyl	**Refraction:** 1–2 drops of 1% solution in each eye, repeat in 5 min; if patient is not seen within 20–30 min, an additional drop may be instilled. **Examination of Fundus:** 1–2 drops of 0.5% solution in each eye 15–20 min prior to examination; may repeat q30min if necessary.	
Vasoconstrictor; Decongestant **Prototype for classification:** Naphazoline HCl		**USE** Ocular vasoconstrictor.	**Contraindicated in:** narrow-angle glaucoma; concomitant use with MAOIs or tricyclic antidepressants. **Cautious use in:** hypertension; cardiac irregularities; advanced arteriosclerosis; diabetes; hyperthyroidism; elderly patients. **ADVERSE/SIDE EFFECTS** Pupillary dilation, increased intraocular pressure, rebound redness of the eye, headache, hypertension, nausea,
Naphazoline HCl	Ak-Con, Albalon, Allerest, Clear Eyes, Comfort, Degest-2, Muro's Opcon, Nafazair, Naphcon, Privine, VasoClear, Vasocon	**Ophthalmic:** 1–3 drops of 0.1% solution q3–4h prn or 1–2 drops of a 0.01–0.03% solution q4h prn.	

*Clinical implications apply to all drugs in the group unless otherwise noted.

GENERIC NAME	BRAND NAMES	INDICATIONS/ADULT DOSE	CLINICAL IMPLICATIONS*
Tetrahydrozoline HCl	Collyrium, Malazine, Murine Plus, Optigene, Soothe, Tyzine, Visine	1–2 drops of 0.05% solution in eye b.i.d. or t.i.d.	weakness, sweating. **Overdosage:** drowsiness, hypothermia, bradycardia, shock-like hypotension, coma.
Corticosteroid, Antiinflammatory **Prototype for classification:** Hydrocortisone		**USE** Inflammation. **Unlabeled use:** anterior uveitis.	**Contraindicated in:** ocular fungal diseases, herpes simplex keratitis, ocular infections, ocular mycobacterial infections, viral disease of cornea or conjunctiva such as vaccina, varicella. **ADVERSE/SIDE EFFECTS Ocular:** blurred vision, photophobia, conjunctival edema, corneal edema, erosion, eye discharge, dryness, irritation, pain; prolonged use: glaucoma, ocular hypertension, damage to optic nerve, defects in visual acuity and visual fields, posterior subcapsular cataract formation, secondary ocular infections. **Other:** headache, taste perversion. Shake all products well before use.
Dexamethasone sodium phosphate	Decadron Maxidex	**Ophthalmic:** 1–2 drops in conjunctival sac up to 4–6 times/d; may instill hourly for severe disease.	
Fluorometholone	Fluor-Op, FML Forte, FML Liquifilm	**Ophthalmic:** *Adult/Child >2 y:* 1–2 drops of suspension in conjunctival sac q.h. for the first 24–48 h; then b.i.d. to q.i.d.; *or* a thin strip of ointment q4h for the first 24–48 h; then 1–3 times/d.	
Loteprednol Etabonate	Alrex, Lotemax	1–2 drops in conjunctival sac q.i.d. during initial treatment; may increase to q1h if necessary.	

Prenisolone sodium phosphate	Inflamase, Inflamase Mild, Pred Mild, Inflamase Forte	1–2 drops in conjunctival sac q.h. during the day; then q2h at night; may decrease to 1 drop t.i.d. or q.i.d.	
Rimexolone	Vexol	**Postoperative Ocular Inflammation:** 1–2 drops q.i.d. beginning 24 h after surgery, continue through first 2 wk postoperatively. **Anterior Uveitis:** 1–2 drops in affected eye q.h. while awake for first week, then q2h for second week, then taper frequency until uveitis resolves.	
Ocular Antihistamines		**USE** Relief of S&S of allergic conjunctivitis.	
Emedastine difumarate	Emadine	*Adult/Child >1 y:* 1 drop in affected eye up to q.i.d.	Wait 10 min after instilling emedastine before inserting soft contact lenses.

*Clinical implications apply to all drugs in the group unless otherwise noted.

GENERIC NAME	BRAND NAMES	INDICATIONS/ADULT DOSE	CLINICAL IMPLICATIONS*
Anticoagulant, Low-Molecular-Weight Heparin **Prototype for classification:** Heparin		**USES** Prevention of DVT following hip or knee replacement or abdominal surgery.	**Contraindicated in:** hypersensitivity to ardeparin, other low-molecular-weight heparins, pork products, or parabens; active major bleeding; thrombocytopenia that is positive for antiplatelet antibodies with ardeparin; uncontrolled hypertension; nursing mothers. **Cautious use in:** hypersensitivity to heparin; history of heparin-induced thrombocytopenia; bacterial endocarditis; severe and uncontrolled hypertension, cerebral aneurysm or hemorrhagic stroke, bleeding disorders, recent GI bleeding or associated GI disorders (e.g., ulcerative colitis), thrombocytopenia, or platelet disorders; severe liver or renal disease, diabetic retinopathy, hypertensive retinopathy, invasive procedures; pregnancy (category C). **ADVERSE/SIDE EFFECTS Body as whole:** allergic reactions (rash, urticaria), arthralgia, pain and inflammation at injection site, peripheral edema, arthralgia, fever. **CNS:** CVA, dizziness, headache, insomnia. **CV:** chest pain. **GI:** nausea, vomiting. **Hematologic:** hemorrhage, thrombocytopenia, ecchymoses, anemia. **Respiratory:** dyspnea. **Skin:** rash, pruritus.
Ardeparin sodium	Normiflo	**Knee Surgery: SC** 50 anti-Xa U/kg q12h starting the evening of the day of surgery or the morning after, for up to 14 d or until the patient is fully ambulatory.	
Dalteparin sodium	Fragmin	**DVT Prophylaxis, Abdominal Surgery: SC** 2500 IU (16 mg) q.d. starting 1–2 h prior to surgery and continuing for 5–10 d postoperatively. **DVT Prophylaxis, Total Hip Arthroplasty: SC** 2500–5000 IU q.d. starting 1–2 h prior to surgery and continuing for 5–13 d postoperatively. **Acute Thromboembolism: SC** 120 IU/kg b.i.d. for at least 5 d. **Recurrent Thromboembolism: SC** 5000 IU b.i.d.for 3–6 mo.	

Danaparoid sodium	Orgaran	**DVT/PE Prophylaxis: SC** 750 anti-Xa units b.i.d. beginning 1–4 h presurgery and restarting 2 h postsurgery. Continue 7–10 d (up to 14 d).	**DRUG INTERACTIONS Aspirin,** NSAIDs, **warfarin** can increase risk of hemorrhage. Alternate injection sites using the abdomen, anterior thigh, or outer aspect of upper arms.
Enoxaparin	Lovenox	**Prevention of DVT after Hip or Knee Surgery: SC** 30 mg SC b.i.d. for 10–14 d starting 12–24 h postsurgery. **Prevention of DVT after Abdominal Surgery: SC** 40 mg q.d. starting 2 h before surgery and continuing for 7–10 d (max 12 d). **Treatment of DVT and Pulmonary Embolus: SC** 1 mg/kg b.i.d.; monitor anti-Xa activity to determine appropriate dose. **Acute Coronary Syndrome: SC** 1 mg/kg q12 h × 2–8 d. Give concurrently with aspirin 100–325 mg/d.	Patient should be sitting or lying supine for injection. Inject deep SC with entire length of needle inserted into skinfold. Aspirate to avoid accidental IM injection. Hold skinfold gently throughout injection and do not rub site after injection. **Lab tests:** CBC with platelet count, urinalysis, and stool for occult blood should be tested throughout therapy. Routine coagulation tests are not required. Carefully monitor for and immediately report S&S of excessive anticoagulation (e.g., bleeding at venipuncture sites or surgical site) or hemorrhage (e.g., drop in BP or Hct). Patients on oral anticoagulants, on platelet inhibitors, or with impaired renal function must be very carefully monitored for hemorrhage.

*Clinical implications apply to all drugs in the group unless otherwise noted.

INHALED CORTICOSTEROIDS (oral and nasal inhalation)

GENERIC NAME	BRAND NAMES	INDICATIONS/ADULT DOSE	CLINICAL IMPLICATIONS*
Corticosteroid, Antiinflammatory **Prototype for classification:** Hydrocortisone		**USES** Oral inhalation to treat steroid-dependent asthma, nasal inhalation for the management of symptoms of seasonal or perennial rhinitis.	**Contraindicated in:** nonasthmatic bronchitis, primary treatment of status asthmaticus, acute attack of asthma. **Cautious use in:** patients receiving systemic corticosteroids; use with extreme caution if at all in respiratory tuberculosis, untreated fungal, bacterial, or viral infections, and ocular herpes simplex; nasal inhalation therapy for nasal septal ulcers, nasal trauma, or surgery.
Beclomethasone dipropionate	Beclovent, Beconase Nasal Inhaler, Vancenase Nasal Inhaler, Vanceril, Vanceril D, Vancenase AQ	**Asthma:** *Adult:* **Oral inhaler** 2 inhalations t.i.d. or q.i.d. up to 20 inhalations/d; may try to reduce systemic steroids after 1 wk of concomitant therapy. *Child:* **Oral inhaler** 1–2 inhalations t.i.d. or q.i.d. up to 10 inhalations/d. **Allergic Rhinitis:** *Adult:* **Nasal inhaler** 1 spray in each nostril b.i.d. to q.i.d. *Child >6 y:* 1 spray q.d.	**ADVERSE/SIDE EFFECTS Oral inhalation:** *candidal infection of oropharynx* and occasionally larynx, hoarseness, dry mouth, sore throat, sore mouth. **Nasal (inhaler):** *transient nasal irritation, burning, sneezing,* epistaxis, bloody mucus, nasopharyngeal itching, dryness, crusting, and ulceration; headache, nausea, vomiting. **Other:** with excessive doses, symptoms of hypercorticism. Note that oral inhalation and nasal inhalation products are not to be used interchangeably.
Budesonide	Pulmicort Turbuhaler, Rhinocort, Rhinocort Turbuhaler	**Asthma, Maintenance Therapy:** *Adult:* **Oral inhalation** 1 or 2 inhalations (200 µg/inhalation) q.d.–b.i.d. (max 800 µg b.i.d.).	**Oral inhaler:** emphasize the following: (1) Shake inhaler well before using. (2) After exhaling fully, place mouthpiece well into mouth with lips closed firmly around it. (3) Inhale slowly

		Child ≥6 *y:* **Oral inhalation** 1 inhalation (200 μg/inhalation) q.d.–b.i.d. (max 400 μg b.i.d.). **Rhinitis:** *Adult/Child* >6 *y:* **Intranasal** 2 sprays in each nostril in the morning and evening or 4 sprays in each nostril in the morning.	through mouth while activating the inhaler. (4) Hold breath 5–10 s, if possible, then exhale slowly. (5) Wait 1 min between puffs. Clean inhaler daily. Separate parts as directed in package insert, rinse them with warm water, and dry them thoroughly. Rinsing mouth and gargling with warm water after each oral inhalation removes residual medication from oropharyngeal area. Mouth care may also delay or prevent onset of oral dryness, hoarseness, and candidiasis. **Nasal inhaler:** directions for use of nasal inhaler provided by manufacturer should be carefully reviewed with patient. Emphasize the following points: (1) Gently blow nose to clear nostrils. (2) Shake inhaler well before using. (3) If 2 sprays in each are prescribed, direct 1 spray toward upper, and the other toward lower part of nostril. (4) Wash cap and plastic nosepiece daily with warm water; dry thoroughly. Inhaled steroids do not provide immediate symptomatic relief and are not prescribed for this purpose.
Dexamethasone sodium phosphate	Aeroseb-Dex, Decadron, Decaspray	*Adult:* **Oral inhalation** Up to 3 inhalations t.i.d. or q.i.d. (max 12 inhalations/d). **Intranasal** 2 sprays in each nostril b.i.d. or t.i.d. (max 12 sprays/d). *Child:* **Oral inhalation** Up to 2 inhalations q.i.d. (max 8 inhalations/d). **Intranasal** 1 or 2 sprays in each nostril b.i.d. (max 8 sprays/d).	
Flunisolide	AeroBid, Nasalide, Nasarel	**Allergic Rhinitis:** *Adult:* **Inhaled/Intranasal** 2 sprays orally, or intranasally in each nostril, b.i.d.; may increase to t.i.d. if needed. *Child 6–14 y:* **Inhaled/Intranasal** 1 spray orally, or intranasally in each nostril t.i.d. *or* 2 sprays b.i.d.	

*Clinical implications apply to all drugs in the group unless otherwise noted.

INHALED CORTICOSTEROIDS (oral and nasal inhalation)

GENERIC NAME	BRAND NAMES	INDICATIONS/ADULT DOSE	CLINICAL IMPLICATIONS*
Fluticasone	Flonase, Flovent	**Seasonal Allergic Rhinitis:** *Adult:* **Intranasal** 100 μg (1 inhalation) in each nostril 1–2 times daily (max 4 times daily). **Inhalation** 1–2 inhalations b.i.d. *Child ≥4 y:* **Intranasal** 1 spray in each nostril once daily. May increase to 2 sprays in each nostril once daily if inadequate response, then decrease to 1 spray in each nostril once daily when control is achieved.	
Mometasone furoate monohydrate	Nasonex	*Adult:* **Intranasal** 2 sprays (50 μg each) in each nostril once daily	
Triamcinolone acetonide	Azmacort	*Adult:* **Inhalation** 2 puffs 3–4 times/d (max 16 puffs/d) or 4 puffs b.i.d. *Child 6–12 y:* **Inhalation** 1–2 sprays t.i.d. or q.i.d. (max 12 sprays/d) or 2–4 sprays b.i.d.	

*Clinical implications apply to all drugs in the group unless otherwise noted.

GENERIC NAME	BRAND NAMES	INDICATIONS/ADULT DOSE	CLINICAL IMPLICATIONS*
Corticosteroid, Antiinflammatory **Prototype for classification:** Hydrocortisone		**USE** Relief of inflammatory and pruritic manifestations of corticosteroid-responsive dermatoses.	**Contraindicated in:** topical steroids contraindicated in presence of varicella, vaccinia, on surfaces with compromised circulation, and in children <2 y. **Cautious use in:** children; diabetes mellitus; stromal herpes simplex; glaucoma, tuberculosis of eye; osteoporosis; untreated fungal, bacterial, or viral infections. **ADVERSE/SIDE EFFECTS Skin:** skin thinning and atrophy, *acne, impaired wound healing;* petechiae, ecchymosis, easy bruising; suppression of skin test reaction; hypopigmentation or hyperpigmentation, hirsutism, acneiform eruptions, subcutaneous fat atrophy; allergic dermatitis, urticaria, angioneurotic edema, increased sweating.
Hydrocortisone	Aeroseb-HC, Alphaderm, Cetacort, Cortaid, Cort-Dome, Cortenema, Cortril, DermaCort, Dermolate, Hydrocortone,	*Adult:* apply a small amount to the affected area 1–4 times/d. **PR** insert 1% cream, 10% foam, 10–25 mg suppository, or 100-mg enema nightly.	Administer retention enema preferably after a bowel movement. The enema should be retained at least 1 h or all night if possible.
Hydrocortisone acetate	Hytone, Proctocort, RectocortA, Synacort Anusol HC, CaldeCort, Carmol HC, Colifoam, Cortaid, Cortamed, Cort-Dome, Cortef Acetate, Corticaine, Cortifoam, CortimentA Epifoam, Hydrocortone Acetate		If an occlusive dressing is to be used, apply medication sparingly, rub until it disappears, and then reapply, leaving a thin coat over lesion. Completely cover area with transparent plastic or other occlusive device or vehicle.

*Clinical implications apply to all drugs in the group unless otherwise noted.

GENERIC NAME	BRAND NAMES	INDICATIONS/ADULT DOSE	CLINICAL IMPLICATIONS*
Aclometasone dipropionate	Alclovate	0.05% cream or ointment applied sparingly b.i.d. or t.i.d.; may use occlusive dressing for resistant dermatoses.	Avoid covering a weeping or exudative lesion. Usually, occlusive dressings are not applied to face, scalp, scrotum, axilla, and groin.
Amcinonide	Cyclocort	Apply thin film b.i.d. or t.i.d.	Inspect skin carefully between applications for ecchymotic, petechial, and purpuric signs, maceration, secondary infection, skin atrophy, striae or miliaria; if present, stop medication and notify physician.
Clobetasol propionate	Dermovate, Temovate	Apply sparingly b.i.d. (max 50 g/wk), or b.i.d. 3 d/wk or 1–2 times/wk for up to 6 mo.	
Clocortolone pivalate	Cloderm	Apply thin layer 1–4 times/d	Warn patient not to self-dose with OTC topical preparations of a corticosteroid more than 7 d. They should not be used for children <2 y. If symptoms do not abate, consult physician.
Desonide	DesOwen, Tridesilon	Apply thin layer b.i.d. to q.i.d.	
Desoximetasone	Topicort, Topicort-LP	Apply thin layer b.i.d.	
Dexamethasone	Decaderm, Decadron	Apply thin layer t.i.d. or q.i.d.	Usually, topical preparations are applied after a shower or bath when skin is damp or wet.
			Cleansing and application of prescribed preparation should be done with extreme gentleness because of fragility, easy bruisability, and poor healing skin.
			Hazard of systemic toxicity is higher in small children because of the greater ratio of skin surface area to body weight. Apply sparingly.
			Urge patient on long-term therapy with topical corticosterone to check shelf-life date.

Diflorasone diacetate	Florone, Florone E, Maxiflor, Psorcon	Apply thin layer of ointment 1–3 times/d or cream 2–4 times/d
Fluocinolone acetonide	FluodermA, Fluolar, Fluonid, Flurosyn, Synalar, Synalar-HP, Synemol	Apply thin layer b.i.d. to q.i.d.
Fluocinonide	Lidemol, Lidex, Lidex-E, Lyderm, Topsyn	Apply thin layer b.i.d. to q.i.d.
Fluandrenolide	Cordran, Cordran SP, DrenisonA	*Adult:* apply thin layer b.i.d. or t.i.d.; apply tape 1–2 times/d at 12-h intervals. *Child:* apply thin layer 1–2 times/d; apply tape once/d.
Fluticasone	Flonase	Apply thin film of cream or ointment to affected area once or twice daily.
Mometasone furoate	Elocon	Apply a thin film of cream or ointment or a few drops of lotion to affected area once daily.
Triamcinolone	Aristocort, Atolone, Kenacort, Kenalog, Kenalog-E	Apply sparingly b.i.d. or t.i.d.

*Clinical implications apply to all drugs in the group unless otherwise noted.

Schedule I

High potential for abuse and of no currently accepted medical use. Examples: heroin, LSD, marijuana, mescaline, peyote. Not obtainable by prescription but may be legally procured for research, study, or instructional use.

Schedule II

High abuse potential and high liability for severe psychlogical or physical dependence. Prescription required and cannot be renewed.[a] Includes opium derivatives, other opioids, and short-acting barbiturates. Examples: amphetamine, cocaine, meperidine, morphine, secobarbital.

Schedule III

Potential for abuse is less than that for drugs in Schedules I and II. Moderate to low physical dependence and high psychological dependence. Includes certain stimulants and depressants not included in the above schedules and preparations containing limited quantities of certain opioids. Examples: chlorphentermine, glutethimide, mazindol, paregoric, phendimetrazine. Prescription required.[b]

Schedule IV

Lower potential for abuse than Schedule III drugs. Examples: certain psychotropics (tranquilizers), chloral hydrate, chlordiazepoxide, diazepam, meprobamate, phenobarbital. Prescription required.[a]

Schedule V

Abuse potential less than that for Schedule IV drugs. Preparations contain limited quantities of certain narcotic drugs; generally intended for antitussive and antidiarrheal purposes and may be distributed without a prescription provided that:

1. Such distribution is made only by a pharmacist.
2. Not more than 240 ml or not more than 48 solid dosage units of any substance containing opium, nor more than 120 ml or not more than 24 solid dosage units of any other controlled substance may be distributed at retail to the same purchaser in any given 48-hour period without a valid prescription order.
3. The purchaser is at least 18 years old.
4. The pharmacist knows the purchaser or requests suitable identification.
5. The pharmacist keeps an official written record of: name and address of purchaser, name and quantity of controlled substance purchased, date of sale, initials of dispensing pharmacist. This record is to be made available for inspection

and copying by U.S. officers authorized by the Attorney General.
6. Other federal, state, or local law does not require a prescription order.

Under jurisdiction of the Federal Controlled Substances Act.
[a]Except when dispensed directly by a practitioner, other than a pharmacist, to an ultimate user, no controlled substance in Schedule II may be dispensed without a *written* prescription, except that in emergency situations such drug may be dispensed upon oral prescription and a written prescription must be obtained within the time frame prescribed by law. No prescription for a controlled substance in Schedule II may be refilled.
[b]Refillable up to 5 times within 6 mo, but only if so indicated by physician.

◆ APPENDIX C CANADIAN CONTROLLED SUBSTANCE CLASSIFICATIONS

Narcotics (N)

Includes products containing a narcotic. Within this broad classification are several levels of regulatory control. These levels range from strict controls for the most abusable of the substances (for example, single-entity narcotics; products containing a narcotic with one active nonnarcotic ingredient; any preparation containing heroin, hydrocodone, or oxycodone) to lesser controls for preparations containing one narcotic and two active nonnarcotic ingredients and exempt codeine preparations (those containing a limited amount of codeine plus two active nonnarcotic ingredients).

Controlled Drugs (C)

Includes nonnarcotic preparations with abuse potential. As with narcotics, different regulations apply, depending on specific content. C drugs include drugs such as amphetamines and barbiturates.

The specific drugs listed under any given controlled substance level within each classification are determined by the individual provinces.

◆ APPENDIX D FDA PREGNANCY CATEGORIES

The FDA requires that all prescription drugs absorbed systemically or known to be potentially harmful to the fetus be classified according to one of five pregnancy categories (A, B, C, D, X). The identifying letter signifies the level of risk to the fetus and is to appear in the precautions section of the package insert. The categories described by the FDA are as follows:

Category A

Controlled studies in women fail to demonstrate a risk to the fetus in the first trimester (and there is no evidence of risk in later trimesters), and the possibility of fetal harm appears remote.

Category B

Either animal-reproduction studies have not demonstrated a fetal risk but there are no controlled studies in pregnant women, or animal-reproduction studies have shown an adverse effect (other than a decrease in fertility) that was not confirmed in controlled studies in women in the first trimester (and there is no evidence of a risk in later trimesters).

Category C

Either studies in animals have revealed adverse effects on the fetus (teratogenic or embryocidal effects or other) and there are no controlled studies in women, or studies in women and animals are not available. Drugs should be given only if the potential benefit justifies the potential risk to the fetus.

Category D

There is positive evidence of human fetal risk, but the benefits from use in pregnant women may be acceptable despite the risk (e.g., if the drug is needed in a life-threatening situation or for a serious disease for which safer drugs cannot be used or are ineffective). There will be an appropriate statement in the "warnings" section of the labeling.

Category X

Studies in animals or human beings have demonstrated fetal abnormalities or there is evidence of fetal risk based on human experience, or both, and the risk of the use of the drug in pregnant women clearly outweighs any possible benefit. The drug is contraindicated in women who are or may become pregnant. There will be an appropriate statement in the "contraindications" section of the labeling.

◆ APPENDIX E ORAL DOSAGE FORMS THAT SHOULD NOT BE CRUSHED

Some oral dosage forms should not be crushed or chewed. These dosage forms have been specially designed to release the drug slowly over several hours, to protect the drug from the low pH of the stomach, and/or to protect the stomach from the irritating effects of the drug.

Drugs may have an **enteric coating** which is designed to allow the drug to pass through the stomach intact with the drug being released in the intestines. This protects the stomach from the irritating effects of the drug, protects the drug from being destroyed by the acid pH of the stomach, and can delay the onset of action.

Extended-release (slow release, SR) formulations are designed to release the drug over an extended period of time. These formulations can include multiple-layer compressed tablets where drug is released as each layer dissolves, mixed-release pellets that dissolve at different time intervals, and special tablets that are themselves inert but are designed to release drug slowly from the formulation. Some extended-release dosage forms are scored and may be broken in half without affecting the release mechanism but still should not be crushed or chewed. Some mixed-release capsule formulations can be opened and the contents sprinkled on food. However, the pellets should not be crushed or chewed. Some extended-release formulations can be identified by common abbreviations used in their brand names. These abbreviations include: CR (controlled release), CRT (controlled-release tablet), LA (long acting), SR (sustained release), TR (time release), SA (sustained action), and XL or XR (extended release).

Occasionally, drugs should not be crushed because they are oral mucosa irritants, are extremely bitter, or contain dyes that may stain teeth or mucosal tissue.

The table contains a list of drugs found in the Guide that should not be crushed or chewed. A liquid dosage form may be available for many of these drugs. However, the dose or frequency of administration may be different from the slow-release product. Check with your pharmacist for liquid availability and dosing conversions.

	Generic Name	Comments
Accutane	isotretinoin	mucous membrane irritant
Acutrim	phenylpropanolamine	slow release
Adalat CC	nifedipine	slow release
Allerest 12 Hour	chlorpheniramine, phenylpropanolamine	slow release
Artane Sequels	trihexyphenydil	slow release; capsules may be opened and contents taken without chewing or crushing
Azulfidine Entabs	sulfasalazine	enteric coated

	Generic Name	Comments
Bayer Extra Strength Enteric 500	aspirin, enteric coated	enteric coated; slow release
Bayer Low Adult 81 mg	aspirin, enteric coated	enteric coated
Bayer Caplet	aspirin, enteric coated	enteric coated
Biphetamine	amphetamine, dextro-amphetamine	slow release
Bisacodyl	bisacodyl	enteric coated
Biscolax	bisacodyl	enteric coated
Bromfed, Bromfed-PD	brompheniramine, pseudoephedrine	slow release
Calan SR	verapamil	slow release
Cama Arthritis Strength	aspirin, magnesium oxide, aluminum hydroxide	special table formulation
Cardizem, Cardizem CD, Cardizem SR	diltiazem	slow release; capsules may be opened and contents taken without chewing or crushing
Chloral Hydrate	chloral hydrate	liquid-filled capsule
Chlor-Trimeton Repetab	chlorpheniramine	slow release
Choledyl SA	oxytriphylline	slow release
Compazine Spansule	prochlorperazine	slow release; capsules may be opened and contents taken without chewing or crushing
Constant T	theophylline	slow release; capsules may be opened and contents taken without chewing or crushing
Contac	chlorpheniramine, phenylpropanolamine	slow release; capsules may be opened and contents taken without chewing or crushing
Cotazym S	pancrelipase	enteric coated; capsules may be opened and contents taken without chewing or crushing
Covera-HS	verapamil	slow release
Deconamine SR	chlorpheniramine, pseudoephedrine	slow release
Depakene	valproic acid	slow release; mucous membrane irritant
Depakote	valproate disodium	enteric coated

	Generic Name	Comments
Desoxyn Gradumets	methamphetamine	slow release
Dexatrim Max Strength	phenylpropanolamine	slow release
Dexedrine Spansule	dextroamphetamine	slow release
Diamox Sequels	acetazolamide	slow release
Dilacor XR	diltiazem	slow release
Dilatrate SR	isosorbide dinitrate	slow release
Dimetane Extentab	brompheniramine, phenylephrine	slow release
Disophrol Chronotab	dexbrompheniramine, pseudoephedrine	slow release
Donnatol Extentab	atropine, scopolamine, hyoscyamine, phenobarbital	slow release
Donnazyme	pancreatin, pepsin, bile salts, atropine, scopolamine, hyoscyamine, phenobarbital	slow release
Drixoral	dexbrompheniramine, pseudoephedrine	slow release
Dulcolax	bisacodyl	enteric coated
Easprin	aspirin	enteric coated
Ecotrin	aspirin	enteric coated
E.E.S 400	erythromycin ethylsuccinate	enteric coated
Elixophyllin SR	theophylline	slow release; capsules may be opened and contents taken without chewing or crushing
E-Mycin	erythromycin	enteric coated
Ergostat	ergotamine	sublingual tablet
Eryc	erythromycin	enteric coated; capsules may be opened and contents taken without chewing or crushing
Ery-tab	erythromycin	enteric coated
Erythromycin Stearate	erythromycin	enteric coated
Erythromycin Base	erythromycin	enteric coated
Eskalith CR	lithium	slow release

	Generic Name	Comments
Fedahist Timecaps	chlorpheniramine, pseudoephedrine	slow release
Feldene	piroxicam	mucous membrane irritant
Feosol	ferrous sulfate	enteric coated
Feosol Spansule	ferrous sulfate	slow release; capsules may be opened and contents taken without chewing or crushing
Fergon	ferrous gluconate	slow release; capsules may be opened and contents taken without chewing or crushing
Ferro-Sequels	ferrous fumarate, docusate	slow release
Fero-Gradumet	ferrous sulfate	slow release
Festal II	pancrelipase	enteric coated
Glucotrol XL	glyburide	slow release
Gris-Peg	griseofulvin	crushing may result in precipitation of drug as larger particles
Ilotycin	erythromycin	enteric coated
Inderal LA	propranolol	slow release
Inderide LA	propranolol, hydro-chlorothiazide	slow release
Indocin SR	indomethacin	slow release; capsules may be opened and contents taken without chewing or crushing
Isoptin SR	verapamil	slow release
Isordil Tembid	isosorbide dinitrate	slow release
Iso-Bid	isosorbide dinitrate	slow release
Isosorbide dinitrate SR	isosorbide dinitrate	slow release
Isuprel Glossets	isoproterenol	sublingual
Kaon CL 10	postassium chloride	slow release
Klor-Con	postassium chloride	slow release
Klotrix	postassium chloride	slow release
K-Tab	postassium chloride	slow release
Levsinex Timecaps	hyoscyamine	slow release
Lithobid	lithium	slow release
Meprospan	meprobamate	slow release; capsules may be opened and contents taken without chewing or crushing

	Generic Name	Comments
Mestinon Timespan	pyridostigmine	slow release
Micro K	postassium chloride	slow release
MS Contin	morphine	slow release
Naldecon	phenylepherine, phenylpropanolamine, chlorpheniramine, phenyltoloxamine	slow release
Nico 400	niacin	slow release
Nicobid	niacin	slow release
Nitro Bid	nitroglycerin	slow release; capsules may be opened and contents taken without chewing or crushing
Nitroglyn	nitroglycerin	slow release; capsules may be opened and contents taken without chewing or crushing
Nitrong SR	nitroglycerin	slow release
Nolamine	phenylpropanolamine, chlorpheniramine, phenindamine	slow release
Norflex	orphenadrine	slow release
Norpace CR	disopyramide	slow release
Novafed A	pseudoephedrine, chlorpheniramine	slow release
Oramorph SR	morphine	slow release
Ornade Spansule	phenylpropanolamine, chlorpheniramine	slow release
Pancrease	pancrelipase	enteric coated
Papaverine Sustained Action	papaverine	slow release
Pavabid	papaverine	slow release
Pavabid Plateau	papaverine	slow release; capsules may be opened and contents taken without chewing or crushing
PBZ-SR	tripelenamine	slow release
Perdiem	psyllium hydrophilic mucioid	wax coated
Peritrate SA	pentaerythritol tetranitrate	slow release
Permitil Chronotab	fluphenazine	slow release

	Generic Name	Comments
Phazyme, Phazyme 95	simethicone	slow release
Phyllocontin	aminophylline	slow release
Plendil	felodipine	slow release
Polaramine Repetabs	dexchlorpheniramine	slow release
Prevacid	lansoprazole	slow release; capsules may be opened and contents taken without chewing or crushing
Prilosec	omeprazole	slow release
Procainamide HCl SR	procainamide	slow release
Procan SR	procainamide	slow release
Procardia XL	nifedipine	slow release
Pronestyl SR	procainamide	slow release
Proventil Repetabs	albuterol	slow release
Prozac	fluoxetine	slow release; capsules may be opened and contents taken without chewing or crushing
Quibron-T SR	theophylline	slow release
Quinaglute Dura Tabs	quinidine gluconate	slow release
Quinidex Extentabs	quinidine sulfate	slow release
Respid	theophylline	slow release
Ritalin SR	methylphenidate	slow release
Robimycin Robitab	erythromycin	enteric coated
Rondec TR	pseudoephedrine, carbinoxamine	slow release
Roxanol SR	morphine	slow release
Sinemet CR	levodopa, carbidopa	slow release; tablet is scored and may be broken in half
Slo-Bid Gyrocaps	theophylline	slow release; capsules may be opened and contents taken without chewing or crushing
Slo-Phyllin Gyrocaps	theophylline	slow release; capsules may be opened and contents taken without chewing or crushing
Slow-Fe	ferrous sulfate	slow release

	Generic Name	Comments
Slow-K	potassium chloride	slow release
Sorbitrate SA	isosorbide dinitrate	slow release
Sudafed 12 hour	pseudoephedrine	slow release
Tavist-D	phenylpropanolamine, clemastine	multiple compressed tablet
Teldrin	chlorpheniramine	slow release; capsules may be opened and contents taken without chewing or crushing
Tepanil Ten-Tab	diethylpropion	slow release
Tessalon Perles	benzonatate	slow release
Theo-24	theophylline	slow release
Theobid, Theobid Jr.	theophylline	slow release
Theo-Dur	theophylline	slow release
Theo-Dur Sprinkle	theophylline	slow release; capsules may be opened and contents taken without chewing or crushing
Theolair SR	theophylline	slow release
Thorazine Spansule	chlorpromazine	slow release
Toprol XL	metaprolol	slow release
Trental	pentoxifylline	slow release
Triaminic	phenylpropanolamine, chlorpheniramine	enteric coated
Triaminic 12	phenylpropanolamine, chlorpheniramine	slow release
Triaminic TR	phenylpropanolamine, pyrilamine, pheniramine	multiple compressed tablet
Trilafon Repetabs	perphenazine	slow release
Triptone Caplets	scopolamine	slow release
Uniphyl	theophylline	slow release
Valrelease	diazepam	slow release
Verelan	verapamil	slow release; capsules may be opened and contents taken without chewing or crushing
Volmax	albuterol	slow release
Welbutrin SR	bupropion	slow release
Wyamycin S	erythromycin stearate	slow release
ZORprin	aspirin	slow release

Actifed (DECONGESTANT [ADRENERGIC]) *capsule or tablet:* pseudoephedrine hydrochloride 60 mg, triprolidine hydrochloride 2.5 mg; *syrup (per 5 ml):* pseudoephedrine hydrochloride 30 mg, triprolidine hydrochloride 1.25 mg.

Agoral (LAXATIVE [LUBRICANT]) *emulsion (per 15 ml):* mineral oil 4.2 g, phenolphthalein 0.2 g with agar, tragacanth, egg albumin, acacia, and glycerin.

Agoral, Plain (LAXATIVE [LUBRICANT]) *emulsion (per 15 ml):* mineral oil 4.2 g with agar, tragacanth, egg albumin, acacia, and glycerin.

Aladrine* (ANTIASTHMATIC) *tablet:* ephedrine sulfate 8.1 mg, secobarbital sodium 16.2 mg.

Alazide* (DIURETIC) *tablet:* spironolactone 25 mg, hydrochlorothiazide 25 mg.

Aldactazide 25/25* (DIURETIC) *tablet:* spironolactone 25 mg, hydrochlorothiazide 25 mg.

Aldactazide 50/50* (DIURETIC) *tablet:* spironolactone 50 mg, hydrochlorothiazide 50 mg.

Aldoclor-150* (ANTIHYPERTENSIVE) *tablet:* chlorothiazide 150 mg, methyldopa 250 mg.

Aldoclor-250* (ANTIHYPERTENSIVE) *tablet:* chlorothiazide 250 mg, methyldopa 250 mg.

Aldoril-15* (ANTIHYPERTENSIVE) *tablet:* hydrochlorothiazide 15 mg, methyldopa 250 mg.

Aldoril-25* (ANTIHYPERTENSIVE) *tablet:* hydrochlorothiazide 25 mg, methyldopa 250 mg.

Aldoril D30* (ANTIHYPERTENSIVE) *tablet:* hydrochlorothiazide 30 mg, methyldopa 500 mg.

Aldoril D50* (ANTIHYPERTENSIVE) *tablet:* hydrochlorothiazide 50 mg, methyldopa 500 mg.

Alka Seltzer (with Aspirin) (ANALGESIC, ANTACID) *effervescent tablet:* aspirin 324 mg with sodium bicarbonate 1.9 g and citric acid 1 g; sodium content 567 mg/tablet, ANC 17.2 mEq/tablet.

Alka Seltzer (without Aspirin) (ANTACID) *effervescent tablet:* sodium bicarbonate 958 mg, citric acid 832 mg, potassium bicarbonate 312 mg; sodium content 284 mg, ANC 10.6 mEq/tablet.

Allegra-D* (ANTIHISTAMINE–DECONGESTANT) *extended-release tablet:* fexofenadine HCl 60 mg, pseudoephedrine HCl 120 mg.

Allerest Tablets (Adults) (DECONGESTANT, ANTIHISTAMINE) *tablet:* phenylpropanolamine hydrochloride 18.7 mg, chlorpheniramine maleate 2 mg.

Allerest Tablets (Children) (DECONGESTANT, ANTIHISTAMINE) *tablet:* phenylpropanolamine hydrochloride 9.4 mg, chlorpheniramine maleate 1 mg.

Allerest 12 Hour Capsules (DECONGESTANT, ANTIHISTAMINE) *sustained-release capsule:* phenylpropanolamine hydrochloride 75 mg, chlorpheniramine maleate 8 mg.

Alma-Mag Improved (ANTACID) *chewable tablet, liquid (per 5 ml):* aluminum hydroxide 200 mg, magnesium hydroxide 200 mg, simethicone 20 mg.

Aludrox (ANTACID) *suspension (per 5 ml):* aluminum hydroxide 307 mg, magnesium hydroxide 103 mg, saccharin, sorbitol, sodium content 2.3 mg, ANC 12 mEq; *chewable tablet:* aluminum hydroxide 233 mg, magnesium hydroxide 83 mg, saccharin, sodium content 1.4 mg, ANC 10 mEq/tablet.

Amacodone C* (NARCOTIC AGONIST ANALGESIC [schedule III]) *tablet:* hy-

*Prescription drug.

drocodone bitartrate 5 mg, acetaminophen 500 mg.

Amaphen* (NONNARCOTIC AGONIST ANALGESIC) *capsule:* acetaminophen 325 mg, caffeine 40 mg, butalbital 50 mg.

Amaphen with Codeine* (NARCOTIC AGONIST ANALGESIC [schedule III]) *capsule:* codeine phosphate 30 mg, acetaminophen 325 mg, caffeine 40 mg, butalbital 50 mg.

Ambenyl Cough Syrup* (ANTITUSSIVE) *syrup:* bromodiphenhydramine hydrochloride 12.5 mg, codeine phosphate 10 mg, alcohol 5%.

Amesec (ANTIASTHMATIC) ephedrine 25 mg, theophylline 104 mg.

Anacin (NONNARCOTIC AGONIST ANALGESIC) *caplet, tablet:* aspirin 400 mg, caffeine 32 mg.

Anatuss Syrup (ANTITUSSIVE) *syrup:* phenylpropanolamine 25 mg, dextromethorphan 15 mg, guaifenesin 100 mg.

Anatuss Tablets (ANTITUSSIVE) *tablet:* phenylpropanolamine 25 mg, dextromethorphan 15 mg, guaifenesin 100 mg, acetaminophen 325 mg.

Anbesol (LOCAL ANESTHETIC) benzocaine 6.3%, phenol 0.5%, alcohol 70%.

Anexsia 5/500* (NARCOTIC ANALGESIC [schedule III]) hydrocodone 5 mg, acetaminophen 500 mg.

Anexsia 7.5/650* (NARCOTIC ANALGESIC [schedule III]) hydrocodone 7.5 mg, acetaminophen 650 mg.

Anodynos-DHC* (NARCOTIC ANALGESIC [schedule III]) hydrocodone 5 mg, acetaminophen 500 mg.

Anoquan* (NONNARCOTIC AGONIST ANALGESIC) *capsule:* acetaminophen 325 mg, caffeine 40 mg, butalbital 50 mg.

Antrocol* (GASTROINTESTINAL ANTICHOLINERGIC, SEDATIVE) *capsule, tablet:* atropine sulfate 0.195 mg, phenobarbital 16 mg.

Apresazide 25/25* (ANTIHYPERTENSIVE) *capsule:* hydralazine hydrochloride 25 mg, hydrochlorothiazide 25 mg.

Apresazide 50/50* (ANTIHYPERTENSIVE) *capsule:* hydralazine hydrochloride 50 mg, hydrochlorothiazide 50 mg.

Apresazide 100/50* (ANTIHYPERTENSIVE) *capsule:* hydralazine hydrochloride 100 mg, hydrochlorothiazide 50 mg.

Apresodex* (ANTIHYPERTENSIVE) *tablet:* hydralazine hydrochloride 25 mg, hydrochlorothiazide 15 mg.

Apresoline-Esidrex* (ANTIHYPERTENSIVE) *tablet:* hydralazine hydrochloride 25 mg, hydrochlorothiazide 15 mg.

Aprodine Syrup (ANTIHISTAMINE, DECONGESTANT) *syrup:* pseudoephedrine 60 mg, triprolidine 2.5 mg.

Aprozide 25/25* (ANTIHYPERTENSIVE) hydralazine 25 mg, hydrochlorothiazide 25 mg.

Aprozide 50/50* (ANTIHYPERTENSIVE) hydralazine 50 mg, hydrochlorothiazide 50 mg.

Aprozide 100/50* (ANTIHYPERTENSIVE) hydralazine 100 mg, hydrochlorothiazide 50 mg.

Aralen Phosphate with Primaquine Phosphate* (ANTIMALARIAL) *tablet:* chloroquine phosphate 500 mg (300 mg base), primaquine phosphate 79 mg (45 mg base).

Arthrotec 50* (NSAID) *tablet:* diclofenac sodium 50 mg, misoprostol 200 µg.

Arthrotec 75* (NSAID) *tablet:* diclofenac sodium 75 mg, misoprostol 200 µg.

Ascriptin (NONNARCOTIC AGONIST ANALGESIC) *tablet:* aspirin 325 mg, magnesium hydroxide 75 mg, aluminum hydroxide 75 mg.

Auralgan Otic* (OTIC PREPARATION: DECONGESTANT, ANALGESIC) *solution:* benzocaine 1.4%, antipyrine 5.4%, glycerin, oxyquinoline sulfate.

Axotal* (NONNARCOTIC AGONIST ANAL-

GESIC) *tablet:* aspirin 650 mg, butalbital 50 mg.

Azdone* (NARCOTIC AGONIST ANALGESIC [schedule III]) *tablet:* hydrocodone bitartrate 5 mg, aspirin 500 mg.

Azo Gantanol* (URINARY ANTIINFECTIVE, ANALGESIC) *tablet:* sulfamethoxazole 500 mg, phenazopyridine hydrochloride 100 mg.

Azo Gantrisin* (URINARY ANTIINFECTIVE, ANALGESIC) *tablet:* sulfisoxazole 500 mg, phenazopyridine hydrochloride 50 mg.

B-A-C* (ANALGESIC) acetaminophen 650 mg, caffeine 40 mg, butalbital 50 mg.

Bacticort Ophthalmic* (ANTIINFLAMMATORY) *suspension:* hydrocortisone 1%, neomycin sulfate 0.35%, polymyxin B 10,000 units.

Bancap* (NONNARCOTIC AGONIST ANALGESIC) *capsule:* acetaminophen 325 mg, butalbital 50 mg.

Bancap HC* (NARCOTIC AGONIST ANALGESIC [schedule III]) *capsule:* hydrocodone bitartrate 5 mg, acetaminophen 500 mg.

Barbidonna Elixir* (GASTROINTESTINAL ANTICHOLINERGIC, SEDATIVE) *syrup:* atropine sulfate 0.034 mg, scopolamine hydrobromide 0.01 mg, hyoscyamine hydrobromide or sulfate 0.174 mg, phenobarbital 21.6 mg per 5 ml, alcohol 15%.

Barbidonna Tablets* (GASTROINTESTINAL ANTICHOLINERGIC, SEDATIVE) *tablet:* atropine sulfate 0.025 mg, scopolamine hydrobromide 0.0074 mg, hyoscyamine hydrobromide or sulfate 0.1286 mg, phenobarbital 16 mg/tablet.

Barbidonna #2 Tablets* (GASTROINTESTINAL ANTICHOLINERGIC, SEDATIVE) *tablet:* atropine sulfate 0.025 mg, scopolamine hydrobromide 0.0074 mg, hyoscyamine hydrobromide or sulfate 0.1286 mg, phenobarbital 32 mg/tablet.

BC Powder (NONNARCOTIC AGONIST ANALGESIC) *powder:* aspirin 650 mg, salicylamide 195 mg, caffeine 32 mg/powder packet.

BC Tablets (NONNARCOTIC AGONIST ANALGESIC) *tablet:* aspirin 325 mg, salicylamide 95 mg, caffeine 16 mg/tablet.

Bellafoline* (GASTROINTESTINAL ANTICHOLINERGIC, SEDATIVE) *tablet:* levorotatory alkaloids of belladonna 0.25 mg; *injection:* levorotatory alkaloids of belladonna 0.5 mg/ml.

Bellergal-S* (GASTROINTESTINAL ANTICHOLINERGIC, SEDATIVE) *tablet:* l-alkaloids of belladonna 0.2 mg, phenobarbital 40 mg, ergotamine tartrate 0.6 mg, *tartrazine.*

Betoptic Pilo Suspension* (ANTIGLAUCOMA) Betaxolol 0.25%, pilocarpine 1.75%.

Biphetamine 12$^{1}/_{(2)}$* (AMPHETAMINE [schedule II]) *capsule:* dextroamphetamine 6.25 mg, amphetamine 6.25 mg.

Biphetamine 20* (AMPHETAMINE [schedule II]) *capsule:* dextroamphetamine 10 mg, amphetamine 10 mg.

Bisodol (ANTACID) *chewable tablet:* magnesium hydroxide 178 mg, calcium carbonate 194 mg, saccharin, sorbitol; *powder:* sodium bicarbonate 644 mg, magnesium carbonate 475 mg; sodium content: 157 mg/5 g, ANC 15 mEq.

Blephamide* (OPHTHALMIC STEROID, SULFONAMIDE) *suspension:* prednisolone acetate 0.2%, sodium sulfacetamide 10%, EDTA, polyvinyl alcohol 1.4%, polysorbate 80, sodium thiosulfate, benzalkonium chloride.

Blephamide S.O.P.* (OPHTHALMIC STEROID, SULFONAMIDE) *ointment:* prednisolone acetate 0.2%, sodium sulfacetamide 10%, phenylmercuric acetate, mineral oil, white petrolatum, nonionic lanolin derivatives.

Brevicon* (MONOPHASIC ORAL CONTRA-

CEPTIVE [ESTROGEN, PROGESTIN]) *tablet:* estrogen: ethinyl estradiol 35 µg; progestin: norethindrone 0.5 mg.

Bromfed* (DECONGESTANT, ANTIHISTAMINE) *sustained-released capsule:* pseudoephedrine hydrochloride 120 mg, brompheniramine maleate 12 mg.

Bromfed-PD* (DECONGESTANT, ANTIHISTAMINE) *sustained-release capsule:* pseudoephedrine hydrochloride 60 mg, brompheniramine maleate 6 mg.

Bromo Seltzer (ANALGESIC, ANTACID) *effervescent granules:* acetaminophen 325 mg, sodium bicarbonate 2.781 g, citric acid 2.224 g/capful measure, sodium content 761 mg/dosage measure.

Bronchial Capsules* (ANTIASTHMATIC) *capsule:* theophylline 150 mg, guaifenesin 90 mg/capsule.

Brondecon* (ANTIASTHMATIC) *tablet:* oxtriphylline 200 mg, guaifenesin 100 mg, saccharin.

Bronkaid Tablets (ANTIASTHMATIC) *tablet:* theophylline 100 mg, ephedrine sulfate 24 mg, guaifenesin 100 mg.

Bufferin (ANALGESIC, ANTACID) *tablet:* aspirin 324 mg, magnesium carbonate, aluminum glycinate.

Butace* (ANALGESIC) acetaminophen 325 mg, caffeine 40 mg, butalbital 50 mg.

Butibel* (GASTROINTESTINAL ANTICHOLINERGIC, SEDATIVE) *elixir:* belladonna extract 15 mg, butabarbital sodium 15 mg, alcohol 7% per 5 ml, *tartrazine; tablet:* belladonna extract 15 mg, butabarbital sodium 15 mg.

Cafergot Suppositories* (ANTIMIGRAINE) *suppository:* ergotamine tartrate 2 mg, caffeine 100 mg/suppository.

Cafergot P-B Suppositories* (ANTIMIGRAINE) *suppository:* ergotamine tartrate 2 mg, caffeine 100 mg, l-alkaloids of belladonna 0.25 mg, pentobarbital 60 mg/suppository.

Caladryl (TOPICAL ANTIHISTAMINE) *cream:* diphenhydramine hydrochloride 1%, calamine, camphor; *lotion:* diphenhydramine hydrochloride 1%, calamine, camphor, alcohol 2%.

Calcet (CALCIUM SUPPLEMENT) Calcium 153 mg, vitamin D 100 IU.

Calcidrine Syrup* (ANTITUSSIVE [schedule V]) *syrup:* codeine 8.4 mg, calcium iodide 152 mg, alcohol 6%.

Cama Arthritis Strength (NONNARCOTIC ANALGESIC, ANTACID) *tablet:* aspirin 500 mg, magnesium oxide 150 mg, aluminum hydroxide 150 mg.

Camalox (ANTACID) *suspension, chewable tablet:* aluminum hydroxide 225 mg, magnesium hydroxide 200 mg, calcium carbonate 250 mg, saccharin, sorbitol; sodium content (suspension): 1.2 mg, ANC 18.5 mEq, sodium content (tablet) 1 mg, ANC 18 mEq/ml.

Cam-ap-es* (ANTIHYPERTENSIVE) *suspension, tablet:* hydrochlorothiazide 15 mg, reserpine 0.1 mg, hydralazine hydrochloride 25 mg.

Capital with Codeine* (NARCOTIC ANALGESIC [schedule V]) *suspension:* codeine phosphate 12 mg, acetaminophen 120 mg/5 ml.

Capozide 25/15* (ANTIHYPERTENSIVE) *tablet:* captopril 25 mg, hydrochlorothiazide 15 mg.

Capozide 25/25* (ANTIHYPERTENSIVE) *tablet:* captopril 25 mg, hydrochlorothiazide 25 mg.

Capozide 50/15* (ANTIHYPERTENSIVE) *tablet:* captopril 50 mg, hydrochlorothiazide 15 mg.

Capozide 50/25* (ANTIHYPERTENSIVE) *tablet:* captopril 50 mg, hydrochlorothiazide 25 mg.

Carisoprodol Compound* (SKELETAL MUSCLE RELAXANT, ANALGESIC) *tablet:* carisoprodol 200 mg, aspirin 325 mg.

Carmol HC* (ANTIINFLAMMATORY) *cream:* hydrocortisone acetate 1%, urea 10%.

Celestone-Soluspan* (GLUCOCORTICOID) *injection (suspension):* betamethasone acetate 3 mg, betamethasone sodium phosphate 3 mg/ml.

Cetacaine* (TOPICAL ANESTHETIC) *gel, liquid, ointment, aerosol:* benzocaine 14%, tetracaine hydrochloride 2%, butamben 2%, benzalkonium chloride 0.5% with cetyldimethylethylammonium bromide.

Cetapred* (STEROID, SULFONAMIDE) *ophthalmic ointment:* prednisolone acetate 0.25%, sodium sulfacetamide 10%, mineral oil, white petrolatum, liquid lanolin, parabens.

Chardonna-2* (GASTROINTESTINAL ANTICHOLINERGIC, SEDATIVE) *tablet:* belladonna extract 15 mg, phenobarbital 15 mg.

Cheracol D Cough Liquid (NONNARCOTIC ANTITUSSIVE, EXPECTORANT) *syrup:* dextromethorphan hydrobromide 10 mg, guaifenesin 100 mg/5 ml, alcohol 4.75%.

Cheracol Plus Liquid (ANTITUSSIVE) *syrup:* phenylpropanolamine hydrochloride 8.3 mg, chlorpheniramine maleate 1.3 mg, dextromethorphan hydrobromide 6.7 mg/5 ml, sorbitol, alcohol 4.75%.

Cheracol Syrup* (NARCOTIC ANTITUSSIVE, EXPECTORANT [schedule V]) *syrup:* codeine phosphate 10 mg, guaifenesin 100 mg/5 ml, alcohol 4.75%.

Chloromycetin Hydrocortisone* (OPHTHALMIC STEROID, ANTIBIOTIC) *solution:* hydrocortisone acetate 8.5%, chloramphenicol 0.25%, cholesterol, methylcellulose, benzethonium chloride 0.01%.

Chloroserpine* (ANTIHYPERTENSIVE) chlorothiazide 500 mg, reserpine 0.125 mg.

Chlor-trimeton Decongestant (DECONGESTANT, ANTIHISTAMINE) *tablet:* pseudoephedrine sulfate 60 mg, chlorpheniramine maleate 4 mg.

Chlor-trimeton Decongestant Repetabs (DECONGESTANT, ANTIHISTAMINE) *sustained-release tablet:* pseudoephedrine sulfate 120 mg, chlorpheniramine maleate 8 mg.

Chlorzoxazone with APAP* (SKELETAL MUSCLE RELAXANT, ANALGESIC) *tablet:* chlorzoxazone 250 mg, acetaminophen 300 mg.

Claritin D* (ANTIHISTAMINE, DECONGESTANT) loratidine, 5 mg, pseudoephedrine 120 mg, loratidine 10 mg, pseudoephedrine 240 mg.

Clindex* (ANTISPASMODIC) clidinium 2.5 mg, chlordiazepoxide 5 mg.

Clinoxide* (ANTISPASMODIC) clidinium 2.5 mg, chlordiazepoxide 5 mg.

Clipoxide* (ANTISPASMODIC) clidinium 2.5 mg, chlordiazepoxide 5 mg.

Co-Apap (ANTIHISTAMINE, DECONGESTANT) pseudoephedrine 30 mg, chlorpheniramine 2 mg, dextromethorphan 15 mg, acetaminophen 325 mg.

Codamine Syrup* (ANTITUSSIVE [schedule III]) *syrup:* phenylpropanolamine 25 mg, hydrocodone 5 mg.

Codiclear DH Syrup* (ANTITUSSIVE [schedule III]) *syrup:* hydrocodone 5 mg, guaifenesin 100 mg, alcohol 10%.

Codimal DH* (ANTITUSSIVE [schedule III]) *syrup:* phenylephrine hydrochloride 5 mg, pyrilamine maleate 8.33 mg, hydrocodone bitartrate 1.66 mg/5 ml.

Codimal LA* (ANTIHISTAMINE, DECONGESTANT) pseudoephedrine 120 mg, chlorpheniramine 8 mg.

Co-Gesic* (NARCOTIC ANALGESIC [schedule III]) hydrocodone 5 mg, acetaminophen 500 mg.

Colabid* (ANTIGOUT) probenecid 500 mg, colchicine 0.5 mg.

ColBenemid* (ANTIGOUT) *tablet:* probenecid 500 mg, colchicine 0.5 mg.

Coldrine (DECONGESTANT) pseudoephedrine 30 mg, acetaminophen 325 mg.

Col-Probenecid* (ANTIGOUT) *tablet:* probenecid 500 mg, colchicine 0.5 mg.

Coly-Mycin S Otic* (OTIC: STEROID, ANTIBIOTIC) *suspension:* hydrocortisone acetate 1%, neomycin sulfate 3.3 mg, colistin sulfate 3 mg, thonzonium bromide 0.05%/ml, polysorbate 80, acetic acid, sodium acetate, thimerosal.

Combipres 0.1* (ANTIHYPERTENSIVE) *tablet:* chlorthalidone 15 mg, clonidine hydrochloride 0.1 mg.

Combipres 0.2* (ANTIHYPERTENSIVE) *tablet:* chlorthalidone 15 mg, clonidine hydrochloride 0.2 mg.

Combipres 0.3* (ANTIHYPERTENSIVE) *tablet:* chlorthalidone 15 mg, clonidine hydrochloride 0.3 mg.

Combivir* (ANTIVIRAL) zidovudine 300 mg, lamivudine 150 mg.

Comtrex (ANTIHISTAMINE, DECONGESTANT) pseudoephedrine 30 mg, chlorpheniramine 2 mg, dextromethorphan 10 mg, acetaminophen 325 mg.

Condrin-LA* (DECONGESTANT, ANTIHISTAMINE) *capsule:* phenylpropanolamine hydrochloride 75 mg, chlorpheniramine maleate 12 mg.

Congespirin Cold Tablets for Children (DECONGESTANT) *chewable tablet:* acetaminophen 81 mg, phenylephrine hydrochloride 1.25 mg, saccharin.

Contac 12 Hour (DECONGESTANT, ANTIHISTAMINE) *caplet, tablet:* phenylpropanolamine hydrochloride 75 mg, chlorpheniramine maleate 12 mg.

Cope (NONNARCOTIC AGONIST ANALGESIC, ANTACID) *tablet:* aspirin 421 mg, caffeine 32 mg, magnesium hydroxide 50 mg, aluminum hydroxide 25 mg.

Cordran-N* (CORTICOSTEROID, ANTIBIOTIC) *cream, ointment:* neomycin sulfate 0.5%, flurandrenolide 0.05%.

Coricidin (ANTIHISTAMINE) *tablet:* chlorpheniramine maleate 2 mg, acetaminophen 325 mg.

Correctol (LAXATIVE [STIMULANT, STOOL SOFTENER]) *tablet:* docusate sodium 100 mg, phenolphthalein 65 mg.

Cortisporin* (OPHTHALMIC STEROID, ANTIBIOTIC) *suspension:* hydrocortisone 1%, neomycin sulfate equivalent to 0.35% neomycin base, polymyxin B sulfate 10,000 units/ml, thimerosal cetyl alcohol 0.001%, glyceryl monostearate, polyoxyl 40 stearate, propylene glycol, mineral oil.

Cortisporin Ointment* (OPHTHALMIC STEROID, ANTIBIOTIC) *ointment:* hydrocortisone 1%, neomycin sulfate equivalent to 0.35% neomycin base, bacitracin zinc 400 units, polymyxin B sulfate 10,000 units/g, white petrolatum.

Corzide 40/5* (ANTIHYPERTENSIVE) *tablet:* nadolol 40 mg, bendroflumethiazide 5 mg.

Corzide 80/5* (ANTIHYPERTENSIVE) *tablet:* nadolol 80 mg, bendroflumethiazide 5 mg.

Cosopt* (OPHTHALMIC, GLAUCOMA) dorzolamide, timolol.

Cotrim* (ANTIINFECTIVE) *tablet:* trimethoprim 80 mg, sulfamethoxazole 400 mg.

Cotrim DS (Double Strength)* (ANTIINFECTIVE) *tablet:* trimethoprim 160 mg, sulfamethoxazole 800 mg.

Cotrim Pediatric* (ANTIINFECTIVE) *suspension:* trimethoprim 40 mg, sulfamethoxazole 200 mg/5 ml.

Cyclomydril* (OPHTHALMIC DECONGESTANT) *ophthalmic solution:* cyclopentolate hydrochloride 0.2%, phenylephrine hydrochloride 0.1%.

Cystex (URINARY ANTIINFECTIVE) *tablet:* methenamine 162 mg, sodium salicylate 97 mg, salicylamide 65 mg, benzoic acid 32 mg.

Damason-P* (NARCOTIC ANALGESIC [schedule III]) hydrocodone 5 mg, aspirin 224 mg, caffeine 32 mg.

Darvocet-N 50* (NARCOTIC AGONIST ANALGESIC [schedule IV]) *tablet:* propoxyphene napsylate 50 mg, acetaminophen 325 mg.

Darvocet-N 100* (NARCOTIC AGONIST ANALGESIC [schedule IV]) *tablet:* propoxyphene napsylate 100 mg, acetaminophen 650 mg.

Darvon Compound-65* (NARCOTIC AGONIST ANALGESIC [schedule IV]) *pulvule (capsule):* propoxyphene hydrochloride 65 mg, aspirin 389 mg, caffeine 32.4 mg.

Decadron with Xylocaine* (GLUCOCORTICOID) *injection:* dexamethasone sodium phosphate 4 mg, lidocaine hydrochloride 10 mg/ml, EDTA, parabens, sodium bisulfite.

Deconamine* (DECONGESTANT, ANTIHISTAMINE) *syrup:* pseudoephedrine hydrochloride 30 mg, chlorpheniramine maleate 2 mg/5 ml, sorbitol; *tablet:* pseudoephedrine hydrochloride 60 mg, chlorpheniramine maleate 4 mg.

Demerol APAP* (NARCOTIC AGONIST ANALGESIC [schedule II]) *tablet:* meperidine hydrochloride 50 mg, acetaminophen 300 mg.

Demi-Regroton* (ANTIHYPERTENSIVE) *injection:* chlorthalidone 25 mg, reserpine 0.125 mg.

Demulen 1/50* (ORAL CONTRACEPTIVE) ethinyl estradiol 50 μg, norethindrone 1 mg.

Depo-Testadiol* (ESTROGEN, ANDROGEN) *injection:* estradiol cypionate 2 mg, testosterone cypionate 50 mg/ml, chlorobutanol in cottonseed oil.

Deprol* (PSYCHOTHERAPEUTIC [schedule IV]) *tablet:* meprobamate 400 mg, benactyzine hydrochloride 1 mg, *tartrazine*.

Dermoplast (TOPICAL ANESTHETIC) *solution:* benzocaine 20%, menthol 0.5%, methylparaben.

Dialose Plus (LAXATIVE [STIMULANT, STOOL SOFTENER]) *capsule:* docusate potassium 100 mg, casanthrol 30 mg.

DiGel (ANTACID) *chewable tablet:* magnesium hydroxide 85 mg, aluminum hydroxide and magnesium carbonate 282 mg, simethicone 25 mg; sodium content: <5 mg, ANC 9 mEq; *liquid:* aluminum hydroxide 200 mg, magnesium hydroxide 200 mg, simethicone 20 mg/5 ml, saccharin, sorbitol, sodium content <5 mg, ANC 10.5 mEq.

Dilantin with Phenobarbital* (ANTICONVULSANT) *capsule:* phenytoin 100 mg, phenobarbital 16 or 32 mg.

Dilaudid Cough Syrup* (NARCOTIC ANTITUSSIVE [schedule II]) *syrup:* hydromorphone 1 mg, guaifenesin 100 mg, alcohol 5%.

Dilor G* (ANTIASTHMATIC) *tablet:* dyphylline 200 mg, guaifenesin 200 mg; *liquid:* dyphylline 100 mg, guaifenesin 100 mg/5 ml, saccharin, sorbitol.

Dimetane Decongestant (DECONGESTANT) phenylephrine 5 mg, brompheniramine maleate 2 mg.

Dimetapp Extentabs (DECONGESTANT, ANTIHISTAMINE) *tablet:* phenylpropanolamine hydrochloride 75 mg, brompheniramine maleate 12 mg.

Disophrol Chronotabs (DECONGESTANT, ANTIHISTAMINE) *tablet:* pseudoephedrine sulfate 120 mg, dexbrompheniramine maleate 6 mg.

Diupres 250* (ANTIHYPERTENSIVE) *tablet:* chlorothiazide 250 mg, reserpine 0.125 mg.

Diupres 500* (ANTIHYPERTENSIVE)

tablet: chlorothiazide 500 mg, reserpine 0.125 mg.

Diurese-R* (ANTIHYPERTENSIVE) *tablet:* trichlormethiazide 4 mg, reserpine 0.1 mg.

Diurigen with Reserpine* (ANTIHYPERTENSIVE) chlorothiazide 250 mg, reserpine 0.125 mg.

Diutensin-R* (ANTIHYPERTENSIVE) *tablet:* methyclothiazide 2.5 mg, reserpine 0.1 mg.

Dolacet* (NARCOTIC AGONIST ANALGESIC [schedule III]) *capsule:* hydrocodone bitartrate 5 mg, acetaminophen 500 mg.

Dolene AP-65* (NARCOTIC AGONIST ANALGESIC [schedule IV]) *tablet:* propoxyphene hydrochloride 65 mg, acetaminophen 650 mg.

Dolene Compound-65* (NARCOTIC AGONIST ANALGESIC [schedule IV]) *capsule:* propoxyphene hydrochloride 65 mg, aspirin 389 mg, caffeine 32.4 mg.

Donnagel (ANTIDIARRHEAL) *suspension:* kaolin 6 g, pectin 142.8 mg, hyoscyamine sulfate 0.1037 mg, atropine sulfate 0.0194 mg, scopalamine hydrobromide 0.0065 mg/30 ml, alcohol 3.8%.

Donnagel-PG* (ANTIDIARRHEAL [schedule V]) *suspension:* powdered opium 24 mg, kaolin 6 g, pectin 142.8 mg, hyoscyamine sulfate 0.1037 mg, atropine sulfate 0.0194 mg, scopolamine hydrobromide 0.0065 mg/30 ml, alcohol 5%.

Donnatal* (GASTROINTESTINAL ANTICHOLINERGIC, SEDATIVE) *capsule, tablet, elixir:* atropine sulfate 0.0194 mg, scopolamine hydrobromide 0.0065 mg, hyoscyamine hydrobromide or sulfate 0.1037 mg, phenobarbital 16.2 mg; the elixir contains alcohol 23%/5 ml.

Donnatal Extentabs* (GASTROINTESTINAL ANTICHOLINERGIC, SEDATIVE) *tablet:* atropine sulfate 0.0582 mg, scopolamine hydrobromide 0.0195 mg, hyoscyamine sulfate 0.3111 mg, phenobarbital 48.6 mg.

Donnatal No. 2* (GASTROINTESTINAL ANTICHOLINERGIC, SEDATIVE) *tablet:* atropine sulfate 0.0194 mg, scopolamine hydrobromide 0.0065 mg, hyoscyamine hydrobromide or sulfate 0.1037 mg, phenobarbital 32.4 mg.

Donnazyme* (DIGESTIVE AID) *elixir:* pancreatin 300 mg, pepsin 150 mg, bile salts 150 mg, hyoscyamine sulfate 0.0518 mg, atropine sulfate 0.0097 mg, scopolamine hydrobromide 0.0033 mg, phenobarbital 8.1 mg.

Doxidan (LAXATIVE [STOOL SOFTENER, STIMULANT]) *capsule:* docusate calcium 60 mg, phenolphthalein 65 mg.

Dristan, Nasal (NASAL DECONGESTANT) *spray solution:* phenylephrine hydrochloride 0.5%, pheniramine maleate 0.2%, alcohol 0.4%, aromatics (menthol, eucalyptol, camphor).

Dristan, Advanced Formula (DECONGESTANT, ANTIHISTAMINE) *tablet:* phenylephrine hydrochloride 5 mg, chlorpheniramine maleate 2 mg, acetaminophen 325 mg.

Drixoral (DECONGESTANT, ANTIHISTAMINE) *sustained-release tablet:* pseudoephedrine sulfate 120 mg, dexbrompheniramine maleate 6 mg; *syrup:* pseudoephedrine hydrochloride 30 mg, brompheniramine maleate 2 mg, sorbitol.

Drize* (DECONGESTANT, ANTIHISTAMINE) *capsule:* phenylpropanolamine hydrochloride 75 mg, chlorpheniramine maleate 12 mg.

D.S.S. Plus (LAXATIVE [STOOL SOFTENER, STIMULANT]) *capsule:* docusate sodium 100 mg, casanthrol 30 mg.

Duo-Medihaler* (BRONCHODILATOR [ADRENERGIC]) *aerosol:* each valve actuation delivers isoproterenol hydrochloride 0.16 mg, phenylephrine bitartrate 0.24 mg.

Duradyne (NONNARCOTIC AGONIST ANALGESIC) *tablet:* acetaminophen 180 mg, aspirin 230 mg, caffeine 15 mg.

Duradyne DHC* (NARCOTIC AGONIST ANALGESIC [schedule III]) *tablet:* hydrocodone bitartrate 5 mg, acetaminophen 500 mg.

Dyazide* (DIURETIC) *capsule:* triamterene 37.5 mg, hydrochlorothiazide 25 mg.

Dyflex-G* (ANTIASTHMATIC) *tablet:* dyphylline 200 mg, guaifenesin 200 mg.

Dyline-GG* (ANTIASTHMATIC) *tablet:* dyphylline 200 mg, guaifenesin 200 mg.

Elase* (TOPICAL ENZYME) *ointment:* fibrinolysin 1 unit, desoxyribonuclease (from bovine pancreas) 666.6 units/g in a liquid petrolatum and polyethylene base.

Elase-Chloromycetin* (TOPICAL ENZYME) *ointment:* chloramphenicol 10 mg, fibrinolysin 1 unit, desoxyribonuclease (from bovine pancreas) 666.6 units/g in a liquid petrolatum and polyethylene base.

Elixophyllin-GG* (ANTIASTHMATIC) theophylline 100 mg, guaifenesin 100 mg.

Empirin with Codeine No. 2* (NARCOTIC AGONIST ANALGESIC [schedule III]) *tablet:* codeine phosphate 15 mg, aspirin 325 mg.

Empirin with Codeine No. 3* (NARCOTIC AGONIST ANALGESIC [schedule III]) *tablet:* codeine phosphate 30 mg, aspirin 325 mg.

Empirin with Codeine No. 4* (NARCOTIC AGONIST ANALGESIC [schedule III]) *tablet:* codeine phosphate 60 mg, aspirin 325 mg.

Endolor* (ANALGESIC) acetaminophen 325 mg, caffeine 40 mg, butalbital 50 mg.

Enduronyl* (ANTIHYPERTENSIVE) *tablet:* methyclothiazide 5 mg, deserpidine 0.25 mg; inactive ingredients: corn starch D&C Yellow No. 10, FD&C Yellow No. 6, lactose, magnesium, stearate, talc, others.

Enduronyl Forte* (ANTIHYPERTENSIVE) *tablet:* methyclothiazide 5 mg, deserpidine 0.5 mg; inactive ingredients: corn starch, iron oxide, lactose, magnesium, stearate, talc, others.

Entozyme* (DIGESTIVE AID) *tablet:* pepsin 250 mg in outer core, pancreatin 300 mg and bile salts 150 mg in enteric-coated inner core.

E-Pilo-1* (ANTIGLAUCOMA) pilocarpine 1%, epinephrine bitartrate 1%.

E-Pilo-2* (ANTIGLAUCOMA) pilocarpine 2%, epinephrine bitartrate 1%.

E-Pilo-3* (ANTIGLAUCOMA) pilocarpine 3%, epinephrine bitartrate 1%.

E-Pilo-4* (ANTIGLAUCOMA) pilocarpine 4%, epinephrine bitartrate 1%.

E-Pilo-6* (ANTIGLAUCOMA) pilocarpine 6%, epinephrine bitartrate 1%.

Equagesic* (NARCOTIC AGONIST ANALGESIC [schedule IV]) *tablet:* aspirin 325 mg, meprobamate 200 mg.

Equazine-M* (ANALGESIC) aspirin 325 mg, meprobamate 200 mg.

Ergo Caff* (ANTIMIGRAINE) *tablet:* ergotamine tartrate 1 mg, caffeine 100 mg.

Esgic* (NONNARCOTIC AGONIST ANALGESIC) *capsule, tablet:* acetaminophen 325 mg, caffeine 40 mg, butalbital 50 mg.

Esimil* (ANTIHYPERTENSIVE) *tablet:* hydrochlorothiazide 25 mg, guanethidine monosulfate 10 mg.

Estratest* (ESTROGEN, ANDROGEN) *tablet:* esterified estrogens 1.25 mg, methyltestosterone 2.5 mg.

Estratest H.S.* (ESTROGEN, ANDROGEN) *tablet:* esterified estrogens 0.625 mg, methyltestosterone 1.25 mg.

Etrafon* (PSYCHOTHERAPEUTIC) *tablet:* perphenazine 2 mg, amitriptyline 25 mg; sugar coated.

Etrafon-A* (PSYCHOTHERAPEUTIC) *tablet:* perphenazine 4 mg, amitriptyline 10 mg; sugar coated.

Etrafon-Forte* (PSYCHOTHERAPEUTIC) *tablet:* perphenazine 4 mg, amitriptyline 25 mg; sugar coated.

Etrafon 2-10* (PSYCHOTHERAPEUTIC) *tablet:* perphenazine 2 mg, amitriptyline 10 mg; sugar coated.

Excedrin (NONNARCOTIC AGONIST ANALGESIC) *caplet, tablet:* acetaminophen 250 mg, aspirin 250 mg, caffeine 65 mg.

Excedrin P.M. (NONNARCOTIC AGONIST ANALGESIC) *tablet:* acetaminophen 500 mg, diphenhydramine citrate 38 mg.

Fansidar* (ANTIMALARIAL [FOLIC ACID ANTAGONISTS]) *tablet:* sulfadoxine 500 mg, pyrimethamine 25 mg.

Fedahist (DECONGESTANT, ANTIHISTAMINE) *tablet:* pseudoephedrine hydrochloride 60 mg, chlorpheniramine maleate 4 mg.

Femcet* (ANALGESIC) acetaminophen 325 mg, caffeine 40 mg, butalbital 50 mg.

Fergon Plus* (IRON SUPPLEMENT) ferrous gluconate 58 mg, ascorbic acid 75 mg.

Fermalox (IRON PREPARATION, ANTACID) *tablet:* ferrous sulfate 200 mg (40 mg iron), magnesium aluminum hydroxide 200 mg.

Ferro-Sequels (IRON PREPARATION, STOOL SOFTENER) *sustained-release tablet:* ferrous fumarate 150 mg (50 mg iron), docusate sodium 100 mg.

Fioricet* (NONNARCOTIC AGONIST ANALGESIC) *tablet:* acetaminophen 325 mg, butalbital 50 mg, caffeine 40 mg.

Fiorinal* (NONNARCOTIC AGONIST ANALGESIC [schedule III]) *capsule, tablet:* aspirin 325 mg, butalbital 50 mg, caffeine 40 mg.

Fiorinal with Codeine No. 1* (NARCOTIC AGONIST ANALGESIC [schedule III]) *capsule:* codeine phosphate 7.5 mg, aspirin 325 mg, caffeine 40 mg, butalbital 50 mg.

Fiorinal with Codeine No. 2* (NARCOTIC AGONIST ANALGESIC [schedule III]) *capsule:* codeine phosphate 15 mg, aspirin 325 mg, caffeine 40 mg, butalbital 50 mg.

Fiorinal with Codeine No. 3* (NARCOTIC AGONIST ANALGESIC [schedule III]) *capsule:* codeine phosphate 30 mg, aspirin 325 mg, caffeine 40 mg, butalbital 50 mg.

Fleet Enema (STIMULANT ENEMA) *squeeze bottle:* sodium phosphate 7 g, sodium biphosphate 19 g/118 ml delivered dose, sodium content 4.4 g/dose.

Flexaphen* (SKELETAL MUSCLE RELAXANT) *capsule:* chlorzoxazone 250 mg, acetaminophen 300 mg.

Fluress* (OPHTHALMIC ANESTHETIC) *ophthalmic solution:* benoxinate hydrochloride 0.4%, fluorescein sodium with povidone 0.25%, chlorobutanol 1%.

4-Way Nasal (NASAL DECONGESTANT) *spray:* phenylephrine hydrochloride 0.5%, naphazoline hydrochloride 0.05%, pyrilamine maleate 0.2%, aromatics (menthol, camphor, eucalyptol).

Gaviscon (ANTACID) *liquid:* aluminum hydroxide 31.7 mg, magnesium carbonate 137 mg/5 ml, sodium alginate, saccharin, sorbitol, sodium content 13 mg, ANC 1 mEq; *chewable tablet:* aluminum hydroxide 80 mg, magnesium trisilicate 30 mg, alginic acid, sodium bicarbonate, sodium content 18.4 mg, ANC 0.5 mEq.

Gaviscon-2 (ANTACID) *chewable tablet:* aluminum hydroxide 160 mg, magnesium trisilicate 40 mg, alginic acid, sodium bicarbonate, sodium content 36.8 mg.

Gelusil (ANTACID) *liquid (per 5 ml), tablet:* aluminum hydroxide 200 mg, magnesium hydroxide 200 mg, simethicone 25 mg/5 ml, sorbitol; sodium content (liquid) 0.7 mg, ANC 12 mEq; sodium content (tablet) 0.8 mg, ANC 11 mEq.

Gelusil-II (ANTACID) *liquid (per 5 ml), chewable tablet:* aluminum hydroxide 400 mg, magnesium hydroxide 400 mg, simethicone 30 mg, saccharin, sorbitol, sodium content (liquid) 1.3 mg, ANC 24 mEq; sodium content (tablet) 2.1 mg, ANC 21 mEq.

Gelusil-M (ANTACID) *liquid (per 5 ml), chewable tablet:* aluminum hydroxide 300 mg, magnesium hydrochloride 200 mg, simethicone 25 mg; sodium content (liquid) 0.7 mg, ANC 12 mEq; sodium content (tablet) 1.3 mg, ANC 12.5 mEq.

Gemnisyn (NONNARCOTIC AGONIST ANALGESIC) *tablet:* acetaminophen 325 mg, aspirin 325 mg.

Genora 0.5/35 (ORAL CONTRACEPTIVE) ethinyl estradiol 35 μg, norethindrone 0.5 mg

Genora 1/35 (ORAL CONTRACEPTIVE) ethinyl estradiol 35 μg, norethindrone 1 mg.

Genora 1/50 (ORAL CONTRACEPTIVE) mestranol 50 μg, norethindrone 1 mg.

Glyceryl-T* (ANTIASTHMATIC) *capsule, liquid (per 5 ml):* theophylline 150 mg, guaifenesin 90 mg.

Granulex* (TOPICAL ENZMYE) *aerosol:* trypsin 0.1 mg, balsam Peru 72.5 mg, castor oil 650 mg/0.82 ml.

Haley's M-O (LAXATIVE [LUBRICANT, SALINE]) *emulsion:* mineral oil 25%, magnesium hydroxide.

Halotussin-DM (ANTITUSSIVE) guaifenesin 100 mg, dextromethorphan 15 mg.

Helidac (ANTIULCER, ANTIINFECTIVE) *tablet:* bismuth subsalicylate 262.4 mg, metronidazole 250 mg, tetracycline 500 mg.

Hexalol* (URINARY ANTIINFECTIVE) *tablet:* methenamine 40.8 mg, phenyl salicylate 18.1 mg, atropine sulfate 0.03 mg, hyoscyamine 0.03 mg, benzoic acid 4.5 mg, methlene blue 5.4 mg.

Hycodan* (ANTITUSSIVE [schedule III]) *tablet:* hydrocodone bitartrate 5 mg, homatropine methylbromide 1.5 mg.

Hycomine Compound* (ANTITUSSIVE [schedule III]) *tablet:* phenylephrine hydrochloride 10 mg, chlorpheniramine maleate 2 mg, hydrocodone bitartrate 5 mg, acetaminophen 250 mg, caffeine 30 mg.

Hycomine Pediatric* (ANTITUSSIVE [schedule III]) *syrup:* phenylpropanolamine hydrochloride 12.5 mg, hydrocodone bitartrate 2.5 mg/5 ml, saccharin, sorbitol.

Hycomine Syrup* (ANTITUSSIVE [schedule III]) *syrup:* phenylpropanolamine hydrochloride 25 mg, hydrocodone bitartrate 5 mg/5 ml.

Hycotuss Expectorant* (ANTITUSSIVE [schedule III]) guaifenesin 100 mg, hydrocodone 5 mg.

Hydrazide 25/25* (ANTIHYPERTENSIVE) hydralazine 25 mg, hydrochlorothiazide 25 mg.

Hydrazide 50/50* (ANTIHYPERTENSIVE) hydralazine 50 mg, hydrochlorothiazide 50 mg.

Hydrocet* (NARCOTIC ANALGESIC [schedule III]) hydrocodone 5 mg, acetaminophen 500 mg.

Hydrogesic* (NARCOTIC ANALGESIC [schedule III]) hydrocodone 5 mg, acetaminophen 500 mg.

Hydromox R* (ANTIHYPERTENSIVE) *tablet:* quinethazone 50 mg, reserpine 0.125 mg.

Hydrophed* (ANTIASTHMATIC) *tablet:* theophylline 130 mg, ephedrine sulfate 25 mg, hydroxyzine hydrochloride 10 mg.

Hydropres 25* (ANTIHYPERTENSIVE) *tablet:* hydrochlorothiazide 25 mg, reserpine 0.125 mg.

Hydropres 50* (ANTIHYPERTENSIVE) *tablet:* hydrochlorothiazide 50 mg, reserpine 0.125 mg.

Hydro-Serp* (ANTIHYPERTENSIVE) *tablet:* hydrochlorothiazide 50 mg, reserpine 0.125 mg.

Hydroserpine* (ANTIHYPERTENSIVE) *tablet:* hydrochlorothiazide 50 mg, reserpine 0.125 mg.

Hydrosine 25* (ANTIHYPERTENSIVE) hydrochlorothiazide 25 mg, reserpine 0.125 mg.

Hydrosine 50* (ANTIHYPERTENSIVE) hydrochlorothiazide 50 mg, reserpine 0.125 mg.

Hyzaar* (ANTIHYPERTENSIVE) losartan 50 mg, hydrochlorothiazide 12.5 mg.

Ilopan-Choline* (GI STIMULANT) *tablet:* dexpanthenol 50 mg, choline bitartrate 25 mg.

Inderide 40/25* (ANTIHYPERTENSIVE) *tablet:* propranolol hydrochloride 40 mg, hydrochlorothiazide 25 mg.

Inderide 80/25* (ANTIHYPERTENSIVE) *tablet:* propranolol hydrochloride 80 mg, hydrochlorothiazide 25 mg.

Inderide LA 80/50* (ANTIHYPERTENSIVE) *long-acting capsule:* propranolol hydrochloride 80 mg, hydrochlorothiazide 50 mg.

Inderide LA 120/50* (ANTIHYPERTENSIVE) *long-acting capsule:* propranolol hydrochloride 120 mg, hydrochlorothiazide 50 mg.

Inderide LA 160/50* (ANTIHYPERTENSIVE) *long-acting capsule:* propranolol hydrochloride 160 mg, hydrochlorothiazide 50 mg.

Innovar* (ANESTHETIC ADJUNCT [schedule II]) *injection:* fentanyl (citrate) 0.05 mg, droperidol 2.5 mg/ml.

Isollyl Improved (NONNARCOTIC AGONIST ANALGESIC) *capsule, tablet:* aspirin 325 mg, caffeine 40 mg, butalbital 50 mg.

Isopto Alkaline (ARTIFICIAL TEAR SOLUTION) *drops:* hydroxypropyl methylcellulose 1%, benzalkonium chloride 0.01%.

Isopto P-ES* (ANTIGLAUCOMA) *solution:* pilocarpine hydrochloride 2%, physostigmine salicylate 0.25%

Kapectolin PG* (ANTIDIARRHEAL [schedule V]) powdered opium 24 mg, kaolin 6 g, pectin 142.8 mg, hyoscyamine 0.1037 mg, atropine 0.0194 mg, scopolamine 0.0065 mg.

Kinesed* (GASTROINTESTINAL ANTICHOLINERGIC, SEDATIVE) *chewable tablet:* atropine sulfate 0.02 mg, scopolamine hydrobromide 0.007 mg, hyoscyamine hydrobromide or sulfate 0.1 mg, phenobarbital 16 mg, saccharin.

Kondremul with Phenolphthalein (LAXATIVE [LUBRICANT, STIMULANT]) *emulsion:* mineral oil 55%, phenolphthalein 150 mg/15 ml, Irish moss as an emulsifier.

Lanophyllin-GG* (ANTIASTHMATIC) *capsule:* theophylline 150 mg, guaifenesin 90 mg.

Levlen* (ORAL CONTRACEPTIVE) ethinyl estradiol 30 μg, levonorgestrel 0.15 mg.

Lexxel* (ANTIHYPERTENSIVE) *tablet:* enalapril 5 mg, felodipine 5 mg.

Librax* (GASTROINTESTINAL ANTICHOLINERGIC) *capsule:* clidinium bromide 2.5 mg, chlordiazepoxide hydrochloride 5 mg.

Lidox* (ANTISPASMODIC) clidinium bromide 2.5 mg, chloridazepoxide 5 mg.

Limbitrol 5-12.5* (PSYCHOTHERAPEUTIC [schedule IV]) *tablet:* chlordiazepoxide 5 mg, amitriptyline (as hydrochloride) 12.5 mg.

Limbitrol DS 10-25* (PSYCHOTHERAPEUTIC [schedule IV]) *tablet:* chlordiazepoxide 10 mg, amitriptyline (as hydrochloride) 25 mg.

Lobac* (SKELETAL MUSCLE RELAXANT, ANALGESIC) *capsule:* chlorzoxazone 250 mg, acetaminophen 300 mg.

Loestrin 1/20* (ORAL CONTRACEPTIVE)

tablet: ethinyl estradiol 20 μg, norethindrone acetate 1 mg.

Loestrin 1/20 Fe* (ORAL CONTRACEPTIVE) *tablet:* ethinyl estradiol 20 μg, norethindrone acetate 1 mg, ferrous fumarate 75 mg in last 7 tablets.

Loestrin 1.5/30* (ORAL CONTRACEPTIVE) *tablet:* ethinyl estradiol 30 μg, norethindrone acetate 1.5 mg.

Loestrin 1.5/30 Fe* (ORAL CONTRACEPTIVE) *tablet:* ethinyl estradiol 30 μg, norethindrone acetate 1.5 mg, ferrous fumarate 75 mg in last 7 tablets.

Lo/Ovral* (ORAL CONTRACEPTIVE) *tablet:* ethinyl estradiol 30 μg, norgestrel 0.3 mg.

Lopressor HCT 50/25* (ANTIHYPERTENSIVE) *tablet:* metoprolol tartrate 50 mg, hydrochlorothiazide 25 mg.

Lopressor HCT 100/25* (ANTIHYPERTENSIVE) *tablet:* metoprolol tartrate 100 mg, hydrochlorothiazide 25 mg.

Lopressor HCT 100/50* (ANTIHYPERTENSIVE) *tablet:* metoprolol tartrate 100 mg, hydrochlorothiazide 50 mg.

Lorcet* (NARCOTIC ANALGESIC [schedule III]) hydrocodone 5 mg, acetaminophen 500 mg.

Lorcet-HD* (NARCOTIC ANALGESIC [schedule III]) hydrocodone 5 mg, acetaminophen 500 mg.

Lortab 5* (NARCOTIC ANALGESIC [schedule III]) hydrocodone 5 mg, acetaminophen 500 mg.

Lortab 7/500* (NARCOTIC ANALGESIC [schedule III]) hydrocodone 7.5 mg, acetaminophen 500 mg.

Lotrel* (ANTIHYPERTENSIVE) amlodipine 5 mg, benazepril 10 mg, *or* amlodipine 5 mg, benazepril 20 mg.

Lotrisone* (CORTICOSTEROID, ANTIFUNGAL) *cream:* betamethasone (as dipropionate) 0.05%, clotrimazole 1% in a hydrophilic emollient base with mineral oil and white petrolatum.

Lufyllin-EPG* (BRONCHODILATOR) dyphylline 100 mg, ephedrine 16 mg, guaifenesin 200 mg, phenobarbital 16 mg.

Lufyllin-GG* (BRONCHODILATOR) dyphylline 100 mg, guaifenesin 100 mg, alcohol 17%.

Maalox No. 1 (ANTACID) *chewable tablet:* aluminum hydroxide 200 mg, magnesium hydroxide 200 mg, saccharin, sorbitol, sodium content 0.7 mg, ANC 9.7 mEq.

Maalox Plus (ANTACID) *chewable tablet:* aluminum hydroxide 200 mg, magnesium hydroxide 200 mg, simethicone 25 mg, saccharin, sorbitol, sodium content 0.8 mg, ANC 11.4 mEq; *suspension:* aluminum hydroxide 225 mg, magnesium hydroxide 200 mg, simethicone 25 mg, sodium content 1.2 mg, ANC 13.3. mEq.

Maalox TC (Therapeutic Concentrate) (ANTACID) *chewable tablet:* aluminum hydroxide 600 mg, magnesium hydroxide 300 mg, sorbitol; sodium content 0.5 mg, ANC 28 mEq.

Magnatril (ANTACID) *chewable tablet:* aluminum hydroxide 260 mg, magnesium hydroxide 130 mg, magnesium trisilicate 455 mg; colloidal suspension: magnesium trisilicate 260 mg, magnesium and aluminum hydroxides.

Marax* (ANTIASTHMATIC, BRONCHODILATOR) *tablet:* theophylline 130 mg, ephedrine sulfate 25 mg, hydroxyzine hydrochloride 10 mg.

Marnal* (ANALGESIC [schedule III]) aspirin 325 mg, caffeine 40 mg, butalbital 50 mg.

Maxitrol* (OPHTHALMIC STEROID, ANTIBIOTIC) *ointment, ophthalmic suspension:* dexamethasone 0.1%, neomycin sulfate equivalent to 0.35% neomycin base, polymyxin B sulfate 10,000 units.

Maxzide* (DIURETIC) *tablet:* triamterene 75 mg, hydrochlorothiazide 50 mg.

Mediatric* (HORMONE, MULTIVITAMIN [schedule III]) *capsule, tablet:* conjugated estrogens 0.25 mg, methyltestosterone 2.5 mg, methamphetamine hydrochloride 1 mg, vitamin B1 10 mg, B2 5 mg, B3 50 mg, B5 20 mg, B6 3 mg, B12 2.5 μg, ascorbic acid 100 mg, ferrous sulfate 9 mg.

Medigesic* (ANALGESIC) acetaminophen 325 mg, caffeine 40 mg, butalbital 50 mg.

Menrium 5-2* (ESTROGEN, PSYCHOTHERAPEUTIC) *tablet:* chlordiazepoxide 5 mg, esterified estrogens 0.2 mg.

Menrium 5-4* (ESTROGEN, PSYCHOTHERAPEUTIC) *tablet:* chlordiazepoxide 5 mg, esterified estrogens 0.4 mg.

Menrium 10-4* (ESTROGEN, PSYCHOTHERAPEUTIC) *tablet:* chlordiazepoxide 10 mg, esterified estrogens 0.4 mg.

Mepergan* (NARCOTIC ANALGESIC [schedule II]) meperidine 25 mg, promethazine 25 mg.

Mepergan Fortis* (NARCOTIC ANALGESIC [schedule II]) meperidine 50 mg, promethazine 25 mg.

Metatensin #2* (ANTIHYPERTENSIVE) *tablet:* trichlormethiazide 2 mg, reserpine 0.1 mg, *tartrazine*.

Metatensin #4* (ANTIHYPERTENSIVE) *tablet:* trichlormethiazide 4 mg, reserpine 0.1 mg.

Metimyd* (STEROID, SULFONAMIDE) *suspension:* prednisolone acetate 0.5%, sodium sulfacetamide 10%, phenylethyl alcohol 0.5%, benzalkonium chloride 0.025%, sodium thiosulfate, EDTA, tyloxapol.

Micrainin* (NARCOTIC AGONIST ANALGESIC [schedule IV]) *tablet:* aspirin 325 mg, meprobamate 200 mg.

Midol Caplets (NONNARCOTIC AGONIST ANALGESIC) *tablet:* aspirin 454 mg, caffeine 32.4 mg, cinnamedrine hydrochloride 14.9 mg.

Midol PMS (NONNARCOTIC AGONIST ANALGESIC) *capsule:* acetaminophen 500 mg, pamabrom 25 mg, pyrilamine maleate 15 mg.

Minizide 1* (ANTIHYPERTENSIVE) *capsule:* polythiazide 0.5 mg, prazosin hydrochloride 1 mg.

Minizide 2* (ANTIHYPERTENSIVE) *capsule:* polythiazide 0.5 mg, prazosin hydrochloride 2 mg.

Minizide 5* (ANTIHYPERTENSIVE) *capsule:* polythiazide 0.5 mg, prazosin hydrochloride 5 mg.

Modane Plus (LAXATIVE) docusate sodium 100 mg, phenolphthalein 65 mg.

Modicon* (ORAL CONTRACEPTIVE) ethinyl estradiol 35 μg, norethindrone 0.5 mg.

Moduretic* (DIURETIC) *tablet:* amiloride hydrochloride 5 mg, hydrochlorothiazide 50 mg.

Murocoll-2* (MYDRIATIC) *ophthalmic drops:* scopolamine hydrobromide 0.3%, phenylephrine hydrochloride 10%/5 ml, benzalkonium chloride 0.01%, sodium metabisulfite, EDTA.

Mus-Lax* (SKELETAL MUSCLE RELAXANT) *capsule:* chlorzoxazone 250 mg, acetaminophen 300 mg.

Mycitracin* (OPHTHALMIC ANTIINFECTIVE) *ophthalmic ointment:* polymyxin B sulfate 10,000 units, neomycin sulfate 3.5 mg, bacitracin 500 units/g; in a lanolin, mineral oil, and white petrolatum base with chlorobutanol 0.65%.

Mycitracin Triple Antibiotic (TOPICAL ANTIINFECTIVE) *topical ointment:* polymyxin B sulfate 5000 units, neomycin sulfate 3.5 mg, bacitracin 500 units/g.

Mycolog II* (CORTICOSTEROID, ANTIFUNGAL) *cream, ointment:* triamcinolone acetonide 0.1%, nystatin 100,000 units/g.

Mylanta (ANTACID) *liquid:* aluminum hydroxide 200 mg, magnesium hydroxide 200 mg, simethicone 20 mg, sorbitol, sodium content 0.68 mg, ANC 12.7 mEq.

Mylanta II (ANTACID) *chewable tablet:* aluminum hydroxide 400 mg, magnesium hydroxide 400 mg, simethicone 40 mg, sodium content 1.3 mg, ANC 23 mEq; *liquid:* aluminum hydroxide 400 mg, magnesium hydroxide 400 mg, simethicone 40 mg, sorbitol, sodium content 1.14 mg, ANC 25.4.

Naldecon* (DECONGESTANT, ANTIHISTAMINE) *sustained-release tablet:* phenylpropanolamine hydrochloride 40 mg, phenylephrine hydrochloride 10 mg, chlorpheniramine maleate 5 mg, phenyltoloxamine citrate 15 mg; *syrup:* phenylpropanolamine hydrochloride 20 mg, phenylephrine hydrochloride 5 mg, chlorpheniramine maleate 2.5 mg, phenyltoloxamine citrate 7.5 mg.

Naldecon Senior DX* (ANTITUSSIVE) dextromethorphan 10 mg, guaifenesin 200 mg.

Nelova 0.5/35 E* (ORAL CONTRACEPTIVE) ethinyl estradiol 35 μg, norethindrone 0.5 mg.

Nelova 1/35 E* (ORAL CONTRACEPTIVE) ethinyl estradiol 35 μg, norethindrone 1 mg.

Nelova 1/50 M* (ORAL CONTRACEPTIVE) mestranol 50 μg, norethindrone 1 mg.

Nelova 10/11* (ORAL CONTRACEPTIVE) ethinyl estradiol 35 μg, norethindrone 0.5 mg|×|10 tablets and 1 mg|×|11 tablets.

Neo-Cortef* (CORTICOSTEROID ANTIBIOTIC) *water-soluble cream, topical ointment:* hydrocortisone acetate 1%, neomycin sulfate 0.5%; ointment has white petrolatum mineral base.

NeoDecadron* (CORTICOSTEROID ANTIBIOTIC) *topical cream:* dexamethasone phosphate 0.1%, neomycin sulfate 0.5% in a greaseless base; *ophthalmic solution:* dexamethasone sodium phosphate 0.1%, neomycin sulfate equivalent to 0.35% base, benzalkonium chloride 0.02%, sodium bisulfite 0.01%; (OPHTHALMIC CORTICOSTEROID ANTIBIOTIC) *ophthalmic ointment:* dexamethasone sodium phosphate 0.05%, neomycin sulfate equivalent to 0.35% base in white petrolatum and mineral oil.

Neosporin* (OPHTHALMIC ANTIINFECTIVE) *ophthalmic drops:* polymyxin B sulfate 10,000 units, neomycin sulfate 1.75 mg, gramicidin 0.025 mg/ml; *ophthalmic ointment:* polymyxin B sulfate 10,000 units, neomycin sulfate 3.5 mg, bacitracin zinc 400 units/g in a white petrolatum base.

Neosporin G.U. Irrigant* (ANTIINFECTIVE) *solution:* neomycin sulfate 40 mg, polymyxin B sulfate 200,000 units/ml, methylparaben.

Neotal* (OPHTHALMIC ANTIINFECTIVE) *ophthalmic ointment:* polymyxin B sulfate 5000 units, neomycin sulfate 5 mg, bacitracin zinc 400 units/g in a white petrolatum and mineral oil base.

Neothylline-GG* (BRONCHODILATOR EXPECTORANT) *tablet:* dyphylline 200 mg, guaifenesin 200 mg.

Neutra-Phos (PHOSPHORUS REPLACEMENT) *capsule, powder:* phosphorous 250 mg, potassium 278 mg, sodium 164 mg; combination of monobasic, dibasic, sodium, and potassium phosphate.

Nolamine* (DECONGESTANT, ANTIHISTAMINE) *tablet:* phenylpropanolamine hydrochloride 50 mg, chlorpheniramine maleate 4 mg, phenindamine tartrate 24 mg.

Norcet* (NARCOTIC ANALGESIC [schedule III]) hydrocodone 5 mg, acetaminophen 500 mg.

Norco* (NARCOTIC AGONIST ANALGESIC [schedule III]) *tablet:* hydrocodone bitartrate 10 mg, acetaminophen 325 mg.

Nordette* (ORAL CONTRACEPTIVE) ethinyl estradiol 30 µg, levonorgestrel 0.15 mg.

Norethin 1/35 E* (ORAL CONTRACEPTIVE) ethinyl estradiol 35 µg, norethindrone 1 mg.

Norethin 1/50 M* (ORAL CONTRACEPTIVE) mestranol 50 µg, norethindrone 1 mg.

Norgesic* (SKELETAL MUSCLE RELAXANT) *tablet:* orphenadrine citrate 25 mg, aspirin 385 mg, caffeine 30 mg.

Norgesic Forte* (SKELETAL MUSCLE RELAXANT, ANALGESIC) *tablet:* orphenadrine citrate 50 mg, aspirin 700 mg, caffeine 60 mg.

Norinyl 1+35* (ORAL CONTRACEPTIVE) ethinyl estradiol 35 µg, norethindrone 1 mg.

Norinyl 1+50* (ORAL CONTRACEPTIVE) mestranol 50 µg, norethindrone 1 mg.

Norlestrin 1/50* (ORAL CONTRACEPTIVE) ethinyl estradiol 50 µg, norethindrone 1 mg.

Norlestrin 2.5/50* (ORAL CONTRACEPTIVE) ethinyl estradiol 50 µg, norethindrone 2.5 mg.

Normozide 100/25* (ANTIHYPERTENSIVE) labetalol 100 mg, hydrochlorothiazide 25 mg.

Normozide 200/25* (ANTIHYPERTENSIVE) labetalol 200 mg, hydrochlorothiazide 25 mg.

Normozide 300/25* (ANTIHYPERTENSIVE) labetalol 300 mg, hydrochlorothiazide 25 mg.

Novafed A* (DECONGESTANT, ANTIHISTAMINE) *capsule:* pseudoephedrine hydrochloride 120 mg, chlorpheniramine maleate 8 mg.

Novahistine DH* (ANTITUSSIVE, DECONGESTANT, ANTIHISTAMINE [schedule V]) *liquid:* codeine phosphate 10 mg, pseudoephedrine hydrochloride 30 mg, chlorpheniramine maleate 2 mg/5 ml, alcohol 5%, saccharin, sorbitol.

Novahistine DMX (DECONGESTANT, ANTIHISTAMINE, EXPECTORANT) *liquid:* dextromethorphan hydrobromide 10 mg, guaifenesin 100 mg, pseudoephedrine hydrochloride 30 mg/5 ml, alcohol 10%.

Novahistine Elixir (ANTIHISTAMINE, EXPECTORANT, DECONGESTANT) *liquid:* chlorphineramine maleate 2 mg, phenylephrine hydrochloride 5 mg/5 ml, alcohol 5%, sorbitol.

Novahistine Expectorant* (ANTITUSSIVE, DECONGESTANT, EXPECTORANT [schedule V]) *liquid:* codeine phosphate 10 mg, pseudoephedrine hydrochloride 30 mg, guaifenesin 100 mg/5 ml, alcohol 7.5%.

Ophtha P/S* (CORTICOSTEROID, SULFONAMIDE) *ophthalmic suspension:* prednisolone acetate 0.5%, sodium sulfacetamide 10%, benzalkonium chloride 0.025%.

Ophthocort* (CORTICOSTEROID, ANTIBIOTIC) *ophthalmic ointment:* hydrocortisone acetate 0.5%, chloramphenicol 1%, polymyxin B sulfate 10,000 units/g, liquid petrolatum and polyethylene.

Optimyd* (CORTICOSTEROID, SULFONAMIDE) *ophthalmic solution:* prednisolone sodium phosphate 0.5%, sodium sulfacetamide 10%, benzalkonium chloride 0.025%, phenylethyl alcohol 0.5%.

Optised* (DECONGESTANT) phenylephrine 0.12%, zinc sulfate 0.25%.

Oreticyl 25* (ANTIHYPERTENSIVE) *tablet:* hydrochlorothiazide 25 mg, deserpidine 0.125 mg.

Oreticyl 50* (ANTIHYPERTENSIVE) *tablet:* hydrochlorothiazide 50 mg, deserpidine 0.125 mg.

Oreticyl Forte* (ANTIHYPERTENSIVE) *tablet:* hydrochlorothiazide 25 mg, deserpidine 0.25 mg.

Ornade Spansules* (DECONGESTANT, ANTIHISTAMINE) *sustained-release capsule:* phenylpropanolamine hydrochloride 75 mg, chlorpheniramine maleate 12 mg.

Ornex (DECONGESTANT, ANALGESIC) *capsule:* phenylpropanolamine hydrochloride 12.5 mg, acetaminophen 325 mg.

PAC (NONNARCOTIC ANALGESIC) *tablet:* aspirin 400 mg, caffeine 32 mg, *tartrazine.*

Pamprin Maximum Cramp Relief (NONNARCOTIC ANALGESIC) *capsule:* acetaminophen 500 mg, pamabrom 25 mg, pyrilamine maleate 15 mg.

Parafon Forte* (SKELETAL MUSCLE RELAXANT) *tablet:* chlorzoxazone 250 mg, acetaminophen 300 mg.

Parepectolin* (ANTIDIARRHEAL [schedule V]) *suspension:* opium 15 mg (equivalent to paregoric 3.7 ml), kaolin 5.5 g, pectin 162 mg/30 ml, alcohol 0.69%, saccharin.

P_1E_1, P_2E_1, P_3E_1, P_6E_1* (ANTIGLAUCOMA) *ophthalmic solution:* epinephrine bitartrate 1%, pilocarpine hydrochloride 1%, 2%, 3%, 4%, or 6%, benzalkonium chloride 0.01%, polyethylene glycol, *sodium bisulfite.*

Percocet* (NARCOTIC ANALGESIC [schedule II]) *tablet:* oxycodone hydrochloride 5 mg, acetaminophen 325 mg.

Percodan* (NARCOTIC ANALGESIC [schedule II]) *tablet:* oxycodone hydrochloride 4.5 mg, oxycodone terephthalate 0.38 mg, aspirin 325 mg.

Percodan-Demi* (NARCOTIC ANALGESIC [schedule II]) *tablet:* oxycodone hydrochloride 2.25 mg, oxycodone terephthalate 0.19 mg, aspirin 325 mg.

Perdiem Granules (LAXATIVE) *granules:* psyllium 3.25 g, senna 0.74 g.

Peri-Colace (LAXATIVE [STOOL SOFTENER, STIMULANT]) *capsule:* docusate sodium 100 mg, casanthrol 30 mg; *syrup:* docusate sodium 60 mg, casanthrol 30 mg/15 ml, alcohol 10%, sorbitol.

Phenaphen-650 with Codeine* (NARCOTIC ANALGESIC [schedule III]) *tablet:* codeine phosphate 30 mg, acetaminophen 650 mg, *sodium bisulfite.*

Phenaphen with Codeine No. 3* (NARCOTIC ANALGESIC [schedule III]) *capsule:* codeine phosphate 30 mg, acetaminophen 325 mg.

Phenaphen with Codeine No. 4* (NARCOTIC ANALGESIC [schedule III]) *tablet:* codeine phosphate 60 mg, acetaminophen 325 mg.

Phenergan with Codeine* (ANTITUSSIVE [schedule V]) promethazine 6.25 mg, codeine 10 mg.

Phenergan-D* (DECONGESTANT, ANTIHISTAMINE) *tablet:* pseudoephedrine hydrochloride 60 mg, promethazine hydrochloride 6.25 mg, saccharin.

Phenylzin (OPHTHALMIC DECONGESTANT) *ophthalmic solution:* phenylephrine hydrochloride 0.12%, zinc sulfate 0.25%, benzalkonium chloride, *sodium bisulfite.*

Phrenilin* (NONNARCOTIC AGONIST ANALGESIC) *tablet:* acetaminophen 325 mg, butalbital 50 mg.

Phrenilin Forte* (NONNARCOTIC AGONIST ANALGESIC) *capsule:* acetaminophen 650 mg, butalbital 50 mg.

PMB 200* (ESTROGEN, ANXIOLYTIC) *tablet:* conjugated estrogens 0.45 mg, meprobamate 200 mg.

PMB 400* (ESTROGEN, ANXIOLYTIC) *tablet:* conjugated estrogens 0.45 mg, meprobamate 400 mg.

Polaramine Expectorant* (DECONGESTANT, ANTIHISTAMINE, EXPECTORANT) *liquid:* pseudoephedrine sulfate 20 mg, dexchlorpheniramine maleate 3 mg, guaifenesin 100 mg/5 ml, alcohol 7.2%.

Polycillin-PRB* (ANTIBIOTIC) *oral suspension:* ampicillin trihydrate 3.5 g, probenecid 1 g/bottle.

Poly-Histine D* (ANTIHISTAMINE, DECONGESTANT) phenylpropanolamine

50 mg, phenyltoloxamine 16 mg, pyrilamine 16 mg, pheniramine 16 mg.

Polysporin (ANTIINFECTIVE [TOPICAL]) *ointment:* polymyxin b sulfate 10,000 units, bacitracin zinc 500 units/g.

Polysporin Ointment* (ANTIINFECTIVE [OPHTHALMIC]) *ophthalmic ointment:* polymyxin B sulfate 10,000 units, bacitracin zinc 500 units/g, white petrolatum, mineral oil.

Prefrin-A* (OPHTHALMIC DECONGESTANT) *ophthalmic solution:* phenylephrine hydrochloride 0.12%, pyrilamine maleate 0.1%, antipyrine 0.1%, benzalkonium chloride, EDTA, *sodium bisulfite.*

Premarin with Methyltestosterone* (ESTROGEN, ANDROGEN) *tablet:* conjugated estrogens 0.625 mg, methyltestosterone 5 mg.

Premphase* (ESTROGEN, PROGESTERONE) *tablet:* conjugated estrogen 0.625 mg, medroxyprogesterone acetate 5 mg.

Prempro* (ESTROGEN, PROGESTERONE) *tablet:* conjugated estrogen 0.625 mg, medroxyprogesterone 2.5 mg; conjugated estrogen 0.625 mg, medroxyprogesterone 5 mg.

Probampacin* (ANTIBIOTIC) *suspension:* ampicillin trihydrate 3.5 g, probenecid 1 g/bottle.

Proben-C* (ANTIGOUT) *tablet:* probenecid 500 mg, colchicine 0.5 mg.

Probenecid with Colchicine* (ANTIGOUT) *tablet:* probenecid 500 mg, colchicine 0.5 mg.

Propacet* (NARCOTIC ANALGESIC) propoxyphene napsalate 100 mg, acetaminophen 650 mg (CIV).

Pseudo-Chlor* (ANTIHISTAMINE, DECONGESTANT) pseudoephedrine 120 mg, chlorpheniramine 8 mg.

Pyridium Plus* (ANALGESIC) *tablet:* phenazopyridine hydrochloride 150 mg, hyoscyamine hydrobromide 0.3 mg, butalbital 15 mg.

Quadrinal* (BRONCHODILATOR, EXPECTORANT) *tablet:* theophylline calcium salicylate 130 mg (63.5 mg of anhydrous theophylline), ephedrine hydrochloride 24 mg, potassium iodide 320 mg, phenobarbital 24 mg.

Quibron* (BRONCHODILATOR, EXPECTORANT) *capsule:* theophylline 150 mg, guaifenesin 90 mg.

Quibron-300* (BRONCHODILATOR, EXPECTORANT) *capsule:* theophylline 300 mg, guaifenesin 180 mg.

Quibron Plus* (ANTIASTHMATIC) theophylline 150 mg, ephedrine 25 mg, guaifenesin 100 mg, butabarbital 20 mg.

Rauzide* (ANTIHYPERTENSIVE) *tablet:* bendroflumethiazide 4 mg, powdered rauwolfia serpentina 50 mg, *tartrazine.*

Rebetron* (INTERFERON, ANTIVIRAL) ribavirin 200-mg capsule; interferon alfa-2b recombinant 3 mU/0.5 ml injection.

Regroton* (ANTIHYPERTENSIVE) *tablet:* chlorthalidone 50 mg, reserpine 0.25 mg.

Renese-R* (ANTIHYPERTENSIVE) *tablet:* polythiazide 2 mg, reserpine 0.25 mg.

Repan* (ANALGESIC) acetaminophen 325 mg, caffeine 40 mg, butalbital 50 mg.

Rifamate* (ANTITUBERCULOSIS) *capsule:* isoniazid 150 mg, rifampin 300 mg.

Rifater* (ANTITUBERCULOSIS) rifampin 120 mg, isoniazid 50 mg, pyrazinamide 300 mg.

Rimactane/INH Dual Pack* (ANTITUBERCULOSIS) *pack:* thirty isoniazid 300 mg tablets, sixty rifampin 300 mg capsules.

Riopan Plus (ANTACID) *suspension:* magaldrate 540 mg, simethicone 20 mg, saccharin, sodium content <0.1 mg, ANC 15 mEq; *chewable tablet:* magaldrate 1080 mg, simethicone 30 mg, saccharin, sorbitol, sodium content not more than 0.3 mg/5 ml or 0.5 mg/tablet, ANC not more than 30 mEq/5 ml or chewable tablet.

Robaxisal* (SKELETAL MUSCLE RELAXANT) *tablet:* methocarbamol 400 mg, aspirin 325 mg.

Robitussin A-C* (ANTITUSSIVE, EXPECTORANT [schedule V]) *syrup:* codeine phosphate 10 mg, guaifenesin 100 mg/5 ml, alcohol 3.5%, saccharin.

Robitussin-CF (ANTITUSSIVE, EXPECTORANT) *syrup:* phenylpropanolamine hydrochloride 12.5 mg, dextromethorphan hydrobromide 10 mg, guaifenesin 100 mg, alcohol 4.75%, saccharin, sorbitol.

Robitussin-DAC* (ANTITUSSIVE, EXPECTORANT [schedule V]) *syrup:* phenylpropanolamine hydrochloride 30 mg, codeine phosphate 10 mg, guaifenesin 100 mg, alcohol 1.4%, saccharin.

Robitussin-DM (ANTITUSSIVE, EXPECTORANT) *syrup:* dextromethorphan hydrobromide 15 mg, guaifenesin 100 mg, alcohol 1.4%, saccharin.

Rondec* (DECONGESTANT, ANTIHISTAMINE) *tablet:* pseudoephedrine hydrochloride 60 mg, carbinoxamine maleate 4 mg; *drops:* pseudoephedrine hydrochloride 25 mg, carbinoxamine maleate 2 mg/ml; *syrup:* pseudoephedrine hydrochloride 60 mg, carbinoxamine maleate 4 mg/ml.

Roxicet* (NARCOTIC ANALGESIC [schedule II]) oxycodone 5 mg, acetaminophen 325 mg.

Roxiprin* (NARCOTIC ANALGESIC [schedule II]) oxycodone 5 mg, aspirin 325 mg.

Rulox (ANTACID) *suspension:* aluminum hydroxide 225 mg, magnesium hydroxide 200 mg, simethicone 25 mg, sodium content 0.82 mg, ANC 12 mg.

Salazide* (ANTIHYPERTENSIVE) hydroflumethiazide 50 mg, reserpine 0.125 mg.

Salutensin* (ANTIHYPERTENSIVE) *tablet:* hydroflumethiazide 50 mg, reserpine 0.125 mg.

Salutensin-Demi* (ANTIHYPERTENSIVE) *tablet:* hydroflumethiazide 25 mg, reserpine 0.125 mg.

Sedapap-10* (ANALGESIC) *tablet:* acetaminophen 650 mg, butalbital 50 mg.

Seldane D (ANTIHISTAMINE, DECONGESTANT) *tablet:* terfenadine 60 mg, pseudoephedrine 120 mg.

Senokot S (LAXATIVE) *tablet:* docusate sodium 50 mg, senna concentrate 187 mg.

Ser-A-Gen* (ANTIHYPERTENSIVE) *tablet:* hydrochlorothiazide 15 mg, reserpine 0.1 mg, hydralazine hydrochloride 25 mg.

Seralazide* (ANTIHYPERTENSIVE) *tablet:* hydrochlorothiazide 15 mg, reserpine 0.1 mg, hydralazine hydrochloride 25 mg.

Ser-Ap-Es* (ANTIHYPERTENSIVE) *tablet:* hydrochlorothiazide 15 mg, reserpine 0.1 mg, hydralazine hydrochloride 25 mg.

Serpasil-Apresoline #1* (ANTIHYPERTENSIVE) *tablet:* reserpine 0.1 mg, hydralazine hydrochloride 25 mg, *tartrazine.*

Serpasil-Apresoline #2* (ANTIHYPERTENSIVE) *tablet:* reserpine 0.2 mg, hydralazine hydrochloride 50 mg, *tartrazine.*

Serpasil-Esidrex #1* (ANTIHYPERTENSIVE) *tablet:* hydrochlorothiazide 25 mg, reserpine 0.1 mg.

Serpasil-Esidrex #2* (ANTIHYPERTENSIVE) *tablet:* hydrochlorothiazide 50 mg, reserpine 0.1 mg.

Serpazide* (ANTIHYPERTENSIVE) hydrochlorothiazide 15 mg, reserpine 0.1 mg, hydralazine 25 mg.

Simron Plus (MULTIVITAMIN, IRON) *capsule:* elemental iron (10 mg), vitamins B_6 (1 mg), B_{12} (3.33 mg), C (50 mg).

Sinutab (DECONGESTANT) *tablet:* pseudoephedrine hydrochloride 30 mg, chlorpheniramine maleate 2 mg, acetaminophen 325 mg.

Sinutab-II Maximum Strength No Drowsiness Formula (DECONGESTANT) *tablet:* pseudoephedrine hydrochloride 30 mg, acetaminophen 500 mg.

Soma Compound* (SKELETAL MUSCLE RELAXANT) *tablet:* carisoprodol 200 mg, aspirin 325 mg.

Soma Compound with Codeine* (SKELETAL MUSCLE RELAXANT [schedule III]) *tablet:* carisoprodol 200 mg, aspirin 325 mg, codeine phosphate 16 mg, sodium metabisulfite.

Spastosed (ANTACID) *chewable tablet:* calcium carbonate 226 mg, magnesium carbonate 162 mg, *tartrazine*.

Spironazide* (DIURETIC) *tablet:* spironolactone 25 mg, hydrochlorothiazide 25 mg.

Spirozide* (DIURETIC) *tablet:* spironolactone 25 mg, hydrochlorothiazide 25 mg.

Statrol* (OPHTHALMIC ANTIBIOTIC) *ophthalmic ointment:* polymyxin B sulfate 10,000 units, neomycin sulfate 3.5 mg, parabens in a white petrolatum and lanolin base; *ophthalmic solution:* polymyxin B sulfate 16,250 units, neomycin sulfate 3.5 mg/ml, benzalkonium chloride 0.004%, hydroxypropyl methylcellulose 0.5%.

Stri-Dex (ANTIACNE) *regular-strength pads:* salicylic acid 0.5%, SD alcohol 28%, citric acid; *maximum-strength pads:* salicylic acid 2%, SD alcohol 44%, citric acid.

Sudafed Plus (DECONGESTANT, ANTIHISTAMINE) *tablet:* pseudoephedrine hydrochloride 60 mg, chlorpheniramine maleate 4 mg; *liquid:* pseudoephedrine hydrochloride 30 mg, chlorpheniramine maleate 2 mg.

Sulfamide* (OCULAR ANTIINFLAMMATORY) prednisolone acetate 0.5%, sulfacetamide 10%.

Sulfoxyl Regular* (ANTIACNE) *lotion:* benzoyl peroxide 5%, sulfur 2%.

Sulfoxyl Strong* (ANTIACNE) *lotion:* benzoyl peroxide 10%, sulfur 5%.

Synalgos-DC* (NARCOTIC AGONIST ANALGESIC [schedule III]) *capsule:* dihydrocodeine bitartrate 16 mg, aspirin 356.4 mg, caffeine 30 mg.

Talacen* (NARCOTIC AGONIST-ANTIAGONIST ANALGESIC [schedule IV]) *tablet:* pentazocine hydrochloride 25 mg, acetaminophen 625 mg.

Talwin Compound* (NARCOTIC ANALGESIC [schedule IV]) pentazocine 12.5 mg, aspirin 325 mg.

Talwin NX* (NARCOTIC ANALGESIC [schedule IV]) pentazocine 50 mg, naloxone 0.5 mg.

Tarka* (ANTIHYPERTENSIVE) *tablet:* trandolapril 2 mg, verapamil HCl 180 mg; trandolapril 4 mg; verapamil HCl 240 mg; trandolapril 1 mg, verapamil HCl 240 mg, trandolapril 2 mg, verapamil HCl 240 mg.

Tavist-D* (DECONGESTANT, ANTIHISTAMINE) *tablet:* phenylpropanolamine hydrochloride 75 mg, clemastine fumarate 1.34 mg.

Teczem* (ANTIHYPERTENSIVE) *tablet:* enalapril 5 mg, diltiazem 180 mg.

Tedral (ANTIASTHMATIC, BRONCHODILATOR) *tablet:* theophylline 118 mg, ephedrine hydrochloride 24 mg, phenobarbital 8 mg.

Tedral SA* (ANTIASTHMATIC, BRONCHODILATOR) *sustained-action tablet:* theophylline 180 mg, ephedrine hydrochloride 48 mg, phenobarbital 25 mg.

Tedrigen (ANTIASTHMATIC) theophylline 125 mg, ephedrine 25 mg, phenobarbital 8 mg.

Teebaconin and Vitamin B_6* (ANTITUBERCULOSIS) *tablet:* isoniazid 300 mg (or 100 mg), pyridoxine hydrochloride 30 mg (or 10 mg), *tartrazine.*

Tega-Tussin Syrup* (ANTITUSSIVE [schedule III]) *syrup:* phenylephrine 5 mg, chlorpheniramine 2 mg, hydrocodone 5 mg.

Tenoretic 50* (ANTIHYPERTENSIVE) *tablet:* chlorthalidone 25 mg, atenolol 50 mg.

Tenoretic 100* (ANTIHYPERTENSIVE) *tablet:* chlorthalidone 25 mg, atenolol 100 mg.

Terra-Cortril Suspension* (OCULAR STEROID AND ANTIBIOTIC) *suspension:* hydrocortisone acetate 1.5%, oxytetracycline 0.5%.

T-Gesic* (NARCOTIC ANALGESIC [schedule III]) hydrocodone 5 mg, acetaminophen 500 mg.

Theodrine (ANTIASTHMATIC) theophylline 125 mg, ephedrine 25 mg, phenobarbital 8 mg.

Theolair-Plus* (ANTIASTHMATIC) *liquid:* theophylline 125 mg, guaifenesin 100 mg/15 ml, menthol; *250 tablet:* theophylline 250 mg, guaifenesin 200 mg; *125 tablet:* theophylline 125 mg, guaifenesin 100 mg.

Timolide* (ANTIHYPERTENSIVE) *tablet:* hydrochlorothiazide 25 mg, timolol maleate 10 mg.

Titralac (ANTACID) *liquid:* calcium carbonate 1000 mg, glycine 300 mg/5 ml; sodium content: 11 mg, ANC 19 mEq; *chewable tablet:* calcium carbonate 420 mg, glycine 150 mg, sodium content <0.3 mg, ANC 7.5 mEq.

Trandate HCT 100/25* (ANTIHYPERTENSIVE) labetalol 100 mg, hydrochlorothiazide 25 mg.

Trandate HCT 200/25* (ANTIHYPERTENSIVE) labetalol 200 mg, hydrochlorothiazide 25 mg.

Trandate HCT 300/25* (ANTIHYPERTENSIVE) labetalol 300 mg, hydrochlorothiazide 25 mg.

Triacin-C Cough Syrup* (ANTITUSSIVE [schedule V]) *syrup:* pseudoephedrine 30 mg, triprolidine 1.25 mg, codeine 10 mg.

Triad* (ANALGESIC) acetaminophen 325 mg, caffeie 40 mg, butalbital 50 mg.

Triaminic Allergy (DECONGESTANT, ANTIHISTAMINE) *tablet:* phenylpropanolamine hydrochloride 25 mg, chlorpheniramine maleate 4 mg.

Triaminic Chewable Tablets (DECONGESTANT, ANTIHISTAMINE) *tablet:* phenylpropanolamine hydrochloride 6.25 mg, chlorpheniramine maleate 0.5 mg, sucrose, saccharin.

Triaminic Expectorant DH* (DECONGESTANT, ANTIHISTAMINE, ANTITUSSIVE, EXPECTORANT [schedule III]) *liquid:* phenylpropanolamine hydrochloride 12.5 mg, pyrilamine maleate 6.25 mg, pheniramine maleate 6.25 mg, hydrocodone bitartrate 1.67 mg, guaifenesin 100 mg/5 ml, alcohol 5%, saccharin, sorbitol.

Triaminic Expectorant with Codeine* (DECONGESTANT, ANTITUSSIVE, EXPECTORANT [schedule V]) *liquid:* phenylpropanolamine hydrochloride 12.5 mg, codeine phosphate 10 mg, guaifenesin 100 mg/5 ml, alcohol 5%, saccharin, sorbitol.

Triaminic Oral Infant Drops* (DECONGESTANT, ANTIHISTAMINE) *liquid:* phenylpropanolamine hydrochloride 20 mg, pyrilamine maleate 10 mg, pheniramine maleate 10 mg/ml, saccharin, sorbitol.

Triaminic TR Tablets* (DECONGESTANT, ANTIHISTAMINE [schedule V]) *timed-release tablet:* phenylpropanolamine hydrochloride 50 mg, pyrilamine maleate 25 mg, pheniramine maleate 25 mg.

Triaminic-12 (DECONGESTANT, ANTIHISTAMINE) *tablet:* phenylpropanolamine hydrochloride 75 mg, chlorpheniramine maleate 12 mg, lactose.

Triaprin* (ANALGESIC) acetaminophen 325 mg, butalbital 50 mg.

Triavil* (PSYCHOTHERAPEUTIC) *2-10 tablet:* perphenazine 2 mg, amitriptyline 10 mg; *2-25 tablet:* perphenazine 2 mg, amitriptyline 25 mg; *4-10 tablet:* perphenazine 4 mg, amitriptyline 10 mg; *4-25 tablet:* perphenazine 4 mg, amitriptyline 25 mg; *4-50 tablet:* perphenazine 4 mg, amitriptyline 50 mg.

Tri-Barbs* (SEDATIVE-HYPNOTIC [schedule II]) *capsule:* phenobarbital 32 mg, butabarbital sodium 32 mg, secobarbital sodium 32 mg.

Trigesic (NONNARCOTIC ANALGESIC) *tablet:* acetaminophen 125 mg, aspirin 230 mg, caffeine 30 mg.

Tri-Hydroserpine* (ANTIHYPERTENSIVE) *tablet:* hydrochlorothiazide 15 mg, reserpine 0.1 mg, hydralazine hydrochloride 25 mg.

Tri-Levlen* (ORAL CONTRACEPTIVE) ethinyl estradiol 30 μg|×|6 d, 40 μg|×|5 d, 30 μg|×|10 d, levonorgestrel 0.05 mg|×|6 d, 0.075 mg|×|5 d, 0.125 mg|×|10 d.

Trinalin Repetabs* (DECONGESTANT, ANTIHISTAMINE) *tablet:* pseudoephedrine sulfate 120 mg, azatadine maleate 1 mg; sugar coated.

Tri-Norinyl* (ORAL CONTRACEPTIVE) ethinyl estradiol 35 μg, norethindrone 0.5 mg|×|7 d, 1 mg|×|9 d, 0.5 mg|×|5 d.

Triphasil* (ORAL CONTRACEPTIVE) ethinyl estradiol 30 μg|×|6 d, 40 μg|×|5 d, 30 μg|×|10 d, levonorgestrel 0.05 mg|×|6 d, 0.075 mg|×|5 d, 0.125 mg|×|10 d.

Triple Antibiotic* (OPHTHALMIC ANTIINFECTIVE) *ophthalmic ointment:* hydrocortisone 1%, neomycin sulfate 0.5%, bacitracin zinc 400 units, polymyxin B sulfate 10,000 units/g.

Triple Antibiotic (TOPICAL ANTIINFECTIVE) *topical ointment:* neomycin sulfate 0.5%, bacitracin zinc 400 units, polymyxin B sulfate 5000 units.

Triple Sulfa* (ANTIINFECTIVE) *tablet:* sulfadiazine 167 mg, sulfamerazine 167 mg, sulfamethazine 167 mg.

Triple Sulfa No. 2* (ANTIINFECTIVE) *tablet:* sulfadiazine 162 mg, sulfamerazine 162 mg, sulfamethazine 162 mg.

Tuinal 100 mg Pulvules* (SEDATIVE-HYPNOTIC [schedule II]) *capsule:* amobarbital sodium 50 mg, secobarbital sodium 50 mg.

Tuinal 200 mg Pulvules* (SEDATIVE-HYPNOTIC [schedule II]) *capsule:* amobarbital sodium 100 mg, secobarbital sodium 100 mg.

Tussionex* (ANTITUSSIVE [schedule III]) chlorpheniramine 8 mg, hydrocodone 10 mg.

Tylenol with Codeine No. 1* (NARCOTIC AGONIST ANALGESIC [schedule III]) *tablet:* acetaminophen 300 mg, codeine phosphate 7.5 mg, sodium *metabisulfite.*

Tylenol with Codeine No. 2* (NARCOTIC AGONIST ANALGESIC [schedule III]) *tablet:* acetaminophen 300 mg, codeine phosphate 15 mg, sodium *metabisulfite.*

Tylenol with Codeine No. 3* (NARCOTIC AGONIST ANALGESIC [schedule III]) *tablet:* acetaminophen 300 mg, codeine phosphate 30 mg, sodium *metabisulfite.*

Tylenol with Codeine No. 4* (NARCOTIC AGONIST ANALGESIC [schedule III]) *tablet:* acetaminophen 300 mg, codeine phosphate 60 mg, sodium *metabisulfite.*

Tylox* (NARCOTIC AGONIST ANALGESIC [schedule II]) *capsule:* oxycodone hydrochloride 5 mg, acetaminophen 500 mg, sodium *metabisulfite.*

Ty-Tab #3* (NARCOTIC AGONIST ANALGESIC [schedule III]) *tablet:* codeine phosphate 30 mg, acetaminophen 300 mg.

Unipres* (ANTIHYPERTENSIVE) *tablet:* hydrochlorothiazide 15 mg, reserpine 0.1 mg, hydralazine hydrochloride 25 mg.

Uniretic* (ANTIHYPERTENSIVE) moexipril 7.5 mg, hydrochlorothiazide 12.5 mg, moexipril 15 mg, hydrochlorothiazide 25 mg.

Urobiotic-250* (URINARY ANTIINFECTIVE) *capsule:* oxytetracycline hydrochloride 250 mg, sulfamethizole 250 mg, phenazopyridine hydrochloride 50 mg.

Uro-Phosphate* (URINARY ANTIINFECTIVE) *tablet:* methenamine 300 mg, sodium acid phosphate 500 mg; sugar coated.

Uroquid-Acid* (URINARY ANTIINFECTIVE) *tablet:* methenamine mandelate 350 mg, sodium acid phosphate 200 mg; sugar coated.

Uroquid-Acid No. 2* (URINARY ANTI-INFECTIVE) *tablet:* methenamine mandelate 500 mg, sodium acid phosphate 500 mg.

Vanoxide-HC* (ANTIACNE) *water-washable lotion:* benzoyl peroxide 5%, hydrocortisone 0.5%, mineral oil, propylene glycol, cetyl alcohol, parabens.

Vanquish (NONNARCOTIC AGONIST ANALGESIC) *capsule (capsule-shaped tablet):* acetaminophen 194 mg, aspirin 277 mg, caffeine 33 mg, magnesium hydroxide 50 mg, aluminum hydroxide 25 mg.

Vaseretic* (ANTIHYPERTENSIVE) *tablet:* enalapril maleate 10 mg, hydrochlorothiazide 25 mg.

Vasocidin* (OPHTHALMIC CORTICOSTEROID, ANTIINFECTIVE) *ophthalmic solution:* prednisolone sodium phosphate 0.25%, sodium sulfacetamide 10%, EDTA, thimerosal 0.001%, polaxamer 407; *ophthalmic ointment:* prednisolone acetate 0.5%, sodium sulfacetamide 10%, mineral oil, white petrolatum.

Vasocon-A* (OPHTHALMIC DECONGESTANT) *ophthalmic solution:* naphazoline hydrochloride 0.05%, antazoline phosphate 0.5%, benzalkonium chloride 0.01%, PEG-8000 polyvinyl alcohol, povidone.

Vasosulf* (SULFONAMIDE DECONGESTANT) *ophthalmic solution:* sodium sulfacetamide 15%, phenylephrine hydrochloride 0.125%.

Veltap* (ANTIHISTAMINE, DECONGESTANT) phenylpropanolamine 5 mg, brompheniramine 4 mg, alcohol 3%.

Vicodin* (NARCOTIC AGONIST ANALGESIC [schedule III]) *tablet:* hydrocodone bitartrate 5 mg, acetaminophen 500 mg.

Vicodin HP* (NARCOTIC AGONIST ANALGESIC [schedule III]) *tablet:* hydrocodone 10 mg, acetaminophen 660 mg.

Vicoprofen* (NARCOTIC AGONIST ANALGESIC C-III) hydrocodone bitartrate 7.5 mg, ibuprofen 200 mg.

Wigraine* (ANTIMIGRAINE) *tablet:* ergotamine tartrate 1 mg, caffeine 100 mg, lactose, magnesium stearate, microcrystalline cellulose, starch; *suppository:* ergotamine tartrate 2 mg, caffeine 100 mg, tartaric acid 21.5 mg, synthetic cocoa butter base.

WinGel (ANTACID) *liquid:* aluminum hydroxide 180 mg, magnesium hydroxide 160 mg, saccharin, sorbitol, sodium content 2.5 mg, ANC 11.6 mEq.

Wygesic* (NARCOTIC AGONIST ANALGESIC [schedule IV]) *tablet:* propoxyphene hydrochloride 65 mg, acetaminophen 650 mg.

Ziac* (ANTIHYPERTENSIVE) *tablet:* bisoprolol 2.5 mg, hydrochlorothiazide 6.25 mg; bisoprolol 5 mg, hydrochlorothiazide 6.25 mg; bisoprolol 10 mg, hydrochlorothiazide 6.25 mg.

Zincfrin (OPHTHALMIC DECONGESTANT) *solution:* phenylephrine hydrochloride 0.12%, zinc sulfate 0.25%, benzalkonium chloride 0.01%.

Zydone* (NARCOTIC AGONIST ANALGESIC [schedule III]) *capsule:* hydrocodone bitartrate 5 mg, acetaminophen 500 mg.

acid-neutralizing capacity (ANC) amount of hydrochloric acid in mEq required to keep an antacid of pH 3 for 2 hours (in vitro).

acid rebound hypersecretion of hydrochloric acid induced by excessive buffering of stomach as with antacid therapy.

acute dystonia extrapyramidal symptom manifested by abnormal posturing, grimacing, spastic torticollis (neck torsion), and oculogyric (eyeball movement) crisis.

adverse effect unintended, unpredictable, and nontherapeutic response to drug action. Adverse effects occur at doses used therapeutically or for prophylaxis or diagnosis. They generally result from drug toxicity, idiosyncrasies, or hypersensitivity reactions caused by the drug itself or by ingredients added during manufacture, e.g., preservatives, dyes, or vehicles.

afterload resistance that ventricles must work against to eject blood into the aorta during systole.

agranulocytosis sudden drop in leukocyte count; often followed by a severe infection manifested by high fever, chills, prostration, and ulcerations of mucous membrane such as in the mouth, rectum, or vagina.

akathisia extrapyramidal symptom manifested by a compelling need to move or pace, without specific pattern, and an inability to be still.

allergic response abnormal and individual hypersensitivity response following exposure to a particular allergen.

analeptic restorative medication that enhances excitation of the CNS without affecting inhibitory impulses.

anaphylactoid reaction excessive allergic response manifested by wheezing, chills, generalized pruritic urticaria, diaphoresis, sense of uneasiness, agitation, flushing, palpitations, coughing, difficulty breathing, and cardiovascular collapse.

anticholinergic actions inhibition of parasympathetic response manifested by dry mouth, decreased peristalsis, constipation, blurred vision, and urinary retention.

bioavailability fraction of active drug that reaches its action sites after administration by any route. Following an IV dose, bioavailability is 100%; however, such factors as first-pass effect, enterohepatic cycling, and biotransformation reduce bioavailability of an orally administered drug.

biotransformation metabolic alterations occurring at some point between absorption and renal elimination and directed toward converting drugs into more polar molecules, hence more readily excretable products. The metabolites produced by enzyme-mediated reactions (oxidation-reduction, hydrolysis, and/or conjugation) are often less active than the parent drug, may be inactive, or may acquire toxic properties including teratogenicity, carcinogenicity, and mutagenicity.

blood dyscrasia pathological condition manifested by fever, sore mouth or throat, unexplained fatigue, easy bruising or bleeding.

bradycardia slowing of the heart, which may result in light-headedness, syncope, and fatigue.

cardiotoxicity impairment of cardiac function manifested by one or more of the following: hypotension, arrhythmias, precordial pain, dyspnea, electrocardiogram (ECG) abnormalities, cardiac dilation, congestive failure.

cholinergic response stimulation of the parasympathetic response manifested by lacrimation, diaphoresis, salivation, abdominal cramps, diarrhea, nausea, and vomiting.

circulatory overload excessive vascular volume manifested by increased central venous pressure (CVP), elevated blood pressure, tachycardia, distended neck veins, peripheral edema, dyspnea, cough, and pulmonary rales.

CNS stimulation excitement of the CNS manifested by hyperactivity, excitement, nervousness, insomnia, and tachycardia.

CNS toxicity impairment of CNS function manifested by ataxia, tremor, incoordination, paresthesias, numbness, impairment of pain or touch sensation, drowsiness, confusion, headache, anxiety, tremors, and behavior changes.

congestive heart failure (CHF) impaired pumping ability of the heart manifested by paroxysmal nocturnal dyspnea, cough, fatigue or dyspnea on exertion, tachycardia, peripheral or pulmonary edema, and weight gain.

cumulative effect increase in drug effect that results when intake of repeated doses exceeds the rate of drug elimination from the body.

Cushing's syndrome fatty swellings in the interscapular area (buffalo hump) and in the facial area (moon face), distension of the abdomen, ecchymoses following even minor trauma, impotence, amenorrhea, high blood pressure, general weakness, loss of muscle mass, osteoporosis, and psychosis.

dehydration decreased intracellular or extracellular fluid manifested by elevated temperature, dry skin and mucous membranes, decrease tissue turgor, sunken eyes, furrowed tongue, low blood pressure, diminished or irregular pulse, muscle or abdominal cramps, thick secretions, hard feces and impaction, scant urinary output, urine specific gravity above 1.030, an elevated hemoglobin.

disulfiram-type reaction Antabuse-type reaction manifested by facial flushing, pounding headache, sweating, slurred speech, abdominal cramps, nausea, vomiting, tachycardia, fever, palpitations, drop in blood pressure, dyspnea, and sense of chest constriction. Symptoms may last up to 24 hours.

drug receptor macromolecule on the cell surface or in the cytoplasm that interacts with a drug, thereby initiating the chain of biochemical events interpreted as drug effects. Because of an affinity for binding a drug, receptors determine quantitative relations between drug dose and effects, direct selectivity of drug action, and mediate action of antagonists.

enterohepatic circulation describes the recycling of a drug or metabolite that is secreted into bile and carried into the duodenum. A portion of this drug may then be reabsorbed from the intestinal lumen to appear unchanged in the blood; the remainder is excreted in feces.

enzyme induction stimulation of microsomal enzymes by a drug resulting in its accelerated metabolism and decreased activity. If reactive intermediates are formed, drug-mediated toxicity may be exacerbated.

first-pass effect reduced bioavailability of an orally administered drug due to metabolism in GI epithelial cells and liver or to biliary excretion. Effect may be avoided by use of sublingual tablets or rectal suppositories.

fixed drug eruption drug-induced circumscribed skin lesion that persists or recurs in the same site. Residual pigmentation may remain following drug withdrawal.

half-life ($t_{1/2}$) time required for concentration of a drug in the body to decrease by 50%. Half-life also represents the time necessary to reach steady state or to decline from steady state after a change (i.e., starting or stopping) in the dosing regimen. Half-life may be affected by a disease state and age of the drug user.

heat stroke a life-threatening condition manifested by absence of sweating; red, dry, hot skin; dilated pupils; dyspnea; full bounding pulse; temperature above 40C (105F); and mental confusion.

hepatic toxicity impairment of liver function manifested by jaundice, dark urine, pruritus, light-colored stools, eosinophilia, itchy skin or rash, and persistently high elevations of alanine amino-transferase (ALT) and aspartate aminotransferase (AST).

hyperammonemia elevated level of ammonia or ammonium in the blood manifested by lethargy, decreased appetite, vomiting, asterixis (flapping tremor), weak pulse, irritability, decreased responsiveness, and seizures.

hypercalcemia elevated serum calcium manifested by deep bone and flank pain, renal calculi, anorexia, nausea, vomiting, thirst, constipation, muscle hypotonicity, pathologic fracture, bradycardia, lethargy, and psychosis.

hyperglycemia elevated blood glucose manifested by flushed, dry skin, low blood pressure and elevated pulse, tachypnea, Kussmaul's respirations, polyuria, polydipsia; polyphagia, lethargy, and drowsiness.

hyperkalemia excessive potassium in blood, which may produce life-threatening cardiac arrhythmias, including bradycardia and heart block, unusual fatigue, weakness or heaviness of limbs, general muscle weakness, muscle cramps, paresthesias, flaccid paralysis of extremities, shortness of breath, nervousness, confusion, diarrhea, and GI distress.

hypermagnesemia excessive magnesium in blood, which may produce cathartic effect, profound thirst, flushing, sedation, confusion, depressed deep tendon reflexes (DTRs), muscle weakness, hypotension, and depressed respirations.

hypernatremia excessive sodium in blood, which may produce confusion, neuromuscular excitability, muscle weakness, seizures, thirst, dry and flushed skin, dry mucous membranes, pyrexia, agitation, and oliguria or anuria.

hypersensitivity reactions excessive and abnormal sensitivity to given agent manifested by urticaria, pruritus, wheezing, edema, redness, and anaphylaxis.

hyperthyroidism excessive secretion by the thyroid glands, which increases basal metabolic rate, resulting in warm, flushed, moist skin; tachycardia, exophthalmos; infrequent lid blinking; lid edema; weight loss despite increased appetite; frequent urination; menstrual irregularity; breathlessness;

hypoventilation; congestive heart failure; excessive sweating.

hyperuricemia excessive uric acid in blood, resulting in pain in flank; stomach, or joints, and changes in intake and output ratio and pattern.

hypocalcemia abnormally low calcium level in blood, which may result in depression; psychosis; hyperreflexia; diarrhea; cardiac arrhythmias; hypotension; muscle spasms; paresthesias of feet, fingers, tongue; positive Chvostek's sign. Severe deficiency (tetany) may result in carpopedal spasms, spasms of face muscle, laryngospasm, and generalized convulsions.

hypoglycemia abnormally low glucose level in the blood, which may result in acute fatigue, restlessness, malaise, marked irritability and weakness, cold sweats, excessive hunger, headache, dizziness, confusion, slurred speech, loss of consciousness, and death.

hypokalemia abnormally low level of potassium in blood, which may result in malaise, fatigue, paresthesias, depressed reflexes, muscle weakness and cramps, rapid, irregular pulse, arrhythmias, hypotension, vomiting, paralytic ileus, mental confusion, depression, delayed thought process, abdominal distension, polyuria, shallow breathing, and shortness of breath.

hypomagnesemia abnormally low level of magnesium in blood, resulting in nausea, vomiting, cardiac arrhythmias, and neuromuscular symptoms (tetany, positive Chvostek's and Trousseau's signs, seizures, tremors, ataxia, vertigo, nystagmus, muscular fasciculations).

hypophosphatemia abnormally low level of phosphates in blood, resulting in muscle weakness, anorexia, malaise, absent deep tendon reflexes, bone pain, paresthesias, tremors, negative calcium balance, osteomalacia, osteoporosis.

hypothyroidism condition caused by thyroid hormone deficiency that lowers basal metabolic rate and may result in periorbital edema, lethargy, puffy hands and feet, cool, pale skin, vertigo, nocturnal cramps, decreased GI motility, constipation, hypotension, slow pulse, depressed muscular activity, and enlarged thyroid gland.

hypoxia insufficient oxygenation in the blood manifested by dyspnea, tachypnea, headache, restlessness, cyanosis, tachycardia, dysrhythmias, confusion, decreased level of consciousness, and euphoria or delirium.

immunomodulation favorable adjustment of the immune system to combat foreign invasion of antigens and viruses.

international normalizing ratio measurement that normalizes for the differences obtained from various laboratory readings in the value for thromboplastin blood level.

jaundice excessive bilirubin in the blood manifested by yellow sclera or skin, dark urine, clay-colored stools, and pruritus.

leukopenia abnormal decrease in number of white blood cells, usually below 5000 per cubic millimeter, resulting in fever, chills, sore mouth or throat, and unexplained fatigue.

liver toxicity manifested by anorexia, nausea, fatigue, lethargy, itching, jaundice, abdominal pain, dark-colored urine, and flu-like symptoms.

loading dose increased initial

dose used to achieve steady state promptly. A loading dose is generally indicated when time to reach steady state is long, as when drug has a long half-life.

metabolic acidosis decrease in pH value of the extracellular fluid caused by either an increase in hydrogen ions or a decrease in bicarbonate ions. It may result in one or more of the following: lethargy, headache, weakness, abdominal pain, nausea, vomiting, dyspnea, hyperpnea progressing to Kussmaul breathing, dehydration, thirst, weakness, flushed face, full bounding pulse, progressive drowsiness, mental confusion, combativeness.

metabolic alkalosis increase in pH value of the extracellular fluid caused by either a loss of acid from the body (e.g., through vomiting) or an increased level of bicarbonate ions (e.g., through ingestion of sodium bicarbonate). It may result in muscle weakness, irritability, confusion, muscle twitching, slow and shallow respirations, and convulsive seizures.

microsomal enzymes drug-metabolizing enzymes located in the endoplasmic reticulum of the liver and other tissues chiefly responsible for oxidative drug metabolism, e.g., cytochrome P450.

myopathy any disease or abnormal condition of striated muscles manifested by muscle weakness, myalgia, diaphoresis, fever, and reddish-brown urine (myoglobinuria) or oliguria.

nadir lowest value or point. For example, thrombocytes and leukocytes reach a nadir in response to cytotoxic drug effects on hematopoietic tissues.

nutriuria excretion of greater than normal amounts of sodium in the urine.

nephrotoxicity impairment of the nephrons of the kidney manifested by one or more of the following: oliguria, urinary frequency, hematuria, cloudy urine, rising BUN and serum creatinine, fever, graft tenderness or enlargement.

neuroleptic malignant syndrome (NMS) potentially fatal complication associated with antipsychotic drugs manifested by hyperpyrexia, altered mental status, muscle rigidity, irregular pulse, fluctuating BP, diaphoresis, and tachycardia.

orphan drug (as defined by the Orphan Drug Act, an amendment of the Federal Food, Drug, and Cosmetic Act which took effect in January 1983): drug or biological product used in the treatment, diagnosis, or prevention of a rare disease. A rare disease or condition is one that affects fewer than 200,000 persons in the United States, or affects more than 200,000 persons but for which there is no reasonable expectation that drug research and development costs can be recovered from sales within the United States.

ototoxicity impairment of the ear manifested by one or more of the following: headache, dizziness or vertigo, nausea and vomiting with motion, ataxia, nystagmus.

paralytic ileus paralysis of the intestinal wall of the ileum manifested by one or more of the following: abdominal distension, constipation, absent bowel sounds usually associated with nausea, vomiting, and epigastric pain.

photosensitivity drug-induced skin changes resulting in unusual susceptibility to effects of sunlight or ultraviolet light; relatively brief exposure to either form of light may cause edema, papules, urticaria, or acute burns.

preload ventricular filling pressure at the end of diastole.

prodrug inactive drug form that becomes pharmacologically active through biotransformation.

protein binding reversible interaction between protein and drug resulting in a drug-protein complex (bound drug) which is in equilibrium with free (active) drug in plasma and tissues. Since only free drug can diffuse to action sites, factors that influence drug-binding (e.g., displacement of bound drug by another drug, or decreased albumin concentration) may potentiate pharmacological effect.

pseudomembranous enterocolitis life-threatening superinfection characterized by severe diarrhea and fever.

pseudoparkinsonism extrapyramidal symptom manifested by slowing of volitional movement (akinesia), mask facies, rigidity and tremor at rest (especially of upper extremities); and pill rolling motion.

pulmonary edema excessive fluid in the lung tissue manifestied by one or more of the following: shortness of breath, cyanosis, persistent productive cough (frothy sputum may be blood tinged), expiratory rales, restlessness, anxiety, increased heart rate, sense of chest pressure.

renal insufficiency reduced capacity of the kidney to perform its functions as manifested by one or more of the following: dysuria, oliguria, hematuria, swelling of lower legs and feet.

serotonin syndrome manifested by restlessness, myoclonus, mental status changes, hyperreflexia, diaphoresis, shivering, and tremor.

Somogyi effect rebound phenomenon clinically manifested by fasting hyperglycemia and worsening of diabetic control in the presence of unnecessarily large insulin doses. Hormonal response to unrecognized hypoglycemia (i.e., release of epinephrine, glucagon, growth hormone, cortisol) causes insensitivity to insulin. Increasing the amount of insulin required to treat the hyperglycemia intensifies the hypoglycemia.

steady-state plasma concentration state reached when the amount of drug absorbed is equivalent to the amount of drug being eliminated; plasma concentration will then fluctuate around a mean or plateau concentration. Full benefit of the drug can be expected when steady state is reached. Drug form, elimination half-life, and renal failure are factors that qualify steady-state concentration.

superinfection new infection by an organism different from the initial infection being treated by antimicrobial therapy manifested by one or more of the following: black, hairy tongue; glossitis, stomatitis; anal itching; loose, foul-smelling stools; vaginal itching or discharge; sudden fever; cough.

tachyphylaxis rapid decrease in response to a drug after administration of a few doses. Initial drug response cannot be restored by an increase in dose.

tardive dyskinesia extrapyramidal symptom manifested by involuntary rhythmic, bizarre movements of face, jaw, mouth, tongue, and sometimes extremities.

therapeutic window range of drug concentration level within which a particular drug has its safest and optimal therapeutic effect, that is, the limits between therapeutic and toxic response to a drug.

thrombocytopenia abnormal reduction in the number of platelets.

thrombophlebitis inflammation of a vein associated with thrombus formation manifested by one or more of the following: arm or leg pain, tenderness or swelling, warmth, Homan's sign, prominence of superficial veins.

tolerance decreased responsiveness to pharmacodynamic action of a drug that occurs during repeated administration of constant drug doses. Larger or more frequent doses, or both, are required to achieve the same effects observed with initial dosing.

urinary tract infection invasion of microorganisms into the urinary tract system as manifested by one or more of the following: fever, polyuria, urgency, frequency, flank pain.

vasovagal symptoms transient vascular and neurogenic reaction marked by pallor, nausea, vomiting, bradycardia, and rapid fall in arterial blood pressure.

water intoxication (dilutional hyponatremia) less than normal concentration of sodium in the blood resulting from excess extracellular and intracellular fluid and producing one or more of the following: lethargy, confusion, headache, decreased skin turgor, tremors, convulsions, coma, anorexia, nausea, vomiting, diarrhea, sternal fingerprinting, weight gain, edema, full bounding pulse, jugular vein distension, rales, signs and symptoms of pulmonary edema.

ABBREVIATIONS

ABGs	arterial blood gases
a.c.	before meals (*ante cibum*)
ACD	acid–citrate–dextrose
ACE	angiotensin-converting enzyme
ACh	acetylcholine
ACIP	Advisory Committee on Immunization Practices
ACLS	advanced cardiac life support
ACS	acute coronary syndrome
ACT	activated clotting time
ACTH	adrenocorticotropic hormone
ADD	attention deficit disorder
ADH	antidiuretic hormone
ADLs	activities of daily living
ad lib	as desired (*ad libitum*)
ADP	adenosine diphosphate
ADT	alternate-day drug (administration)
AIDS	acquired immunodeficiency syndrome
ALT	alanine aminotransferase (formerly SGPT)
AML	acute myelogenous leukemia
AMP	adenosine monophosphate
ANA	antinuclear antibody(ies)
ANC	acid neutralizing capacity
aPTT	activated partial thromboplastin time
ARC	AIDS related complex
ARDS	adult respiratory distress syndrome
ASHD	arteriosclerotic heart disease
AST	aspartate aminotransferase (formerly SGOT)
AT_1	angiotension II receptor
ATP	adenosine triphosphate
AV	atrioventricular
b.i.d.	two times a day (*bis in die*)
BM	bowel movement
BMD	bone mineral density
BMR	basal metabolic rate
BP	blood pressure
bpm	beats per minute
BSA	body surface area
BSP	bromsulphalein
BT	bleeding time
BUN	blood urea nitrogen
C	centigrade, Celsius
CAD	coronary artery disease
cAMP	cyclic adenosine monophosphate
CBC	complete blood count
cc	cubic centimeter
CDC	Centers for Disease Control
CF	cystic fibrosis
CHF	congestive heart failure

Cl_{cr}	creatinine clearance
cm	centimeter
CMV	cytomegalovirus-I
CMVIG	cytomegalovirus immune globulin
CNS	central nervous system
Coll	collyrium (eye wash)
COMT	catecholamine-*o*-methyl transferase
COPD	chronic obstructive pulmonary disease
COX-2	cyclooxygenase-2
CPK	creatinine phosphokinase
CPR	cardiopulmonary resuscitation
CRF	chronic renal failure
C&S	culture and sensitivity
CSF	cerebrospinal fluid
CSP	cellulose sodium phosphate
CT	clotting time
CTZ	chemoreceptor trigger zone
CV	cardiovascular
CVA	cerebrovascular accident
CVP	central venous pressure
d	day
D5W	5% dextrose in water
D&C	dilation and curettage
DIC	disseminated intravascular coagulation
DKA	diabetic keto-acidosis
dl	deciliter (100 ml or 0.1 liter)
DM	diabetes mellitus
DNA	deoxyribonucleic acid
DTRs	deep tendon reflexes
DVT	deep venous thrombosis
ECG, EKG	electrocardiogram
ECT	electroconvulsive therapy
EEG	electroencephalogram
EENT	eye, ear, nose, throat
e.g.	for example (*exempli gratia*)
ENT	ear, nose, throat
EPS	extrapyramidal symptoms (or syndrome)
ER	estrogen receptor
ESR	erythrocyte sedimentation rate
F	Fahrenheit
FBS	fasting blood sugar
FDA	Food and Drug Administration
FSH	follicle-stimulating hormone
FTI	free thyroxine index
5-FU	5-fluorouracil
FUO	fever of unknown origin
g	gram
G6PD	glucose-6-phosphate dehydrogenase
GABA	gamma-aminobutyric acid
G-CSF	granulocyte colony-stimulating factor
GFR	glomerular filtration rate

GH	growth hormone
GI	gastrointestinal
GPIIb/IIIa	glycoprotein IIb/IIIa
GU	genitourinary
h	hour
HCG	human chorionic gonadotropin
Hct	hematocrit
HDL	high density lipoprotein
HDL-C	high-density-lipoprotein cholesterol
HER	human epidermal growth factor
Hgb	hemoglobin
5-HIAA	5-hydroxyindoleacetic acid
HIT	heparin-induced thrombocytopenia
HIV	human immunodeficiency virus
HMG-CoA	3-hydroxy-3-methyl-glutaryl coenzyme A
HPA	hypothalamic–pituitary–adrenocortical (axis)
HPV	human papillomavirus
HR	heart rate
h.s.	nightly or at bedtime (*hora somni*)
HSV-1	herpes simplex virus type 1
HSV-2	herpes simplex virus type 2
5-HT	5-hydroxytryptamine (serotonin receptor)
I&O	intake and output
IBW	ideal body weight
IC	intracoronary
ICP	intracranial pressure
ICU	intensive care unit
ID	intradermal
IDDM	insulin-dependent diabetes mellitus (Type I diabetes)
IFN	interferon
Ig	immunoglobulin
IL	interleukin
IM	intramuscular
INR	international normalizing ratio
IOP	intraocular pressure
IPPB	intermittent positive pressure breathing
IU	international unit
IV	intravenous
kg	kilogram
17-KGS	17-ketogenic steroids
17-KS	17-ketosteroids
KVO	keep vein open
L	liter
LDH	lactic dehydrogenase
LDL	low density lipoprotein
LDL-C	low-density-lipoprotein cholesterol
LE	lupus erythematosus
LFT	liver function test
LH	luteinizing hormone
LSD	lysergic acid diethylamide

LTRA	leukotriene receptor antagonist
M	molar (strength of a solution)
m2	square meter (of body surface area)
MAO	monoamine oxidase
MAOI	monoamine oxidase inhibitor
MBD	minimal brain dysfunction
MCH	mean corpuscular hemoglobin
MCHC	mean corpuscular hemoglobin concentration
mCi	millicurie
μg, mcg	microgram (1/1000 of a milligram)
μm	micrometer
MDI	metered dose inhaler
MDR	minimum daily requirements
mEq	milliequivalent
mg	milligram
min	minute
MI	myocardial infarction
MIC	minimum inhibitory concentration
ml	milliliter (0.001 liter)
mm	millimeter
mo	month
MRSA	methicillin-resistant *Staphylococcus aureus*
MS	multiple sclerosis
N	normal (strength of a solution)
NADH	reduced form of nicotine adenine dinucleotide
NAPA	*N*-acetyl procainamide
nb	note well (*nota bene*)
ng	nanogram (1/1000 of a microgram)
NIDDM	non-insulin-dependent diabetes mellitus (Type II diabetes)
NMS	neuroleptic malignant syndrome
NNRTI	nonnucleoside reverse transcriptase inhibitor
NPN	nonprotein nitrogen
NPO	nothing by mouth
NS	normal saline
NSAID	nonsteroidal antiinflammatory drug
NSR	normal sinus rhythm
OC	oral contraceptive
17-OHCS	17-hydroxycorticosteroids
OTC	over the counter (nonprescription)
PABA	*para*-aminobenzoic acid
PAS	*para*-aminosalicylic acid
PAWP	pulmonary artery wedge pressure
PBI	protein-bound iodine
PBP	penicillin-binding protein
p.c.	after meals (*post cibum*)
PCI	percutaneous coronary intervention
PERLA	pupils equal, react to light and accommodation
PG	prostaglandin
pH	hydrogen ion concentration
PID	pelvic inflammatory disease

PKU	phenylketonuria
PND	paroxysmal nocturnal dyspnea
PO	by mouth or orally (*per os*)
PPM	parts per million
PR	rectally (*per rectum*)
prn	when required (*pro re nata*)
PSA	prostate-specific antigen
PSP	phenolsulfonphthalein
PSVT	paroxysmal supraventricular tachycardia
PT	prothrombin time
PTH	parathyroid hormone
PTT	partial thromboplastin time
PUD	peptic ulcer disease
PVC	premature ventricular contraction
PVD	peripheral vascular disease
PZI	protamine zinc insulin
q	every
q.d.	every day
q.i.d.	four times daily
q.o.d.	every other day
RA	rheumatoid arthritis
RAI	radioactive iodine
RAST	radioallergosorbent test
RBC	red blood (cell) count
RDA	recommended (daily) dietary allowance
RDS	respiratory distress syndrome
REM	rapid eye movement
rem	radiation equivalent man
RIA	radioimmunoassay
RNA	ribonucleic acid
ROM	range of motion
RSV	respiratory syncytial virus
RT_3U	total serum thyroxine concentration
s	second
S&S	signs and symptoms
SA	sinoatrial
SBE	breast self-examination; subacute bacterial endocarditis
SC	subcutaneous
S_{cr}	serum creatinine
SGGT	serum gamma-glutamyl transferase
SGOT	serum glutamic–oxaloacetic transaminase (*see* AST)
SGPT	serum glutamic–pyruvic transaminase (*see* ALT)
SIADH	syndrome of inappropriate antidiuretic hormone
SI Units	International System of Units
SK	streptokinase
SL	sublingual
SLE	systemic lupus erythematosus
SMA	sequential multiple analysis
SOS	if necessary (*si opus cit*)
sp	species

SPF	sun protection factor
sq	square
SR	sedimentation rate
SRS-A	slow-reactive substance of anaphylaxis
SSRI	selective serotonin reuptake inhibitor
stat	immediately
STD	sexually transmitted disease
$t_{1/2}$	half-life
T_3	triiodothyronine
T_4	thyroxine
TCA	tricyclic antidepressant
TG	total triglycerides
TIA	transient ischemic attack
t.i.d.	three times a day (*ter in die*)
TNF	tumor necrosis factor
tPA	tissue plasminogen activator
TPN	total parenteral nutrition
TPR	temperature, pulse, respirations
TSH	thyroid-stimulating hormone
TT	thrombin time
URI	upper respiratory infection
USP	United States Pharmacopeia
USPHS	United States Public Health Service
UTI	urinary tract infection
UV-A, UVA	ultraviolet A wave
VDRL	venereal disease research laboratory
VLDL	very low density lipoprotein
VMA	vanillylmandelic acid
VS	vital signs
wk	week
WBC	white blood (cell) count
WBCT	whole blood clotting time
y	year

BIBLIOGRAPHY

American Hospital Formulary Service (AHFS) Drug Information '99. Bethesda, MD: American Society of Hospital Pharmacists, 1999.

Drug Facts and Comparisons. St. Louis: Facts and Comparisons, 1999.

Gelman CR, Rumack BH, eds. *DrugDex Information System*. Denver: Micromedex, 1999.

King JC. *Guide to Parenteral Admixtures*. St. Louis: Pacemarq, 1996.

Physicians' Desk Reference, 53rd ed. Oradell, NJ: Medical Economics Co., 1999.

Semla TP, Beizer JL, Higbee MD. *Geriatric Dosage Handbook,* 4th ed. Hudson, OH: Lexi-Comp, 1998.

Taketomo CK, Hodding JH, Kraus DM. *Pediatric Dosage Handbook,* 5th ed. Hudson, OH: Lexi-Comp, 1998.

Trissel LA. *Handbook of Injectable Drugs,* 8th ed. Bethesda, MD: American Society of Hospital Pharmacists, 1995.

USP DI: Advice to Patients. Rockville, MD: US Pharmacopeial Convention, 1999.

USP DI: Drug Information for the Health Care Provider. Rockville, MD: US Pharmacopeial Convention, 1999.

INDEX

A

Drug categories are in SMALL CAPS. Prototypes in **bold.**
Generic drug names are given in parentheses.

Drug categories are in SMALL CAPS. Prototypes in **bold.**
Generic drug names are given in parentheses.

Drug categories are in SMALL CAPS. Prototypes in **bold.**
Generic drug names are given in parentheses.

Drug categories are in SMALL CAPS. Prototypes in **bold.**
Generic drug names are given in parentheses.

Drug categories are in SMALL CAPS. Prototypes in **bold.**
Generic drug names are given in parentheses.

Drug categories are in SMALL CAPS. Prototypes in **bold.**
Generic drug names are given in parentheses.

Drug categories are in SMALL CAPS. Prototypes in **bold.**
Generic drug names are given in parentheses.

Drug categories are in SMALL CAPS. Prototypes in **bold.**
Generic drug names are given in parentheses.

Drug categories are in SMALL CAPS. Prototypes in **bold.**
Generic drug names are given in parentheses.

Drug categories are in SMALL CAPS. Prototypes in **bold.**
Generic drug names are given in parentheses.

C

Drug categories are in SMALL CAPS. Prototypes in **bold.**
Generic drug names are given in parentheses.

Drug categories are in SMALL CAPS. Prototypes in **bold.**
Generic drug names are given in parentheses.

D

Drug categories are in SMALL CAPS. Prototypes in **bold.**
Generic drug names are given in parentheses.

Drug categories are in SMALL CAPS. Prototypes in **bold.**
Generic drug names are given in parentheses.

Drug categories are in SMALL CAPS. Prototypes in **bold.**
Generic drug names are given in parentheses.

E

Drug categories are in SMALL CAPS. Prototypes in **bold.**
Generic drug names are given in parentheses.

F

G

Drug categories are in SMALL CAPS. Prototypes in **bold.**
Generic drug names are given in parentheses.

H

Drug categories are in SMALL CAPS. Prototypes in **bold.**
Generic drug names are given in parentheses.

Drug categories are in SMALL CAPS. Prototypes in **bold.**
Generic drug names are given in parentheses.

L

Drug categories are in SMALL CAPS. Prototypes in **bold.**
Generic drug names are given in parentheses.

M

Drug categories are in SMALL CAPS. Prototypes in **bold.**
Generic drug names are given in parentheses.

N

Drug categories are in SMALL CAPS. Prototypes in **bold.**
Generic drug names are given in parentheses.

Drug categories are in SMALL CAPS. Prototypes in **bold.**
Generic drug names are given in parentheses.

P

Drug categories are in SMALL CAPS. Prototypes in **bold.**
Generic drug names are given in parentheses.

Drug categories are in SMALL CAPS. Prototypes in **bold.**
Generic drug names are given in parentheses.

Drug categories are in SMALL CAPS. Prototypes in **bold.**
Generic drug names are given in parentheses.

Drug categories are in SMALL CAPS. Prototypes in **bold.**
Generic drug names are given in parentheses.

S

Drug categories are in SMALL CAPS. Prototypes in **bold.**
Generic drug names are given in parentheses.

Drug categories are in SMALL CAPS. Prototypes in **bold.**
Generic drug names are given in parentheses.

Drug categories are in SMALL CAPS. Prototypes in **bold.**
Generic drug names are given in parentheses.

U

V

Drug categories are in SMALL CAPS. Prototypes in **bold.**
Generic drug names are given in parentheses.

W

insulin	I	I	N	C	C	C	N	N	C
isoproterenol	I	C	N	C	N	N	N	N	C
lorazepam	NN	N	N	NN	C	C	N	I	NN
meperidine	I	C	C	C	C	I	N	C	C
methylprednisolone	C	N	C	C	C	C	N	I	CFC
metoclopramide	C	N	N	C	C	C	N	C	C**
midazolam	N	N	N	N	C	C	N	N	N
morphine	C	C	C	C	I	C	N	C	C
nitroglycerin	C	C	C	C	N	N	N	N	N
ondansetron	I	N	N	C	C	C	N	C	C
phenytoin	I	I	N	I	I	I	I	NN	I
potassium Cl (D5W or NS)	C	C**	C	C	C	C	C	C	C
ranitidine	C	C	C	C	C	C	C	C	C
sargramostim	C	N	C	C	C	I	N	I	CFC

C = Compatible at Y-site; C* = Compatible at Potassium conc. < 80 mEq/L; C** = Compatible at Potassium conc. ≤ 20 mEq/L; CFC = Compatibility depends on fluid and/or concentration; I = Incompatible at Y-site; N = No information available; NN = No information available, probably should NOT mix.

LICENSE AGREEMENT AND LIMITED WARRANTY

READ THE FOLLOWING TERMS AND CONDITIONS CAREFULLY BEFORE OPENING THIS DISK PACKAGE. THIS IS AN AGREEMENT BETWEEN YOU AND APPLETON & LANGE (THE "COMPANY"). BY OPENING THIS SEALED PACKAGE, YOU ARE AGREEING TO BE BOUND BY THESE TERMS AND CONDITIONS. IF YOU DO NOT AGREE WITH THESE TERMS AND CONDTIONS, DO NOT OPEN THE DISK PACKAGE. PROMPTLY RETURN THE DISK PACKAGE AND ALL ACCOMPANYING ITEMS TO THE COMPANY.

1. GRANT OF LICENSE: In consideration of your adoption of textbooks and/or other materials published by the Company, and your agreement to abide by the terms and conditions of this Agreement, the Company grants to you a nonexclusive right to use and display the copy of the enclosed software program (hereinafter the "SOFTWARE") so long as you comply with the terms of this Agreement. The company reserves all rights not expressly granted to you under this Agreement. This license is *not* a sale of the original SOFTWARE or any copy to you.

2. USE RESTRICTIONS: You may *not* sell, license, transfer or distribute copies of the SOFTWARE or Documentation to others. You may *not* reverse engineer, diassemble, decompile, modify, adapt, translate or otherwise reproduce the SOFTWARE or any part of it, or create derivative works based on the SOFTWARE or the Documentation without the prior written consent of the Company.

3. MISCELLANEOUS: This Agreement shall be construed in accordance with the laws of the United States of America and the State of New York, except for that body of law dealing with conflicts of law, and shall benefit the Company, its affiliates and assignees. If any provision of this Agreement is found void or unenforceable, the remainder will remain valid and enforecable according to its terms. Use, duplication or disclosure of the SOFTWARE by the U.S. Government is subject to the restricted rights applicable to commercial computer software under FAR 52.227.19 and DFARS 252.277-7013.

4. LIMITED WARRANTY AND DISCLAIMER OF WARRANTY: Because this SOFTWARE is being given to you without charge, the Company makes no warranties about the SOFTWARE, which is provided "AS-IS." **THE COMPANY DISCLAIMS ALL WARRANTIES, EXPRESS OR IMPLIED, INCLUDING WITHOUT LIMITATION, THE IMPLIED WARRANTIES OF MERCHANTABILITY AND FITNESS FOR A PARTICULAR PURPOSE. THE COMPANY DOES NOT WARRANT, GUARANTEE OR MAKE ANY REPRESENTATION REGARDING THE USE OR THE RESULTS OF THE USE OF THE SOFTWARE. IN NO EVENT, SHALL THE COMPANY, ITS PARENTS, SUBSIDIARIES, AFFILIATES, LICENSORS, DIRECTORS, OFFICERS, EMPLOYEES, AGENTS, SUPPLIERS OR CONTRACTORS BE LIABLE FOR ANY INCIDENTAL, INDIRECT, SPECIAL OR CONSEQUENTIAL DAMAGES ARISING OUT OF OR IN CONNECTION WITH THE LICENSE GRANTED UNDER THIS AGREEMENT INCLUDING, WITHOUT LIMITATION, LOSS OF USE, LOSS OF DATA, LOSS OF INCOME OR PROFIT, OR OTHER LOSSES SUSTAINED AS RESULT OF INJURY TO ANY PERSON, OR LOSS OF OR DAMAGE TO PROPERTY, OR CLAIMS OF THIRD PARTIES, EVEN IF THE COMPANY OR AN AUTHORIZED REPRESENTATIVE OF THE COMPANY HAS BEEN ADVISED OF THE POSSIBILITY OF SUCH DAMAGES.**

SOME JURISDICTIONS DO NOT ALLOW THE EXCLUSION OF IMPLIED WARRANTIES OR THE LIMITATION ON LIABILITY FOR INCIDENTAL, INDIRECT, SPECIAL OR CONSEQUENTIAL DAMAGES, SO THE ABOVE LIMITATIONS MAY NOT ALWAYS APPLY. THE WARRANTIES IN THIS AGREEMENT GIVE YOU SPECIFIC LEGAL RIGHTS AND YOU MAY ALSO HAVE OTHER RIGHTS WHICH VARY IN ACCORDANCE WITH LOCAL LAW.

No sales personnel or other representative of any party involved in the distribution of the software is authorized by the Company to make any warranties with respect to the software beyond what is contained in this agreement. Oral statements do not constitute warranties, shall not be relied upon by you and are not part of this agreement. The entire agreement between you and the Company is embodied herein.

ACKNOWLEDGMENT

YOU ACKNOWLEDGE THAT YOU HAVE READ THIS AGREEMENT, UNDERSTAND IT AND AGREE TO BE BOUND BY ITS TERMS AND CONDITIONS. YOU ALSO AGREE THAT THIS AGREEMENT IS THE COMPLETE AND EXCLUSIVE AGREEMENT BETWEEN YOU AND THE COMPANY.